Campbell's

PHYSICAL THERAPY
for CHILDREN

Fifth
Edition

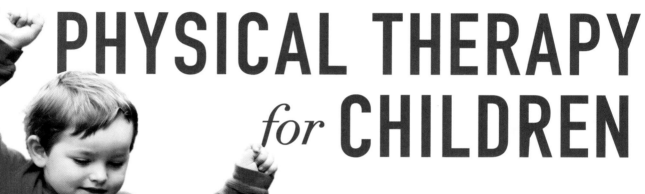

Campbell's
PHYSICAL THERAPY
for CHILDREN

Robert J. Palisano, PT, ScD, FAPTA
Distinguished Professor
Physical Therapy and Rehabilitation Sciences
Drexel University
Philadelphia, Pennsylvania
Scientist
CanChild Centre for Childhood Disability Research
McMaster University
Hamilton, Ontario, Canada

Margo N. Orlin, PT, PhD, FAPTA
Associate Professor
Physical Therapy and Rehabilitation Sciences
Drexel University
Philadelphia, Pennsylvania

Joseph Schreiber, PT, PhD
Professor and Program Director
Physical Therapy Program
Chatham University
Pittsburgh, Pennsylvania

ELSEVIER

ELSEVIER

3251 Riverport Lane
St. Louis, Missouri 63043

Executive Content Strategist: Kathy Falk
Content Development Manager: Jolynn Gower
Senior Content Development Specialist: Courtney Sprehe
Publishing Services Manager: Julie Eddy
Senior Project Manager: Richard Barber
Design Direction: Patrick Ferguson

Printed in Canada

Last digit is the print number: 9 8 7 6 5 4 3

Working together to grow libraries in developing countries

www.elsevier.com • www.bookaid.org

To Suzann K. Campbell and the 126 contributors who have been instrumental to the success of the five editions of Physical Therapy for Children

PREFACE

What makes an outstanding textbook on pediatric physical therapy? First and foremost is the emphasis on clinical reasoning, decision making, family-centered services, and application of knowledge and research to practice. Pediatric physical therapists make numerous clinical decisions, including eligibility and need for services, goals and outcomes, prognosis, intensity of services, and intervention plans. The reasoning and evidence for clinical decisions are emphasized throughout *Campbell's Physical Therapy for Children*. Chapter 1 presents frameworks to guide clinical reasoning and decision making, such as the International Classification of Functioning, Disability and Health (ICF) and the Guide to Physical Therapist Practice, strategies for finding evidence, and criteria for appraisal of evidence. Terms used throughout the book such as *Background* and *Foreground* information are defined.

The editors believe that the priorities, concerns, and aspirations of children and families are integral to pediatric physical therapy practice. Accordingly, the chapters not only address direct interventions, but also child and family goals and information needs; communication and coordination of services as members of healthcare and education teams; and consultation to community agencies, instructors, and coaches. Families of children with disabilities have expressed the importance of planning for the future. To address this priority, key considerations for physical therapy management are presented for infants, children, and adolescents, including the transition to adulthood.

The ability to effectively apply knowledge and research to practice is a characteristic of expert practitioners. Since the publication of the first edition, research pertinent to pediatric physical therapy has dramatically increased. The authors of each chapter have effectively appraised this aspect of pediatric physical therapy, including emerging technologies. Chapters in Sections 2 to 4 feature case scenarios and videos that illustrate application of knowledge and research to practice. Additionally, the cases demonstrate how child and family strengths and preferences, environmental context, and therapist practice knowledge all inform clinical reasoning and the decision making process. These cases and videos are found on the Expert Consult site that accompanies this text (discussed below).

Several new and extensively revised chapters are included in this edition. Chapters have been added on children with autism (Chapter 24), children with cancer (Chapter 16), and measurement (Chapter 2). Content on concussion has been expanded and includes a new case scenario on post-concussion rehabilitation (Chapter 15). Chapter 3, *Motor Development and Control*, integrates content from two previously separate chapters and expands application to practice.

The **45 case scenarios** and **80 videos** on Elsevier's Expert Consult platform are distinctive features of this fifth edition. The cases actively engage readers in clinical reasoning and decision making. The phrase *Pause and Reflect* followed by a question is inserted several times within a case to encourage readers to stop and reflect on what they would do before continuing to read the case. The phrase *Evidence to Practice* is followed by the rationale and evidence for a decision.

We are pleased to provide readers access to videos that illustrate children in their daily lives, examination procedures, and physical therapy interventions. Many of the case scenarios include an accompanying video. Additionally, there are videos on motor development, development of gait, tests and measures, practice in special settings, and transition to adulthood. An introduction to the case scenarios and videos is provided at the end of each chapter. A table of contents for the case scenarios and videos for each chapter is provided for easy reference. We strongly encourage readers to take advantage of these outstanding resources on the Expert Consult website, a user-friendly platform for easy access.

Edition 5 retains the five sections included in previous editions. Section 1, *Understanding Motor Performance in Children*, provides foundation knowledge for pediatric physical therapy practice, including evidence-based decision making, measurement, motor development and control, motor learning, musculoskeletal development and adaptation, and physical fitness. Sections 2 to 4 contain 22 chapters on the management of children with musculoskeletal, neuromuscular, and cardiopulmonary conditions. Chapters are organized by two main headings: *Background Information* (knowledge of the health condition, medical, and pharmacologic management) and *Foreground Information* (evidence-based recommendations for physical therapy management). Text boxes and tables are used to summarize recommendations for tests and measures and evidence for interventions. Section 5, *Special Settings and Special Considerations*, includes chapters on the neonatal intensive care unit, early intervention, the educational environment, transition to adulthood, and assistive technology. Throughout the book, chapters are cross-referenced to integrate content.

Robert J. Palisano
Senior Editor
Drexel University
Philadelphia, Pennsylvania

ACKNOWLEDGMENTS

The fifth edition of *Campbell's Physical Therapy for Children* is dedicated to Suzann K. Campbell and the 126 contributors to one or more editions. Adding Sue's name to the title acknowledges her vision for a comprehensive, evidence-based textbook on pediatric physical therapy and having guided *Physical Therapy for Children* from inception through edition 4. Sue's fingerprints grace the pages of edition 5. Hard to believe (especially for contributors to all five editions) that more than 20 years have passed since publication of the first edition. The key to success has been the expertise of the contributors, including the 73 contributors to edition 5. The contributors are an eclectic mix of pediatric clinical specialists, educators, and clinical researchers. They are distinguished not only by their expertise and leadership but also their commitment to excellence. Contributors have graciously devoted countless hours to their chapters to ensure content is of the highest quality. Collectively, they have made possible a high-quality textbook that spans the breadth and depth of pediatric physical therapy. Their contributions have enriched the education and professional development of countless students and pediatric physical therapists worldwide.

I am extremely grateful to Margo Orlin and Joe Schreiber (co-editors) for their collaboration and innovation in planning and editing the fifth edition. A comprehensive, 34-chapter textbook with extensive resources is a major undertaking—definitely a three-person effort! The editors are appreciative of the support provided by Kathy Falk, Courtney Sprehe, Rich Barber, and the rest of the Elsevier production team. Kathy and Courtney were receptive to the changes we proposed for the fifth edition and made them a reality.

Robert J. Palisano
Senior Editor
Drexel University
Philadelphia, Pennsylvania

CONTRIBUTORS

Jennifer L. Agnew, BHK, BScPT
Physiotherapist
Respiratory Medicine Division
Hospital for Sick Children
Lecturer
Physical Therapy
University of Toronto
Toronto, Ontario
Canada

Yvette Blanchard, PT, ScD, PCS
Professor
Physical Therapy
Sacred Heart University
Fairfield, Connecticut

Brenda Sposato Bonfiglio, MEBME, ATP
Clinical Assistant Professor
Disability and Human Development
University of Illinois at Chicago
Chicago, Illinois

Suzann K. Campbell, PT, PhD, FAPTA
Professor Emerita
Physical Therapy
University of Illinois at Chicago
Managing Partner
Infant Motor Performance Scales, LLC
Chicago, Illinois

Tricia Catalino, PT, DSc, PCS
Assistant Professor
School of Physical Therapy
Touro University Nevada
Henderson, Nevada

Lisa Chiarello, PT, PhD, PCS, FAPTA
Professor
Physical Therapy and Rehabilitation
    Sciences
Drexel University
Philadelphia, Pennsylvania

Nancy Cicirello, PT, MPH, EdD
Professor Emerita
School of Physical Therapy
Pacific University
Hillsboro, Oregon

Colleen Coulter, PT, DPT, PhD, MS, PCS
PT IV
Orthotics and Prosthetics
Children's Healthcare of Atlanta
Adjunct Assistant Professor of Rehabilitation
    Medicine
Division of Physical Therapy
Emory University
Atlanta, Georgia

Robin Lee Dole, PT, DPT, EdD, PCS
Professor of Physical Therapy and Director
Institute for Physical Therapy Education
Widener University
Associate Dean
School of Human Service Professions
Widener University
Chester, Pennsylvania
President
Physical Therapy Consultation and Services
Mount Royal, Pennsylvania

Maureen Donohoe, PT, DPT, PCS
Physical Therapy Clinical Specialist
Therapeutic Services
Nemours/ Alfred I. duPont Hospital
    for Children
Wilmington, Delaware

Antonette Doty, PT, PhD, PCS
School-Based Physical Therapist
Portage County Educational Service Center
Ravenna, Ohio
Adjunct Faculty
Physical Therapy
Walsh University
North Canton, Ohio

Susan V. Duff, PT, EdD, OTR/L, CHT
Adjunct Associate Professor
Physical Therapy
Thomas Jefferson University
Philadelphia, Pennsylvania
Associate Professor
Physical Therapy
Chapman University
Irvine, California

Helene M. Dumas, PT, MS
Manager
Research Center
Franciscan Hospital for Children
Boston, Massachusetts

Stacey Dusing, PhD, PT, PCS
Associate Professor
Physical Therapy
Virginia Commonwealth University
Director
Motor Development Lab
Virginia Commonwealth University
Associate Professor
Pediatrics
Children's Hospital of Richmond at VCU
Richmond, Virginia

Susan Effgen, PT, PhD, FAPTA
Professor
Rehabilitation Sciences
University of Kentucky
Lexington, Kentucky

Heidi Friedman, PT, DPT, PCS
Senior Physical Therapist
Rehabilitation
Ann and Robert H. Lurie Children's Hospital
    of Chicago
Chicago, Illinois
Physical Therapist
Outpatient Rehabilitation
Joe DiMaggio Children's Hospital
Hollywood, Florida

Brian Giavedoni, BSc, MBA, CP, LP
Senior Prosthetist, Assistant Manager
Limb Deficiency Program, Orthotics &
    Prosthetics
Children's Healthcare of Atlanta
Atlanta, Georgia

Allan M. Glanzman, PT, DPT, PCS
Clinical Specialist PT IV
Department of Physical Therapy
The Children's Hospital of Philadelphia
Philadelphia, Pennsylvania

Andrew M. Gordon, BA, MS, PhD
Professor of Movement Sciences
Movement Science Program Coordinator
Teachers College, Columbia University
New York, New York

Suzanne Green, BS
Senior Physical Therapist
Rehabilitation
Ann and Robert H. Lurie Children's Hospital
    of Chicago
Chicago, Illinois

Regina T. Harbourne, PhD, PT
Assistant Professor
Physical Therapy, Rangos School of
    Health Sciences
Duquesne University
Pittsburgh, Pennsylvania

Krystal Hay, PT, DPT
Physical Therapist
Clinical Therapies
Nationwide Children's Hospital
Pediatric Physical Therapy Resident
Nisonger Center
Columbus, Ohio

Paul J.M. Helders Sr., MSc, PhD
Professor Emeritus
Clinical Health Sciences
Utrecht University
Former Director and Medical Physiologist
Child Development and Exercise Center
University Medical Center and Children's
    Hospital
Utrecht, the Netherlands

Kathleen Hinderer, PhD, MS, MPT, PT
Michigan Abilities Center
Physical Therapy, Hippotherapy
Ann Arbor, Michigan

Steven Hinderer, PT, MD
Associate Professor and Residency Program
    Director
Department of Physical Medicine and
    Rehabilitation - Oakwood
Wayne State University School of Medicine
Dearborn, Michigan

Jamie M. Holloway, PT, DPT, PCS
Pre-Doctoral Research Fellow
Departments of Physical & Occupational
    Therapy
University of Alabama at Birmingham
Birmingham, Alabama

Betsy Howell, PT, MS
Physical Therapist
Physical Medicine and Rehabilitation
University of Michigan Medical Center
Ann Arbor, Michigan

Mary Wills Jesse, PT, DHS, OCS
Clinical Specialist
Rehabilitation
Decatur Memorial Hospital
Decatur, Illinois

Therese Johnston, PT, PhD, MBA
Associate Professor
Physical Therapy
Thomas Jefferson University
Philadelphia, Pennsylvania

Maria Jones, PhD, PT
Associate Professor
Rehabilitation Sciences
University of Oklahoma Health Sciences
    Center
Oklahoma City, Oklahoma

Marcia K. Kaminker, PT, DPT, MS, PCS
Physical Therapist
Department of Student Services
South Brunswick School District
South Brunswick, New Jersey

Sandra L. Kaplan, PT, DPT, PhD
Professor and Director of Post-Professional
    Education
Department of Rehabilitation and Movement
    Sciences, Programs in Physical Therapy
Rutgers, The State University of New Jersey
Newark, New Jersey

Michal Katz-Leurer, PhD
Faculty of Medicine
Department of Physical Therapy
Tel Aviv University
Ramat Aviv, Israel

M. Kathleen Kelly, PhD, PT
Associate Professor and Vice Chair
Department of Physical Therapy
University of Pittsburgh
Pittsburgh, Pennsylvania

Christin Krey, PT, MPT
Physical Therapist
Department of Rehabilitation
Shriners Hospital for Children
Philadelphia, Pennsylvania

Amanda Kusler, BS, DPT
Physical Therapy
Children's Hospital of Philadelphia
Philadelphia, Pennsylvania

Toby Long, PhD
Professor
Pediatrics
Associate Director
Center for Child and Human Development
Georgetown University
Washington, D.C.

Linda Pax Lowes, PT, PhD
Center for Gene Therapy
Nationwide Children's Hospital
Columbus, Ohio

Kathryn Lucas, PT, DPT, SCS, CSCS
Physical Therapist II
Occupational Therapy and Physical Therapy
Cincinnati Children's Hospital Medical Center
Cincinnati, Ohio

Richard Magill, PhD, EdM, BS
Visiting Professor
Biobehavioral Sciences
Teachers College, Columbia University
Adjunct Professor
Physical Therapy
New York University
New York, New York

Victoria Marchese, PT, PhD
Associate Professor
Physical Therapy and Rehabilitation Science
University of Maryland, School of Medicine
Baltimore, Maryland

Mary Massery, PT, DPT, DSc
Owner
Massery Physical Therapy
Glenview, Illinois

Melissa Maule, MPT, DPT
Physical Therapist
Mid-Shore Special Education Consortium
Easton, Maryland

Irene McEwen, PT, PhD, DPT
Professor Emerita
Rehabilitation Sciences
University of Oklahoma Health Sciences
    Center
Oklahoma City, Oklahoma

Beth McManus, PT, MPH, ScD
Assistant Professor
Health Systems, Management, and Policy
Colorado School of Public Health
Methodologist
Children's Outcomes Research Program
University of Colorado
Aurora, Colorado

Mary Meiser, BS, MS
Physical Therapist
Mid-Shore Special Education Consortium
Easton, Maryland

Cheryl Missiuna, PhD, OTReg (Ont)
Professor
School of Rehabilitation Science
McMaster University
Hamilton, Ontario, Canada

G. Stephen Morris, PT, PhD, FACSM
President, Oncology Section, APTA
Associate Professor
Wingate University
Department of Physical Therapy
Wingate, North Carolina

Margo N. Orlin, PT, PhD, FAPTA
Associate Professor
Physical Therapy and Rehabilitation
    Sciences
Drexel University
Philadelphia, Pennsylvania

Roberta Kuchler O'Shea, PT, DPT, PhD
Professor
Physical Therapy
Governors State University
University Park, Illinois

Blythe Owen, HBSc, MScPT
Physiotherapist
Rehabilitation Services
The Hospital for Sick Children
Lecturer
Physical Therapy, Faculty of Medicine
University of Toronto
Toronto, Ontario, Canada

Robert J. Palisano, PT, ScD, FAPTA
Distinguished Professor
Physical Therapy and Rehabilitation Sciences
Drexel University
Philadelphia, Pennsylvania
Scientist
CanChild Centre for Childhood Disability
    Research
McMaster University
Hamilton, Ontario, Canada

Mark Paterno, PT, PhD, MBA, SCS, ATC
Associate Professor
Division of Sports Medicine, Department
    of Pediatrics
Cincinnati Children's Hospital Medical
    Center
Cincinnati, Ohio

Nancy Pollock, MSc, BSc
Associate Clinical Professor
School of Rehabilitation Science
McMaster University
Hamilton, Ontario, Canada

Catherine Quatman-Yates, DPT, PhD
Assistant Professor
Sports Medicine
Physical Therapist III
Occupational and Physical Therapy
Cincinnati Children's Hospital Medical
    Center
Cincinnati, Ohio

Lisa Rivard, PT, MSc, PhD(c)
School of Rehabilitation Science
McMaster University
Hamilton, Ontario, Canada

Hemda Rotem, PT
Senior Physical Therapist
Alyn Pediatric and Adolescent Rehabilitation
    Hospital
Jerusalem, Israel

Barbara Sargent, PhD, PT, PCS
Assistant Professor of Clinical Physical Therapy
Division of Biokinesiology and Physical
    Therapy
University of Southern California
Los Angeles, California

Laura Schmitt, BA, MPT, PhD
Assistant Professor of Physical Therapy
School of Health and Rehabilitation Sciences
The Ohio State University
Columbus, Ohio

Joseph Schreiber, PT, PhD
Professor and Program Director
Physical Therapy Program
Chatham University
Pittsburgh, Pennsylvania

Jennifer Siemon, BHSc, MSc(OT)
Coordinator, Behavioural Supports Ontario
Hamilton Health Sciences
Hamilton, Ontario, Canada

David Shurtleff, MD
Professor Emeritus
Pediatrics, Division of Congenital Defects
Children's Hospital and Medical Center
University of Washington
Seattle, Washington

Meg Stanger, MS, PT, PCS
Manager of Physical Therapy and
    Occupational Therapy
Children's Hospital of Pittsburgh of UPMC
Pittsburgh, Pennsylvania

Jean Stout, PT, MS
Research Physical Therapist
James R. Gage Center for Gait and Motion
    Analysis
Gillette Children's Specialty Healthcare
St. Paul, Minnesota

Wayne A. Stuberg, PT, PhD, FAPTA, PCS
Professor and Associate Director
Munroe-Meyer Institute for Genetics and
    Rehabilitation
University of Nebraska Medical Center
Omaha, Nebraska

Lorrie Sylvester, PT, PhD
Clinical Assistant Professor
Rehabilitation Sciences
University of Oklahoma Health Sciences
    Center, College of Allied Health
Oklahoma City, Oklahoma

Tim Takken, PhD
Child Development & Exercise Center
University Medical Center and Children's
    Hospital
Utrecht, the Netherlands

Chris D. Tapley, MSPT
Physical Therapy Clinical Specialist
Department of Physical Medicine and
    Rehabilitation, Occupational and Physical
    Therapy Division
University of Michigan C.S. Mott Children's
    Hospital
Ann Arbor, Michigan

Christina Calhoun Thielen, MSPT
Clinical Research Project Manager
School of Health Professions
Thomas Jefferson University
Philadelphia, Pennsylvania

Kristin M. Thomas, PT, DPT
Physical Therapist
Center for Cancer and Blood Disorders
Children's Hospital Colorado
Aurora, Colorado

Janjaap van der Net, PhD, BSc
Associate Professor
Child Development and Exercise
University Children's Hospital, UMC at
    Utrecht
Associate Professor
Clinical Health Sciences
Utrecht University
Utrecht, the Netherlands

Darl Vander Linden, PT, PhD
Professor
Physical Therapy
Eastern Washington University
Spokane, Washington

William O. Walker, Jr., MD
Chief, Division of Developmental Medicine
Pediatrics
University of Washington School of
    Medicine/Seattle Children's Hospital
Seattle, Washington

Marilyn Wright, BScPT, MEd, MSc
Physical Therapy Discipline Lead
McMaster Children's Hospital
Hamilton Health Sciences
Assistant Clinical Professor
School of Rehabilitation Sciences
McMaster University
Hamilton, Ontario, Canada

CONTENTS

TABLE OF CONTENTS – CASE SCENARIOS

TABLE OF CONTENTS – VIDEOS

Evidence-Based Decision Making in Pediatric Physical Therapy

Joseph Schreiber, Robert J. Palisano

Pediatric physical therapists make multiple complex and challenging clinical decisions on a daily basis. These include determining eligibility and need for services, selecting intervention techniques and strategies to engage and motivate children, deciding the frequency and duration of services including when to discontinue services, and selecting outcome measures and interpretation of findings. An essential aspect of decision making in pediatric physical therapy is effective collaboration with families and children to determine the best course of action for an individual child at a particular point in time. On what basis do we make these important decisions with children and families? Evidence suggests that physical therapists make clinical decisions based primarily on knowledge gained from entry-level education, continuing education conferences, and from peers.[4,6,25,27,53,54,38,24] Although this reliance on professional craft knowledge has historically served us well, it is an expectation in today's health care environment that physical therapists also integrate the best available research evidence into valid and reliable clinical decision making and that decision making be systematic and consistent. The purpose of this chapter is to provide guidance on optimal clinical decision making for pediatric physical therapists. Several overarching frameworks are presented, including the International Classification of Functioning, Disability and Health (ICF), the American Physical Therapy Association (APTA) Guide to Physical Therapy Practice, evidence-based practice, and effective and efficient strategies for knowledge acquisition, analysis, and integration. These frameworks are integrated into a collaborative evidence-informed decision-making model that should serve to optimize outcomes for children and families.

INTERNATIONAL CLASSIFICATION OF FUNCTIONING, DISABILITY AND HEALTH

One important framework to guide clinical decision making is the International Classification of Functioning, Disability and Health (ICF; World Health Organization[55]), which aids in the identification of child and family strengths and needs, along with home and community/environmental considerations, including family resources and availability and accessibility of services. The ICF was developed to provide a scientific basis for understanding and studying health and health-related states, outcomes, and determinants. The ICF also is intended to provide a common language in order to improve communication among people with disabilities, health care providers, researchers, and policy makers. The ICF emphasizes "components of health" rather than "consequences of disease" (i.e., participation rather than disability) and environmental and personal factors as important determinants of health. The ICF model is available on the World Health Organization website (www.who.int/classifications/icf/en). A children and youth version (ICF-CY) was published by the World Health Organization in 2007.[56] The model is the same as the ICF but codes for components of health, personal, and environmental factors were modified and new codes added to reflect development and environments of children and youth from birth to 18 years. A resolution was passed in 2012 to merge the ICF-CY into the ICF. The ICF framework has been incorporated into the third edition of the *Guide to Physical Therapist Practice*[2] and is used throughout this text.

The diagram of the ICF model is presented in Fig. 1.1. The ICF has two parts. Part 1, Functioning and Disability, includes three components of health: body functions and structures, activities, and participation. Part 2, Contextual Factors, includes environmental and personal factors that influence components of health. For example, the impact of activity (ability to walk) and participation (ability to travel with classmates at school when going to lunch) may be influenced by the environment (distance from classroom to cafeteria and time to travel this distance) and personal factors (the child's motivation to walk). The bidirectional arrows in the ICF model are inclusive of all possible relationships. The challenge when applying the ICF is to identify the relationships that are most relevant for an individual child and family.

Body functions are the physiologic and psychological functions of body systems. Physiologic functions include respiration, vision, sensation, muscle performance, and movement. Psychological functions include attention, memory, emotion, thought, and language. *Body structures* are the anatomic parts of the body such as the brain, organs, bones, ligaments, muscles, and tendons. *Impairments* are problems in body functions and structures. Examples of impairments are limited ability to plan and execute movement, poor processing of sensory information, reduced cardiorespiratory endurance, lack of sensation, muscle weakness, balance difficulties, skeletal deformity, and joint contracture. *Activity* is the performance of a task or action by an individual. Activities represent the integrated use of body functions and vary in complexity. Examples of activities are maintaining and changing body positions, walking and moving around, lifting and carrying objects, fine hand use, and self-care. *Activity limitations* are difficulties in performing age-appropriate tasks or actions. *Participation* is involvement in a life situation. Most children participate in home life, school, community activities and organizations, and social relationships with friends. Participation is highly individualized. What is important to one child may be of little consequence to another child. *Participation restrictions* are problems in involvement in life situations. *Environmental factors* make up the physical, social, and attitudinal environments in which people live and conduct their lives. *Personal factors* are the particular background of the individual's life and living that *are not* part of a health condition or disorder. These factors may include gender, race/ethnicity, age, fitness, lifestyle, habits, coping styles, and past and current experiences.[55] Box 1.1 lists considerations for applying the ICF to clinical decision making.

For each of the three components of health and the environment factor, the ICF lists domains, categories within domains, and qualifiers to record the presence and severity of the problem. For example, one domain for Activity and Participation is Mobility, and among the categories of Mobility are Walking and Transportation. Core sets of categories that are considered most relevant for particular health conditions have been developed and include cerebral palsy and autism (http://icf-research-branch.org).

An example of a child with cerebral palsy spastic diplegia, Gross Motor Function Classification System level II, illustrates application of the ICF for clinical decision making (Fig. 1.2).

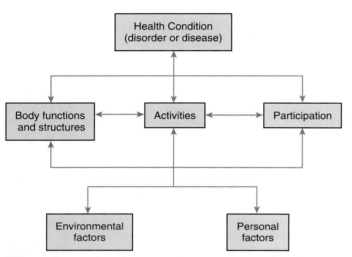

FIG. 1.1 Interactions between the components of the International Classification of Functioning, Disability and Health (IFC). (Courtesy of the World Health Organization: *International classification of functioning, disability and health.* Geneva, Switzerland: WHO; 2002.)

BOX 1.1   Considerations for Using the International Classification of Functioning, Disability and Health as a Framework for Clinical Decision Making

Body Functions and Body Structures
Not all impairments are modified by physical therapy
Not all impairments cause activity limitations and participation restrictions
Relate impairments to activity limitations and participation restrictions
Impairments are identified from examination and evaluation of body functions and structures

Activities
Relate activity limitations to participation restrictions
Activity limitations can cause secondary impairments
Activities are often measured by norm-referenced and criterion-referenced assessments

Participation
Reflects child and family perspectives
Is context dependent (environmental and personal factors)
Is one aspect of health-related quality of life
Is measured by child and parent self-report
Is measured by observations in natural environments as well as parent and child self-report

---

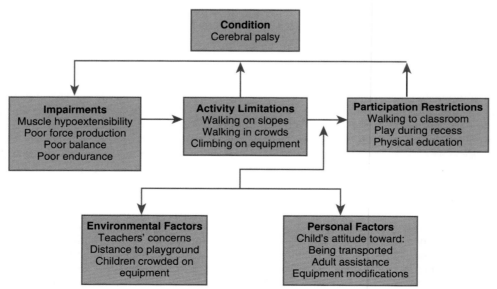

FIG. 1.2 Example of application of the International Classification of Functioning, Disability and Health to clinical decision making.

The child's impairments in the neuromuscular and musculo-skeletal systems include hamstring and gastrocnemius muscle hypoextensibility, reduced muscle force production, poor balance, and limited muscular endurance. The child's activity limitations include difficulties in walking on a sloping surface, walking amid people, and climbing playground equipment. At school, the child occasionally falls when walking from the bus to the classroom. Although the child has several friends and enjoys physical activity, participation in recess and physical education is restricted. Social and physical environmental factors that may contribute to restricted participation include the following: teachers are concerned that the child will get injured; the child's classroom is located at the end of the school most distant from the playground; the terrain of the school yard is uneven; and students are crowded on the playground equipment.

When applying the ICF framework, the therapist is encouraged to identify what the child does (strengths) in addition to impairments, activity limitations, and participation restrictions that limit or restrict what the child wants to or needs to do. The challenge is to hypothesize cause-effect relationships. For example, what are the possible causes of a student's restricted participation during recess and physical education? Will instruction and practice in walking in varied settings and climbing on playground equipment (motor learning) improve participation? A systematic review of interventions for children with cerebral palsy by Novak et al. (2013) reported evidence of effectiveness of interventions that are goal directed and provided in natural environments.[36] Collaboration with the teachers to discuss their safety concerns and the feasibility of modifications to playground equipment are environmental considerations. The child's feelings about energy conservation (e.g., being transported to the playground), modifications of playground equipment, and support from adults are examples of personal factors to consider in formulating an intervention plan. Note that in Fig. 1.2, only the hypothesized interactions are depicted. The arrow from the participation restrictions and activity limitation to impairments represents a secondary impairment.

APTA GUIDE TO PHYSICAL THERAPIST PRACTICE 3.0

The *Guide to Physical Therapist Practice 3.0* (Guide 3.0) provides a framework to inform clinical decision making for patient/client management.[2] At the time this chapter was published, Guide 3.0 was available online at no cost to members of the APTA or by paid subscription for other users. The second edition of the Guide (2001) was designed as a resource not only for physical therapists but also for health care policy makers, administrators, managed care providers, third-party payers, and other professionals. Guide 3.0 is a description of practice intended primarily for physical therapists and physical therapist assistants. The language of the Guide has been modified to be consistent with the ICF, and Review of Symptoms has been added to the Examination. The Preferred Physical Therapist Practice Patterns from earlier editions have been removed. The purposes of Guide 3.0 include description of: a) the roles of physical therapists and physical therapist assistants in different practice settings, including roles in prevention and the promotion of health, wellness, and fitness; b) standardized terminology; c) the clinical decision-making process that occurs as part of patient and client management, including the examination and evaluation process focusing on tests and measures and selection of interventions; and d) measuring outcomes.

Patient/Client Management Model

The model of patient/client management presented in Guide 3.0 is designed to maximize outcomes through a systematic and comprehensive approach to decision making. The model includes six elements: examination, evaluation, diagnosis, prognosis, intervention, and outcomes. The elements are used to organize content throughout the text.

Examination

The physical therapist is required to perform an examination before providing any intervention. The examination consists of the history, systems review, and selected tests and measures. The history is an account of the child's past and current health status, which is obtained through an interview with the child and caregivers and review of medical and educational records. As part of the history, the physical therapist identifies child and family expectations and desired outcomes of physical therapy. A useful means for documenting and quantifying family expectations is the Canadian Occupational Performance Measure.[36] The physical therapist then considers whether these expectations and outcomes are realistic in the context of examination and evaluation data.

The systems review is a brief screening that is intended to help focus the subsequent examination and identify possible health problems that require consultation with or referral to another health care provider. A thorough systems review is critical for managing clients who have direct access to physical therapy services. After analyzing information from the history and systems review, the physical therapist examines the child more closely, selecting tests and measures to obtain sufficient data to make an evaluation, establish a diagnosis and a prognosis, and select appropriate interventions.

Evaluation

Evaluation is a process in which the physical therapist makes judgments about the status of the child based on the information gathered from the examination. Evaluation refers to the process by which the results of the examination are analyzed and interpreted in order to determine a diagnosis within the scope of physical therapist practice; the prognosis, including goals for physical therapy management; and a plan of care. The evaluation process includes judgment of the relationships among impairments in body functions and structures, activity limitations, participation restrictions, and the influence of environmental and personal factors. We encourage therapists to consider child, family, and community strengths as part of the evaluation process. Strength-based and ability-focused interventions build on the strengths and resources of the youth, family, and community.[44]

Diagnosis

The definition of diagnosis as it pertains to physical therapist practice is evolving. Guide 3.0 states: "Physical therapists use labels that identify the impact of a condition on function at the level of the system (especially the movement system) and at the level of the whole person. Physical therapists use a systematic process (sometimes referred to as differential diagnosis) to classify an individual into a diagnostic category."[2] The aim is to identify the capacity of an individual to achieve the desired level of function (achieve goals) and whether this can be accomplished by physical therapy. Physical therapists, therefore, may need to obtain additional information (including diagnostic labels) from physicians and other professionals.

Prognosis

Perhaps the greatest challenge to patient/client management is determination of the likelihood that an individual child or youth will achieve the desired goals of intervention. Prognosis refers to the predicted optimal level of improvement in function and the amount of service needed to reach that level (frequency and duration of intervention). A trend in managed health care is to use periodic and episodic intervals of therapy services based on specific functional problems. This approach is a marked departure for children with developmental disabilities for whom ongoing services have traditionally been reimbursed based on medical diagnosis.

If the examination and evaluation support the need for physical therapy, the therapist's next important decision is the plan of care. What interventions should be implemented, how often, and for how long? Presently, research evidence to guide decisions on amount of service is limited. Outcomes are the changes that are anticipated as a result of implementing the plan of care. Expected outcomes should be measurable and time limited. Outcomes of therapy include changes in health, wellness, and physical fitness, emerging areas of pediatric practice.

Intervention

Intervention is the purposeful and skilled interaction of the physical therapist with the patient/client and, when appropriate, with other individuals involved in patient/client care. Various physical therapy procedures and techniques are used during intervention to enable the child and family to achieve goals and outcomes that are consistent with the child's diagnosis and prognosis. Physical therapy intervention has three components: (1) coordination, communication, and documentation; (2) patient/client instruction; and (3) procedural interventions.

Coordination, communication, and documentation. These services are provided for all children and their families to ensure appropriate, coordinated, comprehensive, and cost-effective care and efficient integration or reintegration into home, community, and work (job/school/play). Services may include (1) case management, (2) coordination of care with family and other professionals, (3) discharge planning, (4) education plans, (5) case conferences, and (6) documentation of patient/client management. Children with disabilities are managed in a variety of settings, from public schools to private offices or rehabilitation facilities to specialty clinics for orthotics, surgery, and assistive technology. Therapists in each of these settings often express frustration regarding the lack of coordination of services and the paucity of effective and timely information sharing among health professionals, teachers, and families.

Patient/client-related instruction. These services are provided for all families to provide information about the child's current condition, the plan of care, and current or future transition to home, work, or community roles. Methods of instruction include demonstration; modeling; verbal, written, or pictorial instruction; and periodic reexamination and reassessment of the home program. The educational backgrounds, needs, and learning styles of family members must be considered during this process. As part of family-centered services, therapists collaborate with children and families to identify how to incorporate exercise and practice of functional movements in daily activities and routines.

Procedural interventions. In the Guide 3.0, physical therapist interventions are organized into 9 categories:

Patient or client instruction (used with every patient and client)
Airway clearance techniques
Assistive technology
Biophysical agents
Functional training in self-care and domestic, work, community, social, and civic life
Integumentary repair and protection techniques
Manual therapy techniques
Motor function training
Therapeutic exercise

The child's response to intervention is closely monitored, and the intervention plan is revised as appropriate. Throughout the text the authors provide recommendations supported by research and best practices for specific procedural interventions based on children's age and health condition.

Outcomes

Outcomes are the results of implementing the plan of care; they indicate the impact of the intervention on functioning (body functions and structures, activities, and participation). Outcomes are essential to evaluate the effect of physical therapy for individual children and evaluate services and programs within a health care organization or education system. Outcome measurement is addressed in Chapter 2, and recommendations are provided in the chapters on management of children with musculoskeletal, neurologic, and cardiopulmonary conditions.

EVIDENCE-BASED PRACTICE

Evidence-based practice is the standard for pediatric physical therapy. Evidence-based physical therapy practice has been defined as "open and thoughtful clinical decision making about the physical therapy management of a patient/client that integrates the best available evidence with clinical judgment and the patient's/client's preferences and values, and that further considers the larger social context in which physical therapy services are provided, to optimize patient/client outcomes and quality of life."[26] This open and thoughtful clinical decision-making paradigm implies a defensible, transparent, and reflective process and requires that practitioners know about and are capable of effectively sharing the best available evidence with patients/clients and caregivers.

Pediatric physical therapists engage in lifelong learning and professional development as ways to know about current best evidence and therefore are faced with an almost constant need to acquire and integrate knowledge. There are a number of challenges and barriers that may impact these processes, including significant time constraints, lack of awareness of the evidence, limited confidence in interpreting and applying research results, disagreement with practice guideline recommendations, and the presence of economic, administrative, and interprofessional constraints.[11,38,41,48] In addition, entrenchment of existing practice behaviors or habits may also limit practice change despite the presence of new knowledge.[16,43,47]

Background and Foreground Information

An essential first step in efficiently acquiring new knowledge occurs during and after interaction with the child and family. Questions naturally arise regarding the best course of action to address problems and concerns. Questions may also arise related to the child's health condition or age group. One way to organize these questions and to guide subsequent searching strategies is to determine whether there is a need for background or foreground information. *Background information* is most often related to a specific diagnostic condition and may include pathology and pathophysiology, etiology, prognosis and natural evolution of the condition, and medical and pharmacologic management. Background information may also include human anatomy, physiology, kinesiology, and neurology. Efforts to gather background information reflect a desire to understand the nature of a patient's/client's health condition, problem, or need. Novices and those lacking experience and expertise with a specific condition are more likely to gather this type of information, but it can also be useful for more experienced practitioners interested in ensuring that knowledge and understanding are up to date.[26,18]

A number of different types of resources may be used to search for and acquire background information. These include consulting with peers or practice leaders, continuing education courses, textbooks, web-based resources, and informal and formal in-services and practice/workshop sessions with colleagues and peers.[50] Research articles often contain information relevant to background questions in their introductory paragraphs.[26] Government agencies, professional societies, and national patient advocacy groups often vet this type of information and publish it for clinicians and consumers in written and electronic formats.[26] In an effort to enhance the organizational structure and to support efficient knowledge gathering for the reader, the chapters in *Physical Therapy for Children* that focus on a health condition are organized by "Background Information" and "Foreground Information." Each background information section includes pathology and pathophysiology, etiology, prognosis and natural evolution, and medical and pharmacologic management, in addition to any other relevant background information pertaining to specific pediatric health conditions.

Practitioners are likely to seek out *foreground information* on a frequent basis. This is due to the ongoing need to acquire new knowledge about the physical therapy management of children who present with specific movement challenges or diagnoses. Foreground information can aid practitioners in identifying, selecting, implementing, and interpreting the most appropriate diagnostic and prognostic tests and measures. In addition, continually building foreground information ensures that practitioners are aware of the most effective intervention strategies and procedures and can therefore collaborate optimally with caregivers and patients/clients to identify the most appropriate intervention for an individual child. Gathering this type of knowledge may be more helpful for practitioners after having acquired background knowledge about a specific health condition.[18,26] In this text, each Foreground Information section includes evidence-based recommendations on physical therapy examination strategies, optimal tests and measures for diagnosis and prognosis, and on physical therapy intervention planning including procedural interventions, coordination and communication, and patient/client/caregiver instruction. Where appropriate, both the Background and Foreground Information will address the implications of life span changes as infants and children grow up and become adolescents and adults.

Declarative and Procedural Knowledge

An interrelated way to organize clinical questions and knowledge gathering is to determine whether there is a need for additional declarative knowledge or procedural knowledge. *Declarative knowledge* can be thought of as "knowing what." The ability to name the bones in the wrist, describe the typical characteristics of an adolescent with Down syndrome, and explain the process of serial casting to a student or novice physical therapist are examples of declarative knowledge. A second type of knowledge is *procedural knowledge,* which involves knowing how and knowing when to apply various procedures, methods, theories, styles, or approaches. For pediatric physical therapists, this might include implementation of standardized testing procedures, modulation of amount of assistance during gait training, and strategies to motivate a child to complete a challenging task.[1] It is common for students and novices to know facts and concepts but not now how or when to apply them. In contrast, practitioners may also be able to perform procedural tasks without being able to articulate a clear understanding of what they are doing and why.[1]

Evidence-Based Resources for Acquiring Knowledge

As noted previously, thoughtful reflection on practice often leads to identification of clinical questions. If the question necessitates obtaining foreground information, an important next step to aid in focusing the search process is to configure the clinical problem into a PICO format, which involves four elements: P = patient, I = intervention, C = comparison intervention, and O = outcome. Examples of PICO questions (or PIO questions, where only one intervention is being investigated) are included in Box 1.2.

Once the question has been refined, the 6S model is a means to enhance efficient knowledge gathering to address the question (Fig. 1.3).[8] This model reflects the evolution over the past decade toward creation and use of "preappraised" resources that facilitate ready access to high-quality research. Preappraised resources can increase the efficiency of searching for and analyzing research evidence because they have undergone a filtering process to include only those studies that are of higher quality. In addition, ideally the resources are updated regularly, which ensures that the evidence is current.[8] The 6S model can aid in gathering background information about a health condition. For foreground information, decision makers should use a PICO question to search for evidence starting at the highest level of the pyramid, and therefore the most synthesized form of evidence, as opposed to beginning the search at the bottom of the pyramid, representing the least synthesized form of evidence. It becomes necessary to move to lower levels in the pyramid only when no evidence exists at a higher level.[42]

At the top of the pyramid are *Computerized Decision Support Systems* that match information from specific clients

---

BOX 1.2   Examples of Clinical Questions Written Using the PICO Format

For (P) children with developmental coordination disorder, is (I) cognitive motor learning more effective than (C) sensory integration in improving (O) motor function?

For children (P) with hemiplegia, is (I) bimanual coordination therapy more effective than (C) constraint-induced movement therapy in improving (O) arm and hand motor function?

For (P) infants with torticollis, what (I) physical therapy interventions improve (O) head and neck alignment and range of motion?

For (P) children with Duchenne muscular dystrophy, is (I) resistive exercise effective in (O) maintaining the ability to walk?

For (P) parents of infants born preterm, does (I) support, education, and instruction in the neonatal intensive care nursery improve (O) confidence and skill in handling and caring for their infants upon discharge to home?

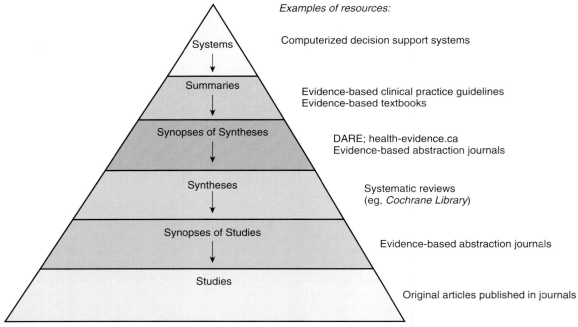

FIG. 1.3 6S hierarchy of preappraised evidence. (From DiCenso A, Bayley L, Haynes RB: Accessing pre-appraised evidence: fine-tuning the 5S model into a 6S model. *Evid Based Nurs* 12(4): 99-101, 2009.)

(individuals, groups, or populations) with the best available evidence that applies. These systems provide suggestions to the clinician for management of the specific patient.[8] Ideally the decision support is provided automatically as part of daily work flow, at the time and location of decision making, and with specific actionable recommendations. Systems represent the ideal resource for evidence-informed decision making because they contain all the research evidence about a specific client or population circumstance, linked to individual client records and to a synopsis of the existing relevant research literature with direct links to the original studies and/or reviews.[42] Although there are efforts currently under way to develop systems level data, it is not expected that these will be readily available in the near future.[42]

The next level of the 6S pyramid is *Summaries,* which integrate the best available evidence from the lower levels (drawing on syntheses [e.g., systematic reviews] as much as possible) to provide a full range of evidence concerning management options for a given health condition.[22] Examples include evidence-informed clinical practice guidelines (CPGs) and electronic textbooks, which can easily be made universally available (e.g., via the Internet), and are more feasible to keep up to date and provide some level of passive decision support. A well-known source for evidence-informed clinical practice guidelines is the National Guidelines Clearinghouse (NGC) (http://guideline.gov). The NGC, an initiative of the Agency for Healthcare Research and Quality (AHRQ), is a repository of clinical practice guidelines. The APTA, in collaboration with a number of sections including the Section on Pediatrics (SOP), also actively supports the development of clinical practice guidelines in order to reduce unwarranted variation in care. An example is a CPG for congenital muscular torticollis published in *Pediatric Physical Therapy* in 2013[28] and also available through the NGC website.

Practitioners accessing CPGs and other summary documents should ensure that they meet the following criteria[15]:
Based on a systematic review of the existing evidence
Developed by a knowledgeable, multidisciplinary panel of experts and representatives from key affected groups
Considers important patient subgroups and patient preferences, as appropriate
Based on an explicit and transparent process that minimizes distortions, biases, and conflicts of interest
Provides a clear explanation of the logical relationships between alternative care options and health outcomes and provides ratings of both the quality of evidence and the strength of the recommendations
Reconsidered and revised as appropriate when important new evidence warrants modifications of recommendations

An additional resource for appraisal of clinical practice guidelines is the Appraisal of Guidelines for Research and Evaluation (AGREE II) collaboration. This collaboration includes members from Denmark, Finland, France, Germany, Italy, the Netherlands, Spain, Switzerland, the United Kingdom, Canada, New Zealand, and the United States. AGREE II is a reliable and valid instrument to assess clinical practice guidelines developed by local, regional, national, or international groups and government organizations and can be used by physical therapists deciding whether to implement recommendations in a practice guideline or pathway. The instrument provides guiding questions and a response scale to assess the scope and purpose of a guideline, the people involved in development, rigor of development, clarity and presentation of recommendations, applicability, and editorial independence. The instrument and training manual are available on the AGREE website (http://www.agreetrust.org).

The next level on the 6S pyramid is *Synopses of Syntheses,* which are defined as succinct descriptions of systematic reviews or meta-analyses that aim to provide the right amount of evidence (not too much nor too little) to inform an intervention.[22] Ideally, these synopses describe the research question, the study groups, the outcomes, and the measure of effect or other results of a body of evidence. These summaries often discuss the methodologic quality of the synthesis and the relevance of the findings to health practice, program development, and policies. Given that many busy clinicians do not have the time to review detailed systematic reviews, a synopsis that summarizes the findings of a high-quality systematic review can often provide sufficient information to support clinical action. One example is the Database of Abstracts of Reviews of Effectiveness (DARE) of the Centre for Review Dissemination (CRD) at the National Institute for Health Research in the United Kingdom. DARE assists decision makers by systematically identifying and describing systematic reviews, appraising their quality, and highlighting their relative strengths and weaknesses.[42]

At the next level, *Syntheses* are synonymous with systematic reviews and meta-analyses and are found in peer-reviewed journals. Syntheses combine, using explicit and rigorous methods, the results of multiple single studies to provide a single set of findings.[22;42] The Cochrane Library (www.thecochranelibrary.com/) houses syntheses about the effectiveness of health care interventions and some diagnostic tests and also includes the DARE database of systematic reviews.[8]

In a well-conducted systematic review, all relevant research is analyzed in an effort to determine the overall evidence. The process involves: (1) a focused clinical question, (2) identification of criteria for inclusion of a study in the review, (3) a comprehensive literature search, (4) appraisal of the internal validity (methodologic quality) of each study included in the review, (5) a description of how results were analyzed, and (6) interpretation of findings in a manner that enhances application to clinical practice.[10] Just as in a research report, therapists must critique a systematic review. A systematic review is only as good as the quality of each study included. Meta-analysis is a mathematical synthesis of the results of two or more research reports. A meta-analysis can be performed on studies that used reliable and valid measures and report some type of inferential statistic (e.g., t-test, analysis of variance). Effect size, odds ratio, and the weighted mean difference are examples of statistics used for meta-analysis.

Effect size is the mean difference of the outcomes of interest between subjects in experimental and comparison/control groups. The most basic measure of effect size is the *d-index*. The d-index is the mean difference between groups divided by the common standard deviation. Cohen[5] provided the following guidelines for interpretation of the d-index: d = 0.2 represents a small effect, d = 0.5 represents a medium effect, and d = 0.8 represents a large effect. Fig. 1.4 and Table 1.1 present the overlap of scores between subjects in the experimental and control group for selected effect sizes. The overlap in distribution of scores has important implications for clinical decision making. A finding that the mean score on the outcome measured was significantly higher for subjects in the experimental group does not indicate that all subjects or even most subjects in the experimental group had better outcomes than subjects in the comparison/control group. As illustrated in Table 1.1, even for a large effect size (0.80), there is a 53% overlap in scores of subjects in the experimental and control groups. Consequently, when applying the evidence to clinical decisions for an individual child, the therapist would not be certain of that child's outcome.

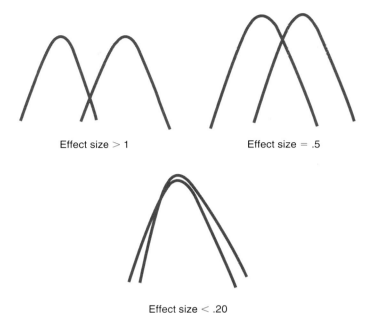

Effect size > 1   Effect size = .5

Effect size < .20

FIG. 1.4 Distribution of scores of subjects in the experimental and control groups for small-, medium-, and large-effect sizes (illustrations not drawn to scale).

TABLE 1.1   Interpretation of Effect Size Based on Cohen's Criteria[5]

Effect Size	Interpretation	Overlap of Scores[a]
0.00	No effect	100%
0.20	Small	85%
0.50	Medium	67%
0.80	Large	53%
1.70		25%

[a]Overlap in individual scores of subjects in the experimental and control groups.

The *Forest Plot Diagram* is used to graphically present the results of a systematic review. Results may be presented as an effect size, weighted mean difference, or odds ratio; however, interpretation is the same. Fig. 1.5 illustrates a Forest Plot Diagram for a meta-analysis of four randomized controlled trials. The odds ratio is used to present the results of each study and the meta-analysis. The odds ratio is presented on a scale of 0.10 to 10.0; 1.00 is the line of no effect. Each study is represented on the graph by a horizontal line. The vertical mark in the middle of the line is the odds ratio, and the diamonds at the far left and right indicate the boundaries of the 95% confidence interval. If a horizontal line crosses the line of no effect, the odds ratio is not significantly greater than 1 (P > 0.05). When the horizontal line is to the right of the line of no effect, the odds ratio is significantly greater than 1 (P > 0.05). In Fig. 1.5 the odds ratio for only one study is significantly greater than 1 (top study). The horizontal lines for the remaining three studies cross the line of no effect, indicating the odds ratio is not significantly greater than 1. The thicker horizontal line at the bottom is the overall odds ratio for the four studies. The overall odds ratio is 0.90 (P > 0.05), indicating that subjects who received the experimental intervention were not more likely to improve compared to subjects who did not receive the experimental intervention (control group). Miser[34] suggested that

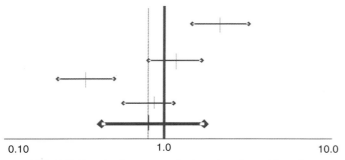

FIG. 1.5 Graph of meta-analysis using the odds ratio.

0.10   1.0   10.0

an odds ratio of 2.0 or greater represents a strong intervention effect. An odds ratio of 2.0 indicates that subjects who received the intervention are two times more likely to have improved on the outcomes measured compared with subjects who did not receive the intervention.

Educators and researchers have responded to the need for systematic reviews and meta-analyses of research on children with developmental conditions. Simple Medline searches in which "cerebral palsy" and "developmental coordination disorder" were each combined with "systematic review" identified 14 systematic reviews of research on children with cerebral palsy and 5 reviews of research on children with developmental coordination disorder published between 2010 and 2015 judged to have application to pediatric physical therapy practice. In most databases, searches can be limited to systematic reviews. This is a good strategy for determining whether a systematic review has been published on the clinical question of interest.

An intermediate level on the 6S pyramid is the *Synopses of Studies*. The synopsis of a single study provides a brief, but often sufficiently detailed, summary of a high-quality study that can inform clinical practice.[8] These synopses will also often include a brief commentary about the clinical applicability of the results of the study. Some relevant resources to obtain these synopses include *Rehab+*, which is a part of McMaster University's evidence-based practice initiative and a subset of *Evidence Updates*. *Rehab+* provides selected abstracts from 130 clinical journals. Each registrant to *Rehab+* receives email alerts with links to the article abstract along with the article's relevance and newsworthiness ratings. In addition, both *Physical Therapy* and *Pediatric Physical Therapy* feature a "Bottom Line" commentary that accompanies many of the clinical research articles in those journals. This commentary asks and answers a number of pertinent questions about the research. A final possible resource for clinicians is to create their own synopses by following a systematic appraisal and documentation process. There are a variety of resources available to aid clinicians in working through this process based on the clinical question and the relevant type of research.[18] The critically appraised topic (CAT) is a one- or two-page summary of a research study that includes implications for practice, the "clinical bottom line." The format is intended to facilitate transfer of research to practice.[10]

The foundation of the pyramid, and the final stop in searching for evidence if none exists at higher levels, is *Individual Studies*. The individual study, published in a peer-reviewed journal, is the most common form of evidence available. Electronic databases are the most efficient method for finding

individual studies in peer-reviewed journals. Electronic databases provide bibliographic references to thousands of peer-reviewed journals and can be searched from a personal computer via the Internet. In addition to the complete reference, databases provide links to the abstract and, increasingly, the full text of published articles. Many journals provide online access to articles before publication in print. Box 1.3 summarizes several commonly used electronic databases. Tutorials are available on each database to aid in conducting efficient and successful searches. Typically, the PICO question provides keywords and phrases that guide the initial search. Each keyword can be used individually or in combination and, depending on the database, can be modified in ways that either expand or narrow the focus of the search.

As with higher levels of the 6S pyramid, physical therapists must use critical analysis skills to ascertain the strength and quality of evidence from individual studies and to determine whether that evidence justifies a change in clinical practice. For example, Harris[20] posed several thought-provoking questions for professionals to ask themselves when analyzing the scientific merit of an intervention. A negative response to one or more of these questions is a warning sign that an intervention is not evidence based.

Is the theory on which the intervention is based consistent with current knowledge?

Is the population for whom the intervention is intended identified?

Are the goals and outcomes of intervention consistent with the needs of the intended population?

Are potential adverse effects of the intervention identified?

Is the overall evidence critiqued?

Are advocates of the intervention open to discussing its limitations?

If these criteria are satisfied, there are a number of strategies to further assess the strength and quality of any evidence.

APPRAISAL OF RESEARCH FROM INDIVIDUAL STUDIES

The paramount questions for applying research evidence from individual studies are whether findings generalize to children who were not in the study and are applicable to the particular child for whom the intervention is a consideration. These are complex issues. To assist practitioners in decision making, systems have been developed to rate the strength of research evidence, methodologic quality (how well the study was conducted), and grade of recommendation.

Strength of Evidence

The levels of evidence framework proposed by Sackett, refined by the Centre for Evidence-Based Medicine (CEBM) at the University of Oxford in 2009 (http://www.cebm.net) and revised in 2011 (Oxford Levels of Evidence 2; http://www.cebm.net), are often used to report the strength of evidence of research on prognosis, diagnosis, differential diagnosis/symptom prevalence, intervention, and economic and decision analyses.[46] Using the CEBM Levels of Evidence (2009) to rate the strength of evidence for therapy interventions, a systematic review of randomized controlled trials (RCTs) provides the strongest evidence (1a), whereas a single RCT of high quality provides 1b evidence. The strength of evidence for studies using observational designs (also referred to as nonexperimental designs) is rated as level 2 or 3. Level 4 evidence is associated with case series (multiple case reports) and poor-quality observational designs. Level 5 evidence is based on expert opinion, general scientific knowledge, or basic science research.

The randomized controlled trial is an experimental design that provides evidence of efficacy (results of interventions provided under randomized and controlled conditions). The feature that distinguishes the RCT from observational designs is random group assignment; subjects have an equal chance of being in the experimental or comparison/control group. In theory, random group assignment controls for variables not measured that may influence intervention outcomes. The RCT therefore provides the strongest evidence of a cause-effect relationship between the experimental intervention (independent variable) and the outcome (dependent variable). Another distinguishing feature of the RCT is that inclusion criteria are usually restrictive in an effort to obtain a sample without characteristics such as co-morbid health conditions that might adversely influence the outcomes. The parameters of the intervention are also specified by the researchers, and the intervention is intended to be provided in the same manner to all subjects.

Although the RCT provides the strongest evidence of a cause-effect relationship between the intervention and outcomes, trials are costly and challenging to implement with children with developmental disabilities. To adhere to the rigor of an experimental design, the intervention is often provided under conditions that are not representative of many practice settings. Consequently, when attempting to apply the results of an RCT, therapists must consider whether subject characteristics generalize to children on their caseloads and whether the intervention is feasible within their practice settings. The *pragmatic clinical trial* is intended to meld the advantages of efficacy and effectiveness research. The pragmatic clinical trial is characterized by random group assignment; however, interventions are clinically feasible, subjects are from diverse populations and practice settings, and a wide range of outcomes are measured.[52]

Observational designs provide evidence of effectiveness (interventions provided under conditions more typical of clinical practice). Cohort, case control, and case series are examples of observational designs. Level 2 evidence is associated with cohort designs, sometimes referred to as quasi-experimental designs. Subjects *are not* randomly assigned to the experimental or comparison/control group. Additionally, subject inclusion criteria and the intervention are usually not controlled by the researchers to the same extent as in the RCT. Level 3 evidence is associated with observational designs where there is no control group or the intervention is not specified by the researchers or both. A *practical clinical trial* refers to a prospective, cohort study designed to analyze variability among patients and interventions on the outcomes of interest.[13]

Clinical practice improvement (CPI) methodology is a type of observational research that is intended to identify specific intervention strategies and procedures that are associated with outcomes and determinants of outcomes.[23] Horn contends that the RCT is designed to investigate a single procedural intervention as opposed to the combination of strategies and procedures that constitutes a typical physical therapy intervention. In clinical practice improvement, standardized forms are created to document intervention strategies and procedures and time spent on each activity. Data are also collected on variables that potentially influence outcomes. Variables might include child characteristics (age, severity of condition, interests, cognition, and communication), family characteristics (family dynamics, interests, resources, supports), and features of the physical, social, and attitudinal environment. Multivariate statistical analyses are used to identify among all of the interventions documented those that are associated with favorable outcomes and child, family, and environment variables that are determinants of outcomes. This type of information is appealing to physical therapists because it informs the decision-making process. Although clinical practice improvement is feasible to implement in practice settings, multivariate analyses require large numbers of subjects.

The CEBM Levels of Evidence 2 differ from the original framework in the definition of levels 1 and 2, removal of subcategories (i.e., 1a, 1b), less technical wording, and the acknowledgement that a "lower level" study with a "dramatic effect" can provide stronger evidence than a "higher level" study. Inclusion of *n*-of-1 trials as level 1 evidence is a marked change from the original framework, which did not address single-subject research designs. The *n*-of-1 trial is similar to the single-subject design; each subject serves as his or her own control. Descriptions of how to conduct *n*-of-1 trials are generally more rigorous that is typical of single-subject designs published in pediatric physical therapy and potentially less feasible to implement in clinical practice.[29]

In the *single-subject design*, outcomes are measured repeatedly during baseline, intervention, and follow-up phases. Within-subject variability between phases is analyzed. This is in contrast to the group design, where between-subject variability is analyzed. The single-subject design is experimental; therefore results can provide evidence of a cause-effect relationship for the subject. Findings, however, should not be generalized to other children. Replication of single-subject designs across subjects and practice settings provides initial evidence of generalizability. Generalization of findings from *n*-of-1 trials is not addressed in Levels of Evidence 2.

Qualitative and Mixed Methods Research

Qualitative and mixed methods of inquiry have been used in nursing and occupational therapy and increasingly more often in physical therapy.[19] Qualitative research is well suited for understanding processes associated with effective communication, coordination, and documentation and child-and family-related instruction, two components of physical therapist interventions. The experiences and values of consumers (e.g., children and families), practitioners, and administrators are integral components of health services research that are too often missing in clinical research. Qualitative research is not addressed in the CEBM Levels of Evidence.

Phenomenology and grounded theory are two qualitative approaches that are frequently used in health care research. Both are concerned with understanding the lived experiences of the population of interest. Themes or theory emerge from analysis of data that are grounded in the social world of the people being studied. This is in contrast to experimental and quantitative research that is based on the researcher's preconceived hypothesis. Participatory action research is a qualitative approach that involves collaboration of consumers, practitioners, and researchers to address specific questions or issues. Children, families, and practitioners are participants or co-researchers who provide input about the questions or issues to address, feasibility of proposed practices, and dissemination of information in usable formats. The preferences and values of consumers and practitioners therefore are incorporated into the design and implementation of research. Schreiber et al.[48] used participatory action research to collaborate with pediatric physical therapists to identify strategies for implementation of evidence-based practice.

Qualitative methods are distinct from those used in experimental research, especially with respect to sample size. Data collection typically involves interviews and focus groups that are recorded and transcribed verbatim. Interviews include neutrally worded, open-ended questions followed by prompts and follow-up questions to encourage participant reflection. Other methods of data collection include observation and examination of artifacts such as medical records and clinical documentation. Data analysis is an iterative process. Procedures to ensure credibility and trustworthiness are used to ensure the themes or therapy that emerges represents the perspectives and lived experiences of study participants. The textbook by Creswell[7] provides a more extensive understanding of qualitative research.

Mixed methods designs, which incorporate both quantitative and qualitative methods, are increasingly being used in rehabilitation research.[39] Depending on a study's aims, the qualitative dimension may proceed or follow the quantitative phase. In outcomes research, qualitative interviews following the intervention are useful in understanding how children, parents, and therapists experienced the intervention and whether the intervention was feasible and acceptable.

Finally, although not a research design per se, the *case report* is a valuable means of communicating practice knowledge including in-depth description of a new, interesting, or unique case and implications for clinical decision making. A case report may also describe innovative approaches to coordination of services, methods of service delivery, and issues germane to a practice setting. McEwen[33] has published an excellent manual for clinicians on how to write case reports.

Methodologic Quality in Individual Research Studies

Methodologic quality is not a primary consideration in systems for rating strength of research evidence in the system developed by the CEBM. Controversy exists as to whether the strength of evidence is greater for a cohort design of high methodologic quality compared with a RCT of poor methodologic quality. The Physiotherapy Evidence Database (PEDro) scale (http://www.pedro.org.au/) is widely used to evaluate the methodologic quality of RCTs. Ten criteria on internal validity (e.g., random allocation to groups, whether subjects, therapists, and assessors were masked to group assignment) and interpretation of results (e.g., between group statistical comparisons, intention to treat analysis) are rated "Yes" or "No."

A Pedro scale score of ≥ 5 or ≥ 6 has been proposed as adequate methodologic quality.[35] Maher et al.[31] reported that the reliability of the PEDro scale varied from "fair" to "substantial" for each criterion and "fair" to "good" for the total score. Macedo et al.[30] found evidence of content and construct validity for 8 of the 10 criteria. The exceptions were "blinding of all therapists" and "blinding of all assessors." Authors are strongly encouraged to report the methodologic quality of each study included in a systematic review and exclude studies with poor methodologic quality. The CONSORT (http://www.consort-statement.org/) and STROBE (http://www.strobe-statement.org/) statements were developed to improve reporting of the results of RCT and observational research respectively. Many peer-reviewed journals require authors to complete the respective checklist when submitting a manuscript to ensure that methodologic strengths and limitations of the study are addressed. Intention to treat analysis is a criterion for rating methodologic quality that has important implications for interpretation of results. Subjects who are enrolled in a clinical trial but do not complete the intervention are included in statistical analysis (potentially reducing the effect size). Not including all subjects in the statistical analysis introduces bias if subjects' reasons for not completing the study are related to group assignment or perceived lack of benefit or progress, compromising the intent of randomized group assignment.

GRADES OF RECOMMENDATIONS

Once new knowledge has been acquired, the GRADE system (Grading of Recommendations Assessment, Development, and Evaluation) is a tool to aid practitioners in determining whether practice change is warranted.[17] An important advantage to this system is that it includes explicit, comprehensive criteria for downgrading and upgrading quality-of-evidence ratings. To achieve transparency and simplicity, the GRADE system classifies the quality of evidence in one of four levels—high, moderate, low, and very low. High-quality evidence indicates that further research is very unlikely to change confidence in the estimate of effect, whereas with low-quality evidence, further research is very likely to have an important impact on confidence in the estimate of the effect and is likely to change the estimate. Evidence from randomized controlled trials may begin as high-quality evidence, but confidence in the evidence may be decreased for several reasons, including study limitations, inconsistency of results, indirectness of evidence, imprecision, and reporting bias. Observational studies start with a low-quality rating, but grading upwards may be warranted if the magnitude of the treatment effect is very large or if there is evidence of a dose-response relation.[17]

An additional important aspect of the GRADE system is that it incorporates a clear separation between quality of evidence and strength of recommendations. Two grades for strength of recommendation are possible: *Strong* and *Weak*. When the desirable effects of an intervention supported by high-quality evidence clearly outweigh the undesirable effects, or clearly do not, this leads to a strong recommendation. On the other hand, when the trade-offs are less certain—either because of low-quality evidence or because evidence suggests that desirable and undesirable effects are closely balanced—weak recommendations are provided. Other factors affecting the strength of recommendation include uncertainty in patient values and preferences and uncertainty about whether the intervention represents a wise use of resources.[17] In the GRADE system a "strong recommendation" implies that all or almost all informed people would make the recommended choice for or against the intervention (*Do it* or *Don't do it*); a "weak recommendation" implies that most informed people would choose the recommended course of action but a substantial number would not (*Probably do it* or *Probably don't do it*)[3]

Novak[37] proposed an *Evidence Alert Traffic Light Grading System* for recommendations on physical therapy and occupational therapy interventions. Based on the amount and quality of evidence, one of three recommendations is made: *Green GO:* High-quality evidence; use this approach. *Yellow MEASURE:* Low-quality or conflicting evidence; measure outcomes carefully to ensure the goal is met. *Red STOP:* High-quality evidence that intervention is ineffective; do not use this approach.[37]

KNOWLEDGE TRANSLATION

If a specific aspect of pediatric physical therapy practice is worthy of a strong recommendation based on the GRADE system, all pediatric physical therapists should strive to integrate this into an evidence-informed decision-making process. In contrast, if there is a strong recommendation to *not* use a specific intervention, this should also be integrated into the evidence-informed decision-making process. If either of these scenarios requires a substantial change from standard practice, either at the individual level or within a group of clinician colleagues, implementing this change is likely to be challenging.

The concept of *knowledge translation (KT)* has recently emerged as a strategy to address this challenge. Knowledge translation is defined as a dynamic and iterative process that includes synthesis, dissemination, exchange, and ethically sound application of knowledge to improve health, provide more effective health services and products, and strengthen the health care system.[40] Graham et al.[14] developed a schematic representation of the knowledge-to-action process (Fig. 1.6). The funnel symbolizes knowledge creation, and the cycle represents the activities and process related to application of knowledge (action).[14] As such, the activities and process cycle is likely to be of more direct relevance to practitioners and others who are attempting to change their own practice behaviors or those of professional colleagues. In an effort to illustrate how this action cycle may be implemented, Table 1.2 presents each phase along with the relevant activities of a recent KT project implemented in a pediatric outpatient facility.[49] The outcomes of this project demonstrated that a comprehensive approach to KT can be effective at supporting behavior change in pediatric physical therapists practicing in an outpatient setting.[49]

EVIDENCE-INFORMED CLINICAL DECISION MAKING

Ultimately, a clinical decision for an individual child and family is guided by a model of evidence-informed decision making.[21] This model, adapted from Haynes et al.[21] and modified for pediatric physical therapy, is presented in Fig. 1.7. Although *evidence-based practice* is a more common term (and is used in the title of this chapter), opinion varies on what constitutes evidence. Initially evidence referred to research. Thus the term *evidence-informed* is used in the model presented in Fig. 1.7 and applied throughout the book to emphasize that factors in addition to research inform decision making. Each of the overarching decision-making frameworks previously described in this chapter contributes to the optimal application of this model. When a clinical question arises, the process must include identification of the child's and family's strengths and needs. This involves systematic data collection at the impairment, activity, and participation levels along with identification of key personal and environmental factors. This data collection may occur during the history, systems review, or tests and measures sections of the physical therapy examination or during the ongoing evaluation of outcomes during intervention within patient/

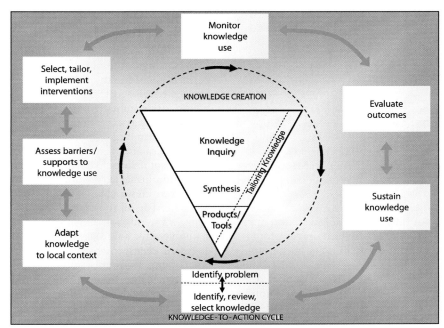

FIG. 1.6 Knowledge-to-action process. (Redrawn from Graham I, Logan J, Harrison MB, et al.: Lost in Knowledge Translation: Time for a Map? *J Contin Educ Health Prof* 26(1):13-24, 2006.)

TABLE 1.2 **Knowledge Translation Example**	
Knowledge-to-Action Cycle Phase	**Project Implementation[49]**
Identify problem: Group or individual identifying a problem or issue that deserves attention or a group or individual becomes aware of knowledge, and then determines whether there is a knowledge-to-practice gap that needs filling with the identified knowledge	Key stakeholders identified inconsistent clinical decision making among staff physical therapists related to frequency and duration of outpatient physical therapy services as a significant clinical problem and that improved selection, administration, interpretation, and sharing of results of pediatric outcome measures was critical to addressing that problem
Identify, review, select knowledge; adapt to local context: A search for knowledge (background) or research (foreground) that might address the problem; this typically will encompass database searches for relevant clinical practice guidelines, systematic reviews, and research articles, appropriate continuing education courses, and reliable web-based resources. Critical appraisal of all evidence then determines validity and usefulness for the identified problem.	Collaboration among senior staff and department administrator to identify appropriate tests/measures for practice setting; database search to ascertain strength of evidence and appropriate use for each outcome measure Note that "adapting to local context" also was incorporated into the intervention stage, where staff members actively practiced with the outcome measures in their workplace and adapted the tests where appropriate to fit within the constraints of each clinic workspace.
Assess barriers to knowledge use so that these may be targeted and hopefully overcome or diminished by intervention strategies; also identify supports or facilitators to address barriers	Lack of knowledge among staff regarding administration and interpretation of key outcome measures; configuration of electronic medical record; access to test/measure materials and equipment; variable space and layout across four separate satellite clinics
Select, tailor, implement interventions based on the identified barriers and audiences; change is more likely to occur with planned and focused interventions	Two-hour workshop led by knowledge broker[45] at each satellite; one-hour follow-up workshop; hard copy and online resource manual (including video demonstrations) with all relevant information about key outcome measures; online discussion board and periodic newsletter updates regarding practice change
Monitor knowledge use to determine how and the extent to which it has diffused among the group; can be used to determine whether interventions have been sufficient or if additional intervention is necessary	Follow-up workshops; mandatory discussion board postings by staff; informal ongoing interaction between knowledge broker, department administrator, and staff; monitoring of data from electronic medical records related to key outcome measures; integration into annual goals for staff
Evaluate outcomes to determine the impact on health and well-being of patients/clients, practitioners, and/or systems	Knowledge assessment related to key outcome measures; a self-report measure of knowledge and performance; electronic medical record review for frequency of test/measure usage before and after the intervention
Sustain knowledge use	Follow-up data collection on outcomes at 10 months post–project implementation date

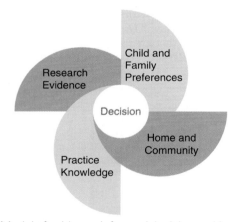

FIG. 1.7 Model of evidence-informed decision making. (Adapted from Haynes RB, Devereaux PJ, Guyatt GH: Clinical expertise in the era of evidence-based medicine and patient choice. *Evid Based Med* 7(2):36-38, 2002.)

client management. The use of valid and reliable tests and measures is an essential aspect of the data collection process.

The practitioner must also identify any additional background and foreground information that may be necessary to address this clinical question and whether additional declarative and procedural knowledge must be obtained. If foreground information is required, practitioners should use the 6S model and the GRADE system to seek out, gather, and evaluate research evidence in order to develop a clinical recommendation. At that point, sharing the findings from the examination or evaluation of outcomes

and offering a GRADE recommendation should incorporate the therapist's practice knowledge and should occur in a way that empowers children and families to integrate their own personal preferences and values to make the best decision at that point in time for that individual child. The statement, "Evidence alone does not make decisions, people do," by Haynes et al.[21] reflects the integral role of the physical therapist in translating and applying research to evidence-informed clinical decisions to achieve optimal participation level outcomes for children and families.

Embedded in the practice knowledge aspect of evidence-informed decision making is clinical reasoning, which has been conceptualized as the process of deciding on the appropriate action for an individual patient at a particular time. Knowledge is viewed as a starting point but not as a strict plan for action. As part of the process of individualizing clinical decisions, the therapist makes judgments and improvises in moving from general practice guidelines to the requirements of a specific situation.[32] Mattingly suggested that judgment and improvisation are often guided by knowledge that is embodied in the therapist's hands or eyes.[32] Part of the therapist's practice knowledge therefore is reflected in implicit thought processes that are translated into habitual ways of observing and interacting with children and families. Pediatric physical therapists are encouraged to strive for better understanding of their thought processes, not only to enhance their own professional development but also to serve their clients and educate physical therapy students more effectively. Understanding how best to integrate child and family strengths and preferences, research evidence, and practice knowledge is essential for the implementation of evidence-based decision making that reflects the broad scope and complexity of

BOX 1.4   Evidence-Informed Decision Making

Clinical Question:

DeMarco is a 5-year-old with a diagnosis of cerebral palsy, level II on the Gross Motor Function Classification System (GMFCS). He has been receiving outpatient physical therapy (2×/week) for the past 2 years. He will be attending kindergarten in the fall. The clinical question is whether DeMarco would benefit from a trial of intensive (5×/week for 4 weeks) outpatient physical therapy this summer in order to maximize his ability to participate in his kindergarten classroom.

Child and Family Strengths, Needs, and Preferences:

Recent re-evaluation data suggest that DeMarco has improved with gross motor function and performance on activity level tasks but that he is well behind age-matched peers in gait velocity and ability to ascend and descend stairs.

DeMarco is willing and able to participate in intensive bouts of activity during weekly physical therapy sessions.

Parents are concerned that DeMarco is becoming isolated from age-matched peers and are strongly invested in doing everything possible to help him succeed both socially and academically in his neighborhood and at school. DeMarco's mother saw a brochure for the intensity program in the waiting room and inquired as to whether this might be an option for him. She expresses some concern that transporting DeMarco to the outpatient clinic 5 days per week would be difficult due to work and family obligations.

Research Evidence:

Two synopses of studies documents were identified.[9,12] The low-quality evidence and the lack of evidence for adverse events suggest a weak recommendation for intensive outpatient therapy for DeMarco.

A synthesis of the evidence suggests that intervention strategies most likely to be effective are goal-directed training/functional training, task-specific practice of child-set goal-based activities using a motor learning approach, and fitness training for improving fitness.[36]

Home and Community:

The family lives in a row home in a city neighborhood. The bathroom and bedrooms are on the second floor. There are two nearby parks within walking distance, and the family frequently visits these parks. DeMarco has one younger sister, age 3 years 2 months.

DeMarco will need to take a school bus to his neighborhood school in the fall. The school building is accessible and all of the kindergarten activities are on one floor. Kindergarten is a full day, and the class has two separate gross motor/free play sessions during the day, either in the school gym or on the playground.

Practice Knowledge:

DeMarco's physical therapist has been working with him for the past 9 months and possesses the knowledge and skills to implement the intensive program with him. She has been in practice for 11 years and is board certified as a pediatric clinical specialist. She has had some success with intensive intervention with other similar children, but most recently one child did not experience any meaningful improvement after participating in this program.

Information Sharing and Decision Making:

A synthesis of the evidence suggests that patients are more likely to understand the research evidence when it is presented in a way that is tailored and interactive.[51] Therefore DeMarco's physical therapist prepared a one-page document that summarizes his current status and recent progress toward goals, along with a bulleted summary of evidence for intensive physical therapy programs. The summary indicated that there is no evidence to date to support a change in participation level outcomes following an intensive program and that the overall recommendation is weak. Several potential adverse events were included.

After some reflection and discussion, the parents decided to continue with DeMarco's 2×/week outpatient program and to reconsider the intensive program at a later date.

---

pediatric physical therapy. A description of evidence-informed clinical decision making is presented in Box 1.4.

SUMMARY

Pediatric physical therapists continually make difficult, complex clinical decisions as part of their daily routine. Historically, most of these decisions were based primarily on experience and practice knowledge. Although there has been an ongoing effort toward incorporating research evidence into clinical decisions, practitioners have benefited recently from the development of a number of overarching frameworks aimed at enhancing efficiency and effectiveness with this process. Thoughtful reflection on practice leads to questions that guide ongoing knowledge acquisition, and critical analysis of that new knowledge determines whether and to what extent it is appropriate to integrate that new knowledge into clinical decisions and recommendations. The PICO format may be used for framing clinical questions. Electronic databases and other web-based resources allow the practitioner to efficiently obtain the highest-level evidence available. The 6S system, CEBM levels of evidence, the GRADE recommendation process, and KT strategies aid in ascertaining whether the evidence merits a change in practice and then in implementing that change. Finally, clinical reasoning strategies allow pediatric physical therapists to effectively integrate new knowledge, practice-based expertise, child and family preferences, and the clinical presentation of the individual child and his or her family into an optimal, collaborative, shared decision that should lead to excellent outcomes for that child.

REFERENCES (NOTE: ASTERISK INDICATES RECOMMENDED READINGS)

1. Ambrose S, Bridges M, DiPietro M, Lovett M, Norman M: *How learning works: 7 research-based principles for smart teaching*, San Francisco, 2010, Josey-Bass.
2. *American Physical Therapy Association: guide to physical therapist practice 3.0*, [website]. Available from: URL: http://guidetoptpractice.apta.org/, 2014.*
3. Andrews J, Schunemann H, Oxman A, et al.: GRADE guidelines: 15. Going from evidence to recommendation—determinants of a recommendation's direction and strength, *J Clin Epidemiol* 66:726–735, 2013.*
4. Carr J, Mungovan S, Shepherd R, et al.: Physiotherapy in stroke rehabilitation: bases for Australian physiotherapists' choice of treatment, *Physiother Theory Pract* 10:201–209, 1994.
5. Cohen J: *Statistical power analyses for the behavioral sciences*, ed 2, Hillsdale, NY, 1988, Lawrence Erlbaum Associates.
6. Connolly B, Lupinnaci M, Bush A: Changes in attitudes and perceptions about research in physical therapy among professional physical therapist students and new graduates, *Phys Ther* 81:1127–1134, 2001.
7. Creswell J: *Qualitative inquiry & research design: choosing among five approaches*, ed 3, Los Angeles, 2013, Sage.
8. DiCenso A, Bayley L, Haynes RB: Accessing pre-appraised evidence: fine-tuning the 5S model into a 6S model, *Evid Based Nurs* 12:99–101, 2009.*
9. Fact Sheet: *Intensity of service in an outpatient setting for children with chronic conditions*, Alexandria, VA, 2012, Section on Pediatrics, American Physical Therapy Association.
10. Fetters L, Figueiredo E, Keane-Miller D, McSweeney D, Tsao C: Critically appraised topics, *Pediatr Phys Ther* 16:19–21, 2004.
11. Fletcher S: *Chairman's Summary of the Conference. Paper presented at: Continuing education in the health professions: improving healthcare through lifelong learning*, Bermuda, New York. 2008.

12. Gannotti M, Christy J, Heathcock J, Kolobe T: A path model for evaluating dosing parameters for children with cerebral palsy, *Phys Ther* 94:411–421, 2014.

13. Glasgow R, Magid D, Beck A, Ritzwoller D, Estabrooks P: Practical clinical trials for translating research to practice: design and measurement recommendations, *Med Care* 43:551–557, 2005.

14. Graham I, Logan JB, Harrison M, et al.: Lost in Knowledge Translation: time for a map? *J Cont Ed Health Prof* 26:13–24, 2006.

15. Graham R, Mancher M, Wolman D, Greenfield S, Steinberg E, editors: *Clinical practice guidelines we can trust*, Washington, DC, 2011, National Academies Press.

16. Grol R, Wensing M: What drives change? Barriers to and incentives for achieving evidence based practice, *Med J Aust* 180:S57, 2004.

17. Guyatt G, Oxman AD, Vist G, et al.: GRADE: an emerging consensus on rating quality of evidence and strength of recommendations, *Br Med J* 336:924–926, 2008.

18. Hack L, Gwyer J: *Evidence into Practice: integrating judgment, values, and research*, Philadelphia, PA, 2013, FA Davis.*

19. Hammel K, Carpenter C: *Evidence-based practice in rehabilitation: informing practice through qualitative research*, Edinburgh, 2004, Elsevier.

20. Harris S: How should treatments be critiqued for scientific merit? *Phys Ther* 76:175–181, 1996.

21. Haynes B, Devereaux P, Guyatt G: Physicians' and patients' choices in evidence-based practice, *Br Med J* 324:1350, 2002.

22. Haynes B: Of Studies, Synthesis, Synopses, Summaries and Sys the 5 S's evolution of Information services for evidence-based healthcare decisions, *Evid Based Nurs* 10:6–7, 2007.

23. Horn S: *Clinical practice improvement methodology: implementation and evaluation*, New York: Faulkner & Gray, 1997.

24. Iles R, Davidson M: Evidence based practice: a survey of physiotherapists' current practice, *Physiother Res Int* 11:93–103, 2006.

25. Jette D, Bacon K, Batty C, et al.: Evidence-based practice: beliefs, attitudes, knowledge, and behaviors of physical therapists, *Phys Ther* 83:786–805, 2003.

26. Jewell D: *Guide to evidence-based physical therapist practice*, ed 3, Burlington, MA, 2015, Jones & Bartlett Learning.

27. Kamwendo K: What do Swedish physiotherapists feel about research? A survey of perceptions, attitudes, intentions, and engagement, *Physiother Res Int* 7:23–34, 2002.

28. Kaplan S, Coulter C, Fetters L: Physical therapy management of congenital muscular torticollis: an evidence-based clinical practice guideline, *Pediatr Phys Ther* 25:348–394, 2013.

29. Lillie E, Patay B, Diamant J, Issell B, Topol E, Schork M: The n-of-1 clinical trial: the ultimate strategy for individualizing medicine? *Personalized Med* 8:161–173, 2011.

30. Macedo L, Elkins M, Maher C, Modeley A, Herbert R, Sherrington C: There was evidence of convergent and construct validity of Physiotherapy Evidence Database quality scale for physiotherapy trials, *J Clin Epidemiol* 63:920–925, 2010.

31. Maher C, Sherrington C, Herbert R, Moseley A, Elkins M: Reliability of the PEDro scale for rating quality of randomized controlled trials, *Phys Ther* 83:713–721, 2003.

32. Mattingly C: What is clinical reasoning? *Am J Occup Ther* 45:979–986, 1991.

33. McEwen I: *Writing case reports: a how-to manual for clinicians*, ed 3, Alexandria, VA, 2009, APTA.*

34. Miser W: Applying a meta-analysis to daily clinical practice. In Geyman J, Deyo R, Ramsey D, editors: *Evidence-based clinical practice: concepts and procedures*, Waltham, MA, 2000, Butterworth-Heinemann, pp 57–64.

35. Moseley A, Herbert R, Maher C, Sherrington C, Elikins M: Reported quality of randomized controlled trials of physiotherapy interventions has improved over time, *J Clin Epidemiol* 64:594–601, 2011.

36. Novak I, Mcintyre S, Morgan S, et al.: A systematic review of interventions for children with cerebral palsy: state of the evidence, *Develop Med Child Neur* 55:885–910, 2013.

37. Novak I: Evidence to practice commentary: the evidence alert traffic light grading system, *Phys Occup Ther Pediatr* 32:256–259, 2012.*

38. Rappolt S, Tassone M: How rehabilitation therapists gather, evaluate, and implement new knowledge, *J Contin Educ Health Prof* 22:170–180, 2002.

39. Rauscher L, Greenfield B: Advancements in contemporary physical therapy research: use of mixed methods designs, *Phys Ther* 89:91–100, 2009.

40. Research CIoH: About knowledge translation. Available from: URL: http://www.cihr-irsc.gc.ca/e/29418.html.

41. Retsas A: Barriers to using research evidence in nursing practice, *J Adv Nur* 31:599–606, 2000.

42. Robeson P, Dobbins M, DeCorby K, Tirilis D: Facilitating access to pre-processed research evidence in public health, *BMC Public Health* 10:1–10, 2010.

43. Rochette A, Korner-Bitensky N, Thomas A: Changing clinicians' habits: is this the hidden challenge to increasing best practices? *Disabil Rehabil* 31:1790–1794, 2009.*

44. Rosenbaum PL, King S, Law M, King G, Evans J, et al.: Family-centered service: a conceptual framework and research review, *Physical and Occupational Therapy in Pediatrics* 18(1):1–20, 1998.

45. Russell D, Rivard L, Walter S, et al.: Using knowledge brokers to facilitate the uptake of pediatric measurement tools into clinical practice: a before-after intervention study, *Implementation Sci* 5:1–17, 2010.

46. Sackett D, Straus S, Richardson W, Rosenberg W, Haynes R: Levels of evidence and grades of recommendations. *Evidence-based medicine: how to practice and teach EBM*, Edinburgh, 2000, Churchill-Livingstone, pp 173–176.

47. Salbach N, Jaglal S, Korner-Bitensky N, Rappolt S, Davis D: Practitioner and organizational barriers to evidence based practice of physical therapists for people with stroke, *Phys Ther* 87:1284–1303, 2007.

48. Schreiber J, Stern P, Marchetti G, Provident I: Strategies to promote evidence-based practice in pediatric physical therapy: a formative evaluation pilot project, *Phys Ther* 89:918–933, 2009.*

49. Schreiber J, Marchetti G, Racicot B, Kaminski E: The use of a knowledge translation program to increase use of standardized outcome measures in an outpatient pediatric physical therapy clinic: administrative case report, *Phys Ther* 95:613–629, 2015.*

50. Thomson-O'Brien MA, Moreland J: Evidence-based information circle, *Physiother Can* 50:171–205, 1998.

51. Trevena L, Davey H, Barratt A, Butow P, Caldwell P: A systematic review on communicating with patients about evidence, *J Eval Clin Pract* 12:13–23, 2006.*

52. Tunis S, Stryer D, Clancy C: Practical clinical trials: increasing the value of clinical research for decision making in clinical and health policy, *JAMA* 290:1624–1632, 2003.

53. Turner P, Whitfield T: Physiotherapists' use of evidence based practice: a cross-national study, *Physiother Res Int* 2:17–29, 1997.

54. Turner P, Whitfield T: Physiotherapists' reasons for selection of treatment techniques: a cross-national survey, *Physiother Theory Pract* 15:235–246, 1999.

55. World Health Organization: *International classification of function, disability, and health*, Geneva, Switzerland, 2001, WHO.*

56. World Health Organization: *International classification of function, disability, and health: children and youth version*, Geneva, Switzerland, 2007, WHO.

2

Measurement

Robin Lee Dole, Joseph Schreiber

INTRODUCTION

Pediatric physical therapists make numerous clinical decisions each day that should be guided by information gathered from standardized outcome measures. Accurate and reliable data collection regarding an individual child and family is essential for optimal decisions about eligibility for services, intervention strategies, meaningful and appropriate goals, and intensity and duration of services. This data should be shared with children and families in a way that encourages and supports collaborative decision making. Pooled data collection from multiple children can also inform decisions about program effectiveness and need for systemwide practice change.

Despite the availability of a wide variety of outcome measures to guide clinical decisions, pediatric physical therapists are not confident with the selection, administration, and interpretation of standardized outcome measures.[30,37,67] This lack of confidence is due to barriers that include lack of time to learn and administer tests, limited knowledge about measures and measurement principles, and inadequate training.[41,66] The purpose of this chapter is to guide clinicians on the effective use of tests and measures in pediatric physical therapy practice. Information will be provided on measurement principles and psychometrics as critical components of the selection, administration, interpretation, and sharing results of appropriate tests and measures. A variety of single and multi-item tests and measures will be presented to aid in identification of body structures and function impairments, activity limitations, and participation restrictions in children. Special emphasis will be placed on use of technology to enhance the feasibility of tests and measures within the daily work routine.

The American Physical Therapy Association's (APTA's) *Standards for Tests and Measurements in Physical Therapy Practice* states that a *measurement* is the "numeral assigned to an object, event, or person, or the class (category) to which an object, event, or person is assigned according to rules."[65] *Tests and measures* are the means of gathering reliable and valid cellular-level to person-level information about the individual's capacity for, and performance during, movement-related functioning. The appropriate selection of tests and measures for a specific child depends on the goals of the child and family, purpose of the testing, and the psychometric properties and clinical utility of the test.[3]

Outcomes are the actual results of implementing the plan of care that indicate the impact on functioning. At the level of pathology, body function, and body structure, outcome measures indicate the success of individual interventions during an episode of care. Outcome measures directed toward activity and participation demonstrate the value of physical therapy in helping individuals achieve their identified *goals,* which are measurable, functionally driven, and time limited and represent the intended results of a plan of care.[3] *Standardized outcome measures* are based on formal descriptions of a conceptual framework and documentation of the development, application, and scoring processes. They are applied within a defined context (e.g., condition, patient characteristics, setting, etc.) and have been reported, critiqued, and substantiated in peer-reviewed forums.[61] Throughout this text, the term *outcome measures* is used synonymously with *tests and measures* and *standardized outcome measures.*

The purpose of testing is a key consideration for pediatric physical therapists when selecting outcome measures. For example, for some children it is necessary to determine eligibility for physical therapy or other services. This is most often based on comparing the child's performance to same-aged peers, which would therefore require administration of a discriminative, norm-referenced outcome measure. A score on a norm-referenced outcome measure is usually expressed as a percentile rank or z-score and therefore identifies children with delays in a specific set of skills as compared to age-matched peers.

In other circumstances, eligibility for services has been established, and the focus of testing is on determining a baseline level of performance related to child and family goals. The child can then be retested over time to identify any change that has occurred and whether goals have been achieved. In this scenario, an evaluative, criterion-referenced outcome measure would be most appropriate. A score on a criterion-referenced outcome measure is most often expressed as a percentage or raw score, or as a scaled score. It is also critical that this type of outcome measure be responsive to change and therefore sensitive to the effects of intervention.

In addition to determining eligibility and accurately measuring change over time, pediatric physical therapists use outcome measures to predict future performance. The results from these tests aid practitioners in anticipating child and family needs and can provide critical support for clinical decisions related to placement, intervention planning, goal setting, environmental adaptations, bracing and orthotics, adaptive equipment, and child and family educational needs. For example, evidence suggests that the Test of Infant Motor Performance (TIMP)[14,33] can predict Peabody Developmental Gross Motor Scale (PDMS-2)[56] scores at preschool age and scores on the Bruininks-Oseretsky (BOT-2)[10] scores at school age.[23,40] Therefore clinicians might expect that infants who score lower on the TIMP are at greater risk for activity and participation restrictions due to suboptimal motor skills. Motor growth curves have been established for children with cerebral palsy based on scores from the Gross

Motor Function Measure (GMFM-66).[26] These growth curves help clinicians and families estimate a child's future motor capabilities including how much independence is likely to be achieved.[63] Practitioners would need to consult the scientific literature and the test manual to determine whether specific outcome measures might be used for prognostic purposes.

Finally, outcome measures may be used to contribute to minimal data sets and score aggregation as part of program evaluation and health services research. Frequently, these measures are based on self- (or parent/caregiver) report, in contrast to performance-based measures that are based on child performance of a particular skill or task.[3] One example of an outcome measure that may be used in this manner is the Patient Reported Outcome Measurement Information System (PROMIS), which is a psychometrically validated, dynamic system to measure patient reported outcomes. The PROMIS initiative is part of the NIH goal to develop systems to support NIH-funded research supported by all of its institutes and centers. PROMIS measures cover physical, mental, and social health and can be used across chronic conditions.[12] A similar tool, Outpatient Physical Therapy Improvement in Movement Assessment Log (OPTIMAL), has been developed by the APTA. This tool integrates patient identification of a primary goal of physical therapy. In addition, OPTIMAL's scoring of the patient's perceived difficulty and confidence in performing a specific activity can help the physical therapist make a clinical judgment on the severity of the impairment limitation restriction.[4] There is potential for use of patient-reported outcome measures to improve quality of care and disease outcomes, to provide patient-centered assessment for comparative effectiveness research, and to enable a common metric for tracking outcomes across providers and medical systems.[12]

MEASUREMENT PRINCIPLES

Norm- Versus Criterion-Referenced Outcome Measures

The two main types of standardized tests or measures, with regard to their scoring and interpretation, are those that are norm referenced and those that are criterion referenced.[11] When the purpose for using a standardized outcome measure is to compare children to a reference group, for example the child's same-aged peers, a norm-referenced test will provide such a comparison. When a therapist desires to know how well a child performs on a specified set of knowledge, skills, or abilities, a criterion-referenced test may be most appropriate. Typically, when the desired information is whether the child performs at, below, or above expectations based on their age, a norm-referenced test is required.[59] Such tests are commonly used to establish eligibility for therapy services when such qualification standards require that a child be below a certain cut-off score when compared to his or her peers. For example, one way to qualify for early intervention services in the United States under Part C of the Individuals with Disabilities Education Act is to have performance that is well below average for age. For some tests and measures this may be defined as a score that is greater than two standard deviations below the mean for a given age.[62]

In the case where a child has a known disability and deficits in knowledge, skills, and abilities have already been established or if eligibility for intervention is based on meeting a set of specific skills, a criterion-referenced test may be of benefit.

A criterion-referenced test may also be an appropriate choice when the purpose of testing is to show whether a child's performance of a set of knowledge, skills, or abilities has changed over a specific period of time.[11] Such an example would be when a therapist desires to document the changes in functional mobility skills for a child who has been receiving intervention to address these skills.

Norm-referenced tests also may be sensitive to changes in knowledge, skills, and abilities over time, but one has to keep in mind that the scores from those tests are always referenced back to the normed group, which in pediatric practice is typically by age. In a situation where the therapist expects the child to "catch up" to same-aged peers with respect to his or her motor skills, changes in scores on a norm-referenced test may be an appropriate way to make that determination. Conversely, when a child who initially scores lower than average for age when compared to peers and on follow-up testing demonstrates no change in standard score performance, it could be evidence that the child is "keeping pace" with their typical peers even if no progress toward catching up to the age-expectations is made. That child has not made progress toward catching up with his or her peers but has not lost any additional ground either. This type of finding may also be an indication that additional data from a criterion-referenced measure is needed to document whether the child has made progress on important skills without reference to age expectations.

Test Development

A brief discussion of how standardized tests are constructed can help illustrate the differences between norm-referenced and criterion-referenced outcome measures. For a more comprehensive review of test development, the reader is referred to the *Standards for Educational and Psychological Testing*[2] and the *Handbook of Test Development*.[20] A measure is considered norm referenced because the test developers seek to create a measure that has enough items to capture the full range of performance on a particular set of knowledge, skills, or abilities and then provide a comparison of how children from the norming group achieve that knowledge, skill, or ability. Test developers also seek to obtain a large enough norming group to record the full range of performance across a variety of relevant demographic variables. Such variables may include age or grade level, gender, ethnicity, race, culture, and level of function. Scores from the norming group are ranked highest to lowest in order to identify average performance based on, in this example, the child's age.[11]

Items for criterion-referenced measures are selected because they are well representative of the domain of content to be measured. For example, for a criterion-referenced measure of gross motor function, the test developers may be less interested in what skills are achieved by a particular age and more concerned about the various elements that contribute to the functional mobility skills of rolling, crawling, cruising, standing, walking, and running. Criterion-referenced measures that are linked to age may do so through standard setting, where individual judgments of or information on expected ages of achievement are the criterion, rather than comparison to a norming group.[22] Both norm-referenced and criterion-referenced measures result in scores that may be interpreted in a diagnostic, predictive, or evaluative manner. Only norm-referenced measures can be used to compare performance to a population or determine difference when compared to same-aged peers through scores referenced to the normal curve, yielding standard scores, T-scores, z-scores, and percentile ranks (Fig. 2.1).[11]

Psychometric Properties

A standardized outcome measure has a specific set of standards for administration, scoring, and interpretation. By adhering to such standards, the stability of the score or outcome is greatly increased. Stability within one test administrator is considered *intrarater reliability* and across multiple administrators is termed *interrater reliability*. The ability of a measure to capture accurately and assess the domain of interest is part of the psychometric property of validity. Both the concepts of reliability and validity, when considering test development, have several levels of complexity. For a more thorough discussion of these concepts the reader is referred to *Foundations of Clinical Research: Applications to Practice*.[59] For consumers of standardized outcome measures, valid use of a test or measure can be ensured when the subject undergoing testing is most like the reference group used in the norming process or population of individuals used to develop and validate the test. According to the test developers, the Gross Motor Function Measure-66 item version (GMFM-66)[26] should only be used with children who have a diagnosis of cerebral palsy. The test developers issue this caution because, at the time of publication of this text, the GMFM-66 has been validated for use only with this population and this measure has been used to develop gross motor curves to assist with making prognoses regarding motor skill abilities based on a child's Gross Motor Function Classification Scale Level (GMFCS).[68] It is important to know how well one's clinical situation fits with the design and purpose of the test as well as the population for which the test was intended.

Another clinical consideration for test validity is the manner in which tests are administered. It is critical for test validity that standardized outcome measures be administered as they were intended, including closely following instructions, using the designated materials, and providing the permitted demonstrations and number of trials that are required of the test.[35] Making modifications to a standardized test diminishes the ability to make judgments from the scores obtained, both for comparison to a reference group and for detecting change in performance of the same individual over time. Therapists may feel compelled to make such modifications because they believe the child's true abilities could be uncovered with such adaptations or that a child's diagnosis or co-occurring condition prevents the child from showing their true performance given the constraints of the test. One way to address this clinically is to administer the test according to the test specifications, including scoring it appropriately, and if the therapist desires to know how well a child could perform on the same item with some form of modification or additional trials, provide that opportunity after the standardized administration of the item or the test is complete. Do not include the performance of this modified item in the scoring and interpretation of the child's performance on the test. The information that has been gathered from modification is less a reflection of how well that child performs on the standardized outcome measure than an indication of how that child might respond to intervention or a method of identifying appropriate strategies to address the child's challenges with a particular skill or ability. One caution here is to refrain from taking specific items from a test and repeatedly practicing those items in therapy or adopting the items as therapy goals for measuring success. Such a practice could also jeopardize the ability to

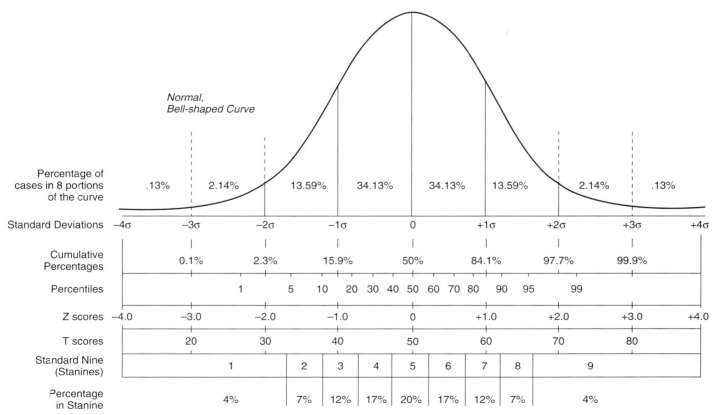

FIG. 2.1 The Normal Distribution.

validly measure performance for comparison to a normed population or to a specific skill criterion. The "Clinical Measurement Practical Guidelines for Service Providers" available through the CanChild Centre for Childhood Disability Research (www.canchild.ca) is a helpful resource for clinicians regarding these issues and their effect on effective use of clinical outcome measures.[29]

For outcome measures designed to screen to predict a condition or diagnosis, the properties of specificity, sensitivity, positive and negative predictive values, and likelihood ratios are important factors to consider for selection and interpretation. Two mnemonics that can be helpful for understanding the importance of specificity and sensitivity are SpPIN: measures with high levels of specificity (true positive rate) indicate that a positive test result will rule in the condition or diagnosis; and SnNOUT: measures with high levels of sensitivity (true negative rate) indicate that a negative test result will rule out the condition or diagnosis.[20] Ideally, measures designed to predict a later outcome should have acceptable measures of specificity and sensitivity; however, how a measure is used can shed light on interpreting the importance of these properties. For example, clinicians using screening measures to help identify those premature infants who would most likely be diagnosed with motor impairment or cerebral palsy at some later point might be willing to accept lower levels of specificity but desire higher levels of sensitivity. This risk of overidentifying children (high false positive rate, 1 − specificity) who may later demonstrate motor impairment and therefore be given early intervention is preferable to having high numbers of children for whom the test incorrectly rules out the likelihood of developing cerebral palsy (false negative rate, 1 − sensitivity) and then are not identified or referred for intervention.[59] The risk of this happening, of course, is low because it would mean that only the score on a single test would be used to identify a condition or diagnosis when clinically it is best practice to use multiple sources of clinical information for decision making. There is the potential, however, that infants may not meet the threshold for developmental differences and still be at risk for later challenges, and early identification and intervention is desired.

Positive and negative predictive values provide an estimate of a test's feasibility in actually identifying that a child who tests positive or negative actually does or does not have the diagnosis or condition of interest. Positive and negative likelihood ratios indicate how much more likely it is that a child may have a particular diagnosis or condition *after* testing positive or negative on a predictive test.[59] These concepts will be discussed further via an example in the section Analysis and Interpretation.

Computer- and Technology-Aided Measures

As computer technology has advanced, options for utilizing more sophisticated test administration and interpretation have been applied to existing pediatric outcome measures and the development of new outcome measures. One way in which technology has enhanced the use of standardized testing is in computer-aided scoring. In this situation, raw scores from a measure are entered into a software program that calculates standard scores, scaled scores, z-scores, percentile ranks, confidence intervals, item maps or other relevant data for interpretation. Such analysis software is specifically applicable to norm-referenced tests and helps to reduce the potential for human error in reading and interpreting scoring tables from a particular test or measure.[69] Some software packages will also print out a report that provides a description of the test, a table

of data, and a first-level analysis of the data. Readers should be cautioned that such reports are based solely on the data that are provided and therefore lack the additional clinical data and impression that can only be provided by the therapist administering the test or measure. Examples of commonly used measures that have this computer-aided scoring are the Peabody Developmental Motor Scales-2 (PDMS-2)[56] and the Bruininks-Oseretsky Test of Motor Proficiency-2 (BOT-2).[10]

Computer-adaptive tests are constructed in such a way as to minimize the number of items that need to be completed in order to arrive at an accurate score that would be comparable to the score achieved if the entire test was administered. The test therefore "adapts" to the responses and performance of the individual being tested.[11] All items on the assessment are ordered by level of difficulty, and the first item administered is in the middle range of difficulty. From there items are selected for administration and scoring based on the response or performance on the item tested, progressing by either increased or decreased difficulty level as appropriate. These measures also have the benefit of computer-based scoring and first level of interpretation of the data. The United States military has heavily supported the development of computer-adaptive testing. It has been using this method for their Armed Services Vocational Aptitude Battery since 1996.[11] Computer-adaptive testing has also been applied to common pediatric assessment tools. An example is the Pediatric Evaluation of Disability Inventory Computer Adaptive Test (PEDI-CAT), which captures functioning in the four domains of daily activities, mobility, social/cognitive, and responsibility.[27] The test developers indicate that the PEDI-CAT is appropriate for all populations of children between the ages of 1 and 21 years and across all settings. The test can be completed by parent or caregiver report or by a practitioner familiar with the child. The PEDI-CAT produces both normed standard scores (percentile and T-scores) and criterion-referenced scaled scores for analysis. The precision version provides a precise score in the quickest fashion and delivers the fewest number of items delivered per domain, and the comprehensive version delivers more items per domain to ensure a more balanced number of items from each domain. The comprehensive version is required if the production of an item map is desired. Item maps show the test items ordered by level of difficulty, which can aid in interpretation and program planning.[27]

Another interesting application of computer technology in testing is the Gross Motor Activity Estimator (GMAE), which can be used in conjunction with the GMFM-66.[26] The GMFM-66 is a criterion-referenced measure and, as such, the scores derived are considered ordinal in nature. The scores have an order to them in that higher numbers indicate better performance but the intervals between the scores are not necessarily equal distance apart.[68] The GMAE provides a manipulation of the scores derived from the GMFM-66, converting those scores to an interval scale. Scores that are considered to be interval can be interpreted differently than scores that are ordinal. When the intervals between two scores are equal distance, it is possible to apply statistical analysis to them and compare scores across individuals.[59,68] See the case of Sophia on Expert Consult for an example of interpretation of the GMFM-66 and GMAE scores.

ANALYSIS AND INTERPRETATION

When choosing tests and measures, therapists should consider the purposes for which they are testing (What type of decision is to be made?), the types of data to be gathered (What information is needed to make that decision?), and the methods to be used to gather the data (How best is the information gathered: by observation, direct assessment of performance, or through self- or caregiver report?). The purpose of testing and the outcome measures that are selected and administered will have a direct impact on the type of analysis and interpretation of results for clinical decision making. Therapists are encouraged to consider collecting data, as appropriate, at all levels of the International Classification of Functioning (ICF).[77a]

Screening and Prediction

When the purpose of testing is to detect the potential for a certain condition or diagnosis either now or in the future, a standardized measure that has been validated for screening or prediction is necessary. Such measures should report the strength of related psychometrics in sensitivity, specificity, positive and negative predictive values, and likelihood ratios. These properties of the measure play a role in selecting appropriate tests to rule or rule out a condition and give an assessment of the strength and quality of the decisions that are made through interpretation of the test results.

Spittle et al[71] investigated the predictive abilities of two motor-related outcome measures, the Alberta Infant Motor Scale (AIMS)[1] and the Neuro-Sensory Motor Developmental Assessment (NSMDA).[48] These tools were used to examine preterm infants at 4, 8, and 12 months (corrected age) and the ability to predict a later diagnosis of cerebral palsy as determined by child's pediatrician and confirmed by a physical therapist. The outcomes were also reviewed for their ability to identify motor impairment based on performance at age 4 years (corrected age) on the Movement Assessment Battery for Children (MABC-2).[46] The specificity related to identification of impairment on both outcome measures assessed during infancy was high for motor impairments at 4 years as assessed by the MABC-2 and for diagnosis of cerebral palsy at 4 years (ranging from 88% to 95%). Sensitivity for predicting motor impairment on the MABC-2 was low (ranging 38% to 56% depending on the cutoff score used), whereas sensitivity for predicting later diagnosis of cerebral palsy was very high (83% at 4 months and 100% at 8 months and 12 months of age). Recall the earlier discussion of sensitivity and specificity. These measures were highly specific for identifying cerebral palsy and later motor impairment, a positive test resulting in a correct identification of children with the condition or impairment. These measures were also highly sensitive for predicting a later diagnosis of cerebral palsy, a negative test resulted in correct identification of the children who did not have the condition. The lower sensitivity for the MABC-2 is concerning in that there may be children who go unidentified. One has to consider that there are limitations, perhaps, with the MABC-2 as a diagnostic tool because all tests have limitations. The authors of the study note that false positives did occur and that serial outcome measurements during follow-up with children at high risk for motor impairment are important.

Positive and negative predictive values (PPVs and NPVs), positive (+LR) and negative likelihood ratios (−LR), and diagnostic accuracy were also reported. Because PPV and NPV take into account the prevalence of the condition under study, these properties provide insight on the clinical utility of the screening measure.[59] In the Spittle et al[71] example, the NPVs for the AIMS and NSMDA are high (82% to 100%) for their probability in identifying infants who did not have motor impairment

as tested on the MABC-2 and did not have diagnosis of cerebral palsy (CP) at age 4. The PPVs, or probability of identifying infants who did have motor impairment as identified by the MABC-2, were higher (54% to 73%) than the PPVs for identifying infants who had a later diagnosis of CP at age 4 (32% to 45%). The study analyzed data on 82 children, of whom only 6 were eventually diagnosed with CP. Just over a quarter had confirmed motor impairment at <15th percentile on the MABC-2. The lower PPVs for the AIMS and NSMDA to estimate the likelihood for an infant who tests as delayed at 4, 8, and/or 12 months to later be diagnosed with CP could have been impacted by a low prevalence for CP among the infants in the study. The positive predictive value answers the question: If the child is identified as positive for the condition on the predictive test, what are the chances that they actually have that condition? However, in studies of predictive tests, if the prevalence of a condition in the general population is low (in this case CP and the overall number of children with identified CP in this sample was low), the positive predictive value will be low as well regardless of how good the sensitivity and specificity of the test. In this study, likelihood ratios (LRs) are independent of prevalence and provide information of the confirming power or certainty of a measure's diagnostic ability. The calculation of positive and negative LRs takes into account sensitivity, specificity, and true and false positive rates (LR+) and true and false negative rates (LR−).[59] In the example discussed here the 11.3 LR+ found for diagnosis of CP indicates that it was 11.3 times more likely that infants with impairment at 4 months would have CP at 4 years than for infants without impairment at 4 months to be later be diagnosed with CP at 4 years.[71]

Determining Difference

Tests and measures may be used in the process of determining whether a child has a motor impairment and may contribute to the determination of a specific diagnosis or determination of eligibility for services. One example where measures of motor skill or impairment may be used to establish evidence for a diagnosis and determine difference is in developmental coordination disorder (DCD). The Developmental Coordination Disorder Questionnaire (DCDQ '07) is a criterion-referenced measure that collects information about a child through parent report to screen for characteristics associated with DCD.[76] In addition, other norm-referenced direct assessments of performance on motor tasks, like the MABC-2 or the BOT-2, may help identify children who perform below their same-aged peers in areas of motor performance that are typically challenging for children with DCD.[8] Measures like these may help to identify whether a child meets the diagnostic criteria for DCD within the *Diagnostic and Statistical Manual of Mental Disorders*, 5th edition (DSM-5).[5,7] When the decision to be made is related to difference, diagnosis, discrimination, or eligibility determination by screening for and confirming a diagnosis, outcome measures that can distinguish those with impairment from those without impairment are needed.[70,74] Parent report measures help to capture the perspective of the parent and may help to ascertain the child's typical performance, whereas direct measures help to identify and quantify which skills may be problematic for the purpose of diagnosis and establishing a baseline of performance for later comparison. The same psychometric properties that were applicable to the screening and predictive measures described earlier are also applicable to measures used for diagnostic or discriminative purposes.[59]

Missiuna and colleagues[45] studied a "staged" approach for the identification of children with DCD, which included using one parent-report measure (DCDQ'07) and one child-report measure (Children's Self Perception of Adequacy in and Predilection for Physical Activity Scale [CSAPPA])[32] as an initial, first-step screening for DCD in over 3000 children. The second stage involved further testing for only those children whose scores on either the DCDQ '07 or CSAPPA were below the 5th percentile as an indication of probable DCD. They also included children known to have ADD/ADHD regardless of their scores on the first step screening due to the high co-incidence of these conditions with DCD. Presence of ADD/ADHD was confirmed using the Conner's Parent Rating Scales (CPRS)[16] during the second stage of the process. Stage 2 also involved direct assessment for motor impairment with the MABC, estimation of cognitive skill with the Kaufman Brief Intelligence Test-2 (KBIT-2),[36] and a structured home interview to assess impact of impaired motor skill on self-care and academic activities. Each of these measures and procedures connected back to one of the diagnostic criteria for DCD set forth in the DSM-5. Children determined to meet criteria for DCD would have motor impairment evidenced by MABC scores below the 15th percentile, typical intelligence evidenced by > 70 on the KBIT-2, and parent confirmation of the impact of motor impairment on daily activities. The results showed that almost 30% of the children initially identified with probable DCD did not go on in stage 2 to demonstrate a significant motor impairment, and about 16% of the children that were not identified during the screening process were later identified as having DCD. Screening processes are not without error and should be used as a part of a system of measurement that identifies difference or diagnosis. The staged approach studied by Missiuna and colleagues[45] also helps to illustrate how important it is to collect information from a variety of measures and perspectives in order to enhance clinical decision-making.

EVALUATING CHANGE

If the decision of interest is whether a child has changed in performance over a specified amount of time, either to track the child's rate of progress or to evaluate the effectiveness of a particular intervention, test results from before and after intervention can be analyzed to help identify change. A measure's ability to detect such change is often referred to as its *responsiveness to change*.[28] To determine if the change in scores from one administration to another is different enough to be true change, it is important to know the minimal detectable change (MDC) for the measure or the smallest amount of change that is reflective of true change and not that which can be accounted for by measurement or test error.[45] Statistical measures are applied to determine the MDC, and most often are reported relative to the confidence interval applied. The MDC90 reflects use of the 90% confidence interval (z score of 1.65); the MDC95 reflects use of the 95% confidence interval (z score of 1.96) in the calculation. The MDC calculation also takes into consideration the coefficient of the measure's established test-retest reliability and the standard error of the measure.[28] The standard error of the measure is a reflection of variability or error in estimating a true score from the observed score on a particular measure. When calculating the 90% or 95% confidence interval, the standard error of the measure is a component of that calculation. If the change in scores from two administrations of a measure exceeds the MDC for that measure, one can conclude that the amount of change beyond the MDC is true change from a statistical

point of view. Therapists should consult the relevant literature for reports of the MDC when available for the outcome measures they commonly use in practice.

Another measure of change is one where clinical meaningfulness is the benchmark for change. The minimal clinical important difference (MCID) has been defined as smallest amount of change that is meaningful from the perspective of a relevant individual, for example a patient or a practitioner. There are multiple ways to determine the MCID; therefore there are some concerns with its use as a measure of meaningful change. The anchor-based method determines the average change of those who have been defined as having improved. The distribution-based method typically takes into consideration effect size. A single measure could have more than one MCID reported in the literature, so when applying this analysis, it is vitally important that the method used to determine the MCID be considered because it can be diagnosis, setting, and population specific.[17]

Iyer, Haley, Watkins and Dumas[34] retrospectively reviewed the inpatient rehabilitation charts from 53 children in order to establish the MCID for the original version of the Pediatric Evaluation of Disability Inventory (PEDI).[57] An anchor-based method was used with the mean change in scores as identified by clinicians as important when comparing admission and discharge summaries. Each clinician rated the level of improvement noted for each subject on both a 0- to 15-cm visual analog scale (VAS) and a 15-point Likert scale. Both scales had extremes from a great deal worse (−7 on the Likert scale) to a great deal better (+7 on the Likert scale) with the middle (0 on the Likert scale) indicating no change. The results of this study identified an 11-point change in a scaled score on the PEDI as the minimal change that can be deemed important in an inpatient rehabilitation setting. For the same measure Haley and Fragala-Pinkham[28] reported the MDC90 to be a 5.1-point scaled score change. It should make sense that the minimal change beyond error is smaller (MDC90 of 5.1 points) than that which might account for clinically important change (MCID of 11 points) A caution with the MCID is that it is likely baseline dependent, meaning that children whose baseline scores are lower performing may need less of a change to be considered meaningful by parents, clinicians, or patients than children whose baseline scores are at the higher end of the performance scale of the measure.[75] A caution with the MDC is that measurement error may not be consistent at all levels across the measure's scaled scores. The standard error of the measure is a component of the 90% confidence interval and therefore a part of the MDC90. Measures that report the standard error of the measure at each point or level of the scale may help offset this concern.[28]

Examples of how to apply analysis and interpretation with outcome measures at the body system and function, activity, and participation levels of the ICF are provided in the case studies on Expert Consult.

SELECTION

A difficult challenge for pediatric physical therapists is the selection of appropriate tests and measures. As noted above, this selection must be based on the purpose of testing and the goals of the child and family. The history and systems review portions of the physical therapy examination process narrow the focus of the examination and guide practitioners in prioritizing tests and measures to obtain data that will inform collaborative clinical decision-making with the child and family. The ICF also provides an organizational framework for this data collection process. The Tests and Measures tables (eTables 2.1 to 2.4) are organized (based on the ICF) into impairment, single-task, multi-item activity, and multi-item participation outcome measures. Relevant information is provided regarding the appropriate clinical circumstances when a specific test might be used, along with information to support accurate analysis and interpretation. Links for many of the tests are also included and allow the reader to obtain more detailed information to guide selection and interpretation.

One additional consideration in selection of tests and measures is the integration of individualized outcome measures into this process. Pediatric physical therapists regularly write individualized outcomes as a way to measure progress toward child and family goals. These outcomes may be at any level of the ICF and should all be related to the parent and child-identified goals at the activity and participation level. Both the Canadian Occupational Performance Measure (COPM)[72] and Goal Attainment Scaling (GAS),[38,39] included in eTable 2.4, Multi-Item Participation Level Tests and Measures, may be used to more precisely measure change in performance on these outcomes. The COPM requires the child and/or family to rank satisfaction and performance on individualized outcomes on a 0–10 scale. With GAS, each individualized outcome is scaled to five levels of attainment: expected level, two outcomes that are less favorable and two outcomes that are more favorable. In addition, with multiple outcomes a T-score can be calculated such that a score > 50 indicates better-than-anticipated performance. Examples of how the COPM and GAS can be integrated into clinical decision making are included in the case studies on Expert Consult.

REPORTING AND SHARING RESULTS

A key responsibility of therapists when using outcome measures in practice is the obligation to report and share results with a variety of stakeholders and through multiple communication methods. Therapists may report results officially in writing as part of documentation, and these reports are likely shared with other professionals, families and caregivers, third-party payers, and (when appropriate) the child. Therapists are often called on to report verbally at team meetings in early intervention, school, hospital or clinic settings. Whenever reporting and sharing results, therapists should adhere to the responsibilities of test users identified in the Standards for Tests and Measurements in Physical Therapy Practice, including using all relevant and available data with appropriate justification for decision making, recognizing the limitations of tests and measures, and identifying any irregularities in the testing protocol or conditions.[65] As routine best practice, therapists should include and share information in ways that are easily understandable by those who will hear or read the report and that allow for collaborative decision-making.[77] Reports should include information about the outcome measures administered, tables or narrative outlining the results, and interpretation of the results within the context of the child and family's needs and goals. Trevena, Davey, Barratt, Butow, and Caldwell[73] found that communication tools in most formats (verbal, written, video, provider delivered, computer based) will increase patients' knowledge and understanding but are more likely to do so if the tools are structured, tailored, and/or interactive. One additional consideration is that some outcome measures may provide age equivalents as a component of analysis of the test results. Therapists should refrain from using age equivalents as a unit of analysis and basis for decision making because age equivalents have significant limitations, including that these scores are ordinal rather than interval, are based on raw scores and not normative or scaled scores, and the likelihood that this data is value laden and therefore easily misinterpreted by children, families, and caregivers.[44]

CASE ILLUSTRATIONS OF ANALYSIS AND INTERPRETATION OF EXAMINATION DATA

This section presents two separate clinical cases to illustrate the use of outcome measures to support evidence-informed and collaborative clinical decision making. The first, Sophia, focuses on the early life span beginning in the neonatal intensive care unit and continuing into early intervention and the elementary school years. The second, Jacob, focuses on the use of outcome measures to make clinical recommendations for intervention, episodes of care, and referral to other health care providers. The case spans Jacob's life between ages 4 years 8 months and 14 years, and many of the outcome measures are appropriate for adolescents and adults as well.

Case 1: Sophia

Sophia was born at 30 weeks gestational age (GA) via emergency C-section and weighing 3 pounds (1361 grams). She spent 8 weeks in the neonatal intensive care unit (NICU), the first week on mechanical ventilation. At 14 days an ultrasound screening revealed a grade II intraventricular hemorrhage (IVH). The first signs that there may be neuromotor challenges were identified when the NICU team assessed Sophia at 34 weeks postmenstrual age (PMA) using the Qualitative Assessment of Generalized Movements (GM).[21,60] This assessment, which requires the tester have formal training, follows a specific protocol for observing infant movements via videotape and classifying those movements (http://general-movements-trust.info/). Sophia's team also administered the Test of Infant Motor Performance (TIMP) as part of its program to identify infants early who may be at risk for later motor impairment.[13,14,33,40] The TIMP assesses functional infant motor behaviors related to posture and movement and can be administered to infants from 34 weeks postconceptual age to 4 months postterm age (or corrected age, CA).[14] Sophia's developmental progress was followed further with the Alberta Infant Motor Scale (AIMS) during NICU follow-up visits at 6 and 12 months.[58] Information on later testing with the Peabody Developmental Motor Scales (PDMS-2), a multi-item assessment of gross and fine motor development, is provided to demonstrate or confirm the presence of motor impairment by age 4 (Table 2.1).[14,24]

Screening and Prediction

How likely is it that Sophia will go on to develop motor impairment? Should intervention be provided?

Eligibility Decisions

Is Sophia's development different enough for her age to warrant the initiation and continuation of early intervention services?

Depending on her state's interpretation of the Individuals with Disabilities Education Act, Sophia may qualify for early intervention services based on her being at risk due to prematurity. If she did not have such a diagnosis, Sophia might qualify based on her developmental status as measured by a standardized outcome measure or by the informed clinical opinion of a practitioner.[62] A targeted evaluation team met with the family at their home and administered the Battelle Developmental Inventory, 2nd edition (BDI-2), a

TABLE 2.1   Various Assessments of Sophia During NICU and Follow-up

Age	Measure	Overall Results	Analysis and Interpretation
34 weeks (PMA)	GM	Cramped synchronized general movements	This movement pattern during the preterm period is associated with a higher likelihood of later diagnosis of motor impairment including cerebral palsy.[9,19,51]
36 weeks (PMA)	TIMP	35 (95% CI 17–53) z score: −.93	TIMP at 3 months (CA) is predictive of motor development on the AIMS at 12 months (CA). Standard error of the measurement (SEM) of the TIMP is 9[18]; 95% CI around the TIMP score is +/− 18 (1.96 × SEM).
2 months (CA)	TIMP	60 (95% CI 42–78) z score: −1.83	For scores at 2 and 4 months, even at the high range of the 95% CI the z score is < the −.05 cutoff point suggested for predictive ability of the TIMP.[13,40]
4 months (CA)	TIMP	90 (95% CI 72–108) z score: −1.88	Even though her scores improved over time, there is evidence that her progress is not keeping pace with expected developmental progress over time. There is ample evidence to make a referral for and continue intervention and follow-up.
6 months (corrected age)	AIMS	20 (95% CI 18.5–21.5) Percentile: between 5th–10th z score: −1.5	AIMS predictive validity at 4 months (cutoff 10th percentile) and 8 months (5th percentile) for identifying infants with poor motor performance at 18 months.[18] Predictive validity studies of the TIMP used AIMS scores <5th percentile at 12 months as an indicator of motor impairment.[13]
12 months (corrected age)	AIMS	43 (95% CI 41.75–44.25) Percentile: below 5th z score: −2.12	Sophia's performance on the TIMP suggested she might have motor impairment at 12 months on the AIMS, which indeed was confirmed. There is continued evidence in support of intervention, and further investigation into a diagnosis of motor impairment may be likely given her inability to keep developmental progress as noted by declining z scores over time.
2 years (corrected age)	PDMS-2 (TMQ)	79 (95% CI 73–85) Percentile: 8th z score: −1.40	Sophia's performance is below her same-aged peers with a z score of −1.4 indicating that she performs at 1.4 standard deviations from mean performance for children her age, which equates to the 8th percentile (92% of children perform better than she does at this age).
4 years (corrected age)	PDMS-2 (TMQ)	66 (95% CI 60–72) Percentile: 1st z score: −2.27	Her performance compared to peers decreased significantly from 2 years to 4 years (SEM for 24–35 and for 48–59 months = 3; 95% CI = 1.96 × SEM). There is no overlap in the two confidence interval ranges, so we can be sure that this difference in performance is not due to potential error or variability of the measure. She continues to perform below her peers and qualifies for therapy services. Should the z score of >1.5 be a cutoff for services, despite her performance at age 2, her therapist can use the 95% CI (the lower bound score of 73 is a z score of −1.8).

Unless otherwise reported from the literature, z scores, percentiles, and SEM to calculate the 95% CI are available in the measure's manual.
AIMS, Alberta Infant Motor Scale; GM, Prechtl's General Movements; PDMS-2, Peabody Developmental Motor Scales (2nd edition); TIMP, Test of Infant Motor Performance; TMC, total motor quotient.

comprehensive assessment of developmental status in a variety of relevant domains (Table 2.2).[49]

Evaluation of Change of Time

How has Sophia's motor function changed over time? What has been the result of intervention?

By the time Sophia reaches school age and enters elementary school, she has officially been diagnosed with cerebral palsy, Gross Motor Classification System level II.[54] She qualifies for special education and related services under the Individuals with Disabilities Education Act based on her diagnosis. Her motor function continues to be below age expectations, and that has a direct impact her participation in school. Results of those outcome measures related to motor function as she progresses through elementary school are presented in Table 2.3.

Case 2: Jacob

Jacob is a 4-year 8-month-old male with a diagnosis of Down syndrome (DS). He has been referred to outpatient physical therapy by the physical therapist at his preschool due to concerns about his gross motor skill in preparation for his attendance at kindergarten within the next 12 months. Jacob's mother and

father identify improved running, jumping, and ability to safely and efficiently walk up and down the stairs as primary goals. During the initial examination the tests and measures collected are shown in Tables 2.4 to 2.7.

Clinical decision: A 6-month episode of care with an emphasis on parent goals.

Measures collected during the initial episode of care are shown in Tables 2.8 to 2.10.

Measures collected during this time are shown in Tables 2.11 to 2.13

The decision to continue with a consultation level of service is based on a comparison of scores to previous performance and to norms for DS where appropriate. It is important to continue to collaborate with the family on goals and to identify community resources and fitness options.

Measures collected during this episode of care are shown in Tables 2.14 to 2.16

This category reflects the decision for a 6-week episode of care, referral for nutrition counseling, focus on fitness-related goals, and preparation for high school.

TABLE 2.2 Results from Two Administrations of the Battelle Developmental Inventory, 2nd Edition (BDI-2), One Year Apart

Age	BDI-2 Domain	Raw Score	Standard Score	Percentile Rank	Z score	Analysis and Interpretation
10 months (7.5 CA)	Adaptive	0	55	0.1	−3.00	Eligibility for EI in Sophia's state: ≤2 standard deviations (SD) below the mean in one domain or 1.5 SDs in two domains; she qualifies based on her motor performance alone but also has significant deficits in adaptive function. Z scores reflect the number of SDs from the mean (see Fig. 2.1).
	Personal-social	31	100	50	0.00	
	Communication	24	89	23	−0.73	
	Motor	24	69	2	−2.07	
	Cognitive	26	90	25	−0.67	
	Total	105	80	9	−1.33	
22 months (19.5 CA)	Adaptive	21	75	5	−1.67	Sophia received intervention for 12 months; increased adaptive function has been noted; new deficits are noted especially in the area of communication that warranted additional evaluation; motor skills have not improved when compared to age, but she has gained skills. Sophia continues to qualify for EI and additional services are provided.
	Personal-social	36	80	9	−1.33	
	Communication	30	63	1	−2.47	
	Motor	60	71	3	−1.93	
	Cognitive	30	77	6	−1.53	
	Total	177	67	1	−2.20	

TABLE 2.3 Results of Outcome Measures through Elementary School

Age Measure	Overall Results	Analysis and Interpretation
4 years PDMS-2 (TMQ)	66 (95% CI 60–72) Percentile: 1st z score: −2.27	• A TIMP cutoff z score of <−0.5 at 3 months correctly identified 87% of children who would later be classified as having motor impairment via a z score of <−2 on the PDMS-2 at 4 years.[40] • Sophia's performance is well below same-aged peers (z score of ≥ −2 at 4 and 5 years).
5 years PDMS-2 (TMQ)	70 (95% CI 68–74) Percentile: 2nd z score: −2	• Her performance compared to peers did not decrease between 4 and 5 years of age and may not have improved enough to be significant; she kept developmental pace with other children her age, but she did not "catch up" to her peers. • 95% confidence intervals (1.96 × SEM) were calculated from the reported SEM (TMQ 48–59 months = 3, 60–71 months = 2); since the 95% CI ranges for 4 years and 5 years overlap, it is possible Sophia's true score could fall in each of those ranges, so these scores do not statistically differ from each other.
4 years GMFM-66 using the GMAE	54 Percentile: 50th	• GMFM-66 scores were converted to interval scores using the GMAE. • Performance on GMFM-66 can be plotted on growth curves for children with CP[64]; changes in percentile scores can vary over time and may not reflect true change in ability; the GMFM-66 score change is a more appropriate assessment of motor ability, as the percentile compares Sophia to other same-aged children with GMFCS level II.[31] Note these percentile ranks are not like others reported for Sophia, as the others compared her to same-aged children without motor impairment. • MCID for large effect sizes for the GMFM-66 with children at GMFCS level II is 1.5[52]; the 6-point change from 4 years to 6 years exceeds the MCID and moves the child from the 50th percentile to 45th when compared to other level II peers; one could argue that the change, though clinically important, also demonstrates that the child kept pace with peers with CP— still very close to "average" expectations given her diagnosis and GMFCS level. • The 1-point change in GMFM-66 score from 6 years to 8 years does not exceed the MCID and the child actually appears to have lost ground when compared to other level II peers, dropping from the 45th percentile to the 25th percentile.
6 years GMFM-66 using the GMAE	60 Percentile: 45th	
8 years GMFM-66 using the GMAE	61 Percentile: 25th	
8 years PEDI-CAT	Daily Activities: • T score: 40 • Percentile: 18 Mobility: • T score: 30 • Percentile: <5	• Daily Activities and Mobility domains of the PEDI-CAT were followed over time as Sophia progressed through elementary school to middle school. • Progression in her skills with respect to how she compares to her peers in daily functional activities are noted in her improvements from a T score of 50 (1 SD below the mean, and just under the 20th percentile for age) to 50 (within average expectations for age at the 50th percentile).
10 years PEDI-CAT	Daily Activities: • T score: 45 • Percentile: 32 Mobility: • T score: 30 • Percentile: <5	• While making marked improvements in her daily activities, Sophia's mobility function was relatively stable from 8 years to 10 years, and a movement from a T score of 30 to a T score of 35 shows a movement from 2 SDs below the mean for age to 1.5 SDs below the mean. • The PEDI-CAT manual[27] notes that T scores between 70 and 30 represent 2 SDs above or below the mean and are within averaged expectations for age. If using T scores or percentiles to qualify for services, either can and should be used in decision making.
12 years PEDI-CAT	Daily Activities: • T score: 50 • Percentile: 50 Mobility: • T score: 35 • Percentile: 7	• Sophia experienced her adolescent growth spurt early and has had challenges with her weight since she entered her preteen years. She has also experienced a decrease in her overall activity level (increase in sedentary time as she became more focused on school and was less involved in recreational activities). These are factors to be considered when interpreting her scores. The fact that her mobility did not decrease but remained stable or slightly increased over time may be attributed to her continued involvement with intervention and home activity programs to maintain her overall fitness and mobility.

Unless otherwise reported from the literature, z scores, percentiles, and SEM to calculate the 95% CI are available in the measures manual.
GMAE, Gross Motor Activity Estimator; GMFM-66, Gross Motor Function Measure (66 item version); PDMS-2, Peabody Developmental Motor Scales (2nd edition); PEDI-CAT, Pediatric Evaluation of Disability Inventory Computer Adaptive Test; TMQ-Total Motor Quotient.

TABLE 2.4 Jacob Baseline-Impairment Level Data

	Baseline Score	Interpretation
Quad Muscle Strength- Dynamometer (Newtons)	49	Well below age- and gender-matched norm[6]
Height (cm)	95	50th percentile
Weight (kg)	12.5	25th percentile
BMI (kg/m²)	13.8	10th percentile

Note: Percentiles are based on the population of children with DS.[47]

TABLE 2.5 Jacob Baseline-Single Task Activity Level Data

	Baseline Score	Interpretation
5× Sit to Stand (sec)	14	
5× Step-ups (sec)	30	
6-Minute Walk (m)	Refuses due to behavior and cognitive limitations	N/A
Standing Broad Jump (cm)	Unable	N/A
30-Yard Running Speed (sec)	16 seconds	Slow, immature, disorganized pattern; norm for age-matched peers is approximately 7 seconds[43]
Timed Up and Down Stairs (sec)	32 seconds for nine stairs (1.78 seconds/stair) Intermittent reciprocal pattern when ascending, step to pattern when descending, with railing	Mean TUDS for chronologic age 8–14 years = 0.58 s• step-1[79]
Timed Up and Go (sec)	13.5 seconds	Norm for age-matched peers = 6.59 +/– 1.36 seconds[50] Norm for children with Down Syndrome who score 50%–69% on Dimension E of the GMFM = 11.24 +/– 2.47 seconds[50]

TABLE 2.6 Jacob Baseline- Multi Item Activity Level Data

	Baseline Score	Interpretation
GMFM 88	73%*	Low for age and diagnosis[55]
Pediatric Balance Scale	34	> 2 standard deviations below mean for age- and gender-matched peers[25]

*GMFM score allows determination of a 34% conditional probability that Jacob will be able to walk up at least two steps from the base of the stairs (alternating feet, without holding on) by age 5 and a 41% conditional probability that he will jump forward (at least 2 inches, both feet simultaneously) by age 5.[55]

TABLE 2.7 Jacob Initial Episode of Care- Goal Attainment Scaling Information

Goal	–2 Score	–1 Score	0 Score	+1 Score	+2 Score
Improve TUDS to 1.4 second/ stair (total)	1.77 (32 seconds)	1.6 (29 seconds)	1.4 (25.2 seconds)	1.25 (22.5 seconds)	1 (18 seconds)
Improve 30-yard running speed to 12 seconds	16	14	12	10	8
Improve standing broad jump to 2 cm	Unable	2-foot take-off and landing	2 cm	4 cm	6 cm

TABLE 2.8 Jacob Initial Episode of Care- Impairment

	Baseline Score	6-Month Score	Interpretation
Quad Muscle Strength- Dynamometer (Newtons)	49	53	Remains well below age- and gender-matched norm[6]
Height (cm)	95	97	50th percentile
Weight (kg)	12.5	13	25th percentile
BMI (kg/m²)	13.8	13.8	10th percentile

Note: Percentiles are based on the population of children with DS.[47]

TABLE 2.9 Jacob Initial Episode of Care- Single Task Activity

	Baseline Score	Biweekly Scores						6-Month Score	Interpretation
5× Sit to Stand (sec)	14	15	21	17	19	16	15	15	No change in this outcome
5× Step-ups (sec)	30	27	26	28	24	22	19	18	Approximately 30% improvement reflects improved motor control with this task
6-Minute Walk (m)	Refuses–due to behavior and cognitive limitations								
Standing Broad Jump (cm)	Unable	0	0	0	0	3	3	4	Achieved this skill; requires continued practice to refine and improve GAS score: +1
30-Yard Running Speed (sec)	16	16	17	16	15	15	14	13	Approximately 20% improvement; still slow compared to age-matched peers[43] GAS score: −1
Timed Up and Down Stairs (sec)	32 Intermittent reciprocal pattern when ascending, step to pattern when descending, with railing	32	31	27	28	31	27	23	Approximately 28% improvement; GAS score: +1
Timed Up and Go (sec)	13.5 seconds	13.5	12	13.1	11.4	12	11	10.8	Approximately 20% improvement exceeds MCID estimate of 2.07 seconds; score is within normal range for age, diagnosis, and current level of gross motor function[50]

TABLE 2.10 Jacob Initial Episode of Care- Multi Item Activity

	Baseline Score	6-Month Score	Interpretation
GMFM 88	73%*	84%	Significant improvement beyond MCID[52]; age-appropriate score for diagnosis[55]–justifies decision to discontinue PT and address GM skills through community-based and age-appropriate programs (e.g., TOP-Soccer, swim club).
Pediatric Balance Scale	34	44	MCID for children with CP = 3.66–5.83.[15] A 30% improvement appears to represent meaningful change; however, the score is approximately 1.5 standard deviations below the mean for age- and gender-matched peers.[25]

*Improvement in goal areas (stairs, running, jumping; GAS T score = 54.57 [score > 50 = better than anticipated change]) along with improvement on GMFM and Pediatric Balance Scale support a change to the consultation service level. Data are provided to the family to share with the school PT; the family is comfortable with the child engaging in community and age-appropriate fitness and recreational opportunities (play in the neighborhood, community swim club, TOPSoccer).

TABLE 2.11   Jacob 6 to 8 Years- Impairment

	Baseline Score: Age 6	Baseline Score: Age 8	Interpretation
Quad Muscle Strength- Dynamometer (Newtons)	79	90	Improving, but still >2 standard deviations below age- and gender-matched norms[6]
Height (cm)	110	120	50th percentile
Weight (kg)	17.5	22.5	25th percentile
BMI (kg/m²)	13.8	14	10th percentile
			Note: percentiles are based on population of children with DS[47]

TABLE 2.12   Jacob 6 to 8 Years- Single Task Activity

	Baseline Score: Age 6	Baseline Score: Age 8	Interpretation
5× Sit to Stand (sec)	15	14	Performance does not merit PT intervention due to ongoing improvement and participation in age-appropriate family and community fitness and recreational activities
5× Step-ups (sec)	16	13	
6-Minute Walk (m)	400	440	
Standing Broad Jump (cm)	20	50	
30-Yard Running Speed (sec)	11	10	
Timed Up and Down Stairs (sec)	18	14	
Timed Up and Go (sec)	9.8	8.5	

TABLE 2.13   Jacob 6-8 Years- Multi Item Activity

	Baseline Score: Age 6	Baseline Score: Age 8	Interpretation
GMFM 88	80	90	Ongoing improvement and performance at level expected for age and diagnosis, thus there is no need for an episode of care
Pediatric Balance Scale	48	55	Ongoing improvement; score at 6 years of age remains 2 standard deviations below the mean for age and gender-matched peers; score at 8 years is at the mean for typically developing children > 7 years of age[25]

TABLE 2.14   Jacob 14 Years- Impairment

	Baseline Score	Interpretation	6-Week Score	Interpretation
Quad Muscle Strength- Dynamometer (Newtons)	150	Improved but > 2 standard deviations below age- and gender-matched norms[6]	152	Focus of episode of care was on aerobic fitness; continue to monitor leg muscle strength and encourage incorporation of resistance exercises into ongoing fitness/exercise program
Height (cm)	155	BMI is at the 90th percentile for age, gender, and diagnosis[47]; physical therapy intervention is appropriate to address this impairment; referral to a nutritionist also initiated	155	BMI remains at the 90th percentile, but the patient and family are committed to regular fitness and improved nutrition; will monitor at follow-up visit in 6 months[47]
Weight (kg)	66		66	
BMI (kg/m²)	27.4		27.4	

TABLE 2.15 Jacob 14 Years- Single Task Activity

	Baseline Score	Interpretation	Biweekly Scores			6-Week Score	Interpretation
5× Sit to Stand	—	—	—	—	—	—	—
5× Step-ups	13	Similar to previous scores	12	12	13	12	Focus of episode of care was on aerobic fitness and collaborating with Jacob and his family to establish a sustainable fitness program
6-Minute Walk	420 (Jacob reports an OMNI RPE[31] of 9 at the conclusion of this walk)	Decreased distance (compared to previous years) and high OMNI RPE indicate concern with level of aerobic fitness	425	435	450	455 (OMNI-RPE = 7)	Steady progress, 30-meter increase, and reduction in OMNI-RPE indicate meaningful improvement
Standing Broad Jump (cm)	55	Skill has plateaued—not an area of emphasis during this episode of care	55	54	55	53	Skill has plateaued—not an area of emphasis during this episode of care
30-Yard Running Speed (sec)	9.8	Limited by fatigue	9.9	12	11.5	9	Approximately 20% improvement, perhaps due to improved endurance; performance is variable due to inconsistent motivation with this task
Timed Up and Down Stairs (sec)	14	Limited by motor control especially when descending	13	13	12	10	Focus of episode of care identified as a goal area by Jacob and his family; improvement on this skill necessary for safety and participation in high school with age-matched peers
Timed Up and Go (sec)	8.5	Norm for age-matched peers = 4.99 +/− 0.87 seconds Norm for children with Down syndrome who score 70%–90% on Dimension E of the GMFM = 9.42 +/− 1.15 seconds[50]	8.7	9	8.5	8.5	Not a focus of episode of care

TABLE 2.16 Jacob 14 Years- Multi Item Activity and Participation

	Baseline Score and Interpretation	6-Week Score and Interpretation
GMFM 88		
Pediatric Balance Scale		
Canadian Occupational Performance Measure (COPM)	Priorities: • Better on stairs satisfaction = 2/10 performance = 3/10 • Better fitness satisfaction = 2/10 performance = 1/10 Faster running speed satisfaction = 2/10 performance = 3/10 • Total satisfaction = 2 • Total performance = 2.3	• Better on stairs satisfaction = 5/10 performance = 6/10 • Better fitness satisfaction = 3/10 performance = 6/10 Faster running speed satisfaction = 4/10 performance = 5/10 • Total satisfaction = 4 Improvement ≥ 2 on satisfaction indicates meaningful change • Total performance = 5.4 Improvement ≥ 2 on performance indicates meaningful change[42]
Activities Scale for Kids (ASK)[78]	70 Not participating in team sports or other community recreational opportunities	85 Some improvement here as a result of collaboration with Jacob and his caregivers on options for participation in the community

Improvement on COPM and ASK following 6-week intervention program justifies resumption of a consultative level of services.

REFERENCES

1. Alberta Infant Motor Scale: Available from: URL: http://www.albertainfant motorscale.com/.

2. American Educational Research Association: *Standards for educational and psychological testing*, Washington, DC, 2014, American Educational Research Association.

3. American Physical Therapy Association: guide to physical therapist practice 3.0. Available from: URL: http://guidetoptpractice.apta.org/.

4. American Physical Therapy Association: OPTIMAL 1.1 Data collection instrument. Available from: URL: http://www.apta.org/OPTIMAL/.

5. American Psychiatric Association: *Diagnostic and statistical manual of mental disorders*, ed 5, Washington, DC, 2013, American Psychiatric Association.

6. Backman E, Odenrick P, Henriksson K, Ledin T: Isometric muscle force and anthropometric values in normal children aged between 3.5 and 15 years, *Scand J Rehabil Med* 1:105–114, 1982.

7. Barnett A: is there a "movement thermometer" for developmental coordination disorder? Curr Dev Disord Rep 20141:132–139.

8. Barnhart R, Davenport M, Epps S, Nordquist V: Developmental coordination disorder, *Phys Ther* 83:722–731, 2003.

9. Bosanquet M, Copeland L, Ware R, Boyd R: A systematic review of tests to predict cerebral palsy in young children, *Dev Med Child Neurol* 55:418–426, 2013.

10. BOT 2: Bruininks-Oseretsky Test of Motor Proficiency, Second Edition. Available from: URL: http://www.pearsonclinical.com/therapy/products/ 100000648/bruininks-oseretsky-test-of-motor-proficiency-second-edition- bot-2.html.

11. Brennan R, editor: *Educational measurement (American Council on Education/ Oryx Press Series on Higher Education)*, Lanham, 2006, Maryland: rowan & Littlefield Publishers.

12. Broderick J, DeWitt E, Rothrock N, Crane P, Forrest C: Advances in patient-reported outcomes: the NIH PROMIS measures, *EGEMS* 1:1–7, 2013.

13. Campbell S, Kolobe T, Wright B, Linacre J: Validity of the Test of Infant Motor Performance for prediction of 6-, 9-, and 12-month scores on the Alberta Infant Motor Scale, *Dev Med Child Neurol* 44:263–272, 2002.

14. Campbell S: *The Test of Infant Motor Performance. Test user's manual version 3.0 for the TIMP Version 5*, Chicago, 2012, Infant Motor Performance Scales. LLC.

15. Chen CL, Wu KP, Liu WY, Cheng HY, Shen IH, Lin KC: Validity and clinometric properties of the Spinal Alignment and Range of Motion Measure in children with cerebral palsy, *Dev Med Child Neurol* 55:745–750, 2013.

16. Connors 3 Rating Scales. Available from: URL: http://addwarehouse.com/ shopsite_sc/store/html/conners-3-manual.html.

17. Copay A, Suback B, Glassman S, Polly D, Schuler T: Understanding the minimum clinically important difference: a review of concepts and methods, *Spine* 7:541–546, 2007.

18. Darrah J, Piper M, Watt M: Assessment of gross motor skills of at-risk infants: predictive validity of the Alberta Infant Motor Scale, *Dev Med Child Neurol* 40:485–491, 1998.

19. Darsaklis V, Snider L, Majnemer A, Mazer B: Predictive validity of Prechtl's Method on the Qualitative Assessment of General Movements: a systematic review of the evidence, *Dev Med Child Neurol* 53:896–906, 2011.

20. Downing S, Haladyna T: *Handbook of test development*, New York, 2006, Routledge.

21. Einspieler C, Prechtl H: Prechtl's assessment of general movements: a diagnostic tool for the functional assessment of the young nervous system, *Ment Retard Dev D R* 11:61–67, 2005.

22. Fein M: *Test development: fundamentals for certification and evaluation*, Alexandria, VA, 2012, ASTD Press.

23. Flegel J, Kolobe T: Predictive validity of the Test of Infant Motor Performance as measured by the Bruininks-Oseretsky Test of Motor Proficiency at school age, *Phys Ther* 82:762–771, 2002.

24. Folio M, Fewell R: *Peabody Developmental Motor Scales*, ed 2, Austin, TX, 2000, Pro-Ed Publishers.

25. Franjoine MR, Darr N, Held SL, Kott K, Young BL: The performance of children developing typically on the pediatric balance scale, *Pediatr Phys Ther* 22:350–359, 2010.

26. Gross Motor Function Measure: Available from: URL: https://canchild. ca/en/resources/44-gross-motor-function-measure-gmfm.

27. Haley S, Coster W, Dumas H, Fragala-Pinkham M, Moed R: *Evaluation of Disability Inventory Computer Adaptive Test: development, standardization and administration manual*, Boston, 2012, Health and Disability Research Institute.

28. Haley S, Fragala-Pinkham M: Interpreting change scores of tests and measures used in physical therapy, *Phys Ther* 86:735–743, 2006.

29. Hanna S, Russell D, Bartlett D, Kertoy M, Rosenbaum P, Swinton M: *Clinical measurement practical guidelines for service providers*, 2005. Available from: URL: http://www.canchild.ca/en/canchildresources/ resources/ClinicalMeasurement.pdf.

30. Hanna S, Russell D, Bartlett D, Kertoy M, Rosenbaum P, Wynn K: Measurement practices in pediatric rehabilitation: a survey of physical therapists, occupational therapists, and speech-language pathologists in Ontario, *Phys Occup Ther Pediatr* 27:25–42, 2007.

31. Hanna SE, Bartlett DJ, Rivard LM, Russell DJ: Reference curves for the Gross Motor Function Measure: percentiles for clinical description and tracking over time among children with cerebral palsy, *Phys Ther* 88:596–607, 2008.

32. Hay J, Hawes R, Faught B: Evaluation of a screening instrument for developmental coordination disorder, *J Adolesc Health* 34:308–313, 2004.

33. IMPS: infant Motor Performance Scales. Available from: URL: http:// thetimp.com/.

34. Iyer L, Haley S, Watkins M, Dumas H: Establishing minimal clinically important differences for scores on the Pediatric Evaluation of Disability Inventory for inpatient rehabilitation, *Phys Ther* 83:888–898, 2003.

35. Jette D, Halbert J, Iverson C, Miceli E, Shah P: Use of standardized outcome measures in physical therapy practice: perceptions and applications, *Phys Ther* 89:125–133, 2009.

36. Kaufman Brief Intelligence Test, Second Edition (KBIT-2). Available from: URL: http://www.pearsonclinical.com/psychology/products/100000390/ kaufman-brief-intelligence-test-second-edition-kbit-2.html.

37. Ketelaar M, Russell D, Gorter JW: The challenge of moving evidence-based measures into clinical practice: lessons in knowledge translation, *Phys Occup Ther Pediatr* 28:191–206, 2008.

38. King GA, McDougall J, Palisano RJ, Gritzan J, Tucker M: Goal attainment scaling: its use in evaluating pediatric therapy programs, *Phys Occup Ther Pediatr* 19:31–52, 1999.

39. Kiresuk T, Sherman R: Goal attainment scaling: a general method for evaluating comprehensive community mental health programs, *Ment Health J* 4:443–453, 1968.

40. Kolobe T, Bulanda M, Susman L: Predicting motor outcome at preschool age for infants tested at 7, 30, 60, and 90 days after term age using the Test of Infant Motor Performance, *Phys Ther* 84:1144–1156, 2004.

41. Law M, King G, Russell D, MacKinnon E, Hurley P, Murphy C: Measuring outcomes in children's rehabilitation: a decision protocol, *Arch Phys Med Rehab* 80:629–636, 1999.

42. Law M, Majnemer A, McColl M, Bosch J, Hanna S, Wilkins S: Home and community occupational therapy for children and youth: a before and after study, *Can J Occupat Ther* 53:289–297, 2005.

43. Malina R, Bouchard C, Bar-Or O: *Growth, maturation, and physical activity*, ed 2, Champaign, IL, 2004, Human Kinetics.

44. Maloney E, Larrivee L: Limitations of age-equivalent scores in reporting the results of norm-referenced tests, *Cont Iss Comm Sci Dis* 34:86–93, 2007.

45. Missiuma C, Cairney J, Pollock N, et al.: A staged approach for identifying children with developmental coordination disorder from the population. *Res Dev Disabil* 32:549–559, 2011.

46. Movement Assessment Battery for Children-Second Edition (Movement ABC-2). Available from: URL: http://www.pearsonclinical.com/therapy/ products/100000433/movement-assessment-battery-for-children-second- edition-movement-abc-2.html.

47. Myrelid A, Gustafsson J, Ollars B, Anneren G: Growth charts for Down syndrome from birth to 18 years of age, *Arch Dis Child* 87:97–103, 2002.

48. NSMDA: Physiotherapy assessment for infants & young children. Available from: URL: http://nsmda.com.au/.

49. Newborg J: *Battelle Developmental Inventory*, ed 2, Itasca, IL, 2005, Riverside Publishing.

50. Nicolini-Panisson RD, Donadio MV: Normative values for the Timed 'Up and Go' test in children and adolescents and validation for individuals with Down syndrome, *Dev Med Child Neurol* 56:490–497, 2014.

51. Øberg GK, Jacobsen BK, Jørgensen L: *Predictive value of general movement assessment for cerebral palsy in routine clinical practice*, *Phys Ther*, 95:1489–1495, 2015.

52. Oeffinger D, Bagley A, Rogers S, et al.: Outcome tools used for ambulatory children with cerebral palsy: responsiveness and minimum clinically important differences, *Dev Med Child Neurol* 50:918–925, 2008.

53. Reference deleted in proofs for 53.

54. Palisano RJ, Rosenbaum P, Bartlett D, Livingstone R: *Gross Motor Function Classification System—expanded and revised*, Hamilton, Ontario, 2007, CanChild Centre for Childhood Disability Research, McMaster University.

55. Palisano RJ, Walter SD, Russell DJ, et al.: Gross motor function of children with down syndrome: creation of motor growth curves, *Arch Phys Med Rehabil* 82:494–500, 2001.

56. Peabody Developmental Motor Scales, Second Edition (PDMS-2): Available from: URL: http://www.pearsonclinical.com/therapy/products/100000249/peabody-developmental-motor-scales-second-edition-pdms-2.html.

57. Pediatric Evaluation of Disability Inventory. Available from: URL: http://www.pearsonclinical.com/childhood/products/100000505/pediatric-evaluation-of-disability-inventory-pedi.html.

58. Piper M, Darrah J: *Motor assessment of the developing infant*, Philadelphia, 1994, WB Saunders.

59. Portney L, Watkins M: *Foundations for clinical research: applications to practice*, ed 3, New Jersey, 2009, Pearson/ Prentice Hall.

60. Prechtl H: Qualitative changes of spontaneous movements in fetus and preterm infant are a marker of neurological dysfunction, *Early Hum Dev* 23:151–158, 1990.

61. Riddle D, Stratford P: *Is this change real? Interpreting patient outcomes in physical therapy*, Philadelphia, 2013, FA Davis.

62. Ringwalt S: Summary table of states' and territories' definitions of /criteria for IDEA Part C eligibility, *Early Childhood Technical Assistance Center*, 2015. Available from: URL: http://ectacenter.org/topics/earlyid/partcelig.asp.

63. Rosenbaum P, Walter S,SH, et al.: Prognosis for gross motor function in Cerebral Palsy: creation of motor development curves, *JAMA* 288: 1357–1363, 2002.

64. Rosenbaum P, Walter SD, Hanna S, et al.: Prognosis for gross motor function in Cerebral Palsy: creation of motor development curves, *JAMA* 288:1357–1363, 2002.

65. Rothstein J, Campbell S, Echternach J, Jette A, Knecht H, Rose S: Standards for tests and measurements in physical therapy practice, *Phys Ther* 71:589–622, 1991.

66. Russek L, Wooden M, Ekedahl S, Bush A: Attitudes toward standardized data collection, *Phys Ther* 77:714–729, 1997.

67. Russell D, Rivard L, Walter S, et al.: Using knowledge brokers to facilitate the uptake of pediatric measurement tools into clinical practice: a before-after intervention study, *Implement Sci* 5:1–17, 2010.

68. Russell D, Rosenbaum P, Wright M: *Gross Motor Function Measure (GMFM-66 and GMFM-88) user's manual*, London, 2013, MacKeith Press.

69. Sampson J: *Computer-assisted testing in counseling and therapy*, ERIC Digest, 1995. Available from: URL: https://www.counseling.org/resources/library/ERIC%20Digests/95-26.pdf.

70. Spironello C, Hay J, Missiuna C, Faught E, Cairney J: Concurrent and construct validation of the short form of the Bruininks-Oseretsky Test of Motor Proficiency and the Movement-ABC when administered under field conditions: implications for screening, *Child Care Health Dev* 36:499–507, 2010.

71. Spittle A, Lee K, Spencer-Smith M, Lorefice M, Anderson P, Doyle L: Accuracy of two motor assessments during the first year of life in preterm infants for predicting motor outcome at preschool age, *PLoS One* 10(5):e0125854, 2015.

72. The Canadian Occupational Performance Measure. Available from: URL: http://www.thecopm.ca/.

73. Trevena LJ, Davey HM, Barratt A, Butow P, Caldwell P: A systematic review on communicating with patients about evidence, *J Eval Clin Pract* 12:13–23, 2006.

74. Venetsanou F, Kambas A, Elinoudis T, Fatouros I, Giannakidou D, Kourtessis T: Movement Assessment Battery for Children test be the "gold standard" for the motor assessment of children with developmental coordination disorder? *Res Dev Disabil* 31:1–10, 2011.

75. Wang Y, Hart D, Stratford P, Mioduski J: Baseline dependency of minimal clinically important improvement, *Phys Ther* 91:675–688, 2011.

76. Wilson B, Crawford S, Green D, Roberts G, Aylott A, Kaplan B: Psychometric properties of the Revised Developmental Coordination Disorder Questionnaire, *Phys Occupat Ther Pediatric* 29:182–202, 2009.

77. Workgroup on Principles and Practices in Natural Environments: *OSEP TA Community of Practice: part C Settings. Agreed upon mission and key principles for providing early intervention services in natural environments*, 2008. Available from: URL: http://ectacenter.org/~pdfs/topics/families/Finalmissionandprinciples3_11_08.pdf.

77a. World Health Organization: *International classification of functioning, disability and health: ICF*, Geneva, Switzerland, 2001, World Health Organization.

78. Young N, Williams I, Yoshida K, Wright J: Measurement properties of the Activities Scale for Kids, *J Clin Epidemiol* 53:125–137, 2000.

79. Zaino CA, Marchese VG, Westcott SL: Timed up and down stairs test: preliminary reliability and validity of a new measure of functional mobility, *Pediatr Phys Ther* 16:90–98, 2004.

SUGGESTED READINGS

Copay A, Suback B, Glassman S, Polly D, Schuler T: Understanding the minimum clinically important difference: a review of concepts and methods, *Spine* 7:541–546, 2007.

Haley S, Fragala-Pinkham M: Interpreting change scores of tests and measures used in physical therapy, *Phys Ther* 86:735–743, 2006.

Hanna S, Russell D, Bartlett D, Kertoy M, Rosenbaum P, Swinton M: *Clinical Measurement Practical Guidelines for Service Providers*, 2005. Available from URL: http://www.canchild.ca/en/canchildresources/resources/ClinicalMeasurement.pdf.

Hanna S, Russell D, Bartlett D, Kertoy M, Rosenbaum P, Wynn K: Measurement practices in pediatric rehabilitation: a survey of physical therapists, occupational therapists, and speech-language pathologists in Ontario, *Phys Occup Ther Pediatr* 27:25–42, 2007.

Oeffinger D, Bagley A, Rogers S, et al.: Outcome tools used for ambulatory children with cerebral palsy: responsiveness and minimum clinically important differences, *Dev Med Child Neurol* 50:918–925, 2008.

Palisano RJ, Walter SD, Russell DJ, et al.: Gross motor function of children with down syndrome: creation of motor growth curves, *Arch Phys Med Rehabil* 82:494–500, 2001.

Rosenbaum P, Walter S,SH, et al.: Prognosis for gross motor function in Cerebral Palsy: creation of motor development curves, *JAMA* 288:1357–1363, 2002.

Russell D, Rivard L, Walter S, et al. Using knowledge brokers to facilitate the uptake of pediatric measurement tools into clinical practice: a before-after intervention study, *Implement Sci* 5:1–17.

Trevena LJ, Davey HM, Barratt A, Butow P, Caldwell P: A systematic review on communicating with patients about evidence, 2010, *J Eval Clin Pract* 12:13–23, 2006.

3

Motor Development and Control

Suzann K. Campbell, Regina T. Harbourne, Stacey Dusing

"Development, then, can be envisioned as a changing landscape of preferred, but not obligatory, behavioral states with varying degrees of stability and instability, rather than as a prescribed series of structurally invariant stages leading to progressive improvement."

Esther Thelen, p 77, Mind as Motion, 1995[313]

Movement expresses our needs, preferences, desires, successes, and interactions with the world. As physical therapists, we are often asked questions about early movement that begin with the word "when." When will my child walk? When will my son sit up by himself? Alternatively, as time passes, the question may be modified from time-based to an absolute: Will my child ever learn to ride a bike? However, as a movement expert the physical therapist must understand much more than the timing of developmental motor milestones. Our questions need to focus on the "how" so that we can provide explanations of *how* a child learns to sit, crawl, stand, and walk. Understanding how a skill emerges benefits us in three ways. First, our predictions become more exact. Knowing the factors contributing to change over time sharpens our estimate of when the next increment of change will occur. Second, understanding how skills emerge allows a therapist to analyze gaps in the contributions to a skill and thus formulate a plan to fill the gap. Finally, understanding the multiple variables that contribute to skill advancement allows versatility in creating intervention suitable to the individual child. In this chapter we will examine in detail the when, how, why, and what of developing motor skill, toward the ultimate goal of building understanding that contributes to effective physical therapy for children with motor needs.

To understand motor development, movement needs to be placed in a context. Motor skill does not develop in a vacuum; motor development depends on individual child factors (physiology, temperament, cognition), and environmental factors such as the immediate microsystem environment (womb, family, home, surroundings, peers), the exosystem environment (extended family, neighborhood, school), as well as the macrosystem environment (community, economic system, culture).[42] Thus the pediatric therapist must consider the layers of influence that build behavior, and she must understand that not all behavior is displayed in every context. For example, a shy child may be unwilling to display her ability to jump or kick a ball in a strange clinical setting, even though she skillfully and delightfully exhibits these skills in her backyard. A hungry infant arching his back and refusing a toy during a testing session might easily sit independently and engage with the same toy once his physiologic needs are met. An infant raised in a culture that does not practice floor play may not exhibit prone skills, even though there is nothing wrong with his extensor musculature. All of these individual, contextual, and cultural factors contribute to wide variability in motor skill development and the variable acquisition of motor control throughout childhood.

Although extensive evidence supports the existence of general developmental trends in motor skill development (Fig. 3.1), strong evidence also reveals wide variability in the acquisition of functional motor skills. What contributes to this variability, and how can therapists capitalize on the flexibility and adaptability of the developing system to build skill within a therapy program? In this chapter we begin by laying a theoretical base for understanding developmental change, with an eye toward historical influences that contribute to ideas that have been evaluated and accepted, rejected, or modified over time based on advances in child development research. We then discuss a current framework for therapeutic motor intervention, which incorporates multiple external factors thought to influence change in children, or the "how" of development. We follow these external factors by detailing the internal factors that influence the child's motor skill: variables within the motor control realm that may be important to consider in determining the "why" questions regarding selection of strategies by children over time. In the third section we describe the acquisition of specific motor skills in greater detail: the "what" and "when" of development. And finally, we provide exemplar stories of children at different ages, with the how, what, why, and when used as a guide to maintain a global view of development within therapeutic practice, yet tailoring that practice toward the needs of the individual child within his or her world.

THEORETICAL BACKGROUND: PERSPECTIVES LEADING TO UNDERSTANDING THE BASICS OF HOW AND WHY MOTOR SKILLS CHANGE OVER TIME

Our understanding of theories of development leads to deeper knowledge of the "how" questions we ask when watching an infant perform a new skill or when we ask "why" a child may not be skillful at a task as we try to create an intervention leading to progress in motor development. Theory drives the way we think and creates the space in which we search for problem solutions. In this section we discuss some major theoretical steps that brought us to currently think in complex ways about development. Importantly, developmental theory springs from contributors outside the motor realm. In fact, much developmental research comes from psychologists and other scientists who are interested in the development of cognition and language and how motor skills contribute to learning.[5] However, early

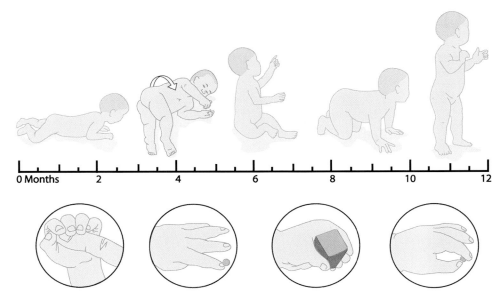

FIG. 3.1 Developmental timeline for several gross and fine motor milestones. (Drawing courtesy Ricardo Solis, Costa Rica.)

theorists used movement and motor skills as a primary means of studying development in all domains. Through movement a child expresses knowledge of the world (cognition), knowledge of how he or she can affect the world (adaptive skills), the exchange of ideas (language), and the connections to others (social/emotional). Thus motor skill reveals much more than simply musculoskeletal information. Movement reveals information about the child's overall development and the effects of other areas on motor skills in a cyclical and ever-changing relationship.

Thelen and colleagues[317] summarized the major theoretical approaches to developmental change as encompassing three world views: (1) neural-maturationist, (2) cognitive, and (3) dynamical systems. Each contributes to a history revealing the strong role that changing biases contribute to the accumulation of new knowledge and the way this knowledge is subsequently interpreted and applied clinically.[19,80,313,314] These theories are reviewed briefly in this chapter, with their major distinguishing features summarized in Table 3.1.

Neural-Maturationist Theories

The neural-maturationist point of view was pioneered by Arnold Gesell,[123,124,125,127,128,126] Shirley,[285] and others. This view proposed that the ontogeny of behavior is "an intrinsic property of the organism, with maturation leading to an unfolding of predetermined patterns, supported, but not fundamentally altered by the environment".[317] According to this approach, functional behaviors appear as the nervous system matures, with more complex behaviors reflecting the activity of progressively higher levels of the nervous system. This theory, therefore, depends on the assumption of a hierarchic maturation of neural control structures. Taking the core concept of the neural-maturationist viewpoint a bit further, one realizes the viewpoint focuses mainly on the child and the child's nervous system. One might even extend the idea to the genetic background of the individual. Thus the roots of this viewpoint, which started in the early 1900s, stem from a worldview that sought to categorize and classify organisms and to predict in a linear fashion what that

organism would be like in the future. These neuromaturational views from developmentalists were linked to discoveries about the way the nervous system controls movement and resulting correlations between changes in behavior and changes in the nervous system.

At the same time neuromaturational theory was prominent advances in techniques to stain neuronal cells helped to shed light on the structures of the motor control system.

The notion of "structure-function" and the maturational-based theory of motor control are two theoretical products of the neuron doctrine. Using staining techniques, anatomists found that structural features distinguish subpopulations of neurons within and between regions of the nervous system and that morphologic changes occur during development. The array of morphologic findings led to the view that structural organization of the nervous system determines behavioral function (structure-function). Physiologists provided evidence for structure-function control of behavior by isolating portions of the nervous system that produced stereotypic movements such as the stretch reflex, the brisk contraction of a muscle in response to a quick stretch of the muscle stimulating its proprioceptors. Based on his many studies of reflex function in the spinal cord of cats, dogs, and monkeys, Sherrington espoused the view that behavior is hierarchically organized and the simple reflex (composed of a receptor, conductor, and effector organ) is the fundamental unit of neural integration.[284] Furthermore, he proposed that motor behavior is the composite coordination of simple reflexes (e.g., reflex chaining) as excitatory and inhibitory actions are summated at the synapse. Sherrington's notion of reflex chaining so dominated the study of physiology in the first half of the 20th century that physiologists gave little attention to other views of motor control in explanations of behavior.[121]

Structure-function organization and reflex chaining were commonly employed rationales in studies of motor development because of timing linkages between emerging stimulus-evoked behavior and anatomic changes in neural pathways.[174] Thus early studies identified the neuroanatomic changes occurring around

TABLE 3.1 Comparison of Developmental Theories

	Neural-Maturationist	Cognitive: Behavioral	Cognitive: Piagetian	Motor Learning Theory	Dynamical Systems
View on "stages"	Stages of motor development occur as a result of CNS maturation	Stages are merely empirical descriptions of behavior	Stages represent alternating periods of equilibrium and disequilibrium	No specific developmental stages. Stages of motor learning: cognitive, associative, and autonomous	Apparent stages of development are actually states of relative stability arising from the self-organizing, emergent properties of a multitude of systems, each developing at its own continuous rate
Driving forces for development	Development spirals with alternating periods of flexor vs. extensor dominance and symmetry vs. asymmetry based on maturation of the CNS	Development occurs through interaction of the individual with the environment	Development occurs through interaction between cognitive-neural structures and environmental opportunities for action	Trial and error practice leads to the development of motor programs	The individual develops as the organism recognizes the affordances of the environment and selects (self-organizes) the most appropriate available responses to tasks
Building blocks of development	Reflexes	Pavlovian and operant responses to environmental stimuli	First actions using reflexes and later from voluntary actions	General motor programs, recall schemas, and recognition schemas are the building blocks of learning that contribute to development	Multiple cooperating systems with individual rates of development and self-motivated exploration of the environment

CNS, central nervous system.

the time a new behavior emerged without considering whether other variables such as environmental enrichment or experience[314] contributed to the behavioral change. Consequently, scientists proposed that certain predictable changes during neural maturation cause behavioral change,[165,226] establishing the foundation for maturational theories. Concurrent with these developments, theories of hierarchic reflex chaining evolved to include the notion that reflex behaviors are expressions of an animal's phylogenetic origins, leading to the use of the term *phylogenetic* for basic and early motor skills in the first year of life, such as rolling and crawling.[174] Such views merged into the notions that the earliest movements are primitive behaviors controlled by phylogenetically older neural structures and that these movements eventually disappear or are inhibited by later differentiating neural structures that are phylogenetically more recent.[319] These notions suggested that the development of control of movement is primarily a reflection of internal neural development. It appears there was little or no scientific challenge of these neuromaturational views into the latter half of the 20th century, perhaps because students of development took little notice of other directions in neurobiologic research that were emerging at the time.[121]

In addition to Sherrington, maturationists such as Gesell were influenced by Darwin[223] (evolution theory, natural selection) and Coghill[72] (general movements are intrinsically driven to differentiate into specific behaviors). These influences led Gesell to his study of detailed descriptions of behaviors as they naturally occurred and an appreciation of the relationship between behaviors and the maturation of the nervous system.[314] Thus the neural-maturationist model reflects the idea that the child's nervous system drives changes in behavior, diminishing any consideration of the role of the external environment.

Gesell's point of view and research findings resulted in the development of important tests of motor milestones and other adaptive behaviors that have had, and continue to have, a monumental influence on practice in the area of diagnosis of developmental delay or deviance.[80,314] Virtually all subsequent tests of development contained items derived from Gesell's work. Item examples that appear in current developmental tests include observations of head in midline at 4 months in supine, head control during pull-to-sit maneuver at 5 months, and pulling a dangling ring to the mouth at 4 months. Gesell emphatically believed in stages of development as biologic imperatives. He ultimately observed that there are individual differences among children and toward the end of his career came to recognize the role of environmental factors in development, particularly for their influence on cognitive development. In spite of that realization, he never completely resolved the paradox between the role of environment and his insistence on maturation as the predominant force driving development.

Pediatric physical therapy originally developed based primarily on a neural-maturationist theoretic model. As a result, emphasis was placed on the examination of stages of reflex development and motor milestones as reflections of increasingly higher levels of neural maturation.[167] Examination of reflexes and motor milestones actually continues to dominate clinical tools of a neurologic exam.[266] The presence or absence of reflexive responses to specific stimuli contributes to decision making about the necessity for further testing or possible follow-up for intervention because of suspected neurologic problems.[303] Treatment of the child with central nervous system (CNS) dysfunction in early approaches was organized around inhibition of primary reflexes that were believed to persist and produce activity limitations, along with facilitation of righting and equilibrium reactions that were supposedly the underlying coordinative structures for development of skilled voluntary motor behavior. It was generally assumed that functional outcomes would naturally follow. However, the utility of examining reflexes to predict future function has been shown to be limited and the evaluation of spontaneous movement to be more accurate in evaluation and prediction of function.[234]

Early pediatric physical therapy approaches to analyzing and treating movement delays or dysfunction, including the Bobath approach, the Rood approach, and the Ayres approach to sensory integration,[322] arose from the neural-maturationist model. The key to recognizing the influence of these approaches lies in their focus on the movement patterns of the child and resulting classification of movement as "primitive" or "abnormal" versus normal. Abnormal movement patterns are interpreted as springing from the excessive influence of an immature, or lower (more primitive), level of the nervous system. Although our purpose here is not to describe therapeutic approaches, an example may clarify the influence of early maturationist theory on the selection of a therapeutic strategy. Imagine a 9-month-old infant being evaluated because of a delay in developing independence in sitting and reaching for toys. The evaluator notes an asymmetrical posture of the infant, such that head turning to the right occurs concurrently with extension of the right arm (a notable tonic reflex in infants around 2 months old). This may be interpreted as an undue influence of a lower level of the brain stem on the infant's movement, blocking the ability of the child to sit and reach (which are considered "higher" level skills in the nervous system). The intervention may be to try and help the infant, through equipment or positioning, to block or inhibit the asymmetrical posture and maintain more midline postures to provoke or stimulate "higher" levels of movement control. These higher levels of the nervous system would inhibit the asymmetrical posture and thus allow the infant to develop sitting and reaching skills over time. From a neural-maturationist viewpoint, milestones would be addressed sequentially, and thus a skill such as standing or walking would not be addressed until "earlier" skills such as sitting and crawling were apparent. This same example of a young child with movement challenges will be used as we briefly review other theoretical viewpoints to illustrate the influence of theory on therapeutic intervention.

Around the same time as Gesell, Skinner[217] popularized his theories of behaviorism. This theory was in opposition to Gesell's because Skinner posited that the environment, via positive or negative reinforcement, was responsible for behavioral change. The driving force was seen as external to the child, rather than the neurologic change within the child. The behavioral approach represented the viewpoint that "nurture," or the external influences on the child, drove changes in behavior and that development was not preordained by genetics or maturational influences, considered "nature." From the behavioral perspective, a child would repeat a movement or action if that action was positively reinforcing in some way. Likewise, if the action elicited a negative reinforcement, the action would be less apt to be repeated. Thus behavioral shaping occurs over time as the environment positively or negatively reinforces specific actions. The behavioral approach of Skinner lies at the roots of approaches currently used today with children diagnosed on the autism spectrum to effect behavioral change.[88] The behaviorist approach does not clearly fit under the neuromaturationist umbrella and could be viewed as a "learning" approach, which may seem to fit under the cognitive umbrella.

However, behaviorists did not credit the cognitive system or the nervous system specifically, rather specifying that behavior could be shaped without indicating the mechanism behind the shaping process. As such, behaviorism pushed the boundaries of the maturationist camp, while still noting changes in behavior, but with an external driving force that somehow caused a change, but without directly addressing the mechanism creating that change.

Another person who pushed the boundaries of the maturationist viewpoint was Myrtle McGraw, who was generally considered a member of the maturationist school. However, she developed a theory of motor development in the 1930s that contained the rudiments of many of the components of the modern dynamical systems approach to understanding motor skill development because she actually considered the maturation of the child together with the effect of environment and experience.[19,80,226] Thus she moved beyond the maturationist views of Gesell and the behaviorist view of Skinner. McGraw was a psychologist who famously studied the effects of intensive longitudinal intervention, beginning at 20 days of age, with Johnny, the weaker of twin boys named Johnny and Jimmy. Her research was conducted at the height of the nature-nurture controversy between maturationists (represented by Gesell) and behaviorists (represented by Skinner). In summary, her work showed that providing up to 7 hours a day of exercise of newly emerging developmental skills in the first year of life did not increase the rate of motor development. Her anecdotal comments, however, indicated that the exercised twin had better coordination of movement than the twin whose movements and exploration had been restricted to a crib for much of the day, with no interaction with people other than for needed care.

McGraw's work was interpreted at the time as supporting the neural-maturationist theory that the environment had little effect on child development. In the second year of his life, however, McGraw provided Johnny (the exercised twin) with a stimulating and challenging environment and extensive practice opportunities (3 hours per day) for developing motor skills that were not otherwise likely to develop in a child younger than 2 years, such as roller skating, climbing inclines of 70°, and jumping off high pedestals. Under these conditions, Johnny excelled in physical growth, problem solving of difficult motor control situations, and attainment of skills that Jimmy refused even to try during the periodic testing sessions that occurred. McGraw also noted the remarkable persistence in tasks demonstrated by Johnny, as well as his extensive visual review of the situation before embarking on a task. Films of the twins at age 40 years, moreover, demonstrated that the twin who exercised intensively during the first 2 years had an impressive physique and elegantly coordinated movement compared with those of his twin. Experience practicing novel motor skills, as well as problem solving, likely enhanced the physical development of the trained twin, and the enhanced skillfulness lasted into adulthood.

Although the results of an analysis of two individual cases cannot be accepted as leading to fundamental laws of motor development, McGraw's study makes it clear that we have little idea of the possibilities inherent in the very young child who is seldom stimulated to achieve the full potential of early motor skill development. By analogy, we can assume that we have barely scratched the surface in our understanding of how therapeutic intervention might be used to mitigate the effects of conditions causing motor dysfunction.

McGraw also described the uneven nature of development, in which a given behavior pattern has a period of "inception, incubation, consummation, and decline".[226] The results of her longitudinal studies on the intratask course of development of important motor patterns were published in 1945 and remain highly informative today. Because of her daily observations, she often saw a movement pattern appear only once or twice (examples of beginner's luck) and then disappear before becoming a stable part of the infant's repertoire. When first becoming stable, the activity seems overworked and exaggerated. Furthermore, she noted that "as the child begins to get control over a pattern or an aspect of a pattern, the activity itself becomes the incentive for repetition".[226] Thus, early in life, movement for the sake of movement is a functional activity. The daily observations of infant development conducted by Adolph and colleagues,[7] generally considered in the dynamic systems camp, confirmed that multiple daily transitions in performance skills are present before a stable new pattern emerges. For example, an individual infant may experiment with different versions of crawling (belly crawling forward, pivoting on belly, rocking on hands and knees and lunging forward) within a day, even from cycle to cycle.[7]

McGraw suggested that a stable movement pattern might seem to disappear as a part of the child's repertoire, becoming superseded by some rapidly developing new behavior. Eventually the "disappearing" movement will reappear and be utilized in its most economic form. She was among the first to note the presence of normal regressions in motor behavior and has been credited as one of the first developmental psychologists to recognize the bidirectionality of neural and behavioral development.[19,27,237,256] A behavior may also become integrated with other behaviors to form a complex activity; thus McGraw noted that the developmental course of a behavior may look quite different during different stages of its maturation. For example, an infant with the new skill of walking may become more bilateral in arm use temporarily during early practice of the walking skill.[74] On the other hand, an infant who has developed some skill in walking may insist on walking during a cognitively challenging task when crawling would be a more efficient choice.[21] Although McGraw discussed regressions in development as well as consuming use of a new skill as normal, recent research reveals that a complex interplay of cognition, perception, and movement may explain an ongoing reallocation of resources for the child. Changing allocation of the child's resources during skill acquisition likely contributes to the apparent temporary regression or stubborn use of a particular skill.[20]

Because McGraw noted these various characteristics across many developing movement patterns, she believed that fits and starts, spurts and regressions, and overlapping of patterns undergoing emergence, development, and decline were firm developmental principles and that snapshots of development, such as motor milestone tests, could not adequately reflect the underlying processes of development.[19] The current work of Adolph and colleagues[7] confirms this belief. McGraw firmly believed that there were sensitive periods (she actually used the term "critical period" but later regretted it because of its "use it or lose it permanently" interpretation in biology) in which interventions could produce the most influence on developing behavioral patterns.[14] During a sensitive period, certain experiences have particularly influential effects on development, although these effects may be modified with subsequent experience.[43] McGraw believed that the period of greatest susceptibility

to exercise was one in which a behavior pattern was entering its most rapid phase of development. Delay did not mean that intervention could no longer affect the behavior pattern (the concept of critical period) but rather that the interference of other ongoing developmental programs, including changes in anthropometric configuration of the body with growth, can decrease effectiveness. McGraw famously detailed progressions of skill within various milestones, such as prone development, sitting development, and standing/walking, which are still utilized today in describing the sequence of development. However, even though McGraw was insightful about the way that environment can change the course of motor development, these progressions of movement were displayed "in air" as though the support surface or any external context, including gravity, did not exist. Thus the interpretation of her contribution to this day focuses on sequences of movement without the advantage of context that supports and shapes motor skill.

In summary, the neuromaturationist perspective provides us with a detailed description of motor milestones in time, or the description of "what" skills change and "when" they change. This knowledge is useful for determining whether a child is progressing in a typical fashion over time. However, to understand the "how" and "why" of motor skill change and provide appropriate intervention, we must delve into other aspects of development. Cognitive theories, in the next section, begin the story of motor skill interaction with other areas of development, an important step toward providing effective developmental care, and determining why skills progress in typical ways.

Cognitive Theories

Movement is observable behavior, prompting early developmental researchers to focus on developmental motor milestones (Gesell, Shirley, McGraw) and relegating specific behaviors and motor acts to a point in developmental time. Perhaps because these motor skills were so carefully mapped to time, the influence of other factors on motor acquisition was ignored as developmental researchers focused on other, "invisible" skills, such as cognition, perception, social understanding and motivation.[246,348] In this section we review two types of cognitive theory. The first originated specifically in regard to a child's development of basic motor skills, or phylogenetic functions (e.g., rolling, sitting, walking). The second, motor learning theory, was developed to explain the basis of new skilled movements in the older child or adult, called ontogenetic skills (e.g., riding a bike, hitting a baseball, shooting a basket). Both perspectives contribute to an overall contemporary knowledge base and theoretical point of view. In addition, both illustrate the intersection of cognition and movement in functional activity.

Developmental Cognitive Theories

Perhaps the most significant contributor to developmental cognitive theory was Jean Piaget (1896-1980).[246] Piaget observed infants in a context and utilized movement to explore what children were thinking. He pioneered the idea of "stages" of development, linking infant overt behavior to stages of cognitive constructs available to the infant. His focus was on understanding how infants think by watching their interaction with objects in the world. Although movement inherently supports the tasks he documented related to cognitive development, the interrelatedness of movement skill to cognition was not described. Piaget described four stages of cognitive development. The first is the sensorimotor stage (0–2 years), followed by the pre-operational stage (2–7 years), then the concrete operational stage (7–11 years), and finally the formal operations stage (11+ years). Each of these stages has substages describing a continuum of constructs that the child understands. Physical therapists likely have application primarily to the sensorimotor stage because of the "motor" influence, but an understanding of the progression of cognitive change through childhood contributes to investigating the "how" of motor skill acquisition at all ages.

In the sensorimotor stage, reflexive schemes are notable in the first month of life, followed by primary circular reactions from 1–4 months, which are simple movements around the infant's own body. Stage 3, labeled secondary circular reactions (4–8 months), focuses on infants' repeating interesting effects of their own movements. This is the stage of repeated movements, such as banging and shaking. And because the infant is fascinated with his or her own movement effects, he or she may shake or bang everything, whether or not the object was meant for that purpose. From 8–12 months infants switch to intentional, goal-directed behavior and develop the concept of object permanence, or the ability to know that an object still exists even when it is out of sight.

Piaget suggested that the experience of acting on the world (assimilation) with whatever sensorimotor schema is currently dominant was frequently met with resistance because the objects of interest were not easily adapted to the current schema (e.g., gently handling a soft cookie when the motor activity of crumpling or shaking is the current schema).[246] This misfit between the child's current sensorimotor functioning and the response of handled objects leads to disequilibrium, which drives developmental progress through the child's persistence in gradually accommodating to the properties of objects eliciting interest. In so doing the child eventually develops a different approach to handling the cookie and thereby alters the cognitive structure as well. Examples of assimilation can be applied to many motor skills. When infants have a stable hand preference at 2 years of age, they persist in using the preferred hand for tool use, even when that might not be the most efficient approach for the task.[77] Infants who are new crawlers plunge recklessly down slopes too steep to negotiate safely toward their waiting mothers at the landing.[1] As they gain more experience in crawling, failures on risky slopes gradually lead to the accidental use of a different, but successful pattern (one that an infant already knows from previous activities), such as sliding down the slope backward or in sitting. The alternative method then becomes one that the child purposely selects for descending slopes perceived to be risky, in a prospective manner. Transitions such as learning about slopes described above are not well explained by developmental theories that suggest that children immediately perceive the affordances of the environment and act on them,[104,105,247,311] but Piaget recognized this type of function and included it in his principle of assimilation.[109] This principle states that when cognitive structures develop a particular schema, it is applied indiscriminately to objects in the environment, assimilating them to the existing cognitive structure. Piaget also posited that repeated experiences with attempted assimilations of inappropriate objects result in gradual *accommodation* to their properties and the appearance of both new behaviors and new cognitive structures.

Piaget's extensive work in the development of cognitive constructs forms the basis of tests and research paradigms used today. Some examples are searching for a hidden object (object permanence concept) and pulling a cloth to obtain a toy (means-end concept).[16] However, the principles of accommodation and assimilation are not applied on a consistent basis to intervention paradigms. Researchers are now beginning to tease apart and understand the interdependence of cognitive change and motor development, an important interaction for the pediatric therapist to understand.[212]

Application of Theory: Recall the 9-month-old infant who presented with a delay in developing independence in sitting and reaching for toys with an asymmetrical posture. From a cognitive theory perspective this infant's lack of exploration of the world through her sensorimotor system prevents advancing to the next stage of development, assimilation (acting on objects in the world). A therapist might provide a variety of sensory experiences to encourage the child to interact with the environment, which the therapist assumes would lead to the next level of motor engagement with the world, handling objects. Alternatively, the therapist might try to engage the child in motor-based interaction with objects by providing direct, hand-over-hand physical guidance to show the child a strategy for interacting with the world and encourage transitions from the assimilation stage to the accommodation stage.

Another theorist in the cognitive camp provides a linkage to sociocultural aspects of learning. Lev Vygotsky[347] championed the important concept of social scaffolding to developmental learning, heralding the necessity of social interaction as a driving force for child learning.[347] He emphasized how social forces shaped the way children think, based on their interaction with more knowledgeable members of the group. At the core of his theory is the construct of the "zone of proximal development," in which a parent supports the child to accomplish skills at successive and slightly advanced levels.[348] This social scaffolding builds incremental skill both cognitively and motorically, as well as socially and emotionally. Thus in our example of a 9-month-old child with delays in sitting and reaching, the adult caregiver constitutes a critical feature of the scenario. The adult's actions to provide an imitative model, the social cues of encouragement given via facial expression and voice, and the ultimate reward of engaging in a joint play experience all drive a child's behavior to new levels. Of course, these same types of social experiences that drive function pertain to siblings, extended family, schoolmates, friends, and the more distant community as the child ages and encounters more challenging functional tasks.

Motor Learning Cognitive Theory

While motor learning theory is covered in depth in Chapter 4 of this text, "learning" in the case of motor skill change certainly falls within the realm of child development. Typically developing infants take over 9000 steps per day and walk over many different surfaces within their home and community.[4] This massive dose of practice allows infants to learn from their experiences. Although the word "learning" was not used as a key component in many developmental theories, learning is implied even in the neuromaturational approaches of Gesell, Skinner, and McGraw. The word *learning*, defined as "the activity or process of gaining knowledge or skill by studying, practicing, being taught, or experiencing something" (*Merriam Webster Dictionary* online), can be applied to the developmental process in multiple ways, including the gradual acquisition of motor skill. The "learning" definition has been used by some to imply a strictly cognitive process, but the actual mechanism of acquiring and improving a skill may involve processes that are not explicitly cognitive.

For example, early neuroscience researchers such as Thorndike extended the notion of response chaining to address how motor skills are learned, and in the law of effect he proposed that skills emerge as we repeat actions that are rewarded, an idea that might sound familiar when considering the ideas of Skinner, McGraw, and Piaget.[277] Fitts and Posner[108] proposed that the first stage of motor learning was cognitive, followed by an associative phase to link component parts into a coordinated whole, culminating in an autonomous, or automatic, stage that frees cognitive processes such as attention.

The importance of repetition of actions is a component of schema theory, one of the most widely embraced of the motor learning theories. Schema theory proposed that motor skill acquisition is a process of learning rules to evaluate, correct, and update memory traces for a given class of movements.[275] This theory extended the idea of learning a specific movement or task to something more general and abstract, which is a set of rules. It is helpful to envision the type of movement imagined within this theoretical approach as a motor act that is goal driven, such as a child trying to bat a ball or learning to hit a target. These higher-level skills were the frequent examples or tasks used to examine the tenets of schema theory; therefore early infant skills such as learning to roll or crawl were not considered, partly because these early skills had been perceived as emerging or developing, rather than being a specific goal-directed task of the infant. Early developmental skills (rolling, sitting, etc.) are likely to be examples of general motor programs from this perspective, and these skills will later be refined within higher level skills.

Schema theory assumes the presence of three constructs: general motor programs and two types of memory traces, recall schema and recognition schema. General motor programs are loosely defined as sets of instructions that are responsible for organizing the invariant or fundamental components of a movement. Recall schemas are defined as memories of relationships between past movement parameters, past initial conditions, and the *movement outcomes* they produced. Recognition schemas are defined as memories of relationships between past movement parameters, past initial conditions, and the *sensory consequences* they produced. It is theorized that recall schemas function to establish rules regarding the relationship between movement parameters of a general motor program, such as force or velocity, and the movement outcome for a given set of initial conditions that can be used to plan similar movements under anticipated conditions. Recognition schema, in turn, are proposed to compare sensory consequences with movement outcome in light of initial conditions to form a second set of rules. The second set of rules can be used to predict the expected sensory consequences for similar movement outcomes during anticipated initial conditions. The expected sensory consequences are proposed to serve as a perceptual memory trace for evaluating new movements. When movements are generated too quickly (ballistically) to be corrected by feedback during the movement (i.e., open loop), it is theorized that after the movement a feedforward motor command is compared with the expected sensory consequences. Schema theory holds that the initial feedforward command given to initiate the movement links to expected sensory consequences. If these expected sensory consequences do not match actual sensory information at the end of the movement, the next attempt will utilize the error information to correct the movement. In this manner the schema are established and refined as a function of practice.

Application of Theory: Recall the 9-month-old infant who presented with a delay in developing independence in sitting and reaching for toys with an asymmetrical posture. From a motor learning–based motor control perspective this child has not developed the motor pattern for sitting. Therapy would focus on providing ample opportunities for trial-and-error learning in a sitting position with as little support as possible, while encouraging symmetry. Intervention would encourage the child to try to sit and expect some variation in sitting control. The assumption would be that the child who practices sitting and reaching would build on a motor program he or she already has, like head control, and develop a new motor program for sitting through the trial-and-error practice. However, in motor learning theory, the context (including the child's motivation to sit, the room, location of nearby toys or siblings) would not be considered.

Schema theory does not attempt to explain the establishment of general motor programs, nor does it attempt to ascribe them to specific neural structures. The term *motor program* is employed in a variety of ways by researchers from a variety of disciplinary backgrounds, which may help explain why there is no consensus as to what constitutes a motor program.[268,283] In motor learning literature, motor programs are commonly invoked to explain the stereotypic attributes of a complex movement pattern that persists as movement parameters or context is altered.[366] For example, it has been suggested that a general motor program for writing our name exists, and its instructions consist of features common to signing our name under different conditions with different tools, different parameters of movement, even different sets of muscles.[258] Motor learning literature also ascribes to motor programs the ability to generate complex movements without benefit of concurrent feedback, such as reaching for a target after administration of a local anesthetic or tourniquet, as well as ballistic movements that may be completed before feedback can contribute to the movement.[276] Although in each of these instances motor programs are viewed as learned sets of instructions, one can see how this idea appears similar to reflexes because of its focus on a pattern of movement that does not require extensive time for processing and that can be "pulled up" immediately for quick access and ease of managing multiple degrees of freedom and limited resources. However, unlike reflexes, motor programs imply learning or the capacity for modification.

Based on more recent motor learning research, the definition of and the presence of general motor programs have been suggested to be outdated.[283] Rather a "scalable response structure" that is not necessarily invariant has been suggested as the more appropriate construct.[283] The notion is that rather than a "memory state" (motor program), we have a "processing mechanism" (scalable response structure) that serves to provide a basic movement that can be altered according to current conditions. Research involving the observation of infant development of walking when presented with various obstacles such as inclines, cliffs, and bridges has supported this notion, suggesting a process of "learning to learn" or a continual process of online problem solving.[2,3]

Although the idea that motor programs account for higher-level behaviors is being challenged, it may be that some basic networks exist. In neurobiology "motor programs" are called "pattern generators" and are viewed as genetically inherited sets of instructions that control the stereotypic features of innate behaviors such as mating, defense, and locomotion.[200] Some of the strongest arguments in neurobiology for the existence of general motor programs refer to the many examples of an animal's ability to execute functional movements in the absence of feedback.[203,250,304,310] Where the movement instructions are stored is yet to be determined, but some investigators implicate the sensorimotor cortex,[12] primary motor cortex,[163] and cerebellum[202,272] for motor learning and the prefrontal association cortex,[120,281] basal ganglia,[280] and subcortical areas[304] for motor memory and planning. Even the spinal cord is implicated as a location for neural circuitry for locomotion patterns.[229]

As theories are tested, the outcomes reveal their shortcomings, clarify the boundaries of our understanding, and raise a new generation of questions. In contrast to maturationist theories, learning-based theories suggest that development of motor skill is the consequence of learning to solve problems by trial and error, in order to master and sequence units of action that are goal directed. Cognitive theories provide additional information to the "what" and "when" of development and begin to answer "how" and "why" skills develop. In the next section, other systems provide building blocks toward a deeper understanding of how functional motor skills are built.

Dynamic Systems

The dynamic systems approach departed from previous theories in a fundamental way. Each prior theoretical viewpoint, although admitting multiple influences on development, stated strongly the existence of a primary driver of the developmental process. For neural-maturationists the nervous system drove change. For cognitive theorists the mind, either via innate learning processes or the external influence of social scaffolding, drove the developmental process. For motor learning theories, trial and error practice modified predetermined motor programs. But in dynamic systems, no primary driving influence leads the developmental charge. Multiple systems engage to produce skill change, and the primary driver role fluidly transfers between systems to allow the emergence of a new behavior. Thus the musculoskeletal system, the environment, social influences, physiologic needs, or many other systems interact to produce behavior, and any system could take the lead in changing the trajectory of development or shifting to a new level of performance.

Any driving influence or factor in the dynamic systems theory is called a control parameter, and these influences or factors may change over time. For example, the stepping movements of a child may cease if the weight of the legs increases too quickly or if weight increases faster than accompanying strength increases.[316] Later in development, increasing height may drive the ability for a child to be able to ascend stairs in a step-over-step fashion because the child's legs reach a critical point of length-to-step-height ratio. Although strength is a critical component of ascending stairs successfully, strength may not be the control parameter depending on the height of the child or the stairs, and the control parameter role may be the height/length of the lower extremities. From a different point of view the control parameter could be step height, a factor external to the child. This is the critical point of the dynamic systems approach: different systems or parameters dynamically interact to adapt the organism to its environmental context and the task at hand.

Along with the idea of multiple systems affecting change, the idea of nonlinearity in development, as part of the dynamic systems approach, challenged the idea of predictable linear milestones occurring in a nonvarying sequence. Wide age ranges of normality of skill acquisition provide a hint that milestone achievement is nonlinear. By nonlinear, we mean that developing motor skills are not smoothly attained on a predictable timetable. Our motor milestone tables average together data from individuals who show great interindividual variability in skill emergence. Although across cultures and generations there is a general pattern of skill achievement (e.g., rolling before sitting, sitting before walking), that pattern appears macroscopically. With microscopic examination, researchers find that infants come into new behavioral states with varying strategies and time scales. There is both intraindividual and interindividual variability, which may average globally to the developmental sequence that appears on norm-referenced tests but which do not explain how novel behaviors emerge in an individual child. Dynamic systems theory posits that factors available to build a level of skill in one position do not transfer to another posture automatically.[22] For example, a body of research by Karen Adolph and colleagues has demonstrated that infants do not use their experience crawling on slopes to alter their approach to walking on slopes until they have experienced walking on the slopes. Differences in the base of support, the forces and joints necessary for the new action, and perception of affordances of the environment require the child to "relearn" the impact of the slopes (environment) on the task (walking). Massive amounts of variable practice, errors, and problem solving are thought to be involved in the transference of skilled navigation when the body posture changes. An example of infants learning to navigate novel surfaces such as slopes in new postures demonstrates a systems approach to skill development and transference because the environment plays just as strong a role in the change of skill over time as the infant's motor skill. Maturation of the nervous system is not the driving force in this theoretical approach, rather it is equal to all other systems.

Adolph's research supports a dynamic systems selectionist view of what infants learn from experience with everyday problem-solving challenges (see following section for more on selectionist theory). Her research paradigm presented young infants with emerging walking skills varying slopes and gaps to navigate. Each new presentation of a slope to the infant presented a choice: to go with the currently preferred mode of locomotion, to choose an alternative (presumably safer) mode of locomotion, or to avoid the situation, using a detour attempt or simply sitting down and waiting for the caretaker to come to the rescue. Notably, the latter was seldom selected with slopes that were moderately risky; it seemed that infants were goal oriented rather than safety oriented. Their choice was made based on, first, visual information and then if still uncertain, tactile and proprioceptive information. The choice was usually their preferred mode of locomotion (walking) until they had many weeks of experience and had, usually accidentally, discovered an already familiar motor strategy (crawling) to be safer or more successful. As they gained experience crawling or walking, their choice was made more and more quickly; after many weeks of practice, a short glance was enough for making a decision. However, near their ability boundary (slopes that generated less than predictable success in descending without falling), they appeared to have less than adequate knowledge of their own motor capabilities and instead made the decision based on their desire to achieve the goal of returning to their caregiver and a quick judgment of whether or not to go based on visual or haptic information. Failure (e.g., falling) did not predict whether infants would choose to go on a subsequent trial, so they appeared to learn little between trials based on successful or unsuccessful outcomes. Adolph concluded that infants have extensive capability to use sensory inputs to make decisions about choice of motor actions, although they are not always right about their motor capabilities for solving the problem at hand. They choose to act rather than avoid a challenging situation, demonstrating the influence of motivation to achieve the goal. At the edge of their abilities, infants do not engage in trial-and-error learning but rather continue to rely on their visual-haptic analysis of whether or not to engage in risky behavior. When useful motor synergies happened serendipitously, however, they seemed to recognize the adaptability of such patterns and used them on subsequent trials as alternatives to generally preferred modes of locomotion that were riskier to use in a given situation. Goldfield[131] summarized Adolph's findings[1] by indicating that "inexperienced infants tend to be drawn inexorably toward the goal, rather than stopping at a choice point, and apparently do not notice the available affordances. Conversely, the experienced infant who has explored the available affordances may be overly conservative because the affordance information about slopes is inherently inhibitory; that is, it specifies ways for slowing, stopping, and changing direction". Thus, it seems that infants generate information visually, use their preferred mode of locomotion if the choice is to go, and then over time learn, accidentally or through a general wealth of experience with variable-level surfaces, to select from a variety of possible choices the most efficacious method of traversing risky terrain. One must conclude that adaptive locomotion (i.e., selecting the most appropriate method for the task at hand) requires exploratory movements to obtain information and a repertoire of available movement synergies from which to select.[1]

Adolph's research once again emphasizes that advances in motor behavior depend on having a variety of movement patterns from which to choose when faced with challenging new opportunities for action. As a result, children with disabilities, who generally have a limited repertoire of movement strategies, are constrained in their motor development by a lack of experience with variable movement and may also have limited perceptual capabilities for making online judgments about the likelihood of successfully accomplishing a motor task even when they have an intense interest in the goal.

Application of Theory: Using the dynamic systems theory viewpoint, the 9-month-old infant with sitting and reaching delays would be analyzed to determine the control parameter most affecting her strategy for reaching. The physical surround would likely be the first factor to be analyzed, and the distance of the object to be reached may be a determining factor in her strategy. If placing objects closer to her body elicited a strategy that was successful, increased practice while slightly varying the placement of the object would be the first suggestion. The child would be allowed to make mistakes, but it would be assumed that the child would eventually stumble upon strategies that worked for her body parameters. Immediate success would not be expected because building the new strategy may take hundreds of attempts.

Neuronal Group Selection Theory

Neuronal group selection theory, or neural Darwinism, is a popular theory that ranges through many disciplines, including psychology, developmental biology, and physiology.[94]

The theory is useful because it helps explain the relationship of brain to behavior. Put simply, the theory utilizes Edelman's prior work in immunology as a framework for understanding nervous system function, based on the concept that a local event and local feedback can create a complex adaptive system. Because the theory incorporates multiple systems, adaptation, and dynamic changes over developmental time, we include it under the general heading of dynamic systems theory.

Edelman argues that popular models describing the brain as analogous to a computer with hardware (neurons) and software (motor programs) bear only superficial resemblance to the actual operation of the brain. He postulates that the nervous system is more akin to the immune system because the immune system must create weapons to attack infectious agents that have not been encountered previously. Thus, like the immune system, the nervous system must continuously solve novel problems. Edelman's theory, called the *neuronal group selection theory*, has three basic tenets. These tenets describe how the anatomy of the brain is produced during development, how experience selects for strengthening certain patterns of responses from the anatomic structures, and how the resulting maps of the brain give rise to uniquely individual behavioral functions through a process called reentry. Sporns and Edelman further described how such a system solves the problem of managing movement in an organism with multiple degrees of freedom.[298]

In Edelman's theory, neuronal groups from various maps throughout the region and the nervous system as a whole combine to produce a particular behavior. The behavior is unique to the individual in whom it occurs because of variations in neuronal maps caused by the effects of individual experience on their development. The combination of neuronal groups used from multiple maps allows the production of a movement that is precisely tuned to the environmental demands for functional performance yet unique to the individual's capacity for processing sensory inputs and his or her individual regional neuronal maps. This neuronal group selectionist system with distributed functions requires a repertoire of variable actions in order to provide adaptability: that is, a variety of means for responding to environmental demands and internal changes such as growth must be available.

Neuronal group selection theory does not hold that preexisting programs are executed by the nervous system; rather, dynamic loops are created that continually match movements and postures to task-related sensory signals of multiple kinds. Functioning is based on statistical probabilities of signals, not coded signals or preformed programs. Edelman further theorized that the system has biologic "values" that are species-specific and drive the selective strengthening of synaptic activities based on experience.[94] These values influence adaptive processes by linkage between the global mappings and activity in pleasure centers and the limbic system of the brain in a way that fulfills homeostatic needs of the organism. For example, in a computer model of Neural Group Selection Theory (NGST), Oztop and colleagues[238] included a variable labeled by the authors "joy of grasping," which modeled the sensory feedback received by the infant from achieving a successful stable grasp and that, in turn, strengthened the future selection of grasping strategies. In a computer model of a visual system with a set "value" that prefers light to no-light conditions in the center of a "visual" field (similar to that produced in humans by evolution), initially nondirected movements of an "arm" were shaped to target an object.[94] If one appreciates that newborn infants possess a primary repertoire that includes moving the hand to the mouth, seeking light, and producing head turns or arm projections in response to moving objects in the visual field, it is not difficult to understand the theory of neuronal group selection as an explanation for the gradual process of learning to reach successfully. In fact, newborn infants will move their hand into a light beam,[327] and early reaching is more likely to be made to a moving object,[345] indicating potential innate value system for neonates. The research of Oztop and colleagues produced the first successful computational model of the process of learning to grasp.[238]

Neuronal map creation through an individual's use of movement to drive brain plasticity can go awry. Byl and colleagues, for example, reported that monkeys trained and reinforced for performing a stereotyped movement thousands of times, using the simultaneous activation of muscles and tactile-kinesthetic receptors, developed degraded primary sensory cortex maps.[48] Neurons in the cortical area related to hand function become responsive to stimulation almost anywhere on the hand (even the back of the hand), a condition Byl and colleagues describe as a dedifferentiation of the normally exquisitely organized response patterns of the sensory cortex. They believe that this animal model may reflect the process of repetitive strain injury with focal dystonia in humans and that the findings support use of a sensorimotor retraining approach to treating this disorder in order to redifferentiate sensory maps in the cerebral cortex. If we think of the constrained and repetitive movements used by infants with CNS dysfunction, it is not hard to conceive of the possibility that they also have a poorly differentiated sensory cortex. The key to understanding and treating this type of problem is recognition that maps are formed connecting various areas of the brain based on the simultaneous activity of sensory and motor systems. We learn (and train the brain to select) what we do. Stereotyped activity leads to poorly differentiated brain maps, whereas learning to use a variety of flexible patterns to accomplish common tasks leads to rich, complex brain organization compatible with adaptability to environmental demands and the internal changes accompanying growth. Thus neuronal group selection theory provides a template for understanding "how" motor skills build over time, as well as how they may be unbuilt or degraded.

Embodied Mind Concept

Another concept that fits within dynamic systems theory and NGST is the concept of the embodied mind. Because the brain is plastic and responds to experience and information gained through movement, the viewpoint that the mind is built via the physical activities of the body within the environment is defined as embodiment. Evidence from infant studies suggests that the mind is embodied, meaning that a strong linkage exists between what we know and what our bodies can do.[50,290] In essence, the interplay between acting on the environment and gathering information about how the world works creates the intellect. Additional research across the life span confirms that movement builds the brain and increases brain volume.[346] The embodied mind concept involves both action and perception, both of which are required to build the brain. Researchers are also investigating the use of models of motor control based on developments in the fields of robotics and neural networks. Both approaches seek to incorporate perception and action to explain control of movement. Robotic models are based on the physics of perception and movement, assigning mathematical values

to known neural and biomechanical relationships to explain movement outcome. For example, as a child begins to explore movement of the arms, he will encounter objects and pick up information about these objects, such as texture, firmness, and shape. The child may grasp the object and wave it around, gaining knowledge about its weight and the forces of the arm required to bring the object into view. In this way, the child's body builds the brain to handle and understand, incrementally, more about the body and the object. Imagine if the child could not reach and handle the object: this rich experience diminishes drastically. Currently, in the area of autonomous robotics there is interest in simulating principles of dynamic systems using a new method called computational neuroethology. The method attempts to account not only for the neural and biomechanical elements of a robot but also for environmental context and any new phenomena that may emerge during action within that environment.[69,220,363] Neural network models are based on the assumption that no simplistic, predictable relationship exists among nerve cells to explain movement, but rather it is the phenomenon of their complex interactions that creates the movement outcome. Thus neural networks focus primarily on specifying the array of cellular and network properties that may govern how a population of neurons will self-assemble under a given set of conditions. Robotics actually utilizes concepts from infant learning and the embodied mind framework to advance artificial intelligence in robots and computing.[290]

Within the dynamic systems theory and embodied mind models, motor control functions are not assumed at successively higher hierarchic levels, leaving behind previously used primitive behaviors and control centers; rather, many levels of the nervous system cooperate in the production of movement behaviors. Typically, no single active site for any particular behavior can be identified; behavior is, rather, an emergent property of the cooperation of various subsystems, with task characteristics organizing the response.[318,24] That is, the characteristics of the task lead the nervous system with its distributed functions to select from a variety of currently available options for assembling a task-related action.

Application of Theory: For our 9-month-old child, NGST adds background justification for allowing the child to find her own unique solution to functional problems. This can be interpreted in multiple ways, and in fact, NGST is used by groups with opposing intervention strategies as justification for an intervention approach. On the one hand, those who utilize NDT have adopted NGST as a theory supporting intervention that discourages "abnormal" movement patterns and encourages "normal" movement patterns in various ways. This justification basically supports the same therapeutic activities seen in the neuromaturational hierarchical approach example. Opposing this viewpoint, NGST can also be used to support an intervention strategy that allows discovery of movements that are unique to the individual, even though the movement may look abnormal. This second interpretation is more in line with the NGST basic theory. Using this second interpretation, the therapist would allow the asymmetrical movement but add supports and environmental cues that continue the basic value-driven behavior while eliciting incrementally variable deviations from that singular strategy to build adaptation and long-range connections between the movement, sensory information, and the accomplishment of the task with the child's own solution (and not a preconceived notion of a normal movement pattern).

Perception Action Theory

Perception-action theory, expressed and researched by Gibson[131] and others, focuses on the relationship between self-generated movement and the child's understanding of properties of the environment in a cyclical pattern that builds skills. No action can be performed without resulting perception, and nothing can be perceived without action. Thus movement plays a central role in what we know and can perceive. Taking an early example, an infant sees a cube in front of him; however, this cube will be a two-dimensional square until it either is touched, to feel the sides and back of the object, or the infant must change the orientation of his body or move the cube to see all sides of the cube. Anyone who has watched an infant grasping a new object delights in the way the baby turns, gazes at, mouths, and touches the object with fasciation in exploiting the details of the object's characteristics. As each action allows a new perception, further exploration is elicited to expand that perception. In fact, Soska and colleagues showed that infants do not understand the spatial properties of an object (such as recognizing a toy from the back versus the front) until they can call upon action to move and handle the object.[292] Thus perception is strongly linked to action, a linkage that should be exploited within physical therapy intervention to advance both motor capacity and the understanding of linkages between movements and perception of how the world works. From a perception-action perspective the focus is on building the perception of affordances, allowing discovery of new actions that inform and build perception of new options.

Application of Theory: In our example of the sitting child with asymmetrical posture with poor reaching ability, the therapist would take some time to explore and understand the strategy the child is using. If the child can reach using an asymmetrical tonic neck reflex (ATNR), the therapist would start there, with a toy that might be mobile, like a small ball with noise and textures to explore. The therapist would encourage small, incremental changes (child initiated) in hand, arm, or head posture, allowing the building of the many actions and postural changes needed to perceive "roundness," the affordance of the chosen surface and gravity to assist or resist movement.

Ecological Theory

Ecological theory is closely related to perception-action theory but takes a broader view by examining behaviors across species and within multiple levels of the environment. Some ideas that evolved from this theory relate specifically to our understanding of prospective control: in other words, how we plan movements based on our understanding of spatial configurations in our world and the medium in which we move.

Ecological theory includes Bronfennbrenner's ideas of the roles of different levels of environmental influence on a child.[42] The theory attempts to explain progressive and mutual accommodations made between an active, growing human and the changing properties of his or her immediate and distant surroundings. This theory also relates to ecological perception and Gibson's[130] ideas of perception being built (as opposed to being innate) as the child experiences the environment. But more importantly, ecological theory presents the idea of an affordance, something in our environment that affords action or a certain type of action or movement. Because we evolved within our environment, ecological theory posits that function stems from the relationship between our body and the properties of things in the world.

Application of Theory: Why is this important to the pediatric physical therapist? Take our earlier example of a 9-month-old infant with an asymmetrical posture and difficulty sitting and reaching. Unlike the hierarchical approach, which would seek to reduce the effect of a "primitive" or lower-level reflex, the ecological approach would examine the affordances available to the child and the current relationship of the child to those affordances. Let's say the child is positioned in a high chair with a flat back, flat tray, and seat belt. The hard back affords pushing against, and flat tray affords leaning on a straight arm, which then supports stability of the child's head and gaze to one side. The ecologic approach, instead of building supports to hold/force the child to midline, might put an inclined, contoured surface in front of the child to afford or invite the child forward and reduce the back of the chair to afford less leaning (or pushing) back. The forward surface also provides a stable base, with gravity assisting, for the child to lean on both arms and learn about the stability that the new orientation lends to the head and gaze. In this way the child discovers and perceives new affordances of a different body configuration.

Theory Summary

In summary, theories of motor learning, motor control, and motor development attempt to explain complex and changing motor behavior and, as theories go, are also not static notions. Theory terminology, which stems from different fields of study, is often obtuse and difficult to understand without intense study. There is no one unifying theory of motor control related to motor development, and there are some overlapping tenets among the broad theoretical positions presented. This likely is influenced by the fact that we may control our movement in a different manner dependent on the type of movement we need. For instance, movements that repeat periodically (e.g., walking) may emerge and evolve differently from skills acquired by following a set of external rules that are learned (e.g., playing a piano) and may not develop from an evolutionary base.[191] Theories, however, guide research and should guide our problem solving when assessing and determining interventions for children with motor dysfunction.

Although no one theory unifies the field of pediatric physical therapy, a blend of dynamic systems, neuronal group selection, perception-action, motor learning, and ecological theories dominate new intervention approaches. This blended theoretical approach supports the use of infant-initiated and infant-directed movements, high dosage and early active experiences, and respect for all the systems that contribute to the acquisition of new skills.

Application of Theory: Take our example of the 9-month-old who has motor asymmetries and is learning to sit. From a blended approach of the various dynamic-based theories, the therapist might present the child with a toy of interest, while using changes in the seat surface (or an adult's lap) and the position of the toy to encourage the child to shift her weight just beyond her current comfort level, increasing the weight borne on one arm while reaching with the other hand. In addition to providing opportunities for new perceptual information and new motor skills, the experience, if repeated in a variable way through infant-directed play, could change the neuronal map used to accomplish this task over time. This would support the infant's development of multiple movement strategies for changing task demands. In the next section, we present a framework that has evolved from the previous perspectives to help therapists build a competent and evidence-based approach to intervention.

CURRENT FRAMEWORK FOR DEVELOPMENTAL INTERVENTION

The most recent approach to theory, under the dynamic systems umbrella, appears compatible with updated research findings in general. Consistent with the dynamic systems approach, therapists should consider the role of both intrinsic and extrinsic factors in the development of each child. Each child presents with different factors influencing his or her particular course of development. Although there is extensive variation in the "typical" course of development, physical therapists play a role in evaluating the influence of intrinsic and extrinsic factors in the development of any child they assess, taking into account not only the what and when of developmental change but also guiding us to answer the how and why questions about skill acquisition.

Although use of dynamical systems theory to drive therapeutic theory and practice in physical therapy is still in its infancy with no large efficacy studies reported to date (Blauw-Hospers et al., 2007; Morgan et al., 2015), it is already clear that this model focuses the attention of the therapist on a number of important aspects of the therapeutic process of facilitating functional activity and participation.[32,227] These aspects include (1) search for the constraints in subsystems that limit motor behavior, such as contractures or weakness, leading to treatment goals related to reduction of impairments; (2) creation of an environment that supports or compensates for weaker (rate-limiting) components of the systems that contribute to development of motor control with a goal of promoting activity and participation; (3) attention to setting up a therapeutic environment that affords opportunities to practice tasks in a meaningful and functional context, especially in the child's home and community, with a high value placed on parent and family interaction for goal setting, activity construction, and social encouragement, as well as a high dosage of practice; (4) use of activities that promote exploration of a variety of movement patterns that might be appropriate for a task; (5) search for control parameters, such as speed of movement or force production, that can be manipulated by intervention to facilitate the attainment of therapeutic goals, especially during sensitive periods of development during which behavior is less stable[104,105,157]; and (6) extensive practice (high dose) to drive developmental learning (Spittle et al., 2015).[297] Thus parents and caregivers must be encouraged and coached in how to provide the multiple and varied repetitions of infant-directed practice needed to advance motor skills. Here we will present some examples of the factors influencing child development. The impact of each factor will vary between children and within one child at various times, which will contribute to the course of development, as do all components within this systems approach.

Factors External to the Nervous System

In the current view of developmental processes, factors external to the nervous system contribute significantly to the emergence of a behavior. These factors may be rate limiting or rate enhancing, depending on other factors within the system of the child and depending on the developmental time being considered.

Anthropometrics, Body Mass, and Nutrition

The emergence of locomotion during development is determined by the interaction of anatomy and the environment during movement. The weight of the child or the child's body parts may be one of those external factors that can affect functional movement. One famous example of the intersection of weight and movement involves infant stepping. Typically, infant stepping is not readily elicited beyond the first to second postnatal month under standard testing conditions, and it was long argued that the behavior disappears as a consequence of encephalization processes (the taking over of control) by maturing higher motor centers.[226] However, the postnatal decreases in rate of stepping temporally correlate with rapid weight gain, suggesting that morphologic changes in body mass may contribute to the "disappearance" of infant stepping. Two lines of evidence support this hypothesis. One, when infants are submerged in water up to chest level, both stepping rate and amplitude increase in comparison with stepping out of water.[315] Two, if weights equivalent to the weight gains at 5 and 6 postnatal weeks are added to the ankles of infants at 4 postnatal weeks, both stepping rate and amplitude decrease in comparison with stepping without ankle weights.[315] Thus buoyancy appears to diminish the damping effect of body mass and gravitational interactions, whereas added weight appears to augment the effect of these interactions. Additionally, weight gain in an infant may not only affect a behavior such as stepping but generally affect the progression of motor development. Infants who are overweight have greater likelihood of delayed motor development,[289] and children classified as overweight are more likely than their normal-weight peers to have motor and mental developmental delays.[57] On the other hand, infants who are premature benefit by additional subcutaneous fat gain; subcutaneous fat addition in premature infants at 3 and 6 months correlated with greater advances in motor skill as infants matured.[186] Thus weight is a factor that interacts with motor skill development at both ends of the spectrum. Related to weight gain, nutrition can be an important factor, with critical nutrients playing a part in overall development. For example, infants with iron deficiency have negatively affected motor skill attainment.[282] Iodide and iron deficiency in early life are linked to impaired brain development affecting both cognitive and motor skills, which may not be reversible.[252]

Musculoskeletal System Factors

In children younger than 4 years of age, some biomechanics can constrain the possible movement options. Most notably, in the first postnatal year, the center of mass is proportionately higher than at any other age because of the combination of a large head and short limbs, requiring large force generation and regulation by neck and upper trunk musculature to counter the inertial forces created by displacements of the head. Likewise, the skeletal alignment of the lower extremity changes significantly between 2 and 10 years of age in typically developing children.[30] Infant growth displays irregularities, and is not a continuous process; there are spurts of growth followed by periods of no growth.[201] These spurts of growth may confound the infant's use of emerging motor skills, either adding to or decreasing difficulties in coordination. Infants who start to pull to stand and walk must generate adequate strength to lift and hold their body up against gravity, which gradually changes the alignment of the hip. It is the interaction between the experience of the child and the developing musculoskeletal system that results in the change in skeletal alignment.

Cultural Differences/Influences on Motor Skill Development

Milestone charts used in all clinics in the United States spring primarily from a European cultural background and grew from the original work by Gesell and McGraw (see theory section). These timetables reflect development of children from a limited scope of cultures. Handling practices for infants and young children vary widely between cultures, and these parenting practices provide for varying amounts of practice of specific motor skills.[166] Some cultures, including some parts of Africa and the Caribbean, do specific exercises with young infants that include practice with sitting and upright postural tasks, as well as stepping and walking. One example is the difference in sitting independently; infants in Cameroon routinely sit well at 5 months such that their parents leave them unattended on elevated surfaces.[187,188] No parent in the United States would assume, at 5 months of age, or even 7 months, that their child would be safe perched alone on an elevated surface. Therefore our milestone guidelines from standardized tests that put independent sitting at 7 months must be understood in the context of our own predominant cultural experience, which stems from the US and Western European culture.[34]

The "Back to Sleep" program, instituted in 1994, was initiated to reduce the numbers of sudden infant death syndrome (SIDS) and is now known as the Safe to Sleep program.[271] The program encouraged parents to position their infants in supine for sleeping, which reduced the incidence of SIDS by 50%. However, infant delays in developmental milestones were suspected as these parenting practices changed.[216] This example shows that a national effort to change one aspect of sleep positioning for infants can affect motor development. Overall, motor skills appear to have changed little due to the supine sleep program.[82] However, deformational plagiocephaly has increased significantly, as well as appearing earlier, related to the supine sleep program.[40]

Some cultures use restrictive positioning in infancy such as swaddling. One such practice is the Ghavora, used in Tajikistan. Infants are bound tightly in the supine position, and as they get older, they have more hours per day out of the restriction. These infants have delayed motor skills compared to our Western norms, with sitting independently occurring at about 1 year of age and walking at about 2 years.[187] Overall, cultural practices may change the trajectory of infant achievement of motor milestones, but these practices do not appear to have long-term consequences. Maternal expectations, related to culture, may affect infant development as well.[195] Pediatric therapists should note these differences in parenting practices and handling and consider culture in assessment and intervention for young children in varying cultures.

Task Demands

Task requirements, which are external to the child, can also be considered to be distinct motor control variables. Task requirements may include any variable that can contribute to or in some way alter movement, including biomechanical requirements, meaningfulness, predictability, or any other variable associated with a given movement context. Physiologic recordings from several sensorimotor centers of the brain indicate that the participation of brain areas in a task is context specific.[78,129,52] Task requirements shape motor strategies. For example, when a person slips, his or her response selection (step/reach/fall) is likely to be contingent on the task he or she was trying to accomplish, (carrying a tray/stepping onto an escalator/playing

in a pool).[44,171] Task requirements can also result in the gating of reflexes; for example, a noxious stimulus applied to the foot may produce a flexor withdrawal response if the leg is in the swing phase of gait, but an extensor "contact" response if the leg is in the stance phase.[270] Evidence suggests that the meaningfulness of the task may enhance or mask performance.[332] The role of meaningfulness is demonstrated by comparing performance when a child is asked to complete a relatively abstract task (e.g., to repetitively pronate and supinate as far as possible) versus a concrete task (e.g., to strike a tambourine, a task requiring repetitive pronation and supination). Children with cerebral palsy (CP) generate larger movement excursions following the concrete instructions than after the abstract instructions.[332] In summary, task requirements, like all other variables we have considered, appear to play a crucial role in the control of movement. There may be multiple possible behavioral outcomes for a given set of centrally generated movement instructions depending on external factors.

For therapists using learning- or dynamic-based theories, thoughtful analyses of task requirements can generate both a deeper understanding of the minimal requirements for completing a task and an array of hypotheses as to why a client cannot complete the task. Analysis can also assist in determining how to modify and reduce task requirements so that a child can successfully complete the modified version of the task.

Internal Child Factors (Related to the Nervous System)

Children have their own personalities and goals from the time of birth. First displayed with the demand for food, caregiving, and sleep, infants express their goals. Some infants are demanding while others are calm with fewer demands. Infants are driven to move and control their bodies, often in an attempt to reach a destination, hold a pacifier in their mouth, roll over to get a toy, or sit up so they can see the world with a different vantage point. The infant's internal drive to achieve movement-related goals can influence development. In this section we discuss subsystems within the child pertaining to neuromuscular control affecting functional movement. These factors can be classified as motor control components, or strategies of control by the nervous system to coordinate the many degrees of freedom of the body, acting in the environment, toward functional movement.

Cognitive and Behavioral Factors

Cognitive factors may include variables that are dependent on conscious and subconscious processes such as reasoning, memory, or judgment to optimize performance. Such variables might include arousal, motivation, anticipatory or feedforward strategies, and the selective use of feedback, practice, and memory. Variations in arousal can probably modify any other control variable, such as pattern generation,[316] or even whether a behavior is demonstrated.[35] Motivation may make multiple contributions to the control of movement and thus development. In some instances motivation may serve primarily to trigger activity, and in other instances motivation may determine the form of the consequent movement.[136] For example, it has been suggested that hand path is straighter during reaches for a moving target than for a stationary one because the infant or child is more motivated to reach and make contact with a moving target.[340] Cognitive-related variables likely emerge with and assist in skill mastery; toddlers as young as 13 to 14 months of age having only a few weeks of standing experience can selectively determine when to use manual assistance for maintaining postural control while standing on an array of support surfaces[301] or when challenged with various obstacles.[2] Cognitive processes associated with action are also important for acquiring spatial maps (memories) of the movement environment,[225] are apparent in the earliest anticipatory behaviors during infancy (such as the anticipatory head and eye turning during games of peekaboo), and may be delayed or differently configured in children with Down syndrome.[11]

Cognitive processes for predicting the postural requirements and selecting timely anticipatory strategies, also called feedforward strategies, are a select form of anticipatory behavior characterized by movement adjustments time locked to voluntary movements.[222] Typically, as we become expert in a movement task, we learn to recognize those sensory cues most reliable for predicting how the environment may change during movement execution, and we learn to ignore less useful cues. Simultaneously, we learn to predict how our movements will change our relationship with respect to a more or less predictable environment and therefore determine the postural requirements for the task. In the control of posture, anticipatory strategies work to minimize equilibrium disturbance and may also assist in completing the desired movement. In other acts, anticipatory strategies minimize the amount of attention dedicated to monitoring feedback and making corrections after initial movement execution. In the adult, for example, when asked to rise onto tiptoes (from a plantigrade to digitigrade posture), ankle dorsiflexor muscles are activated nearly 200 ms before ankle plantar flexors, apparently to shift the center of pressure (COP) at the foot-floor interface a sufficient amount forward before onset of postural elevation.[170] Although anticipatory strategies are not usually conscious cognitive processes, they involve subconscious forecasting processes[222] that are essential for minimizing movement errors during perceptuomotor tasks[334] and sometimes require considerable training such as the anticipatory postural adjustments (APAs) observed in dancers.[228] Indeed, it is argued that anticipatory strategies are learned, that they are relatively fixed under stable conditions, and that they are adapted in less fixed situations only by learning from past movement experiences.[222] Anticipatory strategies are observed in postural adjustments before the onset of whole body movements,[231] postural adjustments prior to onset of arm movements,[170] shaping and orientation of the hand before contact with an object to be grasped,[178] and strategies to time body movements with timing demands of the environment.[334] Anticipatory strategies during preparation to grasp can also be observed as early as 9 months of age[113,334] and appear to be present by 4 postnatal months, as evidenced by postural adjustments in neck and trunk musculature when infants are about to be pulled to sit or picked up from supine[16] and adjustments in gaze as they anticipate an object's trajectory (van der Meer et al., 1994).[328] These anticipatory strategies are built over time through experience and active engagement with the environment.

The amount of attention dedicated to monitoring a movement is also viewed as a variable that can be modified to perfect a motor skill. It has been suggested that during development, children initially execute new movements in a ballistic manner, ignoring feedback, then swing to the opposite extreme attempting to process excessive amounts of feedback, before finally learning to selectively attend to feedback. An example of this transition proposed by Hay[154] is described in the

Reaching section later in this chapter and shown in the videos of the development of reaching on Expert Consult. It is generally thought that once the child (or adult) learns to selectively attend to feedback, more attention (or mental processing) can be assigned to reading the environment and predicting the environmental changes and movement outcome as the movement is executed.[192] Other cognitive variables related to learning, such as form and quantity of practice and the role of memory, are addressed within the context of motor learning in Chapter 4.

Sensory Factors

Infants are born with functional visual, vestibular, auditory, and somatosensory apparatus. However, the use of sensory information likely required practice and is context specific. Thus an infant's ability to look at and track a toy may depend on where she is positioned, how much support she has, and her previous practice with this skill. From a dynamic systems perspective, the sensory system has an equal role in development as all other developing systems. From a motor control perspective, sensory systems have an impact on our ability to control our posture and react to task demands. In this section we will briefly review the role of important sensory systems in typical development.

Vision. The relationship between eye movement and vision is present prior to birth with spontaneous fetal eye movements linked to networks in the frontal and visual cerebrum.[279] At birth vision begins to affect development in multiple systems including: socialization, object interaction, cognition, motivation, and postural control. Infants have the ability to track an object or face and orient to sound within the first hours of life. The opportunity to visualize a face and begin to interact with a caregiver builds early social skills. Infants who are shown toys, even before the onset of reaching, will change their movements in the presence of the toy.[28] Vision can drive complex movement, as when an infant sees a toy just out of reach and transitions to another position to obtain the toy. In relation to movement, vision has been primarily studied for the role it plays in posture.

Vision is perhaps the most powerful sensory system functioning to regulate posture, both for feedback correction and for selection of anticipatory postural strategies.[47,153,207,305] The first to ascribe a proprioceptive function to vision, Gibson[130] suggested that as light from the visual field strikes the retina, changes in light associated with movement create "optical flow patterns" interpreted by the brain to determine the position of the head and body with respect to the surrounding environment. It is argued that the large-amplitude postural sway observed in blind individuals is due to the absence of this optical flow information,[206] although adult individuals blind from birth show little difference in postural adjustments when compared to sighted individuals.[230] This may be due to the dynamic ability of the postural system to adapt during the developmental process. Optical flow patterns can evoke dramatic postural responses in both children and adults. Children begin to demonstrate distinct postural responses to optical flow patterns very early in development, even prior to walking.[47,207,305] Then, they go through several visual dependence periods as they first develop sitting and standing control. Table 3.2 outlines this developmental process. It appears that if children lack visual information during development, they may not minimize their postural sway to the same degree as sighted children.[251,253] Prechtl and colleagues suggested that the visual system exerts a

Components	Age	Skills/Behaviors
Vision	4 to 6 days to 2 months	Activation of neck muscles following visual stimuli from looming visual stimulation in supported sitting[362]
	5 to 13 months	Scaling of postural responses to visual stimulation from moving room[26]
	5 months	Postural response to looming visual stimulation in stance[117]
	13 to 17 months and < 7 months walking experience	Apt to fall in looming moving room[47]
	2 to 10 years	Decreased falls and reaction to eyes closed conditions in moving room, moveable platform, SOT[111,305,358]
Somatosensory		
	> 6 months	Can control head and sitting balance using somatosensory input[207,287]
	4 to 6 years	Beginning ability to use somatosensory input for sensory conflict in standing during SOT[287]
	4 to 10 years	Ability to reweight within visual and somatosensory stimuli of various amplitudes by 4 years old; ability to reweight between visual and somatosensory input by 10 years[287]
	7 to 10 years	Adultlike ability to use somatosensory input to balance during sensory conflicts during SOT[118,287]
Vestibular		
	7 to 10 years	Adultlike ability to use vestibular input to balance during sensory conflict during SOT[67,359]
	12 to 16 years	Adultlike ability to balance during sensory conflict SOT[295,300]

SOT, Sensory Organization Test.

calibrating effect on the proprioceptive and vestibular systems that, when missing in children who are blind from birth, may contribute to early differences in postural control.[253]

In standing and walking the role of vision for posture and control in infants and children is significant. Infants who have recently learned to walk demonstrate an increased gastrocnemius response when perturbed without vision compared to with vision. However, same-aged infants who cannot take independent steps do not demonstrate any change in muscle response without vision.[305] In a now classic set of studies, Lee and Lishman demonstrated that when an adult stands inside a closed space formed by three walls and a ceiling, a forward or backward movement of the wall facing the person (center wall, Fig. 3.2) will trigger a larger sway amplitude (S) than under static visual conditions: a so-called "moving room" paradigm.[208] The effect is greater if the postural task is made more difficult (e.g., standing on one leg) and if the visual stimulus moves along the anterior-posterior (AP) axis of vision (referred to as a looming visual stimulus [A]), and it is least effective if it moves tangential (side to side [B]) to the visual axis. In general, if the subject faces the center wall as it is slowly moved toward the subject, the subject will sway backward; if the wall is moved away from the subject, the subject will lean forward. If the entire enclosure is moved sideways from the subject's left to right (or vice versa), however, little or no change in posture is detected. Clinically, and in research, the Sensory Organization Test (SOT) first suggested by Nashner and colleagues is used to assess the subject's response to visual, vestibular, and proprioceptive feedback, and the visual portion utilizes a "moving room" or "visual surround" to provoke postural responses (Fig. 3.3).[111]

Vision is linked to stability also in terms of perception of stability. In young walkers the actual distance between floor contact and the center of mass is small and results in much higher frequencies of postural sway with relatively larger arcs of motion than at later ages.[260,323] Consequently, younger children sway faster and closer to their limits of stability than older children and adults. Although younger children can produce

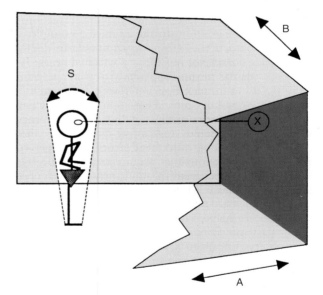

FIG. 3.2 The subject is placed in the center of a partial room formed by three walls and a ceiling that can be slid along in direction A or B. When the subject is facing wall X, room motion in direction A creates a looming visual stimulus and triggers an increase in the magnitude of sway (S) in the anterior-posterior plane. Younger children are likely to sway closer to their limits of stability *(dashed lines)* when presented with a looming visual stimulus but not when the visual stimulus moves side to side (direction B). (Adapted from Lee DN, Aronson E: Visual proprioceptive control of standing in human infants. *Percept Psychophys* 15:529-532, 1974.)

adultlike muscle synergies for postural correction at latencies similar to adult values, given the aforementioned biomechanical constraints, adultlike responses may be too slow for regaining upright posture. Infants learning challenging postures exhibit frequent falls, both in sitting[152] and in standing,[8] which does not appear to deter attempts to continue upright

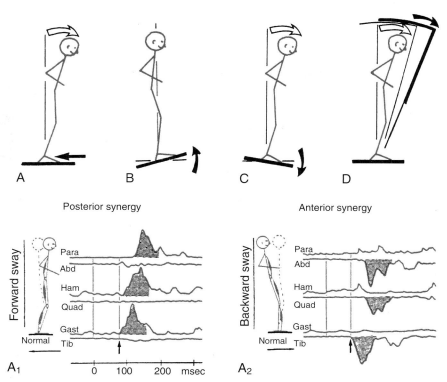

FIG. 3.3 When a child is placed standing on a movable platform that is then displaced in the posterior direction at a fixed rate and duration (computer driven), the child sways forward and the posterior synergy is activated in a distal to proximal sequence over time to realign the head and trunk over the base of support (A_1). Conversely, displacement of the platform in the anterior direction produces a posterior sway that is corrected by activation of the anterior muscle synergy, also in a distal to proximal sequence (A_2). In both conditions illustrated, normal visual, vestibular, and somatosensory inputs are available. If the platform is rapidly rotated to produce ankle dorsiflexion (B) or plantarflexion (not shown), visual and vestibular inputs remain relatively stable throughout the perturbation, whereas somatosensory receptors register displacement. If, however, the platform is rapidly rotated in the same direction and synchronous with normal sway (C), somatosensory input remains relatively stable because the ankle angle changes little during the perturbation, whereas vestibular and visual receptors register the postural sway. Visual information regarding sway can be altered during testing by closing the eyes or by placing a dome around the head to provide a stable visual field (D). If vision is stabilized during platform translations, as in (A), visual inputs will be in conflict with normal vestibular and somatosensory information. If vision is stabilized during platform rotations, as in (B), both visual and vestibular inputs will be in conflict with somatosensory information. Finally, if vision is stabilized during platform rotations synchronized to normal sway (C), visual and somatosensory inputs will be in conflict with normal vestibular information. (Adapted from Nashner LM, Shumway-Cook A, Marin O: Stance posture control in select groups of children with cerebral palsy: deficits in sensory organization and muscular coordination. *Exp Brain Res* 49:393-409, 1983; and Horak FB, Nashner LM: Central programming of postural movements: adaptation to altered support-surface configurations. *J Neurophysiol* 55:1369-1381, 1986.)

activity. Falling from a self-achieved and gaze-directed attempt may assist in calibrating postural adjustments and mapping the child's own parameters for dynamic stability. Thus vision may assist in learning appropriate postural control for the individual child's system.

Vestibular and somatosensory system variables. The vestibular system is activated and drives postural activity to regulate head control and to reference gravitational forces to prevent slow drift of the trunk during complicated postural control tasks early in the first year of life.[58,169,172] The somatosensory system primarily triggers postural activity related to body positioning and righting. When both head and body movement occur, as is common in many functional movements, the two sensory systems appropriately influence the motor outcome based on the various head/body configurations. The location of somatosensory input (i.e., the weight-supporting structure and the use or not of hands to support or balance the body) also greatly influences the postural muscle activity in reaction to or in anticipation of perturbations.[179,257] Further details on the role of the vestibular and somatosensory systems in postural control appear in the following section on motor control of posture.

VARIABLES OF MOTOR CONTROL THAT INFLUENCE DEVELOPMENT

Characteristic of contemporary motor control research is the notion that multiple variables contribute to the initiation and execution of a movement. Thus, it is generally assumed that to understand how movements are controlled, one must be able to identify which variables are important and determine how they interact during movement. Knowledge of this information could be very important for focusing assessment and intervention for children with motor dysfunction. However, one of the challenges of motor control research is that in order to investigate the role of one variable, the others must be held constant, which is not representative of the natural developmental process. Thus when considering the role of motor control in development, the evidence must be interpreted within our contemporary developmental theory of dynamic systems.

We now turn to theory that relates to the older child who has developed basic movements and skills. This section identifies some current hypothesis in motor control followed by motor control variables and research that relate to skill development. Although we describe each variable separately, we encourage the reader to reflect on the role of each variable and the interaction between variables that influence development. For additional motor control theory and background, we encourage the reader to review Shumway-Cook and Woollacott (2011).[286]

Current Hypotheses of Motor Control

While related to development, much of the motor control literature is driven by the implications for adult and older child rehabilitation rather than the generation of new skills during the course of typical development. In addition, many motor control theories exist without a unifying theory. Rather, each theory's hypotheses of motor control attempt to identify controlling variables for specific types of movement. Briefly, we will discuss a few of the most prominent motor control theories that relate to pediatric rehabilitation and development.

A common view of motor control is that movement synergies are the nervous system's solution to controlling the multiple degrees of freedom inherent in coordinating a multisegmented body.[25] Research has supported this hypothesis because relatively few synergies have been identified in frogs' unrestrained kicking[79] and in human movements such as squats, walking, and going up and down a step.[302] Although synergies, such as flexor and extensor synergies, have long been viewed as the stereotypic motoneuron patterns inherent in spinal neural circuitry, current views suggest that movement synergies can be context specific and highly individualistic[193] and can change during the acquisition of coordination.[53]

Current hypotheses of motor control attempt to identify controlling variables for specific types of movement. Central pattern generators (CPGs) are proposed to account for the basic neural organization and function required to execute coordinated, rhythmic movements, such as locomotion, chewing, grooming (e.g., scratching), and respiration, and have been specifically identified in animal models.[221] CPGs are commonly defined as interneuronal networks located in either the spinal cord or brain stem that can order the selection and sequencing of motoneurons independent of descending or peripheral afferent neural input. Under normal conditions, however, neural input from select supraspinal regions, such as the brain stem reticular nuclei, activate CPGs, and peripheral afferents, propriospinal regions, and other supraspinal regions modulate the output of CPGs and adapt the behavior to the movement context. Work in invertebrate species suggests that CPGs can even alter their own configurations (i.e., intrinsic modulation) to produce more than one pattern associated with the same or different behaviors.[190] CPGs can also modulate the inputs they receive, gating potentially disruptive reflex actions such as nociceptive activation of the flexor withdrawal reflex when a limb is fully loaded during the stance phase of locomotion (further review of pattern generators is available in Guertin and Steuer, 2009).[139] A growing body of literature examining the continuum of stepping behaviors in fetuses, premature infants, term infants, and young infants is beginning to make a strong case for the view that human locomotion is also governed by CPGs.[36] Promising research in humans to substantiate the presence of CPGs for locomotion has centered around locomotor recovery studies in adults with spinal cord lesions and hemiplegia.[89,215] Research on infants and children with CP,[81,353] Down syndrome,[321,360] and spinal cord injury[18] who train on treadmills with partial body weight support has also shown positive improvements in these individuals' ability to ambulate faster and without assistive devices, to start walking at a younger age, and to demonstrate some facility in upright ambulation, respectively. Newer studies are documenting changes in cortical activity via functional magnetic resonance imaging[84,245] and changes in short-latency reflexes in the peripheral nervous system.[162] However, evidence of the success of intervention capitalizing on the potential modification of the CPG, such as treadmill training for children with CP, has yet to be produced.

To better understand current concepts of motor control as applied to children, we examine the functions of postural control, reaching, and locomotion.

Postural Control

Postural control is achieved via the cooperative interaction of sensory (e.g., visual, vestibular, and somatosensory systems), musculoskeletal, and motor control systems so as to meet the behavioral goals of postural orientation and stability.[168,170] Although each of the three sensory systems is considered essential to optimal control of both static and dynamic posture, each system can compensate to some extent for the other two, and the relative importance of each system appears to vary with contextual or task demands.[170,288]

The vestibular and somatosensory systems contribute to the generation of directionally appropriate responses in the trunk and legs following anterior posterior displacements in infants and toddlers in sitting[148,159] and in stance.[308] Commonly used testing methods and leg responses are illustrated in Fig. 3.3. It is likely that vestibular and somatosensory systems participate in these postural responses during infancy because directionally appropriate muscle responses are generated even when infants are blindfolded.[358] Variable responses also may be attributed to the availability of vision, for when vision is occluded infants produce more reliable vestibular and somatosensory-evoked neck responses following AP displacements in sitting than when vision is available.[358] These early responses to perturbation are considered by some to be innate building blocks for orientation to vertical and postural skill. However, it is not clear how these early responses to perturbation are related to active, self-initiated movement. Complete developmental information related to use of these systems for postural control is outlined in Table 3.2.

Achievement of postural control is often described in terms that emphasize the closed-loop or sensory feedback aspects of balance correction or reactive postural adjustments (RPAs). Adaptive postural control, however, also employs open loop or anticipatory postural adjustments (APAs). These anticipatory strategies function to minimize potential postural perturbations arising with movement initiation and to assist in achieving the desired movement.

As young infants are exposed to gravity in the extrauterine environment, they must learn to control their bodies and respond to specific task demands. Several common postural control strategies can be observed over the first years of life that many people describe as postural reaction or reflexes. Righting reactions occur when the infant or child moves his or her head to keep his or her eyes on the horizon. Although this reaction has a common goal across tasks, the movements are not stereotypic. When an infant moves from prone to sitting, the infant demonstrates orienting the head to horizontal as the torso moves through a multitude of positions, which we refer to as head righting. The control of the head position is vital to gaze stability and orientation to the environment. However, it is not reflexive because the response is not stereotyped, can be easily interrupted with volitional movement, and may vary from trial to trial or from one child to another. An equilibrium reaction can be observed when the center of mass shifts outside the base of support. In a classic equilibrium reaction the torso elongates on the weight-bearing side and laterally flexes on the non–weight-bearing side. The upper and lower extremity often abduct on the non–weight-bearing side as well. Although this may be the classic description, in daily function equilibrium reactions rarely display the classic pattern because they are not stereotypic movements or typical response-stimulus reflexes. As such the development of the visual, vestibular, and proprioceptive systems, as well as the task or context of the activity, will adapt the degree of equilibrium reaction observed. Equilibrium reactions can be elicited as either a response to an external stimulus such as losing balance on a slippery surface (RPA) or in preparation for a movement such as going into single-limb stance (APA). If a child is unable to maintain his or her balance in response to an external stimulus, a protective reaction results in which the child steps, places a hand down, or grabs for a support. This type of RPA is present in children once they have experience in a position and can determine where their limits of stability are. Righting, equilibrium, and protective reactions can be observed in infants, children, and adults and are often related to the amount of experience the person has controlling his or her center of mass within a given base of support and the speed of movement. For example, a child may be able to stand well while playing with a toy on a flat surface without need for equilibrium or protective reactions. Yet when asked to complete the same task on a dynamic surface, equilibrium reactions are likely to be observed while the child is maintaining his or her balance and protective reactions when the child weight shifts too quickly and cannot maintain his or her balance.

Some mention should be made regarding the failure of researchers to find distinct sequences of development in postural motor responses to RPA.[244] This probably reflects the fact that complex neuromuscular responses are available early in development, and a child's ability to select the most favorable strategy is still developing.[93] In addition, the task requirements and the immediate context in question are critical determinants of any postural response. Infants demonstrate slow and variable reactive muscle responses in sitting, which speed up and become more consistent during development.[143,156,309] The developmental course of RPA in standing is variable, with periods of increasing latency in some children between 4 and 6 years of age and adultlike reactions by 7 to 10 years of age.[287] It has been suggested that the greater variability observed in children 4 to 6 years of age in standing may reflect a period of transition as vision becomes less important and somatosensory information becomes more important in the control of posture.[287,286] During this transition, children may be trying to process excessive amounts of information rather than selectively attending to the most pertinent sensory information, as has been suggested for other types of motor skill acquisition.[154] Children may also attempt to process excessive amounts of information as a strategy for coping with limited ability to anticipate change in the environment.[192] Yet another possible explanation for the variations in children's muscle response patterns may be found in variations in behavioral variables such as restlessness, fatigue, apprehension, and novelty during laboratory testing.[148,161] Finally, several studies have noted that reactive postural responses are task dependent, supporting the idea of a second phase of development.[64,156] See Table 3.3 for detailed developmental information.

Anticipatory activity can be observed in infants when reaching from various lying and sitting positions.[325] Recent research on anticipatory postural control during infancy suggests the importance of exploring variability during the development of optimal postural control.[92] Both too little variability and too much variability may be detrimental to flexible and adaptive control.[149] Sitting development in five infants was examined from the time the infants could prop in sitting using arms on the support surface until they could sit freely using their arms to play.[150] Analyses indicated that, as sitting balance improved, the infant first moved from instability to a period of constraint of the degrees of freedom (i.e., more stability using very consistent unchanging motor coordination patterns). Then the infants moved to a period of releasing the degrees of freedom or using more variable motor coordination patterns, indicating a complex chain of control development. A similar pattern of early postural variability followed by constraint of postural sway was observed during the development of reaching and midline head control in supine as well.[93] Harbourne and Stergiou hypothesized that the increased variability in selection of motor coordination patterns reflects specific individual solutions to solve specific individual problems.[150]

Chen and colleagues examined nine infants' development of standing balance longitudinally from age 6 months until they had been walking for 9 months, while standing with and without support on a forceplate.[65] They found rate-related changes in the children's postural sway. Sway developed toward a lower frequency and a slower, less variable velocity, but the infants did not show overall less amplitude of sway as they developed. This was hypothesized to be due to the child not just controlling sway to remain upright but also using sway to explore the limits of stability and learn about postural control. During the time the infants were tested, they also experienced both growth and development of sensorimotor control mechanisms.[65]

Overall, developmental studies suggest that there is a progression and refinement or modulation of APAs that improves with experience in movement. See Table 3.3 for details on development of the APA. The overlap in refinements of feedback (perturbation-triggered corrections) and feedforward postural

TABLE 3.3 Typical Development of Postural Control: Motor System

Components	Age	Skills/Behaviors
Reactive Postural Adjustments (RPAs)		
Sitting		
	3 to 5 months	Single postural muscle groups activated or antagonist activated rather than an identifiable RPA sequence[141]
	5 to 6 months	Activation of directionally specific motor coordination patterns (agonists opposite to the side the child is falling) Slow and variable timing (cocontractions and reversals of proximal to distal patterns) Poor adaptation to task-specific conditions[41,161]
	7 to 10 months	Decreased timing variability of directionally specific motor coordination patterns (activations of leg, trunk, neck muscles)[141]
	9 months to 3 years	Invariant use of directionally specific motor coordination patterns, some use of co-contractions Good modulation of pelvic muscles at base of support for adaptations to task-specific conditions[141,144] (Hadders-Algra et al., 1998)
	3 years	Variability in directionally specific motor coordination patterns Less co-contraction and use of neck muscles to improve variability of postural control[144] (Hadders-Algra et al., 1998)
Standing		
	7 to 8 months	Infants who pull-to-stand show beginnings of ankle strategies[141,309]
	10 to 12 months	Adultlike RPA with grossly directionally specific (distal to proximal) motor coordination patterns[309] (Hedberg et al., 2007;
	12 to 16 months	More consistent directionally specific motor coordination patterns although onset latencies longer[141]
	3 months walking experience	Compensatory stepping balance responses emerge[267]
	4 to 6 years	Increased variability of motor coordination patterns occurs (perhaps resulting from growth spurts or sensory integration changes)[111] (Shumway-Cook and Woollacott, 2007)
	7 to 10 years	Adultlike use of directionally specific motor coordination patterns (Shumway-Cook and Woollacott, 2007)
Anticipatory Postural Adjustments (APAs)		
Movement in Sitting		
	6 to 8 months	APA in trunk muscles before lifting the arm in sitting[325] (van der Fits et al., 1998) Can adapt to different sitting positions and velocities of reaching movement
	12 to 15 months	Consistent APA, particularly in neck muscles (van der Fits et al., 1998)
	2 to 11 years	APA variable and incomplete by age 11 years when compared to adults[326]
Movement in Standing		
	10 to 17 months	APA activity in gastrocnemius muscles (to counteract the reach and pull movements with arms) in 10- to 13-month-old infants More consistent and temporally specific APAs in 16- to 17-month-olds[356]
	3 to 5 years	APA response variable, with immature as well as adultlike activity[278] Anterior shifts in COP are present before raising an arm while standing, but these are less well coordinated[155] (Raich and Hays, 1990)
	4 to 6 years	APAs recorded in the following tasks: lever pull[115] Voluntary drop weight; raise arm[155,159,160] APA may shift from a supporting function to movement to a compensatory function of postural stability
	6 to 8 years	More continuous, systematic, and harmonious APA during a reaching movement APAs show greater variability of muscle coordination patterns than in 9- to 12-year-olds[351]
	9 to 10 years	Some children exhibit insufficient APA before movement into digitigrade stance[140] APA shown only when postural control disturbances reached "perilous" limits[155] APA less variable during stand and reach[351] Modulation of APA in weighted and unweighted wrist reach task
	12 years	APA with forward leg raising similar to adults and both affected by segmental acceleration (slow vs. fast movement) and sensory context (eyes open vs. closed)[239]
Movement During Gait Initiation		
	1 to 17 months walking experience	Inexperienced walkers use gait initiation APAs involving lateral rather than posterior COP shifts and use both the upper and lower body to make the shifts[13]
	1 to 2.5 years	Variable APA in reaction to a perturbation (holding the limb back) during gait initiation (Woollacott and Assaiante, 2002) APA (posterior COP shift) present, but not coordinated with the velocity of the step forward[205]
	4 to 6 years	Adultlike APA patterns of anterior tibialis activity and posterior COP shifts during gait initiation[218] APA (decrease in latency and increase in amplitude of muscles for push-off) in reaction to a perturbation (holding the limb back) during gait initiation (Woollacott and Assaiante, 2002) With 4 to 5 years walking experience, postural control motor coordination patterns move distally with ability to control gravitational forces with leg muscles during gait (Breniere and Bril, 1998)
	6 to 8 years	APA (posterior COP shift) present and coordinated with the velocity of the step forward[205]

COP, center of pressure.

TABLE 3.4 Age-Related Reaching Development

Age	Skills/Behavior
Newborn period	Arm movements appear to be purposeful (van der Meer et al., 1995) and spatiotemporally structured (von Hofsten and Rönnqvist, 1993) Reaching is visually triggered but not guided (von Hofsten, 1982) Hand is typically open during forward extension of the arm
7 weeks	Rate of reaching briefly decreases Infants seem more interested in looking at the object Hand posture is more likely to be fisted (von Hofsten, 1984)
12 weeks	Frequency of reaching increases Hand prepared for reaching (von Hofsten, 1984; Bhat and Galloway, 2006) Infants acquire ability to visually determine realistic reaching distances (Field, 1977)
12 to 18 weeks	Acquire skill in aiming reaches (von Hofsten and Rönnqvist, 1993) Infants can contact a moving object in as much as 90% of trials Between 15 and 18 weeks, contact shifts from just touching to catching the moving object (von Hofsten, 1979)
19 weeks	Reaches include more movement units that are seen in adults Reaching path is not straight (von Hofsten, 1991)
31 weeks	First movement unit is longer and functions as the transport unit similar to adults Reaching path is straighter (von Hofsten, 1991)
5 to 9 months	Variability in reaching path and movement units while reaching for a stationary object (Fetters and Todd, 1987)

control in children between 1 and 10 years of age suggests that they are two distinct processes that emerge in parallel during development.

Reaching

Reaching is one of the first motor skills infants perform and provides an early window into their motor control and their interactions with the world. (See the video on Expert Consult on the development of reaching from 2 weeks to 6 months.) Table 3.4 is provided to summarize the development of reaching. A growing body of work suggests that arm movements of the neonate, like kicking movements, are rudimentary expressions of skilled reaching that emerge during the first postnatal year. Supported in a semireclined posture, newborns demonstrate rudimentary eye-hand coordination in response to a moving target.[344,329] When infants from 1 to 19 weeks of age are presented with a slowly moving object, they display interest in the object. Prereaching or flapping of the arms during the first months of life is visually guided and often resembles early functional reaching. As infants become more interested in looking at objects, visual attention may inadvertently extinguish neonatal reaching efforts for a brief period of about 1–4 weeks.[23,342] Vision functions to elicit reaching but does not guide the trajectory or help orient the hand during early reaching.[204,213,355] In fact, infants do not appear to require vision of their hands for initiating reaching or contact and grasp of an object.[71] These findings seem to suggest that younger infants initiate reaching using a ballistic strategy to aim the hand toward the target and then switch to a feedback strategy (vision, proprioception, or both) to make corrective movements for grasping once the object is contacted.[71] At 4 to 5 months of age, reaches are as good with vision as when vision is removed after onset of the reach,[71,355] and infants begin to adjust their gaze, anticipating the future trajectory of an object.[328]

During the period from 12 to 36 postnatal weeks, several major changes occur in the form of reaching that suggest the development of a new control strategy.[340] Adult reaches are characterized by 1 to 2 movement units, meaning that there are one or two periods of acceleration and deceleration in a mature reach. The first unit functions to transport the hand 70% to 80% of the distance to the target and is relatively long in duration, and the second unit functions to home in on the object and is relatively short in duration.[178] Between 19 and 31 postnatal weeks, infants progressively restructure reaches for a moving object reducing the number of movement units from an average of 4 movement units per reach to 2 movement units.[340] The sequencing of movement units is also modified. In the younger infant when there are more than 2 movement units per reach, the transport unit can occur as one of the middle movement units rather than the first. In 19-week-old infants, the transport unit is the first movement unit in only half of the reaches, extending an average distance of 80 cm, whereas at 31 weeks, it is the first unit in 84% of reaches and extends 137 cm. Finally, the hand path trajectory straightens with age suggesting that, by 31 weeks, improved spatial planning contributes to advances in aiming skill as the hand is now transported closer to the target in a more efficient manner during the first movement unit, requiring fewer subsequent units to correct for errors.[340] Note the differences in trajectory and movement units between a 9-month-old infant and an adult during reaching in Fig. 3.4.

Experience in reaching is frequently found to be related to an infant's age. But in a series of studies investigating changes in arm movements with and without a toy present, it was found that infants alter the joint kinematics of their spontaneous arm movements in the presence of a toy months before the onset of reaching.[28] Clear stages of prereaching movements can be identified in the coordinated movement patterns of these healthy infants based on their reaching experience, not just their age. Carvalho found that infants with less ability in reaching demonstrated fewer reaching attempts resulting in less practice reaching compared with more skilled reachers of the same age.[55] Thus age alone is not a good indicator of reaching ability; experience must be considered as well.

Another factor influencing the improvements in typical infants' reaching is postural control.[84] As postural control improves in supine between 12 and 24 weeks of age, a decreased number of reaching movement units, a decreased length of the displacement path of the hand, and an increase in the length and duration of the first movement unit have been shown to be correlated.[102] Research on the APAs in preparation for reaching has demonstrated the presence of organized muscle activation patterns before infants are able to successfully reach and during the onset of reaching.[85,325] Muscle activation patterns were less variable by 6 months of age, and infants with a "top-down" or cephalic-caudal temporally ordered recruitment pattern demonstrated a larger percentage of successful reaches than those using a less organized pattern of muscle activation.[85] Although age, reaching experience, posture, and developmental

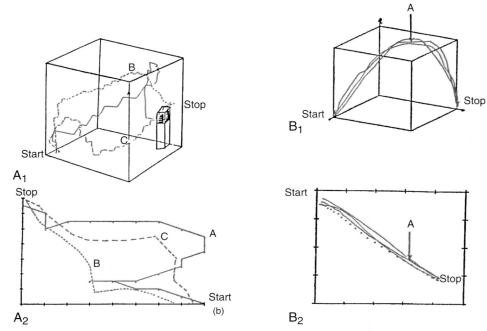

FIG. 3.4 When reaching for a stationary object, infants exhibit reaches containing multiple movement units similar in duration. Three reaches are shown for a 9-month-old infant from a side view (A₁) and an overhead view (A₂). Note the irregularities both within and between reaches as compared with adult performance from the side view (B₁) and overhead view (B₂). (Adapted from Fetters L, Todd J: Quantitative assessment of infant reaching movements. *J Mot Behav* 19:147-166, 1987. Reprinted with permission of the Helen Dwight Reid Educational Foundation. Published by Heldref Publications, 1319 Eighteenth St., NW, Washington, DC 20036-1802. Copyright © 1987.)

delay influence reaching abilities, task demands or extrinsic factors of the task may result in changes in reaching strategies as well.

During the period from 5 to 9 months, infants begin to use visual information at the end of the reach as the hand approaches the target to correct for errors in hand path trajectory.[336] Before 5 months of age, they take little notice of the hand during flight, but thereafter, if vision of the hand is blocked, as when infants reach for a virtual (mirror image) object, performance is frequently disrupted.[204] Although infants continue to use a ballistic reaching strategy well into childhood, withdrawal of visual feedback begins to impair reaching skill at 6 to 7 months of age.[204,355]

During the first postnatal year, interlimb coordination of the arms and hands during reaching is characteristically variable. In a longitudinal case study of one infant from 3 to 52 weeks of age, instances of bimanual reaching appeared to correlate with more variable kinetics, greater limb stiffness, and greater reaching velocities in the following arm as compared with the leading arm. These findings led the investigators to conclude that bimanual reaching predominates until infants learn to differentially control the following arm at approximately 6 to 7 months of age.[76] The degree of coupling between arms during reaching also appears to depend on the complexity of bimanual cooperation required (task demands): that is, whether one hand can remain relatively passive or must produce complementary movement patterns such as when holding a box lid up with one hand while extracting a toy with the other.[100] Complementary bilateral reaching skill emerges at 9 to 10 months of age.[101]

A recent study comparing adults with Down syndrome to typical adults and children found that the individuals with Down syndrome were able to demonstrate stable bimanual coordination during a circle-drawing task that appeared adult-like.[262] In contrast, their unimanual ability was less coordinated and similar to the children examined in the study. This suggests that the individuals with Down syndrome have more mature bilateral reach and fine motor skill and less mature unilateral ability. This may be due to improved postural control via using both sides of the body during the bimanual activity, but this is yet to be examined experimentally.

The influence of object properties on grasping has been well documented (see the next section), but the properties of objects also influence infants' reaching strategies.[75] Infants between 6 and 9 months of age frequently have a preferred reaching strategy, but they may be able to alter that movement strategy based on the task demands. In a study comparing the reaching and grasping strategies of 6- to 9-month-old infants for small balls, large balls, and large pompoms, Corbetta and Snapp-Childs described the infants' ability to use sensorimotor information to alter their preferred reaching strategy.[75] Older infants were better at altering their reaching strategy between unimanual and bimanual based on the task demands than were the younger infants. In addition, handling the object provided more cues to the infant than vision alone, leading to more appropriate changes in reaching strategy.[75]

Reaching in infants is routinely studied in a semireclined seated posture, but several groups have compared the development of reaching among infants in supine, upright, and semireclined postures. An early comparison of reaching in supine and upright sitting at 12 to 19 weeks of age and 20 to 27 weeks of age found that position had little impact on reaching abilities or quality between 20 to 27 weeks of age. Infants in the younger age group, however, demonstrated fewer reaches and grasps, and they had poorer quality of movement in supine.[273] Consistent in the research literature is the finding that younger, less experienced reachers are more influenced by changes in body position that those who have more experience and are older.[54,55,273] Carvalho and colleagues suggested that the similarity of reaching performance of the more experienced reacher in either body position is an indication of the adaptability of the system to new constraints, which is not observed in the less adaptable, less experienced infant.[55]

Locomotive Control

Stepping movements and walking have been studied extensively in both human infants and in developing animals. Animal studies add to our understanding of the control systems for walking as infants develop a more adultlike pattern of movement.

The presence of stepping movements in the human fetus, early onset of infant stepping in premature infants, and rhythmic leg movements of infant kicking provide argument for development of basic stepping circuitry for locomotion in humans during embryogenesis as in other animals.[36] The presence of some potential for locomotion at birth raises the question of whether that potential is established early in fetal development. Here again a parallel may be drawn with animal studies. Ultrasound studies of human fetal movement indicate that isolated kicks are initiated during the 9th embryonic week, and alternating leg movements, reported to resemble neonatal stepping, are initiated with postural changes ("backward somersaults") in utero during the 14th embryonic week.[87] Thus human fetuses appear to exhibit stepping during the first half of the gestational period, about the same portion of the embryonic period when chicks exhibit organized electromyography (EMG) and kinematic features during spontaneous motility.[37,62] Given that low-risk preterm infants born at 34 weeks of gestational age demonstrate orderly kinematic patterns similar to those of full-term newborns and that those features differing from full-term infants appear to be attributable to dynamic interactions emerging during movement,[122,158,180,181,344] the parallel between human fetuses and chick embryos appears reasonable (Fig. 3.5). In other words, the neural foundations for locomotion in humans may be assembled during neurogenesis, as they appear to be in other animals.[37,46]

Several parallels can also be drawn between studies of neonatal animals and rhythmic, locomotor-like leg movements in human infants. When supported on the treadmill, infants perform repetitive leg movements characterized by several kinematic features similar to adult locomotor behavior.[315,320,361] Although infants 6 to 12 months of age become more reliable in producing a sustained pattern of alternating steps that are timed to the treadmill belt speed, even infants as young as 10 days of age occasionally demonstrate these features.[361] Neonatal infant stepping shares many features with early treadmill stepping. Most notably, hip, knee, and ankle joints are synchronously flexed during the swing phase and synchronously extended during the extensor phase; the excursions are accompanied by nonspecific EMG patterns; and there is an absence of both heel strike and push-off at the transitions between swing and stance.[110] These features are also characteristic of infant kicking within the first 1 to 3 postnatal months, further suggesting that

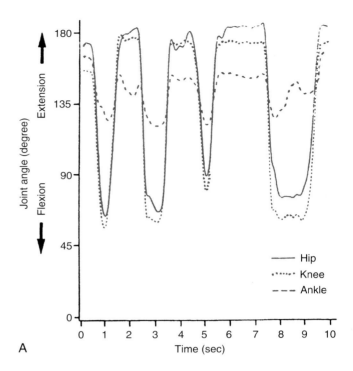

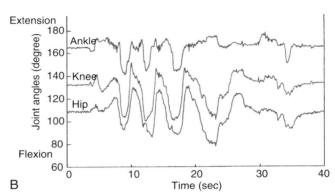

FIG. 3.5 Kinematic analyses indicate that lower extremity movements are organized very early in development. When preterm infants initiate a sequence of several kicks at 40 weeks of gestational age, the alternation of flexion and extension at the hip is synchronous with motions of the knee and ankle in the same direction (A) and is similar to kicking movements during spontaneous motility in chick embryos in ovo at 9 embryonic days of age (B). (Adapted from Heriza, CB. Comparison of leg movements in preterm infants at term with healthy full-term infants. *Phys Ther* 68:1687-1693, 1988.)

some of the mechanisms controlling treadmill stepping, and therefore locomotion, are already functional at birth.[182,183]

Until recently, it was believed that infant locomotion lacked adultlike features typically observed in EMG recordings. Failure to observe adultlike EMG patterns was often attributed to late myelinization of descending paths at caudal spinal levels,[307] late maturation of cortical structures,[110] or late myelination of peripheral nerves.[306] In a study of treadmill locomotion, however, infants as young as 10 days of age occasionally produced steps characterized by alternating activation of antagonist muscles, and the extent of coactivation decreased with practice.[361] The relative duration of flexor and extensor burst durations also varied with treadmill speed in a manner similar to that in adults. Furthermore, it has been demonstrated that prewalking infants, age 4 to 12 months, can respond with adultlike interlimb coordinated responses when given unilateral leg perturbations while supported to walk on a treadmill.[240,241] The failure to observe adultlike EMG patterns for locomotion in previous studies of prewalkers and early walkers may have been the result of adaptive strategies that masked this potential. For example, infants may have coactivated antagonist muscles to increase joint stiffness and stabilize limb posture as a compensation for insufficient postural control or control of force generation for supporting and transporting body mass.[38,236] Also, testing conditions may have masked the potential to generate adultlike locomotor EMG patterns: that is, support in stance or movement against gravity in supine likely altered the task requirements,[320] necessitating a different EMG pattern. Conversely, the testing conditions may have lacked key features for expressing locomotor EMG patterns. For instance, in cats the velocity of limb movements contributes to the generation of certain EMG patterns.[364]

Although there is wide support for the view that basic features of locomotion are spinally mediated,[46,173] some argue that uniquely human features of gait emerge as spinal neural networks are transformed with maturation of higher neural centers.[110] Specifically, it is argued that the basic patterns of alternating flexion and extension observed during neonatal stepping persist with development of locomotion but that maturing sensorimotor input suppresses activation of ankle extensor motoneurons to permit heel contact at the onset of stance. Also, the absence of heel strike in children with CP is thought to occur because cerebral injury impairs development of higher-center control over spinal neural networks for locomotion.[110] As further support for this view, Luo and colleagues studied infants who were born prematurely, compared to a similar group born at full term, in their ability to walk while supported on a treadmill.[214] The factors that contributed across the whole group to earlier attainment of independent walking were a higher percentage of alternating stepping pattern, a decreased association in hip/knee coupling, and an increased association in hip/ankle coupling during swing phase as well as increased interlimb symmetry during stance. A small number of preterm infants were classified as "late walkers," and authors hypothesize that the presence of periventricular leukomalacia—i.e., a neural control deficit and/or chronic lung disease (either linked to muscle weakness and/or to a neural deficit related to poor oxygenation of the brain)—affected the infant's coordination and delayed the development of locomotion.

Conversely, many researchers now speculate that attributes of gait, such as heel strike, need not be specifically dictated by higher neural centers because they may emerge from the inertial interactions and associated feedback among body segments during different types of movement exploration from many practice sessions.[31,63,68,145,164,176,199] For example, when cats walk at relatively fast speeds, the sartorius muscle produces a two-burst pattern, one during late stance and one during late swing, but the second burst does not consistently occur at slower walking speeds. Kinematic and kinetic analyses suggest that the burst in late swing functions to counteract extensor forces at the knee during faster walking speeds, but it is not required and therefore not recruited at slower speeds because viscoelastic properties of knee flexors are sufficient to counter these forces. In adult humans, examination of muscle actions during the walk-to-run transition demonstrates lower swing-related ankle,

knee, and hip flexor muscle activation and higher stance-related activation of the ankle and knee extensors during running than walking.[255] It is suggested that the exaggerated sense of effort in lower extremity flexors during swing of a fast walk may trigger the locomotor pattern to change from the walk to run pattern.

Whether the muscle activity associated with heel strike or other attributes of gait is due to centrally organized neural commands or is an emergent property of movement exploration and motion-dependent feedback has recently received more focused study related to the development of walking in infants. A study of treadmill training in a premature infant who sustained a left grade III/IV intraventricular hemorrhage demonstrated that the infant changed the right and left initial foot contact from a toe touch to either a flat foot or heel strike after 4 months of practice.[33] This improved motor pattern continued for a time after the treadmill training ended, then it reverted to the previous pattern. This finding might suggest that the absolute velocities or rate of change in velocity typically achieved during early over-ground locomotion is insufficient to force the infant to express adultlike ankle control in the step cycle. However, when given the higher velocities of the treadmill to stimulate the walking pattern, the appropriate heel strike pattern emerges even though the infant had early brain damage. From study of early walking development in infants, researchers have demonstrated that the infant's walking pattern related to EMG control,[63] net joint moment control,[146] and coupling of AP and medial-lateral oscillations seems to emerge in a nonlinear manner, requiring cycles of perception and action to self-organize and stabilize.[198]

Heel strike may not be observed until independent walking is established because of immature morphologic characteristics of the infant foot interacting with a support surface. Given the considerable structural change the foot undergoes during the first postnatal year or more, it is conceivable that initial biomechanical features of the foot do not readily afford initiation of heel strike or push-off in the young infant. Recent study would also suggest that strength of the foot/ankle muscles plays a role. Vereijken and colleagues have examined manipulation of body weight during the first 6 months of independent walking.[333] They placed ankle, waist, or shoulder weights on the infant and observed changes in the infant's gait patterns. Ankle weights affected the gait most over these months of development, causing continued slower and shorter stepping patterns. This was hypothesized to occur due to immature strength and control at the ankle.

The gradual refinement of gait is described by Stout in Chapter 34: Development and Analysis of Gait (on Expert Consult).

In summary, during the first several months of walking experience, creeping is gradually abandoned and heel strike in gait develops, allowing faster walking with longer strides. As children become bigger, older, and more experienced, steps become longer, narrower (reflecting a narrowing of the base of support), straighter (reflecting increasing control over the path of progression), and more consistent.[7] Walking practice is a stronger predictor of improvement in walking skill than age and duration of walking experience.[8]

DETAILS OF DEVELOPMENT: WHEN AND WHAT SKILLS ARE ACQUIRED

Because a large number of researchers have documented that the behavior of children varies based on characteristics of tasks and environments,[15,22,211] it has become clear that the apparently invariant sequence of development of motor skills is an artificial creation of the particular tasks chosen by early investigators such as Gesell. Nevertheless, information on when children achieve various skills is of continuing importance in physical therapy and other fields because information about ages and stages of appearance of motor milestones is used in developmental diagnosis of delayed motor performance. Thus this section elaborates on the observable "stages" of gross and fine motor development that represent milestones of developmental progress toward achieving the goals of upright posture, mobility, and manipulation: essential elements of environmental mastery and control. As infants attain and perfect these major developmental motor skills, they are incorporated into functional activities such as self-care, feeding, and play. Important milestones of motor development in later years of childhood will also be briefly addressed.

The major gross motor milestones of the first 12 to 18 months include achieving an indefinitely maintained upright head posture, attaining prone-on-elbows position, rolling from supine to prone, independent sitting, belly crawling, attaining hands-and-knees position, moving from sitting to four-point position and prone, creeping on hands and knees, pulling to a stand, cruising along furniture, crawling up and down stairs, standing independently, and walking independently.[17] As each position or skill is attained, further development will entail the perfecting of postural control in these positions and the ability to make rapid, effortless transitions from one position to another. Table 3.5 compares results for a US sample from Indiana, Pennsylvania, and New York City[22] with those for children from five countries, including Ghana, India, Norway, Oman, and the United States (WHO multicenter growth study, 2006).[352] Ranges for accomplishment of early milestones are narrower than for later milestones, and neither study noted gender differences. Of note, however, is that the order of attainment of mobility skills can vary a great deal. Berger and colleagues found that 64% of their sample used 1 of 8 variations in the order of attainment of skill from belly crawling to stair descent, but in the sample as a whole 57 different orders of attainment were recorded.[22]

Early Development: First Year of Life

The motor skills described in this section are likely to be the most important to a pediatric physical therapist. Changing positions, reaching and attaining objects, and mobilizing through the world are all phylogenetic (basic in all animals) skills needed for survival and self-preservation. Thus pediatric PT is considered necessary if a child is not performing these skills at the expected time, has difficulty with these functions, or has a limited repertoire of movements in the first year of life that may limit exploration and skills development. In addition, early motor delays, reduced strategies of movement, or altered quality of movement may predict future problems in other developmental areas. For example, children with autism often show motor delays that precede delays in communication or social skills.[29,233] Children with developmental coordination disorder (DCD), usually not diagnosed until school age, may display atypical early motor skill in infancy.[296]

Early Neonatal Movement

Skill acquisition starts in utero when a fetus starts to bring hand to mouth, foot to foot, and pushes on the uterine wall. Infants have been observed in utero during real-time ultrasound imaging to perform hand-to-mouth activities, touch other parts of their own bodies, and explore the uterine walls: all, of course, without visual guidance.[294] The first movements are notably general and cause the entire body to move, with lateral bending being the first to appear at around 7 weeks.[86] Isolated arm and leg movement begin around 9 weeks, and breathing movement as early as 10 weeks. Fetuses explore their own body, the umbilical cord, and the uterine wall with their hands.[294] However, there are individual differences, with a wide range of occurrence of any specific movement pattern. As the fetus develops, movement increases so that the child is moving on average of 30% of the day at the height of activity.[86] As the infant reaches the last trimester and becomes constrained by available space, movement decreases and complete positional changes occur infrequently from 26–30 weeks onward.[248] Thus the environmental conditions of the womb also afford ease of movement because of the fluid medium in which the infant resides when size and space allow but then restrict movement toward the end of the pregnancy. Movement in utero not only informs

TABLE 3.5 Average Ages and Ranges of Attainment of Gross Motor Milestones From Two Studies

	BERGER ET AL., 2007 (N 732) (UNITED STATES)		WHO GROWTH STUDY, 2006 (N 816) (GHANA, INDIA, NORWAY, OMAN, AND THE UNITED STATES)	
	Mean Age (mo.)	Range (mo.)	Mean Age (mo.)	1st, 99th Percentile (mo.)
Sitting without support			6.0	3.8, 9.2
Belly crawl	6.8	2.7–11.7		
Stand with assistance			7.6	4.8, 11.4
Hands/knees crawl	8.1	4.6–12.7	8.5	5.2, 13.5
Cruise	9.3	4.3–14.1		
Walk with assistance			9.2	5.9, 13.7
Ascend stairs	11.0	6.1–19.1		
Stand alone			11.0	6.9, 16.9
Walk alone	11.9	8.2–16.8	12.1	8.2, 17.6
Descend stairs	12.5	7.0–20.0		

the infant of consequences of activity but also provides neural feedback that appears to help perpetuate the movement. For example, in experiments with rats, tethering the legs together with a small thread changes kicking patterns from alternating to synchronous. When the thread is removed, the synchronous kicking continues, indicating some type of learning or adaptation within the fetal nervous system.[264] In addition, the musculoskeletal system depends on fetal movement for adequate shaping of the joints; poverty of early fetal movement is associated with congenital joint malformation.[90]

General and variable movement are pervasive in the fetus and young infant, even before goal-directed movements are apparent.[293] In fact, observational tests that focus on detecting variable movement in the early months of life are useful in predicting whether an infant is likely to be diagnosed with cerebral palsy at a later age.[253] This is because a lack of variability of movement, or poverty of movement, is not normally seen in infancy. Following a healthy full-term birth the infant's movements will continue and closely resemble his or her movements in utero. In the extrauterine environment infants must learn to modify their movement in response to gravity and are bombarded with new sensory feedback. Infants engage in many small shifts and wiggles of the body and thus change and shift the weight-bearing surface (even though the infant is unable to support himself in upright postures). This provides a wide array of possibilities for selecting movement strategies for emerging functions.[93] Infants gain experience with postural control and learn to deal with sensory stimulation through their active movements.

Neonatal and Infant Reflexes

Infants are born with the ability to actively select their movement patterns. However, some stereotypic movements, often referred to as primitive or neonatal reflexes, can be elicited in neonates and young infants. In neonates the presence or absence of a reflex may help estimate the infant's gestational age.[91] Neuromaturational theorists assumed that early reflexes diminish as cortical structures take control of active movements. From a dynamic systems perspective, multiple systems contribute to the increasing difficulty in eliciting reflexes with increasing age in infancy. Increased weight, increased engagement with the environment, neural maturation, and increased control of body segments all impact the observation of reflexes. The persistence of reflexes beyond the typical range may indicate a system is not developing typically. Thus many physical therapists and physicians assess primitive reflexes during examinations. Some of the most common primitive reflexes are rooting, plantar and palmar grasp, and stepping. Tonic reflexes including the asymmetric tonic neck reflex (ATNR) and symmetric tonic neck reflex (STNR) and labyrinthine reflex also remain prominent in many children who have neurologic dysfunction. In the section above on postural control is a brief review of the postural control reactions sometimes described as reflexes. Although the functional impact of obligatory reflexes should be documented in physical therapy assessments, treatment based on the current theoretical approaches should not attempt to integrate reflexes. Rather, active movement variability and function are viewed as factors that build motor skill in the child.

Functional Head Control

As an integral component of head control, eye control should be considered in early development. Eye movement early and often contributes to the emergence of movement. Considering that gaze shifts appear at birth and lead the interest of the child even before head control is complete, eye movement should be of interest to anyone hoping to improve a motor skill. Strangely, physical therapists who are concerned with developmental skill building rarely consider the ability of the eyes to shift gaze quickly as necessary groundwork for higher-level skills. In supine, or with the head supported in a reclining position, head turning to either side of midline can usually be elicited by attracting the infant's visual orientation to a moving object. Shifts of gaze are typically preceded by rapid bursts of body movement.[263] Smooth visual pursuit is present by 6 weeks of age and is adultlike by 14 weeks.[341] The ability to move the eyes contributes to cognitive as well as motor advancement and may shift to less skillful levels when a new motor task is emerging. For example, infants learning to sit take longer looks at objects, possibly because they are allocating resources to attending to postural control.[151]

At birth, infants already have the capacity to lift the head from either full flexion or full extension when they are supported in an upright position. A stable vertical head position, however, cannot usually be sustained for more than a second or two, if at all. At about 2 months the infant can sustain the head in midline in the frontal plane during supported sitting but often appears to be looking down at his or her feet so that the eyes are oriented about 30° below the horizontal plane as in Fig. 3.6 (Campbell SK, Kolobe TH, Osten E, Girolami G, Lenke M, unpublished research, 1992). Turning of the unsupported head in the upright position is not usually possible. If the child can be enticed to lift the head to the vertical position, oscillations are typically seen with inability to maintain a stable upright posture. Finer control of neck flexor and extensor muscles typically appears in the third month, when the head is indefinitely stable in a vertical position and can be freely turned to follow visual stimulation, although sometimes with brief oscillations and loss of control. This developmental progression is the product of improving postural control and experience and the use of sensory information such as visually attending to environmental cues. Evidence suggests infants are able to keep their head in midline 2 weeks earlier when an object is in their line of sight.[93] Early complexity supports development of motor behaviors in the first months of life.

When stabilizing control of the head in the upright position has been attained, the infant can typically organize head and trunk activity so that, when placed prone, the child assumes the prone-on-elbows position by lifting the head and extending the thoracic spine while simultaneously bringing both arms up to rest on the forearms (Fig. 3.7). Given the large weight of the head relative to the rest of the body at this age, a stabilizing postural function of the legs and pelvis must provide a stable base of support for simultaneous neck and trunk extension with arm movement. Green and colleagues demonstrated that the developmental progression in both supine and prone positions involves a gradual shifting of the load-bearing surfaces in a caudal direction.[138]

Turning the head to either side while prone on the elbows may still be difficult to coordinate at this stage, and lateral head righting also remains imperfect. Nevertheless, by the end of the third or fourth postnatal month, the head, in conjunction with organized trunk and lower extremity extension, has largely perfected the maintenance of stable positioning in space appropriate for the further development of eye-head-hand control and of

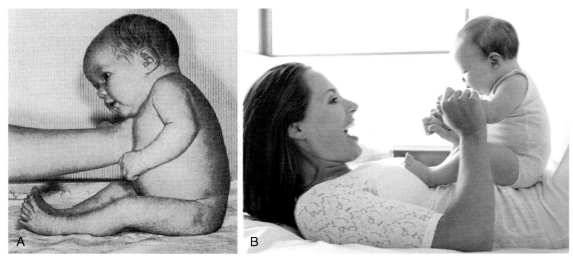

FIG. 3.6 Early head control in space is characterized by the ability to stabilize the head in midline but with eyes angled downward from the vertical. (A) The infant receives support at the trunk in order to exhibit head control. (B) The infant receives support from her mother through the infant's arms to stabilize her upper trunk; she is also assisted by the social interaction and encouragement from her mother, whose face is likely a preferred object of attention for the infant. Notice the slightly rounded trunk in both pictures, indicating a lack of active trunk extension in this position and a reliance on external support from the parent. ([A] From van Blankenstein M, Welbergen UR, de Haas, JH: Le développement du nourrisson: Sa première année en 130 photographies. Paris: Presses Universitaires de France; 1962. p 26. [B] From iStock.com.)

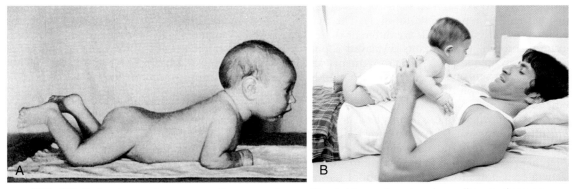

FIG. 3.7 Early stage of prone-on-elbows posture with stable neck extension, elbows close to trunk, and flexed hips and knees. (A) You can see the curvature of the infant's back, which is less than in Figs. 3.8 or 3.9. Also note the significant hip flexion that still exists, driving the pressure at the base of support cephalically. (B) The father assists the infant to shift the weight caudally, allowing for better head lifting, which is also encouraged by the face-to-face interaction of father and child. ([A] From van Blankenstein M, Welbergen UR, de Haas JH: Le développement du nourrisson: Sa première année en 130 photographies. Paris: Presses Universitaires de France; 1962. p 25. [B] From Shutterstock.com.)

independent sitting to come (Fig. 3.8). Bushnell and Boudreau believe that a stable head is a prerequisite for initial ability to perceive depth cues from kinetic information (movement of an object relative to its surroundings or to self), which is present by 3 months of age.[45] Once established by 4 or 5 months of age, binocular vision is used to identify depth cues.

Commensurate with acquisition of functional control of head positioning are important developments in control of the arms that are also related to positioning. For example, the prone position was effective in eliciting hand-to-mouth behavior in 0- to 2-month-old infants, whereas this behavior was elicited more often in sidelying when infants were 3 to 4 months old.[265] During the second and third months, generalized movements of the arms and body have altered their earlier writhing quality.[254] Small, fidgety movements appear throughout the body, the arms and legs may show oscillations during movement, and ballistic swipes and swats with legs or arms appear for the first time.[142] For example, if the legs are flexed up to the chest and then released while the infant is supine, the legs may extend so that the heels pound the supporting surface, or when excited, the infant may make large arm-swiping movements in the air. The first evidence of reciprocal activity of muscular antagonists

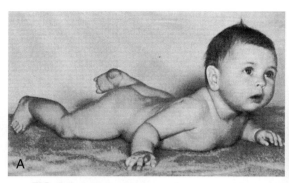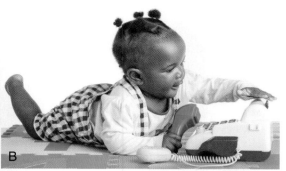

FIG. 3.8 Advanced stage of prone-on-elbows posture, with free movement of head and arms and extended lower extremities. (A) Note that the infant's arms are free to move because the weight of the upper trunk and head is shifted more caudally than in Fig. 3.7. Thus as depicted in (B), infants at this level of skill begin to shift weight to one side and reach to manipulate toys in prone. ([A] From van Blankenstein M, Welbergen UR, de Haas JH: Le développement du nourrisson: Sa première année en 130 photographies. Paris: Presses Universitaires de France; 1962. p 34. [B] From iStock.com.)

about the shoulder underlies the ability to perform these ballistic movements.[142] Ferrari and colleagues suggested the importance of these developing qualitative changes in spontaneous movement by demonstrating that they herald the appearance of goal-directed reaching and by indicating that they do not appear in children destined to be diagnosed as having CP.[103] Children with CNS dysfunction resulting in spasticity also tend to move in tight ranges characterized by simultaneity of activity in multiple limbs, referred to as cramped synchrony, and general movements that tend to repeat monotonously. The characteristics of children with dyskinetic CP are different.[95] Until the second postterm month, these infants displayed a poor repertoire of general movements, circling arm movements, and finger spreading. These movements remained until 5 months, when they became associated with lack of arm and leg movements toward the midline.

It is notable that typically developing infants have an abundance of movement with large variability when awake and alert. Movement is constant, with small shifts of weight and constant orienting to different events or aspects of the environment. This constant self-generated action provides a rich pool of sensory information from which the infant can gain an understanding of the consequences of particular movements and build concepts about the world around him.

Sitting and Transitioning Toward Mobility

Infants are supported in the sitting position by caregivers and in equipment starting at birth. It is not surprising that caregivers encourage sitting, considering the amount of time sitting functions to support everyday activities such as eating, playing, manipulating objects, or just looking and thinking. Sitting "propped" on extended arms after being placed in position by a caregiver begins around month 4 or 5. Prior to maintaining prop sitting, many infants begin to initiate movement toward a more vertical sitting posture when they are in a supported, reclined position, such as in an infant seat or on a parent's lap. Thus head orientation and positioning the arms to access environmental information appears to drive the infant toward sitting. The initial ability to maintain sitting independently on propped arms when placed also co-occurs with the ability to extend the head and trunk in prone position such that the legs and pelvis become load-bearing surfaces (Fig. 3.9). At this time

the infant is also able to control the pelvis and lower extremities while using the arms or moving the head in the supine position, indicating the ability to stabilize the body segments to counteract internally generated forces caused by movement.[138]

Harbourne and Stergiou described the development of sitting independence in three stages.[150] Stage 1 is the prop sitting phase, when the infant begins to explore the limits of the body segments (trunk and head primarily) over a static base of support. The legs are positioned in wide abduction, external rotation, and flexion in a "circle" sit posture. At this point the infant exhibits many "wiggly" movements of the trunk, which appear to be attempts to control the many degrees of freedom of the pelvis, spine, and head. EMG reveals that there is no singular postural pattern of motor control as the infant is placed into the prop sitting position, and variable muscle synergies (muscles that contract in a fixed time sequence) are utilized as the infant goes through a trial-and-error process to find a strategy that successfully controls the posture.[148] Infants at this stage of sitting may attempt to lift the arms to reach, but the effort disrupts the tripod stability of the posture, and the reach appears as primitive batting that does not go above the level of the shoulder.

Typically, in about a month at around 5 months of age, infants progress to Stage 2 of sitting, described as the ability to sit without use of the arms for short periods of time (a minute or two), but the child lacks the skill to maintain the posture while performing ongoing activity such as manipulating objects or looking around the room (Fig. 3.10). Sitting at this time is quite variable as the child attempts to control the body segments from the pelvis on up over the static legs. Trunk movement occurs often in wide excursions, in the infant's attempt to bring his or her center of mass under control. Even turning the head quickly can cause the child to lose balance. During this stage, parents often surround the infant with pillows because movement errors are frequent and falls are inevitable. However, infants persistently reach both within their cone of stability and outside of their stable range, falling and learning with each new reach challenge.[152] Reaching, although expanded to areas outside of the leg boundary of the child and over the level of the shoulder, is now linked to trunk and pelvic movement as the infant freezes degrees of freedom to accomplish the exploration of the surrounding environment. Fewer bilateral reaches are

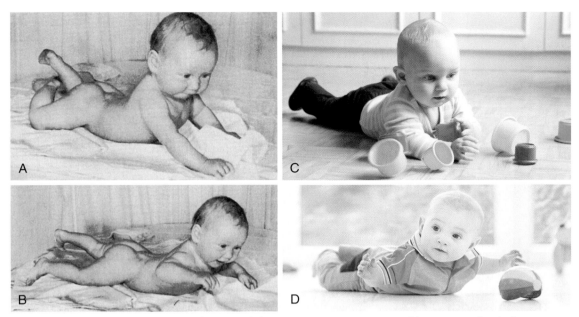

FIG. 3.9 In the most advanced stage of the prone posture, arms and legs move freely from a stable trunk. The skillful control of trunk and hip extension in this position allows the infant to push far up on the arms (A), or to elevate the upper trunk, arms, and legs off the surface in a "superman" pose (B). (C–D) This emerging ability to gain elevation and come off the surface allows engagement with toys and greater visual regard of the environment. ([A–B] From van Blankenstein M, Welbergen UR, de Haas JH: Le développement du nourrisson: Sa première année en 130 photographies. Paris: Presses Universitaires de France; 1962. p 37. [C–D] From iStock.com.)

present at this stage of sitting because the child will attempt to somehow stabilize the body with one arm while reaching with the other. However, once an object is brought close to the center of mass, infants will again resort to bilateral exploration.

Midway through the first year, at about 6–7 months, the average child achieves the ability to sit alone. In this third stage of sitting, infants no longer need to be surrounded by pillows and can sit for extended periods of time without falling. They can reach in all directions and above their head without excessive trunk movement, unless the trunk movement is necessary to extend the reach. The infant can successfully manipulate an object with one hand while the other hand holds it, although sitting and manipulating at once may still be a challenge. Poking fingers explore crevices and crumbs and herald the fine, selective digital control that characterizes the human organism. Strong extension throughout the body in the prone position and caudal shift of the load-bearing surfaces allow significant freedom of action for the arms and head. Bushnell and Boudreau believe that ability to perceive the characteristics of objects through their manipulation now allows the child to use configural cues from objects in depth perception.[45] Despite these developments in arm control, the child in sitting lacks the fine pelvic and lower extremity control needed for moving into and out of the position or for turning the trunk freely on a stable base. However, the legs are no longer fixed in a circle sit position, and infants exhibit variable leg postures, not necessarily symmetrical. The legs can be adjusted to accommodate a shifting center of mass, such as when the infant reaches far beyond his or her base of support. EMG at this stage of sitting reveals that the numerous and widely variable strategies exhibited when in Stages 1 or 2 of sitting have been trimmed to "preferred" or selected strategies that provide a directionally appropriate response to a perturbation.[143,148] EMG also reveals that when infants initiate a forward reach for a toy, they prepare for the disruption to balance by activating the hamstrings and trunk extensors prior to activating arm muscles. Thus the infants have learned, over the past few months of trial and error, the appropriate muscles to activate in the service of efficient reaching and exploration with the hands, a form of anticipatory postural control. Pelvic control notable in sitting is also exhibited in rolling segmentally from the supine to the prone position (Fig. 3.11), pivoting while prone, and playing with the legs and feet while supine.

During the end stage of sitting development, the infant has great variability in arm, trunk, and leg movement. It is during this time that the transition from sitting to prone begins, as the infant leans forward, reaching with one arm while bearing weight on the other arm.[132] The combination of rocking movements, unilateral hand preference for reaching, and increased ability to orient the head and trunk in all directions appears to co-occur with the transition from sitting to crawling. This coalescing of multiple factors fits into the dynamic systems theoretical viewpoint because various systems can contribute to the self-organization of a new pattern of movement.[133]

Upper Extremity Use: Grasping and Object Manipulation

So far we have addressed the use of trunk and lower extremity control in exploratory motor control, but the upper extremity is crucially important to motor exploration. From fetal movements including hand to hand, hand to mouth, and hand to umbilical cord, fetuses are controlling their upper extremity and hand to learn about the world and their own bodies. Following delivery, infants must learn to control their upper extremity and hand in the new environment with gravity, increased visual and auditory stimulus, and more diverse objects to interact with.

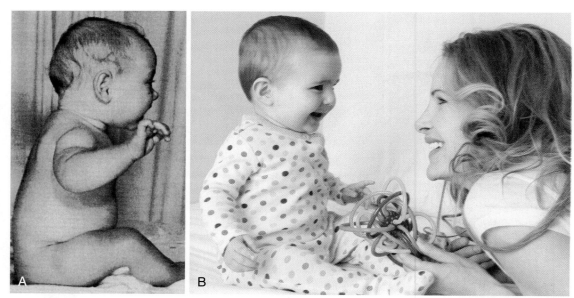

FIG. 3.10 Early stage of independent sitting, with arms used for balance. (A) The infant raises his arms in a "high guard" posture to stabilize the trunk and head; note the trunk is not as curved as in Fig. 3.6. (B) The infant shows his ability to gaze at and interact socially with his mother, as well as having the potential to reach for the toy because the arms are not needed as much for stability. ([A] From van Blankenstein M, Welbergen UR, de Haas JH: Le développement du nourrisson: Sa première année en 130 photographies. Paris: Presses Universitaires de France; 1962. p. 39. [B] From iStock.com.)

While postural control, strength, visual acuity, cognition, and motivation all play a role in the development of reaching and grasping, here we will focus on the control of the upper limb. Upper limb control can be broken into three sections of control development: reaching, object manipulation, and anticipatory grasping. Reaching control was covered in the previous section on motor control; here we move to greater detail about hand use.

As discussed previously, the infant's initial upper extremity goal is to bring the hand to an object or to his or her mouth. Yet the hand's interaction with the target is the true driver of perceptual development, not the reach alone. Early grasping behaviors can be observed in infants during spontaneous movements between 1 and 5 months of age.[350] Infants are observed to open and close their hands and to grasp their clothing and other objects that are near their hands during spontaneous movements. Fisting decreases while preprecision and precision grasp[112] emerge around 2 to 4 months of age. Self-directed grasping and self-exploration increase around 4 months of age in typically developing children.[350] These early grasping behaviors may provide experience and help infants learn to anticipate grasping following reaching at older ages.

Infants use four grasping patterns in the first 5 months, including fisted grasps, preprecision grips (thumb to side of index or middle finger), precision grips of objects, and self-directed grasps of their own body or clothing to explore objects and their own bodies.[350] While Karniol suggested infants move through invariant stages of spontaneous object manipulations,[189] research of Thelen,[311] Thelen and colleagues,[318] Oztop and colleagues,[238] and Keshner and colleagues[194] hypothesizes that, although functional hand use develops in a regular, invariant sequence when tested with a standardized series of tasks, it is likely that each infant uses unique coordinative

patterns and kinetics. Each infant's pattern is developed with a specific manipulative goal circumscribed by individual variations in body structure, experiences, and rate of neural and physical maturation. Karniol suggested that parents and others who choose toys for infants have two important functions: (1) helping infants to master the abilities of each stage by providing objects that are appropriate for emerging skills and (2) facilitating infants' developing sense of capability to control their world by providing objects that are responsive to current manipulative abilities.[189]

Thus the stages of object manipulation presented here as described by Karniol are now considered to be flexible and overlapping, as noted from the dynamic systems perspective.[189] They typically progress from rotation (angular displacement) to translation (movement parallel to the object itself) to vibration (rapid periodic movements of either translation or rotation). Later stages involve combinations of these actions and bimanual activities.[39] One factor that has been shown to affect skill in managing multiple objects during the age range from 7 to 13 months is hand preference.[197] Infants with stable hand-use preference used more sophisticated sequences of activity when presented with multiple objects. Because the task characteristics structure the infant's unique response, parents play an important role in providing opportunities that support development.

Stage 1, rotation of held objects—by 2 months. With improvements in head stability and visual perception, holding objects becomes an intentional act. Objects are first held when they come directly into the infant's reach and are later (by 3 to 4 months) twisted while being held. Karniol indicated that through this action infants learn that objects can be held and their appearance transformed by rotation.[189]

Stage 2, translation of grasped objects—by 3 months. Typical of this stage is reaching for an object while in the prone posi-

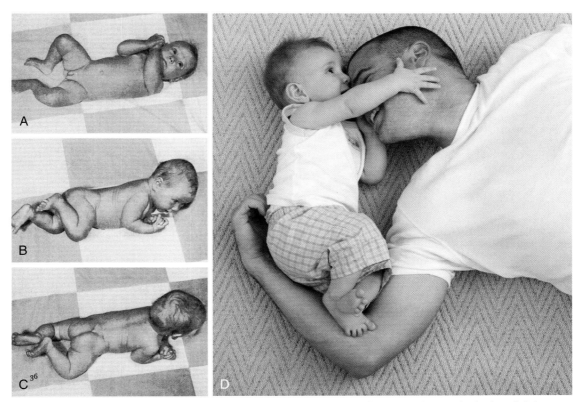

FIG. 3.11 Rolling from supine to prone with head righting. (A–C) These photos depict head righting, or the raising of the head off the surface in the course of rolling over to keep the head aligned to vertical. (D) This photo depicts goal-directed rolling: that is, rolling to interact with a person or an object, as a means of mobility. Note how the infant is reaching toward his father, which would assist the rolling movement as well as provide important interaction with others and with the environment. ([A–C] From van Blankenstein M, Welbergen UR, de Haas JH: Le développement du nourrisson: Sa première année en 130 photographies. Paris: Presses Universitaires de France; 1962. p 36. [D] From ThinkStock.com.)

tion and bringing it to the mouth. The object may also be rotated. What the infant learns through these types of action is that he or she can translate objects in order to look at, or mouth, them and that it is not possible to reach objects farther away than the length of the arm.

Stage 3, vibration (shaking) of held objects—by 4 months. In this stage infants learn that they can make interesting noises by rapidly flexing and extending their arms and can make the noise stop by holding still. If the object does not produce a noise, it may be translated or rotated and examined before being dropped, but visual attention is not a dominant part of this activity.

Stage 4, bilateral hold of two objects—by 4.5 months. The infant may hold an object in one hand and shake an object held in the other; infants thereby learn that it is possible to do more than one thing at a time (Fig. 3.12).

Stage 5, two-handed hold of a single object—by 4.5 months. First use of bimanual holding is to hold an object, such as a bottle, steady, but it rapidly advances to holding (and often rotating) large objects that require the use of two hands. These actions allow the child to learn that two hands can steady and rotate objects better than can one hand, as well as permit the holding of large objects.

Stage 6, hand-to-hand transfer of an object—at 4.5 to 6 months. Transfer is usually followed by repeated actions on the object with the second hand; infants thereby learn that whatever can be done with the right hand can also be done with the left.

Stage 7, coordinated action with a single object in which one hand holds the object while the other manipulates or bangs it—at 5 to 6.5 months. A quintessential example of this type of activity is holding a toy in one hand while picking at it with the other (Fig. 3.13). Displacements of the object caused by handling are followed by rotational readjustments of the hand that holds it. These activities teach the infant that two hands can do more than can one hand alone and that noise can be produced from striking objects that do not respond to vibrating. Infants at this age tend to be unimanual reachers with reaching being space dependent rather than object dependent, and it is not until 6 to 8 months of age that infants can take possession of two objects at the same time.

Stage 8, coordinated action with two objects, such as striking two blocks together—at 6 to 8.5 months. Through these actions, the infant learns to produce interesting effects by moving one object toward another.

Stage 9, deformation of objects—at 7 to 8.5 months. At this stage, the infant learns that it is possible to alter the way things look or sound by ripping, bending, squeezing, or pulling them apart.

Stage 10, instrumental sequential actions—at 7.5 to 9.5 months. These activities involve the sequential use of two hands for

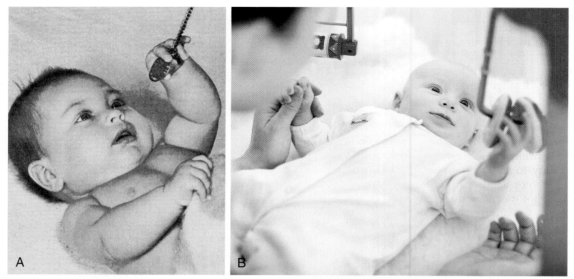

FIG. 3.12 Bilateral hold of two objects. (A) One hand holds the blanket, the other reaches for a keychain (stage 4 of Karniol).[160] Both pictures show bilateral holding action of the infant, but (B) includes the mother within the visual field of the infant. Importantly, the infant can begin to experience joint attention to objects with his mother in such a setup, a critical step in communicating ideas as the infant looks back and forth between mother and object and she reacts with commentary. ([A] From van Blankenstein M, Welbergen UR, de Haas JH: Le développement du nourrisson: Sa première année en 130 photographies. Paris: Presses Universitaires de France; 1962. p 91. [B] iStock.com.)

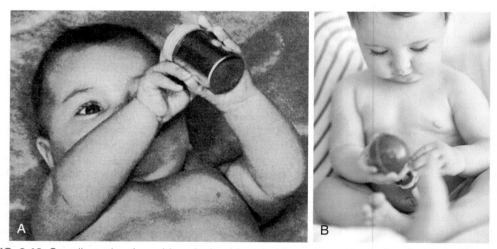

FIG. 3.13 Coordinated action with a single object: holding a toy with one hand while poking at it with another (stage 7 of Karniol) (A).[160] Note in both pictures the infant's visual regard and focus are to the toy and her hands, as eye-hand coordination emerges as the infant learns skillful manipulation of objects. (B) The infant has found an interesting part of the toy that slides and proceeds to explore the sliding motion. ([A] From van Blankenstein M, Welbergen UR, de Haas JH: Le développement du nourrisson: Sa première année en 130 photographies. Paris: Presses Universitaires de France; 1962. p. 93. [B] From iStock.com.)

goal-oriented functions so that the infant learns that coordinated use of the hands leads to desired outcomes. The infant may, for example, open a box with one hand and take out its contents with the other.

Anticipatory Control of the Hand During Grasping

In addition to reaching for or grasping an object placed in front of them, infants must learn to prepare their hand using anticipatory control to grasp an object and learn to grip smaller objects like pencils. Case-Smith and colleagues have shown that the characteristics of objects, such as differences in size and presence of moveable parts, lead to immediate use of distinct actions when grasping that are appropriate to the object's characteristics.[56] For example, a given infant might display more mature patterns of grasp when handling a toy with movable parts than when handling a pellet, so even infants seem to have some capability to recognize the affordances for manipulation offered by different objects despite having preferred modes of operating on items in the environment. Recently Barrett and Needham showed that 11- and 13-month-old infants used visual information from the shape of an object to grasp an asymmetrical object further from its center of mass than a symmetrical object.[15]

As with the development of object manipulation, a general pattern of development can be described that is flexible to the abilities of the child and the constraints in the task. As shown in walking and crawling experiments, we see that infants have extensive capability to use sensory inputs to make decisions about choice of motor actions, although they are not always right about their motor capabilities for solving the problem at hand.[8] They choose to act rather than avoid a challenging situation, do not engage in trial-and-error learning, but rather continue to rely on their visual-haptic analysis of whether or not to engage in risky behavior. While presented with the typical ages of onset, the descriptions of anticipatory control of the hand during grasping are variable, just as many other motor skills vary with experience in the task.

At the onset of functional reaching, infants are not inclined to reach for objects that are placed at the perimeter of their reach.[106] At 5 months of age, they begin to orient their hand toward the object, either just before or at the beginning of the reach,[224] as well as shape the hand in anticipation of object size constraints during manipulation.[232] At this age, infants primarily rely on contact with the object to orient and successfully grasp the object, but over the next 3 months, infants begin to use visual information to both anticipate contact and orient their hand with respect to the object.[213,15]

When adults reach to grasp an object, the distance between index finger and thumb is set with respect to object size at the onset of reaching.[177] Anticipation of object size is similarly observed in the hand posture of 9- to 13-month-old infants during reaching,[344] suggesting that young infants quickly learn to preprogram reaches for object size, location, and distance on the basis of visual information. The grasp of infants older than 9 months continues to exhibit some immature features, one being the relatively constrained range in hand opening when infants are presented with an assortment of objects varying in size.[210]

The infant's hand may open in exaggerated postures. Infants may open the hand widely as a strategy to compensate for limited ability to estimate the task requirements for grasping an object.[344] Finally, this exaggerated hand opening in the infant could be due to the small size of the hand in relation to the object. A body-scaled relation of the grip configuration, based on an equation including the size and mass of the object to be grasped and the length and mass of the grasping hand, has been demonstrated to be invariant across young children (6 to 12 years of age) and adults.[59,60] The force applied during grasp, the duration of the grasp, and displacement phases of prehension have also been shown to adhere to the same body-scaled relationship.[61] These findings support the idea that mature grasp and displacement are ultimately controlled within a single action that relates to body size and object perception.

Becoming Mobile

During the third quarter of the first year, around 7 months, infants begin to explore movement through space and develop movement, freeing them from positioning by others. As infants explore the parameters of their bodies and the affordance of the

environment, new movements emerge. There are many possible patterns of moving within the environment, and not all children choose the same strategy. Some infants drag the belly on the floor in a "combat crawl" style, and other infants scoot along on the bottom in a sitting position alternating with a hands and knees position. Other infants crawl with a reciprocal alternating pattern of the arms and legs. At least 18 different "styles" of crawling have been documented, and some infants use several over the course of becoming mobile.[6]

Context can also dictate a crawling pattern. An infant who normally belly crawls may be forced to crawl on hands and knees if he or she is trying to move in only a diaper on a hot, sticky day when frictional forces prevent dragging the belly on the normally slick tile floor. Although there are many forms of crawling, generally infants converge on a diagonal pattern of limb movement shortly after they have enough control to get their abdomen off the floor.[119] Control of lower trunk and pelvis, combined with previously achieved upper body skills, provides new mobility when prone (Fig. 3.14), crawling and creeping (Fig. 3.15), pulling to a stand, moving from supine to four-point and sitting positions, and moving down to hands and knees or prone position from sitting (Fig. 3.16). Inherent in each activity are freedom from a strong midline symmetry that previously characterized postural control and the continued refinement of rotational abilities within the axis of the trunk.

The presence of oscillations also continues to herald new developments. Rocking on four limbs before launching into creeping[6] and bouncing while standing before beginning to cruise along furniture are examples of self-induced actions that appear to be important precursors of functional skills. These repetitive movements may be a way that the child calibrates the forces needed to control body mass in new positions or a process of perceiving the result of actions that are self-produced.

Once the child has attained competence at standing and cruising along furniture, the legs and feet move toward perfection of selective control because the trunk and pelvis are increasingly reliable supports that permit freedom of lower extremity activities. In creeping, pelvic swiveling motions give way to reciprocal hip flexion and extension activity, and creeping velocity increases because an arm and a leg on the same side of the body can be placed in simultaneous flight. The child can lower himself or herself from standing (Fig. 3.17); bear-walk with dorsiflexed ankles, flexed hips, and partially extended knees (Fig. 3.18); ascend stairs by crawling up at an average age of 11 months with descent several weeks later, usually by backing down;[22] and stand and walk independently at 9 to 15 months of age (Fig. 3.19). As an example of typical regressions in the course of development, the early stage of walking is accompanied by a return to two-handed reaching, which declines again in frequency as balance control improves.[74] Chen and colleagues have also shown that learning to walk affects infants' sitting posture as the internal model for sensorimotor control of posture accommodates to the newly emerging bipedal behavior.[66] Increased postural sway in sitting just prior to or at the onset of walking is commensurate with the idea that new motor behaviors arise during periods of high instability.

Motor Development Beyond the First Year
Functional Motor Skills and Activity Levels in Preschoolers

We turn now to a description of the functional skills of preschool children, combining information on both gross and fine motor function in practical use. Toddlers operate with different

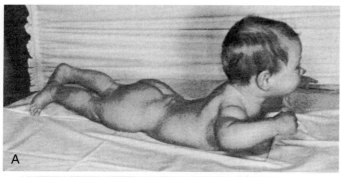

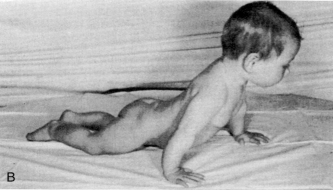

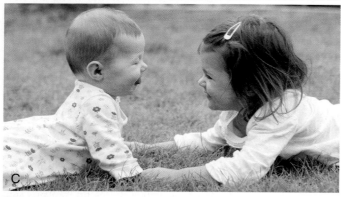

FIG. 3.14 (A–B) Dynamic play in prone position includes "flying" and push-ups on extended arms with strong trunk extension and scapular retraction. These types of movements are often immediate predecessors to rocking in the all fours position. (C) This emerging ability to gain elevation and come off the surface allows eye-to-eye engagement with a sibling and advances social interaction for future communication. ([A–B] From van Blankenstein M, Welbergen UR, de Haas JH: Le développement du nourrisson: Sa première année en 130 photographies. Paris: Presses Universitaires de France; 1962. p 47. [C] From iStock.com.)

anthropometric characteristics than infants. Toddlers gain about 5 pounds in weight and 2.5 inches in height each year, the latter resulting mostly from growth of the lower extremities.[73] Fifty percent of adult height is reached between the ages of 2 and 2.5 years. Children now walk well (although steps are still short and constrained) and enjoy the sheer pleasure of movement through running, climbing up and down stairs independently, and jumping off the bottom step.[10]

The 2-year-old child can kick a ball and steer a push-toy, and by 2.5 years the child can walk on tiptoes, jump with both feet, stand on one foot, and throw and catch a ball using arms and body together. Galloping may appear, but only leading with the preferred foot.[261] The more practical pleasures of dressing independently (pulling on a simple garment at 2 years and pulling off pants and socks by 2.5 years) and eating with a spoon with little spilling also develop.[10] Food preferences can become a touchy subject by around 2.5 years; nevertheless, the toddler is gradually developing impulse control.[73]

Roberton and Halverson hypothesized the following temporal sequence of further development of foot locomotion patterns: walking; running; single leap, jumping down or bounce-jumping, and galloping (in uncertain order, but generally at about 2 to 2.5 years); hopping on dominant foot (seldom before age 3) and then nondominant foot; and skipping and sideways galloping or sliding.[261] Although some children may manage a skip by age 4, many reach an early level of proficiency only by age 7. A rhythmic step-and-hop movement is even more difficult and does not appear until well into the primary school years, when it may be used in many dance forms.

The 3-year-old child can alternate feet easily when ascending stairs, can control speed of movement well, and takes pleasure in riding a tricycle.[10] Hopping may emerge, although it is often a momentary, single hop on the preferred foot.[154] Surprisingly, however, by 3.5 years the child may seem less secure and physically coordinated, stumbling frequently and showing a fear of falling.[10] Hands may show excessive dysmetria during block stacking. Nevertheless, typical 3-year-olds feed themselves well and can hold a glass with only one hand.

At 3.5 years, mealtime may again become trying because the food must be put on the plate in a certain way and the sandwich has to be cut just so. The same may be true of the dressing process, with special objection being expressed against clothing that goes over the head. The typical 3-year-old can put on pants, socks, and shoes, but buttoning may be difficult. Nearly all 3-year-olds are consistently dry during the daytime, and bowel training is well established as the physical skills and the emotional willingness to participate in toilet training come together.[73] The ability to delay gratification is developing, and toddlers strive for autonomy while continuing to intermittently seek reassurance from caregivers to whom they are securely attached.

Despite these generalizations, preschoolers exhibit a variety of individual behavioral styles.[73] About 10% of children are considered "difficult" because of increased levels of activity, emotional negativity, and low adaptability. Another 15% of children are described as "slow to warm up" because they take a long time to adapt to new situations.

Ames and colleagues have described typical 4-year-olds as characteristically out-of-bounds in their exuberance.[10] Behavior in all spheres is frequently wild, and self-confidence and bragging seem endless. The 4-year-old can walk downstairs with one foot per step, catch with hands only, and learn to use roller skates or a small bicycle. (But remember McGraw's experiments demonstrating that learning these skills is possible much earlier.) Athletic activities are particularly enjoyed, especially running, jumping, and climbing. Four-year-olds can button large buttons and lace shoelaces, feed themselves independently except for cutting, and talk and eat at the same time. The average Chinese child can use chopsticks to finish more than half the meal at 4.6 years.[357] Most children can take responsibility for washing hands and face and brushing teeth as well as dressing and undressing without help except

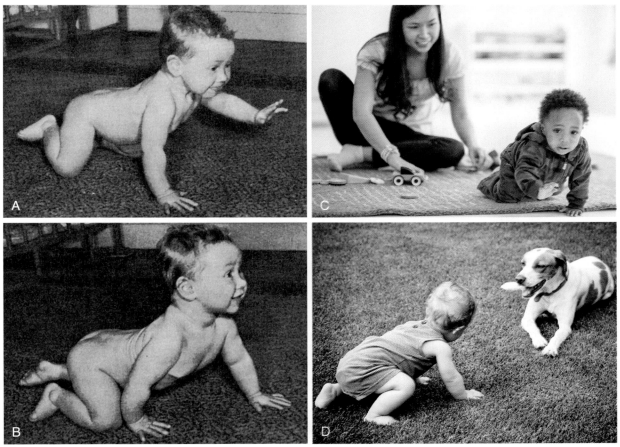

FIG. 3.15 Creeping on hands and knees. (A–B) Coordinated extension of the trunk and head while the legs and arms alternate in flexion. (C–D) This new found mobility allows the child increased exploration and social engagement with people, objects, surfaces, and even pets, providing ample learning situations. ([A–B]From van Blankenstein M, Welbergen UR, de Haas JH: Le développement du nourrisson: Sa première année en 130 photographies. Paris: Presses Universitaires de France; 1962. p 53. [C–D] From iStock.com.)

for tying their shoes or differentiating front from back of some garments.[10]

Early School Years

Five-year-olds tend to be more conforming than the exuberant 4-year-old.[9] Children begin to learn to dodge well at 5 years and can skip, long jump about 2 feet, climb with sureness, jump rope, and do acrobatic tricks.[261] Handedness is well established, and overhand throwing is accomplished.[10] Current research suggests that hand preference is already stable by 12 to 13 months in most children.[101] The 5-year-old likes to help with household tasks, play with blocks, and build houses. Eating is independent, including using a knife except for cutting meat, although dawdling and wriggling in the chair may be trying to parents. The challenge of dressing oneself is past, so children age 5 may ask for more help than they need (usually only for tying shoes or buttoning difficult buttons), and overall, undressing is generally easier than dressing.

At age 6, children are constantly on the go, "lugging, tugging, digging, dancing, climbing, pushing, pulling"(p 49).[10] Six-year-olds seem to be consciously practicing body balance in climbing, crawling over and under things, and dancing about the room. They swing too high, build too tall, and try activities exceeding their ability. Indoors, awkwardness may cause accidents, and the child seems less coordinated than during the previous year. Despite excellent eating skills, falling out of the chair or knocking over full glasses is not uncommon.

Although children may begin to ride a bicycle at age 6, there is wide variability on acquiring this skill due to factors such as access to equipment, location, and child or family interest. Even though a child may learn to ride a bike at this age, even at 12–14 years the child does not have adultlike perception of self versus objects in complex moving environments such as a traffic intersection.[137]

Because of the epidemic levels of obesity in the US population, concern about children's activity levels as an aspect of health has been heightened. In a study of the activity levels of 493 3- to 5-year-old children in 24 preschools, children were found to engage in moderate-to-vigorous physical activity during less than 3% of observations conducted with the Observational System for Recording Physical Activity in Children-Preschool Version.[242] Children were sedentary in more than 80% of the observation intervals. Boys were more active than girls, and younger boys were more active than older boys. An important observation was that activity levels varied by preschool, highlighting the importance of environmental

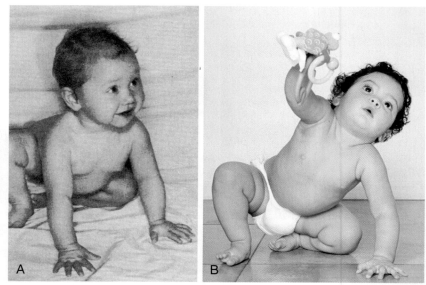

FIG. 3.16 (A) The infant moves from sitting to the four-point position over one leg. Infants transition frequently from sitting to crawling and back to sitting, generally by rocking over one leg and catching or pushing on the arms. (B) This transition comes in handy when the infant wants to socialize with a parent by showing a toy found while crawling or to move quickly out of sitting to reach an object. ([A] From van Blankenstein M, Welbergen UR, de Haas JH: Le développement du nourrisson: Sa première année en 130 photographies. Paris: Presses Universitaires de France; 1962. p 57. [B] From Shutterstock.com.)

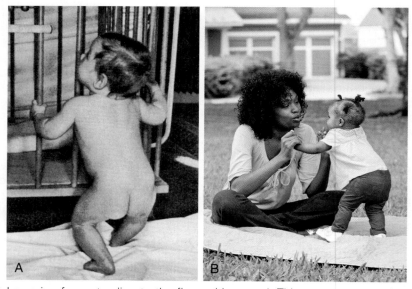

FIG. 3.17 Lowering from standing to the floor with control. This movement requires the affordance of a stable object (A) or the social interaction with an adult (B) to get down from standing. Lowering from standing with control usually develops after the milestone of pulling to stand at a support. ([A] From van Blankenstein M, Welbergen UR, de Haas JH: Le développement du nourrisson: Sa première année en 130 photographies. Paris: Presses Universitaires de France; 1962. p 57. [B] From iStock.com.)

variables in children's opportunities to engage in vigorous activity.

Steps in Motor Skill Development for Older Children

In the various motor skills developed in the preschool and elementary school years, each body segment has its own developmental trajectory within the overall coordinative structure; one part can be at a different level of skill than another, although all parts tend to be at a primitive level early or at an advanced level when skills are well learned.[261] Furthermore, when demands of the task change (increased height, distance, or accuracy requirements) or when fatigue sets in, one body component may regress in its action while another continues to perform at an advanced level of skill. Thus task requirements are once

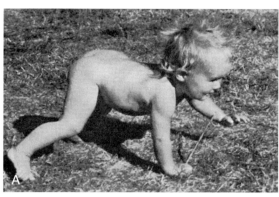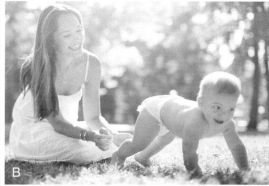

FIG. 3.18 "Bear-walking" on hands and feet. (A) Similar to crawling on hands and knees, this posture is often an option used when the surface either is rough or has added friction. (B) The child obviously enjoys the outing with the family and will adapt his mobility option to his comfort level to play. ([A] From van Blankenstein M, Welbergen UR, de Haas JH: Le développement du nourrisson: Sa première année en 130 photographies. Paris: Presses Universitaires de France; 1962. p 54. [B] From iStock.com.)

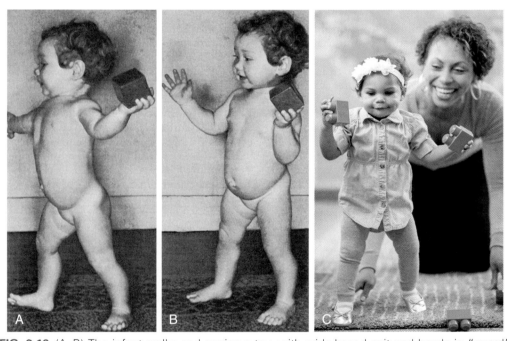

FIG. 3.19 (A–B) The infant walks and carries a toy, with wide-based gait and hands in "guard" position. (C) Early walking is motivated by parental encouragement and by the affordance of being able to carry objects toward and away from others. ([A–B] From van Blankenstein M, Welbergen UR, de Haas JH: Le développement du nourrisson: Sa première année en 130 photographies. Paris: Presses Universitaires de France; 1962. p 64–65. [C] From iStock.com.)

again seen to be influential in determining the characteristics of motor responses. For hopping and other skills, such as catching, throwing, and jumping, Roberton and Halverson provided detailed analyses and photographs of the intratask developmental steps for each critical body component, instruction in how to make detailed observations to categorize the level of skill of body segments, and advice for guiding the learning of these childhood skills.[261]

Physical therapists would find this information useful in planning intervention for children with mild physical disabilities or clumsiness. For example, as children learn to throw, the trunk goes through similar stages of development as those found in early developmental motor activities. The trunk is initially passive, then increasingly a stabilizer for the function of the extremities, and finally a participant in actively imparting force to the flight of the ball. Jumping changes from a functional activity characterized best as falling and catching to one of projection, flight, and landing, each with components that add force and speed or shock absorption to lend elegance and style to the activity.

Although many tests of motor development include assessment of hopping skills, most therapists probably would not view this as a particularly functional activity because children seldom hop spontaneously.[261] Physical educators, however, believe that hopping is an important developmental skill because a hop is often required in situations such as controlling momentum during sudden stops and in handling unexpected perturbations to balance, as well as for pleasurable play activities such as skipping. Hopping is also an excellent activity for describing the development of various strategies leading, finally, to skillful action.

Skillful hopping requires projected flight off the supporting leg and a pumping action of the swinging leg that assist in force production. Initial prehop attempts involve extension of the supporting leg as the child tries to lift off with the nonsupporting leg raised high. The first successful strategy, however, is usually a quick hip-and-knee flexion that pulls the supporting leg off the floor and into momentary flight (actually falling off balance and flexing the leg) while the swing leg remains inactive. At the next level of skill, the supporting leg again extends but with limited range and early timing relative to the point of takeoff. In skillful hopping the swinging leg leads the takeoff, and extension of the supporting leg occurs late; thus the action becomes one of "land, ride, and extend."[261] Just as with infants learning to descend risky slopes, children learn through practice how to control their intrinsic dynamics to produce efficient movements that accomplish intended goals.[1]

Sports and playground games become increasingly important parts of children's motor activities when they enter school and when complex feats of coordination become possible. Children have, however, individual rates of development of the components of motor skill, some undoubtedly innate, some based on cultural characteristics and family interest in development of physical skills. McGraw's work demonstrates, for example, that toddlers can develop motor skills that are usually considered inappropriate, primarily because of safety issues. Furthermore, research has supported the belief that African American children in grade school have superior motor skills, specifically the speed and agility skills on the Bruininks Oseretsky test, relative to white children.[70,249] Most authors have explained these differences on the basis of SES and differences in strategies of child rearing.[51]

Reaching Strategies in School-Age Children

Studies in older children suggest that reaching strategies change very little from 9 months until approximately 7 years of age, at which time there appears to be a transitional period leading to an adult reaching strategy. Five-year-olds continue to use ballistic strategies much like those of older infants, whereas 7-year-olds constantly monitor their movements in a closed-loop strategy to control their reaches. Between 9 and 11 years of age, children begin to combine these strategies to increase the efficiency of their movements and to reduce the amount of attention required.[154,192] These changes in reach strategy appear to coincide with developmental changes in how children utilize sensory information for guiding and adjusting arm position during reach. Based on these studies, the child's ability to understand and utilize sensory information for reach correction continues to develop through at least the first 11 years.[154,196]

In a related vein, one current view of the clumsiness seen in children with mild to moderate movement dysfunction is that a sensory or attention problem hinders the ability of these children to identify or selectively attend to the most pertinent information during a reach.[99,219,274,365] For example, study of

hand paths during movement between two buttons in a repetitive tapping task in 8- to 10-year-olds with minimal neurologic dysfunction (DCD) suggests that these children must constantly monitor and correct their actions. It is believed that using this closed-loop strategy leaves little opportunity to attend to information for executing anticipatory adjustments and minimizing the amount of error correction required. In comparison with age-matched controls, children with minimal neurologic dysfunction also appear to execute more movement units per reach. The first movement unit is less likely to be the longest unit or to achieve the greatest acceleration, and each unit tends to contain more acceleration irregularities.[274] When asked to reach from a starting point to a stationary target, 8- to 10-year-old children with DCD were less accurate than typical peers as a result of spending less time in the deceleration phase of the reach.[291] When the visual conditions were manipulated (vision removed after reach began or only target or target and hand visible), the group with DCD did not seem to take advantage of the visual information available.[330] Similarly, when children with DCD were asked to reach for a target with and without a visual perturbation (prism goggles), they used longer and more curved movement paths than a control group, demonstrating that their response to altered vision was different from typically developing children.[365]

In a different task, manual tracking of a continuously moving stimulus (a coincident-timing task) with a predictable path, children with motor coordination dysfunction (ages 6 and 11 years) were slower than age-matched controls.[330] Their movement distance during an acceleration phase was more variable than that of control children, their tracking motions were more delayed, and they performed more trials with apparently suboptimal attention. As an adaptive strategy, 7-year-olds with minimal brain dysfunction gave themselves more time to cope with less efficient reaching skills by planning a hand trajectory that would intercept a moving target further along its trajectory.[116] When these children were presented with an unpredictable tracking task, they had greater difficulty attending to the task than age-matched controls, perhaps because they could not identify a compensatory strategy.[99,331]

As was suggested for the infant during development, postural control may also affect the reaching behavior of children with DCD. Johnston and colleagues documented differences in the APAs of shoulder and trunk muscles in 8- to 10-year-old children with and without DCD during a goal-directed reaching movement.[185] The children with DCD demonstrated longer reaction times and movement times of their reach as compared to children who were typically developing. From a postural muscle perspective, the DCD group used earlier onsets of shoulder and posterior trunk muscle activity and later than typical activations of the anterior trunk muscles. Johnston and colleagues hypothesized that the altered timing of postural muscle activation influences the speed and quality of the reach movement.[185] Children with myelomeningocele, who frequently have atypical postural control and sensory deficits, used a different strategy for a similar task. The children with myelomeningocele did not alter their movement time while demonstrating a significant decrease in accuracy.[235] Whether the altered postural movements are part of the primary problem or a compensation for difficulty with necessary sensory integration to complete the task is yet to be determined.

In summary, the variables and processes that contribute to an emerging control of reaching skills during infancy and childhood are similar to variables contributing to those for posture and locomotion. In each instance, rudimentary aspects of control can be observed in very young infants if optimal conditions are provided, suggesting that precursors to functional skills may be established at very young ages. Each of these early skills, however, undergoes important transformations as children learn to perceive the task demands, monitor their movements, predict the potential consequences of their actions for a given context, and develop anticipatory strategies for efficient movement execution. As shown in the following section, these variables also contribute to the development of grasp control.

Maturation of Precision Grip and Load Force Control in Preschool and School-Age Children

Once a child's hand comes in contact with an object, he or she must coordinate normal (grip) and frictional (load) forces to grasp and lift an object.[184] Adults coordinate these forces synchronously, whereas infants and young children coordinate them sequentially.[113] To quantitatively examine grip control, infants are encouraged to pick up a toy that is equipped with force transducers to measure the grip forces of the opposing thumb and index finger and the load force necessary to lift the object off the table. During the preload phase (initial contact with the object), infants as young as 8 months contact the object with one finger before the other, creating a latency to onset of grip force that is significantly greater than in infants 18 months of age or older. Infants and young children also tend to press down on the object, creating a negative load force before reversing the direction of force to successfully lift the object off the table. Infants and young children generate a significant portion of the total grip force (often twice the magnitude of adult grasps) for grasping before initiating the load force, and during the load phase they typically exhibit multiple peaks in records for both of these forces. Adults, in contrast, scale the increases in grip and load forces in an economic, synchronous, and nearly linear manner with only a single peak near the middle of the load phase.[113] These findings suggest that the smooth execution of an adult grasp is the consequence of anticipating the object's weight so as to select an appropriate target force magnitude and scaling over time.[184] This anticipation of necessary grip-force adjustments for precision grip to lift, hold, and replace an object has been shown in adults to be related to experience with a predictable stimulus.[354] This collective experience, called central set, appears to affect the response gain of both voluntary and triggered rapid grip force adjustments to be set to a certain extent before perturbation onset in a similar manner as the effects of central set on lower extremity RPAs to platform perturbations. This suggests that in motor control there may be a general rule governing anticipatory processes.

The studies on control of grasp are consistent with a recurring theme of this chapter: infants appear to possess the neural substrate to execute skilled motor patterns early in development, but demonstration of this potential is unreliable.[113,114,115] First, these studies indicate that by 6 to 8 months of age infants can produce each of the actions required for a precision grip, and by 12 months of age infants can occasionally assemble all the components to produce adultlike force patterns, but there is considerable variability in performance across trials.[59] These studies also indicate that infants and young children use far more force than required, a common finding in studies of motor development.[192] Children as young as 2 years of age are able to adjust grip and load forces with respect to the degree of friction or potential slip during repeated lifts of the same object, but when the coefficient of friction is randomized over trials, they cannot adapt grip and load forces effectively. Thus with sufficient practice they can formulate rules for more adultlike performance, but if confronted with uncertainty, they do not know how to draw from limited previous experience.

When typical children 6 to 8 years of age are asked to grasp and lift a 200-g object repeatedly, they initiate nearly synchronous, linear increases in grip and load forces with a single peak in magnitude, as do adults. Children with CP (diplegia or hemiplegia) and autism, in contrast, tend to initiate the forces sequentially, as do younger children with typical development.[83,96] Specifically, it appears that at least some children with CP and autism can produce the requisite forces, but they have difficulty selecting or executing efficient grasp strategies. Available data indicate that these children have difficulty regulating the timing and magnitude of force during both dynamic and static phases, and they tend to bear down on the object before lifting it. When these children are asked to grasp and lift objects of two different weights, presented in blocked and randomized trials, they also have difficulty scaling forces with respect to object weight during both nonrandom and random presentation of the two weights,[97] but if they are given a sufficient number of practice trials, they can anticipate and scale grasp force parameters[98,299] and learn better precision isometric grip force, but not to the same extent of children of the same age who are typically developing.[324] Children with CP may also have difficulty stabilizing their gaze so that they can effectively use the available visual information.[209] Given that the normal acquisition of grasp control has a protracted period of development,[113,114] it is also probable that these children do not experience sufficient amounts and variety of practice to use available information for developing efficient strategies, an issue previously raised by Goodgold-Edwards.[134]

Refinements in the control of grasping continue to occur well into late childhood. Examination of the fine details of grip force amplitude and timing control has suggested that children age 7 to 8 years still do not exhibit finger force components typical of adult skill.[175] By 12 years of age, children approximate adult patterns of control and accuracy of bimanual isometric finger force production for both in-phase (both hands pinching a load cell device at the same time) and antiphase (one hand pinching, then the other) activation.[147] When coordinating grasp and lift of objects, young children execute grasps characterized by multipeaked variations in grip and load forces and do not execute the smooth, coincident increases and decreases in these forces characteristic of adult grasping until approximately 8 years of age.[113] Transitions to smooth, single-peak force patterns may in part be due to gradual improvements in anticipatory strategies.[114] It appears that the scaling of grip and load force rates continues to change until approximately 8 to 15 years of age, depending on the order of presentation of the weights, suggesting that anticipatory skills do not achieve adult levels until some point in this age range.[135]

Collectively, the studies described in this section demonstrate that grasping is a complex skill involving many different aspects of sensorimotor control. Rudimentary skills, biomechanics, experience, and other context-dependent variables probably contribute to the rapid changes in motor control observed in the first year of life. Even during earliest exercise of skill, infants are probably building a database of information for transforming their skills as they become increasingly more intent on shaping their experiences. Probably one of the views enjoying the greatest consensus among researchers in the field of motor control today is that all aspects of movement execution, including the basic physiology, biomechanics, perceptual processing, and development of strategies, must be closely examined under varying movement conditions to better understand the acquisition of motor control during typical development and when it goes awry.

The Role of Play in Development

Research on children's activity memory, or ability to explicitly recall activities they observe or create, is helpful in considering how to structure therapeutic exercise to promote memory regarding what has been experienced. Ratner and Foley reviewed the literature on activity memory and suggested that children remember activities better if (1) there was a clear outcome of the activity, (2) actions within the activity were logically sequenced such that cause and effect were obvious throughout the activity, and (3) the child engaged in planning of the actions involved in the activity in advance of carrying it out (not just mental imaging of it) or was asked to plan to remember what happened.[259] Young children do not always profit from external memory cues, at least not until 3 years of age or older, depending on the type of cue.

Nevertheless, children's behaviors show that they both consciously and verbally anticipate the unfolding and outcomes of activities by at least 2 years of age, even telling themselves "no, no" when about to perform some forbidden action.[259] At this point, imaginary play with objects that are not present appears, and children express surprise when outcomes of actions are not what they expected. Play then provides the opportunity for children to voluntarily act out intentions and to learn the difference between plans and outcomes. By 20 months of age, children are able to work toward a concrete goal, such as building a house from blocks, exhibiting checking behaviors, correcting mistakes, and acknowledging successful achievement of the goal. Repetition of an activity typically enhances memory of it when recall support is provided, and even infants 4 to 6 months of age can be shown to have some retrospective processing of events in that experiments demonstrate that they actively notice properties of an activity that were previously not noticed. Preschoolers allowed to demonstrate what happened will recall far more of an activity than if only verbal recall is elicited. Therapists should consider the mental ages of the children they treat with a mind toward creating therapeutic activities that provide children with disabilities the opportunity to develop cognitive skills such as planning and activity memory as they engage in exercise to reduce impairments.

When seen in its functional context as a learning device, motor activity can also be seen to have a stagelike character. Physical activity play (i.e., play with a vigorous physical component) has three developmental stages.[243] In infancy, babies engage in what Thelen has called rhythmic stereotypies or repetitive gross motor activities without any obvious purpose, including body rocking, foot kicking, and leg waving.[312] Whole-body, self-motion play is also called peragration, and Adolph suggested that such activities are the most direct route to knowledge: infants plunge in and obtain important information as a result.[1] These behaviors peak around the midpoint of the first year of life with as much as 40% of a 1-hour observation at 6 months being composed of such play.[243]

A second stage called exercise play begins at the end of the first year.[243] Such play can be solitary or with others, increases from the toddler to the preschool periods, and then declines during the primary school years. It accounts for about 7% of behavior observed in childcare settings. Activities included in exercise play include running, chasing, and climbing. Children with physical disabilities may need alternatives for participating in such play, particularly with other children.

The third phase of physical activity play is rough-and-tumble play such as wrestling, kicking, and tumbling in a social context. Often this type of play appears first in interaction with a parent, typically a father. Rough-and-tumble play increases through the preschool and primary school years and peaks just before early adolescence. No gender differences are noted in peragration activities, but males engage in more exercise play and rough-and-tumble play than females.

The functional benefits of physical activity play may be deferred or immediate. Pellegrini and Smith suggested that the benefits of rhythmic play in infants are immediate in improving control of specific motor patterns, that is, the primary repertoire in Edelman's terms.[243] Through active self-generated body movement, infants create perturbations to balance for which they gradually learn to accommodate or plan; such play also provides interesting visual and perhaps auditory spectacles for development of perceptual systems. Strength and endurance are also developed through such activities. Pellegrini and Smith posited that the function of exercise play is specifically to promote muscle differentiation, strength, and endurance. Chapter 6 provides further information on health-related physical fitness, which may have its roots in early play behavior. Pellegrini and Smith described animal research on the juvenile period, suggesting that it is a sensitive period for such development (recall McGraw's experiment with Johnny and Jimmy and their respective adult physiques).[243] Play may also have cognitive benefits in terms of providing a break from attention-demanding activities, thus leading to distributed practice and creating an enhanced arousal level of benefit to subsequent engagement in mental activities. Seen in this light, recess becomes something more than a meaningless break in the routine.

Pellegrini and Smith hypothesized that rough-and-tumble play serves a social function, especially for boys, related to establishing and maintaining dominance in social groups (girls are believed to use verbal skills more than boys in establishing dominance hierarchies).[243] As a by-product, children also may use rough-and-tumble play as a way to code and decode social signals. For example, in early rough-and-tumble play with parents, children learn that this is "play" and not aggression. Rosenbaum suggested that this view of motor activity raises the question of what goals we should pursue in therapeutic interventions.[269] Is it more important to provide opportunities to "travel" than to concentrate on improving gait? Do children with disabilities benefit from adapted recreational activities such as horseback riding in terms of social skills and cognitive function, as well as in motor skills per se? What is lost in terms of self-esteem or ability to decode social signals in children with disabilities if they are "protected" from rough-and-tumble play? Such "differentness" begins even in infancy as babies born prematurely are less likely to be included in play date activities in community centers or the homes of other families as much as other babies, in part because of concern for exposure to illness. For children in early intervention services, such isolation may be reinforced by the current emphasis on home-based therapy for the 0 to 3 population.

EXAMPLES OF MULTIFACTORIAL NATURE OF MOTOR DEVELOPMENT: PULLING IT ALL TOGETHER

In this concluding section, we provide examples at different key ages for functional actions and the cooperation of multiple systems for the successful accomplishment of that action. As physical therapists, our understanding of the interaction of multiple systems builds our ability to help new actions emerge. Although understanding of the motor system is important, it is not enough to help build function. We focus here on the first year of life because of the accelerated changes occurring within the child's body during that time.

Nate is a 3-month-old infant who displays indications of need, possibly hunger. His motor system acts by wiggling and twisting toward his mother's breast, while his eye gaze and beginning social understanding get his mother's attention via looking and vocal fussing. As his mother assists him to the food source, early control of the oral system and early reach/grasp orient his body to latch on to eat. Suck and swallow coordinated movement allow successful feeding, which leads to calming of his motor system and beginning understanding of how his motor efforts result in positive reward both socially and physiologically. Think about how the experiences of an infant with movement problems would differ from this typical experience and how the connections between the motor system and other systems might be altered if the infant lacks movement. Alternatively, an infant who is bottle-fed instead of breast-fed may have a different movement strategy of expressing needs, which should be considered in problem solving to assist the development of motor skill.

Katie is a 6-month-old infant who amazes her parents with her newfound interest in objects. Her motor system allows her to reach persistently for objects with her hands and her feet, and her visual system can quickly note novel objects and the details of objects within her view. Her progressing visual, social, and cognitive skill invites adult engagement with her toward an object of interest, heralding the important skill of joint attention, a precursor to language and later speech. She may even vocalize for a toy that is out of reach or object vocally to a toy taken away. High variability in exploration with her motor skills interacts with cognitive skills to begin problem solving and memory of familiar things. She is easy to entertain because she likes to repeat movements like banging a toy, and handling novel objects seems to fascinate her. Imagine how reduced movement would limit the strategies for exploration and learning for Katie. Alternatively, consider the strong implications of environmental context for this child. Without opportunities for both exploration (variety of objects, surfaces, situations) and related movement, cascading effects on cognition and perception can be expected.

Sam is 9 months old and he hears the phone ring in another room. Because he is mobile now via crawling, he can seek the origin of the ringing noise. He expects his mother will begin talking due to his memory of what happens with a phone, and he knows she is in the other room because she just exited his room. He has the object permanence concept now, so he understands his mother still exists even if she walks out of his sight; this concept became solidified when he could move himself and find people and objects that disappeared behind a door. He has

social skills, which have bonded him to close family and friends, and he drags a new toy with him as he crawls to engage in joint attention to the object when he finds his mother. As he finds his mother sitting on the couch, he pulls himself to stand and proudly shows her the toy with a squeal of delight and babbling of consonant-vowel sounds. His mom answers back by labeling the toy, "You found a car!" and they communicate with visual, tactile, and verbal exchanges. This rich learning experience would be significantly limited by a mobility restriction.

Sally is a 12-month-old infant who wants to carry a container of toys from her living room to her room. She has been walking for a couple weeks, and her newfound ability to carry objects with her free arms is a powerful tool. She now can walk on level surfaces easily because she practiced for hundreds of steps per day, and the pattern of stepping is quite automatic unless she comes to a change in surface. However, she knows the route to her room because of her improved memory and spatial skills, related to months of navigating and exploring her house. She can orient her arms and hands around the object (a small bucket of toys) and she has the postural control to maintain upright with this added weight and bulk to her frame. She has visual and prospective control to avoid the sides of the door and the cognitive skill to conceptualize the skill. When she comes to the obstacle of her family dog in the way, she vocalizes to solve the problem by getting her parent's attention. By combining environmental and child factors, Sally is beginning to be in control of her world; her motor development allows this growth to progress and learning to continue.

▌ S U M M A R Y

Theories of motor development have evolved over time, but current thinking suggests that development is a complex outcome of the maturation of multiple physiologic systems in combination with demands placed on children by the environment and task-related experiences. In this chapter, we described developmental principles in combination with motor control theory to provide normative information as a reference for understanding the needs of children facing motor problems. The information provided in this and subsequent chapters will enable pediatric physical therapists to apply current concepts and research for the benefit of our clients—children with disabilities and their families.

REFERENCES

1. Adolph KE: Learning in the development of infant locomotion, *Monogr Soc Res Child Dev* 62(3):1–140, 1997.
2. Adolph KE: Learning to move, *Curr Dir Psycholo Sci* 17(3):213–218, 2008.
3. Adolph KE, Berger SE: Learning and development in infant locomotion, *Prog Brain Res* 164:237–255, 2007.
4. Adolph KE, Berger SE: Motor development, *Handbook of child psychology*, 2006.
5. Adolph KE, Robinson SR: Motor development. In Lerner RM, series editor; Liben L, Muller U, volume editors: *Handbook of child psychology and developmental science, Vol. 2: Cognitive processes*, ed, New York, 2015, Wiley, pp 114–157.
6. Adolph KE, Vereijken B, Denny MA: Learning to crawl, *Child Dev* 69(5):1299–1312, 1998.
7. Adolph KE, Robinson SR, Young JW, Gill-Alvarez F: What is the shape of developmental change? *Psychol Rev* 115:527–543, 2008.

8. Adolph KE, Cole WG, Komati M, Garciaguirre JS, Badaly D, Lingeman JM, Sotsky RB: How do you learn to walk? Thousands of steps and dozens of falls per day, *Psychol Sci* 23(11):1387–1394, 2012.

9. Adolph KE, Berger SE: Physical and motor development. In Bornstein MH, Lamb ME, editors: *Developmental science: an advanced textbook*, ed 7, New York, 2015, Psychology Press/Taylor Francis, pp 261–333.

10. Ames LB, Gillespie C, Haines J, Ilg FL: *The Gesell Institute's child from one to six: evaluating the behavior of the preschool child*, New York, 1979, Harper Row.

11. Aruin AS, Almeida GL: A coactivation strategy in anticipatory postural adjustments in persons with Down syndrome, *Motor Control* 1:178–191, 1997.

12. Asanuma H, Keller A: Neuronal mechanisms of motor learning in mammals, *Neuroreport* 2:217–224, 1991.

13. Assaiante C, Woollacott M, Amblard B: Development of postural adjustment during gait initiation: kinematic and EMG analysis, *J Mot Behav* 32:211–226, 2000.

14. Bailey Jr DB, Bruer JT, Symons FJ, Lichtman JW: *Critical thinking about critical periods*, Baltimore, 2001, Paul H. Brookes.

15. Barrett TM, Needham A: Developmental differences in infants' use of an object's shape to grasp it securely, *Dev Psychobiol* 50:97–106, 2008.

16. Bayley N: *Bayley II*, San Antonio, TX, 1993, Psychological Corporation.

17. Bayley N: *Bayley scales of infant and toddler development*, San Antonio, TX, 2006, Psychological Corporation.

18. Behrman AL, Nair PM, Bowden MG, et al.: Locomotor training restores walking in a nonambulatory child with chronic, severe, incomplete cervical spinal cord injury, *Phys Ther* 88(5):580–590, 2008.

19. Bergenn VW, Dalton TC, Lipsitt LP, McGraw MB: A growth scientist, *Dev Psychol* 28:381–395, 1992.

20. Berger SE: Demands on finite cognitive capacity cause infants' perseverative errors, *Infancy* 5:217–238, 2004.

21. Berger SE: Locomotor expertise predicts infants' perseverative errors, *Dev Psychol* 46:326, 2010.

22. Berger SE, Theuring C, Adolph KE: How and when infants learn to climb stairs, *Infant Behav Dev* 30:36–49, 2007.

23. Bergmeier SA: An investigation of reaching in the neonate, *Pediatr Phys Ther* 4:3–11, 1992.

24. Bernardis P, Bello A, Pettenati P, Stefanini S, Gentilucci M: Manual actions affect vocalizations of infants, *Exp Brain Res*, January 9, 2008. Epub 10.1007/s00221-007-1256-x.

25. Bernstein N: *The coordination and regulation of movements*, London, 1967, Pergamon.

26. Bertenthal BI, Rose JL, Bai DL: Perception-action coupling in the development of visual control of posture, *J Exp Psychol Hum Percept and Perform* 23(6):1631–1643, 1997.

27. Bevor TG: *Regressions in mental development: basic phenomena and theories*, Hillsdale, NJ, 1982, Lawrence Erlbaum Associates.

28. Bhat AN, Galloway JC: Toy-oriented changes during early arm movements: hand kinematics, *Infant Behav Dev* 29(3):358–372, 2006.

29. Bhat AN, Landa RJ, Galloway JC: Current perspectives on motor functioning in infants, children, and adults with autism spectrum disorders, *Phys Ther* 91:1116–1129, 2011.

30. Birkenmaier C, Jorysz G, Jansson V, Heimkes B: Normal development of the hip: a geometrical analysis based on planimetric radiography, *J Pediatr Orthop B* 19(1):1–8, 2010.

31. Black D, Chang CL, Kubo M, Holt K, Ulrich B: Developmental trajectory of dynamic resource utilization during walking: toddlers with and without Down syndrome, *Hum Mov Sci* 28(1):141–154, 2009.

32. Blauw-Hospers CH, de Graaf-Peters VB, Dirks T, Bos AF, Hadders-Algra M: Does early intervention in infants at high risk for a developmental motor disorder improve motor and cognitive development? *Neurosci Biobehav Rev* 31(8):1201–1212, 2007.

33. Bodkin AW, Baxter RS, Heriza CB: Treadmill training for an infant born preterm with a grade III intraventricular hemorrhage, *Phys Ther* 83:1107–1118, 2003.

34. Bornstein MH, Putnick DL, Lansford JE, Deater-Deckard K, Bradley RH: A developmental analysis of caregiving modalities across infancy in 38 low-and middle-income countries, *Child Dev* 86(5):1571–1587, 2015.

35. Bradley NS: What are the principles of motor development? In Forssberg H, Hirschfeld H, editors: *Movement disorders in children medicine and sport science*, Vol. 36. Basel, 1992, Karger, pp 41–49.

36. Bradley NS: Connecting the dots between animal and human studies of locomotion. Focus on "Infants adapt their stepping to repeated trip-inducing stimuli." *J Neurophysiol* 90:2088–2089, 2003.

37. Bradley NS, Bekoff A: Development of coordinated movement in chicks: i. Temporal analysis of hindlimb muscle synergies at embryonic days 9 and 10, *Dev Psychobiol* 23:763–782, 1990.

38. Bradley NS, Smith JL: Neuromuscular patterns of stereotypic hindlimb behaviors in the first two postnatal months. I. Stepping in normal kittens, *Dev Brain Res* 38:37–52, 1988.

39. Brakke K, Fragaszy DM, Simpson K, Hoy E, Cummins-Sebree S: The production of bimanual percussion in 12- to 24-month-old children, *Hum Mov Sci* 30:2–15, 2007.

40. Branch LG, Kesty K, Krebs E, Wright L, Leger S, David LR: Deformational plagiocephaly and craniosynostosis: trends in diagnosis and treatment after the "Back to Sleep" campaign, *J Craniofac Surg* 26(1):147–150, 2015.

41. Brogen E, Hadders-Algra M, Forssberg H: Postural control in sitting children with cerebral palsy, *Neuroscience and Biobehavioral Reviews* 22:591–596, 1998.

42. Bronfenbrenner U: Ecology of the family as a context for human development: research perspectives, *Dev Psychol* 22(6):723, 1986.

43. Bruer JT: A critical and sensitive period primer. In Bailey Jr DB, Bruer JT, Symons FJ, Lichtman JW, editors: *Critical thinking about critical periods*, Baltimore, 2001, Paul H. Brookes, pp 3–26.

44. Burleigh A, Horak F: Influence of instruction, prediction, and afferent sensory information on the postural organization of step initiation, *Journal of Neurophysiology* 75:1619–1627, 1996.

45. Bushnell EW, Boudreau JP: Motor development and the mind: the potential role of motor abilities as a determinant of aspects of perceptual development, *Child Dev* 64:1005–1021, 1993.

46. Butt SJ, Lebret JM, Kiehn O: Organization of left-right coordination in the mammalian locomotor network, *Brain Research and Brain Research Review* 40:107–117, 2002.

47. Butterworth G, Hicks L: Visual proprioception and postural stability in infancy. A developmental study, *Perception* 6(3):255–262, 1977.

48. Byl NN, Merzenich MM, Cheung S, Bedenbaugh P, Nagarajan SS, Jenkins WM: A primate model for studying focal dystonia and repetitive strain injury: effects on the primary somatosensory cortex, *Phys Ther* 77:269–284, 1997.

49. Campbell SK, Kolobe TH, Osten E, Girolami G, Lenke M: *Unpublished research*, 1992.

50. Campos D, Santos DC, Gonçalves VM, et al.: Agreement between scales for screening and diagnosis of motor development at 6 months, *J Pediatr (Rio J)* 82:470–474, 2006.

51. Capute AJ, Shapiro BK, Palmer FB, Ross A, Wachtel RC: Normal gross motor development: the influences of race, sex and socio-economic status, *Dev Med Child Neurol* 27(5):635–643, 1985.

52. Carbonnell L, Hasbroucq T, Grapperon J, Vidal F: Response selection and motor areas: a behavioural and electrophysiological study, *Clinical Neurophysiology* 115(9):2164–2174, 2004.

53. Carson RG, Riek S: Changes in muscle recruitment patterns during skill acquisition, *Experimental Brain Research* 138:71–87, 2001.

54. Carvalho RP, Tudella E, Savelsbergh GJ: Spatio-temporal parameters in infant's reaching movements are influenced by body orientation, *Infant Behav Dev* 30(1):26–35, 2007.

55. Carvalho RP, Tudella E, Caljouw SR, et al.: Early control of reaching: effects of experience and body orientation, *Infant Behav Dev* 31(1):23–33, 2008.

56. Case-Smith J, Bigsby R, Clutter J: Perceptual-motor coupling in the development of grasp, *American Journal of Occupational Therapy* 52:102–110, 1998.

57. Cataldo R, Huang J, Calixte R, Wong AT, Bianchi-Hayes J, Pati S: Effects of overweight and obesity on motor and mental development in infants and toddlers, *Pediatr Obes*, 2015 Oct 21. http://dx.doi.org/10.1111/ijpo.12077. [Epub ahead of print].

58. Cenciarini M, Peterka RJ: Stimulus-dependent changes in the vestibular contribution to human postural control, *J Neurophysiol* 95(5):2733–2750, 2006.

59. Cesari P, Newell KM: The scaling of human grip configurations, *J Exp Psychol Hum Percept Perform* 25:927–935, 1999.

60. Cesari P, Newell KM: The body scaling of grip configurations in children aged 6-12 years, *Dev Psychobiol* 36:301–310, 2000.

61. Cesari P, Newell KM: Scaling the components of prehension, *Motor Control* 6:347–365, 2002.

62. Chambers SH, Bradley NS, Orosz MD: Kinematic analysis of wing and leg movements for type I motility in E9 chick embryos, *Exp Brain Res* 103:218–226, 1995.

63. Chang CL, Kubo M, Ulrich BD: Emergence of neuromuscular patterns during walking in toddlers with typical development and with Down syndrome, *Hum Mov Sci* 28(2):283–296, 2009.

64. Chen J, Woollacott MH: Lower extremity kinetics for balance control in children with cerebral palsy, *J Mot Behav* 39(4):306–316, 2007.

65. Chen LC, Metcalfe JS, Chang TY, Jeka JJ, Clark JE: The development of infant upright posture: sway less or sway differently? *Experimental Brain Research* 186:293–303, 2008.

66. Chen LC, Metcalfe JS, Jeka JJ, Clark JE: Two steps forward and one back: learning to walk affects infants' sitting posture, *Infant Behav Dev* 30:16–25, 2007.

67. Cherng RJ, Chen JJ, Su FC: Vestibular system in performance of standing balance of children and young adults under altered sensory conditions, *Percept Mot Skills* 92(3 Pt 2):1167–1179, 2001.

68. Cheron G, Bengoetxea A, Bouillot E, Lacquaniti F, Dan B: Early emergence of temporal coordination of lower limb segments elevation angles in human locomotion, *Neurosci Letters* 308:123–127, 2001.

69. Chiel H, Beer AR: The brain has a body: adaptive behavior emerges from interactions of nervous system, body and environment, *Trends Neurosci* 20:553–557, 1997.

70. Cintas HM: Cross-cultural variation in infant motor development, *Phys Occupat Ther Pediatr* 8(4):1–20, 1988.

71. Clifton RK, Muir DW, Ashmead DH, Clarkson MG: Is visually guided reaching in early infancy a myth? *Child Dev* 64:1099–1110, 1993.

72. Coghill GE: *Anatomy and the problem of behaviour*, Cambridge University Press, 2015 (original publication 1929).

73. Colson ER, Dworkin PH: Toddler development, *Pediatr Rev* 18:255–259, 1997.

74. Corbetta D, Bojczyk KE: Infants return to two-handed reaching when they are learning to walk, *J Mot Behav* 34:83–95, 2002.

75. Corbetta D, Snapp-Childs W: Seeing and touching: the role of sensory-motor experience on the development of infant reaching, *Infant Behav Dev* 32(1):44–58, 2009.

76. Corbetta D, Thelen E: Shifting patterns of interlimb coordination in infants' reaching: a case study. In Swinnen SP, Heuer H, Massion J, Casaer P, editors: *Interlimb coordination: neural dynamical and cognitive constraints*, San Diego, CA, 1994, Academic Press, pp 413–438.

77. Cox RFA, Smitsman AW: Action planning in young children's tool use, *Dev Sci* 9:628–641, 2006.

78. Crutcher MD, Alexander GE: Movement-related neuronal activity selectively coding either direction or muscle pattern in 3 motor areas of the monkey, *Journal of Neurophysiology* 64:151–163, 1990.

79. d' Avella A, Saltiel P, Bizzi E: Combinations of muscle synergies in the construction of a natural motor behavior, *Nature Neuroscience* 6:300–308, 2003.

80. Dalton TC: Arnold Gesell and the maturation controversy, *Integrat Physiol Behav Sci* 40:182–204, 2005.

81. Damiano DL, DeJong SL: A systematic review of the effectiveness of treadmill training and body weight support in pediatric rehabilitation, *J Neurol Phys Ther* 33(1):27–44, 2009.

82. Darrah J, Bartlett D, Maguire TO, Avison WR, Lacaze-Masmonteil T: Have infant gross motor abilities changed in 20 years? A re-evaluation of the Alberta Infant Motor Scale normative values, *Dev Med Child Neurol* 56(9):877–881, 2014.

83. David FJ, Baranek GT, Giuliani CA, et al.: A pilot study: coordination of precision grip in children and adolescents with high functioning autism, *Pediatr Phys Ther* 21(2):205–211, 2009.

84. de Bode S, Mathern GW, Bookheimer S, Dobkin B: Locomotor training remodels fMRI sensorimotor cortical activations in children after cerebral hemispherectomy, *Neurorehabil Neural Repair* 21(6):497–508, 2007.

85. de Graaf-Peters VB, Bakker H, van Eykern LA, et al.: Postural adjustments and reaching in 4- and 6-month-old infants: an EMG and kinematical study, *Experimental Brain Research* 181(4):647–656, 2007.

86. De Vries JIP, Fong BF: Normal fetal motility: an overview, *Ultrasound Obstet Gynecol* 27(6):701–711, 2006.

87. de Vries JIP, Visser GHA, Prechtl HFR: The emergence of fetal behavior: i. Qualitative aspects, *Early Human Development* 7:301–322, 1982.

88. Dillenburger K, Keenan M: None of the As in ABA stand for autism: dispelling the myths, *J Intellect Dev Disabil* 34(2):193–195, 2009.

89. Dobkin BH: Motor rehabilitation after stroke, traumatic brain, and spinal cord injury: common denominators within recent clinical trials, *Curr Opin Neurol* 22:563–569, 2009.

90. Drachman DB, Sokoloff L: The role of movement in embryonic joint development, *Dev Biol* 14(3):401–420, 1966.

91. Dubowitz LM, Dubowitz V, Palmer P, Verghote M: A new approach to the neurological assessment of the preterm and full-term newborn infant, *Brain and Development* 2(1):3–14, 1980.

92. Dusing SC, Harbourne RT: Variability in postural control during infancy: implications for development, assessment, and intervention, *Phys Ther* 90(12):38–49, 2010.

93. Dusing SC, Thacker LR, Stergiou N, Galloway JC: Early complexity supports development of motor behaviors in the first months of life, *Dev Psychobiol* 55(4):404–414, 2013.

94. Edelman GM: *Bright air brilliant fire: on the matter of the mind*, New York, 1992, Basic Books.

95. Einspieler C, Cioni G, Paolicelli PB, et al.: The early markers for later dyskinetic cerebral palsy are different from those for spastic cerebral palsy, *Neuropediatrics* 33:73–78, 2002.

96. Eliasson AC, Gordon AM, Forssberg H: Basic co-ordination of manipulative forces of children with cerebral palsy, *Dev Med Child Neurol* 33:661–670, 1991.

97. Eliasson AC, Gordon AM, Forssberg H: Impaired anticipatory control of isometric forces during grasping by children with cerebral palsy, *Dev Med Child Neurol* 34:216–225, 1992.

98. Eliasson AC, Gordon AM, Forssberg H: Tactile control of isometric fingertip forces during grasping in children with cerebral palsy, *Dev Med Child Neurol* 37:72–84, 1995.

99. Estil LB, Ingvaldsen RP, Whiting HT: Spatial and temporal constraints on performance in children with movement co-ordination problems, *Exp Brain Res* 147:153–161, 2002.

100. Fagard J: The development of bimanual coordination. In Bard C, Fleury M, Hay L, editors: *Development of eye-hand coordination across the life span*, Columbia, SC, 1990, University of South Carolina Press, pp 262–282.

101. Fagard J, Pezé A: Age changes in interlimb coupling and the development of bimanual coordination, *J Mot Behav* 29:199–208, 1997.

102. Fallang B, Saugstad OD, Hadders-Algra M: Goal directed reaching and postural control in supine position in healthy infants, *Behav Brain Res* 115:9–18, 2000.

103. Ferrari F, Cioni G, Prechtl HRF: Qualitative changes of general movements in preterm infants with brain lesions, *Early Hum Dev* 23:193–231, 1990.

104. Fetters L: Foundations for therapeutic intervention. In Campbell SK, editor: *Pediatric neurologic physical therapy*, New York, 1991, Churchill Livingstone, pp 19–32.

105. Fetters L: Cerebral palsy: contemporary treatment concepts. In Lister MJ, editor: *Contemporary management of motor control problems: proceedings of the II STEP Conference*, Alexandria, VA, 1991, Foundation for Physical Therapy, pp 219–224.

106. Fetters L, Todd J: Quantitative assessment of infant reaching movements, *J Mot Behav* 19:147–166, 1987.

107. Field J: Coordination of vision and prehension in young infants, *Child Dev* 48:97–103, 1977.

108. Fitts PM, Posner MI: *Human performance*, Belmont, CA, 1967, Brooks/Cole.

109. Flavell JH: *The developmental psychology of Jean Piaget*, Princeton, NJ, 1963, VanNostrand.

110. Forssberg H: Ontogeny of human locomotor control. I. Infant stepping, supported locomotion and transition to independent locomotion, *Exp Brain Res* 57:480–493, 1985.

111. Forssberg H, Nashner LM: Ontogenetic development of postural control in man: adaptation to altered support and visual conditions during stance, *J Neurosci* 2(5):545–552, 1982.

112. Forssberg H, Eliasson AC, Kinoshita H, Johansson RS, Westling G: Development of human precision grip. I. Basic coordination of force, *Exp Brain Res* 85:451–457, 1991.

113. Forssberg H, Eliasson AC, Kinoshita H, Johansson RS, Westling G: Development of human precision grip. I. Basic coordination of force, *Exp Brain Res* 85:451–457, 1991.

114. Forssberg H, Eliasson AC, Kinoshita H, Westling G, Johansson RS: Development of human precision grip. IV. Tactile adaptation of isometric finger forces to the frictional condition, *Exp Brain Res* 104:323–330, 1995.

115. Forssberg H, Kinoshita H, Eliasson AC, Johansson RS, Westling G, Gordon AM: Development of human precision grip. II. Anticipatory control of isometric forces targeted for object's weight, *Exp Brain Res* 90:393–398, 1992.

116. Forsström A, von Hofsten C: Visually directed reaching of children with motor impairments, *Dev Med Child Neurol* 24:653–661, 1982.

117. Foster EC, Sveistrup H, Woollacott MH: Transitions in visual proprioception: a cross-sectional developmental study of the effect of visual flow on postural control, *J Mot Behav* 28:101–112, 1996.

118. Foudriat BA, Di Fabio RP, Anderson JH: Sensory organization of balance responses in children 3-6 years of age: a normative study with diagnostic implications, *Int J Pediatr Otorhinolaryngol* 27(3):255–271, 1993.

119. Freedland RL, Bertenthal BI: Developmental changes in interlimb coordination: transition to hands-and-knees crawling, *Psychol Sci* 5(1):26–32, 1994.

120. Fuster JM: Executive frontal functions, *Exp Brain Res* 133:66–70, 2000.

121. Gallistel CR: *The organization of action: a new synthesis*, Hillsdale, NJ, 1980, Lawrence Erlbaum Associates.

122. Geerdink JJ, Hopkins B, Beek WJ, Heriza CB: The organization of leg movements in preterm and full-term infants after term age, *Dev Psychobiol* 29:335–351, 1996.

123. Gesell A: *Infancy and human growth*, New York, 1928, Macmillan.

124. Gesell A: *The mental growth of the pre-school child: a psychological outline of normal development from birth to the sixth year including a system of developmental diagnosis*, New York, 1928, Macmillan.

125. Gesell A: *The embryology of behavior*, New York, 1945, Harper Row.

126. Gesell A, Thompson H, Amatruda CS: *Infant behavior: its genesis and growth*, New York, 1934, McGraw-Hill.

127. Gesell A, Amatruda CS, Castner BM, Thompson H: *Biographies of child development: the mental growth careers of eighty-four infants and children*, New York, 1975, Arno Press.

128. Gesell A, Halverson HM, Thompson H, Ilg FL, Castner BM, Ames LB, Amatruda CS: *The first five years of life*, New York, 1940, Harper Row.

129. Ghez C: Voluntary movements. In Kandel ER, Schwartz JH, Jessell TM, editors: *Principles of neuroscience*, ed 3, New York, 1991, Elsevier, pp 609–625.

130. Gibson JJ: *The senses considered as perceptual systems*, Boston, 1966, Houghton-Mifflin.

131. Goldfield EC: Toward a developmental ecological psychology, *Monogr Soc Res Child Dev* 62(3):152–158, 1997.

132. Goldfield EC: Transition from rocking to crawling: postural constraints on infant movement, *Dev Psychol* 25(6):913, 1989.

133. Goldfield EC, Wolff P: A dynamical systems perspective on infant action and its development, *Theor Infant Dev* 1:3–26, 2004.

134. Goodgold-Edwards SA: Cognitive strategies during coincident timing tasks, *Phys Ther* 71:236–243, 1991.

135. Gordon AM, Forssberg H, Iwasaki N: Formation and lateralization of internal representations underlying motor commands during precision grip, *Neuropsychologia* 32:555–568, 1994.

136. Gottlieb J, Balan P, Oristaglio J, Suzuki M: Parietal control of attentional guidance: the significance of sensory motivational and motor factors, *Neurobiol Learn Mem* 91(2):121–128, 2009.

137. Grechkin TY, Chihak BJ, Cremer JF, Kearney JK, Plumert JM: Perceiving and acting on complex affordances: how children and adults bicycle across two lanes of opposing traffic, *J Exp Psychol Hum Percept Perform* 39:23–36, 2013.

138. Green EM, Mulcahy CM, Pountney TE: An investigation into the development of early postural control, *Dev Med Child Neurol* 37:437–448, 1995.

139. Guertin PA, Steuer I: Key central pattern generators of the spinal cord. A review, *J Neurosci Res* 87(11):2399–2405, 2009.

140. Haas G, Diener HC, Rapp H, Dichgans J: Development of feedback and feedforward control of upright stance, *Dev Med Child Neurol* 31:481–488, 1989.

141. Hadders-Algra M: Development of postural control during the first 18 months of life, *Neural Plasticity* 12:99–108, 2005.

142. Hadders-Algra M, Prechtl HFR: Developmental course of general movements in early infancy. I. Descriptive analysis of change in form, *Early Hum Dev* 28:201–213, 1992.

143. Hadders-Algra M, Brogren E, Forssberg H: Ontogeny of postural adjustments during sitting in infancy: variation, selection and modulation, *J Physiol* 493:273–288, 1996.

144. Hadders-Algra M, Brogren E, Forssberg H: Postural adjustment during sitting at preschool age; presence of a transient toddling phase, *Dev Med Child Neurol* 40(7):436–447, 1998.

145. Hallemans A, Dhanis L, De Clercq D, Aerts P: Changes in mechanical control of movement during the first 5 months of independent walking: a longitudinal study, *J Mot Behav* 39(3):227–238, 2007.

146. Hallemans A, Dhanis L, De Clercq D, Aerts P: Changes in mechanical control of movement during the first 5 months of independent walking: a longitudinal study, *J Mot Behav* 39(3):227–238, 2007.

147. Harabst KB, Lazarus JA, Whitall J: Accuracy of dynamic isometric force production: the influence of age and bimanual activation patterns, *Motor Control* 4:232–256, 2000.

148. Harbourne RT, Giuliani C, Mac Neela J: A kinematic and electromyographic analysis of the development of sitting posture in infants, *Dev Psychobiol* 26:51–64, 1993.

149. Harbourne RT, Stergiou N: Movement variability and the use of nonlinear tools: principles to guide physical therapist practice, *Phys Ther* 89(3):267–282, 2009.

150. Harbourne RT, Stergiou N: Nonlinear analysis of the development of sitting postural control, *Dev Psychobiol* 42(4):368–377, 2003.

151. Harbourne RT, Ryalls B, Stergiou N: Sitting and looking: a comparison of stability and visual exploration in infants with typical development and infants with motor delay, *Phys Occupat Ther Pediatr* 34(2):197–212, 2014.

152. Harbourne RT, Lobo MA, Karst GM, Galloway JC: Sit happens: does sitting development perturb reaching development or vice versa? *Infant Behav Dev* 36(3):438–450, 2013.

153. Hatzitaki V, Zisi V, Kollias I, Kioumourtzoglou E: Perceptual-motor contributions to static and dynamic balance control in children, *J Mot Behav* 34:161–170, 2002.

154. Hay L: Spatial-temporal analysis of movements in children: motor programs versus feedback in the development of reaching, *J Mot Behav* 11:188–200, 1979.

155. Hay L, Redon C: Development of postural adaptation to arm raising, *Exp Brain Res* 139:224–232, 2001.

156. Hedberg A, Forssberg H, Hadders-Algra M: Postural adjustments due to external perturbations during sitting in 1-month-old infants: evidence for the innate origin of direction specificity, *Exp Brain Res* 157:10–17, 2004.

157. Heriza C: Motor development: traditional and contemporary theories. In Lister MJ, editor: *Contemporary management of motor control problems: proceedings of the II STEP Conference*, Alexandria, VA, 1991, Foundation for Physical Therapy, pp 99–106.

158. Heriza CB: Comparison of leg movements in preterm infants at term with healthy full-term infants, *Phys Ther* 68:1687–1693, 1988.

159. Hirschfeld H, Forssberg H: Phase-dependent modulations of anticipatory postural activity during human locomotion, *Journal of Neurophysiology* 66(1):12–19, 1991.

160. Hirschfeld H, Forssberg H: Phase-dependent modulations of anticipatory postural adjustments during locomotion in children, *J Neurophysiol* 68:542–550, 1992.

161. Hirschfeld H, Forssberg H: Epigenetic development of postural responses for sitting during infancy, *Exp Brain Res* 97:528–540, 1994.

162. Hodapp M, Vry J, Mall V, Faist M: Changes in soleus H-reflex modulation after treadmill training in children with cerebral palsy, *Brain* 132 (Pt 1):37–44, 2009.

163. Holdefer RN, Miller LE: Primary motor cortical neurons encode functional muscle synergies, *Exp Brain Res* 146:233–243, 2002.

164. Holt KG, Saltzman E, Ho CL, Ulrich BD: Scaling of dynamics in the earliest stages of walking, *Phys Ther* 87(11):1458–1467, 2007.

165. Hooker D: *Evidence of prenatal function of the central nervous system in man*, New York, 1958, American Museum of Natural History.

166. Hopkins B, Westra T: Maternal expectations of their infants's development: some cultural differences, *Dev Med Child Neurol* 31:384–390, 1989.

167. Horak FB: Assumptions underlying motor control for neurologic rehabilitation. In Lister MJ, editor: *Contemporary management of motor control problems: proceedings of the II STEP Conference*, Alexandria, VA, 1991, Foundation for Physical Therapy, pp 11–27.

168. Horak FB: Postural orientation and equilibrium: what do we need to know about neural control of balance to prevent falls? Review, *Age Ageing* 35(Suppl 2):ii7–ii11, 2006.

169. Horak FB: Postural compensation for vestibular loss, *Review. Ann N Y Acad Sci* 1164:76–81, 2009.

170. Horak FB, MacPherson JM: Postural orientation and equilibrium. In Rowell LB, Sheperd JT, editors: *Handbook of physiology Section 12 exercise: regulation and integration of multiple systems*, New York, 1996, Oxford University Press, pp 255–292.

171. Horak FB, Nashner LM: Central programming of postural movements: adaptation to altered support-surface configurations, *J Neurophysiol* 55:1369–1381, 1986.

172. Horak FB, Buchanan J, Creath R, Jeka J: Vestibulospinal control of posture, *Adv Exp Med Biol* 508:139–145, 2002.

173. Hultborn H, Nielsen JB: Spinal control of locomotion—from cat to man, *Acta Physiol (Oxf)* 189(2):111–121, 2007.

174. Humphrey T: Some correlations between the appearance of human reflexes and the development of the nervous system, *Prog Brain Res* 4:93–135, 1964.

175. Inui N, Katsura Y: Development of force control and timing in a finger-tapping sequence with an attenuated-force tap, *Motor Control* 6:333–346, 2002.

176. Ivanenko YP, Dominici N, Lacquaniti F: Development of independent walking in toddlers, *Exerc Sport Sci Rev* 35(2):67–73, 2007.

177. Jakobson LS, Goodale MA: Factors affecting higher-order movement planning: a kinematic analysis of human prehension, *Experimental Brain Research* 86:199–208, 1991.

178. Jeannerod M: Intersegmental coordination during reaching at natural visual objects in infancy. In Long J, Baddeley A, editors: *Attention and performance IX*, Hillsdale, NJ, 1981, Lawrence Erlbaum Associates, pp 153–168.

179. Jeka JJ, Lackner JR: Fingertip contact influences human postural control, *Exp Brain Res* 100:495–502, 1994.

180. Jeng SF, Chen LC, Yau KI: Kinematic analysis of kicking movements in preterm infants with very low birth weight and full-term infants, *Phys Ther* 82:148–159, 2002.

181. Jeng SF, Yau KI, Chen LC, et al.: Alberta infant motor scale: reliability and validity when used on preterm infants in Taiwan, *Phys Ther* 80(2):168–178, 2000.

182. Jensen JL, Thelen E, Ulrich BD, Schneider K, Zernicke RF: Adaptive dynamics of the leg movement patterns of human infants: III. Age-related differences in limb control, *J Mot Behav* 27:366–374, 1995.

183. Jensen JL, Ulrich BD, Thelen E, Schneider K, Zernicke RF: Adaptive dynamics of the leg movement patterns of human infants: I. The effects of posture on spontaneous kicking, *J Mot Behav* 26:303–312, 1994.

184. Johansson RS, Westling G: Coordinated isometric muscle commands adequately and erroneously programmed for the weight during lifting task with precision grip, *Exp Brain Res* 71:59–71, 1988.

185. Johnston LM, Burns YR, Brauer SG, Richardson CA: Differences in postural control and movement performance during goal directed reaching in children with developmental coordination disorder, *Hum Mov Sci* 21:583–601, 2002.

186. Kanazawa H, et al.: Subcutaneous fat accumulation in early infancy is more strongly associated with motor development and delay than muscle growth, *Acta Paediatr* 103(6):e262–e267, 2014.

187. Karasik LB, Robinson S, et al.: Baby in a bind: traditional cradling practices and infant motor development, *Dev Psychobiol* 57:S19, 2015.

188. Karasik LB, Tamis-LeMonda CS, Adolph KE, Bornstein MH: Places and postures: a cross-cultural comparison of sitting in 5-month-olds, *J Cross Cult Psycho* 46:1023–1038, 2015.

189. Karniol R: The role of manual manipulative stages in the infant's acquisition of perceived control over objects, *Dev Rev* 9:205–233, 1989.

190. Katz PS, Frost WN: Intrinsic neuromodulation: altering neuronal circuits from within, *Trends Neurosc* 19:54–61, 1996.

191. Keele SW: Replies to J. J. Summers: has ecological psychology delivered what it promised? Commentary 1, programming or planning conceptions of motor control speak to different phenomena than dynamical systems conceptions. In Piek JP, editor: *Motor behavior and human skill*, Champaign, IL, 1998, Human Kinetics, pp 403–440.

192. Keogh J, Sugden D: *Movement skill development*, New York, 1985, Macmillan.

193. Keshner EA: Equilibrium and automatic postural reactions as indicators and facilitators in the treatment of balance disorders. In *Touch: topics in pediatrics (Lesson 4)*, Alexandria, VA, 1990, American Physical Therapy Association, pp 1–17.

194. Keshner EA, Campbell D, Katz R, Peterson BW: Neck muscle activation patterns in humans during isometric head stabilization, *Exp Brain Res* 75:335–364, 1989.

195. Kolobe TH: Childrearing practices and developmental expectations for Mexican-American mothers and the developmental status of their infants, *Phys Ther* 84(5):439–453, 2004.

196. Konczak J, Jansen-Osmann P, Kalveram KT: Development of force adaptation during childhood, *J Mot Behav* 35:41–52, 2003.

197. Kotwica KA, Ferre CL, Michel GF: Relation of stable hand-use preferences to the development of skill for managing multiple objects from 7 to 13 months of age, *Dev Psychobiol* 50:519–529, 2008.

198. Kubo M, Ulrich BD: Early stage of walking: development of control in mediolateral and anteroposterior directions, *J Mot Behav* 38(3):229–237, 2006.

199. Kuo AD: The six determinants of gait and the inverted pendulum analogy: a dynamic walking perspective, *Hum Mov Sci* 26(4):617–656, 2007.

200. Kupfermann I: Localization of higher cognitive and affective functions: the association cortices. In Kandel ER, Schwartz JH, Jessell TM, editors: *Principles of neuroscience*, ed 3, New York, 1991, Elsevier, pp 823–838.

201. Lampl M, Johnson ML: Infant growth in length follows prolonged sleep and increased naps, *Sleep* 34(5):641, 2011.

202. Lang CE, Bastian AJ: Cerebellar subjects show impaired adaptation of anticipatory EMG during catching, *Journal of Neurophysiology* 82(5):2108–2119, 1999.

203. Lashley KS: The accuracy of movement in the absence of excitation from the moving organ, *Am J Physiol* 43:169–194, 1917.

204. Lasky RE: The effect of visual feedback of the hand on the reaching and retrieval behavior of young infants, *Child Dev* 48:112–117, 1977.

205. Ledebt A, Blandine B, Breniere Y: The build-up of anticipatory behavior, *Exp Brain Res* 120:9–17, 1998.

206. Lee DN: The optic flow-field: the foundation of vision, *Philos Trans R Soc Lond B Biol Sci* 290:169–179, 1980.

207. Lee DN, Aronson E: Visual proprioceptive control of standing in human infants, *Percept Psychophys* 15:529–532, 1974.

208. Lee DN, Lishman JR: Visual proprioceptive control of stance, *J Hum Mov Stud* 1:87–95, 1975.

209. Lee DN, Daniel BM, Turnbull J, Cook ML: Basic perceptuo-motor dysfunctions in cerebral palsy. In Jeannerod M, editor: *Attention and performance XIII*, Hillsdale, NJ, 1990, Lawrence Erlbaum Associates, pp 583–603.

210. Lee HM, Bhat A, Scholz JP, Galloway JC: Toy-oriented changes during early arm movements IV: shoulder-elbow coordination, *Infant Behav Dev* 31(3):447–469, 2008.

211. Lee M-H, Yeou-Teh L, Newell KM: Longitudinal expressions of infant's prehension as a function of object properties, *Infant Behav Dev* 29(4):481–493, 2006.

212. Lobo MA, Harbourne RT, Dusing SC, McCoy SW: Grounding early intervention: physical therapy cannot just be about motor skills anymore, *Phys Ther* 93(1):94–103, 2013.

213. Lockman JJ, Ashmead DH, Bushnell EW: The development of anticipatory hand orientation during infancy, *J Exp Child Psychol* 37:176–186, 1984.

214. Luo HJ, Chen PS, Hsieh WS, et al.: Associations of supported treadmill stepping with walking attainment in preterm and full-term infants, *Phys Ther* 89(11):1215–1225, 2009.

215. MacKay-Lyons M: Central pattern generation of locomotion: a review of the evidence, *Phys Ther* 82:69–83, 2002.

216. Majnemer A, Barr RG: Influence of supine sleep positioning on early motor milestone acquisition, *Dev Med Child Neurol* 47(06):370–376, 2005.

217. Malone JC, James William, Skinner BF: Behaviorism, reinforcement, and interest, *Behaviorism* 140–151, 1975.

218. Malouin F, Richards CL: Preparatory adjustments during gait initiation in 4 6-year-old children, *Gait Posture* 11:239–253, 2000.

219. Mandich A, Buckolz E, Polatajko H: Children with developmental coordination disorder (DCD) and their ability to disengage ongoing attentional focus: more on inhibitory function, *Brain and Cognition* 51(3):346–356, 2003.

220. Marchal-Crespo L, Reinkensmeyer DJ: Review of control strategies for robotic movement training after neurologic injury, *J Neuroeng Rehabil* 6:20, 2009.

221. Marder E, Rehm KJ: Development of central pattern generating circuits, *Curr Opin Neurobiol* 15(1):86–93, 2005.

222. Massion J: Movement, posture and equilibrium: interaction and coordination, *Prog Neurobiol* 38:35–56, 1992.

223. Mayr E: Darwin's influence on modern thought, *Sci Am* 283(1):66–71, 2000.

224. McCarty ME, et al.: How infants use vision for grasping objects, *Child Dev* 72(4):973–987, 2001.

225. McComas J, Dulberg C, Latter J: Children's memory for locations visited: importance of movement and choice, *J Mot Behav* 29:223–229, 1997.

226. McGraw MB: *The neuromuscular maturation of the human infant*, New York, 1945, Hafner Press.

227. Morgan C, Novak I, Dale RC, Badawi N: Optimising motor learning in infants at high risk of cerebral palsy: a pilot study, *BMC Pediatr* 15(1):30, 2015.

228. Mouchnino L, Aurenty R, Massion J, Pedotti A: Coordinated control of posture and equilibrium during leg movement. In Brandt T, Paulus W, Bles W, et al.: *Disorders of posture and gait*, Stuttgart, 1990, Georg Thieme, pp 68–71.

229. Mui JW, Willis KL, Hao ZZ, Berkowitz A: Distributions of active spinal cord neurons during swimming and scratching motor patterns, *J Comp Physiol A Neuroethol Sens Neural Behav Physiol* 198:877–889, 2012.

230. Nakata H, Kyonosuke Y: Automatic postural response systems in individuals with congenital total blindness, *Gait Posture* 14(1):36–43, 2001.

231. Nashner LM, Forssberg H: Phase-dependent organization of postural adjustments associated with arm movements while walking, *J Neurophysiol* 55:1382–1394, 1986.

232. Newell KM, McDonald PV, Baillargeon R: Body scale and infant grip configurations, *Dev Psychobiol* 26:195–205, 1993.

233. Nickel LR, et al.: Posture development in infants at heightened versus low risk for autism spectrum disorders, *Infancy* 18(5):639–661, 2013.

234. Noble Y, Boyd R: Neonatal assessments for the preterm infant up to 4 months corrected age: a systematic review, *Dev Med Child Neurol* 54(2):129–139, 2012.

235. Norrlin S, Dahl M, Rösblad B: Control of reaching movements in children and young adults with myelomeningocele, *Dev Med Child Neurol* 46(1):28–33, 2004.

236. Okamoto T, Okamoto K: Electromyographic characteristics at the onset of independent walking in infancy, *Electromyogr Clin Neurophysiol* 41:33–41, 2001.

237. Oppenheim RW: Ontogenetic adaptations and retrogressive processes in the development of the nervous system and behavior: a neuroembryological perspective. In Connolly K, Prechtl HFR, editors: *Maturation and development: biological and psychological perspectives*, Philadelphia, 1981, JB Lippincott, pp 73–109.

238. Oztop E, Bradley NS, Arbib MA: Infant grasp learning: a computational model, *Exp Brain Res* 180:480–503, 2004.

239. Palluel E, Ceyte H, Olivier I, Nougier V: Anticipatory postural adjustments associated with a forward leg raising in children: effects of age, segmental acceleration and sensory context, *Clin Neurophysiol* 119(11):2546–2554, 2008.

240. Pang MY, Yang JF: Sensory gating for the initiation of the swing phase in different directions of human infant stepping, *Journal of Neuroscience* 22:5734–5740, 2002.

241. Pang MY, Lam T, Yang JF: Infants adapt their stepping to repeated trip-inducing stimuli, *J Neurophysiol* 90:2731–2740, 2003.

242. Pate RR, McIver K, Dowda M, Brown WH, Addy C: Directly observed physical activity levels in preschool children, *J Sch Health* 78:438–444, 2008.

243. Pellegrini AD, Smith PK: Physical activity play: the nature and function of a neglected aspect of play, *Child Dev* 69:577–598, 1998.

244. Perham H, Smick JE, Hallum A, Nordstrom T: Development of the lateral equilibrium reaction in stance, *Dev Med Child Neurol* 29:758–765, 1987.

245. Phillips JP, Sullivan KJ, Burtner PA, Caprihan A, Provost B, Bernitsky-Beddingfield A: Ankle dorsiflexion fMRI in children with cerebral palsy undergoing intensive body-weight-supported treadmill training: a pilot study, *Dev Med Child Neurol* 49(1):39–44, 2007.

246. Piaget J: *The origins of intelligence in children*, New York, 1952, International Universities Press.

247. Pick Jr HL, Gibson EJ: Learning to perceive and perceiving to learn, *Dev Psychol* 28:787–794, 1992.

248. Piontelli A: *Development of normal fetal movements*, New York, 2014, Springer.

249. Plimpton CE, Regimbal C: Differences in motor proficiency according to gender and race, *Perceptual and Motor Skills* 74:399–402, 1992.

250. Polit A, Bizzi E: Characteristics of motor programs underlying arm movements in monkeys, *J Neurophysiol* 42:183–194, 1979.

251. Portfors-Yeomans CV, Riach CL: Frequency characteristics of postural control of children with and without visual impairment, *Dev Med Child Neurol* 37:456–463, 1995.

252. Prado EL, Dewey KG: Nutrition and brain development in early life, *Nutr Rev* 72(4):267–284, 2014.

253. Prechtl HFR, Cioni G, Einspieler C, Bos AF, Ferrari F: Role of vision on early motor development: lessons from the blind, *Dev Med Child Neurol* 43:198–201, 2001.

254. Prechtl HFR, Heinz FR: General movement assessment as a method of developmental neurology: new paradigms and their consequences The 1999 Ronnie MacKeith Lecture, *Dev Med Child Neurol* 43(12):836–842, 2001.

255. Prilutsky BI, Gregor RJ: Swing- and support-related muscle actions differentially trigger human walk-run and run-walk transitions, *J Exp Biol* 204:2277–2287, 2001.

256. Provost B: Normal development from birth to 4 months: extended use of the NBAS-K. Part II, *Phys Occupat Ther Pediatri* 1(3):19–34, 1981.

257. Rabin E, DiZio P, Ventura J, Lackner JR: Influences of arm proprioception and degrees of freedom on postural control with light touch feedback, *J Neurophysiol* 99:595–604, 2004.

258. Raibert MH: *Motor control and learning by the state-space. Tech. Rep. AI-TR-439*, Cambridge, MA, 1977, Massachusetts Institute of Technology. Artificial Intelligence Laboratory.

259. Ratner HH, Foley MA: A unifying framework for the development of children's activity memory, *Adv Child Dev Behav* 25:33–105, 1994.

260. Riach CL, Hayes KC: Maturation of postural sway in young children, *Dev Med Child Neurol* 29(5):650–658, 1987.

261. Roberton MA, Halverson LE: *Developing children: their changing movement. A guide for teachers*, Philadelphia, 1984, Lea Febiger.

262. Robertson Ringenbach SD, Chua R, Maraj BK, Kao JC, Weeks DJ: Bimanual coordination dynamics in adults with Down syndrome, *Motor Control* 6:388–407, 2002.

263. Robertson SS, Johnson SL, Masnick AM, Weiss SL: Robust coupling of body movement and gaze in young infants, *Dev Psychobiol* 49:208–215, 2007.

264. Robinson SR, Kleven GA, Brumley MR: Prenatal development of interlimb motor learning in the rat fetus, *Infancy* 13:204–228, 2008.

265. Rocha NA, Silva FP, Tudella E: The impact of object size and rigidity on infant reaching, *Infant Behav Devt* 29:251–261, 2006.

266. Romeo DMM, et al.: Neuromotor development in infants with cerebral palsy investigated by the Hammersmith Infant Neurological Examination during the first year of age, *Eur J Paediatr Neurol* 12(1):24–31, 2008.

267. Roncesvalles NC, Woollacott MH, Jensen JL: Development of compensatory stepping skills in children, *J Mot Behav* 32:100–111, 2000.

268. Rosenbaum DA: *Human motor control*, San Diego, CA, 1991, Academic Press.

269. Rosenbaum P: Physical activity play in children with disabilities: a neglected opportunity for research? *Child Dev* 69:607–608, 1998.

270. Rossignol S, Drew T: Phasic modulation of reflexes during rhythmic activity. In Grillner S, Stein PSG, Stuart DG, Forssberg H, Herman RM, editors: *Neurobiology of vertebrate locomotion*, London, 1986, Macmillan, pp 517–534.

271. Safe to Sleep: Website. Available at: https://www.nichd.nih.gov/sts/Pages/default.aspx.

272. Sanes JN, Dimitrov B, Hallett M: Motor learning in patients with cerebellar dysfunction, *Brain* 113:103–120, 1990.

273. Savelsbergh GJ, van der Kamp J: The effect of body orientation to gravity on early infant reaching, *J Exp Child Psychol* 58(3):510–528, 1994.

274. Schellekens JMH, Scholten CA, Kalverboer AF: Visually guided hand movements in children with minor neurological dysfunction: response time and movement organization, *J Child Psychol Psychiatry* 24:89–102, 1983.

275. Schmidt RA: A schema theory of discrete motor skill learning, *Psychol Rev* 82:225–260, 1975.

276. Schmidt RA, Lee TD: *Motor control and learning: a behavioral emphasis*, ed 3, Champaign, IL, 1998, Human Kinetics.

277. Schmidt RA, Lee TD: *Motor control and learning: a behavioral emphasis*, Champaign, IL, 2005, Human Kinetics.

278. Schmitz C, Martin N, Assaiante C: Building anticipatory postural adjustment during childhood: a kinematic and electromyographic analysis of unloading in children from 4 to 8 years of age, *Exp Brain Res* 142:354–364, 2002.

279. Schöpf V, et al.: The relationship between eye movement and vision develops before birth, *Frontiers in human neuroscience* 8, 2014.

280. Seidler RD, Bernard JA, Burutolu TB, et al.: Motor control and aging: links to age-related brain structural, functional, and biochemical effects, *Neurosci Biobehav Rev* 34:721–733, 2010.

281. Seitz RJ, Stephan KM, Binkofski F: Control of action as mediated by the human frontal lobe, *Exp Brain Res* 133:71–80, 2000.

282. Shafir T, et al.: "Iron deficiency and infant motor development." *Early Hum Dev* 84(7):479–485, 2008.

283. Shea CH, Wulf G: Schema theory: a critical appraisal and reevaluation, *J Mot Behav* 37(2):85–101, 2005.

284. Sherrington CS: *The integrative action of the nervous system*, New Haven, 1947, Yale University Press (original work published 1906).

285. Shirley MM: *The first two years: a study of twenty-five babies. Vol. I. Postural and locomotor development*, Minneapolis, MN, 1931, University of Minnesota Press.

286. Shumway-Cook A, Woollacott MH: *Motor control: translating research into clinical practice*, ed 4, Philadelphia, 2011, Lippincott, Williams, Watkins.

287. Shumway-Cook A, Woollacott M: The growth of stability: postural control from a development perspective, *J Mot Behav* 17:131–147, 1985.

288. Shumway-Cook A, Woollacott M: *Motor control theory and practical applications*, Baltimore, 2001, Lippincott Williams Wilkins.

289. Slining M, et al.: Infant overweight is associated with delayed motor development, *J Pediatr* 157(1):20–25, 2010.

290. Smith L, Gasser M: The development of embodied cognition: six lessons from babies, *Artif Life* 11(1-2):13–29, 2005.

291. Smyth MM, Anderson HI, Churchill A: Visual information and the control of reaching in children: a comparison between children with and without developmental coordination disorder, *J Mot Behav* 33:306–320, 2001.

292. Soska KC, Adolph KE, Johnson SP: Systems in development: motor skill acquisition facilitates three-dimensional object completion, *Dev Psychol* 46(1):129, 2010.

293. Sparling JW, editor: *Concepts in fetal movement research*, New York, 1993, Haworth Press.

294. Sparling JW, Van Tol J, Chescheir NC: Fetal and neonatal hand movement, *Phys Ther* 79(1):24–39, 1999.

295. Sparto PJ, Furman JM, Redfern MS: Head sway response to optic flow: effect of age is more important than the presence of unilateral vestibular hypofunction, *J Vestib Res* 16(3):137–145, 2006.

296. Spittle AJ, Orton J: Cerebral palsy and developmental coordination disorder in children born preterm, *Semin Fetal and Neonatal Med* 19(2):84–89, 2014.

297. Spittle A, Orton J, Anderson PJ, Boyd R, Doyle LW: Early developmental intervention programmes provided post hospital discharge to prevent motor and cognitive impairment in preterm infants, *Cochrane Database Syst Rev* 11:CD005495, 2015.

298. Sporns O, Edelman GM: Solving Bernstein's problem: a proposal for the development of coordinated movement by selection, *Child Dev* 64:960–981, 1993.

299. Steenbergen B, Hulstijn W, Lemmens IHL, Meulenbroek RGJ: The timing of prehensile movements in subjects with cerebral palsy, *Dev Med Child Neurol* 40:108–114, 1998.

300. Stendl R, Kunz K, Schrott-Fischer A, Sholtz AW: Effect of age and sex on maturation of sensory systems and balance control, *Dev Med Child Neurol* 48:477–482, 2006.

301. Stoffregen TA, Adolph K, Thelen E, Gorday KM, Sheng YY: Toddlers' postural adaptations to different support surfaces, *Motor Control* 1:119–137, 1997.

302. St-Onge N, Feldman AG: Interjoint coordination in lower limbs during different movements in humans, *Exp Brain Res* 148:139–149, 2003.

303. Sullivan MC, et al.: Refining neurobehavioral assessment of the high-risk infant using the NICU Network Neurobehavioral Scale, *J Obst Gynecol Neonatal Nurs* 41(1):17–23, 2012.

304. Summers JJ, Anson JG: Current status of the motor program: revisited, *Hum Mov Sci* 28(5):566–577, 2009.

305. Sundermier L, Woollacott MH: The influence of vision on the automatic postural muscle responses of newly standing and newly walking infants, *Exp Brain Res* 120:537–540, 1998.

306. Sutherland DH, Olshen RA, Biden EN, Wyatt MP: The development of mature walking, *Clin Developmental Med* 104/105:1–227, 1988.

307. Sutherland DH, Olshen R, Cooper L, Woo SL: The development of mature gait, *J Bone Joint Surg* 62:336–353, 1980.

308. Sveistrup H, Schneiberg S, McKinley PA, et al.: Head, arm and trunk coordination during reaching in children, *Exp Brain Res* 188(2):237–247, 2008.

309. Sveistrup H, Woollacott MH: Longitudinal development of the automatic postural response in infants, *J Mot Behav* 28:58–70, 1996.

310. Taub E, Berman AJ: Movement and learning in the absence of sensory feedback. In Freedman SJ, editor: *The neuropsychology of spatially oriented behavior*, Homewood, IL, 1968, Dorsey Press, pp 173–192.

311. Thelen E: Coupling perception and action in the development of skill: a dynamic approach. In Bloch H, Bertenthal BI, editors: *Sensory-motor organization and development in infancy and early childhood*, Dordrecht, Netherlands, 1990, Kluwer Academic, pp 39–56.

312. Thelen E: Motor development. A new synthesis, *Am Psychol* 50:79–95, 1995.

313. Thelen E: Time-scale dynamics and the development of an embodied cognition. In Port RF, vanGelder T, editors: *Mind as motion: explorations in the dynamics of cognition*, Cambridge, MA, 1995, MIT Press, pp 69–100.

314. Thelen E, Adolph KE, Gesell AL: The paradox of nature and nurture, *Dev Psychol* 28:368–380, 1992.

315. Thelen E, Fisher DM, Ridley-Johnson R: The relationship between physical growth and a newborn reflex, *Infant Behavior Development* 7:479–493, 1984.

316. Thelen E, Fisher DM, Ridley-Johnson R, Griffin NJ: Effects of body build and arousal on newborn infant stepping, *Dev Psychobiol* 15:447–453, 1982.

317. Thelen E, Ulrich BD, Jensen JL: The developmental origins of locomotion. In Woollacott MH, Shumway-Cook A, editors: *Development of posture and gait across the life span*, Columbia, SC, 1989, University of South Carolina Press, pp 23–47.

318. Thelen E, Corbetta D, Kamm K, Spencer JP, Schneider K, Zernicke RF: The transition to reaching: mapping intention and intrinsic dynamics, *Child Dev* 64(4):1058–1098, 1993.

319. Touwen BCL: Primitive reflexes—Conceptual or semantic problem? *Clin Developmental Med* 94:115–125, 1984.

320. Ulrich BD, Jensen JL, Thelen E, Schneider K, Zernicke RF: Adaptive dynamics of the leg movement patterns of human infants: II. Treadmill stepping in infants and adults, *J Mot Behav* 26:313–332, 1994.

321. Ulrich DA, Ulrich BD, Angulo-Kinzler RM, Yun J: Treadmill training of infants with Down syndrome: evidence-based developmental outcomes, *Pediatrics* 108:E84, 2001.

322. Umphred DA, Byl N, Lazaro RT, Roller ML: Chapter 9 Interventions for clients with movement. In Umphred DA, et al, editors: *Neurological rehabilitation*, ed 6, St. Louis, 2013, Elsevier Health Sciences, p 191.

323. Usui N, Maekawa K, Hirasawa Y: Development of the upright postural sway of children, *Dev Med Child Neurol* 37:985–996, 1995.

324. Valvano J, Newell KM: Practice of a precision isometric grip-force task by children with spastic cerebral palsy, *Dev Med Child Neurol* 40:464–473, 1998.

325. van der Fits IB, Hadders-Algra M: The development of postural response patterns during reaching in healthy infants, *Neurosci Biobehav Rev* 22(4):521–526, 1998.

326. van der Heide JC, Otten B, van Eykern LA, Hadders-Algra M: Development of postural adjustments during reaching in sitting children, *Exp Brain Res* 151(1):32–45, 2003.

327. van der Meer AL: Keeping the arm in the limelight: advanced visual control of arm movements in neonates, *Eur J Paediatr Neurol* 1(4):103–108, 1997.

328. van der Meer ALH, van der Weel FR, Lee DN: Prospective control in catching by infants, *Perception* 23:287–302, 1994.

329. van der Meer ALH, van der Weel FR, Lee DN: The functional significance of arm movements in neonates, *Science* 267:693–695, 1995.

330. van der Meulen JHP, Vandergon JJD, Gielen CCA, Gooskens RHJ, Willemse J: Visuomotor performance of normal and clumsy children. 1. Fast goal-directed arm-movements with and without visual feedback, *Dev Med Child Neurol* 33:40–54, 1991.

331. van der Meulen JHP, Vandergon JJD, Gielen CCA, Gooskens RHJ, Willemse J: Visuomotor performance of normal and clumsy children. 2. Arm-tracking with and without visual feedback, *Dev Med Child Neurol* 33:118–129, 1991.

332. van der Weel FR, van der Meer ALH, Lee DH: Effect of task on movement control in cerebral palsy: implications for assessment and therapy, *Dev Med Child Neurol* 33:419–426, 1991.

333. Vereijken B, Pedersen AV, Storksen JH: Early independent walking: a longitudinal study of load perturbation effects, *Dev Psychobiol* 51(4):374–383, 2009.

334. Viviani P, Mounoud P: Perceptuomotor compatibility in pursuit tracking of two-dimensional movements, *J Mot Behav* 22:407–443, 1990.

335. von Hofsten C: Development of visually guided reaching: the approach phase, *J Hum Move Studies* 5:160–178, 1979.

336. Reference deleted in proofs.

337. von Hofsten C: Eye-hand coordination in the newborn, *Dev Psychol* 18:450–461, 1982.

338. von Hofsten C: Developmental changes in the organization of prereaching movements, *Dev Psychol* 20:378–388, 1984.

339. Reference deleted in proofs.

340. von Hofsten C: Structuring of early reaching movements: a longitudinal study, *J Mot Behav* 23:280–292, 1991.

341. Von Hofsten C: Action in development, *Dev Sci* 10:54–60, 2007.

342. von Hofsten C, Fazel-Zandy S: Development of visually guided hand orientation in reaching, *J Exp Child Psychol* 38:208–219, 1984.

343. von Hofsten C, Rönnqvist L: Preparation for grasping an object: a developmental study, *J Exp Psychol Hum Percept Perform* 14:610–621, 1988.

344. von Hofsten C, Rönnqvist L: The structuring of neonatal arm movements, *Child Dev* 64:1046–1057, 1993.

345. von Hofsten C, Vishton P, Spelke ES, Feng Q, Rosander K: Predictive action in infancy: tracking and reaching for moving objects, *Cognition* 67(3):255–285, 1998.

346. Voss MW, et al.: Exercise, brain, and cognition across the life span, *J Appl Physiol* 111(5):1505–1513, 2011.

347. Vygotsky LS: The instrumental method in psychology. In Wertsch JV, editor: *The concept of activity in Soviet psychology*, Armonk, NY, 1981, ME Sharpe.

348. Vygotsky LS: Interaction between learning and development, *Readings Dev Child* 23:34–41, 1978.

349. Reference deleted in proofs.

350. Wallace PS, Whishaw IQ: Independent digit movements and precision grip patterns in 1-5-month-old human infants: hand-babbling, including vacuous then self-directed hand and digit movements, precedes targeted reaching, *Neuropsychologia* 41(14):1912–1918, 2003.

351. Westcott SL, Zaino CA: Comparison and development of postural muscle activity in children during stand and reach from firm and compliant surfaces, *Soc Neurosci Abstr* 23:1565, 1997.

352. WHO Multicentre Growth Reference Study Group: WHO motor development study: windows of achievement for six gross motor development milestones, *Acta Paediatrica* (Suppl 450) 86–95, 2006.

353. Willoughby KL, Dodd KJ, Shields N: A systematic review of the effectiveness of treadmill training for children with cerebral palsy, *Disabil Rehabil* 31(24):1971–1979, 2009.

354. Winstein CJ, Horak FB, Fisher BE: Influence of central set on anticipatory and triggered grip-force adjustments, *Exp Brain Res* 130:298–308, 2000.

355. Wishart JG, Bower TGR, Dunked J: Reaching in the dark, *Perception* 7:507–512, 1978.

356. Witherington DC, von Hofsten C, Rosander K, Robinette A, Woollacott MH, Bertenthal BI: The development of anticipatory postural adjustments in infancy, *Infancy* 3:495–517, 2002.

357. Wong S, Chan K, Wong V, Wong W: Use of chopsticks in Chinese children, *Child Care Health Dev* 28:157–161, 2002.

358. Woollacott M, Debu B, Mowatt M: Neuromuscular control of posture in the infant and child, *J Mot Behav* 19:167–186, 1987.

359. Woollacott MH, Shumway-Cook A: Changes in posture control across the life span: a systems approach, *Phys Ther* 70(12):799–807, 1990.

360. Wu J, Looper J, Ulrich BD, Ulrich DA, Angulo-Barroso RM: Exploring effects of different treadmill interventions on walking onset and gait patterns in infants with Down syndrome, *Dev Med Child Neurol* 49(11):839–845, 2007.

361. Yang JF, Stephens MJ, Vishram R: Transient disturbances to one limb produce coordinated, bilateral responses during infant stepping, *J Neurophysiol* 79:2329–2337, 1998.

362. Yonas A, Bechtold AG, Frankel D, Gordon FR, McRoberts G, Norcia A, Sternfels S: Development of sensitivity to information for impending collision, *Percept Psychophys* 21:97–104, 1977.

363. Zentgraf K, Green N, Munzert J, et al.: How are actions physically implemented? *Prog Brain Res* 174:303–318, 2009.

364. Zernicke RF, Smith JS: Biomechanical insights into neural control of movement. In Rowell LB, Sheperd JT, editors: *Handbook of physiology section 12 exercise: regulation and integration of multiple systems*, New York, 1996, Oxford University Press, pp 293–330.

365. Zoia S, Castiello U, Blason L, et al.: Reaching in children with and without developmental coordination disorder under normal and perturbed vision, *Dev Neuropsychol* 27(2):257–273, 2005.

366. Zwicker JG1, Harris SR: A reflection on motor learning theory in pediatric occupational therapy practice, *Can J Occup Ther* 76:29–37, 2009.

SUGGESTED READINGS

Adolph KE, Robinson SR: Motor development. In Lerner RM, series editor; Liben L, Muller U, volume editors: *Handbook of child psychology and developmental science: vol. 2: cognitive processes.* ed 7, New York: Wiley, 2015. pp 114–157.

Berger SE: Locomotor expertise predicts infants' perseverative errors, *Dev Psychol* 46:326, 2010.

Corbetta D, Snapp-Childs W: Seeing and touching: the role of sensory-motor experience on the development of infant reaching, *Infant Behav Dev* 32(1):44–58, 2009.

De Vries JIP, Fong BF: Normal fetal motility: an overview, *Ultrasound Obstet Gynecol* 27(6):701–711, 2006.

Dusing SC, Harbourne RT: Variability in postural control during infancy: implications for development, assessment, and intervention, *Phys Ther* 90(12):1838–1849, 2010.

Lobo MA, Harbourne RT, Dusing SC, McCoy SW: Grounding early intervention: physical therapy cannot just be about motor skills anymore, *Phys Ther* 93(1):94–103, 2013.

Smith L, Gasser M: The development of embodied cognition: six lessons from babies, *Artif Life* 11(1-2):13–29, 2005.

Spittle A, Orton J, Anderson PJ, Boyd R, Doyle LW: Early developmental intervention programmes provided post hospital discharge to prevent motor and cognitive impairment in preterm infants, *Cochrane Database Syst Rev* 11:CD005495, 2015.

Thelen E: Motor development. A new synthesis, *Am Psychol* 50:79–95, 1995.

Von Hofsten C: Action in development, *Dev Sci* 10:54–60, 2007.

Woollacott M, Assaiante C: Developmental changes in compensatory responses to unexpected resistance of leg lift during gait initiation, *Experimental brain research* 144(3):385–396, 2002.

4

Motor Learning: Application of Principles to Pediatric Rehabilitation

Andrew M. Gordon, Richard Magill

Increasingly, physical therapists are recognizing that effective training of motor function in children requires motor learning. Children need to be active learners to problem-solve how to accomplish a specific task, given their constraints.[2] Such task-oriented approaches[20] are becoming the predominant type of treatment in adult therapy. An important difference among children with disabilities, however, is that unlike adults, children are rarely trying to regain function, and thus they do not have a motor image of how the task should be performed. Rather, their learning must occur in the context of development, whereby age-appropriate skills must be learned for the first time. Such learning can be considered as part of a triad consisting of the person, the task (i.e., skill or activity), and the environmental context in which the child performs the task.

This chapter first discusses this triad and how it applies to adult motor learning, as well as the relevant learning principles derived from studies of adults without disabilities. Specifically, we discuss taxonomies of motor skills in relation to skill progression, types of knowledge gained during motor learning, different types and stages of learning, methods of instructions, feedback types and frequency, types of practice schedules, variability and specificity of training with whole and part practice, and benefits of mental practice. This information provides important theory and context for the training of motor skills in children. Oddly, there is a dearth of good studies on motor learning in typically developing children. We review what is known about motor learning in children and how learning in children may differ from that in adults. We discuss the implications of reduced information-processing capabilities and processing/memory in children and the implications for feedback, along with the type and amount of practice, and will show that skill emerges over enormous amounts of practice and extensive time periods. We continue by discussing the limited research on motor learning in pediatric rehabilitation, with emphasis on cerebral palsy (CP), the most common type of pediatric physical disability. We show that contrary to older notions, CP is not static, but rather motor function improves with development and practice. We provide examples of how intensity matters, models for providing intensive, task-oriented approaches (e.g., constraint-induced movement therapy, bimanual training), and information on how tasks and the environment can be used to optimize learning. We describe the importance of training specificity and provide important clues from the neuroscience literature on how to take advantage of and maximize neuroplasticity. Among these is the fact that neuroplasticity is enhanced when the tasks are meaningful to the performer. Increasingly, this means using video gaming to maintain salience and motivation and to target specific motor impairments. It is suggested that motor learning in the context of gaming can be an important complement to, but not a replacement for, salient task-oriented activities in the real world. Finally, we discuss gaps in the existing knowledge and project where pediatric rehabilitation research needs to be directed to fully incorporate motor learning into practice.

MOTOR LEARNING PRINCIPLES

One way to address the many complexities of the therapist–patient interaction is to consider principles on which to base decisions that must be made during this interaction. One set of principles relevant to this situation relates to learning processes that underlie physical rehabilitation. Patients present not only specific motor skill capabilities and limitations when they initially engage the services of a physical therapist but also future movement goals. The therapist is confronted with the need to determine a plan of action to enable the patient to attain achievable goals given the individual's capabilities and limitations. Implicit in this plan is an understanding of learning processes as they relate to the learning or relearning of motor skills. Accordingly, this section of the chapter provides a foundation on which the therapist can establish knowledge of these processes and apply that knowledge to developing and implementing effective intervention strategies.

Basic Assumptions
General Influences on the Learning of Motor Skills

When a person attempts to learn or relearn a motor skill, at least three sets of characteristics influence that process: the person, the task (i.e., skill or activity), and the environmental context in which the person performs the task (Fig. 4.1). These characteristics interact in ways that influence not only motor skill learning and performance but also the effectiveness of therapeutic intervention strategies. For the physical therapist, this interactive model should provide support for the view that

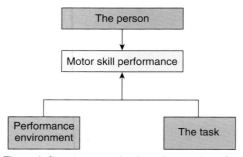

FIG. 4.1 Three influences on the learning and performance of motor skills.

there can be no "one size fits all" approach to creating interventions. As therapists are keenly aware, patients (the "person" part of the model) differ in their capabilities and limitations. However, the intervention planning process for a child must also incorporate specific characteristics of the skills or activities developed and the environmental contexts in which those skills will be performed.

Categories and Taxonomies of Motor Skills

Because the motor skill itself plays an important role in the learning and relearning process, it is important to understand key characteristics of motor skills that influence this process. Several categorization and taxonomy schemes have been developed to identify characteristics of motor skills that make them distinct or similar.[102] The taxonomy that is most relevant to physical therapy is one developed in the United States by A.M. Gentile at Teachers College, Columbia University, which was based on the view that certain characteristics of motor skills place different types and quantities of attention and motor control demands on the person.[57] The full taxonomy consists of the interrelationship of four general characteristics of skills. Rather than discuss all of these categories, we consider only three of the four general characteristics of skills that are especially relevant to the purposes of this chapter.

The first two characteristics concern the environmental context (i.e., all the components of the location and situation in which the skill is performed, such as the supporting surface, objects, and other people). The first of these relates to *whether the skill's regulatory conditions are stationary or in motion.* Gentile defined *regulatory conditions* as those features of the environmental context that specify the movement characteristics needed to achieve the skill's performance goal (note that Gentile used the term *action* goal).[57] Because a person could achieve a specific performance goal with different movement characteristics, the regulatory conditions specify the movement characteristics required to achieve the performance goal in a specific situation. For example, the regulatory conditions associated with walking from one location to another include the surface on which the child walks and the objects or other people in the pathway. These environmental context features influence the person's walking behavior by requiring him or her to alter certain movements to walk from one location to another. Consider, for example, how your movements differ when you walk on a concrete sidewalk, a sandy beach, a moving bus, or a treadmill. Also consider how your movements differ when you walk alone compared to when you walk on a sidewalk that is filled with people walking in various directions and at different speeds. As these examples illustrate, the regulatory conditions of the performance environment influence walking behavior in considerably different ways, depending on the specific characteristic of the regulatory condition and whether or not the regulatory condition is stationary or in motion. Skills for which the regulatory conditions are stationary are commonly referred to as *closed skills*, and skills for which the regulatory conditions are in motion are commonly referred to as *open skills*.

The second general characteristic of a motor skill concerns whether the regulatory conditions are the same or different on successive repetitions of performing the skill. Gentile referred to this characteristic as *intertrial variability*.[57] If the regulatory conditions are the same on successive repetitions, the skill has no intertrial variability. For example, stepping up a series of stair steps when each step is the same height requires repetitions of stepping with each repetition occurring in a performance context in which the regulatory conditions are the same for each repetition. In contrast, if the regulatory conditions are different on successive repetitions, the skill is classified as having intertrial variability. For example, when we drink a glass of water, each successive drink (i.e., repetition) removes some water from the glass, which means that the amount of water in the glass changes on each trial. Although both stair-stepping skills and drinking skills are similar because each is a closed skill, they differ in the demands placed on the performer on succeeding repetitions of the skill. The skill with no intertrial variability (stair-stepping) requires the person to simply repeat each trial's movement characteristics, but the skill with intertrial variability (drinking from a glass) requires the person to adjust specific movement characteristics on each repetition.

The third general characteristic is *whether or not an object must be manipulated* when performing the skill. The same motor skill can place distinctly different attention and motor control demands on the child simply by adding or taking away an object as part of the performance requirement. Consider, for example, the different attention and motor control demands of walking on a sidewalk while carrying or not carrying a book bag.

Gentile organized the taxonomy on the basis of the complexity of each skill.[57] She defined complexity in terms of the amount of attention and motor control demands the skill places on the person performing the skill. The simplest skill, which is the closed skill with no intertrial variability and no object to manipulate, involves the lowest number of these demands. Skill complexity increases with the addition of intertrial variability or an object to manipulate. Because of its systematic basis for identifying the complexity level of a skill, the taxonomy has practical value to the physical therapist. One use of the taxonomy is as a guide for evaluating a patient's movement capabilities and limitations. Another use is for systematically selecting a progression of activities to improve a child's functional capabilities.

Types of Knowledge Acquired During Learning

Learning of motor skills involves the acquisition of two types of knowledge: *explicit* (sometimes referred to as *declarative, or "what to do"*) and *implicit* (sometimes referred to as *procedural, or "how to do" a skill*).[56,57] These types of knowledge are commonly assessed on the basis of how accurately a person can verbally describe the knowledge. For example, if you were asked to provide evidence that you know how to tie your shoes, you could verbally describe how you do it, or you could physically tie them. The verbal description indicates an explicit knowledge of the skill of shoe tying. But if you had difficulty giving this verbal description, it could not be concluded that you do not know how to tie your shoes. Your knowledge may be in an implicit form and therefore difficult, if not impossible, to verbally describe. Evidence of this implicit knowledge of shoe tying would be revealed by physically performing the skill. Although some learning theorists typically view knowledge of how to perform a motor skill as implicit, or procedural, this view is too narrow to present a complete understanding of the knowledge structure underlying motor skill learning. In fact, motor skills involve the acquisition of both explicit and implicit knowledge.[160] Some researchers argue that the acquisition of explicit knowledge precedes that of implicit knowledge; others contend that the two types of knowledge are acquired simultaneously but that certain skill characteristics are acquired explicitly or implicitly.[56,160] Clear evidence that they are separate comes from object rotation experiments. Subjects learn to grasp and lift an object with a symmetrical appearance but whose mass distribution is actually asymmetrical within one or two consecutive lifts by partitioning fingertip load forces asymmetrically before lift-off.[6,131,132] This involves learning to generate a compensatory moment in the opposite direction of the external moment, thus preventing object roll. However, despite subjects' explicit knowledge of the new center of mass (CM) location following object rotation, as determined by verbal cuing, they fail to generate a compensatory moment, resulting in object roll.[6,131,132,170] It is interesting to note that over repeated object rotations and lifts, subjects do reduce object roll through modulation of digit placement along the vertical axis (e.g., thumb lower than index finger when the center of mass is on the left side) but not tangential forces.[170] Thus the explicit knowledge influences the modulation of grasping kinematics but not kinetics. Much remains to be understood about these types of knowledge and their relationship to the skill learning process, but as explored later in the chapter, the type of knowledge acquired has implications for several aspects of the therapist–patient interaction.

Stages of Learning

An important characteristic of the motor skill learning process is that people go through distinct stages, or phases, as they learn. Although several models have been proposed to identify and describe these stages,[102] we consider here one that is especially relevant to physical therapy. Gentile proposed a model of skill learning involving two stages.[54,55,57] The first, which Gentile called the *initial stage,* involves the learner attempting to attain some degree of success at achieving the performance goal of the skill. To do this, the person develops movement characteristics that match the regulatory conditions of the skill. In addition, the person acquires a basic movement coordination pattern that results in reasonably successful achievement of the skill's performance goal, which means that the goal achievement will be inconsistent from trial to trial. In the initial stage, the learner produces movement characteristics that often match, but sometimes do not match, requirements of the regulatory conditions. This stage is therefore characterized by both successful and unsuccessful attempts. Eventually, the learner develops a movement coordination pattern that allows a reasonable amount of performance goal achievement, although the pattern is rather crude and inefficient. As Gentile described it, "Although the learner now has a general concept of an effective approach, he or she is not skilled. The action-goal is not achieved consistently and the movement lacks efficiency" p.[57] An important part of the initial stage is that the learner actively moves to determine the appropriate movements to achieve the action goal.

In the second stage, which Gentile called the *later stages,* the learner needs to acquire three general characteristics: (1) the capability of adapting the movement pattern acquired in the initial stage to specific demands of any performance situation involving that skill; (2) consistency in achieving the performance goal of the skill on each attempt at performing the skill; and (3) efficiency of performance in terms of reducing the energy cost of performing the skill to a level that allows an "economy of effort."[57]

A distinct feature of the second stage is that the learning goals depend on whether the skill being learned is closed or open. Closed skills require what Gentile called *fixation* of the basic movement coordination pattern acquired in the first stage. This means that the learner must refine this pattern so as to achieve the action goal consistently with little, if any, conscious effort and a minimum of physical energy. In contrast, open skills require what Gentile called *diversification* of the basic movement coordination pattern acquired in the first stage. This means that the movement pattern needs to be adaptable to the ever-changing spatial and temporal characteristics of the open-skill performance context.

Another characteristic of Gentile's learning stages model is the involvement of explicit and implicit learning processes in the two stages.[56] Although both types of learning processes occur in both stages, one type predominates in each stage. In the initial stage, explicit learning processes predominate, whereas implicit processes predominate in the later stages. The basis for which type of learning process predominates is the characteristic of the skill being acquired at each stage. For example, Gentile proposed that during the initial stage the learner acquires knowledge about the regulatory conditions that influence the movements required to achieve the skill's performance goal. These conditions and the movements the performer must learn are acquired through explicit learning processes. In contrast, the dynamics of force generation involved in performing a skill are acquired by implicit learning processes and become predominant in terms of what is learned in the later stages of learning.

Practice Conditions Considerations
Generalization: From the Clinic to the Everyday Experience

Physical therapists engage children in specific types of interventions because they want the interventions to ultimately allow patients to function in their everyday world. In the study of motor learning, this clinic-to-everyday-world relationship is known as *generalization,* or *transfer of learning.*[102] Because this type of generalization is such an essential goal of physical therapy practice, it is important to consider the factors that influence it.

The long-standing view is that generalization occurs due to the *similarity between the components of the skills or performance contexts* involved. More generalization occurs with increased amounts of skill or context similarity. Consider first the similarity of skills. If you analyze the movement components of skills or assess the movement goals of skills, you will find similarities as well as differences. For example, reaching for and grasping an object can involve a variety of skills that are distinct according to the characteristics of the object to be grasped and its intended use but are similar in terms of many of the movements required. The context in which a skill or activity is performed also must be considered as a factor influencing generalization, especially if the generalization involves performing a skill or activity in the clinic and then in the daily living environment. Again, more generalization occurs as the degree of similarity increases between these two contexts. Another aspect of why generalization occurs relates to the similarity between the cognitive processes required by the two situations. The more similar the cognitive demands of a practice situation are to the eventual situation, the more generalization can be expected. For example, if the eventual situation demands a high degree of problem solving, such as would be required when a child needs to navigate a crowded room to exit through a door, then the practice situation should require a similar high degree of problem solving. Children typically engage in many problem-solving situations in their everyday environments, which indicates the physical therapy benefits of the inclusion of similar situations in a therapy context.

Taken to its logical conclusion, the greatest amount of generalization of skill performance from a clinical environment to the child's everyday living environment would occur when all the characteristics of the patient's everyday living environment are included in the intervention strategies, wherever they take place. Two implications for physical therapy practice of this view of generalization are the use of simulations in the clinic of a patient's daily living environment and the performance of functional daily living skills in the patient's own home or workplace.

Presenting Instructions About How to Perform a Skill: Demonstration and Verbal Instructions

If you wanted to teach a child how to perform a skill or activity, how would you do it? In any motor skill learning situation, the learner needs to know something about what he or she needs to do to perform the activity. The instructions can be as simple as a verbal description, such as "I want you to walk from this line on the floor to that table" or "I want you to pick up this coin and place it in the jar." This type of instruction works well for motor skills the child can already perform. But, if the person is not familiar with a skill or activity or does not know how to perform it, then some other type of instructions must be provided. The two most common ways therapists provide instructions are by demonstrating the skill or activity and by verbally describing what to do to perform the skill or activity. What do we know about these two forms of presenting instructions?

Demonstration. Sometimes referred to as *modeling*, demonstration is an effective way to communicate how to perform a skill or activity. It is especially effective when the skill or activity involves many movements that must be coordinated or sequenced in a way that the child has not experienced before or if he or she would have difficulty following a long verbal description of the sequence of movements. After demonstration of a complex activity, it is common to observe the person performing a reasonable approximation of the activity on the first attempt. Why does this happen? Most researchers agree that the observation of another person performing an activity engages a part of the brain that involves "mirror neurons."[84,140] These neurons are activated by vision as the person watches the activity being performed. In addition, when engaged in observing an activity, the visual system detects specific movement-related features of the activity that do not change from one performance of the activity to another. These features specify the coordinated movement patterns underlying performance of the activity. For example, if you observe another person walking and running, it is easy to distinguish each skill because each has a unique coordinated movement pattern. The combination of the mirror neurons registering the activity and vision detecting the specific movement pattern associated with the activity allows the observer to form a type of blueprint on which to base his or her own attempt to perform the activity.

Researchers also have shown that novice learners benefit from observing other novice learners.[102] The beneficial learning effect appears to be due to the cognitive problem-solving activity in which the observer engages while watching the novice practice the activity. This means that the observer sees what not to do as well as what to do. One strategy that implements this use of demonstration is the pairing or grouping of children where one of the pair or group practices the activity while the others observe. After a certain number of practice attempts or a specific amount of time, one of the observers practices the activity and the previous performer becomes an observer. This is consistent with the philosophy of conducting intensive therapies such as constraint-induced movement therapy in group or day camp settings,[25,38,61] as described later in the chapter.

Verbal instructions. An alternative to demonstrating how to perform an activity is providing verbal instructions. Although evidence supports the value of verbal instructions, two factors are important to consider. One is that the *amount of instruction* given must be within the limits of the person's capacity to remember and think about when he or she attempts to perform the activity. In general, this means that instructions should be few in number and concise in presentation, particularly when working with children or individuals with limited comprehension.

Another influential factor is where the instructions *focus the person's attention* while performing the activity. Researchers have compared the effects of focusing attention on the movements themselves (i.e., an *internal focus*), such as "be sure that your thigh is parallel to the floor before you place your foot on the step," versus focusing attention on the intended movement outcome (i.e., an *external focus*), such as "be sure to place your foot on the step." Typically better learning occurs with an external focus—that is, when the person's attention is directed to the intended movement outcome. (See Wulf et al.[167] for a review of this research.) Evidence of the benefits of instructing children externally came from a study conducted in Brazil[47] where 6- to 10-year-old children were learning a dynamic balance task, the Pedalo (developed in Germany; for a photo of the device, see Figure 1 in Totsika and Wulf[152]). The device consists of two wheeled platforms, with a foot on each, that moves by alternately pushing the upper platform forward and downward (like pushing the pedals on a bicycle). The typical performance measure is movement time for a specified distance. Internal focus instructions directed the children to push their feet forward to move the Pedalo; external focus instructions directed the children to focus on pushing the platform on which they stood forward. Results showed better learning by those who engaged in the external attention focus.

We commonly think of verbal instructions as words that describe how to perform a skill or activity. But another way to use verbal instructions is to describe a *visual metaphoric image* to help the person determine how to perform the skill. This type of image involves picturing in the mind what the skill or activity is like, rather than the skill itself. For example, the fundamental locomotion movement of hopping with two legs involves a complex array of movements that must be spatially and temporally coordinated. A verbal description of this array of movements may overwhelm the child. Although a demonstration of hopping would be an alternate way to provide information of what to do, telling the child to move from one place to another "like a bunny would move" presents a metaphoric image the child can use to determine how to hop. (For an excellent discussion about the use of imagery in physical therapy, see Dickstein and Deutsch.[34])

Presenting feedback during practice. When a person practices a skill or activity, he or she typically performs some parts correctly and some incorrectly. The therapist supplies essential information about these aspects of the person's performance by providing feedback. Although the term *feedback* is used in various ways, we use it here to denote the information the therapist provides to the child during or after the performance of an activity (sometimes referred to as *augmented, external,* or *extrinsic* feedback to distinguish it from the feedback naturally available through the various sensory systems, such as visual, auditory, or tactile feedback).[102]

Feedback provided by the therapist can refer to the outcome of performing a skill (e.g., "you were 2 inches short of grasping the cup") or the movement characteristics that led to the performance outcome (e.g., "your elbow was not extended enough to allow you to reach the cup"). Motor learning researchers often refer to these two types of feedback as knowledge of results (KR) and knowledge of performance (KP), respectively.[102]

Feedback can play two roles in the motor skill learning process. One is to facilitate achievement of the skill's performance goal. Because feedback provides information about the degree of success achieved while performing a skill (e.g., the errors made or what was done correctly), the learner can determine whether what he or she is doing is appropriate and what he or she should do differently to successfully perform the skill. In this way, feedback can help the person achieve successful performance of the skill more quickly or easily than could occur without the feedback. The second role of feedback is motivational. Feedback can motivate the child to continue striving toward a specific performance goal. In this role, the child uses feedback to compare his or her own performance to a specified performance goal.[26] The person must then decide to continue to pursue that goal, to change the goal, or to stop performing the activity.

Feedback about errors versus correct aspects of performance. An often debated issue is whether the performance information conveyed by feedback should refer to the mistakes the person made or those aspects of the skill or activity that were correctly performed. The consensus appears to be that both types of information are valuable, especially because each relates to a different role of feedback. Research evidence consistently has shown that error information is more effective for facilitating skill learning, especially in the initial stage of learning, and information about correctly performed aspects of an activity serves a motivational role by informing the person that he or she is on track in learning the skill or activity, which should encourage the person to keep trying.[102]

Selecting the skill or activity component for feedback. When performing a skill or activity during a therapy session, a child will undoubtedly make many errors. The challenge for the therapist is determining which error, or errors, to give feedback about. The first step is to acknowledge that the feedback will relate to only one aspect or component of the person's performance. The rationale relates to a similar point made in our earlier discussion about the amount of instruction to present, which emphasized the need to stay within the child's memory and attention limits. To simplify the process of determining how much feedback to give, we recommend that the therapist focus on only one aspect or component of the child's performance.[102]

The therapist should focus on the part of the skill that is most critical for achieving the performance goal. For example, if a child were attempting to step over an object, the most critical part of the skill would be looking at the object. If the child is not looking at the object, the therapist would provide feedback to correct this error. Additional errors to be corrected would be based on a priority list of errors that are most critical for successfully performing the skill.

Frequency of giving feedback. It is not uncommon for therapists to want to give error correction feedback after every attempt a patient makes at performing a skill, or even during the performance itself. However, research shows that giving error correction feedback during or after every practice trial (referred to as 100% frequency) is not optimal for helping a patient to learn motor skills. Rather, a less than 100% frequency optimizes skill learning, at least in healthy adults.[101] The primary problem with 100% frequency is that it engages patients in a fundamentally different, and less effective, learning process than when they receive error correction feedback less frequently. According to the *guidance hypothesis,*[133,161] learners use feedback to guide performance and achieve success, which occurs rather quickly. But there is a negative aspect to this guidance. The benefit experienced during practice creates a dependency on the availability of feedback so that when feedback is not available the performance is poorer. In effect, the feedback becomes a crutch. In contrast, when feedback is available less frequently than on every practice attempt, the learner engages in more active learning strategies on trials. A concern here for pediatric physical therapists is the extent to which the guidance hypothesis, as it relates to feedback frequency, applies to children. As is discussed later in this chapter, some research suggests that the frequency conclusion may not apply to children in the same way as it applies to adults.

Although motor learning scholars have not identified an optimal frequency for giving error correction feedback, they have reported various techniques that reduce the frequency to less than 100%.[102] One is the *fading technique,* which systematically reduces the frequency from high to low as the person progresses in learning the skill. Another technique (referred to as the *self-selection technique*) involves the patient receiving feedback only when he or she requests it. It is interesting to note that research has shown that when novice learners are allowed to request error correction feedback when they want it, they request it at a frequency that is less than 100%. Another technique involves the *interspersing of motivational and error correction feedback* during practice trials. Unfortunately, research has not established an optimal ratio for the interspersing of these two types of feedback.

Practice Structure

In addition to selecting specific activities for each child, an essential part of the physical therapist's decision making involves scheduling the sequence of those activities. Scheduling involves not only the within therapy session activities but also the activities to be completed from the first to the last session. Specific motor learning principles can guide the therapist in making scheduling decisions.

Practice variability. A practice structure characteristic that increases the chances for future performance success is the variability of the learner's experiences during practices. This includes variations in the skill or activity itself, as well as variations in the context in which an activity is practiced. In the motor learning literature, inclusion of these variations is referred to as *practice variability.*[102] A common characteristic of theories of motor skill learning is their emphasis on the learning and performance benefits derived from practice variability. The primary benefit a learner derives from practice experiences that promote movement and context variability is an increased capability to perform a skill or activity in the future. This means that the person has acquired an increased capability not only to perform a practiced skill or activity but also to adapt to performance context conditions that he or she may not have actually experienced.

Practice variability can be included in practice sessions in various ways. One is by directly requiring the child to perform multiple variations of a skill that necessitates different movement patterns or sequences to achieve the same action goal. For example, consider how in a child's daily activities he or she moves to achieve the goal of reaching, grasping, and drinking from a cup. The person may need to use various movement strategies to achieve this goal simply because of the location or shape of the cup, or various movement strategies will be required when the cup is completely full or almost empty. Another way to include variability in practice sessions is to modify the characteristics of the context in which the skill or activity is performed. Using the same reaching-grasping-drinking from a cup example, context characteristics can be varied by using different types and sizes of cups (e.g., cup with sippy cover, one or two handles, with a straw) or different types of contents in the cup. A method of incorporating increased amounts of practice variability in physical therapy sessions is to engage children in *movement exploration*, which some scholars have referred to as *discovery learning*. The benefits of this method for learning motor skills have been provided by much research with infants and children, especially by Adolph[2] and Thelen[147] and their colleagues.

Organizing practice variability. When variations of a skill or activity, or performance context, are included in therapy sessions, the therapist needs to determine how to organize or schedule those variations. Should each variation be practiced separately with a sufficient amount of time or number of practice trials for the person to demonstrate a desired level of improvement? Or should each variation be practiced in such a way that all variations are experienced within each session? Research comparing these organizational schemes has consistently shown the superiority of the latter versus the former approach in terms of learning benefits.[102]

Motor learning research comparing various practice variability schedules has demonstrated the *contextual interference (CI) effect.* The term *contextual interference* refers to the interference (i.e., memory or performance disruption) that results from performing variations of skills or activities within the context of a practice session.[102,103] The CI effect is that higher amounts of CI during practice result in better learning than occurs with lower amounts. In terms of variable practice schedules, this effect translates into schedules that involve more interspersing of skill or activity variations within a practice session, which results in better learning than occurs with schedules that involve less interspersing of variations. The most commonly compared practice schedules have been *blocked* and *random* practice schedules, which are the two extremes of the types of schedules that can be organized within the CI framework.[103] Blocked practice schedules create the lowest amount of CI by engaging the learner in nonrepeated sets of practice trials (or amounts of time) for each skill or activity variation. In contrast, random practice schedules create the highest amount of CI by engaging the learner in performing all skill or activity variations in random order throughout the practice session.

An important characteristic of the CI effect is that performance of the skills or activities is qualitatively different when compared during practice sessions and transfer tests (i.e., performance trials that differ in some way from those experienced during practice sessions). Typically, people perform the skills or activities better during practice in a blocked practice schedule. But an opposite result occurs on transfer tests when people who followed a random practice schedule during practice show superior performance.

Although there is some controversy within the physical rehabilitation community about the applicability of the CI effect to rehabilitation contexts, it is important to note that research in these contexts has been sparse and typically limited to comparisons of only blocked and random schedules. Many alternative practice schedule variations induce different amounts of CI. Unfortunately, too few of these schedules have been investigated to determine the specific application limits for clinical situations. An alternative schedule that shows learning benefits for children involves systematically increasing the amount of CI as practice progresses. This means that early practice involves blocked practice but then as practice continues, smaller block sizes are introduced until a random schedule is experienced when skill level is at a higher level (see an example in a study by Saemi and colleagues[127]).

Practice specificity. The earlier discussion of the generalization of learning emphasized the importance of the degree of similarity between practice conditions and future performance situations. This relationship, often referred to as *practice specificity,* emphasizes the need for comparable conditions in both practice and future performance situations. The practice specificity hypothesis is one of the oldest principles of human learning, with origins that can be traced back to the early 1900s.[149,150] Motor learning researchers since that time have accumulated sufficient evidence to show that practice specificity is especially applicable to the sensory/perceptual characteristics of practice and future performance contexts. According to Proteau, motor skill learning is specific to the sources of sensory/perceptual information available during practice.[120] This conclusion is especially relevant to the availability of visual feedback. Because people use and rely on visual feedback when it is available, it can become a potential problem in practice settings. For example, the use of mirrors as a source of visual feedback to help people learn to move in specified ways can lead to a dependence on the mirrors for performing the skill or activity. When the mirrors are not available, performance is typically poorer than if the mirror is available. In effect, the visual feedback from the mirrors becomes part of what is learned during practice.[100]

The practice specificity and practice variability hypotheses may appear to be at odds, but the two points are actually complementary. Both hypotheses propose that practice conditions can create a dependency on the availability of certain conditions during practice and future performance situations: the more specific the conditions during practice, the more dependent the person becomes on the availability of those conditions. And both hypotheses propose that varying conditions during practice can break this potential dependency.

Massed and Distributed Practice

Another practice structure issue concerns the amount of time to devote to various activities within and across sessions. Included are questions about the length of each session, the amount of engagement in each activity within a session, and the amount of rest between activities within and between sessions. Each of these issues can be addressed by determining whether to use massed or distributed practice conditions. The terms *massed* and *distributed* refer to the amount of time a person actively practices and rests between and during practice sessions. Researchers have not established objective definitions for these terms with respect to amount of time or number of trials. As a result, these terms are operationally defined with respect to the context in which they are used. Massed practice involves longer active practice and shorter rest periods than distributed practice.[102]

One application of massed and distributed practice relates to the *length and distribution of practice sessions*—that is, if a specified amount of time (or number of practice trials) should be devoted to practicing a skill or activity, is it better to schedule longer (and fewer) practice sessions or shorter (and more) practice sessions? In physical therapy settings, this question is often answered by limitations imposed by health care management and financing systems. But when the therapist can set these limits, the decision is made on the basis of evidence from motor learning research. The general principle is that shorter and more practice sessions are preferred to longer and fewer sessions.

The second application of massed and distributed practice relates to the *length of the rest intervals between trials.* For example, if a child is supposed to perform 10 repetitions of an activity, how long should the patient rest between repetitions to maximize the benefit? The answer to this question is not as straightforward as it was for determining the length and distribution of practice sessions. Although the traditional view has been that distributed practice is better than massed, research indicates that distributed practice is better only for learning continuous skills, such as locomotion, cycling, and swimming activities, but massed practice is better for discrete skills, such as reaching, grasping, and limb positioning (e.g., range-of-motion exercises).[99] One factor influencing this effect of the type of skill is the role played by fatigue. Massed practice trials create fatigue problems for continuous skills more than for discrete skills.

Whole and Part Practice

Another of the many decisions the physical therapist must make in a therapy session concerns whether it is better to have the patient initially practice a skill or activity in its entirety or in parts. For example, if a child needs to learn to get out of bed and into a wheelchair, should the child initially practice the entire sequence of the parts of this activity as a whole, or should he or she practice the separate parts before trying the whole activity? One way to answer this question is to analyze the skill in terms of its complexity and organization characteristics. As originally proposed by Naylor and Briggs, *complexity* refers to the number of parts of the skill, as well as the amount of attention demanded by the performer.[109] Complexity increases as the number of parts and the amount of attention demanded increase. The *organization* of a skill is determined by the temporal and spatial relationships of the parts of the skill. Motor skills in which the parts are relatively independent in terms of temporal and spatial relationships between parts are considered to be low in organization. In contrast, skills in which the between-parts relationships are temporally and spatially interdependent have a high level of organization. According to the Naylor and Briggs complexity–organization model, skills that are low in complexity and high in organization should be practiced as whole skills, but skills that are high in complexity and low in organization should be practiced in parts.[109] To apply this model to the skills and activities in physical therapy, the clinician needs to analyze each skill in terms of its levels of complexity and organization

before determining whether the child should initially practice the skill or activity as a whole or in parts.

Most of the functional skills and activities that a physical therapy patient must practice are relatively complex, which means that most of these skills should be practiced in parts before they are practiced as a whole. Now the question becomes which parts should be practiced separately and which should be combined? The answer is determined by the organization characteristic of the parts. Parts that are temporally and spatially interrelated should be grouped together as a natural unit within the skill. For example, research has shown that the reach and grasp components of reaching for and grasping a cup to drink from it are temporally and spatially related, which would indicate a high level of organization for these two parts of the skill.[81] The relationship between these two parts suggests that they should be practiced together as a single natural unit of the skill.

A common strategy for engaging people in practicing individual parts is known as the *progressive part method*. Rather than have people practice each part of a skill separately before performing the whole skill, the progressive part method involves practicing the skill in increasing sizes of sequences of parts. The first part is practiced separately until a certain level of success is achieved, then the second part is added so that the first and second parts are practiced as one unit. Each part is then added progressively until the whole skill is performed.

Reducing difficulty of a skill. For some skills or activities, it may be more desirable to reduce the difficulty of the skill and practice a modified version of the whole skill rather than to practice the skill by parts. This approach to practicing a skill involves at least a two-step sequence. The first step is practicing the simplified version of the skill, which is followed by practicing the actual skill without the modification. Whether additional modifications are needed between these two steps will depend on the skill or activity and the person learning it. Research has shown that several strategies effectively reduce a skill's difficulty and can be employed as an initial practice experience.[102] Each strategy relates to the characteristic of a skill or activity that makes it especially difficult to perform. In addition, each strategy simplifies the performance of the skill or activity in a way that allows the person to practice its basic movement coordination pattern, which is essential in the initial stage of learning. The following three strategies meet these requirements: (1) reduce the speed at which the skill is normally performed to a pace that gives attention to the movement pattern; (2) reduce the difficulty of the object that must be manipulated while performing the skill or activity (e.g., a research investigation in Australia with 6- to 8-year-old children learning a tennis forehand skill found that smaller racquets were superior to regular-sized adult racquets for improving hitting technique and performance[16]); and (3) reduce the attention demands required by the skill, such as by using the body weight support system for performing gait skills. Other effective methods for reducing the complexity and difficulty of skills include the use of virtual reality and simulators. Although physical therapists have increased their use of these devices, research concerning their use and effectiveness is lacking.

Mental Practice

The term *mental practice* refers to the cognitive or mental rehearsal of a physical skill in the absence of overt physical movement. When engaging in mental practice, people may think about the cognitive or procedural aspects of the skill or activity or they may engage in visual or kinesthetic imagery in which they see or feel themselves actually performing the skill or activity. Research concerning the use of mental practice in motor skill learning has established its effectiveness in facilitating skill acquisition in adults and as a means of preparation just before performing a skill or activity.

As an aid to skill acquisition, mental practice is most effective when combined with the actual physical practice of the skill or activity. In some research, the inclusion of mental practice can reduce the need for physical practice by 25% to 50%.[7] This means that 50 physical practice trials combined with 50 mental practice trials are as effective for learning a skill as 100 physical practice trials. Numerous research studies have reported the effectiveness of mental practice in physical rehabilitation settings.[102,111,142]

As a means of skill or activity performance preparation, mental practice involves visually and kinesthetically imagining the performance of the skill in the few minutes or seconds before actually performing the skill. An example in a physical rehabilitation setting would be a situation in which a child must stand up from a seated position. While seated, the child visually sees and kinesthetically feels himself or herself performing the entire sequence of movements required to perform the skill. After engaging in this brief mental imagery experience, the child then physically performs the skill.

Why is mental practice effective for aiding motor skill learning and performance preparation? Researchers have proposed and provided evidence to support several hypotheses. One is the neuromuscular hypothesis, which states that the imaging or visualizing of motor skill performance creates electrical activity in the nerves and musculature involved in performing the skill.[35] Although this activity can be measured by electromyography (EMG), it does not reach a level of intensity that would produce the kind of muscle activity needed to generate observable movement. The brain activity hypothesis involves a similar notion of internal activity that simulates activity that occurs when the skill is actually performed. According to this hypothesis, which is based on the results of brain imaging studies, when a person imagines moving a body part, the brain activity is similar to what occurs when the person physically moves.[116] The third hypothesis, known as the cognitive hypothesis, proposes that mental practice engages the person in the type of cognitive processes in which a person engages before, during, and after physically performing a motor skill.[102] These processes may include cognitive activities such as decision making or developing strategies to correct performance errors. Together the research evidence supporting these three explanations for the effectiveness of mental practice establishes the potential roles that mental practice can play in physical therapy.

MOTOR LEARNING IN TYPICALLY DEVELOPING CHILDREN

Children learn motor skills with astonishing frequency. Functional activities (e.g., crawling, walking, grasping, manipulating), academic skills, and play increasingly involve complex, skilled actions that develop as various cognitive and social skills emerge. Children not only undergo motor learning repeatedly, they also experience changes in cognitive and physical constructs as their bodies change during their development. Thus it is important to consider learning in the context of motor

development of age-appropriate skills. An important aspect is that learning occurs through individual movement exploration, with variations and errors being important features. Furthermore, this learning occurs through astonishing numbers of repetition, with intensive practice involving trial and error as key features of motor learning during development.[2]

Many of the principles derived from the adult studies discussed earlier hold true in children. Although oddly there is a paucity of motor learning studies in children, it is important to note that the nature and capacity of the learner may be quite different, and thus it is important to understand differences in motor learning between adults and children.[148] In this section, we describe key differences between motor learning in children and in adults and discuss how many of the above-described principles may or may not hold true in children.

Children Are Not Simply Little Adults

Perhaps the most important difference between children and adults relates to the concurrent changes in physical structure that provide the ability to learn and also force the child to relearn as his or her body changes. For example, learning to walk can occur only after suitable strength and balance capabilities emerge.[147] Precision grasping can emerge only after the development of finger individuation, which depends on the maturation of the corticospinal tract.[59] That is not to say that learning and development are purely driven by maturation. Rather it is likely epigenetic, where both maturation of physical and neuronal structures and environmental cues and practice influence each other and guide development,[48] just as the person, task, and environment affect adult learning. Furthermore, as changes in body mass and limb length occur, the dynamics required to produce skilled action also change. Thus learning activities must be planned and occur continually in the context of the developing child (see Chapter 3) and motor learning at one time point may not directly transfer to another.

Equally important is the increasing capacity to process and store information. Adults have amazing cognitive processing capabilities, but these emerge slowly throughout development. Children are known to have decreased information-processing capabilities compared with adults.[119,148] This limits the amount and type of information they can process. Children are slower at processing such information and have decreased selective attention to do so. Limited processing and reduced object recognition capabilities affect their ability to copy images.[96] Higher-level attentional focus,[90,104] spatial working memories,[135] and verbal learning and memories[29] all differ between children and adults. This means that the amount of information (e.g., feedback) that children can process and the rate at which they may do so may be limited, and thus many of the principles of motor learning discussed so far may need to be adjusted according to age expectations, as well as any cognitive limitations.

Feedback Schedules

These differences may also bring into question the applicability of some adult learning principles. In fact, in a number of cases, learning indeed has been shown to be quite different in children. One could imagine that slower feedback processing in children could result in information overload, which would interfere with learning; thus like adults, they would benefit from intermittent feedback as described earlier. In contrast, however, reduced feedback has been found to be *less* beneficial than feedback provided after every trial in children.[144] This effect is illustrated in Fig. 4.2, which shows variability during acquisition and retention of an arm movement task in adults (Fig. 4.2, A) and children (Fig. 4.2, B). Specifically, performance accuracy during acquisition was similar in adults regardless of whether or not feedback was reduced. In contrast, reduced feedback in children resulted in more error. This could be due to the reduced attentional capabilities described previously, but it may relate to the fact that children have increased error and movement variability,[12] whereby their signal-to-noise ratio becomes much higher and intrinsic feedback is washed out. Errors may increase disproportionately as accuracy demands increase.[97] Children are also known to rely more on online adjustments during movement, and increased feedback may help calibrate these adjustments.[46,169] Children may require increased feedback to update internal representations, which may interact with information processing.

Early studies on feedback reduction suggested a similarity to adults whereby feedback fading was beneficial as learning progressed in children.[52,136] More recent evidence may suggest that fading of feedback beyond a critical point may in fact be detrimental to learning in children.[144] There may be a critical point in age or skill where feedback reduction interferes, and feedback may need to be withdrawn more gradually. Practice in children can be made more effective with feedback with optimal information without guiding to outcome.[108] Thus a key challenge for the therapist is to monitor how feedback is influencing performance and modify the frequency accordingly. Nevertheless even within a given patient, the optimal feedback frequency may vary, depending on the tasks being learned.

Types of Practice Schedules

The organization of practice variability to modulate contextual interference may also need to differ between children and adults. Some evidence suggests that for children, like adults, random practice is better for learning[88] and retention.[71,119] Yet blocked or mixed practice may be better for some tasks[70] and age groups.[168] Still other studies suggest no difference in practice schedules.[37,87] Blocked practice may be better for younger/less-skilled learners in terms of complex tasks.[76] In this case, random practice schedules may overload the system with too much information, given the reduced and slower information processing. Yet handwriting retention in elementary school kids was found to be better during random practice.[143] And the learning of overarm throwing for accuracy from different distances was best for elementary school children when the practice schedule involved systematically increasing the amount of CI as practice progressed.[127] This means that early practice involves blocked practice but then as practice continues, smaller block sizes are introduced until a random schedule was experienced when skill levels were at a higher level. Thus the type of practice schedule that is most beneficial may in fact depend on age, task complexity, and skill level.[88,168]

Learning Occurs Over Considerable Time and Practice

An important consideration is that unlike many of the laboratory-based tasks used in published research, complex functional motor skills are not learned over short periods. Even in adults, expert typists,[17] chess players, musicians, and athletes[43] engage in immense amounts of practice over long durations to acquire skill. Crawling infants have been shown to practice maintaining balance more than 5 hours per day, equal to approximately 3000 crawling steps.[1] Similarly, emerging (toddler) walkers undergo about 14,000 steps, 46 football fields, and 100 falls per day.[3] Thus hundreds of thousands of trials are spread out over weeks or months during infant development of mobility skills. The naturalistic practice in which these infants and children engaged is not continually the same (blocked); actually a rich variety of events, locations, and surfaces are experienced over an extended time period. This can be considered an exaggerated version of random practice. Thus rather than practicing a solution, this random experience may construct new solutions and dissuade infants from relying on simple stimulus-response learning and instead promote "learning to learn."[1,2,74] This generalization strategy would promote broad transfer of learning within perception action systems (e.g., walking on various surfaces) and narrow specificity between them (walking versus crawling). Rest between learning sets during the development of such skills is intermittent, which may promote the contextual interference effects described earlier in the chapter. Because in most cases physical therapists cannot be with patients over

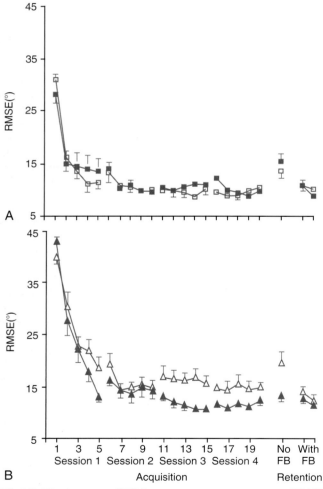

FIG. 4.2 Block means (SE) for root mean square error (RMSE) during acquisition, retention (no feedback), and reacquisition phases (with feedback) for young (A) adults and (B) children. *Filled symbols* denote feedback on all trials; *unfilled symbols* denote feedback on 62% of trials. (Modified from Sullivan KJ, Kantak SS, Burtner PA: Motor learning in children: feedback effects on skill acquisition. Phys Ther 88:720-732, 2008.

such long durations, promoting strategies that will generalize to home environments should be used to facilitate practice in that environment. An example is to use strategies involving active problem solving.[144] Thus the involvement of caregivers is a crucial component of continued learning.

MOTOR LEARNING IN PEDIATRIC REHABILITATION

Although much of pediatric rehabilitation focuses on learning of motor skills, little is known about the learning processes in children with physical or neurologic disabilities. Motor learning in this case is further complicated by the physical constraints involved, as well as by potential sensory impairments that may diminish feedback and affect the updating of internal models used for movement.

In one study of motor learning in typically developing children and children with hemiplegic CP, children were assigned to 100% or reduced (62%) feedback subgroups as they practiced 200 trials of a discrete arm movement task with specified spatiotemporal parameters.[18] Children with hemiplegic CP used their less affected hand. Children in all groups improved in accuracy and consistency. Although typically developing children showed greater accuracy as expected, those who received 100% feedback performed with significantly less error than the 62% feedback group during all phases. In contrast, no statistically significant difference was found between feedback subgroups of children with CP, although the 100% feedback group consistently demonstrated less error. Thus children with CP use feedback in a similar manner as children with typical development when learning new skills with their less involved hand, but they demonstrate less accuracy and consistency.

In terms of efficacious rehabilitation approaches, reviews of all approaches for children with cerebral palsy showed just six with good levels of evidence supporting their implementation.[112,113] These approaches had two commonalities. First, they all involve active movement of the participant using a motor-learning approach to rehabilitation.[20] This approach uses the environment to elicit desired motor behaviors and requires active problem solving. Second, they are all intensive, requiring many hours of training.

The next section of the chapter provides examples of learning in children with physical or neurologic disabilities with a focus on cerebral palsy, which is the most common type of childhood neurologic disability and the focus of most research in pediatric motor learning.

Practice Makes Better

Cerebral palsy (CP) is a developmental disorder of movement and posture that causes limitations in activity and deficits in motor skills (see Chapter 19). CP is attributed to nonprogressive disturbances in the developing fetal or infant brain, and it is the most common pediatric physical disability. Spastic hemiplegia (unilateral CP), characterized by motor impairments mainly affecting one side of the body, is the most common subtype, accounting for 30% to 40% of new cases.[77] Through much of the 20th century, the motor impairments, especially in the upper extremity (UE), were thought to be static, with little potential for rehabilitation. Thus therapy efforts were largely directed at minimizing impairment (e.g., reducing spasticity, preventing contractures). In fact, as recently as the 1990s, studies were suggesting that individuals with CP could reduce unwanted motor activity or spasticity with visual tracking or

biofeedback but that they had little ability to learn appropriate motor commands.[110,114] Early work studying prehensile force control reinforced this view, suggesting that children with CP retain infantile coordination strategies.[59] Subsequent studies, however, provided two separate lines of evidence that these impairments are not static and instead improve with sufficient practice.

First, developmental studies of children with CP have shown that motor function does improve over the course of development. For example, gross motor function has been shown to improve as children with CP get older.[124] Development of hand function has also been observed. For example, Holmefur and colleagues studied the longitudinal development of bimanual UE use in children with hemiplegic CP.[79] Children were followed for 4 to 5 years with the Assisting Hand Assessment (AHA), a Rasch-based measure that describes how the affected UE is used as a nondominant assist during bimanual activities. Investigators found that bimanual proficiency improves during the course of development but that the developmental rate and the subsequent plateau depend on the initial score at 18 months of age (Fig. 4.3, A). Children with hemiplegia with higher bimanual function in early childhood developed bimanual skills faster and reached their limit earlier than children with lower bimanual function. It is interesting to note that the development of bimanual UE use differs from that of gross motor activities in CP,[124] where milder children reach their limit later. During a 13-year follow-up study starting at the age of 6 to 8 years, it was found that hand function in children with CP improves with age.[39] Specifically, time to complete items on the Jebsen-Taylor Test of Hand Function improved in all children, and grip force coordination during grasp improved (Fig. 4.3, B). Thus both gross and fine motor functions do develop, although these two general types of skills seem to develop and reach plateaus differently.

A second line of evidence that motor function is not static in CP comes from systematic studies on the effects of extended practice that have demonstrated that motor performance can indeed improve with practice.[89] In one study, children with CP were asked to repeatedly lift an object of a given weight 25 times.[63] Even though motor learning was considerably slower than in typically developing children, impairments in fine manipulative capabilities and force regulation during grasp were partially ameliorated with this extended practice. This suggests that the initial impaired performance, at least in part, may be due to lack of use, and that many impairments in motor control previously documented may be due to the fact that insufficient practice was provided (i.e., early stages of motor learning rather than motor control capabilities were captured). Similarly, in-hand manipulation has been shown to improve with practice.[38] Such benefit of intensive training has also been documented in postural control in children with CP.[137] It is important to note that these findings suggest intensive practice may provide a window of opportunity for improvement. It is increasingly being recognized that reduction of unwanted tone (i.e., by the use of botulinum toxin) alone does not improve function[121] and that functional or task-oriented approaches and physical conditioning provided with sufficient intensity have the potential to improve motor function in CP.[4,69,91,159] Unlike adults, children with CP may benefit more from concrete instructions than from movement outcome information.[158] Motor learning in this case may require providing careful feedback on knowledge of performance, as well as cognitive strategies to achieve

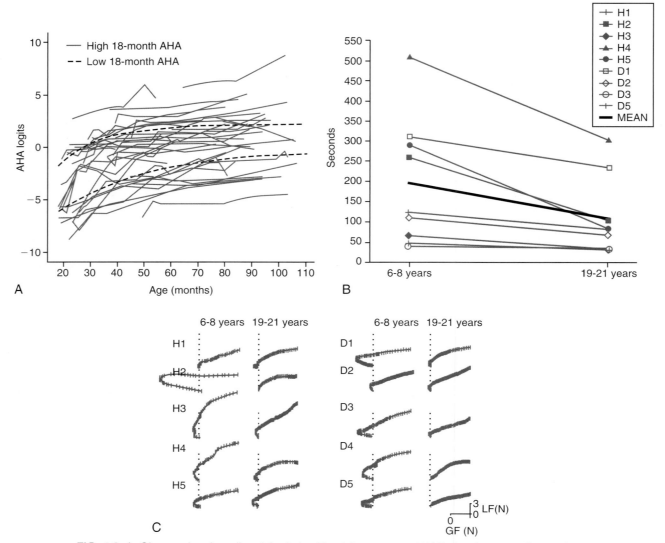

FIG. 4.3 A, Observed and predicted Assisting Hand Assessment (AHA) development. Groups have high (n = 27) or low (n = 16) 18-month score (above or below 3 logits) on the AHA at age 18 months in children with cerebral palsy. Higher scores mean better bimanual performance. B, Time to complete the six timed items (writing excluded) of the Jebsen-Taylor Test of Hand Function for individual participants, as well as mean *(bold line)* from the first (age 6 to 8 years) and second (age 19 to 21 years) data collection sessions. Faster times correspond to better performance. C, Mean grip-force/load-force trajectories for each subject (*A,* hemiplegic subjects; *B,* diplegic subjects) at the ages of 6 to 8 *(left)* and 19 to 21 *(right)* years. The *x* axis corresponds to load force (LF), and the *y* axis represents grip force (GF). *Straighter lines* indicate simultaneous increase in the two forces. *Dn,* diplegic; *Hn,* hemiplegic. (*A,* From Holmefur M, et al.: Longitudinal development of hand function in children with unilateral cerebral palsy, *Dev Med Child Neurol* 52:352–357, 2010. *B* and *C,* From Eliasson AC, Forssberg H, Hung YC, Gordon AM: Development of hand function and precision grip control in individuals with cerebral palsy: a 13-year follow-up study, *Pediatrics* 118:e1226-1236, 2006.)

better performance levels.[151] Thus it is not simply practice of movements, but practice of movements embedded in tasks. The exact dosage of training is unknown and is an important focus of future trials.[94]

Together, these lines of evidence contradict traditional clinical assumptions that motor impairments in CP are static. UE performance in children with CP may improve with practice and development. More important, this implies that hand function in particular may well be amenable to treatment.

So what type of practice schedules may be best for motor learning in children with CP? After a blocked practice schedule over several sessions, children with CP retain the ability to grade isometric grip force (using online visual feedback) after a 5-day delay.[157] Even within a single session of extended blocked practice, children with hemiplegic CP improved their ability to scale fingertip forces to the weight and texture of novel objects.[63] Similar to healthy adults, blocked practice resulted in better acquisition of force scaling to the grip of novel objects in children with CP than did random practice.[37] But both practice schedules resulted in similar retention (Fig. 4.4). These findings suggest that children with CP can form and retain internal representations of novel objects for anticipatory control, irrespective of the type of practice schedule employed. It should be noted, however, that force scaling is a form of parameter learning as opposed to learning a new skill (such as how to grasp). In that sense, the findings are in line with the hypothesis that random practice would not provide an advantage over blocked practice for parameter learning.[103] Thus it is unknown whether one form of practice is more beneficial than the other in this population, although random or mixed practice may resemble naturalistic learning to a greater extent. Nevertheless, it is clear that intensity of practice matters in rehabilitation.[13] An important point is that usual and customary therapy delivery schedules may not be sufficient for providing such intensity. For example, a study of physical therapy and occupational therapy sessions for adults with hemiparesis post stroke showed that the numbers of repetitions of UE movement observed were relatively small.[98] Although it is not known how many repetitions occur in pediatric therapies, one could imagine that this number would be even smaller given the requirement to maintain the interest and attention of children. In fact, one study of intensive constraint-induced movement therapy showed that 4- to 8-year-old children were engaged in tasks over less than 60% of a 6-hour day.[25] This effort is even less than it appears, as this number does not reflect time between trials and time taken to redirect focus as needed. It is interesting to note that children who required less redirection of focus improved to a greater extent than those who required a lot of redirection. Next we consider models for the delivery of intensive practice schedules.

TASK-ORIENTED TRAINING

Unlike neuromuscular reeducation approaches traditionally focused on impairment-level disablement (body functions/structures in International Classification of Functioning, Disability and Health Resources [ICF] language), task-oriented training is a top-down approach that focuses on activity limitations (i.e., an important aspect of CP) rather than on remediation of impairments or correction of movement patterns. Task-oriented training can be considered a motor learning or goal-directed approach to rehabilitation.[20,154,162] The approach is based on integrated models of motor learning and control and behavioral neuroscience focusing on participation and skill acquisition. An important component is the active problem solving described earlier. The associated behavioral demands of the tasks and motor skill training may result in cortical reorganization[118] underlying concurrent functional outcomes. For optimal efficacy, task-oriented training must be challenging, must progressively increase behavioral demands, and must involve active participation. Skilled training in animals shows the plasticity of UE cortical representation, whereas unskilled training does not.[93] The tasks must also have salience to the performer to influence the person–task–environment triad. In fact there may not be a relationship between intensity and

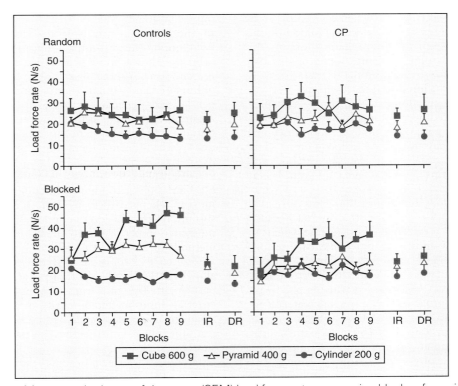

FIG. 4.4 Mean standard error of the mean (SEM) load force rate across nine blocks of acquisition, immediate retention (IR), and delayed retention (DR) during lifts with cylinder *(circle)*, pyramid *(triangle)*, and *cube (square)* for control children *(left)* and children with hemiplegic cerebral palsy (CP) *(right)*. Insets show mean (SEM) single trials from first trial at immediate retention and first trial at delayed retention. Blocked practice resulted in better acquisition of force scaling, but retention was similar for both types of practice. (From Duff SV, Gordon AM: Learning of grasp control in children with hemiplegic cerebral palsy. *Dev Med Child Neurol* 45:746-757, 2003.)

outcome unless the nature of training is considered.[164] Thus at least beyond a certain point, time on task may be less important than what is practiced.

The importance of task-oriented approaches was highlighted in a randomized trial of 55 children with CP comparing functional physical therapy versus a reference group whose therapy was based on the principle of movement normalization (including some aspects of neurodevelopmental treatment [NDT] and the Vojta method).[91] The functional therapy model consisted of the establishment of functional goals, repetitive practice of problematic motor abilities in a meaningful environment, active problem solving, and involvement of caregivers in goal setting, decision making, and implementation in daily life (i.e., many of the motor learning principles described earlier).

Gross motor abilities in a standardized environment were measured with the Gross Motor Function Measure (GMFM).[126] The GMFM is a standardized observational instrument for children with CP, developed to measure change in gross motor function, including lying and rolling, sitting, crawling and kneeling, standing, and walking, running, and jumping. Motor abilities in daily situations were measured using the Pediatric Evaluation of Disability Inventory (PEDI).[73] The PEDI is a judgment-based assessment that uses parent report through a structured interview. Two domains of the PEDI were measured: self-care and mobility. These include independent toileting, brushing teeth, dressing, and so on.

Both measures were taken 6 months, 12 months, and 18 months after implementation of the training programs. Investigators found no group differences in improvement in basic gross motor abilities.[91] However, when examining functional skills in daily situations, they found that children in the functional therapy group improved more than children in the movement normalization group. Thus functional training had the additional benefit of improving motor abilities in the daily environment identified to be important to caregivers.

The efficacy of functional training in CP using varying protocols has been documented by a number of additional investigators.[4,69,159] Treadmill training is another form of functional training that focuses on massed practice of locomotor behaviors. Efficacy in Down syndrome is well established[155]; however, it is not yet clear whether this holds true in CP and other pediatric disabilities.[30,107]

Although evidence for functional and task-oriented approaches is accumulating, evidence for other approaches such as NDT is more limited. An evidence report for the American Academy of Cerebral Palsy and Developmental Medicine concluded that as of 2001, there was not consistent evidence in support of NDT.[19] More than a decade after their report, little evidence supports its efficacy.[112] However, when applied with greater intensity, NDT approaches may provide greater benefit.[9] It should be noted, however, that NDT has been evolving beyond the original concepts introduced by the Bobaths shortly after the Second World War, and more recent NDT approaches appear to incorporate some principles of motor learning.[80]

The examples of task-oriented approaches described earlier highlight the importance of motor learning principles such as intensity, specificity, and task salience. Next we provide several examples of contemporary task-oriented approaches focusing on the upper extremity that further incorporate motor learning approaches, which can be considered use-dependent training as they engage children in activities that necessitate the use to the more affected extremities.

Constraint-Induced Therapy

A rich history of theoretical constructs has been derived from the basic sciences (including neurosciences and motor learning) underlying the application of intensive practice-based models of rehabilitation. For example, it has long been noted that monkeys with unilateral lesions or deafferentation neglect to use their affected UE but indeed will do so if forced by restraint of the contralateral unaffected UE, and that this forced use led to improved use of the affected UE.[145,153] The idea that "residual (masked) capability" could potentially be tapped into by forced use of the deafferentated or impaired limb drove the development of intensive practice-based therapies in humans. This line of research began with studies of forced use in adults with hemiparetic stroke by conducted Wolf and colleagues in the 1980s.[115,163] Subsequently, Taub and coworkers added 6 hours of structured activities using principles of behavioral psychology (shaping).[146] Shaping involves approaching motor activities in small steps by successive approximation to the movement goal or grading of task difficulty based on the patient's capabilities[117,138]; it is similar to part practice described earlier in this chapter. The active intervention involving restraint plus structured practice evolved to become known as *constraint-induced movement therapy (CIMT)*.[146] CIMT can be considered to be a special class of task-oriented training because the triad among person, task, and environment is very much applied, although functional arm use is promoted more than skill. Strong evidence of efficacy has been obtained in adult patients following stroke.[165,166] Although it would be easy to misinterpret this work as suggesting that it is the restraint that is essential, it is important to note that optimal efficacy depends on employing the motor learning principles described so far. An example has been found using an animal model of hemiplegia.[50] One hemisphere of the cat motor cortex is transiently inactivated with muscimol, a GABA agonist, and the cat wears a restraint on the unimpaired limb with no training or receives training for 1 hour per day, 5 days per week, for 4 weeks, along with the restraint. An important finding is that only cats that receive active skilled training have normalization of functional and synaptic plasticity.[50] Thus the ingredients of training matter.

Constraint-Induced Therapy in Children with Hemiparesis

For CIMT to be conducted in children, the overall approach must be changed to focus on age-appropriate activities that sustain interest for long periods, as children are not as easily motivated to perform activities of daily living or part practice methods for sustained periods of time in the way that adults are. Often the duration of restraint wear must be modified along with the type of restraint. These studies differ in age of participants (ranging from 6 months to 18 years), inclusion criteria, duration and intensity of treatment (ranging from usual and customary care schedules to adult models of CIMT), restraint (gloves, mitts, slings, and casts), and outcome measures.[22,40,78] It should be noted that despite these methodologic differences,[42] nearly all of these studies have reported positive outcomes.[8,129]

An important point is that CIMT should not be viewed as a one-time opportunity whereby the less-affected UE is restrained as much as possible (e.g., with a cast) and the highest possible intensity is provided regardless of age. Despite the diversity of approaches, no evidence suggests that one type of restraint is more effective than another; thus comfort and safety should be key factors in restraint selection.[42]

Furthermore, improvements in UE performance in young children have been noted with just 2 hours per day three times per week.[41] Perhaps most important, repeated doses of CIMT have been shown to have an additive effect (Fig. 4.5).[24] This suggests that there is no advantage to maintaining the potentially invasive schedule and restraints, and instead, one could administer CIMT through repeated, and less intensive, bouts. Thus overall, CIMT is just a task-oriented method to induce intensive practice (use-dependent training); it can be considered as part of a child's long-term pediatric rehabilitative care.

CIMT utilizes a number of motor learning principles. These include use of both part and whole practice methods, modifying tasks to ensure success and progression of difficulty as success is achieved, active problem solving, optimal practice and feedback schedules, and the need to generalize learning to performance in everyday environments.

Despite the promise of CIMT, a number of conceptual problems have been noted in applying it to children that need consideration. First, CIMT was developed to overcome learned nonuse in adults with hemiplegia and to promote use over skill. These adults lost UE function and were often highly motivated to regain previously learned functional behaviors. Children, in contrast, must overcome *developmental disuse,* whereby they may have never learned how to effectively use their more affected extremity during many tasks and may need to learn how to use it for the first time. Thus treatment must be developmentally focused and must take into account the principles of motor learning described earlier.

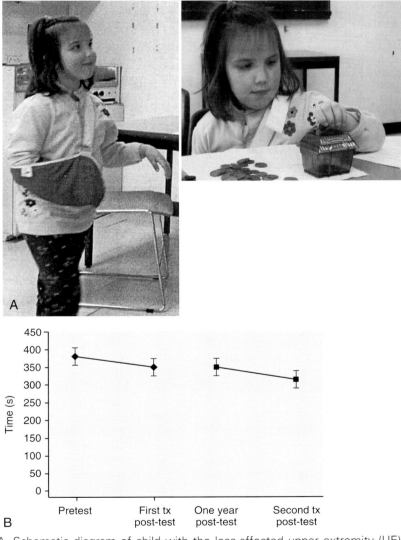

FIG. 4.5 A, Schematic diagram of child with the less-affected upper extremity (UE) restrained with a cotton sling sewn shut, while the more affected UE practices placing coins in a coin bank. B, Mean standard error of the mean (SEM) time to complete the six timed items (writing excluded) of the Jebsen-Taylor Test of Hand Function for eight children before and after 2 weeks of constraint-induced movement therapy (CIMT, 12 months later, and after a second dose of CIMT. Faster times correspond to better performance. The maximum allowable time to complete each item was capped at 120 seconds, resulting in a maximum score of 720 seconds. (*B,* Modified from Charles JR, Gordon AM: A repeated course of constraint-induced movement therapy results in further improvement, *Dev Med Child Neurol* 49:770-773, 2007.)

Second, restraining a child's less-affected extremity (especially with casts) is potentially psychologically and physically invasive and thus should not be performed on young or severely impaired children with the same intensity as in adults. It must be remembered that use of the less-affected side is still developing in children. Neuroanatomic evidence in developing kittens indicates that refinement and maintenance of corticospinal terminations in the spinal cord are activity dependent. Restriction of limb use on one side during a critical period in early development reduces the topographic distribution, branch density, and density of presynaptic boutons on the side of restricted use.[64,105,106] This suggests that there may be a substantial risk of damage to the less affected UE if it is restrained for long periods at too early an age. Thus a greatly modified protocol is required in young children.

Finally, CIMT focuses on unimanual impairments, which do not greatly influence functional independence and quality of life in that children with hemiplegia have a well-functioning (dominant) hand.[139] Training it as a dominant hand while restrained likely will improve manual dexterity, although it lacks specificity of training for how the hand will be used once the restraint is removed, for example, as a nondominant assisting hand during bimanual activities. Children with hemiplegia have impairments in spatial and temporal coordination of the two hands,[65,156] as well as global impairments in motor planning.[141] Constraint therapies cannot address these problems, and thus generalization of training may not be optimal.

Unconstraining the Constraint: Bimanual Training

Development of UE control is the consequence of activity-dependent competition between the two hemispheres, with the more active side winning out over the less active (damaged) side.[44,104] Balancing activity of the two hemispheres after unilateral brain damage may help restore motor function and may establish more normal anatomic organization of the corticospinal tract and motor representational maps in the primary motor cortex.[51] One way to do this is by using noninvasive brain stimulation (NIBS) such as repetitive transmagnetic stimulation (rTMS) and transcranial direct current stimulation (tDCS). These approaches may be used to inhibit activation of ipsilateral pathways and enhance activation of contralateral pathways. Such approaches are promising in adult stroke rehabilitation[49] and may even facilitate motor learning.[122] Evidence supporting NIBS in pediatric populations is more limited.[58,92]

From a functional perspective, principles of practice specificity would suggest that the best way to balance activity of the cerebral cortices and achieve improved bimanual control would be to directly practice bimanual coordination. Bimanual training may be efficacious in adults with hemiparesis.[21,123] A child-appropriate form of task-oriented intensive functional training, hand-arm bimanual intensive therapy (HABIT) was developed, which aims to improve the amount and quality of involved UE use during bimanual tasks.[23] HABIT is a highly structured form of training long used in pediatric rehabilitation, bimanual training that retains the two main elements of pediatric CIMT (intensive structured practice and child-friendliness). Similar to CIMT, this approach engages the child in bimanual activities 6 hours per day for 10 to 15 days in a day camp setting. It is important to note, however, that no physical restraint is used. Rather, bimanual UE coordination is elicited by modifying the environment. Similar to other functional training approaches often used in physical therapy and

occupational therapy, HABIT involves task-oriented training to achieve meaningful goals. However, it differs from these approaches in that intensity is much greater, practice is far more structured, and children problem-solve and focus on how the UE performs at the *end point* of the movement. No attempt to normalize movement is made.

An initial randomized control trial of HABIT was conducted on 20 children with hemiplegic CP between the ages of 3.5 and 14 years.[60] Children who received HABIT had improved scores on the Assisting Hand Assessment, whereas those in the no-treatment control group did not. Frequency of UE use increased for the children who received HABIT. Bimanual coordination, as determined by analysis of the kinematics of a drawer-opening task,[83] showed that children improved temporal coordination of the movements of each extremity after receiving HABIT. Providing HABIT using a magic-themed based approach has also been shown to be efficacious.[72] Part-practice, scaffolding task complexity, and goal training did not have significant effects on unimanual or bimanual performance but did drive the motor learning necessary for improved goal performance.[15] More extensive randomized trials have since been conducted comparing CIMT and HABIT and other variations of bimanual training.[32,45,62,67,128] With small nuances,[14] all of these studies have shown similar improvements in unimanual capacity and bimanual performance.[68] At first glance, these would suggest a lack of training specificity because both approaches yielded unimanual and bimanual improvements. However, follow-up studies suggest caveats. Specifically, 85% of goals identified by children and caregivers were bimanual in nature,[67] and bimanual training (HABIT) resulted in greater gains in performance on these goals.[14,67] Second, kinematic analysis of the drawer-opening task showed greater improvements in spatiotemporal coordination of the two hands following HABIT.[83] It should be noted that although not yet tested, the same logic may hold true for CIMT: greater improvements in unimanual coordination and range of motion. Although these approaches have many similar aspects and may be combined as seen fit,[1,28] it is likely that there may be differential responders to each approach. For example, it has been suggested that children who have a brain reorganization early during development such that one side of the brain controls both hands (ipsilateral corticospinal projections to the spinal cord) appear to respond to a lesser extent than children who maintain normal brain organization.[42,95(but see 85)] Nonetheless, CIMT and bimanual training are not one-time approaches, and thus can each be performed over time on a given individual.

It should be noted that the intensive, motor learning–based approaches described earlier are expensive, logistically challenging, and not likely suited for all children with CP (e.g., younger children). A more distributed model, provided in alternative settings, may be more suitable for some children and families. Both CIMT and HABIT have been shown to elicit greater improvements than NDT-based approaches in a school environment when provided just 2 hours per day.[53] Individualized therapy augmented with a home training program may offer an effective alternative when provided at a sufficient dose.[130] Both CIMT[5,42] and bimanual training have demonstrated efficacy when provided in a home environment. However, this should not be seen as a way to replace therapy delivered by professionals, and its success will likely depend on quality training and supervision by such professionals.

TWO MORE LIMBS

It should be noted that all of the approaches with good levels of evidence are aimed at the upper extremities in children with CP, and there is no evidence yet supporting a given approach for the lower extremities.[113] However, an adaptation of bimanual training, hand-arm bimanual intensive training including the lower extremities (HABIT-ILE)[10] was shown to be promising.[11] This approach simultaneously engaged the upper and lower extremities, with the premise that both are typically performed together in everyday activities. Using a crossover design, children were initially randomized to 90 hours of HABIT-ILE or their usual and customary care as provided in Belgium. The latter largely focused on normalization of movement patterns (i.e., NDT or similar approaches). Each group was then crossed over to receive the other approach. It was found that children in the HABIT-ILE group initially had significant improvements in both upper and lower extremity function, whereas no such changes occurred in the usual and customary care group. When crossed over to HABIT-ILE, the control group then demonstrated improvements in function.

SALIENCE OF MOTOR ACTIVITIES

For rehabilitation to remain effective in light of the importance of task salience (especially protocols involving long hours), it must constantly evolve to include activities that are meaningful and enjoyable, including video gaming. Children play video games on average 8 hours per week.[27] Actional immersion in a video/virtual environment can potentially allow individuals to produce movements that are not feasible in the real world as a result of their motor impairments (e.g., weakness, limited range of motion). This possibility therefore may have novel intriguing consequences and may enhance learning[31] for functional training, as it is therefore possible to provide positive KR for appropriate efforts.

The choice of video game platforms, consoles, and software needs to take into account (1) the initial abilities of the performer, (2) the specific motor impairments targeted, (3) the extent to which therapy is directed to one or both UEs, (4) the ability to attain progress in movement difficulty, and (5) the age and interest of the performer. Although use of virtual reality-based and video gaming protocols is indeed gaining momentum in rehabilitation,[33] presently evidence of the considerable efficacy of gaming by itself is lacking. Like HABIT and CIMT, it is just one means of engaging task-oriented training, but one that is potentially beneficial in maintaining motivation and providing reward, which were shown earlier in the chapter to be important for motor learning and enhancing plasticity.

There are two general approaches to incorporating video-based or virtual reality (VR) training into pediatric rehabilitation protocols.[66] The first is to develop game platforms that target specific impairments or elicit certain movements. This may be particularly useful for eliciting successful movements by altering the gain of required movement to virtual movement provided as feedback. Thus specific impairments could be targeted (e.g., wrist extension) by creating games requiring such movement, again adjusting the gain required to displayed movements. Such approaches are promising and will likely constitute an important part of pediatric rehabilitation in the future. To be successful, however, these forms of pediatric rehabilitation must adhere to the same principles described

earlier (especially salience). A large limitation, meanwhile, is the expense of building and programming devices that are enjoyable and flexible and can progress training suitably with improvements to maintain sufficient challenge. Such activities must address an array of movement impairments across a wide variety of ages. Often there is considerable delay between development and testing and implementation in clinical environments. Even as robotic-assisted therapy becomes more available, the tasks that are employed (often center-out tasks where participants must move a cursor on a screen in a straight line to concentrically arranged targets) are still often unmotivating and thus will not effectively maximize motor learning and generalization. Many robotic-assistive devices are focused on correcting movement patterns (providing templates), and in some cases, passively moving the extremities. Certainly technology does hold promise and will increasingly be part of or supplement therapeutic services. However, for these to work, they need to involve self-initiated movement, the mental and physical effort of the participant, a high intensity of training, and variability of practice including problem solving—all while continuing to be meaningful to the participant.

The second approach is to use or modify commercially available gaming systems (e.g., Nintendo Wii/Wii-Fit, Minami-ku, Kyoto, Japan; Microsoft Kinect, Redmond, WA). Although commercially available motion capture VR systems have been tailored specifically for rehabilitation, the cost may prevent wide-scale application in the near future. Thus commercial, mainstream gaming consoles have the distinct advantage of constantly being updated by game developers to maintain the interest of children and are familiar to most children; also, the initial financial investments are minimal compared with the diversity of devices and games available. A major limitation, however, is that these devices were not created to elicit specific movements that are necessarily impaired in children with disabilities and may not have sensors that are sensitive enough to translate subtle movement improvements into increases in game performance. During free play, children are likely to choose games or consoles that can be performed with one (nonparetic) UE or require minimal (stabilization) movement of the more affected UE.

Paradoxically, because children often already engage in video gaming at home, simply continuing to perform what they do at home may be neither rewarding nor specific enough to elicit movement changes and improvement in gaming ability. Thus therapists must be creative about how the games are used to target movement impairment and elicit motor learning during game play. Rules about how each UE will be used and challenges that progress difficulty of movement beyond speed and accuracy requirements of the game must be considered (e.g., adding wrist weights to promote UE strength, challenging balance by having children sit on a yoga ball while playing). Given these limitations, gaming should be viewed as complementary to, but not as a replacement for, salient task-oriented activities in the real world.

CONSIDERATIONS

It is important to note that an overwhelming majority of motor learning studies in both adults and children have been conducted in carefully controlled laboratory environments. This allows researchers to parcel out important factors that may relate to learning but has limitations in that we do not entirely know what aspects of training transfer to the learning of functional complex tasks. Emphasis in adult motor learning has made use of technology to study center-out tasks or reaching perturbation studies, where subjects need to learn new movement gains. Such paradigms are useful for studying how subjects readapt learned patterns of movement under new conditions, but we do not know how they inform us about learning complex, skilled tasks, especially with the physical constraints present in pediatric patients.

Although training protocols have emphasized intensive practice, it should be noted that the practice of motor skills alone may undershoot the potential for rehabilitation, especially in developing infants. Four interrelated tenants have been suggested to broadly advance future abilities and meet early intervention goals of maximizing children's learning potential: (1) grounded perceptual-motor experiences within cultural/social contexts form cognition, (2) exploration through early behaviors facilitates development, (3) infants and children with limited exploration opportunities are at risk for global developmental impairments, and (4) early interventions targeting exploratory behaviors may be effective for advancing motor abilities. This rationale forms the basis for using mobility devices early during development.[82] Furthermore, through action observation and vigorous action experiences, infants gradually develop more complex action understanding capabilities.[75]

Finally, it should be emphasized that interventions need to be family centered. This approach recognizes that each family is unique, that the family is the constant in the child's life, and that family members are the experts on the child's abilities and needs.[125] Thus the family works in concert with professionals to make informed decisions about the treatments and supports the child and family receive. One such approach, Coping With and Caring for Infants with Special Needs (COPCA), a family-centered program, encourages family members in an equal partnership to discover their own strategies and to decide for themselves about priorities and interventions.[36]

◼ SUMMARY

This chapter described a triad consisting of the person, the task, and the environmental context in which the child performs the task. We discussed this triad in relation to relevant motor learning principles derived from studies of adults and children, mostly without disabilities. This includes taxonomies of motor skills in relation to skill progression, types of knowledge gained during motor learning, different types and stages of learning, methods of instructions, feedback types and frequency, types of practice schedules, variability and specificity of training with whole and part practice, and the benefits of mental practice. We highlighted important differences in motor learning between children and adults. We discussed the implications of reduced information-processing capabilities and processing/memory in children and the implications for feedback and the type and amount of practice, where we showed that skill emerges over enormous amounts of practice and extensive time periods. We demonstrated that although there are certainly many similarities, the way children learn may differ from the way adults learn. More research is required to parcel out these differences.

In the context of rehabilitation, we showed that unlike in adults, learning in children must occur in the context of development, whereby age-appropriate skills are learned for the first time. We showed that intensity of training matters; provided models of intensive, task-oriented approaches such as constraint-induced movement therapy and bimanual training; and discussed how tasks and the environment as part of the triad can be used to optimize learning. We showed the importance of training specificity and provided important clues from the neuroscience literature on how to take advantage of and maximize neuroplasticity. In particular, we showed that neuroplasticity is enhanced when the tasks are meaningful to the performer. Finally we provided an example of a salient task—playing video games targeting specific motor impairments. We discussed the limitations of existing knowledge and projected where pediatric rehabilitation research needs to be directed to fully incorporate motor learning into practice.

Motor learning approaches were slow to gain popularity in pediatric rehabilitation, though there is now considerable evidence supporting their efficacy. Although therapists may be implicitly applying motor learning principles in their treatment protocols, explicit application of these principles is required to determine if this approach is effective. A challenge in coming years to therapists who work with children will be to determine how the principles of motor learning described in this chapter may or may not differ from results of studies performed in adults and void these characteristics. Although intensity of training is one variable that surely will be an important factor in future task-oriented approaches, determining the key intervention ingredients to include in planning intensity will be all the more important.[134]

REFERENCES

1. Aarts PB, et al.: The Pirate group intervention protocol: description and a case report of a modified constraint-induced movement therapy combined with bimanual training for young children with unilateral spastic cerebral palsy, *Occup Ther Int* 19:76–87, 2012.
2. Adolph KE: Learning to move, *Curr Dir Psychol Sci* 17:213–218, 2012.
3. Adolph KE, et al.: How do you learn to walk? Thousands of steps and dozens of falls per day, *Psychol Sci* 23:1387–1394, 2012.
4. Ahl LE, et al.: Functional therapy for children with cerebral palsy: an ecological approach, *Dev Med Child Neurol* 47:613–619, 2004.
5. Al-Oraibi S, Eliasson AC: Implementation of constraint-induced movement therapy for young children with unilateral cerebral palsy in Jordan: a home-based model, *Disabil Rehabil* 33:2006–2012, 2011.
6. Albert F, et al.: Sensorimotor memory of object weight distribution during multidigit grasp, *Neurosci Lett* 463:188–193, 2009.
7. Allami N, et al.: Visuo-motor learning with combination of different rates of motor imagery and physical practice, *Exp Brain Res* 184:105–113, 2008.
8. Andersen J, et al.: Intensive upper extremity training for children with hemiplegia: from science to practice, *Sem Pediatr* 20:100–105, 2013.
9. Anttila H, et al.: Effectiveness of physical therapy interventions for children with cerebral palsy: a systematic review, *BMC Pediatr* 24:8–14, 2008.
10. Bleyenheuft Y, Gordon AM: Precision grip in congenital and acquired hemiparesis: similarities in impairments and implications for neurorehabilitation, *Front Hum Neurosci* 8:459, 2014.
11. Bleyenheuft Y, et al.: Hand and arm bimanual intensive therapy including lower extremity (HABIT-ILE) in children with unilateral spastic cerebral palsy: a randomized trial, *Neurorehabil Neural Repair* 29:645–557, 2015.
12. Bo J, Contreras-Vidal, et al.: Effects of increased complexity of visuo-motor transformations on children's arm movements, *Hum Mov Sci* 25:553–567, 2006.

13. Bower E, et al.: A randomised controlled trial of different intensities of physiotherapy and different goal-setting procedures in 44 children with cerebral palsy, *Dev Med Child Neurol* 38:226–237, 1996.

14. Brandão MB, et al.: Functional impact of constraint-therapy and bimanual training in children with cerebral palsy, *Am J Occup Ther* 66:320–329, 2012.

15. Brandao M, et al.: Comparison of structured skill and unstructured practice during intensive bimanual training in children with unilateral spastic cerebral palsy, *Neurorehabil Neural Repair* 28:452–461, 2014.

16. Buszard T, et al.: Modifying equipment in early skill development: a tennis perspective, *Res Q Exerc Sport* 85:218–225, 2014.

17. Bryan WL, Harter N: Studies on the telegraphic language: the acquisition of a hierarchy of habits, *Psychol Rev* 6:345–375, 1899.

18. Burtner PA, et al.: Motor learning in children with hemiplegic cerebral palsy: feedback effects on skill acquisition, *Dev Med Child Neurol* 56:259–266, 2014.

19. Butler C, Darrah J: Effects of neurodevelopmental treatment (NDT) for cerebral palsy: an AACPDM evidence report, *Dev Med Child Neurol* 43:778–790, 2001.

20. Carr J, Shephert RB: A motor learning model for stroke rehabilitation, *Physiotherapy* 75:372–380, 1989.

21. Cauraugh JH, et al.: Upper extremity improvements in chronic stroke: coupled bilateral load training, *Restor Neurol Neurosci* 27:17–25, 2009.

22. Charles J, Gordon AM: A critical review of constraint-induced movement therapy and forced use in children with hemiplegia, *Neural Plasticit* 12:245–261, 2005.

23. Charles J, Gordon AM: Development of hand-arm bimanual intensive training (HABIT) for improving bimanual coordination in children with hemiplegic cerebral palsy, *Dev Med Child Neurol* 48:931–936, 2006.

24. Charles JR, Gordon AM: A repeated course of constraint-induced movement therapy results in further improvement, *Dev Med Child Neurol* 49:770–773, 2007.

25. Charles J, et al.: Efficacy of a child-friendly form of constraint-induced movement therapy in hemiplegic cerebral palsy: a randomized control trial, *Dev Med Child Neurol* 48:635–642, 2006.

26. Chiviakowsky S, Drews R: Effects of generic versus non-generic feedback on motor learning in children, *PLoS One* 9:e88989, 2014.

27. Cummings HM, Vandewater EA: Relation of adolescent video game play to time spent in other activities, *Arch Pediatr Adolesc Med* 161:684–689, 2007.

28. Cohen-Holzer M, et al.: The effect of combining daily restraint with bimanual intensive therapy in children with hemiparetic cerebral palsy: a self-control study, *NeuroRehabilitation* 29:29–36, 2011.

29. Czernochowski D, et al.: Age-related differences in familiarity and recollection: ERP evidence from a recognition memory study in children and young adults, *Cogn Affect Behav Neurosci* 5:417–433, 2005.

30. Damiano DL, DeJong SL: A systematic review of the effectiveness of treadmill training and body weight support in pediatric rehabilitation, *J Neurol Phys Ther* 33:27–44, 2009.

31. Dede C: Immersive interfaces for engagement and learning, *Science* 323:66–69, 2009.

32. Deppe W, et al.: Modified constraint-induced movement therapy versus intensive bimanual training for children with hemiplegia - a randomized controlled trial, *Clin Rehabil* 27:909–920, 2013.

33. Deutsch JE, et al.: Use of a low-cost, commercially available gaming console (Wii) for rehabilitation of an adolescent with cerebral palsy, *Phys Ther* 88:1196–1207, 2008.

34. Dickstein R, Deutsch JE: Motor imagery in physical therapy, *Phys Ther* 87:942–953, 2007.

35. Dickstein R, et al.: EMG activity in selected target muscles during imagery rising on tiptoes in healthy adults and poststroke hemiparetic patients, *J Mot Behav* 37:475–483, 2005.

36. Dirks T, Hadders Algra M: the role of the family in intervention of infants at high risk of cerebral palsy: a systematic analysis, *Dev Med Child Neurol* 53(Suppl 4):62–67, 2011.

37. Duff SV, Gordon AM: Learning of grasp control in children with hemiplegic cerebral palsy, *Dev Med Child Neurol* 45:746–757, 2003.

38. Eliasson AC, et al.: Clinical experience of constraint induced movement therapy in adolescents with hemiplegic cerebral palsy: a day camp model, *Dev Med Child Neurol* 45:357–359, 2003.

39. Eliasson AC, et al.: Development of hand function and precision grip control in individuals with cerebral palsy: a 13-year follow-up study, *Pediatrics* 118:e1226–e1236, 2006.

40. Eliasson AC, Gordon AM: Constraint-induced movement therapy for children with hemiplegia. In Eliasson AC, Burtner P, editors: *Improving hand function in children with cerebral palsy: theory, evidence and intervention: clinics in developmental medicine*, London, 2008, MacKeith Press, pp 308–319.

41. Eliasson AC, et al.: Effects of constraint-induced movement therapy in young children with hemiplegic cerebral palsy: an adapted model, *Dev Med Child Neurol* 47:266–275, 2005.

42. Eliasson AC, et al.: Guidelines for future research in constraint-induced movement therapy for children with unilateral cerebral palsy: an expert consensus, *Dev Med Child Neurol* 56:125–137, 2014.

43. Ericsson KA, Charness N: Expert performance: its structure and acquisition, *Am Psychologist* 49:725–747, 1994.

44. Eyre JA: Corticospinal tract development and its plasticity after perinatal injury, *Neurosci Biobehav Rev* 31:1136–1149, 2007.

45. Facchin P, et al.: Multisite trial comparing the efficacy of constraint-induced movement therapy with that of bimanual intensive training in children with hemiplegic cerebral palsy: postintervention results, *Am J Phys Med Rehab* 90:539–553, 2011.

46. Ferrel-Chapus C, et al.: Visuomanual coordination in childhood: adaptation to visual distortion, *Exp Brain Res* 144:506–517, 2002.

47. Flores FS, et al.: Benefits of external focus instructions on the learning of a balance task in children of different ages, *Int J Sport Psychol* 46:311–320, 2015.

48. Forssberg H: Neural control of human motor development, *Curr Opin Neurobiol* 9:676–682, 1999.

49. Fregni F, Pascual-Leone A: Technology insight: noninvasive brain stimulation in neurology-perspectives on the therapeutic potential of rTMS and tDCS, *Nat Clin Pract Neurol* 3:383–393, 2007.

50. Friel K, et al.: Using motor behavior during an early critical period to restore skilled limb movement after damage to the corticospinal system during development, *J Neurosci* 23:9265–9276, 2012.

51. Friel KM, Martin JH: Bilateral activity-dependent interactions in the developing corticospinal system, *J Neurosci* 27:11083–11090, 2007.

52. Gallagher JD, Thomas JR: Effects of varying post-KR intervals upon children's motor performance, *J Mot Behav* 12:41–56, 1980.

53. Gelkop N, et al.: Efficacy of constraint-induced movement therapy and bimanual training in children with hemiplegic cerebral palsy in an educational setting, *Phys Occup Ther Pediatr* 35:24–39, 2015.

54. Gentile AM: A working model of skill acquisition with application to teaching, *Quest Monograph* 17:3–23, 1972.

55. Gentile AM: Skill acquisition: action, movement, and neuromotor processes. In Carr JH, et al., editors: *Movement science: foundations for physical therapy in rehabilitation*, Rockville, MD, 1987, Aspen, pp 93–154.

56. Gentile AM: Implicit and explicit processes during acquisition of functional skills, *Scand J Occup Ther* 5:7–16, 1998.

57. Gentile AM: Skill acquisition: action, movement, and neuromotor processes. In Carr JH, Shepherd RB, editors: *Movement science: foundations for physical therapy in rehabilitation*, ed 2, Rockville, MD, 2000, Aspen, pp 111–187.

58. Gillick BT, et al.: Primed low-frequency repetitive transcranial magnetic stimulation and constraint-induced movement therapy in pediatric hemiparesis: a randomized controlled trial, *Dev Med Child Neurol* 56:44–52, 2014.

59. Gordon AM: Development of hand motor control. In Kalverboer AF, Gramsbergen A, editors: *Handbook of brain and behaviour in human development*, Dordrecht, 2001, Kluwer Academic, pp 513–537.

60. Gordon AM, et al.: Efficacy of a hand-arm bimanual intensive therapy (HABIT) for children with hemiplegic cerebral palsy: a randomized control trial, *Dev Med Child Neurol* 49:830–838, 2007.

61. Gordon AM, et al.: Methods of constraint-induced movement therapy for children with hemiplegic cerebral palsy: development of a

child-friendly intervention for improving upper extremity function, *Arch Phys Med Rehabil* 86:837–844, 2005.

62. Gordon AM, et al.: Both constraint-induced movement therapy and bimanual training lead to improved performance of upper extremity function in children with hemiplegia, *Dev Med Child Neurol* 50:957–958, 2008.

63. Gordon AM, Duff SV: Fingertip forces during object manipulation in children with hemiplegic cerebral palsy. I: anticipatory scaling, *Dev Med Child Neurol* 41:166–175, 1999.

64. Gordon AM, Friel K: Intensive training of upper extremity function in children with cerebral palsy. In Hermsdoerfer J, Nowak DA, editors: *Sensorimotor control of grasping: physiology and pathophysiology*, New York, 2008, Cambridge University Press, pp 438–457.

65. Gordon AM, Steenbergen B: Bimanual coordination in children with cerebral palsy. In Eliasson AC, Burtner P, editors: *Improving hand function in children with cerebral palsy: theory, evidence and intervention: clinics in developmental medicine*, London, 2008, MacKeith Press, pp 160–175.

66. Gordon AM, Okita SY: Augmenting pediatric constraint-induced movement therapy and bimanual training with video gaming, *Technol Disabil* 22:179–191, 2010.

67. Gordon AM, et al.: Bimanual training and constraint-induced movement therapy in children with hemiplegic cerebral palsy: a randomized trial, *Neurorehabili Neural Repair* 25:692–702, 2011.

68. Gordon AM: To constrain or not to constrain, and other stories of intensive upper extremity training for children with unilateral cerebral palsy, *Dev Med Child Neurol* 53(S4):56–61, 2011.

69. Gorter H, et al.: Changes in endurance and walking ability through functional physical training in children with cerebral palsy, *Pediatr Phys Ther* 21:31–37, 2009.

70. Granda J, et al.: Effects of different practice conditions on acquisition, retention, and transfer of soccer skills by 9-year-old schoolchildren, *Percept Mot Skills* 106:447–460, 2008.

71. Granda J, Medina MM: Practice schedule and acquisition, retention and transfer of a throwing task in 6 year old children, *Percept Mot Skills* 96:1015–1024, 2003.

72. Green D, et al.: A multi-site study of functional outcomes following a themed approach to hand-arm bimanual intensive therapy (HABIT) for children with hemiplegia, *Dev Med Child Neurol* 55:527–533, 2013.

73. Haley SM, et al.: *Pediatric evaluation of disability inventory (PEDI)*, Boston, MA, 1992, New England Medical Center Hospitals.

74. Harlow HF: The formation of learning sets, *Psychol Rev* 56:51–65, 1949.

75. Hunnius S, Bekkering H: What are you doing? How active and observational experience shape infants' action understanding, *Philos Trans R Soc Lond B Biol Sci* 369:20130490, 2014.

76. Herbert EP, et al.: A comparison of three practice schedules along the contextual interference continuum, *Res Q Exerc Sport* 68:357–361, 1996.

77. Himmelmann K, et al.: The changing panorama of cerebral palsy in Sweden, IX. Prevalence and origin in the birth-year period 1995-1998, *Acta Paediatrica* 94:287–294, 2005.

78. Hoare B, et al.: Constraint-induced movement therapy in the treatment of the upper limb in children with hemiplegic cerebral palsy: a Cochrane systematic review, *Clin Rehabil* 21:675–685, 2007.

79. Holmefur M, et al.: Longitudinal development of hand function in children with unilateral cerebral palsy, *Dev Med Child Neurol* 52:352–357, 2010.

80. Howle JM: *Neuro-developmental treatment approach: theoretical foundations and principles of clinical practice*, Laguna Beach, CA, 2003, Neuro-Developmental Treatment Association.

81. Hu Y: A model of coupling between grip aperture and hand transport during human prehension, *Exp Brain Res* 167:301–304, 2005.

82. Huang HH, et al.: Modified toy cars for mobility and socialization: case report of a child with cerebral palsy, *Pediatr Phys Ther* 26:76–84, 2014.

83. Hung YC, et al.: Bimanual coordination during a goal-directed task in children with hemiplegic cerebral palsy, *Dev Med Child Neurol* 46:746–753, 2004.

84. Iacoboni M, Mazziotta JC: Mirror neuron system: basic findings and clinical applications, *Ann Neurol* 62:213–218, 2007.

85. Islam M, et al.: Is outcome of constraint-induced movement therapy in unilateral cerebral palsy dependent on corticomotor projection pattern and brain lesion characteristics? *Dev Med Child Neurol* 56:252–258, 2014.

86. Hung Y-C, et al.: The effect of training specificity on bimanual coordination in children with hemiplegia, *Res Dev Disabil* 32:2724–2731, 2011.

87. Jarus T, Goverover Y: Effects of contextual interference and age on acquisition, retention and transfer of motor skills, *Percept Mot Skills* 88:437–447, 1999.

88. Jarus T, Gutman T: Effects of cognitive processes and task complexity on acquisition, retention, and transfer of motor skills, *Can J Occup Ther* 68:280–289, 2001.

89. Kantak SS, et al.: Motor learning in children with cerebral palsy: implications for rehabilitation. In Eliasson AC, Burtner P, editors: *Improving hand function in children with cerebral palsy: theory, evidence and intervention. Clinics in developmental medicine*, London, 2008, MacKeith Press, pp 260–275.

90. Karatekin C, et al.: Regulation of cognitive resources during sustained attention and working memory in 10-year-olds and adults, *Psychophysiology* 44:128–144, 2007.

91. Ketelaar M, et al.: Effects of a functional therapy program on motor abilities of children with cerebral palsy, *Phys Ther* 81:1534–1545, 2001.

92. Kirton A, et al.: Cortical excitability and interhemispheric inhibition after subcortical pediatric stroke: plastic organization and effects of rTMS, *Clin Neurophysiol* 121:1922–1929, 2010.

93. Kleim JA, et al.: Functional reorganization of the rat motor cortex following motor skill learning, *J Neurophysiol* 80:3321–3325, 1998.

94. Kolobe TH, et al.: Research Summit III proceedings on dosing in children with an injured brain or cerebral palsy, *Phys Ther* 94:907–920, 2014.

95. Kuhnke N, et al.: Do patients with congenital hemiparesis and ipsilateral corticospinal projections respond differently to constraint-induced movement therapy? *Dev Med Child Neurol* 50:898–903, 2008.

96. Lagers-van Haselen GC, et al.: Copying strategies for patterns by children and adults, *Percept Mot Skills*, 603-615, 2007.

97. Lambert J, Bard C: Acquisition of visual manual skills and improvement of information processing capabilities in 6 to 10 year-old children performing a 2D pointing task, *Neurosci Lett* 377:1–6, 2005.

98. Lang CE, et al.: Counting repetitions: an observational study of outpatient therapy for people with hemiparesis post-stroke, *J Neurol Phys Ther* 31:3–10, 2007.

99. Lee TD, Genovese ED: Distribution of practice in motor skill acquisition: different effects for discrete and continuous tasks, *Res Q Exerc Sport* 59:277–287, 1989.

100. Lynch JA, et al.: Effect on performance of learning a Pilates skill with or without a mirror, *J Bodyw Mov Ther* 13:283–290, 2008.

101. Magill RA: Augmented feedback in motor skill acquisition. In Singer RN, et al., editors: *Handbook of research on sport psychology*, New York, 2001, John Wiley & Sons, pp 86–114.

102. Magill RA, Anderson DA: *Motor learning and control: concepts and applications*, ed 10, New York, 2014, McGraw-Hill.

103. Magill RA, Hall KG: A review of the contextual interference effect in motor skill acquisition, *Hum Mov Sci* 9:241–289, 1990.

104. Mantyla T, et al.: Time monitoring and executive functioning in children and adults, *J Exp Child Psychol* 96:1–19, 2007.

105. Martin JH, et al.: Corticospinal system development depends on motor experience, *J Neurosci* 24:2122–2132, 2004.

106. Martin JH, et al.: Activity- and use-dependent plasticity of the developing corticospinal system, *Neurosci Biobehav Rev* 31:1125–1135, 2007.

107. Mutlu A, et al.: Treadmill training with partial body-weight support in children with cerebral palsy: a systematic review, *Dev Med Child Neurol* 51:268–275, 2009.

108. Naka M: Repeated writing facilitates children's memory for pseudocharacters and foreign letters, *Mem Cognit* 26:804–809, 1998.

109. Naylor J, Briggs G: Effects of task complexity and task organization on the relative efficiency of part and whole training methods, *J Exp Psychol* 65:217–244, 1963.

110. Neilson PD, et al.: Control of isometric muscle activity in cerebral palsy, *Dev Med Child Neurol* 32:778–788, 1990.

111. Nilsen DM, Gillen G, Gordon AM: Use of mental practice to improve upper limb recovery post-stroke: a systematic review, *Am J Occup Ther* 64(5):695–708, 2010.

112. Novak I, et al.: A systematic review of interventions for children with cerebral palsy: state of the evidence, *Dev Med Child Neurol* 55:885–910, 2013.

113. Novak I: Evidence-based diagnosis, health care, and rehabilitation for children with cerebral palsy, *J Child Neurol* 29:1141–1156, 2014.

114. O'Dwyer NJ, Neilson PD: Voluntary muscle control in normal and athetoid dysarthric speakers, *Brain* 111:877–899, 1988.

115. Ostendorf CG, Wolf SL: Effect of forced use of the upper extremity of a hemiplegic patient on changes in function: a single-case design, *Phys Ther* 61:1022–1028, 1981.

116. Page SJ, et al.: Cortical plasticity following motor learning during mental practice in stroke, *Neurorehabil Neural Repair* 23:382–388, 2009.

117. Panyan MC: *How to use shaping*, Lawrence, KS, 1980, H & H Enterprises.

118. Plautz EJ, et al.: Effects of repetitive motor training on movement representations in adult squirrel monkeys: role of use versus learning, *Neurobiol Learn Mem* 74:27–55, 2000.

119. Pollock BJ, Lee TD: Dissociated contextual interference effects in children and adults, *Percept Mot Skills* 84:851–858, 1997.

120. Proteau L: On the specificity of learning and the role of visual information for movement control. In Proteau L, Elliott D, editors: *Vision and motor control*, Amsterdam, 1992, North-Holland, pp 67–103.

121. Rameckers EA, et al.: Botulinum toxin-a in children with congenital spastic hemiplegia does not improve upper extremity motor-related function over rehabilitation alone: a randomized controlled trial, *Neurorehabil Neural Repair* 23:218–225, 2009.

122. Reis J, et al.: Noninvasive cortical stimulation enhances motor skill acquisition over multiple days through an effect on consolidation, *Proc Natl Acad Sci U S A* 106:1590–1595, 2009.

123. Rose DK, Winstein CJ: Bimanual training after stroke: are two hands better than one? *Top Stroke Rehabil* 11:20–30, 2004.

124. Rosenbaum PL, et al.: Prognosis for gross motor function in cerebral palsy: creation of motor development curves, *JAMA* 288:1357–1363, 2002.

125. Rosenbaum P: Family and quality of life: key elements in intervention in children with cerebral palsy, *Devel Med Child Neurol* 53(Suppl 4):68–70, 2011.

126. Russell D, et al.: *Manual for the gross motor function measure*, Hamilton, Ontario, Canada, 1993, McMaster University.

127. Saemi E, et al.: Practicing along the contextual interference continuum: a comparison of three practice schedules in an elementary physical education setting, *Kinesiology* 44:191–198, 2012.

128. Sakzewski L, et al.: Randomized trial of constraint-induced movement therapy and bimanual training on activity outcomes for children with congenital hemiplegia, *Dev Med Child Neurol* 53:313–320, 2011.

129. Sakzewski L, et al.: The state of the evidence for intensive upper limb therapy approaches for children with unilateral cerebral palsy, *J Child Neurol* 11:1077–1090, 2014.

130. Sakzewski L, et al.: Randomized comparison trial of density and context of upper limb intensive group versus individualized occupational therapy for children with unilateral cerebral palsy, *Dev Med Child Neurol* 57:539–547, 2015.

131. Salimi I, et al.: Selective use of visual information signaling objects' center of mass for anticipatory control of manipulative fingertip forces, *Exp Brain Res* 150:9–18, 2003.

132. Salimi I, et al.: Specificity of internal representations underlying grasping, *J Neurophysiol* 84:2390–2397, 2000.

133. Salmoni AW, et al.: Knowledge of results and motor learning: a review and reappraisal, *Psychol Bull* 95:355–386, 1984.

134. Schertz M, Gordon AM: Changing the model: a call for re-examination of intervention approaches & translational research in children with developmental disabilities, *Dev Med Child Neurol* 51:6–7, 2009.

135. Schumann-Hengsteler R: Children's and adults' visuospatial memory: the game concentration, *J Genet Psychol* 157:77–92, 1996.

136. Shapiro DC: Knowledge of results and motor learning in preschool children, *Res Q* 48:154–158, 1977.

137. Shumway-Cook A, et al.: Effect of balance training on recovery of stability in children with cerebral palsy, *Dev Med Child Neurol* 45:591–602, 2003.

138. Skinner B: *The technology of teaching*, New York, 1968, Appleton-Century-Crofts.

139. Sköld A, et al.: Performing bimanual activities: the experiences of young persons with hemiplegic cerebral palsy, *Am J Occup Ther* 58:416–425, 2004.

140. Small SL, et al.: The mirror neuron system and the treatment of stroke, *Dev Psychobiol* 54:293–310, 2012.

141. Steenbergen B, et al.: Motor planning in congenital hemiplegia, *Disabil Res* 29:13–23, 2007.

142. Steenbergen B, et al.: Motor imagery training in hemiplegic cerebral palsy: a potentially useful therapeutic tool for rehabilitation, *Dev Med Child Neurol* 51:690–696, 2009.

143. Ste-Marie DM, et al.: High levels of contextual interference enhance handwriting skill acquisition, *J Mot Behav* 36:115–126, 2004.

144. Sullivan KJ, et al.: Motor learning in children: feedback effects on skill acquisition, *Phys Ther* 88:720–732, 2008.

145. Taub E, Shee LP: *Somatosensory deafferentation research with monkeys: implications for rehabilitation medicine*, Baltimore/London, 1980, Williams & Wilkins.

146. Taub E, Wolf SL: Constraint-induced (CI) movement techniques to facilitate upper extremity use in stroke patients, *Top Stroke Rehabil* 3:38–61, 1997.

147. Thelen E: Motor development: a new synthesis, *Am Psychol* 50:79–95, 1995.

148. Thomas JR: Children's control, learning, and performance of motor skills, *Res Q Exerc Sport* 71:9, 2000.

149. Thorndike EL: *Educational psychology: briefer course*, New York, 1914, Columbia University Press.

150. Thorndike EL, Woodworth RS: The influence of improvement in one mental function upon the efficiency of other functions, *Psychol Rev* 8:247–261, 1901.

151. Thorpe DE, Valvano J: The effects of knowledge of performance and cognitive strategies on motor skill learning in children with cerebral palsy, *Pediatr Phys Ther* 14:2–15, 2002.

152. Totsika V, Wulf G: The influence of external and internal foci of attention on transfer to novel situations and skills, *Res Q Exerc Sport* 74:220–225, 2003.

153. Tower SS: Pyramidal lesion in the monkey, *Brain (London)* 63:36, 1940.

154. Trombly C: Clinical practice guidelines for post-stroke rehabilitation and occupational therapy practice, *Am J Occup Ther* 49:711–714, 1995.

155. Ulrich DA, et al.: Effects of intensity of treadmill training on developmental outcomes and stepping in infants with Down syndrome: a randomized trial, *Phys Ther* 88:114–122, 2008.

156. Utley A, Steenbergen B: Discrete bimanual co-ordination in children and young adolescents with hemiparetic cerebral palsy: recent findings, implications and future research directions, *Pediatr Rehabil* 9:127–136, 2006.

157. Valvano J, Newell KM: Practice of a precision isometric grip-force task by children with spastic cerebral palsy, *Dev Med Child Neurol* 40:464–473, 1998.

158. van der Weel FR, et al.: Effect of task on movement control in cerebral palsy: implications for assessment and therapy, *Dev Med Child Neurol* 33:419–426, 1991.

159. Verschuren O, et al.: Relation between physical fitness and gross motor capacity in children and adolescents with cerebral palsy, *Dev Med Child Neurol* 51:866–871, 2009.

160. Willingham DB: A neuropsychological theory of motor skill learning, *Psychol Rev* 105:558–584, 1998.

161. Winstein CJ, Schmidt RA: Reduced frequency of knowledge of results enhances motor skill learning, *J Exp Psychol* 16:677–691, 1990.

162. Winstein CJ, Wolf SL: Task-oriented training to promote upper extremity recovery. In Stein J, et al., editors: *Stroke recovery and rehabilitation*, New York, 2009, Demos Medical.

163. Wolf SL, et al.: Forced use of hemiplegic upper extremities to reverse the effect of learned nonuse among chronic stroke and head-injured patients, *Exp Neurol* 104:125–132, 1989.

164. Wolf SL, et al.: The Excite trial: relationship of intensity of constraint induced movement therapy to improvement in the Wolf motor function test, *Restor Neurol Neurosci* 25:549–562, 2007.

165. Wolf SL, et al.: Effect of constraint-induced movement therapy on upper extremity function 3 to 9 months after stroke: the EXCITE randomized clinical trial, *JAMA* 296:2095–2104, 2006.

166. Wolf SL, et al.: Retention of upper limb function in stroke survivors who have received constraint-induced movement therapy: the EXCITE randomised trial, *Lancet Neurol* 7:33–40, 2008.

167. Wulf G, et al.: External focus instructions reduce postural stability in individuals with Parkinson disease, *Phys Ther* 89:162–168, 2009.

168. Wulf G, Shea CH: Principles derived from the study of simple skills do not generalize to complex skill learning, *Psychonomic Bull Rev* 9:185–211, 2002.

169. Yan JH, et al.: Developmental differences in children's ballistic aiming movements of the arm, *Percept Mot Skills* 96:589–598, 2002.

170. Zhang W, et al.: Manipulation after object rotation reveals independent sensorimotor memory representations of digit positions and forces, *J Neurophysiol* 103:2953–2964, 2010.

SUGGESTED READINGS

Eliasson AC, et al.: Guidelines for future research in constraint-induced movement therapy for children with unilateral cerebral palsy: an expert consensus, *Dev Med Child Neurol* 56:125–137, 2014.

Gillick BT, et al.: Primed low-frequency repetitive transcranial magnetic stimulation and constraint-induced movement therapy in pediatric hemiparesis: a randomized controlled trial, *Dev Med Child Neurol* 56:44–52, 2014.

Gordon AM: To constrain or not to constrain, and other stories of intensive upper extremity training for children with unilateral cerebral palsy, *Dev Med Child Neurol* 53(S4):56–61, 2011.

Magill RA, Anderson DA: *Motor learning and control: concepts and applications*, ed 10, New York, 2014, McGraw-Hill.

Martin JH, et al.: Activity- and use-dependent plasticity of the developing corticospinal system, *Neurosci Biobehav Rev* 31:1125–1135, 2007.

Novak I, et al.: A systematic review of interventions for children with cerebral palsy: state of the evidence, *Dev Med Child Neurol* 55:885–910, 2013.

Wolf SL, et al.: Effect of constraint-induced movement therapy on upper extremity function 3 to 9 months after stroke: the EXCITE randomized clinical trial, *JAMA* 296:2095–2104, 2006.

5

Musculoskeletal Development and Adaptation

Linda Pax Lowes, Krystal Hay

Pediatric physical therapists routinely work with children whose clinical conditions influence the growth and development of the musculoskeletal system, either directly or indirectly. The musculoskeletal system demonstrates a remarkable ability to adapt to the physical demands, or lack of physical demands, placed on the system. Pathologic conditions may adversely influence the structure and function of any component of the system and may lead to impairments. For example, bone abnormalities due to congenital deformities, disease processes, or abnormal growth can disrupt the normal length/tension relationship of the muscle and result in weakness. Likewise, muscle pathology, such as Duchenne muscular dystrophy (DMD), often leads to secondary adaptations and impairments such as joint contractures. The normal process of adaptation can either enhance function or lead to impairment, activity restriction, and participation limitation.

The musculoskeletal system and the neurologic system are also intertwined. A neurologic insult such as cerebral palsy (CP) frequently leads to muscle contractures and weakness. See Chapter 19 for a complete discussion of cerebral palsy. Neurologic impairments such abnormal neural maturation, insufficient and disorganized motor recruitment, impaired voluntary control, impaired reciprocal inhibition, altered setting of muscle spindles, and reinforcement of abnormal neural circuits[105] can contribute to weakness in individuals with cerebral palsy. In addition to neurologic changes, individuals with cerebral palsy can present with altered muscle tissue and abnormal bone growth. Over time, there is selective atrophy of fast fibers and altered myosin expression, changes in fiber length and cross-sectional area, changes in the length-tension curve, reduced elasticity, and impoverished muscle tissue development.[105] Once considered an isolated neurologic impairment, cerebral palsy is now viewed as a multisystem disease.

Conversely, when a person with an intact nervous system is immobilized in a cast for a musculoskeletal injury such a fracture, the timing and sequencing of muscle activation can change following cast removal due to a newly acquired range-of-motion limitation. Therapeutic interventions are often designed to promote musculoskeletal adaptations in an effort to prevent or correct physical impairments with the hope of enhancing function and participation in daily life activities. Accordingly, knowledge of normal growth and development and of the principles of adaptation of the musculoskeletal system is essential for understanding the efficacy of interventions. This chapter describes (1) the growth and development of muscle and bone and (2) the adaptations of muscle and bone, including the effects of select interventions designed to promote desired adaptations.

MUSCLE HISTOLOGY AND DEVELOPMENT

In the developing vertebrate embryo, two masses of mesoderm cells, called somites, form along the sides of the neural tube. Somites eventually differentiate into dermis (dermatome), skeletal muscle (myotome), and vertebrae (sclerotome). Because the sclerotome differentiates before the other two structures, the term *dermomyotome* refers to the combined dermatome and myotome. Progenitor cells (cells with the ability to differentiate into many types of cells) migrate from the dorsal medial lip of the dermomyotome and differentiate to form primary or secondary myotubes.[9] The primary myotubes are first observed at approximately 5 to 7 weeks' gestational age (GA), and most will eventually differentiate into type I (slow-twitch slow-oxidative) fibers. The three types of fast-twitch fibers (fast-twitch oxidative glycolytic [2A], fast-twitch glycolytic fibers [2B], and fast-twitch intermediate [2X]) primarily develop from the secondary myotubes and are observed at about 30 weeks of gestation.[131] The myofibers are long, cylindrical, multinucleated cells composed of actin and myosin myofibrils repeated as a sarcomere, the basic functional unit of the cell, which is responsible for the striated appearance of skeletal muscle.

A motor unit, consisting of a motoneuron and the muscle fibers it innervates, begins with the development of the neuromuscular junction. The primary myotubes are preferentially innervated first. By 8 weeks of gestation, acetylcholine receptors are dispersed within the myotubular membrane.[63] At this stage in development, multiple motor axons originating from different somites (precursor cells) innervate the developing end plates. These early motor units provide the earliest fetal movement, which is observed in the intercostal muscles. From 18 weeks' GA until several months post term, synaptic elimination occurs until each neuromuscular junction is innervated by only one axon.[30] Synaptic elimination occurs in both the central and peripheral nervous systems and is believed to be influenced by activity.[30] The adult pattern of one axon per muscle fiber permits a reproducible and predictable increase in force during performance of a task. Why fetal muscles are innervated initially by several axons and later undergo the elimination of all but one axon is not well established. It does not appear that the reason is to ensure that every muscle fiber is innervated. In partially denervated muscles of animals, the few remaining muscle fibers still undergo synaptic elimination, thus further reducing the size of the motor unit.[46]

During the last half of gestational growth, the number and size of muscle fibers increase so rapidly that most of the skeletal muscle fibers have developed by birth. This suggests that infants born very prematurely have different muscles from full-term babies. This is also supported by a cohort study that showed that there was a strong correlation between birth weight and adult strength, with other confounding variables accounted for.[83] By the end of the first year of life, the remaining muscle fibers are developed. From this point, new muscle fibers originate from either the division of existing cells or the differentiation of myoblasts into secondary myotubes.[106] During the growing years, muscles increase in length and cross-sectional area through the addition of sarcomeres within individual muscle fibers.[106] Their final size depends on many factors, including blood supply, innervation, nutrition, gender, genetics, and exercise.

The bulk associated with a mature muscle comes from the many multinucleated fibers. Next to these fibers, however, are quiescent satellite cells. Satellite cells are mononucleated, myogenic cells that proliferate in response to stress or injury to aid in muscle regeneration. The satellite cells themselves have the ability to regenerate after restoration of the damaged muscle fibers. In diseases such as DMD, the rate of muscle degeneration greatly exceeds the rate at which the satellite cells can repair tissue and regenerate themselves. This imbalance exhausts the supply of satellite cells, and muscle fibers can no longer be regenerated leading to progressive weakness.[73]

Structure and Function of the Normal Muscle-Tendon Unit

The normal muscle-tendon unit (MTU) is composed of muscle fibers, two cytoskeletal systems within the muscle fibers (exosarcomeric and endosarcomeric), the supportive connective tissues within and around the muscle belly (endomysium, perimysium, and epimysium), and the dense regular connective tissue of the tendon that connects the muscle to the bone. Total muscle force production achieved by an MTU is influenced by many factors, including the size of the muscle fibers, the firing rate of the motor unit action potentials, recruitment and de-recruitment patterns, muscle architecture, the angle of pull, the lever arm, and changes in the length of the muscle. The membrane at the muscle-tendon junction typically has a folded appearance that is thought to reduce membrane stress. With disuse atrophy the amount of folding is decreased and therefore under greater stress. This change is likely why atrophied muscles sustain increased tears.[131]

A passive length-tension curve is developed on the basis of muscle tension that is produced as the muscle is stretched from its resting length to its maximal length. The initial take-up part of the curve (left part of the curve) represents the resting length, and the end point of the curve (right part of the curve) represents the maximal length (Fig. 5.1). The force produced by the active component depends primarily on the amount of overlap of the actin and myosin filaments. The maximum isometric force is produced near the resting length (due to the optimal overlap of the actin and myosin filaments) of an isolated muscle; it decreases as the muscle is lengthened or shortened relative to the resting length. This force-length relationship forms the basis of the sliding filament theory of muscle contraction.[172] The force generated by the active component of the MTU also depends on the integrity of the central and peripheral nervous systems, the excitation-contraction coupling mechanism, and the cross-sectional area of the skeletal muscle tissues. In a completely relaxed skeletal muscle (i.e., when the central nervous system [CNS] is not intact or when no artificial stimulation occurs), no active tension exists.

Passive resistance, which is the equivalent of resting muscle tone, increases exponentially as the muscle is lengthened. When

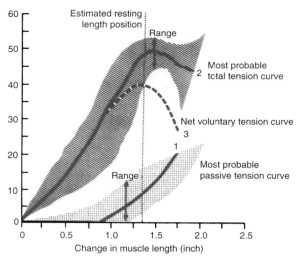

FIG. 5.1 Classic length-tension curves for skeletal muscle. Net voluntary active tension is predicted by subtracting passive tension from total tension. (From Astrand P, Rodahl K, Dahl HA, et al: *Textbook of work physiology*, ed 4, Champaign, IL, 2003, Human Kinetics.)

a resting muscle is passively stretched, the force produced by the passive component of the MTU is thought to be brought about by three mechanisms: (1) stretching stable cross-links between the actin and myosin filaments, (2) stretching proteins within the exosarcomeric and endosarcomeric cytoskeleton (series elastic component), and (3) deformation of the connective tissues of the muscle (parallel elastic component). The passive component accounts for the resistance felt during passive stretch of a fully relaxed muscle. Intracellular and extracellular components are now thought to contribute to passive stiffness. Numerous proteins are believed to play a role in muscle stiffness, but the exact mechanism is unknown.[97,131]

In contrast, tendons, which are made up of dense regular connective tissue, are generally considered noncontributory to the overall passive length-tension relationships of the stretched MTU. Dense regular connective tissues present exceedingly high stiffness and therefore are unlikely to stretch. Passive stiffness can be represented by the ratio of the change in passive torque to the change in the joint angle.

An intermediate-sized protein of the exosarcomeric cytoskeleton known as *desmin* is thought to help reduce passive muscle stiffness. Desmin is the major subunit of the intermediate protein filaments forming the Z-discs. Desmin connects the Z-discs with many cell organelles and also extends longitudinally from Z-disc to Z-disc outside the sarcomere.[172] Because of this longitudinal orientation, desmin lengthens as the sarcomere is stretched. In animal studies, when desmin is removed, the muscle becomes increasingly fibrotic and passive stiffness increases dramatically.[102] Many proteins are present in a sarcomere, other than those discussed here. The absence of or pathology of the sarcomere proteins is responsible for many of the muscular dystrophies.[157]

Adaptations of Muscle Fibers

Muscle fiber types are susceptible to both internal and external influences. In normal muscle, fiber types are randomly distributed to form a mosaic pattern, and little variation in fiber size is noted. In the presence of disease, this pattern is altered and often well documented in adults. Evaluating muscle composition in children, however, is difficult because, unless the sample can be obtained as an adjunct to a surgery, elective biopsy is required. This usually results in small sample sizes, which likely are a cause of the lack of consensus among reports. With this limitation in mind, the following information is presented.

Spasticity is a common impairment seen by physical therapists. Previously, this excessive stiffness was thought to be attributable almost exclusively to a hyperactive stretch reflex. A wider focus is now the current thinking and includes (1) altered muscle fiber size and fiber type distribution, (2) proliferation of extracellular matrix, (3) increased muscle cell, and (4) inferior mechanical properties of extracellular material.[48]

The deep fascicle angle (angle at which fascicles arise from a deep aponeurosis) is also related to stiffness. It is generally believed that the fascicle length of the gastrocnemii and rectus femoris muscles is reduced in CP compared with age-matched peers, but the data are somewhat ambiguous.[98,107,137] It is hypothesized that this angulation contributes to muscle shortening.

Muscle histopathology reports can be inconsistent for children with CP (most likely due to small sample sizes), but researchers agree that spastic muscles vary considerably from typical muscles.[48,50,114,123,138,139] One consistent theme that arises from spastic muscle reports is that the muscles are overall smaller than typically developing peers.[57] In an animal model of young, hypertonic mouse muscles, longitudinal muscle growth has been shown to increase in length at only 55% of the rate of growing bone in contrast to the expected 100%.[180] To keep up with growing bone, the sarcomeres of the spastic muscle stretch to increase to the necessary length. It is generally agreed that this is an important contribution to the muscle weakness and contracture seen in children with cerebral palsy. The reduced growth rate leads to a lower than expected number of in-series sarcomeres and subsequent overstretched length of each individual sarcomere.[98] This shifts the muscle well past the optimal length/tension relationship resulting in a greatly reduced ability to generate force. Longer sarcomeres were also correlated with greater joint contracture. Longer sarcomeres also indicate that there is increased sarcomere strain, resulting in skeletal muscle injury. In turn, repeated strain-induced injuries drastically increase collagen content and fibrosis in skeletal muscle, which will increase stiffness.[140,161] This is an important consideration when intervening to correct a plantar flexion contracture. While lengthening the muscle through a serial casting, the practitioner must be cognizant of the possibility that he or she may be stretching the sarcomeres to an even greater mechanical disadvantage that could result in increased weakness.[98] The pathologic changes in muscle in children with CP also should be considered when contemplating an Achilles tendon lengthening. In many children with CP, the tendon is already longer and the gastrocnemius muscle shorter than in typically developing children.[177] A tendon lengthening will increase the child's range of motion but may decrease the amount of force the child can generate, because the muscles are placed at a decreased mechanical advantage.[177]

Varying degrees of atrophy and hypertrophy of type I and type II fibers have been reported and appear to be dependent on muscle group, severity of CP, and age of the child.[24,48,50,88,123] Moreau and colleagues[107] reported decreased cross-sectional area, muscle thickness, and fascicle length in children with CP compared with typically developing children. Booth[17] found

excessive amounts of collagen and fibrous tissue in older children with CP. The author suggested that collagen and fibrous tissues are irreversible detriments to muscle performance.[17] It is not known whether this is a preventable change.

The clinical application of muscle histology could be enhanced by additional research. One example is the finding by Rose and colleagues[127] that children with spastic diplegia who had a predominance of type I fibers expended more energy and had more prolonged electromyograph (EMG) activity during walking than children with CP and a predominance of type II fibers. There is some evidence that targeted training programs can alter fiber type composition in adults.[37,43,70] Research in children is needed to determine if we could change the muscle composition of our patients and if this would translate to improved function.

FORCE AND LENGTH ADAPTATIONS IN THE MUSCLE-TENDON UNIT

Researchers have used length-tension curves to provide information about histologic and histochemical changes in muscles related to length and stiffness. After intervention, the position and steepness of the curve may change, indicating a change in muscle length or stiffness. For example, a shift of the curve to the left indicates a shorter muscle, and a shift to the right indicates a longer muscle. A steeper curve indicates that the muscle is less compliant (stiffer).

Studies have shown that even short-term casted immobilization can create significant losses in quadriceps strength and cross-sectional area.[41,164] Less than 1 week of immobilization led to a 3.5% to 10% reduction in size and a 9% to 13% strength reduction.[41,148] This was increased to an 8% to 20% decrease in size and a 20% to 23% reduction in strength after 14 days.[148,164] Immobilization for as little as 2 to 3 weeks has been reported to reduce muscle strength by 10% to 47%.[65,111] After 2 weeks of spontaneous activity, an 11% strength deficit was still noted.[65] Similar to casting, bed rest for 28 days or more also consistently shows reduced muscle strength and size.[14]

Although changes in immobilized muscle strength and resting length have been attributed to loss of sarcomeres, changes in passive stiffness following immobilization have been attributed to changes in the connective tissues.[54,173] Early in shortened-position immobilization, an increase in the concentration of hydroxyproline occurs in relation to the total volume of the muscle, indicating an increase in connective tissue. Reorganization of the collagen fibers of the perimysium into more acute angles to the muscle fiber axis was also seen.[71] This resulted in greater tension per unit of passive elongation, otherwise known as increased stiffness. The passive length-tension curves were shifted to the left and appeared steeper, indicating that the muscles were shorter and stiffer after immobilization in the shortened position (Fig. 5.2).

Conversely, animal research suggests that immobilization of muscles in lengthened positions can cause an increase in the number of sarcomeres and therefore in muscle length.[153] However, in animals, the number of sarcomeres will revert to the original number in 4 weeks.[153] The addition of sarcomeres was accompanied by muscle weight gain and increased protein synthesis after immobilization.[142] Similar to immobilization in a shortened position, the change in sarcomeres predominantly occurs at the ends of the muscle fibers, which appear to be the most responsive area, as most of the normal postnatal growth

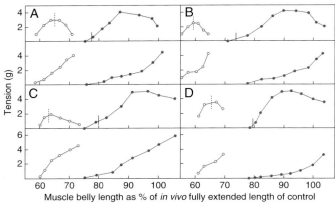

FIG. 5.2 Length-tension curves for young muscles (A to D) immobilized in the shortened position *(red)* and their controls *(blue)*. (From Williams PE, Goldspink G: Changes in sarcomere length and physiologic properties in immobilized muscle. *J Anat* 127(Pt 3): 459–468, 1978.)

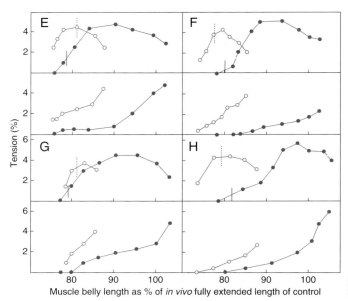

FIG. 5.3 Length-tension curves for young animals (E to H) immobilized in the lengthened position *(red)* and their controls *(blue)*. (From Williams PE, Goldspink G: Changes in sarcomere length and physiologic properties in immobilized muscle, *J Anat* 127(Pt 3): 459–468, 1978.)

of young animals occurs here.[174] As with muscles immobilized in the shortened position, the sarcomere length adapts to maintain optimal actin and myosin overlap. Overall, animal research suggests that immobilization in a shortened position has a more profound change in sarcomeres (40% loss) than immobilization in the lengthened position (19% increase).[153]

Active and passive length-tension curves for adult muscles that were immobilized in a lengthened position were shifted to the right (indicating that they were lengthened) compared with those of adult controls (i.e., nonimmobilized muscle).[173] In young mice, however, muscles immobilized in the shortened or lengthened position resulted in an overall decreased muscle length, with a concomitant increase in tendon length.[173] This caused a shift in the length tension curve to the left, indicating a decline in strength[173] (Fig. 5.3). Evidence suggests that a tendon elongates more readily in young, growing animals than in adult animals. Although this work was performed in animals, it should still be considered when casting to increase range of motion (ROM).

Botulinum toxin (BoNT-A) injections inhibit the release of acetylcholine at the neuromuscular junction, which results in an immobilized portion of the treated muscle.[108] The affected nerve terminals do not degenerate, but the blockage of neurotransmitter release is irreversible. Similar to physical immobilization, this chemical immobilization leads to increased sarcomere length and decreased force production.[156] Initial muscle tissue recovery from a toxin such as BoNT-A is achieved by collateral sprouting from nerve terminals. Sprouting reaches a peak around 8 to 12 weeks post injection. After this time the original function of the neuromotor junction returns and synaptic elimination of excessive neurons begins. This process is similar to the synaptic elimination seen in postnatal development. In animals, the rate of synaptic elimination is dependent on the amount of use the muscle receives.[32] If human muscle responds similarly, this may explain why the addition of BoNT-A to serial casting frequently does not improve outcome.[75]

Skeletal and Articular Structures

Like muscle tissue, both skeletal and articular tissues arise from the mesodermal layer of the embryo (Fig. 5.4). Mesenchymal cells condense to form templates of the skeleton. From this

point, two distinct processes of bone formation take place: (1) endochondral ossification and (2) intramembranous ossification. All bones, with the exception of the clavicle, mandible, and skull, are formed by endochondral ossification (also called intracartilaginous ossification).[106] During the early embryonic period, collagenous and elastic fibers are deposited on the mesenchymal models and form cartilaginous models. Bone minerals are deposited on these new models and gradually replace the cartilage via the process of ossification. Intramembranous ossification occurs directly in the mesenchymal model. Mesenchymal cells differentiate into osteoblasts that deposit a matrix called osteoid tissue. This tissue is organized into bone as calcium phosphate is deposited.[124] Ossification at the primary ossification centers, typically in the center of the diaphysis or body of the bone, commences at the end of the embryonic period (eighth fetal week).[106]

Bone development progresses most rapidly in the prenatal period. By the time of birth, the diaphyses are almost ossified. If a child is born prematurely, however, osteopenia is frequently seen. In the very premature, it may result in bone fragility and must be considered if therapy is being provided to the very young neonate. After birth, long bones grow in length at the epiphyseal plate, which is between the diaphysis and the epiphysis. This cartilaginous plate rapidly proliferates on the diaphyseal side of the bone. The resultant chondrocytes, arranged in parallel columns, become enlarged and are then converted into bone by endochondral ossification.[124] Eventually, the epiphyseal plate is ossified, the diaphyses and epiphyses are joined, and the growth of the bone in length is considered complete. The timing of complete ossification varies with each particular bone. Most bones are fully ossified by 20 years of age, but for a few bones, the process can continue longer into adulthood.[106]

Bone is increased in width through appositional growth, which is the accumulation of new bone on bone surfaces. To keep the bone from becoming too thick and therefore too

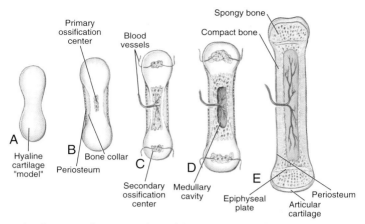

FIG. 5.4 Schematic diagram of progression of bone growth. (From Applegate E: *The anatomy and physiology learning system,* ed 4, St. Louis, 2011, Saunders.)

heavy, osteoblasts on the inside of the bone are reabsorbed as new bone is added on the surface. This results in an increase in thickness and density of the diaphysis without excess weight.

Joint formation also begins as the cartilaginous models are formed. In a specialized area between cartilaginous bone models, the interzonal mesenchyme differentiates to form the joint. The basic structures of the joint are formed during the sixth to seventh weeks of gestation, but the final shape develops throughout early childhood under the influence of the forces of movement and compression.[106] One example of the relationship between joint formation and movement is seen in children with brachial plexus injuries. Pearl and colleagues[117] examined 84 children between the ages of 7 months and 13½ years who had obstetric brachial plexus palsy that resulted in medial rotation contractures of the shoulder. Sixty-one percent had extreme glenohumeral deformities, including flat glenoids, biconcave glenoids, pseudoglenoids, and flattened, oval humeral heads. The mechanical forces created by the unopposed medial rotators had a profound effect on the development of this joint.

Hip joint development is another good example of changes during the fetal period. At 12 weeks of GA, the acetabulum is extremely deep, and the head of the femur is quite round and well covered (Fig. 5.5).[121] As the fetus increases in age, the relative depth of the acetabulum decreases as the head of the femur becomes more hemispheric. At birth, the acetabulum is so shallow that it covers less than half of the femoral head; this results in a relatively unstable hip and is thought to allow for easier passage through the vaginal canal. Because of the combination of shallow acetabulum, flattened femoral head, high neck shaft angle, and a large amount of anteversion, the hip is especially vulnerable to dislocating forces during the third trimester.[121] The risk of dislocation is greatest if the child is delivered in single-breech position (i.e., hips flexed and knees extended).[150] It was postulated that extreme hip flexion combined with knee extension caused the hamstrings to pull the head of the femur downward, stretching the compliant hip capsule. After birth, the femur may be dislocated by the upward pull of the iliopsoas muscle when infants are diapered and wrapped with the hips extended.[150]

During postnatal growth, the forces of compression and movement contribute to an increase in the depth of the acetabulum until the age of 10 years, when the adult level of femoral head coverage is reached.[8] The head of the femur also becomes

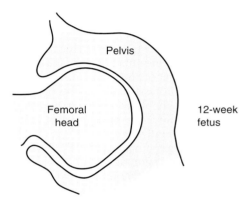

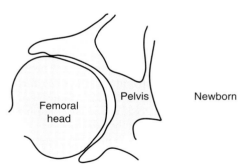

FIG. 5.5 Schematic diagram of the fetal and newborn hip joint, illustrating changes in acetabular coverage of the femoral head. Coverage is extensive in the 12-week fetus, but it is reduced in the newborn.

rounder, but it never achieves the roundness that it had during the early fetal period. A listing of reference values for changing range of motion from birth through 5 years of age can be found in Table 5.1.

Skeletal Adaptations

Although deformities can occur throughout the growing period, the skeleton is most vulnerable during the first few years of life (prenatal and postnatal), when the rate of growth is greatest.[22] Fetal position has been related to various deformities, especially

TABLE 5.1   **Central Tendency Values of Lower Extremity Range of Motion Reported in Degrees for Children Born Full Term, From Birth Through 5 Years Old**

	Birth	6 Weeks	6 Months	1 Year	3 Years	5 Years
Hip extension limitation	34.2	19	7	7	7	7
Hip abduction	55			59	59	54
Hip adduction	6.4			30	31	24
Hip external rotation	90	48	53	58	56	39
Hip internal rotation	33	24	24	38	39	34
Popliteal angle	27		11	0	0	0

From Long TM, Cintas HL, editors: *Handbook of pediatric physical therapy*, Baltimore, MD, 1995, Williams & Wilkins.

those that occur toward the end of pregnancy when the neonate is outgrowing the space in utero. Factors that can increase the risk of prenatal deformities include decreased amniotic fluid, which further limits the space in which the fetus can move, multiple births, and excessive forces from tightly stretched uterine and abdominal walls. Associated deformities include congenital torticollis, plagiocephaly (asymmetrical head), and developmental dysplasia of the hip.[39,84]

After initial development, bone shape can be changed through a process of bone functional adaption, which uses resorption of old or immature bone and formation of new bone to determine its shape. Bone structure adapts in response to the mechanical forces that are placed on the bones.[129] The type of loading and stress (or force per bone area) in different situations affects bones differently.

Loading a bone longitudinally (parallel to the direction of growth) results in compression or tension. Either type of loading, applied intermittently with appropriate force, such as with weight bearing or muscle pull, stimulates bone growth. The *Hueter-Volkmann principle* describes the reaction of bone to excessive force and states that excessive static loading will cause bone material to decrease, which can be detrimental to bone integrity and strength.[124]

Shear forces, which run parallel to the epiphyseal plate, can lead to torsional or twisting changes in the bone. The columns of chondrocytes around the periphery of the plate veer away from the shear forces in a twisting pattern. The normal pull of muscles around a joint contributes to the shear forces, resulting in normal torsional changes in the long bones. For example, at birth, the tibia exhibits 0° to 5° of medial torsion but increases to around 25° of lateral torsion by adulthood.[87]

Just as normal forces shape bones, asymmetrical forces will lead to asymmetrical growth as the growth plates line up perpendicular to the direction of the forces. This can be advantageous during fracture healing, as the bone is able to straighten some degree of malalignment through a process known as *flexure drift*. This remodeling mechanism describes a process whereby strain on a curved bone wall applied by repeated loading tends to move the bone surface in the direction of the concavity to straighten the bone.[87] Bone is resorbed from the convex side and is laid down on the concave side. This process is seen in the femur and tibia as a normal part of development of the position of the knee in the frontal plane. At birth, the infant's knees are bowlegged (genu varum), but they gradually straighten until they reach a neutral alignment between the first and second years. The knee angulation then progresses toward genu valgum, reaching its peak between the ages of 2 and 4 years. After this time, the angle of genu valgum gradually decreases (Fig. 5.6).[130] The final knee angle differs slightly according to race

and gender.[2,20] Typical values vary by author, but in general, by adolescence, Caucasian girls have a tibial angle of between 0° and 5.8° of valgus, and boys range from 5° of valgus to 5° of varus.[20,61] In contrast, Cheng and associates[28] found that Chinese children of both genders progressed to genu varus of less than 5° in the preteen years. The pediatric therapist should be aware that the presence of genu varus between the ages of 2 and 6 years may need a referral to an orthopedic specialist. Artificially applied asymmetrical compression of one epiphyseal plate of the proximal tibia by surgical stapling or a tension band can be used to correct these deformities.[72] For children with leg length differences, surgical staples are applied to both sides of the epiphyseal plate of the longer leg to slow its growth until the shorter leg catches up.[51] The Ilizarov and monolateral devices for limb lengthening use tension to facilitate bone growth.[51] With this technique, the diaphyseal cortex of the bone of the shorter leg is cut, and gradual incremental distraction is applied across the cut ends of the bone. Osteogenesis occurs in the space between the two ends of the cut bone.

Normal developmental changes in the femur illustrate the impact of the muscular system on bone. To understand these changes, the terms *version* and *torsion* require discussion. Torsion refers to the normal amount of twist present in a long bone (Fig. 5.7). Femoral torsion is the angle formed by an axis drawn along the head and neck of the femur and another through the femoral condyles. To visualize this angle, picture a femur with the posterior surfaces of the femoral condyles on a horizontal surface such as a table. When looking up toward the hip, you will notice that the head and neck of the femur are angled upward from the table approximately 15°. This is the angle of torsion.

Antetorsion occurs when the head and neck of the femur are rotated forward in the transverse plane relative to the femoral condyles. If the head and neck of the femur are rotated posteriorly, the femur is said to be in retrotorsion. At birth, the femur has its maximum antetorsion at approximately 30° to 40°.[143] This angle decreases rapidly during the infant's first year, more slowly between 1 and 8 years, and then rapidly again through adolescence to a mean of 16° by age 14 to 16 years.[143] The femur is said to "untwist" through the process of growth, muscle action, reduction of the coxa valga angle, and reduction of the hip flexion contracture. The femoral head, neck, and greater trochanteric areas are made of pliable cartilage and are attached to the rigid osseous diaphysis. As the infant develops, normal torsional forces about this point of fixation cause a decrease in femoral antetorsion. Bleck[12] speculated that the active external hip rotation and extension forces created during walking have a major impact on developmental changes in femoral antetorsion. If active hip motions are minimal or walking is delayed, as

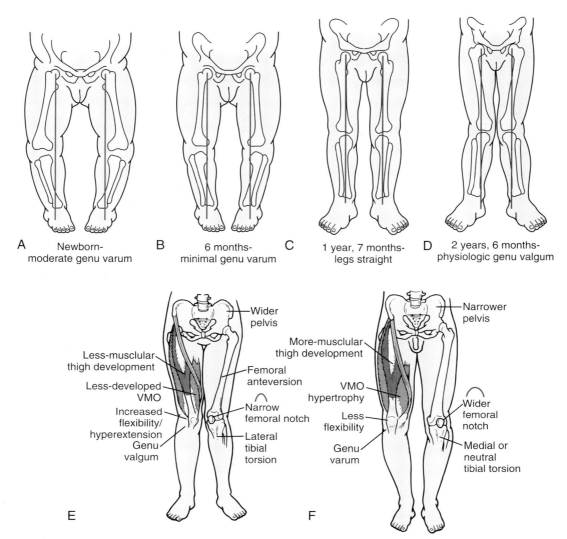

FIG. 5.6 A-D, Physiologic evolution of lower limb alignment at various ages in infancy and childhood. E and F, Alignment differences between teenage female (E) and teenage male (F). (*A-D,* Redrawn from Herring JA: *Tachdjian's pediatric orthopaedics: from the Texas Scottish Rite Hospital for Children Tachdjian's pediatric orthopaedics, ed 5,* Philadelphia, 2014, Saunders. *E and F,* Redrawn from Griffin LY: *Rehabilitation of the injured knee,* ed 2, St. Louis, 1995, Mosby.)

is frequently observed in children with CP, the infantile femoral torsion does not decrease as it should.

Version refers to a position of a segment relative to a plane. Femoral version refers to the position of the head of the femur in the acetabulum (see Fig. 5.7). When the pelvis is visualized in supine, the angle that the head and shaft create relative to the back of the pelvis aligned on the frontal plane is the amount of version. Anteversion positions the head of the femur anteriorly in the acetabulum and results in a position of thigh external rotation. Conversely, retroversion positions the head of the femur posteriorly in the acetabulum, which results in thigh internal rotation. At birth, a neonate has 40° to 60° of anteversion. This gradually resolves over time to 15° to 20° by age 8 to 10 years and down to 12° in adulthood. The externally rotated posture seen in newborns is attributed to the high amount of anteversion. At birth, anteversion (60°) is greater than antetorsion (30°) with a net result of an externally rotated posture.[165]

Excessive or persistent fetal antetorsion can lead to an in-toed gait pattern. In-toeing becomes apparent as the amount of hip

external rotation decreases with age. A majority of otherwise healthy children with persistent fetal antetorsion will improve as the hips spontaneously realign by age 10 years. In less than 1% of these children, antetorsion fails to resolve by age 10 years, and the children warrant treatment.[143] In children with CP, however, persistent fetal antetorsion is a causative factor in the development of hip instability. This is discussed in greater detail later in the chapter.

Atypical pressures, such as those seen in children with obesity or spasticity, can deform the femur and component parts of the hip. Children with obesity are at increased risk of developing a flattened femoral head and a slipped capital epiphysis because of the excessive weight on the developing femoral head.[30] Children with spasticity are at risk for subluxation or dislocation from the asymmetrical pull of spastic muscles around the hip.[179] Buckley and colleagues[19] examined 33 unstable hips in children with these disabilities and found that all had significantly shallower acetabula compared with those of a control group; the hip was most shallow in children with CP.

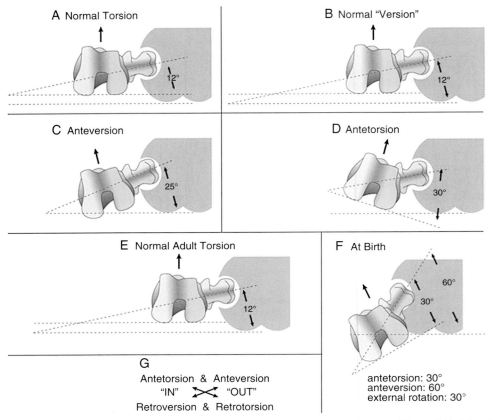

FIG. 5.7 Schematic drawing illustrating femoral version and torsion. (From Effgen, SK: *Meeting the physical therapy needs of children,* ed 2, Philadelphia, 2013, FA Davis Company.)

Five-year outcome of a surveillance program of children and adolescents with cerebral palsy revealed that the incidence of marked hip displacement (migration percentage > 30%) was directly related to gross motor function, classified according to the gross motor function classification system (GMFCS), with distribution of GMFCS I = 10 (3%), II = 40 (13%), III = 53 (43%), IV = 96 (59%), and V = 115 (64%).[79] Ambulation abilities provide the necessary forces to help the hip joint develop properly.

Disuse adversely affects bone by delaying secondary ossification centers and causing the bone to reabsorb. Children with a reduced activity level due to conditions such as CP, myelodysplasia, or arthrogryposis multiplex congenita are at greater risk for fracture because of disuse atrophy of the bones. The diagnosis of CP alone does not increase a child's risk for fractures. In children level GMFCS levels I to III, the risk is similar to that in typically developing children.[68,157] Children classified as GMFCS level IV or V had a twofold increase in the risk of fracture than healthy peers. Researchers have attempted to predict which children with CP are most likely to sustain a fracture.[157] The risk of fractures for those in GMFCS levels IV and V on antiepileptic drug therapy was a twofold increase ($P = 0.004$). The risk for fractures without trauma in children small for their age and those who did not use standing devices was significantly increased: adjusted incidence rate ratio (AIRR) 4.16 ($P = 0.011$) and 3.66 ($P = 0.010$), respectively. The use of a gastrostomy feeding tube produced conflicting results. A reduced risk of fractures with trauma was reported, but an increased risk of fractures without trauma

was also noted (AIRR 0.10, $P = 0.003$, and 4.36, $P = 0.012$, respectively).[45,157]

The increased risk of fracture is assumed to be due to disuse demineralization. Disuse demineralization can occur quickly. One study found a 34% decrease in bone mineralization after non–weight-bearing immobilization following a fracture or surgery in only 4 to 6 weeks.[152]

Decreased bone mineralization is also seen in chronic conditions such as hemophilia,[6] HIV,[25] leukemia,[168] symptomatic epilepsy,[134,135] long-term use of glucocorticoids,[100] growth hormone deficiency, myelomeningocele,[86] and idiopathic scoliosis.[67] Likewise, bone density deficiencies accompany digestive system conditions such as celiac disease,[21] Crohn's disease,[58] and irritable bowel disorder.[132]

Although the literature is inconsistent at times, methods to promote healthy bone mineralization have been documented.[66] A comprehensive review of dietary requirements for bone health is outside the scope of this chapter. The reader is strongly encouraged to review current literature before making any recommendations on supplements.[119] Weight bearing improves bone thickness and density as evidenced by comparing athletes with nonathletes or in individuals who increase their physical activity.[64] An increase in bone density was observed in typically developing children with a consistent program of impact exercise, whereas children who participated in a non–weight-bearing exercise such as swimming did not see an increase in bone density.[34,64]

Parents may be able to help infants with myelomeningocele improve bone mineralization.[86] Parents were asked to help their babies' practice being upright and stepping 10 continuous minutes per day, 5 days per week on an in-home treadmill for 12 months. The results were not statistically significant but were encouraging enough to warrant future research.[86]

There is also evidence that weight-bearing programs improve bone mineral density and promote hip modeling in children with CP.[45,92,170] We do know that mobile children with CP have greater bone mineral density when compared with their less mobile peers.[175,176] In a population-based study, the use of a standing frame was associated with a much lower risk of fracture in children with CP classified as GMFCS levels IV and V.[157] In a review article by Paleg et al.,[114] the authors concluded that standing programs 5 days per week positively affect bone mineral density (60 to 90 min/d); hip stability (60 min/d in 30° to 60° of total bilateral hip abduction); and range of motion of the hip, knee, and ankle (45 to 60 min/d).

Intermittent weight bearing with movement was most beneficial to hip joint modeling.[35,147] Intermittent weight bearing with movement can be accomplished by partial–weight-bearing ambulation with the use of a treadmill or gait trainer. Choosing an appropriate standing frame is also very important. Kecskemethy and colleagues[76] measured the percentage of a child's body weight that was being directed down to the stander and found that it ranged from 37% to 100%. If the goal is to provide weight bearing, then it would be logical to obtain as much weight as the child can tolerate during standing. The authors suggested that the Rifton (Rifton Equipment; PO Box 260, Rifton, New York, 12471-0260) supine stander positioned at an angle of 70° was an appropriate choice.[9] Weight bearing is an important part of physical therapy intervention for young children with neuromuscular diseases that delay the development of stance. The formation, growth, and integrity of articular cartilage are stimulated by compressive forces and movement between bone surfaces. Intermittent joint loading leads to healthy, thick cartilage.

Age and diet also affect bone mass and strength. Children are most at risk for distal forearm fractures during their pubertal growth spurt.[5,125] The rate of increase in the child's height and weight is greater than the rate of increase in the strength of the cortical bone at the radial metaphysis, which puts the bone at a mechanical disadvantage when an adolescent falls onto an outstretched arm.[125] Children who are obese have a higher bone mass density than children of appropriate weight, but not to the extent necessary to support their size. Therefore obese children have a high incidence of upper extremity fractures compared with their lighter-weight peers.[40,169] The overall incidence of forearm fractures in childhood has been increasing; this is postulated to result from the combination of vulnerable bone tissue with changes in diet (i.e., higher soft drink consumption and lower calcium intake) and increases in higher-risk physical activity, such as skate or hover boarding.[31,80]

Changes in the muscular or skeletal system have interactive effects. Understanding the influences of these two systems on the development and final outcome of each system and recognizing the period when these systems are most mutable assist the therapist in designing effective treatment programs, as well as in knowing when to discontinue treatment procedures.

Long-Term Effects of Atypical Musculoskeletal Development

In many neurologic or genetic diseases associated with developmental delay, the initial condition is considered nonprogressive,

but the musculoskeletal impairments that frequently accompany these conditions typically worsen as the child grows. Adults with CP frequently develop a wide range of musculoskeletal issues such as scoliosis, hip dislocation, cervical neck dislocation, contracture, arthritis, patella alta, overuse syndrome, nerve entrapment, and fracture.[151] Discussed here are examples of common developmental musculoskeletal pathologies. More information on specific conditions mentioned can be found in subsequent chapters in this volume.

You have learned that the hip is unstable at birth but undergoes a great deal of normal developmental change, which increases stability. These normal developmental changes result from a combination of muscle pull and weight bearing. Children with CP typically have delayed walking, ROM limitations, and atypical muscular pull/spasticity. Hip subluxation and dislocation therefore are common problems in children with spastic CP. The risk increases dramatically as the level of severity of the cerebral palsy increases. In a surveillance report, the incidence of a migration percentage of greater than 30% was minimal for GMFCS level I and rose to over 80% for level IV (level II = 15%, level III = 40%, level IV = 70%).[178] Adequate ROM allows the hip to move into a stable, well-covered position in the acetabulum. Children with CP tend to lose abduction range and to develop hip flexion contractures, both of which are detrimental to hip stability. Critical ROM values for hip stability include maintaining at least 30° of abduction and avoiding a hip flexion contracture of 20° to 25° or more.[104]

A variety of idiopathic conditions are characterized by a disorder of endochondral ossification. The incidence of many of these conditions is increasing, and the increased obesity rate in children in most often suggested as a cause.[27] See Chapter 14 for a detailed discussion of these orthopedic conditions. Legg-Calvé-Perthes (LCP) disease is a hip disorder that involves repeated episodes of transient synovitis of the hip, usually occurring in boys between the ages of 3 and 12.[62] The synovitis causes an increased joint pressure, which interrupts blood flow in the vessels ascending the femoral neck. This typically results in pain, decreased hip abduction and internal rotation, and an atypical gait pattern, in which patients have a limp and a positive Trendelenburg sign. Roughly 50% of the boys diagnosed with LCP will develop hip arthritis in adulthood.[62]

Slipped capital femoral epiphysis (SCFE) occurs in adolescents between the ages of 12 and 15 when the growth plate of the proximal femoral physis is weak. The subjects in the obese children studies had decreased femoral anteversion. This positioning, along with increased body weight, may account for increased mechanical shear forces acting across the immature hip joint.[27] Patients with SCFE usually have an antalgic gait pattern and pain in the groin. Treatment for SCFE involves keeping the displacement to a minimum, maintaining ROM, and preventing degenerative arthritis. SCFE and Legg-Calvé-Perthes disease are childhood conditions that present a risk factor for the development of osteoarthritis and disability later in life.

Lower extremity rotational and angular problems are common lower extremity abnormalities in children. Rotational problems include in-toeing and out-toeing. In-toeing is caused by metatarsus adductus, increased femoral anteversion, internal tibial torsion, or any combination of the three. Consequently, out-toeing is caused by the opposite factors for in-toeing. Internal tibial torsion is a normal finding in the newborn, but it may pose a problem at walking age if not corrected. Casting can correct metatarsus adductus, but conservative treatments for femoral anteversion and tibial torsion have not been shown to be effective. Angular problems such as genu varus and genu valgum are also common lower extremity abnormalities. Genu varus may lead to Blount's disease, which is a progressive deformity manifested by varus deformity and internal rotation of the tibia in the proximal metaphyseal region immediately below the knee. Blount's disease leads to irreversible pathologic changes at the medial portion of the proximal tibial epiphysis caused by growth disturbances of the subjacent physis.[27,175]

Patella alta is a condition in which the patella is positioned higher than expected on the femur. It frequently presents in early adolescence as anterior knee pain and progresses with age. It is common in individuals who walk with flexed knees, such as adults with CP, or who have overactive quadriceps muscles.[77] Maintaining adequate quadriceps and rectus femoris muscle length may help prevent patella alta. With patella alta, quadriceps strength is compromised and terminal knee extension is difficult. Pain and weakness can result in functional losses during activities such as walking, climbing stairs, or getting out of a chair.

Further study into the causes and prevention of secondary conditions is greatly needed to help guide the treatment of children with developmental disabilities. Pediatric therapists are appropriate professionals to educate parents and children about the lifelong attention that will need to be given to musculoskeletal problems, such as decreased strength and ROM. When appropriate, adolescents should be taught to be responsible for their physical and cardiopulmonary needs. Another role for pediatric therapists is educating their fellow orthopedic physical therapists who treat adults about the musculoskeletal problems in the neglected populations of adults with CP, myelodysplasia, and other developmental disabilities.

Measurement and Effects of Intervention

Fundamental goals of therapeutic intervention for physical disabilities include enhancing participation in daily activities and life roles by preventing or correcting the body structures and function that result from the underlying pathologic condition or from the normal physiologic adaptations superimposed on the pathologic condition. One assumption is that activity and participation will be enhanced if impairments are prevented or corrected. One study found that a moderate correlation existed between rectus femoris size; strength of knee extensors and ankle extensors with the activity; and participation components of the International Classification of Functioning, Disability and Health–Child and Youth.[82] Additional research, however, is needed to establish causation. Achieving functional levels of ROM and strength is a fundamental goal of therapeutic intervention. Accurate assessments of ROM and strength are therefore important components of the physical therapy examination process.

Range-of-Motion Examination

A wide range of methods and instruments have been reported for examining the ROM about a joint or multiple joints, including simple visual estimation, use of various protractors and goniometers, measurements made from still photographs, complex methods using computerized motion analysis systems, and smart phone applications. For most physical therapists, however, the universal goniometer (i.e., full-circle manual goniometer) remains the most versatile and widely used instrument in clinical practice.

Technology is playing a larger role in various aspects of physical therapy including measuring range of motion. When using a smart phone or tablet application to measure ROM, it is important to keep in mind the reliability and validity of the application, which must be redetermined by the developer with each software upgrade. To date, most applications have not been validated for children or for use in dynamic situations such as using a frame of video to measure joint angles during gait.[103]

The reliability of goniometry is based on the reproducibility or stability of ROM measurements in relation to (1) the time intervals between comparable measurements or (2) the use of more than one rater. Many factors influence the reliability and validity of goniometric measurements. These factors include consistency of applied procedures, differences among joint actions and among the structure and function of body regions, passive versus active measurements, intrarater measurements (multiple measurements by one examiner) versus interrater measurements (multiple measurements by two or more examiners), normal day-to-day variations in ROM, and day-to-day variations in different pathologic conditions.[53]

Pandya and colleagues[115] studied seven upper and lower extremity joint limitations in 150 children with DMD and reported that intrarater reliability was high (intraclass correlation coefficient [ICC] range, .81 to .91), but interrater reliability was lower, with wide variation from joint to joint (ICC range, .25 to .91). Reported goniometric reliability in children with CP varies widely. Researchers agree that careful standardized procedures are necessary to ensure reliability and that variances of $\pm 10°$ in ROM over time could be due to measurement error.[60,81,99]

The hip is a particularly difficult joint for which to obtain reliable ROM measures. Bartlett and colleagues[7] compared four methods of measuring hip extension (by prone extension, Thomas test, Mundale method, and pelvic-femoral angle) in 15 children with spastic diplegia, 15 with meningomyelocele, and 15 with no known pathologic condition. They reported that the Thomas test was particularly difficult to apply to patients with spastic diplegia and the least reliable. In the meningomyelocele group the Mundale technique had the lowest reliability. They also reported that the pelvic-femoral angle method is more time consuming and no more accurate than other methods. Considering the ease of measurement and reliability, they recommend the prone hip extension test for patients with cerebral palsy and meningomyelocele and recommend the Thomas test as an alternative for nonspastic patients.

To perform the prone hip extension test, the child is in the prone position on a table with the opposite leg hanging over the edge of the table. In this position, the lumbar spine is flattened. The examiner holds the pelvis down at the level of the posterior superior iliac spines and pulls the leg that is being examined into hip extension until the pelvis begins to move anteriorly. At that point, the angle between the femur and the surface is measured and reflects the degree of hip flexion contracture. One limitation of this test is that it can be difficult to perform with large children because the therapist needs to hold the leg being tested while simultaneously holding the goniometer and measuring the angle.

Physical therapists work to improve a child's range-of-motion limitations, but further research is needed to establish minimum requirements for improved function. In a study by Lowes et al.,[90] strength and to a lesser extent ROM were shown to be accurate predictors of balance and functional skills. Follow-up studies are needed to determine if daily skills require critical ROM values. In other words, can improved ROM guarantee an improved activity level?

Strength Examination

Accurate measurement of strength is important for identifying strength deficits and for documenting changes in strength that result from interventions. See Chapter 2 for additional information on strength testing. Numerous methods of measuring strength are available, including the traditional procedures of manual muscle testing and the use of various handheld force dynamometers[16] and computerized isokinetic testing systems.[78,128] Although manual muscle testing is probably the most versatile and widely used method, evidence indicates that handheld dynamometers may yield more precise measurements and are more sensitive to small changes in strength.[15] Isokinetic systems are effective for quantifying strength in adults, but it can be difficult to adjust the various components to fit children. Another concern is normalizing force measurements to account for differences in size and age.

A therapist must also consider the reliability of methods of strength testing in different patient populations. The reliability of the strength measurements may also vary with the time of day, particularly for patients who are fatigued by the end of the day, and with the level of the child's enthusiasm; with the testing environment; and with the testing clinician's rapport with the child. Children must be able to understand the instructions and follow commands to produce accurate and reliable strength measurements. Some, but not all, children as young as 2 years old with typical development have produced consistent force with a handheld dynamometer.[52] In another sample of children with intellectual difficulties, intrarater and interrater reliability coefficients were all greater than 0.90.[149] Despite these encouraging results, the therapist should be cognizant of the abilities of individual patients. As with goniometry, standardized testing procedures are necessary for optimal reliability of strength measurements. Standardized testing positions for handheld dynamometry are listed in Table 5.2. Taking the average of two measurements rather than a maximum value also improves reliability in children with suspected myopathy and children with CP.[163]

Several authors have reported good consistency when testing the strength of children with DMD using manual muscle testing,[47] isokinetic dynamometers,[141] a handheld dynamometer,[146] and an electronic strain gauge.[44] When strength was measured with a handheld dynamometer, children with meningomyelocele (9–17 years)[94] or with Down syndrome (7–15 years)[101] yielded highly reliable results. The reliability of the measurement of strength in children with CP can be more variable than in some other patient populations, but a review article by Damian and colleagues[36] determines it is still a useful clinical tool. Both handheld dynamometry and isokinetic testing at slower speeds can produce consistent results.[3,10,33,36,90,149,155,163]

In addition to the possibility of objectively measuring the voluntary force produced in spastic muscles, a combination of technologies may now permit objective assessments of the degree of underlying hypertonicity.

Effects of Intervention on the Musculoskeletal System

Objective evidence of the effects of strengthening exercises for particular pediatric conditions is increasing. The recommendation of exercise in children with DMD and other degenerative muscle disorders has changed. A report from a roundtable discussion of experts in the field of DMD suggests that animal models support the idea that submaximal concentric exercise has no negative effect and may be of limited value in increasing strength in DMD.[95] (See Chapter 12 for a more detailed discussion of DMD.) Eccentric contractions should be avoided, as they appear to have the most damaging effect on muscle. The No Use Is Disuse cycling protocol suggests that submaximal stationary bicycle or arm ergometer exercise is safe and may be beneficial in slowing the rate of disease.[69] There are still many unanswered questions regarding the appropriate type, intensity, and duration of exercise that is safe and if it is effective in changing the natural history of the disease.

Two review articles on interventions in CP have suggested that although the data for strength training are incomplete, they appear to be useful not only for improving basic strength but for showing carryover into function and improved gait.[36,42,112,116,122] Additionally resistive strength training regimens have not been shown to adversely affect the level of spasticity.[36] The literature suggests that strength training should be an integral part of an intervention program for children with strength deficits, and we encourage clinicians to continue to document the relationship of strength changes to changes in the activity and participation levels of children.

Botulinum toxin (BoNT-A) injections are often considered to decrease the level of spasticity and increase range of motion. A review article by Strobl et al. suggested that the main decision for the use of BoNT-A is to distinguish whether high muscle tone impedes or improves function.[145] Stiffness may be caused by posturing due to weakened muscles or by simultaneous activity of a group of muscles with high muscle tone. The authors suggest that the decision to administer BoNT-A should be based less on the assessment of individual muscles and more on the general functional impairment. Impairment based assessments such as the Ashworth Scale, Modified Tardieu Scale, or Range of Motion is less important in the use of BoNT than the general functional and developmental assessment and outcome. For this reason, it is essential to define the rehabilitative goal of treatment and to appraise the result with an appropriate assessment rather than evaluating the effect on the injected local muscles only. The author suggests that spastic muscles should only be injected in developing children if the spastic muscle is limiting achievement of the next developmental milestone or putting the child at risk for joint contractures. Controlling spasticity in the very young child may be a method of promoting more normal muscle development, which, in turn, may allow more efficient expenditure of energy and better participation in daily activities. The implication of multiple injections, however, must also be considered. In study of 10 subjects with CP who received multiple BoNT-A injections, neurogenic atrophy in the medial gastrocnemius was seen in 6 participants between 4 months to 3 years post BoNT-A.[161] Type I fiber loss with type II fiber predominance was significantly related to the number of injections.[161]

Limited range of motion is a frequent concern in the children treated by pediatric physical therapists. We have discussed a number of structural changes in spastic muscles that may contribute to loss of motion. The international consensus statement titled *Botulinum toxin assessment, intervention and after-care for lower limb spasticity in children with cerebral palsy* concludes that there is insufficient evidence to determine

TABLE 5.2   Standardized Testing Positions for Handheld Dynamometry

Muscle Group Patient Position	Limb Positions	Manually Stabilized Body Part	Dynamometer Placement
Wrist flexors Supine	Arm beside trunk, elbow flexed 90°, forearm in neutral supination, wrist in neutral flexion	Arm and forearm	Just proximal to metacarpophalangeal joints on extensor surface of hand
Wrist extensors Supine	As wrist flexors	As wrist flexors	Just proximal to metacarpophalangeal joints on flexor surface of hand
Elbow flexors Supine	As wrist flexors	Arm	Just proximal to wrist joint on radial surface of forearm
Elbow extensors Supine	As wrist flexors	Arm	Just proximal to wrist joint on ulnar surface of forearm
Shoulder internal rotators Supine	As wrist flexors	Arm	Just proximal to wrist joint on flexor surface of forearm
Shoulder external rotators Supine	As wrist flexors	Arm	Just proximal to wrist joint on extensor surface of forearm
Shoulder extensors Supine	Shoulder flexed 90°, shoulder in neutral horizontal adduction	Shoulder	Just proximal to elbow on extensor surface of arm
Shoulder flexors Supine	As shoulder extensors	Shoulder	Just proximal to elbow on flexor surface of arm
Shoulder adductors Supine	Elbow extended, shoulder abducted 45°	Trunk	Just proximal to elbow on medial surface of arm
Shoulder abductors Supine	As shoulder adductors	Trunk	Just proximal to elbow on lateral surface of arm
Ankle plantar flexors Supine	Hip and knee extended	Lower limb proximal ankle	Just proximal to metatarsophalangeal joints on plantar surface of foot
Ankle dorsiflexors Supine	As ankle plantar flexors	As ankle plantar flexors	Just proximal to metatarsophalangeal joints on dorsal surface of foot
Knee flexors Sitting	Knee and hip flexed to 90°	Thigh	Just proximal to ankle on posterior surface of leg
Knee extensors Sitting	Knee and hip flexed to 90°	Thigh	Just proximal to ankle on anterior surface of leg
Hip flexors Supine	Hip flexed to 90°, knee relaxed	Trunk	Just proximal to knee on extensor surface of thigh
Hip extensors Supine	As hip flexors	Trunk	Just proximal to knee on flexor surface of thigh
Hip abductors Supine	Knee extended, hip in neutral abduction	Contralateral lower extremity	Just proximal to knee on lateral surface of thigh
Hip adductors Supine	Knee extended, hip in neutral abduction	Contralateral lower extremity	Just proximal to knee on medial surface of thigh

Adapted from Bohannon R: Test-retest reliability of hand-held dynamometry during a single session of strength assessment, *Phys Ther* 66:206-209, 1986.

whether the use of BoNT-A in conjunction with serial casting improves outcomes.[89] Two class II studies showed improvements in the Gross Motor Function Measure walking domain, spasticity, stride length, ankle kinematics, passive ROM, and dorsiflexion strength when BoNT-A was used in conjunction with casting.[1,18] In contrast, a study by Kay[75] revealed that the concurrent addition of BoNT-A to a serial casting regimen led to earlier recurrence of spasticity, contracture, and equinus in gait by 6 months. An explanation of the results was that we as therapists need to strengthen the opposite muscle group to allow for balance. When BoNT-A is combined with serial casting, strengthening cannot occur.

Passive and active slow static stretching exercises are also used routinely to address range-of-motion limitations. De Deyne[38] suggested that muscle adaptation to stretch in healthy, non-neurologically compromised muscles comes from a combination of biomechanical, neurologic, and molecular mechanisms. Short-term improvements in range of motion following short duration stretch, frequently reported as less than 30 seconds, is likely due to the viscoelastic properties of muscle.

The evidence for stretching neurologically compromised muscles is less clear. Despite the widespread use of stretching with children with CP, little is known about its efficacy or effect on activities and participation. Reviews of published literature report that there is insufficient evidence to support/refute manual stretching for lengthening muscles, reducing spasticity, or improving gait.[74,118,171] Limitations that are present in the evidence for stretching spastic muscles include small gains in ROM,[49,74] poor reliability in measuring ROM in spastic muscles discussed earlier in this chapter, and limited carryover to Activities and Participation components of the ICF.[74,118,171]

A classic study by Tardieu,[154] however, supports the use of prolonged stretching. The study found that no progressive contracture was observed after stretching for 6 hours per day, but contractures continued to worsen if stretching was performed for less than 2 hours per day. This would suggest that sustained stretching through the use of night or resting splints is necessary to maintain range of motion.

Serial casting is another way to obtain prolonged stretch on a muscle. A review of the literature completed in 2014[162] concluded that serial casting non-neurologically compromised idiopathic toe walkers did have preliminary evidence of beneficial effects on passive ankle dorsiflexion and gait kinematics. The sustainability of these positive effects after conservative treatment, including casting and physical therapy, was short, up to 1 year.

There is insufficient evidence to support the use of serial casting in children with CP.[11] Some small studies suggest that it can improve range of motion and gait, but there are also concerns about accompanying weakness. BoNT-A injections did not improve the results of casting a neurologically intact muscle system. A review of serial casting, both with and without BoNT-A injections, on individuals with neurologic impairments showed that serial casting with and without BoNT-A had a greater effect on improving range of motion than injections alone,[56] though the effects of BoNT-A when combined with serial casting remain inconclusive. Serial casting a neurologically impaired muscle may improve weight bearing for transfers, relieve pain, and enhance the ability to wear and tolerate orthotics.

The shape and size of the skeletal system are most susceptible to alteration during periods of rapid growth; hence undesirable forces, as well as appropriate corrective forces, are most influential during childhood. Many deformities that occur during the fetal or early postnatal period are more easily corrected in the infant than in the older child. For example, developmentally dislocated hips often readily respond to treatment with a Pavlik harness during the first year of life.[23,144,167] If, however, the dislocated hip is not diagnosed until after 12 months, surgery is often necessary. Similarly, serial casting for wrist deformities in children with distal arthrogryposis was very effective when applied during infancy.[143]

Many parents seek a physical therapist's opinion about what to do if their child has flat feet. Flexible flatfoot is a condition in which the medial longitudinal arch of the foot collapses during weight bearing and restores but is present when the body weight is removed (see Chapter 14 for more detailed information). Most infants are born with flexible flatfoot. Arch development begins between 2 and 6 years of age and becomes structurally mature by 12 or 13 years of age. Prevalence of flexible flatfoot in children 2 to 6 years of age has been reported at between 21% and 57%. Roughly 85% of those with flat feet improve with age, whereas about 15% of the population maintains a flat arch.[136] If flexible flat feet in a typically developing child are producing pain or gait abnormalities, it may be due to heel cord tightness.[59] The presence of risk factors, including ligamentous laxity, obesity, rotational deformities, tibial influence, pathologic tibia varum, equinus, presence of an os tibiale externum, and tarsal coalition, would require further foot evaluation. Treatment of flexible flat feet such as the use of orthotics is controversial and not well researched.[93] Prior to recommending long-term orthotics for flat feet, it is important to remember that cartilage needs movement to survive and repair itself, and joints that are stabilized too long frequently become rigid.

This leads to the question of what to do with asymptomatic flexible flat feet in children with hypotonia. Martin[96] studied 14 children with Down syndrome between the ages of 3.5 and 8 years. Significant improvements on the Gross Motor Function Measure and the Bruininks-Oseretsky Test of Motor Proficiency that could not be attributed solely to maturation were seen with supramalleolar orthoses. During kinematic gait analysis, children with Down syndrome who also had flat feet showed an altered ankle moment and decrease____tion at push-off.[55] This suggests that the child h____ gait pattern.

Submalleolar (below ankle) bracing provide____ with Down syndrome a more neutral foot alignm____ toe-out position during walking, and a more contr____ed walking pattern. Speed, however, did not change.[133]

In general, the decision to brace in the pediatric population is supported in five main areas of documented value: (1) preventing deformity, (2) correcting deformity, (3) promoting a stable base of support, (4) facilitating the development of skills, and (5) improving the efficiency of gait. More evidence is required to determine at what age or developmental functional level bracing is most effective. Orthoses, however, can lead to the development of secondary deformities and disuse atrophy. Lusskin[91] reported two case studies of children with lower extremity paralysis resulting from poliomyelitis. Both children had marked tibial-fibular torsion and were braced in knee-ankle-foot orthoses with the knees and feet facing forward. As a result, a rotational force was placed at the ankle and foot, and these children developed severe metatarsus adductus and heel varus.

Circumferential compressive forces and restriction in active movement can interfere with normal musculoskeletal growth. Pediatric physical therapists have an important responsibility to understand, document, and frequently reevaluate the effects of external devices on the growing child. While trying to solve one problem, intervention may inadvertently create another.

Movement allows compressive forces to be spread throughout the joint surface rather than stay confined to a small area. Combining weight-bearing activities with movement would create more desirable forces for joint formation. Because remodeling of the bone and associated joints takes place most readily during the first few years of life, and because the acetabular shape, for example, is fairly well defined by the age of 3 years,[120] early intervention with weight-bearing activities may have a substantial influence on the shape and function of the joint. To help shape the joint, chronologic age and not developmental age may be more important when determining when to begin weight-bearing activities.

To improve hip stability, Paleg and associates[114] suggested that children with a gross motor delay greater than 25% should begin a supported standing program at around 9 to 10 months of corrected age, as typical children begin pulling to stand at this age. The shape of the acetabulum may not be appropriate for walking, but the hip may be more stable. Over time, this early standing may help prevent or decrease the severity of a dislocated hip. For children with milder delays, less stationary standing time and more weight bearing with movement may help to develop a more normally shaped hip socket. This may contribute to improved gait and a decreased risk of osteoarthritis in adulthood. Careful evaluation of the child's postural alignment when in equipment should be paramount.

Treadmill training has become increasingly popular as an intervention for providing movement and weight-bearing opportunities for children with Down syndrome, spinal cord injury, and CP. Accelerated acquisition of walking was demonstrated in children with Down syndrome when a parent supported the infant on a treadmill for 8 minutes 5 days per week.[158,159] In a randomized, controlled study, 30 children eceived regular physical therapy, but half of them also received the in-home treadmill training program. The experimental group demonstrated the ability to pull to a standing position 60 days earlier than the control group, walked with help 73 days earlier than the control group, and walked independently 101 days earlier than the control group. Despite the documented efficacy of treadmill training in children with Down syndrome, the functional benefit of walking at 20 months versus 24 months is sometimes debated.

A review of the literature completed in 2011[160] found that because of the paucity of large, well-designed clinical trials to support the efficacy of treadmill training for children with CP, evidence for effective programs is inconclusive. This inconsistency might be due to the design of the intervention. Treatment intensity, frequency, and duration are critical to the success of a treadmill program. Traditional exercise training guidelines are explicit in the suggestion that, for fitness to improve, training must occur at a minimum of three times a week and must be sustained for 8 weeks or longer. Several small studies have reported improvements in gait, strength, and function.[26,29,109] Treadmill training can occur in a partial-weight-bearing (PWB) environment in which a therapist uses equipment that includes a harness, overhead support, and a motorized treadmill stimulus. The purpose of the PWB environment is to control body weight, posture, and balance while allowing the child the opportunity for prolonged periods of walking. This allows for strengthening and endurance improvements. Richards et al.[126] performed a 17-week multiple case feasibility study on four children with CP, ranging in age from 1.7 to 2.3 years who were not independent ambulators. They spent 20% to 30% of the time on the PWB treadmill during a 45-minute treatment session four times per week. Support ranged from 40%, 20%, and 0% of body weight with speed ranging from 0.07 m/s to 0.70 m/s. As support decreased throughout the study, the treadmill speed was increased. At the conclusion of the training, two of the children walked independently and one walked with an assistive device. Despite the articles suggesting the potential benefits of PWB therapy for CP, more research is needed to determine the best protocols for frequency, duration, and patient selection.

SUMMARY

This chapter reviewed the normal growth and development of the musculoskeletal system, with emphasis on the adaptations of muscle and bone associated with pathologic conditions encountered by pediatric physical therapists. The microscopic and macroscopic structure and function of the normal MTU and the force and length adaptations to imposed physical changes, such as immobilization and denervation, have been well documented in nonhuman studies using invasive methods of investigation. The results of human studies using noninvasive methods of investigation indicate that the human MTU undergoes adaptations similar to those reported for animals. Clinical evidence for the musculoskeletal adaptations supports these research findings.

In the developing child, atypical changes in the MTU can exert forces on the skeletal system, resulting in bony deformities. Pediatric physical therapists routinely measure physical impairments and develop therapeutic interventions designed to promote musculoskeletal adaptations. To document therapeutic efficacy in relation to specific pediatric disorders,

therapists are encouraged to use objective measures of ROM and strength during specific interventions for correlating changes in musculoskeletal impairment with levels of activity and participation. Additional research is needed to examine the efficacy of therapeutic strengthening and stretching programs and their interrelation with other approaches, such as surgical procedures, casting, and pharmacologic interventions. The application of new research technologies, such as isokinetic dynamometry and EMG, now permits objective measurement of the impairments associated with neuromuscular disorders and the effects of interventions designed to influence these disorders. Additional controlled studies will enhance the scientific basis for using physical therapy to promote participation in life activities.

REFERENCES

1. Ackman JD, Russman BS, Thomas SS, et al.: Comparing botulinum toxin A with casting for treatment of dynamic equinus in children with cerebral palsy, *Dev Med Child Neurol* 47:620–627, 2005.
2. Arazi M, Ogun TC, Memik R: Normal development of the tibiofemoral angle in children: a clinical study of 590 normal subjects from 3 to 17 years of age, *J Pediatr Orthop* 21:264–267, 2001.
3. Ayalon M, Ben-Sira D, Hutzler Y, Gilad T: Reliability of isokinetic strength measurements of the knee in children with cerebral palsy, *Dev Med Child Neurol* 42:398–402, 2000.
4. Reference deleted in proofs.
5. Bailey DA, et al.: Epidemiology of fractures of the distal end of the radius in children as associated with growth, *J Bone Joint Surg Am* 71:1225–1230, 1989.
6. Barnes C, et al.: Reduced bone density among children with severe hemophilia, *Pediatrics* 114:e177–e181, 2004.
7. Bartlett M, Wolf L, Shurtleff D, Stahell L: Hip flexion contractures: a comparison of measurement methods, *Arch Phys Med Rehabil* 66:620–625, 1985.
8. Beals RK, et al.: Developmental changes in the femur and acetabulum in spastic paraplegia and diplegia, *Dev Med Child Neurol* 11:303–313, 1969.
9. Bentzinger CF, Wang YX, Rudnicki MA: Building muscle: molecular regulation of myogenesis, *Cold Spring Harb Perspect Biol* 4, 2012.
10. Berg-Emons RJ, Baak MA, Barbanson DC, et al.: Reliability of tests to determine peak aerobic power, anaerobic power and isokinetic muscle strength in children with spastic cerebral palsy, *Dev Med Child Neurol* 38:1117–1125, 1996.
11. Blackmore A, et al.: A systematic review of the effects of casting on equinus in children with cerebral palsy: an evidence report of the AACPDM, *Dev Med Child Neurol* 49:781–790, 2007.
12. Bleck EE, Michael KAB: *Children's orthopaedics and fractures*, Springer Science & Business Media, 2010.
13. Reference deleted in proofs.
14. Bloomfield SA: Changes in musculoskeletal structure and function with prolonged bed rest, *Med Sci Sports Exerc* 29:197–206, 1997.
15. Bohannon RW: Measurement, nature, and implications of skeletal muscle strength in patients with neurological disorders, *Clin Biomech (Bristol, Avon)* 10:283–292, 1995.
16. Bohannon RW, Andrews AW: Inter-rater reliability of hand-held dynamometer, *Phys Ther* 67:931–933, 1987.
17. Booth CM, et al.: Collagen accumulation in muscles of children with cerebral palsy and correlation with severity of spasticity, *Dev Med Child Neurol* 43:314–320, 2001.
18. Bottos M, Benedetti MG, Salucci P, et al.: Botulinum toxin with and without casting in ambulant children with spastic diplegia: a clinical and functional assessment, *Dev Med Child Neuro!* Nov 45:758–762, 2003.
19. Buckley SL, et al.: The acetabulum in congenital and neuromuscular hip instability, *J Pediatr Orthop* 11:498–501, 1991.

20. Cahuzac JP, Sales de Gauzy D, Vardon J: Development of the clinical tibiofemoral angle in normal adolescents: a study of 427 normal subjects from 10 to 16 years of age, *J Bone Joint Surg Am Br* 77:729–732, 1995.

21. Capriles VD, Martini LA, Areas JA: Metabolic osteopathy in celiac disease: importance of a gluten-free diet, *Nutr Rev* 67:599–606, 2009.

22. Carter DR, Orr TE, Fyhrie DP, Schurman DJ: Influences of mechanical stress on prenatal and postnatal skeletal development, *Clin Orthop Relat Res* 237–250, 1987.

23. Cashman J, Round J, Taylor G, Clarke N: The natural history of developmental dysplasia of the hip after early supervised treatment in the Pavlik harness: a prospective, longitudinal follow-up, *J Bone Joint Surg Br* 84:418–425, 2002.

24. Castle ME, Reyman TA, Schneider M: Pathology of spastic muscle in cerebral palsy, *Clin Orthop Relat Res* 142:223–233, 1979.

25. Cazanave C, Dupon M, Lavignolle-Aurillac V, et al.: Reduced bone mineral density in HIV-infected patients: prevalence and associated factors, *AIDS* 22:395–402, 2008.

26. Cernak K, Stevens V, Price R, Shumway-Cook A: Locomotor training using body-weight support on a treadmill in conjunction with ongoing physical therapy in a child with severe cerebellar ataxia, *Phys Ther* 88:88–97, 2008.

27. Chan G, Chen CT: Musculoskeletal effects of obesity, *Curr Opin Pediatr* 21:65–70, 2009.

28. Cheng JC, Chan PS, Chiang SC, Hui PW: Angular and rotational profile of the lower limb in 2,630 Chinese children, *J Pediatr Orthop* 11:154–161, 1991.

29. Cherng R-J, Liu C-F, Lau T-W, Hong R-B: Effect of treadmill training with body weight support on gait and gross motor function in children with spastic cerebral palsy, *Am J Phys Med Rehabil* 86:548–555, 2007.

30. Chung WS, Barres BA: The role of glial cells in synapse elimination, *Curr Opin Neurobiol* 22:438–445, 2012.

31. Cooper C, Dennison EM, Leufkens HGM, et al.: Epidemiology of childhood fractures in Britain: a study using the general practice research database, *J Bone Miner Res* 19:1976–1981, 2004.

32. Costanzo EM, Barry JA, Ribchester RR: Competition at silent synapses in reinnervated skeletal muscle, *Nat Neurosci* 3:694–700, 2003.

33. Crompton J, Galea MP, Phillips B: Hand-held dynamometry for muscle strength measurement in children with cerebral palsy, *Dev Med Child Neurol* 49:106, 2007.

34. Czeczelewski J, Dlugolecka B, Czeczelewska E, Raczynska B: Intakes of selected nutrients, bone mineralisation and density of adolescent female swimmers over a three-year period, *Biol Sport* 30:17–20, 2013.

35. Damcott M, Blochlinger S, Foulds R: Effects of passive versus dynamic loading interventions on bone health in children who are nonambulatory, *Pediatr Phys Ther* 25:248–255, 2013.

36. Damiano DL, Dodd K, Taylor NF: Should we be testing and training muscle strength in cerebral palsy? *Dev Med Child Neurol* 44:68–72, 2002.

37. Dastmalchi M, Alexanderson H, Loell I, et al.: Effect of physical training on the proportion of slow-twitch type I muscle fibers, a novel nonimmune-mediated mechanism for muscle impairment in polymyositis or dermatomyositis, *Arthritis Care Res* 57:1303–1310, 2007.

38. De Deyne PG: Application of passive stretch and its implications for muscle fibers, *Phys Ther* 81:819–827, 2001.

39. De Hundt M, Vlemmix F, Bais J, et al.: Risk factors for developmental dysplasia of the hip: a meta-analysis, *Eur J Obstet Gynecol Reprod Biol* 165:8–17, 2012.

40. Dimitri P, Wales JK, Bishop N: Fat and bone in children: differential effects of obesity on bone size and mass according to fracture history, *J Bone Miner Res* 25:527–536, 2010.

41. Dirks ML, Wall BT, Snijders T, et al.: Neuromuscular electrical stimulation prevents muscle disuse atrophy during leg immobilization in humans, *Acta Physiol (Oxf)* 210:628–641, 2014.

42. Dodd KJ, Taylor NF, Damiano DL: A systematic review of the effectiveness of strength-training programs for people with cerebral palsy, *Arch Phys Med Rehabil* 83:1157–1164, 2002.

43. Esbjörnsson Liljedahl M, Holm I, Sylvén C, Jansson E: Different responses of skeletal muscle following sprint training in men and women, *Europ J Appl Physiol* 74:375–383, 1996.

44. Escolar D, Henricson E, Mayhew J, et al.: Clinical evaluator reliability for quantitative and manual muscle testing measures of strength in children, *Muscle Nerve* 24:787–793, 2001.

45. Fehlings D, Switzer L, Agarwal P, et al.: Informing evidence-based clinical practice guidelines for children with cerebral palsy at risk of osteoporosis: a systematic review, *Dev Med Child Neurol* 54:106–116, 2012.

46. Fladby T, Jansen JKS: Postnatal loss of synaptic terminals in the partially denervated mouse soleus muscle, *Acta Physiol Scand* 129:239–246, 1987.

47. Florence JM, Pandya S, King WM, et al.: Clinical trials in Duchenne dystrophy standardization and reliability of evaluation procedures, *Phys Ther* 64:41–45, 1984.

48. Foran JRH, Steinman S, Barash I, et al.: Structural and mechanical alterations in spastic skeletal muscle, *Dev Med Child Neurol* 47:713–717, 2005.

49. Franki I, Desloovere K, De Cat J, et al.: The evidence-base for basic physical therapy techniques targeting lower limb function in children with cerebral palsy: a systematic review using the International Classification of Functioning, Disability and Health as a conceptual framework, *J Rehabil Med* 44:385–395, 2012.

50. Fridén J, Lieber RL: Spastic muscle cells are shorter and stiffer than normal cells, *Muscle Nerve* 27:157–164, 2003.

51. Friend L, Widmann RF: Advances in management of limb length discrepancy and lower limb deformity, *Curr Opin Pediatri* 20:46–51, 2003.

52. Gajdosik CG: Ability of very young children to produce reliable isometric force measurements, *Pediatric Phys Ther* 17:251–257, 2005.

53. Gajdosik RL, Bohannon RW: Clinical measurement of range of motion review of goniometry emphasizing reliability and validity, *Phys Ther* 67:1867–1872, 1987.

54. Gajdosik RL: Passive extensibility of skeletal muscle: review of the literature with clinical implications, *Clin Biomech (Bristol, Avon)* 16:87–101, 2001.

55. Galli M, Cimolin V, Pau M, et al.: Relationship between flat foot condition and gait pattern alterations in children with Down syndrome, *J Intellect Disabil Res* 58:269–276, 2014.

56. Glanzman AM, Kim H, Swaminathan K, Beck T: Efficacy of botulinum toxin A, serial casting, and combined treatment for spastic equinus: a retrospective analysis, *Dev Med Child Neurol* 46:807–811, 2004.

57. Gough M, Shortland AP: Could muscle deformity in children with spastic cerebral palsy be related to an impairment of muscle growth and altered adaptation? *Dev Med Child Neurol* 54:495–499, 2012.

58. Harpavat M, et al.: Altered bone mass in children at diagnosis of Crohn disease: a pilot study, *J Pediatr Gastroenterol Nutr* 40:295–300, 2005.

59. Harris EJ: The oblique talus deformity. What is it, and what is its clinical significance in the scheme of pronatory deformities? *Clin Podiatr Med Surg* 17:419–442, 2000.

60. Harris SR, Smith LH, Krukowski L: Goniometric reliability for a child with spastic quadriplegia, *J Pediatr Orthop* 5:348–351, 1985.

61. Heath CH, Staheli LT: Normal limits of knee angle in white children—genu varum and genu valgum, *J Pediatr Orthop* 13:259–262, 1993.

62. Heesakkers N, van Kempen R, Feith R, et al.: The long-term prognosis of Legg-Calvé-Perthes disease: a historical prospective study with a median follow-up of forty one years, *Int Orthop* 39:859–863, 2015.

63. Hesselmans LFGM, Jennekens FGI, Van Den Oord CJM, et al.: Development of innervation of skeletal muscle fibers in man: relation to acetylcholine receptors, *Anat Rec* 236:553–562, 1993.

64. Hind K, Burrows M: Weight-bearing exercise and bone mineral accrual in children and adolescents: a review of controlled trials, *Bone* 40:14–27, 2007.

65. Hortobagyi T, Dempsey L, Fraser D, et al.: Changes in muscle strength, muscle fibre size and myofibrillar gene expression after immobilization and retraining in humans, *J Physiol* 524(Pt 1):293–304, 2000.

66. Hough JP, Boyd RN, Keating JL: Systematic review of interventions for low bone mineral density in children with cerebral palsy, *Pediatrics* 125:e670–e678, 2010.

67. Hung VWY, et al.: Osteopenia: a new prognostic factor of curve progression in adolescent idiopathic scoliosis, *J Bone Joint Surg Am* 87:2709–2716, 2005.

68. Ihkkan KY, Yalcin E: Changes in skeletal maturation and mineralization in children with cerebral palsy and evaluation of related factors, *J Child Neurol* 16:425–430, 2001.

69. Jansen M, de Groot IJ, van Alfen N, Geurts AC: Physical training in boys with Duchenne muscular dystrophy: the protocol of the No Use is Disuse study, *BMC Pediatr* 10:55, 2010.

70. Jansson E, Esbjörnsson M, Holm I, Jacobs I: Increase in the proportion of fast-twitch muscle fibres by sprint training in males, *Acta Physiol Scand* 140:359–363, 1990.

71. Jarvinen TA, Jozsa L, Kannus P, et al.: Organization and distribution of intramuscular connective tissue in normal and immobilized skeletal muscles: an immunohistochemical, polarization and scanning electron microscopic study, *J Muscle Res Cell Motil* 23:245–254, 2002.

72. Jelinek E, Bittersohl B, Martiny F, et al.: The 8-plate versus physeal stapling for temporary hemiepiphyseodesis correcting genu valgum and genu varum: a retrospective analysis of thirty five patients, *Int Orthop* 36:599–605, 2012.

73. Jiang C, Wen Y, Kuroda K, et al.: Notch signaling deficiency underlies age-dependent depletion of satellite cells in muscular dystrophy, *Dis Model Mech* 7:997–1004, 2014.

74. Katalinic OM, Harvey LA, Herbert RD: Effectiveness of stretch for the treatment and prevention of contractures in people with neurological conditions: a systematic review, *Phys Ther* 91:11–24, 2011.

75. Kay RM, Rethlefsen SA, Fern-Buneo A, et al.: Botulinum toxin as an adjunct to serial casting treatment in children with cerebral palsy, *J Bone Joint Surg Am* 86-A:2377–2384, 2004.

76. Kecskemethy HH, Herman D, May R, et al.: Quantifying weight bearing while in passive standers and a comparison of standers, *Dev Med Child Neurol* 50:520–523, 2008.

77. Kedem P, Scher DM: Evaluation and management of crouch gait, *Curr Opin Pediatr* 28:55–59, 2016.

78. Kendall FP, et al.: *Muscles: testing and function, with posture and pain*, Baltimore, MD, 2005, Lippincott Williams & Wilkins.

79. Kentish M, Snapen Wynter M, et al.: Five-year outcome of statewide hip surveillance of children and adolescents with cerebral palsy, *J Pediatr Rehab Med* 413:205–217, 2011.

80. Khosla S, Melton III LJ, Dekutoski MB, et al.: Incidence of childhood distal forearm fractures over 30 years: a population-based study, *JAMA* 290:1479–1485, 2003.

81. Kilgour G, McNair P, Stott NS: Intrarater reliability of lower limb sagittal range-of-motion measures in children with spastic diplegia, *Dev Med Child Neurol* 45:391–399, 2003.

82. Ko I-H, Kim J-H, Lee B-H: Relationships between lower limb muscle architecture and activities and participation of children with cerebral palsy, *J Exerc Rehabil* 9:368, 2013.

83. Kuh D, Bassey J, Hardy R, et al.: Birth weight, childhood size, and muscle strength in adult life: evidence from a birth cohort study, *Am J Epidemiol* 156:627–633, 2002.

84. Kuo AA, Tritasavit S, Graham JM: Congenital muscular torticollis and positional plagiocephaly, *Pediatr Rev* 35:79–87, 2014. quiz 87.

85. Reference deleted in proofs.

86. Lee DK, Muraszko K, Ulrich BD: Bone mineral content in infants with myelomeningocele, with and without treadmill stepping practice, *Pediatr Phys Ther* 28:24–32, 2016.

87. LeVeau BF, Bernhardt DB: Developmental biomechanics: effect of forces on the growth, development, and maintenance of the human body, *Phys Ther* 64:1874–1882, 1984.

88. Lieber RL, Steinman S, Barash IA, Chambers H: Structural and functional changes in spastic skeletal muscle, *Muscle Nerve* 29:615–627, 2004.

89. Love S, Novak I, Kentish M, et al.: Botulinum toxin assessment, intervention and after-care for lower limb spasticity in children with cerebral palsy: international consensus statement, *Eur J Neurol* 17:9–37, 2010.

90. Lowes LP, Westcott SL, Palisano RJ, et al.: Muscle force and range of motion as predictors of standing balance in children with cerebral palsy, *Phys Occup Ther Pediatr* 24:57–77, 2004.

91. Lusskin R: The influence of errors in bracing upon deformity of the lower extremity, *Arch Phys Med Rehabil* 47:520, 1966.

92. Macias-Merlo L, Bagur-Calafat C, Girabent-Farres M, et al.: Effects of the standing program with hip abduction on hip acetabular development in children with spastic diplegia cerebral palsy, *Disabil Rehabil* 38:1075–1081, 2016.

93. MacKenzie AJ, Rome K, Evans AM: The efficacy of nonsurgical interventions for pediatric flexible flat foot: a critical review, *J Pediatr Orthop* 32:830–834, 2012.

94. Mahony K, Hunt A, Daley D, et al.: Inter-tester reliability and precision of manual muscle testing and hand-held dynamometry in lower limb muscles of children with spina bifida, *Phys Occup Ther Pediatr* 29:44–59, 2009.

95. Markert CD, Case LE, Carter GT, et al.: Exercise and Duchenne muscular dystrophy: where we have been and where we need to go, *Muscle Nerve* 45:746–751, 2012.

96. Martin K: Effects of supramalleolar orthoses on postural stability in children with Down syndrome, *Dev Med Child Neurol* 46:406–411, 2004.

97. Mathewson MA, Chambers HG, Girard PJ, et al.: Stiff muscle fibers in calf muscles of patients with cerebral palsy lead to high passive muscle stiffness, *J Orthop Res* 32:1667–1674, 2014.

98. Mathewson MA, Ward SR, Chambers HG, Lieber RL: High resolution muscle measurements provide insights into equinus contractures in patients with cerebral palsy, *J Orthop Res* 33:33–39, 2015.

99. McDowell BC, Hewitt V, Nurse A, et al.: The variability of goniometric measurements in ambulatory children with spastic cerebral palsy, *Gait Posture* 12:114–121, 2000.

100. McMillan HJ, Darras BT, Kang PB: Autoimmune neuromuscular disorders in childhood, *Curr Treat Options Neurol* 13:590–607, 2011.

101. Mercer VS, Lewis CL: Hip abductor and knee extensor muscle strength of children with and without Down syndrome, *Pediatr Phys Ther* 13:18–26, 2001.

102. Meyer GA, Lieber RL: Skeletal muscle fibrosis develops in response to desmin deletion, *Am J Physiol Cell Physiol* 302:C1609–C1620, 2012.

103. Milani P, Coccetta CA, Rabini A, et al.: Mobile smartphone applications for body position measurement in rehabilitation: a review of goniometric tools, *PM&R* 6:1038–1043, 2014.

104. Miller F, Cardoso Dias R, Dabney KW, et al.: Soft-tissue release for spastic hip subluxation in cerebral palsy, *J Pediatr Orthop* 17:571–584, 1997.

105. Mockford M, Caulton JM: The pathophysiological basis of weakness in children with cerebral palsy, *Pediatr Phys Ther* 22:222–233, 2010.

106. Moore KL: Musculoskeletal system. In Keith L, et al.: *Before we are born: essentials of embryology and birth defects*, ed 9, Philadelphia, 2013, Saunders/Elsevier, pp 225–249.

107. Moreau NG, Teefey SA, Damiano DL: In vivo muscle architecture and size of the rectus femoris and vastus lateralis in children and adolescents with cerebral palsy, *Dev Med Child Neurol* 51:800–806, 2009.

108. Münchau A, Bhatia KP: Uses of botulinum toxin injection in medicine today, *BMJ* 320:161–165, 2000.

109. Mutlu A, Krosschell K, Spira DG: Treadmill training with partial body-weight support in children with cerebral palsy: a systematic review, *Dev Med Child Neurol* 51:268–275, 2009.

110. Reference deleted in proofs.

111. Nedergaard A, Jespersen JG, Pingel J, et al.: Effects of 2 weeks lower limb immobilization and two separate rehabilitation regimens on gastrocnemius muscle protein turnover signaling and normalization genes, *BMC Res Notes* 5:166, 2012.

112. Novak I, Mcintyre S, Morgan C, et al.: A systematic review of interventions for children with cerebral palsy: state of the evidence, *Dev Med Child Neurol* 55:885–910, 2013.

113. Reference deleted in proofs.

114. Paleg GS, Smith BA, Glickman LB: Systematic review and evidence-based clinical recommendations for dosing of pediatric supported standing programs, *Pediatr Phys Ther* 25:232–247, 2013.

115. Pandya S, Florence JM, King WM, et al.: Reliability of goniometric measurements in patients with Duchenne muscular dystrophy, *Phys Ther* 65:1339–1342, 1985.

116. Park E-Y, Kim W-H: Meta-analysis of the effect of strengthening interventions in individuals with cerebral palsy, *Res Dev Disabil* 35:239–249, 2014.

117. Pearl ML, et al.: Comparison of arthroscopic findings with magnetic resonance imaging and arthrography in children with glenohumeral deformities secondary to brachial plexus birth palsy, *J Bone Joint Surg Am* 85:890–898, 2003.

118. Pin T, Dyke P, Chan M: The effectiveness of passive stretching in children with cerebral palsy, *Dev Med Child Neurol* 48:855–862, 2006.

119. Price CT, Langford JR, Liporace FA: Essential nutrients for bone health and a review of their availability in the average North American diet, *Open Orthop J* 6:143–149, 2012.

120. Ráliš Z, McKibbin B: Changes in shape of the human hip joint during its development and their relation to its stability, *J Bone Joint Surg Br* 55:780–785, 1973.

121. Ralis Z, McKibbin B: Changes in shape of the human hip joint during its development and their relation to stability, *J Bone Joint Surg Br* 55:780–785, 1973.

122. Rameckers EAA, Janssen-Potten YJM, Essers IMM, Smeets RJEM: Efficacy of upper limb strengthening in children with cerebral palsy: a critical review, *Res Devdisabil* 36:87–101, 2015.

123. Ranatunga KW: Skeletal muscle stiffness and contracture in children with spastic cerebral palsy, *J Physiol* 589(Pt 11):2665, 2011.

124. Rauch F: Bone growth in length and width: the Yin and Yang of bone stability, *J Musculoskelet Neuronal Interact* 5:194–201, 2005.

125. Rauch F, et al.: The development of metaphyseal cortex-implications for distal radius fractures during growth, *J Bone Miner Res* 16:1547–1555, 2001.

126. Richards CL, Malouin F, Dumas F, et al.: Early and intensive treadmill locomotor training for young children with cerebral palsy: a feasibility study, *Pediatr Phys Ther* 9:158–165, 1997.

127. Rose J, et al.: Muscle pathology and clinical measures of disability in children with cerebral palsy, *J Orthop Res* 12:758–768, 1994.

128. Rothstein JM, Rose SJ: Muscle mutability. Part 2, adaptation to drugs, metabolic factors, and aging, *Phys Ther* 62:1788–1798, 1982.

129. Ruff C, Holt B, Trinkaus E: Who's afraid of the big bad Wolff? "Wolff's law" and bone functional adaptation, *Am J Phys Anthropol* 129:484–498, 2006.

130. Sass P, Hassan G: Lower extremity abnormalities in children, *Am Fam Physician* 68:461–468, 2003.

131. Schiaffino S, Reggiani C: Fiber types in mammalian skeletal muscles, *Physiol Rev* 91:1447–1531, 2011.

132. Schmidt S, Mellstrom D, Norjavaara E, et al.: Longitudinal assessment of bone mineral density in children and adolescents with inflammatory bowel disease, *J Pediatr Gastroenterol Nutr* 55:511–518, 2012.

133. Selby-Silverstein L, Hillstrom HJ, Palisano RJ: The effect of foot orthoses on standing foot posture and gait of young children with Down syndrome, *NeuroRehabilitation* 16:183–193, 2000.

134. Sheth RD, Hermann BP: Bone in idiopathic and symptomatic epilepsy, *Epilepsy Res* 78:71–76, 2008.

135. Sheth RD, et al.: Gender differences in bone mineral density in epilepsy, *Epilepsia* 49:125–131, 2008.

136. Shih Y-F, Chen C-Y, Chen W-Y, Lin H-C: Lower extremity kinematics in children with and without flexible flatfoot: a comparative study, *BMC Musculoskel Disord* 13:31, 2012.

137. Shortland AP: In vivo gastrocnemius muscle fascicle length in children with and without diplegic cerebral palsy, *Dev Med Child Neurol* 50:339–340, 2008.

138. Singer BJ, Dunne JW, Singer KP, Allison GT: Velocity dependent passive plantarflexor resistive torque in patients with acquired brain injury, *Clin Biomech (Bristol, Avon)* 18:157–165, 2003.

139. Smith LR, Lee KS, Ward SR, et al.: Hamstring contractures in children with spastic cerebral palsy result from a stiffer extracellular matrix and increased in vivo sarcomere length, *J Physiol* 589(Pt 10):2625–2639, 2011.

140. Smith LR, Lee KS, Ward SR, et al.: Hamstring contractures in children with spastic cerebral palsy result from a stiffer extracellular matrix and increased in vivo sarcomere length, *J Physiol* 589:2625–2639, 2011.

141. Sokolov R, Irwin B, Dressendorfer R, Bernauer E: Exercise performance in 6-to 11-year old boys with Duchenne muscular dystrophy, *Arch Phys Med Rehabil* 58:195–201, 1977.

142. Spector SA, Simard CP, Fournier M, et al.: Architectural alterations of rat hind-limb skeletal muscles immobilized at different lengths, *Exp Neurol* 76:94–110, 1982.

143. Staheli LT: *Fundamentals of pediatric orthopedics*, Philadelphia, PA, 2008, Lippincott Williams & Wilkins.

144. Stevenson RD, Conaway M, Barrington JW, et al.: Fracture rate in children with cerebral palsy, *Dev Neurorehabil* 9:396–403, 2006.

145. Strobl W, Theologis T, Brunner R, et al.: Best clinical practice in botulinum toxin treatment for children with cerebral palsy, *Toxins* 7:1629–1648, 2015.

146. Stuberg WA, Metcalf W: Reliability of quantitative muscle testing in healthy children and in children with Duchenne muscular dystrophy using a hand-held dynamometer, *Phys Ther* 68:977–982, 1988.

147. Stuberg WA: Considerations related to weight-bearing programs in children with developmental disabilities, *Phys Ther* 72:35–40, 1992.

148. Suetta C, Frandsen U, Jensen L, et al.: Aging affects the transcriptional regulation of human skeletal muscle disuse atrophy, *PLoS One* 7:e51238, 2012.

149. Surburg PR, Suomi R, Poppy WK: Validity and reliability of a hand-held dynamometer with two populations, *J Orthop Sports Phys Ther* 16:229–234, 1992.

150. Suzuki S, Yamamuro T: Correlation of fetal posture and congenital dislocation of the hip, *Acta Orthop Scand* 57:81–84, 1986.

151. Svien LR, Berg P, Stephenson C: Issues in aging with cerebral palsy, *Top Geriatr Rehabil* 24:26–40, 2008.

152. Szalay EA, Harriman D, Eastlund B, Mercer D: Quantifying postoperative bone loss in children, *J Pediatr Orthop* 28:320–323, 2008.

153. Tabary J, Tabary C, Tardieu C, et al.: Physiological and structural changes in the cat's soleus muscle due to immobilization at different lengths by plaster casts, *J Physiol* 224:231–244, 1972.

154. Tardieu C, Lespargot A, Tabary C, Bret MD: For how long must the soleus muscle be stretched each day to prevent contracture? *Dev Med Child Neurol* 30:3–10, 1988.

155. Taylor NF, Dodd KJ, Graham HK: Test-retest reliability of hand-held dynamometric strength testing in young people with cerebral palsy, *Arch Phys Med Rehabil* 85:77–80, 2004.

156. Turkoglu AN, Huijing PA, Yucesoy CA: Mechanical principles of effects of botulinum toxin on muscle length-force characteristics: an assessment by finite element modeling, *J Biomechan* 47:1565–1571, 2014.

157. Uddenfeldt Wort U, Nordmark E, Wagner P, et al.: Fractures in children with cerebral palsy: a total population study, *Dev Med Child Neurol* 55:821–826, 2013.

158. Ulrich DA, Lloyd MC, Tiernan CW, et al.: Effects of intensity of treadmill training on developmental outcomes and stepping in infants with Down syndrome: a randomized trial, *Phys Ther* 88:114–122, 2008.

159. Ulrich DA, Ulrich BD, Angulo-Kinzler RM, Yun J: Treadmill training of infants with Down syndrome: evidence-based developmental outcomes, *Pediatrics* 108:e84–e84, 2001.

160. Valentin-Gudiol M, Mattern-Baxter K, Girabent-Farrés M, et al.: Treadmill interventions with partial body weight support in children under six years of age at risk of neuromotor delay, *Cochrane Database Syst Rev* CD009242, 2011.

161. Valentine J, Stannage K, Fabian V, et al.: Muscle histopathology in children with spastic cerebral palsy receiving botulinum toxin type A, *Muscle Nerve* 53:407–414, 2016.

162. van Kuijk AA, Kosters R, Vugts M, Geurts AC: Treatment for idiopathic toe walking: a systematic review of the literature, *J Rehabil Med* 46:945–957, 2014.

163. Van Vulpen L, De Groot S, Becher J, et al.: Feasibility and test-retest reliability of measuring lower-limb strength in young children with cerebral palsy, *Eur J Phys Rehabil Med* 49:803–813, 2013.

164. Wall BT, Snijders T, Senden JM, et al.: Disuse impairs the muscle protein synthetic response to protein ingestion in healthy men, *J Clin Endocrinol Metab* 98:4872–4881, 2013.

165. Wallach DM, Davidson RS: Pediatric lower limb disorders. In Dormans JP, editor: *Pediatric orthopaedics: core knowledge in orthopaedics*, Philadelphia, 2005, Elsevier Mosby.

166. Reference deleted in proofs.

167. Weinstein SL, Flynn JM: *Lovell and Winter's pediatric orthopaedics*, Philadelphia, PA, 2013, Lippincott Williams & Wilkins.

168. White J, et al.: Potential benefits of physical activity for children with acute lymphoblastic leukaemia, *Pediatr Rehabil* 8:53–58, 2005.

169. Surburg PR, Suomi R, Poppy WK: Validity and reliability of a hand-held dynamometer with two populations, *J Orthop Sports Phys Ther* 16(5):229–234, 1992.

170. Whittaker S, Tomlinson R: Question 2: do standing frames and other related physical therapies reduce the risk of fractures in children with cerebral palsy? *Arch Dis Child* 100:1181–1183, 2015.

171. Wiart L, Darrah J, Kembhavi G: Stretching with children with cerebral palsy: what do we know and where are we going? *Pediatr Phys Ther* 20:173–178, 2008.

172. Williams CD, Salcedo MK, Irving TC, et al.: The length-tension curve in muscle depends on lattice spacing, *Proc Biol Sci* 280:20130697, 2013.

173. Williams PE, Goldspink G: Changes in sarcomere length and physiological properties in immobilized muscle, *J Anat* 127(Pt 3):459, 1978.

174. Williams PE, Goldspink G: Longitudinal growth of striated muscle fibres, *J Cell Sci* 9:751–767, 1971.

175. Wills M: Orthopedic complications of childhood obesity, *Pediatr Phys Ther* 16:230–235, 2004.

176. Wilmshurst S, Ward K, Adams J, et al.: Mobility status and bone density in cerebral palsy, *Arch Dis Child* 75:164–165, 1996.

177. Wren TA, Cheatwood AP, Rethlefsen SA, et al.: Achilles tendon length and medial gastrocnemius architecture in children with cerebral palsy and equinus gait, *J Pediatr Orthop* 30:479–484, 2010.

178. Wynter M, Gibson N, Kentish M, et al.: The consensus statement on hip surveillance for children with cerebral palsy: Australian standards of care, *J Pediatr Rehabil Med* 4:183, 2011.

179. Young N, Wright J, Lam T, et al.: Windswept hip deformity in spastic quadriplegic cerebral palsy, *Pediatr Phys Ther* 10:94–100, 1998.

180. Ziv I, Blackburn N, Rang M, Koreska J: Muscle growth in normal and spastic mice, *Dev Med Child Neurol* 26:94–99, 1984.

SUGGESTED READINGS

Castle ME, Reyman TA, Schneider M: Pathology of spastic muscle in cerebral palsy, *Clin Orthop Relat Res* 142:223–233, 1979.

Dodd KJ, Taylor NF, Damiano DL: A systematic review of the effectiveness of strength-training programs for people with cerebral palsy, *Arch Phys Med Rehabil* 83:1157–1164, 2002.

Gajdosik CG: Ability of very young children to produce reliable isometric force measurements, *Pediatr Phys Ther* 17:251–257, 2005.

Gajdosik RL, Bohannon RW: Clinical measurement of range of motion review of goniometry emphasizing reliability and validity, *Phys Ther* 67:1867–1872, 1987.

Katalinic OM, Harvey LA, Herbert RD: Effectiveness of stretch for the treatment and prevention of contractures in people with neurological conditions: a systematic review, *Phys Ther* 91:11–24, 2011.

Kuh D, Bassey J, Hardy R, et al.: Birth weight, childhood size, and muscle strength in adult life: evidence from a birth cohort study, *Am J Epidemiol* 156:627–633, 2002.

LeVeau BF, Bernhardt DB: Developmental biomechanics: effect of forces on the growth, development, and maintenance of the human body, *Phys Ther* 64:1874–1882, 1984.

Lowes LP, Westcott SL, Palisano RJ, et al.: Muscle force and range of motion as predictors of standing balance in children with cerebral palsy, *Phys Occup Ther Pediatr* 24:57–77, 2004.

Münchau A, Bhatia KP: Uses of botulinum toxin injection in medicine today, *BMJ* 320:161–165, 2000.

Stuberg WA: Considerations related to weight-bearing programs in children with developmental disabilities, *Phys Ther* 72:35–40, 1992.

6

Physical Fitness During Childhood and Adolescence

Jean Stout

The International Classification of Functioning, Disability and Health (ICF) emphasizes components of health as important factors related to participation in society.[280] According to its press release, the World Health Organization estimates that as many as 500 million healthy life years are lost each year because of disability associated with health conditions. This statistic includes children. Ensuring physical fitness is one aspect of primary prevention and health promotion upon which the practice of physical therapy is based,[5] and it is a construct that fits appropriately within the ICF model. The scope of pediatric physical therapy in health promotion and physical fitness has explicitly been described.[207] As clinicians who design exercise programs and treat children with disabilities, we have a unique responsibility to understand and promote physical fitness as an aspect of those programs. It is a unique responsibility because we can have a great impact on the exercise lifestyle that children develop and carry with them throughout their lives. We also care for a group of children who might otherwise be physically inactive. Physical fitness is coming to the forefront of pediatric physical therapy practice as focus is directed toward prevention.[207] The research summit devoted to the topic of physical fitness and prevention of secondary conditions for children with cerebral palsy (CP), the defined scope of practice, and the importance of physical activity and fitness for adults with CP underscores the attention and importance that the profession of physical therapy as a whole is placing on this topic.[95,242] It is now well established that promotion of lifelong habits of physical activity in childhood will have direct and indirect effects on health and the prevention of disease in adulthood.[36,79,112] Meanwhile studies based on fitness standards find fewer children are achieving the minimum criterion for activity.[36]

What defines *physical fitness* for typically developing children? Are the criteria for physical fitness different in children with disabilities? How do we help children with physical disabilities incorporate physical fitness into the limitations of their disability? This chapter is designed to answer those questions and to provide an understanding of (1) physical fitness and the cardiopulmonary response to exercise in children of different ages who do not have disabling conditions; (2) the components of physical fitness (cardiorespiratory endurance, muscular strength and endurance, flexibility, and body composition) (Table 6.1); (3) the standards of fitness components consistent with good health; (4) the effects of training and conditioning on overall physical fitness; (5) the components of fitness in various special populations; and (6) guides for program planning. The chapter also includes a review of current physical fitness tests.

HEALTH, PHYSICAL ACTIVITY, AND PHYSICAL FITNESS

Physical fitness is difficult to define because it cannot be measured directly. Physical fitness is generally viewed as having two facets: health-related fitness and the more traditional motor fitness. Motor fitness generally includes physical abilities that relate to athletic performance, agility, and coordination, whereas health-related fitness includes abilities related to daily function and health maintenance. Physical activity is thought to be the path both to physical fitness and to good health and therefore is tightly coupled to fitness, but these are not synonymous terms. *Physical activity* refers to the amount of exercise in which an individual engages. Physical activity does not describe any "level" of physiologic function important to maintain health. Studies suggest that in adults, a positive correlation exists among regular physical activity, cardiovascular fitness, and reduced risk of mortality.[176] Just as in adults, physical inactivity is increasingly being implicated in the escalating "epidemic" of obesity and as a major risk factor for morbidity in children and adolescents.[45,145,157] The current consensus is that physical activity and physical fitness are reciprocally related and each exerts independent effects on health. Physical activity may improve physical fitness and health at the same time, but the improvement in health may be caused by biologic changes different from those responsible for improvement in physical fitness.[36] They are related but distinctly different contributors to health.[62,273] Some of the benefits from physical activity that are important to health and achievement have no relationship to what is defined as *physical fitness* per se.[108,166] One example is the importance of regular exercise to bone health and a reduced risk of osteoporosis; osteoporosis is related to health but not to the components of physical fitness.

Limited information is available regarding how much physical activity is necessary for health and fitness in children. The work of Strong and colleagues outlines the effects of physical activity on health and behavioral outcomes in school-aged youth and offers guidelines for the amount of exercise necessary.[233] The US Department of Health and Human Services published a first-ever Physical Activity Guidelines for Americans, which includes a chapter on children and youth.[193,250] New programs such as the National Football League–sponsored NFL PLAY 60 FITNESSGRAM Partnership project are devoted to promoting physical activity and physical fitness in youth.[12]

TABLE 6.1	Health-Related Fitness Components and the Rationale for Importance to Health Promotion and Disease Prevention
Component	**Rationale**
Cardiorespiratory endurance	Improved physical working capacity
	Reduced fatigue
	Reduced risk of coronary heart disease
	Optimal growth and development
Muscular strength and endurance	Improved functional capacity for lifting and carrying
	Reduced risk of lower back pain
	Optimal posture
	Optimal growth and development
Flexibility	Enhanced functional capacity for bending and twisting
	Reduced risk of lower back pain
	Optimal growth and development
Body composition	Reduced risk of hypertension
	Reduced risk of coronary heart disease
	Reduced risk of diabetes
	Optimal growth and development

Adapted from Pate PR, Shephard RJ: Characteristics of physical fitness in youth. In Gisolfi CV, Lamb DR, editors: *Perspectives in exercise science and sports medicine: youth, exercise, and sport*, vol 2, Indianapolis, IN, 1989, Benchmark Press.[187]

How much physical activity is enough? This question is not easily answered because it depends on many factors. Assessing and understanding physical activity in preschool children relative to child development presents even more challenges.[77] Studies under way, such as the longitudinal Lifestyle Of Our Kids (LOOK) project in Australia, which is investigating how early physical activity contributes to health and development, may also help to answer that question.[240]

The premise that physical activity is the path to both physical fitness and good health has become a primary focus in programs instituted by the US Department of Health and Human Services. As early as 1985, the Centers for Disease Control put forth a specific activity plan for youth through old age to attain specific health fitness goals and achieve optimal health benefits. Developing lifelong physical activity patterns was one of the specific goals for children.[112] In 1990, Healthy Children 2000, a major federal planning document for health promotion and disease prevention for children, was introduced.[246] Originally, eight objectives were outlined to increase the physical activity and fitness levels of youth, with a target date of attainment by the year 2000. Every 10 years, through the Healthy People initiative, the Department of Health and Human Services develops the next iteration of the national objectives for promoting health and preventing disease, which includes physical fitness. Final objectives for Healthy People 2020 retained physical fitness as part of the goal of physical activity but dropped the reference to fitness in the title of the objective[249] (http://www.healthypeople.gov/2020/topics-objectives/topic/physical-activity/objectives).

Progress to targets has been slow. Many of the year 2000 targets were retained in the 2010 objectives, and most of the 2010 objectives remain in the 2020 objectives. Targets directed toward elementary-age and junior high–age children dropped from the 2010 objectives have been reinstated. Eleven objectives for physical activity and fitness are included in Healthy People 2020 (Box 6.1). Plans for 2030 targets have not yet begun.

Physical activity as the path to physical fitness is no less surprising than the relationship of physical activity to improved health and disease prevention. The content of the current nationwide objectives has been guided in part by the concept of health-related fitness. What is different may be the intensity of physical activity required to be physically fit compared with what is necessary to receive benefits to health. Regardless of intensity, both physical fitness and improved health begin with physical activity. The amount and intensity of physical activity were found to be the best predictors of vascular health and function in a group of 10- and 11-year-old children.[114] Evidence of the impact of physical activity and fitness in childhood on fitness, health, and prevention of disease in adulthood is mixed,[36,79,92,123,133,154] but any direct or indirect benefits for the development of lifelong habits of physical activity and fitness in terms of health and disease prevention for typically developing children should be no less true for children with physical disabilities. The concept of physical fitness becomes more important because as individuals become less active in adulthood, the decrease in activity level is more likely to result in loss of function, injury, or both.

Definition of Physical Fitness

As defined previously, *health-related fitness* is a state characterized by (1) an ability to perform daily activities with vigor and (2) traits and capacities that are associated with low risk of premature development of hypokinetic disease (i.e., physical inactivity).[186] Physical fitness is multidimensional. A combination of traits and capacities contributes to physical fitness, and the interaction among them creates true fitness. Each facet is a unique, independent characteristic or ability that is not highly correlated with other components. As the concept of health-related fitness has gained acceptance, four basic components have been identified: cardiorespiratory endurance, muscular strength and endurance, flexibility, and body composition. The rationale for the importance of these parameters in day-to-day functional capacity, health promotion, and disease prevention, and therefore physical fitness, is presented in Table 6.1. The relative independence of the components from one another has been verified by low correlations between components. Of 60 possible correlation coefficients among test items for these components, only 6 were greater than 0.35.[204,206] The conceptual framework developed by the Institute of Medicine Committee on Fitness Measures and Health Outcomes in Youth also highlights the interplay of fitness components, modifying factors, and health markers in the following areas: cardiovascular/respiratory health, metabolic health and obesity, mental and cognitive health, musculoskeletal health, and adverse events.[185]

Cardiopulmonary Response to Exercise

As in adults, the response of a child to exercise (a single event or repeated exercise) includes physiologic changes in the cardiovascular and pulmonary systems, as well as metabolic effects. In children, however, differences in physiologic changes are seen as growth and development occur. Physiologic capacities depend on growth of the myocardium, skeleton, and skeletal muscle. Maturation and improved efficiency of the cardiovascular, pulmonary, metabolic, and musculoskeletal systems are also important. The physical work capacity of children increases approximately eightfold in absolute terms between the ages of

6 and 12 years, partially as a result of growth and maturation.[1] The absolute exercise capacity of children may be less than that of adults, but relative exercise capacity is similar.

Any exercise, in a child or an adult, increases the energy expenditure of the body. The energy for muscle contraction and exercise depends on splitting of adenosine triphosphate (ATP) at the cellular level. ATP is available in small quantities in resting muscle, but once contraction starts, additional sources are required if contraction is to be maintained. Three sources of ATP are available: (1) creatine phosphate (CPh), (2) glycolysis, and (3) the tricarboxylic acid or Krebs cycle. It is beyond the scope of this chapter to describe these mechanisms in detail. The reader is referred to a standard textbook on exercise physiology.[40]

CPh and glycolysis as sources of ATP are referred to as anaerobic pathways because they do not require the presence of oxygen. CPh is found in the sarcoplasm of the muscle cell. During breakdown, it releases a high-energy phosphate bond that can be combined with adenosine diphosphate (ADP) to create ATP:

$$CPh \longrightarrow C + Pi + Energy \qquad [1]$$

$$ADP + Pi + Energy \longrightarrow ATP \qquad [2]$$

CPh breakdown together with ATP production will provide enough energy for 10 to 15 seconds of exercise. Glycolysis, the other anaerobic pathway, breaks down glucose to produce pyruvic acid or lactic acid and ATP. This reaction takes place in the sarcoplasm of the cell. Together, glycolysis and CPh breakdown are methods of anaerobic energy production that can sustain energy for muscle contraction for 40 to 50 seconds.

Energy production by the tricarboxylic acid cycle is called an *aerobic pathway* because it requires oxygen. A supply of oxygen is required for sustained exercise and depends on the aerobic pathway. Most, if not all, activities use both aerobic and anaerobic pathways for the supply of ATP, but often tasks are more highly dependent on one type of pathway than the other.

Because aerobic pathways must be used to sustain exercise, an index of maximal aerobic power is used to reflect the highest metabolic rate made available by aerobic energy. The most common index is maximal oxygen uptake (VO_{2max}), or the highest volume of oxygen that can be consumed per unit time. Oxygen supply to muscle is described by the Fick equation: oxygen uptake (VO_2) is equal to cardiac output (CO) times the difference in oxygen content between arterial (Cao_2) and mixed venous (Cvo_2) blood, or

$$VO_2 = CO\,(Cao_2 - Cvo_2)$$

Because CO is the product of heart rate and stroke volume, the following relationship is also true:

$$VO_2 = \text{Heart rate} \times \text{Stroke volume} \times \text{Arteriovenous} \times O_2 \text{ difference}$$

For VO_2 to increase, one or more of these factors must increase. During exercise, CO is elevated by increases in both heart rate and stroke volume. Elevated blood flow to the muscles increases the difference in oxygen content between arterial and venous blood.

VO_{2max} traditionally implies a plateau in oxygen uptake has been reached despite further exercise. Not all children display a plateau in oxygen uptake during a maximal exercise test to exhaustion. Pediatric exercise science now defines maximal oxygen uptake as VO_{2peak} to indicate that a maximal oxygen uptake may not have reached a plateau.[7,8] Because older literature typically refers to maximal oxygen uptake as VO_{2max} regardless of whether a plateau was reached, this convention will be used to avoid confusion.

VO_{2max} increases throughout childhood from approximately 1 L/min at age 5 years to 3 to 4 L/min at puberty.[8] These changes occur as a result of maturation of the cardiovascular, pulmonary, metabolic, and musculoskeletal systems. As a child grows, the cardiopulmonary and musculoskeletal systems are integrated so that oxygen flow during exercise optimally meets the energy demands of the muscle cells, regardless of body size.[52]

Cardiac Output

CO in children, as in adults, rises at the beginning of exercise or on transition from a lower to a higher level of exercise. CO can increase by an increase in either stroke volume or heart rate. CO in children is similar to that in adults despite the fact that stroke volume in a 5-year-old is about 25% of the stroke volume in an adult.[102] Stroke volume increases parallel to left ventricular size.[208] At all levels of exercise, stroke volume in boys is somewhat higher than in girls.[17] CO levels in children are similar to those in adults because of an increased heart rate throughout childhood. Maximal heart rates in children vary between 195 and 215 beats per minute (bpm) and decrease by 0.7 to 0.8 bpm per year after maturity.[39]

Arteriovenous Difference and Hemoglobin Concentration

At rest, the difference between arterial and mixed venous blood oxygen content is the same in children as in adults.[8,230] Research suggests, however, that children have a higher blood flow to muscles after exercise than do young adults, resulting in a higher arteriovenous oxygen difference.[129] Greater muscle blood flow facilitates increased oxygen transport to exercising muscles and thus a decrease in the oxygen content of the mixed venous blood.

Hemoglobin concentration is lower in children than in the average adult, and this affects the oxygen transport capacity of the blood in children. Studies suggest that children have greater ability to dissociate oxygen from hemoglobin at the tissue level and use a larger percentage of their oxygen-carrying capacity than adults, which partially compensates for the lower hemoglobin concentration.[8]

Arterial Blood Pressure

Lower exercise blood pressure is seen in children than in adults—a finding consistent with lower CO and stroke volume. Blood pressure may also be reduced because of lower peripheral vascular resistance secondary to shorter blood vessels.[17]

Ventilation

Ventilation is the rate of exchange of air between the lungs and ambient air, measured in liters per minute. In absolute terms, ventilation increases with age. Ventilation normalized by body weight is the same for children and adults at maximal activity.[17] At submaximal exercise levels, ventilation is higher in children and decreases with age, suggesting that children have a lower ventilatory reserve than do adults. Studies suggest that children have less efficient ventilation than do adults (i.e., more air is needed to supply 1 L of oxygen in a child than in an adult).[17] Minute ventilation is dependent on a number of factors including neural signals, and it is protocol dependent. Ventilation does not limit the VO_{2max} of healthy children and adolescents.[8]

Vital Capacity

Vital capacity in a 5-year-old child is about 20% of that in an adult and increases with age. It is highly correlated with body size, particularly height,[102] and generally has not been found to be a limiting factor in exercise performance.

Respiratory Rate

Children have a higher respiratory rate than do adults during both maximal and submaximal exercise. A high rate of respiration compensates for decreased lung volume; respiratory rate decreases as lung volume increases.[17]

Blood Lactate

Blood and muscle lactate levels are lower in children than in adults. It has been suggested but not confirmed that lactate production is related to testosterone production and therefore to sexual maturity in boys. Low lactate production in children could limit glycolytic capacity and thus contribute to reduced anaerobic capacity.[8,9,73]

Table 6.2 summarizes comparisons between children and adults for various cardiopulmonary variables. Growth and maturation play a vital part in determining the values of these variables. Despite size differences between adults and children (which might lead one to believe that oxygen transport in children is less efficient because they are smaller), optimal oxygen transport is maintained by highly integrated functions between the cardiopulmonary and musculoskeletal systems.

Review of Tests of Physical Fitness

It has now been longer than 50 years since the first US national youth fitness battery was published.[4] Once emphasizing motor fitness and the readiness of youth for military service, the transition of fitness testing to health-related fitness with a public health emphasis began in the 1970s. The National Children and Youth Fitness Study Tests I and II[203-206] represented the only effort to measure national youth fitness levels for three decades. The prevalence of national physical fitness testing in US schools at the turn of the 21st century was approximately 65% across all school levels.[122,173] Comparison of nationally and regionally used health-related fitness and systematic review of field tests and fitness batteries used worldwide can be found elsewhere.[28,97,185] The FITNESSGRAM/ACTIVITYGRAM[53,169] is now the only national youth fitness test used throughout the United States. The Presidential Youth Fitness Program,[198] which replaced the President's Challenge Youth Fitness Test, has adopted the FITNESSGRAM as its fitness assessment. Together, the FITNESSGRAM and President's Challenge Fitness Test were the basis for the majority of

TABLE 6.2 Cardiopulmonary Function Variables and Response to Exercise in Children

Function	Child Versus Adult Response	Sex Differences
Heart rate (max, submax)	Higher	M = F (max); F > M (submax)
Stroke volume (max, submax)	Lower	M > F
Cardiac output (max, submax)	Lower, similar	
Arteriovenous difference (submax)	Similar	
Blood flow to active muscle	Higher	M = F
Blood pressure	Lower	
Hemoglobin concentration	Lower	
Ventilation/kg body wt (max)	Similar	
Ventilation/kg body wt (submax)	Higher	
Respiratory rate (max, submax)	Higher	
Tidal volume and vital capacity (max)	Lower	
Tidal volume and vital capacity (submax)	Lower	
Blood lactate levels (max, submax)	Similar/lower / Lower	M > F after puberty

max, maximal exercise; *submax*, submaximal exercise.
Adapted from Bar-Or O: *Pediatric sports medicine for the practitioner*, New York, 1963, Springer-Verlag.

scientific decisions over the past half century.[174] A third program, Physical Best,[103] developed concurrently with the others, has since discontinued its assessment component.[173,174] Each test emphasizes health-related fitness components. Most tests provide some information regarding interrater reliability. The validity of health-related fitness components has previously been reviewed.[116,185]

Physical Best Program

This program, originally designed to be both a physical fitness measure and an educational program to promote health and prevent disease, was developed by the American Alliance for Health, Physical Education, Recreation, and Dance (AAHPERD). AAHPERD changed its name to the Society of Health and Physical Educators in 2014, doing business as SHAPE America. The Physical Best Program remains active as a comprehensive health-related fitness education program for physical educators (http://www.shapeamerica.org/prodev/workshops/physicalbest).

FITNESSGRAM Program

This test is a battery that uses criterion-referenced standards that reflect the levels of fitness important for good health. The program was developed by the Cooper Institute for Aerobics Research (https://www.cooperinstitute.org/youth/FITNESSGRAM). Since its initial development, it has been revised three times, most recently in 2010.[53,169] Extensive information on the reliability and validity of the specific standards for all fitness components can be found in the test manual and has been published separately. Development of the standards and the scientific method used to revise the standards is also described. Revised standards for aerobic fitness and body composition using receiver operator characteristic (ROC) curves were completed and published in 2011 as a supplement issue of *American Journal of Preventive Medicine*.[172]

Standards compatible with the FITNESSGRAM for individuals with disabilities have been developed in the Brockport Physical Fitness Test.[276]

National Children, Youth, and Fitness Study I and II

These tests were used in national studies undertaken to assess current levels of physical fitness of children and youth in the United States.[203-206] Until the National Health and Nutrition Examination Survey (NHANES) National Youth Fitness Survey conducted in 2012,[37] these tests represented the only effort to assess youth fitness levels and they remain the basis of most current fitness tests. Initiated by the US Office of Disease Prevention and Health Promotion, the results have been used to set appropriate targets for improved health and fitness. The National Children, Youth, and Fitness Study I (NCYFS I) produced normative data by sex and age and by sex and grade for children and youth age 10 to 18 years, and NCYFS II provided the same information for children age 6 to 9 years. Training procedures were developed for test administrators, and Pearson correlation interrater reliability estimates were found to be .99 for body composition measurements. Concurrent validity of the distance run and VO_{2max} for children of elementary school age had already been established.[117]

Presidential Youth Fitness Program (Replacement for President's Challenge Youth Fitness Test)

The Presidential Youth Fitness Program (PYFP) replaced the President's Challenge Youth Fitness Test (https://www.presidentschallenge.org/challenge/pyfp.shtml) in 2013.[198] A partnership that included the President's Council on Fitness, Sports, and Nutrition, the Amateur Athletic Union, American Alliance for Health, Physical Education, Recreation, and Dance (now SHAPE America), Cooper Institute, and the Centers for Disease Control and Prevention initiated a new focus promoting health among youth versus measuring performance. Fitness within PYFP is assessed using the FITNESSGRAM. The PYFP is a comprehensive program model promoting fitness, physical activity, and education, and its goal is to lead youth to be active throughout life. The President's Challenge Youth Fitness Test has been the most commonly used fitness test among states in the United States that require fitness testing.[173] The change in focus, therefore, has potential for an immediate large-scale impact nationwide. Research on the historical evolution of both the President's Challenge and FITNESSGRAM fitness batteries has been previously published.[185,196]

Brockport Physical Fitness Test

This health-related criterion-referenced test for youth with disabilities was revised in 2014.[276] It offers options for test administrators to individualize testing based on health-related needs and desired fitness profile. The test builds on the framework of the FITNESSGRAM, including the concept of Healthy Fitness Zone, a registered trademark of the Cooper Institute.[169] Target populations for the test include those with visual impairment, intellectual disability, cerebral palsy, spinal cord injury, and amputation, among others. The validity and reliability of the test have been reported separately.[277] The Brockport Physical Fitness Test (BPFT) has been adopted by the Presidential Youth Fitness Program as its assessment program for youth with special needs.[198]

Comparison of Tests

All tests measure similar components of health-related fitness. Each includes items for testing cardiorespiratory endurance, muscular strength and endurance (now sometimes referred to as musculoskeletal fitness), body composition, and flexibility. The tests differ in the reference standard used. Tests are either norm referenced (performance is compared with that of a national US sample of children taking the same test) or criterion referenced (performance is compared with a preset standard consistent with fitness). Criterion-referenced standards are independent of the performance of other children on the same items. The FITNESSGRAM is the only criterion-referenced test. Guidelines for the interpretation of findings with respect to norm-referenced and criterion-referenced evaluations are available.[185]

COMPONENTS OF PHYSICAL FITNESS

The components of health-related fitness, as mentioned earlier, are cardiorespiratory endurance, muscular strength and endurance, flexibility, and body composition. The following information will be reviewed for each component:

- The criterion measure of the component
- Laboratory measurement
- Developmental aspects of the component and standards by age
- Field measurement of the component and its validity in relation to the criterion measure
- Standards by age as determined by the FITNESSGRAM program, a computer-scored fitness test with a health-related focus
- Physical activities with high correlation to the particular fitness component
- Response to training
- Assessment of the component in children with disabilities

Cardiorespiratory Endurance
Criterion Measure

The most widely used criterion measure for cardiorespiratory endurance is directly measured maximal oxygen uptake (VO_{2max} [with a plateau or without a plateau]). This component measures the capabilities of the cardiovascular and pulmonary systems and is significant because oxygen supply to the tissues depends on the efficiency and capacity of these systems. VO_{2max} is the highest rate of oxygen consumed by the body in a given time period during exercise of a significant portion of body muscle mass.[130] It defines the limits of oxygen utilization by exercising muscle and serves as the fundamental marker of physiologic aerobic fitness.[208] Cardiorespiratory endurance is so important to overall fitness that many people view physical fitness as being synonymous with cardiorespiratory endurance.

Laboratory Measurement

Laboratory measurement techniques include measurement of VO_{2max} with the use of an ergometer during progressive exercise to the point of exhaustion. This method is referred to as *direct determination* of VO_{2max}. *Indirect determination* methods predict VO_{2max} from submaximal exercise. A systematic review of reference values of both direct and indirect methods of cardiopulmonary exercise testing in children has been published.[29]

Direct determination. An ergometer is a device that measures the amount of work performed under controlled conditions. The two devices commonly available are a cycle ergometer and

a treadmill. The cycle ergometer has the advantage of being relatively inexpensive and portable, but compared with the treadmill it exercises a smaller total muscle mass. With the cycle ergometer, local fatigue develops (primarily in knee extensors), resulting in premature termination of the testing. Depending on the source, values of VO_{2max} are reported to be 5% to 30% lower on a cycle ergometer than on a treadmill.[17,39,130] For children, the coordination and rhythm, or cadence, required on a cycle ergometer are sometimes difficult to achieve. Both the treadmill and the cycle ergometer present problems when used to test populations with disabilities, in particular those with impairments of balance or coordination.

A variety of protocols for direct determination can be used with children. The most common protocol is one in which resistance, inclination, speed, or height is increased every 1 to 3 minutes without interruption until the child can no longer maintain the activity. In interrupted protocols, which are sometimes used, there is an interruption between each successive increment of exercise. Examples of some common direct determination protocols are given in Table 6.3. The main criterion for indicating that VO_{2max} has been achieved during a progressive protocol is that an increase in power load is not accompanied by an increased VO_2 (usually 2 mL/kg/min or higher).[130] Astrand,[9] however, reported that 5% of all children tested failed to reach a plateau in VO_2, even though evidence from secondary criteria suggested that exhaustion had been reached. This finding in subsequent studies as well has prompted the field to adopt the term VO_{2peak} in children.[7,8]

Despite the difficulty of determining attainment of maximal oxygen uptake, studies suggest that the reliability of direct determination testing with children is high. Coefficients of variation of 3%, 5%, and 8% for VO_{2max} determined by treadmill walk-jogging, running, and walking, respectively, have been reported.[188] A mean variation of 4.5% was reported for children exercising to exhaustion on a cycle ergometer.[272]

TABLE 6.3   Direct Determination All-Out Protocols

BRUCE TREADMILL PROTOCOL			
Stage	Speed, mph	Grade, %	Duration, min
1	1.7	10	3
2	2.5	12	3
3	3.4	14	3
4	4.2	16	3
5	5.0	18	3
6	5.5	20	3
7	6.0	22	3

McMASTER PROGRESSIVE CONTINUOUS CYCLING TEST			
Body Height, cm	Initial Load, watts	Increments, watts	Durations, min
<119.9	12.5	12.5	2
120-139.9	12.5	25.0	2
140-159.9	25.0	25.0	2
>160	25.0	25.0 (F) 50.0 (M)	2

watts, joules per second.
Adapted from Bar-Or O: Appendix II: procedures for exercise testing in children. In Bar-Or O, editor: *Pediatric sports medicine for the practitioner,* New York, 1983, Springer-Verlag.

Indirect determination. Indirect determination methods use submaximal exercise to indirectly predict VO_{2max}. The child is not taken to his or her self-imposed maximum. Heart rate during one or more stages is the variable most commonly used to derive the index of VO_{2max}. Step tests for children are usually submaximal tests, with recovery heart rate used to predict VO_{2max}. Evidence suggests that height-specific step tests can be reliable predictors of VO_{2max}.[96] Important limitations exist, however, in predicting VO_{2max} from submaximal exercise data, and these should always be kept in mind.[282] Examples of test protocols are presented in Table 6.4.

The W_{170} is an index used to predict mechanical power in a submaximal test. Two or more measurements of heart rate are obtained at different powers or workloads, and heart rate is then extrapolated to 170 bpm. The corresponding power is W_{170}. This index, originally described by Wahlund,[263] is based on the assumption that heart rate is linearly related to power at 170 bpm or less. To minimize error, more than two heart rate measurements are taken, one of which is as close as possible to 170 bpm.

More recently, maximal power (as measured during a maximal exercise test on a cycle ergometer) has been advocated, used, and validated as a surrogate for direct measurement of VO_{2max}. This method has been used in children with and without obesity.[66]

Developmental Aspects of Cardiorespiratory Endurance

Maximal oxygen uptake (VO_{2max} or VO_{2peak}) has been extensively studied and documented. Many reviews have combined both cycle ergometer and treadmill data, which has clouded understanding.[8] Maximal oxygen uptake increases with age throughout childhood and is slightly higher in boys than in girls.[8,130,209,221] Initial differences between boys and girls during early childhood are approximately 10%, increasing to 25% by

age 14 years, and exceeding 50% by age 16.[8,130] The development of a greater muscle mass in boys and increasing differences in the amount of time spent in vigorous physical exercise are the most commonly given explanations. Overall, the physical working capacity of children increases approximately eightfold between the ages of 6 and 12 years. Few data are available on VO_{2max} for children younger than age 6.[1,208]

Relative to body weight, only a 1% change in VO_{2max} is noted between the ages of 6 and 16 years for boys (52.8 mL/kg/min at age 6; 53.5 mL/kg/min at age 16), whereas girls display a 12% reduction between the same ages (52 mL/kg/min at age 6; 40.5 mL/kg/min at age 16).[8,130,221] VO_{2max} is highly correlated with lean body mass. The decline in VO_{2max} in girls begins around age 10, when changes in body composition occur as girls develop a relatively increased amount of subcutaneous fat. When VO_{2max} is measured with reference to lean body mass, the difference in values between the sexes disappears.[39] Despite the fact that conventional normalization of VO_{2max} or VO_{2peak} is relative to body mass, the ratios remain size dependent, confounding interpretation.[7,271]

Although the increases in body dimensions of the heart, lungs, and exercising muscle are primarily responsible for the rise in VO_{2max} during the course of childhood, evidence indicates that other factors also contribute. When same-sex adolescents of different ages with identical body weight or body height are compared, the positive relationship with age remains.[231] Functional changes in cardiovascular, pulmonary, hematologic, and musculoskeletal systems resulting in improved efficiency with maturity may play a role. Cooper and colleagues,[52] however, suggested that the functional components of body systems are integrated so that aerobic capacity is optimized throughout the growth process. When cardiovascular responses to exercise are assessed relative to body surface area, they are not substantially different from those measured in adults.[262]

Measurement in the Field

The most common measure of cardiorespiratory fitness in the field is a long-distance run of various structures or lengths. All the physical fitness batteries reviewed previously have a distance run test, commonly a 1-mile run. Test-retest reliability of VO_{2max} during field testing has been shown to be between .60 and .95.[54,212] Construct and concurrent validity with VO_{2max} of 9- and 12-minute run tests in elementary children have also been established.[117,211] Estimation of peak oxygen consumption based on 1-mile run/walk performance is commonly used,[55] but a study has shown that this equation systematically underestimates peak oxygen consumption in endurance-trained children and adolescents with high peak oxygen consumption. This suggests than an alternate method should be applied to children in this category.[48] Prediction models that are independent of body mass index have also shown promise with good criterion-referenced agreement with measured peak VO_2.[43]

The Progressive Aerobic Cardiovascular Endurance Run (PACER) (Fig. 6.1) is an alternative to the 1-mile walk/run test used in the FITNESSGRAM battery. Aerobic performance is estimated on a series of seven 20-meter runs of incrementally increased exercise intensity. Criterion-referenced reliability and equivalency of the PACER were found to be similar to the 1-mile walk/run test in a group of high school students.[24] New minimum Healthy Fit Zones are now available based on the revision of the aerobic capacity standards.[169,268] When examined sequentially by repeated measures, aerobic performance using

TABLE 6.4	Indirect Determination Protocols		
ADAMS SUBMAXIMAL PROGRESSIVE CONTINUOUS CYCLING TEST*			
Body Weight, kg	**Stage 1, watts**	**Stage 2, watts**	**Stage 3, watts**
30	16.5	33.0	50.0
30-39.9	16.5	50.0	83.0
40-59.9	16.5	50.0	100.0
>60	16.5	83.0	133.0
Stage duration = 6/min			
Performance by W_{170}			

MODIFIED 3-MINUTE STEP TEST†		
Stage	**Duration, min**	**Ascent Rate, ascents/min**
1	3	22
2	3	26
3	3	30
Step height dependent on height		
Performance by recovery heart rate		

*Adapted from Bar-Or O: Appendix II: procedures for exercise testing in children. In Bar-Or O, editor: *Pediatric sports medicine for the practitioner*, New York, 1983, Springer-Verlag.
†Adapted and from Francis K, Culpepper M: Height adjusted, rate specific, single stage, step test for predicting maximal oxygen consumption, *South Med J* 82:602-606, 1989.

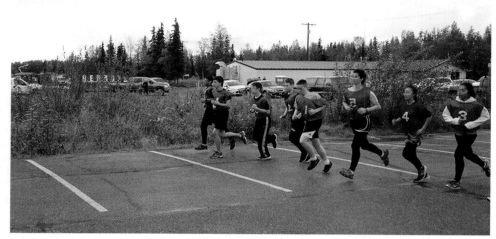

FIG. 6.1 High school students participate in the 20-meter PACER (Progressive Aerobic Cardio-vascular Endurance Run). (Photo taken by Sgt. Brian Ragin.)

the PACER is noted to fluctuate over a 12-month period, likely the result of changing patterns of intensity and type of physical activity.[44] Cross-validation of the PACER with the 1-mile run distances to estimate aerobic capacity is now complete.[33]

Standards by Age

Standards of performance are determined by ranking a child's performance in relation to the performance of a group of children tested on the same test (norm-referenced standard) or against an established criterion found to be consistent with good health (criterion-referenced standard). Criterion-referenced standards are independent of the proportion of the population that meets the standards. A ranking by a norm-referenced standard does not necessarily represent a desirable level of fitness or performance. The limitation of criterion-referenced standards, however, is that they are somewhat arbitrary and the criteria used in the current physical fitness tests differ from one another.[56] Criterion-referenced standards are most accepted today.

FITNESSGRAM has revised criterion-standards for aerobic fitness.[269] The design of new standards is based on receiver operating characteristic curves, an established procedure for establishing clinical thresholds.[270] This is consistent with the current-day emphasis on linking fitness to functional health outcomes. The process of developing new standards also included validation of field tests, as well as classification of students with both old and new standards.[268] A comparison of walk/run standards by age is provided in Table 6.5.

Physical Activities

Activities that are highly correlated with the development of cardiorespiratory endurance are boxing, running, rowing, swimming, cross-country skiing, and bicycling. The common component among these activities is a prolonged, sustained demand on the cardiorespiratory system that requires general stamina.

Response to Training

Debate exists over whether maximal aerobic power of pre-pubescence is a component that can be affected by training. Research results are equivocal. Studies that report improvement

TABLE 6.5   One-Mile Walk/Run Standards

Age, yr	Criterion* Standard		FITNESSGRAM[†] PACER minimum 20-m laps	
	M	F	M	F
5			§	§
6			§	§
7			§	§
8			§	§
9			§	§
10	40.2	40.2	17	17
11	40.2	40.2	20	20
12	40.3	40.1	23	23
13	41.4	39.7	29	25
14	42.5	39.4	36	27
15	43.6	39.1	42	30
16	44.1	38.9	47	32
17	44.2	38.8	50	35
>17	44.3	38.6	54	38

*Criterion standard as set by FITNESSGRAM in ml/kg/min of oxygen uptake. Values reported are minimum for the Healthy Fitness Zone.
[†]Number of 20-m laps to complete on Progressive Aerobic Cardiovascular Endurance Run (PACER). Times reported are minimum for the Healthy Fitness Zone based on 2014 revision standards.
Adapted from Ross JG, the Cooper Institute: *FITNESSGRAM®/ACTIVITYGRAM test administration manual,* updated ed 4, Champaign IL, 2010, Human Kinetics.

in aerobic power with training suggest that the principles of training of children before puberty (i.e., frequency, intensity, and duration) are similar to those for adults. The functional results of conditioning on the cardiorespiratory system include decreased heart rate, increased stroke volume, improved respiratory muscular endurance, and decreased respiration rate.[17,261] A more specific focus on conditioning and training will be found later in this chapter.

Assessment of Cardiorespiratory Endurance in Children With Disabilities

Children with disabilities often exhibit decreased or limited exercise capacity relative to their nondisabled peers. This can result from limited participation in exercise, which leads to

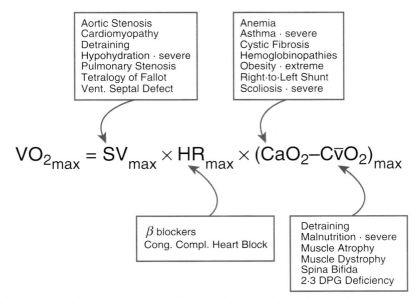

FIG. 6.2 Maximal aerobic power (VO$_{2max}$) and pathology. The Fick equation and specific pathologic conditions that affect its variables and reduce VO$_{2max}$ are shown. (From Bar-Or O, editor: *Pediatric sports medicine for the practitioner*, New York, 1983, Springer-Verlag.)

deconditioning, or the specific pathologic factors of their disability that limit exercise-related functions. Regardless of the cause, children with disabilities often enter a cycle of decreased activity that precipitates loss of fitness and further decreases in activity levels.

Pathophysiologic factors that may limit cardiorespiratory endurance can sometimes be separated by the specific component of the Fick equation that they affect. This provides a convenient way to categorize conditions or diseases by the fitness components they affect most[19,21] (Fig. 6.2). Studies suggest that maximal aerobic uptake is limited not only by central mechanisms of the cardiopulmonary system but also by peripheral mechanisms controlling blood flow, excitation processes in the muscle fiber, local fatigue, and enzyme availability.[214,234] When limitations or reductions in VO$_{2max}$ in children with disabilities are considered, both central and peripheral limitations must be taken into account.

Cerebral palsy. The directly measured maximal aerobic capacity of children and adolescents with cerebral palsy (CP) is 10% to 30% less than that of control subjects. The measurements have been shown to be reliable.[14,139,253] It seems that peripheral mechanisms related to the neuromuscular disorder itself are more likely to contribute to decreased capacity than are central cardiopulmonary mechanisms, although this has not been studied.

When indirectly assessed from submaximal heart rate, the aerobic capacity of adolescents was found to be reduced by 50%.[150] Low mechanical efficiency, however, creates disproportionately high submaximal heart rates in individuals with CP, making submaximal heart rate a poor predictor of maximal aerobic power.[18] Submaximal exercise tests, in general, underestimate aerobic capacity in poorly trained individuals.[9] Numerous studies suggest that heart rate is a good predictor or an appropriate substitute clinical measure of oxygen uptake because of its linear relationship to heart rate.[201,202] It is not a measure of maximal aerobic capacity, however, and therefore it is not an alternative measure of cardiorespiratory fitness.

An increase in blood flow to exercising muscles after conditioning is a response observed in children with CP but not seen in typically developing children without disabilities.[151] Spastic muscles of individuals with adult-onset brain damage exhibit subnormal blood flow during exercise.[134] Whether the rate of blood flow changes after conditioning in individuals with adult-onset brain injury is not known. One hypothesis to explain the increase in blood flow in conditioned individuals with CP is that it results from a decrease in spasticity. More rapid deterioration of maximal aerobic uptake is seen after discontinuation of training in children with CP than in typically developing children.[18]

Functional assessments that relate to the cardiorespiratory fitness of children with various disabilities are becoming more commonplace. The Pediatric Orthopedic Society of North America developed a functional outcomes questionnaire directed toward assessment of pediatric musculoskeletal conditions.[58] Within this questionnaire are queries regarding a child's ability to complete a 1-mile and a 3-mile walk. As more professionals caring for children with disabilities incorporate this assessment and others like it in daily practice, insight will be gained that may assist in determining cardiorespiratory fitness. The 6-minute walk test has been used in children with CP as a submaximal test of capacity.[241] Standards for field testing aerobic capacity in individuals with CP using a long-distance run have been previously published for children age 10 to 17 years.[278]

The Brockport Physical Fitness Test recommends the target aerobic movement test (TAMT) to measure aerobic behavior in children with CP.[276] It measures the aerobic behavior of youngsters and their ability to exercise at or above a recommended target heart rate for 15 minutes. Appropriate activity for the test may include swimming, dancing, running, arm-ergometry, or other aerobic exercise. This test can be used across functional levels for children with CP. The PACER and 1-mile run are also used. See Chapter 19 for more information on CP.

Juvenile idiopathic arthritis. Maximal aerobic capacity measured by cycle ergometry in children with juvenile rheumatoid arthritis has been reported to be 25% to 30% lower when compared to typically developing subjects.[251] No correlation was found between severity of articular disease and aerobic capacity, but it is related to disease duration.[192,237] A randomized controlled trial has demonstrated that exercise programs are safe without and can be performed without disease exacerbation.[223] Physical activity recommendations include radiographic screening for C1-C2 instability before participation in collision/contact sports.[192] Children will have a shorter duration of exercise before exhaustion, which occurs at a lower than normal work rate with a lower peak heart rate. Deficient oxygen extraction from exercising muscles or low blood flow to exercising muscles has been postulated to occur in this population as a result of decreased activity levels.[18,21] See Chapter 7 for more information on juvenile idiopathic arthritis.

Scoliosis. Chest deformity, decreased lung size, and decreased physical activity are believed to contribute to the lower maximal aerobic capacity of children with advanced scoliosis. Peak oxygen uptake during cardiopulmonary exercise testing has been shown to be reduced if compared to healthy individuals at a similar level of peak ventilation.[71] Chronic deconditioning also plays a role in the functional exercise limitations.[229] See Chapter 8 for more information on scoliosis.

Intellectual disabilities. Most studies indicate that individuals with intellectual disabilities display lower VO_{2max} scores than do their peers without disabilities; however, significant variability has been reported among individuals with the same level of disability. Technical problems associated with testing individuals with intellectual disabilities are encountered that create difficulties in establishing reliable and valid information. Treadmill testing appears to be the most reliable form of testing. Despite lower VO_{2max} scores, individuals with intellectual disabilities without Down syndrome have been shown to exhibit similar age-related trends and changes as individuals without disabilities (i.e., decline with age).[23] Field test standards and alternative test items for aerobic capacity in individuals with intellectual and other disabilities are available.[276] See Chapter 18 for more information on children with intellectual disabilities.

Children with obesity. The prevalence of obesity in children age 2 to 19 years designated as overweight by the National Health and Nutrition Examination Survey (2011-2012) was estimated at 16.9%, and 31.8% were estimated to be overweight or obese.[180] Although obesity is not considered a category of "disability" in traditional terms, public health concerns for this group of young people make it worthy of special attention. Field tests of cardiorespiratory endurance in obese youth using the 1-mile walk/run test demonstrate that they perform below typical standards for nonobese peers.[160] Only 34% of obese boys and 38% of obese girls tested fell within the Healthy Fitness Zone of the FITNESSGRAM 1-mile walk/run standards as compared with 73% and 61% of their nonobese counterparts, respectively. Estimation of peak oxygen uptake from the same 1-mile walk/run performance suggested similar results for VO_{2max}.[160] Evidence, however, suggests that VO_{2max} values from prediction equations or submaximal exercise tests overestimate actual VO_{2max} when measured on a maximal exercise test.[10] This suggests that the percentage of obese youth that fall within a zone of healthy fitness may actually be less. Racial differences in obese adolescents have also been reported. Black adolescents had significantly lower VO_{2max} and lower hemoglobin than did white adolescents with no differences in maximal heart rate or respiratory exchange ratio.[6]

Muscular Strength and Endurance

The second component of physical fitness is muscular strength and endurance. Strength is required for movement and has a direct impact on effective performance. Strength is also important for optimal posture and reduced risk of lower back pain, which is the criterion health condition to which this component of physical fitness is linked. Similar to cardiorespiratory endurance, positive relationships between musculoskeletal fitness and health status in adults have been demonstrated.[89,121] The theoretical link between fatigue-resistant trunk muscles (abdominal flexors and trunk extensors) and healthy low back function, however, is stronger than the research evidence between muscular strength and flexibility and the onset or recurrence of low back pain.[194] A growing body of evidence is emerging for children as well as adults that enhanced musculoskeletal fitness is associated with an overall improvement in health status.[195,264,273] No critical level of strength or muscular endurance for good health has been identified.

Muscular strength, muscular endurance, and *muscular power* are not synonymous terms. Muscular strength refers to maximal contractile force. Muscular endurance is the ability of muscles to perform work and assumes some component of muscular strength. Muscular power refers to the ability to release maximal muscular force within a specified time. As velocity increases or time decreases (for maximal muscular force to be obtained), power increases. Because muscular endurance and muscular power have their basis in muscular strength, strength is the primary focus of this discussion.

Laboratory Measurement

The laboratory standard for muscular strength is measurement by dynamometry. Tests include isometric dynamometry, isokinetic dynamometry, and single-repetition maximal isotonic dynamometry. Most measurements are made on specific, selected muscles, then results are extrapolated to give "whole body" strength. The validity of the extrapolation method has been questioned.[195] The deficits not only in reliable, valid laboratory and field standards for musculoskeletal fitness but also the need for scientific links between musculoskeletal fitness and health risk factors/markers have been highlighted.[195] Unfortunately, a limitation for setting standards for strength is that force measurements depend on the type of dynamometer used.[30] The most commonly selected measures are hand grip, elbow flexion and extension, knee flexion and extension, and plantar flexion strength.

Isokinetic strength testing during childhood and adolescence is a relatively new area of study. The reliability of isokinetic testing in children presents unique issues because of the variability of muscle coordination and neuromuscular maturation. Coefficients of variation from 5% to 11% have been reported.[30] Children demonstrate the capacity to perform consistent maximal voluntary contraction under controlled conditions by age 6 to 7 years. Comparative muscle performance data (upper and lower body power and velocity) for children ages 3 to 7 years are now available.[98] The limited amount of research and the lack of available data do not allow definite conclusions on the effects of age and gender differences on isokinetic strength development. Body weight and muscle cross-sectional area, however, appear to correlate positively with isokinetic strength. Gender differences are minimal between ages 3 and 11. After age 13, boys tend to have greater isokinetic strength for the muscles tested than do girls.[15,239]

Developmental aspects and standards by age

Grip strength. Grip strength is the most commonly reported upper extremity strength measure in children. Absolute strength scores, however, are highly sensitive to the type of dynamometer used and to its positioning, making the results of studies difficult to compare. In general, single-hand grip strength increases from an average of approximately 5 kg for children at age 3 years to 45 kg for boys at age 17 and 30 kg for girls at age 17. Bilateral grip strength has been measured at a mean of 25 kg for children at age 7 years, increasing to an average of 95 kg for boys and 50 kg for girls by age 17 years.[30,156] The rate of increase in strength for boys rises dramatically at puberty. This finding is confirmed in the Longitudinal Experimental Growth Study, where a marked acceleration of strength or a strength spurt was noted around the age of peak height velocity. The maximal increase in static strength occurs approximately 1 year later.[239] Absolute values of the developmental range of strength throughout childhood were measured to be slightly larger. Pearson correlations to static strength in adulthood were reported to be fair to high, depending on whether individuals were noted to be early, average, or late maturing.

Elbow flexion and extension. Isometric elbow flexion strength is greater than isometric elbow extension strength throughout childhood and adolescence, and the difference between them increases with increasing age.[279] A 3-year longitudinal study demonstrated that the extension/flexion strength ratio for boys is approximately 0.85 at the age of 13 years and decreases to 0.75 by the age of 15 years. The ratio for girls is less, starting at 0.75 at age 13 years and decreasing to 0.66 by age 15 years.

Knee flexion and extension. Isokinetic knee flexion strength and knee extension strength also increase throughout childhood. Rather than examining each in isolation, studies advocate evaluating reciprocal muscle group ratios to better understand knee function.[63] Eccentric/concentric ratios provide information on knee function, injury risk, and knee stability. Available data for children indicate that during fast velocity movements, prepubescent children have a lower capacity for generating eccentric to concentric torque. Irrespective of age, girls appear to have a reduced capacity for concentric actions, which may make them more susceptible to injury.[64]

Trunk and neck flexion and extension. Few data are available for laboratory dynamometry standards for trunk strength in children. Values for isokinetic trunk flexion and extension strength at varying speeds are available for a group of prepubescent children with and without back pain (mean age 11.9 years).[168] Similar to findings in adults, both extensor and flexor peak torque decreased with increasing speed. Flexor and extensor peak torque were higher in males than females.

Pediatric data are also available for isometric neck strength in children, adolescents, and young adults.[138] Maturation of neck strength increases with age and is modeled as a second-order polynomial. The mismatch between head circumference and muscle strength may implicate susceptibility to injury in prepubertal children. For example, an 8-year-old has an average head circumference that is 91% that of an adult, but strength is only 50%.

Evoked responses. A second method for muscular function assessment in the laboratory is by evoked responses from electrical stimulation. Muscle contractile characteristics, including force production, are studied with this method. Few data are available for children.[30,32]

Developmental Aspects of Muscular Strength and Endurance

A description of the development of the musculoskeletal system is found in Chapter 5. The development of strength depends on the maturation of force production and is influenced by numerous factors, such as the muscle's cross-sectional area.[239] Muscular strength in absolute terms increases linearly with chronologic age from early childhood in both sexes to approximately age 13 to 14 years. Increases in strength are closely related to increases in muscle mass during growth. Boys have greater strength than do girls at all ages (seen as early as age 3 years) and have larger absolute and relative amounts of muscle (kilogram of muscle per kilogram of body weight).[30,239] The sex difference in relative strength (per kilogram of body mass) before puberty is caused at least in part by a higher proportion of body fat in girls from mid-childhood onward—a difference similar to the trend in cardiorespiratory endurance.[91,180] Rarick and Thompson[200] suggested that boys are 11% to 13% stronger than girls during childhood. This value reaches 20% by adulthood for strength per cross-sectional area of muscle.[161] Correlates and determinants of strength are thought to include age, body size, muscle size, muscle fiber type and size, muscle contractile properties, and biomechanical influences.

During adolescence, a marked acceleration in development of strength occurs, particularly in boys. Boys between the ages of 10 and 16 years who were followed longitudinally showed a 23% increase in strength per year. Peak growth in muscle mass occurred during and after peak weight gain, but maximal strength development occurred after peak velocity of growth in height and weight, suggesting that muscle tissue increases first in mass and then in strength.[153,239] Girls generally show peak strength development before peak weight gain.[88] Overall muscle mass increases more than 5 times in males from childhood to adulthood; the increase in females is 3.5 times.

Differentiation in strength between the sexes at puberty is caused, at least in part, by differences in hormonal concentrations, particularly testosterone. Hormones other than the male sex steroids also make an important contribution.[90] Unfortunately, no pediatric studies to date have correlated age-associated changes in endocrinologic function with muscle size and muscular strength.

Measurement in the Field

Strength is considered an important part of physical fitness; however, the standards to meet minimal fitness requirements and the link between musculoskeletal fitness and health are the least clear. Some suggest that the single most pressing research need in this area is to understand which musculoskeletal fitness test items can be unequivocally linked to health risk factors.[194] Field measurements of muscular strength usually entail movement of part or all of the body mass against gravity. The common tests for muscular strength are the flexed arm hang or 90° push-up and the curl-up. The curl-up has replaced the sit-up as the common field test item. The FITNESSGRAM also includes a trunk lift test for back strength (Fig. 6.3). The correlation between abdominal strength and endurance and shoulder girdle strength as measures of absolute strength for physical fitness is not well established. Available data for the reliability and validity of the curl-up and sit-up, tests of trunk extension, and upper arm and shoulder assessments are well outlined by Plowman. Results are variable. In some cases, such as for trunk extension, data on children are lacking.[194]

Curl-ups/sit-ups. The exact relationship between curl-up performance (Fig. 6.4) and abdominal strength and endurance is unclear. How abdominal strength is related to a given number of curl-ups is unknown. Test-retest reliability estimates for curl-ups is well outlined in the FITNESSGRAM reference manual.[194] The most recent study in the series for youth was conducted in 2001 and indicated reliability of between .75 and .89.[190]

Chin-ups/flexed arm hang/90° push-ups. The recommended test for upper body strength and endurance within the FITNESSGRAM is the 90° push-up at a cadence of one repetition every 3 seconds.[194] The flexed arm hang (Fig. 6.5) or chin-up are optional items. The three items are not anatomically interchangeable. Correlations among the field tests exhibit a range from low to high. Concurrent validity has not been established for these tests as definitive measures of strength or muscle endurance. Limited research is available for children.

Standards by Age

The standards of performance by age for the FITNESSGRAM Program are listed in Table 6.6.

Sex differences typically begin at puberty, but each item has slightly different timing when the standards diverge. Modified pull-up standards are the first to diverge between ages 8 and 9 years, followed by 90° push-up standards between age 10 and 11 years, flexed arm hang between standards between 11 and 12 years, and last to diverge are standards for the curl-up, which diverge between age 12 and 13 years. In each case, the standard for boys is higher than it is for girls. The only test item that displays no differentiation by sex is the trunk lift.[169]

Physical Activities

Activities that have a high correlation with muscular strength are gymnastics, jumping, sprinting, weight lifting, and wrestling. Local muscular endurance is affected by cycling, figure skating, and middle-distance running.

Response to Training

Training-induced increases in strength can be influenced by numerous factors, including enhancement of motivation, improvement in coordination, increase in number of contractile proteins per cross-sectional area of muscle, and hypertrophy of muscle.[105] Children can achieve gains in strength and muscle mass with training before or after puberty. Strength improvements in prepubescent children have typically been attributed to neurologic adaptations to training and improved motor unit activation rather than to increased cross-sectional area of muscle,[87,105] but both play a role. Research has demonstrated that a 12-week resistance training program in prepubertal boys was effective in improving both strength and force per unit muscle volume.[72] Direct evidence for the role of neurologic adaptation during strength training has been documented by increases in integrated electromyographic amplitudes and maximal isokinetic strength following an 8-week

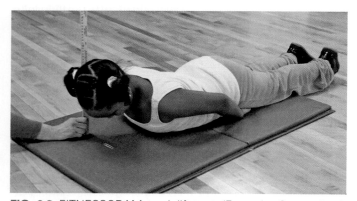

FIG. 6.3 FITNESSGRAM trunk lift test. (From the Cooper Institute, Dallas Texas. Reprinted with permission.)

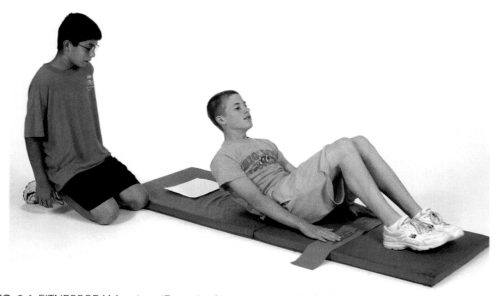

FIG. 6.4 FITNESSGRAM curl-up. (From the Cooper Institute, Dallas Texas. Reprinted with permission.)

strength program.[184] Because the magnitude of change in neuromuscular activation is generally smaller than the observed increase in strength, it has been postulated that improved movement coordination is a contributor to strength gains, particularly in complex multijoint exercises.[25] Neuromuscular maturation in the prepubescent child is therefore an important contributor to strength and should not be underestimated.

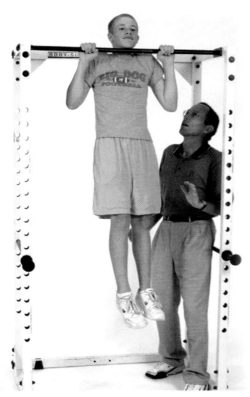

FIG. 6.5 FITNESSGRAM flexed arm-hang test. (From the Cooper Institute, Dallas Texas. Reprinted with permission.)

Controversy has existed for a number of years regarding the safety and efficacy of strength training programs for children and adolescents. The American Academy of Pediatrics Council on Sports Medicine and Fitness guidelines[3] and an international consensus statement from the United Kingdom Strength and Conditioning Association[144] are available for review. The international consensus statement has been endorsed by the American Academy of Pediatrics.

Assessment of Muscular Strength and Endurance in Children With Disabilities

Muscular strength and endurance are crucial fitness components for walking, lifting, and performing most daily functions. Deficits of muscular strength in children with disabilities are a primary focus for the clinician in an attempt to improve (or maintain) maximum function. It is important to keep in mind, however, that strength as measured clinically is not simply the ability of a muscle to generate force. Strength measured clinically is the effectiveness of the muscle force to produce movement of the joint. This encompasses both the ability of the muscle to generate force and appropriate skeletal alignment. In children with disabilities, strength deficits result from the muscles' inability to generate force, malalignment of the skeleton, or a combination of both.

Muscular dystrophy. Strength measurements by dynamometry in children with Duchenne muscular dystrophy (DMD) exhibit progressive deterioration as compared with healthy children.[141] Failure of muscular strength to increase with growth is seen. The result is that the absolute strength in a child with DMD at the age of 16 years is similar to that of a typical 5-year-old.

The use of quantitative muscle testing (QMT) has shown better reliability than manual muscle testing in this population.[162] Longitudinal data have shown increases in QMT in boys up to age 7½ years, followed by substantial decreases. The average 1-year changes were significantly different from those of healthy controls.[141]

Age, yr	FITNESSGRAM Curl-Ups, Number Completed		FITNESSGRAM Modified Pull-Ups, Number Completed		FITNESSGRAM Flexed Arm Hang, Seconds		FITNESSGRAM 90° Push-Ups, Number Completed		FITNESSGRAM Trunk Lift, Inches	
	F	M	F	M	F	M	F	M	F	M
5	≥2	≥2	≥2	≥2	≥2	≥2	≥3	≥3	6-12	6-12
6	≥2	≥2	≥2	≥2	≥2	≥2	≥3	≥3	6-12	6-12
7	≥4	≥4	≥3	≥3	≥3	≥3	≥4	≥4	6-12	6-12
8	≥6	≥6	≥4	≥4	≥3	≥3	≥5	≥5	6-12	6-12
9	≥9	≥9	≥4	≥5	≥4	≥4	≥6	≥6	6-12	6-12
10	≥12	≥12	≥4	≥5	≥4	≥4	≥7	≥7	9-12	9-12
11	≥15	≥15	≥4	≥6	≥6	≥6	≥7	≥8	9-12	9-12
12	≥18	≥18	≥4	≥7	≥7	≥10	≥7	≥10	9-12	9-12
13	≥18	≥21	≥4	≥8	≥8	≥12	≥7	≥12	9-12	9-12
14	≥18	≥24	≥4	≥9	≥8	≥15	≥7	≥14	9-12	9-12
15	≥18	≥24	≥4	≥10	≥8	≥15	≥7	≥16	9-12	9-12
16	≥18	≥24	≥4	≥12	≥8	≥15	≥7	≥18	9-12	9-12
17	≥18	≥24	≥4	≥14	≥8	≥15	≥7	≥18	9-12	9-12
17+	≥18	≥24	≥4	≥14	≥8	≥15	≥7	≥18	9-12	9-12

Data adapted from the Cooper Institute: *FITNESSGRAM®/ACTIVITYGRAM test administration manual,* updated ed 4, Champaign IL, 2010, Human Kinetics.

Muscular endurance (the ability to sustain static or rhythmic contraction for long periods) is also affected in children with DMD. Ninety-two percent of the children tested by Hosking and colleagues scored below the 5th percentile for strength in holding the head 45° off the ground. Measurement on the Wingate anaerobic cycling test indicates that both peak muscular power and mean muscular power output are significantly less than is typical.[21] The test-retest reliability of this test for various neuromuscular and muscular disease conditions has been established.[243] See Chapter 12 for more information on DMD and other types of muscle diseases.

Cerebral palsy. Strength deficits in children with CP are common, and strength profiles for lower extremity muscle groups in children with spastic CP are available.[274] Children with spastic diplegia demonstrated strength values ranging from 16% to 71% of same-age peers depending on the muscle tested. The gluteus maximus and soleus muscles showed the greatest strength deficits. The involved side of children with hemiplegia exhibited values from 22% to 79% of strength values of same-age peers. The gluteus maximus and the anterior tibialis were the weakest muscles. Strength in children with CP is an active area of research. A randomized controlled trial of the efficacy of a 12-week combined functional anaerobic and strength training program on walking ability and gross motor functional capacity is under way.[101]

Inadequate joint moment and power production as measured by computerized gait analysis are seen in children with CP.[100,183] These measures provide indirect evidence in a functional context of decreased strength because strength is a prerequisite for moment and power production. Power production by the ankle plantar flexor muscles in terminal stance phase provides a key source of power for forward motion during the typical walking cycle. Power production in terminal stance phase is often reduced in children with CP. Occasionally, inappropriately timed power production results in excessive, but nonproductive, energy expenditure during gait[99] (Fig. 6.6).

Muscular endurance is also decreased in children with CP. Performance on the Wingate anaerobic test in a group of children with CP resulted in averages that were 30% to 60% lower than typically developing peers.[14,21] The test exhibits moderate reliability in this population.[13]

Modifications for lower and upper extremity strength field test items in children with CP are available within the Brockport Physical Fitness Test manual.[276] Modifications are suggested based on the classification system used by the Cerebral Palsy International Sports and Recreation Association.[49]

Children with obesity. Performance on field tests of abdominal and upper body muscle strength (curl-up and modified pull-up or flexed arm hang) is poorer for children identified as overweight (≥ 95% body mass index). Children who were overweight were 3 times less likely to pass the upper body strength test and 1.5 times less likely to pass the abdominal strength test than children who were not overweight.[126] The negative influences of biomechanical factors related to (1) increased body size such as the need to move fat tissue, which acts as an inert load; (2) weakened force production caused by increased mechanical work and moment of inertia due to a higher trunk mass; and (3) the fact that gravity itself may pull the trunk down; in certain tests, all factors likely contribute to impaired muscle strength and endurance performance.[91] The inverse relationship of obesity to fitness measures of strength is seen across cultures.[38,91,115] An increased incidence of musculoskeletal problems has been reported.[67,131,238]

Flexibility

Inconsistency and controversy exist in how flexibility is classified and its importance as a component of health-related fitness. The Institute of Medicine report maintains fitness as a separate component, consistent with the original categories, but FITNESSGRAM includes flexibility under the umbrella of musculoskeletal fitness along with muscle strength and

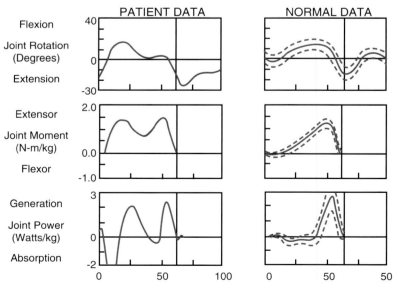

FIG. 6.6 Sagittal plane joint rotation (kinematic), joint moment, and power (kinetics) of a child with cerebral palsy versus a normal child. The child's joint moment is biphasic, and the power graph indicates two distinct bursts of power generation instead of one. The first burst is abnormal and functions to drive the center of gravity upward, not forward, which is nonproductive energy expenditure. (From Gage JR: *Gait analysis in cerebral palsy,* London, 1991, MacKeith Press.)

endurance.[185,194] Evidence supports flexibility as a unique construct of fitness.[76] The definition of flexibility according to the Institute of Medicine report is "the intrinsic property of body tissues including muscle and connective tissues that determines the range of motion achievable without injury at a joint or group of joints."[185] The association to health outcomes has been difficult to clearly demonstrate, but the historical importance of flexibility as a component of health-related fitness is related to the prevention of musculoskeletal impairments later in life, especially lower back pain and posture.[249] The associations have been studied in adults, but the association with flexibility in youth has not been established. As a result, the Institute of Medicine committee did not recommend a flexibility test for a national youth fitness survey. Plowman identified the question of whether flexibility should be part of a health-related fitness assessment as one of the top 10 pressing questions relevant to musculoskeletal fitness testing.[195]

Historically, it is felt that flexible muscles permit proper pelvic rotation, decrease disc compression, and avoid excessive stretch of musculature. Flexibility of the lower back, legs, and shoulders contributes to the prevention of injury. Limitations in spinal mobility can interfere with activities of daily living, such as dressing, turning, and driving. Restrictions in back mobility can also contribute to abnormalities in walking.

Criterion Measure

Joint range of motion (ROM) is the criterion used for standards of flexibility. Although ROM measures for adults are well established and can be found in various textbooks,[178] ROM information for the pediatric population correlated with changes in stature is limited. Upper extremity ROM data for children are not well documented. The typical measurement tool is the universal goniometer. A review of the reliability of goniometry is found in Chapter 5.

Laboratory Measurement and Developmental Aspects of Flexibility

Extremity range of motion. Lower extremity passive ROM measurements have been described in the newborn, infant, and toddler.[75,191,267] Newborns exhibit hypoextensibility of both hip and knee flexor muscles and increased popliteal angles consistent with the flexed posture in utero. Range of motion increases in the first months of life. Ranges of hip abduction and rotation also differ from adult values. See Chapter 5 for information on ROM values for newborns.

Little to no information has been reported for ROM during childhood. Unpublished data from my laboratory on lower extremity ROM measurements in 140 children between the ages of 2 and 18 years suggest variation in some joints throughout childhood and relative stability in others[191] (Table 6.7). Test-retest reliability using Pearson correlations was .95, and interrater reliability was .90. Results suggested age and sex differences, with females exhibiting a trend toward greater flexibility at all ages. Greater flexibility of the hamstring muscles in females is especially apparent during the teenage years in straight leg raising and popliteal angle measurements.

Posture and spinal mobility. Spinal mobility has been measured in both young children and adolescents.[109,170] The technique of measurement of back mobility uses tape measure distance changes in bony landmark relationships before and after a standardized spinal movement. The concurrent validity of this measurement technique with anterior spinal flexion measured radiographically has been established.[152,170] Anterior spinal flexion appears to remain relatively stable throughout childhood and adolescence, but lateral flexion increases linearly with age through adolescence and into early adulthood. Girls were significantly more flexible than boys in both anterior flexion and lateral flexion in the 5- to 9-year-old age group.[109]

The relationship of posture to physical fitness is not often addressed in today's emphasis on health-related fitness. Previous research discussing the relationship of posture to fitness included the importance of posture to trunk strength and the potential for imbalance, back pain, headache, foot pain, and orthopedic deformities.[51,124] Each aspect of posture may be important to mobility in children but becomes of greater importance in adulthood, when impairment can lead to further deformity and loss of function.

Measurement in the Field

The field tests for measurement of flexibility in tests of physical fitness are the sit and reach test or, more recently, the modified sit and reach test—a measure of hamstring muscle and lower back flexibility. This test measures the distance a child can reach forward (shoulders flexed to 90° and elbows extended) from a long-sit position. Starting position is with the back straight, hips at 90°. No field test is available for the assessment of low back flexibility. The back-saver sit and reach test (Fig. 6.7) used in the FITNESSGRAM is similar to the traditional sit and reach test except that the measurement is performed on one side at a time (opposite leg is flexed with opposite foot flat on the floor). The intraclass correlation for test-retest reliability of the sit and reach test was found to be high; coefficients between 0.94 and 0.99 have been reported.[110,118,152] Jackson and Baker[118] assessed

TABLE 6.7	Selected Range-of-Motion Measurements During Childhood					
Mean Range of Motion (Degrees)	**2–5 Years**		**6–12 Years**		**13–19 Years**	
	M	F	M	F	M	F
Straight leg raise	70	75	65	75	60	70
Popliteal angle (unilateral)*	15	10	30	25	40	25
Abduction†	60	60	50	55	45	50
Internal rotation‡	45	50	50	55	45	45
Femoral anteversion§	10	15	7	7	0	0

*Supine position, opposite leg extended. Position from vertical.
†Measured with hip extension.
‡Prone position.
§Prone position by lateral placement of the greater trochanter.
Data from the James R. Gage, Center for Gait and Motion Analysis, Gillette Children's Specialty Healthcare, St. Paul, MN.

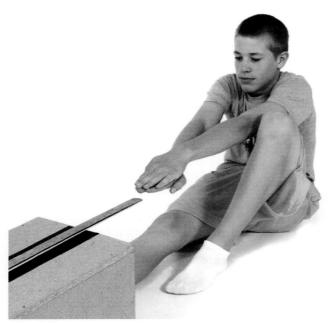

FIG. 6.7 FITNESSGRAM back-saver sit and reach. (From the Cooper Institute, Dallas Texas. Reprinted with permission.)

Assessment of Flexibility in Children with Disabilities

For clinicians involved in the rehabilitation (or habilitation) of children with musculoskeletal disorders, maintenance of flexibility or joint ROM is often a primary concern. Almost any musculoskeletal or neuromuscular disorder for which physical therapy is recommended includes treatment for loss of flexibility. Conditions such as CP, juvenile rheumatoid arthritis, muscular dystrophy (MD), or long bone fracture are common examples.

In Chapter 5, both measurement of and the effects of intervention on improving joint ROM in children were addressed. The challenges of goniometric reliability of joint ROM measurements in children and adults with spasticity are well documented.[35,81,125,164] Similar results have been found in adults.[35,81] Because maintenance of flexibility is an important component of most physical therapy programs for children with disabilities, methods for more reliable assessment of joint ROM are needed.

Field test standards for the back-saver sit and reach test and suggested modifications for test administration have been published for children with visual impairment, mental retardation, and Down syndrome.[276]

Children with obesity. Performance on field tests of flexibility (back-saver sit and reach test) is similar for children identified as overweight (≥ 95% body mass index) compared with typical weight or underweight peers.[126] This finding is supported for adolescents as well.[91]

Body Composition

The term *body composition* is understood to mean total body content of water, protein, fat, and minerals or the components that make up body weight.[65,104] The major contributors are muscle, bone, and fat content, along with organs, skin, and nerve tissue. The importance of body composition to health-related fitness has two components: (1) skeletal muscle, bones, and fluid, the major components of fat-free body mass, are critical to the performance of functional activities, and (2) excessive fat mass (i.e., obesity) is associated with clustering of a number of health risks including coronary artery disease, hypertension, and diabetes mellitus, among others. The relevance of obesity to a child's present and future health cannot be overemphasized. The prevalence of childhood and youth obesity is increasing worldwide. In the United States alone, the prevalence of children classified as overweight increased from 10% in 1988-1994 to 14.4% by 1999-2000 and 16.5% by 2002.[261] Examination of the extent to which children exceed the overweight threshold indicates that the prevalence of overweight children becoming heavier is increasing faster than the prevalence of children becoming overweight.[120] Attainment of appropriate body weight for overweight individuals was an explicit objective of Healthy Children 2000 that has actually moved away from its target.[246,247] Healthy People 2020 has maintained objectives related to the nutritional health of adolescents and youth as one of its focus areas.[248] Large discrepancies continue to exist between current nutrition practices and projected targets.[177]

Laboratory Measurement

The purpose of body composition measurements, whether in the laboratory or in the field, is to obtain a measure of fat-free or lean body mass. Chemical analysis is the only direct method to measure body composition.[128] Because this is expensive and impractical, even laboratory standards of measurement are from indirect assessment. Most standards rely on formulas

the criterion-related validity of the sit and reach test both for hamstring flexibility and for lower, upper, and total back flexibility. A moderate correlation with measurement of straight leg raising using a flexometer was found for hamstring flexibility (0.64). On the other hand, a low correlation with lower back flexibility (0.28) was found with this protocol developed by Macrae and Wright,[152] using tape measure distance changes in bony landmark relationships before and after a standardized spinal movement as the criterion measure (intraclass correlations). Upper back flexibility and total back flexibility were not correlated with the sit and reach scores. The criterion-related validity of the sit and reach test and the modified sit and reach test have been questioned.[47,50,110] Although both tests were found to be related to hamstring flexibility, both hip and low-back flexibility also contribute to the performance of the task.[50] Girls typically show better flexibility than boys at all ages.

Standards by Age

The criterion standard of performance on the FITNESSGRAM Program for the back-saver sit and reach test is 8 inches from the ages of 5 to 17 years in boys. The criterion standard for girls is 9 inches (ages 5-10 years), 10 inches (ages 11-14 years), and 11.5 inches (ages 15-18 years).[169]

Physical Activities

Activities that require a high degree of flexibility include figure skating, gymnastics, jumping (track and field), and judo. Stretching is an important part of any exercise program for general warm-up before vigorous activity and to reduce the potential for injury. Possible physiologic mechanisms for the benefits of stretching include increased blood flow to muscles, increased mechanical efficiency of muscle and tendon, and reduction of viscosity within the muscle.[17] Decreased resistance to extension of connective tissue leads to increased efficiency and power output by muscles. Much of this research is on the adult population, but the same principles are believed to apply to children.[19,132,283]

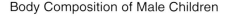

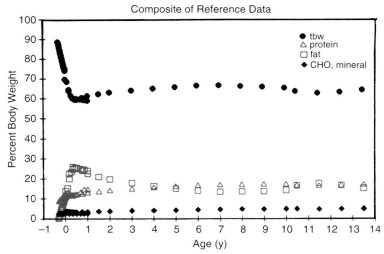

FIG. 6.8 The normal body composition of male children as it changes with age. Derived from data found in descriptions of the reference fetus, infant, male child at 9 years, children from birth to 10 years, and adolescent male. *CHO,* carbohydrate; *tbw,* total body water. (From Spady DW: Normal body composition of infants and children, *98th Ross Laboratories Conference on Pediatric Research,* 98:67-73, 1989. Used with permission of Ross Products Division, Abbott Laboratories, Columbus, OH. ©1989 Ross Products Division, Abbott Laboratories.)

and models of composition, which assume that fat and lean body mass are constant. Because infants and children exhibit variable, not constant, body composition throughout child-hood,[34,111,147,227] numerous problems in determining body composition in children are encountered. Use of adult stan-dards leads to overestimation or underestimation of body fat-ness, depending on the technique.[34] All methods presented have some limitations for use with children, but all have been used. There is no one gold standard for children.

Densitometry. More commonly referred to as underwater or hydrostatic weighing, densitometry determines the density of an individual by dividing actual body weight by the decrease in weight when the person is completely submerged in water. The densities of fat and lean body mass are assumed to be constant and can be calculated for an individual when the density of the whole body is known. Although it is considered the gold standard for measurement of body composition in adults, it has limited applicability to young children because of the requirement for submersion underwater.

Total body water. The measurement of total body water is used as a means of estimating the nonfat portion of the body because neutral fat does not bind water. Stable isotopes of hydrogen or oxygen are administered orally and then measured to determine the amount of dilution in a body fluid.

Bioelectric impedance analysis. This method is based on the principle that impedance to electrical flow varies in proportion to the amount of lean tissue present. A weak electric current is passed through the body, and its impedance is measured. Portable devices are now available that make this method more accessible for clinical and field use.

Dual-energy x-ray absorptiometry. Using dual-energy x-ray absorptiometry (DXA), the body's differential absorption of two low-dose x-rays at different energy levels is measured.

The ratios are used to predict total body mass, lean body mass, and bone mineral density. It has fast become a reference standard for measurement of body composition. Despite its wide use, because of variability of software calculations and instrumentation, the continuous change in body composition of children as they grow suggests that DXA has not yet achieved sufficient reproducibility to be considered the gold standard in pediatric studies.[140,222] Cross-validation between DXA and bioelectric impedance analysis in children and adolescents suggests that the methods are not interchangeable but provide useful and complementary assessments of the percentage of body fat. Less reproducibility is found when younger children are assessed.[78,142]

Developmental Aspects of Body Composition

The influence of rapid growth in fetal and early infancy on fat mass percentage and body composition at 6 months of age has been investigated to gain a better understanding of predictions of obesity later in life. Findings suggest that factors and growth patterns as early as the third trimester of life in utero influence a higher fat mass percentage and body composition at 6 months of age.[11] From prenatal development through adolescence, body composition is constantly changing. Part of this change is caused by chemical maturation as a result of increasing mineral mass and hydration of adipose tissue.[227] Chemical maturation occurs after adolescence, when the constants relating one com-ponent of body composition to another stabilize until the last decades of life.[34,147]

The four major components of body composition are water, protein, mineral, and fat. Reference models describe the body composition of these components in the child at vari-ous ages.[93,94,111,285] A composite of these reference models and changes with growth in males appears in Fig. 6.8.

- Water content: Water content of the body is approximately 89% of body weight at 24 weeks of gestation and drops to 75% at 40 weeks.[227] By 4 months of age, water content stabilizes at approximately 60% to 65% and remains at that level until puberty.
- Protein content: Protein content as a proportion of body weight increases from approximately 13% at birth to 15% to 17% at age 10 years.
- Mineral content: Mineral content of the body rises from 3% at birth to 5% at age 18 years.
- Fat content: Fat is the most variable component of body composition during infancy and childhood. Increases begin in utero when fat content changes from 2.5% at 1 kg of body weight to 12% at term gestation.[227] The proportion of body fat rises from 12% to an average of 25% from birth to 6 months of age. Fat content as a proportion of body weight decreases during early childhood as muscle mass increases. Sex differences are noted early in childhood; girls exhibit a greater percentage of fat content than do boys. At 6 to 8 years of age, the average fat content for boys is 13% to 15%, and for girls it is 16% to 18%.[148] During adolescence, fat content increases in girls so that between the ages of 14 and 16 years the mean percentage of fat content is 21% to 23%.

Differences between the sexes exist in each major component of body composition throughout childhood and are magnified at adolescence. Major changes during adolescence in both sexes consist of a decrease in the percentage of water and an increase in the percentage of osseous minerals.[111,149] These distinct age- and gender-associated variations in body composition have been reaffirmed with the development body fat percentile curves.[135]

Measurement in the Field

Examination of body composition in the field is typically done by measuring skinfold thickness. The validity of this measure is suspect, just as the validity of laboratory methods is in question. The major problem is that skinfold measurement is based on the assumption that body surface measures and body density relationships are stable throughout childhood.[146] Two other threats to the validity of this measurement are (1) that use of skinfold thickness implies that the subcutaneous fat layer reflects the total amount of fat in the body and (2) that selected measurement sites reflect average thickness. These assumptions may not be true.[128] Other researchers have not found large deviations in skinfold thickness distribution across sites.[149,225]

Despite this controversy, measurement of body composition is an important part of almost all health-related fitness tests. Concurrent validity has been demonstrated consistently with moderately high correlations of 0.70 to 0.85 between measurements of skinfolds and densitometry or potassium spectrometry.[103]

Typical sites for measurement of skinfold thickness are the triceps brachii, subscapular area, and calf. Usually these areas are measured in some combination. The method for estimating the percentage of body fatness from skinfold measurement involves estimating density from skinfold measurements and then converting density to the percentage of body fatness. The reader is referred to other sources for more detailed information.[146,147,180] A 3% to 5% error is reported for adults when body fatness is estimated from skinfold measurements.[146]

FITNESSGRAM revised criterion standards for body composition.[269] The design of new standards, like the new standards for aerobic fitness previously described, is based on receiver operating characteristic curves, an established procedure for determining clinical thresholds.[137] This is consistent with the current emphasis on linking fitness to functional health outcomes. The process of developing new standards also included validation of field tests, as well as classification of students with both old and new standards.

Although skinfold measurement and bioelectric impedance remain the preferred methods of assessing body composition, use of body mass index (BMI) has become more prevalent. A major limitation of BMI is the lack of differentiation between fat and lean mass.[197] Classification accuracy using BMI ranges from 87% to 89% when placing subjects into risk categories based on the percentage of body fat.[136]

Standards by Age

The criterion values for ranges of body fatness within the FITNESSGRAM healthy fit zone vary by age and sex.[169] Values for boys range from 8% to 19% at age 5 years to 6% to 22% above age 17 years. Ranges for girls are 9% to 20% at age 5 years to 16% to 30% above age 17 years. Values higher than 25% in boys and 35% in girls are considered to place the child at risk for associated morbidities.

Response to Training

Conditioning and training programs alone may or may not affect body composition. If changes are to occur, the type of exercise must entail high-energy expenditure of intense effort. Appropriate activities include swimming, running, and weight training. Evidence of program effects on body composition is inconclusive in adults. Little information is available on children, but what is available indicates that the percentage of body fatness can be reduced during training for specific sports but rises again when programs are discontinued. Significant changes in body composition with structured physical activity programs are less likely than changes in bone mineral density in both obese and nonobese children.[108,167]

Assessment of Body Composition in Children with Disabilities

Premature infants. Clinicians treat many children with disabilities who were born prematurely. Premature birth has been shown to affect body composition.[228] Compared with a "reference" fetus of similar weight, the infant who was born prematurely has a higher total fat content and a lower total body water content. These differences in composition are probably the result of living outside the womb and being faced with the necessity of increasing body fat for temperature regulation. The implications of this altered body composition during growth have not been studied, nor has body composition been studied in premature infants who experience neonatal complications. There may or may not be effects of premature birth on composition throughout childhood and into adulthood. The previously described pattern of growth changes noted to influence fat mass percentage at 6 months of age may particularly influence children born prematurely, but again this has not been studied.[11]

Cerebral palsy. The importance of body composition measurement has come to the forefront for individuals with CP.[107,179,255] An increased percentage of body fat has been noted.[255] It is postulated that children with CP may have proportionately more subcutaneous fat in the lower extremity skinfold sites because of disuse. More recent work advocates the use of CP-specific equations for clinical assessment.[107,179] Correlations between methods (including DXA) were found to be excellent for determining fat-free body mass and moderate for determining fat mass and percentage of body fat.[143,179] Subject numbers across all studies were relatively small and included children with various types of CP and functional levels. Both type of CP and functional level are likely to be important variables affecting body composition.[179]

Myelomeningocele. The risk of obesity in children with all forms of spina bifida has been a concern of clinicians for decades.[113] Children with myelomeningocele, on average, exhibit decreased stature, reduced fat-free mass, and an increased percentage of body fat compared with typically developing peers.[16,175] The increased total body fat percentage is primarily related to the excess adiposity in the lower extremities. This may reduce the negative health impact.

The percentage of adolescents classified as obese ranged between 29% and 35% as measured by skinfold thickness and BMI.[41,42,252] Nonambulatory individuals had a higher percentage of body fat than those who were ambulatory. However, BMI did not demonstrate a significant correlation with physical activity.

Muscular dystrophy. Regional and whole body composition has been assessed in children with Duchenne muscular dystrophy (DMD) in comparison with typically developing children using DXA.[224] As noted in earlier studies, a decrease in lean tissue mass was observed. Body fat percentage was higher in children with DMD as well. In both cases, regional differences were noted. Trunk and lower leg lean tissue mass differences were not statistically different from those without DMD. Lean tissue mass was found to correlate well with the corresponding regional peak isometric strength for control subjects, but poor correlations were noted for individuals with DMD.[163,224]

CONDITIONING AND TRAINING

Whether physical fitness components can be affected by training programs is an important question, especially to clinicians who are designing programs for children with disabilities. Bar-Or[19] differentiated between the terms *conditioning* and *training*, which are often used interchangeably. *Physical conditioning* is defined as the process by which exercise, repeated over a specified duration, induces morphologic and functional changes in body systems and tissues. The tissues and systems can include skeletal muscles, the myocardium, adipose tissue, bones, tendons, ligaments, the central nervous system, and the endocrine system. Bar-Or considered conditioning to consist of general exercise for overall physical fitness. *Training,* by contrast, is specific exercise designed to promote changes in performance of a particular type of activity. In the context of this chapter, training is discussed in relation to specific fitness components, but overall conditioning is discussed in reference to children with disabilities.

Fitness Components and Training in Children

Many of the physiologic changes that result from training and conditioning in adults also take place during the process of growth and maturation in childhood. These naturally occurring changes make it difficult to study the specific effects of conditioning and training. The primary components of physical fitness of interest to trainers are cardiorespiratory endurance and physical strength.

Cardiorespiratory Endurance

Controversy exists over whether maximal aerobic power or VO_{2max} can be increased by cardiorespiratory training in children.[19,130] Besides the improvements that occur naturally during growth and maturation, other problems in assessing the effects of training include seasonal differences in activity, difficulty in ensuring that a true VO_{2max} has been reached during the testing process, and the already high level of physical activity in young children.

Krahenbuhl and colleagues[130] as early as 1985 concluded that maximal aerobic power can be significantly increased after regular intensive training in children 8 to 14 years of age. A review of the influence of school-based programs continues to demonstrate the positive effects previously noted, especially in adolescence.[68] The long-term impact of such programs is unknown, and only one study reviewed used a direct measurement of VO_{2max}.[46] Endurance exercise appeared more effective than intermittent exercise. General physical education programs alone were not effective in improving VO_{2max}. Effective activities included running, cycle ergometry, and swimming. Increases of 8% to 10% were measured in effective programs. Some studies reported little or no change in VO_{2max} despite improved long-distance running performance after training programs lasting 1 to 9 weeks.[19]

Less controversy exists over whether training improves cardiorespiratory endurance in adolescence. The effects of training in adolescents appear to be similar to those in adults. The functional and morphologic changes of the cardiovascular and pulmonary systems that take place as a result of training are listed in Table 6.8. Training effects usually include increases in myocardial mass, stroke volume, ventilation, and respiratory muscular endurance.

Muscular Strength and Endurance

Muscular strength is a component of fitness that can be affected by training, especially in children at or after puberty. *Resistance strength training (RST)* refers to training for improved muscular strength by repeatedly overcoming heavy resistance. The practice of resistance strength training is problematic in preadolescent

TABLE 6.8 Cardiorespiratory Function Variables and Response to Training in Children

Function Variable	Change With Training
Heart volume	Increase
Blood volume	Increase
Total hemoglobin	Slight increase
Stroke volume (max, submax)	Increase
Cardiac output (max, submax)	Increase, no change, or decrease
Arteriovenous difference (submax)	No change
Blood flow to active muscle	No change
Ventilation/kg body wt (max)	Increase
Ventilation/kg body wt (submax)	Decrease
Respiratory rate (submax)	Decrease
Tidal volume (max)	Increase
Respiratory muscle endurance	Increase

max, maximal exercise; *submax,* submaximal exercise.
Adapted from Bar-Or O: Physiologic responses to exercise in healthy children. In Bar-Or O, editor: *Pediatric sports medicine for the practitioner,* New York, 1983, Springer-Verlag.

children because controversy exists regarding (1) whether children can gain strength and muscle mass, (2) whether gains improve athletic performance, and, particularly, (3) whether children are more susceptible to injury when participating in such training. Despite the controversy, RST has been shown to increase voluntary force production at all ages, may reduce the risk of injury during athletic participation, and may have beneficial effects on important health-related indices such as cardiovascular fitness, body composition, and bone mineral density among others.[32,82,87]

Additionally, it has been reported that the risk of musculoskeletal injury in RST is no greater than for many other sports and recreational activities in which children and adolescents participate.[87] Just as in any exercise program, risks are minimized by appropriate program design, sensible progression, and careful selection of program equipment. Recommendations are available from the American Academy of Pediatrics Council on Sports Medicine and Fitness[3] (http://pediatrics.aappublications.org/cgi/content/abstract/121/4/835), the National Strength and Conditioning Association (http://www.nsca-lift.org/publications/posstatements.shtml)[87] and other sources.[155]

As previously described, the strength increases associated with growth are closely related to increases in muscle mass, including an increase in the numbers of sarcomeres and fibrils per muscle fiber.[153,156] The enhancement of muscular strength caused by growth is estimated to be approximately 1.5 kg per year from age 6 to 14 years. In conjunction with muscular adaptations, neural adaptations associated with improved coordination and motor learning may play a role. For example, the increases in voluntary strength noted with training in prepubescent children have been found to be independent of increased muscle mass or hypertrophy such as that seen in postpubescent children or adults.[31,155,213] Improved motor unit activation and neural adaptations (including more appropriate co-contraction of synergist muscles and inhibition of antagonist muscles, as well as improvements in motor unit recruitment order and firing frequency within the prime movers) are believed to play

a role in producing training effects in both adults and children.[155,171,184,199] It has been suggested that during the early stages of training, neural adaptation predominates in altering performance. Muscular adaptation contributes in the later stages of training[31,213] (Fig. 6.9).

A compelling body of scientific evidence indicates that children and adolescents can significantly increase their strength above and beyond growth and maturation, provided the RST is of sufficient intensity, volume, and duration.[84-87,244] Children show a greater increase in strength than do adults when training-induced strength improvements are expressed as a percentage of change. During maximal voluntary contraction, children can develop the same force per unit of muscle cross-sectional area as adults despite differences in absolute strength and muscle size. Programs that incorporate resistance training with skill-related components of fitness over an 8-week period have also been shown to improve cardiorespiratory endurance.[83] Resistance training programs have been shown to influence tendon properties that may minimize risk of injury.[266]

Principles of Training

The principles of an effective training program include specificity, as well as guidelines for intensity, frequency, and duration of exercise. Rules for children are essentially the same as those for adults.

Specificity

The changes that take place in the body as a result of training are specific to the type of exercise performed and to the tissue involved. Myocardial tissue, for example, is affected by long-distance running but not by RST. The type of contraction (concentric, eccentric, or isometric), the number of repetitions performed, the velocity of muscle contraction, and the particular muscles exercised all influence the results of a strength training program. Different sports develop different components of fitness.

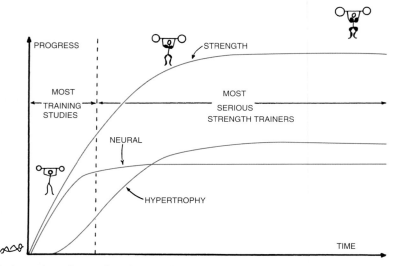

FIG. 6.9 Relative roles of neural and muscular adaptation in strength training. Neural adaptation plays the biggest role in the early phase of training, which can last up to several weeks. Muscular adaptation predominates later and is limited by the extent to which muscles can hypertrophy. (From Sale DG: Strength training in children. In Gisolfi CV, Lamb DR, editors: *Perspectives in exercise science and sports medicine: youth, exercise, and sport*, vol 2, Indianapolis, 1989, Benchmark Press.)

Intensity

Activity at a certain intensity is required to achieve conditioning or training effects. Intensity should be determined as a percentage of the individual's maximum, because the same amount of activity can represent two entirely different levels of intensity for two different individuals. For example, a child with CP who walks at the same velocity as a typically developing child may consume twice as much oxygen, so walking as a form of exercise for the child with CP is more intense. An average 6- to 12-year-old walking at an average velocity consumes about 25% of VO_{2max}; for a child with CP, oxygen uptake can be as high as 75% to 90% of VO_{2max}.[57]

Intensity threshold refers to the intensity of exercise below which few or no training or conditioning effects are observed.[17] The intensity threshold of maximal aerobic power in adults required to produce a training effect is 60% to 70% of VO_{2max}. The threshold for strength is approximately 60% to 65% of maximal voluntary contraction. The principle of overload in strength training is in part related to the intensity threshold of exercise. *Overload* refers to a task that requires considerable voluntary effort to complete. No specific data are available for intensity thresholds in children, but they are thought to be at least equal to those of adults. Whether intensity thresholds for children with various disabilities are the same as those for children without disabilities is also unknown.

Frequency

The optimal frequency of training depends on the type of program, and frequency is interrelated with intensity and duration. Two or three times per week on nonconsecutive days is a general rule of thumb.[3,19,87]

Duration

Any program, whether a therapeutic program or a fitness program, requires a minimum implementation time before benefits are seen. Most effective conditioning programs last at least 6 to 8 weeks. The optimal duration of an exercise session depends on the type of program. In general, the session should consist of a warm-up phase of 10 minutes, an exercise phase above the exercise threshold for 15 to 30 minutes, and a 5- to 7-minute cool-down period. The warm-up phase has been shown to be important for increasing performance of both aerobic and anaerobic tasks in children.[3,19,87] The warm-up period should include (1) activities to raise core body temperature, (2) stretching exercises, and (3) activities specific to the exercise task. The American Academy of Pediatrics[5] recommends that strength training regimens for children include activities to provide strength training for all parts of the body to ensure balanced development.[3]

The duration of the exercise phase in strength training is sometimes associated with the goal of achieving maximal overload. This is usually done in one of two ways: by repeating brief maximal contractions or by repeating submaximal contractions to the point of fatigue.

Progression

A conditioning or training program must be progressive in its demands for continued improvement. The intensity threshold, the duration of exercise sessions, the number of repetitions performed during a session, or the frequency of exercise sessions may need to be increased. All contribute individually and collectively to the progression of the exercise program.

Conditioning in Children with Disabilities
Cerebral Palsy

As children with CP approach and move through adolescence, an important aspect of function is the ability to maintain ambulation. Oxygen uptake during ambulation in preadolescent children with CP (ages 6 to 12 years) is more than twice that of typically developing children walking at the same velocity.[232] If body weight and adiposity increase in adolescence without an increase in muscular strength, maximal aerobic capacity decreases, and the task of walking becomes more and more difficult. Growth in mass is a cubic function (volume), and growth in strength is a function of the square (cross-sectional muscle area). As previously mentioned, muscles increase first in mass, then in strength.[153] During the adolescent growth spurt, mass increases at a faster rate than does strength. For typically developing children, this process occurs without a noticeable deficit or loss of function, but for children with CP, loss of function sometimes occurs because the rate of increase in strength is inadequate to support the rate of increase in muscle mass. A major goal of physical therapy for adolescents with CP is maintenance of the ability to ambulate throughout the growth spurt. If a child has maximal strength and aerobic capacity on entering the growth spurt, function is also likely to be at maximal capacity. Conditioning in a child with CP could play a vital role in the process of maximizing the potential not only of the adolescent but of the preadolescent and school-aged child as well.

The ultimate goal of conditioning programs for children with CP is similar to the goal for all children—to promote life habits and physical health benefits. In addition, children with CP are often faced with deterioration of capacity during adolescence and adulthood. Children who lack the requisite fitness capacity may not be able to achieve their own maximum potential in gross motor activities. Daily physical activity has been found to correlate inversely with the energy cost of walking.[158] Verschuren and colleagues used field tests of physical fitness to assess gross motor capacity and found that performance-related fitness items and functional muscle strength exhibited higher correlations to gross motor capacity than aerobic capacity.[259] This finding supports previous research suggesting that short-term muscle power or anaerobic capacity is a better measure of gross motor capacity than aerobic capacity in children with CP.

The intensity of physical activity is an important aspect of cardiorespiratory fitness in children with CP similar to typically developing children. Children who spend more time in vigorous physically activity (> 3410 counts/min as measured by an accelerometer) have been shown to exhibit greater cardiorespiratory fitness than those who engage in moderate or light physical activity.[210] Current guidelines recommend that children accumulate 60 minutes of moderate to vigorous activity daily. The only guideline for vigorous activity is that "vigorous-intensity activities should be incorporated … at least 3x/week."[281] Children with CP may meet the physical activity guideline with moderate physical activity and may still exhibit low cardiorespiratory fitness. A clinical trial of a high-intensity training program for children with CP and other disabilities is under way.[286] The implications for exercise prescription for programs to increase or improve fitness is clear—to improve outside of cardiorespiratory fitness, vigorous activity must be included. Clinical programs implementing fitness exercise prescription for children with disability including CP are becoming more common with a goal not only to promote wellness but also to reduce/prevent future health risks and prepare for elective surgical procedures.

Along with programs to increase and improve cardiorespiratory fitness, attention is also given to the benefits of strengthening in both children and adolescents with CP. The work of Damiano and colleagues has been instrumental to developing the awareness and benefits of resistance training programs. Functional improvements in both gait and Gross Motor Function Measure scores were noted, as was decreased spasticity.[59-61] A systematic review evaluated 20 studies related to exercise programs for children with cerebral palsy.[260] Of the 20 evaluated, only 5 were randomized controlled trials, which provide the optimal design to test treatment (in this case, training) effects.[69,70,189,245,254] On the basis of the strength training programs reviewed, evidence exists supporting the view that progressive resistance exercise can increase the ability to generate force in children with CP.[260] Functional exercises combining aerobic capacity, anaerobic capacity, and muscle strength have demonstrated a 22% increase in strength in previous studies.[258] Unfortunately, the benefits gained during training often are only partially maintained at follow-up.[254,258] More recent studies of progressive resistive exercise training programs have demonstrated improvements in strength but not improvements in walking ability.[216,217] Context-specific strength training for gait or other functional activities is likely an important factor to consider.

Evidence suggests that neither regular physical education classes nor habitual activities are sufficient to induce conditioning changes in children with CP.[27,74] The program must increase in intensity beyond habitual exercise levels. The duration of the overall program should be longer than 6 weeks; results of 6-week training programs are equivocal.[80] Target heart rate was typically maintained for 15 to 30 minutes in most studies. Longer-duration protocols have been reported.[216] Activities in accordance with the child's ability were used; examples are cycle ergometry, swimming, running, and jogging. Although the importance of increasing vigorous activity in conditioning regimens cannot be overemphasized, decreasing sedentary behavior is imperative as well.[257] Guidelines for activities and field tests are readily available.[14,139,259]

Cystic Fibrosis

Results of studies in children and adolescents with cystic fibrosis (CF) that emphasized aerobic conditioning for 3 to 5 months suggest that VO_{2max}, endurance of respiratory muscles, and pulmonary function all show improvement.[181,284] Jogging, cycling, swimming, weight lifting, and calisthenics of various durations and combinations were used. Statistically significant increases in strength, balance, and submaximal aerobic exercise capacity have also been reported after a 4- to 6-week inpatient rehabilitation program emphasizing sporting-type activities.[106] Based on a growing body of research, it is now well accepted that exercise and exercise training programs are effective therapy methods to improve aerobic exercise capacity and strength as attributes of physical fitness and lung function in individuals with CF.[127,182,215,219]

In addition to the positive effects of conditioning on physical fitness, clinical benefits in the management of the disease have been reported.[20,106] Increased coughing and clearance of mucus may reduce the need for chest therapy to manage secretions.[192]

The effects of exercise on children with CF and other clinical populations must be closely monitored to reduce or avoid potential detrimental effects. Particular concerns in the population with CF are dehydration (especially in high heat) and oxygen desaturation.[192] See Chapter 26 for more information on the management of CF.

Muscular Dystrophy

The role of exercise in DMD continues to be controversial largely due to a lack of evidence. Markert and colleagues summarized potential methods and outcome measures to be used in studying the effects of exercise on the underlying mechanisms.[159]

There appears to be a consensus that low to moderate resistance and aerobic training may be helpful in patients with slowly progressive myopathic disorders.[2,218,235,236,256] A training program instituted for individuals with Becker muscular dystrophy demonstrated improvement in aerobic capacity without rendering patients susceptible to structural or mechanical damage to muscle.[235] Assisted bicycle training was also found to be feasible and safe for boys in one of the first randomized controlled trials in this population.[119] The role of cardiopulmonary exercise testing may offer the potential to detect moderate to severe exercise limitations in participants with only mild functional and motor impairments.[22] Clearly, more work needs to be done in this area.

Children With Obesity

Although addressed elsewhere in this chapter, it is important to highlight known evidence regarding the influence of training and conditioning programs on children with obesity. Studies suggest that resistive training programs are safe and result in positive and significant changes in body composition, strength, and power.[26,165,220,226,265] Most studies found that an 8-week program was sufficient to achieve significant effects. Most resistive exercise programs or aerobic exercise programs did not demonstrate significant changes in peak oxygen uptake.[26,265] As in other areas, better-controlled randomized trials are needed to substantiate evidence.

SUMMARY

This chapter was designed to provide information on physical fitness and conditioning in children with typical development for promoting health and preventing disease. The components of fitness, how they are tested, and how they contribute to health were reviewed. An understanding of physical fitness, physical activity, and conditioning is valuable for appreciating the impact of disabling conditions on these variables, but health-related physical fitness is important for reducing future health risks in every child, regardless of the presence or absence of disability. Preadolescent fitness may be especially important to children with disabilities because of the effects particular disabilities may have on children as they enter puberty and adulthood. The design of exercise programs (their intensity, frequency, and duration) should encompass the minimal requirements for physical fitness, as well as incorporate therapeutic goals. Exercise programs should be designed so that the energy requirements for accomplishing day-to-day activities through the growth period are met. Meeting this goal is likely to require additional exercise beyond current therapy or physical education. One of our goals as pediatric physical therapists should be to ensure, to whatever extent possible, that our clients end their childhood at a fitness level suitable to a healthy adulthood. Research is needed to document the extent to which this goal can be met for specific populations and levels of disability.

Much research remains to be done in those without disabilities as well. Reliability and validity studies must continue on criterion-based measures now being used to determine minimal fitness levels. Research must establish reliable, valid, and universal criteria, both in the laboratory and in the field. Continued identification of the relationship between childhood physical activity and fitness and health in adulthood is vital to our overall understanding of health-related fitness.

Research to benefit those with disabilities has barely begun. With an inadequate base of research in children without disability, developing standards of fitness for those with specific disabilities begins at a disadvantage. A question that remains to be answered is whether the fitness performance criteria for children without disabilities are valid for children with disabilities or special needs. Experience with development of testing and measurement tools for other purposes would suggest that they are not. Are children with disabilities such as CP more fit because they expend in walking an amount of energy equivalent to that of a nondisabled person walking up and down stairs all day long? Are the thresholds and target zones for fitness improvement the same for children with a variety of disabilities as for children with typical development? How are conditioning and training programs best designed for children with disabilities? Do conditioning programs initiated before the onset of puberty help maintain fitness during and after puberty? What physiologic and behavioral factors limit a child's capacity to improve fitness variables or to exercise? How much exercise is detrimental? How do presurgical strengthening programs affect the recovery of strength after surgery? Questions such as these represent only the beginning of our quest for understanding. The journey has just begun.

REFERENCES

1. Adams FH: Factors affecting the working capacity of children and adolescents. In Rarick GL, editor: *Physical activity: human growth and development*, New York, 1973, Academic Press, pp 89–90.
2. Ansved T: Muscular dystrophies: the influence of physical conditioning on disease evolution, *Curr Opin Clin Nutr Metab Care* 6:455–459, 2003.
3. American Academy of Pediatrics Council on Sports Medicine and Fitness: Strength training by children and adolescents: policy statement, *Pediatrics* 121:835–840, 2008.
4. American Association for Health, Physical Education, and Recreation: *AAHPER youth fitness test manual*, Washington, DC, 1958, American Association for Health, Physical Education, and Recreation.
5. American Physical Therapy Association: *Guide to physical therapist practice 3.0*. Alexandria, VA, American Physical Therapy Association. Available at: http://guidetoptpractice.apta.org. Accessed November 14, 2015.
6. Andreacci JL, et al.: Comparison of maximal oxygen consumption between obese black and white adolescents, *Pediatr Res* 58:478–482, 2005.
7. Armstrong N: Aerobic fitness and physical activity in children, *Pediatr Exerc Sci* 25:548–560, 2013.
8. Armstrong N, Welsman JR, et al.: Development of aerobic fitness during childhood and adolescence, *Pediatr Exerc Sci* 12:128–149, 2000.
9. Astrand PO: *Experimental studies of physical working capacity in relation to sex and age*, Copenhagen, 1952, Ejnar Munksgaard.
10. Aucouturier J, et al.: Determination of the maximal fat oxidation point in obese children and adolescents: validity of methods to assess maximal aerobic power, *Eur J Appl Physiol* 105:325–331, 2009.
11. Ay L, et al.: Fetal and postnatal growth and body composition at 6 months of age, *J Clin Endocrinol Metab* 94:2023–2030, 2009.
12. Bai Y, et al.: Prevalence of youth fitness in the United States: baseline results from the NFL PLAY 60 FITNESSGRAM partnership project, *J Pediatr* 167:662–668, 2015.
13. Balemans AC, et al.: Systematic review of the clinimetric properties of laboratory- and field-based aerobic and anaerobic fitness measures in children with cerebral palsy, *Arch Phys Med Rehabil* 94:287–301, 2013.
14. Balemans AC, et al.: Maximal aerobic and anaerobic exercise responses in children with cerebral palsy, *Med Sci Sports Exerc* 45:561–568, 2013.
15. Baltzopoulos V, Kellis E: Isokinetic strength during childhood and adolescence. In Van Praagh E, editor: *Pediatric anaerobic performance*, Champaign, IL, 1998, Human Kinetics, pp 225–240.
16. Bandini LG, et al.: Body composition and energy expenditure in adolescents with cerebral palsy or myelodysplasia, *Pediatr Res* 29:70–77, 1991.
17. Bar-Or O: Appendix II: procedures for exercise testing in children. In Bar-Or O, editor: *Pediatric sports medicine for the practitioner*, New York, 1983, Springer-Verlag, pp 315–341.
18. Bar-Or O: Neuromuscular diseases. In Bar-Or O, editor: *Pediatric sports medicine for the practitioner*, New York, 1983, Springer-Verlag, pp 227–249.
19. Bar-Or O: Physiologic responses to exercise in healthy children. In Bar-Or O, editor: *Pediatric sports medicine for the practitioner*, New York, 1983, Springer-Verlag, pp 1–65.
20. Bar-Or O: Physical conditioning in children with cardiorespiratory disease, *Exerc Sport Sci Rev* 13:305–334, 1985.
21. Bar-Or O: Pathophysiological factors which limit the exercise capacity of the sick child, *Med Sci Sports Exerc* 18:276–282, 1986.
22. Bartels B, et al.: Cardiopulmonary exercise testing in children and adolescents with dystrophinopathies: a pilot study, *Pediatr Phys Ther* 27:227–234, 2015.
23. Baynard T, et al.: Age-related changes in aerobic capacity in individuals with mental retardation: a 20-year review, *Med Sci Sports Exerc* 40:1984–1989, 2008.
24. Beets MW, Pitetti KH: Criterion-referenced reliability and equivalency between the PACER and the 1-mile run/walk for high school students, *J Phys Activ Health* 3(Suppl 2):S21–S33, 2006.
25. Behringer M, et al.: Effects of strength training on motor performance skills in children and adolescents: a meta-analysis, *Pediatr Exerc Sci* 23:186–206, 2011.
26. Benson AC, et al.: The effect of high-intensity progressive resistance training on adiposity in children: a randomized controlled trial, *Int J Obes* 32:1016–1027, 2008.
27. Berg K: Effect of physical training of school children with cerebral palsy, *Acta Paediatr Scand Suppl* 204:27–33, 1970.
28. Bianco A, et al.: A systematic review to determine reliability and usefulness of the field-based test batteries for the assessment of physical fitness in adolescents: the ASSO project, *Int J Occup Med Environ Health* 28:445–478, 2015.
29. Blais S, et al.: A systematic review of reference values in pediatric cardiopulmonary exercise testing, *Pediatr Cardiol* 36:1553–1564, 2015.
30. Blimkie CJR: Age and sex associated variation in strength during childhood: anthropometric, morphologic, neurologic, biomechanical, endocrinologic, genetic, and physical activity correlates. In Gisolfi CV, Lamb DR, editors: *Perspectives in exercise science and sports medicine: youth, exercise, and sport*, vol. 2. Indianapolis, IN, 1989, Benchmark Press, pp 99–163.
31. Blimkie CJR, et al.: Effects of 10 weeks of resistance training on strength development in prepubertal boys. In Osteid S, Carlsen KH, editors: *Children and exercise XIII*, Champaign, IL, 1989, Human Kinetics, pp 183–197.
32. Blimkie CJR, Sale DG: Strength development and trainability during childhood. In Van Praagh E, editor: *Pediatric anaerobic performance*, Champaign, IL, 1998, Human Kinetics, pp 193–224.
33. Boiarskaia EA, et al.: Cross-validation of an equating method linking aerobic FITNESSGRAM® field tests, *Am J Prev Med* 41:S124–S130, 2011.
34. Boileau RA, et al.: Problems associated with determining body composition in maturing youngsters. In Brown EW, Branta CF, editors: *Competitive sports for children and youth: an overview of research and issues*, Champaign, IL, 1988, Human Kinetics, pp 3–16.
35. Boone DC, et al.: Reliability of goniometric measurements, *Phys Ther* 58:1355–1360, 1978.
36. Boreham C, Riddoch C: The physical activity, fitness and health of children, *J Sports Sci* 19:915–929, 2001.
37. Borrud L, et al.: National Health and Nutrition Examination Survey: national youth fitness survey plan, operations, and analysis, *Vital Health Stat* 2(163):1–24, 2014.
38. Bovet P, et al.: Strong inverse association between physical fitness and overweight in adolescents: a large school-based survey, *Int J Behav Nutr Phys Act* 4:24, 2007.
39. Braden DS, Strong WB: Cardiovascular responses to exercise in childhood, *Am J Dis Child* 144:1255–1260, 1990.

40. Brooks GA, et al.: *Exercise physiology: human bioenergetics and its applications*, ed 4, New York, 2004, McGraw-Hill.

41. Buffart LM, et al.: Triad of physical activity, aerobic fitness, and obesity in adolescents and young adults in myelomeningocele, *J Rehabil Med* 40:70–75, 2008.

42. Buffart LM, et al.: Health-related fitness of adolescents and young adults with myelomeningocele, *Eur J Appl Physiol* 103:181–188, 2008.

43. Burns RD, et al.: Development of an aerobic capacity prediction model from one-mile run/walk performance in adolescents aged 13-16 years, *J Sports Sci* 34:18–26, 2016.

44. Butterfield SA, Lehnhrad RA: Aerobic performance by children in grades 4 to 8: a repeated-measures study, *Percept Mot Skills* 107:775–790, 2008.

45. Caballero B: The global epidemic of obesity: an overview, *Epidemiol Rev* 29:1–5, 2007.

46. Carrel AL, et al.: Improvement in fitness, body composition, and insulin sensitivity in overweight children in a school-based exercise program: a randomized controlled study, *Arch Pediatr Adolesc Med* 159:963–968, 2005.

47. Castro-Pinero J, et al.: Criterion-related validity of the sit-and-reach test and the modified sit-and-reach test for estimating hamstring flexibility in children and adolescents aged 6-17 years, *Inter J Sports Med* 30:658–662, 2009.

48. Castro-Pinero J, et al.: Criterion-related validity of the one-mile run/walk test in children aged 8-17 years, *J Sports Sci* 27:405–413, 2009.

49. Cerebral Palsy International Sports and Recreation Association: *CPISRA handbook*, ed 5, Netherlands, 1993, Heteren. Author.

50. Chillon P, et al.: Hip flexibility is the main determinant of the back-saver sit-and-reach test in adolescents, *J Sports Sci* 28:641–648, 2010.

51. Clarke HH: Posture, *Phys Fitness Res Digest* 9:1–23, 1979.

52. Cooper DM, et al.: Growth-related changes in oxygen uptake and heart rate during progressive exercise in children, *Pediatr Res* 18:845–851, 1984.

53. Cooper Institute: *FG10: addendum to the FITNESSGRAM® & ACTIVITYGRAM test administration manual*, Dallas, TX, 2013, Cooper Institute.

54. Cunningham DA, et al.: Reliability and reproducibility of maximal oxygen uptake in children, *Med Sci Sports* 9:104–108, 1977.

55. Cureton KJ, et al.: A generalized equation for prediction of VO_{2peak} from 1-mile run/walk performance, *Med Sci Sports Exerc* 27:445–451, 1995.

56. Cureton KJ, Warren GL: Criterion-referenced standards for youth health-related fitness tests: a tutorial, *Res Q Exerc Sport* 61:7–19, 1990.

57. Dallmeijer AJ, Brehm MA: Physical strain of comfortable walking in children with mild cerebral palsy, *Disabil Rehabil* 33:1351–1357, 2011.

58. Daltroy LH, et al.: The POSNA pediatric musculoskeletal functional health questionnaire: report on reliability, validity, and sensitivity to change, *J Pediatr Orthop* 18:561–571, 1998.

59. Damiano DL, Abel MF: Functional outcomes of strength training in spastic cerebral palsy, *Arch Phys Med Rehabil* 79:119–125, 1998.

60. Damiano DL, et al.: Effects of quadriceps muscle strengthening on crouch gait in children with spastic diplegia, *Phys Ther* 75:668–671, 1995.

61. Damiano DL, et al.: Muscle response to heavy resistance exercise in children with spastic cerebral palsy, *Dev Med Child Neurol* 37:731–739, 1995.

62. DeFina LF, et al.: Physical activity versus cardiorespiratory fitness: two (partly) distinct components of cardiovascular health, *Progress Cardiovasc Dis* 57:324–329, 2015.

63. De Ste Croix M: Advances in paediatric strength assessment: changing our perspective on strength development, *J Sports Sci Medicine* 6:292–304, 2007.

64. De Ste Croix M, et al.: Functional eccentric-concentric ratio of knee extensors and flexors in pre-puberal children, teenagers and adult males and females, *Inter J Sports Med* 28:768–772, 2007.

65. Dell RB: Comparison of densitometric methods applicable to infants and small children for studying body composition, *Ross Laboratories Conference on Pediatric Research* 98:22–30, 1989.

66. Dencker M, et al.: Maximal oxygen uptake versus maximal power output in children, *J Sports Sci* 26:1397–1402, 2008.

67. de Sa Pinto AL, et al.: Musculoskeletal findings in obese children, *J Paediatr Child Health* 42:341–344, 2006.

68. Dobbins M, et al.: School-based physical activity programs for promoting physical activity and fitness in children and adolescents aged 6-18 (Review), *Cochrane Database Syst Rev* 21:CD007651, 2009.

69. Dodd KJ, et al.: A randomized clinical trial of strength in young people with cerebral palsy, *Dev Med Child Neurol* 45:652–657, 2003.

70. Dodd KJ, et al.: Strength training can have unexpected effects on the self-concept of children with cerebral palsy, *Pediatr Phys Ther* 16:99–105, 2004.

71. dos Santos Alves VL, et al.: Impact of a physical rehabilitation program on respiratory function of adolescents with adolescent idiopathic scoliosis, *Chest* 130:500–505, 2006.

72. dos Santos Cunha G, et al.: Physiological adaptations to resistance training in prepubertal boys, *Res Q Exerc Sport* 86:172–181, 2015.

73. Dotan R, et al.: Child-adult differences in muscle activation: a review, *Pediatr Exerc Sci* 24:2–21, 2012.

74. Dresen MHW: Physical and psychological effects of training on handicapped children. In Binkhorst RA, et al, editors: *Children and exercise XI*, Champaign, IL, 1985, Human Kinetics, pp 203–209.

75. Drews J, et al.: Range of motion of the joints of the lower extremities of newborns, *Phys Occup Ther Pediatr* 4:49–62, 1984.

76. Dumith SC, et al.: Physical fitness measures among children and adolescents: are they all necessary? *J Sports Med Phys Fitness* 52:181–189, 2012.

77. Dwyer GM, et al.: The challenge of understanding and assessing physical activity in preschool-age children: thinking beyond the framework of intensity, duration, and frequency of activity, *J Sci Med Sport* 12:534–536, 2009.

78. Eisenmann JC, et al.: Assessing body composition among 3- to 8- year old children: anthropometry, BIA, and DXA, *Obes Res* 12:1633–1640, 2004.

79. Eisenmann JC, et al.: Relationship between adolescent fitness and fatness and cardiovascular disease risk factors in adulthood: the Aerobics Center Longitudinal Study (ACLS), *Am Heart J* 149:46–53, 2005.

80. Ekblom B, Lundberg A: Effect of training on adolescents with severe motor handicaps, *Acta Paediatr Scand* 57:17–23, 1968.

81. Ekstrand J, et al.: Lower extremity goniometric measurements: a study to determine their reliability, *Arch Phys Med Rehabil* 63:171–175, 1982.

82. Faigenbaum A: Strength training for children and adolescents, *Clin J Sports Med* 19:593–619, 2000.

83. Faigenbaum A, et al.: Benefits of strength and skill-based training during primary school physical education, *J Strength Cond Res* 29:1255–1262, 2015.

84. Faigenbaum A, et al.: The effects of different resistance training protocols on upper body strength and endurance development in children, *J Strength Cond Res* 15:459–465, 2001.

85. Faigenbaum A, et al.: Comparison of 1 day and 2 days per week of resistance training in children, *Res Q Exerc Sport* 73:416–424, 2002.

86. Faigenbaum A, et al.: Early muscular fitness adaptations in children in response to two different strength training regimens, *Pediatr Exerc Sci* 17:2337–2348, 2005.

87. Faigenbaum AD, et al.: Youth resistance training: updated position statement paper from the National Strength and Conditioning Association, *J Strength Cond Res* 23(Suppl 5):S60–S79, 2009.

88. Faust MS: Somatic development of adolescent girls, *Soc Res Child Dev* 42:1–90, 1977.

89. FitzGerald SJ, et al.: Muscular fitness and all cause mortality: prospective observations, *J Phys Activ Health* 1:7–18, 2004.

90. Florini JR: Hormonal control of muscle growth, *Muscle Nerve* 10:577–598, 1987.

91. Fogelholm M, et al.: Physical fitness in adolescents with normal weight and overweight, *Scand J Med Sci Sports* 18:162–170, 2008.

92. Foley S, et al.: Measures of childhood fitness and body mass index are associated with bone mass in adulthood: a 20-year prospective study, *J Bone Miner Res* 23:994–1001, 2008.

93. Fomon SJ: Body composition of the male reference infant during the first year of life, *Pediatrics* 40:863–867, 1967.

94. Fomon SJ, et al.: Body composition of reference children from birth to age 10 years, *Am J Clin Nutr* 35:1169–1173, 1982.

95. Fowler EG, et al.: Promotion of physical fitness and prevention of secondary conditions for children with cerebral palsy: section on Pediatrics Research Summit Proceedings, *Phys Ther* 87:1495–1507, 2007.

96. Francis K, Feinstein R: A simple height-specific and rate-specific step test for children, *South Med J* 84:169–174, 1991.

97. Freedson PS, et al.: Status of field-based fitness testing in children and youth, *Prev Med* 31:S77–S85, 2000.

98. Fry AC, et al.: Muscular strength and power in 3- to 7-year-old children, *Pediatr Exerc Sci* 27:345–354, 2015.

99. Gage JR: *Gait analysis in cerebral palsy*, London, 1991, MacKeith Press.

100. Gage JR, Stout JL: Gait analysis: kinematics, kinetics, electromyography, oxygen consumption, and pedobarography. In Gage JR, et al., editors: *The identification and treatment of gait problems in cerebral palsy*, London, 2009, MacKeith Press, pp 260–284.

101. Gillett JG, et al.: FAST CP: protocol of a randomized controlled trial of the efficacy of a 12-week combined functional anaerobic and strength training programme on muscle properties and mechanical gait deficiencies in adolescents and young adults with spastic-type cerebral palsy, *BMJ Open* 5:e008059, 2015.

102. Godfrey S: Growth and development of the cardiopulmonary response to exercise. In Davis JA, Dobbing J, editors: *Scientific foundations in paediatrics*, London, 1981, William Heinemann Medical Books, pp 450–460.

103. Going S: Physical best: body composition in the assessment of youth fitness, *J Phys Educ Recreation Dance* 59:32–36, 1988.

104. Going SB, et al.: Body composition assessment. In Plowman SA, Meredith MD, editors: *FITNESSGRAM®/Activitygram reference guide (pp. Internet resource)*, Dallas, TX, 2013, Cooper Institute.

105. Granacher U, et al.: Effects and mechanisms of strength training in children, *Inter J Sports Med* 35:357–364, 2011.

106. Gruber W, et al.: Health-related fitness and trainability in children with cystic fibrosis, *Pediatr Pulmonol* 43:953–964, 2008.

107. Gurka MJ, et al.: Assessment and correction of skinfold equations in estimating body fat in children with cerebral palsy, *Dev Med Child Neurol* 52:e35–e41, 2010.

108. Gutin B, et al.: Effects of exercise on cardiovascular fitness, total body composition, and visceral adiposity of obese adolescents, *Am J Clin Nutr* 75:818–826, 2002.

109. Haley SM, et al.: Spinal mobility in young children: a normative study, *Phys Ther* 66:1697–1703, 1986.

110. Hartman JG, Looney M: Norm-referenced and criterion-referenced reliability and validity of the back-saver sit-and-reach, *Meas Phys Educ Exerc Sci* 7:71–87, 2003.

111. Haschke F: Body composition during adolescence, *Ross Laboratories Conference on Pediatric Research* 98:76–82, 1989.

112. Haskell WL, et al.: Physical activity: health outcomes and importance for public health policy, *Prev Med* 49:280–282, 2009.

113. Hayes-Allen MC, Tring FC: Obesity: another hazard for spina bifida children, *Br J Prevent Soc Med* 27:192–196, 1973.

114. Hopkins ND, et al.: Relationships between measures of physical fitness, physical activity, body composition and vascular function in children, *Atherosclerosis* 204:244–249, 2009.

115. Huang YC, Malina RM: BMI and health-related fitness in Taiwanese youth 9-18 years, *Med Sci Sports Exerc* 39:701–708, 2007.

116. Jackson AS: The evolution and validity of health-related fitness, *Quest* 58:160–175, 2006.

117. Jackson AS, Coleman AE: Validation of distance run tests for elementary school children, *Res Q* 47:86–94, 1976.

118. Jackson AW, Baker AA: The relationship of the sit and reach test to criterion measures of hamstring and back flexibility in young females, *Res Q Exerc Sport* 57:183–186, 1986.

119. Jansen M, et al.: Assisted bicycle training delays functional deterioration in boys with Duchenne muscular dystrophy: the randomized controlled trial "No use is disuse," *Neurorehabil Neural Repair* 27:816–827, 2004.

120. Jolliffe D: Extent of overweight among US children and adolescents from 1971-2000, *Int J Obes* 28:4–9, 2004.

121. Jurca R, et al.: Association of muscular strength with incidence of metabolic syndrome in men, *Med Sci Sports Exerc* 37:1845–1855, 2005.

122. Keating XD, Silverman S: Teachers' use of fitness tests in school-based physical education programs, *Meas Phys Educ Exerc Sci* 8:145–165, 2004.

123. Kelly RK, et al.: Factors affecting blood pressure from childhood to adulthood: the Childhood Determinants of Adult Health Study, *J Pediatr* 167:1422–1428.e2, 2015.

124. Kendall HO, Kendall FP: *Posture and pain*, Baltimore, 1952, Williams & Wilkins, p 104.

125. Kilgour G, et al.: Intrarater reliability of lower limb sagittal range-of-motion measures in children with spastic diplegia, *Dev Med Child Neurol* 45:391–399, 2003.

126. Kim J, et al.: Relationship of physical fitness to prevalence and incidence of overweight among school children, *Obes Res* 13:1246–1254, 2005.

127. Klijn PH, et al.: Effects of anaerobic training in children with cystic fibrosis, *Chest* 125:1299–1305, 2004.

128. Klish WJ: The "gold standard," *Ross Laboratories Conference on Pediatric Research* 98:4–7, 1989.

129. Koch G: Muscle blood flow after ischemic work during bicycle ergometer work in boys aged 12, *Acta Paediatr Belg* 28(Suppl):29–39, 1974.

130. Krahenbuhl GS: Developmental aspects of maximal aerobic power in children, *Exerc Sport Sci Rev* 13:503–538, 1985.

131. Krul M, et al.: Musculoskeletal problems in obese and overweight children, *Ann Fam Med* 7:352–356, 2009.

132. Kuland DN, Tottossy M: Warm-up strength and power, *Clin Sports Med* 4:137–158, 1985.

133. Kvaavik E, et al.: Physical fitness and physical activity at age 13 as predictors of cardiovascular disease risk factors at ages 15, 25, 33, and 40 years: extended follow-up of the Oslo Youth Study, *Pediatrics* 123:e80–e86, 2009.

134. Landin S, et al.: Muscle metabolism during exercise in hemiparetic patients, *Clin Sci Mol Med* 53:257–269, 1977.

135. Laurson KR, et al.: Body fat percentile curves for U.S. children and adolescents, *Am J Prev Med* 41:S87–S92, 2011.

136. Laurson KR, et al.: Body mass index standards based on agreement with health-related body fat, *Am J Prev Med* 41:S100–S105, 2011.

137. Laurson KR, et al.: Development of youth percent body fat standards using receiver operating characteristic curves, *Am J Prev Med* 41:S93–S99, 2011.

138. Lavallee AV, et al.: Developmental biomechanics of neck musculature, *J Biomech* 46:527–534, 2013.

139. Lennon N, et al.: The clinimetric properties of aerobic and anaerobic fitness measures in adults with cerebral palsy: a systematic review of the literature, *Res Dev Disabil* 45-46:316–328, 2015.

140. Leonard CM, et al.: Reproducibility of DXA measurements of bone mineral density and body composition in children, *Pediatr Radiol* 39:148–154, 2009.

141. Lerario A, et al.: Quantitative muscle strength assessment in Duchenne muscular dystrophy: longitudinal study and correlation with functional measures, *BMC Neurol* 12:91, 2012.

142. Lim JS, et al.: Cross calibration of multi-frequency bioelectric impedance analysis with eight-point electrodes and dual-energy x-ray absorptiometry for assessment of body composition in healthy children ages 6-18 years, *Pediatr Int* 51:263–268, 2009.

143. Liu LF, et al.: Determination of body composition in children with cerebral palsy: bioelectrical impedance analysis and anthropometry vs. dual-energy x-ray absorptiometry, *J Ame Dietetics Assoc* 105:794–797, 2005.

144. Lloyd RS, et al.: Position statement on youth resistance training: the 2014 International consensus, *Br J Sports Med* 48:498–505, 2014.

145. Lobstein T, et al.: editors: Obesity in children and young people: a crisis in public health: report to the World Health Organization, *Obesity Rev* 5(Suppl 1):4–104, 2004.

146. Lohman TG: Measurement of body composition in children, *J Phys Educ Recreation Dance* 53:67–70, 1982.

147. Lohman TG: Applicability of body composition techniques and constants for children and youth, *Exerc Sport Sci Rev* 14:325–357, 1986.

148. Lohman TG: The use of skinfold to estimate body fatness on children and youth, *J Phys Educ Recreation Dance* 58:98–102, 1987.

149. Lohman TG, et al.: Bone mineral measurements and their relation to body density in children, youth, and adults, *Hum Biol* 56:667–679, 1984.

150. Lundberg A, et al.: The effect of physical training on school children with cerebral palsy, *Acta Paediatr Scand* 56:182–188, 1967.

151. Lundberg A, Pernow B: The effect of physical training on oxygen utilization and lactate formation in the exercising muscle of adolescents with motor handicaps, *Scand J Clin Lab Invest* 26:89–96, 1970.

152. Macrae I, Wright V: Measurement of back movement, *Ann Rheum Dis* 52:584–589, 1969.

153. Malina RM: Growth of muscle and muscle mass. In Falkner F, Tanner JM, editors: *Human growth: a comprehensive treatise: postnatal growth*, vol. 2. New York, 1986, Plenum Press, pp 77–99.

154. Malina RM: Physical activity and fitness: pathways from childhood to adulthood, *Am J Hum Biol* 13:162–172, 2001.

155. Malina RM: Weight training in youth-growth, maturation, and safety: an evidenced base review, *Clin J Sports Med* 16:478–487, 2006.

156. Malina RM, et al.: *Growth, maturation, and physical activity*, Champaign, IL, 2004, Human Kinetics.

157. Malina RM, Little BB: Physical activity: the present in the context of the past, *Am J Hum Biol* 20:373–391, 2008.

158. Maltais DB, et al.: Physical activity level is associated with the O_2 cost of walking in cerebral palsy, *Med Sci Sports Exerc* 37:347–353, 2005.

159. Markert CD, et al.: Exercise and Duchenne muscular dystrophy: toward evidence-based exercise prescription, *Muscle Nerve* 43:464–478, 2011.

160. Mastrangelo MA, et al.: Cardiovascular fitness in obese versus nonobese 8-11-year-old boys and girls, *Res Q Exerc Sport* 79:356–362, 2008.

161. Maughan RJ, et al.: Strength and cross-sectional area of human skeletal muscle, *J Physiol* 338:37–49, 1983.

162. Mayhew JE, et al.: Reliable surrogate outcome measures in multicenter clinical trials of Duchenne muscular dystrophy, *Muscle Nerve* 35:36–42, 2007.

163. McDonald CM, et al.: Body composition and water compartment measurements in boys with Duchenne muscular dystrophy, *Am J Phys Med Rehabil* 84:483–491, 2005.

164. McDowell BC, et al.: The variability of goniometric measures in ambulatory children with spastic cerebral palsy, *Gait Posture* 12:114–121, 2000.

165. McGuigan MR, et al.: Eight weeks of resistance training can significantly alter body composition in children who are overweight or obese, *J Strength Cond Res* 23:80–85, 2009.

166. McKay H, Smith E: Winning the battle against childhood physical inactivity: the key to bone strength? *J Bone Miner Res* 23:980–985, 2008.

167. McWhannell N, et al.: The effect of a 9-week physical activity programme on bone and body composition of children aged 10-11 years: an exploratory trial, *Inter J Sports Med* 29:941–947, 2008.

168. Merati G, et al.: Trunk muscular strength in pre-pubertal children with and without back pain, *Pediatr Rehabil* 7:97–103, 2004.

169. Meredith M, Welk GJ, editors: *FITNESSGRAM®-ACTIVITYGRAM test administration manual*, updated ed 4, developed by Cooper Institute (Dallas, TX), Champaign, IL, 2010, Human Kinetics.

170. Moran HM, et al.: Spinal mobility of the adolescent, *Rheumatol Rehabil* 18:181–185, 1979.

171. Moritani T, DeVries HA: Neural factors versus hypertrophy in the time course of muscle strength gain, *Am J Phys Med* 58:115–130, 1979.

172. FITNESSGRAM®: development of criterion-referenced standards for aerobic capacity and body composition, Morrow JR, et al.: *Am J Prev Med* 41:S63–S142, 2001.

173. Morrow Jr JR, et al.: Prevalence and correlates of physical fitness testing in U.S. schools-2000, *Res Q Exerc Sport* 79:141–148, 2008.

174. Morrow Jr JR, et al.: 1958-2008: 50 years of youth fitness testing in the United States, *Res Q Exerc Sport* 80:1–11, 2009.

175. Mueske NM, et al.: Fat distribution in children and adolescents with myelomeningocele, *Dev Med Child Neurol* 57:273–278, 2015.

176. Myers J, et al.: Exercise capacity and mortality among men referred for exercise testing, *N Engl J Med* 346:793–801, 2002.

177. Neumark-Sztainer D, et al.: Overweight status and eating patterns among adolescents: where do youths stand in comparison with the Healthy People 2010 objectives? *Am J Public Health* 92:844–851, 2002.

178. Norkin CC, White DJ: *Measurement of joint motion: a guide to goniometry*, ed 3, Philadelphia, 2003, FA Davis.

179. Oeffinger DJ, et al.: Accuracy of skinfold and bioelectrical impedance assessments of body fat percentage in ambulatory individuals with cerebral palsy, *Dev Med Child Neurol* 56:475–481, 2014.

180. Ogden CL, et al.: Prevalence of childhood and adult obesity in the United States, 2011-2012, *JAMA* 311:806–814, 2014.

181. Orenstein DM, et al.: Exercise conditioning and cardiopulmonary physical fitness in cystic fibrosis: the effects of a three-month supervised running program, *Chest* 80:392–398, 1981.

182. Orenstein DM, Higgins LW: Update on the role of exercise in cystic fibrosis, *Curr Opin Pulmonol Med* 11:519–523, 2005.

183. Ounpuu S: Patterns of gait pathology. In Gage JR, editor: *The treatment of gait problems in cerebral palsy*, London, 2004, MacKeith Press, pp 217–237.

184. Ozmun JC, et al.: Neuromuscular adaptations following prepubescent strength training, *Med Sci Sports Exerc* 26:510–514, 1994.

185. Pate R, et al.: Committee on Fitness Measures and Health Outcome in Youth: *fitness measures and heath outcome in youth*, Institute of Medicine, Washington, DC, 2012, The National Academies Press.

186. Pate RR: A new definition of youth fitness, *Physician Sports Med* 11:77–83, 1983.

187. Pate RR, Shephard RJ: Characteristics of physical fitness in youth. In Gisolfi CV, Lamb DR, editors: *Perspectives in exercise science and sports medicine: youth, exercise, and sport*, vol. 2. Indianapolis, IN, 1989, Benchmark Press, pp 1–45.

188. Paterson DH, Cunningham DA: Maximal oxygen uptake in children: comparison of treadmill protocols at various speeds, *Can J Appl Sport Sci* 3:188, 1978.

189. Patikas M, et al: Effects of a post-operative strength-training program on the walking ability of children with cerebral palsy: a randomized controlled trial, *Arch Phys Med Rehabil* 87:619–6266.

190. Patterson P, et al.: Psychometric properties of child-and-teacher-reported curl-up scores in children ages 10-12 years, *Res Q Exerc Sport* 72:117–124, 2001.

191. Phelps E, et al.: Normal ranges of hip motion of infants between 9 and 24 months of age, *Dev Med Child Neurol* 27:785–792, 1985.

192. Philpott JF, et al.: Physical activity recommendations for children with severe chronic health conditions: juvenile idiopathic arthritis, hemophilia, asthma, and cystic fibrosis, *Clin J Sports Med* 20:167–172, 2010.

193. Physical Activity Guidelines Advisory Committee: Physical Activity Guidelines advisory committee report, 2008, *Nutri Rev* 67:114–120, 2008.

194. Plowman SA: Muscular strength, endurance and flexibility assessments. In Plowman SA, Meredith MD, editors: *FITNESSGRAM®/Activitygram reference guide*, ed 4, Dallas, TX, 2013, Cooper Institute, pp 8–55, (pp. (Internet Resource) 8-1).

195. Plowman SA: Top ten research questions related to musculoskeletal fitness testing in children and adolescents, *Res Q Exerc Sport* 85:174–187, 2014.

196. Plowman SA, et al.: The history of FITNESSGRAM®TM, *J Phys Activ Health* 3(S2):S5–S20, 2006.

197. Prentice AM, Jebb SA: Beyond body mass index, *Obesity Rev* 2:141–147, 2001.

198. Presidential Youth Fitness Program (PYFP): From https://www.presidentschallenge.org/challenge/pyfp.shtml, 2013. Retrieved November 15, 2015.

199. Ramsay J, et al.: Strength training effects in prepubescent boys, *Med Sci Sports Exerc* 22:605–614, 1990.

200. Rarick GL, Thompson JAJ: Roentgenographic measures of leg size and ankle extensor strength of 7 year old children, *Res Q* 27:321–332, 1956.

201. Rose J, et al.: Energy expenditure index of walking for normal children and children with cerebral palsy, *Dev Med Child Neurol* 32:333–340, 1990.

202. Rose J, et al.: Cost of walking in normal children and in those with cerebral palsy: comparison of heart rate and oxygen uptake, *Paediatr Orthop* 9:276–279, 1989.

203. Ross JG, et al.: The National Youth and Fitness Study I: new standards for fitness measurement, *J Phys Educ Recreation Dance* 56:62–66, 1985.

204. Ross JG, Gilbert GG: The National Children and Youth Fitness Study: a summary of findings, *J Phys Educ Recreation Dance* 56:45–50, 1985.

205. Ross JG, Pate RR: The National Children and Youth Fitness Study II: a summary of findings, *J Phys Educ Recreation Dance* 58:51–56, 1987.

206. Ross JG, et al.: The National Children and Youth Fitness Study II: new health related fitness norms, *J Phys Educ Recreation Dance* 58:66–70, 1987.

207. Rowland JL, et al.: The role of pediatric physical therapy practice in health promotion and fitness for youth with disabilities, *Pediatr Phys Ther* 27:2–15, 2015.

208. Rowland TW: Evolution of maximal oxygen uptake in children, *Med Sport Sci* 50:200–209, 2007.

209. Rutenfranz J, et al.: The relationship between changing body height and growth related changes in maximal aerobic power, *Eur J Appl Physiol* 60:282–287, 1990.

210. Ryan JM, et al.: Associations of sedentary behavior, physical activity, blood pressure, and anthropometric measures with cardiorespiratory fitness in children with cerebral palsy, *PLoS One* 10:e0123267, 2015.

211. Safrit MJ: Criterion-referenced measurement: validity. In Safrit MJ, Wood TM, editors: *Measurement concepts in physical education and exercise science*, Champaign, IL, 1989, Human Kinetics, pp 119–135.

212. Safrit MJ: The validity and reliability of fitness tests for children: a review, *Pediatr Exerc Sci* 2:9–28, 1990.

213. Sale DG: Strength training in children. In Gisolfi CV, Lamb DR, editors: *Perspectives in exercise science and sports medicine: youth, exercise, and sport*, vol. 2. Indianapolis IN, 1989, Benchmark Press, pp 165–222.

214. Saltin B, Strange S: Maximal oxygen uptake: old and new arguments for a cardiovascular limitation, *Med Sci Sports Exerc* 24:30–37, 1992.

215. Schneiderman-Walker J, et al.: A randomized controlled trial of a 3-year home exercise program in cystic fibrosis, *J Pediatr* 136:304–310, 2000.

216. Scholtes VA, et al.: Lower limb strength training in children with cerebral palsy: a randomized controlled trial protocol for functional strength training based on progressive resistance exercise principles, *BMC Pediatr* 8:41–51, 2008.

217. Scholtes VA, et al.: Effectiveness of a functional progressive resistance exercise training on walking ability in children with cerebral palsy: a randomized controlled trial, *Res Dev Disabil* 33:181–188, 2012.

218. Scott OM, et al.: Effect of exercise in Duchenne muscular dystrophy, *Physiotherapy* 67:174–176, 1981.

219. Selvadurai HC, et al.: Randomized controlled study of in-hospital exercise training programs in children with cystic fibrosis, *Pediatr Pulmonol* 33:194–200, 2002.

220. Sgro M, et al.: The effect of duration of resistance training interventions in children who are overweight or obese, *J Strength Cond Res* 23:1263–1270, 2009.

221. Shvartz E, Reibold RC: Aerobic fitness norms for males and females aged 6 to 75 years: a review, *Aviat Space Environ Med* 61:3–11, 1990.

222. Shypailo RJ, et al.: DXA: can it be used as a criterion reference for body fat measurements in children? *Obesity* 16:457–462, 2008.

223. Singh-Grewal D, et al.: The effects of vigorous exercise training on physical function in children with arthritis: a randomized controlled, single-blinded trial, *Arthritis Rheum* 57:1202–1210, 2007.

224. Skalsky AJ, et al.: Assessment of regional body composition with dual-energy X-ray absorptiometry in Duchenne muscular dystrophy: correlation of regional lean mass and quantitative strength, *Muscle Nerve* 39:647–651, 2009.

225. Slaughter MH, et al.: Influence of maturation on relationship of skinfolds to body density: a cross-sectional study, *Hum Biol* 56:681–689, 1984.

226. Sothern MS, et al.: Safety, feasibility, and efficacy of a resistance training program in preadolescent obese children, *Am J Med Sci* 319:370–375, 2000.

227. Spady DW: Normal body composition of infants and children, *Ross Laboratories Conference on Pediatric Research* 98:67–73, 1989.

228. Spady DW, et al.: A description of the changing composition of the growing premature infant, *J Pediatr Gastroenterol Nutr* 6:730–738, 1986.

229. Sperandio EF, et al.: Functional aerobic capacity limitation in adolescent idiopathic scoliosis, *Spine J* 14:2366–2372, 2014.

230. Sproul A, Simpson E: Stroke volume and related hemodynamic data in normal children, *Pediatrics* 33:912–916, 1964.

231. Sprynarova S, Reisenauer R: Body dimensions and physiological indicators of physical fitness during adolescence. In Shephard RJ, Lavallee H, editors: *Physical fitness assessment*, Springfield, IL, 1978, Charles C Thomas, pp 32–37.

232. Stout JL, Koop SE: Energy expenditure in cerebral palsy. In Gage JR, editor: *The treatment of gait problems in cerebral palsy*, London, 2004, MacKeith Press, pp 146–164.

233. Strong WB, et al.: Evidence based physical activity for school-age youth, *J Pediatr* 146:732–737, 2005.

234. Sutton JR: VO_{2max}: new concepts on an old theme, *Med Sci Sports Exerc* 24:26–29, 1992.

235. Sveen ML, et al.: Endurance training improves fitness in patients with Becker muscular dystrophy, *Brain* 131:2824–2831, 2008.

236. Sveen ML, et al.: Endurance training: an effective and safe treatment for patients with LGMD2I, *Neurology* 68:59–61, 2007.

237. Takken T, et al.: Aerobic fitness in children with juvenile idiopathic arthritis: a systematic review, *J Rheumatol* 29:2643–2647, 2002.

238. Taylor ED, et al.: Orthopaedic complications of overweight in children and adolescents, *Pediatrics* 117:2167–2174, 2006.

239. Taeymans J, et al.: Developmental changes and predictability of static strength in individuals of different maturity: a 30-year longitudinal study, *J Sports Sci* 27:833–841, 2009.

240. Telford RD, et al.: The lifestyle of our kids (LOOK) project: outline of methods, *J Sci Med Sport* 12:156–163, 2009.

241. Thompson P, et al.: Test-retest reliability of the 10-metre fast walk test and 6-minute walk test in ambulatory school-aged children with cerebral palsy, *Dev Med Child Neurol* 50:370–376, 2008.

242. Thorpe D: The role of fitness in health and disease: status of adults with cerebral palsy, *Dev Med Child Neurol* 51(Suppl 4):52–58, 2009.

243. Tirosh E, et al.: New muscle power test in neuromuscular disease, *Am J Dis Child* 144:1083–1087, 1990.

244. Tsolakis C, et al.: Strength adaptations and hormonal responses to resistance training and detraining in preadolescent males, *J Strength Cond Res* 18:625–629, 2004.

245. Unger M, et al.: Strength training in adolescent learners with cerebral palsy, *Clin Rehabil* 20, 469–467, 2006.

246. United States Department of Health and Human Services: *Healthy Children 2000: national health promotion and disease prevention objectives related to mothers, infants, children, adolescents, and youth*, Washington, DC, 1990, Public Health Service.

247. United States Department of Health and Human Services: *Healthy People 2000: progress report for physical activity and fitness*, Washington, DC, 1995, Public Health Service.

248. United States Department of Health and Health and Health and Human Services: *Nutrition and weight status objectives*, 2009. Retrieved from: http://www.healthypeople.gov/2020/topics-objectives/topic/nutrition-and-weight-status/objectives. Accessed January 25, 2016.

249. United States Department of Health and Health and Health and Human Services: *Physical activity objectives*, 2009. Retrieved from: http://www.healthypeople.gov/2020/topics-objectives/topic/physical-activity/objectives. Accessed November 15, 2015.

250. United States Department of Health and Human Services: *Physical activity guidelines for Americans*, Washington, DC, 2008, United States Department of Health and Human Services.

251. van Brussel M, et al.: Aerobic and anaerobic exercise capacity in children with juvenile idiopathic arthritis, *Arthritis Rheum* 57:891–897, 2007.

252. van den Berg-Emons HJG, et al.: Body fat, fitness, and everyday physical activity in adolescents and young adults with myelomeningocele, *J Rehabil Med* 35:271–275, 2003.

253. van den Berg-Emons RJG, et al.: Reliability of tests to determine peak aerobic power, anaerobic power, and isokinetic muscle strength in children with spastic cerebral palsy, *Dev Med Child Neurol* 38:1117–1125, 1996.

254. van den Berg-Emons RJG, et al.: Physical training of school children with spastic cerebral palsy: effects on daily activity, fat mass, and fitness, *Int J Rehabil Res* 21:179–191, 1998.

255. van den Berg-Emons RJG, et al.: Are skinfold measurements suitable to compare body fat between children with spastic cerebral palsy and healthy controls? *Dev Med Child Neurol* 40:335–339, 1998.

256. van der Kooi EL, et al.: Strength training and aerobic exercise training for muscle disease (Review), *Cochrane Database Syst Rev*, 2005. CD003907.

257. Verschuren O, et al.: Health-enhancing physical activity in children with cerebral palsy: more of the same is not enough, *Phys Ther* 94:297–305, 2014. 265.

258. Verschuren O, et al.: Exercise training program in children and adolescents with cerebral palsy: a randomized controlled trial, *Arch Pediatr Adolesc Med* 161:1075–1081, 2007.

259. Verschuren O, et al.: Identification of a core set of exercise tests for children and adolescents with cerebral palsy: a Delphi survey of researchers and clinicians, *Dev Med Child Neurol* 53:449–456, 2011.

260. Verschuren O, et al.: Exercise programs for children with cerebral palsy: a systematic review of the literature, *Am J Phys Med Rehabil* 87:404–417, 2008.

261. Vincent SD, et al.: Activity levels and body mass index of children in the United States, Sweden, and Australia, *Med Sci Sports Exerc* 35:1367–1373, 2003.

262. Vinet A, et al.: Cardiovascular responses to progressive cycle exercise in healthy children and adults, *Inter J Sports Med* 23:242–246, 2002.

263. Wahlund H: Determination of the physical working capacity, *Acta Med Scand Suppl* 215:5–108, 1948.

264. Warburton DER, et al.: The effects of changes in musculoskeletal fitness on health, *Can J Appl Physiol* 26:161–216, 2001.

265. Watts K, et al.: Exercise training in obese children and adolescents: current concepts, *Sports Med* 35:375–392, 2005.

266. Waugh CM, et al.: Effects of resistance training on tendon mechanical properties and rapid force production in prepubertal children, *J Appl Physiol* 117:257–266, 2014.

267. Waugh KG: Measurement of hip, knee, and ankle joints in newborns, *Phys Ther* 63:1616–1621, 1983.

268. Welk GJ, et al.: Field evaluation of the new FITNESSGRAM® criterion-referenced standards, *Am J Prev Med* 41:S131–S142, 2011.

269. Welk GJ, et al.: Development of new criterion-reference fitness standards in the FITNESSGRAM ® Program: rationale and conceptual overview, *Am J Prev Med* 41:S63–S67, 2011.

270. Welk GJ, et al.: Development of youth aerobic-capacity standards using receiver operating characteristic curves, *Am J Prev Med* 41:S111–S116, 2011.

271. Welsman JR, Armstrong N: Statistical techniques for interpreting body size-related exercise performance during growth, *Pediatr Exerc Sci* 12:112–127, 2000.

272. Welsman J, et al.: Reliability of peak VO_2 and maximal cardiac output assessed through thoracic bioimpedance in children, *Eur J Appl Physiol* 94:228–234, 2005.

273. Westcott WL: Resistance training is medicine: effects of strength training on health, *Curr Sports Med Rep* 11:209–216, 2012.

274. Wiley ME, Damiano DL: Lower extremity strength profiles in spastic cerebral palsy, *Dev Med Child Neurol* 40:100–107, 1998.

275. Reference deleted in proofs.

276. Winnick JP, Short FX: *The Brockport Physical Fitness Test Manual: a health-related assessment for youngsters with disabilities*, Champaign, IL, 2014, Human Kinetics.

277. Winnick JP, Short FX: Brockport Physical Fitness test development, *Adapt Phys Activ Q* 22:315–417, 2005.

278. Winnick JP, Short FX: *Physical fitness testing of the disabled: project UNIQUE*, Champaign, IL, 1985, Human Kinetics, pp 101–104.

279. Wood LE, et al.: Isokinetic elbow torque development in children, *Inter J Sports Med* 29:466–470, 2008.

280. World Health Organization: *International classification of functioning, disability and health*, Geneva, 2001, World Health Organization.

281. World Health Organization: *Global strategy on diet, physical activity and health: physical activity and young people*, . Retrieved from: http://www.who.int/dietphysicalactivity/factsheet_young_people/en/, 2015. Accessed on January 31, 2016.

282. Wyndham C: Submaximal test for estimating maximal oxygen intake, *Can Med Assoc J* 96:736–742, 1976.

283. Yamashita T, et al.: Effect of muscle stretching on the activity of neuromuscular transmission, *Med Sci Sports Exerc* 24:80–84, 1992.

284. Zach MS, et al.: Cystic fibrosis: physical exercise vs chest physiotherapy, *Arch Dis Child* 57:587–589, 1982.

285. Ziegler EE, et al.: Body composition of the reference fetus, *Growth* 40:329–334, 1976.

286. Zwinkels M, et al.: Sport-2-Stay-Fit study: health effects of after-school sport participation in children and adolescents with a chronic disease or physical disability, *BMC Sports Sci Med Rehabil* 7:22, 2015.

SUGGESTED READINGS

Armstrong N, Welsman JR: Development of aerobic fitness during childhood and adolescence, *Pediatr Exerc Sci* 12:128–149, 2000.

Bai Y, et al.: Prevalence of youth fitness in the United States: baseline results from the NFL PLAY 60 FITNESSGRAM partnership project, *J Pediatr* 167:662–668, 2015.

Balemans AC, et al.: Systematic review of the clinimetric properties of laboratory- and field-based aerobic and anaerobic fitness measures in children with cerebral palsy, *Arch Phys Med Rehabil* 94:287–301, 2013.

Balemans AC, et al.: Maximal aerobic and anaerobic exercise responses in children with cerebral palsy, *Med Sci Sports Exerc* 45:561–568, 2013.

Bianco A, et al.: A systematic review to determine reliability and usefulness of the field-based test batteries for the assessment of physical fitness in adolescents: the ASSO project, *Int J Occup Med Environ Health* 28:445–478, 2015.

Blais S, et al.: A systematic review of reference values in pediatric cardiopulmonary exercise testing, *Pediatr Cardiol* 36:1553–1564, 2015.

De Ste Croix M: Advances in paediatric strength assessment: changing our perspective on strength development, *J Sports Sci Med* 6:292–304, 2007.

Fowler EG, et al.: Promotion of physical fitness and prevention of secondary conditions for children with cerebral palsy: section on Pediatrics Research Summit Proceedings, *Phys Ther* 87:1495–1507, 2007.

Granacher U, et al.: Effects and mechanisms of strength training in children, *Inter J Sports Med* 35:357–364, 2011.

Jansen M, et al.: Assisted bicycle training delays functional deterioration in boys with Duchenne muscular dystrophy: the randomized controlled trial "No use is disuse," *Neurorehabil Neural Repair* 27:816–827, 2013.

Lloyd RS, et al.: Position statement on youth resistance training: the 2014 International consensus, *Br J Sports Med* 48:498–505, 2014.

Meredith M, Welk GJ, editors: *FITNESSGRAM®-ACTIVITYGRAM test administration manual*, updated ed 4, developed by Cooper Institute (Dallas, TX), Champaign, IL, 2010, Human Kinetics.

Pate R, Oria M, Pillsbury L, editors: Committee on Fitness Measures and Health Outcome in Youth: *fitness measures and heath outcome in youth, Institute of Medicine*, Washington, DC, 2012, The National Academies Press.

Philpott JF, et al.: Physical activity recommendations for children with severe chronic health conditions: juvenile idiopathic arthritis, hemophilia, asthma, and cystic fibrosis, *Clin J Sports Med* 20:167–172, 2010.

Plowman SA, Meredith MD, editors: *Fitnessgram/Activitygram reference guide*, ed 4, Dallas, TX, 2013, Cooper Institute.

Presidential Youth Fitness Program (PYFP). Retrieved November 15, 2015, from: https://www.presidentschallenge.org/challenge/pyfp.shtml.

Rowland JL, et al.: The role of pediatric physical therapy practice in health promotion and fitness for youth with disabilities, *Pediatr Phys Ther* 27:2–15, 2015.

Ryan JM, et al.: Associations of sedentary behavior, physical activity, blood pressure, and anthropometric measures with cardiorespiratory fitness in children with cerebral palsy, *PLoS One* 10:e0123267, 2015.

Singh-Grewal D, et al.: The effects of vigorous exercise training on physical function in children with arthritis: a randomized controlled, single-blinded trial, *Arthritis Rheum* 57:1202–1210, 2007.

Verschuren O, et al.: Identification of a core set of exercise tests for children and adolescents with cerebral palsy: a Delphi survey of researchers and clinicians, *Dev Med Child Neurol* 53:449–456, 2011.

Waugh CM, et al.: Effects of resistance training on tendon mechanical properties and rapid force production in prepubertal children, *J Appl Physiol* 117:257–266, 2014.

Westcott WL: Resistance training is medicine: effects of strength training on health, *Curr Sports Med Rep* 11:209–216, 2012.

Winnick JP, Short FX: *The Brockport Physical Fitness Test Manual: a health-related assessment for youngsters with disabilities*, Champaign, IL, 2014, Human Kinetics.

Zwinkels M, et al.: Sport-2-Stay-Fit study: health effects of after-school sport participation in children and adolescents with a chronic disease or physical disability, *BMC Sports Sci Med Rehabil* 7:22, 2015.

Juvenile Idiopathic Arthritis

Janjaap van der Net, Paul J.M. Helders, Sr., Tim Takken

Chronic arthritis in childhood can result from any one of a heterogeneous group of diseases, of which juvenile idiopathic arthritis (JIA) is the most common. The disease causes joint swelling, pain, and limited mobility and can significantly restrict a child's activities. Box 7.1 lists the common clinical manifestations of JIA. Other conditions that may cause childhood arthritis include juvenile psoriatic arthritis (JPsA), juvenile ankylosing spondylitis (JAS), and other enthesitis-related arthritides. Arthritis may also be a feature of juvenile scleroderma, systemic lupus erythematosus, and juvenile dermatomyositis.

This chapter provides an overview of the body function and structure impairments, activity limitations, and participation restrictions common to JIA and describes the role of the physical therapist as a member of the rheumatology team in the examination, evaluation, and intervention for the child with arthritis. Outcome instruments appropriate for use in JIA, issues related to school and recreational activities, surgical procedures, and adherence to therapeutic regimens are discussed. Case scenarios illustrate the therapeutic management of a child with JIA.

ROLE OF THE THERAPIST

Physical therapists (PTs) are essential members of the pediatric rheumatology team, which includes the pediatric rheumatologist, nurse, occupational therapist, pediatric ophthalmologist, pediatric orthopedist, and pediatrician. Other pediatric specialists, including dermatologists, cardiologists, orthotists, psychologists, and social workers, provide occasional consultation as needed. After a thorough history the PT conducts a comprehensive examination to identify impairments of body structures and functions relevant to physical therapy intervention and caused by the disease and determines their relationship to observed or reported activity and participation restrictions. Based on an evaluation of these findings, the PT develops a prioritized problem list and an intervention plan to reduce functional limitations, to prevent or minimize secondary problems, and to improve activity and participation levels (Table 7.1). Therapists work with parents and the child to develop a "joint health and self-management" program that includes balanced rest and exercise and to provide guidelines for choosing (extracurricular) physical activities and consult with school personnel to ensure the child's full participation in educational activities.

The role of the therapist varies based on stage and progression of the disease and the care setting; often more than one PT is involved in the child's care. Physical therapists working in a specialized pediatric rheumatology center may perform the initial assessment, set treatment goals, plan a "joint health and self-management" program, and monitor the child's functional status at routine clinic visits. Therapists within the child's home, school, or community usually provide direct services. The frequency of therapy varies widely and depends on the child's physical status, reimbursement for therapy services, and the availability of therapists. Web-based technologies are increasingly utilized, also by PTs, to compensate for limited resources or to increase health service levels such as e-consultation and e-health monitoring or e-learning programs.

BACKGROUND INFORMATION

DIAGNOSIS AND CLASSIFICATION

Three systems are used to diagnose and classify childhood arthritis: the American College of Rheumatology (ACR) criteria for juvenile rheumatoid arthritis (JRA),[8] the European League Against Rheumatism (EULAR) criteria for juvenile chronic arthritis (JCA),[19] and the International League of Associations for Rheumatology (ILAR) criteria for juvenile idiopathic arthritis (JIA).[71] The ILAR criteria are used in this chapter. All three systems are currently based on the disease phenotype; however, increasing insight in the genotype of JIA will gradually lead to new classifications.[72] Juvenile idiopathic arthritis is not a single disease but a term that encompasses all forms of arthritis that begin before the age of 16 years, persist for longer than 6 weeks, and are of unknown cause.[72] The term represents, therefore, an exclusion diagnosis. Because there are no definitive laboratory tests for JIA, the diagnosis is primarily clinical and sometimes is undecided until a clear picture of the disease evolves. Table 7.2 shows the characteristics of the different disease types: systemic arthritis (sJIA), oligoarthritis, polyarthritis (polyJIA), enthesitis-related arthritis, and psoriatic arthritis. All are defined by the clinical signs and symptoms observed during the first 6 months of the disease.

An oligoarticular onset occurs in 27% to 56% of children with JIA, mostly girls between 2 and 4 years of age.[72] Disease signs include low-grade inflammation in four or fewer joints, most often the knee, followed in frequency by the ankles and

BOX 7.1   Primary (P) and Secondary (S) Clinical Manifestations of Juvenile Idiopathic Arthritis (JIA)

Primary

Joint swelling, pain, stiffness
Morning stiffness
Muscle atrophy; weakness; poor muscle endurance
Acute or chronic iridocyclitis (most common in oligoarticular JIA)
Systemic manifestations (may be severe in systemic JIA; mild to moderate in polyarticular JIA)

Secondary

Limited joint motion; soft tissue contracture
Fatigue
Decreased aerobic capacity; reduced exercise tolerance
Growth abnormalities (local and general)
Osteopenia; osteoporosis (increased risk with long-term use of oral corticosteroids)
Difficulties with activities of daily living
Possible activity/participation restrictions

Primary and Secondary

Gait deviations

elbows (Fig. 7.1). The hip and small joints of the hand are usually spared. The joint is swollen and may be warm but is not always painful. Systemic signs such as skin rash or spiking fever are unusual, but about 30% of children develop iridocyclitis, an asymptomatic inflammation of the eye that may lead to functional blindness. These children must have their eyes examined by an ophthalmologist at diagnosis and, depending on the risk, every 3 to 4 or 6 to 12 months. Systemic or topical corticosteroids are used to control the inflammation.

Polyarticular JIA (Fig. 7.2), subdivided into a rheumatoid factor (RF)–positive and an RF factor–negative polyarthritis and defined as arthritis in five or more joints, occurs in 2% to 28% of children with JIA, mostly girls. The RF factor–negative form has an early peak at 2 to 4 years and a later peak at 6 to 12 years, and RF factor–positive polyarthritis has an onset at late childhood or adolescence.[72] Onset is often insidious, with arthritis noted in progressively more joints. Arthritis is symmetrical, affects both large and small joints, and may include the cervical spine and temporomandibular joints. Joints are swollen and warm but rarely red. Systemic symptoms are usually mild and include low-grade fever and mild to moderate hepatosplenomegaly and lymphadenopathy. About 19% develop iridocyclitis. The RF-positive group, mostly females with disease onset

TABLE 7.1   Interventions in Juvenile Idiopathic Arthritis

Outcome	Level of ICF	Intervention	Reference
Physical Function			
Morning stiffness	Function	Movements of any kind, especially in extension direction of joints and stretching biarticular muscles	None
Joint range of motion	Function	Gentle movements of any kind, especially in extension direction of joints and stretching biarticular muscles	None
Muscle strength	Function	Isometric and isokinetic muscle strength exercise	Sandstedt E, 2013
Physical fitness (health related)	Function	Aerobic exercise	Takken et al., 2003
Anaerobic fitness	Function	Anaerobic exercise	Klijn PH, (2004)
Pain behaviors	Function	Relaxation with: Mindfulness, Tai Chi, or Qigong	Stephens (2008)
Gait	Function	Insoles (soft or supinating, retrocapital support) or rocker-bottom external soles	None
Physical Activity and Participation			
Gross and fine motor performance	Activity	Sports and gym activities; play (adapted)	None
School function (writing)	Activity	Pencil thickeners, floating-ball pencils, keyboard and tablet writing	None
Walking	Activity	Nordic walking	None

TABLE 7.2   Frequency, Age at Onset, and Sex Distribution of the International League of Associations for Rheumatology (ILAR) Categories of Juvenile Idiopathic Arthritis

	Frequency[a]	Onset Age	Sex Ratio
Systemic arthritis	4%–17%	Throughout childhood	F > M
Oligoarthritis	27%–56%	Early childhood; peak at 2–4 years	F >>> M
Rheumatoid factor–positive polyarthritis	2%–7%	Late childhood or adolescence	F >> M
Rheumatoid factor–negative polyarthritis	11%–28%	Biphasic distribution; early peak at 2–4 years and later peak at 6–12 years	F >> M
Enthesitis-related arthritis	3%–11%	Late childhood or adolescence	M >> F
Psoriatic arthritis	2%–11%	Biphasic distribution; early peak at 2–4 years and later peak at 9–11 years	F > M
Undifferentiated arthritis	11%–21%	Not known	Not known

[a]Reported frequencies refer to percentage of all juvenile idiopathic arthritis.

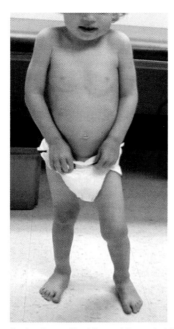

FIG. 7.1 Oligoarticular juvenile idiopathic arthritis causing swelling and flexion contracture of the left knee in a 2-year-old girl. (From Zitelli BJ, McIntire SC, Nowalk AJ: *Zitelli and Davis' atlas of pediatric physical diagnosis.* 6th ed. Philadelphia, Saunders; 2012.)

in late childhood or adolescence, follows a disease course similar to that seen in adults with rheumatoid arthritis. Individuals may have rheumatoid nodules on the elbows, tibial crests, and fingers and may develop erosive synovitis early in the disease course. Nodules are less common in children with RF-negative disease, and fewer joints are affected. Persistent arthritis may occur, causing juxta-articular osteopenia, muscle atrophy, weakness, contractures, and growth disturbances.

Systemic JIA occurs in 4% to 17% of cases. The disease arises as often in boys as in girls and does not know a preferential age onset. The diagnostic marker is a spiking fever of 39°C (102.2°F) or higher that occurs once or twice daily (afternoon or evening) for at least 2 weeks, with a rapid return to normal or below between spikes. The fever is accompanied by a typical evanescent rash (discrete, erythematous macules) that is most often found on the trunk or limbs but may be seen on the face, palms, and soles of the feet (Fig. 7.3). Other systemic signs include pleuritis, pericarditis, myocarditis, hepatosplenomegaly, and lymphadenopathy. Systemic disease may precede arthritis by several months or years. Fever, rash, and pericarditis often subside after the initial disease period but may recur during periods of exacerbation of the arthritis.[12,69,72]

Incidence and Prevalence

Childhood chronic arthritis is not rare. Reported incidence and prevalence vary considerably throughout the world, and the true frequency is unknown. Based on estimations in the industrialized world in an under–18-year-old population of 225 million, the incidence figure is between 11,700–22,500 and prevalence ranges from 186,750–900,000.[11] The reported peak age at onset is still between 1 and 3 years for the total group and for girls, primarily those with oligoJIA and polyJIA.[86] Disease onset for boys showed two peaks, one at 2 years, representing mostly boys with polyJIA, and another between 8 and 10 years

of age that may partially represent children with JAS. Almost twice as many females as males develop JIA. The ratio of girls to boys is 3:1 for oligoJIA (5:1 for those with iridocyclitis) and 2.8:1 for polyJIA.[11]

Origin and Pathogenesis

The cause and pathogenesis of JIA are still poorly understood but seem to include both genetic and environmental components. The prevailing theory is that it is an autoimmune inflammatory disorder, activated by an external trigger, in a genetically predisposed host. A viral or bacterial infection often precedes disease onset. The notion that an infection triggers JIA in genetically susceptible individuals is attractive but not yet fully unraveled.[72] Physical trauma may be associated with onset but may just draw attention to an already inflamed joint. The difference in onset types and disease course, the higher prevalence among girls, the narrow peak age periods of onset for all but systemic JIA, and the extensive immunologic abnormalities suggest that JIA may not be a single disease. Different etiologic vectors may be responsible for each onset type, or a single pathogen may cause distinct clinical patterns as it interacts with the host.

The role of the immune system in the pathogenesis and persistence of inflammation is evident in the altered immunity, abnormal immunoregulation, and cytokine production. The T-cell abnormalities and the pathology of the inflamed synovium suggest a cell-mediated pathogenesis. The presence of multiple autoantibodies and immune complexes and the complement activation indicate humoral abnormalities. The importance of genetic predisposition to JIA is not completely understood. Many of the suspected genetic predispositions are within the major histocompatibility complex (MHC) region of chromosome 6, but the pathogenesis may involve the interactions of multiple genes. Recent studies indicate that correlations found between human leukocyte antigen (HLA) specificities and various types of JIA may have specific risks and protective effects that are age-related for each onset type and some course subtypes.[64]

Pharmacologic Management

The goals of pharmacologic therapy in JIA are to induce remission of the disease and/or control the arthritis, thereby preventing joint erosions, and to manage extra-articular manifestations.[73] Children with severe or persistent disease often require a carefully orchestrated combination of sometimes-aggressive drug therapies, started early in the disease. A core set of six outcome variables is often used in clinical trials to determine subjects' responses to medical therapy.[24] These include physician global assessment of disease activity, parent/patient assessment of overall health status, functional ability, number of joints with active arthritis, number of joints with limited motion, and erythrocyte sedimentation rate (ESR). A positive clinical response is defined as improvement of at least 30% from baseline in at least three of the six variables, with no more than one of the other variables worsening by more than 30%.

Currently (inter-)national consensus on the prescription of medication is published yearly by the Childhood Arthritis and Rheumatology Research Alliance (CARRA). These are referred to as consensus treatment plans (CTPs) and are available on CARRA's website. Because novel therapeutic agents are entering the clinical practice with ever-increasing tempo, it is necessary to review actual consensus statements such as those provided by CARRA. Therefore only a few generic treatment principles are

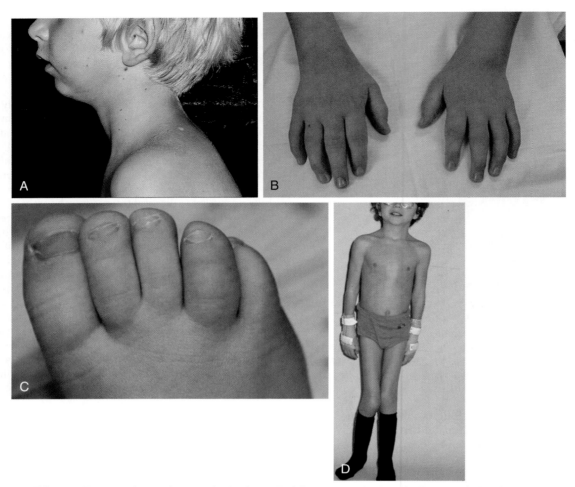

FIG. 7.2 Presentations of polyarticular juvenile idiopathic arthritis. (A) Failure of development of the lower jaw some 5 years after systemic onset of disease. The neck is short and slightly flexed. (B) Polyarthritis affecting the small joints of the hands and wrists. (C) Dactylitis seen in toes of a child with psoriatic juvenile idiopathic arthritis. (D) Severe polyarticular disease. ([A] From Hochberg MC: *Rheumatology.* 6th ed. Philadelphia: Mosby; 2015. [B] From Denman G, Jandial S, Foster H: Diagnosing arthritis in children, *Paediatr Child Health* 25:541-548, 2015. [C] Image courtesy of © UMB Medica/RheumatologyNetwork.com. [D] From Kanski JJ, Bowling B: *Clinical ophthalmology: a systematic approach.* 7th ed. Edinburgh, Saunders; 2011.)

touched on briefly here. The references as well as the websites provide informative algorithms and guidelines for prescription.[76] Nonsteroidal anti-inflammatory drugs (NSAIDs), such naproxen, tolmetin, and ibuprofen, are still the most widely used first-line therapy. The most common adverse effect is gastrointestinal irritation, although NSAIDs that selectively inhibit the cyclo-oxygenase 2 (COX-2) enzyme may limit this problem. Methotrexate (MTX) is the most common disease-modifying antirheumatic drug (DMARD) prescribed for children with polyJIA and sJIA (Fig. 7.4).[73] The drug is usually administered orally once a week, although subcutaneous injection is given if the response is inadequate or if the child experiences adverse effects with the oral dose, including gastrointestinal upset. Although liver toxicity in children taking MTX appears to be rare, physicians check blood counts and liver enzymes periodically. Data on the health risks associated with long-term use of MTX in children are not yet available but expected to be nil.

Patients with a poor prognosis who fail to respond to MTX are treated with one of the so-called biologic medications that

targets the tumor necrosis factor (TNF), a cytokine responsible for many of the effects of inflammation.[60] These drugs include etanercept, infliximab, and adalimumab, but many more enter the market these days. Systemic glucocorticoid drugs are reserved for children, mostly those with sJIA who do not respond to other therapies. Although steroids have a potent anti-inflammatory effect, they do not alter disease course or duration. Serious adverse effects of long-term oral steroids include iatrogenic Cushing's syndrome, myopathy, growth disturbance, osteoporosis and fracture, diabetes mellitus, obesity, and increased susceptibility to infection. For children with refractory disease who are steroid dependent, aggressive therapy with cyclosporin A or cyclophosphamide may provide some benefit.[76] Intra-articular injections of long-acting corticosteroids are used successfully to treat severely inflamed and swollen joints.[76] A study found that intra-articular steroid injections for lower extremity joints decreased the incidence of leg length discrepancies, a major cause of gait and postural abnormalities in children with JIA.[81]

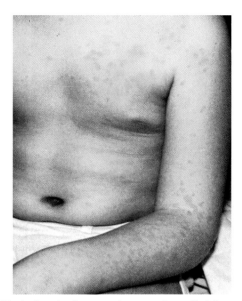

FIG. 7.3 Typical rash of systemic-onset juvenile idiopathic arthritis in a 3-year-old boy. The rash is salmon colored, macular, and nonpruritic. Individual lesions are transient, occur in crops over the trunk and extremities, and may occur in a linear distribution (Koebner's phenomenon) after minor trauma such as a scratch. (From Petty RE, Laxer RM, Lindsley CB, et al., editors: *Textbook of pediatric rheumatology.* 7th ed. Philadelphia, Elsevier; 2016.)

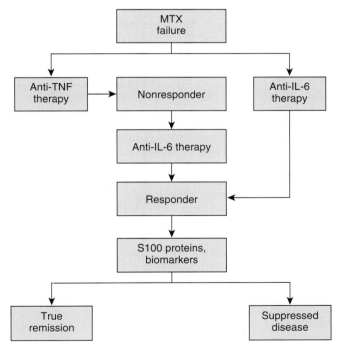

FIG. 7.4 Treatment options for patients with JIA include MTX as well as biologic agents that target TNF or the IL-6 receptor. After clinical remission is achieved, S100 proteins and other biomarkers could help to differentiate between "true" remission and suppressed disease. *JIA*, juvenile idiopathic arthritis; *MTX*, methotrexate. (From Prakken B, Martini A: Paediatric rheumatology in 2014: digging deeper for greater precision and more impact in JIA. *Nat Rev Rheumatol* 11:70-72, 2015.)

PROGNOSIS

Studies assessing outcomes of JIA have provided inconsistent or conflicting results. Studies over the past 10 years have shown that only 40% to 60% of patients had inactive disease or clinical remission at follow-up. Despite long-term persistence of disease activity in most patients, a pronounced improvement in functional outcome has been documented in the past decades.[28,73] Poor articular and functional outcomes in sJIA and polyJIA are linked to the presence of hip involvement and polyarthritis in the first year of disease activity.[83] Children with oligoJIA have the best prognosis for joint preservation and function but may develop contractures during active disease and later degenerative arthritis. They also remain at high risk for inflammatory eye involvement. About 5% to 10% follow an extended disease course, adding multiple joints after the first 6 months. Those who are RF+ often follow a course similar to that of children with RF+ polyJIA, with persistent disease and poor functional outcomes. In contrast, outcome is usually good in boys with disease onset at 9 years of age or older, who are positive for the *HLA-B27* gene, and have arthritis mostly in the hip and sacroiliac joints.

Reports of long-term functional outcomes in JIA vary, possibly because of differences in study methods. And these reports date back to the millennium change, which limit their importance because the treatment paradigm has changed significantly.[73]

BODY FUNCTION AND STRUCTURE

Joint Structure and Function

The cardinal signs of inflammation are swelling, end-range stress pain, stiffness, and loss of full range of joint motion. Swelling around a joint may be the result of intra-articular effusion, synovial hypertrophy, soft tissue edema, or periarticular tenosynovitis. The anatomic bony landmarks of the joint may also be enlarged as a result of bony overgrowth due to increased blood supply to the inflamed area. Swelling and protective muscle spasm contribute to pain. This muscle spasm is referred to as a contraction deformity, in contrast with the more common conception contracture, which refers to a morphologic change in the periarticular soft tissue. Inactivity stiffness most noted upon awakening (also referred to as "morning stiffness") and after periods of prolonged sitting is a common indicator of disease activity.

Chronic inflammation causes abnormalities in joint structure and function. Increased production of synovial fluid stretches and weakens the joint capsule and adjacent structures, leading to ligamentous laxity and joint instability. Massive overgrowth of the synovium, called pannus, spreads over and invades the articular cartilage, releasing inflammatory enzymes into the synovial fluid. In some patients, erosions in the articular cartilage and subchondral bone cause irregularities in the joint surface, compromising alignment, congruency, and stability.[11] Early radiographs show periarticular swelling with widening of the joint space, juxta-articular osteopenia, and periosteal new bone.[74] Radiographs of joints placed under physiologic strain (i.e., tested in function) provide a more precise indication of the quality of the periarticular soft tissue condition (e.g., laxity of wrist ligaments may be visualized in the translation of carpal bones).[33] General demineralization, thinning and loss of articular cartilage, marginal erosions, and osteophytes occur with persistent disease.[11] Nutritional deficiencies, low body weight, and decreased physical activity may result in low bone density and risk for fracture. This will be exacerbated in case of long-term use of systemic corticosteroids.[56] Joint contractures usually result from intra-articular adhesions and fibrosis of adjacent tendons.

The therapist should be aware of possible patterns of joint restriction in JIA and their potential effects on function (Table 7.3). Arthritis may occur in any joint, but the large joints are affected most often. Hip arthritis occurs in 30% to 50% of children, mostly those with sJIA and polyJIA.[83] Early signs of hip disease may include leg length inequality, pain in the groin, buttocks, medial thigh, or knee, and a gluteus medius limp. A child may compensate for a mild hip flexion contracture with increased lumbar lordosis. Children with oligoJIA may lose hip motion secondary to knee flexion contracture and leg length discrepancy. The knee is the joint most often affected in oligoJIA, but it is also involved in other disease types. Flexion contracture may result from intra-articular swelling, joint immobility, spasm of the hamstrings, and shortening of the tensor fasciae latae. Chronic synovitis, with overgrowth of the medial femoral condyle, results in a valgus deformity that is exaggerated by tightness in the iliotibial band (ITB) (see Fig. 7.2). Ankle arthritis occurs in all disease types, but involvement of the small joints of the feet is more common in polyJIA. Problems may initially include loss of ankle dorsiflexion or of plantar flexion and metatarsalgia. In prolonged disease subluxation of the metatarsophalangeal joints, hallux valgus, hallux rigidus, hammer toes, and overlapping toes may become prominent. Arthritis of the subtalar joint may result in hindfoot valgus with forefoot pronation (Fig. 7.5), although some children develop calcaneal varus and a forefoot cavus deformity. Both result in a walking pattern with toeing in or toeing out respectively.

The cervical spine and the temporomandibular joints are frequently involved. Early signs of neck involvement include pain and stiffness in the back of the neck, with loss of extension and limitations in rotation and lateral flexion or restricted shoulder elevation. Atlantoaxial subluxation may occur early in the disease, placing the child at risk for injury from trauma or during intubation for surgery. Cervical spine ankylosis is sometimes seen and can cause similar problems during surgery.

Temporomandibular joint involvement includes difficulties in chewing food, loss of range of motion as shown by a restriction in mouth opening, and pain in the ear region. Chronic involvement of temporomandibular joints will lead to an overgrowth of the jaw or to micrognathia (undergrowth of the mandible) and difficulties in mouth closure. Even the joints of the larynx and the area of the vocal cords can be affected, leading to hoarseness of the voice.

Restrictions in shoulder rotation, flexion, and abduction may occur with arthritis in the glenohumeral joint, as well as in the acromioclavicular, sternoclavicular, and manubriosternal joints. Elbow flexion contractures occur early and may be accompanied by loss of forearm supination. Arthritis in the wrist and small joints of the hands is most common in polyJIA. The pattern and extent of involvement are related to disease type, the child's age, and maturation of the epiphyses at disease onset. Wrist malalignment associated with subluxation and undergrowth of the ulna, with ulnar deviation, occurs in children with disease onset at a young age. Those 12 years or older at onset have a pattern typical of adults, with radial deviation. The metacarpophalangeal (MCP) and proximal interphalangeal (PIP) joints are also involved, either directly by synovitis or indirectly as a result of inflammation in adjacent joints or tendon sheaths.

Muscular Structure and Function

The different stages of the disease will show a difference in muscular structures and functions.

In the acute phase of the disease, periarticular musculature of the affected joints will show spasm and hypertonus, also referred to as contraction deformity.

In subacute and chronic stages of the disease, muscle atrophy and weakness are more pronounced, especially near the affected joints. This also may occur in distant areas and can persist long after remission of the arthritis.[10,24,35] Contributing factors to an altered muscle structure and function include alterations in anabolic hormones, production of inflammatory cytokines and high resting energy metabolism,[48] abnormal protein metabolism,[34] motor unit inhibition from pain and swelling, and disuse. Also a disease onset very early in life, with long periods of active arthritis, may negatively affect muscle development.[103]

Systemic muscle flexibility, tested with a sit-and-reach test, may also be limited as a result of a decreased level of physical activity.

Growth Disturbances and Postural Abnormalities

Retardation of linear growth is associated with extended periods of active disease and is exacerbated by long-term use of systemic steroids. Accelerated growth may occur during remission if the epiphyses are still open. Puberty and the appearance of secondary sex characteristics may be delayed. Osteopenia, mainly in the appendicular skeleton, may be due to inadequate bone formation for age, low bone turnover, and depressed bone formation.[9,11] These circumstances may contribute to an increased risk of bone fracture. Increased blood supply to the inflamed joint early in the disease may cause accelerated growth of the ossification centers, resulting in bony overgrowth. Leg length discrepancies often occur as a result of unilateral knee arthritis. Growth discrepancies between ulnar and radial bones in wrist arthritis have been reported to contribute to instability and functional loss.[65] Premature closure of the growth plates may also occur. This may be widespread and symmetrical, as seen in the small hands and feet of some children with polyJIA, or isolated to a single digit.[11] Micrognathia may result from temporomandibular joint arthritis.

The therapist should observe the child's postural alignment in sitting and standing. Hip and knee flexion contractures, genu valgus, and foot deformities will affect the child's posture in standing. Children with asymmetrical cervical spine arthritis may present with torticollis. Children with leg length differences may develop a functional scoliosis. Small lifts of known thickness placed under the shorter leg with the child standing will level the pelvis and confirm or rule out idiopathic scoliosis.

Physical Fitness: Health-Related Fitness and Performance-Related Fitness

Physical fitness is known to be limited in a multitude of childhood chronic conditions, among them JIA.[96] Physical fitness can be divided into various components, namely, health-related fitness (peak oxygen uptake [VO_2peak]) and performance-related fitness (muscle strength, anaerobic capacity). The VO_2peak is most frequently assessed using progressively graded exercise

TABLE 7.3 Joint and Soft Tissue Restrictions and Clinical Adaptations in Juvenile Idiopathic Arthritis (JIA)[a] [2,4,17,46,105]

Clinical Manifestations	Restrictions/Adaptations
Cervical Spine	
In polyJIA and sJIA	Loss of EXT, rotation, side FLEX
Inflammation, narrowing, then fusion; observed first in C2-C3, but may progress to involve the entire cervical spine[b]	May develop torticollis if asymmetrical
	Intubation for anesthesia[b]
Dysplasia of vertebral bodies	Eye movements or turning body compensates for ↓ neck ROM
Odontoid process instability (less common than in adult RA)	
Temporomandibular Joint	
Common in polyJIA; less common in oligoJIA; often associated with cervical spine disease	Restriction in opening mouth; pain on chewing; may need orthodontia
Mandibular asymmetry if unilateral involvement	Greater functional restrictions if cervical spine is involved
Undergrowth of the mandible (micrognathia); malocclusion of the teeth	EXT is restricted
Shoulder Complex	
Most common in polyJIA[b]	Loss of active GL-H ABD and IR first limitations noted; limited
Overgrowth of humeral head with irregular shape, shallow glenoid fossa	FLEX, tightening of pectorals and scapular protractors; more dysfunction when elbow and wrist involved
Subluxation may occur	
Elbow	
Involved early in disease course[b]	EXT lost early; eventual limitation in FLEX and forearm rotation
Occurs in all types; symmetrical in polyJIA and sJIA; asymmetrical in oligoJIA[b]	Shoulder ROM initially compensates for ↓ supination; loss of > 45° EXT restricts ability to push off from chair
Overgrowth of radial head restricts ROM	
Proximal radioulnar joint involved[b]	Wrist involvement accentuates loss of pronation and supination
Ulnar nerve entrapment possible	
Wrist	
All types; starts early; symmetrical in polyJIA and sJIA; unilateral in oligoJIA[b]	Rapid loss of EXT; weakness of extensors; FLEX contracture and volar subluxation
Accelerated carpal maturation	Rests in flexion and ulnar deviation with spasm of wrist flexors
Undergrowth of ulna; ulnar shortening; may migrate dorsally	In older-onset or RF+ polyJIA, tendency is toward radial deviation[b]
Radiocarpal and intercarpal fusion	Distal radioulnar disease causes loss of pronation and supination
Flexor tenosynovitis; carpal tunnel syndrome is rare; may occur late in disease	
Hand	
Premature epiphyseal fusion and growth abnormalities	PIP (especially 4th) more common than DIP contractures
Flexor tenosynovitis may be dramatic	Loss of MCP FLEX (especially 2nd digit); loss of MCP hyperextension
Involvement later in polyJIA and sJIA than in oligoJIA	Marked decrease in grip strength
MCP and CMP subluxation deformities	Boutonniere < swan neck
Thoracolumbar Spine	
Unusual site in JIA	Kyphosis in association with neck and shoulder involvement
Steroid drug therapy may cause osteoporosis, wedging of vertebral bodies, small compression fractures	Lumbar lordosis 2° to hip flexion contractures; scoliosis 2° to lower limb asymmetries
	Pain with compression fractures[b]
Hip	
Femoral head overgrowth	Flexion contractures, may be masked by lumbar lordosis
Osteoporosis	May present as pain in the groin, over buttocks, medial thigh, around knee[b]
Trochanteric growth changes	IR and ABD lost early 2° to pain and spasm of FLEXs and ADDs
Shallow acetabulum, ↓ femoral neck angle, especially if weight bearing limited	
Lateral subluxation of femoral head aggravated by tight adductors	May have marked pain on standing
Potential for protrusio acetabuli, avascular necrosis	Gluteus medius weakness may cause Trendelenburg gait deviation[b]
Primary cause of ↓ ROM and dysfunction	Secondary deformities of the contralateral hip, knees, and lumbar spine
Occurs in polyJIA and sJIA after a few years	

Continued

TABLE 7.3   Joint and Soft Tissue Restrictions and Clinical Adaptations in Juvenile Idiopathic Arthritis (JIA)[a][2,4,17,46,105]**—cont'd**

Clinical Manifestations	Restrictions/Adaptations
Potential for regeneration of articular cartilage with fibrocartilage if remission of synovitis[b]	Mobility and weight bearing improve cartilage repair[†]
KNEE	
Most common joint involved early in all types	Rapid development of flexion contracture
Overgrowth of distal femur may cause leg length discrepancy in unilateral disease	Rapid atrophy of quadriceps; loss of patellar mobility due to adhesions
Knee valgus aggravated by tight hamstrings and iliotibial band	Risk of femoral fracture associated with falling due to flexion and osteoporosis
Posterior tibial subluxation 2° to prolonged joint	Loss of flexion (often only to 90°)
Involvement or excessive correction of knee flexion contracture	Secondary hip flexion contracture
Ankle/Foot	
Altered growth causes bony changes in tarsals with potential fusion	Early loss of inversion, eversion
Hindfoot valgus/varus due to ankle joint arthritis or 2° to knee valgus	Later loss of D-FL and PL-FL, especially if ambulation is limited
MTP subluxation	Altered gait, loss of MTP hyperextension affects toe-off
Hallux valgus	Overlapping of IPs, especially with hallux valgus
IPs: growth changes due to premature epiphyseal closure	

[a]Data in this table are summarized from information published in Ansell, 1992; Atwood, 1989; Cassidy and Petty, 1990; Emery, 1993; Libby et al., 1991; Reed and Wilmot, 1991; Rhodes, 1991; White, 1990; and Cassidy JT, Petty RE: Juvenile rheumatoid arthritis. In Cassidy JT, Petty RE, editors: *Textbook of pediatric rheumatology.* 4th ed. Philadelphia: WB Saunders; 2001.
[b]The listing is not inclusive, but the features described are characteristic of juvenile arthritis.
Adapted from Wright FV, Smith E: Physical therapy management of the child and adolescent with juvenile rheumatoid arthritis. In Walker JM, Helewa A, editors: *Physical therapy in arthritis.* Philadelphia: WB Saunders; 1996.
ABD, abduction/abductors; *ADD,* adduction/adductors; *CMP,* carpometacarpal-phalangeal; *D-FL,* dorsiflexion; *DIP,* distal interphalangeal; *EXT,* extension; *FLEX,* flexion, flexors; *GL-H,* glenohumeral; *IP,* interphalangeal; *IR,* internal rotation; *MCP,* metacarpophalangeal; *MTP,* metatarsophalangeal; *polyJIA,* polyarticular JIA; *PL-FL,* plantar flexion; *ROM,* range of motion; *sJIA,* systemic JIA.

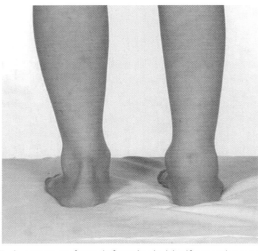

FIG. 7.5 A common foot deformity is hindfoot valgus with pronation. (From Foster HE, Wyllie R: Chronic arthritis in children and adolescents. *Medicine* 34:391-395, 2006.)

tests on a cycle ergometer with respiratory gas analysis in children with JIA,[89] although some researchers have used treadmill testing in children with JIA.[42]

A large body of evidence shows that the peak oxygen uptake of children and adolescents with JIA is lower than that in healthy peers. In the most recent studies in JIA, in the age between 6.7 and 18 years, VO$_2$peak (L/min) and VO$_2$peak corrected for body mass (VO$_2$peak/kg in ml/kg/min) were respectively 69.8% and 74.8% in children and 83% and 80% of predicted for adolescents with JIA.[53,97] These observations confirm the results of a previous meta-analysis showing that VO$_2$peak per kilogram body mass was on average 21.8% lower in children with JIA compared with healthy control subjects or reference values.[89]

Giannini and Protas[25,26] also found that children with JIA had a significantly lower peak work rate (amount of watt that a subject can generate on a cycle ergometer), peak exercise heart rate (HRpeak), and exercise time than healthy control subjects matched for age, gender, and body size. Unpublished observations in 98 children with JIA (Takken et al.) showed that children with JIA had on average an HRpeak of 182 ± 14.7 beats per minute, while healthy children have on average an HRpeak of 193 ± 7 beats per minute. Some of the children with JIA stopped the exercise test because of fatigue and/or musculoskeletal complaints—not because of a cardiopulmonary limitation. In addition, HR and VO$_2$ values during submaximal exercise were higher in subjects with JIA, suggesting that they worked at a higher percentage of their aerobic capacity than did control subjects during routine activities.[15]

Impaired aerobic capacity does not appear to be significantly related to the severity of joint disease but may be due to hypoactivity secondary to disease symptoms, especially in children with long-standing arthritis.[25,26] Physiologic factors, including anemia, muscle atrophy, generalized weakness, and stiffness, resulting in poor mechanical efficiency may also limit the child's performance.

ACTIVITY AND PARTICIPATION RESTRICTIONS

Self-Care and Participation

The impact of JIA on a child's activities depends on the extent and duration of active disease, the child's developmental stage, resiliency, and desire to be independent, and expectations placed on the child by parents and others. Changes in motor activity could very well be the first notable sign of behavioral change in a child. For example, the first sign of wrist involvement in a toddler could be incomplete or compensated palmar support (e.g., when on "all fours"), limiting the ability to crawl during play activities on the floor. Another sign of wrist involvement may be a compensatory pattern of palmar support in which the child does not bear weight on the full palmar part of the hand but only on the palmar part of the fingers, utilizing the ability to hyperextend the MCP joints (which may have a detrimental effect on joint function later in life). A classic example of early impact on motor activities is the change in ambulation in a toddler with arthritis in the knee, leading to a change from walking to bottom shuffling. A child with oligoJIA may demonstrate few functional limitations, but one with severe polyJIA may need assistance with activities of daily living (ADLs) long past the time when other children of the same age are independent. They may have difficulty moving between standing and sitting on the floor, getting into and out of the bed or a bathtub, negotiating steps, and walking long distances. Even children with mild disease may be dependent for some self-care tasks, particularly if parents provide assistance that may be unnecessary. Children may fail to develop gross motor proficiency if parents discourage them from typical childhood activities, such as riding a bike, climbing on playground equipment, or other active play.[63] Most parents are confused as they tend to mix up juvenile idiopathic arthritis with the adult type of rheumatoid arthritis. Research has shown that preschool-age children display greater motor proficiency delays, whereas children at early school age face more delays in activity and participation development.[99] From this cross-sectional study it is not clear if these delays are transient, but clinical observations support the notion that the resilience of children helps them to overcome physical challenges.

The child's participation will also be affected by the extent and quality of supportive services available and utilized by the child and family. Many children who report problems with some aspect of their educational program do not receive related services recommended by the rheumatology team.[57] Tardiness as a result of morning stiffness and frequent absence due to illness or medical appointments may cause the child to miss academic time and social interactions with classmates. Children may feel different and somewhat isolated because they are unable to participate in the same activities as their classmates. Daily fluctuations in disease symptoms may also affect the child's mood and ability to cope.[78] Adolescents with JIA may be unable to gain the same level of independence as their peers because of physical limitations and the need for continued medical care.

FOREGROUND INFORMATION

BODY FUNCTION AND STRUCTURE

Physical Therapy Examination

When examining a child with JIA, the physical therapist has to consider the stage of the disease. In the acute phase the child exhibits a great number of functional limitations, resulting in compensatory motor behavior that will change or disappear when the disease activity is adequately controlled. It is important to understand that physical therapy intervention will be significantly hampered in children with partially controlled or noncontrolled disease. Regular communication between (pediatric) rheumatologist and physical therapist during the acute phase is of utmost importance.

The approach to physical therapy examination in JIA must consider the child's age, motor development before disease onset, and cognitive and emotional development. By first gathering information about the child's activities and participation, the therapist is able to focus the physical examination on impairments that may contribute to the activity limitations or participation restrictions. Monitoring joint motion and integrity is of great importance because loss of range of motion may be the first sign of joint damage and may signal an increased risk for functional decline. Table 7.4 lists standardized outcome instruments that provide quantitative data to guide intervention and evaluate change. A new generation of outcome measures in childhood arthritis has been developed. These are composed of a "composite outcome measure" and a "multidimensional outcome measure"—the Juvenile Arthritis Disease Activity Score (JADAS)[9] and the Juvenile Arthritis Multidimensional Assessment Report (JAMAR),[22] respectively. The JADAS is an outcome measure that scores disease activity on multiple (four) levels. It measures "active joint count," "physician & parent global assessment," and "erythrocyte sedimentation rate" and uses these data to determine one composite score. The JAMAR is a parent- or child-reported measure. It rates the dimensions "well-being," "pain," "functional status," "health-related quality of life," "morning stiffness," "disease activity," "disease status and course," "joint disease," "extra articular symptoms," "side effects of medications," "therapeutic compliance," and "satisfaction with illness outcome" and transfers these into one overall score. The significance of these new outcome measures is that they enable quick and reliable monitoring of both disease status and disease outcome, which is also relevant for the PT.

Pain Examination

Pain is one of the causes of activity restrictions in JIA and is a predictor of the child's adjustment to the disease. Acute pain may result from inflammation and some medical procedures. The cause of chronic pain is less clear, but it may be due at least in part to abnormal joint loading during activity as a result of soft tissue restrictions and muscle imbalance. Older children, especially those with newly diagnosed JIA, report more pain than young children or those with long-standing disease, suggesting that pain perception and report are more closely related to age than to disease severity or duration.[30] Assessment of pain should be ongoing and should include a pain history, a self-report for children over the age of 4 years, a parent report, and behavioral observations. Validated pain behaviors in JIA include bracing, guarding, rubbing, rigidity, and flexing.[40] Self-report tools for young children include the Wong-Baker Faces Rating Scale[108] and the Oucher.[7] The child can also complete a body map, using different colors to represent pain intensity (Fig. 7.6). Children over the age of 7 years can use a numeric rating scale, a horizontal word graphic scale, or a visual analog scale (VAS). This Pain-VAS is also part of Childhood Health Assessment Questionnaire (CHAQ). The Varni/Thompson Pediatric Pain Questionnaire (PPQ)[94] provides a comprehensive assessment with both parent and child reports.

Joint and Muscle Examination

When examining the joints, the physical therapist has to consider the stage of the disease: acute, subacute, or chronic. Each stage of the disease has its typical joint expression. The acute or early phase of the disease is dominated by joint inflammation, joint effusion (fluid can be felt and moved around), ligamentous

TABLE 7.4   Outcome Measurements in Juvenile Idiopathic Arthritis

Outcome	Level of ICF	Measurement	Reference
Disease Activity			
Active joint count	Impairment	ACR joint count	Guzman et al., 1995
Morning stiffness	Impairment	Presence and duration of stiffness	Wright et al., 1996
Global ratings	Impairment	Physician rating on a VAS	Ruperto et al., 1999
Joint range of motion (AAROM or PROM)	Impairment	JC-LOM (ASS) pEPM-ROM GROMS/10-joint GROMS	Klepper et al., 1992; Len et al., 1999; Epps et al., 2002
Muscle strength	Impairment	MMT	Dunn, 1993;
		Handheld dynamometer	Wessel et al., 1999;
		Isokinetic dynamometer	Giannini & Protas, 1993
Grip strength	Impairment	Modified sphygmomanometer or handheld dynamometer	Dunn, 1993
Aerobic fitness	Impairment	Laboratory measures (VO$_2$peak)	Takken et al., 2002
		Standardized walk or run test	Klepper et al., 1992; Takken et al., 2001
Anaerobic fitness	Impairment	Laboratory measures (Wingate Anaerobic Test)	van Brussel et al., 2008
		50-meter sprint	Fan & Wessel, 1998
	Impairment/activity	Physical activity monitoring	Henderson et al., 1995
Gait			
Characteristics of gait pattern	Impairment	Observation	
Time/distance parameters and kinetic parameters	Impairment	Footprint analysis	Wright et al., 1996
		Instrumented gait lab tests	Lechner et al., 1987
Gross and fine motor	Activity	Developmental tests	Morrison et al., 1991; Van der Net et al., 2008
School function	Activity	School checklists	Szer & Wright, 2000
	Activity/participation	School function assessment	Coster et al., 1998
Pain behaviors	Activity	Observation	Jaworski et al., 1995
	Impairment	Child self-report	Beyer et al., 1992; Wong & Baker, 1988; Hester et al., 1990; Thompson & Varni, 1986
	Impairment/activity	Child self-report	Varni et al., 1996
Physical Function			
Parent/child report	Activity	CHAQ	Singh et al., 1994
		JAFAR	Howe et al., 1991
		JASI	Wright et al., 1992
Performance			
Performance	Participation	COPM	Law et al., 2005
Quality of life	Activity	JAFAS	Lovell et al., 1989
Parent/child report	Impairment/activity	JAQQ	Duffy et al., 1997
	Participation	PedsQL	Varni et al., 2002
		QOML scale	Feldman et al., 2000

ACR, American College of Rheumatology; *CHAQ*, Childhood Health Assessment Questionnaire; *COPM*, Canadian Occupational Performance Measure; *GROMS*, Global Range of Motion Scale; *ICF*, International Classification of Functioning, Disability, and Health; *JAFAR*, Juvenile Arthritis Functional Assessment Report; *JAFAS*, Juvenile Arthritis Functional Assessment Scale; *JAQQ*, Juvenile Arthritis Quality of Life Questionnaire; *JASI*, Juvenile Arthritis Functional Status Index; *JC-LOM*, (AS) Joint Count–Limitation of Motion, Articular Severity Score; *MMT*, manual muscle test; *PedsQL*, Pediatric Quality of Life Questionnaire; *pEPM-ROM*, Paediatric Escola Paulista de Medicina–Range of Motion Scale; *QOML*, Quality of MyLife Scale; *VAS*, visual analog scale; VO$_2$peak, peak oxygen uptake.

laxity, and joint instability (can be felt when moving the distal joint parts along its axis). In the subacute and chronic phases, the inflammation has become prolonged (longer than 3 months), leading to joint swelling due to synovial hypertrophy (has a doughy feel) and loss of joint integrity, such as loss of normal joint physiology, erosive changes in cartilage, and loss of joint alignment. During joint examination, special attention should be paid to these typical disease expressions.

Joint counts for swelling (JC-S) and limitation of motion (JC-LOM) are recorded on a stick figure to document disease activity and joint restrictions (Fig. 7.7). Fig. 7.8 shows two methods of verifying a joint effusion by observing fluctuations of fluid from one area of the joint to another, eliciting a bulge

sign. To detect an effusion in the knee, the synovial pouch medial to the patella is emptied by stroking in an upward direction and then is refilled by stroking along the lateral border in an upward or downward direction.

Active joint motion can be estimated by watching the child perform a series of movements during various childhood activities, but goniometric measurement is necessary to document limited joint motion.[31] Two standardized measures of the JC-LOM are the Articular Severity Score (ASS) and the Global Range of Motion Score (GROMS). The ASS scores global range of motion (ROM) for each joint, averaged for the right and left sides, on a 5-point scale (0 = no LOM; 1 = 25% LOM; 2 = 50% LOM; 3 = 75% LOM; and 4 = fused). In contrast, the GROMS

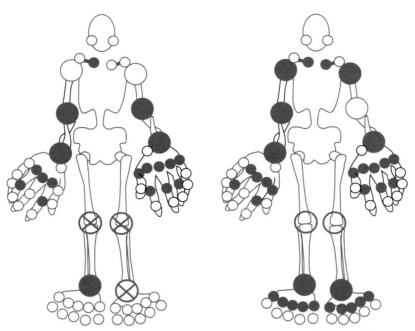

FIG. 7.6 Example of active joint count in a child with polyarticular disease. There are 38 active joints. The left figure shows 22 with effusion *(●)* or soft tissue swelling *(X)*. The right figure shows joints with stress pain or tenderness *(●)*. (From Wright FV, Smith E: Physical therapy management of the child and adolescent with juvenile rheumatoid arthritis. In Walker JM, Helewa A, editors: *Physical therapy in arthritis.* Philadelphia: WB Saunders; 1996. p 215.)

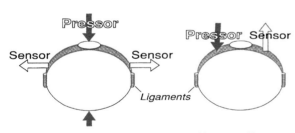

FIG. 7.7 Two ways of detecting joint effusions. Two ways of detecting joint effusions. (From Smythe HA, Helewa A: Assessment of joint disease. In Walker JM, Helewa A, editors: *Physical therapy in arthritis.* Philadelphia: WB Saunders; 1996. p 133.)

provides a single score for global joint function. Each joint movement is weighted from 0 (least important) to 5 (essential), based on expert opinion of its functional importance. The examiner records the mean ROM in degrees for the right and left sides. The ratio of the measured value to the normative value is calculated to obtain the joint movement score. The total GROMS is calculated as the sum for all movements multiplied by 100 and divided by the number of movements (Table 7.5).

A reduced 10-joint version of the GROMS is also available that includes only those joint motions weighted as 5 (essential) on the original GROMS. The total score is calculated using the same method as the full scale. The Pediatric Escola Paulista de Medicina ROM Scale (pEPM-ROM)[54] also includes 10 essential joint movements but uses predetermined cutoff points for scoring (0 = full motion to 3 = severe limitation). The total score (0 to 3) for each side of the body is the sum of all joint scores divided by 10. Each scale demonstrates adequate concurrent validity with other measures of disease status and function in JIA.[18]

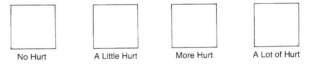

| No Hurt | A Little Hurt | More Hurt | A Lot of Hurt |

Pick the colors that mean *No Hurt, A Little Hurt, More Hurt,* and *A Lot of Hurt* to you and color in the boxes. Now, using those colors, color in the body to show how you feel. Where you have no hurt, use the *No Hurt* color to color in your body. If you have hurt or pain, use the color that tells how much hurt you have.

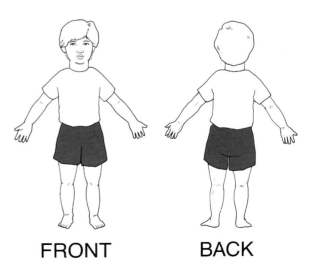

FRONT   BACK

FIG. 7.8 Pain may be assessed by allowing the child to color a body map. Intensity of pain is matched with four different colors.

TABLE 7.5 **Calculating a GROMS Using All Joint Movements Except the Lumbar and Thoracic Spine[a]**

Joint Movement	A Measured	B Normative	C A + B	D Mode	E C × D
Cx spine extension	30	45	0.66	4	2.64
Cx spine rotation	60	80	0.75	4	3
Shoulder flexion	142.5	180	0.79	4	3.16
Shoulder abduction	180	180	1.00	4	4
Shoulder ER	85	85	1.00	3	3
Shoulder IR	70	70	1.00	3	3
Elbow extension	145	145	1.00	3	3
Elbow flexion	145	145	1.00	5	5
R/U supination	90	90	1.00	4	4
R/U pronation	90	90	1.00	4	4
Wrist flexion	67.5	90	0.75	3	2.25
Wrist extension	27.5	90	0.31	5	1.55
MCP (2–5)	68.75	90	0.76	5	3.8
PIP (2–5)	72.5	100	0.73	5	3.65
DIP (2–5)	47.5	90	0.53	4	2.12
Thumb flexion	20	70	0.29	5	1.45
Thumb abduction	30	50	0.60	5	3
Thumb DIP 1	30	90	0.33	2	0.66
Hip flexion	135	135	1.00	5	5
Hip extension	150	155	0.97	5	4.85
Hip abduction	50	50	1.00	4	4
Hip IR	15	45	0.33	2	0.66
Hip ER	40	45	0.88	4	3.52
Knee flexion	145	145	1.00	5	5
Knee extension	145	145	1.00	5	5
Ankle dorsiflexion	20	20	1.00	4	4
Ankle plantar flexion	50	55	0.91	4	3.64

From Epps H, Hurley M, Utley M: Development and evaluation of a single value score to assess global range of motion in juvenile idiopathic arthritis. *Arthritis Care Res* 47:398, 2002. Reprinted by permission of Wiley-Liss Inc, a subsidiary of John Wiley & Sons, Inc.
[a]*GROMS*, Global Range of Motion Scale; *Mode* = weighted value for joint movement based upon experts' opinion of its functional importance.
Cx, cervical; *ER*, external rotation; *IR*, internal rotation; *MCP*, metacarpophalangeal; *PIP*, proximal interphalangeal; *DIP*, distal interphalangeal; *RU*, radio-ulnar.

Excellent test-retest and intertester agreement are reported for the pEPM-ROM.[54] Testing of the 10-joint GROMS continues. Although a reduced JC-LOM saves time during the examination, it may not be appropriate for patients whose arthritis is extensive or does not affect any of the 10 joints measured.

Periarticular muscles may show decreased flexibility due to contractures or "contraction deformities." This can be tested with a "sit-and-reach test" including all lower limb, dorsal trunk, and upper limb muscles in a "functional manner" or per joint. In the latter case it is important to follow the procedures for muscle length testing as described, for example, by Kendall and Kendall.

Physical Fitness Examination

Many centers do not have the equipment to perform respiratory gas analysis to measure VO_2peak. However, peak workload (Wpeak) during a graded bicycle test can be used as a surrogate measure for VO_2peak because an excellent correlation between Wpeak and VO_2peak ($r = 0.95$, $P < 0.0001$) has been observed in 92 children with JIA (Takken et al, unpublished observations). VO_2peak can be predicted from Wpeak, weight, and gender using the following equation (ref 16a):

$$VO_2peak\,(L/min) = 0.308 + 0.146 \times sex\,(0 = female,\ 1 = male) + 0.005 \times weight\,(kg) + 0.008 \times W\,(peak)\,(W)$$

Activity
Performance-Related Fitness Examination
Performance-related fitness includes components like muscle strength and anaerobic capacity. Impairments in muscle strength include weakness in hip extension and abduction, knee extension, plantar flexion, shoulder abduction and flexion, elbow flexion and extension, wrist extension, and grip. Muscle bulk, strength, and endurance should be examined at disease onset and monitored regularly. Bilateral measurements of circumference quantify asymmetries in muscle bulk. Functional muscle strength can be estimated in young children by observing their performance of age-appropriate motor tasks or ADLs. In older children, manual muscle testing can be done to measure isometric strength, especially if the child has pain while moving the limb against resistance. Instrumented measurements using a handheld or isokinetic dynamometer or a modified sphygmomanometer[104] provide consistent and reliable information in individuals with arthritis.

Muscle strength testing in children with JIA, especially handheld dynamometry using the "break" technique, might be problematic in some cases because children might give way as a result of pain instead of the limits in muscle strength.[107]

Dynamic muscle testing of functional muscle groups can be performed when there is no sign of joint inflammation or damage. The maximal weight the child can lift throughout the available ROM for 10 to 15 repetitions (6 to 10 repetition maximum [RM]) is usually sufficient to establish a baseline level of strength and monitor change.[49] An alternative method for children who have pain on movement is to measure isometric strength at multiple angles throughout the ROM. Muscular endurance can be measured by having the child perform as many repetitions as possible at a specified percentage (60% to 80%) of the 6 to 10 RM. A warm-up period of light activity should precede strength testing.

One study suggested that muscle weakness may contribute to activity restrictions in children with arthritis. Fan and colleagues[21] found a significant relationship between 50-meter run times and lower extremity CHAQ scores in girls with JIA.

Two studies investigating anaerobic capacity in children and adolescents with JIA reported significantly lower values of anaerobic capacity in subjects with JIA.[53,97] Anaerobic capacity was reduced to the same extent as aerobic fitness (VO_2peak). Previously, it was found that reduced anaerobic capacity was significantly correlated with CHAQ scores in 18 children with juvenile arthritis, age 7 to 14 years.[93] This is not surprising in that the typical physical activity behavior of children—short bursts of intense activity separated by periods of rest—is anaerobic in nature.[6] Given the apparently similar deficits in anaerobic capacity of youth with JIA, exercise training of the anaerobic energy system (e.g., high-intensity interval training) might be equally as valuable as training of the aerobic system and therefore warranted in children with arthritis. However, this training modality has not yet been studied.

Another widely used performance-related fitness test is the 6-minute walk test (6MWT). In this test, children have to cover as much distance as they can in 6 minutes by walking (not running). This test is used in different patient groups such as JIA, spina bifida, cerebral palsy, and hemophilia.[32,79,95] Lelieveld et al. found a low correlation between walking distance and VO_2peak in children with JIA.[52] In addition, Paap et al. found that children with JIA were exercising at 80% to 85% of their HRpeak and VO_2peak during the 6MWT, indicating that it is an intensive, submaximal exercise test used to measure functional exercise capacity in children with JIA.[68] Furthermore, these data indicate that exercise intensity at the end of the 6MWT can be used for the programming of exercise intensity during aerobic exercise training in children with JIA because this intensity is also sufficient to improve fitness levels.

Activity and Participation
Activity and Participation Examination
Several standardized instruments examine the child's activities. The CHAQ, a measure of physical function designed for children age 1 to 19 years, includes 30 activities organized into eight categories.[82] The respondent (parent or child 9 years or older) scores each item based on how much difficulty the child had performing the task during the past week (0 = without any difficulty; 1 = with some difficulty; 2 = with much difficulty; 3 = unable to do). An item is scored as "not applicable" if the child has difficulty because he is too young. The highest scored item in each section determines the score for that category. If the child needs an assistive device or help from another person to perform a task, the score for that category is at least 2. The Disability Index (DI), calculated as the average score for the eight categories, has a range of 0 to 3. Higher scores indicate greater disability. The CHAQ also includes a question about the presence and duration of morning stiffness and VASs to measure pain intensity and general health status. Recently, the CHAQ has been revised and extended with eight more physically demanding items to meet the challenges of a more physical active lifestyle in children with rheumatic conditions.[50]

Other questionnaires designed to measure physical function include the Juvenile Arthritis Functional Assessment Index (JASI)[110] and the Juvenile Arthritis Functional Assessment Report (JAFAR).[37] A school checklist can be used to examine school-related problems.[87] The School Function Assessment may also be useful[14] (See Chapter 2 for more detail). Two other instruments measure both physical function and quality of life (QOL) in children with JIA. These are the Juvenile Arthritis Quality of Life Questionnaire (JAQQ)[16] and the Pediatric Quality of Life Inventory (PedsQL).[101] The only instrument that measures the child's actual performance is the Juvenile Arthritis Functional Assessment Scale (JAFAS). The child is observed and timed while completing 10 tasks. The score is 0 if the time to complete the task is equal to or less than the criterion time, 1 if the time exceeds the criterion, and 2 if the child cannot perform the task. The test takes 10 minutes and requires a minimum of simple equipment.[59]

PHYSICAL THERAPY INTERVENTION

The focus of physical therapy during the acute stage of the disease is different from that during the subacute and chronic stages. While in the acute phase, efforts are focused on maintaining and preserving joint function; in the subacute and chronic stages, the focus is on restoration and compensation of function and activities.

The overall goals of physical therapy are to restore and optimize the child's activity, participation, and physical health by maintaining or improving function and providing education and support to the child and family. Box 7.2 illustrates the physical therapy intervention in JIA. Intervention is geared to each child's physical, cognitive, and social development and must also consider the family's cultural background. Physical activity and graded exercise are essential to manage the effect of the disease and to maintain optimal health. Exercise in a warm pool, where the buoyancy of the water allows easier movement, is especially recommended during the acute inflammatory stage of joint disease. Most children with mild to moderate JIA can also participate in land-based exercise.

Adherence to the therapeutic regimen is extremely important. Home exercise programs may be necessary but are often a source of conflict between the parent and the child. Giving the child some control over the exercise program—for example, choosing the time and place to exercise—may improve adherence. Older children can collaborate with the parent and therapist to set goals and plan intervention.

Body Function and Structures
Management of Joint Health
Physical measures used in the management of joint health include cold, exercise, and occasional splinting. There is no place for superficial or deep heat application in the management of arthritis. Studies have shown that intra-articular inflammation is increased when these modalities are used.[66,67] Ultrasound and short wave diathermy are not used in children. A study by Wiltink et al.[106] has suggested that these modalities may harm endochondral ossification and the proliferation of epithelial cells.

BOX 7.2   Interventions for Juvenile Idiopathic Arthritis

Coordination, Communication, and Documentation
Anticipated Goals
Care is coordinated with child, family, school, and other professionals.
Insurance payer understands needed rehabilitation services.
Need for modifications in school is determined.
Available resources are maximally utilized.
Decision making regarding child's health, wellness, and fitness needs is enhanced.

Specific Interventions
Communication with community therapist, school personnel, and community resource providers
Prescriptions and letters of medical necessity to support rehabilitation needs
Individualized education plan (IEP); accommodations under Section 504 of Rehabilitation Act

Patient-Related Instruction
Anticipated Goals
Awareness and use of community resources are increased.
Behaviors that protect joints from secondary impairments are enhanced.
Functional independence in activities of daily living (ADLs) is increased.
Patient and family knowledge of the diagnosis, prognosis, interventions, and goals and outcomes are increased.

Specific Interventions
Home exercise program
Instruction regarding joint protection principles
Information from the Arthritis Foundation regarding disease
Referrals to other community resources

Therapeutic Exercise
Anticipated Goals
Ability to perform physical tasks related to self-care, home management, community and school integration, and leisure activities is increased.
Aerobic capacity is increased.
Gait is improved.
Joint and soft tissue swelling, inflammation, or restriction is reduced.
Joint integrity and mobility are improved.
Pain is decreased.
Postural control is improved.
Strength, power, and endurance are improved.

Specific Interventions
Aerobic conditioning
Aquatic exercise
Low-impact weight-bearing exercise
Gait training
Body mechanics training
Postural training
Strengthening, power, and endurance training
Active-assistive, active, and resistive exercise
Task-specific performance training
Flexibility exercise
Muscle lengthening
Range of motion
Static progressive stretching
Balance, coordination, and agility training

Functional Training in Self-Care and Home Management
Anticipated Goals
Ability to perform physical tasks related to self-care and home management is increased.
Level of supervision required for task performance is decreased.
Risk of secondary impairment is reduced.

Specific Interventions
ADL training
Assistive and adaptive device or equipment training
Self-care or home management task adaptation
Leisure and play recommendations
Orthotic, protective, or supportive device or equipment training
Injury prevention training

Functional Training in School, Play, Community, and Leisure Integration
Anticipated Goals
School attendance is improved.
Participation in peer groups for recreation and leisure activity is improved.
Architectural barriers to access home, school, and community resources are removed.

Specific Interventions
Appropriate transportation plan to school identified on IEP
Modifications to school instruction identified on IEP
ADL training
Assistive and adaptive device or equipment training
Adaptation of equipment to allow inclusion in recreation and leisure activity
Home and school site visit to plan for accommodation of any architectural barriers

Prescription, Application, and Fabrication of Devices and Equipment
Anticipated Goals
Ability to perform physical tasks is increased.
Deformities are prevented.
Gait is improved.
Joint stability is increased.
Optimal joint alignment is achieved.
Pain is decreased.
Protection of body parts is increased.

Specific Interventions
Adaptive devices or equipment
Assistive devices or equipment (ambulation aids, wheelchairs, ADL equipment)
Splints and orthotic devices (shoe inserts, resting splints, dynamic splints, braces)
Protective devices (splints, taping, elbow or knee pads)
Supportive devices (compression garments, cervical collars)

Electrotherapeutic Modalities
Anticipated Goals
Muscle performance is increased.
Pain is decreased.

Specific Interventions
Biofeedback

Physical Agents and Mechanical Modalities
Anticipated Goals
Pain is decreased.
Soft tissue swelling, inflammation, or restriction is reduced.
Tolerance to positions and activities is increased.
Joint integrity and mobility are improved.

Specific Interventions
Cryotherapy (RICE—rest, ice, compression, elevation)
Hydrotherapy (aquatic therapy, whirlpool tanks)
Continuous passive motion devices

Modified from Scull S: Juvenile rheumatoid arthritis. In: Campbell S, Vander Linden D, Palisano R, editors: *Physical therapy for children.* 2nd ed. Philadelphia: WB Saunders; 2000. p 245.

Balanced rest and exercise are important in managing joint health and function in JIA. Children who participate in group aquatic or land-based exercise programs report decreased pain.[5,23,44,91] Restful sleep helps to reduce morning stiffness and pain. Sleep time fragmentation is observed to have a relationship with disease symptoms and may corrupt daytime performance.[85] Custom-made resting splints can support joints, may preserve function, and may relieve pain during the night.

When ROM exercises are indicated to preserve joint motion and soft tissue extensibility, active ROM is preferred. Several studies have shown that passive movements of inflamed joints evoke an increase in the release of the proinflammatory peptide substance P,[61] resulting in more pain and inflammation. The child can also be taught combination patterns cloaked in games that encourage motion in several joints at once.

Application of passive corrective modalities demands careful consideration of the biomechanical forces that result from the application. Precautions should be taken not to induce a subluxation or to overload joint parts.

Muscle Strength

Limited evidence suggests the effectiveness of muscle strength training for children with JIA. A recent randomized controlled trial studied muscle strength training in children with JIA within the context of an exercise program.[77] Muscle strength in hip and knee extensors increased after the 12-week program and this was maintained in knee extensors at follow-up.

Strengthening exercises target the muscles surrounding and supporting the joints with arthritis and adjacent areas. During acute joint inflammation, isometric exercise can be used to maintain muscle bulk and strength. Prolonged maximal isometric contractions should be avoided because they may increase intra-articular pressure and constrict blood flow through the muscles.[41] EMG biofeedback may be helpful in training the child to regulate the intensity of the contraction.

Dynamic exercise is added when joint inflammation subsides. Both concentric and eccentric exercises are included. External resistance can be safely added once the child is able to correctly perform light activities against gravity without pain.[62]

Clear directions and illustrations of the exercises are necessary, and training sessions should be supervised. Progression is based on periodic reassessment. Each training session should begin with light aerobic and flexibility activities and end with cool-down and stretching activities. Resistance exercises should be performed twice a week, allowing time between sessions for rest and recovery.[20]

Aerobic Capacity

A Cochrane review identified only three published randomized controlled studies investigating the effects of exercise training for children with JIA.[90] None of these studies found improvements in VO_2peak after the aerobic training program was completed. This lack of effect can be owed to a low exercise frequency (e.g., one time a week), a low exercise intensity (intensity of exercise has to be above the intensity of daily activities), or a low exercise adherence (children often skipped exercise sessions), or it may indicate that children did not perform the prescribed home exercises. However, aerobic fitness is important to improve the child's endurance for routine physical activities and play. In addition, aerobic fitness helps the recovery after intensive exercise. Based on the available literature, it is recommended that children with JIA and a deficit in aerobic fitness should train at least two times a week, with moderate to vigorous intensity (60% to 85% HRpeak), for 45 to 60 minutes per session for at least 6 to 12 weeks.[45,46,88] The specific mode of exercise appears to be less important than the intensity, duration, and frequency. However, weight-bearing exercise is necessary to maintain optimal bone growth and density. Low-impact activities to improve proprioceptive function, balance, and coordination can be incorporated into aerobic fitness training programs. However, not only strenuous activities produce improved aerobic outcome but also more gentle types of exercise such as Qigong, as was shown by Stephens et al.[84]

Anaerobic Capacity

In a study, van Brussel et al.[98] hypothesized that training of the anaerobic energy system (e.g., high-intensity interval training) might be equally valuable as training of the aerobic system and therefore warranted in children with JIA. Although this training modality has not yet been studied in children with JIA, improvements have been observed in function and fitness with anaerobic exercise training in children with other chronic conditions (e.g., cystic fibrosis, cerebral palsy).[47,102] Particularly in children with a larger reduction in anaerobic capacity compared with aerobic capacity, this training modality might be effective. In addition, children prefer this anaerobic type of exercise over the adult type of approach of continuous endurance exercise. The suggested exercise set consists of 15 high-intensity cycling sprints (15 to 30 seconds all out); each sprint is followed by 1 to 2 minutes of active rest (cycling with low resistance). A training session could consist of three of these exercise sets, with 5 minutes of active rest for recovery between the three sets of interval training.

Activity and Participation
Encouraging Active-Healthy Living

Several studies have identified a hypoactive lifestyle of children with JIA.[34,51,92] A significant association has been reported between accelerometry-measured physical activity and health-related fitness (VO_2peak) in children with JIA,[92] suggesting a cause–effect relationship. In addition, no adverse effects of regular sport activity have been observed on joint scores in children with JIA.[43] The link between physical activity levels of children and motor performance[111] suggests that the physical activity levels of children with JIA might be enhanced by improvements in reduced motor proficiency observed in children with JIA.[99] Further, given the fact that adult physical activity levels are established in youth, it is important to encourage children and families of children with JIA to participate in regular physical activity. Regular physical activity can help in the prevention of cardiovascular risk factors, obesity, and reduced bone health, as well as reduced health-related quality of life, in youth with JIA. Physical therapists should reassure parents and stimulate an active-healthy lifestyle as soon as possible.

Self-Care Activities

A primary goal for every child with a chronic condition is to achieve independence in self-care within the home, school, and community. Expectations for independence differ at each age and stage of development. It has been reported that ambulation skills in children with JIA are delayed as early as 4 years of age.[99] This is in contrast with preschool age children, who show more limitations in motor proficiency and in the development of motor milestones.[99] Intervention for an infant with JIA may include suggestions to prevent contractures and facilitate function. A child with limited grasp may benefit from adapted toys. Functional wrist and hand splints can support the joint during hand use, and assistive devices can compensate for a weak grip and reduce hand pain and fatigue. Dressing and hygiene aids include Velcro closures on clothing and shoes, elastic shoelaces, a long-handled shoehorn, a dressing stick, a buttonhook, a zipper pull, and a long-handled bath brush. Built-up handles on grooming items, eating utensils, and writing implements may be necessary for optimal function and independence.

Some modifications within the home may be beneficial, including replacing knobs and faucets with levers, using a jar opener or an electric can opener, adding a raised toilet seat, and installing safety bars in the bathtub. More substantial modifications, including widening doorways and adding a ramp to the entrance, are needed for a child who must use a wheelchair. The therapist must consider the financial, physical, and emotional impact of these changes on the family. The device or adaptation must be affordable and must achieve the stated purpose, be easy to use, and be acceptable to the child and parent. When considering substantial modifications, it is of critical importance to be informed about the prognosis of the course of the disease. Temporary exacerbations may introduce the need for a wheelchair, but most do not need structural changes in and around home.

Functional Mobility

Weight bearing and ambulation are vital for optimal bone growth and density, joint health, and muscle development. Standing, cruising, and walking should be encouraged at the expected age, although the use of infant walkers should be avoided because they may promote an abnormal gait pattern and carry a high risk for injury. Toddlers and preschool-age children should be encouraged to walk within the home and short distances outside. Shoes should support and cushion the joints of the feet and accommodate any deformities. Sneakers with a flexible sole, good arch support, and high heel cup are good choices for most children. A wide, deep toe box may be necessary for a child with swelling in the forefoot joints or hallux valgus, hammer toes, or claw toes. A child with arthritis in the feet and toes should not wear high heels because of the excessive pressure on the MCP joints. A rockerlike addition to the sole of the shoe may provide a mechanical assist at toe-off for a child who has limited or painful toe hyperextension. Custom molded in-shoe orthoses can replace the standard insole to accommodate foot deformities and decrease pressure on those tender joints and provide relief in the majority of the cases.

Few children with JIA require an assistive device for ambulation. However, if a child begins to show problems with weight bearing or difficulty walking, the cause should be determined and addressed. Leg length differences can be accommodated by placing a lift inside the shoe or on the sole of the shoe on the shorter side. A child with unilateral lower extremity pain or weakness can use a cane or elbow crutch on the opposite side to unload the involved limb and increase stability during ambulation. A walker or crutches may be needed if problems are bilateral. Platform attachments can be added if the child has upper limb impairments.

Some children may need to use a form of wheeled mobility for long distances within the school or community environment. A wagon or stroller with a firm seat and back is appropriate for toddlers or preschool-age children. Older children can use a tricycle or a bicycle with training wheels to get around the community. A power-assisted bicycle may facilitate ambulation in the wider neighborhood and allow for peer contact. A nonpowered two-wheeled scooter allows younger children to propel themselves with their feet without weight bearing. A powered scooter or lightweight wheelchair may be necessary for efficient mobility in school. Children with upper extremity arthritis often maneuver the wheelchair with their feet. Powered wheelchairs are usually reserved for children with severe impairments but may be necessary for a college student who must negotiate a large campus. Children who use a wheelchair should spend part of every day out of the chair, standing and walking to preserve bone health, prevent contractures, and maintain walking tolerance.

Issues Related to School

Children with JIA may need occasional modifications to their school program. These might include a second set of books for home, built-up or adapted writing tools, or an easel top for the desk in the classroom. Children with significant hand arthritis may need to record class notes on a tape recorder or word processor and take tests under untimed conditions. Modifications to the school schedule may include time out of the classroom to take medication or rest for brief periods during the day, extra time to travel between classes, or permission to use an elevator if the child is unable to negotiate stairs. Some schools provide these services voluntarily. In other situations, the child may need an individualized educational plan (IEP) or accommodations specified under Section 504 of the Vocational Rehabilitation Act. Vocational counseling is often necessary to prepare adolescents for the transition to higher education and work. Although most states mandate transition planning, Lovell and colleagues[62,64] found that only 8% of children with JIA received vocational counseling. A recent review underlines the paucity of studies examining the early employment experiences of young adults with arthritis. The employment status found in the review ranged from 11% to 71%, and although not always statistically significant, young adults with arthritis were less likely to be employed when compared to their healthy peers. Greater disease severity, less educational attainment, and being female were related to not participating in paid work.[41]

Regular participation in physical education is encouraged. The instructor should be aware of the child's diagnosis and any activity restrictions or precautions. In general, the child should be allowed to monitor his or her own activity level, resting as needed. However, some activities may be strongly discouraged because of their potential for injury or joint damage. These activities include headstands and somersaults; handstands, push-ups, cartwheels, and other similar activities in a child with wrist and hand arthritis; and high-impact running or jumping in a child with spinal or lower extremity arthritis. The therapist can consult with the physical education instructor to modify activities as necessary.

Recreational Activities

Recreational activities provide physical and psychosocial benefits. The choice of activities depends on the child's preferences, physical status, motor skills, and fitness level. Participation on any given day sometimes must be modified to accommodate disease symptoms. Websites such as PRINTO provide updated evidence-based and expert-based recommendations for exercise and sports for parents.[38] Swimming, water or low-impact weight-bearing aerobics, and bicycling provide good cardiovascular exercise. Activities that cause high-impact loading on inflamed or damaged joints should be avoided. Contact sports, including football, hockey, and boxing, and those with a high inherent potential for injury should be carefully evaluated with child and parents and may be ultimately discouraged. Competitive team sports may be physically and emotionally stressful, but each situation should be evaluated individually.

A physical conditioning program before participating in a sport prepares the child for the physical demands of the activity. Warm-up before each practice session or game and a cool-down period after the activity should be encouraged. Instruction in motor skills specific to the sport may be necessary. A sports orthosis or other adaptive equipment may improve joint alignment and stability and is therefore helpful to secure joint health.

ORTHOPEDIC SURGERY AND THE ROLE OF THE PHYSICAL THERAPIST

Orthopedic surgery in children with JIA has become rare over the last decades because more powerful immunosuppressive and immunomodulatory medication results in earlier remission, less extensive joint damage, and fewer growth disturbances in most children.

Total joint arthroplasty (TJA) is considered in the chronic stage of the disease when there is irreversible joint damage and the child has significant pain and functional limitation. The procedure is most frequently performed at the hip and knee, although prostheses are available for other joints. Several factors are considered in the decision, including the child's age, skeletal maturity, general physical status, upper extremity function, and ability to successfully complete the lengthy and intensive postoperative rehabilitation regimen. Customized computer-designed prostheses may be necessary to accommodate changes in joint anatomy, small bone size, and osteoporosis. The longevity of the prosthesis must also be considered, especially when TJA is performed in young children. Procedures are staged if the child requires extensive surgery to ensure the best functional outcome.

■ SUMMARY

JIA is an autoimmune inflammatory disorder and the most common rheumatic disease of childhood. Although the exact cause is unclear, three major distinct onset types are recognized: systemic, polyarticular, and oligoarticular. With advances in the recognition and diagnosis of the disease and more effective medications to treat joint inflammation, most children with JIA do well with early diagnosis and appropriate treatment. However, for many children, JIA results in both short- and long-term problems, including chronic joint swelling, pain, and limited motion, as well as muscle atrophy and weakness, poor aerobic function, and impaired exercise tolerance. General and localized growth disturbances, postural abnormalities, and gait deviations occur with persistent disease. Activity and participation restrictions that result from the arthritis and extra-articular manifestations can negatively affect the child's quality of life. The long-term prognosis depends upon the child's age at disease onset, onset geno- and phenotype, severity and duration of active inflammation, and quality and consistency of medical care and other resources available and utilized by the family.

This chapter reviews the most common characteristics of JIA, standardized examination and outcome measures developed for use in children with arthritis, and current research findings regarding the effects of exercise and physical activity in individuals with chronic inflammatory arthritis. Physical therapists are vital members of the pediatric rheumatology team, providing examination, evaluation, and intervention, and monitoring joint health, physical function, and physical health in a child with JIA. Therapists also serve as an important resource to parents or caregivers and school and community personnel to adapt activities so the child with JIA can participate fully in the home, school, and community environments.

ACKNOWLEDGMENT

Susan E. Klepper, PhD, PT, for her valuable contributions of this chapter in four consecutive editions of this textbook. We have continued to build on her text.

CASE SCENARIOS

Two case scenarios with video are presented. The first case is a toddler with lower extremity involvement. Part 1 of this case illustrates the importance of careful observations during movement to structure the examinations based on the topographic distribution of impaired joints. Part 2 of this illustrates interventions specific to the examination findings with attention to the biomechanical consequences of inflamed joints.

The second case is a teenager with a more severe polyarticular presentation. Examination findings and therapy interventions across ICF domains are discussed.

REFERENCES

1. Reference deleted in proofs.
2. Ansell BM, Rudge S, Schaller JG: *Color atlas of pediatric rheumatology*, London, 1992, Wolfe Publishing Limited, pp 13–75.
3. Reference deleted in proofs.
4. Atwood M: Developmental assessment and integration. In Melvin J, editor: *Rheumatic disease in adult and child: occupational therapy and rehabilitation*, ed 3, Philadelphia, 1989, FA Davis, pp 188–214.
5. Bacon M, Nicholson C, Binder H, White P: Juvenile rheumatoid arthritis: aquatic exercise and lower extremity function, *Arthritis Care Res* 4:102–105, 1991.
6. Bailey RC, Olson J, Pepper SL, Porszasz J, Barstow TJ, Cooper DM: The level and tempo of children's physical activities: an observational study, *Med Sci Sports and Exerc* 27:1033–1041, 1995.
7. Beyer JE, Denyes MJ, Villarruel AM: The creation, validation, and continuing development of the Oucher: a measure of pain intensity in children, *J Pediatr Nurs* 7:335–346, 1992.
8. Brewer EJ, Bass J, Baum J, Cassidy JT, Fink C, Jacobs J, et al.: Current proposed revision of JRA criteria, *Arthritis Rheum* 20(Suppl 2):195–202, 1977.
9. Bulatović Calasan M, de Vries LD, Vastert SJ, Heijstek MW, Wulffraat NM: Interpretation of the Juvenile Arthritis Disease Activity Score: responsiveness, clinically important differences and levels of disease activity in prospective cohorts of patients with juvenile idiopathic arthritis, *Rheumatology (Oxford)* 53:307–312, 2014.
10. Burnham JM, Shults J, Dubner SE, Sembhi H, Zemel BS, Leonard MB: Bone density, structure, and strength in juvenile idiopathic arthritis: importance of disease severity and muscle deficits, *Arthritis Rheum* 58:2518–2527, 2008.
11. Cassidy JT, Petty RE: Juvenile rheumatoid arthritis. In Cassidy JT, Petty RE, Laxer RM, Lindsley CB, editors: *Textbook of pediatric rheumatology*, ed 6, Philadelphia, 2011, WB Saunders, pp 212–297.

12. Childhood Arthritis and Rheumatology Research Alliance (CARRA). Available from: URL:https://www.carragroup.org.

13. Reference deleted in proofs.

14. Coster W, Deeney T, Haltiwanger J, Haley S: *School function assessment*, Boston, MA, 1998, Harcourt Brace.

15. De Backer IC, Singh-Grewal D, Helders PJ, Takken T: Can peak work rate predict peak oxygen uptake in children with juvenile idiopathic arthritis? *Arthritis Care Res (Hoboken)* 62:960–964, 2010.

16. Duffy CM, Arsenault HL, Duffy KN, Paquin JD, Strawczynski H: The Juvenile Arthritis Quality of Life Questionnaire-Development of a new responsive index for juvenile rheumatoid arthritis and juvenile spondyloarthritis, *J Rheumatol* 24:738–746, 1997.

17. Emery HM: The rehabilitation of the child with juvenile chronic arthritis, *Bailliere's Clinical Pediatrics* 1:803–823, 1993.

18. Epps H, Hurley M, Utley M: Development and evaluation of a single score to assess global range of motion in juvenile rheumatoid arthritis, *Arthritis Care Res* 47:398–402, 2002.

19. European League Against Rheumatism: *EULAR bulletin no. 4: nomenclature and classification of arthritis in children*, Basel, 1977, National Zeitung AG.

20. Faigenbaum AD, Milliken LA, Loud RL, Burak BT, Doherty CL, Westcott WL: Comparison of 1 and 2 days per week of strength training in children, *Res Q Exerc Sport* 73:416–424, 2002.

21. Fan J, Wessel J, Ellsworth J: The relationship between strength and function in females with juvenile rheumatoid arthritis, *J Rheumatol* 3:1399–1405, 1998.

22. Filocamo G, Consolaro A, Schiappapietra B, Dalprà S, Lattanzi B, Magni-Manzoni S, et al.: A new approach to clinical care of juvenile idiopathic arthritis: the Juvenile Arthritis Multidimensional Assessment Report, *J Rheumatol* 38:938–953, 2011.

23. Fisher NM, Venkatraman JT, O'Neil K: The effects of resistance exercises on muscle and immune function in juvenile arthritis, *Arthritis Rheum* 44:S276, 2001.

24. Giannini EJ, Ruperto N, Ravelli A, Lovell DJ, Felson DT, Martini A: Preliminary definition of improvement in juvenile arthritis, *Arthritis Rheum* 40:1202–1209, 1997.

25. Giannini MJ, Protas EJ: Aerobic capacity in juvenile rheumatoid arthritis patients and healthy children, *Arthritis Care Res* 4:131–135, 1991.

26. Giannini MJ, Protas EJ: Exercise response in children with and without juvenile rheumatoid arthritis: a case comparison study, *Phys Ther* 72:365–372, 1992.

27. Reference deleted in proofs.

28. Guzman J, Oen K, Tucker LB, et al.: For the ReACCh-investigators. The outcomes of juvenile idiopathic arthritis in children managed with contemporary treatments from the ReACCh-Out cohort, *Ann Rheum Dis* 74:1854–1860, 2015.

29. Reference deleted in proofs.

30. Hagglund KJ, Schopp LM, Alberts KR, Cassidy JT, Frank RG: Predicting pain among children with juvenile rheumatoid arthritis, *Arthritis Care Res* 8:36–42, 1995.

31. Hansmann S, Benseler SM, Kuemmerle-Dreschner JB: Dynamic knee joint function in children with juvenile idiopathic arthritis (JIA), *Pediatr Rheumatol Online J* 13:8, 2015, http://dx.doi.org/10.1186/s12969-015-0004-1.

32. Hassan J, van der Net J, Helders PJ, Prakken BJ, Takken T: Six-minute walk test in children with chronic conditions, *Brit J Sports Med* 44:270–274, 2010.

33. Helders PJ, Nieuwenhuis MK, van der Net J, Kramer PP, Kuis W, Buchanon T: Displacement response of juvenile arthritic wrists during grasp, *Arthritis Care Res* 13:375–381, 2000.

34. Henderson CJ, Lovell DJ, Specker BL, Campaigne BN: Physical activity in children with juvenile rheumatoid arthritis: quantification and evaluation, *Arthritis Care Res* 8:114–119, 1995.

35. Hendrengren E, Knutson LM, Haglund-Akerlind Y, Hagelberg S: Lower extremity isometric torque in children with juvenile chronic arthritis, *Scand J Rheumatol* 30:69–76, 2001.

36. Reference deleted in proofs.

37. Howe S, Levinson J, Shear E, Hartner S, McGirr G, Schulte M, et al.: Development of a disability measurement tool for juvenile rheumatoid arthritis: the Juvenile Arthritis Functional Assessment Report for children and their parents, *Arthritis Rheum* 34:873–880, 1991.

38. IRCCS Istituto G. Gaslini, Università di Genova. Information on Paediatric Rheumatic Diseases. Available froim: URL: http://www.printo.it/pediatric-rheumatology/.

39. Reference deleted in proofs.

40. Jaworski TM, Bradley LA, Heck LW, Roca A, Alarcon GS: Development of an observation method for assessing pain behaviors in children with juvenile rheumatoid arthritis, *Arthritis Rheum* 38:1142–1151, 1995.

41. Jetha A: The impact of arthritis on the early employment experiences of young adults: a literature review, *Disabil Health J* 8:317–324, 2015.

42. Keller-Marchand L, Farpour-Lambert NJ, Hans D, Rizzoli R, Hofer MF: Effects of a weight bearing exercise program in children with juvenile idiopathic arthritis, *Med Sci Sports Exerc* 38(Suppl 5):S93–S94, 2006.

43. Kirchheimer JC, Wanivenhaus A, Engel A: Does sport negatively influence joint scores in patients with juvenile rheumatoid arthritis? An 8-year prospective study, *Rheumatol Internat* 12:239–242, 1993.

44. Klepper S: Effects of an eight-week physical conditioning program on disease signs and symptoms in children with chronic arthritis, *Arthritis Care Res* 12:52–60, 1999.

45. Klepper S: Exercise and fitness in children with arthritis: evidence of benefits for exercise and physical activity, *Arthritis Care Res* 49:435–443, 2003.

46. Klepper SE: Exercise in pediatric rheumatic diseases, *Curr Op Rheumatol* 20:619–624, 2008.

47. Klijn PH, Oudshoorn A, van der Ent CK, van der Net J, Kimpen JL, Helders PJ: Effects of anaerobic training in children with cystic fibrosis: a randomized controlled study. *Chest* 125:1299–1305, 2004

48 2004 Knopps K, Wulffraat N, Lodder S, Houwen R, de Meer K: Resting energy expenditure and nutritional status in children with juvenile rheumatoid arthritis, *J Rheumatol* 26:2039–2043, 1999.

49. Kraemer W, Fleck S: *Strength training for young athletes*, Champaign, IL, 1993, Human Kinetics.

50. Lam C, Young N, Marhawa J, McLimont M, Feldman BM: Revised versions of the Childhood Health Assessment Questionnaire (CHAQ) are more sensitive and suffer less from a ceiling effect, *Arthritis Rheum* 51:881–889, 2004.

51. Lelieveld OT, Armbrust W, van Leeuwen MA, Duppen N, Geertzen JH, Sauer P, et al.: Physical activity in adolescents with juvenile idiopathic arthritis, *Arthritis Rheum* 59:1379–1784, 2008.

52. Lelieveld OT, Takken T, van der Net J, van Weert E: Validity of the 6-minute walking test in juvenile idiopathic arthritis, *Arthritis Rheum* 53:304–307, 2005.

53. Lelieveld OT, van Brussel M, Takken T, van Weert E, van Leeuwen MA, Armbrust W: Aerobic and anaerobic exercise capacity in adolescents with juvenile idiopathic arthritis, *Arthritis Rheum* 57:898–904, 2007.

54. Len C, Ferraz M, Goldenberg J, Oliveira LM, Araujo PP, Rodrigues Q, et al.: Pediatric Escola Paulista de Medicina range of motion scale: a reduced joint count score for general use in juvenile rheumatoid arthritis, *J Rheumatol* 26:909–913, 1999.

55. Reference deleted in proofs.

56. Lien G, Selvaag AM, Flatø B, Haugen M, Vinje O, Sørskaar D, et al.: A two-year prospective controlled study of bone mass and bone turnover in children with early juvenile idiopathic arthritis, *Arthr Rheum* 52:833–840, 2005.

57. Lineker SC, Badley EM, Dalby DM: Unmet service needs of children with rheumatic diseases and their parents in a metropolitan area, *J Rheumatol* 23:1054–1058, 1996.

58. Reference deleted in proofs.

59. Lovell DJ, Howe S, Shear E, Hartner S, McGirr G, Schulte M, et al.: Development of a disability measurement tool for juvenile rheumatoid arthritis: the Juvenile Arthritis Functional Assessment Scale, *Arthritis Rheum* 32:1390–1395, 1989.

60. Mannion ML, Xie F, Curtis JR, Beukelman T: Recent trends in medication usage for the treatment of juvenile idiopathic arthritis and the influence of tumor necrosis factor inhibitors, *J Rheumatol* 41:2078–2084, 2014.

61. McDougall JJ: Arthritis and pain. Neurogenic origin of joint pain, *Arthritis Res Ther* 8:220, 2006.

62. Minor M, Westby D: Rest and exercise. In Robbins L, Burckhardt C, Hannan M, DeHoratius R, editors: *Clinical care in the rheumatic diseases*, ed 2, Atlanta, GA, 2001, American College of Rheumatology, pp 179–184.

63. Morrison CD, Bundy RC, Fisher AG: The contribution of motor skills and playfulness to the play performance of preschoolers, *Am J Occupat Ther* 45:687–694, 1991.

64. Murray KJ, Moroldo MB, Donnelly P, Prahalad S, Passo MH, Giannini EH, et al.: Age-specific effects of juvenile rheumatoid arthritis-associated HLA alleles, *Arthritis Rheum* 42:1843–1853, 1999.

65. Nieuwenhuis MK, van der Net J, Kuis W, Buchanon TS, Helders PJ: Assessment of wrist malalignment in juvenile rheumatoid arthritis, *Advances Physiother* 1:99–109, 1999.

66. Oosterveld FG, Rasker JJ: Effects of local heat and cold treatment on surface and intra-articular temperature of arthritic knees, *Arthritis Rheum* 37:1578–1582, 1994.

67. Oosterveld FG, Rasker JJ, Jacobs JW, Overmars HJ: The effect of local heat and cold therapy on the intra-articular and skin surface temperature of the knee, *Arthritis Rheum* 35:146–151, 1992.

68. Paap E, van der Net J, Helders PJ, Takken T: Physiologic response of the six-minute walk test in children with juvenile idiopathic arthritis, *Arthritis Rheum* 53:351–356, 2005.

69. Pediatric Rheumatology International Trial Organization (PRInTO): information on pediatric rheumatology. Available at: URL: http://www.printo.it/pediatric-rheumatology/.

70. Reference deleted in proofs.

71. Petty RE, Southwood TR, Manners P, et al.: International League of Associations for Rheumatology classification of juvenile idiopathic arthritis, second revision, Edmonton 2001, *J Rheumatol* 31:390–392, 2004.

72. Prakken B, Albani S, Martini A: Juvenile idiopathic arthritis, *Lancet* 377:2138–2149, 2011.

73. Prakken B, Martini A: Paediatric rheumatology in 2014: digging deeper for greater precision and more impact in JIA, *Nat Rev Rheumatol* 11:70–72, 2015.

74. Reed MH, Wilmot DM: The radiology of juvenile rheumatoid arthritis: a review of the English language literature, *J Rheumatol* 31(Suppl):2–22, 1991.

75. Reference deleted in proofs.

76. Ringold S, Weiss PF, Colbert RA, DeWitt EM, Lee T, Onel K, et al.: Juvenile Idiopathic Arthritis Research Committee of the Childhood Arthritis and Rheumatology Research Alliance. Childhood Arthritis and Rheumatology Research Alliance consensus treatment plans for new-onset polyarticular juvenile idiopathic arthritis, *Arthritis Care Res (Hoboken)* 66:1063–1072, 2014.

77. Sandstedt E, Fasth A, Nyström Eek M, Beckung E: Muscle strength, physical fitness and well-being in children and adolescents with juvenile idiopathic arthritis and the effect of an exercise programme: a randomized controlled trial, *Pediatr Rheumatol Online J* 11:7, 2013.

78. Schanberg LE, Sandstrom MJ, Starr K, Gil KM, Lefebvre JC, Keefe FJ, et al.: The relationship of daily mood and stressful events to symptoms in juvenile rheumatic disease, *Arthritis Care Res* 13:33–41, 2000.

79. Schoenmakers MA, de Groot JF, Gorter JW, Hillaert JL, Helders PJ, Takken T: Muscle strength, aerobic capacity and physical activity in independent ambulating children with lumbosacral spina bifida, *Disabil Rehabil* 104:657–665, 2009.

80. Reference deleted in proofs.

81. Sherry DD, Stein LD, Reed AM, Schanberg LE, Kredich DW: Prevention of leg length discrepancy in young children with pauciarticular juvenile rheumatoid arthritis by treatment with intra-articular steroids, *Arthritis Rheum* 42:2330–2334, 1999.

82. Singh G, Athreya B, Fries JF, Goldsmith DP: Measurement of health status in children with juvenile rheumatoid arthritis, *Arthritis Rheum* 37:1761–1769, 1994.

83. Spencer CH, Bernstein BH: Hip disease in juvenile rheumatoid arthritis, *Curr Opin Rheumatol* 4:536–541, 2002.

84. Stephens S, Feldman BM, Bradley N, et al.: Feasibility and effectiveness of an aerobic exercise program in children with fibromyalgia: results of a randomized controlled pilot trial, *Arthritis Care Res* 59:1399–1406, 2008.

85. Stinson JN, Hayden JA, Kohut SA, Soobiah C, Cartwright J, Weiss SK, Witmans MB: Sleep problems and associated factors in children with juvenile idiopathic arthritis: a systematic review, *Pediatr Rheumatol Online J* 12:19, 2014.

86. Sullivan DB, Cassidy JT, Petty RE: Pathogenic implications of age of onset in juvenile rheumatoid arthritis, *Arthritis Rheum* 18:251–255, 1975.

87. Szer IS, Wright FV: School integration. In Melvin J, Wright FV, editors: *Rheumatologic rehabilitation: pediatric rheumatic diseases*, Vol. 3. Philadelphia, 2000, WB Saunders, pp 223–230.

88. Takken T: Exercise testing and training in children with juvenile idiopathic arthritis and dermatomyositis: state of the art, *Ann Rheum Dis* 65:25, 2006.

89. Takken T, Hemel A, van der Net JJ, Helders PJ: Aerobic fitness in children with juvenile idiopathic arthritis: a systematic review, *J Rheumatol* 29:2643–2647, 2002.

90. Takken T, van Brussel M, Engelbert RH, van der Net J, Kuis W, Helders PJ: Exercise therapy in juvenile idiopathic arthritis: a Cochrane review, *Eur J Phys Rehabil Med* 44:287–297, 2008.

91. Takken T, van der Net JJ, Helders PJ: Do juvenile idiopathic arthritis patients benefit from an exercise program? A pilot study, *Arthritis Care Res* 45:81–85, 2001.

92. Takken T, van der Net J, Helders PJ: Relationship between functional ability and physical fitness in juvenile rheumatoid arthritis, *Scandinavian J Rheumatol* 32:174–178, 2003.

93. Takken T, Van der Net J, Kuis W, Helders PJ: Physical activity and health related physical fitness in children with juvenile idiopathic arthritis, *Ann Rheumat Dis* 62:885–889, 2003.

94. Thompson KL, Varni JW: A developmental cognitive-behavioral approach to pediatric pain assessment, *Pain* 25:283–296, 1986.

95. Thompson P, Beath T, Bell J, Jacobson G, Phair T, Salbach NM, et al.: Test-retest reliability of the 10-metre fast walk test and 6-minute walk test in ambulatory school-aged children with cerebral palsy, *Dev Med Child Neurol* 50:370–376, 2008.

96. van Brussel M, van der Net J, Hulzebos E, Helders PJM, Takken T: The Utrecht approach to exercise in chronic childhood conditions: the decade in review, *Ped Phys Ther* 23:2–14, 2011.

97. van Brussel M, Lelieveld OT, van der Net J, Engelbert RH, Helders PJ, Takken T: Aerobic and anaerobic exercise capacity in children with juvenile idiopathic arthritis, *Arthritis Rheum* 57:891–897, 2007.

98. van Brussel M, van Doren L, Timmons BW, Obeid J, van der Net J, Helders PJ, et al.: Anaerobic-to-aerobic power ratio in children with juvenile idiopathic arthritis, *Arthritis Rheum* 61:787–793, 2009.

99. van der Net J, van der Torre P, Engelbert RH, Engelen V, van Zon F, Takken T, et al.: Motor performance and functional ability in preschool- and early school-aged children with juvenile idiopathic arthritis: a cross-sectional study, *Pediatr Rheumatol Online J* 16:6, 2008.

100. Reference deleted in proofs.

101. Reference deleted in proofs.

102. Verschuren O, Ketelaar M, Gorter JW, Helders PJ, Uiterwaal CS, Takken T: Exercise training program in children and adolescents with cerebral palsy: a randomized controlled trial, *Arch Pediatr Adolesc Med* 161:1075–1081, 2007.

103. Vostrejs M, Hollister JR: Muscle atrophy and leg length discrepancies in pauciarticular juvenile rheumatoid arthritis, *Am J Disease Childhood* 142:343–345, 1988.

104. Wessel J, Kaup C, Fan J, Ehalt R, Ellsworth J, Speer C, et al.: Isometric strength measurements in children with arthritis: reliability and relation to function, *Arthritis Care Res* 12:238–246, 1999.

105. White PH: Growth abnormalities in children with juvenile rheumatoid arthritis, *Clin Orthoped Rel Res* 259:46–50, 1990.

106. Wiltink A, Nijweide PJ, Oosterbaan WA, Hekkenberg RT, Helders PJ: Effect of therapeutic ultrasound on endochondral ossification, *Ultrasound Med Biol* 21:121–127, 1995.

107. Wind AE, Takken T, Helders PJ, Engelbert RH: Is grip strength a predictor for total muscle strength in healthy children, adolescents, and young adults? *Euro J Pediatr* 169:281–287, 2010.

108. Wong DL, Baker CM: Pain in children: comparison of assessment scales, *Pediatr Nurs* 14:9–17, 1988.
109. Reference deleted in proofs.
110. Reference deleted in proofs.
111. Wrotniak BH, Epstein LH, Dorn JM, Jones KE, Kondilis VA: The relationship between motor proficiency and physical activity in children, *Pediatrics* 118:1758–1765, 2006.

SUGGESTED READINGS

Background

Prakken B, Albani S, Martini A: Juvenile idiopathic arthritis, *Lancet* 18:2138–2149, 2011.
Prakken B, Martini A: Paediatric rheumatology in 2014: digging deeper for greater precision and more impact in JIA, *Nat Rev Rheumatol* 11:70–72, 2015.
Szer IL, Kimura Y, Malleson P, Southwood TR, editors: *Arthritis in children and adolescents: juvenile idiopathic arthritis*, Oxford University Press, 2006.

Foreground

Eisenberger NI, Inagaki TK, Mashal NM, Irwin MR: Inflammation and social experience: an inflammatory challenge induces feelings of social disconnection in addition to depressed mood, *Brain Behav Immun* 24:558–563, 2010.
Hansmann S, Benseler SM, Kuemmerle-Dreschner JB: Dynamic knee joint function in children with juvenile idiopathic arthritis (JIA), *Pediatr Rheum Online J* 13:8, 2015, http://dx.doi.org/10.1186/s12969-015-0004-1.
Nani Morgan, Irwin Michael R, Chung Mei, Chenchen Wang: The effects of mind-body therapies on the immune system: meta-analysis, *PloS One* 9:e100903, 2014.
Nicassio PM, Ormseth SR, Kay M, Custodio M, Irwin MR, Olmstead R, Weisman Michael H: The contribution of pain and depression to self-reported sleep disturbance in patients with rheumatoid arthritis, *Pain* 153:107–112, 2012.
Nijhof LN, van de Putte EM, Wulffraat NM, Nijhof SL: Prevalence of severe fatigue among adolescents with pediatric rheumatic diseases, *Arthritis Care Res* 68:108–114, 2015.
Sandstedt E, Fasth A, Nyström Eek M, Beckung E: Muscle strength, physical fitness and well-being in children and adolescents with juvenile idiopathic arthritis and the effect of an exercise programme: a randomized controlled trial, *Pediatr Rheumatol* 11:7, 2013.
Stephens S, Feldman B, Bradley N, et al.: Feasibility and effectiveness of an aerobic exercise program in children with fibromyalgia: results of a randomized controlled pilot trial, *Arthritis Care Res* 59:1399–1406, 2008.
Stinson JN, Hayden JA, Kohut SA, et al.: Sleep problems and associated factors in children with juvenile idiopathic arthritis: a systematic review, *Pediatric Rheumatol* 12:19, 2014.
van Brussel M, Lelieveld OT, van der Net J, Engelbert RH, Helders PJ, Takken T: Aerobic and anaerobic exercise capacity in children with juvenile idiopathic arthritis, *Arthritis Rheum* 57:891–897, 2007.
van Brussel M, van der Net J, Hulzebos E, Helders PJM, Takken T: The Utrecht approach to exercise in chronic childhood conditions: the decade in review, *Ped Phys Ther* 23:2–14, 2011.

8

Spinal Conditions

Suzanne Green, Heidi Friedman

The spine is the framework for our posture and our movement. It supports our cranium, extremities, and spinal cord; allows for trunk flexibility; acts as a shock absorber; and provides structural support for normal chest and respiratory development. Orthopedic concerns arise when spinal alignment is altered by congenital or acquired changes, producing scoliosis, kyphosis, or lordosis.

Each one or a combination of these conditions, if left untreated, may affect a child's pulmonary function, psychosocial well-being, potential for back pain, and life expectancy. We, as physical therapists, play a vital role in the detection and treatment of spinal conditions. Two to four percent of the population of school-age children (7–18 years) is at risk for adolescent idiopathic scoliosis, the most common form of scoliosis.[103,107] The prevalence of other spinal conditions varies with the condition and the underlying disease process.[131] This chapter addresses the prevalence and natural history, identification, examination, and treatment of these spinal conditions. Specific cases are presented to discuss impairments and restrictions in activity and participation of children with spinal conditions. Physical therapy intervention is emphasized, along with nonsurgical and surgical management of these spinal conditions.

BACKGROUND INFORMATION

DEVELOPMENT OF THE SPINE

Pathologic spinal conditions are discussed in this chapter, so it is necessary for the reader to have some knowledge of normal spinal development (Fig. 8.1). Therefore a discussion of development in the embryologic, fetal, and childhood stages follows.

Fetal development is divided into three stages. The first 3 weeks after fertilization is termed the preembryonic period. The embryonic period is next, lasting from week 3 to week 8 of gestation; during this stage, the organs of the body develop. The fetal period lasts from week 8 until term, and during this stage, maturation and growth of all structures and organs occur.[93]

Early development of the skeletal, muscular, and neural systems is related to the notochord. Cell proliferation occurs at approximately 3 weeks, forming a trilaminar structure with layers of ectoderm, mesoderm, and endoderm. Proliferation of the mesodermal tissue continues, forming 29 pairs of somites (a pair of blocklike segments that give rise to muscle and vertebrae, which are formed on each side of the notochord[123]) in the fourth week and the remainder (42–44 total) in the fifth week. Differentiation of the somites then occurs, producing 4 occipital, 8 cervical, 12 thoracic, 5 lumbar, 5 sacral, and 8 to 10 coccygeal somites. The occipital somites form a portion of the base of the skull and the articulation between the cranium and the cervical vertebrae, while the last five to seven coccygeal somites disappear. Cervical, thoracic, lumbar, and sacral somites form the structures of the spine.[137]

Proliferation of the somites occurs, leading to the development of three distinct areas. Dorsally, the cells become dermatomes, giving rise to the skin. Medially to the dermatome, cells migrate deep to give rise to skeletal muscle. The ventral and medial cells migrate toward the notochord and the neural tube to form the sclerotome.[93,137]

The sclerotomal cells proliferate and differentiate, giving rise to rudimentary vertebral structures, including rib buds. Chondrification begins at the cervicothoracic level, extending cranially and caudally. Centers of chondrification allow for formation of the solid cartilage model of a vertebra with no line of demarcation between body, neural arch, or rib rudiments.[93]

Ossification occurs at primary and secondary centers. Ossification begins during the late fetal period and continues after birth. Primary centers of ossification extend to the spinous, transverse, and articular processes. Secondary ossification centers develop at the upper and lower portions of the vertebral body, at the tip of the spinous processes, and at each transverse process. These centers expand in late adolescence. Secondary ossification centers also develop in the ribs: one at the head of the rib and two in the tubercle. Ossification of the axis, atlas, and sacrum differs slightly from that of the other vertebrae. The atlas has two primary centers and one secondary center of ossification, and the axis has five primary and two secondary centers of ossification. Ossification of the axis begins near the end of gestation with fusion of the two odontoid centers and is completed in the second decade of life with fusion of the odontoid and centrum. Fusion of the sacrum begins in adolescence and is completed in the third decade of life.[93]

Spinal growth occurs throughout adolescence. Knowledge of spinal growth is essential in nonsurgical and surgical treatment of spinal deformities. Spinal growth studies have demonstrated that there are two periods of rapid spinal growth: the first from birth to age 5 and the second during the adolescent growth spurt. In the years between, growth occurs at a slower rate.[18]

The spinal pubertal growth spurts occur at different chronologic and Tanner ages for females and males. In females the growth spurt coincides with Tanner 2 or a chronologic age of 8 to 14 years, with maximum growth occurring at a mean of 12 years of age. The spurt lasts 2.5 to 3 years. The growth spurt occurs later in males, at Tanner 3 or chronologic age 11 to 16 years, with maximum growth at age 14 years. These values are average values based on white Anglo-Saxon populations.[31]

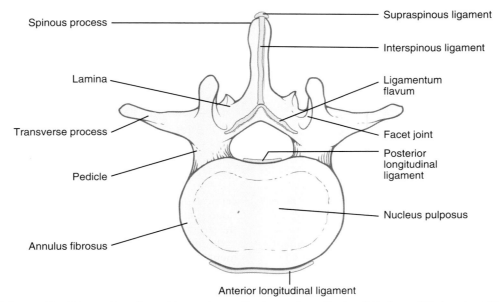

Spinous process

Supraspinous ligament

Interspinous ligament

Lamina

Ligamentum flavum

Transverse process

Facet joint

Posterior longitudinal ligament

Pedicle

Nucleus pulposus

Annulus fibrosus

Anterior longitudinal ligament

FIG. 8.1 The L2 vertebra viewed from above. (Redrawn from Covino BG, Scott DB, Lambert DH: *Handbook of spinal anaesthesia and analgesia.* Philadelphia, WB Saunders, 1994.)

A fused area of the spine does not grow longitudinally, as documented by Moe and colleagues.[92] The surgeon, therefore, considers the information on spinal growth potential for each individual case.

SCOLIOSIS

Background Information

Detection and Clinical Examination

Detection of scoliosis occurs primarily by identification of trunk, shoulder, or pelvic asymmetries. The American Academy of Pediatrics (AAP), American Academy of Orthopaedic Surgeons (AAOS), Scoliosis Research Society (SRS), and Pediatric Orthopaedic Society of North America (POSNA) commissioned a task force to investigate the effectiveness of scoliosis screening. They concluded that the literature does not provide sufficient evidence to merit scoliosis screening of asymptomatic adolescents. However, the societies do not support recommendations against scoliosis screening. The societies acknowledge the benefits of clinical screenings, including the potential to affect curve progression by brace treatment, as well as earlier detection of severe deformities requiring operative correction.[106] Due to gender differences in the onset of puberty and risk of curve progression, the societies recommend that if scoliosis screening is initiated, females should be screened twice, at ages 10 and 12, and males once, around age 13 or 14.[114]

Children with asymmetries should be referred to an orthopedic surgeon with an interest in and knowledge of scoliosis for a baseline evaluation. An examination begins with a complete patient history to obtain information regarding curve detection, familial conditions, general health, and physical maturity. A basic neurologic examination should also be performed on all patients with evidence of scoliosis including strength testing, deep tendon reflexes, and a check for upper motor neuron signs.[111] The physical examination may include assessment of general alignment including shoulder and pelvic symmetry, spinal alignment by forward bend test, trunk compensation using a plumb line, and leg length measurement. The magnitude of a rib hump is quantified using a scoliometer with the forward bend test.[93] The scoliometer, an inclinometer designed by Bunnell,[10] is placed over the spinous process at the apex of the curve to measure the angle of trunk rotation (ATR). The ATR correlates with the severity of the scoliosis.[107] A minimal measurement of at least 5° by the scoliometer is considered a good criterion for identifying lateral curvatures of the spine with Cobb angles of 20° or greater. Therefore, a scoliometer reading of 5° or greater warrants further evaluation[10] and is an indication for a radiograph.[118]

Standing radiographs with two initial views, lateral and anterior-posterior,[108] are used to determine location, type, and magnitude of the curve, as well as skeletal age with anterior-posterior views used at subsequent appointments. Skeletal maturity is determined using the Risser sign, which quantifies the amount of ossification of the iliac crest, using grades 0 to 5. Grade 0 represents absence of ossification. Grades 1 to 4 are excursions from 25% to 100%, starting at the anterior-superior iliac spine.[143] Grade 5 categorizes skeletal maturity. Grades 0, 1, and 2 correlate with the highest risk for curve progression,[108] grade 3 with progressing skeletal maturity, grade 4 with cessation of spinal growth, and grade 5 with cessation of increase in height (Fig. 8.2).

The spinal curvature is measured using the Cobb method. To complete the measurement, one must first identify the end vertebrae. The end vertebrae are described as the most cephalad vertebra of a curve whose upper surface maximally tilts toward the curve's concavity and the most caudal vertebra with maximal tilt toward the convexity. Lines are drawn as extensions of the end vertebrae from end plate or pedicles. The degree of curvature is measured as the angle formed by the intersection of lines perpendicular to these end vertebral lines[118] (Fig. 8.3). Magnetic resonance imaging, computed tomography, myelography, and bone scans can be used to identify subtle central nervous system abnormalities and to provide additional information as necessary to aid in diagnosis and detection of spinal conditions.

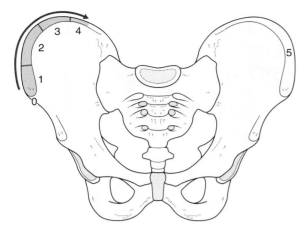

FIG. 8.2 Risser sign, grades 0 to 5. (From Adam A, Dixon AK, Gillard JH, et al, editors: *Grainger & Allison's diagnostic radiology*, ed 6, Edinburgh, 2015, Churchill Livingstone.)

TABLE 8.1 Classification of Spinal Curve Based on Location	
Cervical curve	C1-C6
Cervicothoracic curve	C7-T1
Thoracic curve	T2-T11
Thoracolumbar curve	T12-L1
Lumbar curve	L2-L4
Lumbosacral curve	L5-S1

are most common. Left thoracic curves are not directly linked to a disease process but merit further evaluation, as they are more likely to have an underlying neurologic cause.[111]

There are two major types of curvatures: structural and nonstructural. A nonstructural curve fully corrects clinically and radiographically on lateral bend toward the apex of the curve and lacks vertebral rotation. A nonstructural curve is usually nonprogressive and is most often caused by a shortened lower extremity on the side of the apex of the curve. It is essential, however, to monitor nonstructural curves during growth because they may occasionally develop into structural deformities.

A structural curve cannot be voluntarily, passively, or forcibly fully corrected. Rotation of the vertebrae is toward the convexity of the curve. A fixed thoracic prominence or rib hump in a child with a thoracic deformity or a lumbar paraspinal prominence in a child with a lumbar curve is evidence of rotation when observed on clinical examination.[46]

Idiopathic Scoliosis

Idiopathic scoliosis denotes a lateral curvature of the spine of unknown cause and is the most common form of scoliosis in children. Three strong factors have been identified that correlate with curve progression for idiopathic scoliosis: curve magnitude, Risser sign, and the patient's chronologic age at the time of diagnosis.[77]

Background
Origin, Incidence, and Pathophysiology

In 1954, James, et al. defined three subtypes of idiopathic scoliosis based on the age of onset: infantile, juvenile, and adolescent.[94] These categories correlate to major growth spurts with potential for maximal progression of scoliosis.[19] Infantile idiopathic scoliosis develops in children between birth and 3 years, usually manifesting shortly after birth. This form of scoliosis accounts for less than 1% of all cases in North America.[86,91] Infantile idiopathic scoliosis occurs more frequently in male infants, and most curves are left. Eighty to ninety percent of these curves spontaneously resolve, but many of the remainder of cases will progress throughout childhood resulting in severe deformity. Because infantile idiopathic scoliosis is common in England and northern Europe but rare in the United States, environmental factors have been implicated in the development of the deformity.[46,86]

Juvenile idiopathic scoliosis develops between ages 4 and 9 years.[27] The most common curve is right thoracic, occurring in males and females with equal frequency.[17] It is most often recognized at around 6 years of age. Juvenile idiopathic curves have a high rate of progression and result in severe deformity if untreated. Charles et al.[17] found that curves greater than 30° at onset of the pubertal growth spurt increased rapidly and presented a 100% prognosis for surgery. Curves 21° to 30° also presented a 75% progression risk and would benefit from careful follow-up.

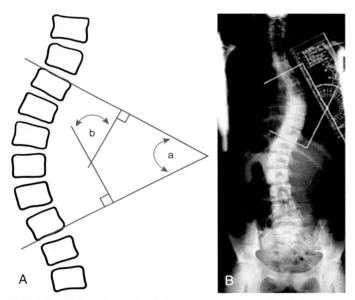

FIG. 8.3 (A) Cobb's method of measuring the angle of the curve in scoliosis (see text). (B) The Cobb method of measuring the curve angle of scoliosis, as seen on a radiograph. ([A] From Evans RC: *Illustrated orthopedic physical assessment.* 3rd ed. St. Louis: Mosby, 2009. [B] From Kim HJ, et al.: Update on the management of idiopathic scoliosis. *Curr Opin Pediatr* 21:55-64, 2009.)

Terminology

Scoliosis refers to a three-dimensional curvature of the spine. To be considered a scoliosis, the curvature in the coronal plane must be greater than 10° with a vertebral rotation component on the radiograph.[5,36] Spinal deformities are classified according to origin, location, magnitude, and direction. Curvatures may be idiopathic, neuromuscular, or congenital and may be further classified by the area of the spine in which the apex of the curve is located, as described in Table 8.1.

Magnitude is measured using the Cobb method as described above. Direction of the curve is designated as right or left by the side of the convexity of the deformity.[108] Right thoracic curves

Adolescent idiopathic scoliosis (AIS) categorizes curves manifesting at or around the onset of puberty and accounts for approximately 80% of all cases of idiopathic scoliosis. The prevalence of idiopathic scoliosis is 2% to 3% of children ages 10 to skeletal maturity.[111] The female-to-male ratio is 1:1 in curves of approximately 10°. With curve magnitude of 10° to 20°, the female-to-male ratio increases to 5:1. For curves greater than 30°, the ratio further increases to 10:1.[111] A greater percentage of curves will progress in the female patient: 19.3% compared with 1.2% of males. A large number of AIS curvatures are structural at the time of detection, although flexibility and the progression of these curves vary. Structural curves have a greater tendency to progress throughout adolescence at an average rate of 1° per month if untreated, whereas nonstructural curves may remain flexible enough to avoid becoming problematic.[46]

Currently in the orthopedic literature there is newer terminology categorizing scoliosis into early-onset scoliosis (EOS) and late-onset scoliosis (LOS), although therapists and families may continue to see previous verbiage in use (infantile, juvenile, and adolescent scoliosis). The Scoliosis Research Society describes EOS as occurring before 10 years of age. Use of this terminology is controversial. People who advocate its use believe that it delineates populations of patients with greater risk of developing pulmonary failure versus LOS patients, for whom that is unlikely.[109] Age of onset is an important factor because major thoracic curves seen prior to the age of 5 years old are more likely to be associated with thoracic insufficiency syndrome (to be discussed later in this chapter) and increased mortality.[94] On the other hand, supporters of the use of the terms *infantile* (0 to three years of age) and *juvenile* (4 to 10 years of age) scoliosis acknowledge that there are increased mortality rates but less so in juvenile than infantile scoliosis, thereby demonstrating the continued relevance of these terms.

Extensive research has been devoted to uncovering the cause of idiopathic scoliosis; still the mechanics and specific origin are not clearly understood. A number of theories have been proposed to attempt to explain the mechanics of vertebral column failure and decompensation of the spine, as seen in idiopathic scoliosis. It is thought that the cause of scoliosis is multifactorial. Current researchers have investigated many areas, including, but not limited to, growth timing in relationship to maturational changes; biomechanics; skeletal framework, specifically, spine slenderness; disproportionate growth of the anterior portion of the vertebrae compared with the posterior portion; melatonin; and genetics.[11] Data from studies by Wynne-Davies[140] and Cowell and colleagues[22] reflect the existence of a familial tendency. Janicki[57] also stated that a genetic component is included, noting that siblings of patients with scoliosis are diagnosed seven times more often and children of patients with scoliosis are diagnosed three times more often. Current research provides strong evidence for a genetic basis for idiopathic scoliosis; however, the specific mode or modes of heritability are still not clear. Understanding the genetic transmission of this disorder would be helpful in determining appropriate intervention approaches, particularly for those who might be at risk for severe disability.[90]

According to Wolff's law, bone remodels over time in response to the loads applied to it. In accordance with the Hueter-Volkmann principle, compressive loading will hinder

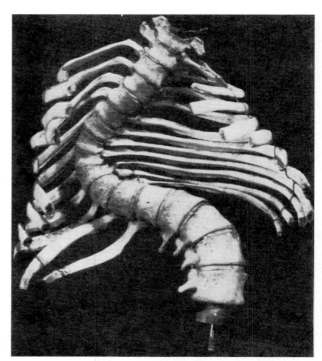

FIG. 8.4 Anatomic specimen of the spine demonstrating structural changes of right thoracic scoliosis. Note vertebral wedging on the concave side and rotation of the vertebral bodies to the convexity of the curve. (From James JIP: *Scoliosis,* ed 2, London, 1976, Churchill Livingstone.)

bone growth, and reduced loading will hasten it.[112] Asymmetrical loading of a growing spine will lead to asymmetrical bony growth, resulting in wedge-shaped vertebrae.[120] Changes occurring on the concave side of the curvature include compression and degenerative changes of intravertebral discs and shortening of muscles and ligaments (Fig. 8.4). Changes in the thoracic spine directly affect the rib cage. The translatory shift of the spine causes an asymmetrically divided thorax, producing decreased pulmonary capacity on the convex side and increased pulmonary capacity on the concave side. Severe curves in the thoracic spine associated with increased angulation of the ribs posteriorly further reduce aeration of the lung on the convex side, potentially causing abnormal stresses on the heart and disturbed cardiac function.[26,50] The pulmonary system may also be affected. Czaprowski D et al.[23] examined the physical capacity of girls with mild and moderate AIS. They found that maximal oxygen intake was lower in the girls with moderate scoliosis (25° to 40° curvature) as compared to the control group, which is an indication of decreased cardiovascular endurance with physical activity.

Investigators have established an association between scoliosis and vestibular dysfunction. Multiple groups have found increased body sway and diminished balance control in situations where there are proprioceptive and visional challenges in patients with scoliosis. Furthermore, cognitive integration of vestibular signals was impaired compared to patients without scoliosis. There are also studies describing anatomic differences in patients having scoliosis from their peers in their vestibular system apparatus.[43] Therefore for the treating clinician, the balance testing during the physical therapy evaluation is warranted.

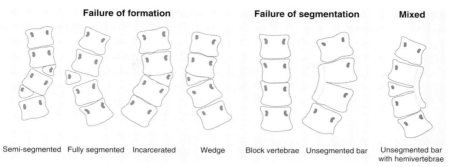

FIG. 8.5 Types of congenital scoliosis. (From Fender D, Purushothaman B: Spinal disorders in childhood II: spinal deformity. *Surgery (Oxford)* 32(1): 39-45, 2014.)

Natural History

A progressive curve is defined as a sustained increase of 5° or more on two consecutive examinations occurring at 4- to 6-month intervals. An untreated progressive curve has the potential to increase in magnitude in adult life. Following are the main factors that influence the probability of progression in the skeletally immature patient[108,111,118]:

The younger the patient at diagnosis, the greater the risk of progression.

Double-curve patterns have a greater risk for progression than single-curve patterns.

The lower the Risser sign, the greater the risk of progression.

Curves that are larger at initial presentation are more likely to progress.

Risk of progression in females is approximately 10 times that in males with curves of comparable magnitude.

Greater risk of progression is present when curves develop before menarche.

Congenital Scoliosis
Origin, Incidence, and Pathophysiology

Congenital scoliosis curves are caused by anomalous vertebral development in utero. Kaplan et al.[58] suggested that congenital scoliosis has both a genetic and environmental basis and that abnormalities appear to be sporadic. The term *congenital scoliosis* should not be confused with *infantile scoliosis*. Clinical manifestations of congenital scoliosis may not be apparent at birth, but the vertebral anomaly is present. Infantile scoliosis will not demonstrate vertebral anomalies upon radiography.[132] Congenital anomalies of the vertebrae can be attributed to failure of vertebral segmentation, failure of vertebral formation, or mixed defect, which is a combination of the two. Both pathologic processes are frequently seen in the same spine and may occur at the same or at different levels. Location of the pathologic process on the vertebrae (anterior, posterior, lateral, or a combination) determines the congenital deformity. Purely lateral deformity produces congenital scoliosis, and anterolateral and posterolateral deformities produce congenital kyphoscoliosis and lordoscoliosis, respectively.[137,138] The male-to-female ratio for congenital scoliosis is 1:1.4.[75]

A defect of segmentation is seen when adjacent vertebrae do not completely separate from one another, thereby producing an unsegmented bar with no growth plate or disk between the adjacent vertebrae. A lateral, one-sided defect of segmentation produces severe progressive congenital scoliosis. Circumferential failure of segmentation produces en bloc vertebrae, an anomaly that results in loss of segmental motion and

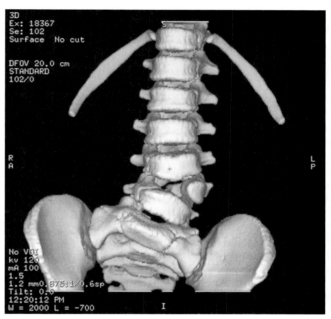

FIG. 8.6 Computed tomography illustrating a hemivertebrae. (From Janicki JA, Alman B: Scoliosis: Review of diagnosis and treatment. *Paediatr Child Health* 12:771-776, 2007.)

loss of longitudinal vertebral growth but no rotational or angular spinal deformity.[137]

Defects of formation may be partial or complete (Fig. 8.5 A–B).[21] Anterior failure of formation of all or part of the vertebral body produces a kyphosis. A partial unilateral defect of formation of a vertebra produces a wedge-shaped hemivertebra (Fig. 8.6) with one pedicle and only one side with growth potential. A nonsegmented hemivertebra is completely fused to the adjacent proximal and distal vertebrae. A semisegmented hemivertebra is fused to only one adjacent vertebra and is separated from the other by a normal end plate and disc. A segmented hemivertebra is separated from proximal and distal vertebrae by a normal end plate and a disc. Hemivertebrae may be unbalanced, with the defect present on one side of the spine, or balanced, with different hemivertebrae present, with defects on opposite sides of the spine compensating for any curves.[137,138]

Abnormalities involving other organ systems have been found in as many as 61% of patients with congenital scoliosis.[45] Multiple organ systems develop while the sclerotomes are differentiating to form vertebral bodies during the embryonic period. Therefore any noxious influence affecting the formation of vertebral structures may also have an adverse effect on the concomitant development of organ systems, including the heart, kidneys, trachea, and esophagus. Cardiac anomalies have been associated with congenital scoliosis of the thoracic spine, and kidney anomalies have been associated with lumbar scoliosis.[75]

The risk of curve progression can be analyzed by examining the growth potential of the congenital anomaly. Many congenital curves become stable and do not progress. The highest risk of progression occurs when asymmetrical growth occurs, in which the convexity outgrows the concavity. This discrepancy usually occurs when the anatomy of the convex side is relatively normal and the concave side is deficient. A shortened trunk may be the main deformity if both convex and concave growth deficiencies occur over multiple levels.[138] Thoracolumbar involvement has the worst prognosis in curves greater than 50° by the age of 2.[58]

Thoracic Insufficiency Syndrome

Growth of the lungs is limited to the anatomic space provided by the boundaries of the thorax. Spinal and rib cage malformations that reduce thoracic volume early in life may have a negative impact on the size of the lungs at skeletal maturity, explaining why patients with congenital scoliosis have lower vital capacities on pulmonary testing than patients with idiopathic scoliosis with equivalent degrees of curvature.[14] The most rapid period of spinal growth is in the first 5 years of life increasing to 50% of its length[18] at a rate of 1.4 cm per year, 0.6 cm per year between the ages of 5 and 10 years old, and increasing in rate again during adolescence to 1.2 cm per year.[59] The greatest increase in alveolar number is within the first 2 years of life and is complete by age 8, although lung volumes continue to increase into adolescence. Pulmonary volumes are expected to begin to decline in the mid-30s.[18]

Thoracic insufficiency syndrome as defined by Campbell et al.[14] is "the inability of the thorax to support normal respiration or lung growth" resulting in lack of pulmonary development. This is correlated to the rib fusions and chest wall anomalies that are associated with congenital scoliosis. If the chest cannot elongate with growth, there will be inadequate space for alveolar growth. Thoracic insufficiency is a combination of two thoracic deficiencies: it must provide support for normal respiration and support normal lung size that is required as an adult. When a child has a thorax that cannot support normal breathing, the child will form compensations that may enable him to appear clinically normal with mild thoracic insufficiency syndrome, but progression of the deformities leads to progression of the syndrome, stressing lung development and function. However, when the child can no longer compensate adequately, clinical signs of respiratory insufficiency may emerge. Dyspnea may appear, with the potential need for supplemental oxygen or ventilatory support to maintain arterial oxygen levels. Recommendations for the treating therapist include monitoring the patient's tolerance to exercise. Items to monitor include facial coloring, heart rate, and respiratory rate. Mild thoracic insufficiency syndrome should be monitored by the child's physician with clinical evaluation of respiratory function, physical examination, radiographs, imaging, and pulmonary function studies. Early intervention during rapid lung growth is preferable.[14]

Congenital scoliosis likely leads to decreased vital capacity because of diminished growth potential of the malformed vertebrae and resultant spinal and chest wall deformity. Also it is known that an increased number of involved vertebrae is related to worsening pulmonary function.[59] Campbell et al.[14] found that even in cases with early spinal surgery children with thoracic spinal deformities may still have hypoplastic thoraxes. During early childhood these children demonstrate nearly typical tolerance to exercise; however, they develop respiratory insufficiency in later adolescence when their body mass increases. People with restrictive lung disease may clinically tolerate it for long periods, but after 40 years of age, some will become oxygen or ventilator dependent with a significant increase in mortality.

Interventions for Idiopathic and Congenital Scoliosis

Treatment decisions are based on the skeletal maturity of the child, as measured by the Risser sign, the growth potential of the child, and the curve magnitude. In addition to surgical intervention, nonsurgical interventions that include serial casting, orthotic treatment, and exercise may be provided.

Surgical Interventions

The major indication for spinal fusion is a documented progressive idiopathic curve with a Cobb angle that reaches 45° or greater in an immature spine. Curves greater than 40° are increasingly difficult to manage with orthotics and have significant risk of progression after skeletal maturity.[67] The main objective of spinal fusion surgery is to obtain a solid arthrodesis because the fusion mass is ultimately what prevents further progression of the deformity.[29,67] The ideal correction system should provide correction in all three planes of the scoliosis, provide rigid fixation, and attain maximal correction with minimal fusion levels.[70]

The classification system that is frequently used when working with children with AIS is the Lenke system, developed in 1983. The main goal of the Lenke system is to categorize surgical curves by analyzing curve pattern similarities to provide comparisons that will ultimately provide the best treatment when making surgical decisions regarding which levels need to be fused.[73] Lenke's system classifies curves into six types[84] with subsets including lumbar and sagittal modifiers.[74] The curve is analyzed looking at upright coronal and sagittal plane x-rays and lateral flexion in supine. The Cobb angles are measured in the proximal thoracic, main thoracic, and thoracolumbar/lumbar regions to determine the major and minor curves, and then they are identified as structural or nonstructural curves. Lenke's recommendations include the major curve and minor structural curves in the instrumentation and exclude nonstructural minor curves.[74]

A posterior surgical procedure, posterior spinal fusion (PSF) with instrumentation, is currently considered to be the gold standard used for spinal fusion.[102,139] The differences among posterior spinal fusion techniques lie with the instrumentation used to obtain correction and protect the fusion.

Spinal instrumentation has evolved since Harrington designed the first generation of posterior instrumentation for scoliosis. Harrington rods correct frontal plane deformities but do not allow for sagittal plane correction and do not address the rotatory components of scoliosis. Further, the placement of Harrington rods calls for postoperative bracing.[105]

The Cotrel-Dubousset (CD) posterior spinal instrumentation (Fig. 8.7) was introduced in the early 1980s and strove for

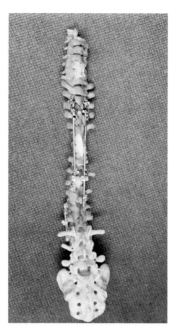

FIG. 8.7 Cotrel-Dubousset instrumentation system implanted on a plastic spine.

a three-dimensional correction of the spinal deformity while avoiding the need for postoperative bracing. A minimum of two parallel rods are used: one on either side of the spine and attached to the spine with hooks or screws. Selective compression or distraction forces may be applied on the rod at any level to correct the deformity.[30] Recent articles have questioned the rotational correction of scoliosis using conventional CD instrumentation.[70,97,121]

In 1999 a new model called direct vertebral rotation (DVR) was introduced. In a prospective study, Lee et al.[70] found improved curve correction as well as correction of apical vertebral rotation when patients with AIS underwent DVR as compared with simple rod derotation. The concept of DVR is to apply both a coronal and a rotational correction. Pedicle screw fixation allows a correcting force to be directed opposite the deformity. The addition of DVR provides the rotational plane correction of the deformity in idiopathic scoliosis.[70]

It is important to treat children with scoliosis while they are still growing, though PSF with instrumentation is generally postponed until the child reaches skeletal maturity in order to preserve spinal growth and ensure adequate space for pulmonary development.[14] Growth-sparing techniques have been developed to manage the scoliotic curve while allowing continued growth of the spine in an effort to delay PSF until the child reaches skeletal maturity. Growth-sparing techniques will be discussed in the next few paragraphs.

Expandable growing spinal rod technique surgery is indicated for children without bony anomaly of the vertebrae or rib cage and with curve flexibility. The mechanism of distraction yields increased growth of the spine and vertebral column. Serial lengthenings must be performed approximately every 6 months during the growing years. Matsumoto et al.[84] report that as the number of rod-lengthening procedures increases, so does the complication rate. Magnetically controlled growing rods (MCGR) have been developed to address this challenge,[84]

as they allow for gradual distraction from an external device.[69] MCGR are now in clinical use and will be an area for further research.[84]

A surgery performed for patients with congenital scoliosis with fused ribs or thoracic insufficiency syndrome is insertion of vertical expandable prosthetic titanium ribs (VEPTR) with an expansion thoracotomy. In this procedure, one or more rib-to-rib or rib-to-spine configurations may be placed.[141] Campbell and Hell-Vocke[13] concluded that growth of the spine approached normal rates after the insertion of VEPTR, including those with bony bars. They believe that the distraction applied by the prosthesis unloads the concave side of the scoliosis, thereby facilitating growth by the Hueter-Volkmann principle. Smith et al.[117] found improvement in lung volume and density, suggesting consequential improved pulmonary function. This is of importance because the lungs are rapidly developing during childhood. A tenfold increase in the number of alveoli occurs by adulthood, but most form within the first 8 years of life.[54] Complications of VEPTR surgery may include brachial plexus injury and multiple outpatient subsequent lengthenings as the child grows.[141]

Vertebral stapling procedures and flexible tethering have been studied to treat AIS. Although these implants vary in flexibility, they are mechanically similar in that they restrict unilateral growth of the convex side of a curvature, accomplished by increasing stress over the growth plates of two adjacent vertebrae, then take advantage of remaining spinal growth to allow the concave side to grow and change over time.[2,20,28] Several studies have noted that various growth-sparing techniques, whether they be tethering,[2,51] growing rods,[113] or fusionless devices in general,[28] focus on coronal plane correction and do not necessarily correct sagittal or transverse plane deformities. Although this is a clear disadvantage of fusionless devices, the benefit of postponing spinal fusion until the child reaches skeletal maturity often outweighs this limitation.

Of note, hospitals are scrutinizing the frequency of readmissions within 90 days of the original surgery because they are now financially accountable for these readmissions under provisions in the Affordable Care Act.[56] This will continue to be an area of continued research going forward.

Nonsurgical Interventions

Idiopathic curves of less than 25°, curves of nonsurgical magnitude of any type in a skeletally mature patient, and nonprogressive congenital curves are evaluated by clinical examination every 4 to 6 months. Radiographs are obtained at each visit; however, unchanged results of a scoliometer examination may reduce the frequency of radiographs to every other visit, depending on individual physician and institution practice.

Serial casting. One technique addressing the treatment of EOS is serial casting. It is theorized that the rapid growth of children in this age group inside the constricted environment of the hard cast allows the Hueter-Volkmann principle to take effect, decreasing curve progression by unloading the growth plates on the concave side of the curvature, therefore fostering growth of the spinal column.[42] The primary goal of casting is to be a growth friendly modality to enhance thoracic spine growth, allowing for closer-to-normal pulmonary function.

During the casting process, children lie on a specially designed frame by the surgeon. Patients are placed under general anesthesia while the plaster or fiberglass cast and traction are applied. The casts are changed every 2 to 3 months.[33]

Serial casting has been shown to preserve thoracic vertebral height growth at the same velocity as the expected norm, having a positive impact on pulmonary function.[4] Authors have reported good results with this technique. In cases of mild to moderate idiopathic EOS with curves of 60° or less, complete resolution has been achieved if started at less than 2 years of age. For older children and for those with more severe curves, recent evidence demonstrates that serial casting may delay surgery, theoretically reducing the potential for complications with recurrent surgical procedures.[24]

Baulesh et al.[4] reported complications from serial casting affected 19% of the children and included nonfatal pulmonary complications that required a break from casting and superficial skin irritation; all complications were resolved without invasive interventions. Hassanzadeh et al.[42] state that the effect of casting on pulmonary function is an area meriting further study.

Orthotic management. The goal of orthotic management is to alter the natural history of curve progression in AIS. Correction of a frontal plane curvature involves application of force in directions opposite to the natural tendency of the curve. Forces are applied at the apex of the curvature, and opposing forces are applied both above and below it.[44]

The indication for orthotic use depends on curve type, magnitude, and location. Orthoses are typically prescribed for children with idiopathic scoliosis who are skeletally immature with a Risser sign of 0, 1, or 2 and have a curve from 25° to 45°[38,60,104] (see Fig. 8.2). A curve with a greater magnitude at the time of detection has an increased risk of progression. Similarly, the effect of an orthosis on prevention of curve progression decreases as the magnitude of the curve increases.[61]

The Milwaukee brace or cervical-thoracic-lumbar-sacral orthosis (CTLSO) remains the gold standard for idiopathic scoliosis in terms of curve correction (based on mechanics), but it is rarely used today in the United States due, in part, to psychosocial stressors associated with brace wear and limited dosage reported by patients. Additionally, the introduction of the thoracolumbosacral orthosis (TLSO) offers a low-profile option for the treatment of curves with an apex as high as T7.[54] There are a number of different TLSO types available, but the goal of the brace design remains the same. Rigid brace design can promote active correction as the patient shifts away from pressure within the brace, or passive correction, preventing curve progression using external forces of the brace on the spine.[134] Appropriate force application is a must. An orthotist molds a prefabricated brace to the patient and customizes the orthosis by adding lumbar pads and relief areas to meet the individual's specific needs. The rigid shell provides a firm support, and the foam lining allows for comfort. A Boston brace is an example of a TLSO and best treats a thoracic curve with an apex of T7 or below.[132] A Boston brace may be modified by the addition of an extension on the concave side with lateral pressure from a convex pad to achieve improved control of curves with an apex at T7 to T9.[62,132] Other TLSO types include the Wilmington and Charleston models. A Wilmington TLSO is a total-contact, custom-molded orthosis that achieves maximal spinal correction by the tight contact and fit, not by pads and relief areas.[62] A Charleston orthosis is used for idiopathic curves and is worn only at night because it is fabricated in the position of maximum side-bend correction.[101]

A recent multicenter trial of the effects of bracing with patients with AIS demonstrated that dosage was the biggest factor when it comes to orthotic management. If a patient wore the brace anywhere from 0–6 hours/day, it was comparable to findings in the observation only group. However, if the patient wore the brace at least 12.9 hours/day, it was associated with success rates of 90% to 93%.[134] The amount of brace wear was logged using thermal indicators. A relatively high success rate with a brace-wearing schedule well below the previously recommended 23 hours/day would likely contribute to improved patient adherence with the recommended dosage and have a subsequent positive impact on patient outcomes.

Margonato et al.[83] suggested that bracing appears to limit maximal exercise performance and recommended moderate physical exercise during brace wear to offset the limitations of the cardiovascular, respiratory, and musculoskeletal systems associated with the brace encompassing the rib cage. Frownfelter et al.[35] found that wearing a TLSO does restrict pulmonary function both at rest and after exercise in healthy adults and suggested adding an abdominal cut out to the TLSO to ease the work of breathing. Further research would be necessary to monitor spinal stability and ensure curve correction is maintained in patients with AIS when using a TLSO with an abdominal cutout.

Orthotic treatment continues until one of two conditions occurs: the curve is no longer controlled (usually at 45° or higher), at which time the patient may become a surgical candidate (treatment failure), or until skeletal maturity occurs, at which time weaning of the brace may begin (treatment success). An orthotic treatment is considered successful if the curve magnitude at the end of treatment is within 5° of the magnitude at the start of the treatment.

FOREGROUND INFORMATION

Physical Therapy Considerations for Postoperative Management

Activity restrictions following spinal fusion surgery are largely anecdotal, although they are often imposed as best practice in an effort to protect the fresh surgical site until the arthrodesis is formed. Activity restrictions are set at the discretion of the orthopedic surgeon and may include avoiding trunk rotation, hip or shoulder flexion greater than 90°, and/or prone activities. A physical therapist's role in the acute postoperative phase includes instruction in body mechanics for bed mobility, transfers, dressing, and ambulation. To avoid trunk rotation, the therapist must instruct the patient in log-rolling and in transitioning from a supine position to sitting without rotation. Shoes and socks are donned or removed with the legs in a "figure four" seated position with negligible forward flexion (patient positioned sitting with the ankle of one leg supported on the distal thigh of the other leg, such that neither lower extremity exceeds hip flexion greater than 90°). If applicable the therapist may also instruct the patient in donning or removing the orthosis while in bed, while from a sidelying to a supine position, or while standing with assistance (if not contraindicated by physician's orders). For the acute stage, donning or removing of the orthosis in bed is preferable. The patient is instructed in general range of motion and strengthening exercises (without resistance) for the extremities such as ankle pumps to promote circulation, isometric quadriceps contractions, supine hip abduction, heel slides, and isometric gluteal sets. Because the patient's functional activities for the first two postoperative weeks are limited to showering and walking, the therapist's role is to encourage ambulation. Not only does this enable the patient to experience fewer side effects from bed rest, it is also beneficial for the development of a strong, healthy fusion mass or arthrodesis.

Formal guidelines to return to sport following spinal fusion are not well established in the literature. Lehman, et al.[71] surveyed experienced surgeons to better describe the variability in practice. Overall, they found that surgeons will allow earlier return to sports after surgery to correct AIS with the use of pedicle screw constructs as compared to hybrid (a combination of pedicle screws and hooks) and hook constructs. According to the survey, most patients with pedicle screw constructs are permitted to return to running by 3 months, both noncontact (e.g., PE class, swimming) and contact sports (soccer, basketball, volleyball) by 6 months, and collision sports (American football, hockey, rugby) by 12 months postoperatively. There are, however, approximately 20% of respondents who reported that they do not permit patients to return to collision sports, regardless of construct. Further research is merited to establish evidence-based guidelines for return to sport.

Exercise

Currently, research is evaluating the potential for physiotherapy scoliosis-specific exercises (PSSE) to play a role in improvement of postural awareness and subsequent spinal alignment in patients with AIS. The characteristics of PSSE include self-correction, elongation, and chest wall expansion with focus on incorporation of the corrected posture into one's daily activities of living.[52] Different PSSE approaches have emerged including, but not limited to, the Scientific Exercise Approach to Scoliosis (SEAS) in Italy and the Schroth technique from Germany. In an effort to investigate optimal treatment techniques for scoliosis that may include both operative and nonoperative treatment strategies, the SRS supports pilot research studies to critically evaluate the efficacy of PSSE in the treatment of AIS. Together with the Society on Scoliosis Orthopedic and Rehabilitative Treatment (SOSORT), the SRS is evaluating current treatment strategies for scoliosis including bracing, PSSE, and other fusionless treatments. The current stance of the SRS (2014) is that, while some evidence has shown that some PSSE programs are superior to programs with nonspecific exercises, it is too soon to comment on their general applicability.

A home exercise program designed to maintain or improve trunk and pelvic strength and flexibility is often prescribed for children with idiopathic or congenital scoliosis. Exercises include spinal stabilization, balance activities, core strengthening, and postural correction, including lateral shifts, flexibility exercises, and respiratory activities. Negrini et al.[98] investigated the SEAS protocol. In this approach the patient actively corrects his own posture with a goal of maximal curve correction and follows a specific exercise program designed to increase spinal stability, improve balance reactions, and retain physiologic sagittal spinal curvatures.

The Schroth method, introduced in the 1930s, also utilizes a personalized exercise protocol tailored to each patient to achieve maximal postural correction. The Schroth method strives to decrease curve progression, reduce pain, increase vital capacity, and improve posture and appearance.[72] The Schroth method has three major contributing concepts: postural correction, correction of breathing patterns, and correction of postural perception. The Schroth school believes that in order to affect postural control one must first change his postural perception.[135] Initially, Schroth addressed large thoracic spine curves (curves exceeding 70° to 80°),[8] but over the past several decades the program has evolved to affect small or moderate curves and to incorporate a focus on activities of daily living (ADLs) training to prevent loss of postural control throughout daily activities.[135] Originally, the program was performed over a period of at least 3 months, but recently shorter programs have been developed.[8] A 2015 study examined patients with AIS dividing them into 3 groups: a group performing Schroth exercises in a clinical setting under direct supervision of a physiotherapist, a home exercise group, and a control group who were observed. The investigators concluded that the exercise group under direct supervision was superior to a home exercise program or to no treatment at all, the latter two showing curve progression. The authors found that the home exercises may affect change in the lateral plane but without change in the rotation component.[7,127]

Borysov and Borysov investigated the effect of the Schroth method on the ATR and vital capacity in 34 children with AIS over 7 days. Both ATR and vital capacity were decreased, indicating improvement. These trials demonstrate that physical therapy may have the potential to effect positive change with idiopathic scoliosis. However, these studies and others are preliminary. Researchers have indicated that there are no mid- or long-term studies and more research is needed, which is in agreement with the statement put out by the SRS. The recommendation for the treating therapist is to incorporate exercises including spinal stabilization, balance activities, core strengthening, and postural correction, including lateral shifts, flexibility exercises, and respiratory activities into the plan of care. It is important to note that the Schroth method is copyrighted and certification is required to practice this technique (Fig. 8.8).

Outcomes for Persons with Idiopathic Scoliosis

Most people with AIS live functional and normal lives and have a mortality rate similar to that of the general population.[130,133] However, Weinstein et al.[130] found that patients with untreated scoliosis not only reported an increased incidence of both chronic and acute back pain but were found to have decreased body image as compared with people of similar age and gender without scoliosis. A Cobb angle greater than 50° at skeletal maturity was identified by Weinstein et al.[130] as a strong predictor of decreased pulmonary function. A curvature with a thoracic apex is also associated with shortness of breath.[130] Severe thoracic curves, greater than 100°, have been shown to decrease pulmonary function with dyspnea upon exertion leading to probable alveolar hypoventilation and chronic respiratory failure.[68]

Merola et al.[88] studied patients' status postsurgical correction of AIS and found statistically significant improvements in general self-image, function from back condition, and level of activity domains as compared with preoperative status but no significant correlation between magnitude of curve correction and outcome scores. Successful outcomes may be correlated with patient perception, such as elimination of the rib hump or restoration of the waistline, rather than focusing on magnitude of curve correction alone.[88]

The natural history of idiopathic scoliosis continues into adult life because curves can progress after skeletal maturity. Risk of progression depends on curve magnitude and location.[79] Curves of greater than 45° at the time of skeletal maturity have a higher risk of progressing and producing complications.

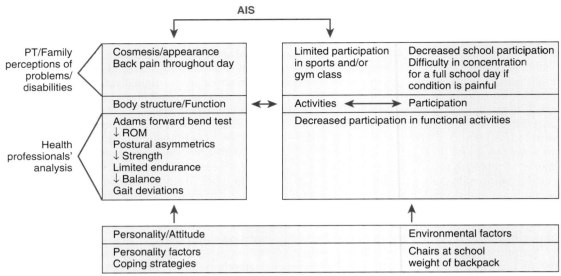

FIG. 8.8 Adolescent idiopathic scoliosis table of interventions. (Created using data from Steiner WA, Ryser L, Huber E, et al.: Use of the ICF model as a clinical problem-solving tool in physical therapy and rehabilitation medicine. *Phys Ther* 82:1098-1107, 2002.)

Although both thoracic and lumbar curves can progress, progression in the thoracic region may cause more significant complications because of its effects on the cardiopulmonary system. Complications of untreated scoliosis include severe cosmetic deformity and major disability, which may include pain, respiratory insufficiency, or right-sided heart failure.[46] Indications for adult treatment include back pain, compromised pulmonary function, psychosocial effects, and an increased risk for premature death. The treatment plan is consistent with that for adolescent idiopathic scoliosis.[131]

BACKGROUND INFORMATION

Neuromuscular Scoliosis

In contrast to idiopathic scoliosis, neuromuscular scoliosis is associated with systemic or chronic diseases and often has a rapid progression.[96] Neuromuscular curves tend to progress more rapidly and to have more disabling outcomes such as decreased ability to sit, diminished hand function, respiratory compromise due to intercostal muscle weakness,[132] and decreased lung capacity[53] and are highly associated with pelvic obliquity.[125] In the general population the prevalence of scoliosis is 1% to 2% while in cerebral palsy (CP) it has a large variance of 15% to 80%. The variance in those with CP is attributable to age, nature of severity of the neurologic impairment, extent of the physical impairment, and whether the child was positioned in supine versus upright when the x-ray was taken. It has been reported that a scoliosis of at least 40° at maturity is present in 30% of people with quadriplegic CP, 10% of those with diplegia, and 2% of those with hemiplegia.[66] See Chapter 19 for more detailed information on cerebral palsy.

In Duchenne muscular dystrophy (DMD) the development of scoliosis is correlated with the ability to ambulate; ambulators do not develop scoliosis. As children with DMD lose their ability to ambulate and become more dependent on their wheelchairs, a scoliotic curve begins to develop, typically in the thoracolumbar region.[95] A correlation between the ability to ambulate and the development of scoliosis has also been noted in those with CP in that the prevalence of scoliosis in nonambulators with total body involvement is also significantly higher than the prevalence in ambulators.[125] Scoliosis affects 100% of patients with spinal muscular atrophy (SMA) type II, typically beginning at about 3 years of age. On average, curves are greater than 54° by 10 years of age, typically with a low thoracic C-curve although 17% will develop an S-curve.[95] See Chapter 12 for more information on Duchenne muscular dystrophy.

The direct cause of neuromuscular scoliosis is not understood; however, Berven and Bradford[5] identified asymmetrical paraplegia, mechanical forces, intraspinal and congenital anomalies, sensory feedback, and control of spinal balance by central pathways as possible contributors in children. Disruption in any one of these areas may lead to spinal deformity. The SRS divides neuromuscular scoliosis into two categories: neuropathic (i.e., cerebral palsy [upper motor neuron] or spinal muscular dystrophy [lower motor neuron]) and myopathic (i.e., Duchenne muscular dystrophy).[132]

Important health issues are associated with neuromuscular conditions that may be influenced by scoliosis. Mullender et al.[95] reported in patients with either DMD or SMA type II, scoliosis is related to a decline in pulmonary function and that the decline in vital capacity is part of the natural history of the condition and not necessarily causally related to DMD or SMA type II. Large curves affect the ability to sit, requiring upper extremity propping and large rib prominences can be susceptible to pressure to the skin and may lead to ulceration and pain in children with cerebral palsy.[66]

An understanding of the orthopedic consequences associated with neuromuscular scoliosis is essential. Physical therapists play an important role in helping to manage and educate families about orthopedic concerns. The curve pattern commonly seen among people with neuromuscular scoliosis is a long C-curve (Fig. 8.9) beginning in the thoracic region and extending into the sacrum.[132] Relationships between the spine, pelvis, and hips have been investigated by several authors. Terjesen, Lange, and Steen[122] found that the severity of the

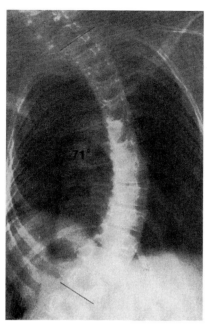

FIG. 8.9 Severe neuromuscular scoliosis. (From Moe JH, Winter RB, Bradford DS, et al.: Scoliosis and other spinal deformities. 2nd ed. Philadelphia: WB Saunders, 1987.)

curve correlated with the severity of the pelvic obliquity. Studies have reported there may be increased potential for hip subluxation in patients with scoliosis,[16,95] while multiple studies have described a link between the direction of a windswept deformity and the curve convexity.[66] Therapists should be aware of these potential consequences. Physical therapists should be monitoring spinal and hip range of motion for changes. They can instruct caregivers in positioning, stretches, and active or assistive-active range-of-motion exercises. Changes in seating in the patient's wheelchair may also be warranted.

Surgical Intervention

Surgical intervention for neuromuscular scoliosis differs from that for idiopathic scoliosis in several ways. In nonambulatory patients with CP the fusion with instrumentation is extended from the upper thoracic spine into the pelvis in order to obtain curve correction and reduce the risk of recurrent deformity. Improved pelvic alignment can also be achieved when the fusion is extended into the pelvis[66] for nonambulators.[125] The goals of the spinal fusion are to attain improvement of the deformity, stability of the new spinal shape, and a safe and tolerable surgery.[66]

Complications in patients undergoing spinal fusion have been shown to be high in children with CP,[66,110] occurring in 40% to 80% of patients. Major complications include blood loss, pulmonary compromise, deep wound infection, spinal cord dysfunction, and pseudoarthrosis.[66] Death occurs in 1% of patients. Pulmonary function is compromised in up to 25% of patients with neuromuscular scoliosis. It is most commonly seen when preoperative testing demonstrates a forced vital capacity of less than 40%.[66,110] Pulmonary function is at increased risk in children with neuromuscular scoliosis for respiratory problems, with pulmonary function being compromised for various reasons that may include weakness and scarring from aspiration or pneumonia. Pulmonary capacity is further compromised

in scoliosis. Flexibility of the rib cage is decreased, restricting chest wall excursion when breathing. Organs contained within the thorax are compressed by shortening of the trunk. These changes result in decreased gas exchange and diffusion capacity and ventilation/perfusion imbalance.[110] It is important that the treating physical therapist keep these limiting factors in mind and adjust intervention as needed.

In children with DMD or SMA the preferred fusion levels are T2 or T3 to L5. Fixation to the sacrum has been associated with loss of function, increased surgery length, and increased blood loss. A more mobile lumbosacral joint may assist functions such as seating and transfers when fusing to L5.[95]

The recommended surgical approach in this condition is to use the Luque segmental spinal instrumentation (SSI)–Galveston procedure. The Luque SSI procedure uses L-shaped rods surgically fixed at each segment with sublaminar wires forming a more rigid fixation in comparison to the Harrington rods due to the correction at each level. The Luque procedure was later modified with the use of intrailiac (Galveston) posts that are long lever arms to reduce lateral bending and flexion-extension movement. This allows the rods to span the sacroiliac joint. Long-term studies have demonstrated that this surgery is efficient and safe in those with DMD. Due to cardiac and respiratory issues it is recommended that spinal fusion be considered earlier than curve progression to 40°. The primary goal of surgery is to stop curve progression to obtain comfortable seating.[53] Healing from the spinal fusion takes an extended period of time; the arthrodesis takes 3 to 9 months to be completely healed. Precautions including spinal rotation and hip flexion beyond 90° are not permitted.[95]

A curve may require both an anterior approach with a discectomy and posterior fusion with instrumentation, although this is no longer the typical surgical approach. The anterior component of the procedure can improve spinal flexibility, minimizing residual curve and helping to achieve a level pelvis in children with CP.[66] Studies demonstrate that there is increased blood loss and length of hospital stay, including time spent in the intensive care unit, for combined anteroposterior spinal fusion compared to posterior only procedures.[126]

The role of the physical therapist is similar to that for postoperative treatment of other curve types. The intervention may have to be modified to adjust to a patient's motor and cognitive abilities.[95] Multiple studies utilizing parent/caregiver questionnaires suggest that spinal fusion surgery is beneficial and has a positive impact on their child's quality of life for children with neuromuscular scoliosis.[87] The parents of children with CP felt that their children had improved trunk balance, sitting, ease of transfers, and personal care.[66,125,126]

Nonsurgical Intervention

Nonsurgical intervention for neuromuscular spinal curvatures includes clinical observation, radiographic examination, and orthotic management.[132] Clinical observation allows a thorough assessment of the child's present and potential function, level of comprehension, and ability to cooperate.[32] Mullender et al.[95] discuss the importance of a well-fitting and supportive seating system as an integral part of the care in this population. This is best addressed by the team approach, including a physical therapist, an occupational therapist, a physician, an equipment vendor, and an orthotist. Please refer to Chapter 33, Assistive Technology, regarding appropriate seating options for this population.

The goal of orthotic management in children with neuromuscular scoliosis is to provide support directly to the trunk and possibly aid in simplifying the required seating.[66] Studies have demonstrated that the use of a spinal orthotic for a neuromuscular scoliosis does not have an impact on curve progression.[89] In DMD, as the spine matures, curve progression is predicted to be 10° per year with the use of bracing.[53] Terjesen, Lange, and Steen[103] found that, despite this, many families and caregivers have remained pleased with the outcome following TLSO use for 2 years, with improvements in sitting stability and overall function being reported. Orthotic management might include the custom-molded, total-contact TLSO; the underarm TLSO; or the Milwaukee brace.[78]

Researchers have studied other methods to manage neuromuscular scoliosis. King et al.[65] evaluated the effects of daily corticosteroid use on orthopedic outcomes in 143 boys with DMD. They found that those treated with steroids not only demonstrated a decreased prevalence of scoliosis, but they also had decreased magnitude of curvatures as compared with the untreated group. However, 32% of the treated group suffered vertebral compression fractures, a serious adverse effect of corticosteroid therapy. Other researchers have looked at the ability to prolong walking in boys with DMD and have seen some boys walk up to the ages of 13 to 15 years old, therefore slowing the rapid development of scoliosis, but this had not been corroborated.[95] Hsu and Quinilvan[53] reported that the lordotic posture present in boys with DMD delays development of spinal collapse while ambulatory. Other researchers have studied the effects of intrathecal baclofen (ITB) on curve progression[115,116] using matched groups for age, functional impairment, and curve magnitude and concluded that ITB does not have a significant effect on curve progression. Curve progression was found to increase compared with the expected natural history after insertion of ITB pumps in nonambulatory children with quadriplegic cerebral palsy and neuromuscular scoliosis.[37]

KYPHOSIS

Background and Foreground Information

A kyphosis is an abnormal posterior convexity of the spine; normal thoracic kyphosis measures 20° to 40° between vertebral segments T5 through T12 with a lumbar lordosis and a Cobb angle typically measuring 20° to 50°.[41] A spinal kyphosis may occur as the result of trauma, congenital conditions, or neuromuscular, post-traumatic (tuberculosis), or Scheuermann disease. The most common causes of an abnormal thoracic kyphosis in children and adolescents are Scheuermann disease and poor posture.[41] The discussion in this section focuses on congenital kyphosis, postural roundback, and Scheuermann disease.

Congenital Kyphosis

Congenital kyphosis is a rare deformity that is typically progressive, consisting of anterior nonsegmentation, centrum deficiencies, and mixed deformities. The exact cause is unknown, although animal studies suggest that there may be a vascular disruption causing centrum defects. Anomalies occur later during the chrondrification and ossification stages of the embryonic period. Additionally, posterior segmentation and block vertebrae defects have been seen. The most frequent defects are multiple hemivertebrae (44%), anterior segment defect (32%), and single hemivertebrae (18%). Up to 60% of patients may have associated anomalies, including the renal and cardiac systems,

or sacral agenesis. Congenital kyphosis typically requires surgical intervention and without surgery the progressive natural history will likely lead to paraplegia or cardiac dysfunction. Studies have demonstrated that orthotics are an ineffective treatment modality. Recommendations for surgery may be as young as prior to 3 years old to reduce possible neurologic sequelae. Posterior spinal arthrodesis can be safely completed in patients as young as 6 months of age. The goals of surgery are to stop deformity progression that leads to unbalanced growth and anterior decompression that places neural structures at risk. Arthrodesis with a posterior spinal fusion is recommended for deformities less than 50° to 60° and an additional anterior release and arthrodesis for larger deformities. In the immature spine, some spontaneous correction can occur after a posterior arthrodesis due to continued growth in the anterior portion of the vertebral body.[64] Basu et al.[3] studied the incidence of defects of other organ systems in patients with both congenital kyphosis and scoliosis and found it to be high, concluding that an essential part of patient evaluation is MRI and echocardiography. Zeng Y et al.[144] stated that there is an incidence of 20% to 40% of intraspinal anomaly associated with congenital spine deformity and therefore this must also be evaluated.

The spine is angled in congenital kyphosis and kyphoscoliosis compressing the rib cage forward on both sides, therefore impairing movement of the diaphragm when this compression occurs in the thoracic spine. A cross-sectional study demonstrated that with a more severe kyphosis, respiratory function became more impaired.[85]

Postural Roundback

Differential diagnosis of Scheuermann disease includes postural roundback. In this condition the thoracic kyphosis is up to 60°. It is flexible and will correct with hyperextension; it is smooth and nonprogressive. There is no disc involvement, and the vertebrae have a normal appearance.[124] The hallmark sign that distinguishes postural roundback from Scheuermann disease is a rigid spine.[41] Exercise alone as described below for Scheuermann disease is the treatment of choice. If the kyphosis progresses beyond 60°, the patient may be treated with a Milwaukee brace to prevent permanent structural changes.[93]

Scheuermann Disease

Scheuermann disease is a rigid form of postural kyphosis. It often is neglected, developing during childhood and adolescence, and usually is ascribed to poor posture[132] resulting in delayed referral to the appropriate clinician, diagnosis, and initiation of treatment.[1] Scheuermann kyphosis is the most common type of kyphosis in the adolescent population. The a rate of incidence ranges from 1% to 8% with nearly equal incidence in males and females.[80] Onset typically occurs during the prepubescent growth spurt becoming clinically apparent between the ages of 11 and 14 years of age.[41] In most cases progression is slow and stops when axial skeletal growth is completed.[34] Diagnosis is made by radiographic criteria including: (1) anterior wedging of 5° or more for at least three or more contiguous vertebrae, (2) narrowing of the intervertebral disc space,[76,80] (3) kyphosis greater than 45°[124] between vertebral segments T5 and T12 coupled with compensatory cervical and/or lumbar hyperlordosis[41] that is uncorrected on active hyperextension,[1] and (4) irregular vertebral end plates with Schmorl nodules, which are disc protrusions of the nucleus pulposus through the end plate into the vertebral body appearing as incongruent depressions.[9]

One third of patients have a mild scoliosis measuring 25° or less with minimal vertebral rotation[9,41,124] and varying degrees of spondylolysis and spondylolisthesis.[1,9,124] Back pain is an associated component typically occurring at the apex of the kyphosis, but occasionally in the low back. It is commonly aggravated with sitting, standing, and strenuous activities.[1] The pain is dull and nonradiating in nature.[124] Scheuermann disease also has thoracolumbar and lumbar variants. Gradual disc degeneration may be seen at the apex of the kyphosis[9,124] correlating the acute angulation and short segmented curves.[124]

Further research on the origin of Scheuermann kyphosis is needed. Studies demonstrate a strong genetic prevalence inherited though an autosomal dominant gene confirming a familial aggregation[142] with a less significant environmental component.[80] Relatives who were examined at age 40 or older presented with osteochondrosis (78%), spondylosis (56%), and arthrosis (33%), all of which are considered to be secondary changes.[142] Histologic studies have shown disorganized endochondral ossification, reduced amounts of collagen with thinner fibers, and increases in end plate mucopolysaccharides.[80,132] One theory based on examination of the mechanical factors suggests that some kyphosis is likely present from early in life, which leads to vertebral wedging caused by anterior pressure exerted upon the vertebrae.[132]

Clinical findings include tight pectoral, hamstring and iliopsoas muscles,[124,132] increased thoracic kyphosis with a compensatory increased lumbar lordosis, and forward head posture. Furthermore, 38% of patients with Scheuermann kyphosis had pain and worked in lighter-duty jobs than controls.[80]

Intervention

Surgical intervention is controversial because of the limited evidence on the natural history of Scheuermann disease. Surgical correction can be recommended for patients with curves greater than 70° that bracing does not control; those with disabling pain that is resistant to nonoperative measures including activity modification and exercises; those who have used anti-inflamatories for at least 6 months; or those who have concerns regarding their appearance.[124] Surgical management of a less rigid curve often includes a posterior spinal fusion, although more rigid curves also require an anterior fusion.[49,124]

Orthotic treatment is used when the kyphosis is between 45° and 65°. A modified Milwaukee-type brace is used. The reported success rate is high in the skeletally immature patient; however, skeletally mature patients do not respond to this treatment.[1,49] A modified Milwaukee brace is worn full time (22 hours per day) for 18 months.[80] Once patients have reached skeletal maturity, it may be used part-time at night for maintenance. The brace works as a three-point dynamic system and promotes thoracic extension.[1,132] Posterior pads apply pressure at the apex of the kyphosis, and pelvic pads stabilize the lumbar spine, decreasing the lordosis.[132] Brace use has been shown to decrease vertebral wedging with 12–18 months of full-time wear 22 hours per day followed by part-time wear of 12 hours per day to maintain the correction. Patients allowed 2 to 4 hours out of their brace to participate in sports generally have better acceptability of use of the brace and compromise of curve improvements were not seen.[1] It has been observed that the anterior longitudinal ligament may thicken and partial reversal of vertebral wedging may occur with use of a brace.[132] Predictors of poor outcomes to bracing include: a rigid kyphosis of greater than 65°, vertebral

wedging of greater than 10°, and limited or no remaining spinal growth. Whether a scoliosis is present does not impact the outcome of bracing. With appropriate patient selection, kyphosis can be improved. However, even with the most adherent patients, partial correction of an average of 30° can be expected once the brace is discontinued.[124]

Exercise plays an integral role in the treatment of patients with Scheuermann disease. The prescribed exercises are specific for active trunk extensor strengthening, general postural exercise, and hamstring stretches (Fig. 8.10). Sports that have a trunk extensor component such as volleyball or swimming and aerobic exercise are recommended. The goals of physical therapy are to improve postural alignment and to increase flexibility and extensor strength.[132] The progression of the kyphosis is not affected by physical therapy, but it is recommended for symptomatic patients as an adjunct to bracing to prevent increased stiffening of their spines. Studies have demonstrated that pain can be lessened with exercise.[124]

LORDOSIS

Background and Foreground Information

An anterior convexity (or a posterior concavity) of a segment of spine is termed a *lordosis*. Congenital lordosis is the result of bilateral posterior failure of segmentation.[137] Lordosis, both fixed and flexible, may be found in children with a variety of diagnoses. Lordosis in children with myelomeningocele usually occurs in the lumbar spine secondary to use of a tripod gait pattern. A lordosis may develop in the thoracic vertebrae to compensate for an increased lumbar kyphosis.[46] Hahn et al.[40] stated that a lumbar lordosis facilitates balanced sitting in the DMD population. In children with DMD the postural control muscles are weakened; therefore support for the vertebral column and upright control are affected. Hip flexion contractures, which are often present in individuals with DMD, mechanically pull the pelvis anteriorly, thereby leading to an increased lumbar lordosis. Kerr et al.[63] found that lordosis improved stability of the lumbar spine through locking of the articular facet joints.

Children without motor deficits may have an increased lumbar lordosis. Assessment includes testing of lower extremity ROM, spinal flexibility, trunk and lower extremity strength, posture, and gait. Interventions include abdominal strengthening (curls, crunches, and pelvic lifts), pelvic tilts in supine and standing positions, trunk extensor strengthening, and appropriate lower extremity stretching.

Spondylolysis and Spondylolisthesis

Spondylolysis is a defect of the pars interarticularis (Fig. 8.11). Herman, Pizzutillo, and Cavalier[48] suggest that upright, bipedal position, genetic predisposition, and repetitive loading of the lumbar spine are possible causative factors. Athletes involved in sports with repetitive hyperextension and rotational loading on the lumbar spine, such as gymnastics and diving, are noted to have a higher incidence of spondylolysis and spondylolisthesis than the general population.[15,47] Spondylolisthesis is the forward translatory displacement of one vertebra on another, usually occurring at the fifth lumbar vertebra (see Fig. 8.11). Multiple classification systems have been proposed for spondylolysis and spondylolisthesis; however, the Wiltse-Newman method remains the most widely utilized.[15] Five types of spondylolysis and spondylolisthesis have been classified by Wiltse and associates[136] as follows:

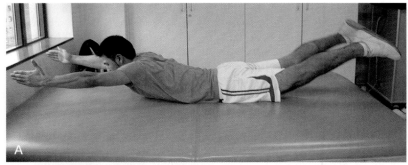

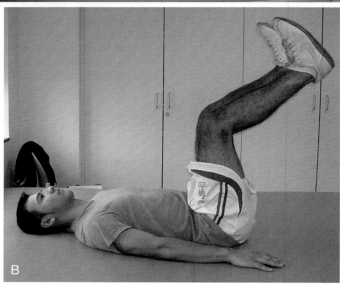

FIG. 8.10 (A) Active trunk extensor strengthening by prone lifts. (B) Lower abdominal strengthening exercises.

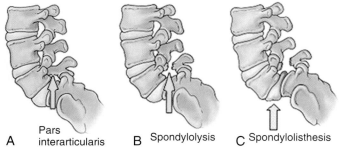

A Pars interarticularis   B Spondylolysis   C Spondylolisthesis

FIG. 8.11 (A) The pars interarticularis is the bony segment between the inferior and superior articular facets in the lumbar spine. (B) Spondylolysis, depicting a fracture of the pars interarticularis. (C) Depiction of spondylolisthesis, anterior slippage of one vertebra on another. (Courtesy of John Killian, MD, Birmingham, AL.)

Dysplastic malformations develop secondary to congenital malformations of the sacrum and posterior vertebral arch of L5. These malformations may include hypoplasia of the superior surface of the body of S1, hypoplasia-aplasia of the facets, elongation of the pars interarticularis, and spina bifida. The malformations decrease the efficiency of the posterior stabilizing system.[136] The degree of slippage is usually severe and may produce neurologic deficits as the laminae of L5 are pulled against the dural sac.[50]

Isthmic describes spondylolisthesis in the setting of spondylolysis. It describes the anterior slip of a vertebrae relative to the next caudal segment, often occurring at L5 over S1, related to a defect in the pars interarticularis.[47] Isthmic is divided into Type II A, lytic-fatigue fracture of the pars, Type II B, elongated but pars intact (pathogenic factors cause elongation of the pars secondary to repeated microfractures that heal with the pars in an attenuated-elongated position),[50] and Type II C, acute pars fracture.[47]

A degenerative type occurs in adults older than age 50 and is caused by the structural destruction of the capsule and ligaments of the posterior joints, producing hypermobility of the segment.

A traumatic type, more correctly defined as a fracture, is caused by a sudden fracture of the posterior arch of a vertebral segment. The fracture may occur at the pedicle, laminae, or facet, leaving the pars interarticularis intact.

Pathologic spondylolisthesis occurs most often secondary to an infectious disease that destroys the posterior arch of the vertebra.[136]

Dysplastic and isthmic spondylolisthesis types are the most common types seen in the pediatric population. Spondylolisthesis is further described by the degree of severity as characterized by percentage of slippage. According to the Meyerding classification system, grade I is the mildest slippage at less than 25%, grade II is 25% to 50% slippage, grade III is slippage of 50% to 75%, grade IV is 75% to 100% slippage,[50,136] and grade V refers to the ptosis of the cranial vertebra.[99]

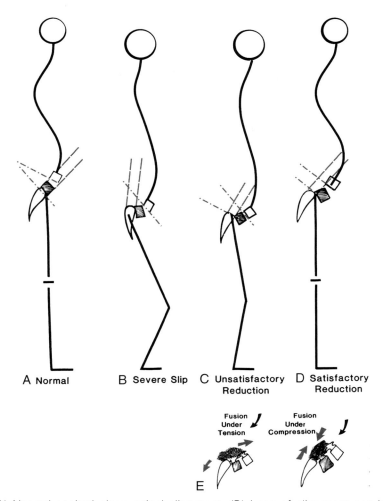

FIG. 8.12 (A) Normal sagittal plane spinal alignment. (B) Loss of alignment can be visualized after a severe L5 spondylolisthesis. The sacrum becomes vertical, and the resultant lumbosacral kyphosis "pushes" the lumbar spine forward. (C) An unsatisfactory reduction occurs when L5 has little mobility and L4 lies anterior to the "anatomic zone" and is kyphotic in relationship to the sacrum. The fusion in this case will be under tension and less likely to hold. (D) A satisfactory reduction occurs when L4 can be placed in the anatomic zone and oriented lordotic in relation to the sacrum. (E) The more L4 can be positioned over the sacrum, the more posterior compressive forces will be directed across the fusion. In this position, sagittal plane alignment and hence deformity will be corrected. (From Moe JH, Winter RB, Bradford DS, et al.: *Scoliosis and other spinal deformities.* 2nd ed. Philadelphia: WB Saunders, 1987.)

Clinical Symptoms

A spondylolisthesis is often an incidental finding, discovered on a radiograph taken for some other purpose. The clinical picture includes poor posture and increased lumbar lordosis in mild slippage. Higher-grade slippage may produce a flattened lumbar spine, a vertically oriented sacrum, and a visible or palpable step-off at the involved level.[47,48] (Fig. 8.12). Symptoms may include low back pain relieved by rest, sciatic-type pain, local tenderness, hamstring spasm or tightness, and, in severe cases, torso shortening.[50]

Risk of Progression

The risk of progression of spondylolysis and low-grade spondylolisthesis is low, occurring in less than 3% of skeletally immature children or adolescents.[47] Clinically, adolescents who are symptomatic are at a higher risk for increased slippage during their growth spurt. Females are at greater risk than males, as are patients with increased ligament laxity, including those with Down syndrome or Marfan syndrome. Presently, the best radiographic measure to help guide prognosis appears to be the slip angle.[81] Positive slip angles appear as kyphotic slips while negative slip angles appear as lordotic slips.[81] Radiographically, dysplastic types or patients with a 50% slippage, with a slip angle greater than 55° (kyphotic) in a skeletally immature patient (normal: −10° to 0° [lordotic] as identified by Mac-Thiong and Labelle)[82] or with bony instabilities or decreased anatomic stability of L5 and S1 are at greater risk for increased slippage.[50,93]

Surgical Intervention

Indications for surgery include persistent back pain despite conservative measures such as physical therapy, as well as gait deviations, greater than 50% slippage, marked instability of the defect with slip progression, neurologic deficit/radiculopathy, and hamstring contracture.[47,50] Surgery is recommended for patients with high-grade spondylolisthesis (grades III–V), even for asymptomatic patients due to the high risk of neurologic compromise if left untreated.[81] The goals of surgery are to prevent further slippage, immobilize the unstable segment, prevent further neurologic deficit, relieve any nerve root irritation, and correct clinical symptoms of poor posture, gait, and decreased hamstring length.[50]

Surgical options include posterolateral arthrodesis, anterior arthrodesis, decompression, and reduction with instrumentation. The surgical procedure most often performed is a bilateral posterolateral arthrodesis in situ. The fusion usually extends from L4 to S1 and is performed with an iliac bone graft.[39] Physical therapy is indicated for bed mobility, gait training, and activities of daily living and may be initiated to regain normal hamstring flexibility.

A neurologic deficit is the most common reason to perform a decompression. A decompression consists of removal of the bony anatomy that is causing nerve root irritation. The segments are then fused posteriorly to prevent further slippage.[128,129]

A reduction of the spondylolisthesis is indicated in cases in which the sacrum is in a vertical position, causing a severe lumbosacral kyphosis that displaces the lumbar spine anteriorly (see Fig. 8.12). The result is a marked compensatory lumbar lordosis. An open reduction technique can be anterior or posterior, with or without instrumentation, or a combination of surgical approaches may be used. An anterior fibular strut graft may be used for severe slips.[55] Circumferential fusion may also be performed. This technique improves stability of the fusion and provides increased surface area for loading the joint surface.[82]

Nonsurgical Intervention

Observation is the treatment of choice with asymptomatic low-grade spondylolisthesis (less than 50% slippage). These children are routinely followed two times per year with clinical and radiographic examinations. Patients presenting with symptomatic spondylolysis or low-grade spondylolisthesis often respond well to activity restriction, physical therapy, and spinal bracing.[47] Upon referral to physical therapy, patients learn lumbar stabilization exercises, in which they are taught to maintain pain-free, neutral alignment of the pelvis and lumbar spine while they vary their positions.[100] O'Sullivan et al.[100] emphasized the importance of strength training of the transverse abdominis, lumbar multifidus, and internal oblique muscles. They recommended incorporating cocontraction of these stabilizers into functional activities to support the lumbar spine and decrease low back pain in patients with spondylolysis and spondylolisthesis. Exercises may include bridging, wall squats, abdominal strengthening, prone gluteal strengthening, and other stabilization exercises in supine as well as exercises targeting hamstring flexibility. A therapeutic exercise ball may be incorporated into the exercise session to allow patients to achieve and maintain neutral lumbar spine stabilization on a mobile surface.

Immobilization using a TLSO is indicated following a stress fracture of the pars or with a well-defined spondylytic defect, although the goals of treatment differ: namely, healing of the pars defect in the former and alleviation of symptoms in the latter. Brace wear ranges from 6 to 12 weeks, depending on the goal of treatment, and may continue for up to 6 months if radiographs reveal incomplete healing of the pars stress injury. Return-to-play guidelines for the young athlete include painless spinal mobility, resolved hamstring spasm and contracture, and return to activities without pain.[48] If symptoms persist, surgery is indicated.

SUMMARY

Scoliosis, kyphosis, and lordosis are common pediatric orthopedic conditions of the spine. We, as pediatric physical therapists, often concentrate our therapy for many types of patients on the trunk for midline activities, symmetry, and stability for movement; therefore we can play a vital role in early detection of spinal deformities. We encourage children to become active to improve their cardiorespiratory function, muscle strength, and endurance. We can provide a referral source for families, instruction in home exercises, input for selecting appropriate adaptive equipment and seating, and rehabilitative intervention following injury or surgery. We address issues concerning the spine on a daily basis and play an important role in achieving and maintaining good health by maximizing proper alignment and function.

Case Scenario on Expert Consult

The case scenario related to this chapter uses the ICF model to detail the physiology of spondylolysis and spondylolisthesis and to discuss how it impacts a 9-year-old girl's participation in her daily activities. A video is also included to illustrate the examination and intervention details that can be applied to this case.

REFERENCES

1. Ali RM, Green DW, Patel TC: Scheuermann's kyphosis, *Curr Opin Pediatr* 11:131–136, 2000.
2. Aronsson DD, Stokes IA: Nonfusion treatment of adolescent idiopathic scoliosis by growth modulation and remodeling, *J Pediatr Orthop* 31(1):S99–S106, 2011.
3. Basu PS, Hazem E: Congenital spinal deformity: a comprehensive assessment at presentation, *Spine* 27:2255–2259, 2002.
4. Baulesh DM, Huh J, Judkins T, et al.: The role of serial casting in early-onset scoliosis, *J Pediatr Orthop* 7(32):658–663, 2012.
5. Berven S, Bradford DS: Neuromuscular scoliosis: causes of deformity and principles for evaluation and management, *Semin Neurol* 22:167–178, 2002.
6. Reference deleted in proofs.
7. Borysov M, Borysov A: Scoliosis short-term rehabilitation (SSTR) according to 'best practice' standards—are the results repeatable? *Scoliosis* 7(1), 2012.
8. Reference deleted in proofs.
9. Bowles AO, King JC: Scheuermann's disease: the lumbar variant, *Am J Phys Med Rehabil* 83:467, 2004.
10. Bunnell W: An objective criterion for scoliosis screening, *J Bone Joint Surg Am* 66:1381–1387, 1984.
11. Burwell RG: Aetiology of idiopathic scoliosis: current concepts, *Pediatr Rehabil* 6:137–170, 2003.
12. Reference deleted in proofs.
13. Campbell RM, Hell-Vocke AK: Growth of the thoracic spine in congenital scoliosis after expansion thoracoplasty, *J Bone Joint Surg Am* 85:409–420, 2003.
14. Campbell RM, Smith M, Mayes TC, et al.: The characteristics of thoracic insufficiency syndrome associated with fused ribs and congenital scoliosis, *J Bone Joint Surg Am* 85(3):399–408, 2003.
15. Cavalier R, Herman MJ, Cheung EV, et al.: Spondylolysis and spondylolisthesis in children and adolescents: I. Diagnosis, natural history, and nonsurgical management, *J Am Acad Orthop Surg* 14:417–424, 2006.

16. Chan KG, Galasko CSB, Delaney C: Hip subluxation and dislocation in Duchene muscular dystrophy, *J Pediatr Orthrop B* 10:219–225, 2001.

17. Charles YP, Daures JP, deRosa V, et al.: Progression risk of idiopathic juvenile scoliosis during pubertal growth, *Spine* 31:1933–1942, 2006.

18. Cheung JPY, Samartzis D, Cheung KMC: management of early-onset scoliosis, *J Bone Joint Surg* 1–5, 2013.

19. Cheung WY, Luk KDK: classification of adolescent idiopathic scoliosis, *Retrieved August 10* (2015).

20. Clin J, Aubin C, Parent S: Biomechanical stimulation and analysis of scoliosis correction using a fusionless intravertebral epiphyseal device, *Spine* 40(6):369–376, 2015.

21. Congenital scoliosis. Available from: URL: https://www.srs.org/patients-and-families/conditions-and-treatments/parents/scoliosis/early-onset-scoliosis/congenital-scoliosis.

22. Cowell HR, Hall JN, MacEwen GD: Genetic aspects of idiopathic scoliosis, *Clinic Orthop* 86:121–132, 1972.

23. Czaprowski D, Kotwicki T, Biernat R, et al.: Physical capacity of girls with mild and moderate idiopathic scoliosis; influence of the size, length and number of curves, *Eur Spine J* 21(6):1099–1105, 2012.

24. Demirkiran HG, Bekmez S, Celilov R, et al.: Serial derotation casting in congenital scoliosis and a time-buying strategy, *J Pediatr Orthop* 35(1):43–49, 2015.

25. Reference deleted in proofs.

26. Dickson RA, Lawton JD, Archer JA, et al.: The pathogenesis of idiopathic scoliosis, *J Bone Joint Surg Br* 66:8–15, 1984.

27. Dobbs MB, Weinstein SL: Infantile and juvenile scoliosis, *Orthop Clin North Am* 30:331–341, 1999.

28. Driscoll M, Aubin C, Moreau A, et al.: Biomechanical comparison of fusionless growth modulation corrective techniques in pediatric scoliosis, *Med Biol Eng Comput* 49:1437–1445, 2011.

29. Drummond DS: A perspective on recent trends for scoliosis correction, *Clin Orthop Rel Res* 264:90–102, 1991.

30. Dubousset J, Cotrel Y: Application technique of Cotrel-Dubousset instrumentation for scoliosis deformities, *Clin Orthop Rel Res* 264:103–110, 1991.

31. Duval-Beaupere G: The growth of scoliosis patients: hypothesis and preliminary study, *Acta Orthopaedica Belgica* 38:365–376, 1972.

32. Fisk JR, Bunch WH: Scoliosis in neuromuscular disease, *Orthop Clin North Am* 10:863–875, 1979.

33. Fletcher ND, McClung A, Rathjen KE, et al.: Serial casting as a delay tactic in the treatment of moderate-to-severe early-onset scoliosis, *J Pediatr Orthop* 32(7):664–671, 2012.

34. Fotiadis E, Grigoriadou A, Kapetanos G, et al.: The role of sternum on the etiopathogenesis of Scheuermann's disease of the thoracic spine, *Spine* 33(1):E21–E24, 2008.

35. Frownfelter D, Stevens K, Massery M, et al.: Do abdominal cutouts in thoracolumbosacral orthoses increase pulmonary function? *Clin Orthop Rel Res* 472:720–726, 2014.

36. Giampietro PF, Blank RD, Raggio CL, et al.: Congenital and idiopathic scoliosis: clinical and genetic aspects, *Clin Med Res* 1:125–136, 2003.

37. Ginsburg GM, Lauder AJ: Progression of scoliosis in patients with spastic quadriplegia after the insertion of an intrathecal baclofen pump, *Spine* 32:2745–2750, 2007.

38. Green NE: Part-time bracing of adolescent idiopathic scoliosis, *J Bone Joint Surg Am* 68:738–742, 1986.

39. Grzegorzewski A, Kumar SJ: In situ posterolateral spine arthrodesis for grades III, IV, and V spondylolisthesis in children and adolescents, *J Pediatr Orthop* 20:506–511, 2000.

40. Hahn F, Hauser D, Espinosa N, et al.: Scoliosis correction with pedicle screws in Duchenne muscular dystrophy, *Eur Spine J* 17:255–261, 2008.

41. Hart ES, Merlin G, Harisiades J, et al.: Scheuermann's thoracic kyphosis in the adolescent patient, *Orthop Nurs* 29(6):365–371, 2010.

42. Hassanzadeh H, Nandyala SV, Puvanesarajah V, et al.: Serial mehta cast utilization in infantile idiopathic scoliosis: evaluation of radiographic predictors, *J Pediatr Orthop* 0(0):1–5, 2015, Nov 17. Epub ahead of print.

43. Hawasli AH, Hullar TE, Dorward IG: Idiopathic scoliosis and the vestibular system, *Eur Spine J* 24(2):227–233, 2015.

44. Heary RF, Bono CM, Kumar S: Bracing for scoliosis, *Neurosurgery* 63:A125–A130, 2008.

45. Hedequist D, Emans J: Congenital scoliosis, *J Am Acad Orthop Surg* 12:266–275, 2004.

46. Herkowitz HN, Gardfin SR, Balderson RA, et al.: *Rothman-Simeone: the spine*, Philadelphia, 1999, WB Saunders.

47. Herman MJ, Pizzutillo PD: Spondylolysis and spondylolisthesis in the child and adolescent: a new classification, *Clin Orthop Rel Res* 434:46–54, 2005.

48. Herman MJ, Pizzutillo PD, Cavalier R: Spondylolysis and spondylolisthesis in the child and adolescent athlete, *Orthop Clin North Am* 34:461–467, 2003.

49. Herrera-Soto JA, Parikh SN, Al-Sayyad MJ, et al.: Experience with combined video-assisted thoracoscopic surgery (VATS) anterior spinal release and posterior spinal fusion in Scheuermann's kyphosis, *Spine* 30:2176–2181, 2005.

50. Herring JA: *Tachdjian's pediatric orthopedics*, ed 3, Philadelphia, 2002, WB Saunders, pp 213–312, 323-349, 1279–1291.

51. Hershman SH, Park JJ, Lonner BS: Fusionless surgery for scoliosis, *Bull Hosp Jt Dis* 71(1):49–53, 2013.

52. Hresko MT: SRS statement on Physiotherapy Scoliosis Specific Exercises, *Scoliosis Research Society*, 2014. Available from: URL: www.srs.org.

53. Hsu JD, Quinlivan R: Scoliosis in Duchene muscular dystrophy (DMD), *Neuromuscul Disord* 23(8):611–617, 2013.

54. Hsu JD, Michael JW, Fisk JR: *AAOS atlas of orthoses and assistive devices*, ed 4, Philadelphia, 2008, Mosby Elsevier.

55. Hu SS, Bradford DS, Transfeldt EE, et al.: Reduction of high-grade spondylolisthesis using Edwards instrumentation, *Spine* 21:367–371, 1996.

56. Jain A, Puvanesarajah V, Emmanuel N, et al.: Unplanned hospital readmissions and reoperations after pediatric spinal fusion surgery, *Spine* 40(11):856–862, 2015.

57. Janicki JA, Alman B: Scoliosis: review of diagnosis and treatment, *Paediatr Child Health* 12:771–776, 2007.

58. Kaplan KM, Spivak JM, Bendo JA: Embryology of the spine and associated abnormalities, *Spine J* 5:564–576, 2005.

59. Karol LA, Johnston C, Mladenov K, et al.: Pulmonary function following early thoracic fusion in non-neuromuscular scoliosis, *J Bone Joint Surg Am* 90(6):1272–1281, 2008.

60. Katz DE, Durrani AA: Factors that influence outcome in bracing large curve in patients with adolescent idiopathic scoliosis, *Spine* 26:2354–2361, 2001.

61. Katz DE, Richards BS, Browne RH, et al.: A comparison between the Boston brace and the Charleston bending brace in adolescent idiopathic scoliosis, *Spine* 22:1302–1312, 1997.

62. Kehl DK, Morrissy RT: Brace treatment in adolescent idiopathic scoliosis: an update on concepts and technique, *Clin Orthop Rel Res* 229:34–43, 1988.

63. Kerr TP, Lin JP, Gresty MA, et al.: Spinal stability is improved by inducing a lumbar lordosis in boys with Duchenne muscular dystrophy: a pilot study, *Gait Posture* 28:108–112, 2008.

64. Kim Y, Otsuka NY, Flynn JM, et al.: Surgical treatment of congenital kyphosis, *Spine* 26(20):2251–2257, 2001.

65. King WM, Ruttencutter R, Nagaraja HN, et al.: Orthopedic outcomes of long-term daily corticosteroid treatment in Duchenne muscular dystrophy, *Neurology* 68:1607–1613, 2007.

66. Koop S: Scoliosis in cerebral palsy, *Dev Med Child Neurol* 51(Suppl l4):92–98, 2009.

67. Kostuik JP: Current concepts review operative treatment of idiopathic scoliosis, *J Bone Joint Surg Am* 72:1108–1113, 1990.

68. Koumbourlis AC: Scoliosis and the respiratory system, *Paediatr Respir Rev* 7:152–160, 2006.

69. LaRosa G, Oggiano L, Ruzzini L: Magnetically controlled growing rods for the management of early-onset scoliosis: a preliminary report, *J Pediatr Orthop* July 17 (Epub ahead of print), 2015.

70. Lee SM, Suk SI, Chung ER: Direct vertebral rotation: a new technique of three-dimensional deformity correction with segmental pedical screw fixation in adolescent idiopathic scoliosis, *Spine* 29:343–349, 2004.

71. Lehman RA, Kang DG, Lenke LG, et al.: Return to sports after surgery to correct adolescent idiopathic scoliosis: a survey of the Spinal Deformity Study Group, *Spine J* 15:951–958, 2015.

72. Lehnert-Schroth C: Introduction to the three-dimensional scoliosis treatment according to Schroth, *Physiotherapy* 78:810–815, 1992.

73. Lenke LG: The Lenke classification system of operative adolescent idiopathic scoliosis, *Neurosurg Clin North Am* 18(2):199–206, 2007.

74. Lenke LG: Lenke classification system of adolescent idiopathic scoliosis: treatment recommendations, *Instr Course Lect* 54:537–542, 2005.

75. Letts RM, Jawadi AH: Congenital spinal deformity. Available from: URL: http://emedicine.medscape.com/article/1260442-overview.

76. Lonner BS, Newton P, Betz R, et al.: Operative management of Scheuermann's kyphosis in 78 patients: radiographic outcomes, complications, and technique, *Spine* 32:2644–2652, 2007.

77. Lonstein JE, Carlson JM: The prediction of curve progression in untreated idiopathic scoliosis during growth, *J Bone Joint Surg Am* 66:1061–1071, 1984.

78. Lonstein JE, Renshaw TS: *Neuromuscular spine deformities: instructional course lectures*, vol. 36. St. Louis, 1987, Mosby, pp 285–304.

79. Lonstein JE, Winter RB: Adolescent idiopathic scoliosis, *Orthop Clin North Am* 19:239–246, 1988.

80. Lowe TG, Line BG: Evidence based medicine analysis of Scheuermann kyphosis, *Spine* 32:S115–S119, 2007.

81. Lundine KM, Lewis SJ, Al-Aubaidi Z, et al.: Patient outcomes in the operative and nonoperative management of high-grade spondylolisthesis in children, *J Pediatr Orthop* 34(5):483–489, 2014.

82. Mac-Thiong J, Labelle H: A proposal for a surgical classification of pediatric lumbosacral spondylolisthesis based on current literature, *Eur Spine J* 15:1425–1435, 2006.

83. Margonato V, Fronte F, Rainero G, et al.: Effects of short term cast wearing on respiratory and cardiac responses to submaximal exercise in adolescents with idiopathic scoliosis, *Eura Medicophys* 41:135–140, 2005.

84. Matsumoto M, Watanabe K, Hosogane N, et al.: Updates on surgical treatments for pediatric scoliosis, *J Orthop Sci* 19:6–14, 2014.

85. McMaster MJ, Glasby MA, Singh H, et al.: Lung function in congenital kyphosis and kyphoscoliosis, *J Spinal Disord Tech* 20(3):203–208, 2007.

86. Mehlman CT: Idiopathic scoliosis. Available from: URL: http://emedicine.medscape.com/article/1265794-overview treatment of adolescent idiopathic scoliosis using the Scoliosis Research Society (SRS) outcome instrument. *Spine* 27:2046–2051, 2008.

87. Mercado E, Alman B, Wright J: Does spinal fusion influence quality of life in neuromuscular scoliosis? "multiple studies utilizing parent/caregiver questionnaires..." *Spine* 32(19) (Suppl):S120–S125, 2007.

88. Merola AA, Haher TR, Brkaric M, et al.: A multicenter study of the outcomes of the surgical treatment of adolescent idiopathic scoliosis using the Scoliosis Research Society (SRS) outcome instrument, *Spine* 27:2046–2051, 2002.

89. Miller A, Temple T, Miller F: Impact of orthoses on the rate of scoliosis progression in children with cerebral palsy, *J Pediatr Orthop* 16:332–335, 1996.

90. Miller NH: Genetics of familial idiopathic scoliosis, *Clin Orthop Rel Res* 462:6–10, 2007.

91. Miller NH: Cause and natural history of adolescent idiopathic scoliosis, *Orthop Clin North Am* 30:343–352, 1999.

92. Moe JH, Sundberg AB, Gustlio R: A clinical study of spine fusion in the growing child, *J Bone Joint Surg Br* 46:784–785, 1964.

93. Moe JH, Winter RB, Bradford DS, et al.: *Scoliosis and other spinal deformities*, ed 2, Philadelphia, 1987, WB Saunders, pp 162–228, 237–261, 347-368, 403–434.

94. Moreau S, Lonjon G, Mazda K, et al.: Derotation night-time bracing for the treatment of early onset idiopathic scoliosis, *Orthop Traumatol Surg Res* 100(8):935–939, 2014.

95. Mullender MG, Blom NA, DeKleuver M, et al.: A Dutch guideline for the treatment of scoliosis in neuromuscular disorders, *Scoliosis* 3(14):1–14, 2008.

96. Murphy NA, Firth S, Jorgensen T, et al.: Spinal surgery in children with idiopathic and neuromuscular scoliosis. What's the difference? *Spine* 26:216–220, 2006.

97. Muschik M, Schlenzka D, Robinson PN, et al.: Dorsal instrumentation for idiopathic adolescent thoracic scoliosis: rod rotation versus translation, *Eur Spine J* 8:93–99, 1999.

98. Negrini S, Zaina F, Romano M, et al.: Specific exercises reduce brace prescription in adolescent idiopathic scoliosis: a prospective controlled cohort study with worst-case analysis, *J Rehabil Med* 40:451–455, 2008.

99. Niggeman P, Kuchta J, Grosskurth D, et al.: Spondylolysis and isthmic spondylolisthesis: impact of vertebral hypoplasia on the use of the Meyerding classification, *Br J Radiol* 85:358–362, 2012.

100. O'Sullivan PB, Twomey LT, Allison GT: Evaluation of specific stabilizing exercise in the treatment of chronic low back pain with radiologic diagnosis of spondylolysis and spondylolisthesis, *Spine* 22:2959–2967, 1997.

101. Price CT, Scott DS, Reed Jr FR, et al.: Nighttime bracing for adolescent idiopathic scoliosis with the Charleston bending brace: preliminary report, *Spine* 15:1294–1299, 1990.

102. Puttlitz CM, Masaru F, Barkley A, et al.: A biomechanical assessment of thoracic spine stapling, *Spine* 32:756–761, 2007.

103. Reamy BV, Slakey JB: Adolescent idiopathic scoliosis: review and current concepts, *Am Fam Phys* 64:111–116, 2001.

104. Renshaw TS: *Orthotic treatment of idiopathic scoliosis and kyphosis: instructional course lectures*, vol. 34. St. Louis, 1985, Mosby, pp 110–118.

105. Renshaw TS: The role of Harrington instrumentation and posterior spine fusion in the management of adolescent idiopathic scoliosis, *Orthop Clin North Am* 19:257–267, 1988.

106. Richards BS, Vitale MG: Screening for idiopathic scoliosis in adolescents: an information statement, *J Bone Joint Surg Am* 90:195–198, 2008.

107. Roach JW: Adolescent idiopathic scoliosis, *Orthop Clin North Am* 30:353–365, 1999.

108. Roltan D, Nnadi C, Fairbanks J: Scoliosis: a review, *Paediatr Child Health* 24(5):197–203, 2013. 85b.

109. Sanders JO, D'Astous J, Fitzgerald M, et al.: Derotational casting for progressive infantile scoliosis, *J Pediatr Orthop* 29(6):581–587, 2009.

110. Sarwahi V, Sarwark JF, Schafer MF, et al.: Standards in anterior spine surgery in pediatric patients with neuromuscular scoliosis, *J Pediatr Orthop* 21(6):756–760, 2001.

111. Sarwark JF, LaBella CR: *Pediatric orthopaedics and sports injuries: a quick reference guide*, ed 2, Elk Grove, 2014, American Academy of Pediatrics.

112. Sarwark JF, Aubin CE: Growth considerations of the immature spine, *J Bone Joint Surg* 89(Supp 1):8–13, 2007.

113. Schroerlucke SR, Akbarnia BA, Pawelek JB, et al.: How does thoracic kyphosis affect patient outcomes in growing rod surgery? *Spine* 37(15):1303–1309, 2012.

114. Scoliosis Research Society. SRS-AAOS position statement. Available from: URL: www.srs.org.

115. Senaran H, Shah SA, Presedo A, et al.: The risk of progression of scoliosis in cerebral palsy patients after intrathecal baclofen therapy, *Spine* 32:2348–2354, 2007.

116. Shilt JS, Lai LP, Cabrera MN, et al.: The impact of intrathecal baclofen on the natural history of scoliosis in cerebral palsy, *J Pediatr Orthop* 28:684–687, 2008.

117. Smith JT, Jerman J, Stringham J, et al.: Does expansion thoracoplasty improve the volume of the convex lung in a windswept thorax? *J Pediatr Orthop* 29:944–947, 2009.

118. Staheli LT: *Practice of pediatric orthopedics*, ed 4, Philadelphia, 2008, Lippincott Williams Wilkins.

119. Steiner WA, Ryser L, Huber E, et al.: Use of the ICF model as a clinical problem-solving tool in physical therapy and rehabilitation medicine, *Phys Ther* 82:1098–1107, 2002.

120. Stokes I: Analysis and simulation of progressive adolescent scoliosis by biomechanical growth modulation, *Eur Spine J* 16:1621–1628, 2007.

121. Suk SI, Choon KL, Kim WJ, et al.: Segmental pedicle screw fixation in the treatment of thoracic idiopathic scoliosis, *Spine* 20:1399–1405, 1995.

122. Terjesen T, Lange JE, Steen H: Treatment of scoliosis with spinal bracing in quadriplegic cerebral palsy, *Dev Med Child Neurol* 42:448–454, 2000.

123. Thomas CL, editor: *Taber's cyclopedic medical dictionary*, ed 16, Philadelphia, 1989, FA Davis.

124. Tsirikos AI, Jain AK: Instructional review: spine Scheuermann's kyphosis; current controversies, *J Bone Jt Surg Br* 93-B 857–864, 2011.

125. Tsirikos AI, Chang W, Shah SA, et al.: Preserving ambulatory potential in pediatric patients with cerebral palsy who undergo spinal fusion using unit rod instrumentation, *Spine* 28(5):480–483, 2003.

126. Tsirikos AI, Lipton G, Chang W, et al.: Surgical correction of scoliosis in pediatric patients with cerebral palsy using unit rod instrumentation, *Spine* 33(10):1133–1140, 2008.

127. Kuru T, Yelden I, Dereli EE, et al.: The efficacy of three-dimensional Scroth exercises in adolescent idiopathic scoliosis: a randomised controlled clinical trial, *Clin Rehabil* 30(2):181–190, 2015.

128. Van Rens TG, Van Horn JR: Long-term results in lumbosacral interbody fusion for spondylolisthesis, *Acta Orthopaedica Scand* 53:383–392, 1982.

129. Verbeist H: The treatment of lumbar spondyloptosis or impending lumbar spondyloptosis accompanied by neurologic deficit and/or neurogenic intermittent claudication, *Spine* 4:68–77, 1979.

130. Weinstein SL, Dolan LA, Spratt KF, et al.: Health and function of patients with untreated idiopathic scoliosis: a 50-year natural history study, *JAMA* 289:559–567, 2003.

131. Weinstein SL: *Adolescent idiopathic scoliosis: prevalence and natural history: instructional course lectures*, vol. 38. St. Louis, 1989, Mosby.

132. Weinstein SL: *The pediatric spine: principles and practice*, ed 2, Philadelphia, 2001, Lippincott Williams Wilkins.

133. Weinstein SL, Zavala DC, Ponseti IV: Idiopathic scoliosis: long-term follow-up and prognosis in untreated patients, *J Bone Joint Surg Am* 63:702–712, 1981.

134. Weinstein SL, Dolan LA, Wright JG, et al.: Effects of bracing in adolescents with idiopathic scoliosis, *N Engl J Med* 369(16):1512–1521, 2013.

135. Weiss HR: The method of Katharina Schroth—history, principles, and current development, *Scoliosis* 6(17), 2011.

136. Wiltse LL, Newman PH, MacNab I: Classification of spondylolysis and spondylolisthesis, *Clin Orthop* 117:23–29, 1976.

137. Winter RB: *Congenital deformities of the spine*. New York, 1983, Thieme-Stratton, pp 6-10, 43–49.

138. Winter RB: Congenital scoliosis, *Orthop Clin North Am* 19:395–408, 1988.

139. Wong HK, Hee H-T, Yu Z, et al.: Results of thoracoscopic instrumented fusion versus convention posterior instrumented fusion in adolescent idiopathic scoliosis undergoing selective thoracic fusion, *Spine* 29:2031–2038, 2004.

140. Wynne-Davies R: Familial (idiopathic) scoliosis, *J Bone Joint Surg Br* 50:24–30, 1968.

141. Yazici M, Emans J: Fusionless instrumentation systems for congenital scoliosis: expandable spinal rods and vertical expandable prosthetic titanium rib in the management of congenital spine deformities in the growing child, *Spine* 34:1800–1807, 2009.

142. Zaidman AM, Zaidman MN, Strokova EI, et al.: The mode of inheritance of Scheuermann's disease, *Biomed Res Int* 973716, 2013, http://dx.doi.org/10.1155/2013/973716. Epub 2013 Sep 12.

143. Zaouss AL, James JIP: The iliac apophysis and the evolution of curves in scoliosis, *J Bone Joint Surg Br* 40:442–453, 1958.

144. Zeng Y, Chen Z, Qi Q, et al.: The posterior surgical correction of congenital kyphosis and kyphoscoliosis: 23 cases with minimum 2 years follow-up, *Eur Spine J* 22(2):372–378, 2013.

SUGGESTED READINGS

Background

Campbell RM, Smith M, Mayes TC, et al.: The characteristics of thoracic insufficiency syndrome associated with fused ribs and congenital scoliosis, *J Bone Joint Surg Am* 85(3):399–408, 2003.

Cavalier R, Herman MJ, Cheung EV, et al.: Spondylolysis and spondylolisthesis in children and adolescents: i. Diagnosis, natural history, and nonsurgical management, *J Am Acad Orthop Surg* 14:417–424, 2006.

Hassanzadeh H, Nandyala SV, Puvanesarajah V, et al.: Serial mehta cast utilization in infantile idiopathic scoliosis: evaluation of radiographic predictors, *J Pediatr Orthop* 0(0):1–5, 2015, Nov 17. Epub ahead of print.

Kaplan KM, Spivak JM, Bendo JA: Embryology of the spine and associated abnormalities. *Spine J* 5(5):564–57, 2005.

Koumbourlis AC: Scoliosis and the respiratory system, *Paediatr Respir Rev* 7:152–160, 2006.

McMaster MJ, Glasby MA, Singh H, et al.: Lung function in congenital kyphosis and kyphoscoliosis, *J Spinal Disord Tech* 20(3):203–208, 2007.

Foreground

Ali RM, Green DW, Patel TC: Scheuermann's kyphosis, *Curr Opin Orthop* 11:131–136, 2000.

Borysov M, Borysov A: Scoliosis short-term rehabilitation (SSTR) according to 'best practice' standards—are the results repeatable? *Scoliosis* 7(1), 2012.

Czaprowski D, Kotwicki T, Biernat R, et al.: Physical capacity of girls with mild and moderate idiopathic scoliosis; influence of the size, length and number of curves, *Eur Spine J* 21(6):1099–1105, 2012.

Koop S: Scoliosis in cerebral palsy, *Dev Med Child Neurol* 51(Suppl 4):92–98, 2009.

Mullender MG, Blom NA, DeKleuver M, et al.: A Dutch guideline for the treatment of scoliosis in neuromuscular disorders, *Scoliosis* 3(14), 2008.

Negrini S, Zaina F, Romano M, et al.: Specific exercises reduce brace prescription in adolescent idiopathic scoliosis: a prospective controlled cohort study with worst-case analysis, *J Rehabil Med* 40:451–455, 2008.

O'Sullivan PB, Twomey LT, Allison GT: Evaluation of specific stabilizing exercise in the treatment of chronic low back pain with radiologic diagnosis of spondylolysis and spondylolisthesis, *Spine* 22:2959–2967, 1997.

Roltan D, Nnadi C, Fairbanks J: Scoliosis: a review, *Paediatr Child Health* 24(5):197–203, 2013. 85b.

Tsirikos AI, Jain AK: Instructional review: spine Scheuermann's kyphosis; current controversies, *J Bone Joint Surg Br* 93-B:857–864, 2011.

Weinstein SL, Dolan LA, Wright JG, et al.: Effects of bracing in adolescents with idiopathic scoliosis, *N Engl J Med* 369(16):1512–1521, 2013.

9

Congenital Muscular Torticollis

Sandra L. Kaplan, Barbara Sargent, Colleen Coulter

Congenital muscular torticollis (CMT) and cranial deformation (CD) are commonly seen in infants at birth or soon after. CMT results from unilateral shortening of the sternocleidomastoid (SCM) muscle and is named for the side of the involved SCM muscle. It is characterized by a lateral head tilt toward and chin rotation away from the involved side. Fig. 9.1 illustrates a right CMT with head tilt to the right and rotation of the chin to the left secondary to a tight right SCM. Reports of incidence vary from 0.3% to 16% of newborns.[143] It is the third most common congenital musculoskeletal condition after hip dislocation and clubfoot.[17] CMT is associated with mandibular asymmetry, craniofacial asymmetry including deformational plagiocephaly,[26,165] eye and mouth displacement,[26] scoliosis,[13,21] brachial plexus injury,[10] pelvic asymmetry, congenital hip dysplasia, foot deformity,[26] muscle[109] and functional asymmetry,[13] and greater use of related services in early school years.[158] Synonyms for CMT include fibromatosis colli, wry neck, or twisted neck.[74]

CD is a distortion of the shape of the skull resulting from mechanical forces that occur pre- or postnatally.[127] It is different from craniosynostosis, defined as cranial asymmetry resulting from premature closure of one or more of the cranial sutures.[72] CD is a coexisting impairment in up to 90.1%[26] of infants with CMT and increases the risk of facial,[7] ear,[7,99] and mandibular asymmetry.[73,140] Prevalence of CD is age dependent and ranges from 6%[160] to 61%[143] at birth, 16%[61] to 46.6%[98] from 1.5 to 4 months, 6.8% at 1 year,[61] 3.3% at 2 years[61] and 2% at 12–17 years.[126] Synonyms for CD include positional deformation, deformational cranial flattening, or nonsynostotic head asymmetry.

Physical therapy intervention is highly effective in resolving CMT and CD when initiated early in infancy.[86,120] This chapter discusses the etiology and pathophysiology, screening and examination, intervention, and expected outcomes for CMT and CD.

BACKGROUND INFORMATION

ANATOMY OF THE STERNOCLEIDOMASTOID MUSCLE AND CRANIUM

The SCM illustrated in Fig. 9.2 has two major palpable bands: the medial band originates at the manubrium of the sternum and the lateral band originates from the medial third of the clavicle, with both joining to insert on the ipsilateral mastoid process and the superior nuchal line of the cranium.[102] The SCM muscle is innervated by the second and third cervical nerves for sensation; the spinal portion of the accessory nerve provides motor innervation to both the SCM and the upper trapezius muscle. Infants with CMT present with unilateral tightness of the SCM, a possible mass or nodule in the

muscle and may also have ipsilateral restrictions or tightness of the upper trapezius muscle.[116] The trapezius is a synergist of the ipsilateral SCM muscle for lateral head tilt, and it elevates the scapula. The contour of the upper part of the neck is formed by the fibers of the SCM muscle, and the contour of the lower part of the neck is formed by the fibers of the trapezius muscle.

An infant's cranium is composed of bone plates (frontal, occipital, parietal, temporal) that are separated by fibrous sutures (coronal, lambdoid, metopic, sagittal, squamosal) and fontanelles (anterior, mastoid, posterior, sphenoid), which are soft membrane–covered spaces, often referred to as soft spots. Open sutures and fontanelles, illustrated in Fig. 9.3, give the infant's cranium flexibility to pass through the birth canal and to expand in response to pressure exerted by the rapidly growing infant brain. Head circumference increases considerably over the first year of life: approximately 2 cm per month in the first 3 months, 1 cm per month between 4 and 6 months, and 0.5 per month from 6 to 12 months.[57] Approximately 70% to 80% of skull growth occurs by 2 years of age, and the remaining growth occurs slowly into adulthood.[104]

ETIOLOGY AND PATHOPHYSIOLOGY OF CMT

The etiology of CMT has been attributed to prenatal, perinatal, and postnatal factors. Prenatal factors that might cause CMT include ischemic injury based on abnormal vascular patterns or head position in utero leading to compartment syndrome,[37] intrauterine crowding or persistent malpositioning,[79] rupture of the muscle, infective myositis,[158] and hereditary factors.[138,153] Perinatal factors may include birth trauma from breech presentations or assisted deliveries.[79,146] Postnatal factors associated with CMT, but not necessarily causative, include the presence of hip dysplasia,[163] positional preference,[14] and the presence of deformational plagiocephaly.[38] There are no clear correlations with pre- or perinatal factors and the severity of the CMT that an infant will develop.

Histologic tissue changes of the SCM in infants with CMT include excessive fibrosis, hyperplasia, and atrophy.[24] The degree of fibrosis evident on ultrasound may fluctuate with age but typically decreases over time.[89] In some infants a palpable nodule, illustrated in Fig. 9.4, may be present in the SCM as early as 2–3 weeks[37]; both the degree of fibrotic changes and the location of the nodule are associated with the prognosis for resolution. Nodules in the lower one third of the SCM are most likely to resolve with conservative stretching as compared to nodules that occupy the middle one third or both the lower and middle one third, and those that occupy the length of the SCM are the most recalcitrant.[27,89] Synonyms for the nodule include SCM mass, tumor,[138] or pseudotumor of infancy.[148,165]

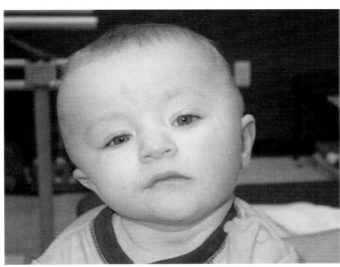

FIG. 9.1 Child with right CMT and CD, left asymmetrical brachycephaly. Note the right lateral flexion, chin turned to the left, asymmetry of the ear pinnae, eyebrows, mandible, and neck folds, wider forehead, right shoulder elevation, and trunk rotation.

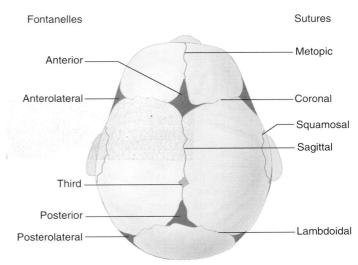

Fontanelles   Sutures

Anterior — — Metopic

Anterolateral — — Coronal

— Squamosal

— Sagittal

Third —

Posterior —

Posterolateral — — Lambdoidal

FIG. 9.3 Fontanelles and cranial suture lines and junctions. (From Graham JM: *Smith's recognizable patterns of human deformation.* 3rd ed. Philadelphia, Saunders, 2007.)

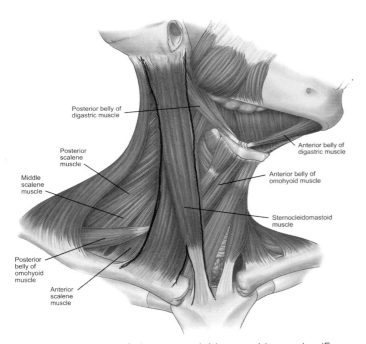

Posterior belly of digastric muscle

Posterior scalene muscle

Middle scalene muscle

Posterior belly of omohyoid muscle

Anterior scalene muscle

Anterior belly of digastric muscle

Anterior belly of omohyoid muscle

Sternocleidomastoid muscle

FIG. 9.2 Anatomy of the sternocleidomastoid muscle. (From Deslauriers J: Anatomy of the neck and cervicothoracic junction. *Thorac Surg Clin* 17:529-547, 2007.)

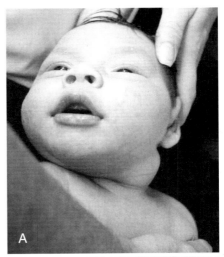
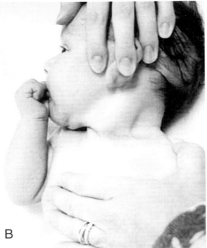

FIG. 9.4 (A) A 2-month-old infant with a fibrotic nodule in the left SCM muscle that involves the whole muscle. (B) Same infant at 3 months of age.

Potential confounding factors to full resolution of CMT are age at which an infant is referred for intervention,[20,120] the severity of the range-of-motion (ROM) limitations,[25,85] the thickness of a SCM nodule,[59] and the variability in foci and dosage of intervention.[114,152]

Postures that can mimic CMT may result from nonmuscular causes, including absence of the SCM,[60] benign paroxysmal torticollis,[155] congenital malformations, bony anomalies, brachial plexus injury, ocular disorders, and

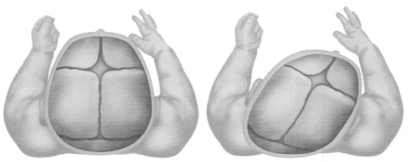

FIG. 9.5 Cranial deformation as a result of persistent asymmetrical pressure. (Redrawn from Mortenson PA, Steinbok P: Quantifying positional plagiocephaly: reliability and validity of anthropometric measurements. *J Craniofac Surg* 17:413-419, 2006.)

neurologic impairments,[10,155,156] so it is important for clinicians to take a detailed history and carefully examine infants who present with asymmetrical postures to rule out causes other than CMT.

ETIOLOGY AND PATHOPHYSIOLOGY OF CD

The etiology of CD has been attributed to intrauterine deformation that worsens postnatally,[118,143] postnatal positioning,[69,160] and cervical muscular imbalance or CMT.[52]

Intrauterine deformation has been theorized to result from uterine constraint that is perpetuated and accentuated postnatally as the infant preferentially lies in supine on the flattened area of the skull.[118,143] Factors associated with increased risk for CD include: male gender, firstborn, delivered with assistance using forceps or vacuum extractor, cumulative exposure to the supine position, and neck problems.[12] Although CD may be present at birth, a relationship between CD at birth and CD after 6 weeks has not been established.[160]

Stronger support exists for the hypothesis that postnatal positioning is a causal factor in CD. An increase in referrals for CD has been noted by craniofacial clinics[16] since the 1992 "Back to Sleep" campaign.[1] The American Academy of Pediatrics recommends that infants be placed on their backs to sleep to prevent sudden infant death syndrome (SIDS).[3] Although this recommendation has resulted in more than a 40% reduction in the incidence of SIDS in the United States, an unintended consequence was the observed increase in CD.[2] Supine sleeping[61,69] is associated with CD, as well as several other postnatal positioning factors including: infrequent tummy time,[66,160] consistent bottle feeding on the same arm,[160] and consistent positioning in a crib.[66,160] Motor development is inversely associated with CD, supporting the theory that earlier achievement of motor milestones, such as head control, may provide a possible preventive effect for CD.[160] This is further supported by the observation that infants whose mothers perceive them as having lower activity levels[61,66] or developmental delays[66] have a higher risk of CD.

Cervical muscular imbalance or CMT has been proposed as a causative factor of CD.[127,129] CD at birth and limited passive cervical rotation[5] or CMT[118] are not associated; however, associations have been established between CD at 6–7 weeks of age and limited newborn passive cervical rotation,[61] positional head preference in supine sleeping during the first 4 weeks of life,[160] and positional head preference at 6 weeks.[66] Furthermore, up

to 75% of infants with CD exhibit SCM imbalance or CMT.[52] Taken together, this evidence suggests that although intrauterine constraint may induce some cases of CD, positional preference from cervical muscular asymmetry and cumulative exposure to the supine position in early infancy likely interact to make a stronger contribution to the development of CD in the majority of infants.

The natural history of CD is characterized by increasing incidence until approximately 4 months of age, when infants independently maintain their head upright, then decreasing incidence until 2 years of age.[61] Controversy exists as to whether CD at 2 years of age persists[35] or further normalizes[126] during childhood and adolescence. Factors that contribute to the degree of resolution of CD are the severity of the CD,[162] age at which an infant begins intervention,[78,133] and type of intervention.[47] Fig. 9.5 illustrates how persistent positional preference to the right in supine can contribute to asymmetrical development of the infant's skull.

COMBINED CONDITIONS OF CMT AND CD

It is not clear in all children whether the CMT yields the CD or whether the CD with a positional preference might lead to CMT. Infants with CMT who spend excessive time with the head turned to one side may develop flattening of the skull on that side. Likewise, an asymmetrical skull may cause the head to persistently tip toward the flattened side when supine, causing ipsilateral adaptive shortening of the SCM. Regardless of cause, many children present with both conditions and both will need to be addressed in the plan of care.

METHODS OF CLASSIFICATION FOR CMT

Infants with CMT have been grouped in many ways, including the age at which their intervention began, severity of the ROM limitations, the presence of deformational plagiocephaly, the muscle fiber qualities based on ultrasound imaging, and the type of CMT.[74]

The three types of CMT commonly described are postural, muscular, and SCM nodule. Postural CMT is the mildest form and presents as a positional preference of the head and neck by the infant without limitations to PROM and without a nodule in the muscle.[14,138] Muscular CMT involves unilateral tightness of the SCM apparent during cervical rotation and/or lateral flexion, without a nodule in the muscle. The most severe form presents with a palpable nodule[50] or fibrous bands[86] in the SCM and limitations in either or both cervical rotation and lateral flexion.[106]

CMT severity can also be classified with ultrasound images based on the degree of muscle fibrosis and fiber orientation.[43,86] In general, larger and thicker nodules and/or higher ultrasound ratings are correlated with more severe presentations and longer treatment durations.[149]

The clinical practice guideline on the management of CMT[74] suggests a classification method that accounts for the type of CMT, the degree of ROM limitations, and the age at which treatment begins. Seven grades of severity are provided with operational definitions that provide greater detail for comparing clinical outcomes (Table 9.1).

TABLE 9.1 Grades of CMT Severity

Grade	Definition
Grade 1: Early Mild	These infants present between 0 and 6 months of age with only postural preference or muscle tightness of less than 15° of cervical rotation.
Grade 2: Early Moderate	These infants present between 0 and 6 months of age with muscle tightness of 15° to 30° of cervical rotation.
Grade 3: Early Severe	These infants present between 0 and 6 months of age with muscle tightness of more than 30° of cervical rotation or an SCM nodule.
Grade 4: Late Mild	These infants present between 7 and 9 months of age with only postural preference or muscle tightness of less than 15° of cervical rotation.
Grade 5: Late Moderate	These infants present between 10 and 12 months of age with only postural or muscle tightness of less than 15° of cervical rotation.
Grade 6: Late Severe	These infants present between 7 and 12 months of age with muscle tightness of more than 15° of cervical rotation.
Grade 7: Late Extreme	These infants present after 7 months of age with an SCM nodule or after 12 months of age with muscle tightness of more than 30° of cervical rotation.

From Kaplan SL, Coulter C, Fetters L: Physical therapy management of congenital muscular torticollis: an evidence-based clinical practice guideline from the section on pediatrics of the American Physical Therapy Association. *Pediatr Phys Ther* 25:348-394, 2013.

METHODS OF CLASSIFICATION FOR CD

CD is classified by the type and severity of the deformation.[91] The three types are plagiocephaly, brachycephaly, and dolichocephaly. Infants may also present with a combination of types.[65,99]

Deformational plagiocephaly (DP), depicted in Fig. 9.6B, is characterized by a parallelogram shape of the skull with ipsilateral occipital flattening and contralateral occipital bossing or bulging. DP is commonly associated with CMT,[26] and the flattened occiput is typically contralateral to the tight SCM; for example, left CMT with a shortened left SCM is associated with right DP. DP is also known as lateral deformational plagiocephaly, nonsynostotic occipital plagiocephaly, and positional plagiocephaly.

Deformational brachycephaly (DB), depicted in Fig. 9.6C, is characterized by central occipital flattening and is commonly associated with prolonged supine positioning.[53,54] DB is also known as posterior deformational plagiocephaly and flat head syndrome. When DB presents asymmetrically with bilateral posterior flattening greater on one side of the skull compared to the other, it is specifically called asymmetrical brachycephaly.

Deformational dolichocephaly, also known as scaphocephaly and depicted in Fig. 9.6D, is characterized by a disproportionately long and narrow skull. It is commonly associated with premature birth.[68]

The severity of CD can be classified by rating scales based on clinical observation.[7,108] Argenta's clinical classification scale[7] is the most frequently reported. It distinguishes five types of DP and three types of DB based on the severity of the asymmetry of the skull, ear position, and face. Refer to Tables 9.2 and 9.3 for definitions and diagrams of each type.

Quantitative measurement techniques for CD include using calipers,[166] digital photographic techniques,[62] or three-dimensional (3D) digital imaging.[9] These techniques are often used in research or by specialized craniofacial clinics. All three techniques measure cranial width, cranial length, and transcranial diagonals as illustrated in Fig. 9.7. DP is quantified by the transcranial diagonal difference (TDD),[141] oblique cranial length ratio (OCLR),[64] and cranial vault asymmetry index (CVAI).[103] These three measures vary in the location of their measurements, but they all measure the ratio of the longer to the shorter transcranial diagonal. Standard cutoff values have not been established but the following have been proposed: TDD of 3–10 mm is mild, 10–12 mm moderate, and > 12 mm severe.[91]

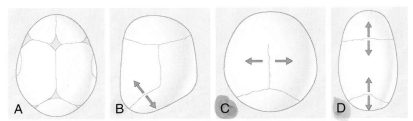

FIG. 9.6 Types of cranial deformation. (A) Typical. (B) Plagiocephaly characterized by ipsilateral occipital flattening. (C) Brachycephaly characterized by central occipital flattening. (D) Dolichocephaly characterized by a long and narrow skull. (From Gilbert-Barnes E, Kapur RP, Oligny LL, et al., editors: *Potter's pathology of the fetus, infant and child.* 2nd ed. St. Louis, Mosby, 2007.)

TABLE 9.2 **Argenta's Clinical Classification of Deformational Plagiocephaly (DP)**

Types	Definition	Diagram
Type I	Cranial deformation limited to posterior skull	
Type II	Adds displacement of the ipsilateral ear forward or downward	
Type III	Adds ipsilateral frontal bone protrusion	
Type IV	Adds ipsilateral facial asymmetry due to excessive fatty tissue and, less frequently, hyperplasia of the ipsilateral zygoma	
Type V	Adds temporal bulging or abnormal vertical growth of the posterior skull	

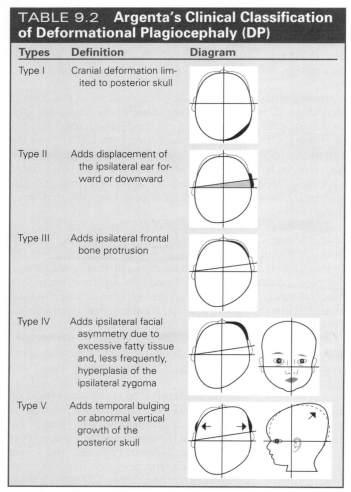

From Argenta L: Clinical classification of positional plagiocephaly. *J Craniofac Surg* 15:368-372, 2004. Illustrations copyright Technology in Motion Ltd.

TABLE 9.3 **Argenta's Clinical Classification of Deformational Brachycephaly (DB)**

Types	Definition	Diagram
Type I	CD limited to posterior skull	
Type II	Adds widening of the posterior skull	
Type III	Adds temporal bulging or abnormal vertical growth of the posterior skull	

From Argenta L: Clinical classification of positional plagiocephaly. *J Craniofac Surg* 15:368-372, 2004. Illustrations copyright Technology in Motion Ltd.

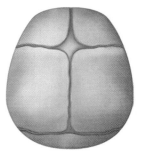

FIG. 9.7 Points of measurement for cranial width, cranial length, and transcranial diagonals to quantify cranial asymmetry (Redrawn from Steinberg JP, Rawlani R, Humphries LS, Rawlani V, Vicari FA: Effectiveness of conservative therapy and helmet therapy for positional cranial deformation. *Plast Reconstr Surg* 135:833-842, 2015.)

DB is quantified by the cephalic or cranial index (CI), the ratio of cranial width to cranial length. Standard cutoff values have not been established, but the following have been proposed: CI of 82% to 90% is mild, 90% to 100% moderate, and > 100% severe.[91] Deformational dolichocephaly is defined as a CI of < 76%.[88] Normative cranial values are available with age- and gender-specific cutoffs for mild, moderate, and severe DP or DB or a combination of DP and DB.[166]

CMT CHANGES IN BODY STRUCTURE AND FUNCTION, ACTIVITY, AND PARTICIPATION

Common body structure and function, activity limitations, and participation restrictions of CMT are listed in Table 9.4. CMT typically presents as a consistent head preference into ipsilateral cervical lateral flexion and contralateral cervical rotation due to unilateral shortening or fibrosis of the involved SCM. Primary impairments include the presence of a tight band or nodule in the involved SCM,[26,28] tightness of the involved SCM and ipsilateral cervical musculature, and decreased PROM into contralateral cervical lateral flexion and ipsilateral cervical rotation of the involved SCM.[26,113] Additionally, muscle imbalance and decreased strength of the cervical musculature may result in decreased active range of motion (AROM) into contralateral cervical lateral flexion and ipsilateral cervical rotation of the involved SCM.[113] Tightness of the SCM and cervical musculature can lead to red, irritated skinfolds of the ipsilateral anterior cervical region.[55] The SCM and cervical musculature tightness can cause discomfort or pain during extremes of passive stretching.[21] As the infant grows and if a positional preference is maintained, the cervical tightness and muscle imbalance can lead to asymmetrical movement of the face, spine, rib cage, and extremities that may lead to secondary tightness, muscle imbalance, and deformities of the cranium and face,[168] or spine and extremities,[55,143] some of which are illustrated in Fig. 9.8. Deformities associated with CMT include facial asymmetry,[168] mandibular hypoplasia,[168] C1-C2 subluxation,[136] mild scoliosis,[13,55] and hip asymmetry.[70]

Consistent positional preference by the infant may lead to activity limitations and participation restrictions resulting from difficulty actively rotating the head toward the side ipsilateral to the involved SCM. Clinical reports describe decreased visual tracking toward the ipsilateral side,[55,82,119] altered midline perceptual motor coordination,[152] decreased tolerance of the prone

TABLE 9.4　Potential Body Structure and Function, Activity, and Participation Limitations of CMT and CD

Medical Condition	Body Structure and Function Limitations	Activity Limitations	Participation Restrictions
CMT	Presence of tight band or nodule in SCM[27]	Restricted neck motion[152]	
	SCM, cervical, or upper trapezius ROM tightness[26]	Positional preference[158] and decreased tolerance to prone positioning[94]	Prefers bottle feeding to one side or difficulty breastfeeding equally on both sides[14]
		Asymmetrical propping on upper extremities[67]	Reduced tolerance of prone positions for play[111]
	SCM, cervical, or upper trapezius weakness[109]		Reduced tolerance to prone positions for play[111]
	Asymmetrical postures in all positions[159]	Asymmetrical movements and transitions: rolling, sitting, quadruped, kneel, one-half kneel, and standing[67]	Possible delays in development[111,130]
	Possible hip dysplasia[163]		
	Red, irritated skinfolds[55]		Difficulty cleaning infant's neck
	Pain during stretches[21]	Resistance to stretching that increases with head control	
	Cervical and thoracic scoliosis[21]	Asymmetrical sitting, standing postures	
CD	Lateral or bilateral occipital flattening[7]	Visual tracking in supine	
	Widening of the posterior skull or cranial base[7]		Teasing by peers due to craniofacial asymmetry[134,142]
	Frontal bossing and/or temporal bulging[7]		
	Abnormal vertical growth of the posterior skull[7]		
	Facial and ear asymmetry[7,168]	Difficulty fitting eyeglasses[124]	
	Mandible asymmetry[140,73]		Difficulty bottle or breastfeeding equally on both sides[164]

position,[111] asymmetry in head turning in all developmental positions,[55] delayed rolling,[55] and asymmetrical or delayed protective and righting reactions of the head, neck, and trunk.[67] Participation restrictions include a preference for side-of-bottle feeding[81,161,160] and nursing,[164] preference to look toward one side during play, and preference to look toward one side while sleeping.[101,121] In addition, CMT is associated with delays in gross motor development at 2 and 6 months of age.[111,130,131] For most children, the delays resolve by 10 months,[111] but for others, delays may persist into early childhood.[130]

CD CHANGES IN BODY STRUCTURE AND FUNCTION, ACTIVITY, AND PARTICIPATION

Common body structure and function, activity limitations, and participation restrictions of CD are listed in Table 9.4. Craniofacial asymmetries observed in infants with CD are specific to the type of deformation. DP is characterized by asymmetry of the posterior cranium with lateral occipital flattening.[7,16] As the severity of the deformity increases, the following may be observed: cranial base deformation[7]; ear asymmetry with the ear ipsilateral to the posterior flattening displaced anteriorly, inferiorly, or both[7]; protrusion of the frontal bone ipsilateral to the posterior flattening (frontal bossing)[7]; facial asymmetry[7]; and temporal bulging or abnormal vertical growth of the posterior skull.[7] Fig. 9.9A–D illustrates cranial asymmetry consistent with DP. Activity limitations and participation restrictions associated with DP include difficulty with visual tracking to the contralateral side of the posterior flattening, particularly when supine or in equipment that supports the head in a reclined sitting position, e.g. car seats and infant swings. If ear asymmetry is present, DP may also result in difficulty fitting glasses.[124] Peer

teasing about head shape has been reported by 5% to 10% of elementary school children with CD.[134,142]

DB is characterized by central occipital flattening.[7] As the severity of the deformity increases, the following may be observed: widening of the posterior half of the skull and temporal bulging or abnormal vertical growth of the posterior skull.[7,90] DB has not been reported in the literature to be associated with specific secondary impairments, activity limitations, and participation restrictions; however, clinical presentations may include excessive use of supine-supported positioning devices,[90] bilateral shoulder hiking and decreased active and passive cervical ROM in rotation and lateral flexion, and reduced cervical flexion due to upper trapezius muscle tightness. Reflux may contribute to the severity of DB if infants require prolonged upright positioning after feeding; reflux discomfort may cause trunk and neck arching[87] with increased pressure against the supporting surface. Infants with DB may have decreased tolerance to prone positions for play if they have not had supervised prone positioning from early infancy (see Fig. 9.6C).[54,101]

Deformational dolichocephaly is characterized by a disproportionately long and narrow skull.[68] It may result in activity limitations and participation restrictions associated with difficulty maintaining the head in midline when supine or in equipment that supports the head in a reclined sitting position (see Fig. 9.6D).

CD has traditionally been regarded as a cosmetic condition with benign neurodevelopmental sequelae.[124] However, recent evidence demonstrates an increased prevalence of gross motor delay in infants with CD,[63,117] lower developmental scores in preschool children with CD,[30] and an increased use of special education and therapy services in school-aged children with a history of CD.[100] Although it cannot be ruled out that CD is the

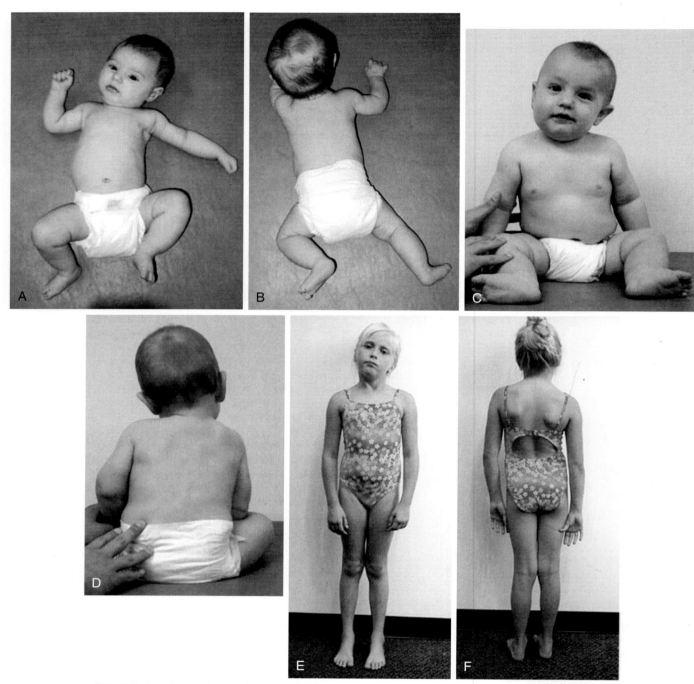

FIG. 9.8 Anterior and posterior views of characteristic asymmetric postural deformities shown in a 3-month-old infant (A–B), an 8-month-old infant (C–D), and an untreated 8-year-old child (E–F). All have left congenital muscular torticollis (CMT) and deformational plagiocephaly (DP). (A) 3-month-old in supine with incurvation of the entire vertebral column. (B) Same 3-month-old infant in prone. Note little change in the postural alignment. (C) 8-month-old in sitting exhibiting postural asymmetry. (D) 8-month-old in sitting exhibiting ipsilateral shortening of the posterior cervical muscles, shoulder elevation, and rotation of the thorax. (E–F) Untreated 8-year-old in standing with long-term functional consequences of CMT and DP, including postural asymmetries.

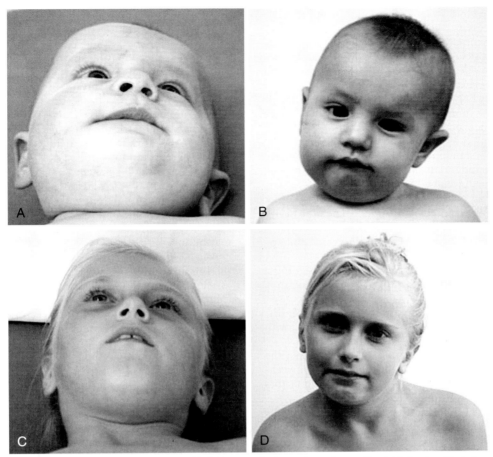

FIG. 9.9 Craniofacial asymmetries. (A) Submental view of an 8-month-old infant with left congenital muscular torticollis (CMT) and deformational plagiocephaly (DP). Note recession of the frontal bone, eyebrow, and zygoma on the ipsilateral side and inferiorly and posteriorly positioned ipsilateral ear. (B) En face view shows hemihypoplasia of the face, decreased vertical facial height on the left, asymmetry of the eyes with the ipsilateral eye smaller, inferior orbital dystopia, canting of the mandible, and deviation of chin and nasal tip. (C) Submental view of an 8-year-old with untreated left CMT and DP demonstrating the same facial asymmetries as the 8-month-old infant. (D) En face view of same 8-year-old demonstrates similar cranial facial asymmetries and shortening of the left sternocleidomastoid muscle.

cause of the delays, it may be that infants with early neurodevelopmental concerns are at increased risk for developing CD[30,125] due to abnormal muscle tone[49] and decreased activity levels.[61]

FOREGROUND INFORMATION

PHYSICAL THERAPY MANAGEMENT OF CMT AND CD

The overall management of CMT and CD begins with prevention of limitations and deformities by repositioning to facilitate symmetrical movement and head shaping; clinicians can provide prevention education to caregivers, professional staff, and the community. Physical therapy intervention is highly effective in resolving CMT and CD when initiated early in infancy[86,120]; therefore, it is imperative that infants receive a physical therapy evaluation and therapeutic intervention as soon as asymmetries are identified. Management follows the American Physical Therapy Association (APTA) patient management model,[6] beginning with screening to rule out potential causes of asymmetry that are not CMT; conducting a full

examination; diagnosing the limitations in body structure and function, activities, and participation; providing a prognosis based on the severity of the conditions; providing intervention to correct the conditions; and all the while, reexamining to determine if progress is adequate, if discharge criteria are met, or whether referrals to other specialists are needed. The following examination and intervention descriptions follow the 2013 CMT clinical practice guideline (CMT CPG),[74] augmented by the literature on CD.

Screening and Differential Diagnosis for Confounding Conditions

The purpose of screening is to rule out conditions that mimic CMT postures, to determine if the asymmetrical posture is congenital or acquired, and to determine the risk for or the presence of CD. Infants with suspected CMT require a thorough history and screening for neurologic, musculoskeletal, visual, gastrointestinal, integumentary, and cardiopulmonary integrity. This is necessary to identify possible conditions other than CMT that could cause asymmetrical posturing and for which consultation with the child's pediatrician and/or appropriate specialists may be necessary.

The typical history of CMT begins with the parent reporting or pediatrician noticing a persistent positional preference of tilting or turning to one side, or resistance to passive cervical rotation. Parents report challenges with cleaning under their infant's chin, breastfeeding on one side more than the other, or positioning the infant symmetrically in car seats, or they notice the infant's asymmetrical posture in pictures. Action Statement 3 of the CMT CPG[74] specifies nine health history factors to document, in addition to standard intake information. Standard intake information includes date of birth, date of examination, gender, birth order, birth weight, birth length, reason for referral or parental concerns, general health of the infant, and other health care providers who are seeing the infant. The nine health history factors include items that are known to be associated with CMT and/or are typically included in a physical therapy history. They are:

1. Age at initial visit[20,93] because this assists with assigning a severity grade and determining a prognosis for the episode of care.
2. Age of onset of symptoms[26,44] because this assists with distinguishing between acquired torticollis and CMT and with determining a prognosis for the episode of care.
3. Pregnancy history, including maternal sense of whether the infant was "stuck" in one position during the final 6 weeks of pregnancy[144] because this assists with identifying factors associated with CMT and CD.
4. Delivery history including birth presentation (cephalic or breech)[26] or multiple births[79] because this assists with understanding possible causes of CMT and CD.
5. Use of assistance during delivery such as forceps or vacuum suction[143,150] because these methods may be a cause of CMT if the SCM was strained during delivery.
6. Head posture/preference[14,160] and changes in the head/face[25,143] because these asymmetries are classic presentations of CMT and possible CD.
7. Family history of torticollis or any other congenital or developmental conditions[138,153] because there may be a genetic component to the condition.
8. Other known or suspected medical conditions[10] because they may be a cause of asymmetries.
9. Developmental milestones appropriate for age because delays may signal other contributing factors to asymmetries or may be a consequence of CMT.[130,152]

Following the history, the clinician continues a systems-based screen for neurologic, musculoskeletal, visual, gastrointestinal, integumentary, and cardiopulmonary integrity. Up to 18% of children presenting with a torticollis posture may have a nonmuscular etiology.[10] Thus the differential diagnostic process requires screening for possible conditions that may cause posturing that mimics CMT and taking an accurate history of the onset of asymmetrical posturing to rule out an acquired torticollis.

Neurologic causes of asymmetrical posturing include brachial plexus injuries, central nervous system (CNS) lesions, astrocytomas, brain stem or cerebellar gliomas, agenesis of CNS structures,[10,106] and hearing deficits.[83] CMT is not typically associated with pain or discomfort at rest or during PROM within the bounds of muscle tightness; thus the presence of pain may indicate an acute condition needing medical referral.[10,155] The clinician will need to distinguish between infant crying due to pain and stranger or setting anxiety. Screen for the following

red flags: abnormal or asymmetrical tone, retention of primitive reflexes, resistance to movement, cranial nerve integrity, brachial plexus injury, and pain signals during movement; a neurologic consult may be appropriate.

Musculoskeletal conditions that mimic CMT include Klippel-Feil syndrome (fusion of cervical vertebrae), clavicle fracture, congenital scoliosis, or C1-C2 rotary subluxation.[10] Screen for the following: asymmetry of the face, neck, spine, and hips, asymmetrical passive neck rotation, the presence of masses in the SCM. Red flags include: atypical positions, such as right cervical rotation with a right lateral flexion, asymmetrical cervical vertebrae on palpation, acute pain responses on cervical movement, tissue masses outside of the SCM or in other areas of the body, children with Down syndrome, C1-C2 cervical spine instability, and late onset of a head tilt with known symmetry for the first few months of life; an orthopedic consult may be appropriate.

Visual conditions may cause asymmetrical posturing as the infant attempts to stabilize his or her focus and include ocular apraxia, strabismus, ocular muscle imbalances, and nystagmus.[10,106] Screen for the following: asymmetrical and discoordinated visual tracking in any direction or clinician inability to distinguish between limitations due to ocular control versus neck rotation; an ophthalmologic consult may be appropriate.

Gastrointestinal conditions include Sandifer syndrome, a hiatal hernia with gastroesophageal reflux[105] that typically causes trunk arching and neck flexion to the right following eating,[42] a history of reflux or constipation,[155] and easier or preferred feeding to one side.[14] Through parental report and observing the infant's behavior before, during, and after feeding, screen for the following red flag: curvature or arching of the trunk and head turning as a means of extending away from the esophagus, usually accompanied by crying; a gastrointestinal consult may be appropriate.

Integumentary conditions include redness or irritation in the folds of the neck, asymmetry of the skinfolds about the neck, asymmetry of the skinfolds of the hips as a sign of hip dysplasia,[107] and color of the skin that might suggest trauma as a cause of asymmetry.[107] Screen for the following red flags by inspecting the skin and ROM with clothing removed: asymmetrical skinfolds, bruising, raw skin breakdown, or purulent exudate; a medical consult is appropriate.

Cardiopulmonary conditions include asymmetric expansion and appearance of the rib cage and respiratory distress.[107,155] Screen by observation of the chest wall during breathing at rest and when active or crying. Red flags include: stridor, wheezing, shortness of breath, cyanotic lips; a consult with the child's pediatrician or a cardiologist is appropriate.

Acquired torticollis, in contrast to congenital torticollis, may occur in older babies and children and be caused by ocular lesions, benign paroxysmal torticollis, dystonic syndromes, infections, Arnold-Chiari malformation, syringomyelia,[33] posterior fossa tumors,[157] and trauma.[107,138] The natural history of these conditions includes a more acute onset, a red flag that should be discussed with the child's pediatrician and that may require immediate medical attention.

Cranial deformation screening identifies cranial asymmetries and differentiates them from pathologic craniosynostosis, or premature closure of one or more cranial sutures. Craniosynostosis results in characteristic head shape asymmetries due to restriction of growth perpendicular to the fused suture. Although craniosynostosis is rare (approximately 0.04%

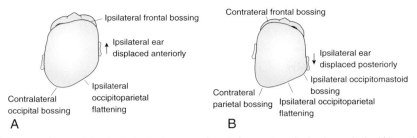

FIG. 9.10 Comparison of typical skull changes for deformational plagiocephaly (A) and unilambdoid synostosis (B). (From Kabbani H, Raghuveer TS: *Craniosynostosis, American Family Physician* 69(12):2863-2870, 2004.)

of births[15]), early identification is critical because craniosynostosis may restrict brain growth and increase intracranial pressure necessitating surgical intervention to prevent neurologic complications.[34,46] Screen for head shape asymmetries not consistent with DP, DB, or deformational dolichocephaly by observing the symmetry of the skull from the front, top, and sides, noting symmetry of the ears and eyes and midline alignment of the chin and nose relative to the perimeter of the face. Premature closure of one lambdoid suture results in the plagiocephalic head shape commonly associated with CMT. Fig. 9.10 illustrates a way to differentiate between DP and unilambdoid synostosis: posterior displacement of the ear ipsilateral to occipital flattening is indicative of unilambdoid synostosis, whereas anterior ear displacement is more consistent with DP. If craniosynostosis is suspected, prompt referral to a craniofacial specialist is recommended.[34,46] See e-fig. 9-1 for greater detail on characteristics of craniosynostosis.

Consistent with the CMT CPG,[74] the physical therapist should request copies of x-ray, ultrasound, computerized tomography (CAT), or magnetic resonance imaging (MRI) images or image reports from the child's parents or guardians that may have been performed prior to the physical therapy screening. These will provide additional details about the infant's physical status and, in the case of ultrasound images or reports, may help the clinician to visualize the location and extent of any existing nodule(s).

If no unusual signs or symptoms are identified through screening, the clinician may proceed with a more detailed examination. If there are red flags that the asymmetrical posture may not be caused by CMT or CD, the clinician will need to determine whether to refer the infant back to his or her primary physician for immediate care, for further consultation, or whether to consult with the physician but also proceed with conservative intervention.

Physical Therapy Examination

The detailed physical therapy examination should evaluate and document across the three International Classification of Functioning, Disability and Health (ICF) domains of body structure and function, activities, and participation (Tables 9.5 and 9.6). The exam is typically organized to maximize the infant's ability to cooperate throughout the full exam, although documentation may reflect a different order of information. (See e-fig. 9-2 for a sample CMT/CD initial evaluation form.[58]) This means engaging the infant in play to assess participation and functional mobility before conducting measures of impairments, when greater handling and movement restrictions are required.

TABLE 9.5	**Key Examination Tools for CMT**
Limitation	**PT Measurement**
Cervical PROM	Arthrodial protractor measurement of PROM
Cervical AROM	Arthrodial protractor or seated swivel test
Prone tolerance	Time per episode and episodes per day in prone
Gross motor function	TIMP for < 4 months old; AIMS for > 4 months to 1 year
Pain	FLACC
Cervical strength	Muscle Function Scale

AIMS, Alberta Infant Motor Scale; *AROM*, Active Range of Motion; *CMT*, Congenital Muscular Torticollis; *FLACC*, Face, Legs, Activity, Cry, Consolability scale; *PROM*, ; *PT*, Physical Therapist; *TIMP*, Test of Infant Motor Performance.

TABLE 9.6	**Key Examination Tools for CD**
Limitation	**PT Measurement**
Cranial shape	Argenta Clinical Classification Scales of DB and DP
Cervical AROM	Arthrodial protractor or seated swivel test

AROM, Active Range of Motion; *CD*, Cranial Deformation; *DB*, Deformational Brachycephaly; *DP*, Deformational Plagiocepahly.

Participation

Participation for young infants includes their ability to pose for pictures, symmetrically explore their immediate surroundings both visually and physically, alternate sides easily during breast or bottle feeding, and tolerate playing while prone for increasingly longer periods of time. Time spent in supported supine-positioning devices, such as car seats, strollers, bouncers or infant swings, should allow for symmetrical positioning. Examination of participation is through parent interview and observation of the infant during these activities.

Parents may first suspect a problem when trying to pose their infant for photographs, when positioning him or her in car seats, or when observing him or her during diaper changes. Perusing photos on a parent's smartphone of the infant's earliest days may help to pinpoint when the asymmetry first appeared. Preference for or more efficient feeding to one side may be a subtle accommodation to limited neck rotation or an asymmetrical mandible.[164] Purposive positioning of the young infant is a critical intervention for correcting CMT, preventing CD if it is not present, and correcting CD if it is present.[161] Questions should be asked about sleep position, head rotation or turning preference when sleeping, sleeping surface, and tolerance to prone positioning. Understanding the amount of time the infant spends in passive positioning devices versus time in prone play is important for parental education and for designing an intervention approach.

Activities

Infant activities focus on acquisition of developmental milestones and symmetrical exploration of their own movements and their immediate environment. Full and active range of the neck, spine, and extremities is critical for exploring surfaces, visually tracking activity around them, and moving through space. Activity limitations and developmental milestones should be documented at each visit, including changing tolerances to positions, acquisition of or delays in milestones, presence, absence, or asymmetry in reflex postures or protective reaction patterns, and asymmetry of volitional movements and positions. Development should be assessed with an age-appropriate, standardized valid and reliable tool. Examples of such tests that can assist with early identification of delays during the age range when CMT is often evident include the Test of Infant Motor Performance (http://thetimp.com/) for infants who are 34 weeks postconception to 4 months postterm, the Harris Infant Neuromotor Test (HINT, http://thetimp.com/) for infants 2.5–12.5 months old, and the Alberta Infant Motor Scale (AIMS, http://www.albertainfantmotorscale.com/) for infants who are 0–18 months old. More information on these tests can be found in Chapter 2.

Body Function and Body Structures

The CMT CPG[74] describes seven key body function and body structure items to examine. They are presented in order from the most active to most passive in terms of an infant's ability to cooperate. Infant posture in supine, prone, sitting, and standing, with or without support as appropriate for age, is assessed for symmetry and tolerance for the position. Parents can assist in this portion of the examination by placing their infant in these positions to mitigate stranger anxiety and to allow for a therapeutic trust to build among the infant, the parent/caretaker, and the clinician. In supine and prone, document the side of CMT and any asymmetries of the shoulders, spine, hips, or legs. In prone, document the infant's tolerance to the position as an indicator as to whether prone play is a natural part of the infant's experiences. In sitting and standing, whether supported or independent, document the child's ability to maintain the position and any postural asymmetries. If feasible and permitted by the clinic, digital images in these positions can provide accurate measures of the observed asymmetries.[123] Specifically, the following impairments should be documented at the initial examination and routinely until discharge.

Bilateral active cervical rotation, lateral flexion, and diagonal movements. Rotation should be measured in supine for infants under 3 months; for infants > 3 months, it should be measured while sitting on the parent's lap using the rotating stool test,[82] by enticing the infant to follow toys or sounds in all directions. Lateral flexion should be measured with the Muscle Function Scale[113,115] by holding the infant vertically in front of a mirror and tipping her horizontally 90° to each side, observing for the amount of active neck righting from the horizontal line. The Muscle Function Scale is reliably scored with a picture scale (ICC ≥ 0.94)[115] as 0 = with the head below horizontal, 1 = with the head on the horizontal line, 2 = with the head slightly over the horizontal line, 3 = with the head high over the horizontal line, and 4 = with the head very high over the line approaching vertical.[113] Active neck extension and rotation should be assessed in prone to determine whether the infant has enough AROM to clear the airway and face; this is critical for safety during prone play.

Passive and AROM of the upper and lower extremities, including screening for hip dysplasia. Passively move the upper and lower extremities through full range to examine for brachial plexus injuries, clavicle fractures, abnormal tone, neurologic impairments, or CNS lesions.[107] Assess for tightness of the upper trapezius, scalene, and posterior neck muscles of the ipsilateral side. Use the Ortolani and Barlow maneuvers in infants < 3 months old to screen for hip dysplasia.[145] For infants > 3 months, the Galeazzi sign, asymmetrical posturing, or hip abduction limitations may be stronger indicators of hip dysplasia.[32] Observe active movement of the extremities for symmetrical and reciprocal use, particularly bilateral hand exploration and upper extremity (UE) midline play to assess for hemi-neglect. More information on the Ortolani and Barlow maneuvers is located in Chapter 14.

Bilateral passive cervical rotation and lateral flexion should be measured with an arthrodial protractor. Reference values for typically developing infants are 110 ± 6.2° for cervical rotation and 70 ± 2.4° for lateral flexion.[113] Cervical neutral should be maintained in all measures.[48]

For cervical rotation, infants and young toddlers should be measured in supine; children older than 2 years can be measured in sitting if they are able to cooperate.[77] Measuring with a clear arthrodial protractor requires a minimum of two adults with a mounted protractor, one to stabilize the infant (usually the parent) and one to rotate the head while maintaining cervical neutral and to read the measures. If the protractor is not securely positioned on a wall, plinth, or in a frame, an additional adult may be needed to hold the protractor above the infant, as depicted in Fig. 9.11A. Testing in supine may require elevating the infant's torso on a blanket or 2-in mat, or extending the infant's head beyond the edge of the mat table, to allow for clearance of the rotating occiput and to ensure a cervical neutral position. Visually assess for symmetry of the nose, chin, and ear placement to ensure that the head is in neutral and the nose is aligned to 90° as the starting reference point.

Lateral flexion is measured in supine with the arthrodial protractor laid in the same plane as the infant, as depicted in Fig. 9.11B. A parent/caregiver can stabilize the infant's torso while the clinician supports the head laterally over each ear or under the occiput while moving into the end ranges. Again, care should be taken to test in cervical neutral; raising the trunk with a blanket or 2-inch mat may be required.

Whatever measurement approach is chosen, measurement procedures should be consistent within each child and across children within a practice setting.

Pain or discomfort at rest and during passive or active ROM, using the Faces, Legs, Activity, Cry, Consolability (FLACC) scale.[96] Pain is not a typical sign or symptom of CMT. It can be associated with skinfold irritation or acute or acquired asymmetries, for which immediate medical attention is appropriate. Pain, exhibited as facial grimacing or crying, may be observed during stretching or positioning out of the infant's preferred postures. The revised FLACC tool rates facial expressions, movement, and behavior states on a 3-point scale of 0 for no expression or a quiet state, 1 for occasional expressions or movements, and 2 for frequent grimacing or large movements. Discriminating whether crying is a sign of pain, versus stranger or clinic anxiety, is most easily accomplished by handing the infant to the parent and observing the speed with which the infant stops crying.

Integumentary evaluation of the infant's cervical skin and hip folds. This includes assessment of skin integrity; symmetry of skinfolds; the presence and location of a SCM nodule or

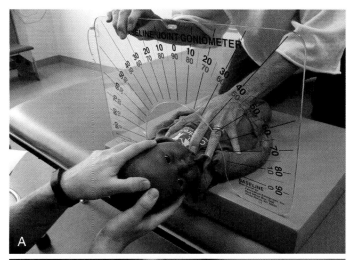

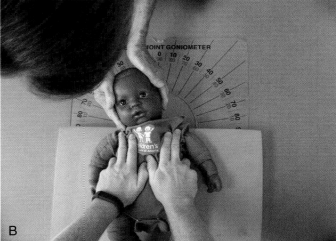

FIG. 9.11 Measuring with an arthrodial protractor. (A) Position of the arthrodial protractor for measuring neck rotation. (B) Placement of the protractor for measuring lateral neck flexion.

fibrous band; and size, shape, and elasticity of the SCM capital and trapezius muscles. Evaluate skin integrity by noting areas of discoloration, reddening, skin breakdown, irritation, or rashes. Observe for symmetry of the skinfolds about the neck for consistency with CMT and the hip joints or inguinal folds for potential hip dysplasia. Palpate the SCM to determine the quality of tightness and pliability of the muscle and to identify the presence, size, and location within the SCM of any nodule. Nodules that are higher up or less than one third of the muscle length tend to resolve more quickly than those that extend through a greater proportion of the muscle or are located in the lower one third.[27,28] Redness and deeper skinfolds along the anterior lateral side of the neck are characteristic of SCM tightness. Redness and deeper posterior neck skinfolds are an indication of tightness in the upper trapezius muscle.

Craniofacial assessment for asymmetries. This includes palpation of the anterior and posterior fontanelles for size, shape, position, and fullness; palpation of cranial sutures to assess for ridging over each suture; and visual assessment of craniofacial symmetry with photo documentation.[34,91] The assessment of craniofacial symmetry is done in six views, depicted in Fig. 9.12A–F: an anterior view to assess symmetry of

the cheek, eyes, ears, and nose (Fig. 9.12A); a vertex (top down) view to assess symmetry of the frontal bones and occiput, width of the biparietal diameter, skull length, shape of the forehead, and relative anteroposterior position of the ears (placing one index finger in each of the infant's ears and viewing from above can aid in detecting anterior or posterior displacement of one ear [Fig. 9.12B]); a posterior view to assess whether the skull base is level and to identify the presence of a temporal bulge and/or vertical displacement of an ear (Fig. 9.12C); two lateral views to evaluate the presence of a high sloping forehead or abnormal vertical growth of the posterior skull (Fig. 9.12D–E); and an inferior or submental view to evaluate symmetry of the forehead, ears, eyes, and cheek (Fig. 9.12F).

Physical Therapy Classification and Prognosis for Clinical Management

Based on the results of the examination, the clinician should classify each condition's severity. Classification supports more accurate prognoses of the expected outcomes and episode of care and more appropriate alignment of interventions to achieve the expected outcomes. For both CMT and CD the key factors that impact classification and prognosis are the age at which the infant presents for intervention and the severity of the impairments.

The prognosis for infants with CMT, with or without CD, should address the potential for resolution of CMT and/or CD relative to the grade of severity and the options for intervention, the estimated episode of care to reach resolution relative to different intervention approaches, and the potential benefits, harms, and/or costs of implementing each approach.[74] This should be communicated clearly to the parents/caregivers to facilitate shared decision making about the frequency of clinical visits, the dosage of home exercise programs, the use of cranial remolding therapy, the potential for more invasive interventions if conservative management is ineffective, and concerns about the social, functional, and developmental implications of watchful waiting.

CMT Classification and Prognosis

Table 9.1 describes the seven grades of CMT severity recommended by the CMT CPG[74]; they account for the age at which the infant is initially evaluated, the limits of cervical rotation, and the presence or absence of an SCM nodule. Assigning a grade of severity can assist with estimating the length of the episode of care; lower grades are associated with faster impairment resolution.[120] Assigning grades can also assist with measuring service outcomes because infants can be compared to others with the same severity grades rather than being grouped together.

The prognosis for full resolution of CMT is 100% for infants < 3 months of age, if they are referred early and caregivers are adherent with conservative intervention. The prognosis for full resolution drops to 75% for infants referred between 3 to 6 months of age, and 30% for toddlers between 6 to 18 months of age.[41] Because the potential for full resolution reduces with increasing age of treatment initiation, the potential for surgical release increases with later ages of referral.[41,120]

CD Classification and Prognosis

Tables 9.2 and 9.3 describe the Argenta Clinical Classification Scales for DP and DB[7] recommended by the CMT CPG[74] for documenting the severity of CD in clinical settings. These scales are clinically practical, easily understood by families, do

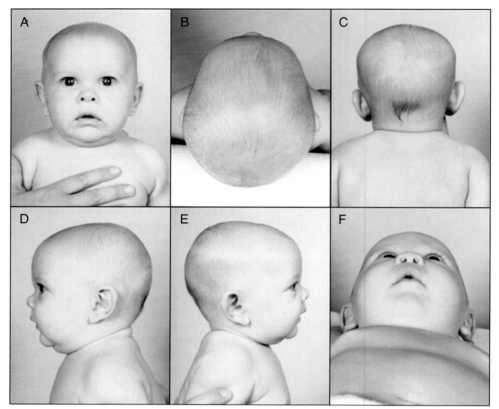

FIG. 9.12 Six craniofacial views to assess for asymmetries (3-month-old infant without CD). (A) Anterior. (B) Vertex. (C) Posterior. (D) Left lateral. (E) Right lateral. (F) Inferior or mental. (Copyright © 2016 Cranial Technologies, Inc.)

not require time-intensive measurements or use specialized equipment,[7] and demonstrate moderate interrater (weighted kappa = 0.51–0.66) and intrarater (weighted kappa = 0.6–0.85) reliability.[139]

The prognosis for full resolution of CD is 77% after parent education in repositioning and 94% to 96% after cranial remolding therapy, whether or not it is preceded by parent education in repositioning.[141] Risk factors for moderate to severe CD after parent education in repositioning with or without physical therapy include poor adherence, initiating intervention after 3 months of age, persistence of CMT beyond 6 months of age, developmental delay, and severity of initial CD.[141] Risk factors for moderate to severe CD after cranial remolding therapy include poor adherence with wearing the helmet and initiating intervention after 9 months of age.[141] Surgical management of CD is considered in only very severe cases because outcomes are inconsistent and high rates of complications have been reported.[36,97]

Conservative Interventions for CMT and CD

Currently, most authors advocate conservative, nonoperative interventions for CMT and CD, and those interventions can be divided into first-choice interventions with strong and consistent evidence for effectiveness and supplemental interventions with weaker or less consistent evidence of effectiveness (Tables 9.7 and 9.8).

First-Choice Interventions

The conservative first-choice interventions for CMT consist of five components: parent/caregiver education, environmental

TABLE 9.7	Key Interventions for CMT
Limitation	**PT Intervention**
Decreased cervical rotation	Manual stretching of tight musculature, active cervical rotation toward nonpreferred side, strengthening of cervical musculature, passive positioning to stretch tight tissues
Head tilt	Manual stretching of tight musculature, active cervical lateral flexion away from head tilt, strengthening of cervical musculature, passive positioning to stretch tight tissues
Positional preference and/or trunk asymmetry	Active movement and strengthening opposite of the preferred side or asymmetry
Prone position intolerance	Increase use of prone positioning to strengthen capital muscles and facilitate symmetrical trunk and head alignment
Asymmetrical postures	Active movement and strengthening opposite of the asymmetry
Developmental delay	Facilitate equal use of all extremities and head turning to both directions during daily activities and play

adaptations, passive neck ROM exercises, neck and trunk AROM, and facilitation of symmetrical movement activities.[74] The conservative interventions for CD include parent/caregiver instruction in repositioning and environmental adaptations for CD under 6 months of age and cranial remolding therapy for severe CD after 4 months of age.[47,125]

TABLE 9.8	Key Interventions for CD
Limitation	**PT Intervention**
Brachycephaly	Increase prone positioning to relieve pressure on occiput to allow for reshaping. Refer severe cases for cranial orthotic assessment at 4 months of age and moderate cases for cranial orthotic assessment at 6 months of age.
Plagiocephaly	Head turning and positioning opposite of preferred position, increased time in prone, facilitation of development to encourage overall movement away from the flattened side. Refer severe cases for cranial orthotic assessment at 4 months of age and moderate cases for cranial orthotic assessment at 6 months of age.

Parent/caregiver education. Parent/caregiver daily adherence to the home program is critical to the success for remediating CMT and CD; it must be stressed to the caregivers that they are the primary interventionists for these conditions and that the role of the clinician is to help guide and advance the home program.

Prevention of CMT and CD through early parental education and active infant repositioning, including the use of prone positioning and unfettered movement, can effectively reduce the incidence of either or both CMT from positional preference and postnatal CD.[22,159] The American Academy of Pediatrics recommends counseling of all parents during the newborn period (by 2 to 4 weeks of age) in active infant repositioning and environmental adaptations to prevent CD,[82] and increasing evidence supports that parent guidance before discharge from the maternity ward may reduce the prevalence and severity of CD in early infancy.[4,22] Reinforcing or improving neck ROM, strength, and postural control can be accomplished in any number of ways throughout the day. In infants without CMT or CD, caregivers should be aware to change the infant's position throughout the day and present voice and objects of interest equally to the right and left sides. Midline development should be stressed.

In infants with CMT and/or CD, caregivers should be taught to purposefully carry, hold, and position the infant in ways that create a prolonged stretch of the tight muscles and promote midline development and symmetry of movements.[13,152] Toys should be presented to the nonpreferred side to facilitate head turning and reaching in all planes.[13] Caregivers should also be taught to approach and feed the infant to promote looking toward the nonpreferred side[160] or by alternating sides for feedings.[92] Home exercise programs should include eliciting balance reactions for strength development of the neck and trunk muscles, specifically cervical lateral flexion away from the preferred head tilt. Once an adequate amount of neck muscle strength is obtained, the exercises should be task specific to encourage the infant to use that strength to lift the head against gravity during pull to sit, in prone play, and for visual tracking in all directions.[152] Strengthening neck and trunk rotator muscles promotes development of transitional movements such as rolling and coming to sit from prone and supine.

Caregivers providing ROM exercises should be instructed to observe for changes in the infant's behavioral and physiologic states and to discontinue exercises if the following occur: changes in face color, breathing rate, or heart rate; increased hand and foot movement; plantar or palmar sweating; eye squeezing; perspiration; nasal flaring or brow bulging; mouth gaping; and crying.[11] Passive movement should be done slowly, and stretching should not be done against an infant actively resisting the stretch.

Parent education to prevent and minimize CD includes repositioning to decrease pressure on the flattened area of the skull when sleeping in supine and during bottle and breastfeeding and supervised prone positioning for play[4,47] with a goal of at least 30–60 min a day.[82]

Environmental adaptations for CMT and CD. Adaptations to the infant's environment can support the home exercise program and facilitate goal attainment. Attention should be paid to the type of positioning devices used by the family and the amount of time an infant spends in those devices.[82,119] Parents should be aware that car seats, infant swings, and bouncy seats that rely on semireclined supine positioning need to be used with correct postural alignment to prevent reinforcement of CMT and that time in those devices should be minimized in favor of supervised prone play.[82] Environmental adaptations to correct CMT, or to prevent and minimize CD, include limiting time in supported supine positions such as car safety seats, infant swings, and infant carriers and environmental modifications to encourage the infant to rotate the head toward the nonpreferred side, including changing toy positions and the position of the infant's crib relative to the door and reversing the head-to-toe position of the infant in the crib and on the changing table.[4,47]

PROM of the neck. The origin, insertion, and biomechanics of the SCM muscle, and the location of any nodules or fibrous bands, dictate the angles of stretching necessary to elongate the muscle to correct CMT. The elongated position can be attained with ipsilateral rotation, contralateral lateral flexion, and contralateral asymmetric extension from a starting point of neutral cervical spine alignment. In younger infants stretching can be accomplished in most positions, including when carried prone on the caregiver's forearm, up against the chest wall, in supine, or supervised prone lying, as illustrated in Figs. 9.13 for cervical rotation and Figs. 9.14A–C for lateral flexion. To maximize stretching routines in the older infant, placing the infant supine on the parent's lap or in a reclined sitting position may be more comfortable and acceptable to the infant. Regardless of the chosen position, the clinician should consider the following factors:

Starting position: Place the infant in a comfortable position, either supine or reclined sitting on the caregiver's lap, with the head and neck in midline, aligned as possible with the trunk and pelvis. Use the infant's nose and umbilicus as landmarks for midline alignment.

Identify the tight muscles and their line of pull to maximize stretching biomechanics.

Stabilize the shoulders. Stretching should be isolated to the tight muscles. Differentiate between cervical and shoulder tightness in order to determine the correct stretch.

Check for skin irritation and redness. These may be indicators of muscle tightness.

Do not force the stretch. PROM should not be painful. Low-intensity, sustained holding at the end of range will avoid microtrauma of the muscle[159]; positioning and handling to facilitate passive elongation are also effective.[110,151] PROM through passive positioning or manual stretching while walking around or rocking the infant provides multiple sensory stimuli to the infant and may distract him or her from resisting the stretch sensation.

Contraindications for passive neck ROM include Klippel-Feil syndrome, bony abnormalities, fractures (particularly of

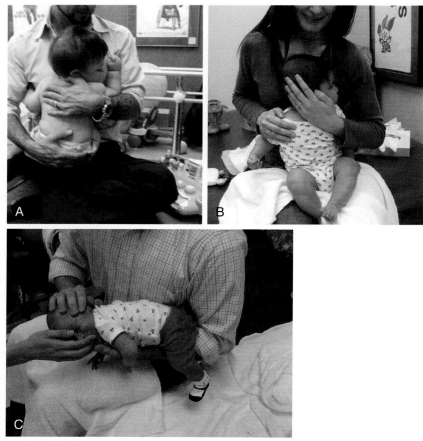

FIG. 9.13 Positions to encourage cervical rotation. (A) Chest hold for trunk and neck rotation to the right. (B) Supported sitting with right shoulder stabilization and stretching to the left. (C) Football style support with head turned toward the shortened side.

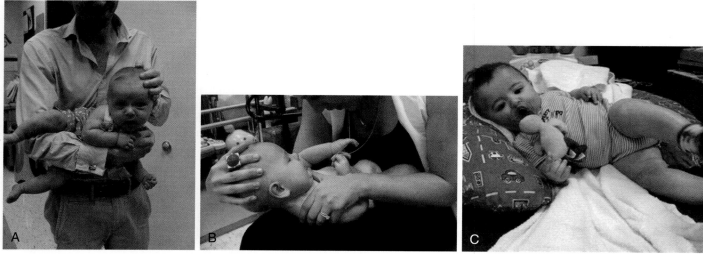

FIG. 9.14 Positions to encourage cervical lateral flexion. (A) PROM into right lateral flexion to stretch the left in a modified football carry. (B) PROM into left lateral flexion and right cervical rotation in supported supine, with gentle stretch to right upper trapezius. (C) PROM during supported sidelying to stretch the right lateral cervical and trunk flexors.

the clavicle), C1-C2 subluxation, odontoid abnormalities, CNS or bone tumors, or brain stem malformations (e.g., Arnold-Chiari malformation).[106,137] Caregivers providing ROM exercises should be instructed to observe for changes in physical appearances such as worried facial expressions, chin quivering, nasal flaring, and increased body tone and physiologic signs such as changes in color, breathing, or heart rate[8] and to consult with the clinician on how to continue a safe home program.

AROM of the neck and trunk. The focus of AROM is to strengthen weak neck and trunk muscles. This can be achieved through positioning, handling, and carrying during care and play,[110] offering food from the nonpreferred side to encourage active cervical rotation,[155] and using righting reactions to activate weaker muscles[110,155] as depicted in Fig. 9.15A–C. Active play in prone may need to be modeled for the parent/caregiver who is wary of placing the infant prone or who is not sure how to modify the prone position so that the infant can tolerate it. Prone play is critical for elongating the neck flexors and strengthening capital muscles.[45,95]

Symmetrical motor development. In addition to remediating impairments about the neck, the clinician should facilitate development of age-appropriate function, inclusive of rolling, creeping, crawling, sitting, and standing, as well as active and symmetrical play within each of those positions. There are several studies supporting a possible association between CMT and delayed development,[111,130,131] and any postural preference to one side may bias an infant for associated rotation along the spine, resulting in asymmetrical postures.[152,158]

Intervention dosage. The duration of physical therapy intervention and outcomes of intervention depend on the cause of the torticollis, the initial deficit of passive cervical rotation, and the age of the infant when intervention is initiated. Published intervention protocols for CMT vary considerably and are often standardized to fit research protocols. They range from cervical stretching done 2 to 3 times daily, repeating each

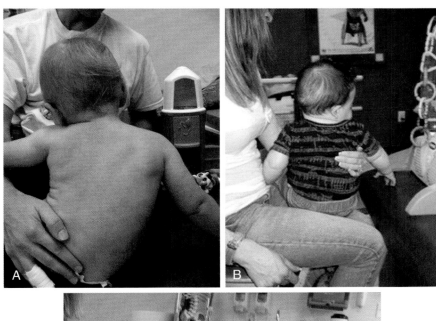
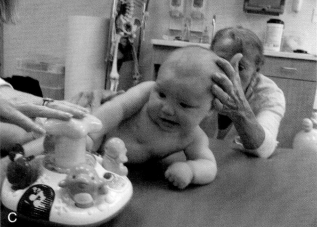

FIG. 9.15 Positions for AROM, strengthening, and midline orientation. (A) Sitting on parent's lap using weight shifting on right to encourage active left cervical and trunk lateral flexion via righting reactions. (B) Sitting on parent's lap to encourage active right cervical rotation to interact with toys. Notice the parent stabilizing the trunk. (C) Facilitated sidelying play with intermittent manual assist to encourage prolonged antigravity activation of right cervical lateral flexors.

stretch 5 to 15 times with 1- to 10-second holds,[28,44] to two-person passive neck stretching exercises carried out 4 to 8 times daily with at least 30 to 40 repetitions in each set.[23,41] The exact intervention dosage for clinical use will depend on the level of severity, the ability of the family to adhere to the recommended stretching protocols, and the age of the infant and his or her ability to tolerate intervention. Younger infants tolerate stretching better because they have less neck strength; infants 3 to 4 months or older are developing sufficient neck strength and willpower to resist passive stretching if they are not comfortable with the sensation or if they are intent on looking at something on the preferred side. The overall consensus across studies is that stretching should be done frequently across the day and should be tied to routines of infant carrying, playtime, diaper changes, feedings, bath times, and position changes.

Supplemental Physical Therapy Interventions with Evidence for CMT

CMT and mild CD in most infants will respond to the first-choice interventions, but for infants with slower resolution or more severe presentations, there are other approaches described in the literature but for which the body of evidence is smaller, the study designs are less rigorous, or there may be conflicting evidence. Nevertheless, these approaches may provide useful additions to the first-choice interventions to support CMT or CD resolution. The choice of a supplemental intervention should be based on discussions with the family, the child's current rate of improvement, the family's ability to adhere to additional or different protocols, the family's perceived acceptance of the approach, the clinician's skill or training to provide the approach, potential additional costs, and the likelihood of the child's improvement.

Clinicians who use these approaches should be vigilant to document objective measures to determine their effectiveness on the degree and speed of resolution because they may add to the cost of care. Clinicians who choose to use approaches that have no peer-reviewed publications that describe foundational principles and provide evidence of effectiveness should be conscientious about receiving the informed consent of the caregivers and documenting objective measures at baseline and throughout care. All clinicians are encouraged to publish cases that are emblematic of new approaches or unusual outcomes.

Microcurrent for CMT

Low-intensity alternating current (200 μA) is applied superficially over the involved SCM such that the infant does not perceive the current; stretching follows the treatment. Two small randomized controlled trials (RCTs)[76,80] have demonstrated similar outcomes of increased ROM in significantly less time than with passive stretching alone or stretching combined with ultrasound diathermy. The overall episodes of care averaged 2.6 months for infants receiving microcurrent and 6.3 for those who received only stretching.[80] Infants receiving microcurrent cried less during treatment than infants who did not receive it,[76] and ultrasound imaging of the SCM posttreatment demonstrated significantly less tissue thickness of the involved SCM.[80] Replication of this approach with larger sample sizes is appropriate, but microcurrent appears to be a promising approach with strong evidence for shortening the episode of care without

adverse reactions. Clinicians will need to be comfortable with administering microcurrent and have the proper type and size of equipment to provide this intervention.

Myokinetic Stretching for CMT

This technique consists of applying mild overpressure with 1 or 2 fingers on the SCM while it is in its lengthened position.[29] PTs provided 60 repetitions over 30-minute treatment sessions, 5 times week on infants less than 50 days old; parents additionally performed home stretching, massage, and positioning. Given the young age of the subjects and the confounding factor of a home program, it is not clear if this particular technique is significantly different from any other strategy of SCM intervention; however, if other approaches are not tolerated, this study provides moderate evidence for an alternative stretching technique. Clinicians will need postgraduate training to provide this approach.

Kinesiologic Taping for CMT

Stretchable tape is applied to supporting muscles to provide sensory feedback. A retrospective study provides weak but promising evidence that when kinesiologic tape is applied for the purpose of relaxing the affected side, immediate Muscle Function Scale gains were significantly greater[112]; long-term benefits have not been reported. The approach requires postgraduate training, and some infants may have skin sensitivity to the tape.

Tscharnuter Akademie for Motor Organization (TAMO) Approach for CMT

A single case study describes this approach as using light touch and the infant's responses to gravity and support surfaces to facilitate movement exploration.[122] The approach was mixed with AROM, home programming, carrying techniques for passive positioning, and head righting, so it is not clear how much the TAMO approach contributed to the resolution of CMT, but there was a notable absence of PROM as an intervention. Clinicians will need postgraduate training to provide this approach.

Cervical Collars for CMT

Several versions of neck orthoses are described in case reports but have not been rigorously assessed as to their comparative benefits over conservative management alone. All are intended to facilitate active movement within a corrected range and are not meant to be passive supports for the neck. As with other supplemental approaches, cervical orthoses may be an appropriate adjunct to conservative care if changes are occurring slowly, but they require careful application, supervision, and monitoring by the caregiver. As with all cervical collars, remove the collars immediately if there are any concerns about fit, skin irritation, or development of pressure areas. Clinicians may need postgraduate and/or supervised training to properly fit and apply selected collars.

The Tubular Orthosis for Torticollis (TOT collar)[44] is a cervical orthosis designed to decrease head tilt posture, assist in midline head control, and stimulate movement away from the tilted head position[55] in infants with adequate head control and who demonstrate more than 5° of head tilt. The TOT collar is worn during waking hours when the infant is moving, playing, and even feeding. The clinician must be knowledgeable of the indications for, fitting of, and modifications to the TOT collar before fitting it to an infant. For example see eFig. 9-3.

Soft cervical foam collars may be used for immediate post-operative management following SCM release,[138] post-SCM release with physical therapy,[83,84] and after Botox injections[71] to protect the surgical site and facilitate movements away from the side of released SCM. The use of soft felt cervical collars was described by Binder et al.[13] in infants with a persistent head tilt and restrictions in active cervical rotation.

Cranial Remolding Therapy and Positioning Devices for CD

Cranial Remolding Therapy for CD

Cranial remolding therapy uses cranial orthoses, helmets, or bands. Cranial orthoses are constructed from high-temperature thermoplastic materials, and most are lined with high-density, hypoallergenic medical grade foam.[39] Cranial orthoses do not restrict cranial growth but rather redirect subsequent cranial growth into voided areas facilitating a symmetrical shape,[75] as illustrated in Fig. 9.16A–B. Most cranial orthoses are custom fabricated, but soft shell helmets in generic sizes with custom foam padding are commercially available.[154]

Cranial orthoses are initiated from 4 to 6 months of age and worn 20 to 23.5 hours a day for 2 to 7 months for optimal outcomes.[47,51] Duration of cranial remolding therapy varies based on the age of the child and severity of the CD because the rate of correction decreases logarithmically with increasing age.[133] At 5 months of age, the rate of cranial asymmetry improvement is 0.93 mm per week, whereas at 8 to 11 months of age the rate of improvement stabilizes at 0.41 to 0.42 mm per week.[133] Cranial remolding therapy results in more complete correction and shorter treatment duration when initiated before 6 months of age,[78] but correction can occur up to 15 to 18 months of age although the correction will likely be incomplete and require a substantially longer treatment duration.[75,133] After 12 months of age the rate of correction decreases due to reduced rate of skull growth and adherence issues as older infants may adamantly refuse the cranial orthotic and independently remove it.[82,133] Adverse effects associated with cranial orthoses are low but include occasional malodorous perspiration, minor skin irritations and fungal infections, poor helmet fit with severe DB, nonreimbursable cost, social stigma of cranial orthotic use, and unsatisfactory cosmetic results.[56] Daily cleaning of the cranial orthotic is critical to avoid skin irritations and fungal infections.

Assessment for cranial remolding therapy is indicated based on the age of the child and the severity of the CD.[47] It is not indicated for infants under the age of 4 months or infants at any age with mild CD that is limited to the posterior skull (Argenta DP Type I, Argenta DB Type I).[47,82] Cranial orthotic assessment is indicated for infants over 4 months with severe CD that includes facial asymmetry (Argenta DP Type IV) and temporal bulging and abnormal vertical growth of the skull (Argenta DP Type V, Argenta DB Type III).[82] Cranial orthotic assessment is also indicated for infants over 6 months with moderate CD that includes ear displacement (Argenta DP Type II), frontal bone protrusion (Argenta DP Type III), or widening of the posterior skull (Argenta DB Type II).[47,82] At the cranial orthotic assessment, quantitative measures of CD are taken and a decision is made as to whether cranial remolding therapy is warranted. Some practitioners recommend an objective assessment of the infant with moderate CD

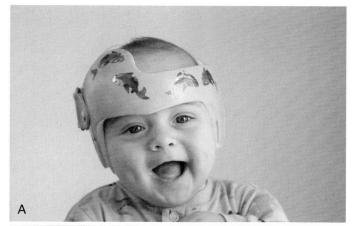

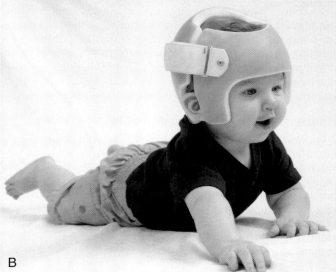

FIG. 9.16 Examples of custom cranial orthoses. (A) En face view of a 4-month-old infant with right congenital muscular torticollis and deformational plagiocephaly wearing a cranial band (B) 8-month-old infant with DP wearing a cranial helmet. ([A] Courtesy iStock.com. [B] From STARband Orthomerica, Orlando FL.)

at 4 months and again at 6 months to document whether 2 months of repositioning was effective in reshaping the skull; this will assist with the determination of whether cranial remolding therapy is warranted at 6 months. Refer to eFig. 9-4 for a clinical decision tree for managing CD.[47]

Consistent and strong evidence supports that cranial remolding therapy is effective in reducing cranial asymmetry in infants with moderate to severe CD when implemented by 6 months of age and parents/caregivers diligently follow the prescribed wearing schedule.[47,51] However, it is unknown whether cranial remolding therapy, as compared to parent education in repositioning, results in a clinically significant difference in cranial shape that affects long-term satisfaction and quality of life.[47,51] The only RCT to compare cranial remolding therapy with parent education in repositioning in 5- to 6-month-old infants with moderate to severe CD did not find a statistically significant difference in cranial asymmetry between the two interventions when children were 2 years of age.[162] However, only 23% to 26%

of children in both groups obtained complete correction at 2 years of age, a much smaller percentage than in previous studies, perhaps because the study's criteria for complete correction was more stringent than previous studies.[162] Further high-quality evidence is needed to determine the efficacy of cranial remolding therapy as compared to parent education in repositioning.

Positioning Devices

Positioning devices that alter the shape of the surface an infant lies on have been investigated as a means to prevent or minimize CD. These devices rest the infant's head into a depression to redistribute contact pressure between the surface and the cranium. Although some devices have shown favorable results, such as bedding pillows,[167] passive orthotic mattresses,[135] cranial cups,[40,128] and Plagio Cradle orthotics (Boston Brace, Avon, MA),[132] others such as the Safe T Sleep Sleepwrap positioning wrap (safetsleep.com)[64] have not. Although the evidence is weak and does not support that these devices are more effective than repositioning alone for most infants, these devices may be promising for infants with severe CD who are younger than 4 months or whose development is compromised. Additional studies are needed to determine their effectiveness as compared to conscientious repositioning, as well as the cost-effectiveness of available devices.

Nonconservative Interventions for CMT

Nonconservative interventions for CMT should be considered for infants who are not progressing after 6 months of conservative intervention or for children initially referred after 1 year of age and who have Grade 7 severity.[74] These options include surgery or botulinum toxin type A (Botox) for CMT. The clinician should collaborate with the infant's primary or referring physician for follow-up care if these approaches are being considered. This form eliminates any misinterpretation that the PT is doing these interventions.

Surgery

Surgical options range from tendon lengthening to unipolar or bipolar release of the SCM. Indications for surgery include persistent residual tightness of > 15°[18] or progressing ROM limitations.[159] The goals of surgery are to normalize neck ROM and to improve or prevent additional craniofacial asymmetry resulting from persistent asymmetrical posturing. Concerns with surgical interventions include potential damage to the facial, greater auricular, or spinal accessory nerves, visible scars, recurrent muscle band formation, loss of neck contour, and the recurrence of SCM contracture.[18,19] Endoscopic surgery by an experienced surgeon avoids many of these complications by improving the operative field view with magnification, ensuring precise muscle fiber transection, and preserving the neurovascular structures.[18] Children who have releases before 1 year of age have the best chance of reversing their facial and skull deformities[19]; however, older children and untreated adults can benefit from the procedure as well.[147]

Botox

This neurotoxin is injected into the SCM and is presumed to either relax the tight muscle by inhibiting acetylcholine release or by causing muscle atrophy that allows for easier stretching.[116] The use of Botox is considered off label for infants; however, there is a growing body of support for its use with recalcitrant CMT to reduce the need for surgical correction.[31,71,116]

ANTICIPATED OUTCOMES AND DISCHARGE CRITERIA

If left untreated, CMT is a condition that will persist and possibly progress. As the infant grows older, growth of the surrounding musculoskeletal structures can be impacted by the SCM tightness causing further restriction of range or CD.[137] Infants who are discharged from physical therapy for CMT should be monitored throughout their early childhood to observe for return of tightness as they go through growth spurts; achieve antigravity milestones such as crawling or walking; during higher-stress activities such as climbing, pulling, or other resisted sporting activities; or when ill or teething.[79] Parents should be alerted that temporary asymmetrical presentations will most likely resolve when the challenging factor is resolved but that a physical therapy examination may be indicated if the postural preference persists. A longer treatment duration of cranial remolding therapy may be indicated if the infant's CD has resolved but the CMT has not; repositioning and use of a cranial orthotic during sleep may be continued until the CMT is resolved to prevent reoccurrence of cranial asymmetry.

The anticipated outcomes and criteria for discharge from physical therapy intervention are:
1. Full PROM of neck, trunk, and extremities to within 5° of the nonaffected side
2. Symmetrical movement patterns throughout the passive range
3. Age-appropriate gross motor development including symmetrical movement patterns between the left and right sides during static, dynamic, and reflexive movements
4. Improved skull symmetry to Argenta Type I or referred for further management of CD
5. No visible head tilt
6. Parents/caregivers understand what to monitor as the child grows

■ SUMMARY

This chapter discussed the management of CMT and CD. They are often comorbidities, and physical therapy is highly effective in resolving both CMT and CD when initiated early in infancy. A fibrotic and shortened SCM muscle is the most typical finding in CMT, resulting in rotation away from and a lateral head tilt toward the involved SCM muscle. The "back-to-sleep" campaign is thought to have spurred a growing incidence of CMT and CD. Differential diagnosis is critical to rule out other causes of asymmetrical posturing, such as neurologic, visual, or orthopedic conditions. Most infants with CMT can be successfully managed with first-choice conservative treatments including parent/caregiver education, environmental adaptations, passive neck ROM exercises, neck and trunk AROM, and facilitation of symmetrical movement activities. The CMT severity grade assists with prognosis for the episode of care to achieve resolution. CD is typically responsive to repositioning during the early months, but cranial remolding interventions may be necessary to correct moderate to severe CD in infants older than 4 to 6 months. Physical therapy for both CMT and CD should address all aspects of the ICF framework. Evidence-based objective measures should be documented at baseline and on subsequent visits to monitor the effectiveness of home programming. Collaboration with the family and caregivers is critical for successful outcomes; referrals for specialist consults when an infant is not progressing or when red flags are identified should be coordinated with the infant's primary physician.

ACKNOWLEDGMENT

Karen Karmel-Ross, PT, PCS, LMT for her valuable contributions to this chapter in all previous editions of this book.

Case Scenario on Expert Consult

The case scenario for this chapter describes "Riley," an infant with a classical presentation of CMT combined with CD. Data are provided for the initial evaluation and subsequent measures at 4–6 weeks, 16 weeks, and 24 weeks in the hopes of portraying typical resolution of both conditions. Shared decision making throughout the episode of care strongly influences the choice of interventions and the manner of their delivery, beginning with the immediate family and eventually extending to Riley's day care providers.

REFERENCES

1. AAP Task Force on Infant Positioning: SIDS: positioning and SIDS, *Pediatrics* 89:1120–1126, 1992.
2. AAP Task Force on Infant Sleep Position and Sudden Infant Death Syndrome: Changing concepts of sudden infant death syndrome: implications for infant sleeping environment and sleep position. *Pediatrics* 105:650–656, 2000.
3. AAP Task Force on Sudden Infant Death Syndrome: SIDS and other sleep-related infant deaths: expansion of recommendations for a safe infant sleeping environment, *Pediatrics* 128:1030–1039, 2011.
4. Aarnivala H, Vuollo V, Harila V, Heikkinen T: Preventing deformational plagiocephaly through parent guidance: a randomized, controlled trial, *Eur J Pediatr* 174:1197–1198, 2015.
5. Aarnivala HEI, Valkama AM, Pirttiniemi PM: Cranial shape, size and cervical motion in normal newborns, *Early Hum Dev* 90:425–424, 2014.
6. APTA: Guide to physical therapist practice, *Phys Ther* 81:1–768, 2001.
7. Argenta L: Clinical classification of positional plagiocephaly, *J Craniofac Surg* 15:368–372, 2004.
8. Arif-Rahu M, Fisher D, Matsuda Y: Biobehavioral measures for pain in the pediatric patient, *Pain Manag Nurs* 13:157–168, 2012.
9. Atmosukarto MS, Shapiro LG, Starr JR, Heike CL, et al.: 3D head shape quantification for infants with and without deformational plagiocephaly, *Cleft Palate Craniofac J* 47:368–377, 2010.
10. Ballock RT, Song KM: The prevalence of nonmuscular causes of torticollis in children, *J Pediatr Orthopaed* 16:500–505, 1996.
11. Bellieni CV: Pain assessment in human fetus and infants, *AAPS J* 14:456–461, 2012.
12. Bialocerkowski AE, Vladusic SL, Ng CW: Prevalence, risk factors, and natural history of positional plagiocephaly: a systematic review, *Dev Med Child Neurol* 50:577–586, 2008.
13. Binder H, Eng GD, Gaiser JF, Koch B: Congenital muscular torticollis: results of conservative management with long-term follow-up in 85 cases, *Arch Phys Med Rehab* 68:222–225, 1987.
14. Boere-Boonekamp MM, van der Linden-Kuiper LT: Positional preference: prevalence in infants and follow-up after two years, *Pediatrics* 107:339–343, 2001.
15. Boulet SL, Rasmussen SA, Honein MA: A population-based study of craniosynostosis in metropolitan Atlanta, 1989, *Am J Med Genetics Part A* 146A:984–991, 2008.
16. Branch LG, Kesty K, Krebs E, Wright L, et al.: Deformational plagiocephaly and craniosynostosis: trends in diagnosis and treatment after the "back to sleep" campaign, *J Craniofac Surg* 26:147–150, 2015.
17. Bredenkamp JK, Hoover LA, Berke GS, Shaw A: Congenital muscular torticollis. A spectrum of disease, *Arch Otolaryngol Head Neck Surg* 116:12–16, 1990.
18. Burstein FD: Long-term experience with endoscopic surgical treatment for congenital muscular torticollis in infants and children: a review of 85 cases, *Plast Reconstr Surg* 114:491–493, 2004.
19. Burstein FD, Cohen SR: Endoscopic surgical treatment for congenital muscular torticollis, *Plast Reconstr Surg* 101:20–24, 1998.
20. Cameron BHLJC, Cameron GS: Success of nonoperative treatment for congenital muscular torticollis is dependent on early therapy, *J Pediatr Surg* 9:391–393, 1994.
21. Canale ST, Griffin DW, Hubbard CN: Congenital muscular torticollis. A long-term follow-up, *J Bone Joint Surg* 64:810–816, 1982.
22. Cavalier A, Picot MC, Artiaga C, Mazurier E, et al.: Prevention of deformational plagiocephaly in neonates, *Early Hum Dev* 87:537–543, 2011.
23. Celayir AC: Congenital muscular torticollis: early and intensive treatment is critical. A prospective study, *Pediatr Int* 42:504–507, 2000.
24. Chen HX, Tang SP, Gao FT, Xu JL, et al.: Fibrosis, adipogenesis, and muscle atrophy in congenital muscular torticollis, *Medicine (Baltimore)* 93(23):e138, 2014.
25. Cheng JC, Tang SP, Chen TM: Sternocleidomastoid pseudotumor and congenital muscular torticollis in infants: a prospective study of 510 cases, *J Pediatr* 134:712–716, 1999.
26. Cheng JC, Tang SP, Chen TM, Wong MW, et al.: The clinical presentation and outcome of treatment of congenital muscular torticollis in infants—a study of 1,086 cases, *J Pediatr Surg* 35:1091–1096, 2000.
27. Cheng JC-Y, Metreweli C, Chen TM-K, Tang S-P: Correlation of ultrasonographic imaging of congenital muscular torticollis with clinical assessment in infants, *Ultrasound Med Biol* 26:1237–1241, 2000.
28. Cheng JCY, Wong MWN, Tang SP, Chen TM, et al.: Clinical determinants of the outcome of manual stretching in the treatment of congenital muscular torticollis in infants: a prospective study of eight hundred and twenty-one cases, *J Bone Joint Surg* 83:679–687, 2001.
29. Chon SC, Yoon SI, You JH: Use of the novel myokinetic stretching technique to ameliorate fibrotic mass in congenital muscular torticollis: an experimenter-blinded study with 1-year follow-up, *J Back Musculoskel Rehab* 23:63–68, 2010.
30. Collett BR, Gray KE, Starr JR, Heike CL, et al.: Development at age 36 months in children with deformational plagiocephaly, *Pediatrics* 131:e109–e115, 2013.
31. Collins A, Jankovic J: Botulinum toxin injection for congenital muscular torticollis presenting in children and adults, *Neurology* 67:1083–1085, 2006.
32. Committee on Quality Improvement-Subcommittee on Developmental Dysplasia of the Hip: Clinical practice guideline: early detection of developmental dysplasia, *Pediatrics* 105(4):896–905, 2000.
33. Coventry MB, Harris LE: Congenital muscular torticollis in infancy some observations regarding treatment, *J Bone Joint Surg* 41:815–822, 1959.
34. Cunningham ML, Heike CL: Evaluation of the infant with an abnormal skull shape, *Curr Opin Pediatr* 19:645–651, 2007.
35. Danby PM: Plagiocephaly in some 10-year-old children, *Arch Dis Child* 37:500–504, 1962.
36. David DJ, Menard RM: Occipital plagiocephaly, *Brit J Plast Surg* 53:367–377, 2000.
37. Davids JR, Wenger DR, Mubarak SJ: Congenital muscular torticollis: sequela of intrauterine or perinatal compartment syndrome, *J Pediatr Orthoped* 13:141–147, 1993.
38. de Chalain TMB, Park S: Torticollis associated with positional plagiocephaly: a growing epidemic, *J Craniofac Surg* 16:411–418, 2010.
39. de Ribaupierre S, Vernet O, Rilliet B, Cavin B, et al.: Posterior positional plagiocephaly treated by cranial remodelling orthosis, *Swiss Med Weekly* 137:368–372, 2007.
40. Degrazia M, Giambanco D, Hamn G, Ditzel A, et al.: Prevention of deformational plagiocephaly in hospitalized infants using a new orthotic device, *J Obst Gynecol Neonat Nurs* 44:28–41, 2015.
41. Demirbilek S, Atayurt HF: Congenital muscular torticollis and sternomastoid tumor: results of nonoperative treatment, *J Pediatr Surg* 34:549–551, 1999.
42. Deskin RW: Sandifer syndrome: a cause of torticollis in infancy, *Int J Pediatr Otorhinolaryngol* 32:183–185, 1995.
43. Dudkiewicz I, Ganel A, Blankstein A: Congenital muscular torticollis in infants: ultrasound-assisted diagnosis and evaluation. *J Pediatr Orthop* 25:812–814.
44. Emery C: The determinants of treatment duration for congenital muscular torticollis, *Phys Ther* 74:921–929, 1994.

45. Emery C: Conservative management of congenital muscular torticollis: a literature review, *Phys Occupat Ther Pediatr* 17:13–20, 1997.

46. Fearon JA: Evidence-based medicine: craniosynostosis, *Plast Reconstr Surg* 133:1261–1275, 2014.

47. Flannery ABK, Looman WS, Kemper K: Evidence-based care of the child with deformational plagiocephaly. Part II: management, *J Pediatr Health Care* 26:320–321, 2012.

48. Fletcher JP, Bandy WD: Intrarater reliability of CROM measurement of cervical spine active range of motion in persons with and without neck pain, *J Orthopaed Sports Phys Ther* 38:640–645, 2008.

49. Fowler EA, Becker DB, Pilgram TK, Noetzel M, et al.: Neurologic findings in infants with deformational plagiocephaly, *J Child Neurology* 23:742–747, 2008.

50. Freed SS, Coulter-O'Berry C: Identification and treatment of congenital muscular torticollis in infants, *J Prosthet Orthot* 16:S18–S23, 2004.

51. Goh JL, Bauer DF, Sr Durham, Stotland MA: Orthotic (helmet) therapy in the treatment of plagiocephaly, *Neurosurg Focus* 35:1–6, 2013.

52. Golden KA, Beals SP, Littlefield TR, Pomatto JK: Sternocleidomastoid imbalance versus congenital muscular torticollis: their relationship to positional plagiocephaly, *Cleft Palate Craniofac J* 36:256–261, 1999.

53. Graham JM, Gomez M, Halberg A, Earl DL, et al.: Management of deformational plagiocephaly: repositioning versus orthotic therapy, *J Pediatr* 146:258–262, 2005.

54. Graham JM, Kreutzman J, Earl D, Halberg A, et al.: Deformational brachycephaly in supine-sleeping infants, *J Pediatr* 146:253–257, 2005.

55. Gray GM, Tasso KH: Differential diagnosis of torticollis: a case report, *Pediatr Phys Ther* 21:369–374, 2009.

56. Gump WC, Mutchnick IS, Moriarty TM: Complications associated with molding helmet therapy for positional plagiocephaly: a review, *Neurosurg Focus* 35:1–3, 2013.

57. Guo S, Roche AF, Moore WM: Reference data for head circumference and 1-month increments from 1 to 12 months of age, *J Pediatr* 113:490–494, 1988.

58. Gutierrez D, Kaplan SL: Aligning documentation with congenital muscular torticollis clinical practice guidelines: administrative case report, *Phys Ther* 96:111–120, 2016.

59. Han JD, Kim SH, Lee SJ, Park MC, et al.: The thickness of the sternocleidomastoid muscle as a prognostic factor for congenital muscular torticollis, *Ann Rehabil Med* 35:361–368, 2011.

60. Haroon S, Beverley D: Congenital absence of the left sternomastoid muscle, *Arch Dis Child Fetal Neonatal Ed* 90:F102, 2004.

61. Hutchison BL, Hutchison LAD, Thompson JMD, Mitchell EA: Plagiocephaly and brachycephaly in the first two years of life: a prospective cohort study, *Pediatrics* 114:970–980, 2004.

62. Hutchison BL, Hutchison LAD, Thompson JMD, Mitchell EA: Quantification of plagiocephaly and brachycephaly in infants using a digital photographic technique, *Cleft Palate Craniofac J* 42:539–547, 2005.

63. Hutchison BL, Stewart AW, Chalain TD, Mitchell EA: Serial developmental assessments in infants with deformational plagiocephaly, *J Paediatr Child Health* 48:274–278, 2012.

64. Hutchison BL, Stewart AW, de Chalain TB, Mitchell EA: A randomized controlled trial of positioning treatments in infants with positional head shape deformities, *Acta Paediatr* 99:1556–1560, 2010.

65. Hutchison BL, Stewart AW, Mitchell EA: Characteristics, head shape measurements and developmental delay in 287 consecutive infants attending a plagiocephaly clinic, *Acta Paediatr* 98:1494–1499, 2009.

66. Hutchison BL, Thompson JMD, Mitchell EA: Determinants of nonsynostotic plagiocephaly: a case-control study, *Pediatrics* 112:e316–e322, 2003.

67. Hylton N: Infants with torticollis: the relationship between asymmetric head and neck positioning and postural development, *Phys Occupat Ther Pediatr* 17:91–117, 1997.

68. Ifflaender S, Rüdiger M, Konstantelos D, Lange U, et al.: Individual course of cranial symmetry and proportion in preterm infants up to 6 months of corrected age, *Early Hum Dev* 90:511–515, 2014.

69. Joganic JL, Lynch JM, Littlefield TR, Verrelli BC: Risk factors associated with deformational plagiocephaly, *Pediatrics* 124:e1126–e1133, 2009.

70. Joiner ERA, Andras LM, Skaggs DL: Screening for hip dysplasia in congenital muscular torticollis: is physical exam enough? *J Child Orthop* 8:115–119, 2014.

71. Joyce MB, de Chalain TM: Treatment of recalcitrant idiopathic muscular torticollis in infants with botulinum toxin type A, *J Craniofac Surg* 16:321–327, 2005.

72. Kabbani H, Raghuveer TS: Craniosynostosis. *Am Fam Phys* 69:2863–2870, 2004.

73. Kane AA, Lo L-J, Vannier MW, Marsh JL: Mandibular dysmorphology in unicoronal synostosis and plagiocephaly without synostosis, *Cleft Palate Craniofac J* 33:418–423, 1996.

74. Kaplan SL, Coulter C, Fetters L: Physical therapy management of congenital muscular torticollis: an evidence-based clinical practice guideline from the section on pediatrics of the American Physical Therapy Association, *Pediatr Phys Ther* 25:348–394, 2013.

75. Kelly KM, Littlefield TR, Pomatto JK, Manwaring KH, et al.: Cranial growth unrestricted during treatment of deformational plagiocephaly, *Pediatr Neurosurg* 30:193–199, 1999.

76. Kim MY, Kwon DR, Lee HI: Therapeutic effect of microcurrent therapy in infants with congenital muscular torticollis, *Phys Med Rehab* 1:736–739, 2009.

77. Klackenberg EP, Elfving B, Haglund-Åkerlind Y, Carlberg EB: Intra-rater reliability in measuring range of motion in infants with congenital muscular torticollis, *Advances Physiother* 7:84–91, 2005.

78. Kluba S, Kraut W, Reinert S, Krimmel M: What is the optimal time to start helmet therapy in positional plagiocephaly? *Plast Reconstr Surg* 128:492–498, 2011.

79. Kuo AA, Tritasavit S, Graham Jr JM: Congenital muscular torticollis and positional plagiocephaly, *Pediatr Rev* 35:79–86, 2014.

80. Kwon DR, Park GY: Efficacy of microcurrent therapy in infants with congenital muscular torticollis involving the entire sternocleidomastoid muscle: a randomized placebo-controlled trial, *Clin Rehab* 10:983–991, 2014.

81. Lal S, Abbasi AS, Jamro S: Response of primary torticollis to physiotherapy, *J Surg Pakistan* 16:153–156, 2011.

82. Laughlin J, Luerssen TG, Dias MS: Prevention and management of positional skull deformities in infants, *Pediatrics* 128:1236–1241, 2011.

83. Lee IJ, Lim SY, Song HS, Park MC: Complete tight fibrous band release and resection in congenital muscular torticollis, *J Plast Reconstr Aesthet Surg* 63:947–953, 2010.

84. Lee J, Moon H, Park M, Yoo W, et al.: Change of craniofacial deformity after sternocleidomastoid muscle release in pediatric patients with congenital muscular torticollis, *J Bone Joint Surg* 94:e93–e97, 2012.

85. Lee J-Y, Koh S-E, Lee I-S, Jung H, et al.: The cervical range of motion as a factor affecting outcome in patients with congenital muscular torticollis, *Ann Rehabil Med* 37:183–190, 2013.

86. Lee Y-T, Yoon K, Kim Y-B, Chung P-W, et al.: Clinical features and outcome of physiotherapy in early presenting congenital muscular torticollis with severe fibrosis on ultrasonography: a prospective study, *J Pediatr Surg* 46:1526–1531, 2011.

87. Lightdale JR, Gremse DA: Gastroesophageal reflux: management guidance for the pediatrician, *Pediatrics* 131:e1684–e1695, 2013.

88. Likus W, Bajor G, Gruszczynska K, Baron J, et al.: Cephalic index in the first three years of life: study of children with normal brain development based on computed tomography, *Sci World J* 2014:1–6, 2014.

89. Lin J-N, Chou M-L: Ultrasonographic study of the sternocleidomastoid muscle in the management of congenital muscular torticollis, *J Pediatr Surg* 32:1648–1651, 1997.

90. Littlefield TR, Kelly KM, Reiff JL, Pomatto JK: Car seats, infant carriers, and swings: their role in deformational plagiocephaly, *J Prosthet Orthot* 15:102–106, 2003.

91. Looman WS, Flannery ABK: Evidence-based care of the child with deformational plagiocephaly. Part I: assessment and diagnosis, *J Pediatr Health Care* 26:242–250, 2012.

92. Losee JE, Mason AC, Dudas J, Hua LB, et al.: Nonsynostotic occipital plagiocephaly: factors impacting onset, treatment, and outcomes, *J Plast Reconstr Surgery* 119:1866–1873, 2007.

93. Luxford BK: The physiotherapy management of infants with congenital muscular torticollis: a survey of current practice in New Zealand, *New Zeal J Physioth er* 37:127–135, 2009.

94. Majnemer A, Barr RG: Influence of supine sleep positioning on early motor milestone acquisition, *Dev Med Child Neurol* 47:370–376, 2005.

95. Majnemer A, Barr RG: Association between sleep position and early motor development, *J Pediatr* 149:623–629, 2006.

96. Malviya S, Voepel-Lewis T, Burke C, Merkel S, et al.: The revised FLACC observational pain tool: improved reliability and validity for pain assessment in children with cognitive impairment, *Paediatr Anaesth* 16:258–265, 2006.

97. Marchac A, Arnaud E, Di Rocco F, Michienzi J, et al.: Severe deformational plagiocephaly: long-term results of surgical treatment, *J Craniofac Surg* 22:24–29, 2011.

98. Mawji A, Robinson Bollman A, Hatfield J, McNeil DA, et al.: The incidence of positional plagiocephaly: a cohort study, *Pediatrics* 132:298–304, 2013.

99. Meyer-Marcotty P, Bohm H, Linz C, Kochel J, et al.: Spectrum of positional deformities - is there a real difference between plagiocephaly and brachycephaly? *J Cranio Maxillofac Surg* 42:1010–1016, 2014.

100. Miller RI, Clarren SK: Long-term developmental outcomes in patients with deformational plagiocephaly, *Pediatrics* 105:e26–e30, 2000.

101. Monson RM, Deitz J, Kartin D: The relationship between awake positioning and motor performance among infants who slept supine, *Pediatr Phys Ther* 15:196–203, 2003.

102. Moore KL, Dalley AF: *Clinically oriented anatomy*, ed 5, Baltimore, 2006, Lippincott Williams & Wilkins.

103. Mortenson PA, Steinbok P: Quantifying positional plagiocephaly: reliability and validity of anthropometric measurements, *J Craniofac Surg* 17:413–419, 2006.

104. Nellhaus G: Head circumference from birth to eighteen years: practical composite international and interracial graphs, *Pediatrics* 41:106–114, 1968.

105. Nucci P, Curiel B: Abnormal head posture due to ocular problems: a review, *Curr Pediatr Rev* 5:105–111, 2009.

106. Nucci P, Kushner BJ, Serafino M, Orzalesi N: A multi-disciplinary study of the ocular, orthopedic, and neurologic causes of abnormal head postures in children, *Am J Ophthalmol* 140:65–68, 2005.

107. Nuysink J, van Haastert IC, Takken T, Helders PJM: Symptomatic asymmetry in the first six months of life: differential diagnosis, *Eur J Pediatr* 167:613–619, 2008.

108. Ohman A: The inter-rater and intra-rater reliability of a modified "severity scale for assessment of plagiocephaly" among physical therapists, *Physiother Theory Prac* 28:402–406, 2012.

109. Öhman A, Beckung E: Functional and cosmetic status in children treated for congenital muscular torticollis as infants, *Adv Physiother* 7:135–140, 2005.

110. Öhman A, Mardbrink E-L, Stensby J, Beckung E: Evaluation of treatment strategies for muscle function, *Physiother Theory Pract* 27:463–470, 2011.

111. Öhman A, Nilsson S, Lagerkvist A, Beckung ERE: Are infants with torticollis at risk of a delay in early motor milestones compared with a control group of healthy infants? *Dev Med Child Neurol* 51:545–550, 2009.

112. Öhman AM: The immediate effect of kinesiology taping on muscular imbalance for infants with congenital muscular torticollis, *Phys Med Rehab* 4:504–508, 2012.

113. Öhman AM, Beckung ERE: Reference values for range of motion and muscle function of the neck in infants, *Pediatr Phys Ther* 20:53–58, 2008.

114. Öhman AM, Mårdbrink E-l, Orefelt C, Seager A, et al.: The physical therapy assessment and management of infants with congenital muscular torticollis. A survey and a suggested assessment protocol for CMT, *J Novel Physiother* 3:165, 2013.

115. Öhman AM, Nilsson S, Beckung ER: Validity and reliability of the muscle function scale, aimed to assess the lateral flexors of the neck in infants, *Physiother Theory Pract* 25:129–137, 2009.

116. Oleszek JL, Chang N, Apkon SD, Wilson PE: Botulinum toxin type A in the treatment of children with congenital muscular torticollis, *Am J Physical Med Rehab* 84:813–816, 2005.

117. Panchal J, Amirsheybani H, Gurwitch R, Cook V, et al.: Neurodevelopment in children with single-suture craniosynostosis and plagiocephaly without synostosis, *Plast Reconstr Surg* 108:1492–1498, 2001.

118. Peitsch WK, Keefer CH, LaBrie RA & Mulliken JB: Incidence of cranial asymmetry in healthy newborns, *Pediatrics* 110(6): e72–e72, 2002.

119. Persing J, James H, Swanson J, Kattwinkel J, et al.: Prevention and management of positional skull deformities in infants, *Pediatrics* 112:199–202, 2003.

120. Petronic I, Brdar R, Cirovic D, Nikolic D, et al.: Congenital muscular torticollis in children: distribution, treatment duration and outcome, *Eur J Phys Rehabil Med* 45:153–188, 2010.

121. Pin T, Eldridge B, Galea MP: A review of the effects of sleep position, play position, and equipment use on motor development in infants, *Dev Med Child Neurol* 49:858–867, 2007.

122. Rahlin M: TAMO therapy as a major component of physical therapy intervention for an infant with congenital muscular torticollis: a case report, *Pediatr Phys Ther* 17:209–218, 2005.

123. Rahlin M, Sarmiento B: Reliability of still photography measuring habitual head deviation from midline in infants with congenital muscular torticollis, *Pediatr Phys Ther* 22:399–406, 2010.

124. Rekate HL: Occipital plagiocephaly: a critical review of the literature, *J Neurosurg* 89:24–30, 1998.

125. Robinson S, Proctor M: Diagnosis and management of deformational plagiocephaly, *J Neurosurg Pediatr* 3:284–295, 2009.

126. Roby BB, Finkelstein M, Tibesar RJ, Sidman JD: Prevalence of positional plagiocephaly in teens born after the "back to sleep" campaign, *Ped Otolaryngol* 146:823–828, 2012.

127. Rogers GF: Deformational plagiocephaly, brachycephaly, and scaphocephaly. Part II: prevention and treatment, *J Craniofac Surg* 22:17–23, 2011.

128. Rogers GF, Miller J, Mulliken JB: Comparison of a modifiable cranial cup versus repositioning and cervical stretching for the early correction of deformational posterior plagiocephaly, *Plast Reconstr Surg* 121:941–947, 2008.

129. Rogers GF, Oh AK, Mulliken JB: The role of congenital muscular torticollis in the development of deformational plagiocephaly, *Plast Reconstr Surg* 123:643–652, 2009.

130. Schertz M, Zuk L, Green D: Long-term neurodevelopmental follow-up of children with congenital muscular torticollis, *J Child Neurol* 28(10):1215–1221, 2012.

131. Schertz M, Zuk L, Zin S, Nadam L, et al.: Motor and cognitive development at one-year follow-up in infants with torticollis, *Early Hum Dev* 84:9–14, 2008.

132. Seruya M, Oh AK, Sauerhammer TM, Taylor JH, et al.: Correction of deformational plagiocephaly in early infancy using the plagio cradle orthotic, *J Craniofac Surg* 24:376–379, 2013.

133. Seruya M, Oh AK, Taylor JH, Sauerhammer TM, et al.: Helmet treatment of deformational plagiocephaly: the relationship between age at initiation and rate of correction, *Plast Reconstr Surg* 131:55–61, 2013.

134. Shamji MF, Fric-Shamji EC, Merchant P, Vassilyadi M: Cosmetic and cognitive outcomes of positional plagiocephaly treatment, *Clin Invest Med* 35:E246–E270, 2012.

135. Sillifant P, Vaiude P, Bruce S, Quirk D, et al.: Positional plagiocephaly: experience with a passive orthotic mattress, *J Craniofac Surg* 25:1365–1368, 2014.

136. Slate RK, Posnick JC, Armstrong DC, Buncie JR: Cervical spine subluxation associated with congenital muscular torticollis and craniofacial asymmetry, *Plast Reconstr Surg* 91:1187–1195, 1993.

137. Snyder EM, Coley BD: Limited value of plain radiographs in infant torticollis, *Pediatrics* 118:e1779–e1784, 2006.

138. Sönmez K, Turkiyilmaz Z, Demirogullari B, Ozen IO, et al.: Congenital muscular torticollis in children. [review] [16 refs], *J Oto-Rhino-Laryngol* 67:344–347, 2005.

139. Spermon J, Spermon-Marijnen R, Scholten-Peeters W: Clinical classification of deformational plagiocephaly according to Argenta: a reliability study, *J Craniofac Surg* 19:664–668, 2008.

140. St John D, Mulliken JB, Kaban LB, Padwa BL: Anthropometric analysis of mandibular deformational posterior plagiocephaly, *J Oral Maxillofac Surg* 60:873–877, 2002.

141. Steinberg JP, Rawlani R, Humphries LS, Rawlani V, et al.: Effectiveness of conservative therapy and helmet therapy for positional cranial deformation, *Plast Reconstr Surg* 135:833–842, 2015.

142. Steinbok P, Lam D, Singh S, Mortenson PA, et al.: Long-term outcome of infants with positional occipital plagiocephaly, *Child Nerv Sys* 23:1275–1283, 2007.

143. Stellwagen LM, Hubbard E, Chambers C, Jones KL: Torticollis, facial asymmetry and plagiocephaly in normal newborns, *Arch Dis Child* 93:827–831, 2008.

144. Stellwagen LM, Hubbard E, Vaux K: Look for the "stuck baby" to identify congenital torticollis, *Contemp Pediatr* 21:55–65, 2004.

145. Storer SK, Dimaggio J, Skaggs DL, Angeles CHL, et al.: Developmental dysplasia of the hip, *Am Fam Phys* 74:1310–1316, 2006.

146. Suzuki S, Yamamuro T, Fujita A: The aetiological relationship between congenital torticollis and obstetrical paralysis, *Intl Orthopaed* 8:175–181, 1984.

147. Swain B: Transaxillary endoscopic release of restricting bands in congenital muscular torticollis—a novel technique, *J Plast ReconstrAesth Surg* 60:95–98, 2007.

148. Tang S, Liu Z, Quan X, Qin J, et al.: Sternocleidomastoid pseudotumor of infants and congenital muscular torticollis: fine-structure research, *J Pediatr Orthoped* 18:214–218, 1998.

149. Tang SFT, Hsu K-H, Wong AMK, Hsu C-C, et al.: Longitudinal followup study of ultrasonography in congenital muscular torticollis, *Clin Orthopaed Related Res* 403:179–185, 2002.

150. Tatli B, Aydinli N, Caliskan M, Ozmen M, et al.: Congenital muscular torticollis: evaluation and classification, *Pediatr Neurolo* 34:41–44, 2006.

151. Taylor JL, Norton ES: Developmental muscular torticollis: outcomes in young children treated by physical therapy, *Pediatr Phys Ther* 9:173–178, 1997.

152. Tessmer A, Mooney P, Pelland L: A developmental perspective on congenital muscular torticollis: a critical appraisal of the evidence, *Pediatr Phys Ther* 22:378–383, 2010.

153. Thompson F, McManus S, Colville J: Familial congenital muscular torticollis: case report and review of the literature, *Clini Orthopaed Rel Res* 202:193–196, 1986.

154. Thompson JT, David LR, Wood B, Argenta A, et al.: Outcome analysis of helmet therapy for positional plagiocephaly using a three-dimensional surface scanning laser, *J Craniofac Surg* 20:362–365, 2009.

155. Tomczak KK, Rosman NP: Torticollis. *J Child Neurol*, 28:365–378, 2013.

156. Tumturk A, Ozcora GK, Bayram AK, Kabaklioglu M, et al.: Torticollis in children: an alert symptom not to be turned away, *Child Nerv Sys* 31:1461–1470, 2015.

157. Turgut M, Akalan N, Bertan V, Erbengi A, et al.: Acquired torticollis as the only presenting symptom in children with posterior fossa tumors, *Child Nerv Sys* 11:6–8, 1995.

158. van Vlimmeren LA, Helders PJ, van Adrichem LN, Engelbert RH: Diagnostic strategies for the evaluation of asymmetry in infancy-a review, *Eur J Pediatr* 163:185–191, 2004.

159. van Vlimmeren LA, Helders PJM, van Adrichem LNA, Engelbert RHH: Torticollis and plagiocephaly in infancy: therapeutic strategies, *Pediatr Rehabil* 9:40–46, 2006.

160. van Vlimmeren LA, van der Graaf Y, Boere-Boonekamp MM, L'Hoir MP, et al.: Risk factors for deformational plagiocephaly at birth and at 7 weeks of age: a prospective cohort study, *Pediatrics* 119:e408–e418, 2007.

161. van Vlimmeren La, van der Graaf Y, Boere-Boonekamp MM, L'Hoir MP, et al.: Effect of pediatric physical therapy on deformational plagiocephaly in children with positional preference: a randomized controlled trial, *Arch PediatrAdolesc Med* 162:712–718, 2008.

162. van Wijk RM, van Vlimmeren LA, Groothuis-Oudshoorn CG, Van der Ploeg CP, et al.: Helmet therapy in infants with positional skull deformation: randomised controlled trial, *Brit Med J* 348:g2741, 2014.

163. von Heideken J, Green DW, Burke SW, Sindle K, et al.: The relationship between developmental dysplasia of the hip and congenital muscular torticollis, *J Pediatr Orthoped* 26:805–808, 2006.

164. Wall V, Glass R: Mandibular asymmetry and breastfeeding problems: experience from 11 cases, *J Hum Lactat* 22:328–334, 2006.

165. Wei JL, Schwartz KM, Weaver AL, Orvidas LJ: Pseudotumor of infancy and congenital muscular torticollis: 170 cases, *Laryngoscope* 111(4 Pt 1): 688–695, 2001.

166. Wilbrand J-F, Schmidtberg K, Bierther U, Streckbein P, et al.: Clinical classification of infant nonsynostotic cranial deformity, *J Pediatr* 161:1120–1125, 2012.

167. Wilbrand J-F, Seidl M, Wilbrand M, Streckbein P, et al.: A prospective randomized trial on preventative methods for positional head deformity: physiotherapy versus a positioning pillow, *J Pediatr* 162:1216–1221, 2013.

168. Yu C-C, Wong F-H, Lo L-J, Chen Y-R: Craniofacial deformity in patients with uncorrected congenital muscular torticollis: an assessment from three-dimensional computed tomography imaging, *Plast Reconstr Surg* 113:24–33, 2004.

SUGGESTED READINGS

Background

Cunningham ML, Heike CL: Evaluation of the infant with an abnormal skull shape, *Curr Opin Pediatr* 19:645–651, 2007.

Steinberg JP, Rawlani R, Humphries LS, Rawlani V, et al.: Effectiveness of conservative therapy and helmet therapy for positional cranial deformation. *Plast Reconstr Surg* 135:833–842, 2015.

Suhr MC, Oledzka M: Considerations and intervention in congenital muscular torticollis, *Curr Opin Pediatr* 27:75–81, 2015.

Task Force on Sudden Infant Death Syndrome: SIDS and other sleep-related infant deaths: expansion of recommendations for a safe infant sleeping environment, *Pediatrics* 128:1030–1039, 2011.

Tessmer A, Mooney P, Pelland L: A developmental perspective on congenital muscular torticollis: a critical appraisal of the evidence, *Pediatr Phys Ther* 22:378–383, 2010.

Foreground

Ballock RT, Song KM: The prevalence of nonmuscular causes of torticollis in children, *J Pediatr Orthopaed* 16:500–504, 1996.

Flannery ABK, Looman WS, Kemper K: Evidence-based care of the child with deformational plagiocephaly. Part II: management, *J Pediatr Health Care* 26:320–331, 2012.

Gutierrez D, Kaplan SL: Aligning documentation with congenital muscular torticollis clinical practice guidelines: administrative case report, *Phys Ther* 96:111–120, 2016.

Kaplan SL, Coulter C, Fetters L: Physical therapy management of congenital muscular torticollis: an evidence-based clinical practice guideline from the Section on Pediatrics of the American Physical Therapy Association, *Pediatr Phys Ther* 25:348–394, 2013.

Looman WS, Flannery ABK: Evidence-based care of the child with deformational plagiocephaly, Part 1: assessment and diagnosis, *J Pediatr Health Care* 26:242–250, 2012.

10

Arthrogryposis Multiplex Congenita

Maureen Donohoe

Arthrogryposis multiplex congenita (AMC) is a nonprogressive neuromuscular syndrome that is present at birth. AMC is characterized by severe joint contractures, muscle weakness, and fibrosis. Although the child's condition does not deteriorate as a result of the primary diagnosis, the long-term sequelae of AMC can be very disabling. Activity limitations in mobility and self-care skills can lead to varying degrees of participation restriction.

Working with children with AMC presents the physical therapist with a variety of challenges. Many children who have AMC are bright and motivated. Physical therapists must use their knowledge of biomechanics and normal development to maximize functional skills. Proper timing for therapeutic and medical interventions helps maximize the child's opportunities for independence. Creativity is needed to adapt equipment and the environment to allow the child with AMC to be able to participate in life roles to the fullest extent possible.

In this chapter, we address the pathophysiology of AMC, its management from a medical and surgical perspective, physical therapy examination and evaluation, and specific physical therapy and team interventions used for children with AMC from infancy to adulthood.

BACKGROUND INFORMATION

INCIDENCE AND ETIOLOGY

Arthrogryposis, which is defined by the presence of contractures in two or more body areas, is diagnosed in 1 of every 3000 to 5000 live births.[4,28,56] Many times the cause of AMC is unknown; however, the insult is believed to occur during the first trimester of pregnancy.[16,26,72] It is believed insults occurring early in the first trimester have the potential for creating greater involvement of the child than those occurring late in the first trimester. The basic pathophysiologic mechanism for multiple joint contractures appears to be fetal akinesia.[19,27,66] More than 150 different contracture syndromes have been mapped to specific genes. Over 400 specific conditions have been identified that relate to gene mutations and chromosomal abnormalities.[21,27]

Various forms of arthrogryposis are known; amyoplasia is the most commonly recognized. Newborns with congenital contractures fall evenly into three groups: one consists of amyoplasia, the second is related to the central nervous system and is lethal, and the third is a heterogeneous group. The heterogeneous group includes neuromuscular syndromes, congenital anomalies, chromosomal abnormalities, contracture syndromes, and skeletal dysplasia. Distal arthrogryposis, which affects primarily the hands and feet and is highly responsive to treatment, has a genetic basis and is inherited as an autosomal dominant trait.[21,22] Gene mapping has been helpful in identifying those with arthrogryposis. Neuropathic arthrogryposis is found on chromosome 5 and can have survival motor neuron gene deletion.[12,58] Distal arthrogryposis type I maps to chromosome 9.[3,5]

AMC is associated with neurogenic and myopathic disorders in which motor weakness immobilizes the fetal joints, leading to joint contractures. It is not known whether all those with the neuropathic form of AMC have degeneration of the anterior horn cell, but of those studied postmortem, this is a consistent finding. A neurogenic disorder of the anterior horn cell is believed to cause muscle weakness with subsequent periarticular soft tissue fibrosis.[20,25,70,72] Because of failure of the muscle to function, the joints in the developing fetus lack movement, which probably explains the stiffness and deformities of the newborn's joints. The fetus may have an imbalance in strength of oppositional muscle groups, creating the tendency toward a certain posture. For example, the fetus with good strength in the hamstrings and triceps brachii but weakness in the quadriceps and biceps brachii will have a flexed knee and extended elbow posture in utero. Decreased amniotic fluid throughout the pregnancy, but especially during the last trimester when the fetus is largest, may further inhibit freedom of movement in utero.

Although the cause of AMC remains unknown, several factors have been implicated. Hyperthermia of the fetus is caused by a maternal fever greater than 37.8°C (100°F). Some mothers of children with AMC report having an illness with a fever for 1 to 2 days during the first trimester. Prenatal viral infection, vascular compromise of the blood supply between mother and fetus, uterine fibroid tumors, and a septum in the uterus have all been proposed as causes of AMC.[26,27,28,57,72]

PROGRESS IN PRIMARY PREVENTION

Arthrogryposis has been documented in artwork as early as the 1700s, although medical literature did not begin to address it until nearly the 1950s. Eight major categories of problems can occur during a pregnancy that could precipitate the lack of movement associated with congenital contractures; these include maternal illness or exposures, fetal crowding, neurologic deficits, vascular compromise, metabolic disturbances, neuromuscular end plate abnormalities, connective tissue abnormalities/skeletal defects, and muscle defects.[28] Given its nonspecific origin, little progress has been made in prevention of this rare disorder. However, significant improvements have been made in the management of children with AMC.

DIAGNOSIS

No definitive laboratory studies can diagnose AMC prenatally, unless a familial trait is documented. Some forms of arthrogryposis have been mapped to chromosomes 5, 9, or 11.[5,47,58] Most AMC cases occur sporadically with no known familial trait; therefore prenatal testing beyond ultrasound studies is inconsequential. Over 70% of cases of amyoplasia were missed on prenatal testing.[22] If a parent or physician suspects that something is amiss, a detailed ultrasound evaluation can be helpful in identifying anomalies and decreased fetal movements. Real-time ultrasound studies lasting up to 45 minutes, repeated several times during the pregnancy, are most useful. Having an ultrasound track movement over a longer period of time helps to identify if there are limitations in movement or movement biases due to position of the fetus. Repeating this test several times helps to identify if the same movement issues are persisting throughout the pregnancy. Clues that are looked for include nuchal edema; thin, undercalcified bones; small lungs; decreased movement time after 11 weeks of gestation; limitations in the diaphragm; and structural or space limitations.[21,22,27] If arthrogryposis is diagnosed during pregnancy, the mother can do some things to help exercise the baby as long as she is cleared by her physician from a health standpoint.[28] These activities include deep breathing, light exercise, and daily caffeine intake to help stimulate the baby.

Blood tests including a genetic microarray can be helpful in finding genetic alterations associated with arthrogryposis.[4] Muscle biopsy in AMC varies with the muscle under study. Histologic analysis reveals that relatively strong muscles appear virtually normal, and very weak muscles reveal fibrofatty changes but may have normal muscle spindles. Embryologically, the muscles are formed normally, but they are replaced by fibrous and fatty tissue during fetal development.[24, 26] With electromyographic testing, neuropathic and myopathic changes can be seen in different muscles in the same patient.[53,58] Muscle biopsies along with blood tests and clinical findings rule out progressive and fatal disorders, while providing evidence to support the diagnosis of AMC.

CLINICAL MANIFESTATIONS

Clinical manifestations of AMC demonstrate great variability but generally include severe joint contractures and lack of muscle development or amyoplasia. The typical severely affected body parts in the AMC population include, in decreasing order of prevalence, the foot (78%–95%), the hip (55%–90%), the wrist (43%–81%), the knee (38%–90%), the elbow (35%–92%), and the shoulder (20%–92%).[41,48,64]

Two commonly seen variations of AMC have been noted. In one type the child has flexed and dislocated hips, extended knees, clubfeet (equinovarus), internally rotated shoulders, flexed elbows, and flexed and ulnarly deviated wrists (Fig. 10.1). In another type the child has abducted and externally rotated hips, flexed knees, clubfeet, internally rotated shoulders, extended elbows, and flexed and ulnarly deviated wrists (Fig. 10.2). Parents often describe the legs in the first type as jackknifed, and in the second type as froglike. Because of the stiffness of the joints, extremity movements are described as wooden or marionette-like. The position of the upper extremities in the second type is described as the "waiter's tip" position owing to the internally rotated shoulder, extended elbow, pronated forearm,

and flexed wrist. Common to both types are clubfeet, flexed and ulnarly deviated wrists, and internally rotated shoulders. Other associated characteristics may include scoliosis, dimpling of skin over joints, hemangiomas, absent or decreased finger creases, congenital heart disease, facial abnormalities, respiratory problems, and abdominal hernias. Intelligence and speech are usually normal. Many arthrogrypotic syndromes occur that have the main characteristics of AMC but may also involve abnormal muscle tone, webbing at contracted joints, changes in cognition, seizure activity, feeding issues not related to muscle strength or jaw opening, and limited visual skills.[54,70]

MEDICAL MANAGEMENT

The main component of medical treatment includes well-timed surgical management.[25,51] Orthopedic treatment should be timed so that the child benefits optimally from the procedure. For example, clubfoot management with minimally invasive surgical techniques such as the Ponseti method should start approximately 1 month after the child is born. This allows the child to naturally stretch out and the family to become accustomed to the therapy routine before embarking on months of serial casting and positioning devices, allowing for plantigrade feet in time for developmentally appropriate upright activity.[8,38,46,69] Ponseti method is frequently being used to address relapsing clubfeet through serial casting and minimally invasive soft tissue lengthening.[50]

Although becoming less common, some continue to have open surgical techniques such as the posteromediolateral release (PMLR) for clubfoot. The entire hindfoot is opened during surgery so as to shorten the lateral column, lengthen the medial column, and lengthen the tendo Achillis.[49,53] Occasionally, wires are used to realign the talus and the calcaneus. If the clubfoot recurs and does not respond to serial casting, a second PMLR involves shortening the cuboid bone to help improve forefoot alignment. If the foot is tight just in the hindfoot and no forefoot adductus is noted, a distal tibial wedge osteotomy is done to realign the foot in reference to the floor. Later in life, when the child is near the end of growth, a triple arthrodesis can be performed to prevent future inversion of the foot. This involves fusing the calcaneus to the cuboid, the talus to the navicular, and the talus to the calcaneus. Use of an external fixator such as an Ilizarov procedure to address recurrent clubfoot problems has had some promising results, although no data from long-term outcome studies are presently available.[11,14] Historically, in severe cases of equinovarus and in cases in which the Ilizarov procedure fails, a talectomy may be performed.[13,43] Salvage procedures to correct recurrent problems are difficult, however, when a talectomy has been previously performed.[42,49,63] Research supports that invasive surgical correction of feet results in stiff painful feet in adulthood.[35,42]

Children with AMC often have subluxed or dislocated hips. Dislocation is as frequently bilateral as unilateral. One dislocated hip is usually relocated to prevent secondary pelvic obliquity and scoliosis, unless the hip is extremely stiff.[55,62] Given that these hips tend to have poor acetabular development, if both hips are dislocated, they are not always surgically reduced because of the risk of continued unilateral dislocation even after open reduction. Careful evaluation of dislocated hips is necessary before surgical intervention is undertaken because if the hips are very tight into extension, limiting sitting ability, they will be even tighter after surgery. If the hips are dislocated high

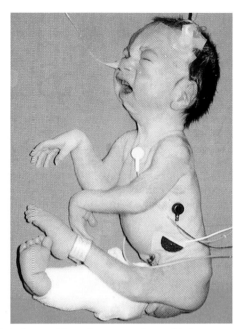

FIG. 10.1 Infant with arthrogryposis multiplex congenita with flexed and dislocated hips, extended knees, clubfeet (equinovarus), internally rotated shoulders, flexed elbows, and flexed and ulnarly deviated wrists. (From Moore KL, Persaud TVN, Torchia MG: The developing human. 9th ed. Philadelphia, Saunders, 2013. Courtesy of Dr. AE Chudley, Section of Genetics and Metabolism, Department of Pediatrics and Child Health, Children's Hospital and University of Manitoba, Winnipeg, Manitoba, Canada.)

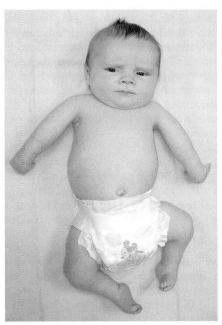

FIG. 10.2 Infant with arthrogryposis multiplex congenita with abducted and externally rotated hips, flexed knees, clubfeet, internally rotated shoulders, extended elbows, and flexed and ulnarly deviated wrists. (From Bamshad M, Van Heest AE, Pleasure D: Arthrogryposis: a review and update, *J Bone Joint Surg Am* 91[Suppl 4]:40-46, 2009.)

and posterior, with poor bony elements for the acetabulum, satisfactory surgical reduction may not be possible. Those who surgically reduce arthrogrypotic dislocated hips most commonly perform the surgery during the first year of life and use an anterolateral approach.[44,55,62,64,65] Szoke and colleagues[65] advocate early open reduction with a medial approach because resultant hip stiffness was greater for those who were older at the initial surgery. Yau and colleagues[73] found that open reduction was necessary to have success in treating dislocated hips because closed reduction in children with AMC was never successful. It may be more important to have mobile, painless, yet dislocated hips than to have very stiff but located ones. Prolonged immobilization following open or closed techniques can lead to the serious sequelae of fused or stiff hips.[1]

Moderate to severe contractures of the knee joint can be addressed surgically, but through the conservative approach, one waits until the child is ambulating comfortably before performing surgical correction. Knee flexion contractures are most commonly associated with capsular changes within the joint. Medial and lateral hamstring lengthening or sectioning (if the muscle is fibrosed), along with a posterior capsulotomy of the knee joint, may be performed.[48,66] These contractures respond inconsistently to hamstring lengthening and posterior capsulotomy because subsequent loss of muscle strength and risk of scar tissue lead to further joint stiffness and recurrence of the contracture. A distal femoral osteotomy is more frequently successful in realigning the joint and changes the arc of motion without risk of increased scar tissue and loss of strength[17] (Fig. 10.3). Growing children with moderate knee flexion contractures do well with distal femoral anterior epiphysiodesis. This procedure is done when the child is large enough to accept the surgical hardware but small enough to have adequate growth available, usually after the child is 5 years old but before 11 years of age. It allows the posterior aspect of the femur to continue to grow while the anterior aspect remains unchanged (Fig. 10.4). The angle of the femur results in apparent knee straightening.[37,40,52] Severe knee flexion contractures are often addressed through the use of external fixators to distract the joint and slowly elongate the tissues.[11,34,68]

Knee extension contractures frequently have associated patellar subluxation.[10] Patellar realignment is done before the fifth birthday to allow the femoral groove to develop with growth.[10] Later in life, extension contractures are addressed by quadriceps lengthening if at least 25° of range of motion (ROM) is observed in the knee. Intra-articular procedures such as a capsulotomy may be necessary if the knee is stiff.[33] Some evidence suggests that surgery to address knee extension contractures results in better outcomes than surgery to address knee flexion contractures.[61] An important consideration before surgical intervention is determination of whether the limitation in ROM is creating problems with sitting or walking and, if so, if surgical intervention will likely improve the child's function. For example, if the legs extend straight out when sitting, this position may interfere with activities such as sitting at school desks or riding in a car and as a result may decrease participation at school and in the community. The child should participate in decisions regarding surgical interventions as appropriate for his or her age.

Restrictions in shoulder movement are rarely addressed through surgical interventions such as capsular or soft tissue release because the musculature is usually inappropriate for transfer. If adequate muscle strength and control are present,

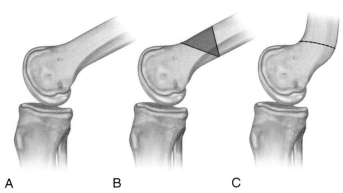

FIG. 10.3 Diagram of a distal femoral wedge osteotomy performed to realign the contracted knee joint. (A) Knee flexion contracture deformity before surgery. (B) Distal femoral wedge osteotomy for reduction of the knee flexion deformity. (C) Realignment after surgery.

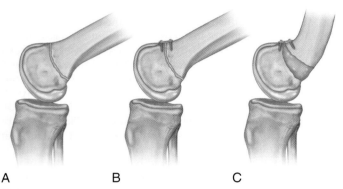

FIG. 10.4 Diagram of guided growth for knee contracture management. (A) Knee flexion contracture deformity before surgery. (B) Distal femoral anterior epiphysiodesis for reduction of the knee flexion deformity. (C) Realignment after surgery.

surgery may be indicated to place wrists and elbows in positions of optimal function. One scenario involves a child with symmetrical weakness or severe contractures of the upper extremities. In this case a dominant arm can be identified for feeding (postured in flexion) and the other arm for hygiene care (postured in extension).[71] If both arms were postured in extension, surgery would be necessary to position one arm in a functional flexion position. Such surgical considerations would include a pectoralis or triceps brachii transfer to give a child active elbow flexion with a posterior capsulotomy to allow for elbow flexion.[2,66] The muscle under consideration for transfer would need to be strong before transfer with adequate passive elbow flexion could present. A consistent passive ROM and stretching program from birth is essential to maintain elbow motion for this type of surgery to be successful.

Wrists can be fused in positions for function if conservative splinting and stretching management have been unsuccessful. Wrists are fused in dissimilar positions. Before a surgical wrist fusion, casting of the wrist for 1 week in the position of the potential fusion is suggested. During this time, the child's functional ADL (activity of daily living) skills are assessed while the child is wearing the cast to ascertain the

appropriateness of this potential surgery. Surgical management through carpectomies or dorsal wedge osteotomies of the carpal bones should be considered only if finger function will be enhanced.[2]

Scoliosis is frequently managed conservatively with bracing. In about one fifth of children and adolescents with AMC, a long C-shaped thoracolumbar scoliosis develops.[66] If the curve continues to progress, surgical fusion should be considered. Those with a progressive congenital scoliosis have done well with the use of the vertical expandable prosthetic titanium rib implant for correcting scoliosis while allowing a significant amount of growth.[31] Most commonly, a posterior spinal fusion is performed when the child is close to puberty. On large stiff curves, an anterior release of structures limiting spinal mobility may be necessary before posterior spinal fusion to obtain satisfactory results.[74] The type of fixation used is based on the preference of the orthopedic surgeon (see Chapter 8).

FOREGROUND INFORMATION

BODY STRUCTURES AND FUNCTIONS

Diagnosis and Problem Identification

The primary impairments in the child with AMC are limitations of joint movement and decreased muscle strength and bulk. Joint contractures are evident at birth, although a formal diagnosis of AMC may not be given at that time. In AMC, limitation of movement typically is seen in two or more joints in different body areas.[27] In the amyoplasia form of arthrogryposis, 85% have symmetrical presentation of contractures.[27,28]

Contractures can develop from an imbalance in muscle pull of agonist and antagonist muscles but also occur when symmetrical weakness is present on all sides of the joint, thus hindering movement. Theoretically, this may be indicative of the point in fetal development at which the insult occurs. For example, because flexors develop before extensors in the upper extremity, a child may develop elbow flexion contractures but does not develop the usual strength in either the biceps or the triceps brachii subsequent to the time of insult.

Decreased muscle bulk is evidence of muscle weakness secondary to decreased functioning motor units in a muscle. Histologic analysis of muscles reveals nonspecific changes in the muscle such as fibrofatty scar tissue. Weakened muscles often have a fat layer around the muscle with dimpling of the skin. A muscle with a contracture but of normal strength through its available ROM may not have normal muscle bulk secondary to its inability to be active throughout the entire ROM.

Problem Identification by the Team

The team evaluation establishes a baseline from which to set realistic and functional goals. In addition to physical therapists, the primary intervention team consists of patients and their families and such medical professionals as orthopedists and geneticists, occupational therapists, and orthotists. Occasionally, speech pathologists, dentists or oral surgeons, neurologists, neurosurgeons, and ophthalmologists are consulted as well. One of the goals of the primary team is to educate the family about AMC. Families are taught that arthrogryposis is a nonprogressive disorder but that without positioning, stretching, and strengthening, or possible surgery, the child's

TABLE 10.1 International Classification of Functioning, Health, and Disability for Children With Arthrogryposis Multiplex Congenita

Changes in Body Structure	Changes in Body Functions	Activity	Participation
Prenatal damage to the anterior horn cells, resulting in neurogenic and myopathic disorder	Multiple joint contractures Fibrotic joint capsule	Limited functional mobility skills, including rolling, creeping, and feeding, transitional movements, and high-level mobility skills	Limited opportunity for play with young peers Inability to live independently Limited access to educational and work opportunities
Decreased number of motor units within a muscle	Strength limitations, frequently imbalance of oppositional muscles with stronger muscles often shortened	Limited ability to transfer Dependence for transfers for ADL including toileting Limited independence in self-care skills, including dressing Limited ambulation Inability to manage uneven terrain	Need to learn how to adapt for new alignment once allowed to mobilize Limited access to a wide range of environments Health insurance may not pay for adaptive equipment necessary for least restrictive mobility device.
Scar tissue and fibrotic tissue do not grow and stretch to the same extent as healthy muscles.	Joint contractures can be progressive with growth.	Immobilization during periods of orthopedic management Increased limitations in mobility while immobilized Limited independence in wheelchair mobility without costly adaptations Decreased endurance	Limited participation in physical activities because of endurance and safety issues Social isolation

impairments could lead to further activity limitations and participation restrictions in later life (Table 10.1).

During the initial examination by the team, photographs and videos are taken of the child, illustrating the child's position of comfort and specific contractures such as clubfeet. This is an objective way to document changes that occur during growth and throughout splinting procedures and should be repeated every 4 months for the first 2 years.

In physical therapy, baseline goniometry is performed, documenting passive ROM and the resting position of each joint. ROM can be measured with a standard goniometer cut down to pediatric size. Active ROM is measured at the hips, knees, shoulders, elbows, and wrists. If possible, the same therapist consistently measures ROM for the child. Intratester and intertester reliability is determined for all therapists who evaluate children with AMC and should be checked annually. Functional active ROM is also assessed to assist with visualizing the whole composite of motions and evaluating functional abilities. For example, functional active ranges include assessment of hand to mouth, ear, forehead, top of head, and back of neck.

A formal manual muscle test is performed when appropriate. Muscle grades for infants and very young children are ascertained by using palpation, observing the ability of extremities to move against gravity, and evaluating gross motor function. The strength of the extensor muscles of the lower extremities is especially important in determining the appropriate level of bracing. Less than fair (grade 3/5) muscle strength in hip extensors will require bracing above the hip. Less than fair (grade 3/5) strength in knee extensors will require bracing above the knee. Corrected clubfeet require molded braces during growth to minimize problems of recurrent clubfeet. Children with poor upper extremity function and weak lower extremities may not be functional community ambulators as a result of decreased motor control and protective responses. Power mobility may be the most appropriate means of community locomotion.

Gross motor skills and functional levels of mobility and ADL are assessed. No current developmental tests have been designed specifically for children with AMC, but these children usually score lower than average on formal gross motor tests secondary to inadequate strength and ROM in their extremities. Certain gross motor skills may never be attained owing to physical limitations. For example, some developmental milestones such as creeping may not be attained, even though the child is able to stand and is beginning to walk. Cognitively, children with AMC tend to score average to above average in formal developmental tests.[55,60]

The physical therapist assesses the child for current and potential modes of functional mobility. This may include ambulation with assistive devices or the use of a manual or power wheelchair or mobility devices. The therapist evaluates movement patterns and muscle substitutions used to accomplish each motor task or ADL skill. Therapists should address a child with AMC from a biomechanical approach because having limb segments aligned for mechanical advantage maximizes function and ultimately participation.

Following the examination, short-term and long-term goals are developed by the team related to splinting, stretching, developmental stimulation, orthopedic management including a surgical plan, and bracing. Incorporating the family early on as part of the team is important to maximize the child's independence in ADL and mobility.

PHYSICAL THERAPY IN INFANCY

Babies born with contracture syndromes have most significant involvement in the newborn period because they have had limited mobility in utero, so benefit from early opportunities to stretch out and remold. It is important to be aware that a large population of newborns have early feeding issues caused by structural abnormalities at the jaw and tongue.[54]

Great variability can be seen in the presentation of contractures; however, two more common body types have been noted. One body type involves clubfeet, hip flexion contractures, knee extension contractures, shoulder tightness (especially internal rotation), and elbow and wrist flexion contractures. At birth, these children are commonly breech presentations. Another body type often associated with the amyoplasia type of AMC exhibits posturing of hips widely abducted, flexed, and externally rotated, flexed knees, clubfeet, internally rotated shoulders, extended and pronated elbows, and flexed wrists. Asymmetrical posturing of the extremities, which is especially problematic at the hip when dislocation of only one hip is present, occurs. The resulting asymmetry makes surgical correction the treatment of choice to relocate the hip and secondarily prevent pelvic obliquity and scoliosis. Children who are born with rocker-bottom feet and multiple contractures often have a syndrome with associated arthrogryposis and benefit from further genetic workup to possibly identify the specific contracture syndrome.

Examination

Formal assessment of an infant with arthrogryposis begins as soon as possible after birth. The assessment consists of goniometry of passive ROM with reevaluation of ROM done on a monthly basis during this period. The therapist also documents the presence and strength of muscles based on observation of the child's movements and palpation of muscle contractions. Muscles of the trunk and upper and lower extremities are evaluated. Formal developmental assessment tools are used occasionally but reflect poorly on a child with contractures because strength and ROM limitations preclude the achievement of many motor milestones. Delayed motor milestones may result in activity limitations and participation restrictions when children with AMC are compared with healthy peers on standardized developmental tests.

Motor milestones in these children are often delayed or skipped. For example, good trunk control and balance, coupled with weak upper extremities in compromised positions, results in development of the ability to sit-scoot rather than creep for early floor mobility. Functional mobility and the mechanism used in attaining this mobility are more important to evaluate than is assignment of a developmental level or score. The therapist assesses activities such as rolling, prone tolerance, sitting control, scooting, creeping, crawling, transitional movements, and standing tolerance and upright mobility. Occupational therapy (OT) plays a key role in assessing feeding, ADL skills, and manipulation of objects. Physical therapists also assess the fit of any supportive or assistive devices that may be used. Another key role of therapists dealing with young children who have arthrogryposis is to track clubfoot alignment. Early recognition and aggressive treatment of clubfoot relapse may limit immobilization time.

Although it is not imperative to use formal scales in assessing motor development and documenting activity restrictions, some useful tests include the Alberta Infant Motor Scale, the Bayley Scales of Infant Development, and the Peabody Developmental Motor Scales. The Pediatric Evaluation of Disability Inventory (PEDI), Patient Reported Outcomes Measurement Information System (PROMIS), and the WeeFIM (Functional Independence Measure for Children) may be used to measure activity and participation (see Chapter 2 for more information on these measurement tools). Use of such tools helps to identify baseline skills and areas of need for treatment planning. Use of standardized testing helps not only for baseline but allows for tracking change over time, qualifying a child for support services, and identifying if therapeutic intervention is making a measureable change in functional skills. See Chapter 2 for more specific information on these and other tests and measures.

Physical therapy goals for very young children include maximizing strength, improving ROM, and enhancing general sensorimotor development. Education of the family emphasizes instruction in proper positioning, stretching techniques, and the avoidance of potentially harmful activities that feed into deformity.

Intervention Strategies

Intervention strategies focus on improving alignment to maximize the biomechanical advantage for strengthening and reducing the joint contracture through stretching, serial casting, foot abduction braces, thermoplastic serial splinting, and positioning activities. Interventions address developmental skills and teaching compensatory strategies) especially in ADL and alternative modes of mobility) to maximize participation in age-appropriate activities.

Development, Strength, and Mobility

Infants with the first type of AMC described earlier begin life with limited positioning options as a result of hip flexion contractures. Consequently, stretching hip flexors and prone positioning are encouraged within the first 3 months of life. Developmentally, these infants learn to roll or scoot on their bottoms as their primary means of floor mobility because it is nearly impossible to comfortably assume the quadruped position without reinforcing a flexed posture of the upper extremities. Although delayed in their ability to attain sitting independently, they are often able to do so by 15 months of age using trunk flexion and rotation. These children typically are able to stand when placed well before they initiate pulling to stand. If the child has dislocated hips that have been surgically reduced in the first year, the child may have significant stiffness initially, limiting willingness to change position from sitting to standing. Usually, the child begins to walk with assistance, an assistive device, and lower extremity orthotics around 18 months of age; most are independent ambulators by the middle of their second year of life.

Initially, infants with the amyoplasia type of AMC have more positioning options due to their hip and knee flexion contractures. Some have difficulty with prone positioning because of elbow extension contractures that limit their ability to comfortably prop. A towel roll or wedge under the infant's chest assists with increasing tolerance for this position. Positioning the hips in neutral rotation and neutral abduction is encouraged. Towel rolls can be placed along the lateral aspect of the thighs when the infant is sitting, and a wide Velcro band can be strapped around the thigh when the child is lying supine to keep the legs in more neutral alignment (Fig. 10.5).

Developmentally, these children tend to be a little slower in attaining rolling but faster in attaining sitting and scooting than children with the first type of posturing. Although assuming the quadruped position and creeping are often feasible for this type of child, sitting and scooting are more energy efficient. Depending on muscle strength and the amount of bracing needed for standing, these children may never perform transitional movements from sitting on the floor to standing independently. They begin ambulating by the middle of their second year but require a significant amount of bracing for success. Independence with ambulation may take years and sometimes is not fully accomplished. Therapy focuses on addressing some key functional motor skills, such as rolling,

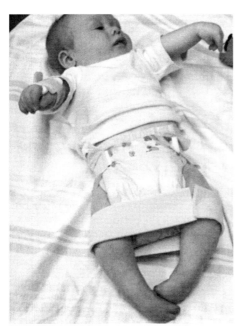

FIG. 10.5 This child with arthrogryposis multiplex congenita is wearing a wide Velcro band strapped around the thigh to keep the legs in more neutral alignment.

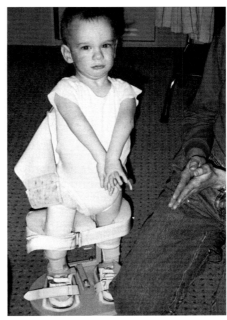

FIG. 10.6 Child who has arthrogryposis multiplex congenita in a standing frame.

sitting, sit-scooting, standing, and strengthening those muscles that assist in maintaining posture. The goal is to maximize mobility to enhance participation in age-appropriate activities but with an eye toward skills necessary for lifelong independence.

Strengthening during the first 2 to 3 years is most frequently addressed through developmental facilitation and play. Dynamic strengthening of the trunk can be achieved by having the child reach for, swipe at, or roll toys in the positions of sitting and static standing or while straddling the therapist's leg so that the child must rotate the trunk. These maneuvers incorporate stretching and strengthening into the therapeutic play activity. Aquatic therapy is often helpful for strengthening and developing functional mobility skills. If working on upright control in the pool, knee splints, specifically for use in the water, are helpful when bracing is needed on land, too. One way to determine whether functional training is having a strengthening effect is to ascertain the child's improved ability to perform the task.

Self-care skills, feeding, and manipulation of objects are dependent on hand function and elbow flexibility. Children with limited upper extremity strength may have decreased ability to manipulate objects. Fortunately, these children tend to be resourceful in using other body parts, such as their feet or mouth, to manipulate objects when hands have inadequate strength and ROM. These skills are quite useful early in life but not as useful in an older child. If the child has adequate ROM but inadequate strength, the child learns to support the arm on a leg or a table to assist in bringing hand to mouth. If the child is unable to get hand to mouth, adaptive equipment may make it possible to do some self-feeding. For example, if shoulder strength is absent, overhead arm slings are fashioned out of polyvinyl chloride piping and added to the high chair to permit finger feeding. If the upper extremities are postured in elbow extension, a typical and effective method of grasping an object

is with a hand crossover maneuver, which affords some control and strength in holding or lifting an object. Electronic toys can be adapted so that the child can operate them via switches that can be activated by movement of the head, hand, or foot. These compensatory intervention strategies help to enhance skills needed for independence in ADL.

Standing is an important component of physical therapy during the first and second years. Families are encouraged to begin standing the child at approximately 6 months of age, as is normally done with children without physical limitations. If a child is in casts with knees flexed, upright positioning continues to be an important component of therapy because it helps to strengthen the trunk for standing once casts are removed. Standing is best completely upright rather than angled toward supine or prone because it helps develop skill in the biomechanical alignment necessary to stand without external support. During standing, splints can be used to maintain the lower extremities in adequate alignment. Shoes can be wedged to accommodate plantar flexion deformities and to allow the child to bear weight throughout the plantar surface of the foot.

Standing is initiated in a standing frame and progresses to independent static standing in the frame (Fig. 10.6). A therapist may need to be creative to work on standing with a child who is wearing a foot abduction brace, but use of the brace should not limit work on standing skills. By 1 year of age, a child should be able to tolerate a total of 2 hours a day in the standing frame. This standing helps the child begin self-stretching of the feet and encourages emerging independent standing and walking skills. Use of a prone stander is usually avoided because this type of stander does not encourage dynamic trunk control, and therefore the child is less likely to be working on the skills needed to stand outside the stander. Dynamic standing is encouraged through ball games such as kicking a soccer ball or batting a ball off a tee. Floor-to-stand activities usually do not begin to emerge until the child is ambulating securely, and sit-to-stand activities from a low chair usually begin to emerge when ambulation begins. Limitations in lower extremity strength and ROM can be addressed through splinting and bracing while the child is standing. Knee extension splints may be worn to compensate for weakness of knee extensors and mediolateral instability of the knees.

Stretching and Splinting

Stretching programs for joint contractures are imperative and should be taught to parents and caregivers from the time of the initial examination. This intervention strategy addresses one of the primary impairments of AMC. A stretching program is divided into 3 to 5 sets a day with three to five repetitions during each set. Each stretch is held for 20 to 30 seconds. With the realization that this is a significant time commitment, families are taught to incorporate stretching into times when the child would normally have one-on-one time with the caregiver, such as performing lower extremity stretches during diaper changes and upper extremity stretches during feeding. Dressing and bath times also provide good opportunities for stretching, especially once the child is self-feeding and out of diapers. Stretching must be a daily lifelong commitment for a person with arthrogryposis, but consistent stretching is most critical during the growing years and especially within the first 2 years of life.[63]

To maintain the prolonged effect of the stretch, the extremity is maintained in a comfortable position of stretch with thermoplastic splints. Attempting to maintain the maximum stretch, rather than a comfortable position, over prolonged periods will cause skin breakdown and intolerance to splints. Splints are adjusted for growth and improvements in ROM, usually every 4 to 6 weeks during infancy. When ankle-foot orthoses (AFOs) are fabricated for clubfeet, the calcaneus must be aligned in a neutral position because this will affect the position of the entire foot. If the calcaneus is allowed to move medially with respect to the talus, the forefoot will fall into an undesirable varus position. When the hindfoot and the forefoot are in a neutral position between varus and valgus, splinting can address insufficient dorsiflexion of the hindfoot rather than forefoot. This will prevent the potential problem of a midfoot break resulting in a rocker-bottom foot. To be maximally effective, AFOs are worn 22 hours per day.

Knee contractures are addressed early using splinting and stretching. For the first 3 to 4 months, anterior thermoplastic knee flexion splints for extension contractures or posterior knee extension splints for knee flexion contractures are worn up to 20 hours per day. For an older infant with knee extension contractures, it is advised that children not wear a knee flexion splint at greater than 50° of flexion for sleeping because this may encourage hip flexion contractures. Older babies with knee extension contractures should use the knee flexion splints for activities that require flexion, such as sitting in the car seat or the high chair, or when positioned in prone, utilizing knee flexion and the splint to enhance the quadruped position. Knee extension splints, which control knee flexion contractures or medial-lateral instability, are initially worn up to 18 hours a day, especially during sleep. Once the child is older than 6 months of age, the knee extension splints can be used for standing activities because they encourage optimal lower extremity alignment during upright activity. Splints to control knee flexion contractures should be off 6 hours a day to allow floor mobility in a child with emerging skills.

Newborns are provided with cock-up wrist splints, but splints for hands are generally provided only after 3 months of age. This allows the child to integrate the normal physiologic flexion before placing a stimulus across the palm. Two sets of hand splints are fabricated. For day use the child wears dorsal cock-up splints with a palmar arch in a position of neutral deviation and a slight stretch into extension as tolerated. This allows the child to have fingers available to manipulate toys. For night wear, the splint is a dorsal cock-up splint with a pan to allow finger stretching when the child is sleeping.

When considering elbow splinting, note that function and independence in ADL are improved when one elbow is able to flex adequately to reach the mouth and one elbow is in adequate extension to reach the perineum. Other factors to consider include available muscle strength and ROM, response to stretching, and potential future surgical procedures. Elbow extension splints are best worn while sleeping, but elbow flexion splints and elbow flexion-assist splints tend to be most functional when worn during the day. This allows the child to experiment with the hand in a more functional position for most play activities.[39]

Young children respond most readily to conservative treatment using serial splinting, frequent stretching, and proper positioning. In Fig. 10.7A, the infant's posture is shown without leg splints. In Fig. 10.7B, the infant's lower leg is held out of the deforming postures through molded thermoplastic knee and AFO splints. The key to successful intervention for contractures is family education. Family education begins during the initial evaluation as caretakers not only are given general information about arthrogryposis but also receive information regarding their child's specific needs. Appropriate stretching exercises for involved joints are given with sketches or photographs to supplement the verbal instructions. Subsequent visits to the physical therapist allow work on splint fabrication and modification and positioning. Developmental play ideas are incorporated into the exercises to help the child progress developmentally. Physical therapists also work with the family to adapt age-appropriate toys to stimulate the child both physically and cognitively.

PHYSICAL THERAPY IN THE PRESCHOOL PERIOD

During the preschool period, the child's functional abilities and age-appropriate participation vary according to the degree of involvement. Poor upper extremity function from the contractures and lack of muscle strength may limit the child's independence in feeding, dressing, and playing, at a time when typical peers are relishing their independence. This may be particularly distressing for the parents, who become more aware of the magnitude of their child's limitations when the child is no longer an infant in whom dependency is expected.

Structural limitations impeding participation in age-appropriate activities during this stage are similar to those found in the younger child. Restriction in joint ROM continues to be a problem secondary to rapid growth changes. Independent ambulation is often limited by poor protective responses of the upper extremities.

Examination

Passive and active ROM continues to be closely monitored by the physical therapist and caregivers. Proper fit of orthotics and splints is imperative in providing adequate stretch and positioning to impede the development of further deformities.

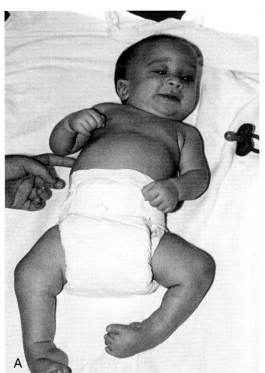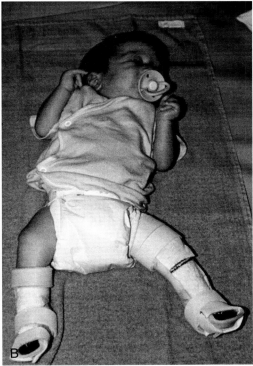

FIG. 10.7 (A) A child who has arthrogryposis multiplex congenita without leg splints. (B) The same child's lower extremity is held out of the deforming positions through the use of molded thermoplastic knee splints and ankle-foot orthoses.

Functional muscle strength is an important component in the preschooler because it determines to a great degree the extent of bracing necessary and the level of independence in self-care skills. Formal manual muscle testing[32,36] becomes more appropriate during this period because the child can comprehend verbal instructions. When testing strength, it is important to grade the resistance throughout the arc of motion because the child with AMC will frequently be strong in the midrange but unable to move the extremity to the shortened end range. This finding is significant because the end range is where the child needs to work the muscle to maintain stretch of the antagonist muscles.

Examination of gait function should include distance, use of assistive devices (including braces and shoe adaptations, as well as upper extremity support), speed, symmetry of step length, gait deviations, and muscle activity. Increased lateral trunk sway is not uncommon with arthrogryposis.[9] Some children ambulate as their primary means of locomotion; others rely on a stroller for community mobility. Despite research that supports powered mobility for the very young,[56,67] mobility with wheelchairs is not usually addressed until school age, when slow speed of ambulation, endurance, and safety concerns may preclude the child from interacting with peers. These children are bright and will often forgo ambulation for power mobility if it is presented too early. Forgoing ambulation early may limit standing for functional activities later in life.

Goals

Ability rather than disability must be stressed, with a strong emphasis on assisting the child through problem solving rather than through physical assistance. The ultimate goals for this age are to reduce the disability and enhance independent ambulation and mobility with minimum bracing and use of assistive devices. Physical and environmental structural barriers may limit achievement of some fine and gross motor skills, but social skill attainment is paramount. Another goal is for the team to work together to improve the child's function in basic ADL skills.

Intervention Strategies

The team will work together during the preschool period to solve basic ADL challenges, such as independent feeding and toileting. For example, the use of a lightweight reacher may assist with dressing skills. Preschoolers usually can self-feed with adaptive equipment.[30] These children are often toilet trained but lack the ability to perform the task independently. At times, orthopedic surgical intervention will be used to help gain better biomechanical alignment of joints. These surgeries initially may change the focus of the therapeutic intervention, but ultimately, the focus and the goal remain the same because surgical intervention is done to enhance position and function.

Stretching

The need for stretching at this age continues to be addressed despite the preschooler's decreased tolerance to passive stretching three to five times a day. Two times a day for the stretching program is more realistic and appears to maintain ROM adequately in most cases. Families report that the best time for this is during dressing and bathing, which incorporates the program into an automatic part of the daily routine. Children can be taught how to assist with stretching through positioning. The child is also encouraged to verbally participate in the program, for example, by counting the number of repetitions. AFOs and positional splints continue to be worn to maintain the achieved positions.

Independent mobility in a safe and efficient manner is important for the preschooler to achieve and enhance social skills, as well as allow functional mobility. Independent ambulation with supportive bracing and with as few assistive devices as possible is stressed. Children with adequate strength and ROM who do not require bracing to walk generally need an AFO to prevent recurring clubfoot deformities. Older preschoolers with AMC are generally at the level of bracing that will be continued throughout school age.

Orthotics

Most orthotics are fabricated from lightweight polypropylene although those with less foot deformity may use carbon fiber braces. Children with knee extension contractures tend to require less bracing than those with knee flexion contractures. If there is any question about the child's ability to maintain an upright position without hip support, the child's first set of long leg braces, a hip-knee-ankle-foot orthosis, will include a pelvic band. This type of orthosis is used for several reasons. The family may perceive that the child is regressing if initially unsuccessful ambulating occurs without the pelvic band, and later a band is added for ambulation success. The pelvic band encourages neutral rotation and abduction of the lower extremities. The pelvic band can also facilitate full available hip extension, and the hips can be locked in that position for prolonged standing. Use of a pelvic band allows a pivot point for the trunk to move into extension to help with posterior weight shift on the stance side during gait. Once the child is ambulating with both hips unlocked, without jackknifing at the hips during stance, the pelvic band can be removed.

Maintaining hip strength, especially when the pelvic band is removed, continues to be important. One activity is to have the child begin static and dynamic standing on the tilt board. The child also begins taking steps forward, backward, and sideways. Strengthening, as with progressive resistive exercises, may be appropriate at this time. Clinical experience suggests that muscles may increase in strength by one half to a full muscle grade with exercise.

Ideally, the least amount of bracing is optimal, but if decreasing the bracing requires the child to use an assistive device that was previously unnecessary, increased bracing may be more appropriate. A child with strong extensors such as the gluteus maximus and quadriceps is more functional than a child who requires bracing as a functional substitute for the extensors. The child with a good deal of bracing has difficulty donning and removing braces and usually is dependent for locking and unlocking hip and knee joints for standing and sitting.

Those children who learn to walk may be limited in their independence if they do not have adequate strength and ROM to manipulate the assistive device, such as a walker, that is required to ambulate. Walkers are often heavy and cumbersome for the child, who may have inadequate protective responses in standing and upper extremity limitations. Thermoplastic material can be molded to the walker for forearm support when hand function is limited, affording the child added support and control (Fig. 10.8). Many children prefer to walk with someone rather than use a walker while they are gaining confidence in ambulatory skills. When learning to stand and walk, it is of utmost importance that the child learn how to use the

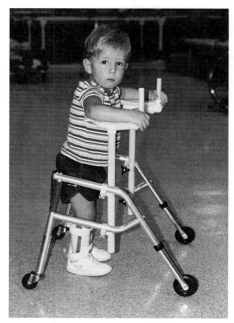

FIG. 10.8 Thermoplastic forearm supports can be customized to the walker.

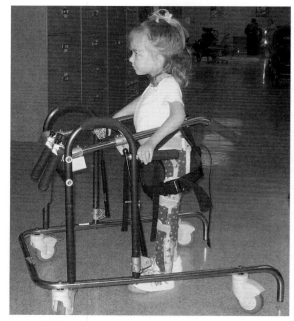

FIG. 10.9 Child with arthrogryposis multiplex congenita wearing polypropylene hip-knee-ankle orthosis and using a gait trainer that allows dynamic weight shift.

head and trunk to stand and balance and then to weight shift for limb advancement. If a child uses a gait trainer and leans on the device to move it, without regaining balance, he or she may not be training in the skills necessary to stand and balance for functional transfers for a lifetime. Use of a gait trainer that enhances the opportunity to stand upright and weight shift (Fig. 10.9) while relying on the support as a "safety net," rather than leaning into it, may produce better long-term functional outcomes in upright for transfers and ADL. Careful evaluation of ambulation potential is needed when one is deciding on an assistive device for ambulation. Some walkers will give independence in exercise walking but will not translate into greater independence outside the walker.

Children with weak quadriceps and knee flexion contractures tend to ambulate with locked knee and ankle-foot orthoses. These braces can be fabricated with dial knee locks so that the knee position can be adjusted to coincide with the changing state of the knee flexion contracture. This will afford the ongoing opportunity to stretch out the contracture. Shoes may need external wedges to compensate for hip and knee flexion contractures that interfere with static standing.[7] If the brace cannot stand in the wedged shoe, the child cannot be expected to balance in the brace with the shoes. The child should be able to comfortably balance with the feet plantigrade without upper extremity support.

Families may require assistance in identifying and removing environmental barriers that impede the child's independence both in the home and in the preschool environment.

Children in this age group are encouraged to participate in activities with children the same age in preschool, day care, and swimming classes and in other peer group activities. They are encouraged to develop relationships with children who do not have disabilities, as well as with those who do. These early relationships help to enhance lifelong participation in integrated activities with peers. During the preschool period, many states mandate therapy services for children with special needs. Preschool services, as well as additional therapy services, are imperative for maximizing these children's skills for the demands they will encounter during school.

PHYSICAL THERAPY DURING THE SCHOOL-AGE AND ADOLESCENT PERIODS

The focus of physical therapy moves from the outpatient clinic into the classroom at this stage. Most children are enrolled in regular classrooms in their neighborhood schools, although they may have adaptive physical education, physical therapy, occupational therapy, and speech services to enhance the educational process.

Participation in school and classroom activities may be impeded by limitations in mobility. At school, children have increased demands to travel longer distances and move in groups under limited time frames. Alternative means of mobility such as a motorized wheelchair or a scooter may be needed to enhance independence while managing materials (such as books and personal effects) with minimal outside assistance. Efficient and independent dressing, feeding, and toileting abilities take on a more compelling nature. Joint contractures continue to be problematic, especially through the last few growth spurts. This is a time when the adolescent is becoming more independent in self-care, and adult monitoring of contractures tends to decrease.

Examination

The school therapist acts as a team member, addressing goals of the child and family with regard to enhancing the child's educational experience. The physical therapy examination determines what types of training and adaptive equipment are needed to achieve educational objectives. Functional ADL skills are assessed to ascertain how efficiency and independence can be improved. The School Function Assessment (SFA)[15,45]

is a tool that is helpful in identifying functional skill levels in the school environment and in identifying activities for individualized educational plan (IEP) goals so that physical therapy interventions can ultimately allow for greater participation of the child at school. The Activity Scale for Kids (ASK) is a self-report tool that may be helpful in defining where a child is having greatest limitations in functional skills at home and in the community.[75] See Chapter 2 for more information on these examination tools.

Goals

During this period the child with AMC must be responsible for self-care and for an exercise program to be performed to the best of the child's ability. If the child is physically unable to do these tasks, it is still important to be able to orchestrate care through verbal instructions to a caregiver. The family must also become more responsible for expecting and allowing the child to be more independent. The goal of independence in mobility and keeping up with friends is important in the development of peer relationships. Early school-based goals should include ability to independently participate in one to three playground activities during recess.

ROM is not an educational goal, but it continues to be a focus to maximize long-term function. The child with AMC will lose motion if he or she does not continue to stretch throughout the growing years. As sitting requirements for education increase, hip and knee flexion contractures also can increase if positioning options to enhance extension are not addressed. Final growth spurts, coupled with increased sitting requirements for education, can result in a significant loss of extension at the knees and the hips. If the school-age child is not conscientious about night splint use and positioning for stretch, the ability to walk may be lost during the teen years. Surgical intervention to regain ambulation skill during the second decade of life is not always an option.

Intervention Strategies

Dressing, toileting, and feeding may require adaptive equipment or setup for the child to be independent. Children with AMC require some selective pieces of adaptive equipment for achieving independence, but most are adaptable and innovative in using compensatory strategies rather than relying on assistive devices to achieve their goals. Frequently, classroom chairs and tables must be at custom-made heights to accommodate rising from a chair without manipulating brace knee locks. The desktop may need to be adjusted so that the child, by using a mouth stick or a wrist aid to hold writing implements, can maneuver items on the desk or write (Fig. 10.10). Assistive technology is quite helpful for those with limited hand function to perform school work on a computer, although management of the computer may be challenging for a child who changes classes. Implementation of ideas such as these limits disability by providing the child with successful compensatory strategies (Table 10.2).

Continued adherence with the customized splinting and stretching program is expected. Children at this age may lose a few degrees of motion during growth, but further regression may result in loss of skills that previously were not a problem when more motion was available. Surgical intervention is sometimes helpful for improving joint position. A self-stretching program, utilizing assistive straps, braces, and positioning, can be incorporated into the child's routine to promote independence in attaining goals. The adolescent must be permitted to

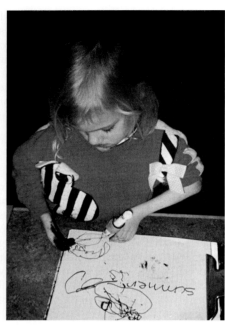

FIG. 10.10 Child who has arthrogryposis multiplex congenita using a wrist aid to hold a crayon.

help plan his or her schedule, or adherence can be expected to be poor. Adaptive physical education in school, as well as adaptive sports programs outside school, can be adjunctive to physical therapy for promoting strength, endurance, and mobility.[23] During adolescence and through adulthood, the importance of maintaining a healthy weight is imperative because weight gain can significantly limit one's mobility and ultimately one's independence. Vocational rehabilitation may be a helpful adjunct in assisting those with physical limitations to access future employment opportunities.

Speed and safety in independent mobility are important in the development of peer relationships. Families may be advised during this time to consider powered mobility devices as an adjunct to manual mobility devices. Cumbersome bracing, inefficient gait, and poor upper extremity function can limit a child's ability to participate in playground or social activities.[18] Alternative modes of mobility may allow the child to participate safely. Use of alternative modes need not preclude ambulation but rather provides supplemental mobility for safety and energy conservation. Most children can achieve functional household ambulation but may require a wheelchair for efficient community mobility. The importance of standing and walking skills for maximal independence in the bathroom cannot be overstressed.

TABLE 10.2	**Recommended Measures for Children with Arthrogryposis**		
	Test Information	**Considerations for Arthrogryposis**	**Reference**
Body Structures and Function			
Range of motion	Goniometer can be used to identify range of motion as well as resting posture of the limbs.	May need to cut down a goniometer to allow reliable use with a small child.	Clarkson HM: *Musculoskeletal assessment: joint motion and muscle testing.* 3rd ed. Baltimore, Lippincott, Williams & Wilkins, 2012.
Strength	Observation, palpation, and hand pressure are used to determine muscle strength.	In the young child, one must identify bony landmarks when testing because rotational differences influence the biomechanics of the muscles.	Hislop HJ, Montgomery J, editors: *Daniels & Worthingham's muscle testing: techniques of manual examination.* 8th ed. Philadelphia, Elsevier Science, 2007.
Activity: Single Task			
Timed standing balance	Documentation of amount of time the individual can stand statically.	No norms for this population. Tracks change over time for the individual. Able to compare with and without orthotic support as well as with and without heel wedges. Translates to functional skills such as transfers and self-care.	
Gait speed	Documentation of speed traveling a specific distance. Document for bracing and assistive device during testing.	No norms for this population. Can track change over time for the individual.	Lythgo N, Wilson C, Galea M: Basic gait and symmetry measures for primary school-aged children and young adults. II: Walking at slow, free and fast speed. *Gait Posture* 33:29-35, 2011.
6-minute walk test	The individual walks as far as possible in a 6-minute period.	No norms for this population including level of bracing necessary and assistive device. Can track change over time for the individual.	Please refer to Chapter 2 for more information.
Timed up and go	Individual rises from a standardized chair height, walks 3 meters, turns around, and returns to sitting in the chair.	No norms for this population. Child may be too small to safely get in and out of the standardized chair height. Tracks change over time for the individual. Record chair height for the individual if not using the standardized chair height and replicate height during future testing.	Please refer to Chapter 2 for more information.

TABLE 10.2 Recommended Measures for Children with Arthrogryposis—cont'd			
	Test Information	**Considerations for Arthrogryposis**	**Reference**
Activity: Multiple Items			
Peabody Developmental Motor Scale	Fine and gross motor assessments compare skills to those of typically developing peers aged birth to 72 months.	Due to limited motion and strength, some children may never attain some of the skills on this test.	Please refer to Chapter 2 for more information.
Patient Reported Outcomes Measurement Information System (PROMIS)	Parent and/or child report. Multiple dimensions to help tease out perceived strengths and needs. Helpful in therapy goal establishment.	Short and long forms available. Can be reported on paper or via computer access. PROMIS has pediatric and adult versions.	Please refer to Chapter 2 for more information.
School Function Assessment	Educational staff report on child's abilities. Helpful in identifying needs within the educational environment.	Some children will need assistance with skills but should learn to how to orchestrate care.	Please refer to Chapter 2 for more information.
Pediatric Evaluation of Disability Inventory (PEDI and PEDI-CAT)	Self or caregiver report tool designed to identify functional delay in areas of daily activities, mobility, social/cognitive, and responsibility.	The PEDI takes 1 hour to administer while the PEDI-CAT is a shorter, more intuitive computerized version.	Please refer to Chapter 2 for more information.

TRANSITION TO ADULTHOOD

Little has been published about the transition from childhood to adulthood for the person who has arthrogryposis. Several authors[29,59] have published surveys focused on issues related to aging. Results indicated that activity limitations during adulthood were related to continued problems with ROM and strength that consequently limited independence in ADL, ambulation, and mobility. Those who required assistance with ADL during their school-age years continued to require assistance throughout their lifetime but were able to achieve a degree of independence with feeding, dressing, and grooming using selected assistive ADL devices. Those with severe joint involvement had long-term dependency on others for ADLs.[18,29,60]

Pain appears to be a significant issue that occurs with aging. Most survey respondents reported difficulty with back and neck pain and increased discomfort in other joints as well.[59] Those who have had surgical intervention for clubfeet can expect pain and stiffness to develop during the adult years.[35] Some specific problems that occur in adults include arthritic changes in weight-bearing joints and overuse syndromes in muscles and joints that are used for compensation or unique postures. Osteoarthritis, carpal tunnel problems, and neuropathies may develop as a result of prolonged joint constrictions and deformities. Increasing muscle weakness with increasing age has been found to occur, starting in early adulthood.[59] Mobility problems emerging later in life may stem from secondary degenerative changes and muscle overuse syndromes.[25,53] Manual or power wheelchairs may be used more commonly by adults than by adolescents and teenagers. Adults with AMC often use a wheelchair as their primary mode of mobility for long distances.

Advanced education is of utmost importance so that the adult with AMC becomes trained in a specialized skill or field. The type of work chosen will depend on the degree of activity limitations, education, and marketable skills. Computer-related work and occupations that do not rely on manual labor should be considered as employment options. Advancements in technology allow those with arthrogryposis to have opportunities that enhance their freedom of mobility and their career options. Assistive technology, including computers and voice-activated equipment, can be of value in helping the individual safely and efficiently achieve work and leisure goals. Many people who have arthrogryposis who are artistically talented use their skills in painting and drawing for vocation and avocation.

Many of the barriers that the adult with AMC will meet are physical barriers. Although the Americans with Disabilities Act has helped, transportation continues to limit access to vocational and avocational activities. Those who live near strong public transportation systems or who have access to an automobile with proper adaptations have better opportunities for participation in activities outside the home. Personnel at adult rehabilitation facilities are probably unfamiliar with AMC owing to the small number of adults who consistently seek care during adulthood. These facilities can provide services regarding assistive technology, seating systems, and orthotics, as well as help in funding for supportive equipment and services.

Intervention Strategies

Once skeletal growth has stopped, stretching is not as imperative, but maintaining flexibility and proper positioning is encouraged to impede the further development of deformities. Those with AMC who used orthoses during the school-age years typically continue to do so throughout adulthood. Those who used only AFOs for clubfoot control tend not to need these orthoses once growth is complete. Dressing and, most important, donning of shoes are often the last skills achieved because abandoning bracing allows for easier dressing of the lower body.

Information about the long-term sequelae of AMC in relation to degenerative changes, mobility levels, and use of adaptive ADL devices is critical to providing the most effective therapy to persons with AMC. Joint conservation and addressing the secondary impairments resulting from degenerative changes that occur in adulthood are necessary to maximize long-term independence.

Research regarding the extent of independence of children, adolescents, and adults who have AMC is lacking in the areas of ADL, use of manual or power wheelchairs, and ambulation ability. This lack of data may be a result of the fact that children are followed early on within a medical model that addresses their primary orthopedic concerns, but when they transfer to the educational setting and require less medical intervention, they are lost to follow-up. To meet the objective of providing the most appropriate intervention to this population, a nationwide database on functional outcomes, mobility, and associated long-term problems should be established. Those who do enter the physical therapy system are often referred because of pain management issues. Pain is most likely due to overuse injuries, as well as to inefficient strategies for ADL. The emphasis of therapy should be placed on energy conservation, assistive devices to enhance efficiency, and the primary issue leading to the referral. As adults who have contracture syndromes age, they have secondary complications of being sedentary; therefore education on lifelong fitness opportunities needs to be investigated to help with cardiovascular fitness and weight management (Table 10.3).

TABLE 10.3 Interventions Based on International Classification of Functioning, Health, and Disability for Individuals With Arthrogryposis

	Activities Across the Life Span	Early Intervention through School Age	School Age Through Adulthood	Adolescence Through Adulthood	Other
Body Structure	Joint contracture bias will continue throughout lifetime if left untreated.	Treatments focus on putting limbs in a position of biomechanical advantage for function.	Muscle transfer surgery will give power to joints that were not previously strong.		Due to limited number of motor units supplying the strength to the muscle, with aging, fatigue of motor units is noted similar to post-polio syndrome.
Body Functions	Bracing is important to assist with upright mobility and standing. Shoe wedges help to balance the individual when full extension or dorsiflexion is not available when braced.	Emphasis on range of motion for upright mobility. Serial casting and management of clubfeet, bracing to get end range alignment for antigravity extension of hip and knee. Focus on standing balance with progression to ambulation.	Surgical management to align joints in alignment for lifetime independence in motor skills, coupled with therapeutic exercise to maximize surgical outcome. Bracing to support muscles not strong enough to maintain upright alignment against gravity with weight shift. Biomechanically, addressing alignment with shoe wedges to bring heel to the floor while allowing end range hip extension.	This is an age when bracing is often not as readily accepted. In this situation, strategies for independence using bias of contractures is important. Once in adulthood, progression of contractures is not as big an issue, but ability to use alignment will be important.	Weight management is important. Obesity negatively impacts on transfers and independent mobility.
Activity	Identify equipment needs to enhance independence.	Joint contractures and limitations in muscle strength may limit ability to achieve all motor milestones. Emphasis on rolling, scooting, standing balance, and ambulation. Use of an assistive device for endurance but short distance ambulation without an assistive device will translate to better independence for ADLs in the future including toilet transfers and dressing.	Emphasis on independent mobility both from a wheelchair level and from a functional mobility standpoint. Emphasis on reaching for highest level of functional mobility with independence.	Work toward mobility in the community. Identify self-care limitations and work toward highest level of independence.	Adapt environment as necessary to help with independence. Some with joint contractures and muscle weakness in all extremities will need external support for ADLs throughout the life span.
Participation	At each age group, focus needs to be on age-appropriate peer participation.	Playground and gym-related play is imperative in preschool and school age, working to find activities that allow independent participation as well as fitness opportunities.	Identify physical activities allowing for lifelong exercise and recreation participation and peer groups.	Work on strategies to enhance community participation with focus on activities addressing positive quality of life including but not limited to employment and recreation.	Teach self-advocacy. Those who cannot do for themselves need to be able to orchestrate their own care.

SUMMARY

Arthrogryposis poses a variety of challenges for the health care team throughout the patient's lifetime. Although AMC is non-progressive, its sequelae can limit participation in even basic ADLs. Variability in clinical manifestations has been noted, but severe joint contractures and lack of muscle development are hallmarks of the disease. Each stage of development requires special attention for maximizing the child's function. An early goal of the team is to educate the family about AMC and to create the understanding that, without intervention, the child's body structure and functional skills could lead to further limitation in activity throughout a lifetime. Early medical and therapeutic management includes vigorous stretching, splinting, positioning, and strengthening, all of which will allow the child to develop optimal positions for functional ADL and will enhance motor skill development. Timing of surgical procedures is critical to minimize intervention while maximizing benefit.

Each age has challenges on which physical therapy can have a positive impact. During infancy, motor milestones are often delayed or skipped, and determining functional mobility is more important than ascribing a developmental level. Intervention strategies focus on maximizing postural alignment through serial splinting and strengthening and on facilitating developmental activities. Ambulation is a preliminary primary goal, but once the child reaches school age, the focus shifts toward more independent, functional, and safe mobility. During the school-age years, the child must become more responsible for stretching exercises because stretching is an integral part of the program throughout the growing years. The team emphasizes assisting the child with problem solving and working toward independent mobility. Adaptive equipment is often necessary to allow the child with AMC to be independent in mobility and self-care. A comprehensive and integrated team approach is critical in developing strategies to meet these challenges. Ultimately, the goal is to have the child who has arthrogryposis grow to be an adult who is as independent as possible and an active participant in the community.

Case Scenarios on Expert Consult

The case scenarios related to this chapter address two case scenarios. Both focus on management over time, emphasizing mobility and function. They also highlight episodic care and educationally based services. Will's case begins as an infant and progresses to age 18 and Joseph, with video as a younger child, is followed from early intervention through early school age.

ACKNOWLEDGMENT

Special thanks to Dr. Robert Wellmon for insight, support, and a view on the diagnosis that is forever helpful.

REFERENCES

1. Asif S, Umer M, Beg R, Umar M: Operative treatment of bilateral hip dislocation in children with arthrogryposis multiplex congenita, *J Orthop Surg* 12:4–9, 2004.
2. Axt MW, Niethard FU, Doderlein L, Weber M: Principles of treatment of the upper extremity in arthrogryposis multiplex congenita type I, *J Pediatr Orthop B* 6:179–185, 1997.
3. Bamshad M, Bohnsack JF, Jorde LB, Carey JC: Distal arthrogryposis type 1: clinical analysis of a large kindred, *Am J Med Genet* 65:282–285, 1996.
4. Bamshad M, Van Heest AE, Pleasure D: Arthrogryposis: a review and update, *J Bone Joint Surg Am* 91(Suppl 4):40–46, 2009.
5. Bamshad M, Watkins WS, Zenger RK, Bohnsack JF, Carey JC, Otterud B, et al.: A gene for distal arthrogryposis type I maps to the pericentromeric region of chromosome 9, *Am J Genet* 55:1153–1158, 1994.
6. Reference deleted in proofs.
7. Bartonek A, Lidbeck CM, Pettersson R, Weidenhielm EB, Eriksson M, Gutierrez-Farewik E: Influence of heel lifts during standing in children with motor disorders, *Gait Posture* 34(3):426–431, 2011.
8. Boehm S, Limpaphayom N, Alaee F, Sinclair MF, Dobbs MB: Early results of the Ponseti method for the treatment of clubfoot in distal arthrogryposis, *J Bone Joint Surg Am* 90:1501–1507, 2008.
9. Bohm H, Dussa CU, Multerer C, Doderlein L: Pathological trunk motion during walking in children with amyoplasia: is it caused by muscular weakness or joint contractures? *Res Dev Disabil* 34(11):4286–4292, 2013.
10. Borowski A, Grissom L, Littleton AG, Donohoe M, King M, Kumar SJ: Diagnostic imaging of the knee in children with arthrogryposis and knee extension or hyperextension contracture, *J Pediatr Orthop* 28:466–470, 2008.
11. Brunner R, Hefti F, Tgetgel JD: Arthrogrypotic joint contracture at the knee and the foot: correction with a circular frame, *J Pediatr Orthop B* 6:192–197, 1997.
12. Burglen L, Amiel J, Viollet L, Lefebvre S, Burlet P, Clermont O, et al.: Survival motor neuron gene deletion in arthrogryposis multiplex congenita-Spinal Muscular Atrophy Association, *J Clin Invest* 98:1130–1132, 1996.
13. Cassis N, Capdevila R: Talectomy for clubfoot in arthrogryposis, *J Pediatr Orthop* 20:652–655, 2000.
14. Choi IH, Yang MS, Chung CY, Cho TJ, Sohn YJ: The treatment of recurrent arthrogrypotic club foot in children by the Ilizarov method, *J Bone Joint Surg Br* 83B:731–737, 2001.
15. Coster WJ, Deeney T, Haltiwanger J, Haley SM: *School function assessment*, San Antonio, TX, 1998, The Psychological Corporation.
16. Darin N, Kimber E, Kroksmark A, Tulinius M: Multiple congenital contractures: birth prevalence, etiology, and outcome, *J Pediatr* 140:61–67, 2002.
17. DelBello DA, Watts HG: Distal femoral extension osteotomy for knee flexion contracture in patients with arthrogryposis, *J Pediatr Orthop* 16:122–126, 1996.
18. Dillon ER, Bjornson KF, Jaffe KM, Hall JG, Song K: Ambulatory activity in youth with arthrogryposis: a cohort study, *J Pediatr Orthop* 29:214–217, 2009.
19. Dimitraki M, Tsikouras P, Bouchlariotou S, Dafopoulos A, Konstantou E, Liberis V: Prenatal assessment of arthrogryposis. A review of the literature, *J Matern Fetal Neonatal Med* 24(1):32–36, 2011.
20. Drummond DS, Siller TN, Cruess RL: Management of arthrogryposis multiplex congenita. In *AAOS instructional lectures*, vol. 23. St. Louis, 1974, Mosby, pp 79–95.
21. Fassier A, Wicart P, Dubousset J, Seringe R: Arthrogryposis multiplex congenita: long-term follow-up from birth until skeletal maturity, *J Child Orthop* 3:383–390, 2009.
22. Filges I, Hall JG: Failure to identify antenatal multiple congenital contractures and fetal akinesia—proposal of guidelines to improve diagnosis, *Prenat Diagn* 33(1):61–74, 2013.
23. George CL, Oriel KN, Blatt PJ, Marchese V: Impact of a community-based exercise program on children and adolescents with disabilities, *J Allied Health* 40(4):e55–e60, 2011.
24. Hall JG: Genetic aspects of arthrogryposis, *Clin Orthop* 194:44–53, 1985.
25. Hall JG: Arthrogryposis. *Am Fam Phys* 39:113–119, 1989.
26. Hall JG: Arthrogryposis multiplex congenita: etiology, genetics, classification, diagnostic approach, and general aspects, *J Pediatr Orthop B* 6:157–166, 1997.
27. Hall JG, Aldinger KA, Tanaka KI: Amyoplasia revisited, *Am J Med Genet A* 164A(3):700–730, 2014.
28. Hall JG: Arthrogryposis (multiple congenital contractures): diagnostic approach to etiology, classification, genetics, and general principals, *Eur J Genet* 57:464–472, 2014.

29. Hartley J, Baker S, Whittaker K: Living with arthrogryposis multiplex congenita: a survey, *APCP J* 4(1):19–26, 2013.

30. Haumont T, Rahman T, Sample W, King MM, Church C, Henley J, Jayakumar S: Wilmington robotic exoskeleton: a novel device to maintain arm improvement in muscular disease, *J Pediatr Orthop* 31(5):e44–e49, 2011.

31. Hell AK, Campbell RM, Hefti F: The vertical expandable prosthetic titanium rib implant for the treatment of thoracic insufficiency syndrome associated with congenital and neuromuscular scoliosis in young children, *J Pediatr Orthop B* 14:287–293, 2005.

32. Hislop HJ, Montgomery J, editors: *Daniels Worthingham's muscle testing: techniques of manual examination*, ed 8, Philadelphia, 2007, Elsevier Science.

33. Ho CA, Karol LA: The utility of knee releases in arthrogryposis, *J Pediatr Orthop* 28:307–313, 2008.

34. Hosny GA, Fadel M: Managing flexion knee deformity using a circular frame, *Clin Orthop Rel Res* 466:2995–3002, 2008.

35. Ippolito E, Farsetti P, Caterini R, Tudisco C: Long-term comparative results in patients with congenital clubfoot treated with two different protocols, *J Bone Joint Surg Am* 85A:1286–1294, 2003.

36. Kendall FP, McCreary EK, Provance PG: *Muscle testing and function*, ed 5, Baltimore, 2005, Lippincott, Williams Wilkins.

37. Klatt J, Stevens PM: Guided growth for fixed knee flexion deformity, *J Pediatr Orthop* 28:626–631, 2008.

38. Kowalczyk B, Lejman T: Short-term experience with Ponseti casting and the Achilles tenotomy method for clubfeet treatment in arthrogryposis multiplex congenita, *J Child Orthop* 2:365–371, 2008.

39. Kozin SH: Congenital differences about the elbow, *Hand Clin* 91:277–291, 2009.

40. Kramer A, Stevens PM: Anterior femoral stapling, *J Pediatr Orthop* 21:804–807, 2001.

41. Lampasi M, Antonioli D, Donzelli O: Management of knee deformities in children with arthrogryposis, *Musculoskelet Surg* 96(3):161–169, 2012.

42. Legaspi J, Li YH, Chow W, Leong JC: Talectomy in patients with recurrent deformity in clubfoot, *J Bone Joint Surg Br* 83B:384–387, 2001.

43. Letts M, Davidson D: The role of bilateral talectomy in the management of bilateral rigid clubfeet, *Am J Orthop* 28:106–110, 1999.

44. MacEwen GD, Gale DI: Hip disorders in arthrogryposis multiplex congenita. In Katz J, Siffert R, editors: *Management of hip disorders in children*, Philadelphia, 1983, JB Lippincott, pp 209–228.

45. Mancini MC, Coster W, Trombly CA, Heeren TC: Predicting participation in elementary school of children with disabilities, *Arch Phys Med Rehabil* 81:339–347, 2000.

46. Morcuende JA, Dobbs MB, Frick SL: Results of the Ponseti method in patients with clubfoot associated with arthrogryposis, *Iowa Orthop J* 28:22–26, 2008.

47. Moynihan LM, Bundey SE, Heath D, et al.: Autozygosity mapping, to chromosome 11q25, of a rare autosomal recessive syndrome causing histiocytosis, joint contractures, and sensorineural deafness, *Am J Hum Genet* 62:1123–1128, 1998.

48. Murray C, Fixsen JA: Management of knee deformity in classical arthrogryposis multiplex congenita (amyoplasia congenita), *J Pediatr Orthop B* 6:186–191, 1997.

49. Niki H, Staheli L, Mosca VS: Management of clubfoot deformity in amyoplasia, *J Pediatr Orthop* 17:803–807, 1997.

50. Nogueira MP1, Ey Batlle AM, Alves CG: Is it possible to treat recurrent clubfoot with the Ponseti technique after posteromedial release? A preliminary study, *Clin Orthop Relat Res* 467(5):1298–1305, 2009.

51. Palmer PM, MacEwen GD, Bowen JR, Matthews PA: Passive motion therapy for infants with arthrogryposis, *Clinic Orthop Rel Res* 194:54–59, 1985.

52. Palocaren T, Thabet A, Rogers K, Holmes L, Donohoe M, King M, Kumar SJ: Anterior distal femoral stapling for correcting knee flexion contracture in children with arthrogryposis-preliminary results, *J Pediatr Orthop* 30:169–173, 2010.

53. Riemer G, Steen U: Amyoplasia: a case report of an old woman, *Disabil Rehabil* 35(11), 2013.

54. Robinson RO: AMC: feeding, language and other health problems, *Neuropediatrics* 21:177–178, 1990.

55. Sarwark JF, MacEwen GD, Scott CI: Amyoplasia (a common form of arthrogryposis), *J Bone Joint Surg Am* 72:465–469, 1990.

56. Schiulli C, Corradi-Scalise D, Donatelli-Schulthiss ML: Powered mobility vehicles as aides in independent locomotion for very young children, *Phys Ther* 68:997–999, 1988.

57. Sells JM, Jaffe KM, Hall JG: Amyoplasia, the most common type of arthrogryposis: the potential for good outcome, *Pediatrics* 97:225–231, 1996.

58. Shohat M, Lotan R, Magal N, Shohat T, Fishel-Ghodsian N, Rotter J, Jaber L: A gene for arthrogryposis multiplex congenita neuropathic type is linked to D5S394 on chromosome 5qter, *Am J Hum Genet* 61:1139–1143, 1997.

59. Sneddon J: AMC aging survey, *Avenues* 10:1–3, 1999.

60. Sodergard J, Ryoppy S: The knee in arthrogryposis multiplex congenita, *J Pediatr Orthop* 10:177–182, 1990.

61. Sodergard J, Hakamies-Blomqvist L, Sainio K, Ryoppy S, Vuorinen R: Arthrogryposis multiplex congenital: perinatal and electromyographic findings, disability, and psychosocial outcome, *J Pediatr Orthop B* 6:167–171, 1997.

62. Staheli LT, Chew DE, Elliot JS, Mosca VS: Management of hip dislocations in children with AMC, *J Pediatr Orthop* 7:681–685, 1987.

63. Staheli LT, Hall JG, Jaffe KM, Paholke DO: *Arthrogryposis: a text atlas*, New York, 1998, Cambridge Press.

64. Stilli S, Antonioli D, Lampasi M, Donzelli O: Management of hip contractures and dislocations in arthrogryposis, *Musculoskelet Surg* 96(1):17–21, 2012.

65. Szoke G, Staheli LT, Jaffe K, Hall J: Medial-approach open reduction of hip dislocation in amyoplasia-type arthrogryposis, *J Pediatr Orthop* 16:127–130, 1996.

66. Tachdjian MO: Arthrogryposis multiplex congenita (multiple congenital contractures). In Tachdjian M, editor: *Pediatric orthopedics*, Philadelphia, 1990, WB Saunders, pp 2086–2114.

67. Tefft D, Guerette P, Furumasu J: Cognitive predictors of young children's readiness for powered mobility, *Dev Med Child Neurol* 41:665–670, 1999.

68. van Bosse HJ, Feldman DS, Anavian J, Sala DA: Treatment of knee flexion contractures in patients with arthrogryposis, *J Pediatr Orthop* 27:930–937, 2007.

69. van Bosse HJ, Marangoz S, Lehman WB, Sala DA: Correction of arthrogrypotic clubfoot with a modified Ponseti technique, *Clin Orthop Rel Res* 467:1283–1293, 2009.

70. Vanpaelmel L, Schoenmakers M, van Nesselrooij B, Pruijs H, Helders P: Multiple congenital contractures, *J Pediatr Orthop B* 6:172–178, 1997.

71. Williams PF: The elbow in arthrogryposis, *J Bone Joint Surg Br* 55:834–840, 1973.

72. Wynne-Davies R, Williams PF, O'Conner JCB: The 1960s epidemic of arthrogryposis multiplex congenita, *J Bone Joint Surg Br* 63:76–82, 1981.

73. Yau PW, Chow W, Li YH, Leong JC: Twenty-year follow up of hip problems in arthrogryposis multiplex congenita, *J Pediatr Orthop* 22:359–363, 2002.

74. Yingsakmongkol W, Kumar SJ: Scoliosis in arthrogryposis multiplex congenita: results after nonsurgical and surgical treatment, *J Pediatr Orthop* 20:656–661, 2000.

75. Young NL, Williams JI, Yoshida KK, Wright JG: Measurement properties of the Activities Scale for Kids, *J Clin Epidemiol* 53:125–137, 2000.

SUGGESTED READINGS

Background

Bamshad M, Van Heest AE, Pleasure D: Arthrogryposis: a review and update, *J Bone Joint Surg Am* 91(Suppl 4):40–46, 2009.

Hall JG: Arthrogryposis (multiple congenital contractures): diagnostic approach to etiology, classification, genetics, and general principals, *Eur J Genet* 57:464–472, 2014.

Hall JG, Aldinger KA, Tanaka KI: Amyoplasia revisited, *Am J Med Genet A* 164a(3):700–730, 2014.

Foreground

Azbell K, Dannemiller L: A case report of an infant with arthrogryposis, *Pediatr Phys Ther* 27(3):293–301, 2015.

Bartonek A, Lidbeck CM, Pettersson R, Weidenhielm EB, Eriksson M, Gutierrez-Farewik E: Influence of heel lifts during standing in children with motor disorders, *Gait Posture* 34(3):426–431, 2011.

Bohm H, Dussa CJ, Multerer C, Doderlein L: Pathological trunk motion during walking in children with amyoplasia: is it caused by muscular weakness or joint contractures? *Res Dev Disabil* 34(11):4286–4292, 2013.

Dillon ER, Bjornson KF, Jaffe KM, Hall JG, Song K: Ambulatory activity in youth with arthrogryposis: a cohort study, *J Pediatr Orthop* 29:214–217, 2009.

Fassier A, Wicart P, Dubousset J, Seringe R: Arthrogryposis multiplex congenita: long-term follow-up from birth until skeletal maturity, *J Child Orthop* 3:383–390, 2009.

Haumont T, Rahman T, Sample W, M King M, Church C, Henley J, Jayakumar S: Wilmington robotic exoskeleton: a novel device to maintain arm improvement in muscular disease, *J Pediatr Orthop* 31(5):e44–e49, 2011.

Lampasi M, Antonioli D, Donzelli O: Management of knee deformities in children with arthrogryposis, *Musculoskelet Surg* 96(3):161–169, 2012.

Mancini MC, Coster W, Trombly CA, Heeren TC: Predicting participation in elementary school of children with disabilities, *Arch Phys Med Rehabil* 81:339–347, 2000.

Sawatzky B: Long term outcomes of individuals born with arthrogryposis. Available at: URL: http://icord.org/studies/2015/02/long-term-outcomes-of-individuals-born-with-arthrogryposis/.

van Bosse HJ, Marangoz S, Lehman WB, Sala DA: Correction of arthrogrypotic clubfoot with a modified Ponseti technique, *Clin Orthop Rel Res* 467:1283–1293, 2009.

ADDITIONAL RESOURCES

Arthrogryposis Multiplex Congenita Support, Inc: www.AMCsupport.org

Avenues: TAG: The Arthrogryposis Group: www.TAGonline.org/uk

11

Osteogenesis Imperfecta

Maureen Donohoe

Osteogenesis imperfecta (OI) is an inherited disorder of connective tissue. Other terms in the literature used to describe OI include *fragilitas ossium* and *brittle bones*. OI has an incidence of 1 in 10,000–20,000 births.[57,75] This disorder comprises a number of distinct syndromes and has great variability in its manifestations. The salient impairments of OI are lax joints, weak muscles, and diffuse osteoporosis, which result in multiple recurrent fractures. These recurring fractures, which can be sustained from even minimal trauma, when coupled with weak muscles and lax joints, result in major deformity. Additional impairments in OI with variable presentation include blue sclerae, dentinogenesis imperfecta, deafness, hernias, easy bruising, and excessive sweating. Dentinogenesis imperfecta is a defect in the dentin and the dentinoenamel junction of the tooth. Often the enamel is normal, but teeth initially look gray, bluish, or brown because of the dentin defect. These teeth have a higher incidence of cracking, wear, and decay as the enamel cracks away from the dentin. Primary teeth are often more affected than adult teeth.[62]

Without early and adequate intervention, these problems in children with OI may lead to irreversible deformities and disability. Physical therapy can have a positive impact on these children and their families. Therapists can accomplish this through strengthening exercises, conditioning activities, adapting the environment, educating caregivers, and encouraging activity participation across a lifetime. Early physical therapy and medical interventions help prevent deformities and long-term functional limitations.

Children and adolescents with OI are often overprotected as a result of recurring fractures, which can contribute to social isolation. Some have difficulty interacting in peer play, adjusting to regular school, and achieving an independence level necessary to accomplish vocational goals. Most children with OI have average or above-average intelligence and greatly benefit from a stimulating educational environment. These children become adults who are usually productive members of society.[79] Management of their disabilities should be directed toward obtaining optimal independence, social integration, and educational achievement. The overall prognosis of OI and its long-term sequelae depend on the severity of the disease, which ranges from very mild to severe. Likewise, disability ranges from relatively mild with no deformities to extremely severe, with death occurring at birth or shortly thereafter.

In this chapter, we address the classification and pathophysiology of OI, medical and surgical interventions, physical therapy examination, evaluation, and interventions from infancy through adulthood. A case scenario of a child with OI is presented on Expert Consult.

BACKGROUND INFORMATION

CLASSIFICATION

OI is a heterogeneous collection of impairments with varying severity, marked by fragility of bone. Clinically, many types of OI present similarly. Despite this, OI is not a single genetic disorder but rather an array of different disorders based on a complement of information, including clinical presentation, genetic testing, and histologic analysis.

Prior to gene mapping, classification was based on clinical presentations and historically divided into three classifications, OI congenita (OIC) and OI tarda type I (OIT type I) and OI tarda type II (OIT type II), with OIC being the most severe and disabling form.[26,43,64,68] It is characterized by numerous fractures at birth, dwarfism, bowing or deformities of the long bones, blue sclerae (80% of cases), and dentinogenesis imperfecta (80% of cases). Infants with OIC have a poor prognosis, with a high mortality rate resulting from intracranial hemorrhage at birth or recurring respiratory tract infections during infancy.[74]

OIT is considered the milder form of OI, in which fractures occur after birth. It has been subclassified on the basis of the degree of bowing of the extremities or the number of fractures.[74] Clinical characteristics of OIT type I include dentinogenesis imperfecta, short stature, and bowing of only the lower extremities. Most with OIT type I can ambulate but may need external support such as orthotics. Surgery is often indicated for correction of the long bone deformity. OIT type II is the least disabling form of OI, where fractures are not associated with bowing of the bones. Most of these children approach average height and have an excellent prognosis for ambulation.

In 1978, Sillence and Danks delineated four distinct genetic types of OI. This numeric classification system is based on clinical presentation, radiologic criteria, and mode of inheritance and is generally well accepted by clinicians, as well as basic scientists.[69] The Sillence Classification uses a numeric system that correlates with morphologic and biochemical studies of OI.[68] With the onset of gene mapping and better databases for tracking the OI population, Glorieux expanded the classification to 11 distinct categories that help with medical management of the individual with OI.[6,32,75]

Most of the first four types of OI are considered autosomal dominant in inheritance.[68–70] The first four types of OI are caused by a defect in type I collagen structure that can be tracked back to a mutation in the genes *COL1A1* and *COL1A2* located on chromosomes 7 and 17. These genes are responsible for encoding the two alpha chains that make up type I collagen genes.[29,60] The other classifications of OI, types V through VIII, do not have a type I collagen defect but do have significant bone fragility and present clinically similar to types with the collagen defect.[31,33,35,61] Physical therapists are most likely to see types I, III, IV, V, VI, XI, mild versions of VII, as well as possibly the severe forms of type VIII, IX, and X. Types II, VII, VIII, IX, and X have lethal versions where some therapists may meet the baby briefly in the NICU.

OI Type I

OI type I makes up 50% of the total OI population.[31] It is characterized by markedly blue sclerae throughout life, generalized osteoporosis with bone fragility, joint hyperlaxity, and presenile conductive hearing loss. Patients are generally short but are not as short as those with other forms of OI. At birth, weight and length are normal; short stature occurs postnatally. Dentinogenesis imperfecta is variably present. Those with OI type IA have normal teeth, and those with OI type IB have dentinogenesis imperfecta. Fractures may be present at birth (10%) or may appear at any time during infancy and childhood.[68] The frequency and development of skeletal deformity are also variable.

OI Type II

Based on the Sillence Classification, OI type II is not compatible with life, and infants may be stillborn or may die within a few weeks. Extreme bone fragility occurs with minimal calvarial mineralization. Marked delay of ossification of the skull and facial bones is noted, and the long bones are crumbled.[74] Infants are small for their gestational age and have characteristic short, curved, and deformed limbs.

OI Type III

According to the Sillence Classification, OI type III usually is autosomal dominant, but on the rare occasion it is recessive. This form is severe, with progressive deformity of the long bones, skull, and spine, resulting in very short stature. Abnormal growth plate lines give the long bones a popcorn-like appearance.[53] Usually, severe bone fragility, moderate bone deformity at birth, multiple fractures, and severe growth retardation are noted. OI type III appears similar to OI type II, except that the lack of skull ossification is not as marked, and birth weight and length are within normal range. Sclerae in OI type III have a variable hue, tending to be bluish at birth and becoming less so with age. Dentinogenesis imperfecta occurs in 45% of patients with OI type III, and hearing loss is common. As a result of the complications of severe kyphoscoliosis and resulting respiratory compromise, death may occur in childhood.

OI Type IV

OI type IV is characterized by mild to moderate deformity and postnatal short stature. Bone fragility and deformities of the long bones of variable severity are noted. Dentinogenesis imperfecta is common in type IV while hearing loss is variable. The prognosis for ambulation in this population is excellent.[12]

OI Type V

In 2000, Glorieux first described the autosomal dominant OI type V. It is characterized by hypertrophic calcification of fractures and surgical osteotomies. Many patients have calcification of the interosseous membrane of the radius and ulna, ultimately limiting supination/pronation of the forearm. OI type V represents 5% of the moderate-to-severe cases of OI.[31-33,61]

OI Type VI

OI type VI is autosomal recessive and extremely rare and presents with moderate-to-severe deformity, similar to OI type IV, but with normal teeth and sclera. No abnormality of calcium, phosphate, parathyroid hormone, vitamin D metabolism, or growth plate mineralization is noted.[31,33,61]

OI Type VII

OI type VII is presumed autosomal recessive and is associated with a gene defect mapped to chromosome 3p22-24.1. This mutation affects the translation of the collagen with mutations in the cartilage-associated protein gene (CRTAP) and the prolyl 3-hydroxylase-1 gene (LEPRE1).[6,31,77] No type I collagen defect is noted in this form of OI, rather the defect involves how the collagen is translated to create bone.

With this gene defect, there is moderate-to-severe bone fragility and shortening of the humerus and femur.[40] Those with partial expression of CRTAP have moderate bone dysplasia similar to OI type IV; all cases with absence of CRTAP have been lethal.[31]

OI Type VIII

OI type VIII is presumed autosomal recessive and caused by mutations of genes that affect the translation of the collagen with mutations in the CRTAP and the LEPRE1.[6,46] No type I collagen defect is noted in this form of OI, rather the defect involves how the collagen is translated to create bone.

The absence or severe deficiency of prolyl-3-hydroxylase activity due to the LEPRE1 gene results in lethal to severe osteochondrodystrophy. Osteochondrodystrophy is a disorder of skeletal growth due to a bone and cartilage malformation resulting in severe growth deficiency and bone fragility in those who survive into the teen years. Those affected have flattened, long bones, slender ribs without beading, and small-to-normal head circumference.[45,53] OI type VIII is clinically similar to OI types II and III.

OI Type IX

OI type IX is clinically similar to Sillence Classification, OI type II, or a severe type III with extreme bone fragility. The gene mutation is on chromosome 15q22.31. This PPIB mutation is responsible for how protein folds when it creates collagen resulting in severe skeletal dysplasia.[29,75]

OI Type X

OI type X is clinically similar to Sillence Classification, OI type II or a severe type III with extreme bone fragility. The gene mutation is on chromosome 11q12.5. This SERPINH1 mutation is responsible for matching up with another protein and "chaperoning" it to encode with another collagen binding protein to create collagen. The defect in the gene results in severe skeletal dysplasia due to lack of collagen type 1 formation.[29,75]

OI Type XI

OI type XI is clinically similar to Sillence Classification, OI type III with extreme bone fragility. The gene mutation is on chromosome 17q21. The FKBP10 gene causes delayed collagen secretion, resulting in progressive deformity including joint contractures as well as bone fragility. Histologically, the bone looks similar to type VI with a fish scale–like appearance on the bone lamellae.

With the rapid rate of gene mapping and the dedication of the Osteogenesis Imperfecta Foundation to maintaining a patient database, it is expected that new information on classification of OI will continue to grow. Many of the classifications defined beyond Sillence's initial four types resemble the first four types clinically, but molecularly, the bone fragility is vastly different (Table 11.1).[29,31,81] Knowing how the bone disease presents genetically helps in planning treatments because some disorders do not respond to the bisphosphonates. With the expansion of the classification via genetic testing, the need for grouping based on clinical presentation has again become important from a rehabilitation and functional skill level.

PATHOPHYSIOLOGY

In the first four types of OI a defect in collagen synthesis results from an abnormality in processing procollagen to type I collagen, apparently causing the bones to be brittle. This defect affects the formation of both enchondral and intramembranous bone. Collagen fibers fail to mature beyond the reticular fiber stage. Studies show that osteoblasts have normal or increased activity but fail to produce and organize the collagen.[59] Although similar bone fragility is found with OI types VI, VII, and VIII, the defect lies in how the normally developed type I collagen is translated into bone.[32] Histological variability is evident among the different types of OI. With OI type I, morphologic findings include an increased amount of glycogen in osteoblasts, mild hypercellularity of bone,[1] and no abnormality in collagen fiber diameter.[18] Those with OI type II have abnormally thin corneal and skin collagen fibers.[11] Bone histology reveals decreased trabeculae and cortical bone thickness.[61] In types III and IV, morphologic findings include an increased amount of woven bone, increased cellularity, an increased number of resorption surfaces, and wide osteoid seams.[25] Histologically, OI type V has lamellar organization in an irregular meshlike pattern.[61] OI types VI and XI have a unique fish scale–like appearance of the lamellae. The appearance of a mineralization defect similar to osteomalacia is apparent with osteoid accumulation histologically, although no defects are associated with calcium, phosphate, parathyroid hormone, or vitamin D metabolism.[29,61]

OI type VII is histologically similar to OI type I, and it is not until analysis of the collagen and the genes is done that it can be differentiated. Both have decreased cortical width and trabecular number with increased bone turnover.[76] The lethal forms of OI types VIII, IX, and X are similar to OI type II because bone histology has decreased trabeculae and cortical bone thickness.[61]

Persons who have inherited OI tend to have the same type of mutation through the family, although clinical manifestations within that type may be variable. First-generation OI tends to be caused by a novel mutation of the gene. This specific gene mutation can then be passed to offspring. Genetic counseling when OI is found gives parents an accurate estimate of the risk of recurrence and an understanding of clinical variability in the family.[55,80]

MEDICAL MANAGEMENT

No cure for OI is known. Historically, no consistently effective medications were available to strengthen skeletal structures and prevent fractures until the bisphosphonate class of drugs was introduced to this population in the late 1990s.[3,4,41] Since then the direction of OI management has dramatically changed, especially for individuals with moderate to severe bone fragility.[2]

Bisphosphonates are having promising effects. Positive results such as reducing fractures and improving bone density have been reported from such pharmacologic agents as bisphosphonates,[41] including pamidronate and alendronate.[24,48,56] Bisphosphonates work by reducing normal bone turnover. They inhibit osteoclast activity; therefore the osteoblasts are not destroyed as rapidly by the osteoclasts.

Despite significant improvements that have resulted from the use of bisphosphonates, great debate continues over long-term use and implications of use around the time of orthopedic surgery.[45,50,51,60,78]

Another aspect of care with OI is ensuring adequate vitamin D level. Vitamin D allows the body to absorb calcium. Inadequate vitamin D limits the body's ability to form the hormone calcitriol, leading to insufficient calcium absorption from the diet; therefore the body must take calcium from the skeleton.[42] If vitamin D deficiency is established, vitamin supplementation, as well as calcium supplementation, is recommended.

Bone marrow transplant and stem cell therapy have been used sparingly. Transplantation of normal mesenchymal stem cells with the potential to differentiate into mature osteoblasts may result in significant improvement in bone collagen and mineral content. The therapeutic effect is possibly due to the selective growth advantage of normal cells over diseased host cells. Some research is being directed toward transplanting bone marrow cells with osteogenic potential with the collagen gene.[13,36,52,58]

The use of whole body vibration (WBV) is being researched as a minimally invasive technique to improve bone density and strength in children and adolescents with significant motor impairment. The child is on a vibrating platform on a tilt table. Increased bone density and improved function, based on the Brief Assessment of Motor Function and the Gross Motor Function Measurement, occurred in children who participated in vibration studies. Those who have telescoping rods and/or a history of joint subluxation are not good candidates for this treatment.[37,65–67] There is some concern that the vibration may be too stressful across instable joints and may create movement in the hardware of the telescoping rods.

Once a fracture occurs, the bone is more susceptible to refracture. The already weakened structure predisposes the child to limb deformities from bowing of the long bones. Immobilization to assist in setting the bone in proper alignment can cause disuse osteoporosis, causing greater risk of future fractures. A vicious circle is created: osteoporosis leads to fracture, and then immobilization for the fracture creates disuse osteoporosis, putting one at risk for further fracture. The goal is to limit immobilization of the extremities as much as possible to reduce osteopenia and risk of additional fractures.

Fractures in patients with OI generally heal within the normal healing time, although the resultant callus may be large but of poor quality. These fractures must be immobilized for pain relief and to promote healing in the correct alignment. Pseudarthrosis may occur when the fracture is not immobilized. Immobilization may occur in the form of splinting with thermoplastic materials, orthoses, hip spica posterior shells, or

TABLE. 11.1 Classification of Osteogenesis Imperfecta

Classification	Inheritance	Genetic/Histologic Information	CLINICAL FEATURES							
			Fractures	Radiographic Features	Stature	Dentin	Sclerae	Hearing	Ambulation	Other
Osteogenesis imperfecta type I (A, B)	Autosomal dominant	Lower than normal type I collagen, but structure of collagen is normal because of frameshift in COL1A1	Mild to severe bone fragility	Multiple fractures of long bones, compression fractures of vertebrae	Average or slightly shorter than average stature	Normal: IA Dentinogenesis imperfecta: IB	Blue	Hearing loss	Ambulation without assistive devices	50% of the total OI population Triangular face noted
Osteogenesis imperfecta type II (A, B, C)	New autosomal dominant mutation	Mutation in COL1A1 and COL1A2, which encode for type I collagen	Extreme bone fragility	Absent or limited calvarial mineralization, flat vertebral bodies, crumpled long bones, beaded ribs	Very short stature		Normal: IIA, IIB Blue: IIC		Nonambulatory	Lethal form of OI. Infants have low birth weight. Most have respiratory, swallowing problems. Some may have cardiac impairment.
Osteogenesis imperfecta type III	Autosomal dominant (usual) Autosomal recessive (rare)	Mutation in COL1A1 and COL1A2, which encode for type I collagen, reduced amounts of bone matrix	Variable bone fragility (often severe)	Progressive skeletal deformity (bowing), abnormal growth plates give long bones popcorn-like appearance	Very short stature	Variable dentin abnormality	Variable; blue at birth	Hearing loss	Nonambulatory to ambulation for exercise and transfers, usually relies on an assistive device for support	Rib fractures in infants can cause life-threatening breathing problems. Increasing scoliosis is noted with age. Loose joints and triangular face are present.
Osteogenesis imperfecta type IV	Autosomal dominant	Mutation in COL1A1 and COL1A2, which encode for type I collagen, reduced amounts of bone matrix	Bone fragility	Variable deformity	Short stature	Normal/dentinogenesis imperfecta	Normal	Variable	Ambulatory but may use an assistive device	Triangular face and progressive scoliosis noted Most fractures occur before puberty.
Osteogenesis imperfecta type V	Autosomal dominant	No type I collagen defect, lamellae of bone have mesh-like appearance, decreased cortical and cancellous bone	Moderate to severe bone fragility	Hypertrophic callus formation, calcification of the interosseous membrane between radius and ulna	Short stature	Normal	Normal		Ambulatory	5% of the moderate to severe cases of OI. Resembles type IV in clinical presentation

Continued

TABLE. 11.1   Classification of Osteogenesis Imperfecta—cont'd

Classification	Inheritance	Genetic/Histologic Information	Fractures	Radiographic Features	CLINICAL FEATURES					
					Stature	Dentin	Sclerae	Hearing	Ambulation	Other
Osteogenesis imperfecta type VI	Autosomal recessive	No type I collagen defect, fish scale-like appearance on the bone lamellae	Bone fragility, moderate severity	Variable deformity, vertebral compression fractures	Short stature	Normal	Normal	Variable	Ambulatory but may use an assistive device	Extremely rare, resembles type IV in clinical presentation
Osteogenesis imperfecta type VII	Autosomal recessive	Mutation in gene for cartilage-associated protein (*CRTAP*) on chromosome 3p22-24.1	Bone fragility	Variable deformity, short humeri and femora, coxa vara common	Short stature	Normal/dentinogenesis imperfecta	Normal	Variable	Mild: ambulatory Severe: nonambulatory	Mild cases clinically resemble OI type IV; severe cases resemble OI type II and are lethal.
Osteogenesis imperfecta type VIII	Autosomal recessive	Absence or severe deficiency of prolyl3-hydroxylase activity due to *LEPRE1* gene	Variable bone fragility (often severe)	Progressive skeletal deformity (bowing), may have popcorn calcifications on long bones	Very short stature		Normal			Presents similarly to the lethal forms of OI type II or III
Osteogenesis imperfecta type IX	Autosomal recessive	Homozygous mutations of *PPIB* gene in chromosome 15q22.31	Severe bone dysplasia	Severe bowing of extremities, wide flat bones with popcorn lesions	Very short stature	Normal			Nonambulatory	Severe to lethal similar to OI type II or III
Osteogenesis imperfecta type X	Autosomal recessive	Homozygous mutations of *SERPINH1* gene in chromosome 11q13.5. Do not produce type 1 collagen	Bone deformity and fracture	Osteopenia, fractures	Very short stature	Dentinogenesis imperfecta	Blue		Nonambulatory	Severe to lethal similar to OI type II or III
Osteogenesis imperfecta type XI	Autosomal recessive	Homozygous mutations of *FKBP10* gene in chromosome 17q21. Fish scale-like appearance on the bone lamellae.		Long bone fractures, ligamentous laxity, flat vertebral bodies, scoliosis	Short, bowed extremities	Normal	Normal			Severe, progressive deformity/contractures

casting. With malunion of fractures, angulation and bowing of the long bones occur, frequently accompanied by joint contractures. The physis may be disrupted, resulting in asymmetrical growth and deformity. When angulation occurs, mechanical forces tend to increase the deformity, aggravating the overall problem.[1] The cartilaginous ends of the long bones are disproportionately large and have irregular articular surfaces. Fortunately, in nearly all patients with OI the fracture rate diminishes near or after puberty.

The most successful means of fracture stabilization in long bones in OI is internal fixation with intramedullary rods.[38] Consensus indicates that intramedullary rods are advantageous, although significant debate continues over the type of internal fixation to be used in terms of material (steel versus titanium) and fixation (static rod versus telescoping rod). Although use of the intramedullary rod is not without complications, it can be helpful in preventing long bones from bowing after fracture. The rod provides internal support to prevent additional fractures. Indications for stabilization with rods include multiple recurring fractures and increasing long bone deformity that is interfering with orthotic fit and impairing function.[38] The age of the patient and the size of the bone determine the type and timing of surgery. Intramedullary rod fixation of the femur is best done after 4 or 5 years of age, when the thigh is not so short as to complicate surgery by compounding the technical difficulty. Surgical insertion of the rod in thin bones is also technically difficult.

The type of rod used depends on the type and severity of fracture. When a solid rod is used, bone growth may occur beyond the ends of the rods, necessitating subsequent surgery later for placement of a longer rod. Because children with severe OI are at greater than normal anesthetic risk from potential respiratory compromise, the number of operative procedures is best kept to a minimum. Special instrumentation has been designed that "elongates" with the child's growth, eliminating the need for multiple surgical revisions as the bone grows (Fig. 11.1).[29]

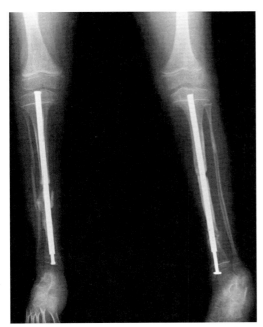

FIG. 11.1 Extensible intramedullary fixation rods that elongate as the bone grows in a child with osteogenesis imperfecta.

Telescoping rods are most frequently used in the femur but also may be used in the humerus, tibia, and forearm. Problems with intramedullary rods involve the control of rotation and migration when extensible rods are used; thus postoperative casting may be necessary.[38] Orthoses may be needed after insertion of the rod for further external support. Early weight bearing with orthotic support is initiated as soon as possible. With internal fixation a risk of osteopenia around the rod is present, especially with telescoping rods.

Spinal deformities, including scoliosis and kyphosis, occur in 50% of patients with OI as a result of osteoporosis and vertebral compression fractures. Progressive spinal deformities such as scoliosis and pathologic kyphosis are more likely to occur in children with types III and IV OI than in those with type I OI.[20] Kyphoscoliosis can be disabling and may be present in 20% to 40% of patients.[74] Unlike in the typical population, kyphoscoliosis in those with OI can be progressive over a lifetime, which further compounds the patient's short stature. The most common curve is that of thoracic scoliosis. Scoliotic and kyphotic curves in patients with OI are not usually amenable to conservative bracing. The incidence of a scoliosis developing in adolescents and adults with severe OI is 80% to 90%. Surgical stabilization is often advocated for the management of these deformities because the greater the curve, the greater the difficulty involved in meeting motor milestones.[22]

IMPAIRMENT

Diagnosis and Problem Identification

In the most severe forms of OI, the infant is born with multiple fractures sustained in utero or during the birth process. The prognosis of OI depends on its type. In its most severe forms, including types II, VII, VIII, IX, and X, multiple fractures noted prenatally and developed during delivery are associated with a high mortality rate. Prognostic indicators concerning survival and ambulation include the time of the initial fracture and the radiologic appearance of long bones and ribs at the time of the initial fracture. Spranger and associates[71] devised a scoring system for providing an accurate prognosis for newborns with OI. This system coded the degree of skeletal changes based on clinical and radiographic findings in 47 cases. These investigators found that newborns who had marked bowing of their lower extremities but less severe changes in the skull, ribs, vertebrae, and arms and normal sclera survived and had fewer fractures as they grew older. For the moderate and mild types, although the prognosis varies, a gradual tendency toward improvement has been noted when fracture incidence decreases after puberty.

If a family is known to be at risk of having a child with OI and the collagen defect or if the genetic mutation has been identified in the parent, human chorionic villous biopsy can be done prenatally at 10 weeks of gestation to determine whether the child has the same defect. A prenatal ultrasound examination in the second trimester of pregnancy can be helpful in identifying skeletal dysplasia and associated fractures.[39]

The infant is usually of normal size at birth, but postnatal growth is impaired. Although no conclusive causative factors for this impaired growth are known, possible factors include the deformities themselves or abnormalities in the epiphyseal growth plates. The radiologic appearance of long bones associated with the most severe cases indicates bones with a thin radiolucent appearance. The malformed ribs affect respiratory function, which may lead to respiratory tract infection and reduced functional potential of the child.

Children with moderate OI are often identified after several fractures have resulted from seemingly slight trauma. An example is a fractured humerus caused by the child holding on to a car seat while the caretaker is trying to get the child out of the car. Those children who begin to have fractures of unknown origin at a young age can have collagen and biochemical studies done, usually from a skin biopsy. These tests can also be helpful in ruling out other disorders, such as idiopathic juvenile osteoporosis, leukemia, and congenital hypophosphatasia. Genetic testing can be done to identify if the child has one of the identified forms of OI, although not all forms of bone fragility have been specifically mapped at this time. Infants with large heads and short limbs may be initially misdiagnosed because OI and achondroplasia are often confused. Radiographic reports, however, easily distinguish between the two.

Dual-energy x-ray absorptiometry (DEXA) is a helpful evaluation tool in the detection of low bone density. It is most useful in those children with milder forms of OI because it can detect changes more specifically than traditional radiographs.[49] DEXA scans are also helpful in tracking drug efficacy in gaining bone density.

Collagen and biochemical studies can assist in differentiating a battered infant from an infant with OI. Radiographic studies are helpful because fractures at the epiphysis are rare in OI but common in child abuse in which soft tissue trauma is also evident. Bruising is common to both the infant with OI and the battered infant, but the bruising will disappear when the battered infant is in a safe environment. Three of the most helpful radiographic views in diagnosing OI are those of the skull (wormian bones), the lateral view of the spine (biconcave vertebrae or platyspondyly), and the pelvis (the beginnings of protrusio acetabuli).[83]

In moderate-to-severe forms of OI, early childhood fractures lead to multiple recurring fractures caused by the already weakened structure. The child develops limb deformities from bowing, which leads to impairment of mobility and of other functional skills. In the least severe forms of OI, because the first pathologic fractures occur later in childhood, recurring fractures with associated long bone deformities are less likely, and the overall prognosis is improved.

Engelbert and colleagues,[23] in a cross-sectional study of 54 children with OI, analyzed range of motion (ROM) and muscle strength for different types of OI. In OI type I, generalized hypermobility of the joints occurred without a decrease in ROM. In OI type III, extremities, especially the lower extremities, were severely malaligned. In OI type IV, upper and lower extremities were equally malaligned. Muscle strength in OI type I was normal except in periarticular muscles at the hip joint. In OI type III, however, muscle strength was severely decreased, especially around the hip joint. In OI type IV, the proximal muscles of both upper and lower extremities were weak.

Team members other than physical therapists who have an important role in the management of OI include orthopedists, orthotists, occupational therapists, audiologists, dentists, and geneticists. Little progress has been made in the primary prevention of this disorder, but much improvement in medical management is evident in recent years.

FOREGROUND INFORMATION

EXAMINATION, EVALUATION, AND INTERVENTION TABLES 11.2 TO 11.4

Infancy

Typical participation restrictions for an infant with OI depend on the severity of the case. In severe cases the most serious impairments are those of rib and skull fractures, which may compromise pulmonary status and neural status, respectively. Because of possible cardiopulmonary compromise, time may be spent in the neonatal intensive care unit; this could lead to decreased parental interaction and bonding. If OI is moderate to severe, parents have increased anxiety about holding the infant for fear of fracturing the infant's bones. This may result in minimal contact and may decrease the mutually nurturing interaction vital to both parent and child. Children with severe OI who have reduced mobility from skeletal deformities may be unable to achieve age-appropriate activities of daily living (ADLs) or to play in the normal peer environment.

Infants with OI are at a very delicate stage of life. They have special needs regarding handling, positioning, and playing. During this stage, the role of caregivers is paramount in minimizing fractures, thereby limiting further muscle weakness and joint laxity. This is accomplished primarily through a physical therapy home program and caregiver education involving proper positioning and handling, which begin as soon as the child has been recognized as an infant with fragile bones.

At birth the infant may be of normal size, but postnatal growth is almost always stunted. Typical deformities of the infant include a relatively large head with a soft and membranous skull and bowed limbs, which usually are short in the more severe forms of OI. Other features include a broad forehead and faciocranial disproportion, which give the face a triangular shape. Radiographically, fractures present at birth may be at varying stages of healing. The bones of infants with severe OI are short and wide with thin cortices, and the diaphyses are as wide as the metaphyses. Crepitation can be palpated at fracture sites.

The physical therapist should be aware of the infant's medical history of past and present fractures and should know the types of immobilizations employed before beginning the examination. Assessing pain is important when working with this population because it can establish baseline comfort and anticipated changes with intervention. The FLACC (face, legs, activity, cry, and consolability) Scale is an observational scale that is used to quantitatively assess pain behaviors in preverbal patients.[44,47]

Assessment of the caregiver's handling and positioning techniques during dressing, diapering, and bathing is necessary. Therapists can be helpful in identifying and modifying techniques that put the child at fracture risk. If the baby is hospitalized, it is imperative that all caregivers be educated in proper handling techniques.

Therapy assesses active, but not passive, ROM in the young child with OI because passive stretching is contraindicated in most cases. A standard goniometer can be used for measuring active ROM but may need to be cut down to a size suitable for the infant. This active ROM can be translated to functional ROM, useful in visualizing the whole composite of motions needed in functional abilities. For example, functional active ranges include the extent to which the child can bring the hand

TABLE. 11.2 International Classification of Functioning, Health, and Disability for Children With Osteogenesis Imperfecta

Changes in Body Structure	Changes in Body Functions	Activity	Participation
Connective tissue disorder secondary to defect in collagen synthesis	Diffuse osteoporosis resulting in multiple recurrent fractures	Limited functional mobility skills, including rolling, creeping, transitional movements, and higher-level mobility skills	Limited participation in physical activities caused by endurance limitations and safety concerns
Brittle bones	Weak muscles	Limited ability to transfer	Limited peer play
	Joint laxity	Limited ambulation	Infantilization
	Bowing of long bones	Decreased endurance	Limited access to educational and work opportunities
	Scoliosis	Limited independence in self-care skills, including dressing and feeding	Limited access to wide range of environments
	Kyphosis	Limited ability for ambulation on uneven terrain	Limited independent living
		Limited independence in wheelchair mobility	Social isolation

TABLE. 11.3 Recommended for Children With Osteogenesis Imperfecta

	Test Information	Considerations for Osteogenesis Imperfecta	Reference
Body Structures and Function			
Range of motion	Goniometer can be used to identify range of motion as well as resting posture of the limbs.	May need to cut down a goniometer to allow reliable use with a small child.	Clarkson HM: *Musculoskeletal assessment: joint motion and muscle testing.* 3rd ed. Baltimore, Lippincott, Williams & Wilkins, 2012.
Strength	Observation, palpation, and hand pressure are used to determine muscle strength.	Extreme caution is necessary when testing across long bones. Manual muscle testing is more a guideline of strength above or below antigravity strength.	Hislop HJ, Montgomery J, editors: *Daniels & Worthingham's muscle testing: techniques of manual examination.* 8th ed. Philadelphia, Elsevier Science, 2007.
Activity: Single Task			
Timed standing balance	Documentation of amount of time the individual can stand statically.	No norms for this population. Can track change over time for the individual. Can look at stand on one foot and compare symmetry.	
Gait speed	Documentation of speed traveling a specific distance. Document for bracing and assistive device during testing.	No norms for this population. Can track change over time for the individual. Can also be used to monitor manual wheelchair speed.	Lythgo N, Wilson C, Galea M: Basic gait and symmetry measures for primary school-aged children and young adults. II: Walking at slow, free and fast speed, *Gait Posture* 33:29-35, 2011.
6-minute walk test	The individual walks as far as possible in a 6-minute period.	No norms for this population including assistive device. Useful to track change over time for the individual.	Please refer to Chapter 2 for more information.
Timed up and go	Individual rises from a standardized chair height, walks 3 meters, turns around, and returns to sitting in the chair.	No norms for this population. Child may be too small to safely get in and out of the standardized chair height. Tracks change over time for the individual. Record chair height for the individual if not using the standardized chair height and replicate height during future testing.	Please refer to Chapter 2 for more information.
Activity: Multiple Items			
Peabody Developmental Motor Scale	Fine and gross motor assessments compare skills to typically developing peers aged birth to 72 months.	Higher-level locomotor skills and object manipulation skills should be approached with caution because these activities could put a child at risk for fracture.	Please refer to Chapter 2 for more information.
Brief Assessment of Motor Function (BAMF)	Test specifically designed for OI population. Predictive of ambulation potential.		Cintas HL, Siegel KL, Furst GP, Gerber LH: Brief assessment of motor function: reliability and concurrent validity of the Gross Motor Scale, *Am J Phys Med Rehabil* 82:33-41, 2003.

Continued

TABLE. 11.3 Recommended for Children With Osteogenesis Imperfecta—cont'd

	Test Information	Considerations for Osteogenesis Imperfecta	Reference
Patient Reported Outcomes Measurement Information System (PROMIS)	Parent and/or child report. Multiple dimensions to help tease out perceived strengths and needs to help with goal establishment.	Short and long forms available. Can be reported on paper or via computer access. PROMIS has pediatric and adult versions.	Please refer to Chapter 2 for more information.
School Function Assessment	Educational staff report on child's abilities. Helpful in identifying needs within the educational environment	Some children will need assistance with skills but should learn to how to orchestrate care.	Please refer to Chapter 2 for more information.
Pediatric Evaluation of Disability Inventory (PEDI and PEDI-CAT)	Self-report or caregiver report tool designed to identify functional delay in areas of daily activities, mobility, social/cognitive, and responsibility.	The PEDI takes 1 hour to administer while the PEDI-CAT is a shorter, more intuitive computerized version.	Please refer to Chapter 2 for more information.

TABLE. 11.4 Interventions Based on International Classification of Functioning, Health, and Disability for Individuals With Osteogenesis Imperfecta

	Activities Across the Life Span	Early Intervention Through School Age	School Age Through Adulthood	Adolescence Through Adulthood	Other
Body Structure	Postfracture management for strength and motion.				Have a fracture plan in place for home/school/community/work.
Body Function	When working on rehabilitation from fracture or surgery, providing intervention in an aquatic medium is often helpful to address strength and mobility prior to achieving the same skills on land.	Encourage child to avoid rotational and deforming forces across joints when learning postural transitions. Position with neutral alignment of hips when possible.	Equalize leg length for those who are standing and/or walking. Work on trunk strength and overhead reaching to help limit the progression of scoliosis.	Lifetime participation in some type of cardiovascular fitness is important.	Weight management is important. Obesity negatively impacts on transfers and independent mobility.
Activity	Identify equipment needs to enhance independence.	Work developmental sequence to help enhance transfers and potential for ambulation.	Emphasis on independent mobility both from a wheelchair level and from a functional mobility standpoint. Emphasis on reaching for highest level of functional mobility with independence.	Work toward mobility in the community. Identify self-care limitations and work toward highest level of independence.	Adapt environment as necessary to help with independence.
Participation	At each age group, focus needs to be on age-appropriate peer participation.	Playground and gym-related play is imperative in preschool and school age, working to find activities that allow independent participation as well as fitness opportunities.	Identify physical activities that allow for lifelong participation and peer groups.	Work on strategies to enhance community participation with focus on activities to address improvement in quality of life including but not limited to employment and recreation.	Teach self-advocacy, especially during emergency situations. School and work need to have an action plan in place prior to an emergency. This may include whom to call, splinting of fractures, and triage prior to calling an ambulance to send the individual to the emergency room.

to the mouth, reach hands to midline, and reach toward the top of the head. If possible, the same therapist measures ROM during reevaluations. Intrarater and interrater reliability of goniometry should be determined for therapists and should be checked annually if more than one therapist examines the child.

Muscle strength is assessed through observation of the infant's movements and palpation of contracting muscles, rather than with the use of formal muscle tests.

A gross motor developmental evaluation should also be performed because these children often have delayed development of gross motor skills secondary to fractures and muscular weakness. Delayed gross motor skills are manifested as activity limitations involving impaired achievement of motor milestones. Sitting by the age of 10 months is a good predictor of future walking ability.[16] Formal tests used include the Peabody Developmental Motor Scales, 2nd edition[28]; the Pediatric Evaluation of Disability Inventory[34]; the Bayley Scales of Infant Development II[9]; and the Brief Assessment of Motor Function, which can be used to obtain a quick description of gross, fine, and oral motor performance.[15,54] See Chapter 2 for more information on examination tools. Finally, it is important to assess the appropriateness of equipment used for seating, transporting, and encouraging independent mobility of the infant.

Physical therapy includes early parent education on proper handling and positioning techniques. Safe bathing, dressing, and carrying of an infant with OI are critical to reduce the risk of fracture.[8] When handling the infant, it is important that forces not be put across the long bones; instead the head and trunk should be supported with the arms and legs gently draped across the supporting arm. Some parents feel most comfortable supporting the infant on a standard-sized bed pillow for carrying at home. It is important to have a repertoire of carrying positions for the infant, so the baby can develop strength by accommodating to postural changes. Holding and carrying positions that safely challenge head control are important in that head control is a hallmark of function over time. Loose clothing and front snaps, side snaps, or Velcro closures can facilitate dressing and undressing. Overdressing should be avoided to reduce excessive sweating. Proper diapering includes a technique of rolling the infant off the diaper and supporting the buttocks with one hand with the infant's legs supported on the caregiver's forearm, while the other hand positions the diaper. The infant should never be lifted by the ankles. Bathing is done in a padded, preferably plastic, basin. Infant carriers that are designed to safely support the head, trunk, and extremities are frequently used for household transporting. For the very fragile infant, the carrier can be customized, as with a one-piece molded thoracolumbosacral orthosis, which incorporates the legs so they will not dangle and sustain injury. This carrier minimizes stresses to the fragile bones while it aids in positioning and transporting the infant. Physical therapy can play a role in educating families on the proper car seat, even before the child is initially discharged from the hospital. Early on, an infant may need a car bed (Fig. 11.2) if a rear-facing infant seat is too large or if the risk of fracture while getting into and out of the seat is too great during the first few months. Extra padding may have to be added between the child and the transportation device, allowing a snug fit without putting undue stress on the fragile child through the strap systems. Families need to be trained on how to rearrange padding in the seat to accommodate the various devices the child may be placed in for immobilization of

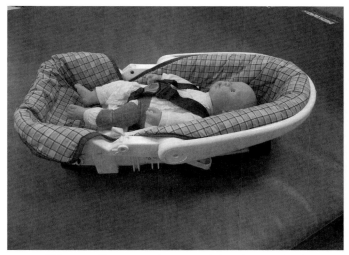

FIG. 11.2 Example of a young infant in a car bed.

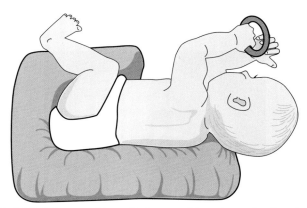

FIG. 11.3 Infant positioned lying on side using rolls. Emphasis is on maintaining trunk alignment while allowing for active and spontaneous but safe movement.

fracture sites. Given the low bone density and the high risk for fracture, the child should use a rear-facing car seat for as long as possible to maximize safety in the car.

Proper positioning is a critical component of the home program and management of the infant with OI. One position that offers good support is sidelying with towel rolls along the spine and extremities, so they are aligned and protected while allowing the child to be active (Fig. 11.3).

Prone positioning should start with the baby on the caregiver, where the child is well supported and most comfortable when being challenged. As the child gains skill in prone, the baby can be positioned over a towel roll or with a soft wedge under the chest as an alternative. Prone positioning is helpful for improving head control, strengthening back extensors, and molding the anterior chest wall. When supine, the infant needs support for the arms, and the hips should be in neutral rotation with the knees over a roll (Fig. 11.4). Positions should be changed frequently and should not restrict active spontaneous movement because spontaneous movement enhances muscle strengthening and bone mineralization.[8] Positioning is useful not only for the purpose of protecting from fracture but also for minimizing joint malalignment and deformities. Fig. 11.5 shows an infant's legs being poorly positioned in an infant carrier. The

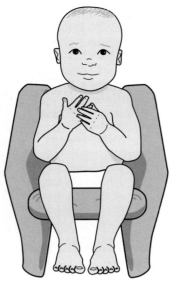

FIG. 11.4 Infant positioned supine with hips in neutral rotation and knees flexed and supported through the trunk.

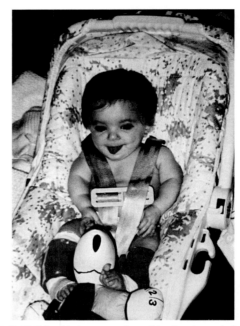

FIG. 11.6 Child with improved positioning in an infant seat.

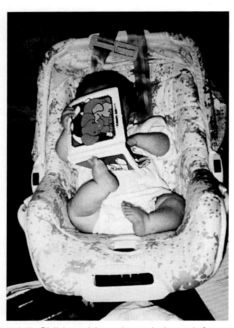

FIG. 11.5 Child positioned poorly in an infant seat.

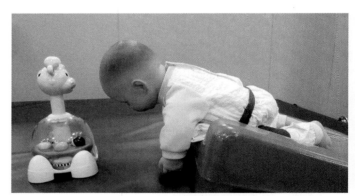

FIG. 11.7 Infant positioned prone over a bolster encourages weight bearing, extremity and trunk alignment, and strengthening of extensor musculature during developmental play.

same seat is modified with lateral leg pads to keep the infant's hips and legs in neutral alignment, along with lower leg molded plastic splints (Fig. 11.6). Varying the position of the infant promotes the development of age-appropriate developmental skills.

Promotion of sensorimotor developmental skills is an ongoing component in the management of the infant and child. Identification of appropriate and safe toys for a child and of comfortable play positions that promote development is often addressed jointly by the occupational therapist and the physical therapist. For example, lying prone on a soft roll or over a parent's leg allows weight-bearing use of the arms with cocontraction of the shoulder musculature, which promotes active neck and back extensor muscle control (Fig. 11.7). Increasing muscle strength and support around the joint in activities such as this is

especially important because the joint ligaments are lax. Prone positioning may be most comfortable over an elevated surface such as a wedge, a sofa cushion, or a roll, but just as important is lower extremity positioning with hips in neutral rotation and maximal hip extension.

Developmental activities such as rolling and supported sitting should be encouraged as tolerated by the child. When rolling is encouraged, the infant's arm is placed alongside his or her head, and then he or she attempts to roll over. Supported sitting is accomplished with seat inserts or corner chairs. Upright unsupported sitting can begin on the parent's lap with a pillow. When the child exhibits appropriate head control, short-sit and straddle activities can be done over the caregiver's leg or a roll but with avoidance of rotation across the lower extremity. These activities promote the development of protective and equilibrium responses and the beginning of protected weight bearing of the lower extremities. Many children with OI spend much time scooting on their buttocks before crawling is accomplished. Many children develop sitting skill and mobility in sitting long before they develop consistent ability to move from horizontal prone or supine to sitting. This is due to short arms in relation to body length and can be adapted for by giving a child a raised surface to push off of, such as a pillow, as the child is learning to move into a sitting position.

Proper handling while encouraging developmental skills is of key importance. For instance, a pull-to-sit maneuver is contraindicated when a distraction pull on the hands is used. Rather, this maneuver should be modified and facilitated by supporting the child around the shoulders while the child attempts to sit up. In working on trunk control over a ball, the therapist's hands are positioned on the pelvis and trunk rather than supporting or facilitating movement from the legs. Parents should be cautioned against using devices that support a baby upright in standing such as baby walkers or jumping seats. These devices put unnecessary stress on the legs where the child fits through the sling, and if the baby has difficulty controlling the device, devastating torque to the bone may result. These devices do not foster proper positioning and weight bearing for these fragile children. Such upright activities can give parents a false sense that the infant is protected. Active, spontaneous activity and exercise are encouraged in sidelying and supine positions and in supported sitting, with the child reaching for, swiping at, rolling, and lifting lightweight toys of different textures. Pool exercises may begin as early as 6 months of age with the goals of promoting active exercise and weight bearing.[8] Extremity movement may occur unobstructed in the water as the child is supported in a flotation device accompanied by a parent or the therapist.

At this stage, goals include teaching safe handling and positioning techniques to caregivers and providing opportunities for development of age-appropriate skills. The intensity of treatment varies with the individual needs of the infant and family, but providing a home program and regular home visits by a physical therapist at least weekly is essential to ensuring that the environment is suitable for sensorimotor and cognitive development. The therapist can act as a resource and support for the caregivers as together they develop strategies to meet the challenges of safe caregiver handling, mobility, and developmental facilitation. Another important role for early intervention therapists in the home is to help families develop a repertoire of positioning and activity options for the child. This is most important when the child recovers from fractures.

When fractures do occur, they may require splinting with materials such as thermoplastic materials or fiberglass. Ace wraps have been used to support and protect a limb in mild cases and in young infants. Fractures may heal within 2 weeks in the newborn and generally within the same time frame as other fractures in infancy (usually 6 weeks).

Preschool Period

Bone fragility, joint laxity, and reduced muscle strength continue to be present in the preschool period but are now accompanied by secondary impairments of disuse atrophy and osteoporosis from fracture immobilization (Fig. 11.8). At this point, if a child has had issues with recurrent fractures, treatment with bisphosphonates has begun to help decrease the fracture cycle. Structural changes and secondary impairments from fractures may limit mobility and subsequently restrict participation in play and socialization for the child with OI. This may affect the child's adjustment to regular school and may hinder academic progress. The temperament of the child with OI may

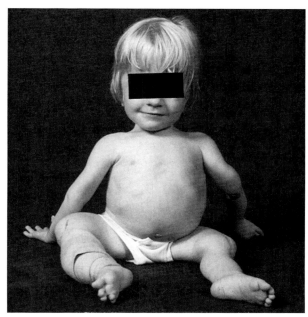

FIG. 11.8 Child with osteogenesis imperfecta showing joint laxity and bony deformities: femoral anterolateral bowing and tibial anterior bowing.

play a role in his ability to adjust to his activity limitations and participation restrictions. Cintas and colleagues[15] demonstrated that the temperament of children with OI was comparable with that of children without disability except for having lower activity scores. Temperament was significantly and positively related to motor performance in terms of persistence, approach, and activity.

At this stage, muscles are usually weakened and developmental motor skills are lagging as a result of frequent immobilization and relative disuse. Despite this, cognitive skills should be appropriate for the child's age. When a fracture is sustained, children with OI typically complain little of pain and usually have minimal soft tissue trauma.[84]

If the child begins to walk without adequate support, further bending of the long bones occurs as a result of abnormal stress on the weakened structure. Bowing occurs in the anterolateral direction in the femur and anteriorly in the tibia. In those children who do not walk, lack of normal weight-bearing stress leads to a honeycomb pattern of osteoporosis in the long bones.

Emphasis at this stage is on protected weight bearing and self-mobility for enhanced independence. Although proper positioning, handling, and transferring are still important, the focus shifts to the child's active participation in his or her care. During this period the child with OI should have adequate upright control to begin bearing weight and, at the very least, should be held in a standing position because early weight bearing appears to have some beneficial effect.[30] When radiographs of children with OI from the time of birth and several years later are compared, the changing levels of bone density suggest that progressive osteoporosis has been superimposed on the basic bone defect.[10] Upper extremity bones were frequently denser than those of the lower limbs and were less likely to fracture. This finding may be related to the use and stress placed on upper extremity bones during self-care and play activities.

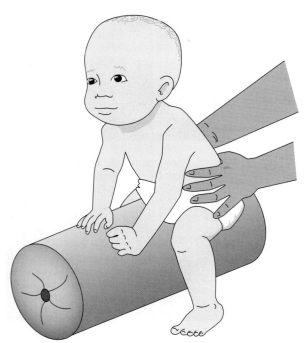

FIG. 11.9 Straddle roll activity of supported sit-to-stand for lower extremity strengthening and weight bearing.

For the preschool child an evaluation of modes of mobility and adapted equipment is essential to promote supported sitting functional mobility and independence. Equipment requires constant updating because of changing positional needs related to mobilization-immobilization status. Splinting needs and adaptive ADL equipment are assessed for fit and function to allow optimal levels of independence.

Developmental assessment tools that are appropriate include the Peabody Developmental Motor Scales II, the Brief Assessment of Motor Function, and the Pediatric Evaluation of Disability Inventory to assess gross motor function and activity limitations in children with OI. Pain should continue to be assessed in the preschool-age child. Appropriate pain assessments include the FLACC Behavioral Scale and the self-report Numeric or Wong-Baker Faces Scale.[44,82] Active exercise continues to be emphasized to increase muscle strength of weakened muscles, most typically, hip extensor and abductor muscles. Active exercise can be achieved primarily through developmental play. One developmental activity to increase weight bearing and maintain or increase strength in the quadriceps and hip extensor musculature involves having the child straddle a roll and come to stand, with the therapist supporting the child's pelvis (Fig. 11.9). The therapist begins with the child sitting on a high roll that requires a small excursion of movement to go from sitting to standing and then gradually changes to using a lower roll. An active-resistive program graded for the patient's tolerance should be cautiously established. Use of light weights may be incrementally increased, but they should be attached close to large joints so as to avoid a long lever arm, which increases the potential for fracture.

Early gym-related activities that can be introduced at this age may include scooter board activities, riding tricycles, and playground games such as Simon Says, Red Light Green Light, and Follow the Leader. Activities that encourage overhead reaching are helpful in maximizing trunk extension. These activities can

include modified basketball activities when the ball is light and the child uses low-speed passing. Racket sports using a tethered tennis ball help to build upper body strength. A responsible adult to ensure safety should closely monitor all activities. If the child is attending preschool, all members of the team should have a basic emergency plan if fractures occur at school. This plan would include but is not limited to notification of family and splinting of involved extremities while awaiting supportive medical intervention.

An aquatic exercise program is excellent for the child with OI. It can be started at an early age and continue for a lifetime. Aquatic therapy benefits include the opportunity to socialize with peers in a safe environment, a safe method of strengthening muscles through resistance and assistance of the water, and the opportunity to improve cardiovascular fitness and bear weight in a protected environment. The therapist can finely grade the progression of exercises in the pool by first using the buoyancy effect of the water to assist weak movements, then supporting the movements, and finally, using water to resist active movements. Exercises can be modified with floats by changing the length of the lever arm of the moving body part through the use of turbulence and by altering the speed and direction of the movement.[19]

Pool exercises can enhance deep breathing to facilitate chest expansion and enhance overall respiratory function, which are especially important because chest deformities that compromise breathing capacity are common. Certain precautions should be taken when pool therapy is considered for the child with OI. The heat of the water creates a rise in body temperature and increases metabolism, which is frequently already elevated in these children. It is suggested, therefore, that time in the water, water temperature, and activity level be closely monitored for each child. Initially, pool sessions are generally limited to 20 to 30 minutes.[14]

Pool exercise therapy may interrupt the cycle of further disuse and secondary complications from immobilization. Not only is aquatic therapy an ideal therapeutic modality for the child with OI, it also can be a therapeutic, lifelong avocational activity that can ameliorate the effects of the disabling process.

One key goal and big challenge for the preschool child who has frequent fractures is safe, independent mobility. The aim is to prevent an activity limitation of reduced mobility resulting from the initial impairment. Research has linked limited mobility opportunities in the first few years with later life problem-solving skill difficulties.[72] Opportunities for multiple safe modes of mobility should be explored to expand the child's repertoire of environmental experiences. A scooter for sitting propelled with legs or hands may be useful (Fig. 11.10). Families should be encouraged to investigate ride-on toys that can be purchased at a toy store. It is often a challenge to get a device that accommodates the child's shortened femurs and shortened arms yet gives enough weight-bearing surface to enhance trunk control. Sometimes handlebars need to be adapted to allow the child to steer effectively. A ride-on toy may give the child safe mobility without the rotational components of sit-scooting.

The degree of ambulation attainable varies for preschool children with OI. Those children with limited ambulatory skills may need formal gait training as well as the instruction of family members. Interest in standing often occurs in the child's second year of life. Factors affecting the ability to stand and ambulate include the degree of bowing in the extremities and the muscle strength of the limbs. Ambulation is often introduced in the

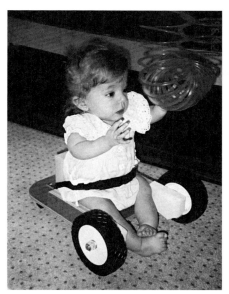

FIG. 11.10 Scooter used for mobility that can be propelled by a child's legs or arms.

pool, for protected weight bearing. Because the buoyancy of water provides support for the body, weight bearing on weakened extremities and unstable joints can be gradually introduced without fear of causing trauma.

Weight relief depends on the proportion of the body that is below the water level. For maximum weight relief for ambulation, the child begins standing in the pool where the water level is at the child's neck. Over time, the child gradually progresses to bearing more weight in shallow water. If the child with OI is recovering from a fracture, it is recommended that thermoplastic splints be used to further protect the extremity while in the pool during early weight bearing. General guidelines for walking reeducation in water according to Duffield[19] suggest that a patient start in parallel bars or a walking frame, with the therapist initially supporting the pelvis from the front. The patient practices weight shifts from side to side, forward, and backward and progresses to walking forward. The therapist cues the patient to lean slightly forward to counteract the upthrust of buoyancy, which tends to cause the child to overbalance backward. In this manner, protected walking for a child with OI can start much earlier than on a solid surface. Unsupported standing on solid ground is not recommended because it leads to rapid bowing of the long bones. When severe bowing of the extremities occurs, the child usually undergoes orthopedic surgery in the form of osteotomies. Age-appropriate lower extremity weight bearing is encouraged, although the child with moderate to severe OI needs external devices such as splints or braces to protect fragile long bones.

In moderate-to-severe OI, braces and splints are usually required to begin standing activities on solid surfaces. Use of orthotics provides the protected weight bearing needed to reduce the impact of stress on osteoporotic bony deformities. Braces or splints may be used first in conjunction with a standing frame if the child has significant lower extremity bowing and does not have standing skill.

The child who does not naturally embark on a standing program can use a standing device for support. An air splint can be used to prevent fractures and to temporarily manage fractures.

Use of such a device may be a nice stepping stone between using a stander for weight bearing and standing freely without support.[63] Many children begin early ambulation with sit-to-stand activities and cruising along furniture. Air splints can be helpful to institute graded weight bearing and gait training in a child with OI. Drawbacks of air splints are that they may be bulky and hot, so the child may not always tolerate them well.

Once a child graduates from a stander, ambulation may be protected through the use of parallel bars or a walker. A walker that supports the majority of body weight through the trunk and pelvis is often used to assist in weight bearing during initial overland ambulation. This walker supports weight by means of a trunk support cuff and a padded pommel that is positioned between the child's legs. Rear-wheeled and four-point walkers followed by canes or crutches (depending on the type and severity of OI) also may be used. Forearm attachments to walkers or crutches afford a degree of weight bearing distributed throughout the forearm to reduce stress on the arm and wrist, as well as to relieve some weight bearing on the lower extremities. Older preschoolers who use a walker may benefit from a walker with a seat, so they can easily rest between walking activities and can fully participate in preschool-related play. Most children ambulate without braces when the fracture rate decreases. Although bracing of the lower extremity is not as prevalent as it had been before the use of bisphosphonates, many benefit from orthotics in the shoe to support the longitudinal arch that often collapses as the result of ligamentous laxity.

Families often will invest in a lightweight wheelchair the child can self-propel during times of fracture recovery. For those who have significant bone fragility, a motorized wheelchair is a consideration at this age. With training, the child could safely handle a mobility device allowing age-appropriate peer-related play. These alternative mobility modes do not preclude ambulation but are useful additional mobility options. Regardless of the mode of mobility used, it is imperative to provide the child with a degree of functional independence in the home and in the preschool environment that will promote participation in social activities.

Physical therapists are often consulted on seating issues with children who have OI. Given that most states mandate child safety seats in cars for children younger than 8 years of age, it is important to assist families in proper seating choices once the child has outgrown the infant car seat. Children with the most severe forms of OI are safest in rear-facing seating devices for as long as possible. A five-point harness rather than a seat belt helps to distribute pressure from accidents more evenly. Booster seats should be used until the child meets the size restrictions for the seating; the age restrictions of the law should not be the only focus in these decisions.

School Age and Adolescence

Due to reduced mobility and limited independence in ADLs, school-age children and adolescents often have limited ability to participate in peer-related activities (Table 11.2). Social skill development also may be hampered if the school-age child has been overprotected by caregivers because of overwhelming fear and anxiety regarding fractures. This may have an impact on the school-age child's scholastic endeavors and future vocational achievements. Studies have shown that children with OI tend to have similar temperament to typically developing peers.[73] The child who has negative behavior, including negative moods and high intensity of expression, influences the parent's perception of the difficulty related to dealing with the care of and individual with bone fragility. The severity of the child's disease does not have as big an impact on parental coping as does the child's temperament.[73] Parents and educators should encourage a positive attitude and excellence in school performance to prepare the child for a productive future.

At this age the spine may exhibit varying degrees of deformity. Usually, scoliosis, kyphosis, or both are present, resulting from compression fractures of the vertebrae, osteoporosis, and ligamentous laxity. The child with moderate-to-severe OI typically has marked bowing of the long bones from multiple fractures and growth arrest at the epiphyseal plates. In the femur the neck-shaft angle may be decreased with a coxa vara deformity and acetabular protrusion. The tibia is anteriorly angulated, which, in combination with the angulation of the femur, results in an apparent knee flexion contracture. The patellofemoral joint frequently dislocates, predisposing the patient to falls and fractures. Pes valgus frequently occurs at the ankle. In the upper extremities the humerus is angulated laterally or anterolaterally and the forearms are limited in supination and pronation. The elbows often exhibit cubitus varus deformities, and elbow flexion contractures may be present.

The frequency of fracture tends to decrease markedly after puberty. Possible causes include hormonal changes, increased awareness of how to prevent fractures, improvement in coordination, and increasing bone strength.[31] Paradoxically, the adolescent who senses his or her increased stability and emerging independence may maximize involvement in activities, which increases the risk of more severe types of fractures. In an effort not to discourage these activities and independence, ongoing use of safe methods of mobility, caution, and responsible behavior should be stressed in patient instruction throughout childhood.

Physical therapy management at this stage involves other team members, including professionals in orthopedics, orthotics, occupational therapy, and rehabilitation engineering, to maximize the child's independence in ADLs, mobility, endurance, problem solving, and adjustment to the school environment.

Children and adolescents should be encouraged to be active family members. They should have a share in home-related chores and responsibilities within their functional capacity. This is important because it helps the child learn a level of independence for a lifetime, allows the child to feel valued, and may lessen sibling rivalry.

In this period, physical therapy may be helpful in returning the child to premorbid mobility status after a series of immobilizations from prepubertal fractures. Weight management and physical activity are important at this age.

Management of scoliosis and kyphosis is usually addressed by a spinal fusion, but the long-term results in maintaining alignment are questionable. Back braces have been shown to be ineffective in controlling scoliosis and kyphosis.[7]

Along with occupational therapy, physical therapy can help to maximize the child's independence by identifying safe, energy-efficient positions in which the child can work. Adaptive equipment is imperative for those with severe involvement. Occupational therapists, physical therapists, and rehabilitation engineers work together to adapt wheelchairs and seating and mobility devices to accommodate skeletal deformity, scoliosis, and kyphosis. A variety of lightweight and easily maneuverable manual wheelchairs can be adapted with seating inserts for

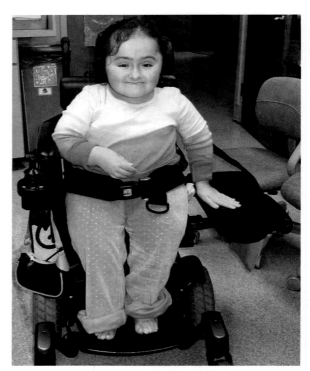

FIG. 11.11 Adolescent using power mobility with a seat elevator and a motorized transfer arm.

trunk control and proper positioning. Vinyl upholstery is usually unsatisfactory for the child with OI because of the propensity for excessive perspiration. Proper wheelchair positioning is critical for prevention of further disabling deformity and for protection of exposed extremities from trauma. Those who do rely on power mobility may benefit from a seat elevator and a motorized transfer arm to allow independence in transfers and ability to access all work surfaces in the home and at school (Fig. 11.11).

The adolescent continues physical therapy to work on ambulation, endurance, and strength. Household ambulation is usually achieved with assistive devices if adequate upper extremity strength is present. Walkers with progression to canes or crutches may be used.

Many children with OI who have primarily used the wheelchair for mobility are now able to ambulate about the house without any special change in their program. It is important to emphasize the maintenance of adequate skeletal alignment and maximal muscular strength throughout childhood to prepare for this improved function as an adolescent and adult. Community ambulation, however, is not practical given the patient's short stature, the energy expenditure required, and the reduced muscle power. Most school-age and older children with OI use wheelchairs for community ambulation.[10] Independence in mobility is paramount because it has been shown to correlate with the degree of adaptation to the community environment. Bachman[5] found that independence in travel away from home was the most important factor in an adolescent's ability to participate successfully outside the school environment.

Strengthening and endurance programs can be most successful when the child participates in developing a program that suits his or her interests and schedule. Of key importance at this age for those who are not ambulatory population is core strength and the ability to sit-scoot. Adequate trunk strength will positively affect the child's ability to assist with transfer and self-care skills throughout adulthood. Programs can consist of progressive resistive exercises using incremental weights, aquatic activity, adaptive sport activities, or computer-assisted physical activity. Enjoyable avocational activities that incorporate functional strengthening and mobility also must be stressed at this age. Although contact sports, such as football, soccer, and baseball, must be avoided, customized athletic and fitness programs are vital for youngsters with OI. These adaptive physical education activities can assist in improving physical health, finding a competitive outlet, helping to discover one's potential, and providing an opportunity to make friends.[17] Sports and recreation activities should be encouraged as an adjunct to therapy. These activities will assist children to develop lifelong fitness interests. Adaptive sports that are available to the child who is interested include swimming, challenger baseball, cycling, boating, non-contact martial arts, adaptive dance, billiards, golf, wheelchair sports, racket sports, and even sled hockey. It is important to keep an open mind when helping a child develop fitness interests. Weigh the benefits against the risks when helping a child make choices. The physical therapist's role is to set appropriate parameters for participation, to provide precautions, and to upgrade the level of activity progressively. Volunteer jobs and social opportunities, such as Boy Scouts and Girl Scouts, encourage emotional growth and develop leadership skills. Experience in a volunteer capacity can be helpful to the adolescent when applying for employment in the future.[27]

Transition to Adulthood

In the transition to adulthood, emphasis needs to be placed on the skills necessary for independent living. Identifying personal goals for education and employment is important for the physical therapist to help to establish a plan of care. Once personal goals are established, the therapist can assist the young adult in problem-solving aspects of the activity to allow participation. The mildly involved person with OI tends not to seek assistance; more involved individuals may need support to address specific goals such as transfers for toileting in public or gaining the skills necessary to run a household without outside assistance. Strategies need to be established to maximize independence with and without the presence of fractures. In the transition to adulthood, appropriate career placement is important, while taking into consideration the patient's intellectual capacity and physical constraints. Because most patients with OI become productive members of society, optimal academic, social, and physical development will enhance their opportunities to succeed in a competitive job market.[10]

In addition to functional independence, those who have OI need to participate in behaviors to enhance lifelong health. These involve regular exercise, weight management, a healthy calcium-rich diet, limited caffeine consumption, and avoidance of smoking tobacco. Therapists need to review how each aspect influences overall health and, more important, the management of osteoporosis.

Some encounter problems with deafness in adult life. Scoliotic curves may be severe and may continue to progress. The incidence of scoliosis approaches 80% to 90% in teenagers and adults.[1] Patients who have OI are especially susceptible to postmenopausal osteoporosis or the osteoporosis of immobilization,[68] when more fractures may occur.[55] Adults with OI also report problems with arthritic changes and back pain.

By the time these children reach adulthood, most moderately involved persons use either manual or power wheelchairs for community mobility. Ambulation consists of household walking with an assistive device.

Case Scenario on Expert Consult

The case scenario related to this chapter illustrates issues related to the many episodes of care children with OI will have secondary to frequent fractures. "Jenna's" needs for mobility are the focus of this case, in which she is followed from early childhood to middle school.

REFERENCES

1. Albright JA: Management overview of osteogenesis imperfecta, *Clin Orthop* 159:80–87, 1981.
2. Alharbi M, Pinto G, Finidori G, et al.: Pamidronate treatment of children with moderate-to-severe osteogenesis imperfecta: a note of caution, *Horm Res* 71:38–44, 2009.
3. Astrom E, Soderhall S: Beneficial effect of bisphosphonate during five years of treatment of severe osteogenesis imperfecta, *Acta Paediatr* 87:64–68, 1998.
4. Astrom E, Soderhall S: Beneficial effect of long term intravenous bisphosphonate treatment of osteogenesis imperfecta, *Arch Dis Child* 86:356–364, 2002.
5. Bachman WH: Variables affecting post school economic adaptation of orthopedically handicapped and other health-impaired students, *Rehabil Lit* 3:98, 1972.
6. Basel D, Steiner RD: Osteogenesis imperfecta: recent findings shed new light on this once well-understood condition, *Genet Med* 11:375–385, 2009.
7. Benson DR, Newman DC: The spine and surgical treatment in osteogenesis imperfecta, *Clin Orthop* 159:147–153, 1981.
8. Binder H, Hawkes L, Graybill G, Gerber NL, Weintrob JC: Osteogenesis imperfecta: rehabilitation approach with infants and young children, *Arch Phys Med Rehabil* 65:537–541, 1984.
9. Black MM, Matula K: *Essentials of Bayley Scales of Infant Development II assessment*, New York, 1999, John Wiley Sons.
10. Bleck EE: Nonoperative treatment of osteogenesis imperfecta: orthotic and mobility management, *Clin Orthop* 159:111–122, 1981.
11. Bluemcke S, Niedorf HR, Thiel HJ, Langness U: Histochemical and fine structural studies on the cornea in osteogenesis imperfecta, *Virchows Arch B Cell Pathol* 11:124–132, 1972.
12. Byers PH: *Osteogenesis imperfecta: an update: growth, genetics and hormones*, vol. 4. New York, 1988, McGraw-Hill. Part 2.
13. Chamberlain JR, Schwarze U, Wang PR, et al.: Gene targeting in stem cells from individuals with osteogenesis imperfecta, *Science* 303:1198–1201, 2004.
14. Cintas HL: Aquatics. In Cintas HL, Gerber LH, editors: *Children with osteogenesis imperfecta: strategies to enhance performance*, Gaithersburg, MD, 2005, Osteogenesis Imperfecta Foundation, pp. 101–121.
15. Cintas HL, Siegel KL, Furst GP, Gerber LH: Brief assessment of motor function: reliability and concurrent validity of the Gross Motor Scale, *Am J Phys Med Rehabil* 82:33–41, 2003.
16. Daly K, Wisbeach A, Sampera Jr I, Fixsen JA: The prognosis for walking in osteogenesis imperfecta, *J Bone Joint Surg Br* 78:477–480, 1996.
17. Donohoe M: Sports and recreation. Chapter 6. In Cintas HL, Gerber LH, editors: *Children with osteogenesis imperfecta: strategies to enhance performance*, Gaithersburg, MD, 2005, Osteogenesis Imperfecta Foundation, pp. 122–160.
18. Doty SB, Matthews RS: Electron microscopic and histochemical investigation of osteogenesis imperfecta tarda, *Clin Orthop* 80:191–201, 1971.
19. Duffield MH: Physiological and therapeutic effects of exercise in warm water. In Skinner AT, Thomson AM, editors: *Duffield's exercise in water*, ed 3, London, 1983, Bailliere Tindall.

20. Engelbert RHH, Gerver WJM, Breslau-Siderius LJ, van der Graaf Y, Pruijs HEH, van Doorne JM: Spinal complication in osteogenesis imperfecta: 47 patients 1-16 years of age, *Acta Orthop Scand* 69:283–286, 1998.

21. Reference deleted in Proofs.

22. Engelbert RH, Uiterwaal CS, van der Hulst A, Witjes B, Helders PJ, Pruijs HE: Scoliosis in children with osteogenesis imperfecta: influence of severity of disease and age of reaching motor milestones, *Eur Spine J* 12:130–134, 2003.

23. Engelbert RH, van der Graaf Y, van Empelen MA, Beemer A, Helders PJM: Osteogenesis imperfecta in childhood: impairment and disability, *Pediatrics* 99:E3, 1997.

24. Falk MJ, Heeger S, Lynch KA, DeCaro KR, Bohach D, Gibson KS, Warman ML: Intravenous biophosphate therapy in children with osteogenesis imperfecta, *Pediatrics* 111:573–578, 2003.

25. Falvo KA, Bullough PG: Osteogenesis imperfecta: a histometric analysis, *J Bone Joint Surg Am* 55:275–286, 1973.

26. Falvo KA, Root L, Bullough PG: Osteogenesis imperfecta: a clinical evaluation and management, *J Bone Joint Surg Am* 56:783–793, 1974.

27. Fehribach G: *Independent living*, Pittsburgh, PA, 1990, Presented before the Osteogenesis Imperfecta Foundation National Convention, August 9, 1990.

28. Folio M, Fewell R: *Peabody Developmental Motor Scales and activity cards*, Allen, TX, 1983, DLM Teaching Resources.

29. Forlino A, Cabral WA, Barnes AM, Marnini JC: New perspectives on osteogenesis imperfecta, *Nat Rev Endocrinol* 7:540–557, 2012.

30. Gerber LH, Binder H, Weintrob J, Grenge DK, Shapiro J, Fromherz W, et al.: Rehabilitation of children and infants with osteogenesis imperfecta: a program for ambulation, *Clin Orthop Rel Res* 251:254–262, 1990.

31. Glorieux F: *Guide to osteogenesis imperfecta for pediatricians and family practice physicians*, Bethesda, MD, 2007, National Institutes of Health Osteoporosis and Related Bone Diseases National Resource Center.

32. Glorieux FH, Rauch F, Plotkin H, Ward L, Travers R, Roughley P, et al.: Type V osteogenesis imperfecta: a new form of brittle bone disease, *J Bone Miner Res* 15:1650–1658, 2000.

33. Glorieux FH, Ward LM, Rauch F, Lalic L, Roughley PJ, Travers R: Osteogenesis imperfecta type VI: a form of brittle bone disease with a mineralization defect, *J Bone Miner Res* 17:30–38, 2002.

34. Haley SM, Faas RM, Coster WJ, Webster H, Gans BM: *Pediatric Evaluation of Disability Inventory*, Boston, 1989, New England Medical Center.

35. Harrington J, Sochett E, Howard A: Update on the evaluation and treatment of osteogenesis imperfecta, *Pediatr Clin North Am* 61:1243–1257, 2014.

36. Horwitz EM, Prockop DJ, Gordon PL, et al.: Clinical responses to bone marrow transplantation in children with severe osteogenesis imperfecta, *Blood* 97:1227–1231, 2001.

37. Hoyer-Kuhn H, Semler O, Stark C, et al.: A specialized rehabilitation approach improves mobility in children with osteogenesis imperfecta, *J Musculoskelet Neuronal Interact* 14(4):445–453, 2014.

38. Jerosch J, Mazzotti I, Tomasvic M: Complications after treatment of patients with osteogenesis imperfecta with a Bailey-Dubow rod, *Arch Orthop Trauma Surg* 117:240–245, 1998.

39. Krakow D, Alanay Y, Rimoin LP, et al.: Evaluation of prenatal-onset osteochondrodysplasias by ultrasonography: a retrospective and prospective analysis, *Am J Med Genet* 146:1917–1924, 2008.

40. Labuda M, Morissette J, Ward LM, et al.: Osteogenesis imperfecta type VII maps to the short arm of chromosome 3, *Bone* 31:19–25, 2002.

41. Landsmeer-Beker EA: Treatment of osteogenesis imperfecta with the bisphosphonate olpadronate (dimethylaminohydroxypropylidene bisphosphonate), *Eur J Pediatr* 156:792–794, 1997.

42. Lips P, Bouillon R, van Schoor NM, Vanderschueren D, Verschueren S, Kuchuk N, et al.: Reducing fracture risk with calcium and vitamin D, *Clin Endocrinol* 73:277–285, 2010.

43. Looser E: Zur Kenntnis der Osteogenesis imperfecta congenita und tardannte idiopathische Osteopsathyrosis, *Mitteilungen Grenzgebieten Medizin Chirurgie* 15:161, 1906 (Translation: Toward an understanding of osteogenesis imperfecta and tarda [also known as idiopathic osteopsathyrosis]. *Transactions of Frontiers of Medicine and Surgery*).

44. Manworren RC, Hynan LS: Clinical validation of FLACC: preverbal patient pain scale, *Pediatr Nurs* 29:140–146, 2003.

45. Marini JC: Should children with osteogenesis imperfecta be treated with bisphosphonates? *Nature Clin Pract Endocrinol Metabol* 2:14–15, 2006.

46. Marini JC, Cabral WA, Barnes AM: Null mutations in LEPRE1 and CRTAP cause severe recessive osteogenesis imperfecta, *Cell Tissues Res* 339:59–70, 2010.

47. Merkel S, Voepel-Lewis T, Malviya S: Pain assessment in infants and young children: FLACC scale, *Am J Nurs* 102:55–58, 2002.

48. Montpetit K, Plotkin H, Pauch F, Bilodeau N, Cloutier S, Rabzel M, Glorieux FH: Rapid increase in grip force after start of pamidronate therapy in children and adolescents with severe osteogenesis imperfecta, *Pediatrics* 111:601–603, 2003.

49. Moore MS, Minch CM, Kruse RW, Harke HT, Jacobson L, Taylor A: The role of dual energy x-ray absorptiometry in aiding the diagnosis of pediatric osteogenesis imperfecta, *Am J Orthop* 27:797–801, 1998.

50. Morris CD, Einhorn TA: Bisphosphonates in orthopaedic surgery, *J Bone Joint Surg Am* 87:1609–1618, 2005.

51. Munns CF, Rauch F, Zeitlin L, Fassier F, Glorieux FH: Delayed osteotomy but not fracture healing in pediatric osteogenesis imperfecta patients receiving pamidronate, *J Bone Miner Res* 19:1779–1786, 2004.

52. Niyibizi C, Wang S, Mi Z, Robbins PD: Gene therapy approaches for osteogenesis imperfecta, *Gene Ther* 11:408–416, 2004.

53. Obafemi AA, Bulas DI, Troendle J, Marini JC: Popcorn calcification in osteogenesis imperfecta: incidence, progression, and molecular correlation, *Am J Med Genet A* 146A:2725–2732, 2008.

54. Parks R, Cintas HL, Chaffin MC, Gerber L: Brief assessment of motor function: content validity and reliability of the fine motor scale, *Pediatr Phys Ther* 19:315–325, 2007.

55. Paterson CR: Clinical variability and life expectancy in osteogenesis imperfecta, *Clin Rheumatol* 14:228, 1995.

56. Poyrazoglu S, Gunoz H, Darendeliler F, et al.: Successful results of pamidronate treatment in children with osteogenesis imperfecta with emphasis on the interpretation of bone mineral density for local standards, *J Pediatr Orthop* 28:483–487, 2008.

57. Primorac D, Rowe DW, Mottes M, Barisic I, Anticevic D, Mirandola S, et al.: Osteogenesis imperfecta at the beginning of bone and joint decade, *Croat Med J* 4:393–415, 2001.

58. Prockop DJ: Targeting gene therapy for osteogenesis imperfecta, *N Engl J Med* 350:2302–2304, 2004.

59. Ramser JR, Frost HM: The study of a rib biopsy from a patient with osteogenesis imperfecta: a method using in vivo tetracycline labeling, *Acta Orthop Scand* 37:229–240, 1966.

60. Rauch F, Glorieux FH: Bisphosphonate treatment in osteogenesis imperfecta: which drug, for whom, for how long? *Ann Med* 37:295–302, 2005.

61. Roughley PJ, Rauch F, Glorieux FH: Osteogenesis imperfecta—clinical and molecular diversity, *Eur Cell Mater* 5:41–47, 2003.

62. Schwartz S: Dental care for children with osteogenesis imperfecta. In Chiasson R, Munns C, Zeitlin L, editors: *Interdisciplinary treatment approach for children with osteogenesis imperfecta*, Canada, 2004, Shriners Hospital for Children, pp 137–150.

63. Scott EF: The use of air splints for mobility training in osteogenesis imperfecta, *Clin Suggest* 2:52–53, 1990.

64. Seedorf KS: Osteogenesis imperfecta: a study of clinical features and heredity based on 55 Danish families comprising 180 affected members, *Opera ex Domo Biologiae Hereditariae Humanae Universitatis Hafniensis* 20:1–229, 1949.

65. Semler O, Fricke O, Vezyroglou K, Stark C, Schoenau E: Improvement of individual mobility in patients with osteogenesis imperfecta by whole body vibration powered by Galileo-System, *Bone* 40:S77, 2007.

66. Semler O, Fricke O, Vezyroglou K, Stark C, Schoenau E: Preliminary results on the mobility after whole body vibration in immobilized children and adolescents, *J Musculoskelet Neuronal Interact* 7:77–81, 2007.

67. Semler O, Fricke O, Vezyroglou K, Stark C, Schoenau E: Results of a prospective pilot trial on mobility after whole body vibration in immobilized children and adolescents with osteogenesis imperfecta, *Clin Rehabil* 22:387–394, 2008.

68. Sillence DO: Osteogenesis imperfecta: expanding panorama of variants, *Clin Orthop Rel Res* 159:11–25, 1981.

69. Sillence DO, Danks DM: The differentiation of genetically distinct varieties of osteogenesis imperfecta in the newborn period, *Clin Res* 26:178A, 1978.

70. Sillence DO, Senn A, Danks DM: Genetic heterogeneity in osteogenesis imperfecta, *J Med Genet* 16:101–116, 1979.

71. Spranger J, Cremin B, Beighton P: Osteogenesis imperfecta congenita, *Pediatr Radiol* 12:21–27, 1982.

72. Stanton D, Wilson PN, Foreman N: Effects of early mobility on shortcut performance in a simulated maze, *Behav Brain Res* 136:61–66, 2002.

73. Suskauer SJ, Cintas HL, Marini JC, Gerber LH: Temperament and physical performance in children with osteogenesis imperfecta, *Pediatrics* 111:E153–E161, 2003.

74. Tachdjian MC: *Pediatric orthopedics*, ed 3, vol. 2. Philadelphia, 2002, WB Saunders.

75. Valadares ER, Carneiro TB, Santos PM, Oliveira AC, Zabel B: What is new in genetics and osteogenesis imperfecta classification? *J Pediatr (Rio J)* 90:536–541, 2014.

76. Van Brussel M, Takken T, Uiterwaal C, Pruijs HJ, Van der Net J, Helders PJM: Physical training in children with osteogenesis imperfecta, *J Pediatr* 152:111–116, 2008.

77. Ward LM, Rauch F, Travers R, et al.: Osteogenesis imperfecta type VII: an autosomal recessive form of brittle bone disease, *Bone* 31:12–18, 2003.

78. Weber M, Roschger P, Fratzl-Zelman N, et al.: Pamidronate does not adversely affect bone intrinsic material properties in children with osteogenesis imperfecta, *Bone* 39:616–622, 2006.

79. Wekre LL1, Froslie KF, Haugen L, Falch JA: A population-based study of demographical variables and ability to perform activities of daily living in adults with osteogenesis imperfecta, *Disabil Rehabil* 32:579–587, 2010.

80. Widmann RF, Laplaza FJ, Bitan FD, Brooks CE, Root L: Quality of life in osteogenesis imperfecta, *Int Orthop* 26:3–6, 2002.

81. Womack J: Osteogenesis imperfecta types I-XI: implications for the neonatal nurse, *Adv Neonat Care* 14:309–315, 2014.

82. Wong D, Baker C: Pain in children: comparison of assessment scales, *Pediatr Nurs* 14:9–17, 1988.

83. Wynne-Davies R, Gormley J: Clinical and genetic patterns in osteogenesis imperfecta, *Clin Orthop Rel Res* 159:26–35, 1981.

84. Zack P, Franck L, Devile C, Clark C: Fracture and non-fracture pain in children with osteogenesis imperfecta, *Acta Paediatr* 94:1238–1242, 2005.

SUGGESTED READINGS

Background

Marini JC: Should children with osteogenesis imperfecta be treated with bisphosphonates? *Nature Clin Prac Endocrinol Metabol* 2:14–15, 2006.

Valadares ER, Carneiro TB, Santos PM, Oliveira AC, Zabel B: What is new in genetics and osteogenesis imperfecta classification? *J Pediatr (Rio J)* 90:536–541, 2014.

Foreground

Brizola E, Staub AL, Felix TM: Muscle strength, joint range of motion, and gait in children and adolescents with osteogenesis imperfecta, *Pediatr Phys Ther* 26(2):245–252, 2014.

Cintas HL, Segel KL, Furst GP, Gerber LH: Brief assessment of motor function: reliability and concurrent validity of the Gross Motor Scale, *Am J Phys Med Rehabil* 82:33–41, 2003.

Engelbert RH, Gulmans VA, Uiterwaal CS, Helders PJ: Osteogenesis imperfecta in childhood: perceived competence in relation to impairment and disability, *Arch Phys Med Rehabil* 82:943–948, 2001.

Hill CL, Baird WO, Walters SJ: Quality of life in children and adolescents with osteogenesis imperfecta: a qualitative interview based study, *Health Qual Life Outcomes* 12:54, 2014. http://doi.org/10.1186/1477-7525-12-54.

Semler O, Fricke O, Vezyroglou K, Stark C, Schoenau E: Results of a prospective pilot trial on mobility after whole body vibration in immobilized children and adolescents with osteogenesis imperfecta, *Clin Rehabil* 22:387–394, 2008.

Suskauer SJ, Cintas HL, Marini JC, Gerber LH: Temperament and physical performance in children with osteogenesis imperfecta, *Pediatrics* 111:E153–E161, 2003.

Van Brussel M, Takken T, Uiterwaal C, Pruijs HJ, Van der Net J, Helders PJM: Physical training in children with osteogenesis imperfecta, *J Pediatr* 152:111–116, 2008.

Wekre LL1, Froslie KF, Haugen L, Falch JA: A population-based study of demographical variables and ability to perform activities of daily living in adults with osteogenesis imperfecta, *Disabil Rehabil* 32:579–587, 2010.

RESOURCES

Osteogenesis Imperfecta Foundation
804 W Diamond Avenue, Suite 210
Gaithersburg, MD 20878
www.oif.org

12

Muscular Dystrophies and Spinal Muscular Atrophy

Allan M. Glanzman, Amanda Kusler, Wayne A. Stuberg

Neuromuscular diseases include disorders of the motor neuron (anterior horn cells and peripheral nerves), neuromuscular junction, and muscle. Duchenne muscular dystrophy (DMD) and spinal muscular atrophy (SMA) are two prevalent, progressive neuromuscular diseases that require physical therapy. Progressive weakness, muscle atrophy, contracture, deformity, and progressive disability characterize both diseases. No cure is available for either disease. Incurable, however, is not synonymous with untreatable, and the physical therapist can be influential in prevention of complications, preservation of function, and maximizing quality of life.

The objective of this chapter is to present an overview of childhood neuromuscular disorders and to discuss the role of the physical therapist as a member of the management team. The clinical presentation of these diseases is reviewed and examination procedures are presented to assist the clinician in identifying impairments and limitations in activity and participation associated with diseases of the muscle and nerve. Guidelines for physical therapy management are outlined and reflect our clinical experience and review of related literature. Background and foreground information are presented throughout, in each of the following condition-specific sections.

ROLE OF THE PHYSICAL THERAPIST

As a member of the management team in the educational or medical setting, the physical therapist assists in identification and amelioration of impairments, as well as in promotion of activity and participation for persons with neuromuscular disorders. The team often includes physician(s) (neurologist, orthopedist, or physiatrist), physical therapist, occupational therapist, nutritionist, speech therapist, educator, social worker, genetic counselor, psychologist, and orthotist. Because therapists typically maintain a higher frequency of contact with families, referral to and ongoing communication with other team members becomes an important part of maintaining continuity of care.

The team approach should be family centered with a focus on collaborative goal setting among affected individuals, family members, and professionals to ensure optimal care.[277] When care is provided using a family-centered philosophy, the pivotal role of the family is recognized and respected in the lives of people with special health care needs.

Prevention is an important role of the physical therapist. Stress on the child/individual and family can be reduced and coping facilitated through accurate prognostic information and recognition of signs that portend changing status and a resultant increase in disability. Examples of status change are seen in the period before the loss of walking, before the need for architectural modifications to accommodate adaptive equipment for mobility, during transition from the educational to the vocational/avocational environment, and during the terminal stages of the disease, when the decision to use mechanical ventilation becomes a major issue.

Providing information to the patient, family, and team regarding physical limitations and expected participation restrictions is an important role of the physical therapist. Many resource materials are available online through the national Muscular Dystrophy Association (MDA) or through Parent Project Muscular Dystrophy for DMD and Cure SMA.

PHYSICAL THERAPY EXAMINATION AND EVALUATION

The progression of the more common neuromuscular disorders is relatively well known, but many of those that are less common can be quite variable and the natural history is often less known. A full understanding of the expected clinical progression is critical to providing quality patient care and being able to anticipate and address the evolution of impairments and their expected functional impacts. The clinician must carefully monitor the child for changes that require intervention and modifications in the context of the expected natural history. As stated by Thomas McCrae (1870–1935), "More is missed by not looking than by not knowing,"[241] but clearly both are important. Ongoing dialogue with families is invaluable in identifying family-centered goals and the need for program modification.

The physical therapy examination is the initial step in management of the child with neuromuscular disorders and should include those components identified in the *Guide to Physical Therapist Practice*.[4] The following domains should be carefully considered and used as appropriate. Please see Chapter 2 for more details on selected measures in these domains.

1. History with family concerns
2. Aerobic capacity and endurance
3. Assistive and adaptive devices
4. Community and work (job/school/play) integration
5. Environmental, home, and job/school/play barriers
6. Gait, locomotion, and balance
7. Integumentary status (when using orthoses, adaptive equipment, or wheelchair)
8. Muscle performance and strength
9. Neuromotor development
10. Orthotic, protective, and supportive devices
11. Posture
12. Range of motion
13. Self-care and home management
14. Ventilation/respiration

Systematic documentation of disease progression is essential for timing interventions during transitions from one functional status to another or during times of increased family need.

DISEASES OF THE MUSCLE

The most prevalent types of muscle disease that typically exhibit initial clinical signs in infancy, childhood, or adolescence are listed in Table 12.1. Emery-Dreifuss muscular dystrophy (humeroperoneal) is very rare and will be discussed only briefly. Limb-girdle muscular dystrophy may exhibit signs late in the first decade or in the second decade of life, and at times the onset of symptoms can occur in early adulthood; therefore along with the adult-onset forms of MD, it is not discussed in this chapter.

Most diseases of the muscle are the result of single gene defects and often have either recessive or dominant inheritance patterns. Here DMD and Becker muscular dystrophy (BMD) will be used as examples of dystrophic muscle disease. The diagnosis of the specific muscle disease is confirmed by genetic testing that identifies a causative gene mutation or by muscle biopsy where an absence of or decrease in the specific protein is noted. The process of diagnosis may include a history, clinical examination, electromyography, muscle ultrasound, blood levels of the muscle enzyme creatine phosphokinase, muscle biopsy, and DNA analysis.[126] Criteria for classification of the various forms of muscular dystrophy (MD) have changed over the years, and various classification systems have been suggested. When the first forms of muscular dystrophy were identified in the 1800s, phenotypic classification was the standard with distribution of weakness, age of onset, and mode of inheritance driving classification. With the growth of light microscopy, various microscopically descriptive diagnostic categorizations invaded the lexicon. In the age of genetics and identified protein products, identifying diagnosis based on the defective protein has become more prevalent.

The primary impairment in all forms of muscular dystrophy is insidious weakness. In congenital forms of muscular dystrophy, the weakness is pronounced at birth and is easily recognizable. In DMD, the weakness becomes evident between age 3 and 5 years. In most diseases of the muscle cognitive function is preserved; however, there are a few exceptions to this. The incidence of intellectual disability is highest in congenital myotonic dystrophy with impairment correlating with physical symptomatology.[26] Cognitive delay is also noted in DMD but it is less frequent.

Secondary impairments in all forms of MD include the development of contractures and postural malalignment. Postural malalignment is seen in antigravity positions of sitting and standing and often includes development of scoliosis. Other secondary impairments include decreased respiratory capacity, cardiac dysfunction, easy fatigability, and, occasionally, obesity, oral motor dysfunction, and impaired GI motility. Although significant intellectual impairment is not usual in DMD, IQ commonly averages 85; 30% of boys with DMD have an IQ below 70.[3] This finding is related to a loss of dystrophin in the brain and is more common with mutations in the region of exons 45–52.[6,52] Learning difficulties are reported in more than 40% and ADHD in almost a third of boys with DMD while cognitive impairment is found in both DMD and BMD although those with BMD appear less impaired.[21,45,285]

With the progression of muscle weakness, increasing caregiver assistance is required for people with DMD to carry out activities of daily living (ADLs). Progressive disability is a hallmark of DMD and requires multidisciplinary team management to maximize participation through the use of adaptive equipment and environmental adaptations.

Physical management is a key intervention in the treatment of DMD because no therapy has been found to be curative.[115,175,191,258] Physical therapy has been used to prolong the child's independence, slow the progression of complications, and improve quality of life.

DYSTROPHIN-ASSOCIATED PROTEINS AND MUSCULAR DYSTROPHY

Over the past 10 years, significant advances have been made in the molecular genetics and pathophysiology of the muscular dystrophies. These advances have followed identification of the genetic defect behind DMD and the missing protein dystrophin. The pathology underlying these diseases results from a fragility in muscle membrane stability during muscle contraction and relative muscle hypoxia as a result of an aberrant vascular response to exercise. This combination results in a progressive loss of muscle contractility caused by the destruction of myofibrils and replacement with fat and connective tissue that can be seen on muscle biopsy as characteristic dystrophic changes.

Dystrophin is present within the muscle cell and has functional attachments to both actin and the transmembrane proteins alpha and beta dystroglycan that allow the transmission of force to the extracellular matrix. These transmembrane proteins along with the sarcoglycans are termed *dystrophin-associated proteins (DAPs).*[27] The DAPs form a complex of extracellular, transmembrane, and intracellular proteins, which are represented in Fig. 12.1.[54,118]

TABLE 12.1	**Muscle Disease Characteristics**		
Type	**Typical Onset**	**Inheritance**	**Course**
Duchenne muscular dystrophy	1–5 years	X-linked	Rapidly progressive; loss of walking typically by 9 to 10 years; death in late teens
Becker muscular dystrophy	5–10 years	X-linked	Slowly progressive; maintain walking past 16; life span into third decade or beyond
Congenital muscular dystrophy	Birth	Recessive	Course dependent on specific genetics variable severity; shortened life span
Congenital myotonic dystrophy	Birth	Dominant	Typically slow with significant intellectual impairment
Childhood-onset facioscapulohumeral	First decade	Dominant/ Recessive	Slowly progressive loss of walking in later life; variable life expectancy
Emery-Dreifuss muscular dystrophy	Childhood to early teens	X-linked	Slowly progressive with cardiac abnormality and normal life span

Dystrophin and the DAP complex as a whole act as an anchor in the intracellular lattice to enhance and transmit tensile strength. The other proteins are thought to act as a physical pathway where various transmembrane signaling molecules anchor.[118] This includes alpha1 syntrophin, which is required for nitric oxide synthase regulation of muscle-specific adrenergic vasoconstriction allowing for appropriate adjustments in blood flow in the face of the metabolic demands experienced during exercise and daily activity. In addition, nitric oxide synthase, which impacts blood flow regulation, also binds with dystrophin. Alpha1 syntrophin also plays a role in regulation of sodium channels, which initiates calcium release and excitation-contraction coupling.[54]

Absence of dystrophin or any of the transmembrane proteins results in suboptimal integration of the complex as a whole and faulty mechanics of the cell membrane and intolerance of the mechanical forces that are experienced during muscle contraction.

DUCHENNE MUSCULAR DYSTROPHY

Background Information

The muscular dystrophies as a group have a prevalence of between 19.8 and 25.1 per 100,000.[259] DMD is the most common X-linked disorder known, with an incidence of about 1 in 3500 live male births.[187] The prevalence of DMD in the general population is reportedly between 1.7 and 4.2 cases per 100,000.[68,187,259] Initial diagnosis in families without a genetic history typically occurs around 5 years of age, although symptoms are often seen earlier and may be attributed to developmental delay.[51] Longevity is variable, from the late teens to the end of the third or into the fourth decade, depending on the rate of disease progression, the presence of complications, and the aggressiveness of cardiopulmonary care, including the use of assisted ventilation.[78]

In the late 1980s Kunkel and associates[141] identified the gene on the X chromosome (Xp21) that, when mutated, causes DMD and BMD; Hoffman and associates[116] then identified the protein (dystrophin). Cloning of the dystrophin gene was the next major accomplishment. These seminal accomplishments provided a mechanism for prenatal or postnatal diagnosis and the differentiation of DMD and BMD from other phenotypically similar limb girdle syndromes.[137]

Muscle cell destruction in DMD and BMD is caused by abnormal or missing dystrophin and its effect at the muscle cell membrane and associated proteins. Mechanical weakening of the sarcolemma, inappropriate calcium influx, aberrant signaling, increased oxidative stress, and recurrent muscle ischemia all combine as mechanisms associated with myofibril damage.[210]

The focus of research for the treatment of DMD is on exploring genetic or molecular, cellular, and pharmacologic therapies that either promote the production of dystrophin or diminish the secondary pathophysiologic consequences including hypoxia and fibrosis.[44,75,191] These interventions include gene- and cell-based replacement therapy, attempts to increase production of other dystrophin-related sarcolemmal proteins such as utrophin, and use of drugs such as steroids. All therapies are in the experimental stage, and the only one that is shown to modify the natural history of the disease is steroid therapy.

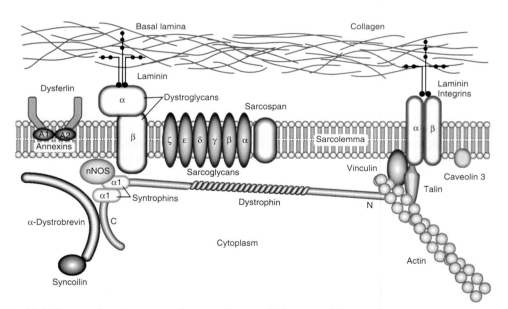

FIG. 12.1 Connections between the muscle cytoskeleton and the extracellular matrix. Actin is linked through integrins to the matrix, as in many cell types. Dystrophin forms an extra link through the dystroglycan-sarcoglycan complex of glycosylated proteins. The helical section of dystrophin is homologous to spectrin and may form homodimers or oligomers. Dystrophin links two intricate systems: the sarcolemma and the basal lamina. The COOH-terminus of dystrophin is associated with the sarcoglycans, dystroglycans, dystrobrevin, syncoilin, nNos, and the syntrophins. The NH 3-terminus links actin, vinculin, and the integrins with laminin and the basil lamina. These two adhesion systems provide a supportive substructure to maintain the integrity of the sarcolemma. The annexins and dysferlin have a role in muscle regeneration. (From Firestein GS, Budd RC, Gabriel SE, et al., editors: *Kelley's textbook of rheumatology.* 9th ed. Philadelphia, Saunders, 2013.)

Genetic therapy research involves exon skipping and stop codon readthrough. Exon skipping involves the use of medication that removes entire exons from the RNA that is used to make the final protein and medication for stop codon readthrough acts to make the ribosome ignore premature stop codon signals during reading of the RNA. Exon skipping with antisense oligonucleotides can cause the damaged exon to be excluded during the splicing process, removing the damaged exon and reestablishing the reading frame. When the abnormal exon is removed, the reading frame of the ribosome is reestablished and a partially functional protein is produced.[172] In the case of mutations that cause a stop codon, medications that promote the ribosome to continue reading despite the premature stop codon facilitate the production of dystrophin.

Another strategy for genetic therapy is the introduction of a custom-made mini dystrophin gene that is delivered in a viral vector. The gene must be modified because of dystrophins' large size so it fits in the vector. It is also important that it is modified to retain the functional binding domains of dystrophin but is small enough to be packaged in a virus. Pharmacologic approaches can focus on protein upregulation as a replacement for dystrophin; primarily these have focused on utrophin. Utrophin is a muscle protein that has molecular similarity to dystrophin. Utrophin levels in the muscle are high in the fetus and newborn but gradually diminish. Utrophin is found primarily at the neuromuscular or musculotendinous junction in adults and in children with DMD. Utrophin levels have been shown to increase in the mouse model of DMD through upregulation.[56,260] It is hypothesized that utrophin might act as a substitute for abnormal or missing dystrophin.[209] Upregulation of other compensatory proteins such as integrin and sarcospan has been reported in animal models, but human clinical trials have not yet begun.[158,191]

Pharmacologic approaches can also focus on ameliorating the downstream mechanisms that are at the heart of the impairment in individuals with DMD. This includes muscle fiber necrosis, fibrosis, and calcification in addition to muscle inflammation and hypoxia.[139] Currently there is preliminary support for the roll of tadalafil in alleviating muscle hypoxia in boys with DMD, and clinical trials are ongoing to evaluate the impact of this on function.[190] The use of creatine in boys with DMD has demonstrated improved muscle strength and endurance and a reduction in joint stiffness.[20,73,136,148] Louis and colleagues also reported improved bone mineral density in boys who were wheelchair users, suggesting that the negative effects of steroids on bone mineral density might be offset by the use of creatine. However, the impact is small: on the order of less than 9% in terms of muscle. Other downstream mechanistic targets are in various stages of evaluation and many show promise but have yet to reach clinical trials.

Long-term steroid use (prednisone and deflazacort) has been shown to improve outcomes, including prolonged walking by up to 3 years, improved isometric muscle strength by 60% in the arms and 85% in the legs when compared with untreated control subjects, and improved pulmonary function and possibly even cognitive skills.[22,24,28,115,175,229,284] Reported side effects, however, include weight gain (particularly with prednisone), growth suppression, cataracts, and osteoporosis. Strict dietary controls to offset the side effects are recommended.[284] Deflazacort is available outside of the United States, although it has not been approved by the FDA.

Although it is commonly agreed that the prevention of contractures and the preservation of independent mobility are primary goals of a physical management program,[266] the prolongation of ambulation through surgery remains controversial. Some authors promote the use of surgery and lightweight knee-ankle-foot orthoses (KAFO)[13,18,111,120,178,256]; others express skepticism about prolonging the inevitable in a progressive disease, when the financial and emotional costs to the family may be very high.[88] Evidence is available that the use of steroids and supported walking and standing with KAFOs are associated with reduced risk of scoliosis development and later onset of scoliosis.[134] A decreasing trend in the use of KAFOs from 69% of the MDA clinics surveyed in 1989 to 27% in 2000 has been reported[12] and would suggest a trend of less aggressive orthotic management in this population. Consistent recommendations regarding the use of KAFOs for prolonged walking or standing are important, and a recognition of and discussion of the characteristics of ambulation with KAFOs are often helpful in guiding the parents in this choice. Ambulation with KAFOs is always exercise ambulation and not functional because assistance will be needed transferring to and from standing.

Surgical management has focused on control of lower extremity contractures, use of orthoses in conjunction with surgery to prolong ambulation, and spinal stabilization for control of scoliosis. Achilles tendon lengthening and fasciotomy of the tensor fasciae latae and iliotibial bands are two procedures commonly reported to be used either in conjunction with KAFOs and physical therapy to prolong ambulation or maintain standing[13,81,105,120,155] or early in the course of the disease to correct initial onset of contracture. The latter approach has been accompanied by occasional loss of ambulation if the musculotendinous unit is overlengthened and ground reaction forces are diminished. Posterior tibialis transfer into the third cuneiform to reverse equinovarus deformity has also been reported.[120]

Surgical management of scoliosis typically includes the use of spinal instrumentation with segmental fixation.[157] With the increased prevalence of steroid treatment, the incidence of scoliosis has declined[142]; however, boys with DMD still have an increased risk of developing severe scoliosis.[217] Orthotic management has not been shown to stop the progression of the curve,[112] but fusion to avoid development of a significant curve may allow some functional benefit related to sitting balance and comfort.[134,252] For many boys, spinal fusion is also met with some functional challenges that the physical therapist needs to be aware of and address proactively. All boys have a lack of spinal motion as a result of the fusion, and often when they rely on spinal (and neck) flexion to bring their mouth to their hand when feeding this can be a challenge following surgery and use of a ball bearing feeder, of which there are many kinds. Some feeders have elastic properties that drive a 4-bar linkage to unweight the arm, like the Wilmington Robotic ExoSkeleton, and to assist with antigravity movement while others are of a more basic design.[74,110] Ball bearing feeders are helpful following surgery and should be in place prior to spine surgery so that the individual can become accustomed to use of the device.

Impairments, Activity Limitations, and Participation Restrictions

Examination of the 4- to 5-year-old child demonstrates the onset of classical clinical features of DMD and primary impairment of muscle weakness. The posterior calf is usually enlarged as a result of fatty and connective tissue infiltration, which is the origin of the term *pseudohypertrophic muscular*

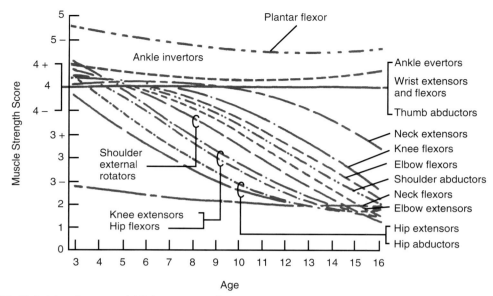

FIG. 12.2 Muscle strength 50th percentile lines plotted against age of 150 children with Duchenne muscular dystrophy (Redrawn from Brooke, MH: *A clinician's view of neuromuscular diseases.* 2nd ed. Baltimore, Williams & Wilkins, 1986.)

dystrophy. Pseudohypertrophy occasionally can be seen to affect the deltoid, quadriceps, or forearm extensor muscle groups. Initial weakness of the neck flexor, abdominal, interscapular, and hip extensor musculature can be noted, with a more generalized distribution with progression of the disease. Fig. 12.2 demonstrates the trends of muscle strength decline up to age 16 years from a study by Brooke.[34] These data were obtained in a multiclinic study of 150 children with DMD over a follow-up period of 3 to 4 years. The data represent approximately 15 data points per boy, as recorded during follow-up visits. Similar findings on anthropometric data, range of motion, spinal deformity, pulmonary function, and functional skills were reported by McDonald and colleagues[167] in a cohort of 162 boys with DMD followed over a 3-year period and for the 6-minute walk test and dynamometry in over 400 boys.[96,166]

Muscle strength can be documented using manual muscle testing (MMT), which has been reported to have acceptable intrarater reliability,[80] although it is not as sensitive as using specialized devices such as a dynamometer. Instruments such as a handheld dynamometer[248] or strain gauge devices[37] can be used to obtain objective strength recordings in the older child to assist in monitoring the progression of the disease process. Timed functional activities have also been shown to be closely correlated to muscle strength and are predictive of loss of ambulation. Ten-meter walk/run time more than 9 seconds and inability to rise from the floor predict loss of ambulation within 2 years, and a 10-meter time of more than 12 seconds predicts loss of ambulation loss within 1 year.[164]

No limitations in range of motion (ROM) are typically noted before 5 years of age in DMD. Mild tightness of the gastrocnemius-soleus and tensor fasciae latae muscles usually occurs first. The normal lordotic standing posture is increased, and mild winging of the scapulae is then seen as compensation to keep the center of mass behind the hip joint to promote standing stability (Fig. 12.3). Scoliosis typically develops just before or during adolescence.

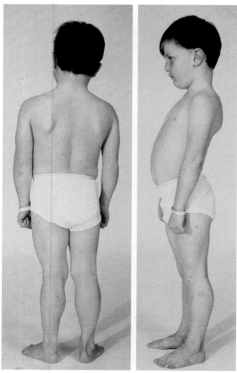

FIG. 12.3 A patient with typical Duchenne dystrophy; notice prominent lordosis and winging of the scapulae and mild calf muscle enlargement. (From Bertorini TE: *Neuromuscular case studies.* Philadelphia, Butterworth-Heineman/Elsevier, 2008.)

Foreground Information
Management Considerations

An international collaboration recently published a consensus document on the management and outcome measurement for patients with DMD.[39,40] More specific information related to

---

BOX 12.1   Evidence-Based Tests and Measures

Duchenne Muscular Dystrophy
Body Functions and Body Structures
Goniometry
Handheld myometry
Manual muscle testing
Quantitative muscle testing (for DMD)
Pulmonary function testing

Activity: Single Task
6-minute walk test
Timed testing (10-m walk/run, time up 4 steps, timed Gowers', timed sit-to-stand)
9-hole peg test

Activity: Multiple Items
Northstar ambulatory assessment
The Performance of Upper Limb for Duchenne
Motor function measure
Brook Scale (classification)
Vignos Scale (classification)

Participation: Multiple Items
Health Utilities Index Questionnaire
PEDS QL
Egen Klassifikation Scale

Spinal Muscular Atrophy
Body Functions and Body Structures
Goniometry
Handheld myometry
Manual muscle testing
Quantitative muscle testing (for SMA)
Pulmonary function testing

Activity: Single Task
6-minute walk test

Activity: Multiple Items
Northstar ambulatory assessment
Revised upper limb module for SMA
Motor function measure

Participation: Multiple Items
Pediatric Evaluation of Disability Index
PEDS QL
Egen Klassifikation Scale

---

physical therapy management by age and progression follows. See Box 12.1 for key tests and measures.

Infancy to Preschool-Age Period. Impairments, activity limitations, and participation restrictions typically seen in the infant or toddler with DMD are related to delayed development. Gardner-Medwin[89] reported that half of the children fail to walk until 18 months of age. Delay in walking, however, rarely leads to the diagnosis of DMD. Symptoms of obvious weakness are seldom noted before age 3 to 5 years unless the family history is positive and caregivers are looking for early signs. The mean age at diagnosis is usually reported to be around 5 years.[178]

Although no significant disability occurs in early childhood, many disability-related issues must be addressed. The family will have questions regarding peer interaction, routine activity level for the child, and the prognosis. The therapist must be aware of each family's coping response, goals, and needed supports, to provide family-centered care. This is the appropriate time to discuss with the family the social aspects of the disability and to answer questions without portraying a future without hope. Given the established natural history related to contracture of the ankle anticipatory guidance related to early night splinting and range of motion can be considered at this time.

Early School-Age Period. Initial limitations in activity in DMD typically become more apparent by age 5 years and include clumsiness, falling, and inability to keep up with peers while playing. The young child's gait pattern is only slightly atypical, with an increased lateral trunk sway (compensated Trendelenburg). Attempts at running, however, accentuate the waddling pattern, and running is marked by a high step pattern with limited push off. Gowers' sign (through plantar grade using the arms to push on the thighs to attain standing) is usually present when the child transitions from the floor to assuming a standing position (Fig. 12.4).

Stair climbing and arising to standing from the floor become progressively more difficult and signal the first significant functional limitation by age 6 to 8 years. Progressive changes in the gait pattern include deviations of an increased base of support, pronounced lateral trunk sway (compensated Trendelenburg), toe-walking, and lordosis with retraction of the shoulders with lack of reciprocal arm swing. Toe-walking initially may be a compensation for weakness of the abdominal and hip extensor muscles or may be related to limited ankle range of motion and the inability to attain a comfortable plantar grade posture. A restrictive pattern of pulmonary impairment and progressive decline in maximal vital capacity also becomes increasingly evident.[87]

Physical therapy management typically begins when the child is initially diagnosed at age 3 to 5 years. Goals of the program are to provide family support and education, obtain baseline data on muscle strength and ROM, monitor for the progression of muscle weakness that will lead to limitations in activity and participation, and, most importantly, maintain flexibility. Initial therapeutic input should not be burdensome to the child or family and is typically limited to ankle stretches and night splinting because the child is usually independent in all ADLs before the age of 5 years.

Information should be provided to the family pertaining to the therapist's role as a member of the management team. An appropriate activity level to avoid fatigue should be discussed with the family and school staff. Information on services available through the local MDA office should be provided, including identification of support groups or contact families.

Strength and exercise. Muscle weakness is apparent in the school-age child by age 6 to 8 years and should be objectively documented using a handheld dynamometer,[248] electrodynamometer,[228] isokinetic dynamometer,[180,231] or other device. Use of a dynamometer in conjunction with manual muscle testing has been shown to provide reliable information on the progression of weakness in key muscle groups.[37,83,248] Contracture development should be documented using goniometry and a standardized protocol. Intrarater reliability of measurements has been shown to be acceptable in

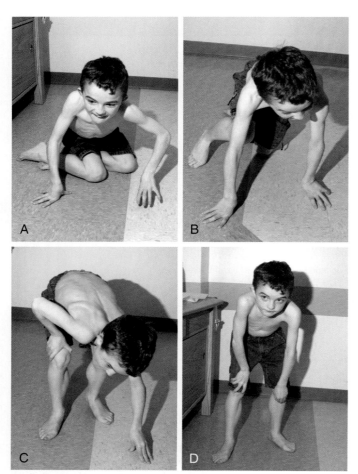

FIG. 12.4 Gowers' sign in a boy with hip girdle weakness due to Duchenne muscular dystrophy. When asked to rise from a prone position (A), the patient uses his hands to walk up his legs to compensate for proximal lower extremity weakness (C–D). (From Kliegman RM, Stanton B, St. Geme J, et al., editors: *Nelson textbook of pediatrics*. 20th ed. Philadelphia, Elsevier, 2016.)

providing objective information for program planning when a standardized measurement protocol is used.[199]

The role of exercise in the treatment of DMD is controversial.[7,8,82,104,266] It is widely accepted that both eccentric strenthening[48,121,125,269] and immobilization[269] are detrimental. The use of graded resistive exercise has been reported to have a range of results from good[268] to limited[59] to adverse.[7] Resistive exercise theoretically would be indicated with the disproportionate loss of type II (fast-twitch) muscle fibers in DMD.[67] However, the use of resistive exercise in the young school-age child with DMD should not be universally prescribed. An early submaximal endurance exercise program has been shown to have beneficial effects.[84,97] However, the optimal characteristics of exercise and intensity are not well understood and such an approach should be offered only to families who have a specific desire to include it in the child's program.[123] Consideration should be given to the fact that significant muscle weakness is not seen in the early stage of the disease, and the use of an exercise program may be burdensome to the child and family.

If exercise is initiated early, the key muscle groups to be included are the abdominal, hip extensor and abductor, and knee extensor groups. Cycling and swimming are excellent activities for overall conditioning and are often preferred over formal exercise programs.[3,8,89,124,266] Standing or walking for a minimum of 2 to 3 hours daily has also been recommended.[240,286] High-resistance and eccentric exercise should be avoided; however, the characteristics required to optimize exercise are clearly still controversial.[7,8,9,43]

Range of motion. One of the primary considerations in the early management program of the young school-age child is to slow the development of contractures. Contractures have not been shown to be preventable, but their progression can be slowed with positioning and a ROM program.[122,232,234,283] The initial ROM program should include stretching the gastrocnemius-soleus and, later, the hamstrings and tensor fasciae latae. Progressive contracture of the gastrocnemius-soleus and tensor fasciae latae corresponds to gait deviations of toe-walking and increased base of support. Stretching for the gastrocnemius-soleus for older children can be done using a standing runner's stretch. The child stands on a supportive surface, places one leg back at a time with the knee straight, and leans forward. The position also assists with maintenance of hip flexor flexibility; however, specific stretching for the hip flexors should be included when any limitation is noted. Having the child lie supine with one thigh off the edge of a mat or bed and the other held to the chest (Thomas test position) can be used to stretch the hip flexors initially. An alternative method is discussed later for use as progression of hip extensor weakness evolves. A standing stretch for the tensor is accomplished by having the child stand with one side toward the supportive surface with the feet away from the wall and with the knee kept straight while leaning sideways toward the supportive surface.

A home ROM program should be emphasized for the young child, and the family should be instructed in the stretching activities because self-stretch in young children is often not effective. Agreement is lacking as to the frequency and duration of the stretching program. Suggested frequency of the program varies from once daily[89,178,232] to twice daily,[269,286] and duration from 1 repetition up to 10; however, total end range time is likely an important factor as well.[269] Other authors have suggested a time frame of 10[283] to 20[89] minutes to complete the stretching exercises. As a general recommendation, each movement should be repeated for five repetitions with a 30- to 60-second hold in the stretched position. The stretch should be done slowly and should not be painful. A good rule is to use the child's tolerance to guide the program because stretching needs to be a continuous process over the life span. Developing a good relationship with the child and allowing him or her a degree of control over what can be at times uncomfortable are important factors in successful implementation. Reassessment of the contracture progression should be used as the final guide to stretching frequency and duration.

The ROM program can often be part of the physical education program at school. Instruction should be provided to the physical education teacher to develop an adapted program, particularly if the teacher does not have an adapted physical education endorsement. General physical education activities will require modification for the child's participation and should not be exhaustive. Physical fitness test activities such as push-ups, sit-ups, or timed running for long time periods should be modified or excluded to avoid fatigue or overwork weakness.

Night splints are helpful for slowing the progression of ankle contractures and should allow positioning at comfortable end range. Scott and associates[232] studied the efficacy of night splints and a home ROM program in a group of 59 boys diagnosed with MD and ranging in age from 4 to 12 years. Subjects were categorized into three groups on the basis of adherence with splint wear and use of stretching. The group that followed through on the daily passive stretching program and the use of below-knee splints over the 2 years of the study demonstrated significantly less progression of Achilles tendon contractures and less deterioration in functional skills, leading to a longer period of independent walking. Boys in the group who did not follow through on the stretching or splint program lost independent walking at a younger age. In a randomized study comparing the effects of ROM exercise versus ROM and night splints, the combined intervention was found to be 23% more effective than ROM alone in slowing the progression of posterior calf contracture.[122] Similar findings were reported in a study by Seeger and colleagues,[234] which compared the use of night splints, stretching, and surgery. For those who are unable to adhere to night splinting and stretching regimens, serial casting is an option to improve range of motion. However, one must be cognizant of the fact that the gain in range of motion in this population is slower and the risk of tendonitis and falls is greater than other populations that use serial casting. Therefore it should be reserved for individuals who are relatively more functional and can rise from the floor without assistance.[92,153]

The use of prone positioning at night to slow the progression of hip and knee flexion contractures may be possible if tolerated by the child. The recommendation to have the child sleep prone with the ankles off the edge of the bed has not been shown to affect the progression of knee flexion contractures but is theoretically beneficial. Additionally, the progression of knee flexion contractures is slow prior to loss of ambulation and therefore generally does not impact function until the child is using a wheelchair full time.

Respiratory function and spinal alignment. A clinical estimate of respiratory function can be obtained through measurement of respiratory rate and chest wall excursion (using a tape measure) and by noting the child's ability to cough and clear secretions. A portable spirometer is recommended to obtain a more direct and objective reading of expiratory capacity before formal pulmonary function testing is needed. Breathing exercises have been shown to slow the loss of vital capacity and forced expiratory flow rate.[138,160,222] Game activities such as inflating balloons or using blow-bottles to maintain pulmonary function can easily be included in a home program and will decrease the severity of symptoms during episodes of colds or other pulmonary infections. Inspiratory muscle training has also been investigated in patients with DMD and has good support in the literature with short-term follow-up.[261]

Scoliosis is not common when the child is ambulatory, but the spine should be checked routinely.[134] Kinali and associates[134] report an incidence of scoliosis ranging from 68% to 90% in boys with DMD who are not on steroids. Onset is typically seen after cessation of standing at around 12 years; however, this has become significantly more variable with the increased use of steroids in this population and many boys don't develop scoliosis. Postural analysis using the forward bend test is recommended to monitor spinal alignment for scoliosis. The presence of a rib hump with the forward bend test verifies a structural versus functional curve of the spine. Amendt and colleagues[1] demonstrated that a rib hump measuring at least 5° of inclination with a scoliometer is a reliable method and can be correlated with radiographic assessment. Although the study by Amendt and colleagues[1] was not inclusive of children with DMD, it demonstrates an objective method of performing noninvasive screening for scoliosis. Orthopedic referral is indicated if a rib hump is documented. Surgical intervention for scoliosis is ideally completed while the curve is still flexible and pulmonary function relatively intact and may not be possible for individuals when vital capacity values fall below 30% of age norm values.[156]

Functional mobility, equipment, and participation. An examination to document limitations in activity and participation is essential. Various formats have been reported[245,270] that are variations of the guidelines initially published by Swinyard and associates.[255] A classification system published by Vignos and colleagues[269] is outlined in Box 12.2. A more detailed examination format for DMD published by Brooke and associates[35] includes pulmonary function and timed performance of activities, the latter of which along with the 6-minute walk test (6MWT) (see Chapter 2) has become a standard measurement tool in patients with DMD.[201] Normative data for DMD have been published using the clinical protocol of Brooke and associates.[34] A similar assessment called the North Star Ambulatory Assessment (NSAA) has been devised and reliability established for use in multicenter clinical trials.[60,163] The assessment tool chosen will depend on the diagnosis because tools vary in their responsiveness depending on the rate of progression and pattern of progression of the various types of muscular dystrophy.[39,149] Other functional assessment tools, such as the Performance of Upper Limb (PUL) for DMD, Pediatric Evaluation of Disability Inventory (PEDI)[107,200] (see Chapter 2), the School Function Assessment (SFA)[55] (see Chapter 2), the Egen Klassifikation (EK) Scale,[245] or the Barthel Index,[189] should also be considered to obtain more specific information on the child's functional skills. The EK Scale, which was recently validated for DMD and SMA, includes ordinal scoring of 10 categories, including items on mobility, transfers, ability to cough/speak, and physical well-being and reflects the untreated natural history of the disease. The PEDI, the SFA, or

---

BOX 12.2   Vignos Functional Rating Scale for Duchenne Muscular Dystrophy

1. Walks and climbs stairs without assistance
2. Walks and climbs stairs with aid of railing
3. Walks and climbs stairs slowly with aid of railing (over 25 seconds for eight standard steps)
4. Walks, but cannot climb stairs
5. Walks assisted, but cannot climb stairs or get out of chair
6. Walks only with assistance or with braces
7. In wheelchair: Sits erect and can roll chair and perform bed and wheelchair ADLs
8. In wheelchair: Sits erect and is unable to perform bed and wheelchair ADLs without assistance
9. In wheelchair: Sits erect only with support and is able to do only minimal ADLs
10. In bed: Can do no ADLs without assistance

Data from Vignos PJ, Spencer GE, Archibald KC: Management of progressive muscular dystrophy. *JAMA* 184:103-112, 1963. Copyright © 1963, American Medical Association.

the Vignos (Brooke) functional testing format can be used for diagnosis of other types of MD or SMA.

Falls and complaints of fatigue while walking become increasingly more frequent as the child reaches age 8 to 10 years. Guarding during stair climbing or during general walking should be considered to ensure safety as balance becomes tenuous. As weakness progresses it is important to maintain an open dialogue with the family regarding the risk of falls and potentially fractures. This discussion should also focus on the risks of restricting mobility to prevent falls, recognizing the disuse atrophy that can accompany restriction beyond what is necessary for safety. Each parent will balance the risks and benefits of end-stage ambulation differently and needs to be supported through this process. A manual wheelchair, stroller, or scooter with appropriate fit and accessories will allow for limited mobility as walking becomes more difficult. As progression of weakness in the trunk and hip girdle begins to make walking difficult, a similar amount of weakness of the shoulder girdle musculature is also present, making propulsion of a manual wheelchair difficult, except on level and smooth surfaces such as linoleum. A motorized scooter should be considered to provide the child with independence provided that access is available in the home and school (Fig. 12.5). Ideally a scooter (or stroller) is obtained well in advance of loss of ambulation, when there are many years of walking ahead. It is often used for long community trips and should be considered when the family begins to select options for entertainment based on what activities the child has the endurance to participate in. When this is the case, a mobility device can help the child regain access to those marginal activities, which is emotionally positive for the child and family because loss of ambulation is not a risk at that stage.

Information should be made available to families concerning recreational activities provided through the local chapter of the MDA or other groups. Summer MDA camp is a wonderful experience for most children, and a support group is often developed for the child or family through participation in MDA and other group activities that provide both physical and emotional support (Boxes 12.3 and 12.4).

Adolescent Period. Adolescence marks a time of significant progression of physical symptomatology that results from the combined impact of muscle weakness and contractures. Walking is typically lost as a means of mobility, and increasing difficulty in mobility and transfers is seen. Use of powered mobility becomes necessary during adolescence. When powered mobility is used, assistance with finances for the purchase of equipment or home modifications for access is typically needed, with coordination through a social worker or an MDA patient services coordinator. Many MDA offices have equipment pools that allow families to borrow equipment, including power chairs, at no cost. Changes in physical capacity such as muscle strength and pulmonary function using the EK Scale have been reported among adolescents by Steffensen and colleagues.[244] Muscle weakness leads to increasing difficulty with ADLs, including dressing, transfers, bathing, grooming, and feeding. Physical and occupational therapists can help during this time by providing adaptive equipment or alternate strategies. Surgical intervention may be considered for the management of scoliosis[47] or contractures or to prolong exercise ambulation with the use of orthoses if this is the family's choice.[18]

Exercise and range of motion. With the cessation of walking in late childhood or early adolescence, the emphasis

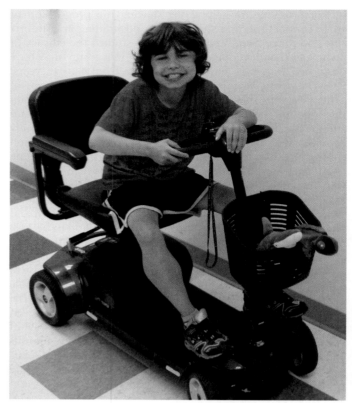

FIG. 12.5 Motorized three-wheeled scooter for independence in distance mobility as an adjunct to walking.

BOX 12.3 **Evidence-Based Examinations for Children With DMD**

Body Functions and Body Structures
Goniometry
Handheld myometry
Manual muscle testing
Quantitative muscle testing
Pulmonary function testing

Activity: Single Task
6-minute walk test

Timed Testing (Time and Grade)
Timed up/down 4 steps
Timed Gowers'
Timed 10-m run/walk

Activity: Multiple Items
Northstar ambulatory assessment
Performance Upper Limb Module for DMD
Motor function measure

Participation: Multiple Items
Pediatric Evaluation of Disability Index
PEDS QL
Egen Klassifikation Scale
Health Utilities Index Questionnaire

From Brooke MH, Griggs RC, Mendell JR, Fenichel GM, Shumate JB, Pellegrino RJ: Clinical trial in Duchenne dystrophy: I. The design of the protocol. *Muscle Nerve* 4:186-197, 1981.

BOX 12.4 Evidence-Based Interventions for Children With DMD

Body Functions and Body Structures

Stretching
Night splinting at end range
Concentric endurance exercise (pool, bike, non–weight bearing)
Inspiratory muscle training
Cough assist/BiPAP with respiratory insufficiency (per pulmonary)
Percussion and postural drainage (with upper respiratory infection)

Activity

Standing program prior to or at cessation of ambulation
Mobile arm support with feeding difficulty or prior to spinal fusion

Participation

Power mobility
Environmental modification
Ramps
Bathroom adaptation or equipment
Van with lift/tie down
Assistive tech for computer access (onscreen keyboard dictation programs etc.)
Adapted gym/sport activity

---

of an endurance exercise program should shift from the lower extremities to the upper extremities. More important, however, active endurance exercise should be encouraged by having the adolescent assist as much as possible in ADLs such as grooming, upper body dressing, and feeding through consultation with an occupational therapist and by either a pool or upper extremity ergometry program.[3] Key muscle groups for maintenance of strength for transfers include the shoulder depressors and triceps. The shoulder flexor and abductor and elbow flexor muscle groups are key areas for exercises to maintain routine ADLs such as self-feeding and hygiene. Weakness of the upper arm musculature by 16 years of age makes ADLs extremely difficult, and consideration of mobile arm support is important when these activities are effortful in advance of a complete inability to participate in feeding and grooming.

The ROM program will require further modification as the adolescent becomes nonambulatory. Gentle stretching of the ankle, hamstrings, hip flexors, and iliotibial band that were initiated in the school-age child should be continued to maintain flexibility. Additionally, stretching of the long finger flexors, shoulder, and elbow should be included as indicated. Limitations in shoulder flexion and abduction, elbow extension, forearm supination, and wrist extension are most common.

Once ambulation is lost, the focus of manual stretching often needs to shift. Contracture of the ankle and knee that typically accompanies the loss of ambulation can be diminished with the use of a standing program, and splinting can be used either in the daytime or night depending on preference. Contractures should continue to be monitored to ensure that they do not become an obstacle to routine ADLs, and the focus of the range of motion and splinting programs needs to be shifted to maintaining upper extremity flexibility and functional skills. Typical upper extremity contractures that begin to develop at this stage include the forearm pronators, elbow flexors, and long finger flexors. Later in the course of the disease the thumb adductors also become affected. The shoulder musculature is also at risk

for contracture but is much less functionally relevant due to the severe proximal weakness that is present. However, maintenance of shoulder ROM might be important in the context of any shoulder pain that might develop later in the course of the disease.

Respiratory function and spinal alignment. Maintaining the spine in a neutral or slightly extended position is essential to slow the formation of a scoliosis. The spine should be in slight extension to increase weight bearing through the facet joints, minimize truncal rotation and lateral flexion, and slow the progression of scoliosis formation.[90] The lordotic posture in the ambulant child is suggested to delay development of spinal collapse, and prolonging ambulation can slow the development of scoliosis.[119] Spinal orthoses have not been shown to prevent development of a significant scoliotic curve.[41,53] Custom-molded seating inserts, corsets, and modular seating inserts are options to provide trunk support in an attempt to slow the progression of the scoliosis. However, studies comparing the three methods of spinal control in DMD have concluded that the progression of the curvature was not significantly changed by any of them.[53,235]

With the use of corticosteroids the risk of developing scoliosis that requires surgical intervention has been reduced from 90% to only 15% to 20% of patients.[119,142] When necessary, early surgical intervention is recommended for the control of scoliosis through the use of segmental spinal instrumentation with Luque rods or similar techniques.[157,177,237] Miller and associates[177] have reported improved quality of life, attainment of a balanced sitting posture, and more normal alignment following surgical intervention for scoliosis.[119,142,143] Suk and colleagues[252] have reported reduced rates of pulmonary function decline following spinal fusion as compared to no surgical intervention. Pulmonary complications are reported as minimal if forced vital capacity is at least 30% of normal age-predicted values.[5]

Continuation of standing or walking. As muscle weakness becomes more pronounced in the trunk and hip musculature and as contractures of the hip flexors, tensor fasciae latae, and gastrocnemius-soleus progress, walking becomes increasingly difficult until cessation of independent walking occurs, usually by age 10 to 12. If orthoses or a stander is used to maintain a standing or walking program, it should be initiated before the child reaches the stage of being nonambulatory. If a stander is the choice, one might consider ordering one when the 10-meter walk time falls below about 9 seconds so that the child can begin a standing program prior to the loss of ambulation.

The use of orthoses for a standing program or continuation of supported walking is not appropriate for all individuals; in fact, this should be considered a personal rather than a therapeutic decision. Although a standing program may be useful to slow the progression of contractures, a braced walking program has little long-term functional or practical application aside from contracture prevention. The child will eventually use a wheelchair, so it is often easier for the child to accept this transition rather than hold on to ambulation when it is no longer functional. Continuation of standing through use of a standing frame, knee immobilizers, or KAFOs is a goal at our facility to address the issue of decreased bone mineral density[168] and subsequent increased risk of contracture and fracture.[23] Because surgery is often required in addition to orthotics for prolonged ambulation, there are additional risks associated with this option. The parents and the adolescent must agree to balance these risks with a realistic informed view of the characteristics and functionality of ambulation that will be gained. Prolongation of ambulation through surgery and orthotics is not a common goal. More typically, power mobility, adaptive equipment, and environmental adaptations provide for a more functional experience and tend to optimize quality of life.

Prognostic factors for success that should be considered in making the decision to use orthoses to prolong walking include residual muscle strength (approximately 50%)[266]; absence of severe contractures; timely application of braces[13]; residual walking ability[267]; and motivation of the child and family.[32] The degree of cognitive impairment and obesity should also be considered. The timely use of orthoses has been shown to prolong walking.[13,32,111]

If the decision to use orthoses to prolong standing or walking is made, KAFOs should be prescribed (Fig. 12.6).[18,32] The characteristics of ambulation with KAFOs should be reviewed with the patient and family including the need for assistance with transferring from sitting to standing so that an informed choice can be made before pursuing these devices. Ankle-foot orthoses (AFOs) are appropriate for positioning but do not provide the knee stability required to avoid falls while walking. Although the use of AFOs to control equinus is common for other diagnoses such as cerebral palsy, with DMD the orthoses often interfere with walking speed and step length.[263] Assistive devices such as standard walkers, crutches, or canes are seldom functional because of the degree of proximal shoulder girdle and upper extremity muscle weakness that is present. Standby assistance

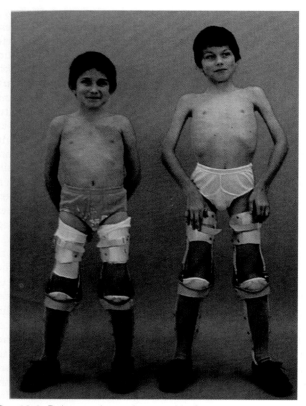

FIG. 12.6 Polypropylene knee-ankle-foot orthosis on two brothers (ages 12 yr and 9 yr) with Duchenne muscular dystrophy. They had continued ambulation in orthoses 2 years and 6 months, respectively, after provision of orthoses. (From Dubowitz V: Deformities in Duchenne dystrophy. *Neuromuscul Disord* 20[4]:282, 2010.)

should be provided when KAFOs are used owing to the risk of injury from falls. Closer guarding and increased assistance will be needed as the weakness progresses. Transfers to and from standing are dependent because the knee joints of the KAFO must be locked to provide stability. KAFOs or standers that can accommodate ankle, knee, and hip contractures and allow for a lateral transfer in sitting and a transition to standing in the device can be used for continuation of a standing program even after walking is no longer possible.

The patient may prefer surgical intervention and braced ambulation. Indications for surgery include ankle plantar flexion contractures greater than 10°, iliotibial band contractures greater than 20°, or knee-hip flexion contractures greater than 20° but less than 45°.[32] Subcutaneous tenotomy of the Achilles tendon or more commonly gastrocnemius facia lengthening and fasciotomy of the iliotibial bands are the most commonly reported surgical procedures.[13,32,120,266] Transfer of the posterior tibialis tendon is occasionally used for correction of equinovarus foot posture.[120,230]

An intensive postoperative management program is essential to minimize the effects of immobilization.[241] Standing in the plaster casts can be done on the first or second postoperative day. Gait training is begun as tolerated, and general conditioning exercises for the hips, trunk, and upper extremities are recommended. Breathing exercises and aggressive pulmonary management should also be stressed with any surgical procedure to minimize the chance of postoperative atelectasis and pneumonia.[179] A smooth transition to bracing is ensured by having the child fitted for the KAFOs before hospitalization for surgery.

Functional mobility and equipment. Various methods to predict the termination of walking have been reported, including 50% reduction in leg strength,[231,267] manual muscle test grade below grade 3 for hip extensors or below grade 4 for ankle dorsiflexors,[167] or inability to climb steps. Brooke and colleagues[34] reported the cessation of unassisted walking within 2.4 years (range, 1.2–4.1 years) when 5 to 12 seconds was required to climb four standard steps, or within 1.5 years (range, 0.6–2.2 years) when longer than 12 seconds was required. Monitoring and management of contractures become a key element in maintaining walking when the older child spends more time in a sitting position. Because the hip extensor musculature is significantly weak in the early stage of the disease and weakness of the quadriceps muscles becomes pronounced by age 8 to 10 years, inability to maintain the center of gravity behind the hip joint or in front of the knee joint during stance will lead to loss of the ability to stand.

Standing pivot transfers eventually will be replaced by one- or two-person lifts or use of a patient lift because of the development of knee and hip flexion contractures and the pronounced weakness of the lower extremities. Transfers to and from the wheelchair, toilet, tub, car, and furniture usually become dependent shortly after the loss of ambulation. A sliding board typically is not functional due to the significant upper extremity weakness, and hydraulic lift can help during transfers. Parents typically prefer manual lifting with either a one-person or two-person lift for as long as one of them is able. Despite this, having an hydraulic lift in place so both parents can participate in transfers or in case one parent becomes injured is important to consider. Proper instruction for transfers is also needed because the degree of trunk muscle weakness makes sitting balance more and more tenuous as the child ages. If the caregiver is using manual lifting for transfers, he or she should be observed for and instructed in proper body mechanics and safety. A hydraulic lift can be used for transfers to and from the wheelchair, particularly when the adolescent is large or obese or when the caregiver cannot safely perform a manual lift. A U-style divided leg sling with headrest extension should be used with the lift to provide adequate head and trunk support during transfers and to allow the sling to be removed from under the child after the transfer.

Hydraulic lifts cannot be used for transfer to the tub or shower. If the parents are unable to lift the child to a bath bench, either a dedicated tub lift or sliding-style shower commode that can roll over the toilet and then attach to a base in the shower or tub and slide onto the secondary base for bathing can provide a solution for limited bathroom transfers. Some families will have the resources to construct a barrier-free shower for bathing for which they will need a wheeled rehabilitation shower commode. Depending on bathroom accessibility and the amount of renovation that is done, a review of the bathroom size and layout is necessary to ensure that the chosen equipment will fit in the existing space. Many bathrooms are small, and sliding-style shower commodes do not fit, so alternative systems may need to be considered.

A power scooter like the one shown in Fig. 12.5 should be considered as an initial power wheelchair prescription for the child who is having difficulty for longer distances in the community. This transition is often easier when ambulation is still secure and limitations are related to endurance. The power scooter can be presented as an opportunity to access social and community activities that the child no longer chooses to participate in because ambulation has become limited either from a stability or endurance point of view. Because the child no longer chooses to participate in the activities, he or she will be less concerned with substituting power mobility for ambulation and more accepting of now having access to an activity that he or she has since abandoned. The scooter is also often more easily accepted by the child and may be used as an initial step in the transition to a standard power wheelchair because it can fold and stow in the trunk of a car. One needs to be aware that the scooter will not be able to be used for transport on a bus to and from school, and the child will need to be able to transfer out of the scooter to a standard bus or car seat or obtain a wheelchair that is crash tested for transit. If a power scooter is used initially, transition to a power wheelchair will be necessary when the adolescent is seen propping on the arm rests for trunk control or is no longer able to maintain contact with the tiller to drive. Asymmetric sitting postures should be aggressively managed owing to the correlation of increased sitting time and asymmetric sitting posture with the onset of scoliosis.

A manual wheelchair or stroller can be considered as a backup to the primary power mobility device if resources allow and can be used for nonaccessible areas in the usual environment. Architectural barriers in the home or inability to transport a power wheelchair may also necessitate the use of a manual wheelchair, manual wheelchair with power assist, or a scooter, all of which can be stowed in the trunk of a car. However, ramps or lifts for the home are the best long-term solution to accessibility barriers because they allow full use of the power wheelchair. Additionally, if an adapted van is not available, an alternative device as a backup should be considered and is often available through insurance or as a loaner from some parent organizations such as the MDA.

Fit of the wheelchair must be closely monitored to provide adequate support. The reader should refer to Chapter 33: Assistive Technology for information on wheelchairs and postural support systems. Special attention should be given to alignment of the spine and alignment and pressure relief for the pelvis. Accessories to be considered for the manual or power wheelchair prescription should include a solid back and seat, lateral trunk support on the side of the joystick, adductor pads, seat belt, and chest strap. The angle adjustable footrests should be modified to support the ankle in a neutral position. Additional items that may be appropriate include a tray, head support, or coated push rims, if the child has the strength to propel the wheelchair. A reclining back will allow a position change for toileting or changing while sitting in the wheelchair and will help deter flexion contracture formation at the hip, and a tilt-in-space option can be considered to allow for pressure relief. Midline placement of the control stick on a power wheelchair may be considered to assist in symmetrical trunk alignment if the child chooses to have a tray in place most of the time. However, many children will prefer to have a joystick with a quad link mount that they can push out of the way, allowing them to roll up to a table.

The seating evaluation should start with the base of support and evaluation of the pelvis. It is important to note where the weight line falls within the base of support and how this impacts pressure distribution. The patient's weight line must be assessed both in the frontal and sagittal plane; this becomes more critical the weaker the boy and the more tenuous the head control becomes. The younger patient who has relatively good sitting balance will do well with a cushion with a foam base and flow lite pressure-relieving gel. For individuals in the later stage of disease or those with more rigid pelvic obliquity, often the high side of the pelvis will need to be supported either with a foam obliquity insert in the cushion or with an air-filled cushion that allows the four quadrants of the cushion's pressure to be adjusted. This will provide for accommodation of the fixed pelvic deformity, as might be the case following spinal fusion. In the sagittal plane, most boys will sit forward with an anterior pelvic tilt that allows them to rely on the contracted posterior neck ligaments to aid in head control. This forward posture also aids in allowing the patient to shift his weight because there is no friction with the wheelchair back and the patient's center of gravity is directly over the base of support. Some boys will prefer a chest strap to lean on while others will need this only for stability around corners in a vehicle. It is important to recognize this is not a crash-tested restraint and that the wheelchair and child need to be secured in the vehicle with an appropriate crash-tested restraint.

Management of lower extremity positioning in the wheelchair needs to account for the tendency for patients to assume a hip-abducted, ankle planovarus posture. The use of hip adductors mounted on the wheelchair to maintain alignment is important, and footrests that allow plantarflexion adjustment are also helpful. The headrest is less critical and typically is used only when the tilt function of the wheelchair is accessed unless the patient sits back in the chair.

The family will need to consider additional equipment or home modifications as the child reaches adolescence. A van with a lift or ramp will be needed to transport a power wheelchair. Modification of the bathroom can significantly assist the family when a wheeled commode chair is used for toileting and bathing with a handheld shower. A slider-style bath system is a second option for bathing. Both systems will allow the child to use a mechanical lift in the bedroom, roll over the toilet, and then either roll into an adapted shower or slide over the tub or into a stall shower without necessitating an additional transfer. A urinal should be available at home and at school to decrease the frequency of transfers to the toilet, and some are specifically molded for use in a wheelchair. Modifications of the bed are also frequently required because the adolescent is unable to change position. An airflow mattress, egg-crate or memory foam cushion, and hospital bed are all possibilities to be considered. A positioning program to include position changes at night is necessary for adolescents who are thin in order to provide comfort and prevent skin breakdown. Customized foam wedges fabricated by the therapist or moldable pillows may also be helpful in positioning at night.

Transition to Adulthood. The transition to adulthood marks a time of continued progression of disability with greater reliance on assistive technology for environmental access and increased need for assistance to carry out routine ADLs.[247] Mobility using a power wheelchair is necessary because upper extremity and truncal weakness typically will not allow use of a motorized scooter once weakness progresses. Assistance with ADLs, including dressing, transfers, and bathing, is now required. Hygiene about the face and feeding become increasingly difficult but usually remain manageable for a period of time. Many social issues also arise with the completion of educational programming and transition to a prevocational, vocational, or home environment on a more full-time basis. Another major issue that requires thoughtful consideration by the family, individual, and management team is the utilization of assisted ventilation with progressive respiratory involvement at the terminal stage of the disease.

Although it may be assumed by care providers that the quality of life and therefore satisfaction are significantly reduced for severely disabled individuals with DMD, this notion may be incorrect. In a survey of 82 ventilator-assisted individuals with DMD, Bach and colleagues[15] concluded that a vast majority of individuals had a positive outlook and were satisfied with life despite the physical dependence. Furthermore, it was found in a survey of 273 physically intact health care professionals that they significantly underestimated patient life satisfaction scores, and therefore they may make patient management recommendations based on their attitudes rather than on the patient's wishes. Bach and colleagues[15] strongly recommended that we as professionals need to objectively assess family and individual needs when interacting to provide therapeutic programs and the inclusion of social work and psychosocial support in this process may be helpful. With the early use of steroids and intervention with ventilator assistance, longevity has been reported to increase into the third or fourth decade.[188]

The physical therapist should be aware of the stages of disease progression and especially the preterminal signs to avoid making inappropriate comments concerning prognosis. Often little needs to be said, but rather a good listening ear is needed to help the family work through the crisis that is ever pending. The person with DMD and his family members may indicate the need for additional support, and if issues are not being resolved adequately by the support that is available, consideration for involvement by a social worker, psychologist, counselor, clergy member, MDA support group, or other trained professional is indicated. Literature is available through the MDA to comfort family members, and texts are available if the family is interested.[46,188,220]

Respiratory function. Progressive muscular weakness results in decreased ventilatory volumes caused by restriction of chest wall excursion both as a result of weakness and contracture. Forced vital capacity and peak expiratory flow typically improve in absolute value until the age of 10, and after the age of 18 typically both FVC and PEF show a decline over time.[161] Coordination of care with the respiratory therapist is essential when clinical findings of respiratory muscle weakness, inability to cough, or chest wall restrictions are observed. Close monitoring of respiratory function should become routine with increasing age because respiratory failure or pulmonary infection is the major contributing factor to death in children with DMD.[91] Longevity in DMD can be significantly prolonged by assisted ventilation.[16,65] A 1997 survey of MDA-sponsored clinics reported that 88% of clinic directors offered noninvasive ventilatory aid for acute respiratory failure.[12] Bach and Chaudhry[12] stressed the need for health care professionals to explore attitudes toward mechanical ventilation because our perceived impression of patient desires may often be incorrect. The use of daytime intermittent positive-pressure ventilation via mask or nasal cannula, nocturnal bilevel positive airway pressure (BiPAP), negative-pressure ventilators, and suctioning should be considered for the chronic hypoventilation related to weakness of respiratory musculature.[12]

Breathing exercises, postural drainage, or intermittent pressure breathing treatments should be included in the management program based on results of pulmonary evaluation and sleep studies that should be considered in the second decade of life.[222] Specific tests of pulmonary function that document respiratory status include forced vital capacity (FVC = amount of air expired following a maximal inspiration) and peak expiratory flow rate (highest flow rate sustained for 10 ms during maximal expiration). BiPAP is recommended for nighttime use when indicated by sleep study.[150,244] Assisted ventilation with tracheostomy or by mask or sip is recommended when respiratory insufficiency is present with abnormal blood gas levels during the day or night.[244,271] In addition to breathing exercises and assisted coughing, the family and caregivers should be instructed in the technique of postural drainage. For additional details, the reader should refer to the American Thoracic Society consensus statement on the care of individuals with DMD or the report from the DMD working group.[5,40,65]

Functional mobility and equipment. By late adolescence assistance is required for transfers. The use of a hydraulic or other mechanical lift should be considered depending on the patient's weight and the parent's comfort. A divided leg sling with headrest extension, to allow it to be removed after the transfer, is indicated because head and trunk control are minimal at this stage of the disease.

A power recline and tilt feature on the power wheelchair may be desirable, depending on accessibility and family choice, if funding is available. If not, a regular schedule for pressure relief through lateral weight shifting with assistance is needed. A properly fitted and well-tolerated cushion to avoid skin breakdown becomes an important area of intervention with loss of the ability to weight shift in the wheelchair. Skin breakdown is not a typical problem in DMD, but a cushion should be considered. A Jay Medical cushion (Jay Medical, Boulder, CO) is often well tolerated and provides a firm base of support to control pelvic obliquity, yet the gel inserts can be adjusted to allow for adequate pressure distribution. A customized insert will be needed if deformity becomes severe (e.g., severe scoliosis without surgical stabilization). If the firmer cushion is not tolerated well, then use of a Roho quatro cushion (The Roho Group, Belleville, IL) is recommended because it will allow for greater pressure relief.

A ball bearing feeder may be considered to assist arm movement when progression of upper extremity weakness makes independent feeding difficult.[50] The device can also be used to assist with general use of the arms in conjunction with activities at a table, such as when using a computer, or to maintain the ability to self-feed. Trial use of a mobile arm support is recommended, and a mobile arm support with elastic assist like the WREX (Wilmington Robotic Exoskeleton) could be considered. Coordination of planning with an occupational therapist to address feeding and dressing issues is needed to identify solutions to increased dependence in the areas of feeding, dressing, and hygiene.

A power-controlled bed to allow elevation of the head for respiratory management should be considered. Use of a bed with elevating capability also allows for greater ease in transfers, and height adjustment promotes use of proper body mechanics by family members for activities that require assistance such as dressing; however, some insurance companies will view this as a convenience for the family and will not cover the cost. Mattress selection should also be reviewed with the family because an airflow mattress or memory foam mattress may be needed when increasing dependence for bed mobility is encountered. Use of a mattress with deep pressure relief may decrease the frequency of need for turning and repositioning at night. If sitting in a wheelchair is no longer tolerated in the later stages of the disease, which may occur if severe scoliosis and back pain are present, elevation of the head of the bed becomes beneficial for reading or watching television. An easel will be required for reading.

To maintain independence in environmental access, consideration should be given to using environmental control devices. An environmental control unit included on the power wheelchair can be used to independently access lights, telephone, television, motors on doors, or a computer, to name just a few applications. Computer access for vocational applications such as word processing or avocational activities such as games is available.

BECKER MUSCULAR DYSTROPHY

Background Information

Becker muscular dystrophy (BMD), a more slowly progressive variant of DMD, has an incidence of about 1 in 20,000 births and a prevalence of 2 to 3 cases per 100,000 population.[68] The impairments and participation restrictions of BMD closely resemble those of DMD; however, the progression is slower, with a longevity into the forties.[70,91] The genetic defect for BMD is located on the same gene as that for DMD. Dystrophin is present in reduced amounts or inconsistently integrated into the muscle cell structure rather than completely absent as in DMD, which may explain the slower progression of clinical symptoms.[146]

Initial clinical symptoms typically are not identified in boys with BMD before late childhood or early adolescence except for families with a history of the disease. Emery and Skinner[70] found the mean age at onset of symptoms to be 11 years, inability to

walk at 27 years, and death at 42 years although this has changed with the increased use of steroids for muscle strength and medication for the associated cardiac comorbidities. The authors pointed out that the range of walking cessation is very wide, but by definition to be classified as having BMD one needs to continue independent bracefree ambulation beyond the 16th birthday.

The impairments of BMD are the same as in DMD, although less severe, and initial clinical signs include gastrocsoleus contracture and proximal weakness in the mid to late teens. The exception is the increased presence of cardiac involvement in BMD that is not necessarily correlated with the degree of weakness. Dilated cardiac myopathy is more prevalent with BMD because of the longer life span, and routine cardiac screening is recommended.[129] The pattern of weakness is the same as in DMD, and pseudohypertrophy of the calves may be present. The incidence of contracture, scoliosis, and other skeletal deformities is lower in BMD. Although not as severe as in DMD, hip, knee, and ankle plantar flexor muscle contractures can be present when walking is no longer possible. The use of night splints to maintain ankle dorsiflexion ROM is often indicated, along with a home program of posterior calf stretching. Significant disability may develop by the mid-20s in most individuals, although this is variable. As weakness progresses, the use of power mobility may be required. KAFOs can also be used to prolong walking; however, braced ambulation will not be functional for community access but rather as a means of exercise.

Foreground Information

The general goals and management procedures for BMD are the same for as those for DMD, including the progression from walking to use of power mobility, although the predictive guidelines may differ because the rate of progression in BMD is slower. Although the precautions against eccentric exercise, excessive fatigue, and delayed-onset muscle soreness should be followed with BMD as with DMD, because of the milder phenotype of individuals with BMD, endurance training has been found to be beneficial.[253] Sveen and colleagues reported on a cohort of 11 individuals with BMD who participated in a cycling program of 50 30-minute sessions at 65% of their maximal oxygen uptake level over 12 weeks. The group demonstrated 47% improvement in maximum oxygen uptake and an 80% increase in maximal workload with no evidence of increased serum creatine phosphokinase levels and no presence of necrotic or increased numbers of central nuclei on muscle biopsy. The exercise group also demonstrated a significant increase in strength in select lower extremity muscles. Sveen and colleagues also reported that endurance training may be beneficial for increasing strength in these individuals without leading to increased muscle damage; however, more research is needed to determine the most appropriate intensity of training.[254]

Transition planning following completion of school and assistance with living arrangements to accommodate the progressive nature of the disability into adulthood become major issues in this population. Longevity is commonly reported into the mid-40s, with complications from dilated cardiac myopathy being the limiting factor on longevity.[58] Vocational or avocational choices should be made with the disease progression and disability level in mind. Vocational rehabilitation services should be initiated before completion of high school to allow adequate time for evaluation and transition plan development. Governmental support through Medicaid, Social Security, or other sources may be needed to offset expenses to allow for independent living and access to post-secondary education. Typically, both adaptive equipment and an attendant will be needed in addition to an environmental evaluation and modification. No data are available regarding the number of individuals who go to college or become employed following high school, but with the assistive technology available to promote independence, either option can be explored.

CONGENITAL MUSCULAR DYSTROPHY

Background Information

Congenital MD is a heterogeneous group of muscle disorders with onset in utero or during the first year of life that are characterized by delayed motor development and early onset of weakness.[214] The mode of inheritance in congenital MD is reported as autosomal recessive.[69,187] Although all forms are rare, the range of severity and disability varies significantly among types. Recent advances have led to the identification of several new genes associated with forms of congenital MD. A new classification system reports forms based on genetic, clinical, and pathologic characteristics along the spectrum of the disease. Reported forms of congenital MD include (1) defects of dystroglycan associated with central nervous system (CNS) disease (Fukuyama syndrome, Walker-Warburg disease, and muscle-eye-brain disease); (2) defects of structural proteins, including merosin-deficient congenital MD and collagenopathies (Ullrich MD Bethlem myopathy); (3) defects of the endoplasmic reticulum and nucleu (rigid spine syndrome); and (4) defects of the mitochondria merosin-deficient, Ullrich, and Fukuyama forms.[169,174,242] The reader should refer to the review chapter by Sparks and Escolar for additional information.[242] Other valuable resources for information are the Online Mendelian Inheritance of Man (OMIM) website of the National Center for Biotechnology (www.ncbi.nlm.nih.gov/omim) and GeneReviews (www.genereviews.org).

Congenital MD with complete merosin deficiency (MDC1A) is the most common form, affecting approximately 30% to 40% of the children in European countries but is less reported in North America.[242] Onset is at birth, and children never attain the ability to walk unsupported in contrast to children with partial merosin deficiency, for which onset is during the first decade and children typically are able to walk by the age of 2 to 3 years. Children with congenital MD typically have decreased respiratory function observed by the end of the first decade and often require overnight ventilator support. Feeding difficulties are also frequently reported.

In children with merosin-absent or partial merosin-deficient MD, abnormalities on brain imaging are reported, but with infrequent reduction in IQ. Thirty percent are reported to develop epilepsy.[113] Contractures and scoliosis are common, along with early breathing difficulties that may require assisted ventilation. Children with the merosin-deficient form of MD are reported to have cardiac involvement. In congenital MD with partial merosin deficiency, a delay in walking, with acquisition of walking ranging from 13 months to 6 years, is reported.[193]

Progressive contractures may be present, and in most cases of merosin-deficient congenital MD the child never attains the

ability to walk independently. Twenty-five percent of children are reported to be able to walk with support. Longevity ranges from 15 to 30 years. Pegorago and associates[208] reported on a cohort of 22 children with merosin-deficient congenital MD. All children demonstrated severe floppiness at birth, normal intelligence, and delay in achievement of motor milestones. Merosin-deficient congenital MD is due to a defect in the *LAMA2* gene at chromosome 6q22.

Muscle weakness and contractures are the primary impairment in merosin-deficient congenital MD, with scoliosis common in merosin-absent MD. Brain malformations can include cobblestone type II lissencephaly or polymicrogyria as pathologic features of the CNS portion of the disease. Weakness is more pronounced in proximal muscles. Feeding delays are common with lesser involvement of the bulbar muscular than is generally observed with weakness of the trunk and axial musculature, requiring a feeding program that should be coordinated with occupational therapy. Contractures must be managed aggressively with a home ROM program that includes manual stretching, positioning, and splinting. Although children with partial merosin-deficient MD can develop walking, ankle plantar flexion contractures that cannot be managed conservatively may require orthopedic intervention.

Another more prevalent form of congenital MD is Ullrich MD, due to a collagen VI defect. It is characterized by hypotonia and weakness with distal joint hyperlaxity. Proximal joint contractures and skeletal abnormalities may also be observed. Hip dysplasia is seen in about 50% of cases. Delayed milestones can be the first symptom leading to diagnosis, and usually this clinically manifests around 12 months of age. Most patients achieve independent walking; however, this skill is often lost by the teen years. Children also develop respiratory insufficiency, often requiring the use of noninvasive ventilator support overnight. Characteristic facial features include rounded face, drooping of lower eyelids, and prominent ears. Intelligence is normal in these children, and longevity has been described well into adulthood. Early management of these children includes mobilization and maintenance of ROM. Gait is marked by crouch and progressive knee flexion contracture and/or ankle contractures. Standing frames, orthotics, and ambulatory aides may be prescribed. As contractures progress over time, surgical intervention may also be indicated. A milder phenotype is Bethlem myopathy. Mild weakness and laxity may be observed in childhood with contracture development at the end of the first decade. Weakness becomes more pronounced in the third and fourth decades and many require assistance to walk around the age of 60 years.[30]

In congenital MD with associated CNS disease (Fukuyama type), intellectual disabilities and seizures are common, along with moderate to severe weakness at birth and the presence of contractures.[86] Magnetic resonance imaging reveals cerebral malformations and occasionally cobblestone type II lissencephaly as pathologic features of the CNS disease. Contractures typically involve the lower extremities (hips, knees, and ankles) and elbows. Other commonly reported dysmorphic features include torticollis, congenital dislocation of the hips, pectus excavatum, pes cavus, and kyphoscoliosis. Facial weakness and ptosis are common, and weakness of the extraocular muscles, optic atrophy, and nystagmus has also been reported.[214] Children with this type of MD rarely attain the ability to walk; however, milder phenotypes have been identified and present as a limb girdle phenotype.[69,98] The genetic defect is at chromosome 9q31-q33 with the missing protein fukutin.

Foreground Information

The early management program in children with congenital MD with central nervous system disease should focus on family instruction, developmental activities to address delays in gross motor skill development, and aggressive management of contractures. Attention to positioning is necessary to guard against secondary deformity resulting from gravitational effects on the trunk with the presence of moderate to severe weakness. Early intervention by an occupational or speech therapist to address feeding and oral motor control issues is commonly coordinated with physical therapy to help with positioning the upper trunk and neck and adjusting the body position with respect to gravity to aid in oral motor control and optimize the chances of success. Impaired respiratory function and pulmonary complications are hallmark features of congenital MD. The family should be instructed in airway clearance techniques including percussion and postural drainage, and consultation with a respiratory therapist and pulmonologist may be needed on an ongoing basis.

Because many children with congenital MD and associated nervous system disease do not attain walking, maximizing functional skills in sitting becomes a primary goal of the physical therapy management program as the child ages. Therapeutic exercise to improve head and trunk control should be aggressively addressed with use of adaptive equipment to slow the progression of spinal deformity and contractures and to maximize access to the environment. Because intellectual disabilities are common, power mobility may not be an option. Additional management issues for children with significant weakness are discussed later in the chapter in the section on acute SMA.

Activity limitations, such as delayed acquisition of gross motor skills, should be managed with an understanding of the natural progression of the diagnosis because a slower rate of skill progression is expected. Because these children vary in their rate of motor skill development, information can be provided to the family concerning probable rates of motor skill acquisition, but unrealistic therapeutic expectations should be avoided. Because children with congenital MD have a wide range of functional deficits, care must be taken in predicting functional gross motor outcomes or level of participation at home and school.

CHILDHOOD-ONSET FACIOSCAPULOHUMERAL MUSCULAR DYSTROPHY

Background

Facioscapulohumeral MD is rare, with an incidence of 1 in 10,000 to 21,000, and typically demonstrates onset in adulthood.[198] The disorder is inherited as autosomal dominant disorder that is unique in that it results from a contraction of a triple repeat found in the gene.[227] In addition, there is a high rate of new mutation. The genetic defect is on chromosome 4q35 in the case of *FSHD1*, which accounts for 95% of cases with the remaining cases classified as *FSHD2*. The disorder affects males and females equally. Childhood-onset facioscapulohumeral MD typically results in the onset of clinical signs within the first 2 years but without significant impairment or disability until later in the first decade. Contractures are seldom a problem for mobility.

Foreground
Infancy and Preschool-Age Period

The impairment of muscle weakness about the face and shoulder girdle is typically the only prominent feature of the disease during the infant and preschool-age period. Parents report that the child may sleep with the eyes partially open, and on physical examination weakness of the facial musculature is predominant although from a functional mobility point of view the weakness of the trunk muscles, plantarflexors, and sometimes quadriceps can be the most impairing.[10,218,219] Children frequently are unable to whistle, and drinking with a straw may be difficult due to the facial weakness. When asked to purse the lips together and puff the cheeks out, the child is unable to maintain the cheeks out when even the slightest pressure is applied. The child's smile may also be masked because of the weakness, thereby hindering communication as a result of inconsistency between what is spoken and the affect displayed.

Children with childhood-onset facioscapulohumeral MD typically develop independence in walking without significant delay. An excessive lordotic posture during walking is a classic clinical feature with progression of weakness, and the plantarflexor and quadriceps weakness often lead to hyperextension of the knee to maintain stability in stance. The scapulae are widely abducted and outwardly rotated, giving evidence of the degree of interscapular muscle weakness and winging that can be elicited by a number of maneuvers.[132]

School-Age Period

Progressive activity limitations occur during the school-age period, with weakness becoming more generalized throughout the trunk, shoulder, and pelvic girdle musculature. Progression of childhood-onset facioscapulohumeral MD is more insidious than in the adult form, and independent walking may be lost by the end of the first decade.[89]

Severe winging of the scapula, a hallmark feature of the adult form of the disease, becomes more prominent with age in activities such as reaching overhead. Management should focus on instruction to the child and family on activities to avoid that may cause fatigue, and endurance training should be considered for this population.[36,125,196,272]

As weakness of the hip and knee extensors progresses, the use of lightweight carbon fiber AFOs that resist dorsiflexion and stabilize the knee with a ground reaction force can be considered, and eventually KAFOs for assisted walking and transfers may be beneficial. When walking becomes increasingly difficult, power mobility using a scooter or power wheelchair should be considered because the degree of upper extremity weakness will not allow independence in propulsion of a manual wheelchair.

Transition to Adulthood

No specific prognostic information on the longevity of individuals with childhood-onset facioscapulohumeral MD is available; therefore transition planning from the educational environment should be a goal of the therapy program, and standard of care documents and the available natural history experience should be considered to guide management.[249,257] If severe weakness is present and significant assistance from the family is needed, individuals may not desire to plan for living outside the family home. If independent living is desired, coordination of planning with vocational rehabilitation services and an attendant may be necessary and accessibility issues will need to be evaluated. The wide variability of severity and pattern of weakness in this population even between family members needs to be considered in terms of the expected prognosis when planning for the future; however, progression over time in each individual is often uniform and slow with long periods of stability and most patients remain ambulatory.[249] The reader is referred to an excellent review by Shree Pandya for an overview of the phenotypic presentation and functional considerations one must be aware of in this population.[198]

MYOTONIC DYSTROPHY

Background

Myotonic dystrophy is the most common adult-onset neuromuscular disease, with an incidence of 1 in 8000 births.[109] Congenital myotonic dystrophy is rare and demonstrates severe clinical features of the adult-onset diagnosis (see OMIM, myotonic dystrophy type 1). Inheritance is reported as autosomal dominant with a genetic defect of chromosome 19q13.3 affecting males and females equally. A second form of myotonic dystrophy (myotonic dystrophy type 2) (proximal myotonic myopathy, or PROMM) has been reported and linked to chromosome 3q21.[216]

Children with congenital myotonic dystrophy are almost exclusively born to mothers with myotonic dystrophy who have the chromosome 19 defect. Approximately 25% of children born to mothers with myotonic dystrophy will have congenital myotonic dystrophy.[26,109] Most children demonstrate severe weakness at birth; however, a few children have no significant motor impairments as infants and first show signs of intellectual disability only by age 5 years as the cognitive demands increase at school age. Because the children who initially have only intellectual impairment follow a progression of motor impairment similar to that of adult-onset myotonic dystrophy, the infant-onset form is the primary focus of discussion in this section of the chapter.

Intellectual disability in congenital myotonic dystrophy is common, affecting 50% to 60% of the children. An average IQ of 74 is typically reported for children with cognitive impairment with verbal IQ higher than performance; however, like the motor phenotype there is wide variability among the population.[62,223,243] No evidence of progressive deterioration of cognitive function has been found. A study by Rutherford and coworkers[226] of 14 children provided prognostic information regarding survival and its relationship to mechanical ventilation at birth.

In children with congenital myotonic dystrophy survival beyond the early weeks of life indicates a prognosis of steady improvement in motor function over the first decade, with most children developing independent walking after age 2.[66,111,128,223] A follow-up study by O'Brien and Harper[194] of 46 children reported only 4 children who died outside the neonatal period at ages 4, 18, 19, and 22 years. Four additional children demonstrated significant disability associated with a poor prognosis, and none was older than age 30 years. In a study of 115 children with congenital myotonic dystrophy, Reardon and colleagues[213] reported that 25% of the children lived to age 18 months, and of those who survived infancy, 50% lived into their mid-30s. The use of noninvasive ventilation has improved this number significantly, but there may still be a 25% mortality rate in the first year.[42]

Severe weakness and partial paralysis of the diaphragm at birth are clinical features that often suggest the diagnosis of congenital myotonic dystrophy. Myotonia (delay in relaxation after muscular contraction) is a hallmark feature of myotonic dystrophy. Myotonia in congenital myotonic dystrophy typically is not considered to be a significant impairment or a cause of functional limitations in comparison with the degree of weakness that is present. The symptoms of myotonia, however, are increased with fatigue, cold, or stress. Typical facial features include a tented V-shaped upper lip. Facial movements are limited with a typical pattern of a myopathic face. Severe respiratory impairment is prominent in the newborn period, requiring resuscitation and assisted ventilation in the most severe cases. Cardiac involvement is common, and there have been reports of arrhythmias in up to 90% of patients with some requiring the insertion of pacemakers.[26] It is recommended that cardiac consults be obtained for young adults who are engaging in sports activities.[66] Talipes equinovarus contractures are reported in more than 50% of children, and a general arthrogrypotic pattern with contracture of more than one joint at birth occurring in less than 5%.[109]

Foreground
Infancy

Talipes equinovarus contractures should be aggressively managed in infancy with Ponseti casting and stretching exercise but may ultimately require surgical orthopedic intervention to facilitate optimal weight-bearing foot position for walking.[213] Ankle-foot orthoses and/or night splints are indicated on the basis of individual needs to maintain correction. In addition to home instruction for ROM activities to manage contractures, the family should be provided with a general program of activities to promote gross motor skill development.

Consultation with a respiratory therapist on pulmonary care will be needed until the infant is weaned from assisted ventilation. Feeding may require the use of a nasogastric tube during the newborn period or early infancy, and initiation of a feeding program should be coordinated with an occupational or speech therapist. A swallowing study may be indicated when the feeding program is initiated to evaluate potential for aspiration. If the newborn survives early respiratory difficulties, progressive improvement in pulmonary function is usually seen without the need for ongoing intervention.

School-Age Period

Progressive improvement in gross motor skills can be expected if the child survives the newborn period. The degree of intellectual impairment becomes a major factor in the progression of milestone acquisition as the child ages.

Children typically develop walking, but further activity limitations follow the clinical progression of adult-onset disease. In some cases, progressive weakness may occur in the second decade, leading to a loss of ambulation. However, it is most frequently reported that activity limitations remain steady and slight throughout childhood and later progress in the third or fourth decades of life.[66] Patients present with the typical impairments of ligamentous laxity, generalized weakness, and a drop foot during the swing phase of gait that often will benefit from a lightweight AFO.[109]

Consultation for development of adaptive physical education participation will be needed during the school-age period. Other physical therapy–related activities will depend on the use of orthoses and the progression of gross motor skill development. Specific therapeutic exercise programs for

ROM and strengthening have not been reported but may be indicated.

Transition to Adulthood

The natural progression of myotonic dystrophy is insidious weakness of the distal upper and lower extremity musculature and myotonia, leading to activity limitations and participation restrictions; however, in the moderately affected group the cognitive findings are often the most impactful as adolescents transition to adulthood. Children with congenital myotonic dystrophy will demonstrate progression in the disease as described for adults, but typically at an earlier stage. The severity of disease represents the full spectrum from adults with very mild impairments to infants with very severe disability.[66] The reader should refer to references on adult myotonic dystrophy for further information on clinical course and management.[109]

EMERY-DREIFUSS MUSCULAR DYSTROPHY

Background

The most common form of Emery-Dreifuss muscular dystrophy (EMD), known as XL-EMD or EDMD1, is inherited as an X-linked recessive disorder at gene locus Xq28 resulting in the absence of the protein emerin. Another identified form of EMD can also be inherited, but as either an autosomal dominant (AD-EMD) or recessive (AR-EMD) disorder with a defect on chromosome 1q21.2 and a defect of the protein lamin.[29] The dominant form is more common, with the recessive form only reported in one case of a family with a severe phenotype.

The clinical features of Emery-Dreifuss vary widely but consist of a pattern of contractures, slowly progressing muscle weakness, and cardiac disease.[239] The clinical pictures of XL-EMD and AD-EMD are similar but have some differences. Typically, in XL-EMD joint contractures precede signs of weakness, whereas in AD-EMD there is pronounced muscle weakness prior to the development of contractures. Loss of ambulation can occur in AD-EMD but is not common in XL-EMD. The risk of cardiac involvement is also higher in XL-EMD. A very characteristic pattern of contractures includes contracture of the posterior neck and spinal extensors, elbow flexors, pectoral muscles, and ankle plantar flexors. A prominence of contracture over weakness in the presentation of the phenotype is common. A humeroperoneal pattern of muscle weakness is observed with usual onset in the teen years but ranges from neonatal to the third decade. Progression of weakness to the legs with a peroneal weakness pattern is reported with a drop foot in the swing phase of gait.

Cardiac evaluation with Holter monitoring is advised to identify cardiac abnormalities, and pacemakers are often needed to control rhythm. Sudden death has been reported in persons ranging in age from 25 to 56 years[211] in a large family cohort with bradyarrhythmias; all patients should be screened by Holter monitoring at diagnosis.

Foreground

Physical therapy management is often focused on maintaining flexibility during the childhood period because contracture is the most common impairment. Independent walking is typically maintained into adulthood. A ROM program for contracture prevention is advised, and serial casting and orthopedic intervention are common to correct the posterior calf contractures.[159]

BACKGROUND INFORMATION

SPINAL MUSCULAR ATROPHY

Classification of SMA into four groups is based on clinical presentation and progression (Table 12.2). Historically the four groups have been referred to in various ways. Type I can also be referred to as Werdnig-Hoffmann disease, type II as chronic SMA, type III as Kugelberg-Welander disease, and type IV as adult-onset SMA. This latter group frequently has a different genetic basis and overlaps with motor neuronopathies. These are also often classified with Charcot-Marie-Tooth disease and present with different phenotypic patterns and genetic causes and will not be discussed here.

Standards of care have been developed, and as part of that effort we have included the most up-to-date rehabilitation literature available.[182] The standard of care document that has been in place is currently in the process of being revised in light of advances that have occurred in the intervening years.[173] Information regarding the functional status of children with SMA and the overall disease progression is now more readily available as the result of international collaborations that have allowed the collection of large data sets for this relatively rare disease.[49,79,130,131] There is currently no cure, but various compounds have been evaluated in clinical trials with some limited success.[135,203]

Diagnosis and Pathophysiology

SMA represents the second most common group of fatal recessive diseases after cystic fibrosis.[157] The primary pathologic feature of SMA is loss of the anterior horn cells in the spinal cord. The diagnosis of SMA is often suspected based on clinical examination and laboratory procedures, including electromyography, muscle ultrasound, and muscle biopsy, and is ultimately confirmed by genetic testing.[151] Electromyographic findings include decreased combined motor unit action potentials and spinal H reflexes, positive sharp waves, fibrillation potentials,

TABLE 12.2	Classification of Spinal Muscle Atrophy		
Type	Typical Onset	Inheritance	Course
SMA type I, Werdnig-Hoffmann, acute	0–4 mo	Recessive	Rapidly progressive; severe weakness; mortality dependent on aggressiveness or respiratory support, typically 1–10 years
SMA type II, childhood-onset	6–12 mo	Recessive	Initial progression that becomes slowly progressive over years; moderate to severe weakness
SMA type III, Kugelberg-Welander, juvenile-onset	1–10 yr	Recessive	Slowly progressive; mild impairment

and a decrease in the number of motor units by EMG estimation. Sensory and motor nerve conduction velocities are both normal. Muscle biopsy demonstrates changes that are typical of a disease involving denervation (i.e., large groups of atrophic fibers dispersed among groups of normal or hypertrophic fibers).

SMA is typically inherited as autosomal recessive with the genetic defect on chromosome 5q11.2-13.[144,170,171,236] The gene for SMA, termed survival motor neuron *(SMN1)*, is found on chromosome 5q13. An almost identical copy of *SMN1*, thought to be a paralog, is found just proximal to *SMN1*. This almost identical copy is termed *SMN2*. These two genes are responsible for the production of a protein bearing the same name.[212,225] The SMN protein is involved in a number of basic cellular functions, including axonal transport and most notably the splicing of pre-mRNA into mRNA. Ultimately, as the result of defective splicing of a number of lower motor neuron–specific genes, the anterior horn cell and the spinal reflex arc are impacted leading to apoptosis (programmed cell death).[76] The primary modifying gene in SMA is *SMN2*. *SMN2* produces a smaller amount of SMN and acts to modify the phenotype with more full-length protein being produced the more copies of *SMN2* that are present. In addition to the *SMN2* gene, there are other modifiers of the phenotype including plastin 3[281] and another gene in a near locus that that codes for neuronal apoptosis inhibitory protein (NAIP), which is thought to play a role in SMA.[59,221,264]

The incidence of SMA as a whole is between 1 in 6000 and 1 in 10,000 live births.[236] The majority of cases are children with SMA type I (60%) with type II accounting for about 27% of cases and SMA type III representing the smallest group.[195,251] Classification of SMA is based on the highest level of functional ability achieved.[63] Despite the classification into various types, SMA is now viewed more as a continuum of involvement. Here we will use this rubric because it helps to clarify management goals and guide intervention. Patients with genetically confirmed SMA can be classified into three categories based on the maximal motor skill achieved. Those with SMA type III have been able to ambulate without assistance or bracing at some point in their lives, patients with SMA type II have been able to sit independently at some point, and those with SMA type I have never been able to sit independently. SMA (type I) was first reported by Werdnig and Hoffmann in the late 1800s.[117,278] A more slowly progressive form of SMA (type III) with onset usually between the ages of 2 and 9 years was reported by Kugelberg and Welander[140] and also by Wohlfart and colleagues.[282] Werdnig-Hoffmann disease and Kugelberg-Welander disease have therefore become the eponyms for infantile-onset and juvenile-onset SMA; however, most authors prefer to use the numeric classification system as outlined in Table 12.2.

No cure is available for SMA, but physical therapy is commonly advocated.[159,276] Poor prognosticators for long-term survival include early age at onset, which is often noted as weak fetal movement or onset of weakness in the first months of life. More recent evidence has shown that children with SMA type I and severe onset of symptoms may survive up to their fifth birthday and beyond with proactive pulmonary management and noninvasive ventilation with two thirds surviving to 4 years of age and half to 10 years of age in some series; however, this is accompanied by severe physical impairment.[31,197] The cranial nerves are occasionally involved in SMA type II. Contractures may be a presenting feature in the most severe forms of SMA that present at birth or in utero, with reports of talipes equinovarus or other intrauterine deformities secondary to limited fetal movement. Some authors will term this SMA type 0 referring the prenatal onset of symptoms.[212,225]

SPINAL MUSCULAR ATROPHY (TYPE I)

Background

Impairments, Activity Limitations, and Participation Restrictions

The primary impairment in all forms of SMA is muscle weakness secondary to progressive loss of anterior horn cells in the spinal cord. Weakness is particularly pronounced in the acute and chronic childhood forms (types I and II). Muscle fasciculations, including fasciculations of the tongue, are most commonly reported in children with SMA type I.[159] Unlike the faces of children with myotonic dystrophy or facioscapulohumeral MD, children with SMA type I appear alert and responsive. Respiratory distress presents after limb weakness but is present early, and significant effort to augment breathing by the infant is typical with a paradoxical pattern characteristic of a reliance on the diaphragm and associated collapse of the thoracic cavity and expansion of the abdomen with each breath.

Secondary impairments in SMA type I include the development of scoliosis and contractures. It is widely reported in the literature that all children with SMA develop scoliosis, and surgical intervention is an option depending on the aggressiveness that families choose for treatment.[103,147] Other secondary impairments include decreased respiratory capacity and increased fatigability of muscle. Treatment should begin early with a focus on feeding, ROM, positioning, respiratory care, and selected developmental activities (Boxes 12.5 and 12.6).

Range of motion should be monitored by goniometry, and muscle strength can be measured in the context of functional

---

BOX 12.5 Evidence-Based Examinations for Children With SMA

Body Functions and Body Structures
Goniometry
Handheld myometry
Manual muscle testing
Quantitative muscle testing
Pulmonary function testing

Activity – Single Task:
6-minute walk test
Timed testing (time and grade)
Timed up/down 4 steps
Timed Gowers'
Timed 10-m run/walk

Activity – Multiple Items:
The Children's Hospital of Philadelphia Infant Test of Neuromuscular Disorders –CHOP INTEND (type I)
The Expanded Hammersmith Functional Motor Scale (type II or III)
Revised Upper Limb Module for SMA
Motor function measure

Participation – Multiple Items:
Pediatric Evaluation of Disability Index
PEDS QL
Health Utilities Index Questionnaire

antigravity extremity movement and head control in various postures. The Children's Hospital of Philadelphia Infant Test of Neuromuscular Disorders (CHOP INTEND) can be used to monitor motor activity over time.[93,94]

Foreground
Infancy
In SMA type 1, weak or absent fetal movement during the last months of pregnancy can be reported by the mother with some authors classifying this as SMA type 0. Significant weakness typically develops within the first 2 weeks to 4 months; this manifests as inability to perform antigravity movements with the pelvic more than shoulder girdle

---

BOX 12.6   Evidence-Based Interventions for Children With SMA

Body Functions and Body Structures
Stretching
Night splinting at end range
Concentric endurance and strength training exercise
Inspiratory muscle training with respiratory insufficiency
Cough assist/BiFAP with respiratory insufficiency (per pulmonary)
Percussion and postural drainage (with upper respiratory infection)

Activity
Standing program with ischial weight-bearing KAFOs at cessation of ambulation or if nonambulatory
Mobile arm support (or slings and springs) with feeding difficulty or for function/play

Participation
Power mobility
Environmental modification
Ramps
Bathroom adaptation or equipment
Van with lift/tie down
Assistive tech and switch toys
Adapted gym/sport activity

---

musculature and typical posturing in a gravity-dependent position (Fig. 12.7).

Respiratory care is one focus of the therapy program in acute childhood SMA. The aggressiveness of supportive care in this population is an individual choice. The medical team needs to discuss the options with the family related to the child's therapy program as well as medical care and maintain an open dialogue about their expectations and choices regarding the aggressiveness of care in the context of a disease with a limited life expectancy.[224] Children frequently require intubation in the context of intercurrent illness and then, when they are well, often can be weaned. However, for more chronic respiratory distress some will consider use of a tracheostomy, although use of noninvasive ventilatory support is frequently advocated to allow for the development of language skills.[11,17] The use of ventilatory support with either tracheostomy or noninvasive mechanical ventilation has been shown to prolong survival in children with SMA type I.[17] Coordination with nurses and respiratory therapists on a program that includes suctioning, mechanical cough assist, and percussion and postural drainage is necessary. The use of supported sitting should be closely monitored for spinal alignment and respiratory response because, as the children become weaker, sitting may be accompanied by respiratory decompensation.

The proximal musculature of the neck, trunk, and pelvic and shoulder girdles demonstrates the greatest weakness. Limited antigravity movement of upper and lower extremity musculature is present, and a positioning program is necessary in the newborn period or at the onset of symptoms. Use of wedges should be considered to avoid supine positioning in the presence of reflux; however, respiratory distress can be an issue in the more advanced stages, and upright posture will be less well tolerated due to the effects of gravity on the diaphragm. If the supine position is used, rolled towels or bolsters are needed to keep the upper extremities positioned in midline and to prevent lower extremity abduction and external rotation. The sidelying position allows midline head and hand use for play without having to work against gravity. Prone positioning even on wedges

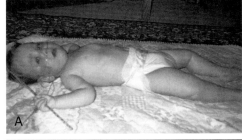
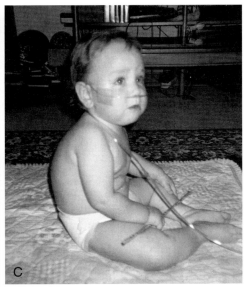
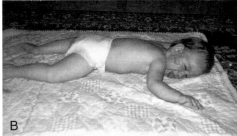

FIG. 12.7 Typical postures seen in a young child with spinal muscular atrophy in supine (A), prone (B), and sitting (C) positions. Note the limited antigravity control and dependent posturing.

TABLE 12.3 **Handheld Dynamometry Scores Recorded With a Standardized Protocol With Isometric Contraction**

Measurement	Position	Right, lb		Left, lb	
		7 yr–2 mo	8 yr–4 mo	8 yr–4 mo	7 yr–2 mo
Hip flexion	Supine, 90°	9	15	7	13
Hip extension	Supine, 90°	28	26	29	28
Hip abduction	Supine, 0°	9	17	8	16
Knee flexion	Sitting, 90°	13	16	11	16
Knee extension	Sitting, 90°	20	23	19	23
Ankle dorsiflexion	Supine, 90°	10	9	9	12
Ankle plantar flexion	Supine, 90°	52	54	50	56

should be limited or not used, owing to the effort required for head righting to interact with the environment and due to the inhibition of abdominal expansion and diaphragmatic depression thus limiting respiratory function.

Head control fails to develop or is significantly impaired in those with SMA type I. Early developmental postures such as prone on elbows are not attained. The use of developmental exercise in type I SMA should be considered if the child tolerates and enjoys the activities. ROM exercises with proper positioning should be carried out to ensure maintenance of flexibility and comfort. Flexion contractures of the hips, knees, and elbows, hip abductors, ankle plantar flexors, and positional torticollis are deformities that can be minimized with a comprehensive ROM and positioning program.[25] The exercise program should also include limited activities to encourage active movement and for strengthening, such as lightweight toys or rattles with Velcro straps around the wrists or mobiles positioned close to the hands for easy access. The use of slings and springs has also been advocated to counteract the impact of gravity and provide the child with the opportunity for movement with only slight movements of the body.[71,72] Developmental activities such as the use of supported sitting for the development of head control should be of short duration to avoid fatigue.

In conjunction with an occupational or speech therapist, a feeding program that is safe and not excessively exhausting should be implemented, but the risk of aspiration needs to be closely monitored due to the rapidly changing status of these patients. The medical team should discuss the parents' expectations regarding the aggressiveness of care. Once symptoms related to feeding are noted, more frequent feedings are necessary, and referral to a GI physician is often considered for a G-tube and Nissan fundoplication should the parents want this type of treatment. Breastfeeding may be difficult in this population due to the strength needed to develop sufficient suction.[72] Special care with feeding is necessary to avoid aspiration and secondary respiratory problems.

Death secondary to pneumonia or other respiratory complications is common in the absence of medical supportive care within a few months to few years of diagnosis in SMA type I owing to the degree of weakness and apnea.[72] The mean age of death is widely variable depending on the aggressiveness of care but many children with aggressive care can live well into the first decade of life albeit with significant functional impairment.[176,197] Counseling related to end-of-life issues and treatment choices as well as support for the

parents and family is an extremely important component in the management of this condition, and often a hospice team will be involved in counseling the family alongside the neuromuscular team.

SPINAL MUSCULAR ATROPHY (TYPE II)

Background

Impairments, Activity Limitations, and Participation Restrictions

The onset of weakness in SMA type II usually appears within the first year, with the course of the disease somewhat variable. Muscle strength testing in children and adults with SMA type II has been evaluated using handheld dynamometry (Table 12.3),[77] manual muscle testing,[279] and qualitative muscle testing with a tensiometer.[215] Forced vital capacity[279] data are also available. Progressive loss of strength and pulmonary function have been consistently reported.[274] However, the overall course of the disease can be stable over long periods of time with progression detectable over periods upwards of a year.[131] The Hammersmith Functional Motor Scale for Children with SMA has also been developed by Marion Main at the Hammersmith in London as a specific functional skills rating tool for children with SMA type II. It has been expanded to allow evaluation of patients with SMA type III and is part of the SMA Functional Composite score, which includes evaluation of gross motor function, upper extremity function, and ambulatory ability.[95,154,184] The functional composite could be used to monitor upper extremity and gross motor function or ambulation and muscle fatigue in response to a strength-based treatment approach or to monitor recovery following a hospitalization or surgery to determine when return to full baseline status is achieved.

Contractures are frequently an impairment in SMA type II and often develop within the first decade of life. They frequently limit the ability to stand either in a stander or in KAFOs if the contracture becomes severe. The distribution of weakness is similar to SMA types I and III with primary proximal involvement. Weakness is usually greatest in the hip, knee extensors, and elbow extensors with the hamstrings, biceps, and hip adductors being relatively preserved. Involvement of the distal musculature appears later in the course of the disease and is less severe than the proximal involvement. Involvement of the cranial nerves has been reported but is not considered to be a typical feature of SMA. Fasciculations of the tongue have been reported in approximately one half of the children and can be seen by muscle ultrasound almost uniformly. Minimyoclonus (a fine tremor) of the hands is also often noted. Fatigue is a significant impairment for these patients, and endurance training has been shown to have an impact on oxidative capacity but with an increase in fatigue related to the training that can limit the application of an endurance exercise program.[152]

Foreground

Infancy

Because the clinical presentation and progression of SMA type II are somewhat variable, the management program must address the major impairments, activity limitations, and participation restrictions as they are manifested. Typically, presentation is during the second half of the first year of life with some of the children with mild SMA type II presenting after a year with delay in ambulation onset. Some children may develop the ability to stand but lose this ability quickly after the onset of weakness; a few are able to ambulate with KAFOs.

Sitting posture is an area of primary concern in the management program for children who demonstrate significant weakness, and external head and trunk support in antigravity positions are sometimes required. A thoracolumbosacral orthosis (TLSO, or "body jacket") for support in sitting can be used; however, this is not universally recommended due to the increased work of breathing required. It is important to make sure there is a generous abdominal cutout to allow abdominal expansion if one is prescribed. Developmental activities provided on an ongoing basis are indicated to develop gross motor skills. Therapy sessions should be monitored, and an awareness of fatigue and function following exercise is important. An ergometer can be considered, and swimming has been reported to be beneficial in maintaining muscle strength and functional skills.[57] Instruction to the family in the use of adaptive equipment for proper positioning is crucial in slowing the deforming effects of gravity on the spine when the child is sitting or standing.

Standing by the age of 12 to 18 months should be initiated prior to the onset of contractures. The adaptive equipment necessary for standing should be considered.[100,197] Merlini favored the use of KAFOs with the proximal rim fitted in a similar way to a quadrilateral socket with ischial weight bearing. It should be aligned in enough dorsiflexion (or posted at the heel) to allow the weight line to fall toward the anterior portion of the base of support and posterior to the hip. With this type of bracing patients with a milder presentation of SMA type II will be able to take some steps while those with a more severe presentation will require either parapodiums or A-frame standers. The rate of fracture incidence in SMA has been reported to be increased and falls within a wide range. Weight bearing is an important modality to maintain bone stock in those who are not able to ambulate.[19,85,238] A supine stander is recommended for children without adequate head control, and vertical standers or KAFOs as described above are appropriate for patients with better head and trunk control. Orthopedic consultation for a corset or TLSO (with abdominal cutout) should be considered for use in standing to maintain trunk alignment if the adaptive equipment does not provide adequate control.

Preschool-Age and School-Age Period

In the toddler, orthotics for standing might also be considered (lightweight KAFOs); however, the progression of weakness and contracture may make walking an unrealistic goal. In a report of promotion of walking in 12 children with intermediate SMA or SMA type II (ages 13 months to 3 years), Granata and associates[101] described success in attaining assisted ambulation, with 58% of the children using KAFOs. This has not been the experience of all investigators, but standing is nonetheless an important goal. Although only a small number of children were studied, these investigators also reported less severe scoliotic curves in the children who used the orthoses in comparison with a control group of children with SMA.

If a walking program is initiated and successful, training in the parallel bars followed by use of a walker or other device to allow greater independence is desired. Close monitoring of safety with supported walking is necessary owing to the degree of weakness present and the potential for injury from a fall. The incidence of hip dislocation and contractures has also been reported as less when a supported walking program is used.[102]

Independence with mobility other than walking is a primary goal for the child with SMA type II who typically will not develop independence in walking.[127] Because most power scooters do not provide adequate trunk support, use of a power wheelchair is indicated. Many children with SMA type II will become independent in a power wheelchair between 1 and 2 years of age and some of the stronger patients will be able to push a lightweight manual wheelchair (Fig. 12.8A) for short distances on tile floors. This is often not functional over the long term, however, and typically, a power wheelchair is needed also for longer distances (Fig. 12.8B). If a TLSO is not used to support the trunk, close attention to fit is needed with use of lateral trunk supports. Severe contractures as a result of prolonged sitting and progression of scoliosis are experienced in all children, necessitating implementation of a consistent ROM program.[85] Surgical intervention for spinal stabilization is indicated if the curve progresses.[2] A variety of internal fixation methods are available that will allow the thoracic cavity and trunk to grow yet stabilize the progression of the curve. Orthosis have not been shown to change the progression of the curve but have been helpful with sitting balance and comfort in sitting.[212]

Exercise in patients with SMA type II appears to be safe and from a practical point of view possible. There is some suggestion that endurance training can impact endurance capacity, but there is a risk of fatigue that might limit the acceptability of this to the patient, and there is limited data to suggest functional gains can be expected.[106,145,152,181]

Transition to Adulthood

Survival into adulthood is typical in SMA type II and depends on aggressive respiratory management and the progression of muscle weakness and secondary deformities.[99] Because of the significant degree of muscle weakness, assistance is typically required for transfers and ADLs. An attendant or family member is needed to provide assistance for general ADLs. Intelligence is rarely affected; therefore vocational goals in areas of interest should be explored through vocational rehabilitation services.

An aggressive program of pulmonary care is required, including breathing exercises and percussion and postural

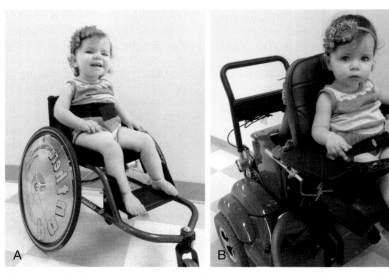

FIG. 12.8 Child with SMA type II shown in a lightweight manual wheelchair (A) and a power wheelchair (B).

drainage with illness. Forced vital capacity has been shown to decrease by about 1.1% per year, but mechanical ventilation is seldom needed.[244] The ROM and bracing program should also be continued to control progression of the contractures with the goal of maintaining a pattern of stability over time with growth.

SPINAL MUSCULAR ATROPHY (TYPE III)

Background

SMA type III (Kugelberg-Welander disease) typically demonstrates symptoms of weakness shortly after the onset of ambulation. Barry Russman and others have divided this group into two categories: type IIIA (onset of weakness prior to 2 years of age) and type IIIB (onset of weakness after 2 years of age).[225] Of the patients in the SMA type IIIA group, 50% retained the ability to walk past the age of 12; in the type IIIB group, 50% retained the ability to walk passed the 44th birthday. Fasciculations, most easily observed in the tongue, are noted in about half of the individuals, and minimyoclonus (a fine tremor) may be a primary impairment noted on examination, but it rarely interferes with function.[61]

Impairments, Activity Limitations, and Participation Restrictions

In a study by Dorscher and colleagues[61] reviewing the status of 31 patients with Kugelberg-Welander disease, or SMA type III, proximal lower extremity weakness was the most common impairment reported, but for these patients fatigue is also a significant functional impairment.[181,182,185] Secondary impairments included postural compensations resulting from muscle weakness and contractures; in about half of patients, scoliosis develops later in the first or early in the second decade.[250] An increased lumbar lordosis and compensated Trendelenburg gait pattern are common postural compensations for proximal muscle weakness of the lower extremities. Ankle plantar flexion contractures are occasionally reported but not with the frequency seen in DMD. In adolescents with type III SMA, the incidence of scoliosis and its severity are related to the degree of weakness and functional status.[85] Individuals who maintain

independent walking have a lower incidence of scoliosis and less severe curves if scoliosis develops.

Foreground
School-Age Period

The initial disability in SMA type III usually becomes apparent within the first decade and includes difficulty in arising from the floor, climbing stairs, and keeping up with peers during play. A compensated Trendelenburg or waddling gait, which becomes more pronounced with attempts at running, will also be observed. Upper extremity function is usually less prominent, and proximal upper extremity strength can be somewhat preserved.[184] Walking can in some cases be maintained lifelong as the primary means of mobility. In those cases when weakness is noted before 2 years of age, however, a manual wheelchair or scooter may ultimately be required for mobility over long distances during the school-age period as their gait becomes more inconsistent and unsteady and falls increase.[181,182,183,185,186] A significant percentage of these children will also lose ambulation through puberty.

Management for the adolescent with SMA type III is consistent with the concepts previously presented in this chapter. ROM exercises should be prescribed as appropriate, and selected strengthening and or endurance exercises may be indicated to maintain functional skills. Adaptive equipment for mobility is indicated based on functional demands, and a power scooter for long-distance mobility or manual wheelchair may be needed in certain cases. If performance of ADLs becomes a problem, collaboration with an occupational therapist to address concerns may be needed.

Transition to Adulthood

Difficulty in ADLs that require overhead lifting can be expected, and vocational activities that involve manual labor or long periods of standing are not recommended. Because the life span is not significantly shortened, vocational planning is needed. Adaptive equipment and environmental access requirements are dependent on functional needs that, unlike DMD, are more slowly progressive, leaving more time for appropriate planning. In milder cases these may not be required until later in adulthood.

SUMMARY

Muscle weakness and contracture are hallmark features of the childhood neuromuscular disorders. Background knowledge of therapeutic exercise, functional use of orthoses and adaptive equipment, and strategies to minimize disabilities secondary to the primary impairments in strength, endurance, muscle length, and cardiopulmonary function allow the physical therapist to bring unique information and skills to the management team.

Many of the disorders significantly reduce longevity. Therefore the patient's quality of life and attention to how the family copes with the stress should be included in the team's intervention program. Providing the children and families with anticipatory guidance and support as well as realistic expectations is an important goal. Connection with support groups or contact with other families that have had a similar experience should be arranged with the help of social work and can often help the family work through crisis periods, particularly when extended family support is not available.

Through the combined perspectives and innovative solutions of team members, a comprehensive program can be provided that takes into consideration the multifaceted demands of each individual and family. A philosophy of using a family-centered approach to care will help ensure that needs are met to the best of the team's ability.

Case Scenarios on Expert Consult

The case scenarios related to this chapter look at two patients. The first is "Donald," and video examples of the issues demonstrated by Donald's case are also included. The case presents Donald's issues as the disease progresses over time from diagnosis to death. The case illustrates the role of the physical therapist as addressed in the chapter. The second case, "Derek," is a child with a dystrophinopathy and focuses on management during early childhood.

ACKNOWLEDGMENTS

Our personal thanks goes to the children and their families who contributed to our knowledge of MD and SMA. Special thanks to Donald and Derek and their families for sharing their stories. Support from the SMA Foundation to AG is acknowledged.

REFERENCES

1. Amendt LE, Ause-Ellias KL, Eybers JL, Wadsworth CT, Nielsen DH, Weinstein SL: Validity and reliability testing of the scoliometer, *Phys Ther* 70:108–117, 1990.
2. Reference deleted in proofs.
3. Alemdaroğlu I, Karaduman A, Yilmaz OT, Topaloğlu H: Different types of upper extremity exercise training in Duchenne muscular dystrophy: effects on functional performance, strength, endurance, and ambulation, *Muscle Nerve* 51(5):697–705, 2014.
4. American Physical Therapy Association: *Physical therapist examination and evaluation: focus on tests and measures. Guide to physical therapist practice 3.0*, Alexandria, VA, 2014, American Physical Therapy Association. Available at http://guidetoptpractice.apta.org/content/1/SEC4.body.
5. American Thoracic Society Documents: Respiratory care of the patient with Duchenne muscular dystrophy, *Am J Respir Crit Care Med* 170:456–465, 2004.
6. Anderson JL, Head SI, Rae C, Morley JW: Brian function in Duchenne muscular dystrophy, *Brain* 125:4–14, 2002.
7. Ansved T: Muscle training in muscular dystrophies, *Acta Physiol Scand* 171:359–366, 2001.
8. Ansved T: Muscular dystrophies: influence of physical conditioning on the disease evolution, *Curr Opin Clin Nutr Metab Care* 6:435–439, 2003.
9. Anziska Y, Inan S: Exercise in neuromuscular disease, *Semin Neurol* 34(5):542–556, 2014.
10. Aprile I, Padua L, Iosa M, Gilardi A, Bordieri C, Frusciante R, et al.: Balance and walking in facioscapulohumeral muscular dystrophy: multi-perspective assessment, *Eur J Phys Rehabil Med* 48(3):393–402, 2012.
11. Bach JR: The use of mechanical ventilation is appropriate in children with genetically proven spinal muscular atrophy type 1: the motion for, *Paediatr Respir Rev* 9:45–50, 2008.
12. Bach JR, Chaudhry SS: Standards of care in MDA clinics, *Am J Phys Med Rehab* 79:193–196, 2000.
13. Bach JR, McKeon J: Orthopaedic surgery and rehabilitation for the prolongation of brace-free ambulation of patients with Duchenne muscular dystrophy, *Am J Phys Med Rehab* 70:323–331, 1991.
14. Reference deleted in proofs.
15. Bach JR, Campagnolo DI, Hoeman S: Life satisfaction of individuals with Duchenne muscular dystrophy using long-term mechanical ventilatory support, *Am J Phys Med Rehab* 70:129–135, 1991.
16. Bach JR, O'Brien J, Krotenberg R, Alba AS: Management of end stage respiratory failure in Duchenne muscular dystrophy, *Muscle Nerve* 10:177–182, 1987.
17. Bach JR, Saltstein K, Sinquee D, Weaver B, Komaroff E: Long-term survival in Werdnig-Hoffmann disease, *Am J Phys Med Rehab* 86:339–345, 2007.
18. Bakker JP, deGroot IJ, Beckerman H, deJong BA, Lankhorst GJ: The effects of knee-ankle-foot orthoses in the treatment of Duchenne muscular dystrophy: review of the literature, *Clin Rehabil* 14:343–359, 2000.
19. Ballestrazzi A, Gnudi A, Magni E, Granata C: Osteopenia in spinal muscular atrophy. In Merlini L, Granata C, Dubowitz V, editors: *Current concepts in childhood spinal muscular atrophy*, New York, 1989, Springer-Verlag, pp 215–219.
20. Banerjee B, Sharma U, Balasubramanian K, Kalaivani M, Kalra V, Jagannathan NR: Effect of creatine monohydrate in improving cellular energetics and muscle strength in ambulatory Duchenne muscular dystrophy patients: a randomized, placebo-controlled 31P MRS study, *Magn Reson Imaging* 28(5):698–707, 2010.
21. Banihani R, Smile S, Yoon G, Dupuis A, Mosleh M, Snider A, McAdam L: Cognitive and neurobehavioral profile in boys with Duchenne muscular dystrophy, *J Child Neurol* 30(11):1472–1482, 2015.
22. Beenakker EA, Fock JM, Van Tol MJ, Maurits NM, Koopman HM, Brouwer OF, Van der Hoeven JH: Intermittent prednisone therapy in Duchenne muscular dystrophy: a randomized controlled trial, *Arch Neurol* 62:128–132, 2005.
23. Bianchi ML, Mazzanti A, Galbiati E, Saraifoger S, Dubini A, Cornelio F, Morandi L: Bone mineral density and bone metabolism in Duchenne muscular dystrophy, *Osteoporos Int* 14:761–767, 2003.
24. Biggar WD, Gingras M, Fehlings DL, Harris VA, Steele CA: Deflazacort treatment of Duchenne muscular dystrophy, *J Pediatr* 138:45–50, 2001.
25. Binder H: New ideas in the rehabilitation of children with spinal muscular atrophy. In Merlini L, Granata C, Dubowitz V, editors: *Current concepts in childhood spinal muscular atrophy*, New York, 1989, Springer-Verlag, pp 117–128.
26. Bird TD: Myotonic muscular dystrophy type 1, *GeneReviews*, 2015. Available at: URL: www.genereview.org.
27. Blake DS, Weir A, Newey SE, Davis KE: Function and genetics of dystrophia and dystrophia related proteins in muscle, *Phys Rev* 82:291–329, 2002.
28. Bonifati MD, Ruzza G, Bonometto P, Berardinelli A, Gorni K, Orcesi S, et al.: A multicenter, double-blind, randomized trial of deflazacort versus prednisone in Duchenne muscular dystrophy, *Muscle Nerve* 23:1344–1347, 2000.
29. Bonne G, Quijano-Roy S: Emery-Dreifuss muscular dystrophy, laminopathies, and other nuclear envelopathies, *Handb Clin Neurol* 113:1367–1376, 2013.
30. Bönnemann CG: The collagen VI-related myopathies Ullrich congenital muscular dystrophy and Bethlem myopathy, *Handb Clin Neurol* 101:81–96, 2011.
31. Borkowska J, Rudhik-Schoneborn S, Hausmanowa-Petrusewicz I, Zerre K: Early infantile form of spinal muscle atrophy, *Folia Neuropathol* 40:19–26, 2002.

32. Bowker JH, Halpin PJ: Factors determining success in reambulation of the child with progressive muscular dystrophy, *Orthop Clin North Am* 9:431–436, 1978.

33. Reference deleted in proofs.

34. Brooke MH, Fenichel GM, Griggs RC, et al.: Duchenne muscular dystrophy: patterns of clinical progression and effects of supportive therapy, *Neurology* 39:475–481, 1989.

35. Brooke MH, Griggs RC, Mendell JR, et al.: Clinical trial in Duchenne dystrophy: I. The design of the protocol, *Muscle Nerve* 4:186–197, 1981.

36. Brouwer OF, Paderg GW, Van Der Ploeg RJO, Ruys CJM, Brand R: The influence of handedness on the distribution of muscular weakness of the arm in facioscapulohumeral muscular dystrophy, *Brain* 115:1587–1598, 1992.

37. Brussock CM, Haley SM, Munsat TL, Bernhardt DB: Measurement of isometric force in children with and without Duchenne's muscular dystrophy, *Phys Ther* 72:105–114, 1992.

38. Reference deleted in proofs.

39. Bushby K, Connor E: Clinical outcome measures for trials in Duchenne muscular dystrophy: report from International Working Group meetings, *Clin Investig (Lond)* 1(9):1217–1235, 2011.

40. Bushby K, Finkel R, Birnkrant DJ, et al.: Diagnosis and management of Duchenne muscular dystrophy, part 2: implementation of multidisciplinary care, *Lancet Neurol* 9:177–189, 2010.

41. Cambridge W, Drennan JC: Scoliosis associated with Duchenne muscular dystrophy, *J Pediatr Orthop* 7:436–440, 1987.

42. Campbell C, Sherlock R, Jacob P, Blayney M: Congenital myotonic dystrophy: assisted ventilation duration and outcome, *Pediatrics* 113(4):811–816, 2004.

43. Carter GT, Abresch RT, Fowler Jr WM: Adaptations to exercise training and contraction-induced muscle injury in animal models of muscular dystrophy, *Am J Phys Med Rehabil* 81(Suppl 11):S151–S161, 2002.

44. Chakkalakal JV, Thompson J, Parks RJ, Jasmin BJ: Molecular, cellular, and pharmacological therapies for Duchenne/Becker muscular dystrophies, *FASEB J* 19:880–891, 2005.

45. Chamova T, Guergueltcheva V, Raycheva M, Todorov T, Genova J, Bichev S, et al.: Association between loss of dp140 and cognitive impairment in Duchenne and Becker dystrophies, *Balkan J Med Genet* 16(1):21–30, 2013.

46. Charash LI, Lovelace RE, Wolfe SG, Kutscher AH, Price D, Leach R, Leach CF: *Realities in coping with progressive neuromuscular disease*, Philadelphia, 1987, Charles Press Publishers.

47. Cheuk DK, Wong V, Wraige E, Baxter P, Cole A, N'Diaye T, Mayowe V: Surgery for scoliosis in Duchenne muscular dystrophy, *Cochrane Database Syst Rev* 24, 2007. CD005375.

48. Childers MK, Okamura CS, Bogan DJ, Bogan JR, Petroski GF, McDonald K, Kornegay JN: Eccentric contraction injury in dystrophic canine muscle, *Arch Phys Med Rehabil* 83(11):1572–1578, 2002.

49. Chung BH, Wong VC, Ip P: Spinal muscular atrophy: survival pattern and functional status, *Pediatrics* 114:e548–e553, 2004.

50. Chyatte SB, Long C, Vignos PJ: Balanced forearm orthosis in muscular dystrophy, *Arch Phys Med Rehabil* 46:633–636, 1965.

51. Ciafaloni E, Fox DJ, Pandya S, Westfield CP, Puzhankara S, Romitti PA, et al.: Delayed diagnosis in Duchenne muscular dystrophy: data from the Muscular Dystrophy Surveillance, Tracking, and Research Network (MD STARnet), *J Pediatr* 155:380–385, 2009.

52. Cohen EJ, Quarta E, Fulgenzi G, Minciacchi D: Acetylcholine, GABA and neuronal networks: a working hypothesis for compensations in the dystrophic brain, *Brain Res Bull* 110:1–13, 2015.

53. Colbert AP, Craig C: Scoliosis management in Duchenne muscular dystrophy: prospective study of modified Jewett hyperextension brace, *Arch Phys Med Rehabil* 68:302–304, 1987.

54. Constantin B: Dystrophin complex functions as a scaffold for signalling proteins, *Biochim Biophys Acta* 1838(2):635–642, 2014.

55. Coster W, Deeney T, Haltiwanger J, Haley S: *School function assessment*, San Antonio, TX, 1998, Therapy Skill Builders.

56. Courdier-Fruh I, Barman L, Briguet A, Meier T: Glucocorticoid-mediated regulation of utrophin levels in human muscle fibers, *Neuromuscul Disord* 12(Suppl 1):S95–S104, 2002.

57. Cunha MC, Oliveira AS, Labronici RH, Gabbai AA: Spinal muscular atrophy type II and III: evolution of 50 patients with physiotherapy and hydrotherapy in a swimming pool, *Arq Neuropsiquiatr* 54:402–406, 1996.

58. Darras BT, Korf BR, Urion DK: Dystrophinopathies, *GeneReviews*. Available at: URL: www.genereviews.org.

59. Dastur RS, Gaitonde PS, Khadilkar SV, Udani VP, Nadkarni JJ: Correlation between deletion patterns of SMN and NAIP genes and the clinical features of spinal muscular atrophy in Indian patients, *Neurol India* 54(3):255–259, 2006.

60. De Sanctis R, Pane M, Sivo S, et al.: Suitability of North Star Ambulatory Assessment in young boys with Duchenne muscular dystrophy, *Neuromuscul Disord* 1:14–18, 2015.

61. Dorscher PT, Mehrsheed S, Mulder DW, Litchy WJ, Ilstrup DM: Wohlfart-Kugelberg-Welander syndrome: serum creatine kinase and functional outcome, *Arch Phys Med Rehabil* 72:587–591, 1991.

62. Douniol M, Jacquette A, Cohen D, Bodeau N, Rachidi L, Angeard N, et al.: Psychiatric and cognitive phenotype of childhood myotonic dystrophy type 1, *Dev Med Child Neurol* 54(10):905–911, 2012.

63. Dubowitz V: The clinical picture of spinal muscular atrophy. In Merlini L, Granata C, Dubowitz V, editors: *Current concepts in childhood spinal muscular atrophy*, New York, 1989, Springer-Verlag, pp 13–19.

64. Reference deleted in proofs.

65. Eagle M, Baudouin SV, Chandler C, Giddings DR, Bullock R, Bushby K: Survival in Duchenne muscular dystrophy: improvements in life expectancy since 1967 and the impact of home nocturnal ventilation, *Neuromuscul Disord* 12:926–929, 2002.

66. Echenne B, Bassez G: Congenital and infantile myotonic dystrophy, *Handb Clin Neurol* 113:1387–1393, 2013.

67. Edwards RHT: Studies of muscular performance in normal and dystrophic subjects, *Br Med Bull* 36:159–164, 1980.

68. Emery AEH: *Duchenne muscular dystrophy*, Oxford, 1993, Oxford University Press.

69. Emery AEH: The muscular dystrophies, *Lancet* 359:687–695, 2002.

70. Emery AEH, Skinner R: Clinical studies in benign (Becker-type) X-linked muscular dystrophy, *Clinic Genet* 10:189–201, 1976.

71. Eng GD: Therapy and rehabilitation of the floppy infant, *R I Med J* 72:367–370, 1989.

72. Eng GD: Rehabilitation of the child with a severe form of spinal muscular atrophy (type I, infantile or Werdnig-Hoffman disease). In Merlini L, Granata C, Dubowitz V, editors: *Current concepts in childhood spinal muscular atrophy*, New York, 1989, Springer-Verlag, pp 113–115.

73. Escolar DM, Buyse G, Henricson E, et al.: CINRG randomized controlled trial of creatine and glutamine in Duchenne muscular dystrophy, *Ann Neurol* 58:151–155, 2005.

74. Estilow T, Glanzman A, Flickinger J, Powers KM, Medne L, Tennekoon G, Yum SW: The Wilmington robotic exoskeleton (WREX) improves upper extremity function in patients with Duchenne muscular dystrophy, *Poster presentation, MDA Scientific Conference*, 2014.

75. Farini A, Razini P, Erratico S, Torrente Y, Meregalli M: Cell based therapy for Duchenne muscular dystrophy, *J Cell Physiol* 221:526–534, 2009.

76. Farrar MA, Kiernan MC: The genetics of spinal muscular atrophy: progress and challenges, *Neurotherapeutics* 12(2):290–302, 2015.

77. Febrer A, Rodriguez N, Alias L, Tizzano E: Measurement of muscle strength with a handheld dynamometer in patients with chronic spinal muscular atrophy, *J Rehabil Med* 42:228–231, 2010.

78. Finder JDA: Perspective on the 2004 American Thoracic Society statement, "respiratory care of the patient with Duchenne muscular dystrophy." *Pediatrics* 123(Suppl 4):S239–S241, 2009.

79. Finkel RS, McDermott MP, Kaufmann P, Darras BT, Chung WK, Sproule DM, et al.: Observational study of spinal muscular atrophy type I and implications for clinical trials, *Neurology* 83(9):810–817, 2014.

80. Florence JM, Pandya S, King WM, Robinson JD, Baty J, Miller JP, et al.: Intrarater reliability of manual muscle test (Medical Research Council Scale) grades in Duchenne's muscular dystrophy, *Phys Ther* 72:115–122, 1992.

81. Forst J, Forst R: Surgical treatment of Duchenne muscular dystrophy patients in Germany: the present situation, *Acta Myol* 31(1):21–23, 2012.

82. Fowler WM: Rehabilitation management of muscular dystrophy and related disorders: I. The role of exercise, *Arch Phys Med Rehabil* 63:208–210, 1982.

83. Fowler WM, Gardner GW: Quantitative strength measurements in muscular dystrophy, *Arch Phys Med Rehabil* 48:629–644, 1967.

84. Frinchi M, Macaluso F, Licciardi A, Perciavalle V, Coco M, Belluardo N, et al.: Recovery of damaged skeletal muscle in mdx mice through low-intensity endurance exercise, *Int J Sports Med* 35(1):19–27, 2014.

85. Fujak A, Kopschina C, Forst R, Gras F, Mueller LA, Forst J: Fractures in proximal spinal muscular atrophy, *Arch Orthop Trauma Surg* 130(6):775–730, 2010.

86. Fukuyama Y, Osaw M, Suzuki H: Congenital muscular dystrophy of the Fukuyama type: clinical, genetic and pathological considerations, *Brain Dev* 3:1–29, 1981.

87. Galasko CSB, Williamson JB, Delany CM: Lung function in Duchenne muscular dystrophy, *Eur Spine J* 4:263–267, 1995.

88. Gardner-Medwin D: Controversies about Duchenne muscular dystrophy: II. Bracing for ambulation, *Dev Med Child Neurol* 21:659–662, 1979.

89. Gardner-Medwin D: Clinical features and classification of the muscular dystrophies, *Br Med Bull* 36:109–115, 1980.

90. Gibson DA, Koreska J, Robertson D: The management of spinal deformity in Duchenne's muscular dystrophy, *Clin Orthop* 9:437–450, 1978.

91. Gilroy J, Holliday P: *Basic neurology*, New York, 1982, Macmillan.

92. Glanzman AM, Flickinger JM, Dholakia KH, Bönnemann CG, Finkel RS: Serial casting for the management of ankle contracture in Duchenne muscular dystrophy, *Pediatr Phys Ther* 23(3):275–279, 2011.

93. Glanzman AM, Mazzone E, Main M, Pelliccioni M, Wood J, Swoboda KJ, et al.: The Children's Hospital of Philadelphia Infant Test of Neuromuscular Disorders (CHOP INTEND): test development and reliability, *Neuromuscul Disord* 20(3):155–161, 2010.

94. Glanzman AM, McDermott MP, Montes J, et al.: Validation of the Children's Hospital of Philadelphia Infant Test of Neuromuscular Disorders (CHOP INTEND), *Pediatr Phys Ther* 23(4):322–326, 2011.

95. Glanzman AM, O'Hagen JM, McDermott MP, Martens WB, Flickinger J, Riley S, et al.: Pediatric Neuromuscular Clinical Research Network for Spinal Muscular Atrophy Muscle Study Group (MSG), validation of the Expanded Hammersmith Functional Motor Scale in spinal muscular atrophy type II and III, *J Child Neurol* 26(12):1499–1507, 2011. PNCR.

96. Goemans N, Klingels K, van den Hauwe M, Boons S, Verstraete L, Peeters C, et al.: Six-minute walk test: reference values and prediction equation in healthy boys aged 5 to 12 years, *PLoS One* 8(12), e84120. 2013.

97. Gordon BS, Lowe DA, Kostek MC: Exercise increases utrophin protein expression in the mdx mouse model of Duchenne muscular dystrophy, *Muscle Nerve* 49(6):915–918, 2014.

98. Gordon E, Hoffman EP, Pegoraro E: Congenital muscular dystrophy overview, *GeneReviews*, 2006. Available at: URL: www.genereviews.org.

99. Gormley MC: Respiratory management of spinal muscular atrophy type 2, *J Neurosci Nurs* 46(6):E33–E41, 2014.

100. Granata C, Cornelio F, Bonfiglioli S, Mattutini P, Merlini L: Promotion of ambulation of patients with spinal muscular atrophy by early fitting of knee-ankle-foot orthoses, *Dev Med Child Neurol* 29(2):221–224, 1987.

101. Granata C, Magni E, Sabattini L, Colombo C, Merlini L: Promotion of ambulation in intermediate spinal muscle atrophy. In Merlini L, Granata C, Dubowitz V, editors: *Current concepts in childhood spinal muscular atrophy*, New York, 1989, Springer-Verlag, pp 127–132.

102. Granata C, Marini ML, Capelli T, Merlini L: Natural history of scoliosis in spinal muscular atrophy and results of orthopaedic treatment. In Merlini L, Granata C, Dubowitz V, editors: *Current concepts in childhood spinal muscular atrophy*, New York, 1989, Springer-Verlag, pp 153–164.

103. Granata C, Merlini L, Magni E, Marini ML, Stagni SB: Spinal muscular atrophy: natural history and orthopaedic treatment of scoliosis, *Spine* 14:760–762, 1989.

104. Grange RW, Call JA: Recommendations to define exercise prescription for Duchenne muscular dystrophy, *Exer Sport Sci Rev* 35:12–17, 2007.

105. Griffet J, Decrocq L, Rauscent H, Richelme C, Fournier M: Lower extremity surgery in muscular dystrophy, *Orthop Traumatol Surg Res* 97(6):634–638, 2011.

106. Grondard C, Biondi O, Armand AS, Lécolle S, Della Gaspera B, Pariset C, et al.: Regular exercise prolongs survival in a type 2 spinal muscular atrophy model mouse, *J Neurosci* 25(33):7615–7622, 2005.

107. Haley SM, Coster WJ, Ludlow LH, Haltiwanger JT: *Pediatric Evaluation of Disability Inventory (PEDI): development, standardization and administration manual*, Boston, 1992, New England Medical Center Hospital.

108. Reference deleted in proofs.

109. Harper PS: *Myotonic dystrophy: major problems in neurology*, ed 2, vol. 21. Philadelphia, 1989, WB Saunders.

110. T1 Haumont, Rahman T, Sample W,M, King M, Church C, Henley J, Jayakumar S: Wilmington robotic exoskeleton: a novel device to maintain arm improvement in muscular disease, *J Pediatr Orthop* 31(5):e44–e49, 2011.

111. Heckmatt JZ, Dubowitz V, Hyde SA: Prolongation of walking in Duchenne muscular dystrophy with lightweight orthoses: review of 57 cases, *Dev Med Child Neurol* 27:149–154, 1985.

112. Heller KD, Forst R, Forst J, Hengstler K: Scoliosis in Duchenne muscular dystrophy, *Prosthet Orthot Int* 21:202–209, 1997.

113. Herrmann R, Straub V, Meyer K, Kahn T, Wagner M, Voit T: Congenital muscular dystrophy with laminin alpha 2 chain deficiency: identification of a new intermediate phenotype and correlation of clinical findings to muscle immunohistochemistry, *Eur J Paediatr* 155:968–976, 1996.

114. Reference deleted in proofs.

115. Hoffman EP, Reeves E, Damsker J, Nagaraju K, McCall JM, Connor EM, Bushby K: Novel approaches to corticosteroid treatment in Duchenne muscular dystrophy, *Phys Med Rehabil Clin N Am* 23(4):821–828, 2012.

116. Hoffman EP, Brown RH, Kunkel LM: Dystrophin: the protein product of the Duchenne muscular dystrophy locus, *Cell* 51:919–928, 1987.

117. Hoffmann J: Ueber chronische spinale Muskelatrophie im Kindesalter, auf familiar Basis, *Deutsche Zeitschrift fur Nervenheilkunde* 3:427, 1893.

118. Holland A, Carberry S: Ohlendieck K1: proteomics of the dystrophin-glycoprotein complex and dystrophinopathy, *Curr Protein Pept Sci* 8:680–697, 2013.

119. Hsu JD, Quinlivan R: Scoliosis in Duchenne muscular dystrophy, *Neuromuscul Disord* 23(8):611–617, 2013.

120. Hsu JD: Orthopedic approaches for the treatment of lower extremity contractures in the Duchenne muscular dystrophy patient in the United States and Canada, *Semin Neurol* 15:6–8, 1995.

121. Hu X, Blemker SS: Musculoskeletal simulation can help explain selective muscle degeneration in Duchenne muscular dystrophy, *Muscle Nerve* 52(2):174–182, 2015.

122. Hyde SA, Floytrup I, Glent S, Kroksmark A, Salling B: A randomized comparative study using two methods for controlling tendo Achilles contracture in Duchenne muscular dystrophy, *Neuromuscul Disord* 10:257–263, 2000.

123. Hyzewicz J, Tanihata J, Kuraoka M, Ito N, Miyagoe-Suzuki Y, Takeda S: Low intensity training of mdx mice reduces carbonylation and increases expression levels of proteins involved in energy metabolism and muscle contraction, *Free Radic Biol Med* 82:122–136, 2015.

124. Jansen M, van Alfen N, Geurts AC, de Groot IJ: Assisted bicycle training delays functional deterioration in boys with Duchenne muscular dystrophy: the randomized controlled trial "no use is disuse." *Neurorehabil Neural Repair* 27(9):816–827, 2013.

125. Johnson EW, Braddom R: Over-work weakness in facioscapulohumeral muscular dystrophy, *Arch Phys Med Rehabil* 52:333–336, 1971.

126. Jones KJ, North KN: Recent advances in diagnosis of the childhood muscular dystrophies, *J Paediatr Child Health* 33:195–201, 1997.

127. Jones MA, McEwen IR, Hansen L: Use of power mobility for a young child with spinal muscular atrophy, *Phys Ther* 83:253–262, 2003.

128. Joseph JT, Richards CS, Anthony DC, Upton M, Perez-Atayde AR, Greenstein P: Congenital myotonic dystrophy pathology and somatic mosaicism, *Neurology* 49:1457–1460, 1997.

129. Kaspar RW, Allen HD, Montanaro F: Current understanding and management of dilated cardiomyopathy in Duchenne and Becker muscular dystrophy, *J Am Acad Nurse Pract* 21:241–249, 2009.

130. Kaufmann P, McDermott MP, Darras BT, et al.: Observational study of spinal muscular atrophy type 2 and 3: functional outcomes over 1 year, *Arch Neurol* 68(6):779–786, 2011.

131. Kaufmann P, McDermott MP, Darras BT, et al.: Prospective cohort study of spinal muscular atrophy types 2 and 3, *Neurology* 79(18):1889–1897, 2012.

132. Khadilkar SV, Chaudhari CR, Soni G, Bhutada A: Is pushing the wall, the best known method for scapular winging, really the best? A Comparative analysis of various methods in neuromuscular disorders, *J Neurol Sci* 351(1-2):179–183, 2015.

133. Reference deleted in proofs.

134. Kinali M, Main M, Eliahoo J, Messina S, Knight RK, Lehovsky J, et al.: Predictive factors for the development of scoliosis in Duchenne muscular dystrophy, *Eur J Paediatr Neurol* 11:160–166, 2007.

135. Kissel JT, Scott CB, Reyna SP, Crawford TO, Simard LR, Krosschell KJ, et al.: Project Cure Spinal Muscular Atrophy Investigators' Network. SMA CARNIVAL TRIAL PART II: a prospective, single-armed trial of L-carnitine and valproic acid in ambulatory children with spinal muscular atrophy, *PLoS One* 6(7):e21296, 2011.

136. Kley RA, Tarnopolsky MA, Vorgerd M: Creatine for treating muscle disorders, *Cochrane Database Syst Rev* 6, 2013.

137. Koenig M, Hoffmann EP, Pertelson CK: Complete cloning of the Duchenne muscular dystrophy (DMD) cDNA and preliminary genomic organization of the DMD gene in mouse and affected individuals, *Cell* 50:509–517, 1987.

138. Koessler W, Wanke T, Winkler G, Nader A, Toifl K, Kurz H, Zwick H: 2 years' experience with inspiratory muscle training in patients with neuromuscular disorders, *Chest* 120:765–769, 2001.

139. Kornegay JN, Spurney CF, Nghiem PP, Brinkmeyer-Langford CL, Hoffman EP, Nagaraju K: Pharmacologic management of Duchenne muscular dystrophy: target identification and preclinical trials, *ILAR J* 55(1):119–149, 2014.

140. Kugelberg E, Welander L: Heredofamilial juvenile muscular atrophy simulating muscular dystrophy, *AMA Arch Neurol Psychiatry* 75:500, 1956.

141. Kunkel LM, Monaco AP, Middlesworth W, Ochs SD, Latt SA: Specific cloning of DNA fragments absent from the DNA of a male patient with an X chromosome deletion, *Proc Nat Acad Sci USA* 82:4778–4782, 1985.

142. Lebel DE, Corston JA, McAdam LC, Biggar WD, Alman BA: Glucocorticoid treatment for the prevention of scoliosis in children with Duchenne muscular dystrophy: long-term follow-up, *J Bone Joint Surg Am* 95(12):1057–1061, 2013.

143. Lee CC, Pearlman JA, Chamberlain JS, Caskey CT: Expression of recombinant dystrophin and its localization to the cell membrane, *Nature* 349:334–336, 1991.

144. Lefebvre S, Bürglen L, Reboullet S, Clermont O, Burlet P, Viollet L, et al.: Identification and characterization of a spinal muscular atrophy-determining gene, *Cell* 80(1):155–165, 1995.

145. Lewelt A, Krosschell KJ, Stoddard GJ, Weng C, Xue M, Marcus RL, et al.: Resistance strength training exercise in children with spinal muscular atrophy, *Muscle Nerve* 52(4):559–567, 2015.

146. Liechti-Gallati S, Koenig M, Kunkel LM, Frey D, Boltshauser E, Schneider V, et al.: Molecular deletion patterns in Duchenne and Becker type muscular dystrophy, *Human Genet* 81:343–348, 1989.

147. Lonstein JE: Management of spinal deformity in spinal muscular atrophy. In Merlini L, Granata C, Dubowitz V, editors: *Current concepts in childhood spinal muscular atrophy*, New York, 1989, Springer-Verlag, pp 165–173.

148. Louis M, Lebacq J, Poortmans JR, Belpaire-Dethiou MC, Devogelaer J, Van Hecke P, et al.: Beneficial effects of creatine supplementation in dystrophic patients, *Muscle Nerve* 27:604–610, 2003.

149. Lue YJ, Lin RF, Chen SS, Lu YM: Measurement of the functional status of patients with different types of muscular dystrophy, *Kaohsiung J Med Sci* 25:325–333, 2009.

150. Lyager S, Steffensen B, Juhl B: Indicators of need for mechanical ventilation in Duchenne muscular dystrophy and spinal muscular atrophy, *Chest* 108:779–785, 1995.

151. MacKenzie AE, Jacob P, Surh L, Besner A: Genetic heterogeneity in spinal muscle atrophy: a linkage analysis-based assessment, *Neurology* 44:919–924, 1994.

152. Madsen KL, Hansen RS, Preisler N, Thøgersen F, Berthelsen MP, Vissing J: Training improves oxidative capacity, but not function in spinal muscular atrophy type III, *Muscle Nerve* 52(2):240–244, 2015.

153. Main M, Mercuri E, Haliloglu G, Baker R, Kinali M, Muntoni F: Serial casting of the ankles in Duchenne muscular dystrophy: can it be an alternative to surgery? *Neuromuscul Disord* 17(3):227–230, 2007.

154. Main M, Kairon H, Mercuri E, Muntoni F: The Hammersmith functional motor scale for children with spinal muscular atrophy: a scale to test ability and monitor progress in children with limited ambulation, *Eur J Paediatr Neurol* 7:155–159, 2003.

155. Manzur AY, Hyde SA, Rodillo E, Heckmatt JZ, Bentley G, Dubowitz V: A randomized controlled trial of early surgery in Duchenne muscular dystrophy, *Neuromuscul Disord* 2(5-6):379–387, 1992.

156. Manzur AY, Kinali M, Muntoni F: Update on the management of Duchenne muscular dystrophy, *Arch Dis Child* 93:986–990, 2008.

157. Marchesi D, Arlet V, Stricker U, Aeibi M: Modification of the original Luque technique in the treatment of Duchenne's neuromuscular scoliosis, *J Pediatr Orthop* 17:743–749, 1997.

158. Marshall JL, Kwok Y, McMorran BJ, Baum LG, Crosbie-Watson RH: The potential of sarcospan in adhesion complex replacement therapeutics for the treatment of muscular dystrophy, *FEBS J* 280(17):4210–4229, 2013.

159. Marshall CR: Medical treatment of spinal muscular atrophy. In Gamstorp I, Sarnat HB, editors: *Progressive spinal muscular atrophies: International Review of Child Neurology series*, New York, 1984, Raven Press, pp 163–171.

160. Matsumura T, Saito T, Fujimura H, Shinno S, Sakoda S: Lung inflation training using a positive end-expiratory pressure valve in neuromuscular disorders, *Intern Med* 51(7):711–716, 2012.

161. Mayer OH, Finkel RS, Rummey C, Benton MJ, Glanzman AM, Flickinger J, et al.: Characterization of pulmonary function in Duchenne muscular dystrophy, *Pediatr Pulmonol* 50(5):487–494, 2015.

162. Mazzone E, Martinelli D, Berardinelli A, et al.: North Star Ambulatory Assessment, 6-minute walk test and timed items in ambulant boys with Duchenne muscular dystrophy, *Neuromuscul Disord* 20(11):712–716, 2010.

163. Mazzone ES, Messina S, Vasco G, et al.: Reliability of the North Star Ambulatory Assessment in a multicentric setting, *Neuromuscul Disord* 19:458–461, 2009.

164. McDonald CM, Abresch RT, Carter GT, Fowler Jr WM, Johnson ER, Kilmer DD, Sigford BJ: Profiles of neuromuscular diseases. Duchenne muscular dystrophy, *Am J Phys Med Rehabil* 74(Suppl 5):S70–S92, 1995.

165. McDonald CM, Henricson EK, Abresch RT, Florence J, Eagle M, Gappmaier E, Glanzman AM, et al.: The 6-minute walk test and other clinical endpoints in Duchenne muscular dystrophy: reliability, concurrent validity, and minimal clinically important differences from a multicenter study, *Muscle Nerve* 48(3):357–368, 2013.

166. McDonald CM, Henricson EK, Abresch RT, Florence JM, Eagle M, Gappmaier E, et al.: The 6-minute walk test and other endpoints in Duchenne muscular dystrophy: longitudinal natural history observations over 48 weeks from a multicenter study, *Muscle Nerve* 48(3):343–356, 2013.

167. McDonald CM, Abresch RT, Carter GT, Fowler WM, Johnson ER, Kilmer DMD, Sigford BJ: Profiles of neuromuscular diseases: Duchenne muscular dystrophy, *Am J Phys Med Rehab* 74(Suppl):S70–S92, 1995.

168. McDonald DG, Kinali M, Gallagher AC, Mercuri E, Muntoni F, Roper H, et al.: Fracture prevalence in Duchenne muscular dystrophy, *Dev Med Child Neurol* 44:695–698, 2002.

169. McMillan HJ: Congenital muscular dystrophies: new evidence-based guidelines for the diagnosis and management of this evolving group of muscle disorders, *Muscle Nerve* 51(6):791–792, 2015.

170. Melki J, Lefebvre S, Burglen L, Burlet P, Clermont O, Millasseau P, et al.: De novo and inherited deletions of the 5q13 region in spinal muscular atrophies, *Science* 264(5164):1474–1477, 1994.

171. Melki J, Sheth P, Abdelhak S, Burlet P, Bachelot MF, Lathrop MG, et al.: Mapping of acute (type I) spinal muscular atrophy to chromosome 5q12-q14. The French Spinal Muscular Atrophy Investigators, *Lancet* 336(8710):271–273, 1990.

172. Mendell JR, Rodino-Klapac LR, Sahenk Z, et al.: Eteplirsen for the treatment of Duchenne muscular dystrophy, *Ann Neurol* 74(5):637–647, 2013.

173. Mercuri E, Bertini E, Iannaccone ST: Childhood spinal muscular atrophy: controversies and challenges, *Lancet Neurol* 11(5):443–452, 2012.

174. Mercuri E, Muntoni F: The ever-expanding spectrum of congenital muscular dystrophies, *Ann Neurol* 72(1):9–17, 2012.

175. Merlini L, Cicognani A, Malaspina E, Gennari M, Gnudi S, Talim B, Franzoni E: Early prednisone treatment in Duchenne muscular dystrophy, *Muscle Nerve* 27:222–227, 2003.

176. Merlini L, Granata C, Capelli T, Mattutini P, Colombo C: Natural history of infantile and childhood spinal muscular atrophy. In Merlini L, Granata C, Dubowitz V, editors: *Current concepts in childhood spinal muscular atrophy*, New York, 1989, Springer-Verlag, pp 95–100.

177. Miller F, Moseley CF, Koreska J: Spinal fusion in Duchenne muscular dystrophy, *Dev Med Child Neurol* 34:775–786, 1992.

178. Miller G, Dunn N: An outline of the management and prognosis of Duchenne muscular dystrophy in Western Australia, *Aust Pediatr J* 82:277–282, 1982.

179. Mills B, Bach JR, Zhao C, Saporito L, Sabharwal S: Posterior spinal fusion in children with flaccid neuromuscular scoliosis: the role of noninvasive positive pressure ventilatory support, *J Pediatr Orthop* 33(5):488–493, 2013.

180. Molnar GE, Alexander J: Objective, quantitative muscle testing in children: a pilot study, *Arch Phys Med Rehabil* 54:224–228, 1973.

181. Montes J, Blumenschine M, Dunaway S, Alter AS, Engelstad K, Rao AK, et al.: Weakness and fatigue in diverse neuromuscular diseases, *J Child Neurol* 28(10):1277–1283, 2013.

182. Montes J, Dunaway S, Garber CE, Chiriboga CA, De Vivo DC, Rao AK: Leg muscle function and fatigue during walking in spinal muscular atrophy type 3, *Muscle Nerve* 50(1):34–39, 2014.

183. Montes J, Dunaway S, Montgomery MJ, Sproule D, Kaufmann P, De Vivo DC, Rao AK: Fatigue leads to gait changes in spinal muscular atrophy, *Muscle Nerve* 43(4):485–488, 2011.

184. Montes J, Glanzman AM, Mazzone ES, et al.: SMA functional composite score: a functional measure in spinal muscular atrophy, *Muscle Nerve* 52(6):942–947, 2015.

185. Montes J, McDermott MP, Martens WB, et al.: Six-Minute Walk Test demonstrates motor fatigue in spinal muscular atrophy, *Neurology* 74(10):833–838, 2010.

186. Montes J, McIsaac TL, Dunaway S, Kamil-Rosenberg S, Sproule D, Garber CE, et al.: Falls and spinal muscular atrophy: exploring cause and prevention, *Muscle Nerve* 47(1):118–123, 2013.

187. Muscular Dystrophy Association: *Facts about muscular dystrophy*, Tucson, AZ, 2010, Muscular Dystrophy Association.

188. Muscular Dystrophy Association: Learning to live with neuromuscular disease. Available at: URL: http://www.mda.org/sites/default/files/publication/Learning_to_Live_P-195.pdf.

189. Nair KP, Vasanth A, Gourie-Devi M, Taly AB, Rao S, Gayathri N, Murali T: Disabilities in children with Duchenne muscular dystrophy: a profile, *J Rehabil Med* 33:147–149, 2001.

190. Nelson MD, Rader F, Tang X, et al.: PDE5 inhibition alleviates functional muscle ischemia in boys with Duchenne muscular dystrophy, *Neurology* 82(23):2085–2091, 2014.

191. Nelson SF, Crosbie RH, Miceli MC, Spencer MJ: Emerging genetic therapies to treat Duchenne muscular dystrophy, *Curr Opin Neurol* 22:532–538, 2009.

192. Reference deleted in proofs.

193. North KN, Specht LA, Sethi RK, Shapiro F, Beggs AH: Congenital muscular dystrophy associated with merosin deficiency, *J Child Neurol* 11:291–295, 1996.

194. O'Brien T, Harper PS: Course, prognosis and complications of childhood-onset myotonic dystrophy, *Dev Med Child Neurol* 26:62–67, 1984.

195. Ogino S, Wilson RB, Gold B: New insights on the evolution of the SMN1 and SMN2 region: simulation and meta-analysis for allele and haplotype frequency calculations, *Eur J Hum Genet* 12(12):1015–1023, 2004.

196. Olsen DB, Orngreen MC, Vissing J: Aerobic training improves exercise performance in facioscapulohumeral muscular dystrophy, *Neurology* 64:1064–1066, 2005.

197. Oskoui M, Levy G, Garland CJ, Gray JM, O'Hagen J, De Vivo DC, Kaufmann P: The changing natural history of spinal muscular atrophy type 1, *Neurology* 69(20):1931–1936, 2007.

198. Pandya S, King WM, Tawil R: Facioscapulohumeral dystrophy, *Phys Ther* 88(1):105–113, 2008.

199. Pandya A, Florence JM, King WM, Robinson JD, Oxman M, Province MA: Reliability of goniometric measurements in patients with Duchenne muscular dystrophy, *Phys Ther* 65:1339–1342, 1985.

200. Pane M, Mazzone ES, Fanelli L, et al.: Reliability of the Performance of Upper Limb assessment in Duchenne muscular dystrophy, *Neuromuscl Disord* 24(3):201–206, 2014.

201. Pane M, Mazzone ES, Sivo S, et al.: Long term natural history data in ambulant boys with Duchenne muscular dystrophy: 36-month changes, *PLoS One* 9(10):e108205, 2014.

202. Pane M, Mazzone ES, Sivo S, et al.: The 6 minute walk test and performance of upper limb in ambulant Duchenne muscular dystrophy boys, *PLoS Curr* 6, 2014. http://dx.doi.org/10.1371/currents.md.a93d9904d57dcb08936f2ea89bca6fe6. pii: ecurrents. md.a93d9904d57dcb08936f2ea89bca6fe6.

203. Pane M, Staccioli S, Messina S, et al.: Daily salbutamol in young patients with SMA type II, *Neuromuscul Disord* 18(7):536–540, 2008.

204. Reference deleted in proofs.

205. Reference deleted in proofs.

206. Reference deleted in proofs.

207. Reference deleted in proofs.

208. Pegoraro E, Marks H, Garcia CA, Crawford T, Connolly AM: Laminin alpha2 muscular dystrophy: genotype/phenotype studies of 22 patients, *Neurology* 51:101–110, 1998.

209. Perkins KJ, Davies KE: The role of utrophin in the potential therapy of Duchenne muscular dystrophy, *Neuromuscl Disord* 12:S78–S89, 2002.

210. Petrof BJ: Molecular pathophysiology of myofiber injury in deficiencies of the dystrophin-glycoprotein complex, *Am J Phys Med Rehab* 81:S162–S174, 2002, 2002.

211. Pinelli G, Dominici P, Merlini L, DiPasquale G, Granata C, Bonfiglioli S: Cardiologic evaluation in a family with Emery-Dreifus muscular dystrophy, *G Ital Cardiol* 17:589–593, 1987.

212. Prior TW, Russman BS: Spinal muscular atrophy, *GeneReviews*, 2013. Available at: URL: www.genereviews.org.

213. Reardon W, Newcombe R, Fenton I, Sibert J, Harper PS: The natural history of congenital myotonic muscular dystrophy: mortality and long term clinical aspects, *Arch Dis Child* 68:177–181, 1993.

214. Reed UC: Congenital muscular dystrophy. Part I: a review of phenotypical and diagnostic aspects, *Arq Neuro-Psiquiatr* 67:144–168, 2009.

215. Rhodes LE, Freeman BK, Auh S, Kokkinis AD, La Pean A, Chen C, et al.: Clinical features of spinal and bulbar muscular atrophy, *Brain* 132:3242–3251, 2009.

216. Ricker K: The expanding clinical and genetic spectrum of the myotonic dystrophies, *Acta Neurol Belg* 100:151–155, 2000.

217. Rideau Y, Glorion B, Delaubier A, Tarle O, Bach J: The treatment of scoliosis in Duchenne muscular dystrophy, *Muscle Nerve* 7:281–286, 1984.

218. Rijken NH, van Engelen BG, de Rooy JW, Geurts AC, Weerdesteyn V: Trunk muscle involvement is most critical for the loss of balance control in patients with facioscapulohumeral muscular dystrophy, *Clin Biomech (Bristol, Avon)* 29(8):855–860, 2014.

219. Rijken NH, van Engelen BG, de Rooy JW, Weerdesteyn V, Geurts AC: Gait propulsion in patients with facioscapulohumeral muscular dystrophy and ankle plantarflexor weakness, *Gait Posture* 41(2):476–481, 2015.

220. Ringel SP: *Neuromuscular disorders: a guide for patient and family*, New York, 1987, Raven Press.

221. Robinson A: Programmed cell death and the gene behind spinal muscle atrophy, *Can Med Assoc J* 153:1459–1462, 1995.

222. Rodillo E, Noble-Jamieson CM, Aber V, Heckmatt JZ, Muntoni F, Dubowitz V: Respiratory muscle training in Duchenne muscular dystrophy, *Arch Dis Child* 64:736–738, 1989.

223. Roig M, Balliu PR, Navarro C, Brugera R, Losada M: Presentation, clinical course and outcome of the congenital form of myotonic dystrophy, *Pediatr Neurol* 11:208–213, 1994.

224. Roper H, Quinlivan R: Workshop participants. Implementation of "the consensus statement for the standard of care in spinal muscular atrophy" when applied to infants with severe type 1 SMA in the UK, *Arch Dis Child* 95(10):845–849, 2010.

225. Russman BS, Buncher CR, White M, Samaha FJ, Iannaccone ST: Function changes in spinal muscular atrophy II and III. The DCN/SMA Group, *Neurology* 47(4):973–976, 1996.

226. Rutherford MA, Heckmatt JZ, Dubowitz V: Congenital myotonic dystrophy: respiratory function at birth determines survival, *Arch Dis Child* 64:191–195, 1989.

227. Sacconi S, Salviati L, Desnuelle C: Facioscapulohumeral muscular dystrophy, *Biochim Biophys Acta* 1852(4):607–614, 2015.

228. Saranti AJ, Gleim GW, Melvin M: The relationship between subjective and objective measurements of strength, *J Orthop Sports Phys Ther* 2:15–19, 1980.

229. Sato Y, Yamauchi A, Urano M, Kondo E, Saito K: Corticosteroid therapy for Duchenne muscular dystrophy: improvement of psychomotor function, *Pediatr Neurol* 50(1):31–37, 2014.

230. Scher DM, Mubarak SJ: Surgical prevention of foot deformity in patients with Duchenne muscular dystrophy, *J Pediatr Orthop* 22:348–391, 2002.

231. Scott OM, Hyde SA, Goddard E: Quantification of muscle function in children: a prospective study in Duchenne muscular dystrophy, *Muscle Nerve* 5:291–301, 1982.

232. Scott OM, Hyde SA, Goddard C, Dubowitz V: Prevention of deformity in Duchenne muscular dystrophy: a prospective study of passive stretching and splintage, *Physiotherapy* 67:177–180, 1981.

233. Reference deleted in proofs.

234. Seeger BR, Caudrey DJ, Little JD: Progression of equinus deformity in Duchenne muscular dystrophy, *Arch Phys Med Rehabil* 66:286–288, 1985.

235. Seeger BR, Sutherland AD, Clark MS: Orthotic management of scoliosis in Duchenne muscular dystrophy, *Arch Phys Med Rehabil* 65:83–86, 1984.

236. Semprini L, Tacconelli A, Capon F, Brancati F, Dallapiccola B, Novelli C: A single strand conformation polymorphism-based carrier test for spinal muscle atrophy, *Genet Test* 5:33–37, 2001.

237. Sengupta SK, Mehdian SH, McConnell JR, Eisenstein SM, Webb JK: Pelvic or lumbar fixation for the surgical management of scoliosis in Duchenne muscular dystrophy, *Spine* 27:2072–2079, 2002.

238. Shanmugarajan S, Swoboda KJ, Iannaccone ST, Ries WL, Maria BL, Reddy SV: Congenital bone fractures in spinal muscular atrophy: functional role for SMN protein in bone remodeling, *J Child Neurol* 22(8):967–973, 2007.

239. Shapiro F, Specht L: Orthopaedic deformities in Emery-Dreifus muscular dystrophy, *J Pediatr Orthop* 11:336–340, 1991.

240. Siegel IM: The management of muscular dystrophy: a clinical review, *Muscle Nerve* 1:453–460, 1978.

241. Siegel IM: *Muscle and its diseases: an outline primer of basic science and clinical method*, Chicago, 1986, Year Book Medical Publishers.

242. Sparks SE, Escolar DM: Congenital muscular dystrophies, *Handb Clin Neurol* 101:47–79, 2011.

243. Spranger M, Spranger S, Tischendorf M, Meinck HM, Cremer M: Myotonic dystrophy: the role of large triplet repeat length in the development of mental retardation, *Arch Neurol* 54:251–254, 1997.

244. Steffensen BF, Lyager S, Werge B, Rahbek J, Mattsson E: Physical capacity in non-ambulatory people with Duchenne muscular dystrophy or spinal muscular atrophy: a longitudinal study, *Dev Med Child Neurol* 44:623–632, 2002.

245. Steffensen B, HYDE S: VALIDITY OF THE EK SCALE: A FUNCTIONAL ASSESSMENT OF NON-AMBULatory individuals with Duchenne muscular dystrophy, *Physiother Res Int* 6:119–134, 2001.

246. Reference deleted in proofs.

247. Stuberg WA: Home accessibility and adaptive equipment in Duchenne muscular dystrophy: a case report, *Pediatr Phys Ther* 13:169–174, 2001.

248. Stuberg WA, Metcalf WM: Reliability of quantitative muscle testing in healthy children and in children with Duchenne muscular dystrophy using a hand-held dynamometer, *Phys Ther* 68:977–982, 1988.

249. Stübgen JP, Stipp A: Facioscapulohumeral muscular dystrophy: a prospective study of weakness and functional impairment, *J Neurol* 257(9):1457–1464, 2010.

250. Sucato DJ: Spine deformity in spinal muscular atrophy, *J Bone Joint Surg Am* 89(Suppl 1):148–154, 2007.

251. Sugarman EA, Nagan N, Zhu H, Akmaev VR, Zhou Z, Rohlfs EM, et al.: Pan-ethnic carrier screening and prenatal diagnosis for spinal muscular atrophy: clinical laboratory analysis of >72,400 specimens, *Eur J Hum Genet* 20(1):27–32, 2012.

252. Suk KS, Lee BH, Lee HM, Moon SH, Choi YC, Shin DE, et al.: Functional outcomes in Duchenne muscular dystrophy scoliosis: comparison of the differences between surgical and nonsurgical treatment, *J Bone Joint Surg Am* 96(5):409–415, 2014.

253. Sveen ML, Jeppesen TD, Hauerslev S, Køber L, Krag TO, Vissing J: Endurance training improves fitness and strength in patients with Becker muscular dystrophy, *Brain* 131:2824–2831, 2008.

254. Sveen ML, Andersen SP, Ingelsrud LH, Blichter S, Olsen NE, Jønck S, et al.: Resistance training in patients with limb-girdle and Becker muscular dystrophies, *Muscle Nerve* 47(2):163–169, 2013.

255. Swinyard CA, Deaver GG, Greenspan L: Gradients of functional ability of importance in rehabilitation of patients with progressive muscular and neuromuscular diseases, *Arch Phys Med Rehabil* 38:574–579, 1957.

256. Taktak DM, Bowker P: Lightweight, modular knee-ankle-foot-orthosis for Duchenne muscular dystrophy: design, development, and evaluation, *Arch Phys Med Rehabil* 76:1156–1262, 1995.

257. Tawil R, van der Maarel S, Padberg GW, van Engelen BG: 171st ENMC international workshop: standards of care and management of facioscapulohumeral muscular dystrophy, *Neuromuscul Disord* 20(7):471–475, 2010.

258. Tedesco FS, Dellavalle A, Diaz-Manera J, Messina G, Cossu G: Repairing skeletal muscle: regenerative potential of skeletal muscle stem cells, *J Clin Invest* 120:11–19, 2010.

259. Theadom A, Rodrigues M, Roxburgh R, Balalla S, Higgins C, Bhattacharjee R, et al.: Prevalence of muscular dystrophies: a systematic literature review, *Neuroepidemiology* 43:259–268, 2014.

260. Tinsley JM, Fairclough RJ, Storer R, Wilkes FJ, Potter AC, Squire SE, et al.: Daily treatment with SMTC1100, a novel small molecule utrophin upregulator, dramatically reduces the dystrophic symptoms in the mdx mouse, *PLoS One* 6(5), 2011.

261. Topin N, Matecki S, Le Bris S, Rivier F, Echenne B, Prefaut C, Ramonatxo M: Dose-dependent effect of individualized respiratory muscle training in children with Duchenne muscular dystrophy, *Neuromuscl Disord* 12(6):576–583, 2002.

262. Reference deleted in proofs.

263. Townsend EL, Tamhane H, Gross KD: Effects of AFO use on walking in boys with Duchenne muscular dystrophy: a pilot study, *Pediatr Phys Ther* 27(1):24–29, 2015.

264. Tran VK, Sasongko TH, Hong DD, Hoan NT, Dung VC, Lee MJ, Gunadi, et al.: SMN2 and NAIP gene dosages in Vietnamese patients with spinal muscular atrophy, *Pediatr Int* 50(3):346–351, 2008.

265. Reference deleted in proofs.

266. Vignos PJ: Physical models of rehabilitation in neuromuscular disease, *Muscle Nerve* 6:323–338, 1983.

267. Vignos PJ, Archibald KC: Maintenance of ambulation in childhood muscular dystrophy, *J Chron Dis* 12:273–290, 1960.

268. Vignos PJ, Watkins MP: The effect of exercise in muscular dystrophy, *JAMA* 197:121–126, 1966.

269. Vignos PJ, Spencer GE, Archibald KC: Management of progressive muscular dystrophy, *JAMA* 184:103–112, 1963.

270. Vignos PJ, Wagner MB, Karlinchak B, Katirji B: Evaluation of a program for long-term treatment of Duchenne muscular dystrophy, *J Bone Joint Surg Am* 78:1844–1852, 1996.

271. Villanova M, Brancalion B, Mehta AD: Duchenne muscular dystrophy: life prolongation by noninvasive ventilatory support, *Am J Phys Med Rehabil* 93(7):595–599, 2014.

272. Voet N, Bleijenberg G, Hendriks J, de Groot I, Padberg G, van Engelen B, Geurts A: Both aerobic exercise and cognitive-behavioral therapy reduce chronic fatigue in FSHD: an RCT, *Neurology* 83(21):1914–1922, 2014.

273. Reference deleted in proofs.

274. Wang HY, Yang YH, Jong YJ: Correlations between change scores of measures for muscle strength and motor function in individuals with spinal muscular atrophy types 2 and 3, *Am J Phys Med Rehabil* 92(4):335–342, 2013.

275. Reference deleted in proofs.

276. Watt JM, Greenhill B: Commentary: rehabilitation and orthopaedic management of spinal muscle atrophy. In Gamstorp I, Sarnat HB, editors: *Progressive spinal muscular atrophies: International Review of Child Neurology series*, New York, 1984, Raven Press.

277. Weidner NJ: Developing an interdisciplinary palliative care plan for the patient with muscular dystrophy, *Pediatr Ann* 34:546–552, 2005.

278. Werdnig G: Eine fruhinfantile progressive spinale Amyotrophie, *Arch Psychiatrie Nervenkrank* 26:706–744, 1894.

279. Werlauff U, Steffensen BF, Bertelsen S, Fløytrup I, Kristensen B, Werge B: Physical characteristics and applicability of standard assessment methods in a total population of spinal muscular atrophy type II patients, *Neuromuscul Disord* 20:34–43, 2010.

280. Reference deleted in proofs.

281. Wirth B, Garbes L, Riessland M: How genetic modifiers influence the phenotype of spinal muscular atrophy and suggest future therapeutic approaches, *Curr Opin Genet Dev* 23(3):330–338, 2013.

282. Wohlfart G, Fex J, Eliasson S: Hereditary proximal spinal muscular atrophy: a clinical entity simulating progressive muscular dystrophy, *Acta Psychiatrica Neurol Scand* 30:395–406, 1955.

283. Wong CK, Wade CK: Reducing iliotibial band contractures in patients with muscular dystrophy using custom dry floatation cushions, *Arch Phys Med Rehabil* 76:695–700, 1995.

284. Wong LY, Christopher C: Corticosteroids in Duchenne muscular dystrophy: a reappraisal, *J Child Neurol* 17:184–190, 2002.

285. Young HK, Barton BA, Waisbren S, Portales Dale L, Ryan MM, et al.: Cognitive and psychological profile of males with Becker muscular dystrophy, *J Child Neurol* 23:155–162, 2009.

286. Ziter FA, Allsop KG: The diagnosis and management of childhood muscular dystrophy, *Clin Pediatr* 15:540–548, 1976.

SUGGESTED READINGS

Al-Zaidy S, Rodino-Klapac L, Mendell JR: Gene therapy for muscular dystrophy: moving the field forward, *Pediatr Neurol* 51(5):607–618, 2014.

Angelini C: Neuromuscular disease: diagnosis and discovery in limb-girdle muscular dystrophy, *Nat Rev Neurol* 12(1):6–8, 2016.

Brandsema JF, Darras BT: Dystrophinopathies. *Semin Neurol* 35(4):369–384, 2015.

Bushby K, Finkel R, Birnkrant DJ, et al.: Diagnosis and management of Duchenne muscular dystrophy, part 1: diagnosis, and pharmacological and psychosocial management, *Lancet Neurol* 9(1):77–93, 2010.

Bushby K, Finkel R, Birnkrant DJ, et al.: Diagnosis and management of Duchenne muscular dystrophy, part 2: implementation of multidisciplinary care, *Lancet Neurol* 9(2):177–189, 2010.

Donkervoort S, Bonnemann CG, Loeys B, Jungbluth H, Voermans NC: The neuromuscular differential diagnosis of joint hypermobility, *Am J Med Genet C Semin Med Genet* 169C(1):23–42, 2015.

Dubowitz V: The muscular dystrophies, Postgrad, *Med J* 68:500–506, 1992.

Finkel RS, McDermott MP, Kaufmann P, et al.: Observational study of spinal muscular atrophy type I and implications for clinical trials, *Neurology* 83(9):810–817, 2014.

Kang PB, Morrison L, Iannaccone ST, et al.: Guideline Development Subcommittee of the American Academy of Neurology and the Practice Issues Review Panel of the American Association of Neuromuscular Electrodiagnostic Medicine: evidence-based guideline summary: evaluation, diagnosis, and management of congenital muscular dystrophy: report of the Guideline Development Subcommittee of the American Academy of Neurology and the Practice Issues Review Panel of the American Association of Neuromuscular & Electrodiagnostic Medicine, *Neurology* 84(13):1369–1378, 2015.

Kaufmann P, McDermott MP, Darras BT, et al.: Pediatric Neuromuscular Clinical Research Network for Spinal Muscular Atrophy (PNCR): prospective cohort study of spinal muscular atrophy types 2 and 3, *Neurology* 79(18):1889–1897, 2012.

Montes J, Dunaway S, Garber CE, Chiriboga CA, De Vivo DC, Rao AK: Leg muscle function and fatigue during walking in spinal muscular atrophy type 3, *Muscle Nerve* 50(1):34–39, 2014.

Wang CH, Finkel RS, Bertini ES, et al.: Participants of the International Conference on SMA Standard of Care, *J Child Neurol* 22(8):1027–1049, 2007.

Wang CH, Dowling JJ, North K, et al.: Consensus statement on standard of care for congenital myopathies, *J Child Neurol* 27(3):363–382, 2012.

13

Limb Deficiencies and Amputations

Meg Stanger, Colleen Coulter, Brian Giavedoni

The child with an amputation is defined as a person with an amputation who is skeletally immature because the epiphyses of the long bones are still open.[1] Amputations can be classified as congenital or acquired. Many different factors must be considered in the management of children with a limb deficiency or amputation. These factors differ from those involved in the management of adults with a limb deficiency or amputation because as children grow their musculoskeletal systems continue to develop. Children also are emotionally immature and variably dependent on adults for care and decision making regarding surgical and prosthetic issues.

In this chapter the causes of limb deficiencies and amputations in children, surgical management, physical therapy intervention relative to a child's age and developmental function, and pediatric prosthetic options are discussed. Emphasis is on the aspects of management that differ from those encountered by adults with amputations. The role of the physical therapist includes education of parents of infants and children with limb deficiencies, development and progression of postoperative exercise programs, training in mobility and self-care skills, and providing input to both parents and the child or adolescent regarding prosthetic options. Studies have shown that children with limb deficiencies who participated in extensive rehabilitation programs have vocational skills with high employment potential.[92]

BACKGROUND INFORMATION

CONGENITAL LIMB DEFICIENCIES

Classification

Various classification systems of congenital limb deficiencies have been developed. Greek terminology has been used to describe various deficiencies but is often inaccurate and ambiguous.[17] Frantz and O'Rahilly[25] developed a classification system based on embryologic considerations and the absent skeletal portions. Swanson and colleagues[91] modified that system with a classification system of seven categories based on embryologic failure: (1) Failure of formation of parts (arrest of development), (2) failure of differentiation (separation of parts), (3) duplication, (4) overgrowth, (5) undergrowth (hypoplasia), (6) congenital constriction band syndrome, and (7) generalized skeletal deformities. The International Society for Prosthetics and Orthotics (ISPO) and the International Federation of Societies on Surgeries of the Hand (IFSSH) made additional modifications to this classification system in 1973 and 1989. The classification developed by the ISPO and IFSSH has been published as an international standard, International Standards Organization (ISO) 8548-1:1989, "Method of Describing Limb Deficiencies Present at Birth."[17]

The ISO classification of congenital limb deficiency is restricted to skeletal deficiencies described on anatomic and radiologic bases only; Greek terminology, such as *hemimelia* and *phocomelia* is avoided because of its lack of precision and difficulty of translation into languages that are not related to Greek.[17] Deficiencies are described as transverse or longitudinal. In transverse deficiencies the limb has developed normally to a particular level beyond which no skeletal elements exist, although digital buds may be present. A transverse deficiency is described by naming the segment in which the limb terminates and then describing the level within the segment beyond which no skeletal elements exist[17] (Fig. 13.1).

In longitudinal deficiencies reduction or absence of an element or elements occurs within the long axis of a limb. Normal skeletal elements may be present, distal to the affected bones. A longitudinal deficiency is described by naming the bones affected in a proximal-to-distal sequence and stating whether each affected bone is totally or partially absent[17] (Fig. 13.2).

One of the purposes of an international classification system is to provide a common language for accuracy when reporting statistics and research. However, because the ISO system does not specifically characterize common clinical manifestations of limb deficiencies, other terminology persists, such as proximal femoral focal deficiency or fibular deficiency. Additional classifications have been proposed to further define this broad spectrum of limb deficiencies. The additional classifications may be etiologically, radiologically, anatomically, or functionally based and are often developed to guide medical interventions and decision making. Basic knowledge of the various classification systems is important because much of the literature published prior to 1989 will often use the older classification systems.

Origin

To fully understand the causes of congenital limb deficiencies, a basic knowledge of embryonic skeletal development is necessary. Limb buds first appear at the end of the fourth week of embryonic development, arising from mesenchymal tissue. During the next 3 weeks the limb buds grow and differentiate into identifiable limb segments. Development of limb buds occurs in a proximodistal sequence, with upper limb development preceding lower limb development by several days. The mesenchymal tissue undergoes chondrification to become cartilaginous models of individual bones. By the end of the seventh week, a recognizable embryonic skeleton is present. The entire process of limb development is very complex and involves precise timing of events as well as the interaction of genetics and molecular control from signaling centers in the developing limb.[82,84]

Causative factors for congenital limb deficiencies include genetic, vascular, teratogenic, and amniotic bands, but for

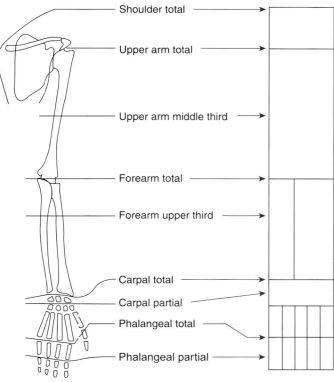

FIG. 13.1 Examples of transverse deficiencies at various levels of the upper extremity. (From Day HJ: The ISO/ISPO classification of congenital limb deficiency. In Bowker JH, Michael JW, editors: *Atlas of limb prosthetics: surgical, prosthetic, and rehabilitation principles.* 2nd ed. St. Louis, Mosby-Year Book, 1992.)

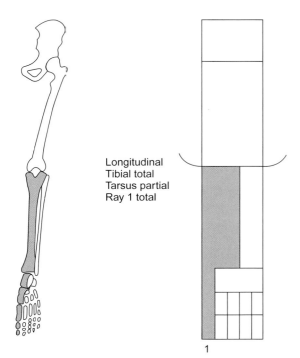

FIG. 13.2 Example of a longitudinal deficiency of the lower extremity. (From Day HJ: The ISO/ISPO classification of congenital limb deficiency. In Bowker JH, Michael JW, editors: *Atlas of limb prosthetics: Surgical, prosthetic, and rehabilitation principles.* 2nd ed. St Louis: Mosby-Year Book; 1992. p 748)

many children, the exact cause is unknown. A genetic link may be associated with a few limb anomalies, but most limb deficiencies are the result of sporadic genetic mutation.[46] Limb deficiencies, especially of the upper extremity, may be associated with other congenital anomalies such as Holt-Oram, Fanconi, Poland, thrombocytopenia-absent radius, and VATER syndromes. Several teratogenic factors (e.g., medications such as thalidomide and misoprostol, irradiation) have been indicated as possible causative factors for congenital limb deficiencies but account for only 4% of cases in a study conducted by McGuirk.[60] McGuirk[60] reported that the cause of congenital limb deficiencies was vascular disruption in 34% of cases and unknown in 32% of cases. A study by Robitaille et al. found that low maternal intake of riboflavin was associated with transverse limb deficiencies.[80] Teratogenic and vascular disruption factors must be present at some time between the third and seventh weeks of embryonic development to produce a limb deficiency.

Levels of Limb Deficiency

The incidence of congenital limb deficiencies ranges from 2 to 7 per 10,000 live births and has been relatively unchanged over time.[21] The US Centers for Disease Control reports an incidence of 6 in 10,000 live births per year with limb deficiencies of the upper extremity occurring twice as frequently as those involving the lower extremity.[14] The clinical presentation of a child with a congenital limb deficiency depends on the type, level, and number of deficiencies. Almost any combination or variety of limb deficiency is possible. However, some are more common, and these are discussed in this chapter in detail. Approximately 20% of children present with limb deficiencies affecting more than one limb[18] (Fig. 13.3). Longitudinal deficiencies occur more frequently than transverse deficiencies with no strong difference between left- and right-sided prevalence.[7,35] Many

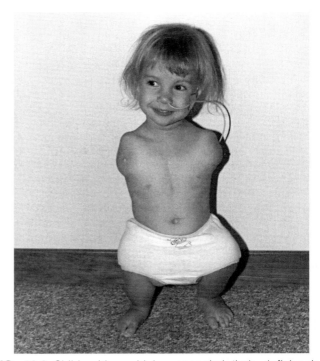

FIG. 13.3 Child with multiple congenital limb deficiencies, including bilateral transverse upper arm deficiency and bilateral proximal femoral focal deficiency.

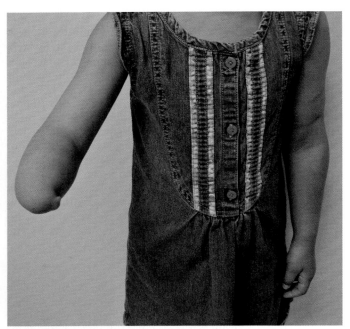

FIG. 13.4 Child with congenital transverse upper limb difference. (From Le JT, Scott-Wyard PR: Pediatric limb differences and amputations. *Phys Med Rehabil Clin N Am* 2015 Feb;26[1]:95-108.)

transverse deficiencies proximal to the wrist and ankle are unilateral and frequently include rudimentary vestiges called nubbins (Fig. 13.4).

A complex lower extremity longitudinal limb deficiency has been termed *proximal femoral focal deficiency (PFFD)*. Aitken[2] first described this deficiency, which includes absence or hypoplasia of the proximal femur with varying degrees of involvement of the acetabulum, femoral head, patella, tibia, and fibula. The deficiency may be unilateral or bilateral. If the deficiency is unilateral, the contralateral limb often exhibits subtle deficiencies such as hypoplasia of the femur that may not be initially recognized. Aitken described four classes of severity—A through D—with class A exhibiting the least involvement based on radiographic findings (Fig. 13.5). Gillespie[32] has developed a classification system for PFFD based on the complexity of medical intervention. Children classified into group A may require only limb lengthening, and those in groups B and C may require some level of amputation or surgical revision and prosthetic fitting.

The clinical manifestations of a child with PFFD are relatively consistent. They include a shortened thigh that is held in flexion, abduction, and external rotation; hip and knee flexion contracture; and severe leg length discrepancy, with the foot often at the level of the opposite knee. These children also have instability of the knee joint secondary to absent or deficient cruciate ligaments and a 70% to 80% incidence of total longitudinal deficiency of the fibula. Fifteen percent of children with PFFD have bilateral involvement.[62] The incidence of PFFD is reported to be 1 per 50,000 live births and it is usually of unknown origin.[62]

ACQUIRED AMPUTATIONS

Acquired amputations most frequently occur as the result of trauma or disease, with trauma being twice as common as disease-related factors.[55] Disease-related factors are most frequently tumors but also include infections and vascular malformations.

Ninety percent of acquired amputations involve only one limb, and the lower extremity is involved in 60% of cases.[19]

Traumatic Amputations

Males, especially in the adolescent age ranges, account for a larger percentage of traumatic amputations in children.[48,56]

Accidents involving farm machinery and household power tools are the leading cause of acquired amputations in the pediatric population, followed closely by vehicular accidents, gunshot wounds, and railroad accidents.[56] Incidences vary according to age and geographic location. When amputations of the digits are included in the data, the highest incidence of amputations is seen in the fingers of children younger than 2 years of age secondary to closing a door on the child's finger.[48] Vehicular accidents, farm machinery, gunshot wounds, and trains are more common causes of traumatic amputations in the older child.[56] Loder documented a seasonal trend with childhood amputations that could influence community prevention and education programs. It is no surprise that most traumatic amputations occur in the summer, with lawn mower injuries peaking in June, motor vehicle accidents in July, and farm machinery accidents in September.[56]

Disease-Related Amputations
Sarcoma of Bone
Primary bone tumors are rare in children, accounting for only 6% of cancers in children younger than 20 years of age. Osteosarcoma and Ewing's sarcoma are the most common of the primary bone tumors, with an annual incidence in the United States of 8.7 per million children younger than 20 years of age.[13]

Osteosarcoma
Osteosarcoma is a primary malignant tumor of bone derived from bone-forming mesenchyme in which the malignant proliferating spindle cell stroma produces osteoid tissue or immature bone. The peak incidence of osteosarcoma coincides with the pubertal growth spurt, and it occurs most frequently at the metaphyseal portion of the most rapidly growing bones in adolescence. As a result, the distal femur, proximal tibia, and proximal humerus are the most common sites for osteosarcoma. This finding supports the theory that these rapidly growing cells are susceptible to oncogenic agents or mitotic errors and that osteosarcoma is the result of an aberration of the normal process of bone growth and bone turnover.[37]

Ewing's Sarcoma Family of Tumors
The Ewing's sarcoma family of tumors (ESFT) includes a spectrum of neuroepithelial tumors ranging from the undifferentiated round cell tumor of Ewing's sarcoma of bone (ES) to the neural differentiated peripheral primitive neuroectodermal tumor (PNET). Ewing's tumors often involve both bone and soft tissue by the time of diagnosis, including infiltration into the medullary cavity and bone marrow. The most common primary sites are the flat bones of the pelvis and chest and the long bones of the lower extremities. Ewing's sarcoma is also seen during times of peak growth rates with the highest number seen in the second decade of life.[43]

Diagnosis
The initial complaint for both osteosarcoma and Ewing's sarcoma is pain at the site of the tumor with or without a palpable mass. Localized swelling or the complaint of a palpable mass is seen with both osteosarcoma and Ewing's sarcoma. Systemic

Type		Femoral Head	Acetabulum	Femoral Segment	Relationship Among Components of Femur and Acetabulum at Skeletal Maturity
A	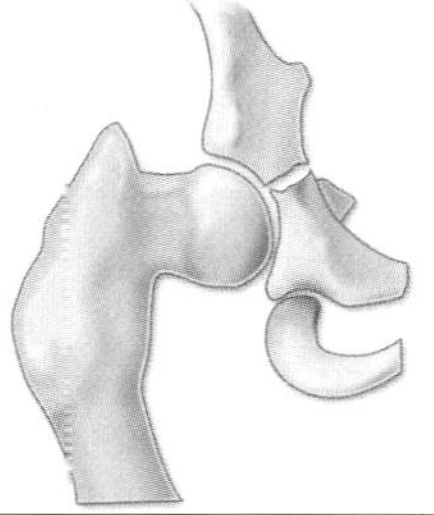	Present	Normal	Short	Bony connection between components of femur Femoral head in acetabulum Subtrochanteric varus angulation, often with pseudarthrosis
B	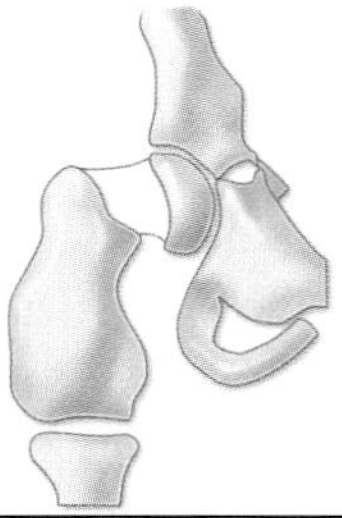	Present	Adequate or moderately dysplastic	Short, usually proximal bony tuft	No osseous connection between head and shaft Femoral head in acetabulum
C	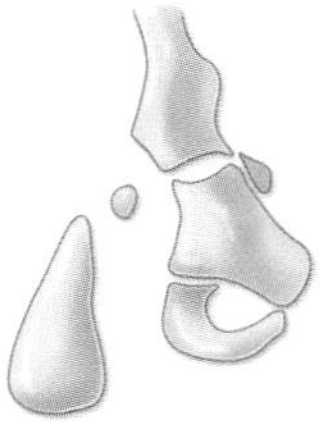	Absent or represented by ossicle	Severely dysplastic	Short, usually proximally tapered	May be osseous connection between shaft and proximal ossicle No articular relation between femur and acetabulum
D	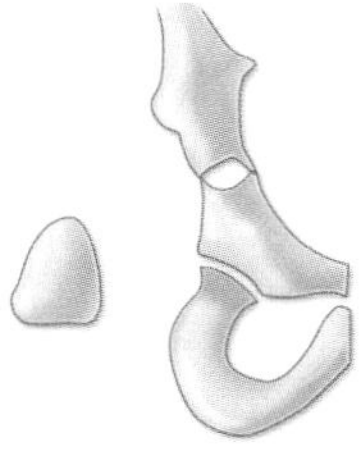	Absent	Absent Obturator foramen enlarged Pelvis squared in bilateral cases	Short, deformed	None

FIG. 13.5 Aitken classification of proximal femoral focal deficiency. (From Herring JA: *Tachdjian's pediatric orthopaedics: from the Texas Scottish Rite Hospital for Children.* 5th ed. Philadelphia: Saunders; 2014, Elsevier.)

symptoms are rare in osteosarcoma unless widespread metastatic disease is present. On the other hand, systemic symptoms, most commonly fever and weight loss, are complaints with large Ewing's tumors.[44] Because the initial complaint for both osteosarcoma and Ewing's sarcoma is pain at the site of the tumor, diagnosis is often delayed. Children presenting to a physical therapist with a complaint of pain that is often chronic, a negative history of injury, and no evidence of musculoskeletal abnormalities should be referred for further medical workup to rule out a malignant bone tumor.

The key to diagnosis of a bone tumor is radiologic evaluation. Plain-view radiographs will reveal evidence of a mass and bony destruction; however, a definitive diagnosis is made through biopsy and histologic examination. The extent of the tumor is more precisely defined through magnetic resonance imaging. To complete the workup, a radionuclide bone scan and chest computed tomography are performed to determine the extent of metastasis.[41]

Medical Management of Malignancies

Medical intervention for children with sarcomas typically includes a multimodality approach with chemotherapy to eradicate systemic disease and surgery and/or radiation therapy to control local disease. Medical management of bony tumors and neoplasms is based on the following goals: (1) complete and permanent control of the primary tumor, (2) control and prevention of microstatic and metastatic disease, and (3) preservation of function to the greatest degree possible. Local control of the primary tumor is most often achieved through surgery and radiation therapy. Surgical options include amputation, limb-sparing procedures, and rotationplasty. Control of microstatic and metastatic disease is achieved through radiation therapy and chemotherapy. Surgical options and use of radiation therapy are based on the type of tumor, location and extent of the tumor, age of the child, and child and family beliefs and their activities. See Chapter 16 for more information.

Radiation Therapy

Osteosarcoma is generally unresponsive to radiation therapy and is typically used only if adequate surgical margins were unable to be achieved. Ewing's sarcoma is highly responsive to radiation therapy; consequently, it has been utilized for local control of the tumor. However, improvement with surgical techniques and recognition of the long-term effects of radiation therapy has decreased the use of radiation therapy in pediatrics. As with osteosarcoma, radiation therapy is utilized for Ewing's sarcoma when full resection of the tumor is not a reasonable option.[41]

The side effects of radiation therapy are related to tumor location, dose rate and duration, age of the patient, and use of chemotherapy. Acute side effects are seen in rapidly dividing tissues such as the skin, bone marrow, and gut. Common side effects are red and tender skin, mouth sores from irradiation to mucous membranes, and nausea and vomiting from irradiation to the abdomen.[53] Children receiving radiation therapy may exhibit a decreased activity level secondary to nausea and vomiting, poor appetite secondary to mouth sores, and generalized malaise. Their physical therapy sessions may need to be altered on a daily basis to accommodate their changing energy levels. Children wearing prostheses must be monitored closely for skin irritation and breakdown.

Late side effects of radiation include fibrosis of soft tissues, bony changes ranging from osteoporosis to fractures, and growth disturbances, including damage to the epiphyseal plate and bowing of the metaphysis. Butler and colleagues[12] reported that 77% of patients with Ewing's sarcoma who received radiation therapy developed a leg length discrepancy; in 58% of these patients, the leg length discrepancy was significant enough to require treatment. Advances in surgical options have minimized the need for radiation therapy at the site of the primary tumor. If radiation therapy is indicated, attempts are made to shield the epiphyseal plate at the opposite end of the involved bone to minimize radiation-linked growth retardation and still allow for some growth of the extremity. For some young children an amputation may produce a more functional extremity than an extremity that is significantly shortened as a result of radiation therapy.

Chemotherapy

Chemotherapy is administered according to several principles, including the use of multiple drug combinations, administration of chemotherapy agents at maximally tolerated doses, and administration before the development of detectable micrometastatic disease (adjuvant chemotherapy). Most chemotherapy agents interfere with the function of DNA and RNA. However, these agents are nonselective and cause damage to both malignant and normal cells, resulting in undesirable and at times toxic side effects.[86] Physical therapists working with children receiving chemotherapy should know the specific agents being used with the child and the side effects. Typical side effects of chemotherapy can include nausea and vomiting, hair loss, diarrhea, and constipation. Other potential side effects consist of blood-related concerns such as anemia, neutropenia, and thrombocytopenia or neurologic issues such as peripheral neuropathies. The physical therapy interventions may need to be altered or limited depending on the child's status and development of potentially serious side effects.

The introduction of adjuvant chemotherapy, given preoperatively and postsurgically, in the 1970s and early 1980s increased the survival rates for both osteosarcoma and Ewing's sarcoma. Survival rates are dependent upon age, location of the tumor, and the presence and location of metastatic disease at the time of diagnosis. Three-year event-free survival (EFS) rates for children with Ewing's sarcoma treated with a combination of radiation therapy, chemotherapy, and surgery have improved to 65% to 70% for patients with nonmetastatic disease.[39] Overall 5-year event-free survival rates for children with osteosarcoma treated with a combination of surgery and chemotherapy also drastically improved from 20% in the 1970s to 65% to 70%. Children with nonmetastatic osteosarcoma of the extremity are more likely to have a favorable outcome than children with more proximal tumors and the presence of metastatic disease.[36] However, the survival rates for both Ewing's sarcoma and osteosarcoma are relatively unchanged since the mid-1980s.[28]

SURGICAL OPTIONS IN THE MANAGEMENT OF ACQUIRED AND CONGENITAL LIMB DEFICIENCIES

The goal of any surgical intervention is to improve the function of the child and, in the case of bone sarcoma, to not alter the child's chance of survival. Traditionally, amputation has been the typical approach for children with bone sarcoma. It has also been used to modify the lower extremities of children with congenital limb deficiencies for improved prosthetic fit and function. However, with improved survival rates of children with bone tumors, the long-term function and comfort of the child must also be considered. Limb-sparing procedures, including rotationplasty, are viable options for many children with congenital limb deficiencies and for those previously considered to be candidates for amputation secondary to a bone tumor. Each of these procedures offers advantages and disadvantages, and functional outcome, psychological impact, and long-term survival all must be considered in the surgical decision. This section discusses the surgical options of amputation, rotationplasty, and various limb-sparing procedures for children with congenital limb deficiencies, as well as those with a diagnosis of bone sarcoma.

Amputation as a General Surgical Option

Although most of the basic premises related to management of adults with amputations also apply to children, important differences may be noted. First, skeletal immaturity and future growth are important factors when surgical alternatives are considered. Physes should be preserved whenever possible to ensure continued growth of the limb. For the upper extremity, most growth occurs in physes around the shoulder and wrist, whereas in the lower extremity the physes around the knee account for most of the growth.[45] If an amputation will result in a significantly short residual limb, a limb-sparing procedure may offer better function and improved cosmesis for the child.

Second, the fact that amputation through long bones may result in terminal overgrowth is an important point that should not be overlooked. Terminal or bony overgrowth is a painful, spikelike prominence of new growth on the transected end of the residual limb. Significant pain can interfere with weight bearing and wearing of the prosthesis. The spikelike growth is not well understood but is seen more frequently in children under the age of 12 years.[85] Terminal overgrowth can occur in any long bone but is most frequently in the tibia. Bone capping consists of excision of the overgrowth spike and fixation of a graft on the end of the residual limb in an attempt to prevent future terminal overgrowth. Multiple surgical revisions to remove an overgrowth spike may result in a shorter residual limb. Surgical options include revisions and bone capping. Surgical revision and bone capping with biologic materials result in frequent complications including high recurrence rates for revision and infection with biologic capping materials. More recently, surgeons have been utilizing autologous caps, specifically the proximal fibula, with promising results of decreased rates of infection and recurrence of the bony overgrowth.[23] An amputation through a joint such as a knee disarticulation eliminates the possibility of bony overgrowth. As in adults, length of the lever arm, function of the extremity, and prosthetic fit remain important considerations when deciding on the level of amputation. Saving the child's life is, of course, the most important consideration, whether the amputation is the result of a malignancy or trauma.

Finally, wound healing in children is rarely a concern as it may be in adults with peripheral vascular disease. Skin grafts therefore may be used to close the amputation site in preference to performing a higher-level amputation for a child with a traumatic injury.

Amputation to Revise Congenital Limb Deficiencies to Improve Function

Amputation and surgical reconstruction are rarely necessary with upper extremity limb deficiencies but may be indicated for some children with lower extremity limb deficiencies. Children with bilateral PFFD and equal leg lengths, however, may be more functional without any surgery. They will be of short stature but will walk quite well.[62] For cosmesis or to equalize leg lengths and stability in standing and walking, an extension prosthesis may be an option for some children with bilateral PFFD.

The surgical treatment of a child with unilateral PFFD is case-specific. If the child has a stable hip and foot and a significant portion of normal femur is present, one of the limb-lengthening procedures may be appropriate. Most surgeons agree that 60% of predicted femoral length must be present for a lengthening procedure to be a viable alternative.[31,46] If limb lengthening is not an option, surgical options for PFFD include femoral osteotomy, a knee arthrodesis, and foot amputation or a rotationplasty. Usually the Syme or Boyd amputation of the foot is recommended. A Syme amputation involves complete removal of the foot, including the calcaneus, but the Boyd amputation preserves the calcaneus. The Boyd procedure requires an arthrodesis of the calcaneus and the tibia, which adds length to the limb.[62] The knee is usually fused to form one long bone for fitting of an above-knee prosthesis[46,62] (Fig. 13.6).

Amputation may also be an option for a child with a longitudinal tibial or fibular total deficiency in which a significant limb length difference exists along with deformity of the foot. Frequently, the foot is positioned in equinovarus with a tibial deficiency or equinovalgus with a fibular deficiency, and both may include absent rays. If the tibia is completely absent, a knee disarticulation and fitting with a prosthesis will provide a very functional lower extremity for the child. If the leg length difference is too significant for limb-lengthening techniques or epiphysiodesis of the uninvolved leg, or if the ankle is significantly unstable, a Syme or Boyd amputation may lead to a more functional lower extremity with the addition of a prosthesis for a child with partial absence of the fibula. When an amputation is being considered for a child, it is important that alternatives are discussed with the family and child and that the ultimate lifestyle goals are known.

Amputation in the Management of Traumatic Injuries and Malignant Tumors

Amputations secondary to trauma may result in a short residual limb if the child has significant growth remaining. This is especially true of an above-knee amputation in which the distal physes around the knee have been resected. It may be possible to increase the length of a residual limb in older children by using one of the limb-lengthening techniques (see Chapter 14).

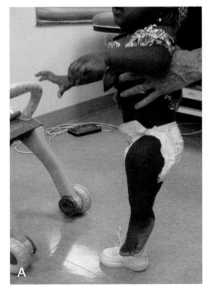 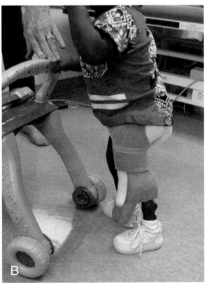

FIG. 13.6 (A) Child with unilateral proximal femoral focal deficiency (PFFD) without any surgical modifications to her leg. (B) Same child wearing a prosthesis to equalize limb lengths for weight bearing. Initial surgery has not yet occurred.

Lengthening of a short residual limb may increase the efficiency of gait and promote a better prosthetic fit.

The traditional approach for malignant bone tumors had been amputation of the limb in which the tumor is found. A wide surgical margin for an amputation is utilized to achieve local control of the tumor. Amputation for tumors of the pelvis or proximal femur results in complete loss of the limb or a very short residual limb, which makes functional ambulation with a prosthesis difficult. Limb-sparing procedures may result in a more functional extremity than a proximal amputation without decreasing the expected rate of survival for the child. Due to the short length of the residual limb and advances in chemotherapy since the 1970s, limb-sparing procedures have become the preferred surgical approach for both Ewing's sarcoma and osteosarcoma in the pediatric population.[43] The decision regarding an amputation is based on expectations regarding control of the primary tumor, survival of the child, and functional use of the extremity.

Rotationplasty

Rotationplasty (also called the Van Nes procedure) is an option for children with congenital limb deficiencies, specifically PFFD, as well as for those with bony tumors of the proximal tibia or distal femur. For PFFD this procedure involves excision of the distal femur and proximal tibia; 180° rotation of the residual lower limb, including the distal femur and proximal tibia, ankle joint, foot, and neurovascular supply; and reattachment to the proximal femur (Fig. 13.7). The ankle then functions as a knee joint, with ankle plantar flexion used to extend the "knee" and ankle dorsiflexion to flex the "knee"[52] (Fig. 13.8). Rotationplasty requires a functioning hip joint and ankle joint. For children with PFFD the residual foot must be adequately aligned anatomically for active plantar flexion and dorsiflexion to power the prosthetic knee. If the fibula is absent, alignment of the foot will not be adequate for a successful rotationplasty.

In the case of malignant tumors, the site of rotation is dependent on the location of the tumor. Rotation at the level of the femur proximally may have a greater effect on the function and power of the hip muscles. Rotation at the level of the distal femur or proximal tibia may have a greater effect on the

muscles and function of the foot and ankle complex required to power the prosthetic knee.[40] Rotationplasty is possible only if the tumor has not invaded the surrounding soft tissue, especially the neurovascular supply.

The advantages of a rotationplasty include increased limb length, improved prosthetic function with the ankle serving as a knee joint, improved weight-bearing capacity, and elimination of the problems of terminal overgrowth and pain from neuromas or phantom limb sensations.[51] Weight is borne through the heel, which is more suitable for weight bearing than the end of a residual limb. Rotationplasty also allows for some growth of the leg. With an appropriate prosthesis, children who have had a rotationplasty procedure can functionally participate in running, jumping, and playing with their peers and can participate in high-impact sports and activities.

Disadvantages of rotationplasty are cosmesis and derotation of the limb. Critics cite poor cosmesis and psychological issues as a deterrent to the procedure. In our experience with children who underwent a rotationplasty for a tumor or for congenital PFFD, cosmesis was not a complaint from the child or the child's parents. Krajbich and Bochmann[51] cite their experience of 27 children with osteosarcoma who underwent a rotationplasty. Twenty-two of these children are alive with no evidence of metastatic disease. No long-term complications related to cosmesis and psychological decompensation were reported; in fact, virtually all of the children with a rotationplasty now actively participate in sports and other activities with their peers. When a rotationplasty is being considered as a surgical option, it may be helpful for parents and the child to meet another child who has had the rotationplasty performed. Certainly, the cosmetic disadvantages must be discussed. Additional studies have shown that children with PFFD who underwent a rotationplasty demonstrated a higher walking speed with less oxygen consumption and fewer compensatory gait deviations than children who underwent a foot amputation and foot and knee arthrodesis.[24,68]

When the procedure is performed on young children, derotation of the limb may occur, requiring rerotation of the limb. The limb may derotate secondary to the spiral pull of the muscles proximal and distal to the osteotomy.[46] Both Krajbich[52] and Gillespie[31] discussed surgical options to limit derotation of the limb after a rotationplasty. Derotation is more common in children younger than 10 years of age and is most frequently seen in children when a rotationplasty is performed at 3 or 4 years of age.[31] Concern has also been raised about the long-term consequences of the altered weight bearing on the ankle joint. A study by Akahane[4] assessed 21 patients at a mean follow-up of 13.5 years post rotationplasty and found no evidence at that point of joint arthrodesis or degenerative joint changes.

Limb-Sparing Procedures

With the use of chemotherapy, improvements in diagnostic imaging to determine tumor margins, and new techniques of reconstruction, amputation is not always the treatment of choice for children with bony malignancies. Limb-sparing procedures may be an alternative to amputation for many children with malignant bone tumors. Limb-sparing procedures involve resection of the tumor and reconstruction of the limb to preserve function without amputation of the limb. Reconstruction of the limb may include excision of bone without replacement of the excised area or replacement with an allograft or endoprosthetic implant.

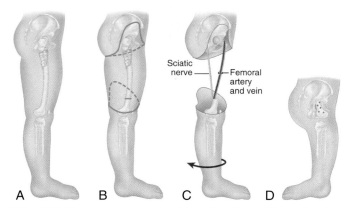

Sciatic nerve — Femoral artery and vein

A   B   C   D

FIG. 13.7 Technique of type BI rotationplasty. (From Toy PC, Heck RK: General principles of tumors. In Canale ST, Beaty JH, editors: Campbell's *operative orthopaedics*, 12th ed. Philadelphia: Mosby; 2013. Redrawn from Winkelmann WW: Hip rotationplasty for malignant tumors of the proximal part of the femur, *J Bone Joint Surg* 68A:362, 1986.)

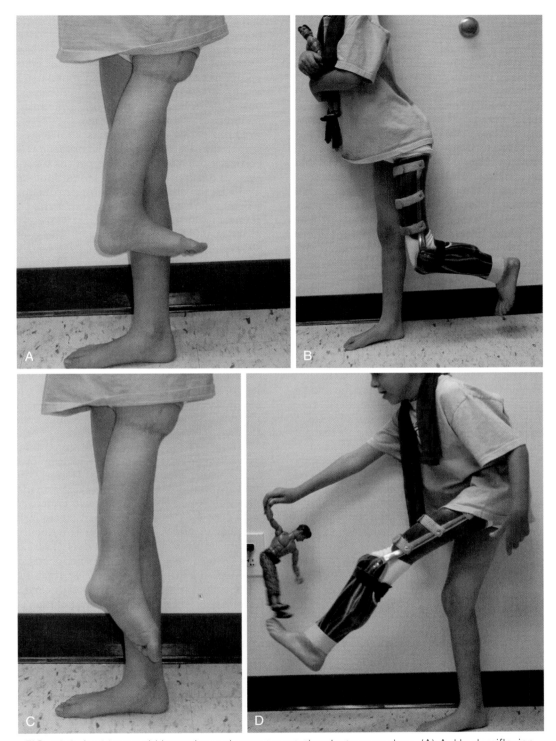

FIG. 13.8 An 11-year-old boy who underwent a rotationplasty procedure. (A) Ankle dorsiflexion. (B) Ankle dorsiflexion produces prosthetic knee flexion. (C) Ankle plantar flexion. (D) Ankle plantar flexion produces prosthetic knee extension.

Appropriate selection of children for limb-sparing surgery is critical. The goal of saving the limb should never compromise the goal of removing all gross and microscopic tumor. Limb-sparing surgery is contraindicated if the tumor has invaded the surrounding soft tissue to a large extent, if it involves the neurovascular supply, or if the tumor has invaded the intramedullary cavity.[43] In addition, limb-sparing surgery for the lower extremity of a young child may not be beneficial when the child is skeletally immature and may be left with a severe leg length discrepancy and a nonfunctional lower extremity. In these cases, amputation may be a better choice than limb-sparing surgery.

Autologous grafts are rarely appropriate because long segments of bone usually must be excised. Replacement of the excised bone with a near-equal length of noninvolved bone from another portion of the body often is not possible. Cadaver structural allografts, intercalary or osteoarticular, are another option. They involve resection of the tumor and surrounding bone and implantation of a section of cadaver bone. Osteoarticular allografts can preserve some growth plates, especially those of the distal femur and proximal tibia, if the tumor resection involves the proximal femur. The grafts are stabilized with plates or intramedullary rods until osteosynthesis has occurred. Once osteosynthesis has occurred and the child's bone has formed a latticework within the implanted bone, the graft is very stable and may last a lifetime. Complications of allografts include infection, nonunion, and fracture, all of which may compromise the long-term integrity of the implant. Infections and nonunions are early-onset complications that are seen with greater frequency in children receiving chemotherapy.[37] As is true with most limb-sparing procedures, high-intensity activities such as athletic participation are limited for the child with an osteoarticular allograft.

At times a tumor may be excised without replacing the excised bone. The proximal fibula may be resected if the soft tissue involvement is minimal and the peroneal nerve is not included in the soft tissue involvement. The biceps femoris tendon and the fibular collateral ligament are reattached to the lateral condyle of the tibia.[45] After healing, full knee motion and a normal gait pattern can be expected. Endoprosthetic devices are ultimately an extension of joint arthroplasty procedures. These manufactured devices consist of modular components that are implanted in the area of the excised bone such as the proximal humerus, elbow, proximal and distal femur, and proximal tibia. These modular components may be periodically replaced surgically to compensate for the child's growth. This surgical exchange of components involves multiple surgical procedures for the skeletally immature child, and each procedure predisposes the child to complications of infection, pain, and vigorous postoperative physical therapy to restore function and mobility.[64] Endoprosthetic designs often incorporate a telescoping unit that can be expanded to accommodate growth. Expansion of the prosthesis typically involves a surgical procedure at periodic intervals. Complications of expansion include loosening of the prosthesis, infection after lengthening procedures, mechanical failure, and fracture. The need for repeat surgical procedures to expand or grow the device is costly and inconvenient for the child, and the risk for infection is increased with each procedure. A review by Eckardt and colleagues[20] of 32 patients with expandable prostheses included patients ranging from 3 to 15 years of age. Fourteen of the 32 patients had no complications; 18 patients had 27 complications, including infection, loosening of the device, mechanical failure, fracture, knee flexion contracture, and prosthetic shoulder joint subluxation; and 1 patient died of a pulmonary embolism. The authors stressed the need for strong family participation during rehabilitation to avoid knee flexion contractures in skeletally immature patients. Effective growth of the child's limb of 7 to 9 cm with the use of an endoprosthetic device has been reported.[20]

To avoid the multiple surgical procedures involved with the modular devices and the early telescoping units, an endoprosthesis that can be expanded with the use of an external electromagnetic field was developed. Exposure of the limb to the electromagnetic field unlocks an energy-stored spring and allows for controlled lengthening without a surgical procedure.[94] Early studies showed decreased rates of infection and more frequent but smaller adjustments in length that were less disruptive to gait and possible range of motion (ROM) complications.[8,65] Ness and colleagues found that similar functional results were achieved with the noninvasive expandable endoprosthetic device compared with a modular device requiring periodic surgical procedures.[67]

Limb-sparing surgery yields similar recurrence rates as amputation when adjuvant chemotherapy is used and when particular attention is given to patient selection, surgical margins, and surgical techniques.[81] A limb-sparing procedure involving the distal femur and/or proximal tibia may result in a significant leg length difference in a child 10 years of age or younger because growth will be lost with excision of the growth plates around the knee. Futani and colleagues[26] retrospectively assessed 40 children younger than 11 years who underwent a limb-sparing procedure secondary to a bone sarcoma. They determined that a limb-sparing procedure could provide good functional outcomes in this younger population. The authors did caution that the functional outcome often was the result of multiple procedures and revisions, including limb lengthenings for expandable prostheses.[26] A long-term complication of lower extremity limb-sparing procedures is reduced ROM, especially at the knee.[10] The ROM deficits, specifically at the hip and knee, that are frequently seen after a limb-sparing procedure are correlated with deficits in mobility.[58] Children with knee flexion ROM deficits exhibited greater difficulty with timed up and down stairs, timed up and go, and a 9-minute run-walk distance.

Lifestyle of the child is another important presurgical consideration because many limb-sparing procedures such as osteoarticular allografts and endoprosthetic implants may limit participation in competitive physical activities. Recent studies have shown that young adults who underwent a limb-sparing procedure for a bone tumor participate in fitness and sports activities regularly. Participation is influenced by presurgical activity level as well as type and level of surgical procedure and long-term complications such as peripheral nerve damage.[47,54] Limb-sparing procedures such as rotationplasty and limb lengthening are increasingly used with children with congenital limb deficiencies to avoid an amputation and often result in excellent function for the child.

Comparison of Surgical Options

With improved survival rates of children with bone sarcomas since the 1970s and the increased use of limb-sparing procedures, it is important to assess the functional outcomes of the various surgical options and to understand the role of physical therapy in successful rehabilitation of these children. Limb-sparing procedures were developed to provide alternatives that spare the child's limb and minimize the functional limitations associated with high-level amputations. However, most of the outcome studies have not demonstrated the marked advantage of limb-sparing procedures that was expected because of some of the complications associated with these procedures.

To compare outcomes, it is best to differentiate between below- and above-knee amputations, as well as between femur and tibia limb-sparing procedures. Ginsberg et al.[34] compared functional outcomes and quality of life among children who had an amputation, limb-sparing, or rotationplasty procedure. They utilized a newer assessment tool, the Functional

Mobility Assessment (FMA), which measures pain, timed up and down stairs, timed up and go, use of ambulation supports, satisfaction of walking quality, participation in work and sports, and endurance.[57] Adolescents and young adults who underwent a femur limb-sparing surgery scored significantly higher on the FMA than those who had an above-knee amputation. However, those who underwent a below-knee amputation scored higher on quality of life measures than those patients who had a limb-sparing procedure of the tibia. Pardasaney[70] and colleagues found that individuals who had undergone an above-knee amputation used an assistive device and walked with a limp more frequently and had higher anxiety levels than those had a femur limb-sparing procedure. However, employment status and ability to participate in sports were not significantly different between the two groups. Researchers also reported that no significant physical functioning or psychological differences were noted between individuals who had a below-knee amputation and those who had a tibia limb-sparing procedure.

Limb Replantation

For children with traumatic amputations, limb replantation may be a surgical option. As with other surgical options, the goal of replantation is directed not only at preserving the amputated limb but also at restoring pain-free function to the extremity that is superior to the function obtained with a prosthesis. For an upper extremity replantation to be considered successful, function of the elbow and hand and distal sensation must be restored. Replantation of a lower extremity must provide a painless, sensate extremity capable of bearing weight during normal daily activities.[9]

Distal replantations of an upper extremity usually result in a more favorable outcome than proximal replantations and are performed more frequently. Digit replantation occurs in approximately 40% of pediatric finger amputations.[87] Proximal replantations are often associated with a violent mechanism of injury that results in damage to the nerves, blood vessels, and muscles. A proximal replantation also necessitates a longer distance for the nerves to regenerate for functional use of the hand. Physical therapy is indicated for these children for wound care, control of edema, joint ROM, strengthening, gait training, and self-care activities. Rehabilitation will include close communication with the physician regarding precautions and progression of activities and family instruction while the child is in the hospital and is treated as an outpatient.

Osseointegration

Osseointegration is the direct attachment of a prosthesis to the end of the bone of the residual limb. The prosthesis attaches to an abutment that has been surgically attached to the bone and protrudes through the skin. The concept of directly attaching a prosthesis to the bone is not new, but the technology to enable the interface of a foreign material with the bone and yet protrude through the skin has expanded the clinical application of this technique. Osseointegration is a long process that requires multiple surgical procedures. The first surgical stage involves the implant of a threaded cylinder directly into the end of the residual bone. At least 6 months later a metal abutment is threaded onto the existing cylinder at the second surgical stage. The metal abutment protrudes through the skin at the distal end of the residual limb and will eventually receive the prosthesis. During the last but lengthy stage, weight-bearing loads on the abutment are gradually increased through the use of a temporary and then a permanent prosthesis. To allow for secure integration of the abutment with the skeleton, this last stage of gradually increasing weight-bearing loads can take well over a year.[71,79]

The purported advantages of osseointegration are the elimination of a socket and the inherent problems associated with poorly fitting sockets and suspension methods. Because the prosthesis is directly attached to the bone through the abutment, some sensation is preserved such as the ability to perceive stepping on a stone or an uneven surface.[71] This procedure is still in its early stages and is not indicated at this time for children or adolescents who are skeletally immature.

Phantom Limb Sensations

Phantom limb sensations are an occurrence in many adults with amputations, but fewer reports are available concerning children with phantom limb sensations. Some persons may believe that if young children do not complain of phantom limb pain, they therefore must not have any pain. Melzack and colleagues[61] reported that 20% of individuals with a congenital limb deficiency and 50% of those with an acquired amputation before 6 years of age experienced phantom limb sensations. However, most of the individuals reporting phantom limb sensations reported not pain but rather the perceived ability to voluntarily move the phantom limb.[61] A study from St Jude Children's Research Hospital found that 70% of children and young adults experienced phantom limb pain at some point during their first year after a cancer-related amputation.[11]

The phantom limb sensations and pain of adolescents can become intense. If left untreated, phantom limb sensations can become debilitating and interfere with prosthetic wear and daily activities. Some teenagers are able to control the sensations through rubbing or massaging the uninvolved limb at similar points to those in which they are experiencing the phantom limb sensations of the amputated limb. Others feel more in control by keeping a daily log of their sensations and reporting the pain intensity on one of a variety of pain scales. Mirror therapy has been proposed as an effective intervention to reduce phantom limb pain through the facilitation of an illusion of an unaffected limb. Mirror therapy theorizes that this illusion of two unaffected limbs fosters reorganization of the somatosensory cortex of the brain to reduce phantom limb pain.[77] For some adolescents the use of analgesics may be beneficial. If available, a referral to a pain management team should be instituted for children undergoing amputations.

OVERVIEW OF PROSTHETICS

Upper Extremity Prosthetics

Upper extremity prosthetic systems may be body powered or externally powered. Externally powered prosthetic devices are typically referred to as myoelectric devices. Body-powered components include a terminal device, a wrist unit, possibly an elbow unit, and a socket and are operated by a harness and cable system. With a myoelectric system a muscle contraction activates electrodes placed in the direction of the muscle fibers in the socket on designated muscles, which act to control the terminal device, wrist, or elbow. Children may also utilize a prosthesis that is a combination of body-powered and externally powered components. For example, the child may operate

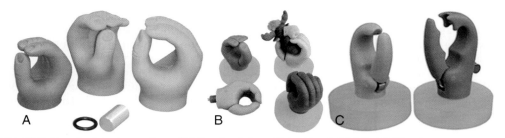

FIG. 13.9 Terminal device options: (A) Passive Infant Alpha Hand. (B) L'IL E-Z Hand promotes grasping when the thumb is moved. (C) ADEPT voluntary closing hand. (Courtesy TRS, Boulder, CO.)

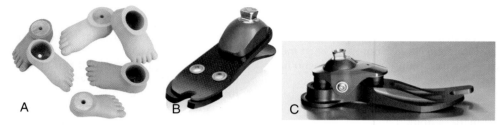

FIG. 13.10 Prosthetic feet options: (A) Little Feet. (B) Flex-Foot Junior. (C) Truper Foot. ([A] Courtesy TRS, Boulder, CO. [B] Courtesy Össur Americas, Foothill Ranch, CA. [C] College Park Industries, Warren MI.)

the elbow using a body-powered cable system and operate the hand with a myoelectric system.[22]

Terminal devices range from the passive hand or fist to a myoelectric hand. Terminal devices often used in pediatrics include the passive fist or hand, the CAPP (Child Amputee Prosthetics Project [Hosmer Dorrance, Campbell, CA]), various hooks, including the Dorrance and ADEPT (Anatomically Designed-Engineered Polymer Technology [Therapeutic Recreation Systems, Boulder, CO]) models, and myoelectric hands such as the Ottobock Electrohand (Ottobock Orthopedic, Plymouth, MN) and the New York Mechanical Hand (Hosmer Dorrance) (Fig. 13.9). The child's age and size, as well as the parents' and child's desires and functional goals, determine the appropriate terminal device. The wrist unit allows forearm pronation and supination and accommodates the terminal device.

As a child's activities change, different terminal devices may be needed. Various recreational terminal devices are available to allow participation in a variety of sports activities.[16,22] Teenagers may desire a cosmetic hand for social activities and a functional terminal device for daily activities.

Suspension systems generally fall into two categories. The first is a harnessed system that is used to suspend a prosthesis or to control a terminal device. Both above-elbow and below-elbow amputation levels can use this type of suspension. The figure 8 and the chest strap are two harness configurations that can be used to suspend and/or control a terminal device.

The figure 8 harness and chest strap fit over the shoulder of the involved limb and around the chest to secure the prosthesis without limiting shoulder movement. The figure 8 harness securely anchors the prosthesis, so the child may activate the cable system of an above-elbow prosthesis. Self-suspending sockets are available for young children. A simple self-suspending socket may be all that is necessary to suspend a below-elbow prosthesis of an infant or toddler. If additional suspension is required, a small silicone sleeve can be rolled over the prosthesis and onto the humeral area. This affords added suspension

without any additional restriction of movement. When the cable for the terminal device is added to the prosthesis, a triceps pad or cuff to secure the cable can be incorporated. A shoulder disarticulation prosthesis is secured with a chest strap. A prosthesis at this level is often very difficult to fit and now is most commonly restricted to myoelectric or hybrid control.

With recent developments in upper extremity research, an increasing number of options are becoming available to the child amputee. Electrodes embedded into silicone liners allow the prosthesis to be both self-suspending and myoelectrically controlled. Recent technological enhancements to electrodes now allow the fitting of children with heavy scarring or weak signal strength so they can benefit from a myocontrolled prosthesis.

Lower Extremity Prosthetics

The fact that children are growing and may be facing several surgical interventions makes fitting a child with a prosthesis very different from fitting an adult with a prosthesis. In addition, angular deformities associated with various congenital deficiencies result in gait and alignment challenges not generally seen in the adult traumatic population. Consequently, many prosthetists will fit a child with a prosthesis that accommodates some growth, stage the introduction of components, and utilize components that can be replaced as the child grows. The variety of components available to the pediatric population continues to expand but does not yet compare with the wide variety available for the adolescent or adult population.

The SACH (Solid Ankle Cushion Heel) (Ottobock) foot has long been the mainstay for pediatric prosthetic feet and continues, in various forms, to be used for young toddlers. The L'IL foot (TRS Industries, Fargo, ND) is a variation of the SACH foot. The entire foot is made of a more flexible plastic that allows a better response during kneeling and pulling to stand. However, young children can now be fitted with dynamic-response or energy-storing feet (Fig. 13.10). In two separate

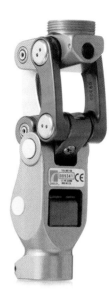

FIG. 13.11 Total Knee Junior is a polycentric knee that provides stability and aids in the initiation of a smooth gait pattern. (Courtesy Össur Americas, Foothill Ranch, CA.)

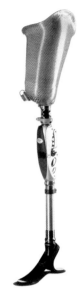

FIG. 13.12 Example of a lower extremity prosthetic system, including socket; 3R60 is a polycentric knee joint and 1C30 Trias is a prosthetic foot. (Courtesy Ottobock HealthCare LP, Austin, TX.)

retrospective analyses, Anderson found that parents and children preferred the cosmetic appearance of dynamic response feet and stated that these feet improved their child's endurance and possibly stability.[3]

The shank of a lower extremity prosthesis has either an exoskeletal or an endoskeletal design. Exoskeletal shanks are fabricated of a rigid polyurethane foam and are laminated to form a hard outer covering. Endoskeletal shanks consist of a pylon made of ultralight material, such as graphite or titanium, and covered with foam. Teenagers often prefer endoskeletal shanks because of their cosmesis and decreased weight. The durability of exoskeletal shanks is often more appropriate for the younger child. Exoskeletal shanks can then be finished with various patterns or designs that are appropriate for the younger amputee.

A wider variety of prosthetic knees are now available for the pediatric population, including toddlers just beginning to pull to stand. A single-axis constant-friction knee is set to function at a certain walking speed. If the speed of walking increases, the prosthesis lags behind because the shank cannot swing through as quickly as the uninvolved limb. In addition, this type of knee is not very stable and buckles quickly if the ground reaction force is not anterior to the knee joint. When the young toddler who is only beginning to stand is fitted, the socket is aligned anterior to the knee center to increase stability. Another type of knee joint available for the pediatric population is a polycentric knee with a four-bar linkage mechanism (Fig. 13.11). A polycentric knee mimics the anatomic knee joint to increase stability. The axis of motion is posterior during stance to provide added stability and anterior during swing to shorten the shank and assist with clearance. A lower extremity prosthesis with a polycentric knee is shown in Fig. 13.12. Polycentric knees are now available for use with toddlers, leading some centers to incorporate a prosthetic knee into a child's first prosthesis.

A larger variety of knee units are available for teenagers, including hydraulic, pneumatic, and microprocessor-controlled knees. Hydraulic and pneumatic knee units are variable-friction units that allow variable walking and running speeds. Variable-friction units are equipped with a swing control mechanism that sets the drag of the shank through swing phase and a stance control unit that permits knee flexion during stance without collapse of the leg. Swing and stance control mechanisms are excellent options for active teenagers, especially those engaged in physical activities. Drawbacks of hydraulic and pneumatic knees are the added weight to the prosthesis, cost, and the intricacy of adjustments. Recent advances in technology have reduced the size and weight of hydraulic systems, resulting in a more functional option for the child amputee.

Like adult sockets, pediatric socket design has changed over the past 15 years. Children with a transfemoral amputation can be fitted with a narrowed medial-lateral ischial containment socket or an anatomically correct socket design. The narrowed medial-lateral socket with ischial containment more evenly distributes weight-bearing pressures and allows less lateral movement of the distal femur, thereby providing greater stability during stance. Adolescents with a below-knee or transtibial amputation may be fitted with the standard patellar tendon–bearing socket or total surface-bearing design. However, younger children may require a supracondylar socket that offers greater suspension. Because most congenital deficiencies result in disarticulations, the Syme prosthesis is the most common lower extremity socket design in the pediatric population. The bulbous end present in most Syme revisions allows for a suspension point just proximal to the distal end. The bladder or segmented socket design is then used to increase independence and eliminate additional suspension systems. These designs are often referred to as self-suspending.

Infants and toddlers will require some type of suspension to secure their prosthesis. A Silesian belt or total elastic suspension (TES) belt works well for younger children with an above-knee amputation or PFFD, and preschoolers can become independent in their use (Fig. 13.13). Neoprene sleeves and silicone liners with a locking mechanism are additional suspension methods commonly used with young children. The silicone liner is rolled on the residual limb, and the pin on the end of

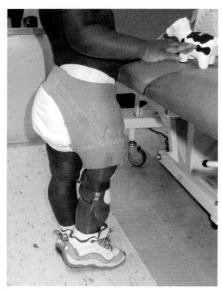

FIG. 13.13 Toddler with a right proximal femoral focal deficiency fitted with a prosthesis before any surgical procedures were performed to modify her leg. A neoprene total elastic suspension belt is used as the suspension method to secure the prosthesis.

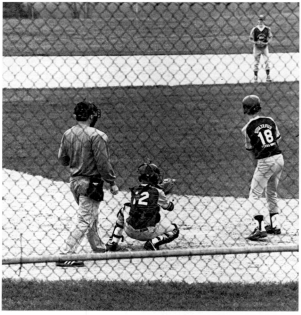

FIG. 13.15 Catcher is an adolescent with a left below-knee amputation.

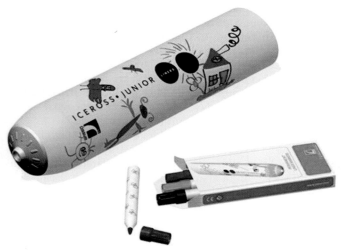

FIG. 13.14 Suspension systems may utilize a silicone liner that is rolled onto the residual limb and attached to the distal end of the socket with a pin-locking mechanism. (Courtesy Össur Americas, Foothill Ranch, CA.)

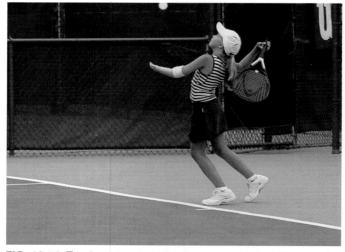

FIG. 13.16 Tossing a tennis ball using a prosthesis with a passive hand.

the sleeve is threaded into the prosthesis and locked in place. To remove the prosthesis, the pin is released by pushing a button on the distal end of the socket[16] (Fig. 13.14).

Suction sockets are appropriate for the older child who is not growing rapidly or is undergoing weight fluctuations secondary to chemotherapy treatment. Suction sockets utilize negative pressure as air is expelled through a distal valve and surface tension between the skin and socket to maintain the suspension.[16] Advances in silicone liners allow a suction fit over the liner with various design elements that may include a ring seal. A ring seal and other design elements aim to improve the suction and mechanical suspension of the socket as well as to reduce rotation and pistoning of the socket.

Children with a rotationplasty use a prosthesis that incorporates the plantarflexed foot in the socket. The socket is essentially a below-knee socket with a thigh cuff attachment and external hinges for the knee joint. A Silesian or TES belt may be needed for suspension.

Children of all ages with a limb deficiency or amputation should be encouraged to participate in activities with their peers. Many children may want to participate in sports at a recreational or a competitive level (Fig. 13.15). Many prosthetic options are available that promote participation in various sports. Recreational prosthetics options are too numerous to mention for this discussion, and the reader is referred to other resources.[76] Ultimately, any prosthesis for a child should allow the opportunity for age-appropriate function and be cosmetically appealing to the child and family (Fig. 13.16). Decision making for infants' and toddlers' prosthetic needs should include the parents, orthopedist, prosthetist, and physical therapist. The older child should be included in the decision-making process.

Appropriate prosthetic components are costly, and a full prosthesis must be replaced at least every 12 to 18 months for growing children and adolescents. If an adolescent chooses to participate in sports or swimming activities, an additional prosthesis or components may be required. Third-party payers are reluctant to pay for multiple prostheses or myoelectric devices. Currently, some health maintenance organizations will pay for only one prosthesis in a lifetime.

Studies are beginning to examine the cost-effectiveness of surgical procedures and various prosthetic options. Grimer and colleagues[38] compared long-term costs of limb-sparing procedures versus amputation with a prosthesis. Limb-sparing procedures are more costly initially, but amputations for children or adolescents are very costly over time because of the need for multiple and sophisticated prostheses.

FOREGROUND INFORMATION

PHYSICAL THERAPY INTERVENTION FOR THE CHILD WITH A LIMB DEFICIENCY OR AN ACQUIRED AMPUTATION

The parents are an integral part of the rehabilitation team for a child with an amputation or a limb deficiency. The rehabilitation team should also include an orthopedist, a prosthetist, and a physical therapist who are experienced in the management of children with amputations. This may often mean traveling to a major medical center for periodic assessments and prosthetic adjustments. Physical therapy can be delivered in the local community if available, but the therapist must be in communication with the managing rehabilitation team.

The overall goals of physical therapy are to facilitate as normal a sequence of development as possible for the child and to prevent or minimize the development of impairments, activity limitations, and participation restrictions. Impairments can include joint contractures and weakness with resultant activity limitations of reduced mobility and a lack of independence in self-care skills. Physical therapy goals are directed toward preventing joint contractures, minimizing muscle strength imbalances, preventing skin breakdown, and developing independence with mobility and self-care skills. Ideally these goals are accomplished through physical therapy intervention for the child, child or parent instruction, and follow-up of a child's progress and functional outcomes. The child's age, type of limb deficiency, or level of amputation, as well as other medical factors, will influence the intensity of physical therapy needed.

The physical therapy examination should follow the components listed in the *Guide to Physical Therapist Practice*.[5] A thorough examination of joint integrity and mobility and range of motion is important for the child with a limb deficiency. Some children with a congenital limb deficiency may have other associated musculoskeletal impairments, as well as other syndromes that affect the integrity of the musculoskeletal system. Integumentary integrity will be important postsurgery and for the child with a prosthesis. Examination of gait and balance, neuromotor development, aerobic capacity and endurance, community and work integration, and self-care will begin to highlight the child's functional abilities (Box 13.1).

BOX 13.1 Recommended Measures for Children With Limb Deficiencies or Amputations

Body Functions and Structures
Pain
Skin integrity
Anthropometric measures
Range of motion
Strength

Activity – Single Task
6-minute walk test
Timed up and down steps

Activity – Multiple Items
Peabody Developmental Motor Scales
Pediatric Balance Scale
Functional Mobility Assessment (FMA)
Child Amputee Prosthetics Project – Functional Status Inventory (CAPP-FSI)

Participation
Pediatric Quality of Life Inventory (PedsQL)
Pediatric Evaluation of Disability Index (PEDI)

Functional outcomes can be assessed using current assessment tools. However, these assessment tools may not be able to determine the functional effectiveness of various prosthetic options. Third-party payers and state-funded programs will opt for the prosthetic options that are less costly if outcomes are not present to justify the more expensive options. Pruitt and colleagues (1996) developed and tested an outcome measure for children with limb deficiencies. The Child Amputee Prosthetics Project—Functional Status Inventory (CAPP-FSI) assesses 40 activities on two scales to determine whether the child performs the activity with or without a prosthesis. The child is also rated for the severity of his or her limb loss. Internal reliability for the two scales that compose the CAPP-FSI was 0.96.[73] The CAPP-FSIP and the CAPP-FSIT were developed to assess the functional outcomes of preschoolers age 4 to 7 years and toddlers age 1 to 4 years, respectively.[74,75] The FMA is a more recently developed functional outcome measure that has been validated for children and young adults with bone sarcomas. The FMA comprises six categories: (1) pain, (2) function as measured by the timed up and down stairs (TUDS) and the timed up and go (TUG), (3) use of supports or assistive devices, (4) satisfaction with quality of walking, (5) participation in work, school, and sports, and (6) endurance as measured by a 9-minute walk/run test.[57]

Infancy and Toddler Period

An infant with a limb deficiency should be referred for an initial examination by a pediatric orthopedist and a physical therapist shortly after birth. Monitoring by the physical therapist with suggestions to parents regarding positioning and ROM exercises may be all that is needed initially. The motor development of children with multiple limb deficiencies or upper extremity deficiencies may become delayed or impaired owing to their inability to use their arms for such activities as pushing up to sit, crawling, and pulling to stand. Physical therapy is necessary to monitor the infant's developmental progress, ROM, and strength needed for later prosthetic use. The physical therapist should also teach the parent or caregiver how to incorporate physical therapy goals into the child's daily activities. This can be accomplished through periodic physical therapy examinations and evaluations, optimally at 1-month intervals, with updated parent instruction provided.

Generally, infants with limb deficiencies do not develop contractures after birth, but ROM should be carefully monitored according to individual needs. The parents of a child with a PFFD may benefit from instruction to decrease the hip flexion and abduction contractures that are typically noted at birth and will later interfere with prosthetic fit. Most children with upper extremity limb deficiencies will maintain ROM and strength through their developmental activities.

Careful monitoring of the developing infant is necessary to evaluate ROM, functional strength, weight-bearing capabilities, and posture while prone, sitting, and standing. Often a child with a limb deficiency will tend to bear weight asymmetrically in prone and during sitting activities. Some children will take increased weight on their limb-deficient side to free their uninvolved side for reaching and movement. Other children may take more weight through their uninvolved side because of weight-shifting and balance difficulties. Suggestions may be given to the parents and therapy provided to encourage weight-shifting activities to improve symmetry. For the child with an upper limb deficiency, this will encourage cocontraction of the shoulder musculature as needed later for prosthetic use. For the child with a lower limb deficiency, this encourages assumption of an erect trunk with normal balance reactions. Shifting weight to the limb-deficient side is also important for the preprosthetic training needed for standing and ambulation activities.

If an infant is not progressing developmentally, physical therapy intervention may be warranted to provide alternative methods of achieving the normal developmental sequence. For example, a child with bilateral upper extremity limb deficiencies may need assistance to learn to stand from sitting or to safely learn to balance in standing.

A child is usually fitted with a prosthesis at a developmentally appropriate age. A child with a lower extremity deficiency will be fitted for a prosthesis when weight bearing is appropriate and the child is beginning to pull to stand (between 8 and 10 months of age depending on the child's developmental progress). A child with a unilateral PFFD may initially be fit with an extension prosthesis to equalize limb lengths as soon as transitioning into and out of standing while biding time to allow for skeletal development that will determine the surgical options.[62] A child with an upper extremity limb deficiency may be fitted with a prosthesis to assist with early playing skills in sitting or even as early as 3 months to assist with weight-bearing skills while prone. Children are typically fitted with an upper extremity prosthesis between 5 and 7 months, when they are able to sit independently.[83]

When a child first receives a prosthesis, the fit and alignment as well as the overall function of the prosthesis are assessed. The initial session is spent on instructing the parents in properly donning the prosthesis, checking the skin, and developing a wear schedule. The initial goal is to have the infant or toddler wear the prosthesis comfortably for as many hours a day as possible and for the parents to be comfortable in donning and removing the prosthesis. The prosthesis may be removed for naps and should be removed when the child sleeps at night.

A child with an upper extremity prosthesis may initially ignore it. The focus of therapy should be on having the child wear the prosthesis while playing and to begin to use it for

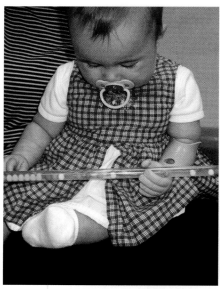

FIG. 13.17 Toddler holding a toy in the passive hand of her prosthesis.

bimanual play such as manipulating and holding large toys and during gross motor activities such as pushing up to sitting or quadruped, protective reactions, and propping in sitting.

The child's first upper extremity prosthesis may have one of several terminal device options (see Fig. 13.9). A young infant may have a nonarticulating hand that is cosmetically appealing but has limited movement (Fig. 13.17). As the child begins to engage in bimanual play, reaching, and propping activities, the decision to use a body-powered or an externally powered myoelectric device is made. Body-powered devices may be a simple split hook terminal device or a CAPP voluntary opening device. The split hook is similar to that used with adult prosthetics, except it is smaller. The CAPP was designed specifically for children, is cosmetically more appealing than a hook terminal device, is safer than a hook for a young child, and provides an efficient grip without requiring great operating force. The goal for the young child at this time is to adjust to the weight of a prosthesis, to begin to use it to manipulate larger toys, and to shake or remove toys placed in the terminal device by an adult.

Children are not expected to begin to operate the terminal device until 18 months of age or later, when they understand simple commands and cause and effect.[83] Training to operate the terminal device is dependent on the child's developmental level. Generally, children are taught to open the terminal device, place objects in it, and then release them, in that order. This corresponds with the normal developmental sequence of learning to grasp before learning to release objects.[72] The therapist must be familiar with the mechanism that controls the terminal device because this can differ from child to child, depending on the design of the device. The CAPP and Hosmer Dorrance hook are voluntary-opening terminal devices; forward reaching of the arm pulls the cable tight and activates opening of the terminal device. Children with a transverse deficiency of the upper arm will need to use scapular abduction to activate opening of the terminal device with the elbow locked; control of the prosthetic elbow comes at a later age. The ADEPT hook is a voluntary-closing terminal device designed to mimic forward reaching to grasp or close on an object (Fig. 13.18).

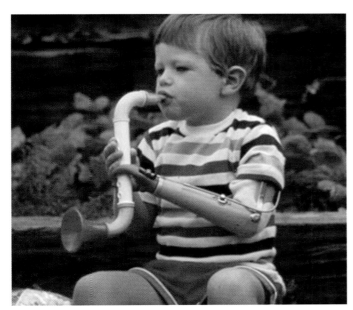

FIG. 13.18 Child engaging in bimanual play wearing a forearm prosthesis with an ADEPT voluntary closing hook. (Courtesy TRS, Boulder, CO.)

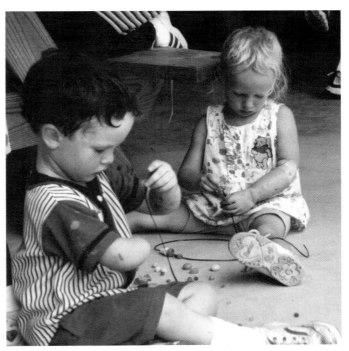

FIG. 13.19 Young girl using her myoelectric single-site prosthesis to complete a bimanual activity.

If the decision is made to fit the child with an externally powered prosthesis, the New York Hand (Hosmer Dorrance) or the Ottobock Electrohand is commonly used with young children. Children typically are fitted initially with a myoelectric hand with only one electrode. When this electrode is activated through muscle contraction, the hand opens. When the child relaxes the muscle, the hand closes. Typically, by 3 to 4 years of age the child's myoelectric device can be converted to two electrodes, two sites, so that opening and closing the hand are controlled by the child[16] (Fig. 13.19).

Recent evidence indicates that children younger than 2 years with a lower limb deficiency or above-knee amputation can be fit with a prosthesis that incorporates a prosthetic knee. Infants and toddlers demonstrated the ability to transition into and out of positions, crawl, squat, and play in kneeling and tall kneeling incorporating the prosthetic knee[29,30] (Fig. 13.20). The principle for fitting a young child with a knee component is that knee flexion during gait simulates a more normal gait pattern and may therefore eliminate some of the gait deviations, such as vaulting on the uninvolved limb and circumduction of the prosthetic limb that may develop and become ingrained after ambulating with a prosthesis without a knee.[15] When toddlers are fitted with a lower extremity prosthesis, normal stance and gait patterns for their developmental age should be kept in mind. Children 1 year of age stand and walk with a wide base of support and exhibit increased hip external rotation during the swing phase.[90] For this reason, a toddler's prosthesis may need to be aligned with greater hip abduction than is provided to an older child.

Because a goal of physical therapy is symmetry of posture and movement during developmental activities, proper alignment and controlled weight-shifting and balance activities are emphasized for children with a lower limb prosthesis. Many children with a lower limb prosthesis do not require an assistive device for ambulation; however, initial gait training with an assistive device promotes a reciprocal gait pattern and an

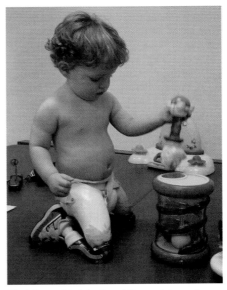

FIG. 13.20 Toddler with his first bilateral transfemoral prosthesis with knee joint to promote age-appropriate ambulation skills and play activities on the floor.

erect trunk. As the child develops balance and is able to control weight shifting, he or she will naturally discard the assistive device when comfortable with independent ambulation.

Preschool- and School-Age Period

When a child attends a preschool or kindergarten class for the first time, many anxieties may resurface for the parents of a child with a limb deficiency. Parents will worry that their child may not fit in or will look different from his or her peers. This is also an age by which typical children have achieved independence with ADL skills such as eating and dressing, and their social relationships with peers increase. The preschool years should emphasize development of independence in self-care skills and mobility and acquisition of school skills such as coloring, cutting, and writing. If these skills are achieved during the preschool years, the child will enter school with minimal or no activity limitations or participation restrictions.

The child with an upper limb deficiency should be able to activate the terminal device of the prosthesis by this age. Children using above-elbow prostheses can begin to learn to control the elbow by 3 or 4 years of age. Most above-elbow body-powered prostheses have a dual cable system that allows the child to control elbow flexion and extension and forearm pronation and supination. With control of the elbow and forearm, the terminal device of the prosthesis becomes more functional in a variety of positions.

Emphasis should always be on assisting the child to learn skills that are appropriate for his or her age. Play skills involving manipulation of smaller objects, using the prosthesis to hold and turn paper for coloring and cutting activities, holding the handlebars of a tricycle, and self-dressing and feeding skills are important. A child with a unilateral upper limb prosthesis will always use it as a helper hand and not as the dominant hand.

For those children with bilateral upper limb deficiencies, the use of a prosthesis should be carefully monitored. These children should always be allowed to use their feet or mouth for play and self-care activities. A prosthesis may aid these children for only some periods of the day and may actually limit their function during some activities. Children with lower limb deficiencies requiring the use of prostheses, including those children with unilateral PFFD, should be functional ambulators at this age. During the preschool years, some surgery is usually necessary for the child with a unilateral PFFD. Femoral osteotomy, arthrodesis of the knee joint, and foot ablation are usually performed between 2.5 and 4 years of age. These procedures increase the lever arm of the thigh and eliminate any knee instability.[31,62] Femoral or tibial epiphysiodesis may be performed at the time of knee arthrodesis. The ultimate goal is for limb length on the prosthetic side to be 5 cm shorter than on the contralateral femur. This enables the prosthetic knee joint to be at approximately the same level as the contralateral knee joint at maturity. Placement of the prosthetic knee joint at the same level as the contralateral knee joint allows for improved cosmesis and improved gait.

For the child with an acquired lower extremity amputation, an immediate postoperative fit prosthesis (IPOP) or preparatory prosthesis is typically prescribed. This may not be the case if significant trauma to the surrounding tissue was present or if skin grafting was necessary after the injury. The physical therapy examination and evaluation focuses on sensitivity of the residual limb, active movement, strength, bed mobility, transfers for toileting and getting out of bed, and ambulation. The goals of postoperative physical therapy are similar to those for an adult with an amputation.

Children are more likely than an adult to move about after an amputation, so contractures are less likely to occur. However, some children undergoing chemotherapy are extremely ill and weak and may tend to lie in bed with their residual limb propped on pillows. They must be monitored for developing contractures, and parents and nursing staff must be instructed in ROM exercises and positioning of the residual limb.

Gait training should begin as soon as cleared by the physician. Young children can safely learn to ambulate with their preparatory prosthesis using a walker or crutches. If a child has been hospitalized for a period of time, strengthening exercises for the uninvolved leg and the residual limb may be necessary.

After removal of the preparatory prosthesis, the child is fitted with a definitive prosthesis. The exception to this would be a child who is undergoing chemotherapy. Weight gain and weight fluctuations are common, and these children tend to remain in their preparatory prosthesis for a longer period of time to allow their limb size to stabilize before moving on to their definitive prosthesis. Children with above-knee amputations should be fitted with a prosthesis with a knee joint. Most children with an above-knee amputation will require a suspension method to help hold the prosthesis in place. Instruction must be given to both the parents and the child in donning and removing the prosthesis, care of the prosthesis, skin checks, and wear schedule.

For the child who undergoes a rotationplasty, gentle active and active-assisted hip, ankle, and foot exercises should be initiated per the surgeon's or team protocol. For ambulation and sitting, 0° to 20° of ankle dorsiflexion is more than adequate. Some children will be able to achieve 30° of ankle dorsiflexion, which will allow for some squatting activities and facilitate bike riding. Maximal plantar flexion will allow for greater extension of the leg in stance. Optimal plantar flexion ROM is at least 45° to 50°; the prosthetist can align the prosthesis to achieve an additional few degrees of plantar flexion for stance. Exercises should begin gently and progress to active and resistive exercises.

The child who undergoes a rotationplasty is fitted with a custom-made prosthesis that incorporates the foot in a position of maximum plantar flexion and allows it to act as a knee joint. An external knee hinge joint with an attached thigh cuff may be used for suspension, or the prosthesis may incorporate a laminar thigh socket and utilize a TES or Silesian belt for suspension. A child who has had a limb-sparing procedure will also require physical therapy after surgery. Lower extremity procedures usually require a period of non–weight bearing. Rehabilitation for children with a limb-sparing procedure to the upper or lower extremity includes exercise through active movement with progression to strengthening exercises. The progression of the intervention is dictated by the procedure that was performed, the surgeon's protocols, and the amount of bone replaced. Children who have had a limb-sparing procedure involving the femur will also frequently require physical therapy after a lengthening procedure of the endoprosthetic implant. ROM of the knee often becomes restricted, similar to what is seen with children who undergo limb-lengthening techniques (see Chapter 14).

Gait training for all children at this age will focus on symmetry and the normal characteristics of gait, such as stride length, step length, and velocity, as well as all skills that the child needs to participate in play and games with other children. When initially learning to ambulate or after a surgical procedure, most children will use an assistive device. As balance and ambulation speed improve and postsurgical limitations are lifted, many children will begin to discard the assistive device. The assistive device should be discarded, however, only if the child's ambulation is safe and speed is functional to keep pace with the child's peers.

During the school-age years the physical therapist should instruct the child in running techniques so that he or she may participate in play and games with her or his peers. This is the age at which the child may also show an interest in participating in various sports or recreational programs designed for persons with amputations.

When attending school for the first time, the child will be questioned about the prosthesis and assistive devices. This is especially true of a child with an upper limb deficiency. A meeting before the beginning of school with the child and his or her parents, the child's teacher, and perhaps the child's physical therapist may be helpful to allay any concerns and to answer or develop a way to answer the questions of the child's peers. The child with a unilateral limb deficiency or amputation should succeed in school with minimal adaptations.

The child with bilateral upper limb deficiencies may need to use voice-activated technology or a computer to assist with writing skills. In school a child with bilateral upper limb deficiencies may be able to carry papers or books in the classroom between the chin and shoulder. The child may use the mouth for manipulating and holding objects such as pencils. Whether the child uses his or her feet in school for manipulation or grasping is something that should be clearly discussed with the child, parents, and teacher before school entrance. Many children opt not to use their feet for grasping objects in public as they get older; however, this can limit their independence, especially with toileting and feeding. If a child is adept with the use of his or her feet and is independent and chooses to use the feet, this should not be discouraged. If the teacher displays a supportive attitude toward the child's use of the feet, the child's classroom peers will soon view this as usual procedure in their classroom. The ultimate outcome is for the child to be functional in our society as an adult; this may mean use of the feet or a combination of use of the feet and prostheses.

Adolescence and Transition to Adulthood

Adolescence, with its hallmark concerns of appearance and acceptance by peers, relationships with the opposite sex, career decisions, and the struggle for independence, can be a trying time for anyone. Restrictions on participation for the child with a limb deficiency may become more apparent during adolescence. Most teenagers with a congenital limb deficiency have been adjusting both functionally and emotionally from birth. At this point in their lives, they are part of a social network of friends, realize the support of their families, and have attempted and succeeded at various activities in school and the community. They will be dealing with these adolescent issues right alongside their peers, although increased fears concerning dating and social acceptance can be typical at this time, and participation in school athletic activities may be limited. A higher percentage of children and adolescents with congenital limb deficiencies exhibit greater behavioral and emotional problems and lower social competence than their peers without a disability.[93]

Amputation of a limb during the adolescent years adds quite an emotional burden to a teenager, who must deal with the loss of a body part and the grieving process and may be facing the possibility of death. Added to the physical appearance difficulties are possible side effects such as hair loss from chemotherapy. A teenager who is facing a possible amputation as the result of cancer should be included, if he or she desires, in discussions of treatment options, including surgical options. Obviously, this is not possible if the amputation is the result of sudden trauma.

The immediate postoperative concerns and physical therapy interventions for adolescents undergoing an amputation or a limb-sparing procedure are similar to those described for school-age children. If an immediate-fit prosthesis is not used, teenagers are more likely to develop edema of their residual limb following surgery. In this case, wrapping of the residual limb or fitting with a shrinker sock should be instituted.

Teenagers who sustain a lower extremity amputation are fitted with a prosthesis when the residual limb has stabilized. They should be involved in the fitting of the prosthesis and in deciding on the design of the socket and the type of knee joint and foot to be used. For most teenagers, a large variety of prosthetic options are available. These should be fully discussed with the teenager and parents, and the choice should complement the lifestyle of the user. Both the teenager and his or her family should be cautioned that the prosthesis will not function and will not look exactly like the contralateral limb.

Many teenagers with a high above-knee amputation will attempt to ambulate with a prosthesis but may opt for no prosthesis and crutches because ambulation with crutches is faster and more energy efficient. The decision to use or not to use a prosthesis should be the child's and should not be based on society's idea of the most appropriate physical appearance. Some teenagers use a prosthesis for certain activities and not for others. Advances in microprocessor knee and ankle technology can optimize function in adolescents with complex and higher levels of limb loss. The ultimate outcome is for them to be comfortable with their peers and to interact socially with their peers at school and in the community.

The use of prosthetics varies for teenagers with upper limb deficiencies. Those who have become adept with a prosthesis since early childhood probably will continue to use their prosthesis. The teenager who has an upper limb amputation may learn to operate a body-powered above- or below-elbow prosthesis. Microprocessor partial hand and digit prostheses are being developed that offer adolescents grasp and manipulation functions. Examples of these are the i-limb and i-digits (Touch Bionics, Mansfield, MA) and Michelangelo prosthetic hand (Ottobock, Austin, TX). To become functional with the prosthesis requires much practice, and the teenager may opt not to use one. An outcome study assessed the function and quality of life of 489 children with a transverse below-elbow limb deficiency, comparing 321 children who wore a prosthesis and 168 who did not wear a prosthesis. Researchers found small differences between the two groups, but they were not significant enough to meet the definition of a clinically important difference in the Pediatric Quality of Life Inventory.[50]

One major milestone for teenagers is the acquisition of a driver's license. Nearly all teenagers with a limb deficiency or amputation can learn to drive. Hand controls can be used for the teenager with bilateral PFFD or with bilateral lower extremity amputation as the result of trauma. For the teenager with a unilateral upper limb deficiency or amputation, minimal adjustments will be necessary. Driving can be done by using the sound hand, or a driving ring can be attached to the steering wheel. The prosthetic terminal device, preferably a hook, slips into the ring to assist with controlling the steering wheel and easily slips out of the ring in emergencies. Driving becomes more difficult for the teenager with bilateral upper limb deficiencies or amputations. A driving ring may be used by the dominant limb. Controls such as light switches or turn signals may need to be moved to the dominant side and within reach of the limb or can be operated by the driver's knee. Unless specifically trained in the area of driver education, physical therapists should assist the teenager and his or her parents to seek information and driver training from a local rehabilitation center.

Career and college decisions are also made during adolescence. Some teenagers may work at a part-time job during high school. Most teenagers with limb deficiencies or amputations eventually seek employment. At times, adjustments must be made to a prosthesis, such as a specific terminal device, to assist the young adult in his or her particular career area. Going to college is a true test of independence with self-care skills. Some individuals with bilateral upper limb deficiencies or multiple limb deficiencies will always require some degree of assistance with self-care activities. Toileting, especially wiping after defecation, and dressing, specifically managing underpants and bras, are self-care activities for which it is difficult for anyone with bilateral upper limb deficiencies or short above-elbow amputations to achieve total independence. This does not preclude attending college or independent living, but an aide or other arrangements may be needed. Creativity, experimentation, and talking with other teenagers or adults with limb deficiencies can often produce strategies for accomplishing difficult tasks. Quality of life outcomes for young adults who have survived a childhood bone sarcoma with either an amputation or limb-sparing procedure are very diverse. Some studies report high employment rates, active lifestyles, and marriage for adults who underwent an amputation as a child or adolescent.[63,92] However, survivors of childhood bone tumors are more likely to have a physical limitation than those from other groups of childhood cancer, and those survivors with physical limitations are less likely to be employed, married, and/or earning an annual income greater than $20,000.[66] The data are conflicting on quality of life outcomes comparing adults who underwent a childhood amputation with those who had a limb-sparing procedure for a childhood bone sarcoma.[59] With the improvements in prosthetic design that are available as well as the limb-sparing procedures, further research is needed to follow the functional and overall satisfaction of these individuals as adults in society (Box 13.2).

BOX 13.2 Interventions: Child and Caregiver Communication and Education Across All Three Domains

Body Functions and Structures
Desensitization techniques
Massage
Strengthening

Activity
Developmental activities training
Transfer and gait training
Training with prosthetic device for ADLs

Participation
Training with prosthetic device for IADLs (school, play, driving, sports, work)
Education regarding environmental and prosthetic adaptations for activities and sports

---

■ SUMMARY

The origin and classification of congenital limb deficiencies and the causes of acquired amputations were reviewed in this chapter. An overview of the medical and surgical management of congenital limb deficiencies and amputations was presented. Treatment of a child with a congenital limb deficiency or amputation is complex and must involve a team of professionals who recognize the impact of various treatment options on the child's functioning in both home and school environments and ultimately as an independent adult. Careful planning and thoughtful discussions with the family regarding expected outcomes, goals of physical therapy, surgical options, and prosthetic options are necessary. Each child must be assessed as an individual, with consideration given to the child's age and musculoskeletal development and immediate and long-term functional abilities, the family's and child's activity level and lifestyle choices, and prosthetic and physical therapy interventions needed to meet the child's goals.

The continued proliferation of prosthetic designs, along with advances in microprocessor technology and materials available to the pediatric population, has opened up many options for recreation and sports, vocation, and self-care, as well as early fitting of infants and toddlers with prostheses.

Case Scenarios on Expert Consult

The case scenarios related to this chapter address three patients:

"Becca": Child With PFFD (Proximal Focal Femoral Deficiency)

This case reviews the prosthetic prescription for an infant with a congenital limb deficiency and the physical therapy interventions to facilitate her developmental skills and provision of initial caregiver education. The case study follows her for several years, including a surgical revision for her involved leg and the subsequent prosthetic and physical therapy needs.

"Andrew": Child With Cancer, Osteosarcoma Right Distal Femur

The focus of this case is on the surgical options available for a very young, skeletally immature child with a bony tumor. The rationale for choosing a rotationplasty is discussed as well as the focus of his physical therapy postoperatively. Andrew is followed for several years after his initial diagnosis and surgery to demonstrate the impact of the surgical procedure on his ultimate function and participation in activities with his peers.

"Anthony": Child With Traumatic Amputation

This case scenario focuses on the acute physical therapy intervention of an adolescent with a traumatic amputation and follows his rehabilitation through the fitting of his first prosthesis.

Two video cases are also presented. The first describes a teenager who sustained a traumatic mutilating lower extremity injury, and the second shows a preschool aged child with a congenital longitudinal tibial deficiency.

REFERENCES

1. Aitken GT: Surgical amputation in children, *J Bone Joint Surg Am* 45:1735–1741, 1963.
2. Aitken GT: Proximal femoral focal deficiency: definition, classification, and management. In *Proximal femoral focal deficiency: a congenital anomaly*, Washington, DC, 1969, National Academy of Sciences.
3. Anderson TF: Aspects of sports and recreation for the child with a limb deficiency. In Herring JA, Birch JG, editors: *The child with a limb deficiency*. Rosemont, IL, American Academy of Orthopedic Surgeons, 1998.

4. Akahane T, Shimizu T, Isobe K, Yoshimura Y, Fujioka F, Kato H: Evaluation of postoperative general quality of life for patients with osteosarcoma around the knee joint, *J Pediatr Orthop B* 16:269–272, 2007.

5. American Physical Therapy Association: *Guide to physical therapist practice*, revised second edition, Alexandria, VA: APTA; 2003.

6. Reference deleted in proofs.

7. Bedard T, Lowry RB, Sibbald B, Kiefer GN, Metcalfe A: Congenital limb deficiencies in Alberta-a review of 33 years from the Alberta congenital anomalies surveillance system, *Am J Med Genet A* 2599–2609, 2015.

8. Beebe K, Song KJ, Ross E, Tuy B, Patterson F, Benevenia J: Functional outcomes after limb-salvage surgery and endoprosthetic reconstruction with an expandable prosthesis: a report of 4 cases, *Arch Phys Med Rehabil* 90:1039–1047, 2009.

9. Beris AE, Soucacos PN, Malizos KN, Mitsionis GJ, Soucacos PR: Major limb replantation in children, *Microsurgery* 15:474–478, 1994.

10. Buchner M, Zeifang F, Bernd L: Medial gastrocnemius muscle flap in limb-sparing surgery of malignant bone tumors of the proximal tibia: mid-term results in 25 patients, *Ann Plast Surg* 51:266–272, 2003.

11. Burgoyne LL, Billups CA, Jiron JL: Phantom limb pain in young cancer-related amputees: recent experience at St Jude Children's Research Hospital, *Clin J Pain* 28(3):222–225, 2012.

12. Butler MS, Robertson WW, Rate W, D'Angio GJ, Drummond DS: Skeletal sequelae of radiation therapy for malignant tumors, *Clin Orthop Rel Res* 251:235–239, 1990.

13. Caudill JS, Arndt CA: Diagnosis and management of bone malignancy in adolescents, *Adolesc Med State Art Rev* 18:62–78, 2007.

14. Centers for Disease Control and Prevention: Facts about upper lower limb reduction defects. Website. Available at http://www.cdc.From.gov/ncbddd/birthdefects/ul-limbreductiondefects.html.

15. Coulter-O'Berry C: Physical therapy. In Smith DG, Michael JW, Bowker JH, editors: *Atlas of limb amputations and limb deficiencies*, ed 3, Rosemont, IL, 2004, American Academy of Orthopedic Surgeons, pp 831–840.

16. Cummings DR: Pediatric prosthetics, current trends and future possibilities, *Phys Med Rehabil Clin N Am* 11:653–679, 2000.

17. Day HJB: The ISO/ISPO classification of congenital limb deficiency, *Prosthet Orthot Int* 15:67–69, 1991.

18. Dillingham TR, Pezzin LE, MacKenzie EJ: Limb amputation and limb deficiency: epidemiology and recent trends in the United States, *South Med J* 95:875–883, 2002.

19. Dormans JP, Erol B, Nelson CB: Acquired amputations in children. In Smith DG, Michael JW, Bowker JH, editors: *Atlas of limb amputations and limb deficiencies*, ed 3, Rosemont, IL, 2004, American Academy of Orthopedic Surgeons, pp 841–852.

20. Eckhardt JJ, Kabo JM, Kelley CM, Ward WG, Asavamongkolkul A, Wirganowics PZ, et al.: Expandable endoprosthesis reconstruction in skeletally immature patients with tumors, *Clin Orthop Rel Res* 373:51–61, 2000.

21. Ephraim PL, Dillingham TR, Sector M, Pezzin LE, MacKenzie EJ: Epidemiology of limb loss and congenital limb deficiency: a review of the literature, *Arch Phys Med Rehabil* 84:747–761, 2003.

22. Farnsworth T: The call to arms, overview of upper limb prosthetic options, *Active Living, Health and Activity for the O P Community* 12:43–45, 2003.

23. Fedorak GT, Watts HG, Cuomo AV, Ballesteros JP, Grant HJ, Bowen HE, Scaduto AA: Osteocartilaginous transfer of the proximal part of the fibula for osseous overgrowth in children with congenital or acquired tibial amputation, *J Bone Joint Surg Am* 97:574–581, 2015.

24. Fowler E, Zernicke R, Setoguchi Y: Energy expenditure during walking by children who have proximal femoral focal deficiency, *J Bone Joint Surg Am* 78:1857–1862 1996.

25. Frantz CH, O'Rahilly R: Congenital skeletal limb deficiencies, *J Bone Joint Surg Am* 43:1202–1204, 1961.

26. Futani H, Miramaki T, Nishimoto Y, Abe S, Yabe H, Ueda T: Long-term follow-up after limb salvage in skeletally immature children with a primary malignant tumor of the distal end of the femur, *J Bone Joint Surg Am* 88:595–603, 2006.

27. Reference deleted in proofs.

28. Gasper N, Hawkins DS, Dirksen U, Lewis IJ, Ferrari S, et al.: Ewing sarcoma: current management and future approaches through collaboration, *J Clin Oncol* 33:3036–3048, 2015.

29. Geil MD, Coulter-O'Berry C, Schmitz M, Heriza C: Crawling kinematics in an early knee protocol for pediatric prosthetic prescription, *J Prosthet Orthot* 25(1):22–29, 2013.

30. Geil MD, Coulter CP: Analysis of locomotor adaptations in young children with limb loss in an early knee prescription protocol, *Prosthet Orthot Int* 38(1):54–61, 2014.

31. Gillespie R: Principles of amputation surgery in children with longitudinal deficiencies of the femur, *Clin Orthop Rel Res* 256:29–38, 1990.

32. Gillespie R: Classification of congenital abnormalities of the femur. In Herring JA, Birch JG, editors: *The child with a limb deficiency*, Rosemont, IL, 1998, American Academy of Orthopedic Surgeons, pp 63–72.

33. Reference deleted in proofs.

34. Ginsberg JP, Rai SN, Carlson CA, Meadows AT, Hinds PS, Spearing EM, et al.: A comparative analysis of functional outcomes in adolescents and young adults with lower-extremity bone sarcoma, *Pediatr Blood Cancer* 49:964–969, 2007.

35. Gold NB, Westgate MN, Holmes LB: Anatomic and etiological classification of congenital limb deficiencies, *Am J Med Genet A* 1225–1235, 2011.

36. Goorin AM, Schwartzentruber DJ, Devidas M, Gebhardt MC, Ayala AC, Harris MB, et al.: Presurgical chemotherapy compared with immediate surgery and adjuvant chemotherapy for nonmetastatic osteosarcoma: pediatric oncology group study pog-8651, *J Clin Oncol* 21:1574–1580, 2003.

37. Gorlick R, Bielack S, Teot L, et al.: Osteosarcoma: biology, diagnosis, treatment, and remaining challenges. In Pizzo PA, Poplack DG, editors: *Principles and practice of pediatric oncology*, Philadelphia, 2011, Lippincott Williams Wilkins, pp 1015–1044.

38. Grimer RJ, Carter SR, Pynsent PB: Cost-effectiveness of limb salvage for bone tumors, *J Bone Joint Surg Br* 79:558–561, 1997.

39. Gupta AA, Pappo A, Saunders N, Hopyan S, Ferguson P, Wunder J, et al.: Clinical outcome of children and adults with localized Ewing sarcoma, *Cancer* 3189–3194, 2010.

40. Gupta SK, Alassaf A, Harrop AR, Kiefer GN: Principles of rotationplasty, *J Am Acad Orthop Surg* (20):657–667, 2012.

41. Haduong JH, Martin AA, Skapek SX, Mascarenhas L: Sarcomas, *Pediatr Clin N Am* 62:179–200, 2015.

42. Reference deleted in proofs.

43. Hawkins DS, Bolling T, Dubois S, et al.: Ewing sarcoma. In Pizzo PA, Poplack DG, editors: *Principles and practice of pediatric oncology*, Philadelphia, 2011, Lippincott Williams Wilkins, pp 987–1014.

44. Heare T, Hensley MA, Dell'Orfano S: Bone tumors: osteosarcoma and Ewing's sarcoma, *Curr Opin Pediatr* 21:365–372, 2009.

45. Herring JA: Growth and development. In Herring JA, editor: *Tachdjian's pediatric orthopedics*, ed 3, Philadelphia, 2002, WB Saunders, pp 3–21.

46. Herring JA: Limb deficiencies. In Herring JA, editor: *Tachdjian's pediatric orthopedics*, ed 3, Philadelphia, 2002, WB Saunders, pp 1745–1810.

47. Hobusch GM, Lang N, Schuh R, Windhager R, Hofstaetter JG: Do patients with Ewing's sarcoma continue with sports activities after limb salvage surgery of the lower extremity? *Clin Orthop Rel Res* 473:839–846, 2015.

48. Hostetler SG, Schwartz L, Shields BJ, Xiang H, Smith GA: Characteristics of pediatric traumatic amputations treated in hospital emergency departments: United States, 1990-2002, *Pediatrics* 116:667–674, 2005.

49. Reference deleted in proofs.

50. James MA, Bagley AM, Brasington K, Lutz C, McConnell S, Molitor F: Impact of prostheses on function and quality of life for children with unilateral congenital below-the-elbow deficiency, *J Bone Joint Surg Am* 88:2356–2365, 2006.

51. Krajbich JI, Bochmann D: Van Nes rotation-plasty in tumor surgery. In Bowker JH, Michael JW, editors: *Atlas of limb prosthetics: surgical, prosthetic, and rehabilitation principles*, ed 2, St. Louis, 1992, Mosby, pp 885–899.

52. Krajbich JL: Rotationplasty in the management of proximal femoral focal deficiency. In Herring JA, Birch JG, editors: *The child with a limb deficiency*, Rosemont, IL, 1998, American Academy of Orthopedic Surgeons, p 87.

53. Kun LE: General principles of radiation oncology. In Pizzo PA, Poplack DG, editors: *Principles and practice of pediatric oncology*, Philadelphia, 2011, Lippincott Williams Wilkins, pp 406–425.

54. Lang N, Hobusch GM, Funovics PT, Windhager R, Hofstaetter JG: What sports activity levels are achieved in patients with modular tumor endoprostheses of osteosarcoma about the knee? *Clin Orthop Rel Res* 473:847–854, 2015.

55. Le JT, Scott-Weyward PR: Pediatric limb deficiencies and amputations, *Phys Med Rehabil Clin N Am* 26:95–108, 2015.

56. Loder RT: Demographics of traumatic amputations in children, *J Bone Joint Surg Am* 86:923–928, 2004.

57. Marchese VG, Rai SN, Carlson CA, Hinds PS, Spearing EM, Zhang L, et al.: Assessing functional mobility in survivors of lower-extremity sarcoma: reliability and validity of a new assessment tool, *Pediatr Blood Cancer* 49:183–189, 2007.

58. Marchese VG, Spearing E, Callaway L, Rai SN, Zhang L, Hinds PS, et al.: Relationships among range of motion, functional mobility, and quality of life in children and adolescents after limb-sparing surgery for lower-extremity sarcoma, *Peditr Phys Ther* 18:238–244, 2006.

59. Mason GE, Aung L, Gall S, Meyers PA, Butler R, Krug S, et al.: Quality of life following amputation or limb preservation in patients with lower extremity bone sarcoma, *Front Oncol* 3:1–6, 2013.

60. McGuirk CK, Westgate MN, Holmes LB: Limb deficiencies in the newborn infants, *Pediatrics* 108:E64, 2001.

61. Melzack R, Israel R, Lacroix R, Schultz G: Phantom limbs in people with congenital deficiency or amputation in early childhood, *Brain* 120:1603–1620, 1997.

62. Morrissy RT, Giavedoni BJ, Coulter-O'Berry C: The limb-deficient child. In Morrissy RT, Weinstein SL, editors: *Lovell Winter pediatric orthopedics*, ed 6, Philadelphia, 2006, Lippincott Williams Wilkins, pp 1333–1382.

63. Nagarajan R, Neglia JP, Clohisy DR, Yasui Y, Greenberg M, Hudson M, et al.: Education, employment, insurance, and marital status among 694 survivors of pediatric lower extremity bone tumors, *Cancer* 97:2554–2564, 2003.

64. Nagarajan R, Clohisy DR, Neglia JP, Yasui Y, Mitby PA, Sklar C, et al.: Function and quality-of-life of survivors of pelvic and lower extremity osteosarcoma and Ewing's sarcoma: the childhood cancer survivor study, *Br J Cancer* 91(11):1858–1865, 2004.

65. Neel MD, Wilkins RM, Rao BN, Kelly CM: Early multicenter experience with a noninvasive expandable prosthesis, *Clin Orthop Rel Res* 415:72–81, 2003.

66. Ness KK, Hudson MM, Ginsberg JP, Nagarajan R, Kaste SC, Marina N, et al.: Physical performance limitations in the childhood cancer survivor study cohort, *J Clin Oncol* 27:2382–2389, 2009.

67. Ness KK, Neel MD, Kaste SC, Billips CA, Marchese VG, Rao BN, Daw NC: A comparison of function after limb salvage with non-invasive expandable or modular prostheses in children, *Eur J Cancer* 50:3212–3220, 2014.

68. Oppenheim WL, Setoguchi Y, Fowler E: Overview and comparison of Syme amputation and knee fusion with the Van Nesrotationplasty in proximal femoral focal deficiency. In Herring JA, Birch JG, editors: *The child with a limb deficiency*, Rosemont, IL, 1998, American Academy of Orthopedic Surgeons, pp 73–86.

69. Reference deleted in proofs.

70. Pardasaney PK, Sullivan PE, Portney LG, Mankin HJ: Advantage of limb salvage over amputation in proximal lower extremity tumors, *Clin Orthop Rel Res* 444:201–208, 2006.

71. Parente MA, Geil M: In the future: surgical and educational advances and challenges. In Carroll K, Edelstein JE, editors: *Prosthetics and patient management: a comprehensive clinical approach*, Thorofare, NJ, 2006, Slack Publishing, pp 233–241.

72. Patton JG: Occupational therapy. In Smith DG, Michael JW, Bowker JH, editors: *Atlas of limb amputations and limb deficiencies*, ed 3, Rosemont, IL, 2004, American Academy of Orthopedic Surgeons, pp 813–830.

73. Pruitt SD, Varni JW, Setoguchi Y: Functional status in children with limb deficiency: development and initial validation of an outcome measure, *Arch Phys Med Rehabil* 77:1233–1238, 1996.

74. Pruitt SD, Varni JW, Seid M, Setoguchi Y: Functional status in limb deficiency: development of an outcome measure for preschool children, *Arch Phys Med Rehail* 79:405–411, 1998.

75. Pruitt SD, Seid M, Varni JW, Setoguchi Y: Toddlers with limb deficiency: conceptual basis and initial application of a functional status outcome measure, *Arch Phys Med Rehabil* 80:819–824, 1999.

76. Radocy R: Prosthetic adaptations in competitive sports and recreation. In Smith DG, Michael JW, Bowker JH, editors: *Atlas of limb amputations and limb deficiencies*, ed 3, Rosemont, IL, 2004, American Academy of Orthopedic Surgeons, pp 327–338.

77. Rothgangel A, Braun S, deWitte L, Beurskens A, Smeets R: Development of a clinical framework for mirror therapy in patients with phantom limb pain: an evidence-based practice approach, *Pain Pract* 16:1–13, 2015.

78. Reference deleted in proofs.

79. Robinson KP, Branemark R, Ward DA: Future developments: osseointegration in transfemoral amputees. In Smith DG, Michael JW, Bowker JH, editors: *Atlas of limb amputations and limb deficiencies*, ed 3, Rosemont, IL, 2004, American Academy of Orthopedic Surgeons, pp 841–852.

80. Robitaille J, Carmichael SL, Shaw GM, Olney RS: Maternal nutrient intake and risks for transverse and longitudinal limb deficiencies: data from the national birth defects prevention study, 1997-2003, *Birth Defects Res A Clin Mol Teratol* 85:773–779, 2009.

81. Rougraff BT, Simon MA, Kneisel JS: Limb salvage compared with amputation for osteosarcoma of the distal end of the femur: a long-term oncological, functional and quality of life study, *J Bone Joint Surg Am* 163:1171–1175, 1994.

82. Sammer DM, Chung KC: Congenital hand differences: embryology and classification, *Hand Clin* 25:151–156, 2009.

83. Shaperman J, Landsberger SE, Setoguchi Y: Early upper extremity prosthesis fitting: when and what do we fit, *J Prosthet Orthot* 15:11–17, 2003.

84. Shimizu H, Yokoyama S, Asahara H: Growth and differentiation of the developing limb bud from the perspective of chondrogenesis, *Dev Growth Differ* 49:449–454, 2007.

85. Soldado F, Kozin SH: Bony overgrowth in children after amputation, *J Pediatr Rehabil Med* 2:235–239, 2009.

86. Sparreboom A, Evans WE, Baker SD: Chemotherapy in the pediatric patient. In Orkin SH, Fisher DE, Look AT, et al, editors: *Oncology of infancy childhood*, Philadelphia, 2007, Saunders Elsevier, pp 175–207.

87. Squitieri L, Reichert H, Kim HM, Steggerda J, Chung KC: Patterns of surgical care and health disparities of treating finger amputation injuries in the United States, *J Am Coll Surg* 213:475–485, 2011.

88. Reference deleted in proofs.

89. Reference deleted in proofs.

90. Sutherland DH: *Gait disorders in childhood and adolescence*, Baltimore, 1984, Williams Wilkins, pp 14–27.

91. Swanson AB, Barsky AJ, Entin MA: Classification of limb malformations on the basis of embryological failures, *Surg Clin N Am* 48:1169–1179, 1968.

92. Tebbi CK: Psychological effects of amputation in sarcoma. In Humphrey GB, Koops HS, Molenaar WM, Postma A, editors: *Osteosarcoma in adolescents and young adults*, Boston, 1993, Kluwer Academic, pp 39–44.

93. Varni JW, Setoguchi Y: Screening for behavioral and emotional problems in children and adolescents with congenital or acquired limb deficiencies, *Am J Dis Child* 146:103–107, 1992.

94. Wilkins RM, Soubeiran A: The Phoenix expandable prosthesis: early American experience, *Clin Orthop Rel Res* 382:51–58, 2001.

SUGGESTED READINGS

Background

Gold NB, Westgate MN, Holmes LB: Anatomic and etiological classification of congenital limb deficiencies, *Am J Med Genet A* 155A:1225–1235, 2011.

Haduong JH, Martin AA, Skapek SX, Mascarenhas L: Sarcomas. *Pediatr Clin N Am* 62:179–200, 2015.

Hawkins DS, Bolling T, Dubois S, et al.: Ewing sarcoma. In Pizzo PA, Poplack DG, editors: *Principles and practice of pediatric oncology*, Philadelphia, 2011, Lippincott Williams Wilkins, pp 987–1014.

Isakaff MS, Bielack SS, Meltzer P, Gorlick R: Osteosarcoma: current treatment and a collaborative pathway to success, *J Clin Oncol* 33:3029–3036, 2015.

Sammer DM, Chung KC: Congenital hand differences: embryology and classification, *Hand Clin* 25:151–156, 2009.

Foreground

Geil MD, Coulter CP: Analysis of locomotor adaptations in young children with limb loss in an early knee prescription protocol, *Prosthet Orthot Int* 38(1):54–56, 2014.

Gupta SK, Alassaf A, Harrop AR, Kiefer GN: Principles of rotationplasty, *J Am Acad Orthop Surg* 20:657–667, 2012.

James MA, Bagley AM, Brasington K, Lutz C, McConnell S, Molitor F: Impact of prostheses on function and quality of life for children with unilateral congenital below-the-elbow deficiency, *J Bone Joint Surg Am* 88:2356–2365, 2006.

Lang N, Hobusch GM, Funovics PT, Windhager R, Hofstaetter JG: What sports activity levels are achieved in patients with modular tumor endoprostheses of osteosarcoma about the knee? *Clin Orthop Rel Res* 473:847–854, 2015.

Le JT, Scott-Weyward PR: Pediatric limb deficiencies and amputations, *Phys Med Rehabil Clin N Am* 26:95–108, 2015.

Marchese VG, Rai SN, Carlson CA, Hinds PS, Spearing EM, Zhang L, et al.: Assessing functional mobility in survivors of lower-extremity sarcoma: reliability and validity of a new assessment tool, *Pediatr Blood Cancer* 49:183–189, 2007.

Ness KK, Neel MD, Kaste SC, Billips CA, Marchese VG, Rao BN, Daw NC: A comparison of function after limb salvage with non-invasive expandable or modular prostheses in children, *Eur J Cancer* 50:3212–3220, 2014.

Ottaviani G, Robert RS, Huh WW, PallaS Jaffe N: Sociooccupational and physical outcomes more than 20 years after the diagnosis of osteosarcoma in children and adolescents, *Cancer* 119:3727–3736, 2013.

Stokke J, Sung L, Gupta A, Lindberg A, Rosenberg AR: Systematic review and meta-analysis of objective and subjective quality of life among pediatric, adolescent, and young adult bone tumor survivors, *Pediatr Blood Cancer* (62):1616–1629, 2015.

14

Orthopedic Conditions

Mary Wills Jesse

Physical therapists working with the pediatric population may not frequently intervene with patients with primary orthopedic diagnosis; however, general knowledge of orthopedics is important throughout the intervention process. This becomes even more challenging in the pediatric population as the musculoskeletal system grows and changes with age. What may be considered "typical" at one age may be significantly atypical at another.

Additionally, as physical therapist practice becomes more autonomous, we are challenged to identify problems that may be outside the scope of our practice and make appropriate referrals for care. We have a responsibility as therapists to have the knowledge base to determine these conditions in children.

Space in this chapter will not allow an exhaustive review of all the orthopedic conditions that affect children. Many references are provided throughout the text for further study, however. This chapter presents information on conditions commonly seen; specific areas of concern to the physical therapist will be highlighted to provide a basic framework for the practicing clinician. Background and foreground information will be presented together in each of the following condition-specific sections.

TORSIONAL CONDITIONS (IN-TOEING AND OUT-TOEING)

In-toeing and out-toeing are visible conditions in children that often raise much concern for parents and family members. They are also a common reason for elective referral of a child to an orthopedist. Even though these rotational conditions usually do not require any intervention, concern often escalates with comments from neighbors, teachers, and strangers on the street: "Why does your child walk funny?" This group of children has been described by Dr. Mercer Rang as "the worried well," a phrase that indicates the strong concern of the family and others involved with the child over alignment conditions that are often part of the spectrum of normal musculoskeletal development.

Differing opinions exist on how to define torsional conditions, how to measure them, and especially how to intervene for correction, or if they should receive intervention at all. An understanding of the normal growth and development of the lower extremity is imperative in evaluating a child's rotational alignment as normal changes occur during the growth process. Further description of the normal process may be found in Chapter 5. Interventions, such as orthotic shoes, casting, and bracing, have previously been used in early childhood without success and in many of these cases, unnecessarily because the child's positioning would have corrected spontaneously over time. Often, rotational deformities are seen in typically developing children and rarely persist into adolescence. Knowledge of normal growth and development will assist therapists in making better clinical judgments as well as educating parents and family members of whether there is a need for concern. Education should also be given to the caregivers about the normal changes in alignment to help them monitor the child for changes that are occurring abnormally. As always, neuromuscular dysfunctions or other serious conditions should be ruled out.

In-toeing and out-toeing are both clinical symptoms and do not define the etiology or provide a diagnosis of the underlying problem. By definition, in-toeing is a rotational variation of the lower extremity alignment where the feet or toes point toward the midline during gait. Out-toeing is a rotational variation of the lower extremity alignment where the feet or toes point away from the midline during gait. Through clinical history and physical evaluation, the cause of the rotation can be determined.

Clinical History

A specific history provides a wealth of information regarding possible causative factors and indications for possible intervention. Specific information obtained may also direct the examiner to expand the examination to rule out other, more severe conditions that may initially produce a chief complaint of in-toeing or out-toeing. Relevant information to be elicited from the parents includes the following:

1. Birth history. Was the infant full-term or premature? Was it a vaginal or cesarean delivery? Was oligohydramnios (deficiency of amniotic fluid) present? How many times has the mother been pregnant? What is the birth order of the parent? Many of the torsional problems seen in infants are "packaging" defects (i.e., caused by a restricted intrauterine environment). It is easy to imagine that an infant's lower limbs may "grow" into a particular position as one visualizes a full-term 9-pound fetus in the womb of a gravida 1, para 1 mother.
2. Age. At what age was the in-toeing or out-toeing noted? Has it improved or worsened since first noted? Was any previous intervention provided? For the walking child, at what age did the child start to walk independently? In the differential diagnosis the index of suspicion should be increased when a child has a history or prematurity, difficult birth, or delayed motor milestones or has significant in-toeing or out-toeing that is worsening with time or is very asymmetrical. Children with mild spastic diplegia may have in-toeing, and children with Duchenne muscular dystrophy may have out-toeing and flat feet. Conditions such as these must be ruled out.

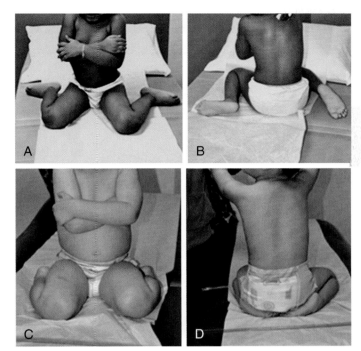

FIG. 14.1 (A–E) The W-sitting or television-sitting position with the legs externally rotated. (C–D) A similar position with the feet tucked under the buttocks accentuating the internal tibial torsion as well as metatarsus adductus. (From Harris E: The intoeing child: etiology, prognosis, and current treatment options. *Clin Podiatr Med Surg* 30:531-65, 2013.)

3. Family history. In many cases, a positive family history for in-toeing or out-toeing is reported, and this should be noted, especially if intervention was undertaken for other family member(s).
4. Sleeping and sitting positions. The natural positions that a child lies and sits also provide information. Sleeping prone and sitting on feet encourages internal tibial torsion.[186] Sitting in a W-sit position may encourage the persistence of femoral anteversion (Fig. 14.1).

Torsional Profile

The torsional profile is a composite of measurements of the lower extremities.[202] It differentiates thigh, leg, and foot variations as the anatomic basis of torsional deformity. It also documents the severity of the abnormality. Each segment needs to be evaluated to determine the cause of the abnormality so that intervention can be appropriately prescribed. Rotational alignment of the lower extremity is determined by the alignment of the foot, the rotation of the tibia in relation to the transcondylar axis of the femur (tibial torsion), and the rotation of the neck of the femur in relation to the transcondylar axis of the femur (femoral version). The examination usually begins with clinical observation of the child's gait pattern and progresses to evaluation from proximal to distal body segments.[42] The torsional profile generally consists of six measurements with normative data available for the first five variables. These are: foot progression angle (FPA), lateral hip rotation (LHR), medial hip rotation (MHR), thigh-foot angle (TFA), transmalleolar axis (TMA), and forefoot alignment. Also added to this description are trochanteric prominence angle test as an alternate way to

examine femoral version and flexibility of forefoot to determine the rigidity of the position. Table 14.1 gives a description of these components and the method of measuring each.

Foot Progression Angle

The FPA, or "the angle of gait," is defined as the angular difference between the axis of the foot and the line of progression during gait.[201] The child is observed while walking, and a value is assigned to the angle of both the right and the left foot. This is a subjective determination and represents an average of the angle noted on multiple steps. Various footprint techniques can be used to measure FPA, but these are time consuming and may not be practical in the clinical situation. In-toeing is expressed as a negative value, and out-toeing is expressed as a positive value. This angle gives an overall view of the degree of in-toeing of out-toeing in the walking child. The FPA can also be examined in supported stance for the child who is not yet walking independently. FPA is variable during infancy. During childhood and adult life, it shows little change, with a mean of +10° and a normal range of −3° to +20°.[202] In-toeing of −5° to −10° is considered mild, −10° to −15° is considered moderate, and more than −15° is considered severe.[201] When a child toes in or toes out, the condition is usually bilateral, but occasionally one sees "windswept" lower extremities, with one limb toeing in and the other limb toeing out. Normative values can be found in Fig. 14.2.

Although this gives a composite view of the lower extremity, measurement of each segment is recommended because compensations may occur that affect the FPA. For example, significant femoral anteversion at the hip may be balanced by external tibial torsion with a straight foot (no metatarsus adductus or calcaneovalgus). The foot progression angle would be 0°/0° (right/left) with the feet pointing straight ahead even though abnormalities are present.

Hip Rotation

In order to correctly explain clinical findings at the hip, terminology in the literature should be understood. Version describes the position of the femoral head in the frontal plane. If the head lies anterior to the plane, it is anteverted, with the average angle being 14° to 20°.[34] A head that is positioned posterior to this normal average angle is retroverted.[34] Torsion describes the osseous position of the bone in its longitudinal axis, or "twist." It is measured by the angle formed at the intersection of the axis of the head and neck and the axis of the femoral condyles.[34] The difference could also be explained by femoral torsion being the osseous "twist" between the upper femur and lower femur and femoral version being the momentary position of the femur in the acetabulum or the relative position of the acetabulum on the pelvis.[77] The measurement of hip internal and external rotation will include both torsion between the femoral head and femur and also the inclination of the femoral head to the acetabulum (version).[113] Fig. 14.3 demonstrates these differences.

Hip rotation range of motion (ROM) is measured most accurately in the prone position, with the hip in a position of neutral flexion/extension and knee flexed to 90°. Femoral anteversion will be indicated by an increase in internal rotation compared to external rotation. If the differences between internal and external rotation measurements are 45° or more, this indicates an abnormally high anteversion angle at the hip.[73] Femoral retroversion is indicated by increased external rotation compared to very little internal rotation. An

TABLE 14.1   Measurements for Torsional Profile

Measurement	Technique	Documentation	Visual
Foot progression angle	Child is observed while walking with subjective determination of in-toeing and out-toeing Footprint technique can be used to measure	In-toeing is expressed as negative value and out-toeing is expressed as positive value	
Femoral Version Hip rotation ROM	Child in prone position with the hip in a position of neutral flexion/extension and knee flexed to 90°	Femoral anteversion indicated by an increase in internal rotation compared to external rotation	
Trochanteric prominence angle test	Child lies prone with knees flexed to 90° Examiner stands on the contralateral side and uses the left hand to palpate the greater trochanter while the right hand internally rotates the hip At point of maximum trochanter prominence, the femoral neck is horizontal	If the tibia is externally rotated, this corresponds to an antetorsion value If the tibia is internally rotated, it corresponds to a retrotorsion value	
Tibial Torsion Thigh-foot angle	Child prone with knees flexed to 90° Measure the angle of the long axis of the foot against the axis of the thigh	If line of the heel points toward the midline relative to the thigh, an internal torsion is present and is given a negative value If line of the heel points away from the midline relative to the thigh, external torsion is present and is given a positive value	
Transmalleolar angle: prone	Child prone with knees flexed to 90° Measure the angle of the line that bisects the malleoli against the axis of the thigh	Measurement is the angular difference between a line projected toward the heel at right angles to the transmalleolar axis and the axis of the thigh Positive value is external torsion	

Continued

TABLE 14.1	**Measurements for Torsional Profile—cont'd**		
Measurement	**Technique**	**Documentation**	**Visual**
Transmalleolar angle: sitting	Patient seated with knee flexed and leg hanging from the edge of the table with the thigh directly in front of the hip joint and heel against vertical surface Measurements are made from each malleolus to the back wall Measurement is also made of the width of the ankle (intermalleolar distance)	Internal tibial torsion is present if the medial malleolus is level with or posterior to the lateral malleolus Use grid established by Staheli and Engel to determine the transmalleolar axis angle	

Foot Alignment	**Technique**	**Measurements**	**Visual**
Heel bisector method	Child prone with knees flexed to 90° with plantar surface of foot parallel to the ceiling Line is visually drawn to bisect the heel	Normal: heel bisector line through second and third webspace Mild MTA: heel bisector line through third toe Moderate MTA: heel bisector line through third and fourth toe webspace Severe MTA: heel bisector line through fourth and fifth toe webspace	 Normal Valgus Mild Moderate Severe
Flexibility of forefoot	Lateral force is applied to the great toe attempting to reduce the heel bisector line back to the second toe (arrow shows hand position for evaluation)	Determines flexibility of deformity with more rigid feet sometimes needing corrective treatment	

MTA, metatarsus adductus; *ROM*, range of motion.

Foot progression angle. Redrawn from Kliegman RM, editor: *Practical strategies in pediatric diagnosis and therapy.* Philadelphia, Saunders, 2004.
Hip rotation ROM. From Kliegman RM, editor: *Practical strategies in pediatric diagnosis and therapy.* Philadelphia, Saunders, 2004.
Trochanteric prominence angle test. From Harris E: The intoeing child: etiology, prognosis, and current treatment options. *Clin Podiatr Med Surg* 30:531-565, 2013.
Thigh-foot angle. From Smith BG: Lower extremity disorders in children and adolescents. *Pediatr Rev* 30:287-294, 2009.
Transmalleolar angle: prone. From Kwon OY, Tuttle LJ, Commean PK, et al.: Reliability and validity of measures of hammer toe deformity angle and tibial torsion. *Foot (Edinb)* 19:149-155, 2009.
Heel bisector method. From Jones S, Khandekar S, Tolessa E: Normal variants of the lower limbs in pediatric orthopedics. *Int J of Clin Med* 4:12-17, 2013.
Flexibility of forefoot. From Rosenfeld SB: Approach to the child with in-toeing. In: UpToDate, Phillips W (Section Ed),Torchia MM (Deputy Ed), UpToDate, Waltham, MA (http://www.uptodate.com/contents/approach-to-the-child-with-in-toeing?source=machineLearning&search=phillips+W%2C+Torchina+MM+in-toeing&selectedTitle=2%7E150&section-Rank=1&anchor=H21546646#H21546681 Accessed on January 7, 2016).

abnormally low anteversion angle would be indicated by the external rotation being at least 50° higher than the internal rotation measurement.[73] This is not an accurate test in children below 3 years of age because of the limitation in internal rotation by factors extrinsic to the hip joint.[73] Normative values can be found in Figs. 14.4 to 14.6.

Another way to clinically examine femoral neck anteversion is the trochanteric prominence angle test (TPAT).[180] This test is also known as the Ryder test or the Craig test. A child lies prone. The examiner stands on the contralateral side and uses the left hand to palpate the greater trochanter while the right hand internally rotates the hip, with the patient's knee flexed to 90°. At the point of maximum trochanter prominence, the femoral neck is assumed to be horizontal. If the tibia is externally rotated, this corresponds to an antetorsion value; if it is internally rotated, it corresponds to a retrotorsion value. Reliability of this method has been questioned.[135,234]

When the hip is in anteversion (or "anteverted") because of the femoral head being positioned on the frontal plane, the

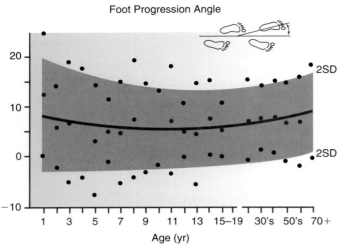

FIG. 14.2 Foot progression angle. Mean values, plus or minus two standard deviations for each of the 22 age groups. The solid lines show the mean changes with age; the shaded areas, the normal ranges; the solid blue circles, the mean measurements for the different age groups; and the solid black circles, plus or minus two standard deviations for the same mean measurements. (Redrawn from Staheli LT, Corbett M, Wyss C, et al.: Lower-extremity rotational problems in children. Normal values to guide management. *J Bone Joint Surg Am* 67:39-47, 1985.)

patient will usually have more hip medial rotation than lateral rotation ROM, assuming no soft tissue tightness. If hip medial rotation is measured at 70° and lateral rotation is 25°, for example, the child is said to have femoral anteversion (FA) and may in-toe when walking (Fig. 14.7). In retroversion the femoral head is positioned posterior to the frontal plane when the knee is aligned straight ahead, and the patient will have greater lateral rotation range. These describe positions in the child who matures without neurologic disorders such as cerebral palsy. The neonatal biomechanics and typical skeletal maturational changes in the child are presented in greater detail in Chapter 5.

Thigh-Foot Angle

The TFA, transmalleolar angle, and FPA are methods used to measure tibial torsion. The TFA is evaluated by placing the child prone, flexing the knee to 90°, and then measuring the angle of the long axis of the foot against the axis of the thigh.[113,201] If the line of the heel points toward the midline relative to the thigh, an internal torsion is present and is given a negative value. If the line of the heel points away from the midline relative to the thigh, external torsion is present and is given a positive value.[201] Changes in these values occur normally with development; from the middle of childhood on, the mean angle remains approximately 10°.[202] Normative values are shown in Fig. 14.8.

Transmalleolar Axis

The transmalleolar angle may be preferred over the thigh-foot angle because hindfoot varus or valgus and foot adduction or abduction will not affect results.[101] The TMA-thigh angle can be measured in the same position as the thigh-foot angle. Measurement is made between the angle of the line bisecting the thigh and the line that bisects the malleoli on the plantar surface of the foot. Normative values are in Fig. 14.9.

Another method for the TMA has the patient seated with knee flexed and leg hanging from the edge of the table with the thigh directly in front of the hip joint and heels against a flat vertical surface.[203] With the foot held in neutral position, the medial malleolus is held between the thumb and index finger and the center point is marked. The lateral malleolus is marked in a similar manner. With the heel resting comfortably against the back wall of the platform, measurements are made of the distance between the marks over the medial malleolus and the back wall (A) and the distance between the marks over the lateral malleolus and the back wall (B). The difference between these two measurements is then calculated (A−B). The inter-malleolar distance is measured (width of the ankle between malleoli). Using the grid established by Staheli and Engel, the TMA can be established.[203] This method demonstrates that the TMA angle averages about 5° of external rotation during the first year, 10° during midchildhood and 14° in older children and adults.[203] Normative data and a conversion grid can be found in Figs. 14.10 and 14.11.

Others have measured the TMA by the footprint method. In this test the patient sits with his hip and knee at 90° of flexion with the hip in neutral rotation and the tibial tubercle facing forward. The foot is set on a piece of lined paper so that the lines are parallel to the knee axis. The footprint is traced, and two marks are made vertically below the centers of the malleoli. A line drawn between this line and any line on the paper will provide the TMA.[80]

Foot Alignment

Foot alignment is best documented using the Bleck heel bisector method.[38] The heel bisector line is measured with the child prone with the knee flexed and ankle dorsiflexed so that the plantar surface of the foot is parallel to the ceiling. A line is visualized parallel to the heel and extended distally to the toes. A normal heel bisector line goes through the second toe. The line passes more laterally in those with metatarsus adductus (medial deviation of the forefoot). Also, flexibility of the foot position should be determined by applying lateral force to the great toe and attempting to reduce the heel bisector line back to the second toe. The degree of metatarsus adductus can be graded as (I) flexible with the ability to correct beyond midline, (II) moderately flexible with the ability to correct to midline, or (III) severe with the inability to achieve midline.[18]

Radiographs may be used to evaluate the position of the foot but are not considered imperative and, in some cases, are difficult to reproduce.[95] The age and flexibility of the deformity are considered better predictors of outcome although the radiologic examination may help determine the presence of complex deformities or the presence of rearfoot compensation.[95]

In-Toeing

Although in-toeing is a common problem that causes parents to seek medical care, very few require medical intervention. A study of 202 children who were referred to a pediatric orthopedic clinic found that none of these children (median age of 4 years) had significant pathology.[17] Another study of 720 children below the age of 8 years referred for in-toeing found only one required an osteotomy.[110] The components that may contribute to in-toeing are femoral anteversion, internal tibial torsion, and metatarsus adductus (Table 14.2).

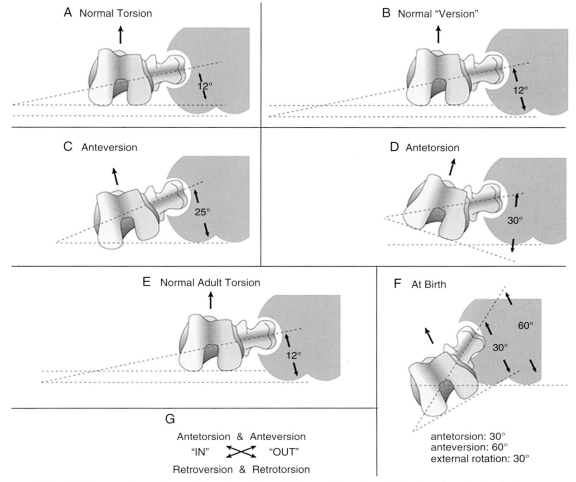

A Normal Torsion	B Normal "Version"
12°	12°
C Anteversion	D Antetorsion
25°	30°
E Normal Adult Torsion	F At Birth
12°	60° / 30°

G

Antetorsion & Anteversion
"IN" ✕ "OUT"
Retroversion & Retrotorsion

antetorsion: 30°
anteversion: 60°
external rotation: 30°

FIG. 14.3 Femoral version and torsion. (From Effgen SK, editor: *Meeting the physical therapy needs of children.* Philadelphia, FA Davis, 2005.)

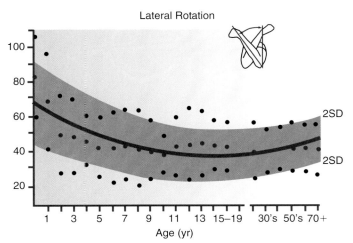

Lateral Rotation

FIG. 14.4 Lateral rotation of the hip in male and female subjects combined. Mean values, plus or minus two standard deviations for each of the 22 age groups. The solid lines show the mean changes with age; the shaded areas, the normal ranges; the solid blue circles, the mean measurements for the different age groups; and the solid black circles, plus or minus two standard deviations for the same mean measurements. (Redrawn from Staheli LT, Corbett M, Wyss C, et al.: Lower-extremity rotational problems in children. Normal values to guide management. *J Bone Joint Surg Am* 67:39-47, 1985.)

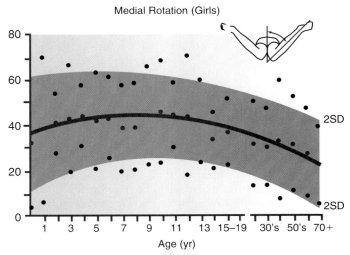

Medial Rotation (Girls)

FIG. 14.5 Medial rotation of the hip in female subjects. Mean values, plus or minus two standard deviations for each of the 22 age groups. The solid lines show the mean changes with age; the shaded areas, the normal ranges; the solid blue circles, the mean measurements for the different age groups; and the solid black circles, plus or minus two standard deviations for the same mean measurements. (Redrawn from Staheli LT, Corbett M, Wyss C, et al.: Lower-extremity rotational problems in children. Normal values to guide management. *J Bone Joint Surg Am* 67:39-47, 1985.)

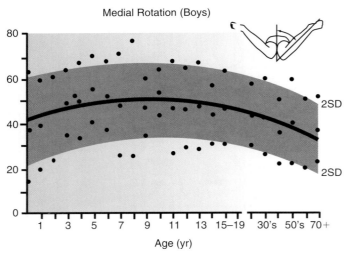

FIG. 14.6 Medial rotation of the hip in male subjects. Mean values, plus or minus two standard deviations for each of the 22 age groups. The solid lines show the mean changes with age; the shaded areas, the normal ranges; the solid blue circles, the mean measurements for the different age groups; and the solid black circles, plus or minus two standard deviations for the same mean measurements. (Redrawn from Staheli LT, Corbett M, Wyss C, et al.: Lower-extremity rotational problems in children. Normal values to guide management. *J Bone Joint Surg Am* 67:39-47, 1985.)

Femoral Antetorsion and Anteversion

One specific cause of in-toeing is FA. Although most of these cases will normalize spontaneously by age 8 years,[70] some cases require medical attention. Neurologically typical children are likely to spontaneously correct while those with neurologic abnormalities have a lower incidence of spontaneous correction.[77] Abnormal antetorsion is more frequently seen in females and also has been found to possibly have a genetic component because it seems to run in some families.[77]

The history of the onset is generally an observation of the child's gait being normal until age 2 years. At that time the family notices the in-toeing. This observation would go along with the changes occurring in the child's gait; hip rotation in extension is changing from relative external rotation to internal rotation, which allows the abnormal FA to be noticed.[77] The child also favors the W-sitting position as seen in Fig. 14.1.

Measurement of the abnormality will be achieved through completion of the torsional profile. Internal rotation measuring between 70° and 90° is evidence of femoral torsion.[174] In an infant, tightness in the hip external rotation muscles and capsular ligaments results in a laterally rotated position, masking the femoral anteversion. The tightness of the hip soft tissues gradually stretches out, and the true anteversion of the femur becomes apparent. This process is often described incorrectly as "femoral anteversion increases"; the amount of femoral version is actually decreasing but is more easily visualized because the muscle tightness of the external rotators is decreasing. The FA becomes increasingly more apparent clinically as the child approaches 5 to 6 years of age, with this decrease in soft tissue tightness. Studies have shown a gradual decrease in FA with age: 40° at birth to between 15° and 20° by 8 to 10 years of age.[222] Femoral antetorsion is mild if internal hip rotation is 70° to 80°, moderate if 80° to 90°, and severe if 90° plus in childhood.[201] By midchildhood, the femoral head and neck have

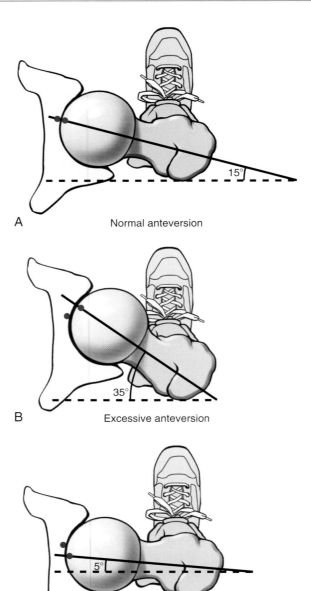

FIG. 14.7 In the femur, version is the angular difference between the transcondylar axis of the knee (the horizontal line in this drawing) and the axis of the femoral neck. These two lines form an angle and document whether the femur is in anteversion or retroversion. (A) Normal anteversion: with this small amount of anteversion, the individual can walk comfortably with the foot pointed straight ahead (i.e., a neutral angle of foot progression). (B) Excessive anteversion with in-toeing: when a large amount of anteversion is present, the individual must internally rotate the femur to seat the femoral head in the acetabulum and achieve improved joint congruity. This results in a negative foot progression angle, and the foot is pointed in during gait (in-toeing). (C) Retroversion: in this drawing, significant reduction can be seen in the angle formed between the two axes, depicting retroversion. If this were excessive, the individual would need to externally rotate the femur to seat the femoral head in the acetabulum and would have a positive angle of foot progression (out-toeing). (From Neumann DA: *Kinesiology of the musculoskeletal system: foundations in rehabilitation.* 2nd ed. St. Louis, Mosby; 2010.)

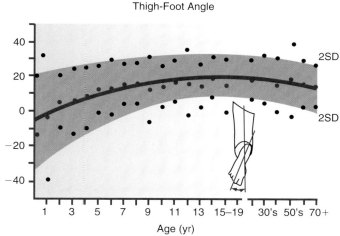

FIG. 14.8 Thigh-foot angle. Mean values, plus or minus two standard deviations for each of the 22 age groups. The solid lines show the mean changes with age; the shaded areas, the normal ranges; the solid blue circles, the mean measurements for the different age groups; and the solid black circles, plus or minus two standard deviations for the same mean measurements. (Redrawn from Staheli LT, Corbett M, Wyss C, et al.: Lower-extremity rotational problems in children. Normal values to guide management. *J Bone Joint Surg Am* 67:39-47, 1985.)

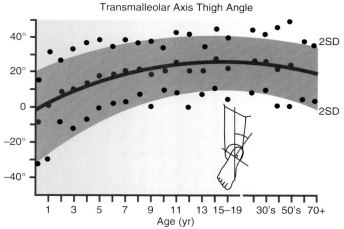

FIG. 14.9 Transmalleolar axis thigh angle. Mean values, plus or minus two standard deviations for each of the 22 age groups. The solid lines show the mean changes with age; the shaded areas, the normal ranges; the solid blue circles, the mean measurements for the different age groups; and the solid black circles, plus or minus two standard deviations for the same mean measurements. (Redrawn from Staheli LT, Corbett M, Wyss C, et al.: Lower-extremity rotational problems in children. Normal values to guide management. *J Bone Joint Surg Am* 67:39-47, 1985.)

usually assumed a relatively more neutral position in relationship to the femoral shaft, and children typically have approximately equal amounts of hip medial and lateral rotation. Clinical measurement of rotation underestimates the true value of the medial twist of the femur that would be measured by computed tomography (CT) scan by 10° to 15°.[208] Therefore radiographic measurement may need to be pursued in cases that do not resolve spontaneously. Femoral and tibial torsions are generally measured on axial CT images. In consideration of dosages of radiation, low-dose simultaneous perpendicular biplanar radiography scanners and magnetic resonance imaging are options that are now being used.[118,179]

Many types of interventions have been tried to correct FA, including braces, twister cables, shoe modifications, or orthotic devices. These have not been proven to be effective.[218] Anecdotal findings may note the efficacy of these conservative methods, although spontaneous improvement occurs naturally in most cases. One reasonable recommendation is to have the child avoid W-sitting (reverse tailor sitting) and to encourage tailor sitting in maximum hip lateral rotation. If significant FA is still present at age 10 to 14 years and is resulting in cosmetically unappealing in-toeing, surgical correction in the form of femoral derotation osteotomies may be considered, although the possible risks of the operation may outweigh the benefits of realignment. In the adult, FA does not cause degenerative arthritis and rarely causes any disability.[201] Surgical intervention may be warranted and has proven successful in children with severe symptomatic torsional malalignment with excessive FA or external tibial torsion (ETT) associated with patellofemoral pathology when conservative intervention has failed.[204]

Internal Tibial Torsion

Internal tibial torsion (ITT) in infancy often is not apparent to the parents or the casual examiner because the hips have

external rotation muscle contractures and the infant's legs tend to assume abducted and externally rotated position. The ITT may become noticeable only as the hip contractures stretch out, resulting in a more neutral position of the hip, especially when the child begins to walk independently. One interesting note is the effect of in-toeing with sprinting. Fuchs and Staheli[62] studied high school students (50 sprinters and 50 control subjects) and found that the sprinters tended to have low normal thigh-foot angles and in-toed when sprinting.

Controversy exists regarding appropriate intervention of ITT as it does in FA. Many orthopedists believe that it should not receive intervention at all because the natural history of the condition is gradual improvement. The very small percentage of children who do not improve and who have a significant functional deficit as a result of ITT can receive surgical intervention at a later date with external rotational osteotomy of the tibia and fibula. A different school of thought relies on natural improvement up to about 18 months of age and at that age advocates intervention for persistent ITT with a Friedman counter splint (Universal Shoe Splint Assembly, United States), a flexible leather strap, or a Denis Browne bar, a metal bar, for night wear, usually for about 6 months. These devices attach to shoes and hold the feet in an externally rotated position. The Denis Browne bar is an uncomfortable intervention that, because of adherence difficulties, is sometimes limited. Also, with the knees extended, the torque applied by the bar may be directed to the hips because the knees are extended. The Wheaton brace with an upper component has also been developed to isolate the correction to the tibia, not to apply torque to the hip. With this device, the knee is flexed to 90°, and improved comfort with this device may improve adherence. Another option is the Tibia Counter Rotator with toe-out gait plate (Biomechanics Technology Co Ltd, Goyang, Korea).

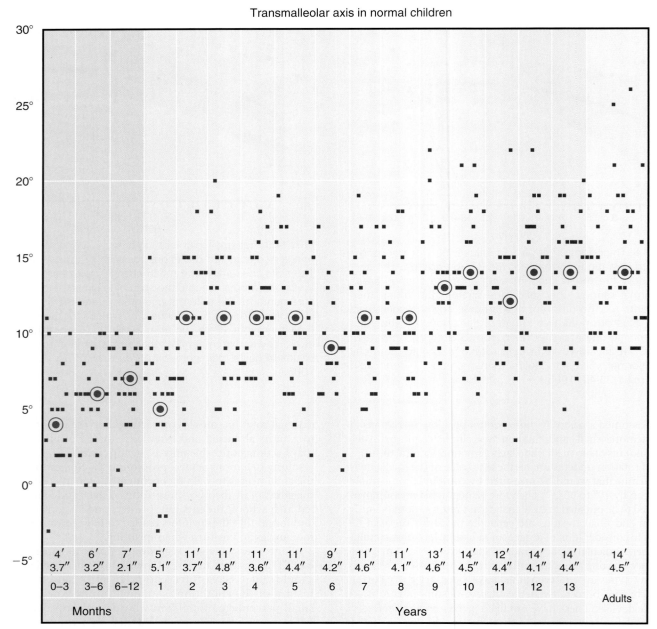

FIG. 14.10 Transmalleolar axis in normal children and adults. The mean in each age group is indicated by the larger dot and circle. ′ = the mean age group. ″ = the standard deviation. (Redrawn from Staheli LT, Engel GM: Tibial torsion: a method of assessment and a survey of normal children. *Clin Orthop Rel Res* 86:183-186, 1972.)

It consists of well-padded straps, foot plate, and metal brace (Fig. 14.12). This device is considered more comfortable because it allows complete freedom of hip motion. It does accommodate the amount of torsion and can be adjusted periodically to continue improvement over time. Significant improvements have been seen in early studies.[198,199]

Surgical correction is a supported option in a minority of cases, where there is severe cosmetic or functional deformity or a TFA over three standard deviations from the mean.[52,186] No surgical intervention should be considered under the age of 10 years, with surgery associated with a high complication rate (avascular necrosis, osteomyelitis, overcorrection, nonunion, etc.).[201] Successful approaches have included supramalleolar tibial rotation osteotomy[44] and Haas's multiple-longitudinal osteotomy technique.[48] Correction can occur at the proximal tibia but has more risk of complication (compartment syndrome, damage to the common peroneal nerve and major neurovascular structures posterior to the upper tibia).[77]

Metatarsus Adductus

The infant foot is malleable, making it susceptible to deformation and compression from intrauterine positioning.

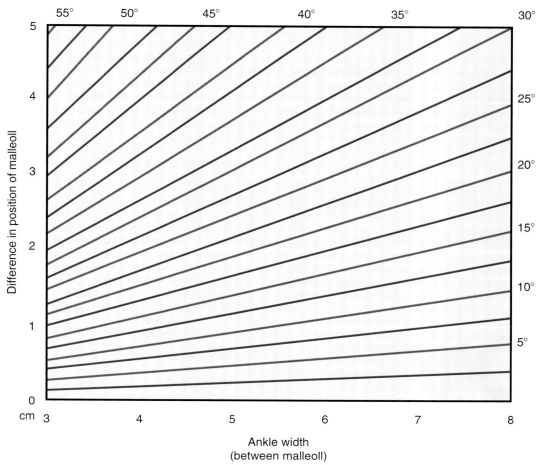

FIG. 14.11 Conversion grid for the transmalleolar axis. (Redrawn from Staheli LT, Engel GM: Tibial torsion: a method of assessment and a survey of normal children. *Clin Orthop Rel Res* 86:183-186, 1972.)

TABLE 14.2	**Clinical Features of Common Causes of In-Toeing in Children**		
	Metatarsus Adductus	**Internal Tibial Torsion**	**Increased Femoral Anteversion**
Age of noticed onset	Birth to 1 year	1 to 3 or 4 years	> 3 years
Laterality	Usually bilateral; may be unilateral with left > right[51]	Usually bilateral; may be unilateral with left > right[58]	Bilateral; other conditions should be considered if unilateral[51]
Natural history	Resolves by age 1 year	Resolves by age 5 years	Resolves by age 11 years

Alterations in alignment of the foot can be a result of increased intrauterine pressure, osseous abnormality, or abnormal muscle attachments.[230] Metatarsus varus, also called metatarsus adductus (MTA), is one of the most commonly seen positional conditions in infants (occurs in 1 per 1000 live births).[46] MTA is solely a forefoot deformity and because of this can be distinguished from talipes equinovarus and skewfoot, which involve the hindfoot structures.[230] The deformity is at the tarsometatarsal joints (Lisfranc joint) of the foot, which results in contracture of the soft tissues around this joint. The forefoot is then adducted in relationship to the hindfoot. In some cases a dynamic deformity is seen only during the child's gait, called "searching great toe." The foot appears straight at rest, but

forefoot varus as a result of muscle action occurs with medial motion of the great toe. This usually corrects spontaneously.[201] Patients under 3 years old have a flexible or semiflexible metatarsus adductus. Patients over 4 years old tend to develop a progressively more rigid deformity.[223]

Intervention is rarely required for mild cases (grade I), which usually resolve on their own by about 4 to 6 months. Moderate cases (grade II) may receive intervention with stretching exercises and corrective shoes (straight-last or reverse-last shoes or both). A recommended stretching technique is to face the child, cup the heel of the foot with the left hand (if right foot MTA), and abduct the foot with the right hand while keeping the heel in varus. Pressure should be applied gently across the metatarsals.[222] Severe cases may warrant manipulation and serial casting, followed by corrective shoes. Surgery is not considered before 4 years to allow for spontaneous resolution.[222] Although surgery should be used selectively, correction may be important in prevention of further problems as the child reaches adulthood.[214] An increased risk of stress fractures in those with MTA has been documented. [214] Patients ages 25 to 61 years who experienced metatarsal fractures had a forefoot adductor angle of 21° to 37° (normal range, 8° to 14°).[214]

Out-Toeing

Components that may contribute to out-toeing are external rotation contractures of the hip (and, rarely, femoral retroversion), external tibial torsion, and calcaneovalgus (Table 14.3).

External Rotation Contractures of the Hip/True Femoral Retroversion

True femoral retroversion in an infant is rare; it is usually tightness in the hip external rotation muscles and capsular

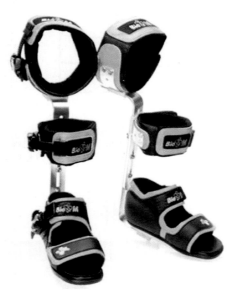

FIG. 14.12 Tibia Counter Rotator with toe-out gait plate. (From Son SM, Ahn SH, Jung GS, et al.: The therapeutic effect of tibia counter rotator with toe-out gait plate in the treatment of tibial internal torsion in children. *Ann Rehabil Med* 38:218-225, 2014.)

ligaments that is producing the externally rotated position, masking the femoral anteversion.[168] In utero the hips are laterally rotated, making this a normal position in infancy. When the infant is positioned upright, the feet may turn out. If only one foot turns out, usually the turned-out foot is the normal one.[201] If this continues into the second year of life, further evaluation may be needed because retrotorsion may increase the risk of slipped capital femoral epiphysis[201] and has also been associated with degenerative arthritis of the hip[201] and stress fracture.[68]

External Tibial Torsion

ETT usually becomes worse with time because the tibia normally rotates laterally with growth[201] and becomes most problematic in late childhood and adolescence. It is the rotational deformity most likely to require operative correction.[201] ETT is most problematic and noticeable when present in combination with increased FA (malalignment syndrome).[201] The knee is internally rotated and ankle externally rotated.[201] This combination results in an inefficient gait, patellofemoral joint pain,[201] and osteochondritis dessicans.[21] Derotational tibial osteotomy is the only effective intervention but should be reserved for patients with knee pain, severe cosmetic and functional deformity, and an external TFA greater than 40°.[200]

Calcaneovalgus

Calcaneovalgus is a common positional foot problem in newborns, and more than 30% of neonates have bilateral calcaneovalgus.[209] This is an example of an intrauterine "packaging" deformity. The ankle is in excessive dorsiflexion, the forefoot is curved out laterally, and the hindfoot is in valgus. The dorsum of the foot may actually be touching the anterior surface of the leg at birth. The positional calcaneovalgus foot corrects spontaneously and does not require intervention. In cases where ankle plantar flexion limitation is more severe, casting may be an option if stretching fails.[71] Calcaneovalgus may also rarely be caused by a vertical talus. Congenital vertical talus is a very rare condition that is generally found along with other abnormalities[100] and is characterized by the talus in a vertical orientation and the navicular displaced onto the dorsal surface of the talus. The forefoot is dorsiflexed but the hindfoot is plantarflexed, and the foot bends at the instep. This characteristic position is described as a "rocker-bottom" deformity of the foot, and the foot is much more rigid than the typical calcaneovalgus foot. This may more commonly be seen in association with other

TABLE 14.3	Clinical Features of Common Causes of Out-Toeing in Children			
	External Rotation Contracture of the Hip	**Femoral Retroversion**	**External Tibial Torsion**	**Calcaneovalgus**
Age of noticed onset	Birth to 1 year	Older than 3 years	Late childhood, early adolescence	Newborn
Laterality	Usually bilateral and symmetrical	Usually bilateral and symmetrical; when unilateral the right side is more often affected[51]	Often unilateral with the right side more often affected[51]	Bilateral
Natural history	Usually resolves by 12 months	Does not improve spontaneously; may be associated with hip or knee arthritis, stress fractures, and slipped capital femoral epiphysis	Usually does not correct spontaneously; may worsen over time, but rarely causes problems of sequelae such as patellofemoral pain or instability, arthritis of the knee	Recovers spontaneously[7]

conditions such as neural tube defects, neuromuscular disorders, or congenital malformation syndromes.[49] Without intervention, this leads to progressive foot pain in all sensate ambulators.[222] Nonambulators may be fitted for shoes that accommodate their deformity because surgery is considered the only corrective intervention.[222]

ANGULAR CONDITIONS

Genu varum (bowlegs) and genu valgum (knock-knees) are similar to torsional conditions in that they are commonly seen in developing children, and a specific natural history has been described that results in normal skeletal alignment at maturity (Fig. 14.13). A description of the natural growth and development process is in Chapter 5. Generally, the presentation of valgus is considered normal up to an age of 7 years.[182,133] After the age of 8 years, pathologic conditions should be considered if deviations from this norm are present.[15]

Clinical Examination

Subjective history of any problems will again provide valuable information.
1. Ask about noticed onset. Was there an injury or illness?
2. Is the deformity progressing? Are there old photographs that would show progression?
3. Tell me about your child's general health. Have there been any other health concerns or problems with muscles or bones? Specific pathologic disorders have been identified with genu varum and valgum. Pathologic problems are generally indicated by: asymmetrical deformity, inconsistency with the normal sequence of angular development, stature less than the 5th percentile for age, severe deformity (> 10 cm intermalleolar or intercondylar distance), history of rapid progression, or presence of other musculoskeletal abnormalities.[57,15]

Measurement of the Hip-Knee-Ankle Angle

Both clinical and radiographic documentation of the degree of varus and valgus will help provide baseline information for

Development of the HKA in Children

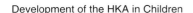

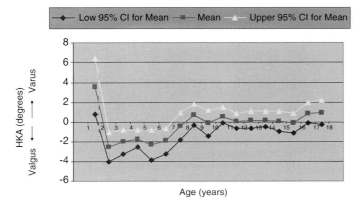

FIG. 14.13 Graphic representation of the development of the tibiofemoral angle during growth. (Redrawn from Sabharwal S, Zhao C: The hip-knee-ankle angle in children: reference values based on a full-length standing radiograph. *J Bone Joint Surg Am* 91:2461-2468, 2009.)

later comparison. For clinical measurement the child must be undressed with diaper removed for accurate documentation. For genu varum the child is placed with the medial malleoli approximated. The distance between femoral condyles is measured. Some clinicians use the distance between the knees at the knee joint line. A plastic triangle with centimeters marked on both sides is useful, allowing the examiner to easily obtain accurate measurements, especially of a wiggling child. Measurement of genu valgum can be performed with the child supine or standing, with the medial aspects of the knees lightly touching each other. The intermalleolar distance is documented. Radiographically, an anteroposterior view can be taken with the full length of the femur and tibia. The hip-knee-ankle angle is measured to document the amount of varum or valgum at the knee.[201] Other pathologic conditions may be noted on the films also.

Genu Varum

When a child develops severe genu varum, especially after 4 years of age or worsening over time, pathologic disorders should be ruled out. Documented causes of pathologic genu varum are congenital tibial hemimelia, osteochondrodysplasia, partial physeal arrest related to trauma, rickets, growth plate injury due to infection, tibial vara (Blount's disease), or excessive prenatal fluoride ingestion.[15,201] Also, the presence of an anterolateral bow of the tibia should be noted and can be confirmed on radiograph.[201] This is the sign of a serious condition because the sclerotic intramedullary canal puts the tibia at severe risk of fracture in the first year of life. The tibial and fibula may fail to unite in these cases, resulting in a condition called "pseudoarthrosis of the tibia." Protective bracing and surgical intervention may be helpful, but amputation may eventually be required because of persistent pseudoarthrosis.[201]

Infants usually have ITT and genu varum, and this combination tends to make the child look "bowlegged and pigeon-toed," causing many parents and others great concern. Even when the genu varum has resolved and the child may actually have developed genu valgum, the presence of ITT may make the child look bowlegged.

Physiologic genu varum does not usually require intervention unless it persists after age 2 years and either shows no tendency to correct or is actually worsening. This latter condition may require bracing in hip-knee-ankle-foot orthoses (HKAFOs) or knee-ankle-foot orthoses (KAFOs) with no knee joint or a hinged knee joint that can be locked. Surgical correction is sometimes required, although this is rare.

Genu Valgum

Genu valgum can occasionally persist beyond the age range when one expects the legs to become generally straight. Many of the children with persistent genu valgum are overweight and have an out-toeing foot progression angle, an awkward gait, and flat feet. Causes of pathologic valgum include: congenital fibular hemimelia, osteochondrodysplasia, overgrowth or partial physeal arrest related to trauma, rickets, osteogenesis imperfecta, growth plate injury related to infection, rheumatoid arthritis of knee, or paralytic conditions such as polio or cerebral palsy leading to contracture of the iliotibial band.[15,201]

Children with significant femoral anteversion may often appear knock-kneed. Once again, a clear understanding of the three-level concept of torsional conditions and the angular conditions is necessary to isolate the problem. Athletes have been noted to be predisposed to overuse injuries from both extrinsic factors (e.g., training errors) and intrinsic or anatomic factors, such as malalignment of the lower extremities. Variations in alignment may predispose athletes to knee extensor mechanism injuries, iliotibial band syndrome, stress fractures, and plantar fasciitis. Some adolescents with genu valgum present with anterior knee pain, patellofemoral instability, circumduction gait, and difficulty running.[205] Genu valgum can also be seen in multiple epiphyseal dysplasia.[184] Asymmetrical genu valgum may result from trauma or fracture of the lateral distal femoral epiphysis.

If severe, physiologic genu valgum can be safely and effectively corrected in the teenage years by stapling of the medial femoral growth plate and genu varum by leg stapling of the lateral growth plate.[97] This allows the unstapled side of the femoral growth plate to continue growing, and the leg gradually grows into better alignment. A second option for surgical intervention is femoral osteotomy.

FLAT FOOT

A flatfoot is considered normal during at least the first 2 years of life and often is still present at age 6 years.[157] Almost all children will demonstrate a flatfoot when they begin ambulating. Intrinsic laxity and a lack of neuromuscular control result in flattening of the arch when weight bearing.[153] With weight bearing the ligaments stretch and allow mild subluxation of the tarsal bones. Morley[145] documented flat feet in 97 percent of 18-month-olds. In a study of 835 children the incidence of flatfoot in 3-year-old children was 54 percent and in 6-year-old children was 24 percent.[166] Most will develop an arch in the first decade of life (4 percent incidence of flat feet by age 10 years).[145] After age 10 years, natural resolution is not likely and family history may be a factor.[43]

In a large population-based interview study of prevalence of flat foot, the odds ratio for prevalence of flatfoot in adults in fourth decade was 1.02 although this increased to 1.04 in the group with body mass index 26 pounds/in² and higher.[191] This observation may be trivial but might also be noted clinically when a higher body mass index is present. Many parents will request medical consultation for their child when he or she begins to bear weight; because the normal development demonstrates changes through ages 8 to 10 years, no intervention is generally recommended until after this time period, especially when the child is asymptomatic.[43,201] The pediatric flatfoot can be divided into two categories: flexible or rigid.

Flexible Flatfoot

Flexible flatfoot is characterized by a normal arch during non–weight bearing and a flattening of the arch on stance that may be symptomatic or asymptomatic. At birth, infants have a physiologic ligamentous laxity and lack a medial arch. A fat pad is also present underneath the medial longitudinal arch and resolves between the ages of 2 and 5 years as the arch forms.[147] Children often will also demonstrate more mobility of other joints as well, such as hyperextension of the fingers, elbows, and knees.[157] In these cases the child can form an arch when asked to stand on tiptoe. The heels will roll into a varus position, and good strength of the ankle and foot muscles is measurable[43] (Fig. 14.14).

Besides ligament laxity, other factors have been identified as affecting the presence of a flexible flatfoot. Shoe wear was found to be an influence on the presence of flat feet in a study by Rao et al.[172] of 2300 children between the ages of 4 and 13 years. Those who did not wear shoes had a 2.8% prevalence while those who wore closed-toe shoes had a 13.2% prevalence of flatfoot. Shoe wear was not found to be a significant factor in a study of 560 children (ages 6 to 12 years) in Nigeria, however.[1]

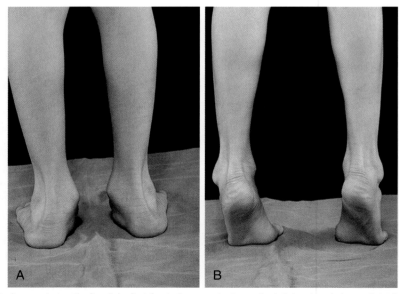

FIG. 14.14 Asymptomatic flexible flat feet demonstrate a diminished arch in weight bearing with hindfoot valgus present (A). Upon weight bearing on toes, the arch reconstructs and the hindfoot moves into varus (B). (From Chaudhry B, Harvey D: *Mosby's color atlas and text of pediatrics and child health*, St. Louis: 2001; Mosby.)

Another factor that is found more often in children with bilateral flatfoot is obesity. In children 6 years and younger, the incidence was found to be higher by Dowling et al.[47] and Chen et al.[30] Others have found that children (ages 7 to 15 years) who are more physically active have a lower arch than those who are less active.[163] Also, children who habitually sit in the W-position have a higher rate of flat-footedness.[30] Boys are more likely to be flat-footed than girls as well.[163,166]

It has been widely documented that a low arch usually is less of a problem in adulthood than high-arched (cavus) feet. Michelson et al.[140] studied 196 college athletes with flat feet who had 227 episodes of lower extremity injury. Pes planus was not a risk factor for any lower extremity injury; therefore the use of orthotics to prevent further injury was discouraged. In a retrospective study of 97,279 military recruits, mild pes planus resulted in no greater incidence of anterior knee pain or intermittent low back pain when compared with controls.[119] Athletic performance was not hindered by flat-footedness in children 11 to 15 years in a study comparing arch height and ability to perform motor skills.[217]

Intervention of the flexible flat foot generally is not necessary.[43,157,201] Shoe modifications or inserts have been used, although studies have not shown these to be beneficial.[43] Some pediatric orthopedists who counsel parents regarding the natural history of improvement in flat feet through childhood advise the use of a lightweight running shoe as the only recommendation. Using shoes with an arch support and a strong counter will not correct the flatfoot but can help decrease wear on the medial border of the shoes, thereby decreasing the expense of frequent shoe purchase.

In order to rule out rheumatologic, inflammatory, neoplastic, or neurologic disease, the presence of morning stiffness, night pain, pain at rest, numbness, weakness, muscle wasting, constitutional symptoms, and polyarticular pain or swelling should be documented.[43] Family history of hyperlaxity or syndromes associated with flat feet, such as Ehler-Danlos or Marfan syndrome should be considered.

Children occasionally have an extra ossicle located at the medial border of the navicular, called an accessory navicular, that is frequently associated with flat feet. This condition may become symptomatic in late childhood or early adolescence, resulting in pain over the ossicle and along the medial arch, and can be corrected surgically.

Rigid Flat Feet

Rigid flat feet are present in only about 1% of flat feet in children.[221] Primary causes of this are tarsal coalition, congenital vertical talus, and neurologic, neoplastic, or post-traumatic pathologies.[43] As with asymptomatic flexible flat feet, asymptomatic rigid flat feet do not require any intervention.[43] When the hindfoot is fixed in a valgus position, symptoms such as pain, callus, ulceration, poor brace tolerance, and excessive shoe wear can be relieved by lengthening of the Achilles tendon and other surgical soft tissue and osseous procedures.[43,221]

Tarsal coalition involves two or more tarsal bones that are joined by fibrous, cartilaginous, or bony material.[43,221] This connection will reduce movement, generally at the calcaneonavicular or talocalcaneal joints. Usually, this results in a flat foot, although normal alignment or cavus can occur.[43] Passive or active hindfoot inversion results in a painful spasm of peroneal muscles so that it sometimes is called spastic peroneal flatfoot.[221] Many coalitions are asymptomatic and no intervention is necessary.[43] Symptoms may include foot pain, difficulties in walking on uneven ground, feeling of local fatigue, and peroneal spasm.[221] In these cases, casting, splints, orthoses, and modified weight bearing may be needed, and in cases where conservative measures fail, surgical options of removal of the soft tissue interposition or arthrodesis are available.[43,221]

Congenital vertical talus typically presents in infancy as a rigid rocker-bottom foot.[43] Primarily, the talus is in a plantarflexed position and the navicular is dislocated dorsally on the talus.[43] Contractures of the Achilles tendon and the extensor digitorum longus muscle support these positions.[221] Reduction of the deformity is not possible without serial casting and corrective surgeries.[43,221] This is often seen along with myelomeningocele, arthrogryposis, and congenital hip dislocation.[221]

CLUBFOOT

Clubfoot, or congenital talipes equinovarus, is a common congenital deformity affecting approximately 1–2 in 1000 births.[72] The components include forefoot adductus, hindfoot varus, and ankle equinus (Fig. 14.15). Anatomically, the talus is smaller in clubfoot than a normal foot and has a flattened superior surface with consequent decreases in talocalcaneal angle.[232] The subtalar joint facets are misshapen, and the navicular is oriented more downward and medial than in the normal foot.[232] Deformities of the tarsal bones are considered to be the primary cause while ligament and joint capsule changes adjust to the distorted position.[232] The ligaments are generally thickened and muscles hypoplastic, resulting in generalized hypoplasia of the limb with shortening of the foot and smallness of the calf.[201] The foot appears smaller as the result of a flexible, softer heel caused by the hypoplastic calcaneus.[71] Ankle valgus may evolve with growth and may be mistaken for "overcorrected clubfoot," or hindfoot valgus.[206] Severe cases of metatarsus adductus may be confused with this, but the equinus component differentiates the diagnosis.

Other musculoskeletal abnormalities commonly occur in conjunction with idiopathic clubfoot. Tibial shortening, ITT (or decreased external tibial torsion), and increased internal hip rotation have been documented.[92,175] These changes may not

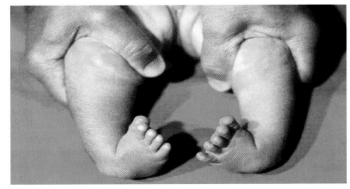

FIG. 14.15 Child with clubfoot with hindfoot varus, hindfoot equinus, and forefoot varus. (Pisani G: "Coxa Pedis" today. *Foot Ankle Surg* 22:78-84, 2016.)

be significant in some because the external tibial torsion may increase with age and the internal hip rotation may decrease with age.[41,175] Also a factor may be the manipulation technique used to correct clubfoot; external tibial torsion increases if the corrective technique does not allow a progressive eversion of the talus underneath the calcaneus.[58] Therefore rotational malalignment should be examined and monitored, although operative correction generally is not recommended until after 7 years of age because alignment may spontaneously correct with growth.[175]

The cause of clubfoot is considered to be a combination of genetic and environmental factors.[201,222] A genetic influence is suggested because siblings have up to 30 times the risk of developing clubfoot deformity and monozygotic twins have a 33% concordance rate.[66,14,201,222] Also, a male predominance (2:1 ratio) is present although affected females are more likely to pass on the trait to their children and have siblings with clubfoot than males.[121] Higher incidence is also seen in Hispanics and a lower incidence in Asians.[201] Environmental factors have also been identified.[14,66,201] These include factors during pregnancy such as cigarette smoking, early amniocentesis, or viral infection.[66,14] Cases of clubfoot related to intrauterine positioning are generally mild and correct rapidly with intervention.[201] More severe cases are thought to be from factors occurring earlier in fetal life, while idiopathic cases are generally in the middle range of the severity spectrum.[201] Histologic anomalies have been identified in every tissue in the clubfoot, including muscle, nerve, vessels, tendon insertions, ligaments, fascia, and tendon sheaths.[98] In addition, Loren et al.[130] found congenital muscle fiber type disproportion or fiber size variation in 50 percent of peroneus brevis muscle biopsies performed at the time of posteromedial release, and those feet with such muscle variation had a significantly greater incidence of recurrent equinovarus deformity.

The goal of intervention of clubfoot is to correct the deformity and retain mobility and strength.[201] The foot needs to be plantigrade and must have a normal load-bearing area.[201] Also included in the objectives are the ability to wear normal shoes, satisfactory appearance, and avoidance of unnecessary complicated or prolonged interventions.[201] Extrinsic clubfoot (severe positional or soft tissue deformity that is supple) can often be successfully corrected with conservative intervention such as serial casting, which should be started as soon after birth as possible,[40,171,236] although some have used up to 9 years of age.[14] Casts are changed in the Ponsetti method semiweekly or weekly, and the foot should be positioned so that it can be corrected in an orderly sequence by first correcting the cavus, rotating the foot from under the talus, and finally correcting the equinus.[201] After four to six castings, many may require an Achilles tenotomy to lengthen the tendon. Most can change to a brace for 3 months at that time, followed by a sleep brace for 2 to 4 years.[66,222] This method is considered the standard approach throughout the world.[201] A second method, the French method, involves daily manipulations of the foot by a therapist, stimulation of the muscles around the foot, and temporary immobilization of the foot with plaster cast.[40] Duration of the intervention is generally 2 months[14,40] and has been found to be effective in varying stages of severity.[40] Some may require a tibialis anterior tendon transfer, usually between 3 and 5 years of age, to control dynamic forefoot supination or recurrent deformity.[66] This is considered to be a minor procedure as it does not affect the joints of the foot.[66]

In cases of intrinsic (rigid) clubfoot, manual reduction and surgery may be required.[71] Surgical techniques include Z lengthening of the Achilles and posterior tibiotalar and talocalcaneal capsulotomy to correct equinus, posteromedial talocalcaneal capsulotomy and/or subtalar release to correct hindfoot varus, release of the abductor hallucis and talonavicular joint for midfoot adduction, and plantar fascia release for cavus deformity.[222]

BLOUNT'S DISEASE/TIBIA VARA

Blount's disease, or tibia vara, is a developmental condition resulting from a deceleration of growth at the posteromedial proximal tibial physis that ultimately results in a varus deformity of the tibia, along with flexion and internal rotation of the tibia and relative limb shortening in unilateral cases.[16,181] Clinically, this disorder has been classified into three forms: infantile (onset 0 to 4 years), juvenile (onset 4 to 10 years), and adolescent (onset after 10 years).[181] The etiology of Blount's disease is unknown, but some predisposing factors have been identified.[16,181] Boys are more affected than girls, and approximately 50% of the cases are bilateral but not always symmetrical.[16] The growth inhibition at the proximal tibia may be related to excessive compressive forces medially. In infantile forms, an early walking age, large stature, obesity, or a combination of these factors has been suggested.[16] Others have suggested that various genetic, medical, biomechanical, and environmental factors contribute.[181] In adolescent forms the likely cause is a mechanical injury to the medial tibial physis, with or without a preexisting varus deformity.[16] Differential diagnoses that should be considered are rickets, renal osteodystrophy, focal fibrocartilaginous defect, and proximal tibial physeal injury.[16]

The influence of obesity should be considered in this population. In a child with genu varum, obesity will cause an increased compressive force at the medial tibia.[181] Also of note are gait deviations caused by obesity related to increased thigh girth.[181] When the thigh girth limits adduction of the hips, a varus moment results at the knees and increases the pressure at the medial part of the proximal tibial physis. Therefore late-onset Blount's disease may result from these mechanical factors and not a preexisting varus alignment.[16,181]

In children younger than 2 years of age, it sometimes is difficult to distinguish between physiologic genu varum and Blount's disease.[222] Physiologic genu varum will be demonstrated by angular deformity from the femur and the tibia, and infantile Blount's disease involves deformity isolated to the proximal tibia.[222] Radiographic findings will show varus angulation centered at the knee, mild metaphyseal beaking (appearance similar to a bird's beak), thickening of the medial tibial cortices, and tilted ankle joints. Six stages of infantile Blount's disease (from 1 through 6, least to more involved) have been described on the basis of this radiographic appearance[16,201,222] (Fig. 14.16). Also useful in the diagnosis of and choice of intervention for infantile Blount's disease is the metaphyseal-diaphyseal angle.[201,222] If the angle exceeds 16°, Blount's disease is likely to develop.[16,201] Radiographs are performed every 3 to 6 months, and improvement will be seen with physiologic varus after the child's second birthday; however, Blount's disease will progress and show metaphyseal changes.[201] In adolescent Blount's disease, the distal femur may also be angulated, and radiographs will demonstrate medial physeal and epiphyseal

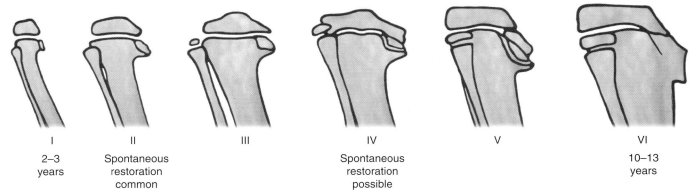

I	II	III	IV	V	VI
2–3 years	Spontaneous restoration common		Spontaneous restoration possible		10–13 years

FIG. 14.16 Langenskiold's radiographic classification system describes the six stages of infantile Blount's disease. (Redrawn from Langeskiöld A: Tibia vara [osteochondrosis deformans tibiae]: a survey of 23 cases. *Acta Chir Scand* 103:1-22, 1952.)

hypoplasia of the proximal tibia.[222] Also, a lateral or varus thrust during gait may be seen.[222]

Intervention is based on the stage of tibia vara and age of the child.[16,181,201] In children younger than 3 years of age, observation is very important, with bracing prescribed in the presence of a lateral thrust[201] or in stages 1 and 2.[222] Richards et al.[176] found a 70 percent success rate with bracing in this group. During this study, three different types of orthoses were used and included conventional HKAFOs, conventional KAFOs, and elastic Blount KAFOs (medial upright design that uses a wide elastic band just inferior to the knee joint) and the elastic Blount brace has been the choice at this clinic since its development in 1987. Surgery is recommended if the tibia vara progresses or is initially seen in stage 3 or 4.[16,181,201] This option is considered if conservative intervention has failed by the fourth birthday.[222] Surgery may be needed to correct the varus deformity, correct the ITT, restore normal joint congruity, and prevent or correct limb length discrepancy.[2] Better outcomes with operative realignment were found when surgery was performed before 4 years of age.[181,222] Also, better outcomes were documented when surgery was performed before permanent physeal damage had occurred.[88] Late-onset Blount's disease is corrected surgically with proximal tibial osteotomy and/or lateral physeal hemiepiphysiodesis (selective closure of half of the growth plate to allow the contralateral portion of the physis to correct with growth).[222]

DEVELOPMENTAL DYSPLASIA OF THE HIP

Developmental dysplasia of the hip (DDH) is a term used to describe a wide-ranging spectrum of disorders from minor acetabular dysplasia to irreducible dislocation of the femoral head, with the primary cause being instability of the hip.[39,107] It may also include hips that may have been normal or were believed to be normal at birth but subsequently were documented to have dysplasia.[170]

The term *dysplasia* describes abnormal development or growth. Normal muscle balance and a femoral head that is concentric, congruent with, and seated deep within the acetabulum are necessary prerequisites for normal hip development. The concave acetabulum develops in response to a spherical femoral head, and the depth normally increases with growth.

The incidence of hip dysplasia in the United States is 5.5 per 1000 for full-term babies within the first 2 days of life.[6] The incidence dropped to 0.5 per 1000 after 2 weeks of age, indicating that many cases improve without intervention.[6] Prompt recognition of and initiation of intervention for DDH, preferably in the newborn period, provide the best chance for subsequent optimal hip development and a normal hip at skeletal maturity, especially in those cases that do not resolve spontaneously. Ideally, DDH will be identified in the neonatal screening, but cases have been found that were clinically stable in the neonatal period but subluxed or dislocated later.[170] This finding would encourage clinicians to evaluate the hip beyond the neonatal period until the child begins to walk.[170]

The origin of DDH is thought to be multifactorial. The Subcommittee on Developmental Dysplasia of the Hip of the American Academy of Pediatrics[37] has identified four periods during which the hip is at risk. If a dislocation occurs as the fetal lower limb rotates medially during the 12th week of gestation, all elements of the hip joint develop abnormally.[37] During the 18th gestational week, the hip muscles are developing, and neuromuscular problems occurring at this time, such as myelodysplasia and arthrogryposis, can lead to dislocation.[37] During the final 4 weeks of pregnancy, dislocation can occur as the result of mechanical forces.[37] Most noted in this time frame is breech positioning, as DDH occurs in as many as 23% of breech presentations.[37] The breech position puts the child at high risk by placing the hip in flexion and the knee in extension.[37] The left hip is involved three times more often than the right hip because of intrauterine positioning with the left hip positioned posteriorly against the mother's spine, potentially limiting abduction.[37] Also related to intrauterine positioning is the increased incidence seen in firstborn children[173,188] as well as babies with high birth weights.[188] Because these are related to positioning due to limited space in the uterus, other abnormalities may coexist with DDH including torticollis, metatarsus adductus, and oligohydramnios.[188] In the postnatal period, positioning such as swaddling, combined with ligament laxity, can have a role.[37] Girls are more susceptible to the maternal hormone relaxin, which may contribute to ligament laxity[37] and possibly account for the five times higher frequency in females.[188] Also of interest is the reduced incidence of DDH among cultures in which infants are routinely carried with their hips in flexion and wide abduction in cloth slings on the mother's back or astride her hips[54] along with the increase in dysplasia noted in children who are swaddled in the first few months of life.[36] Although risk factors have been identified, all children should be considered because the majority of cases of DDH have no identifiable risk factors.[193]

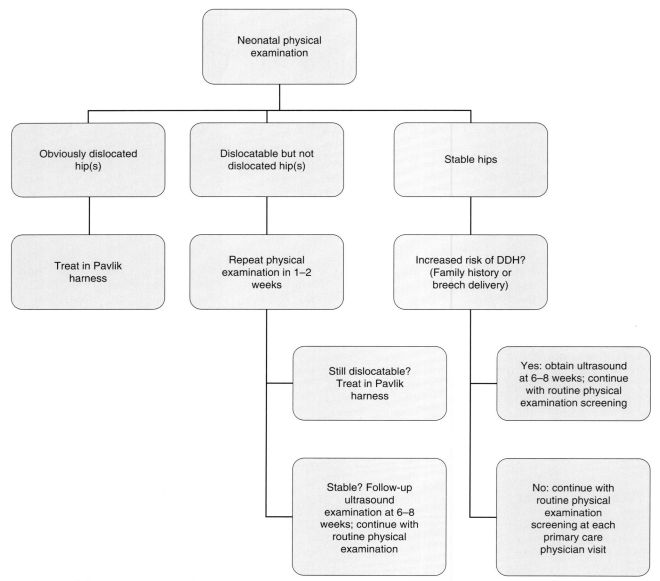

FIG. 14.17 Algorithm for neonatal physical examination screening for hip dysplasia. *DDH,* developmental dysplasia of the hip. (From Mahan ST, Katz JN, Kim YJ: To screen or not to screen? A decision analysis of the utility of screening for developmental dysplasia of the hip. *J Bone Joint Surg Am* 91:1705-1719, 2009.)

Clinical Examination

Screening for DDH has been the focus of many studies and reviews for the purpose of developing protocols that allow for early intervention when needed.[90,94,134,193,211] Generally, the accepted practice is clinical screening of all newborns and ultrasound screening on all newborns with identified risk factors.[90,94,134] An algorithm of this process is in Fig. 14.17.

Clinical screening includes performance of the Ortolani test (reduction test) and the Barlow test (stress test). Description of these tests is in Fig. 14.18. The child needs to be completely relaxed for these maneuvers to have reliable diagnostic value. Every slight muscular contraction around the hip can obscure the instability and negate the examination. The experience of the clinician with these tests has been shown to be a strong predictor of the test results.[193] Pediatricians have been shown to have a case identification rate of 8 per 1000, while orthopedists

identify 11 per 1000.[126] The Ortolani and Barlow tests are often negative by 2 to 3 months of age because the hip improves in stability and stays in the socket or becomes fixed in a dislocated position. Positive tests will continue to be the most reliable clinical findings in older infants and toddlers with dysplasia. Other clinical signs at greater than 3 months of age are restricted hip abduction (<60 degrees with infant supine and knees flexed to 90 degrees), leg length discrepancy (prone and with Galeazzi test), and asymmetrical thigh and gluteal skin folds.[94]

Diagnostic studies are considered appropriate when clinical testing is positive and even with a normal clinical examination if risk factors are present. Ultrasound during the first 3 months of life is the most appropriate test due to the incomplete ossification of the femoral head.[193] Any child with a breech delivery or a family history (parent or sibling) of DDH should be considered for an ultrasound screening even

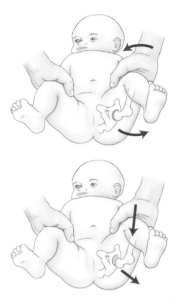

FIG. 14.18 Barlow maneuver. The hip is first flexed and abducted, then is gradually adducted, with pressure exerted in a posterior direction. Dislocation of the femoral head over the posterior acetabular rim indicates an unstable hip. The head may slide to the edge of the socket (subluxatable) or may dislocate out of the acetabulum (dislocatable). In the Ortolani-positive hip, the hip is dislocated in a position of flexion and adduction. Gentle flexion, abduction, and slight traction (the Ortolani maneuver) reduce the hip. A positive Ortolani sign indicates a more unstable hip than a positive Barlow sign. (From Hagen-Ansert SL: *Textbook of diagnostic sonography.* 7th ed. St. Louis, Mosby, 2012.)

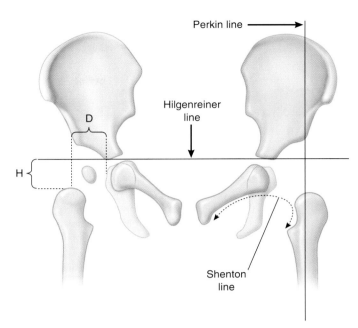

FIG. 14.19 Radiographic measurements that are useful for evaluating developmental dysplasia of the hip. The Hilgenreiner line is drawn through the triradiate cartilates. The Perkin line is drawn perpendicular to the Hilgenreiner line at the margin of the bony acetabulum. The Shenton line curves along the femoral metaphysic and connects smoothly to the inner margin of the pubis. Dimension H (height) is measured from the top of the ossified femur to the Hilgenreiner line. Dimension D (distance) is measured from the inner border of the teardrop to the center of the upper tip of the ossified femur. Dimensions H and D are measured to quantify proximal and lateral displacement of the hip and are most useful when the head is not ossified. (From Herring JA: *Tachdjian's pediatric orthopaedics: from the Texas Scottish Rite Hospital for Children.* 5th ed. Philadelphia, Saunders, 2014.)

if the clinical exam is normal.[94,134] Ultrasound may also be a good option if four or more of the following risk factors are identified: breech presentation, family history, female baby, large baby (> 4 kg), overdue (> 42 weeks), oligohydramnios, presence of plagiocephaly, torticollis, or foot deformities, or firstborn baby or multiple pregnancies (decreased intrauterine space).[94] Ultrasonography allows examination of the cartilaginous structures not visualized on plain radiographs and allows stress testing (to document instability), with the additional advantage of no radiation exposure. It is also useful in the management of DDH, documenting reduction of the dislocated hip in the Pavlik harness[213] and providing information on the status of the hip to aid decisions on altering or stopping intervention (Fig. 14.19). The Graf classification system is used in classifying hips with DDH (Fig. 14.20). At age 5 months and older, radiographs are the more appropriate screening tool.[94,193] Because of the need for a radiograph of the uninvolved side for comparison and because of the frequency of bilateral involvement, the standard radiograph is an anteroposterior view of the pelvis. The benefits of x-ray to monitor DDH through walking age outweigh the risks of radiation exposure.[185] The acetabular index (Fig. 14.21) can be monitored through the radiographs as well as an early finding of the "teardrop" indicating a stable, concentric reduction of the hip has been achieved.[196] The "teardrop" is a landmark in the inferior medial acetabulum on an anteroposterior radiograph.[196] Many parameters of hip development can be measured on hip radiographs.

When the clinical finding is hip instability (either reducible dislocation or dislocatable hip), the hip becomes stable spontaneously in about half the cases.[188] The other cases can be classified as dysplasia, subluxation, or dislocation.[81] Dysplasia describes a radiographic finding of increased obliquity and the loss of the concavity of the acetabulum, with an intact Shenton line. The Shenton line should be continuous with no breaks. It is drawn on radiographs along the inferior border of the superior pubic ramus and then continues along the inferomedial border of the neck of the femur.[81] A superolateral migration of the proximal femur results in a discontinuous Shenton line. Subluxation describes when the femoral head is not in full contact with the acetabulum with the presentation of a widened teardrop femoral head distance, a reduced center-edge angle, and a break in the Shenton line.[81] In these cases the femoral head is in the socket but can be partially displaced out of the acetabular rim. Dislocation refers to the femoral head not in contact with the acetabulum.[81] This can include cases where the femoral head is reduced but can be dislocated with a Barlow maneuver, dislocated but reducible (where the femoral head is out of the acetabulum at rest but can be reduced with an Ortolani maneuver), or dislocated but not reducible (which is generally related to other medical issues occurring before birth). Both subluxated and dislocated hips

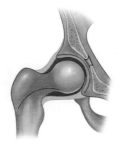
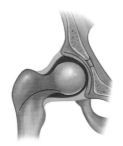
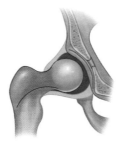
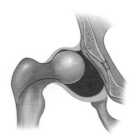

FIG. 14.20 Graf classification of infant hips based on the depth and shape of the acetabulum as seen on coronal ultrasonograms. Type I: normal; characterized by a well-formed acetabular cup with the femoral head beneath the acetabular roof. Type II: immature in infants less than 3 months of age and mildly dysplastic in infants older than 3 months of age; characterized by a shallow acetabulum with a rounded rim. Type III: subluxated; characterized by a very shallow acetabulum with some displacement of the femoral head. Type IV: dislocated; characterized by a flat acetabular cup and loss of contact with the femoral head. (Redrawn from French LM: Screening for developmental dysplasia of the hip. *Am Fam Physician* 60:177-184, 1999. © 1999 David Klem.)

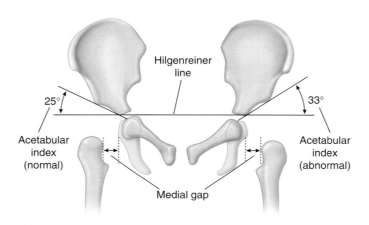

FIG. 14.21 Acetabular index. The acetabular index is the angle between a line drawn along the margin of the acetabulum and the Hilgenreiner line; it averages 27.5° in normal newborns, and it decreases with age. (From Herring JA: *Tachdjian's pediatric orthopaedics: from the Texas Scottish Rite Hospital for Children.* 5th ed. Philadelphia, Saunders, 2014.)

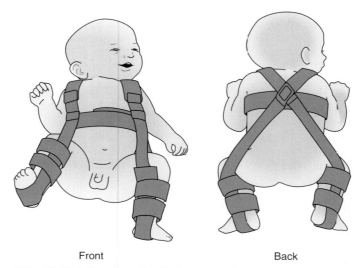

Front   Back

FIG. 14.22 Infant in a Pavlik harness. (From Ball J: *Mosby's pediatric patient teaching guides.* St. Louis, Mosby, 1998.)

have dysplastic changes.[81] Over time, the stresses on the joints will cause further problems if left without correction. Dysplastic hips without subluxation will usually become painful and develop degenerative changes. Often they will become subluxed as the degenerative disease progresses.[81] The subluxed hip will lead to symptomatic degenerative disease with gradual increasing pain starting as early as the second decade of life in severe cases and the fifth and sixth decades in the least severe cases.[81] A completely dislocated hip will demonstrate symptoms later than a subluxed hip and, in some, never become symptomatic.[81]

Intervention for DDH

Goals for Intervention

The basic goal for intervention of DDH is the same regardless of the age of the patient: reduce and maintain the reduction to provide an optimal position for the development of the femoral head and acetabulum.[224] If this reduction is maintained, the femoral head and femoral anteversion can remodel.[224] The

intervention to achieve this position becomes more complex as the child ages. Also, with increasing age and complexity come more risks of complications and the likelihood of the development of degenerative joint disease.[224]

Birth to 6 months old. The Pavlik harness is the primary method of correcting DDH during infancy. The Pavlik harness was first described by Dr. Arnol Pavlik, who originally called his intervention device "stirrups." Modifications have been made in the design of the device, but the principles of intervention and the requirements of the harness remain essentially the same as described by him over 50 years ago.[164] Pavlik stressed that one of the main advantages of the harness over casts is that it allows active motion, thereby decreasing the incidence of avascular necrosis (AVN) of the femoral head.[165]

The Pavlik harness restricts hip extension and adduction that can lead to redislocation, but it allows further flexion and abduction, which lead to reduction and stabilization (Fig. 14.22). The position of flexion and abduction enhances normal acetabular development, and the kicking motion allowed in this position stretches the contracted hip adductors and promotes

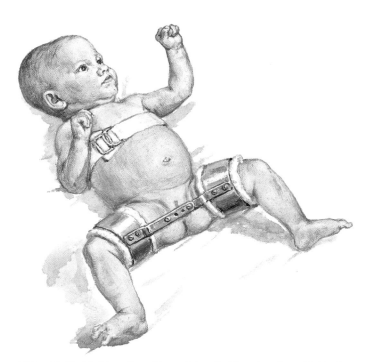

FIG. 14.23 Ilfeld splint. (Copyright © Elsevier, Inc: NetterImages.com.)

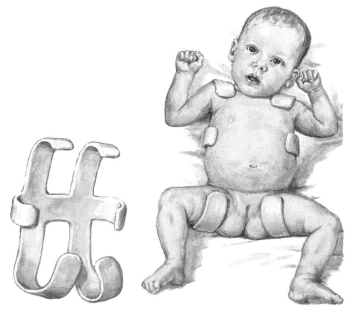

FIG. 14.24 The Von Rosen splint. (Copyright © Elsevier, Inc: NetterImages.com.)

spontaneous reduction of the dislocated hip. By maintaining the Ortolani-positive hip in a Pavlik harness continually for 6 weeks, hip instability resolves in 90% to 95% of the cases of subluxation and dysplasia, and there is approximately 85% success in cases of dislocation.[150,224] The overall success rate has been described as 91.5% at a minimum of 14 years' follow-up.[150] Ultrasonography is an important tool to monitor intervention (after initial 7 to 10 days and every 3 weeks thereafter)[81,224] and to determine when intervention should be discontinued either because of successful or unsuccessful results.[39] Failure of the harness is generally thought to be from inappropriate application or persistence of intervention when not effective.[224] Complications can occur if a child is positioned in greater than 12° flexion (femoral nerve palsy or dislocation of femoral head inferiorly).[81,224] After 6 months of age, the failure rate for the Pavlik harness is over 50 percent because the active and crawling child is difficult to maintain in position in the harness.[224] The harness is contraindicated in patients with significant muscle imbalance (myelodysplasia or cerebral palsy), significant stiffness of joints (arthrogryposis), and excessive ligament laxity (Ehlers-Danlos syndrome).[224] Use of an abduction splint following the use of the Pavlik harness is advocated by some to allow further development of the acetabulum.[81] The Ilfeld splint (Fig. 14.23) and the von Rosen splint (Fig. 14.24) have shown high success rates for this.[81] Triple diapering has not shown positive effects.[81]

If the use of the Pavlik harness is not successful in reducing a dislocated hip, surgical intervention is indicated. This may include a period of 2 to 3 weeks of traction to reduce the incidence of AVN of the femoral head. Home traction is a safe, effective, and much less expensive alternative to performing traction in the hospital.[115] Surgery includes an arthrogram to define the anatomic landmarks of the femoral head and acetabulum and to detect the presence of soft tissue (pulvinar) interposition between the head and acetabulum; adductor tenotomy; closed

or (if necessary) open reduction of the hip; and application of a spica cast. Luhmann and colleagues[131] reported that delaying reduction of a dislocated hip until the appearance of an ossification nucleus more than doubled the need for additional reconstructive procedures, advocating early intervention.

6 months to 2 years old. The child who is between 6 months and 2 years old who presents with a newly dislocated hip and the child who has failed conservative care to this point is managed in similar ways.[81,224] In these patients the obstacles to maintaining reduction are different, the intervention has greater risks, and the end results are less predictable.[224] The goal is still to achieve reduction, maintain that reduction to provide an environment for the development of the femoral head and acetabulum, and avoid proximal femoral growth disturbance.[81,224] The two primary methods of intervention will be closed reduction or open reduction, either of which may be preceded by traction.[81,224]

The need for the use of traction is a choice that may vary among physicians.[81,224] The purpose of traction prior to a reduction is to stretch contracted muscles, allowing the reduction to be performed without excessive force decreasing the incidence of avascular necrosis and open reduction.[224] The use for traction has been challenged because studies have shown conflicting results on its benefits when compared to no traction prior to closed reduction.[122,194] Also debated has been the effect of traction on the rate of open reductions needed.[81] In fact, this practice of traction seems to have changed significantly over the last 20 years with fewer surgeons using it routinely presurgically.[224] For those who would benefit from it, home traction is an option because it may be applied for 2 to 3 weeks, and this would allow decreased hospital admission time, although adherence of the family and patient is essential to this option.[81,224]

Closed reductions are performed with general anesthesia or deep sedation. The hip is reduced as it would be in the Ortolani maneuver with minimal force applied. The ROM that is allowed while the hip remains reduced is compared to normal ROM and a "safe zone" is determined[81] (Fig. 14.25). If the reduction is determined to be stable, the child is immobilized in a hip spica

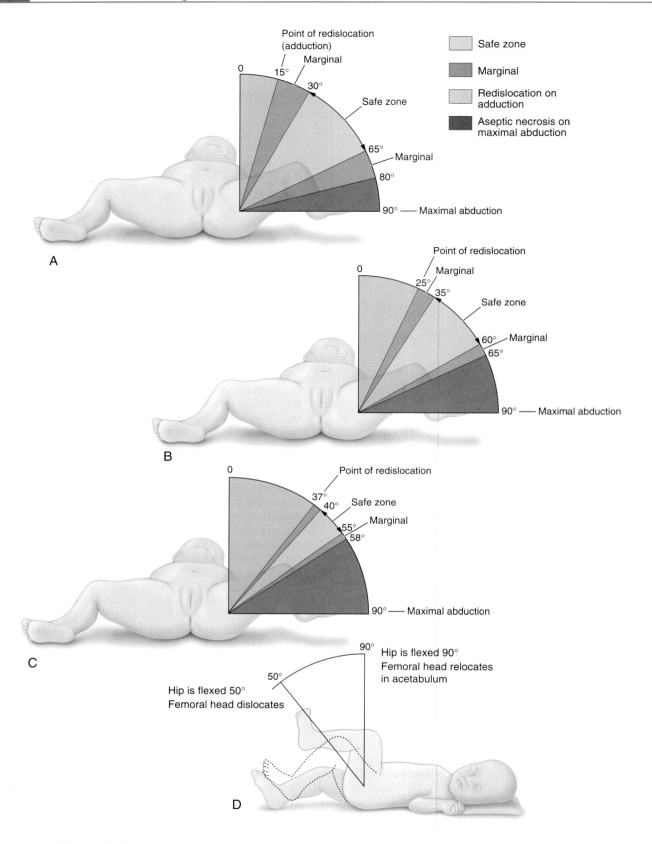

FIG. 14.25 Examination of the hip with developmental dysplasia. (A) Wide zone of safety. (B) Moderate zone of safety. (C) Narrow zone of safety. (D) Femoral head dislocation. (From Herring JA: *Tachdjian's pediatric orthopaedics: from the Texas Scottish Rite Hospital for Children.* 5th ed. Philadelphia, Saunders, 2014.)

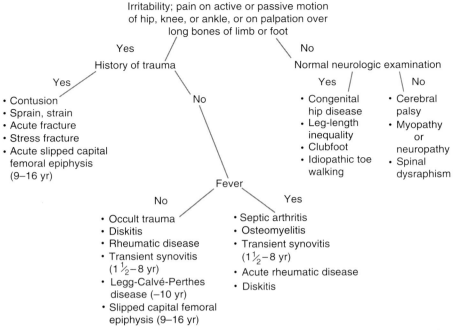

FIG. 14.26 A clinical decision tree for children with a limp. (From Scoles PV: *Pediatric orthopedics in clinical practice.* 2nd ed. Chicago, Year Book Medical Publishers, 1988.)

cast. The length of time in the cast will vary with each patient, but generally the first cast is applied for 6 weeks with examination at that time followed by a second cast for 6 weeks. Further immobilization will be determined at that time depending on the stability of the joint. Some will continue with abduction splinting following the casting.[81,224]

Open reduction is indicated when closed reduction fails to obtain a stable hip. This may be determined at the time of the initial closed reduction or may become evident at the cast change. The surgical procedure can be performed from an anterior or medial approach to perform a capsulorrhaphy, capsular repair, and pelvic osteotomy, if needed.[81,224] Following the surgery, casting will be applied as done with a closed reduction.[81]

Two years old and older. Intervention for older children with hip dislocation becomes more challenging. The femoral head is usually in a more proximal location, and the muscles that cross the hip are generally more contracted. Generally, a femoral shortening will need to be performed because this has shown better results than skeletal traction in this age group. Also, an acetabular reshaping osteotomy will be needed.[81] A potential complication is posterior dislocation of the hip. Good results have been reported with this intervention with low rates of avascular necrosis.[81] The upper age at which this should be performed has been debated. It may be appropriate for children up to 9 or 10 years old in unilateral cases and up to age 8 years in bilateral cases.[81] When children reach late juvenile and adolescent age, a triple pelvic osteotomy is often required for intervention.[227]

A number of children with acetabular dysplasia are never diagnosed as infants or toddlers. With mild dysplasia, they will walk without a limp, will have essentially normal hip ROM, and can actively participate in all childhood activities, including sports. However, the hip is like a tire that is out of alignment: you can drive on it for quite a few miles, but uneven wear will occur. The dysplastic hip, especially the one with subluxation, also develops uneven wear with subsequent articular cartilage damage. The person may develop degenerative arthritis, hip

pain, and limp as early as the late teens. Very mild dysplasia may go undetected for many decades and may be diagnosed later in life when the patient develops degenerative hip joint disease. One area of discussion is the presence of acetabular retroversion and/or femoral acetabular impingement as a long-term outcome for those with hip dysplasia or as a result of intervention.[224] Femoral acetabular impingement can further lead to acetabular cartilage delamination and degenerative joint disease over time.[224]

CAUSES OF LIMPING IN CHILDREN

The acute onset of limp in a child is a condition that warrants evaluation. In this section chronic causes of limp, such as those due to muscle weakness, will not be addressed. Orthopedic conditions that can result in acute limping will be reviewed. Although some of these are transitory and benign, some can result in lifelong impairments, especially if not corrected promptly and effectively. Fig. 14.26 and Box 14.1 provide useful information for the initial evaluation and assist in confirming a differential diagnosis. It is important to identify those who need immediate medical or surgical attention to prevent complications. Especially for those working in a direct access situation, attention to the history and systemic symptoms are important in the determination of referral to other professionals.

History and Physical Examination

When a child has a limp, a complete and thorough evaluation is recommended. A detailed history should be taken and should include a description of any recent illness or injury that may be a contributory factor. The clinician should be aware, however, that children do fall frequently, and a fall could be related to the onset of the limp or other injury, even though it may be incidental and unrelated.

Physical examination should include an observational gait analysis. This should allow the clinician to determine which leg is involved and perhaps the location within the leg. Gait analysis can provide much assistance in the direction of further testing. The algorithm in Fig. 14.27 demonstrates the process of generally categorizing the gait by observation with further physical examination and diagnostic testing used as confirmation.

The physical examination should also include a complete examination of the spine, hips, thighs, knees, lower legs, ankles, and feet, including the uninvolved side for comparison. Objective measurements of ROM and strength should be taken, as should observations of the presence of muscle atrophy, swelling, redness, and difference in temperature between limbs. Also, the child's subjective response of pain with palpation and with movement and muscle contraction is important. Much information can be gathered from the way a child performs functional activities, which is especially important when a child's cooperation might limit a formalized evaluation. Observation of the child moving from the floor to standing or crawling or achieving a comfortable sitting position can provide usable information. For example, a child may refuse to walk because of pain but may crawl easily, indicating that the problem is probably evident in the lower part of the leg, rather than in the hip or knee. A child might also demonstrate the use of his hands to "walk" up his body to rise to standing from the floor (Gowers' sign) because of hip and thigh muscle weakness, which could be related to neurologic disorders or other conditions causing proximal muscle weakness.

One consideration should be the various types of osteochondroses that are common causes of limp in the 5- to 10-year-old group and in the 10- to 15-year-old age group (Table 14.4). The

---

BOX 14.1   Diagnoses of Limping Commonly Found in Various Age Groups

Birth to Age 5 Years
Osteomyelitis
Septic arthritis
Transient synovitis
Occult fractures
Kohler syndrome

Child (4–10 Years)
Transient synovitis
Legg-Calvé-Perthes disease
Discoid lateral meniscus
Sever disease
Growing pains

Adolescent (11–15 Years)
Slipped capital femoral epiphysis
Osgood-Schlatter syndrome
Osteochondritis dissecans
Tarsal coalition
Freiberg disease
Accessory navicular

TABLE 14.4   Conditions of Osteochondroses

Ossification Center	Eponym	Typical Age (Years)
Tarsal navicular	Kohler disease	3–8
Capital femoral	Legg-Calvé-Perthes disease	4–8
Calcaneus	Sever disease	8–15
Tibial tubercle	Osgood-Schlatter syndrome	Boys 12–15; girls 8–12
Second metatarsal head	Freiberg disease	13–18
Vertebral ring	Scheuermann disease	10–12
Capitellum	Panner disease	< 10

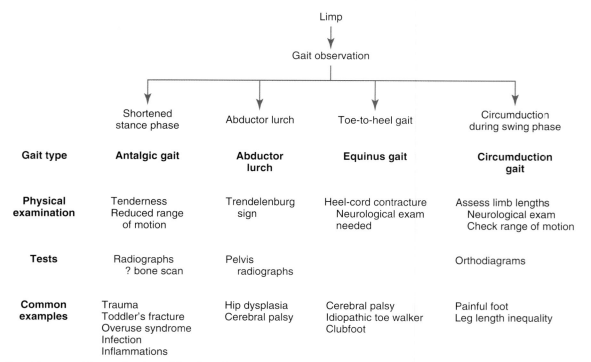

Gait type	Antalgic gait	Abductor lurch	Equinus gait	Circumduction gait
Physical examination	Tenderness Reduced range of motion	Trendelenburg sign	Heel-cord contracture Neurological exam needed	Assess limb lengths Neurological exam Check range of motion
Tests	Radiographs ? bone scan	Pelvis radiographs		Orthodiagrams
Common examples	Trauma Toddler's fracture Overuse syndrome Infection Inflammations	Hip dysplasia Cerebral palsy	Cerebral palsy Idiopathic toe walker Clubfoot	Painful foot Leg length inequality

FIG. 14.27 Algorithm used for evaluation of limping. A general category can be determined by observation with physical examination and tests used to confirm the problem. (From Staheli LT: *Practice of pediatric orthopedics.* 2nd ed. Philadelphia, Lippincott Williams and Wilkins, 2006.)

osteochondroses represent a group of disease of children and adolescents in which localized tissue death (necrosis) occurs, usually followed by full regeneration of healthy bone tissue.[51] During the years of rapid bone growth, blood supply to the epiphyses (growing ends of bones) may be compromised, resulting in necrotic bone, usually near joints.[51] Because bone is undergoing a continuous rebuilding process, the necrotic areas are often self-repaired over a period of weeks or months.[51] Osteochondrosis is generally divided into three locations: physeal, articular, and nonarticular. Physeal osteochondrosis (Scheuermann disease) occurs at the intervertebral joints.[51] Articular diseases occur at the joints (articulations), with common forms occurring at the hip, foot, and elbow.[51] Nonarticular osteochondrosis occurs at any other skeletal location, with one example being Osgood-Schlatter disease, which occurs at the tibia.[51] Many cases are idiopathic although stress related; repetitive trauma and infection are noted causes, and occurrence generally is more frequent at times of rapid growth of the epiphysis.[51]

Other Diagnostic Tests

In addition to a careful clinical examination, other tests are often indicated. Radiographs can document fractures or other bony abnormalities, although some occult fractures are not identifiable on radiography until 10 to 14 days after onset, when a repeat radiograph may document formation of callus. Laboratory examination of blood samples provides information regarding the presence of infection or other acute processes. The erythrocyte sedimentation rate (ESR) and C-reactive protein (CRP) can indicate the presence of acute inflammation, as well as response to intervention. More complex diagnostic studies may also be needed to define the problem or evaluate the efficacy of interventions. These studies include bone scans, magnetic resonance imaging (MRI) (for soft tissue), and CT (for bony structures).

The cause of a limp in a child may be as simple as a foreign object in the shoe or as complex as osteogenic sarcoma. Therefore generalizations regarding management should not be made, and a diagnosis should be established as quickly as possible. Many cases may be easily corrected, and some require no intervention beyond observation. Many causes of limp are associated with specific age groups, specifically one of three groups: birth to 5 years, 5 to 10 years, and 10 to 15 years. Soft tissue injuries (i.e., contusion, ligaments, and tendon injuries) and fractures are found in all age groups.

Osteomyelitis

Osteomyelitis has the highest incidence in children under the age of 3 years.[177] It can be classified as acute (< 14 days' disease duration) or subacute (> 14 days' disease duration). Also, occurring rarely is chronic recurrent multifocal osteomyelitis (CRMO), which is an autoinflammatory bone disease that may present with pain and signs of inflammation over months or years without responding to intervention.[3,7] The incidence rate can vary regionally with approximate values of 8 per 100,000 for acute osteomyelitis and 5 per 100,000 for subacute osteomyelitis (13 per 100,000 combined).[177] The incidence of CRMO is 1 in 1 million.[7] Most commonly, osteomyelitis in children is hematogenous, which means circulating pathogenic organisms settle in the metaphyses of long bones due to slower circulation in these regions.[169] In the United States, the incidence of acute hematogenous osteomyelitis is 1 in 5000 children under the age of 13 years.[133] Nonhematogenous

osteomyelitis is the result from direct inoculation of organisms into the bone due to conditions such as penetrating trauma or open fractures.[169] When trauma occurs, local edema may alter the blood flow, and the formation of a hematoma may provide a good environment for bacterial proliferation.[229] In some instances a history of recent respiratory infection, otitis media, or an infected wound is reported.[45] Boys are more susceptible than girls with an approximate ratio of 2:1.[158] When the infection spreads to the adjacent joint, septic arthritis may result, which is a more likely complication in neonates.[156] This is related to the vascular anatomy of the epiphyses in neonates; before the secondary ossification center forms, the cartilaginous epiphyses receive their blood supply directly from metaphyseal blood vessels.[156] In joints such as the hip, where the metaphysis is intracapsular, the spread of infection to the joint occurs.[156] In neonatal osteomyelitis, infection leads to damage to the epiphysis or septic arthritis in 76% of the cases.[156] CRMO will generally resolve postpubertally,[141] although long-term studies have shown that up to 25 percent have persistent disease, with complications including risk of permanent bone deformities, poorer quality of life, and difficulty in achieving vocational goals.[89,93,137,167]

The most common etiology of hematogenous osteomyelitis in children is *Staphylococcus aureus*[79,156,158] although occasionally fungi, viruses, or parasites may be involved, especially in the immunocompromised.[10,69] Since the introduction of the *Haemophilus influenzae* type b (Hib) vaccine in 1992, the incidence of *Haemophilus influenzae* infection in infants and older children is much less.[91] Of noted concern at this time is the virulent strains of methicillin-resistant *Staphylococcus aureus* (MRSA).[79] The prevalence of osteomyelitis caused by MRSA increased from 0.3 to 1.4 per 1000 hospital admissions from 2002 to 2007 in a survey of 20 metropolitan hospitals in the United States.[64] When MRSA is the etiology of osteomyelitis in children, more severe bone infection has been documented with more aggressive surgical and medical management required.[79] Another cause is *Kingella kingae*.[76] This organism has been found in several geographical regions and is difficult to culture, requiring specific testing techniques.[76,158] Some differences between the clinical findings in the presence of *Staphylococcus aureus* and *Kingella kingae* can be found in Table 14.5.[158]

Clinically, the onset of osteomyelitis is generally sudden, and the rapid progression can cause permanent damage and later consequences in the child.[45] The most common sites of osteomyelitis are the rapidly growing ends of long bones; the condition is more common in the lower extremity.[45] Therefore the metaphyses of the distal femur and of the proximal tibia are the most common sites of infection.[45,156]

TABLE 14.5	**Characteristics of *Staphylococcus Aureus* Versus *Kingella Kingae***	
	Staphylococcus Aureus	**Kingella Kingae**
Age	Any age group	Often < 4 years
Fever	> 38°C	Afebrile on admission
C-reactive protein (CRP)	Elevated	May be normal
White blood cell count (WBC)	Elevated	May be normal

From Pääkkönen M, Peltola H: Bone and joint infections. *Pediatr Clin N Am* 2013;60:425-436.

The signs and symptoms of acute hematogenous osteomyelitis are variable, according to factors such as age of the patient, site of infection, resistance of the child, and virulence of the affecting organism.[45] Generally, however, onset is sudden, with localized bone tenderness, swelling, and pain over the metaphysis of the involved bone.[45] A high fever and chills are often present, and the patient is often unwilling to use the affected limb.[45] Frequently, the child will refuse to walk when the lower extremity is affected.[45] Neonates often do not demonstrate signs of systemic illness, and signs of pseudoparalysis and pain with passive motion are difficult to detect.[45]

Initial routine blood tests, such as ESR, C-reactive protein (CRP), and white blood count (WBC), are used to determine the extent of the inflammation and also help monitor the response to antibiotic therapy.[158] All of these levels are elevated in the presence of osteomyelitis. With intervention, ESR and CRP will normalize, although the CRP value normalizes in 7 to 10 days while the ESR takes 3 to 4 weeks.[45,158] The signs and symptoms, routine blood tests, and vaccination history against Hib or pneumococcus will help in the speculation of the causative organism, but the gold standard for identification is a bacterial culture.[76,158] These should include bone samples and blood cultures.[76,158] For accuracy the blood cultures should be obtained before antibiotic therapy is initiated.[45]

Imaging can provide further information in cases of osteomyelitis. Plain radiographs are important for the purpose of excluding other diagnoses such as fracture.[76] Deep soft tissue swelling can be seen within the first few days of onset.[76,156] Osteopenia or osteolytic lesions from destruction of bone or periosteal new bone formation will not be visible until 2 to 3 weeks after onset.[76,156] Therefore other imaging techniques may be helpful. Ultrasound allows the detection of subperiosteal collections and joint effusions as early as 48 hours although it does not determine the presence or absence of infection.[156] Skeletal scintigraphy allows for a whole-body survey, which is especially helpful in those with poorly localized symptoms or if multiple foci of infection are suspected.[76,156] It does, however, require exposure to ionizing radiation and the sensitivity is lower in neonates.[76] Differentiation of the cause of the osteomyelitis as well as limited ability to diagnose community-acquired *Staphylococcus aureus* osteomyelitis are issues with scintigraphy.[76] Magnetic resonance imaging (MRI) is helpful in identifying intra osseous, subperiosteal and soft-tissue abscesses but does not differentiate these conditions from similar ones found with fracture and infarct.[76] CT is helpful in detecting sequestra (indicative of chronic osteomyelitis) and intraosseous gas and can define subperiosteal abscesses, all of which should be considered in intervention.[76,156] Also, CT may help guide aspiration and biopsy.[156]

The identification of the source of the infection is important for successful intervention. Generally, antibiotic therapy will range from 4 to 6 weeks in duration[76,156] but will be individualized according to the severity of the infection, the time elapsed between onset of the disease and initiation of intervention, the extent of bone involvement, and laboratory responses after the initial intervention.[152] Surgical intervention may be needed in cases where an abscess or a sequestra has developed, but guidelines are subjective because some of these have resolved with antibiotic course.[158] The decision to intervene will be based on the clinical presentation and response to antibiotic therapy. Persistent fevers and persistent elevation of the CRP in a patient with a periosteal abscess would be indications for surgical drainage.[158] This is more often needed when the onset of symptoms is more than a week prior to intervention.[158] Other surgical procedures may be needed if damage to the involved bone occurs (pathologic fracture, premature/asymmetrical closure of growth plate, angular deformities of bone).[76]

Septic Arthritis

Septic arthritis (pyogenic arthritis) is defined as an infection of a joint caused by bacterial organisms. This is an extremely threatening condition because a joint may be destroyed within 48 hours of onset of symptoms. Septic arthritis causes destruction of articular cartilage and long-term growth arrest. The resulting deformities may be permanent and may have a wide-ranging, lifelong impact, affecting the person's gait, participation in sports, and choice of occupation and leisure activities.

As described previously in the osteomyelitis section, septic arthritis results from osteomyelitis in 76% of the cases in neonates.[156] Septic arthritis generally causes a rapid inflammatory response.[45] The synovial membrane responds with a hyperemia followed by excessive production of fluid and pus.[45] Pus contains enzymes that rapidly destroy articular cartilage, causing irreversible joint damage.[45] Permanent joint destruction can result in as little as 3 days.[45] Any joint may be affected, but about 80% of cases are located in the lower extremity with the hip (in the young child) and the knee (in the older child) being the most common locations.[65,109,138] Because of the lax nature of the surrounding musculature in neonates, the presence of joint effusion may lead to subluxation or dislocation of the affected joint.[156] In a newborn the cartilaginous femoral head can be completely destroyed, requiring salvage procedures later in life. Damage to the epiphysis may cause trochanteric overgrowth and leg length discrepancy when the growth plate is damaged.[45] Also, the intra-articular pressure may be increased by the accumulation of inflammatory exudate causing vascular compression that occludes the blood supply to the femoral head, causing avascular necrosis.[156]

The diagnosis of septic arthritis is based on clinical findings. Septic arthritis is most common in children ages 2 years and younger.[156] Clinical presentation for septic arthritis may have many of the same characteristics as osteomyelitis: high fever and chills, unwillingness to use the affected limb, and absence of spontaneous movement, as well as refusal to bear weight on the affected limb.[45,158] The affected joint will demonstrate swelling, redness, warmth, and local tenderness.[45] Generally, those with septic arthritis are more ill than those with osteomyelitis.[158] Table 14.6 describes the different characteristics of osteomyelitis and septic arthritis.[158]

Laboratory tests of ESR, CRP, and WBC are commonly used tools to diagnose septic arthritis.[144] Others have suggested that

TABLE 14.6 Characteristics of Osteomyelitis Versus Septic Arthritis		
	Osteomyelitis	Septic Arthritis
Fever > 38.5°C	Suggestive if present	Suggestive
Malaise	Usually	Usually
Swollen joint/limited motion	Not unless concurrent arthritis	Nearly always
Edema overlying bone	Often	Absent
Back pain	Suggestive of spinal osteomyelitis	Rare
Difficulty weight bearing	Lower limb affected	Lower limb affected

From Pääkkönen M, Peltola H: Bone and joint infections. *Pediatr Clin N Am* 2013;60:425-436.

measuring the presence of procalcitonin (PCT) is helpful in differentiating noninfectious inflammation and bacterial infections.[144] Chloe et al.[31] found the specificity and sensitivity of diagnosis of septic arthritis were greater with PCT and PCT was also 100% accurate in differentiation between gram-negative and gram-positive infections, helping guide antibiotic therapy more quickly. This tool may be more useful, especially in cases involving *Kingella kingae*.[144]

Radiographs are of lesser importance in septic arthritis because they will show an enlarged joint space at most.[158] Ultrasonography is helpful to identify small joint effusions and can guide joint aspiration.[45] A bone scan may also help diagnostically to determine diffuse uptake within the joint in the early phase or a rise in intra-articular pressure.[45] The MRI is considered the most accurate diagnostic tool and provides the best anatomic detail.[144,158]

Joint aspiration is imperative for the diagnosis and should not be delayed if septic arthritis is suspected.[158] The aspirated fluid should be cultured, and drainage and appropriate intravenous antibiotics should be started quickly.[45,133] Intravenous antibiotic therapy is recommended until improvement in clinical signs is seen; at that time, oral antibiotics may be used.[133]

Transient Synovitis

Transient synovitis of the joint is a common cause of lower extremity pain, specifically the hip, in children between the ages of 3 and 8 years. It presents itself as a rapid onset of hip pain, limited joint ROM, and limping (or an inability to walk, if the condition is severe).[85] The child may have a history of an antecedent viral illness,[85] and the resulting effusion of the joint leads to a position of hip flexion and external rotation.[11] Reports have also shown referred pain in the knee with transient synovitis.[120] Males are also more likely to develop transient synovitis.[11]

In 1999, Kocher et al.[117] established a clinical algorithm to differentiate cases of septic arthritis from those of transient synovitis in 99.6% of cases. These variables were confirmed as highly predictive in a separate study published in 2004.[116] This clinical algorithm found that when four specific variables were all present, the diagnosis of septic arthritis could be confirmed at a very high rate. When only some of the variables were present, there was less certainty in diagnosing septic arthritis versus transient synovitis. These four variables are: history of fever of ≥ 38.5°C, inability to bear weight, ESR ≥ 40 mm/hr, and serum WBC of > 12,000 cells/liter.[117] A fifth predictor, CRP ≥ 20 mg/L was later also used.[210] Sultan and Hughes[210] have since found a lower rate (59.9%) of success using this algorithm, although fever was still the best predictor. Radiographs are normally unremarkable, and ultrasound examination of the affected hip may show effusion.[85] The concern is that septic arthritis and transient synovitis could present very similarly, and caution and care should be used in diagnosing the problem. Some children will have recurrent problems, and a small percentage will develop Legg-Calvé-Perthes disease.[123,219]

Intervention is generally symptomatic, consisting of limitation of activity, bed rest, and avoidance of weight bearing in combination with the use of nonsteroidal anti-inflammatory medications. Light traction during bed rest may be of benefit, and routine aspiration of the joint has also been beneficial.[85] Clinical symptoms will usually resolve within 10 days.[85]

Occult Fractures

By definition an occult fracture is a fracture that cannot be detected by standard radiographic examination until weeks after the onset.[146] In children, several variables may limit the finding of the problem: minor trauma that may not be merited consideration by the parents, poor localization of pain by young children, difficulty with communication with child, unexplained trauma history, and physician oversight.[32] Common areas of involvement are elbow, knee, ischium, distal fibula, proximal femur, and humeral shaft.[32] Upon presentation, pain and swelling may be present; generally, radiographs are negative for 2 to 3 weeks. Ultrasound has been found to be advantageous in the early diagnosis of both soft tissue and bone injuries.[32,151] Especially in the skeletally immature, ultrasound can identify discontinuity in the cortex but cannot visualize intraosseous deformities.[32] Also, the ultrasound can be done without sedation and with some movement by the child, making it clinically less difficult than an MRI, the gold standard.[32] Diagnosing the fracture early will allow for better intervention and prevention of complications such as slower healing times, growth arrest, fracture deformity, and pain.[32]

Kohler Disease

Kohler disease is an osteochondrosis of the navicular bone of the foot. Generally, patients present between 2 and 8 years of age, and boys are 3 to 5 times more likely to be affected.[215,216] It was first described by Alban Kohler, a German radiologist.[228] The condition occurs when the navicular bone temporarily loses its blood supply. The child usually has localized pain in the area of the navicular bone and a limp. There is usually no history of previous trauma. Point tenderness may be present over the navicular bone on examination.[216] There may also be mild swelling and warmth over the dorsal midfoot.[19] Radiographic changes may be visible and include navicular sclerosis, flattening, and fragmentation.[19] These cases have all shown good resolution, with no clinical or radiologic abnormalities seen in adulthood.[190] A short leg cast for up to 8 weeks may accelerate the resolution of symptoms, although long-term outcomes are good regardless of intervention.[216]

Legg-Calvé-Perthes Disease (LCPD)

Legg-Calvé-Perthes disease (LCPD) is a condition that occurs in children, who may receive referrals for physical therapy for resulting muscle weakness, ROM limitations, and gait deviations. By definition, LCPD is a condition in which an avascular event affects the capital epiphysis (head) of the immature femur. After this event, growth of the ossific nucleus stops and the bone becomes dense. This dense bone is then resorbed and replaced by new bone. As this occurs the mechanical properties of the femoral head change such that the head tends to flatten and enlarge. Once new bone is in place, the head slowly remodels until skeletal maturity is achieved.[82]

The onset of LCPD is between 18 months and skeletal maturity with cases most often between 4 and 8 years of age.[12,225] Boys are 4 to 5 times more likely to develop the disease than girls.[12,82,225] It is found bilaterally in 10 to 12 percent of patients.[82,225] About 35% of children with unilateral Perthes disease also demonstrate changes in the unaffected proximal femur on radiographs, including small epiphysis, flattening of the epiphysis, contour irregularities, and changes in the growth plate.[108] Recurrent cases of LCPD have been noted and generally will have a poor prognosis because the entire femoral head is generally involved and recurrence occurs when the child is older.[226]

The etiology of LCPD is multifactorial.[82,225] Vascular factors include both arterial supply and venous drainage.[82,225]

The medial femoral circumflex artery is the principal vessel in the complex vascular distribution in the neck and head of the femur. Also, the vessel advances between the trochanter and the capsule, which is a narrow passage and is particularly constricted in children less than 8 years of age.[82] A synovial intracapsular ring comprised of four ascending cervical arterial groups has also been found to be incomplete in the younger group as well.[82] When the arterial flow is obstructed or compromised, as has been noted in patients with LCPD, avascular necrosis will obviously occur at the femoral head. An abnormal venous drainage through the medial circumflex vein of the head and neck of the femur has also been noted with LCPD.[82] Findings of an increased venous pressure in the affected femoral neck and associated venous congestion in the metaphysis as well as more distal exit of venous outflow through the diaphyseal veins have also been noted in cases of LCPD.[82] The presence of this obstruction in the venous flow in this population would suggest it is at least a contributing factor in LCPD.[82] Coagulation factors also contribute to blood flow in this population.[82,225] Children with changes in clotting properties commonly show avascular changes at the femur including hemoglobinopathies (i.e., sickle cell disease, thalassemia), leukemia, lymphoma, idiopathic thrombocytopenic purpura, and hemophilia.[82] Also, increased blood viscosity has been noted in patients with LCPD.[82] Abnormal thrombus formation has been documented in LCPD, specifically with deficiencies in proteins C and S and in the presence of hypofibrinolysis, which then results in venous hypertension and hypoxic bone death.[82]

Children with LCPD also seem to present with similar growth and development abnormalities.[82,225] Most commonly a delay in bone age relative to the child's chronologic age is seen.[82,225] Those who are diagnosed with the disease before age 5 years tend to normalize during adolescence while those diagnosed at an older age tend to have a smaller stature throughout life.[225] Also, the birth weight of children with LCPD is lower than unaffected children.[82] Growth hormone, specifically somatomedin C insulin-like growth factor-1 (which is responsible for postnatal skeletal bone maturation), has also been noted to be lower in those with LCPD.[82,225] These levels generally increase as children age, but this increase is not seen in the group with LCPD.[82]

Other common influences have also been noted. Trauma may be a factor in the child who may already have some predisposition to LCPD (17%).[82,225] Many of the children have been noted as hyperactive or having attention deficit hyperactivity disorder.[82,225] Environmental commonalities of urban living and lower socioeconomic groups have been found with possible link to nutrition status and secondhand smoke, which are known to affect stature and growth.[82,225] A higher frequency of occurrence is found among the Japanese, other Asians, Eskimos, and Central Europeans, and a lower frequency in native Australians, Americans, Indians, Polynesians, and persons of African origin.[225] Genetic factors have been speculated but not conclusive of effect of heredity versus environment.[82] Perinatal HIV infection is also a risk factor for osteonecrosis.[59]

Further examination of affected femurs has shown the epiphyseal cartilage to contain high proteoglycan content, a decrease in structural glycoproteins, and different size collagen fibrils compared with normal tissue, suggesting that the disease could be a localized expression of a generalized transient disorder responsible for delayed skeletal maturation.[226] These abnormalities can be primary or secondary to the ischemia, but collapse and necrosis of the femoral head could result from the breakdown and disorganization of the matrix of the epiphyseal cartilage, followed by abnormal ossification.[226] The exact cause is unknown, but it occasionally follows repeated episodes of transient synovitis of the hip. Increased joint pressure secondary to synovitis may be one of the pathologic processes that causes an interruption of blood flow in vessels ascending the femoral neck.

Patients most commonly present with an insidious onset of limp, demonstrating an abductor limp. Pain will be described as activity related and relieved by rest. Commonly, pain is localized to the groin, anterior hip region, or laterally around the greater trochanter and may be referred to the anteromedial thigh or knee. Knee involvement when pain is present should be ruled out in a clinical examination because pain in the knee is a fairly common pattern with hip issues. Because of the mild nature of the symptoms, patients may not present for medical evaluation for weeks or months after the onset. ROM is limited in the directions of abduction and internal rotation. Early in the course of the symptoms the limited motion is related to synovitis and spasms in the adductor group, but the limitation may progress with tightening of the soft tissue structures.[225] Limb shortening will be present in cases of significant collapse of the femoral head[225] and with premature closure of the proximal growth plate of the femur.[162]

In order to best predict the prognosis and make decisions on necessary interventions, classification of the hip is of great value.[139] Currently, the Herring lateral pillar classification is commonly used and demonstrates strong predictive value.[86] Using this system, patients are placed in categories of group A, B, or C based on the involvement of the lateral pillar (the lateral 5 to 30 percent of the femoral head on an AP radiograph).[29] Group A hips do not involve the lateral pillar, group B hips have limited involvement with maintenance of over 50% of the lateral pillar, and group C hips have over 50% collapse of pillar height.[29] Group B/C has also been added, defining the lateral pillar as narrowed or poorly ossified with approximately 50% of height maintained. The Stulberg classification system is used to describe the hip at skeletal maturity.[29,139] This system is based on the deformity of the femoral head and congruity in relation with the acetabulum.[29,139] Class I is defined by a normal spherical head, class II by a spherical head with coxa magna/breva or steep acetabulum, class III by nonspherical head, class IV by a flat head and flat acetabulum, and class V by aspherical incongruence.[139]

Also, four stages of LCPD can be described radiographically.[82] These can be described as follows:

Initial stage: Early signs include lateralization of the femoral head with widening of the medial joint space and a smaller ossific nucleus. Later signs include subchondral fractures and physeal irregularity. This phase normally lasts a mean of 6 months.

Fragmentation stage: Radiolucencies develop in the ossific nucleus; a central dense fragment becomes demarcated from the medial and lateral segments of the femoral head. End of the stage shows appearance of new bone in the subchondral sections of the femoral head. This phase lasts a mean of 8 months.

Reossification (healing) stage: New subchondral bone is seen in the femoral head. Reossification starts medially and expands laterally. This phase lasts until the entire head has reossified and lasts a mean of 51 months.

Residual stage: Femoral head is fully reossified with gradual remodeling of the head shape until skeletal maturity. This shape may vary from completely normal to extremely flat and aspherical. Overgrowth of the greater trochanter may be seen because the disease has disrupted growth of the capital physis.

Intervention of LCPD depends on the age and stage of presentation. The primary goals are to prevent deformity and stop growth disturbance and consequently prevent degenerative joint disease.[225] Some speculation is used in the formulation of intervention algorithms because the natural history of the condition is not well known.[29,225] Generally, 60% of patient with LCPD do not need intervention.[225] Those with early onset have a better prognosis.[29] A study by Herring et al.[182] identified three prognostic conclusions in a study of 438 patients:

1. Children with symptom onset prior to 8 years of age have good results regardless of intervention.
2. In children with onset after 8 years of age with at least 50% lateral pillar height maintenance (Herring groups B and B/C), operatively managed hips had better outcomes than nonoperatively managed hips.
3. Children with hips in Herring group C with greater than 50% collapse of lateral pillar height had poor outcomes regardless of intervention.

Prior to age 4 years, observation is generally recommended.[29] Most children will present at 4 years or older.[29] In these cases the first goal is to reduce the synovitis and symptoms.[82,29] One primary focus during this time is to restore motion.[225] Interventions to assist in this stage include limitation of activity, nonsteroidal anti-inflammatory drugs, light skeletal traction, and physical therapy for ROM.[29,82,225] Most see resolution of symptoms in 7 to 10 days.[225] This may be the only intervention needed in those patients with group A disease or those with group B disease who are under 8 years (Herring lateral pillar classification).[82,225] For those in the fragmentation and reossification stages, impaired hip motion is often due to deformity of the femoral head, and further intervention may be needed.[82]

Containment is an important principle of intervention for LCPD.[225] This describes preventing deformities of the diseased epiphysis by containing the anterolateral part of the avascular capital femoral epiphysis within the depths of the acetabulum, thereby equalizing the pressure on the head and allowing the molding action of the acetabulum to occur.[225] If supported in the acetabulum, weightbearing forces and muscular stresses across the femoral rim will not deform the femoral head.[106] It reduces the forces through the hip joint by actual or relative varus positioning.[225] Full abduction to 45° is recommended for containment, although at least 30° may show favorable results in those with limitations.[25] Containment can be achieved through nonoperative or operative methods.[82,225]

One method of nonoperative containment is bracing. Currently, this is being chosen less by orthopedic surgeons.[82,139,225] The literature has not supported its efficacy.[139] In cases where it is still used, the Atlanta Scottish Rite brace (Fig. 14.28) is generally used. It consists of a metal pelvic band, hip hinges, thigh cuffs, and an extensible bar between the thigh cuffs permitting abduction of the limb but restricting adduction.[82] For mild cases the protocol is to wear the brace during the day and remove it at night, and in more advanced cases the brace may be worn 24 hours a day until there is evidence of new bone formation.[82,225] Casting the lower extremities and using bars between the legs so that the hips are abducted to 45° and rotated internally 5° to 10° is another option.[82] The casts would need to be changed every 3 to 4 months until the femoral head was in the healing stage, possibly 19 months. This may be most useful in older patients whose ROM is too restricted and painful to allow proper positioning of the femoral head in a brace.[82]

Surgical containment is advocated by many studies due to positive results as well as the advantage of early mobilization and the avoidance of prolonged bracing or casting.[225] This seems to be the preferred intervention in those who have a group B or B/C lateral pillar classification and those who are over 8 years of age.[114,139] The timing of the surgery should also be considered. Some recommend that surgery be performed within 8 months of the onset of symptoms.[129] Others have reported that premature physeal closure may occur if the femoral osteotomy is performed too early or too late in the

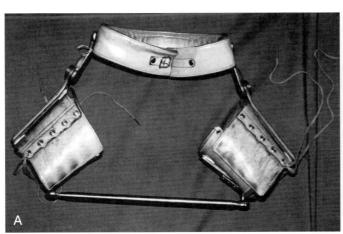
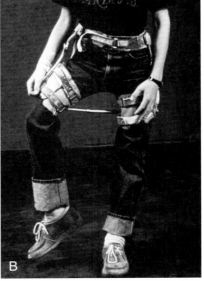

FIG. 14.28 (A–B) Atlanta Scottish Rite orthosis used for treatment of LCPD. (From Hsu JD, Michael J, Fisk J: *AAOS atlas of orthoses and assistive devices.* 4th ed. Philadelphia, Mosby, 2008.)

process.[13] Femoral osteotomies have the best results when performed in the initial or fragmentation stage of the disease.[82,225] In cases of hinge abduction, the femoral head cannot be contained conservatively, and serious damage may occur if this is attempted.[225] Hinge abduction occurs when the deformed femoral head impinges on the lateral margin of the acetabulum during abduction of the hip. Performance of femoral osteotomy can reduce the impingement.[139] During this procedure, trochanteric epiphysiodesis is also recommended to prevent overgrowth and resulting abductor weakness.[29,82]

Performance of an innominate osteotomy has a smaller result of limb shortening compared to femoral osteotomy.[82] This procedure assists with recontainment by redirecting the acetabulum, providing better coverage for the anterolateral portion of the femoral head.[225] For best results the femoral head should be minimally deformed, no significant restriction of ROM should be present at the hip, and it should be early in the course of the disease.[82,225] A procedure combining femoral and innominate osteotomy is an option in severely affected hips.[82,225] The dual approach may provide better containment than either procedure alone.[82] Another option is shelf arthroplasty. This option is being proposed as a primary method of management in children over 8 years of age in groups B or C with a reducible subluxation.[225] The advantage of this procedure may be better coverage of the anterolateral portion of the head allowing better remodeling, prevention of subluxation, and prevention of lateral overgrowth of the epiphysis.[225]

Generally, the time frame from initiation to complete healing is a median of 2.8 years.[106] Many progress through the stages of this disease without complications in later life, although deformation of the epiphysis can occur during the process of revascularization, resulting in degenerative arthritis in later years.[106] The physical therapist should be in communication with the orthopedist during the course of this child's treatment to determine if any precautions should be taken. Intervention will generally focus on mobility, strength, and gait.

Discoid Lateral Meniscus

Menisci are C-shaped fibrocartilaginous structures between the tibial plateau and the femoral condyles that are important for shock absorption, load sharing, reduction of contact stresses, and stability within the knee joint.[192] The lateral meniscus generally covers a larger portion of the tibial plateau than the medial side.[35] A discoid lateral meniscus is an abnormal variant in which the central area is completely filled rather than the normal C shape.[78] Also, the outer rim of the discoid meniscus is much thicker than the normal meniscal rim.[78] This condition is

present in 1% to 3% of the pediatric population and is bilateral in 10% to 20%.[78] A discoid medial meniscus is much less common, with an occurrence of 0.12%.[61] The cause of a discoid meniscus is thought to be multifactorial.[78] It may simply be a congenital anomaly or malformation, but a genetic factor does seem present as well as a higher incidence in the Asian population.[61,78]

Generally, children with a discoid meniscus will present between the ages of 5 and 10 years with a snapping knee joint that is both heard and felt by the child or parent.[78] This may coexist with any combination of pain, giving way, effusion, quadriceps atrophy, limitation of motion, clicking, or locking.[78] More acute symptoms such as significant pain, knee locking, and inability to put weight on the affected extremity are most likely due to a tear in the discoid meniscus.[78] Plain radiographs may show small widening of the lateral joint space but may be normal.[78] MRI would be needed for confirmation.[78]

An asymptomatic knee with an incidental detected discoid meniscus does not require intervention.[78] Arthroscopic surgery is usually recommended in cases of mechanical symptoms with emphasis on meniscal preservation and salvage to prevent degenerative changes in the future.[78]

Sever Disease

Sever disease, or calcaneal apophysitis, is an overuse syndrome caused by repetitive microtrauma at the insertion of the Achilles tendon at the calcaneal apophysis.[103,215] Inflammation results from traction between the Achilles tendon and the plantar fascia and aponeurosis and can also involve the bursa.[104,215] In rare cases, calcaneal apophysitis without intervention can cause calcaneal apophyseal avulsion fractures at the point of attachment.[104] This painful condition generally presents in children ages 8 to 15 years but can be present as young as 6 years.[104] This timing coincides with the presence of the calcaneal growth apophysis, which appears at about 7 years of age and fuses in girls at approximately 13 years and in boys at 15 years.[103]

Symptoms are generally pain in the heel, especially with activity and greater with running and jumping with more strain at the Achilles applied. Local tenderness is present at the heel and pain may be reproduced with resistance of plantar flexion. Factors that may predispose the development of this disorder include: growth and gastrocnemius/soleus tightness with more tension at the Achilles; cavus or planus foot type causing more strain due to harder heel strike, infection, trauma, and obesity.[103]

The condition is usually self-limiting. Conservative intervention is recommended and includes rest, ice, heel cups, heel lifts, reduced activity, and Achilles tendon stretching exercises. In cases of severe pain a short leg walking cast may be helpful.

TABLE 14.7   Diagnostic Criteria for Growing Pains[197,198]

Characteristics of Pain	Inclusion Criteria	Exclusion Criteria
Nature of pain	Intermittent	Persistent
	Some pain-free days and nights; generally occurs once or twice per week with duration of 30–120 min	Increases in severity with time
	Totally pain free between the episodes	
Unilateral or bilateral	Bilateral	Unilateral
Location of pain	Anterior thigh, calf, popliteal fossa, shins	Pain in joints
Time of day	Evening and nights	Night pain that remains in morning
Physical examination	Normal	Signs of inflammation: swelling, tenderness, local trauma or infection, reduced joint ROM, limping
Diagnostic tests	Normal	Objective findings on x-ray, bone scan, or laboratory testing
Limitation of activity	None	Reduced physical activity

ROM, range of motion.

Growing Pains

By definition, growing pains are a clinical presentation of pain in the legs.[55,145] The diagnosis is made by several inclusion and exclusion criteria (Table 14.7). No specific testing is recommended but used to rule out more serious conditions. The prevalence rate of growing pains has varied with many variables in the reporting standards. Kaspiris and Zafiropoulou[111] found a prevalence of 24.5% among 532 children of age 4 to 12 years. Evans and Scutter[56] found a rate of 36.9% in children aged 4 to 6 years. No specific etiologies of growing pains have been identified but theoretical factors include: anatomic factors (e.g., posture, flat feet, genu valgus, scoliosis, decreased bone strength, altered vascular perfusion, joint hypermobility), fatigue or local overuse syndrome, psychological factors, and lower pain threshold.[55,143] Reassurance of the benign nature of the condition, symptomatic intervention using massage, nonsteroidal anti-inflammatory medications, muscle stretching, and time usually resolve the symptoms.[55,143] Another intervention theory is the use of vitamin supplementation in areas of deficiency.[143]

Slipped Capital Femoral Epiphysis (SCFE)

Slipped capital femoral epiphysis (SCFE) is the displacement of the femoral head relative to the femoral neck and shaft. The term *slipped capital femoral epiphysis* is technically incorrect because the femoral epiphysis maintains its normal relationship within the acetabulum but the femoral neck and shaft move relative to the femoral epiphysis and acetabulum.[84,112] The femoral proximal femoral neck and shaft generally displace anteriorly and superiorly (externally rotate) in relation to the femoral head.[34,112]

The incidence rate of SCFE is 2 per 100,000 globally[54] and 10.80 per 100,000 in the United States.[125] Also, in the United States there is a 3.94 times higher rate in black children and 2.53 higher rate in Hispanic children when compared to white children.[125] The presence in boys (13.35 per 100,000) is higher than girls (8.07 per 100,000).[125] Another factor found in the demographic data was climate.[23,125] An increased incidence is noted north of 40° latitude during the summer and south of 40° latitude during the winter.[125] Possible reasons for this include seasonal changes in activity, seasonal patterns of growth and weight gain in adolescence, and vitamin D deficiency caused by decreased cutaneous synthesis during the winter.[23,125] The age on onset is peripubertal. The average age of onset in boys is 14 years and in girls is 12 years.[84] If an onset occurs before the age of 10 years or after the age of 14 years in girls and 16 years in boys, the clinician should suspect an underlying metabolic or systemic condition as a causative factor.[112,125] Also of note is that older children generally have more severe slips.[128] The trend has been for the onset to be at a younger age, which is postulated to correlate with earlier children maturation.[161] Eighty percent of cases are unilateral.[112,125] More than 80 percent of the children diagnosed with SCFE are reportedly obese (body mass index greater than the 95th percentile).[136] This factor is of great concern because of the increasing rates of childhood obesity that are present and may affect the increasing incidence of SCFE.[149] Obesity may increase the risk of SCFE as a result of both higher mechanical loads across the femoral physis and a metabolic disorder.[154] Obese children are noted to have decreased femoral anteversion[63] and a more vertical-oriented proximal femoral physis.[142]

SCFE may be classified by the onset of symptoms or the degree of displacement of the capital femoral epiphysis on the femoral neck.[84] Classification by onset of symptoms is divided into three subtypes[84]:

1. Acute: Occurs suddenly with trauma generally not considered significant enough to result in fracture (e.g., twist of fall). Patient experiences pain in groin, thigh, or knee. This is usually a severe, fracturelike pain. Usually the patient is unable to bear weight and will report quickly for medical care. The position of comfort is usually lying with the affected limb in external rotation. Moderate shortening of the limb is apparent upon examination. Symptoms must be present for less than 3 weeks to be considered acute.

2. Chronic: This is the most frequent form. Adolescent presents with a few months' history of vague groin pain, upper or lower thigh pain, and a limp. Pain may be intermittent or constant and is exacerbated by running or sport activity. The patient generally holds the affected limb in position of external rotation. Thigh atrophy may be apparent in unilateral cases. Local tenderness will be present anteriorly over the hip joint. Loss of hip motion, especially hip internal rotation, flexion, and abduction, may be present although hip extension, external rotation, and adduction may be increased. Shortening of the limb by 1 to 2 cm may be noted.

3. Acute-on-chronic: The patient has already experienced some aching in the hip, thigh, or knee for weeks or even months as a result of a slip. Then, a sudden exacerbation of pain occurs with a further displacement of the epiphysis.

The presence of these symptoms when presenting to a rehabilitation professional warrants significant concern. Some advise that any patient between the ages of 10 and 16 years who presents with a limp and pain in the groin, hip, thigh, or knee should be considered to have an SCFE until a differential diagnosis is made.[112] No weight bearing should be allowed until a medical examination and definitive diagnosis can take place.[112] When the child presents in this manner, the clinician should limit the PT examination in order to limit the possibility of further damage. As with LCPD, the presentation of knee pain may be the primary complaint due to referral from the hip.

A second classification categorizes SCFE by the degree of displacement of the capital femoral epiphysis on the femoral neck.[84] By the Southwick method, mild slips are defined as a head-shaft angle less than 30°, moderate slips are angles between 30 and 60°, and severe slips have an angle more than 60° from the contralateral normal side.[84] Fig. 14.29 demonstrates this measurement.

The etiology of SCFE is multifactorial. Three mechanical factors are thought to predispose a child to SCFE.[84] The first of these is the thinning of the perichondral ring complex (structure surrounding the physis) that occurs with maturation. The strength of this structure may be affected by endocrinopathies (most commonly hypothyroidism), abnormalities requiring growth hormone administration, and chronic renal failure (with secondary hyperparathyroidism).[84,112] A second mechanical factor is relative or absolute femoral retroversion.[84,112] With this position an increased shear force is present across the proximal femoral physis.[84,112] A third factor is a decreased femoral neck-shaft angle with a more vertical physis present. This position increases the shear force across the physis.[84,112] A deeper acetabulum seems to also be a risk factor.[112] When the capital femoral epiphysis is anchored more deeply in the acetabulum, forces across the physis may be increased, especially at the extremes of motion. Another factor may be genetics, but this has not been confirmed.[112] Obesity is a factor that must be considered also.[84,112] Some of the endocrine changes may increase the presence of obesity and add to the risk. Chung et al.[33] found

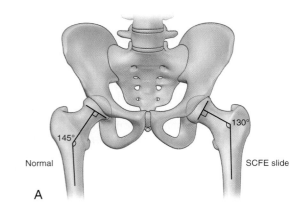

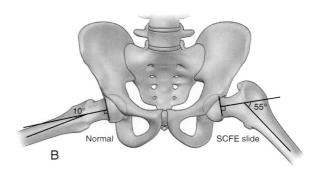

FIG. 14.29 Southwick method of measuring the head-shaft angle for determination of the severity of SCFE. (From Herring JA: *Tachdjian's pediatric orthopaedics: from the Texas Scottish Rite Hospital for Children.* 5th ed. Philadelphia, Saunders, 2014.)

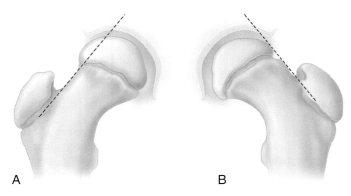

FIG. 14.30 Anteroposterior radiographic findings of a normal hip (A) and a hip with mild chronic slip (B). (From Herring JA: *Tachdjian's pediatric orthopaedics: from the Texas Scottish Rite Hospital for Children.* 5th ed. Philadelphia, Saunders, 2014.)

that mechanical forces across the femoral head during gait reach as high as 6.5 times body weight, and these forces may result in SCFE in a patient who is obese. Also, others report that the combination of proximal femoral varus and retroversion in a child who is overweight could result in forces leading to SCFE.[60]

In most cases, plain anteroposterior and lateral radiographs will confirm the diagnosis of SCFE.[84,112] On the anteroposterior view, widening and irregularity of the physis will be seen early, even before much displacement of the femoral neck and shaft (sometimes termed "preslip").[84,112] A decreased height of the capital femoral epiphysis when the epiphysis lies posterior to the femoral neck may also be visible.[112] In a normal hip a line drawn tangential to the superior femoral neck (Klein line) intersects a small portion of the lateral capital epiphysis.[84] When a slip occurs, this line will intersect a small portion of the epiphysis or not at all.[84] This can be viewed in Fig. 14.30. Lateral views may be more useful in detecting smaller slips.[112] The frog-leg lateral view may be difficult due to pain when positioning the child.[112] When the slip is acute, little or no remodeling of the femoral neck is present on radiographs and only the displacement will be visible.[84] CT of the upper femur may be helpful in identifying the anatomy and the decreased upper femoral neck anteversion or true retroversion.[84,112] CT may be helpful throughout the intervention process in determining if physeal closure has occurred and also postoperatively to determine whether penetration of the hip joint has occurred with the fixation devices.[84,112] Ultrasound is not commonly used for

SCFE but may be an option in the absence of radiographic findings, although an MRI is often chosen.[112] An MRI does have a high specificity for finding avascular necrosis and also is helpful in identifying physeal widening, osseous edema adjacent in the physis, and anatomic deformities.[112] Bone scans also can identify avascular necrosis and chondrolysis.

The goals of intervention for SCFE are to keep the displacement to a minimum, maintain motion, and delay or prevent premature degenerative arthritis. When a child is suspected to have SCFE, immediate referral with radiology testing is recommended.[84,112] Once the diagnosis has been confirmed, absolutely no weight bearing is recommended because this can lead to osteonecrosis.[112] Spica casting is rarely used currently due to the difficulty with stabilization, the length of the intervention (over 100 days), and the complications.[112] Options for surgical management include in situ internal fixation or pinning, bone graft epiphysiodesis, and primary osteotomy through the apex or base of the femoral neck or intertrochanteric area (with or without fixation of the epiphysis to the femoral neck).[84,112] The goal of in situ pinning is to prevent slip progression.[84,112] This procedure may use one or multiple pins to provide stabilization. The screws should be placed as close to the center of the capital epiphysis as possible but remain extra-articular (Fig. 14.31). The screws do not have to routinely be removed and are generally left when asymptomatic. This is considered the intervention of choice in cases of stable SCFE regardless of the severity and also in unstable slips although the exact placement and number of pins may be altered.[84,112] Postoperative management allows those with stable slips to bear weight as tolerated and use crutches as needed. Limited weight bearing is recommended for 3 to 6 weeks in those with unstable slips. These patients can be monitored by radiographs to confirm physeal closure, and return to sporting activities is generally allowed between 3 and 6 months for stable slips and 4 and 6 months for unstable slips.[84,112]

Bone graft epiphysiodesis may be considered in more severe cases in which the insertion of the screw would require exiting the posterior femoral neck and reentering the capital epiphysis to stabilize.[84] Recovery for those with acute slips includes the possibility of traction or hip spica cast until early healing is present, possibly 3 to 6 weeks, with no weight bearing for 6 to 8 weeks.[84,112] In those who have stable slips, toe-touch weight bearing with crutches may begin 2 to 3 days postoperatively and

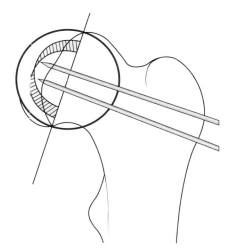

FIG. 14.31 Placement of screws in the treatment of SCFE should be near the center of the epiphysis but remain extraarticular. (From Herring JA: *Tachdjian's pediatric orthopaedics: from the Texas Scottish Rite Hospital for Children.* 5th ed. Philadelphia, Saunders, 2014.)

progressed with physeal healing (6 to 12 weeks).[84,112] An osteotomy may be chosen when a chronic or healed slip has resulted in a head-shaft deformity between 30° and 70° as this allows correction.[84] Following this procedure, patients are allowed protected toe-touch weight bearing until healed.[84]

Complications of SCFE are avascular necrosis and chondrolysis.[54,201] Avascular necrosis of the femoral head is more frequently associated with acute and unstable slips and is most likely due to vascular injury associated with the initial femoral head displacement, with more severe steps exhibiting greater involvement of the vascular supply.[201] Additional problems can occur with aggressive manipulation of the femoral head or penetration of the fixation device in the posterior cortex of the femoral head or articular surface.[201] Intervention should be directed at maintaining motion and preventing collapse by decreasing weight bearing until healing occurs.[201] Chondrolysis is an acute dissolution of articular cartilage in association with rapid progressive joint stiffness and pain.[201] Although this can occur in the uncorrected hip,[54,201] it has been most often found with manipulative reduction, prolonged immobilization, realignment osteotomies, and pin penetration of the femoral head.[201] The rate of these problems has decreased significantly in recent years with improved screw placement.[201] The joint space narrows, hip motion decreases, and an abduction contracture may develop.[54] Intervention should include modification of activities, use of crutches, gentle ROM to maintain motion, and anti-inflammatory medications.[201] Physical therapy may be helpful during this time to keep the patient mobile. A combination of avascular necrosis and chondrolysis is extremely devastating and usually results in hip fusion.[54]

The risk for development of degenerative arthritis in the hip with SCFE is directly related to the severity of the residual deformity at skeletal maturity.[84] Most conditions that do or do not receive intervention will result in some degree of osteoarthritis because of the presence of some biomechanical derangement.[112] The complications of avascular necrosis and chondrolysis greatly accelerate the development of osteoarthritis (OA) and may even lead to end-stage OA in adolescence.[112] Some studies

are being performed to determine if OA may be prevented by restoring more normal proximal femoral anatomy by performing proximal femoral redirectional osteotomies, although long-term follow-up is not available at this time.[8]

Osgood-Schlatter Syndrome

Osgood-Schlatter disease, or syndrome, is characterized by activity-related pain at the anterior knee due to repetitive traction of the patellar tendon on the tibial tubercle ossification center or apophysis, resulting in inflammation and pain.[12] Radiographically, the severity can be classified into three grades: grade I shows slight elevation of the tibial tubercle, grade II shows radiolucency of the tibial tubercle, and grade III shows fragmentation of the tibial tubercle.[75] Several contributory factors have been suggested, including trauma, local alterations of the chondral tissue,[50] and mechanical overpull by the extensor muscles of the knee, which can result in patella alta and traction apophysitis,[9,102] eccentric muscle pull and muscle tightness,[96] reduced width of the patellar angle,[187] and increased external tibial torsion.[67]

Generally, this condition is seen in the apophyseal stage when the secondary ossification center of the tibial tuberosity appears.[75] Because this stage differs in the development of boys and girls, some differences are seen in the age of onset of Osgood-Schlatter syndrome. For boys, common ages are between 12 and 15 years and for girls common ages are between the 8 and 12 years.[75] Up to 30% may have bilateral involvement.[27] About 50% of all cases are involved in regular athletic activity.[12] Osgood-Schlatter syndrome may present as acute, severe pain, causing a child to limp, or may be noted by the child over a period of months as low-grade discomfort, usually brought on by running, jumping, or participation in sports. Direct pressure, such as kneeling, is also painful. Clinically, tenderness at the tibial tubercle and swelling may be seen. This is a self-limiting process that responds to activity modification, nonsteroidal anti-inflammatory medications, and application of ice. Stretching to improve flexibility of hamstrings and quadriceps may reduce symptoms.[12] In more severe cases, immobilization for 7 to 10 days may alleviate symptoms.[201] The symptoms will generally resolve when the tubercle fuses to the main body of the tibia, usually at around 15 years of age. For those with persistent problems after skeletal maturity, excision of the ossicle and prominence is an option.[201]

Osteochondritis Dissecans

Osteochondritis dissecans (OD or OCD) describes the separation of subchondral bone from the articular surface. It is characterized by a localized necrosis of the subchondral bone, which later revascularizes, reabsorbing and reossifying the bone necrosis.[28] Joint damage may occur because these lesions are adjacent to articular cartilage.[51] The fragment of bone can also detach, becoming a loose body in the joint.[51] The actual cause of osteochondritis dissecans is not known although several theories and factors have been proposed.[24,233] Repetitive microtrauma, including shear and compressive forces, leads to subchondral bone stress, especially in athletic persons.[155] Other factors such as genetic predisposition, ischemia that may be caused by vascular spasm, fat emboli, infection thrombosis, and abnormal ossification seem to play a causative role.[87] Patients are typically 12 to 20 years of age[87] and the male-to-female ratio is 2:1.[178] The most commonly affected areas are the knee (medial femoral condyle), the elbow joint (capitellum), and the talus (superior lateral dome).[51] The classic location is the lateral aspect of the medial femoral condyle, possibly a result of the repetitive impingement against the prominent tibial spine.[24] Symptoms are a vague, poorly localized knee pain, with recurrent effusion.[233] Also loose bodies may result as articular cartilage breaks off causing mechanical symptoms of locking or catching of the knee.[233] Antalgic gait and an externally rotated gait pattern may also present.[24] Clinical exam may show atrophy of the quadriceps and tenderness along the surface of the affected chondral area with palpation (distal aspect of the medial femoral condyle with the knee flexed to 90°).[233]

OCD can be diagnosed with radiographs with a radiolucent area identifying an area of the lesion. Multiple views are typically recommended (anteroposterior, lateral, merchant, and notch or tunnel views) because the posterior aspect of the medial femoral condyle is more difficult to visualize.[233] MRI is useful in detecting the lesion and also in staging the lesion for determination of intervention.[24,233]

The preferred intervention in skeletally immature patients with symptomatic yet stable OCD lesions is limitation of weight bearing or even immobilization for 6 to 8 weeks followed by unloader bracing and activity restriction.[233] The important thing to communicate to the athlete is that if pain is not eliminated, the lesion is not healing.[24] Up to 90 percent of small lesions may heal spontaneously.[201] Lesions that fail conservative intervention, large lesions, or unstable OCD lesions may require surgical intervention.[233] Surgery may be needed to remove loose fragments.[51] Also, drilling the necrotic fragment may allow more rapid vascular ingrowth and replacement.[51] The drilling provides channels for adequate revascularization and healing. Fixation with hardware and bone graft are also options for stabilization.[51,201,233] In lesions that involve a large portion of weight-bearing area, OA is a risk in future years.[51]

Tarsal Coalition

Tarsal coalition is a failure of segmentation between adjoining tarsal bones. Coalitions may exist between all of the tarsal bones, but talocalcaneal and calcaneonavicular coalitions are the most common.[26] The etiology seems to have a congenital factor.[26,235] It has been found to be bilateral 50% to 80% of the time and occurs in both sexes equally.[26] It occurs in less than 1% of the population.[26] Symptoms generally present in early adolescence,[201] when the abnormal cartilaginous bar begins to ossify. The resulting fusion imposes stress on adjacent joints and consequently may result in degenerative arthritis, pain, and peroneal spasm.[201] Specifically, subtalar motion is greatly restricted in the talocalcaneal conditions and moderately limited in calcaneonavicular and talonavicular coalitions.[235] This leads to a rigid flatfoot deformity, with significant restriction of inversion.[26,235] Radiographs will generally show the bony coalitions with the three standard views of the foot.[235] In the fibrous or cartilaginous stages a CT or MRI allows for better definition and also can provide delineation of the extent of joint involvement as well as degenerative changes.[235] The goal of intervention is to limit joint ROM to reduce pain and muscle spasms.[235] Conservative intervention may include arch supports, short leg walking casts, immobilization in neutral or slight varus positions, and NSAIDs.[235] Surgical resection is an option in those who fail conservative intervention.[235]

Freiberg Disease

Freiberg disease is an idiopathic segmental avascular necrosis of the head of a metatarsal.[201] Most commonly, this occurs in adolescent girls, ages 13 to 18 years, and involves the second metatarsal.[201] It is unilateral in 90% of the cases.[12] The etiology is unknown, but factors such as trauma, repetitive stress, disruption in blood supply, or improper shoe wear may affect ossification.[12] Structural deformities, such as hallux valgus or hallux rigidus, may transfer the weight lateral to the second metatarsal increasing stress as well.[189] When microfractures occur at the junction of the metaphysis and growth plate, inadequate circulation to the epiphysis results.[222] Clinical presentation generally consists of pain in the forefoot, localized to the head of the second metatarsal, and localized swelling and limitation of motion in the metacarpophalangeal (MP) joint.[201,222] Early stages of the disease may not be detected on standard radiographs, and advanced imaging such as MRI or CT may be needed.[189,201,222] Later radiographs will show the stages of irregularity of the articular surface, sclerosis, fragmentation, and finally re-formation.[189,201,222] Conservative intervention includes offloading the metatarsal with orthotics, metatarsal pads, modified shoe gear, and removable walking boots.[189] Generally, this may take a course of 4 to 6 weeks.[201,222] If conservative intervention fails, surgical resection of the metatarsal heads is an option.[201,222]

Accessory Navicular

Accessory navicular is an extra bone that develops on the medial side of the tarsal navicular, either within the posterior tibial tendon or as a separate bone.[127,201] It is a result of the failure of the secondary ossification center of the navicular to unite during childhood.[127] This occurs in about 10% of the population.[201] Classification consists of three types:
1. Type I is a small oval to round ossicle within the posterior tibialis tendon that is seldom symptomatic.[189,201,222]
2. Type II is a larger lateral projection from the medial aspect of the navicular with a clear separation from the navicular.[189,222] The fibrocartilaginous connection between the tuberosity from the navicular is disrupted and may be mistaken for a fracture.[127,201] These are often symptomatic, and disruptions commonly occur during adolescence in relation to repetitive trauma.[127,201]
3. Type III occurs when a bony bridge is present between the accessory navicular and the navicular.[127] This may represent an end stage of type II[127] and may be prominent enough to cause irritation of the overlying skin.[201,222]

Symptoms often begin in childhood with medial pressure of the accessory navicular against the shoe.[127] Commonly, the patient will report pain and tenderness along the medial midfoot region.[127] Swelling and erythema may also present.[127] The symptoms are usually exacerbated with weight-bearing activity.[127] Often radiographs are the only imaging modality needed for diagnosis.[127] Conservative intervention is directed toward relief of symptoms. Wider, more comfortable shoes to off-load the medial midfoot as well as orthotics may be helpful. Casting can limit pull of the posterior tibial tendon.[127] Activity modification is also recommended along with NSAIDs.[127] Surgical excision of the accessory navicular can be performed in extreme cases.[127]

Additional Causes of Limp

Other orthopedic conditions that can cause an acute limp in children from birth to age 5 years include juvenile idiopathic arthritis (see Chapter 7), nonaccidental trauma (fractures or soft tissue injuries), hemophilia, discitis, discoid meniscus, popliteal cysts, foreign bodies, and bone tumors.

Patellofemoral pain and recurrent patellar subluxation or dislocations are common causes of limp in ages 10 to 15 years (see Chapter 15 for a more detailed discussion). Monoarticular inflammatory arthritis and gonococcal arthritis also can cause acute onset of limp in a child.

Many types of neoplasms and related bone lesions can cause a child to limp. Commonly seen conditions include osteoid osteoma, unicameral bone cyst, osteochondroma (single or multiple), enchondroma, aneurysmal bone cyst, eosinophilic granuloma, and nonossifying fibroma. Symptoms may include limp, pain, and pathologic fracture through the lesion.[201,222]

HEMANGIOMA/VASCULAR MALFORMATION

A hemangioma is an abnormal proliferation of blood vessels that may occur in any vascularized tissue. Hemangiomas that affect the musculoskeletal system are more accurately termed vascular malformations. Vascular malformations are rare congenital lesions that are caused by a defect during vascular embryogenesis. By definition, they are always present at birth but are not always clinically evident until later in life.[124,132] Skeletal changes are commonly seen with vascular malformations, although they are rarely seen with hemangiomas.[132]

At birth, vascular formations are fully formed, although the lesion may not be clinically apparent.[124,132] This type of lesion may appear later because of vessel dilation or hematoma formation, resulting in rapid enlargement.[132] Males and females are equally affected.[132] Vascular malformations can be subclassified by the predominant type of vessels found within the lesion (i.e., venous, arterial, lymphatic, capillary, or mixed) and by blood flow within the lesion (i.e., high flow versus low flow).[132] Venous malformations often remain asymptomatic although complications may include pain secondary to vessel dilation, bleeding, and hematoma formation, as well as intra-articular involvement, hemarthrosis, pathologic fractures of bone, and compression of adjacent structures.[124,132] They may also result in skeletal and soft tissue undergrowth or overgrowth in an affected limb.[132] Deep arteriovenous malformations can progress to distal ischemia, pain, and necrosis, with consequent risk for fracture, related to arterial steal of the bone.[132] The involvement of bone occurs in 20% of those with vascular malformations.[22]

Diagnostically, the first step in the imaging workup should be an ultrasound and Doppler examination.[124] This testing will allow immediate differentiation of the type of blood flow in the lesion.[124] In cases of low-flow malformations, an MRI is recommended, which helps confirm, characterize, and differentiate the malformation for planning of intervention.[124] If a high-flow lesion is detected, CT or CT angiography (CTA) may be used because they allow for accurate measurement and mapping of the feeding and draining structures and involvement of adjacent structures, which will help in interventional radiologic or surgical planning.[124] Intervention of these lesions varies widely with the extent of involvement. Conservative intervention is recommended when possible and included symptomatic intervention with compression stockings and analgesia.[22] Some cases may require surgical resection and/or intralesional transarterial embolization and amputation when involvement of muscle or bone has resulted in pain, functional impairment, or pathologic fracture.[22] Epiphysiodesis may be required in cases of skeletal overgrowth to correct for leg length discrepancy.[132]

MISCELLANEOUS CONDITIONS

Back Pain

The presence of back pain in children should be considered carefully because it can indicate serious disease in children.[212] Besides mechanical causes, pain could be the result of infection (including discitis related to bacteria), bony and spinal neoplasms, autoinflammatory and autoimmune causes such as chronic recurrent multifocal osteomyelitis, spondyloarthropathies that could progress to ankylosing spondylitis, vasculitis, or reflex neurovascular dystrophy that can manifest as back pain.[212] Findings that indicate further investigation include fever, weight loss, nighttime pain or pain that awakens the child from sleep, neurologic deficits, worsening pain over time, or inflammatory back pain.[212]

The incidence of nonspecific low back pain in adolescents has been reported as high as 74%.[105] Among mechanical causes that should be considered are spondylolysis (unilateral fracture of the pars interarticularis), Scheuermann disease (increasing thoracic or thoracolumbar kyphosis with tightness of the hamstrings and iliopsoas), sacroiliac dysfunction, and apophysitis (growth plate irritation from chronic repetitive stress localized to the iliac crests or ischial tuberosity).[212] Specifically, Scheuermann disease is a disturbance of the vertebral end plates causing anterior vertebral body wedging that results in kyphosis during a growth spurt.[12] Surgery is considered only in severe cases (greater than 75°, pain, unacceptable appearance).[12]

Another factor that has been found to directly affect the incidence of low back pain is BMI.[5,197] Akdag et al.[5] found that a BMI of 19.84 kg/m² was a significant factor for pain intensity in a population of children ages 10 to 18 years. Others determined that the likelihood of joint pain increased by 10% for every 10-kilogram increase of weight and an increase of 3 percent for every unit increase in BMI.[207] A detailed review of spinal conditions may be found in Chapter 8.

Idiopathic Toe-Walking

Toe-walking that persists after the age of 2 years in the absence of neurologic or orthopedic abnormalities is termed idiopathic toe walking (ITW).[220] The incidence of ITW has been reported as nearly 5%.[53] Generally, it is a diagnosis of exclusion, ruling out neurologic involvement (ankylosing spondylitis, cerebral palsy, Charcot-Marie-Tooth disease, muscular dystrophy, spina bifida, tethered cord syndrome, transient focal dystonia), neurogenic and developmental disabilities (Angelman syndrome, autism spectrum disorders, developmental coordination disorder, global developmental delay, schizophrenia), and traumatic or biomechanical conditions (soft tissue injuries, congenital talipes equinus, leg length discrepancy, puncture wounds, scarring, tumor in belly of gastrocnemius muscle, venous malformation of the gastrocnemius muscle, viruses).[231] No known cause has been identified for ITW but a family history is common[220,231] and a possible autosomal dominant genetic link has been suggested.[231] Initially, children with ITW walk on their toes but can bear weight with their foot flat on request and with concentration on their gait.[220] Over time, an equinus contracture, defined as a limitation of at least 10° of passive ankle dorsiflexion with the knee extended and the ankle in neutral position, may develop.[220] If not corrected, the contracture can develop into acquired flatfoot, metatarsalgia, diabetic foot ulceration, and plantar fasciitis.[220]

Intervention for ITW may vary due to lack of evidence for effectiveness of intervention.[85,220] Generally, it improves without intervention.[85,220] Conservative measures may include stretching of the plantar flexors including passive stretching, prolonged ankle foot orthosis, serial casting, and/or Botox injections.[220,231] Surgical lengthening of the Achilles tendon may often be performed in cases that persist.[85,220,231]

Achondroplasia

Achondroplasia (dwarfism) is the most common of a large group of conditions known as the osteochondrodysplasias, a heterogenous group of disorders characterized by abnormal growth and remodeling of cartilage and bone.[160] Prevalence for achondroplasia is 0.36 to 0.6 per 10,000 live births.[99] The disorder is an autosomal dominant trait, but 80 percent of cases are the result of a random mutation.[160] The typical presentation of achondroplasia is obvious at birth.[160] Features include:

- symmetric shortening of all long bones with proximal portions more affected and lower limb more affected than upper limb;
- epiphysis is closer to metaphyses resulting in apparent increase in the depth of the articular cartilage space; results in chevron or ball and socket relationship deformity, commonly at lower end of femur;
- hand bones appear thick and tubular with widely separated second and third digits of the hands and inability to approximate them in extension;
- pelvic cavity is short and broad;
- vertebral bodies that are cuboid shaped, which may cause narrowing of the spinal canal and cord compression, with short pedicles and associated dorso-lumbar lordosis;
- skull base that is narrowed, with narrowing of foramen magnum with relative midface hypoplasia and depressed nasal bones.[160]

Neurologic impairments and complications are possible with 10% of children showing neurologic signs by 10 years of age.[99] The altered body position does affect developmental motor skill sequencing but is consistent within this group and milestone reference tables do exist.[99] Positioning should be considered and restricted time in sitting is advised to avoid development of a fixed thoracolumbar kyphosis.[99]

Counseling to maintain appropriate weight for height is helpful in controlling orthopedic injuries.[99]

LEG LENGTH INEQUALITY

Leg length inequality (LLI) may also be called leg length discrepancy (LLD) and is often defined as a 2.5 cm or greater difference in leg length. Differences smaller than this tend not to cause clinical problems. Differences in leg length may be due to relative overgrowth or shortening.

Origin

The origin of LLI is divided into a number of categories: trauma; congenital, neuromuscular, or acquired disease; infections causing physeal growth arrest; tumors; and vascular disorders. Types of trauma include epiphyseal and diaphyseal injuries. Epiphyseal injuries with growth plate closure may be asymmetrical, as in fracture involving the medial epiphysis of the distal femur. This type of injury can result in an angular deformity (varus), as well as shortening of the femur.

Congenital disorders include hemihypertrophy, in which one half of the body (the arm and leg) is larger than the other. Conversely, in hemiatrophy, one half of the body is smaller than the other. These sometimes can be difficult to distinguish, necessitating a decision on which arm and leg best "match" the rest of the body. Proximal focal femoral deficiency, congenital coax vara, fibular and tibial hemimelia, and other focal dysplasias are additional causes of LLI (see Chapter 13). DDH can also cause a leg length discrepancy as the result of an apparent femoral shortening noted when the hip is dislocated or actual shortening caused by femoral head AVN. Surgical interventions for DDH can change the leg length; these include use of a varus derotation osteotomy (VDRO), which shortens the femur, and pelvic osteotomies, which may add up to one inch to the height of the pelvis.

Neuromuscular disorders can cause asymmetrical growth of lower extremity bones. Decreased growth in the affected leg may be due to decreased muscle forces in weak or paralyzed muscles. Examples include myelodysplasia, poliomyelitis, and hemiplegia caused by congenital or acquired cerebral palsy. However, not all cases of LLI should be corrected. A child with hemiplegia can have a short lower limb on the affected side. With weakness and spasticity in that leg, foot clearance may be difficult as a result of decreased hip and knee flexion and equinus. The shortness of the leg makes foot clearance in swing easier.

Acquired conditions such as LCPD and SCFE can also result in shortened lower extremity, usually as a result of AVN of the femoral head, or occasionally as the result of surgical intervention. Fibrous dysplasia and tumors, including benign bone cysts and malignant neoplasms, can change leg length by interfering with growth centers or secondarily as a result of fracture or surgical intervention.

Impairments

The effects of LLI vary widely among patients because of the actual amount of difference and how well the patient physically compensates for it, the possibility of progression of the inequality, the patient's perception of the problem, and the overall picture of muscle strength, motor control, and ROM. If the discrepancy is marked or compensation is limited, poor cosmesis may be evident, and a significant increase in work by the muscles may be required to walk.[4] Musculoskeletal adaptations and compensations may result. These secondary impairments include pelvic obliquity, which requires more effort by the abductor muscles of the hip and lumbar paraspinal muscles, placing more strain on the spinal ligament.[4] Others have reported the development of scoliosis, low back pain, sciatica, excessive stress on hip of knee joints, and lower extremity dysfunction such as stress fracture, plantar fasciitis, or parapatellar knee pain.[83] The development of osteoarthritis with LLI has been shown.[4] In children a gait strategy is used that puts more work on the longer limb, which may be associated with the higher number of cases of OA in the longer limbs.[4] Compensatory patterns include circumduction of persistent flexion of the longer limb, vaulting over the longer limb, toe-walking on the shorter limb, and a greater vertical displacement of the center of body mass.[4] Consequently, musculoskeletal adaptations may be observed that include pelvic tilt, knee flexion, and equinus. These problems may be significant but easily accommodated because of the inherent energy and motivation usually present in children. In adulthood, however, factors of increased size and weight, increased energy expenditure to walk, increased sensitivity regarding the poor cosmesis of a lurching gait, and long-term effects of asymmetrical lumbosacral spinal alignment may combine to significantly reduce the ability to walk and even render a person nonambulatory.

Clinical Examination

The physical therapy examination for patients with LLI starts with obtaining a complete history, including any previous intervention. The physical examination incorporates the following elements:

Measurement of ROM, joint stability, and muscle strength of the trunk, hips, knees, ankles, and feet

Sensation of the lower extremities

Anthropometric measurements: sitting and standing height, weight, and arm span; girth of thighs and calves; leg lengths

Functional activities such as rising from a chair to standing and moving down to the floor and back up

Clinical analysis of posture and gait, including observation of the spine and lower extremity alignment and substitution patterns; observations of the patient with and without assistive devices and shoe lift during gait on level ground, ramps, and stairs.

These tests will help determine if the LLI is structural due to a measurable difference in a lower extremity segment, functional due to asymmetry in the positioning of one lower extremity relative to the other, or a combination of these.[83]

Different methods of clinical measurement of leg length are used. One is to level the pelvis in standing, using graduated blocks under the short leg, and then to measure the height of the blocks. This method is pictured in Fig. 14.32. Measurements with a tape measure may also be taken with the child supine on an examining table from the superior iliac spine to the medial joint line and the medial malleolus or from the umbilicus to the medial malleolus (Fig. 14.33). A third method has been described by Smith[195] and labeled the thigh-leg technique. The patient is placed supine on an examining table with the hips and knee flexed 90°. Discrepancies are measured between the table and the thigh, between the thighs at the knees, and between the soles with the knees even (Fig. 14.34). Caution should be used when correcting LLI of less than 5 mm when only clinical examination methods have been used because of the inaccuracy and lack of reliability of the techniques.[20]

Radiographic measurement of leg length will provide more accurate measurements of an inequality. Computed tomography scanogram is currently used by many.[74,83] The radiation dosage for this procedure is 1% of the exposure with conventional radiography.[83] This method is quicker, which better accommodates small children, and also can be used when contractures or external fixators are present.[74,83] This compares to the standard x-ray technique in which the patient is positioned on the x-ray table with a ruler alongside the legs, and three radiographs are taken at the level of the hips, knees, and ankles, with the patient held motionless. These three views with the ruler markings next to them allow the examiner to measure the length of the femur and tibia and combine them for the total leg length. Landmarks commonly used are the top of the femoral head, the bottom of the medial femoral condyle, and the tibial plafond. A film of the left wrist and hand may also be performed at the same time for determination of skeletal age of the patient.

Measurement error is present in any of these techniques, making both clinical and radiographic leg length determinations an inexact science. Determining the percentage of growth

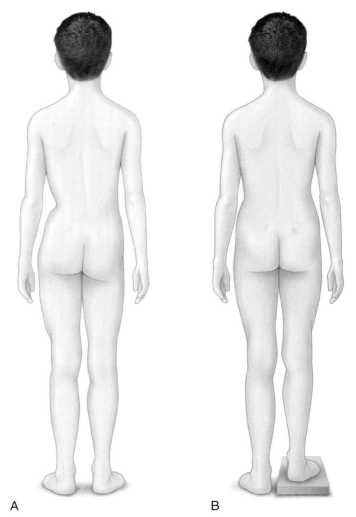

A   B

FIG. 14.32 Clinical measurement of leg length inequality using graduated blocks. (A) Leg length inequality in standing can be viewed with asymmetric iliac crest or posterior iliac spine heights with the patient standing erect. The patient must be standing evenly on the legs, with knees straight and feet flat on the floor. (B) A measurement of inequality can be made by using graduated blocks until the pelvis is level. (From Herring JA: *Tachdjian's pediatric orthopaedics: from the Texas Scottish Rite Hospital for Children.* 5th ed. Philadelphia, Saunders, 2014.)

inhibition assists in estimating the eventual discrepancy at skeletal maturity. For example, a 10% inhibition of growth in the short leg may result in minor discrepancy when the child is quite young. When the leg is 20 cm long, a 10 percent shortening is only 2 cm. However, as the child matures, when the unaffected leg is 70 cm long, a 10% inhibition of growth on the involved side will result in a shortening of 7 cm, which is significant.

If the patient can be followed with serial measurement over time, scanogram measurement of total length of both the long and the short leg and skeletal age at the time of each scanogram can be plotted on the Moseley graph, which depicts past growth and predicts future growth[148] (Fig. 14.35). Timing of epiphysiodesis is based on the predicted LLI at skeletal maturity. The effects of surgery can also be plotted on the graph to predict alteration in leg lengths and the eventual impact on discrepancy

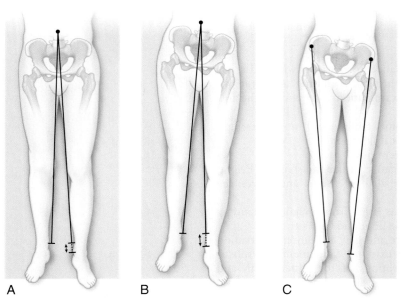

FIG. 14.33 Assessment of functional and actual leg length inequality while supine using a tape measure. Figure A represents one patient and Figures B and C represent a second patient. (A) With the legs in an extended and neutral position, lengths are uneven when measured from the umbilicus to the medial malleolus (left leg longer than right) and from the anterior iliac spine to the medial malleolus in a patient with structural leg length discrepancy. (B) In a patient with fixed pelvic obliquity but no true limb length inequality, asymmetry is noted on the measurement from the umbilicus. In this measurement, the adducted left leg is longer than the right. (C) Measurement from the anterior iliac spine to the medial malleolus demonstrates no structural length inequality. (From Herring JA: *Tachdjian's pediatric orthopaedics: from the Texas Scottish Rite Hospital for Children.* 5th ed. Philadelphia, Saunders, 2014.)

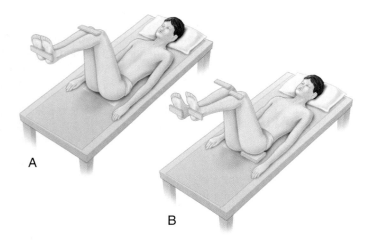

FIG. 14.34 Thigh-leg technique for measurement of leg length inequality. (A) Patient is positioned supine with the hips and knees flexed to 90°. Discrepancy between the sides is noted between the table and thigh, between the thighs and knees, and between the soles with the knees even. Figure A shows no discrepancy. (B) Discrepancy in leg length is seen with use of graduated blocks to determine amount. (From Herring JA: *Tachdjian's pediatric orthopaedics: from the Texas Scottish Rite Hospital for Children.* 5th ed. Philadelphia, Saunders, 2014.)

at skeletal maturity. Paley et al.[159] have developed a mathematical formula that allows these predictions to be accurately based on as few as one or two measurements (Table 14.8).

Intervention

Intervention for LLI is affected by the patient's age, current discrepancy, and the projected discrepancy at maturity.[74] During growth the family and surgeon may conservatively intervene with shoe lifts or other prosthetic devices. The three final options for intervention after skeletal maturity are: continue the prosthetic or orthotic resources as in the childhood years, shorten the long limb, or lengthen the short limb. The general guideline is:

    0–2 cm: No intervention
    2–6 cm: Orthotic use, epiphysiodesis, skeletal shortening
    6–20 cm: Limb reconstruction (limb lengthening with or without adjunctive procedures)
    > 20 cm: Prosthetic fitting (with or without surgical optimization)[74]

Another consideration is the contribution of growth by each growth center (Table 14.9).

Orthotic Intervention

Lifts inside the shoe of the short limb are usually effective for 1.5- to 2-cm correction.[74] For larger discrepancies, lifts may be applied to the outside of the shoe.[74] Lifts higher than 5 cm are not tolerated well with the weight of the lift being one factor.

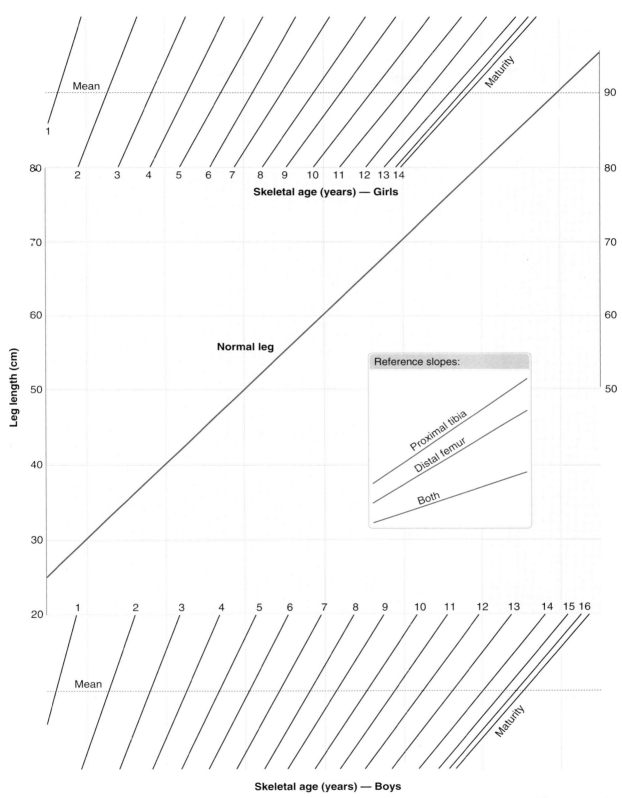

FIG. 14.35 Moseley graph used to plot a patient's serial scanogram measurements and bone ages to determine the discrepancy at maturity and the possibilities for surgical intervention. Growth of a short leg would be depicted by a line below the normal leg line. The surgical increase in the length of the short leg would allow the two legs to be approximately equal at skeletal maturity. (Redrawn from Moseley CE: A straight-line graph for leg-length discrepancies. *J Bone Joint Surg Am* 59:174-179, 1977.)

TABLE 14.8 Lower Limb Multipliers for Boys and Girls Used to Predict the Limb Length Discrepancy and the Amount of Growth Remaining

| Age (yrs + mos) | MULTIPLIER | |
	Boys	Girls
Birth	5.080	4.630
0 + 3	4.550	4.155
0 + 6	4.050	3.725
0 + 9	3.600	3.300
1 + 0	3.240	2.970
1 + 3	2.975	2.750
1 + 6	2.825	2.600
1 + 9	2.700	2.490
2 + 0	2.590	2.390
2 + 3	2.480	2.295
2 + 6	2.385	2.200
2 + 9	2.300	2.125
3 + 0	2.230	2.050
3 + 6	2.110	1.925
4 + 0	2.000	1.830
4 + 6	1.890	1.740
5 + 0	1.820	1.660
5 + 6	1.740	1.580
6 + 0	1.670	1.510
6 + 6	1.620	1.460
7 + 0	1.570	1.430
7 + 6	1.520	1.370
8 + 0	1.470	1.330
8 + 6	1.420	1.290
9 + 0	1.380	1.260
9 + 6	1.340	1.220
10 + 0	1.310	1.190
10 + 6	1.280	1.160
11 + 0	1.240	1.130
11 + 6	1.220	1.100
12 + 0	1.180	1.070
12 + 6	1.160	1.050
13 + 0	1.130	1.030
13 + 6	1.100	1.010
14 + 0	1.080	1.000
14 + 6	1.060	NA
15 + 0	1.040	NA
15 + 6	1.020	NA
16 + 0	1.010	NA
16 + 6	1.010	NA
17 + 0	1.000	NA

NA, not applicable.
From Paley D, Bhave A, Herzenberg JE, et al.: Multiplier method for predicting limb-length discrepancy. *J Bone Joint Surg Am* 82:1432, 2000.

TABLE 14.9 Percentage of Growth for Each Growth Center in the Femur and Tibia

Growth Center	For Entire Leg	Total Length of Femur	Total Length of Tibia
Proximal femur	15%	30%	–
Distal femur	35%	70%	–
Proximal tibia	30%	–	60%
Distal tibia	20%	–	40%

Also, the weakness of the legs does not counter the inversion stress, and frequent ankle strains may result. More stability can be achieved by an orthotic extension up the posterior calf or above the malleoli.[74] A prosthesis is an option for those with a congenital amputation.[74] Also, amputation is sometimes chosen in cases where the femur is less than half the length of the contralateral side, if the length is projected to be > 15 to 20 cm and especially if the foot is not functional.[74] The decision for amputation is difficult for families but those who undergo surgery and prosthetic early in life show very good results with adaptation to a prosthesis.[74] Discussion with families and children who have undergone this intervention may be helpful for families making this decision.[74]

Shortening the long limb. Shortening of the longer limb in the growing child can be achieved through epiphysiodesis, the surgical physeal arrest of one or more growth centers in the long leg, which allows the short leg to "catch up" in length. This is a good way to intervene with mild to moderate discrepancy. In order for this to be an option, the child must have enough growth remaining to recoup the differences in length.[74] It is especially helpful in cases of overgrowth from fracture, inflammation, or overgrowth syndromes.[74]

Timing of the epiphysiodesis is obviously crucial. Future growth of each leg must be predicted and the surgery performed at a time when the amount of growth denied the long leg will match the amount of growth still available in the short leg, allowing them to be approximately equal in length at skeletal maturity. If the epiphysiodesis if performed too early, the long leg may actually become the short leg, with an obviously less than optimal surgical result. Epiphysiodesis can also be performed on only the medial or lateral growth part of the growth plate to correct angular deformities. For example, a fracture of the distal femur may cause damage to the medial aspect of the distal femoral growth plate. The lateral part of the growth plate continues to function normally, and the leg grows into varus, which also produces a functional shortening.

Another option for shortening the long leg is a shortening osteotomy, usually considered in a skeletally mature patient who is not a candidate for epiphysiodesis. A second option for correction of angular deformities is to staple the medial or lateral growth plate; for the limb that is in varus in the growing child, the lateral portion of the growth plate can be stapled to stop growth while the medial side continues to grow.

Lengthening the short limb. Surgical lengthening of the short leg has appeal because the surgery is performed on the affected leg, not the "normal" leg, and opportunity exists for correction of discrepancies of much greater magnitude. Criteria for leg lengthening include a discrepancy of greater than 4 to 6 cm, adequate soft tissue mobility available to allow correction, and a stable joint above and below, although unstable joints can be protected with an external frame. The femur and tibia can each be lengthened or both. The final goal is equal leg length with equal knee heights in standing.

Corrections up to 15 to 20 cm are now possible with technology.[74] Corrections can be very involved and time consuming and this should be well explained to the patient and family. Lengthening often consists of a series of operations to optimize the results with each increasing the length 10 to 20 percent of the original bone length.[74] Each lengthening attempt will require at least 1 month of fixator time for every centimeter of length gained followed by an external fixator for 6 months with rehabilitation following.[74] Opinions vary as to the best timing for this procedure. Some support delaying limb lengthening until 10 to 12 years so that the patient can comprehend the task ahead while others suggest that lengthening at an earlier age (5 to 7 years) may allow for more normal growth post lengthening and perhaps less ultimate discrepancy.[74] Other osseous or joint deformities (e.g., hip dysplasia, ankle valgus) should be addressed prior to initiating this procedure.[74]

Methods of lengthening include distraction osteogenesis, limb lengthening with external fixation, distraction epiphysiolysis, lengthening over intramedullary rod, and intramedullary lengthening device.[74] With distraction osteogenesis, an osteotomy is performed and the bone ends are approximated for 3 to 14 days. After this period of time in which the inflammatory phase of fracture healing occurs, the osteotomy then enters the reparative stage of fracture healing and the site is distracted 1 mm per day. Maintaining motion is very important during this procedure, with some recommending discontinuation if a knee extension contracture of $> 30°$ occurs.[74] Distraction will be continued until the goal is achieved. The patient is then in the consolidation phase and full weight bearing is allowed. The device remains on the leg until radiographs determine the strength of the bone is adequate for weight bearing.[74]

An external fixator can also be used for limb lengthening. There are several types of external fixators and techniques. One of note is the Ilizarov technique. An osteotomy is performed as described above. In this procedure, fixation is achieved by tensioned through-and-through wires attached to complete or partial rings that are attached to the limb by multiple bone pins.[74] The lengthening is performed through turning the device at a rate of 1 mm per day.

Distraction epiphysiolysis is designed to correct growth at the physis. A distraction force is applied across the physis until it fractures. Lengthening is then achieved through gradual distraction. This method is more painful, and complications of further damage to the physis are possible. It is generally used for children who are very near the end of growth.[74]

Lengthening over an intramedullary rod has the advantage of removal of the external fixator earlier and quicker recovery of knee motion.[74] The rod maintains alignment during the distraction and the consolidation phases. With the rod providing stability, the external fixator can be removed after lengthening is complete. Because the femur remains stabilized, progressive weight bearing and restoration of motion can begin.[74] The risks are damage to the femoral physis and AVN as well as the knee having a more medial placement relative to the femur during the process due to the lengthening being performed along the anatomic axis of the femur.[74] Changes in knee positioning could affect distribution of weight.[74] Infection is also a concern.[74]

Intramedullary nailing allows lengthening and stabilization without the risks of an external fixator.[74] These are not as widely used for children because of risk of damage to the growth plates.[74] This may be the best option in those who have already experienced damage.[74]

The list of complications for limb lengthening include hypertension during lengthening, device malfunction, pin failure, pin tract infection, osteomyelitis, premature consolidation, poor bone formation, fracture after device removal, decreased growth of the limb, malalignment during lengthening, pain, soft tissue scarring, muscle tightness leading to joint stiffness contracture, dislocation, stretch paralysis of the nerves, and joint damage.[74]

Children undergoing leg lengthening as well as the family may need guidance because of the pain that may be experienced as well as the length of the process. The child may experience frustration, anger, and fear because of the temporary loss of independence inherent in the procedure. Difficult behavior may require intervention by a psychologist to assist the child and family in developing appropriate coping strategies. Candidates for surgical lengthening must be extremely motivated, with a supportive and committed family. Successful limb lengthening also mandates a comprehensive medical care system, with knowledgeable, experienced physicians, nurses, and therapists to guide the patient and family through the process.

Physical therapy may be helpful preoperatively to perform crutch-fitting and instruction in restricted weight bearing on the involved leg, instruction in home exercises, and postoperative positioning and splinting in conjunction with the patient, parents, and other caregivers, and stretching and strengthening exercises to use in preparation for surgery. Much of this may be possible through a home exercise program. Postoperatively, therapy may include instruction in functional activities, active assistive and isometric exercise, proper positioning of the extremity, gait training with progressive weight bearing as tolerated, and pin care. Modalities such as ice or transcutaneous electrical nerve stimulation (TENS) may be useful for pain management. Dynamic splinting may be used in the limb-lengthening stage to provide low-intensity, prolonged stretch to joints with significantly limited ROM. Exercise techniques that may be useful throughout the Ilizarov lengthening include closed- and open-chain exercises for strengthening and active-assistive or passive exercises for ROM. A stationary bicycle and a treadmill may be used. After removal of the fixator, the patient may require additional gait training, monitoring, and adjusting of the exercise program and possible refitting and retraining, with orthotic or prosthetic devices worn preoperatively. Throughout the course of intervention, children are encouraged to participate in their usual school and leisure activities to the fullest extent possible.

SUMMARY

The pediatric orthopedic conditions presented in this chapter represent a wide range of problems that may be encountered by physical therapists in children referred to them for a specific problem (e.g., clumsy gait) or perhaps a specific complaint that turns out to be a "red herring." An example of this is a child referred to physical therapy for intervention for knee pain who in fact has a slipped capital femoral epiphysis. Alternatively, a child might be referred from a primary care physician or a neurologist to a physical therapist with one diagnosis (e.g., gross motor developmental delay) but also may be receiving intervention by an orthopedist for developmental dysplasia of the hip. In all these various scenarios, it is essential that the physical therapist be knowledgeable about various pediatric orthopedic conditions, including their signs, symptoms, differential diagnoses, and intervention. Physical therapists must be well informed regarding when to refer to other practitioners, such as the orthopedic surgeon in the case of a child with a suspected acute SCFE. As physical therapists, we often have the advantage of following a child intensively over a period of time, as opposed to a physician's visit once every 6 months, and thereby have unique insights into the child's condition and the family dynamics surrounding it. The well-informed physical therapist can often serve to bridge the gap that sometimes occurs between various specialists following a child, including primary care physicians, orthopedists, neurologists, and physiatrists.

RECOMMENDED MEASURES FOR CHILDREN RECEIVING ORTHOPEDIC EVALUATION

Body Functions and Structures

Torsional profile of lower extremity
Hip-knee-ankle joint ROM
Ortolani test
Barlow test
Leg length
Strength
Pain
Foot progression angle
Normal progression of physical changes with growth and development (e.g., flatfoot, genu valgum, torsion of lower extremity)

Activities and Participation

Gait assessment
Physical participation in play
Self-chosen position in play

Case Scenarios on Expert Consult

The case scenarios related to this chapter address a patient with Sever disease and a patient with a vascular malformation of the lower extremity. The case with Sever disease focuses on the evaluation and treatment process, and the case with the vascular malformation focuses on the process involved with differential diagnosis of this disorder.

REFERENCES

1. Abolarin T, Aiyegbusi A, Tella A, et al.: Predictive factors for flatfoot: the role of age and footwear in children in urban and rural communities in South West Nigeria, *Foot (Edinburgh)* 21:188, 2011.
2. Accadbled F, Laville JM, Harper L: One-step treatment of evolved Blount's disease: four cases and review of the literature, *J Pediatr Orthop* 23:747, 2003.
3. Acikgoz G, Averill LW: Chronic recurrent multifocal osteomyelitis: typical patterns of bone involvement in whole-body bone scintigraphy, *Nucl Med Commun* 35:797, 2014.
4. Aiona M, Do KP, Emara K, et al.: Gait patterns in children with limb length discrepancy. *J Pediatr Orthop* Jul 29, 2014.
5. Akdag B, Cavlak U, Cimbiz A, et al.: Determination of pain intensity risk factors among school children with nonspecific low back pain, *Med Sci Monit* 17:PH12, 2011.
6. Alsaleem M, Set KK, Saadeh L: Developmental dysplasia of hip: a review, *Clin Pediatr* Nov 6, 2014.
7. Alshammari A, Usmani S, Elgazzar AH, et al.: Chronic recurrent multifocal osteomyelitis in children: a multidisciplinary approach is needed to establish a diagnosis, *World J Nucl Med* 12:120, 2013.
8. Anderson LA, Gililland J, Pelt C, et al.: Subcapital correction osteotomy for malunited slipped capital femoral epiphysis, *J Pediatr Orthop* 33:345, 2013.
9. Aparicio G, Abril JC, Calvo E, et al.: Radiologic study of patellar height in Osgood-Schlatter disease, *J Pediatr Orthop* 17:63, 1997.
10. Arkun R: Parasitic and fungal disease of bones and joints, *Semin Musculoskelet Radiol* 8:231, 2004.
11. Asche SS, van Rijn RM, Bessems JHJM, et al.: What is the clinical course of transient synovitis in children: a systematic review of the literature, *Chiropr Man Ther* 21:39, 2013.
12. Atanda A, Shah SA, O'Brien K: Osteochondrosis: common causes of pain in growing bones, *Am Fam Physician* 83:285, 2011.
13. Barnes JM: Premature epiphysial closure in Perthes' disease, *J Bone Joint Surg, Br* 62:432, 1980.
14. Bergerault F, Fournier J, Bonnard C: *Orthop Traumatol Surg Res*, pp 99S–S150, 2012.
15. Berkowitz CD: Angular deformities of the lower extremity: bowlets and knock-knees. In Berkowitz CD, editor: *Berkowitz's pediatrics: a primary care approach*, ed 3, Elk Grove Village, IL, 2008, American Academy of Pediatrics.
16. Birch JG: Review article: Blount disease, *J Am Acad Orthop Surg* 21:408, 2013.
17. Blackmur JP, Murray AW: Do children who in-toe need to be referred to an orthopaedic clinic? *J Pediatr Orthop B* 19:415, 2010.
18. Bleck EE: Metatarsus adductus: classification and relationship to outcomes of treatment, *J Pediatr Orthop* 3:2, 1983.
19. Borges JL, Guille JT, Bowen J: Kohler's bone disease of the tarsal navicular, *J Pediatr Orthop* 15:596, 1995.
20. Brady RJ, Dean JB, Skinner TM, et al.: Limb length inequality: clinical implications for assessment and intervention, *J Orthop Sports Phys Ther* 33:221, 2003.
21. Bramer JA, Maas M, Dallinga RJ, et al.: Increased external tibial torsion and osteochondritis dessicans of the knee, *Clin Orthop Rel Res* 422:175, 2004.
22. Breugem CC, Maas M, Breugem SJM, et al.: Vascular malformations of the lower limb with osseous involvement, *J Bone Joint Surg* 85:399, 2003.
23. Brown D: Seasonal variation of slipped capital femoral epiphysis in the United States, *J Pediatr Orthop* 24:139, 2004.
24. Carey JL, Grimm NL: Treatment algorithm for osteochondritis dissecans of the knee, *Orthop Clin N Am* 46:141, 2015.
25. Carney BT, Minter CL: Nonsurgical treatment to regain hip abduction motion in Perthes disease: a retrospective review, *South Med J* 97:485, 2004.
26. Cass AD, Camasta CA: A review of tarsal coalition and pes planovalgus: clinical examination, diagnostic imaging, and surgical planning, *J Foot Ankle Surg* 49:274, 2010.
27. Cassas KJ, Cassettari-Wayhs A: Childhood and adolescent sports-related overuse injuries, *Am Fam Phys* 73:1014, 2006.
28. Cepero S, Ullot R, Sastre S: Osteochondritis of the femoral condyles in children and adolescents: our experience over the last 28 years, *J Pediatr Orthop B* 14:24, 2005.
29. Chaudhry S, Phillips D, Feldman D: Legg-Calve-Perthes disease: an overview with recent literature, *Bull Hosp Joint Dis* 72:18, 2014.
30. Chen KC, Yeh CJ, Tung LC, et al.: Relevant factors influencing flatfoot in preschool-aged children, *Eur J Pediatr* 170:931, 2011.
31. Chloe H, Inaba Y, Kobayashi N, et al.: Use of real-time polymerase chain reaction for the diagnosis of infection and differentiation between gram-positive and gram-negative septic arthritis in children, *J Pediatr Orthop* 33:e28, 2013.
32. Cho KH, Lee SM, Lee YH, et al.: Ultrasound diagnosis of either an occult or missed fracture of an extremity in pediatric-aged children, *Korean J Radiol* 11:84, 2010.
33. Chung SM, Batterman SC, Brighton CT: Shear strength of the human femoral capital epiphyseal plate, *J Bone Joint Surg Am* 58:94, 1976.
34. Cibulka MT: Determination and significance of femoral neck anteversion, *Phys Ther* 84:550, 2004.
35. Clark C, Ogden J: Development of the menisci of the human joint: morphologic changes and their potential role in childhood meniscal injury, *J Bone Joint Surg Am* 65:538, 1983.
36. Clarke NMP: Swaddling and hip dysplasia: an orthopaedic perspective, *Arch Dis Child* 99:5, 2014.
37. Committee on Quality Improvement, Subcommittee on Developmental Dysplasia of the hip: clinical practice guideline: early detection of developmental dysplasia of the hip, *Pediatrics* 105:896, 2000.
38. Connors JF, Wernick E, Lowy LI, et al.: Guidelines for evaluation and management of five common podopediatric conditions, *J Am Podiatr Med Assoc* 88:206, 1998.
39. Cooper AP, Doddabasappa SN, Mulpuri K: Evidence-based management of developmental dysplasia of the hip, *Orthop Clin North Am* 45:341, 2014.

40. Cosma D, Paraian I, Vasilescu D: Results of the conservative treatment in clubfoot using the French method, *J Pediatr Surg Spec* 8:1, 2014.

41. Cuevas de Alba C, Buille JT, Bowen JR: Computed tomography for femoral and tibial torsion in children with clubfoot, *Clin Orthop Rel Res* 353:203, 1998.

42. Cusick BD, Stuberg WA: Assessment of lower-extremity alignment in the transverse plane: implications for management of children with neuromotor dysfunction, *Phys Ther* 72:3, 1992.

43. Dare DM, Dodwell ER: Pediatric flatfoot: cause, epidemiology, assessment, and treatment, *Curr Opin Pediatr* 26:93, 2014.

44. Davids JR, Davis RB, Jameson C, et al.: Surgical management of persistent intoeing gait due to increased internal tibial torsion in children, *J Pediatr Orthop* 34:467, 2014.

45. De Boeck H: Osteomyelitis and septic arthritis in children, *Acta Orthop Belg* 71:505, 2005.

46. Dietz FR: Intoeing—fact, fiction and opinion, *Am Fam Physician* 5, 1249, 1994.

47. Dowling AM, Steele JR, Barr LA: Does obesity influence foot structure and plantar pressure patterns in prepubescent children? *Int J Obes Relat Metab Disord* 25:845, 2001.

48. Dror L, Alan A, Leonel C: The Haas procedure for the treatment of tibial torsional deformits, *J Pedatric Orthop B* 16:120, 2007.

49. Eberhardt O, Fernandez FF, Wirth T: The talar axis-first metatarsal base angle in CVT treatment: a comparison of idiopathic and non-idiopathic cases treated with the Dobbs method, *J Child Orthop* 6:491, 2012.

50. Ehrenborg G, Engfeldt B: Histologic changes in the Osgood-Schlatter lesion, *Acta Chir Scand* 121:328, 1961.

51. Eilert RE: Orthopedics. In Hay Jr WW, Levin MJ, Sondheimer JM, et al., editors: *Current pediatric diagnosis and treatment*, ed 17, Chicago, 2005, Lange Medical Books/McGraw-Hill.

52. Engel GM, Staheli T: The natural history of torsion and other factors influencing gait in childhood, *Clin Orthop Rel Res* 99:12, 1974.

53. Engstom P, Tedroff K: The prevalence and course of idiopathic toe-walking in 5-year-old children, *Pediatrics* 130:279, 2012.

54. Erol B, Dormans JP: Hip disorders. In Dormans JP, editor: *Pediatric orthopaedics: core knowledge in orthopaedics*, ed 1, Philadelphia, 2005, Mosby.

55. Evans AM: Growing pains: contemporary knowledge and recommended practice, *J Foot Ankle Res* 1:4, 2008.

56. Evans AM, Scutter SD: Prevalence of "growing pains" in young children, *J Pediatr* 145:255, 2004.

57. Farr S, Danzl A, Pablik E, et al.: Functional and radiographic consideration of lower limb malalignment in children and adolescents with idiopathic genu valgum, *J Orthop Res* 32:1362, 2014.

58. Farsetti P, Dragoni M, Ippolito E: Tibiofibular torsion in congenital clubfoot, *J Pediatr Orthop B* 21:47, 2012.

59. Faughan DM, Mofeson LM, Hughes MD, et al.: AIDS Clinical Trials Group Protocol 219 Team. Osteonecrosis of the hip (Legg-Calve-Perthes disease) in human immunodeficiency virus-infected children, *Pediatrics* 109:E74, 2002.

60. Fishkin Z, Armstrong DG, Shah H, Patra A, et al.: Proximal femoral physis shear in slipped capital femoral epiphysis—a finite element study, *J Pediatr Orthop* 26:291, 2006.

61. Flouzat-Lachaniette CH, Pujol N, Boisrenoult P, et al.: Discoid medial meniscus: report of four cases and literature review, *Orthop Traumatol Surg Res* 97:826, 2011.

62. Fuchs R, Staheli LT: Sprinting and intoeing, *J Pediatr Orthop* 16:489, 1996.

63. Galbraith RT, Gelberman RH, Hajek PC, et al.: Obesity and decreased femoral anteversion in adolescence, *J Orthop Res* 5:523, 1987.

64. Gerber JS, Doffin SE, Smathers SA, et al.: Trends in the incidence of methicillin-resistant *Staphylococcus aureus* infection in children's hospitals in the United States, *Clin Infect Dis* 49:65, 2009.

65. Goergens ED, McEvoy A, Watson M, et al.: Acute osteomyelitis and septic arthritis in children, *J Paediatr Child Health* 41:59, 2005.

66. Gibbons PJ, Gray K: Update on clubfoot, *J Paediatr Child Health* 49:E434, 2013.

67. Gigante A, Bevilacqua C, Bonetti MB, et al.: Increased external tibial torsion in Osgood Schlatter disease, *Acta Orthop Scand* 74:431, 2003.

68. Giladi M, Milgrom C, Stein M, et al.: External rotation of the hip. A predictor of risk for stress fractures, *Clin Orthop Rel Res* 216:131, 1987.

69. Gold R: Diagnosis of osteomyelitis, *Pediatr Rev* 12:292, 1991.

70. Gordon JE, Pappademos PC, Schoenecker PL, et al.: Diaphyseal derotational osteotomy with intramedullary fixation for correction of excessive femoral anteversion in children, *J Pediatr Orthop* 25:548, 2005.

71. Gore AI, Spencer JP: The newborn foot, *Am Fam Phys* 69:865, 2004.

72. Graf A, Wu KW, Smith PA, et al.: Comprehensive review of the functional outcome evaluation of clubfoot treatment: a preferred methodology, *J Pediatr Orthop B* 21:20, 2012.

73. Gulan G, Matoviniovic D, Nemee B, et al.: Femoral neck anteversion: values, development, measurement, common problems, *Coll Antropol* 24:521, 2000.

74. Halanski MA, Noonan KJ: Limb-length discrepancy. In Weinstein SL, Flynn JM, editors: *Lovell and Winter's pediatric orthopaedics*, ed 7, vol. 2. Philadelphia, 2013, Lippincott Williams & Wilkins.

75. Hanada M, Koyama H, Takahashi M, et al.: Relationship between the clinical findings and radiographic severity in Osgood-Schlatter disease, *Open Access J Sports Med* 3:17, 2012.

76. Harik NS, Smeltzer MS: Management of acute hematogenous osteomyelitis in children, *Expert Rev Anti Infect Ther* 8:175, 2010.

77. Harris E: The intoeing child: etiology, prognosis, and current treatment options, *Clin Podiatr Med Surg* 30:531, 2013.

78. Hart ES, Kalra KP, Grottkau BE, et al.: Discoid lateral meniscus in children, *Orthop Nurs* 27:174, 2008.

79. Hawkshead III JJ, Patel NB, Steele RW, et al.: Comparative severity of pediatric osteomyelitis attributable to methicillin-resistant versus methicillin-sensitive *Staphylococcus aureus*, *J Pediatr Orthop* 29:85, 2009.

80. Hazlewood ME, Simmons AN, Johnson WT, et al.: The footprint method to assess transmalleolar axis, *Gait Posture* 25:597, 2007.

81. Herring JA: Developmental dysplasia of the hip. In Herring J, editor: *Tachdjian's pediatric orthopaedics*, ed 5, vol. 1. Philadelphia, 2008, Elsevier Saunders.

82. Herring JA: Legg-Calve-Perthes disease. In Herring J, editor: *Tachdjian's pediatric orthopaedics*, ed 5, vol. 1. Philadelphia, 2008, Elsevier Saunders.

83. Herring JA: Limb length discrepancy. In Herring J, editor: *Tachdjian's pediatric orthopaedics*, ed 5, vol. 1. Philadelphia, 2008, Elsevier Saunders.

84. Herring JA: Slipped capital femoral epiphysis. In Herring J, editor: *Tachdjian's pediatric orthopaedics*, ed 5, vol. 1. Philadelphia, 2008, Elsevier Saunders.

85. Herring JA, Birch JG: The limping child. In Herring J, editor: *Tachdjian's pediatric orthopaedics*, ed 5, vol. 1. Philadelphia, 2008, Elsevier Saunders.

86. Herring JA, Kim HT, Browne R: Part I: classification of radiographs with use of the modified lateral pillar and Stulberg classifications, *J Bone Joint Surg Am* 86:2103, 2004.

87. Hixon AL, Gibbs LM: Osteochondritis dissecans: a diagnosis not to miss, *Am Fam Phys* 61:151, 2000.

88. Hofmann A, Jones RE, Herring JA: Blount's disease after skeletal maturity, *J Bone Joint Surg Am* 64:1004, 1982.

89. Holden W, David J: Chronic recurrent multifocal osteomyelitis: two cases of sacral disease responsive to corticosteroids, *Clin Infect Dis* 40:616, 2005.

90. Holen KJ, Tengagnder A, Bredland T, et al.: Universal or selective screening of the neonatal hip using ultrasound? A prospective, randomised trial of 15,529 newborn infants, *J Bone Joint Surg Br* 84:886, 2002.

91. Howard AW, Viskontas D, Sabbagh C: Reduction in osteomyelitis and septic arthritis related to *H. influenzae* type B vaccination, *J Pediatr Orthop* 19:705, 1999.

92. Howlett JP, Mosca BS, Bjornson K: The association between idiopathic clubfoot and increased internal hip rotation, *Clin Orthop Rel Res* 467:1231, 2009.

93. Huber AM, Lam PY, Duffy CM, et al.: Chronic recurrent multifocal osteomyelitis: clincial outcomes after more than five years of follow-up, *J Pediatr Orthop* 141:198, 2002.

94. Hunter New England NSW Health: Screening, assessment and management of developmental dysplasia of the hip (DDH), Clinical Guidelines for Hunter New England NSW Health, *HNEH CG 10_10*, 2010.

95. Hutchinson B: Pediatric metatarsus adductus and skewfoot deformity, *Clin Podiatr Med Surg* 27:93, 2010.

96. Ikeda H, Yamauchi Y, Saluraba K, et al.: Etiologic factor of Osgood-Schlatter disease in young sports players. In *Proceedings of the 20th Congress of the SICOT Amsterdam*, 1996, The Netherlands.

97. Inan M, Chan G, Bowen JR: Correction of angular deformities of the knee by percutaneous hemiepiphysiodesis, *Clin Orthop Rel Res* 456:164, 2007.

98. Ippolito E, Panseti IV: Congenital clubfoot in the human fetus: a histological study, *J Bone Joint Surg Am* 62:8, 1980.

99. Ireland PJ, Pacey V, Zankl A, et al.: Optimal management of complications associated with achondroplasia, *Appl Clin Genet* 7:117, 2014.

100. Jacobsen ST, Crawford AH: Congenital vertical talus, *J Pediatr Orthop* 3:306, 1983.

101. Jacquemier M, Glard Y, Pomero V, et al.: Rotational profile of the lower limb in 1319 healthy children, *Gait Posture* 28:187, 2008.

102. Jakob RP, von Gumppenberg S, Englehardt P: Does Osgood-Schlatter disease influence the position of the patella? *J Bone Joint Surg Br* 63:579, 1981.

103. James AM, Williams CM, Haines TP: Heel raises versus prefabricated orthoses in the treatment of posterior heel pain associated with calcaneal apophysitis (Sever's Disease): study protocol for a randomized controlled trial, *J Foot Ankle Res* 3:3, 2010.

104. James AM, Williams CM, Haines TP: Effectiveness of interventions in reducing pain and maintaining physical activity in children and adolescents with calcaneal apophysitis (Sever's disease): a systematic review, *J Foot Ankle Res* 6:16, 2013.

105. Jeffries LJ, Milanese SF, Grimmer-Somers KA: Epidemiology of adolescent spinal pain: a systematic overview of the research literature, *Spine (Phila Pa 1976)* 32:2630, 2007.

106. Joseph B, Varghese G, Mulpuri K, et al.: Natural evolution of Perthes disease: a study of 610 children under 12 years of age at disease onset, *J Pediatr Orthop* 23:590, 2003.

107. Judd J, Clarke NMP: Treatment and prevention of hip dysplasia in infants and young children, *Early Hum Dev* 90:731, 2014.

108. Kandzierski G, Karski T, Kozlowske K: Capital femoral epiphysis and growth plate of the asymptomatic hip joint in unilateral Perthes disease, *J Pediatr Orthop B* 12:380, 2003.

109. Kao HC, Huang YC, Chiu CH, et al.: Acute hematogenous osteomyelitis and septic arthritis in children, *J Microbiol Immunol Infect* 36:260, 2003.

110. Karol LA: Rotational deformities in the lower extremities, *Curr Opin Pediatr* 9:77, 1997.

111. Kaspiris A, Zafiropoulou C: Growing pains in children: epidemiological analysis in a Mediterranean population, *Joint Bone Spine* 76:486, 2009.

112. Kay RM, Kim YJ: Slipped capital femoral epiphysis. In Weinstein SL, Flynn JM, editors: *Lovell and Winter's Pediatric orthopaedics*, ed 7, vol. 2. Philadelphia, 2013, Lippincott Williams & Wilkins,.

113. Kim HD, Lee DS, Eom MJ, et al.: Relationship between physical examinations and two-dimensional computed tomographic findings in children with intoeing gait, *Ann Rehabil Med* 35:491, 2011.

114. Kim HK: Legg-Calve-Perthes disease, *J Am Acad Orthop Surg* 18:676, 2010.

115. Kitakoji T, Kitoh H, Katoh M, et al.: Home traction in the treatment schedule of overhead traction for developmental dysplasia of the hip, *J Orthop Sci* 10:475, 2005.

116. Kocher MS, Mandiga R, Aurakowski D, et al.: Validation of a clinical prediction rule for the differentiation between septic arthritis and transient synovitis of the hip in children, *J Bone Joint Surg Am* 86:1629, 2004.

117. Kocher MS, Zurakowski D, Kasser JR: Differentiating between septic arthritis and transient synovitis of the hip in children: an evidence-based clinical prediction algorithm, *J Bone Joint Surg Am* 81:1662, 1999.

118. Koenig JK, Pring ME, Dwek JR: MR evaluation of femoral neck version and tibial torsion, *Pediatr Radiol* 42:113, 2012.

119. Kosahvili Y, Fridman T, Backstein D, et al.: The correlation between pes planus and anterior knee pain or intermittent low back pain, *Foot Ankle Int* 29:910, 2008.

120. Krul M, van der Wouden JC, Schellevis FG, et al.: Acute non-traumatic hip pathology in children: incidence and presentation in family practice, *Fam Pract* 27:166, 2010.

121. Kruse LM, Dobbs MB, Gurnett CA: Polygenic threshold model with sex dimorphism in clubfoot inheritance: the Carter effect, *J Bone Joint Surg Am* 90:2688, 2008.

122. Kutlu A, Ayata C, Ogun TC, et al.: Preliminary traction as a single determinant of avascular necrosis in developmental dislocation of the hip, *J Pediatr Orthop* 20:579, 2000.

123. Landin LA, Danielsson LG, Wattsgard C: Transient synovitis of the hip, *J Bone Joint Surg Br* 69:238, 1987.

124. Legiehn GM, Heran MKS: A step-by-step practical approach to imaging diagnosis and interventional radiologic therapy in vascular malformations, *Semin Intervent Radiol* 27:209, 2010.

125. Lehmann CL, Arons RR, Loder RT, et al.: The epidemiology of slipped capital femoral epiphysis: an update, *J Pediatr Orthop* 26:286, 2006.

126. Lehmann HP, Hinton R, Morello P, et al.: Developmental dysplasia of the hip practice guideline: technical report, Committee on Quality Improvement and Subcommittee on Developmental Dysplasia of the Hip, *Pediatrics* 105:E57, 2000.

127. Leonard Z, Fortin PT: Adolescent accessory navicular, *Foot Ankle Clin North Am* 15:337, 2010.

128. Loder RT, Starnes T, Dikos G, et al.: Demographic predictors of severity of stable slipped capital femoral epiphyses, *J Bone Joint Surg Am* 88:97, 2006.

129. Lloyd-Roberts GC, Catterall A, Salamon PB: A controlled study of the indications for and the results of femoral osteotomy in Perthes'disease, *J Bone Joint Surg Br* 13:598, 1976.

130. Loren GJ, Karpinski NC, Mubarak SJ: Clinical implications of clubfoot histopathology, *J Pediatr Orthop* 18:765, 1998.

131. Luhmann SJ, Bassett GS, Gordon JE, et al.: Reduction of a dislocation of the hip due to developmental dysplasia: implications for the need of future surgery, *J Bone Joint Surg Am* 85:239, 2003.

132. McCarron JA, Johnston DR, Hanna BG, et al.: Evaluation and treatment of musculoskeletal vascular anomalies in children: an update and summary for orthopaedic surgeons, *Univ Penn Orthop J* 14:15, 2001.

133. McCarthy JJ, Dormans JP, Kozin SH, et al.: Musculoskeletal infections in children: basic treatment principles and recent advancements, *J Bone Joint Surg Am* 86:850, 2004.

134. Mahan ST, Katz JN, Kim YJ: To screen or not to screen? A decision analysis of the utility of screening for developmental dysplasia of the hip, *J Bone Joint Surg Am* 91:1705, 2009.

135. Maier C, Zingg P, Seifert B, et al.: Femoral torsion: reliability and validity of the trochanteric prominence angle test, *Hip Int* 22:534, 2012.

136. Manoff EM, Banffy MB, Winell JJ: Relationship between body mass index and slipped capital femoral epiphysis, *J Pediatr Orthop* 25:744, 2005.

137. Manson D, Wilmot DM, King S, et al.: Physeal involvement in chronic recurrent multifocal osteomyelitis, *Pediatr Radiol* 20:76, 1989.

138. Maraqa NE, Gomez MM, Rathore MH: Outpatient parenteral antimicrobial therapy in osteoarticular infections in children, *J Pediatr Orthop* 22:506, 2002.

139. Mazloumi SM, Ebrahimzadeh MH, Kachooei AR: Evolution in diagnosis and treatment of Legg-Calve-Perthes disease, *Arch Bone Joint Surg* 2:86, 2014.

140. Michelson JD, Durant DM, McFarland E: The injury risk associated with pes planus in athletes, *Foot Ankle Int* 23:629, 2002.

141. Miettunun PMH, Wei X, Kaura D, et al.: Dramatic pain relief and resolution of bone inflammation following pamidronate in 9 pediatric patients with persistent chronic recurrent multifocal osteomyelitis (CRMO), *Pediatr Rheumatol* 7:2, 2009.

142. Mirkopulos N, Weiner DS, Askew M: The evolving slope of the proximal femoral growth plate relationship to slipped capital femoral epiphysis, *J Pediatr Orthop* 8:268, 1988.

143. Mohanta MP: Growing pains: practitioners' dilemma, *Indian Pediatr* 51:379, 2014.

144. Montgomery NI, Rosenfeld S: Pediatric osteoarticular infection update, *J Pediatr Orthop* 00:00, 2014.

145. Morley AJ: Knock-knee in children, *Br Med J* 2:976, 1957.

146. Occult fracture. Mosby's Medical Dictionary. 8th ed. Available at: http://medical-dictionary.thefreedictionary.com/occult+fracture.

147. Mosca VS: Flexible flatfoot in children and adolescents, *J Child Orthop* 4:107, 2010.

148. Moseley CE: A straight-line graph for leg-length discrepancies, *J Bone Joint Surg Am* 59:174, 1977.

149. Murray AW, Wilson NI: Changing incidence of slipped capital femoral epiphysis: a relationship with obesity? *J Bone Joint Surg Br* 90:92, 2008.

150. Nakumura J, Kamegaya M, Saisu T, et al.: Treatment for developmental dysplasia of the hip using the Pavlik harness: long-term results, *J Bone Joint Surg Br* 89:230, 2007.

151. Najaf-Zadeh A, Nectoux E, Dubos F, et al.: Prevalence and clinical significance of occult fractures in children with radiograph-negative acute ankle injury: a meta-analysis, *Acta Orthop* 85:518, 2014.

152. Nelson JD: Toward simple but safe management of osteomyelitis, *Pediatrics* 99:883, 1997.

153. Nemeth B: The diagnosis and management of common childhood orthopedic disorders, *Cur Probl Pediatr Adolesc Health Care* 41:2, 2011.

154. Novais EN, Millis MB: Slipped capital femoral epiphysis: prevalence, pathogenesis, and natural history, *Clin Orthop Relat Res* 470:3432, 2012.

155. Obedian RS, Grelsamer RP: Osteochondritis dissecans of the distal femur and patella, *Clin Sports Med* 16:157, 1997.

156. Offiah AC: Acute osteomyelitis, septic arthritic and discitis: differences between neonates and older children, *Eur J Radiol* 60:221, 2006.

157. Ozlem EI, Akcali O, Losay C, et al.: Flexible flatfoot and related factors in primary school children: a report of a screening study, *Rheumatol Int* 26:1050, 2006.

158. Paakkonen M, Peltola H: Bone and joint infections, *Pediatr Clin North Am* 60:425, 2013.

159. Paley D, Bhave A, Herzenberg JE, et al.: Multiplier method for predicting limb-length discrepancy, *J Bone Joint Surg Am* 82:1432, 2000.

160. Panda A, Gamanagatti S, Jana M, et al.: Skeletal dysplasias: a radiographic approach and review of common non-lethal skeletal dysplasias, *World J Radiol* 6:808, 2014.

161. Parent AS, Teilman G, Juul A, Skakkebaek LE, et al.: The timing of normal puberty and the age limits of sexual precocity: variations around the world, secular trends, and changes after migration, *Endocr Rev* 24:668, 2003.

162. Park KW, Jang KS, Song HR: Can residual leg shortening be predicted in patients with Legg-Calve-Perthes' disease? *Clin Orthop Rel Res* 471:2570, 2013.

163. Pauk J, Ezerskiy V, Raso JV, et al.: Epidemiologic factors affecting plantar arch development in children with flat feet, *J Am Podiatr Med Assoc* 102:114, 2012.

164. Pavlik A: Stirrups as an aid in the treatment of congenital dysplasias of the hip in children. *LeKarskeListy* 5:81, 1950 (Translated by Bialik V, Reis ND: *J Pediatr Orthop* 9:157, 1989).

165. Pavlik A: The functional method of treatment using a harness with stirrups as the primary method of conservative therapy for infants with congenital dislocation of the hip. *Zeitschrift fur Orthopadie und Ihre Grenzgeneit* 89:341, 1957 (Translated by Peltier LF: *Clin Orthop Rel Res* 281:4, 1992).

166. Pfeiffer M, Kotz R, Ledi T, et al.: Prevalence of flat foot in preschool-aged children, *Pediatrics* 118:634, 2006.

167. Piddo C, Reed MH, Black GB: Premature epiphyseal fusion and degenerative arthritis in chronic recurrent multifocal osteomyelitis, *Skel Radiol* 29:94, 2000.

168. Pitkow RB: External rotation contracture of the extended hip, *Clin Orthop Rel Res* 110:139, 1975.

169. Pugmire BS, Shailam R, Gee MS: Role of MRI in the diagnosis and treatment of osteomyelitis in pediatric patients, *World J Radiol* 6:530, 2014.

170. Raimann A, Baar A, Raimann R, et al.: Late developmental dislocation of the hip after initial normal evaluation: a report of five cases, *J Pediatr Orthop* 27:32, 2007.

171. Rampal V, Chamond C, Barthes X, et al.: Long-term results of treatment of congenital idiopathic clubfoot in outcome of the functional "French" method if necessary completed by soft-tissue release, *J Pediatr Orthop* 33:48, 2013.

172. Rao UB, Joseph B: The influence of footwear on the prevalence of flat foot. A survey of 2300 children, *J Bone Joint Surg Br* 74:525, 1992.

173. Redjal HR, Zamorano DP: Developmental hip dysplasia. In Berkowitz CD, editor: *Berkowitz's pediatrics: a primary care approach*, ed 3, Elk Grove Village, IL, 2008, American Academy of Pediatrics.

174. Redjal HR, Zamorano DP: Rotational problems of the lower extremity: in-toeing and out-toeing. In Berkowitz CD, editor: *Berkowitz's pediatrics: a primary care approach*, ed 3, Elk Grove Village, IL, 2008, American Academy of Pediatrics.

175. Reikeras O, Kristiansen LP, Gunderson R, et al.: Reduced tibial torsion in congenital clubfoot, *Acta Orthop Scand* 72:53, 2001.

176. Richards BS, Katz DF, Sims JB: Effectiveness of brace treatment in early infantile Blount's disease, *J Pediatr Orthop* 18:374, 1998.

177. Riise OR, Kirkhus E, Handeland KS, et al.: Childhood osteomyelitis-incidence and differentiation from other acute onset musculoskeletal features in a population-based study, *BMC Pediatr* 8:45, 2008.

178. Robertson W, Kelly BT, Green DW: Osteochondritis dissecans of the knee in children, *Curr Opin Pediatr* 15:38, 2003.

179. Rosskopf AB, Ramseier LE, Sutter R, et al.: Femoral and tibial torsion measurement in children and adolescents: comparison of 3D models based on low-dose biplanar radiography and low-dose CT, *Am J Roentgenol* 202:W285, 2014.

180. Ruwe PA, Agae JR, Ozhonoff MB, et al.: Clinical determination of femoral anteversion. A comparison with established techniques, *J Bone Joint Surg Am* 74:820, 1992.

181. Sabharwal S: Current concepts review: Blount disease, *J Bone Joint Surg* 91:1758, 2009.

182. Sabharwal S, Zhao C: The hip-knee-ankle angle in children: reference values based on a full-length standing radiograph, *J Bone Joint Surg Am* 91:2461, 2009.

183. Salenius P, Vankka E: The development of the tibiofemoral angle in children, *J Bone Joint Surg Am* 57:259, 1975.

184. Sang GS, Song HR, Kim HW, et al.: Comparison of orthopaedic manifestations of multiple epiphyseal dysplasias caused by MATN3 versus COMP mutations: a case controls study, *BMC Musculoskel Disord* 15:84, 2014.

185. Sarkisson EJ, Sankar WN, Zhu L, et al.: Radiographic follow-up of DDH in infants: are x-rays necessary after a normalized ultrasound? *J Pediatr Orthop* 35(6):551–555, 2014.

186. Sass P, Hassan G: Lower extremity abnormalities in children, *Am Fam Phys* 68:461, 2003.

187. Sen RK, Sharma LR, Thakur SR, et al.: Patellar angle in Osgood-Schlatter disease, *Acta Orthop Scand* 60:26, 1989.

188. Seringe R, Bonnet JC, Katti E: Pathogeny and natural history of congenital dislocation of the hip, *Orthop Traumatol* 100:59, 2014.

189. Shane A, Reeves C, Wobst G, et al.: Second metatarsophalangeal joint pathology and Freiberg disease, *Clin Podiatr Med Surg* 30:313, 2013.

190. Sharp RJ, Calder JD, Saxby TS: Osteochondritis of the navicular: a case report, *Foot Ankle Int* 24:509, 2003.

191. Shibuya N, Jupiter DC, Ciliberti LJ, et al.: Characteristics of adult flatfoot in the United States, *J Foot Ankle Surg* 49:363, 2010.

192. Shieh A, Bastrom T, Roocroft J, et al.: Meniscus tear patterns in relation to skeletal maturity: children versus adolescents, *Am J Sports Med* 41:2779, 2013.

193. Shipman SA, Helfand M, Moyer VA, et al.: Screening for developmental dysplasia of the hip: a systematic literature review for the US preventive services task force, *Pediatrics* 117:e557, 2006.

194. Sibinski M, Murnaghan C, Synder, M: The value of preliminary overhead traction in the closed managment of DDH, *Int Orthop* 30:268, 2006.

195. Smith CF: Instantaneous leg length discrepancy determination by "thigh-leg" technique, *Orthopedics* 19:955, 1996.

196. Smith JT, Matan A, Coleman SS, et al.: The predictive value of the development of the acetabular teardrop figure in developmental dysplasia of the hip, *J Pediatr Orthop* 17:165, 1997.

197. Smith SM, Sumar B, Dixon KA: Musculoskeletal pain in overweight and obese children, *Int J Obes* 38:11, 2014.

198. Son SM, Ahn SH, Jung GS, et al.: The therapeutic effect of tibia counter rotator with toe-out gait plate in the treatment of tibial internal torsion in children, *Ann Rehabil Med* 38:218, 2014.

199. Song DH, Lee Y, Eun BL, et al.: Usefulness of tibia counter rotator (TCR) for treatment of tibial internal torsion in children, *Korean J Pediatr* 50:79, 2007.

200. Staheli LT: Rotational problems in children, *Instr Course Lect* 43:199, 1994.

201. Staheli LT: *Practice of pediatric orthopedics*, ed 2, Philadelphia, 2006, Lippincott Williams and Wilkins.

202. Staheli LT, Corbett M, Wyss C, et al.: Lower-extremity rotational problems in children. Normal values to guide management, *J Bone Joint Surg Am* 67:39, 1985.

203. Staheli LT, Engel GM: Tibial torsion: a method of assessment and a survey of normal children, *Clin Orthop Rel Res* 86:183, 1972.

204. Stevens PM, Gilliland JM, Anderson LA, et al.: Success of torsional correction surgery after failed surgeries for patellofemoral pain and instability, *Strategies Trauma Limb Reconstr* 9:5, 2014.

205. Stevens PM, MacWiliams B, Mohr RA: Gait analysis of stapling for genu valgum, *J Pediatr Orthop* 24:70, 2004.

206. Stevens PM, Otis S: Ankle valgus and clubfeet, *J Pediatr Orthop* 19:515, 1999.

207. Stovitz SD, Pardee PE, Vazquez G, et al.: Musculoskeletal pain in obese children and adolescents, *Acta Paediatr* 97:489, 2008.

208. Stuberg WA, Koehler A, Wichita M, et al.: Comparison of femoral torsion assessment using goniometry and computerized tomography, *Pediatr Phys Ther* 3:115, 1989.

209. Sullivan JA: Pediatric flatfoot: evaluation and management, *J Amer Acad Orthop Surg* 7:44, 1999.

210. Sultan J, Hughes PJ: Septic arthritis or transient synovitis of the hip in children: the value of clinical prediction algorithms, *J Bone Joint Surg Br* 92:1289, 2010.

211. Talbot CL, Paton RW: Screening of selected risk factors in developmental dysplasia of the hip: an observational study, *Arch Dis Child* 98:692, 2013.

212. Taxter AJ, Chauvin NA, Weiss PF: Diagnosis and treatment of low back pain in the pediatric population, *Phys Sportsmed* 42:94, 2014.

213. Taylor GR, Clarke NM: Monitoring the treatment of developmental dysplasia of the hip with the Pavlik harness: the role of ultrasound, *J Bone Joint Surg Br* 79:719, 1997.

214. Theodorou DJ, Theodorou SJ, Boutin RD, et al.: Stress fractures of the lateral metatarsal bones in metatarsus adductus foot deformity: a previously unrecognized association, *Skeletal Radiol* 28:679, 1999.

215. Trott AW: Developmental disorders. In Jahss MH, editor: *Disorders of the foot and ankle*, Philadelphia, 1991, WB Saunders.

216. Tsirikos A, Riddle EC, Kruse R: Bilateral Kohler's disease in identical twins, *Clin Orthop Relat Res* 409:195, 2003.

217. Tudor A, Ruzic L, Sestan B, et al.: Flat-footedness is not a disadvantage for athletic performance in children aged 11 to 15 years, *Pediatrics* 123:e386, 2009.

218. Uden H, Kumar S: Non-surgical management of a pediatric "intoed" gait pattern—a systematic review of the current best evidence, *J Multidiscip Healthc* 5:27, 2012.

219. Uziel Y, Bubbul-Aviel Y, Barash J, et al.: Recurrent transient synovitis of the hip in childhood: longterm outcome among 29 patients, *J Rheumatol* 33:810, 2006.

220. van Bemmel AF, van de Graaf VA, van den Bekerom MPJ, et al.: Outcome after conservative and operative treatment of children with idiopathic toe walking: a systematic review of literature, *Musculoskel Surg* 98:87, 2014.

221. Vukasinovic ZS, Spasovski DV, Matanovic DD, et al.: Flatfoot in children, *Acta Chir Iugosi* 58:103, 2011.

222. Wallach DM, Davidson RS: Pediatric lower limb disorders. In Dormans JP, editor: *Pediatric orthopaedics: core knowledge in orthopaedics*. Philadelphia: Elsevier Mosby,.

223. Wan SC: Metatarsus adductus and skewfoot deformity, *Clin Podiatr Med Surg* 23:23, 2006.

224. Weinstein SL: Developmental hip dysplasia and dislocation. In Weinstein SL, Flynn JM, editors: *Lovell and Winter's pediatric orthopaedics*, ed 7, vol. 2. Philadelphia, 2013, Lippincott Williams & Wilkins.

225. Weinstein SL: Legg-Calve-Perthes Syndrome. In Weinstein SL, Flynn JM, editors: *Lovell and Winter's pediatric orthopaedics*, ed 7, vol. 2. Philadelphia, 2013, Lippincott Williams & Wilkins.

226. Weinstein SL: Long-term follow-up of pediatric orthopedic conditions, *J Bone Joint Surg Am* 82:980, 2000.

227. Wenger DR: Surgical treatment of developmental dysplasia of the hip, *Instr Course Lect* 63:313, 2014.

228. Wenger D, Rang M: *The art of pediatric orthopedics*, New York, 1993, Raven Press.

229. Whalen JL, Fitzgerald Jr RH, Morrisy RT: A histological study of acute hematogenous osteomyelitis following physeal injuries in rabbits, *J Bone Joint Surg Am* 70:1383, 1988.

230. Williams CM, James AM, Tran T: Metatarsus adductus: development of a non-surgical treatment pathway, *J Paediatr Child Health* 49:E428, 2013.

231. Williams CM, Tinley P, Rawicki B: Idiopathic toe-walking: have we progressed in our knowledge of the causality and treatment of this gait type? *J Am Podiatr Med Assoc* 104:253, 2014.

232. Windisch G, Ander Huber F, Haldi-Brandle V, et al.: Anatomical study for an update comprehension of clubfeet. Part I: bones and joints, *J Child Orthop* 1:69, 2007.

233. Yen YM: Assessment and treatment of knee pain in the child and adolescent athlete, *Pediatr Clin North Am* 61:1155, 2014.

234. Yoon TL, Park KM, Choi SA, et al.: A comparison of the reliability of the trochanteric prominence angle test and the alternative method in healthy subjects, *Manual Ther* 19:97, 2014.

235. Zhou B, Tang K, Hardy M: Talocalcaneal coalition combined with flatfoot in children: diagnosis and treatment: a review, *J Orthop Surg Res* 9:129, 2014.

236. Zionts LE: What's new in idiopathic clubfoot? *J Pediatr Orthop*, 2014.

SUGGESTED READINGS

Background

Dormans JP, editor: *Pediatric orthopaedics: core knowledge in orthopaedics*, Philadelphia, 2005, Mosby.

Herring J, editor: *Tachdjian's pediatric orthopaedics*, ed 5, vol. 1. Philadelphia, 2005, Elsevier Saunders.

Staheli LT: *Practice of pediatric orthopedics*, ed 2, Philadelphia, 2006, Lippincott Williams and Wilkins.

Weinstein SL, Flynn JM, editors: *Lovell and Winter's pediatric orthopaedics*, ed 7, vol. 2. Philadelphia, 2013, Lippincott Williams & Wilkins.

Foreground

Blackmur JP, Murray AW: Do children who in-toe need to be referred to an orthopaedic clinic? *J Pediatr Orthop B* 19:415, 2010.

Brady RJ, Dean JB, Skinner TM et al.: Limb length inequality: clinical implications for assessment and intervention, *J Orthop Sports Phys Ther* 33:221, 2003.

Committee on Quality Improvement: Subcommittee on Developmental Dysplasia of the hip: Clinical practice guideline: early detection of developmental dysplasia of the hip, *Pediatrics* 105:896, 2000.

Cooper AP, Doddabasappa SN, Mulpuri K: Evidence-based management of developmental dysplasia of the hip, *Orthop Clin North Am* 45:341, 2014.

Graf A, Wu KW, Smith PA, et al.: Comprehensive review of the functional outcome evaluation of clubfoot treatment: a preferred methodology, *J Pediatr Orthop B* 21:20, 2012.

Stovitz SD, Pardee PE, Vazquez G, et al.: Musculoskeletal pain in obese children and adolescents, *Acta Paediatr* 97:489–493, 2008.

Zionts LE: What's new in idiopathic clubfoot? *J Pediatric Orthop* 35(6): 547–550, 2015.

15

Sports Injuries in Children

Mark Paterno, Laura Schmitt, Catherine Quatman-Yates, Kathryn Lucas

Youth participation in sports is growing at an exponential rate. Current estimates suggest greater than 30 million to 45 million youths between the ages of 5 and 17 years of age participate in community-sponsored athletic programs.[4,321] This represents an increase from roughly 5 million participants in 1970. More than 7.6 million teenagers regularly participate in competitive high school team sports.[402]

Participation in athletics is a means for our youth to remain physically active and reap the many health benefits of activity. In 2001 the Surgeon General[396] reported the incidence of obesity in our youth was reaching epidemic proportions as approximately 15% of children ages 6 to 19 years old are classified as obese and 30% are classified as overweight.[309] More recent evidence suggests obesity rates for children between the ages of 2 and 19 years old is now 17%.[308] This resulted in a health care expense in excess of $117 billion.[131]

Current estimates from the Centers for Disease Control and Prevention (CDC) suggest fewer than 65% of adolescents participate in regular physical activity and fewer than 45% are enrolled in a physical education class at their school. Participation in sports likely increases physical activity levels, which is critical to the long-term health of our youth. In addition, participation in athletics provides children with an opportunity to enhance their physical abilities and skills as well as for social interaction with their peers. Participation in sports is linked to positive aspects of individual development and academic performance, including higher grade point averages, lower school absentee rates, and overall better behavior.

Coinciding with increased participation is the potential for increases in sports-related injury in children. Emergency room data acquired since the later 1990s suggest more than 3.5 million children between the ages of 5 and 14 years old require medical attention for acute, sports-related injuries. In 2008, one study reported nearly 500,000 sports-related injuries requiring an emergency department visit in patients between the ages of 13 and 19 years old in 1 year.[296] More concerning is the fact that more than 50% of sports-related injuries in children are likely overuse injuries[298] and would not be included in these data. Furthermore, the progression of many children to become specialized in a singular sport early in their life has raised concerns from the American Academy of Pediatrics and other health care organizations about the safety of year-round participation in a single sport with infrequent rest periods and a lack of diversity in activity.[11] Attention must be given to the management of unique injuries in this population. However, the child cannot be considered simply a small adult. Children have different structural and physiologic components that must be specifically addressed.[393] This chapter provides an extensive overview of sports medicine in children and youth for the pediatric physical therapist. The purposes of the chapter are to review the elements of injury prevention/risk reduction and to discuss those factors that increase risk for sports-related injury in children with and without disabilities. The chapter addresses the types and sites of sports injuries unique to the child and provides considerations for rehabilitation.

BACKGROUND INFORMATION

INCIDENCE OF INJURY

Appreciating the true incidence of sports-related injuries in a young, active population is a challenge because of the varying methodologies in current research. Injury incidence is defined as the number of new cases of a disease (or injury) during a specific period of time, such as an athletic season or a year.[211] Incidence can be further subdivided into clinical incidence, which reports the percentage of new cases within a defined population, and incidence rate, which describes the rate of injuries per unit of exposure to activity.[68] Incidence rate is a much more powerful descriptor of the risk of injury in a population or within a certain activity and is necessary to accurately compare the rate of injury, normalized to exposure, between populations. Unfortunately, these data in the pediatric sports medicine literature are lacking. Varying methodologies and definitions of injury have hindered development of broad epidemiologic data accurately reporting the incidence of injuries in this population. In addition, many sports with high participation rates have little or no epidemiologic reports in the literature, which limits the ability to assess a documented risk in sports participation.

A summary of studies reporting incidence rates for males and females, separated by sport, is listed in Tables 15.1 and 15.2. The highest rate of injuries in males per 1000 hours of exposure occurs in ice hockey, rugby, and soccer. Females experience the highest rate of injury per 1000 hours of exposure in basketball and gymnastics. When injury data are normalized to the number of athletic exposures rather than hours of exposure, higher incidence rates are noted in cross-country running for males and soccer and cross-country running for females.[69] With respect to age and participation level, young males appear to experience higher rates of injury as they age.[68] Authors theorized that as males grow in body mass, strength, and speed, they have the ability to create greater forces and increase the risk of injury.[68,69] Females also grow with respect to height and mass through pubertal maturation, but they may not experience the coinciding development of strength and speed at the same pace as males. This may result in a similar change in risk of injury; however, the increase may be derived from a different mechanism than that theorized in males.

TABLE 15.1   Summary of Incidence Rates in Boys' Sports

Study	Study Design[a]/ Country	Data Collection[b]	Duration of Injury Surveillance	Team Type or Age(s)	Number of Injuries	Number of Exposures (Hours)	Number of Exposures (AEs)[c]	Rate: Number of Injuries per 1000 Hours	Rate: Number of Injuries per 1000 AEs	95% CI (Low/ High)
Baseball										
Knowles et al.	P (United States)	DM	3 years	HS	94				0.95	0.61/1.47
Comstock et al.	P (United States)	DM	1 year	HS					1.19	
Radelet et al.	P (United States)	Q	2 years	7–13 years	128		6913		17.0	
Powell and Barber-Foss	P (United States)	Q	3 seasons	HS	861		311,295		2.8	
Basketball										
Knowles et al.	P (United States)	DM	3 years	HS	186				2.32	1.45/3.71
Comstock et al.	P (United States)	DM	1 year	HS					1.89	
Powell and Barber-Foss	P (United States)	DM	3 seasons	HS	1933		444,338		4.8	
Messina et al.	P (United States)	DM	1 season	HS	543	169,885		3.2		
Cross-Country Running										
Rauh et al.	P (United States)	DM	1 season	HS	159		10,600		15.0	
Rauh et al.	P (United States)	DM	15 seasons	HS	846		77,491		10.9	
Football										
Knowles et al.	P (United States)	DM	3 years	HS	909				3.54	2.86/4.37
Comstock et al.	P (United States)	DM	1 year	HS					4.36	
Malina et al.	P (United States)	DM	2 seasons	Youth	259				10.4	9.2/11.8
				4th–5th grades	58				6.6	5.1/8.6
				6th grade	61				9.8	7.6/12.7
				7th grade	90				13.4	10.8/16.5
				8th grade	50				16.2	12.2/21.5
Turbeville et al.	P (United States)	DM	2 seasons	HS	132				3.2	2.7/3.3
Turbeville et al.	P (United States)	DM	2 seasons	MS	64				2.0	
Radelet et al.	P (United States)	Q	2 years	7–13 years	129		8462		15.0	
Powell and Barber-Foss	P (United States)	DM	3 seasons	HS	10,557		1,300,446		8.1	
Gymnastics										
Bak et al.	P (Denmark)	Q	1 year	Club	26			1.0		
Ice Hockey										
Emery and Meeuwisse	P (Canada)	DM	1 season	All minor	296			4.13		3.67/4.62

TABLE 15.1   Summary of Incidence Rates in Boys' Sports—cont'd

Study	Study Design[a]/ Country	Data Collection[b]	Duration of Injury Surveillance	Team Type or Age(s)	Number of Injuries	Number of Exposures (Hours)	Number of Exposures (AEs)[c]	Rate: Number of Injuries per 1000 Hours	Rate: Number of Injuries per 1000 AEs	95% CI (Low/ High)
				Atom	14			1.12		0.61/1.87
				Pee Wee	53			3.32		2.49/4.34
				Bantam	73			4.16		3.26/5.23
	296			Midget	156			6.07		5.16/7.1
Smith et al.	P (United States)	DM	1 season	HS	27			34.4		
Gerberich et al.	R (United States)	Q	1 season	HS				5		
Rugby										
McManus and Cross	P (Australia)	DM	1 season	Junior Elite	84			13.3		
Garraway and Macleod	P (United Kingdom)		1 season	Less than 16 years	26			3.4		2.1/4.8
				16–19 years	72			8.7		6.5/10.8
Roux et al.	P (France)	Q	1 season	HS	495			7.0	1.6	
Soccer										
Knowles et al.	P (United States)	DM	3 years	HS	252				2.81	2.03/3.90
Comstock et al.	P (United States)	DM	1 year	HS					2.43	
Le Gall et al.	P	DM	10 seasons	All	1152			4.8		
				U16	371			5.2		
				U15	361			4.6		
	1152			U14	420			4.9		
Kucera et al.	P (United States)	Q	3 years	U12–18	467		109,957		4.3	3.9/4.7
Emery et al.	P (Canada)	DM	1 season	Overall					5.5	
				U18	16	2030		3.2		
				U16	16	2817		5.7		
	16			U14	7	2177		7.9		
Radelet et al.	P (United States)	Q	2 years	7–13 years Alsace	47		2799		17	
Junge et al.	P (Europe)	DM	1 year	14–18 years Czech Republic	57			2.3		
				14–18 years	130			2.6		
Powell and Barber-Foss	P (United States)	DM	3 seasons	HS	1765		385,443		4.6	
Backous et al.	P (United States)	Q	1 week	6–17 years					7.3	
Wrestling										
Knowles et al.	P (United States)	DM	3 years	HS	154				1.49	0.85/2.62
Comstock et al.	P (United States)	DM	1 year	HS					2.5	

Continued

TABLE 15.1	Summary of Incidence Rates in Boys' Sports—cont'd								
Study	Study Design[a]/ Country	Data Collection[b]	Duration of Injury Surveillance	Team Type or Age(s)	Number of Injuries	Number of Exposures (Hours)	Number of Exposures (AEs)[c]	Rate: Number of Injuries per 1000 Hours	Rate: Number of Injuries per 1000 AEs	95% CI (Low/ High)
Pasque and Hewett	P (United States)	I, Q	1 season		219				6.0	
Powell and Bar-ber-Foss	P (United States)	DM	3 seasons	HS	2910	522,608			5.6	
Hoffman and Powell	P (United States)	DM	2 seasons				36,262		7.6	

[a]Design: *P*, prospective cohort; *R*, retrospective cohort.
[b]Data collection: *DM*, direct monitor; *HS*, high school; *IR*, insurance records; *MS*, middle school; *Q*, questionnaire; *RR*, record review.
[c]*AE*, one athlete participating in one practice or game in which the athlete is exposed to the possibility of athletic injury.
From Caine D, Maffulli N, Caine C: Epidemiology of injury in child and adolescent sports: injury rates, risk factors and prevention. *Clin Sports Medicine* 27:22-25, 2008.

Anatomic Location

In regard to anatomic location, the incidence of lower extremity injury in children is greatest across many sports, including basketball, football, gymnastics, soccer, and track and field.[68] Other sports, such as baseball,[68] snowboarding,[169] judo,[332] and tennis,[206] result in a greater incidence of upper extremity injuries. Still others, such as wrestling, result in a higher incidence of head injuries.[182] Collectively, the anatomic location with the greatest incidence of injury in children is the lower extremity, particularly the knee and ankle.[68]

Incidence of Acute Injuries

Acute injuries, often from emergency room visit data, have been reported in the epidemiologic literature for years. Taylor and Attia[399] reviewed all sports-related injuries in children between 5 and 18 years of age seen in an emergency room over a 2-year period. They reported 677 injuries, 71% in males. Sports most commonly implicated were basketball (19.5%), football (17.1%), baseball/softball (14.9%), soccer (14.2%), inline skating (5.7%), and hockey (4.6%). Sprains and strains were the most frequent types of injuries, followed by fracture, contusions, and lacerations; these accounted for 90% of all injuries. The National Health Interview Survey estimated that the sports-related injury rate for 5- to 24-year-olds was 42% higher than the estimates based on emergency room visits. The highest rate (59.3%) was for 5- to 14-year-olds.[96] Lenaway and colleagues[234] noted that middle school/junior high students had the highest injury rate, followed by elementary school students and then high school students. Sports, which accounted for 53% of all injuries, were an increasing cause of injury as grade level increased. Location of injury was the playground for elementary ages, the athletic field for middle school students, and the gym for high school students.

Incidence of Overuse Injuries

Of more recent concern is the rising incidence of overuse injuries in the pediatric population. Once thought to be a rare occurrence in children, overuse injuries are now estimated to make up more than 50% of injuries in this population.[298] This measure is likely a conservative estimate because, unlike acute injuries, which often require immediate medical attention and facilitate data tracking, overuse injuries are often self-managed and as a result are typically underreported. Micheli and Nielson[277] reported the mechanism behind this increase in overuse injury is likely due to increased participation in sports and, more specifically, a tendency toward sports specialization in greater numbers of children. Other factors may include an increase in complexity and duration of training at a young age, which increases stress to a growing body, and a lack of appropriate coaching and skill training. Specific risk factors for stress fractures and other overuse injuries typically seen in a younger, athletic population are outlined later in this chapter.

Alternative Sports

Children and adolescents are becoming more involved in extreme variations of sports as well as increased risk-taking with everyday sports. Various authors have noted significant injury rates with cycling,[150,430] exer-cycling,[40] riding in all-terrain vehicles,[60,204,289] diving,[102] snowboarding and skiing,[117,177,297,387] and inline skate, skateboard, or scooter use.[255,297,301,338] Although many of these injuries are contusions, fractures, and sprains/strains, authors noted significant cases of abdominal trauma with damage to the kidney, pancreas, or liver; head and neck injury; and hand trauma. A multicenter study[235] evaluating pediatric cervical spine injuries reported that sports accounted for as many cervical spine injuries as motor vehicle crashes among 8- to 15-year-olds.

Catastrophic Injuries

The incidence of catastrophic injuries and fatalities at the high school and college level has been documented for the years 1982 through 2013, with 2101 catastrophic sports-related injuries and illnesses.[288] The majority of these injuries were at the high school level (80.8%) and directly attributed to the sport-related activities (66.3% acute traumatic). Of these injuries, nearly 42% were fatal with the remaining nonfatal injuries (1221) leading to permanent functional disability or dysfunction (47%) or full recovery (53%). The most recent data from the National Center for Catastrophic Sport Injury Research report 41 catastrophic injuries in high school (n = 29) and college (n = 12) level sports, a rate of 0.53 injuries per 100,000 participants.[288] Football is associated with the greatest

TABLE 15.2 Summary of Incidence Rates in Girls' Sports

Study	Study Design[a]	Data Collection[b]	Duration of Injury Surveillance	Team Type or Age(s)	Number of Injuries	Number of Exposures (Hours)	Number of Exposures (AEs)[c]	Rate: Number of Injuries per 1000 Hours	Rate: Number of Injuries per 1000 AEs	95% CI (Low/High)
Basketball										
Knowles et al.	P (United States)	DM	3 years	HS	151				1.28	0.88/1.86
Comstock et al.	P (United States)	DM	1 year	HS					2.01	
Powell and Barber-Foss	P (United States)	DM	3 seasons	HS	1748		394,143		4.4	
Messina et al.	P (United States)	DM	1 season	HS	543		120,751	3.6		
Gomez et al.	P (United States)	DM	1 year	HS	436	107,353		4.1		
Cross-Country Running										
Rauh et al.	P (United States)	DM	1 season	HS	157		8008		19.6	
Rauh et al.	P (United States)	DM	15 seasons	HS	776		46,572		16.7	
Field Hockey										
Powell and Barber-Foss	P (United States)	DM	3 seasons	HS	510		138,073		3.7	
Gymnastics										
Caine et al.	P (United States)	DM	3 years	All levels	192	76,919.5	22,584	2.5	8.5	
				Top	125	36,040.0		3.5		
				Beginning	67	40,879.5		1.6		
Kolt and Kirkby	PR (Australia)	Q	18 months	All levels	349	105,583		3.3		
				Elite	151	57,383		2.6		
				Subelite	198	48,200		4.1		
Kolt and Kirkby	R (Australia)	Q	1 year	All levels	321	163,920		2.0		
				Elite	111			1.6		
				Subelite	210			2.2		
Bak et al.	P (Denmark)	Q	1 year	Club	41			1.4		
Lindner and Caine	P (Canada)	QI	3 seasons	Club	90	173,263		0.5		
Caine et al.	P (United States)	IR	1 year	All levels	147	40,127		3.7		
				Top	83	22,536		3.7		
				Middle	64	20,591		3.1		
Soccer										
Knowles et al.	P (United States)	DM	3 years	HS	121				2.35	1.55/3.55
Comstock et al.	P (United States)	DM	1 year	HS					2.36	
Kucara et al.	P (United States)	Q	3 seasons	12–18 years	320	60,166		5.3		4.7/6.0
Emery et al.	P (Canada)	DM	1 season	Overall	20	2526		5.6		
				U14	14	2440		7.9		
				U16	5	1976		5.7		
				U18				2.5		

Continued

TABLE 15.2 Summary of Incidence Rates in Girls' Sports—cont'd

Study	Study Design[a]	Data Collection[b]	Duration of Injury Surveillance	Team Type or Age(s)	Number of Injuries	Number of Exposures (Hours)	Number of Exposures (AEs)[c]	Rate: Number of Injuries per 1000 Hours	Rate: Number of Injuries per 1000 AEs	95% CI (Low/High)
Soderman et al.	P (Sweden)	DM	1 season	14–19 years	79			6.8		
Radelet et al.	P (United States)	Q	2 years	Community	16		1637		23.0	
Powell and Barber-Foss	P (United States)	DM	3 seasons	HS	1771		355,512		5.3	
Backous et al.	P (United States)	Q	1 week	6–17 years				10.6		
Softball										
Knowles et al.	P (United States)	DM	3 years	HS	71				.96	0.61/1.42
Comstock et al.	P (United States)	DM	1 year	HS					1.13	
Radelet et al.	P (United States)	Q	2 years	Community	37		3807		10.0	
Powell and Barber-Foss]	P (United States)	DM	3 seasons	HS	910				3.5	
Volleyball										
Comstock et al.	P (United States)	DM	1 year	HS					1.64	
Powell and Barber-Foss	P (United States)	DM	3 seasons	HS	601		359,547		1.7	

[a]Design: *P*, prospective cohort; *R*, retrospective cohort.
[b]Data collection: *DM*, direct monitor; *HS*, high school; *IR*, insurance records; *Q*, questionnaire; *RR*, record review.
[c]*AE*, one athlete participating in one practice or game in which the athlete is exposed to the possibility of athletic injury.
From Caine D, Maffulli N, Caine C: Epidemiology of injury in child and adolescent sports: injury rates, risk factors and prevention. *Clin Sports Medicine* 27:26-28, 2008.

number of catastrophic injuries, although data from the 2012 season indicate lower numbers of catastrophic injuries compared to previous seasons. Brain and cervical spine injuries account for most direct injures, with heart and heat-related illness as the major causes of indirect deaths. Head injuries are the primary anatomic area injured in ice hockey at the high school level, with body checking being the primary mechanism for all ice hockey injuries.[39] National Amateur Baseball Catastrophic Injury Surveillance Program data showed annual fatality, nonfatal catastrophic injury, and serious catastrophic injury rates of between 0.03 to 0.05 per 100,000 participants, with an average of 2 deaths per year in youth baseball from 1996–2006.[351] These deaths resulted from impact to the head and from blunt chest impact.[351]

Sex Differences in Injury Rates

Significant attention has been directed to differences in types and rates of injuries in males and females. A recent study[395] compared differences between males and females in pediatric sports-related injuries that included a random sample of 2133 medical records of children aged 5 to 17 years from 2000 to 2009 at a large pediatric hospital. Female athletes had a higher percentage of overuse injuries (62.5%) compared with traumatic injuries (37.5%), whereas the opposite was observed in male athletes (41.9% vs. 58.2%, respectively).[395] By body

region, females sustained more injuries to the lower extremity (65.8%) and spine (11.3%) compared to males (53.7% and 8.2%, respectively).[395] In the upper extremity, males had a greater percentage of injuries compared to females (29.8% vs. 15.1%, respectively).[395] At the hip/pelvis, female athletes sustained more overuse (90.9%) and soft tissue (75.3%) injuries compared to males, who sustained more traumatic (58.3%) and bony (55.6%) injuries.[395] In particular, the percentage of females with patellofemoral pain was approximately three times greater than males (14.3% vs. 4.0%, respectively), while males were twice as likely to be diagnosed with osteochondritis dissecans (8.6% vs. 4.3%, respectively) and fractures (19.5% vs. 8.2%, respectively).[395] The percentage of males and females who sustained anterior cruciate ligament injury was nearly equal (10.0% vs. 8.9%).[395] When evaluating injury rates between males and females by sport, Loes and colleagues[111] reported that the risk of knee injury was significantly higher for women ages 14 to 20 years than men of the same age in cross-country and downhill skiing, gymnastics, volleyball, basketball, and handball. Hosea and colleagues[186] reported increased risk for grade 1 ankle sprains in women basketball players.

Sex differences in incidents of anterior cruciate ligament (ACL) injuries have been a focus of pediatric sports-related research. There has been an increase in the incidence of ACL rupture in skeletally immature athletes over the past 20 years.[126,212,213,382,383] Among skeletally immature athletes, ACL tears are more common in males. It is thought that this is a result of males participating in more demanding organized sports at an earlier age than females.[342] However, this trend reverses upon reaching skeletal maturity, with females sustaining more complete ACL tears than males.[342] Skeletally mature females are 2 to 10 times more likely to sustain an ACL injury than their male counterparts.[349] The underlying mechanism of female sex disparity in ACL injury risk may be rooted in sex-specific changes that occur during pubertal development. Risk factors for primary ACL noncontact injury, specifically for the female athlete, include structural/anatomic,[180] hormonal,[183] biomechanical, and neuromuscular factors.[181]

PREVENTION OF INJURIES

The key to management of sports injuries in children is prevention. As discussed in Chapter 6, children need proper physiologic conditioning, strength, and flexibility to participate safely in an organized or recreational athletic endeavor. Although lack of fitness, strength, and flexibility does not preclude participation, remediation must be built into conditioning and training programs to decrease the risk of injury. The major elements in the process of injury risk management are preparticipation examination, conditioning and training, proper supervision, protection of the body, and environmental control.[391]

Preparticipation Examination

The preparticipation examination (PPE) is a step in the process of injury prevention. The American Medical Association Committee on Medical Aspects of Sports constructed a Bill of Rights for the Athlete, one part of which is a thorough preseason history and medical examination.[16] The underlying goal of a PPE is to ensure the safety and health of athletes during training and athletic participation.[388] The original primary objectives of the PPE were to (1) determine the general health of the athlete and detect conditions that place the participant at additional risk, (2) identify relative or absolute medical contraindications to participation, (3) identify sports that may be played safely by the individual, (4) serve as a limited general health screening, (5) fulfill legal and insurance requirements, and (6) evaluate physical maturation.[245] Although the goals and implementation of the PPE have evolved over the years, and continue to do so, most agree that they involve the "attempt (of the PPE) to identify those conditions that may place an athlete at increased risk and affect safe participation in organized sports."[95]

The fourth edition of the Preparticipation Physical Evaluation (PPE-4)[10] contains the most current guidelines for implementation of the PPE, with the primary objectives of screening for conditions that may be life threatening or disabling and screening for conditions that may predispose to injury or illness.[270,367] Although the efficacy of the PPE pertaining to these objectives is debated,[95] recent work[429] highlights the need for a comprehensive and uniformly administered approach to PPE, thought to allow for the best opportunity to screen health risk.[10,367] Most states require either an individual examination or a multistation screening, with a protocol that should be comprehensive within available resources.[10] The primary physician performing an individual examination knows or has access to the athlete's health records, can discuss sensitive health or personal issues, and may be most qualified to oversee any necessary follow-up care. The time and cost are a disadvantage of the individual examination.

TABLE 15.3 Preparticipation Physical Examination Stations and Professional Experts for Athlete Assessment

Station	Personnel
Sign-in/instructions	Ancillary personnel/coach
Height/weight/vital signs	Nurse, nurse practitioner, exercise physiologist, athletic trainer, or physical therapist
Visual examination	Nurse, nurse practitioner, or coach
Dental examination	Dentist
Medical examination	Internist or family practitioner
Orthopedic evaluation	Physician or physical therapist
Flexibility assessment	Physical therapist or athletic trainer
Strength evaluation	Physical therapist, athletic trainer, or exercise physiologist
Body composition	Exercise physiologist, physical therapist, or athletic trainer
Speed, agility, power, balance, endurance	Exercise physiologist, coach, or athletic trainer
Assessment/clearance	Physician

Additionally, disparate knowledge and interest among physicians regarding sports and the requirements to participate may hinder effective evaluation for all participants. The multistation approach to PPE is more cost and time efficient and provides a thorough and appropriate screening for all potential participants. Professional experts assess each athlete in the area of her or his specialization (Table 15.3), with the team physician consulting the appropriate specializations.[367] State regulations may dictate which medical has the final decision for clearing an athlete for participation, as well as what other providers, aside from physicians, can perform evaluations.[367] The timing and frequency of the PPE are often debated and vary depending on level of the athlete. PPE should be performed with enough time prior to the athletic season to allow for the treatment or rehabilitation of identified problems,[367] with recommendations of at least 6 weeks prior to the start of participation.[245,324] At the collegiate level, athletes often undergo a comprehensive health examination prior to entry with annual examinations thereafter, as dictated by university/college policy.[367] Younger athletes may be required to participate in a comprehensive PPE annually, or every 2 to 3 years with annual updates.[10,367] In this model a complete entry-level examination and evaluation are followed by annual reevaluation that includes a brief physical examination, a physical maturity assessment, and an examination/evaluation of all new problems. The American Academy of Pediatrics[12] has recommended a biannual complete evaluation followed by an interim history before each season. The schedule that meets the primary objectives of the academy, however, is a complete entry-level evaluation followed by a limited annual reevaluation that includes a brief medical examination (to evaluate height, weight, blood pressure, and pulse; perform auscultation; examine the skin; and test visual acuity) and an evaluation of all new problems.

The components of the PPE are the medical history; the medical examination, including cardiovascular and eye examinations; a musculoskeletal assessment; body composition and height and weight determination; specific field testing; and an assessment of readiness, both physical and psychological. Research has identified alterations in movement mechanics, landing patterns, and functional performance that are associated with increased risk of sports-related injuries.[322] As such, dynamic functional performance assessments may be implemented into PPE, although this is not standard practice. The components of the examination should be tailored to the specific demands of the sport.

History

The medical history is the cornerstone of the medical evaluation [85,245] and identifies the majority of problems affecting athletes.[157] Short forms that are easy to complete, written in lay terms, and understandable to young athletes are preferable. Forms should be completed by both the athlete and parent/guardian to obtain an accurate and complete history.[85] Content areas that should be particularly noted include exercise-induced syncope or asthma; family history of cardiac problems including heart disease or sudden death; history of loss of consciousness, concussion, or neurologic conditions; history of heat injury or stroke; medications; allergies; history of musculoskeletal dysfunction or activity-related injury or joint trauma; history of acute illness; dates of hospitalizations or surgery; absence or loss of a paired organ; immunizations; female maturation including menstrual history; and eating/dieting patterns. A standard form is recommended by the PPE-4.[10]

Medical Examination

The medical examination is used to evaluate areas of concern identified in the history.[17] The minimally sufficient examination includes cardiovascular (including blood pressure, pulse, respiration) and eye examinations, and a review of all body systems. Both the American Heart Association[258] and PPE-4[10] describe cardiovascular screening procedures and recommendations. It is recommended that athletes with heart rate over 120 beats/minute, arrhythmias, or systolic or diastolic murmurs be referred for further examination.[367] Asthma screening should also be completed, including documentation of medications.

Visual acuity is often tested using a Snelling chart and should be correctable to 20/200. Any inequality of pupil diameter or reactivity should be noted so responses after potential injury can be compared with this baseline value. Uncorrectable legal blindness (acuity less than 20/200 or absence of an eye) requires counseling regarding participation in collision or contact sports. The importance of protective eyewear for athletes who wear glasses or have unilateral vision should be stressed.[33]

Abdominal assessment determines rigidity, tenderness, organomegaly, or the presence of masses. Participation by any athlete with organomegaly is restricted until further tests determine the cause of the enlarged organ.[33]

Careful examination of the skin is vital in examination of all persons, but it is particularly important for those who will participate in contact sports. Participation in these sports should be deferred for children with evidence of any communicable skin disease, such as impetigo, carbuncles, herpes, scabies, and louse or fungal infections.[245]

Genitourinary examination of males is used to assess the child for testicular presence, descended testicles, and possible inguinal hernia. The genital examination is deferred in girls unless a history of amenorrhea or menstrual irregularity warrants referral. A maturational index, such as Tanner staging, is no longer recommended as part of a routine PPE because there are no data to indicate this leads to injury reduction.[91]

A more thorough neurologic examination is performed in athletes with a history of head injuries or neuropraxias.[324] Documentation of baseline values is important should a

subsequent injury occur. Examination may include neck/upper extremity range of motion, strength, sensation, reflexes, and other special tests.[10,324]

A musculoskeletal and orthopaedic screening and examination may be combined for asymptomatic athletes with no history of previous injuries.[95] If an athlete has an injury history or other signs of symptoms during a general screening, a more site-specific examination should be performed.[95]

Musculoskeletal Examination

Although no specific components are required, tests/examinations of flexibility, gait, muscle performance, and joint laxity, as well as a review of prior injury, are frequently included.[367] Assessment of posture with particular attention to atrophy, spinal asymmetry, pelvic level, discrepancy of leg lengths, and lower extremity deformities such as genu valgus or varus, patellar deformities, and pes planus is also part of a musculoskeletal examination. Gait should be examined with the athlete walking and running, as well as walking on toes and heels. Passive range of motion and two-joint musculotendinous flexibility should be screened. Muscle strength can be assessed using a manual muscle test, handheld dynamometer, or isokinetic device. Special stability testing of the shoulders, knees, and ankles should be conducted if the child has had a previous injury or if the current assessment indicates that instability may be present. Dynamic functional performance assessments, general and sports specific, may also be implemented to identify potential injury risk.

Medication Use

The PPE can be utilized to screen for involvement in risky health behaviors such as tobacco and alcohol use and use of recreational drugs or ergogenic aids. All medications and supplements currently used by the athlete should be reviewed by the examiner.[95]

From 3% to 12% of adolescent males and 1% to 2% of females report having used steroids.[24,432] The most compelling reasons for taking steroids are to increase body weight and muscle mass, decrease fatigue, and increase aggressive behavior. The adverse effects of steroid use include hypertension, hepatitis, testicular atrophy, loss of libido, hepatic carcinoma, and premature epiphyseal closure.[48] Warning signs of steroid abuse include irritability; sudden mood swings; puffiness in face, upper arms, and chest; sudden increases in blood pressure and weight; yellowish coloration around the fingernails and eyes; hirsutism; and deepening of voice and acne in girls.[262] Other substances that have been utilized to increase muscle performance include DHEA (dehydroepiandrosterone), branched chain and essential amino acids, creatine, growth hormone, and dietary supplements containing nandrolone and testosterone. Designer steroids have been introduced to provide the effects of steroid use but avoid detection. Other dietary substances including ephedra and carnitine have been utilized to increase energy and endurance, suppress appetite, and promote weight loss.[38,170] These natural elements have been touted in popular literature as aids for growth, performance, immunity, and healing and are used by both high school and college athletes, as well as professional athletes. Research has not supported the efficacy of these substances for performance enhancement with the exception of creatine[378] and carnitine.[218] Existing research has examined these substances in young adults; no research has been done in the pediatric population under the age of 18 years. Research has reported potential risk and harm with ingestion of substantial amounts of several substances, including steroids and nandrolone, ephedra, and branched chain amino acids. The use of ephedrine-containing compounds has been banned by most professional and collegiate sports organizations, as well as the National Federation of State High School Associations.

Diuretics are frequently used to "make weight" for an event or to mask drug usage. Performance may, however, decrease as a result of dehydration or electrolyte losses.[48,262] Likewise, stimulants such as caffeine and amphetamines are commonly abused in an effort to increase performance in sports. They serve only to mask normal fatigue and to increase aggression, hostility, and uncooperativeness and can lead to addiction and death.[419]

The use of barbiturates, antidepressants, and beta-blockers has been noted in sports in which fine control is required, such as shooting and archery. Although they do calm the nervous system and lower heart rate, even therapeutic doses may cause bronchospasm, hypotension, and bradycardia.[280]

The use of recreational drugs, including nicotine, smokeless tobacco, alcohol, marijuana, cocaine, and even heroin, is increasing among youth. Symptoms such as agitation, restlessness, insomnia, difficulty with short-term memory or concentration, and decline in performance might signal behavior indicative of substance abuse.[89,160]

Specific Field Tests

Field testing is done to assess specific athletic potential in a specific sport. The components assessed are muscle strength, muscle power, endurance, speed, agility and flexibility, and cardiovascular performance. Field test performance has been shown to identify deficits from previous injury that standard physical examination may not define.[295]

General muscle strength can be assessed with a maximal activity pertinent to the sport, such as bench presses, pull-ups, or push-ups for the upper extremities and leg presses or sit-ups for the lower extremities. Endurance can be assessed by performing as many repetitions of the task as possible. Muscle power can be evaluated with vertical jumping, performing a standing long jump, or throwing a medicine ball, as appropriate.

Speed is evaluated using a 40- or 50-yard dash, and agility can be assessed with the Vodak agility test[147] or a similar battery of tests. The most common, standardized methods of assessing flexibility are the sit and reach test, which has norms for children, and active knee extension performed in a supine position with the hips flexed to 90°.[189] Cardiovascular performance is most easily assessed using a submaximal test on an appropriate device, such as a cycle ergometer, treadmill, or upper-body ergometer. A field test for cardiovascular performance is the 12-minute run or the timed 1.5-mile run.[33,65,229] Field tests that involve jumping and sprinting have been correlated to laboratory results.[29]

Limitations and Outcomes of the PPE

Despite efforts to create a thorough and comprehensive PPE, it is not without limitations. The PPE is designed to identify life-threatening contraindications to sports participation. In addition, the PPE is able to identify various static musculoskeletal deficiencies. However, often some PPE settings do not address more dynamic risk factors. More concerning is the lack of follow-up that may occur if deficits are identified. McKeag et al.[269] reported 10% of athletes receiving a PPE present with a musculoskeletal disorder; however, others have noted that only 1% to 3% of athletes are

referred for intervention following a PPE.[390] Although many athletes are identified with musculoskeletal deficits, the deficits are often not addressed. Future work should focus on increasing the ability of the PPE to identify dynamic risk factors for injury and create a more seamless approach to recommend intervention for those athletes who are identified at risk.

The outcome of the PPE determines the level of clearance to participate in sports. Clearance can be unrestricted for any sport or restricted to specific types of sports in the following manner: (1) no collision (violent, direct impact) or contact (physical touching), (2) limited contact or impact, or (3) noncontact only. The American Academy of Pediatrics has developed a classification system for sports activities and recommendations for restriction of participation that are excellent guides in making decisions for individual athletes.[11]

Training Program

The preseason examination clearly defines the individual athlete's areas of strength and limitations (Fig. 15.1). The next appropriate step in prevention is the development of an individualized training plan designed to address the particular problems of the athlete as they relate to the requirements of the sport(s) (Box 15.1). This program could be developed by a sports physical therapist, athletic trainer, or exercise physiologist involved in the preseason screening. Once developed, it should be taught to the athlete, the parent, and the coach.

The training program should be a systematic, progressive plan to address the athlete's weaknesses and to maximally condition the athlete for participation. Training consists of off-season, preseason, in-season, and postseason programs for year-round conditioning and for development of appropriate peak performance. Components should include energy training (aerobic foundation and anaerobic training), muscle training (strength, endurance, flexibility, and power), speed, and proper nutrition. A well-developed, variable, and well-paced program will help the young athlete to avoid boredom and potential overuse injury. The psychological effects of year-round training, or exercise in general, are controversial and not well documented. The risk-benefit ratio, however, tends to favor exercise for improvement of mood, self-concept, and work behavior when competition is sensibly controlled.[282]

BOX 15.1 Text Box for Examination

Body Functions and Structures
- Range of motion with goniometry
- Muscle strength, power, and endurance with isokinetic assessment
- Ligament integrity/stability with manual assessment
- Joint laxity with the Beighton-Horan screening
- Posture
- Gait with visual observation
- Dynamic movement assessment with visual assessment
- Functional Performance Testing with single-leg hop testing

Activities and Participation
- Tegner Activity Scale
- Marx Activity Scale
- HSS Pedi-FABS

Other (e.g., Environment, QoL when applicable)
- PedsQL

QoL, quality of life.

Athletic fitness scorecard for boys

Test	0 Below average	1 Above average	2 Good	3 Very good	4 Excellent
Strength Pull-ups (no)	Fewer than 7	7 to 9	10 to 12	13 to 14	15 or more
Power Long jump (in)	Fewer than 85	85 to 88	89 to 91	92 to 94	95 or more
Speed 50-yd dash (sec)	Slower than 6.7	6.7 to 6.4	6.3 to 6.0	5.9 to 5.6	5.5 or less
Agility 6-c agility (c)	Fewer than 5-5	5-5 to 6-3	6-4 to 7-2	7-3 to 8-1	8-2 or more
Flexibility Forward flexion (in)	Not reach ruler	1 to 2	3 to 5	6 to 8	9 or more
Muscular endurance Sit-ups (no)	Fewer than 38	38 to 45	46 to 52	53 to 59	60 or more
Cardiorespiratory endurance 12-min run (mi)	Fewer than 1½	1½	1¾	2	2¼ or more

YOUR SCORE

	Strength	Power	Speed	Agility	Flexibility	Muscular endurance	Cardiorespiratory endurance
Your Score							
Rating (0–4)							

Athletic fitness scorecard for girls

Test	0 Below average	1 Above average	2 Good	3 Very good	4 Excellent
Strength Pull-ups (no)	Fewer than 2	2 to 3	4 to 5	6 to 7	8 or more
Power Long jump (in)	Fewer than 63	63 to 65	66 to 68	69 to 71	72 or more
Speed 50-yd dash (sec)	Slower than 8.2	8.2 to 7.9	7.8 to 7.1	6.9 to 6.0	5.9 or less
Agility 6-c agility (c)	Fewer than 3-5	3-5 to 4-3	4-4 to 5-2	5-3 to 6-2	6-3 or more
Flexibility Forward flexion (in)	Fewer than 3	3 to 5	6 to 8	9 to 11	12 or more
Muscular endurance Sit-ups (no)	Fewer than 26	26 to 31	32 to 38	39 to 45	46 or more
Cardiorespiratory endurance 12-min run (mi)	Fewer than 1¼	1¼	1½	1¾	2 or more

YOUR SCORE

	Strength	Power	Speed	Agility	Flexibility	Muscular endurance	Cardiorespiratory endurance
Your Score							
Rating (0–4)							

FIG. 15.1 Athletic fitness for boys and girls. (From Gaillard B, Haskell W, Smith N, et al.: *Handbook for the young athlete*. Palo Alto, CA, Bull Publishing, 1978.)

Energy Training

The basis of energy training, a strong aerobic base, should be developed during the off-season. Good training consists of low-intensity, long-duration activity with natural intervals of low- and moderate-intensity work that is sport-specific. Swimming would be a good choice for the field athlete, and cycling or running is appropriate for those in track, soccer, and football. Training on hills or performance of similar resistance efforts should be executed in moderation or in an interval fashion with other activities. Children exhibit less efficient movement patterns and a lower maximal acidosis level. Their greater surface area–to–body mass ratio facilitates greater heat gain on hot days and greater heat loss on colder days. Children produce less sweat and less total evaporative heat loss. Children produce more metabolic heat per pound of body weight during exercises, such as walking and running. Finally, although children can acclimatize, they do so at a slower rate than adults.[125] Consequently, intense training in the extreme heat and hard training involving long durations should be minimized until puberty.

Anaerobic training programs consist of exertion at 85% to 90% of maximal heart rate for short periods. Anaerobic fitness is a person's ability to generate a high level of mechanical power over a short period of time. Optimal training levels to achieve peak anaerobic fitness are often debated; however, biweekly anaerobic training is often recommended for maximal benefit. Methods including interval training, fartlek (speed play, or alternate fast and slow running in natural terrain), and pace training are variations of the anaerobic method. Sport-specific anaerobic skills should be developed during preseason and early-season activities.[288] Young children are less capable to see significant increases in anaerobic fitness due to anatomic and physiologic differences in the skeletally immature athlete. As a result, this training is difficult for young athletes and has less impactful fitness benefits until they mature. Some training should be used, however, to achieve relaxation and mechanical efficiency at these levels.

Resistance Training (Strength Training)

The use of resistance training (strength training) in prepubertal children has been controversial. Historically, clinicians and researchers believed individuals with growing bones and open growth plates should not participate in resistance training because it could potentially place the open growth plates at risk for injury. In 1983 the American Academy of Pediatrics issued a position statement that suggested that resistance training in a prepubescent athlete may not only be a high-risk activity but also may be unlikely to result in a significant increase in strength because of the lack of circulating androgens in this population. Importantly, recent evidence suggests both of these fears are unfounded, and several professional organizations now advocate appropriately implemented resistance training as an intervention for young athletes.[243]

With regard to efficacy of resistance training, several research studies have demonstrated that strength can be improved by systematic overload of muscle in postpubescent athletes with results similar to training in adults.[42,282] The mechanism of this gain in strength is likely related to neural adaptations in the muscle and not secondary to an increase in cross-sectional area or hypertrophy of muscle tissue.[122] Similar to an adult who initiates a resistance training program, initial gains in strength in the first 4 to 5 weeks after onset of training are due to neural adaptations in the muscle. Only after this initial neuromuscular change do adults see a change in their muscle diameter, which may result in continued progression of strength. Children have the potential to experience a similar neuromuscular adaptation, which can increase strength despite the absence of circulating androgens, once thought to be necessary to see any increase in strength.[123,167]

Safety during resistance training is a priority in a population of young athletes. Initial epidemiology data regarding injuries during resistance training suggested a high incidence of injury in a population of young individuals. However, more recent evidence suggests the incidence of injury is relatively low and, with certain precautions, this risk can be reduced even further.[290] Many of the injuries reported by Myer and colleagues identify accidents as the primary cause of injury in the weight room with a young population. As a result, current guidelines regarding resistance training in young athletes suggest appropriate supervision be present at all times to minimize the chance of these accidental injuries. In fact, professional organizations such as the American College of Sports Medicine, the National Strength and Conditioning Association, and the American Academy of Pediatrics suggest that resistance training is a safe and effective intervention in young athletes.[122] Furthermore, resistance training has also been shown to be effective in reducing various lower extremity injuries.[233]

Through the joint contributions of these professional organizations, a general consensus on the safe initiation of resistance training in a young population has been issued.[290] These recommendations suggest a young athlete should have sufficient emotional maturity to accept and follow directions prior to initiating a resistance training program. Appropriate supervision should be available at all times to reduce the risk of accidental injuries and also to provide regular feedback regarding the "technique" of each lift. A primary goal of the onset of a resistance training program is to develop good lifting technique at an early age. Supervision is necessary to ensure this development. Finally, a dynamic warm-up is always recommended, and an appropriate volume and intensity of each activity should be initiated and monitored. Specifically, young athletes should avoid executing one maximum repetition and should focus on the use of lighter weight with higher sets and repetitions rather than using lower sets and striving to gain power. Together, these factors have resulted in a safer and more efficacious algorithm for resistance training participation by young athletes.

Speed

Current evidence suggests the proportion of fast twitch fibers in muscle is largely determined by genetic code, with little potential to change fiber type. Hence speed is somewhat genetically determined. All athletes, however, can train the intermediate muscle fibers and improve the components of reaction and movement time. This can result in relative improvements in speed and quickness.[227] Faster reactions are taught in sport-specific practice drills, such as starts, acceleration drills, or play drills, that gradually narrow choice. Movement time is enhanced from a base of flexibility and strength with ballistic motions, sprint loading (explosive jump or throw), overspeed, or resisted sprinting.[381]

Proper Supervision

The first in the series of supervisors is the coach, the key to a successful sports program. However, 2.5 million adult volunteers with varying levels of expertise coach approximately 20 million children. The American Academy of Pediatrics has stated that coaches should encourage preparticipation screenings annually, enforce use of warm-up procedures, require suitable protective equipment, and enforce rules concerning safety. In addition, it recommends completion of a certification program that covers teaching techniques, basic sports skills, fitness, first aid, sportsmanship, enhancement of self-image, and motivational skills.[12]

Qualified officials and professional medical personnel at games and practices are the second level of supervision. These individuals provide game control and immediate injury containment onsite. Medical personnel could include physicians, physical therapists, or athletic trainers who have certification in basic first aid and cardiopulmonary resuscitation techniques in addition to their medical skills.[12,343]

Protection

Outfitting the child athlete with proper equipment should be mandated and enforced for the protection of the participants. Equipment must be appropriate for the sport. High quality and proper fit are essential to correct function. Proper footwear with adequate cushioning, rearfoot control, and sole flexibility for the sport should be required.[282] Protective padding in contact or kicking sports, such as shoulder and shin pads, should be required.

Protective headgear for contact and collision in football, baseball, and hockey is necessary to limit the number of head and neck injuries. Schuller and colleagues[375] have demonstrated a lower risk of auricular damage in wrestlers wearing headgear (26% incidence) versus those with no headgear (52% incidence). Helmets should be approved by the National Operating Committee on Standards for Athletic Equipment (NOCSAE) and the American National Safety Institute.[307,327]

Eye injuries remain a common occurrence in athletics with nearly 40,000 sports-related eye injuries reported in the National Electronic Injury Surveillance System Database.[416] It is estimated that as many as 90% are preventable.[331] Eye protectors that dissipate injury to a wider area without reducing visual field should be required in racquet sports, ice hockey, baseball, basketball, and football and during use of air-powered weapons. They should be cosmetically and functionally acceptable and made of impact-resistant material. Polycarbonate is the most impact- and scratch-resistant material. A list of high-risk sports and recommended protection is given in Table 15.4. All eye protectors should be approved by either the Canadian Standards Association or the American Society for Testing and Materials.

Studies have highlighted the incidence of oral and facial injuries in many sports, particularly football, hockey, baseball, basketball, wrestling, and boxing.[148] Before mandatory use of mouthguards, oral trauma constituted 50% of all football injuries.[272] The mandatory use of mouthguards has cut the injury rate of oral trauma in football to fewer than 1% of all injuries.[205] The mouth protector serves to prevent injury to the teeth and lacerations of the mouth. Because it absorbs blows to the oral and facial structures, it also prevents fractures and dislocations. It should position the bite so the condyles of the mandible do not contact the fossae of the joints. These mouthguards should be inexpensive, strong, and easy to clean and should not interfere with speech or breathing. They should be used alone in field hockey, rugby, wrestling, basketball, and other field events and used in conjunction with face protectors in football, ice hockey, baseball, and lacrosse.

Environmental Control

Assessment and control of the environment are also vital to the safety of the child athlete. The playing area should have adequate lighting and be maintained for safety. Surfaces should be free from obstacles and smooth and even, with good shock-absorbing qualities (wood as opposed to concrete). Modifications of equipment that have been shown to decrease injury (e.g., breakaway bases) should be installed. Sports equipment and playing environments should be scaled down to the size of the athlete.[282]

TABLE 15.4 Risk Level for Eye Injury With Recommendations for Protective Eyewear

Risk	Sport	Protective Wear
Unacceptable	Boxing	Not applicable
Very high	Ice hockey	Helmet with full visor
	Squash	Polycarbonate sports protector
	Badminton	Polycarbonate sports protector
	Basketball	Polycarbonate sports protector
	Men's lacrosse	Helmet with full visor
High	Racquetball	Polycarbonate sports protector
	Baseball	Polycarbonate sports protector
	Cricket	Helmet with full visor
	Field hockey	Helmet with full visor
	Rugby football	Debatable
	Soccer	Debatable
	Water polo	Polycarbonate goggles
	Shooting	Polycarbonate sports protector
	Women's lacrosse	Helmet with full visor
Moderate	Tennis	Plastic lens spectacles
	American football	Helmet with polycarbonate visor
Low	Golf	Sports protector if one-eyed
	Volleyball	Sports protector if one-eyed
	Skiing	UV filter goggles ± helmet
	Cycling	Sports protector ± helmet
	Fishing	Polycarbonate protector if one-eyed
	Swimming	Goggles if in water for long periods
	High diving	Not feasible
	Track and field	None required

From Jones N: Eye injury in sport. *Sports Med* 7:163-181, 1989.

Ambient temperature and humidity should be carefully monitored. During exercise, children require more fluid replacement per kilogram of body weight than adults to avoid dehydration. Children have a greater surface area per body weight, so their rate of heat exchange is greater with lower ability to endure exercise in climatic extremes. They also have a distinctly deficient ability to perspire, so they carry a larger heat load. They acclimatize less efficiently and require more "exposures" for acclimatization to occur.[350] Exercise should be modified if the wet bulb temperature (an index of climatic heat stress) is above 75°F.[13]

Dehydration can be avoided by drinking plenty of liquid before, during, and after play. Thirst is not a valid indicator of the amount of water needed, so every pound (16 oz) lost should be replaced with two cups (16 oz) of water.[329] The American College of Sports Medicine[8] recommends that 400 to 500 mL of water be ingested before distance running. It further recommends water intake every 35 to 45 minutes of football practice and nude weighing before and after practice. If residual weight loss from day to day exceeds 2 to 3 lb, practice is restricted until water is replenished. Recommendations for hydration include prehydration of 3 to 12 oz (3 to 6 oz for < 90 lb; 6 to 12 oz for > 90 lb weight) 1 hour before activity, and 3 to 6 oz just prior to activity. During activity 3 to 9 oz (3 to 5 oz for < 90 lb; 6 to 9 oz for > 90 lb) should be ingested every 10 to 20 minutes relative to the temperature and humidity. Eight to 12 oz should be consumed for each pound of weight lost in 2 to 4 hours following activity (Table 15.5).[75]

TABLE 15.5 Recommended Fluid Intake and Availability for a 90-Minute Practice

WEIGHT LOSS		Minutes Between Water Break	FLUID PER BREAK	
Lb	Kg		Oz	Ml
8	3.6	*		
7.5	3.4	*		
7	3.2	10	8–10	266
6.5	3.0	10	8–9	251
6	2.7	10	8–9	251
5.5	2.5	15	10–12	325
5	2.3	15	10–11	311
4.5	2.1	15	9–10	281
4	1.8	15	8–9	251
3.5	1.6	20	10–11	311
3	1.4	20	9–10	281
2.5	1.1	20	7–8	222
2	0.9	30	8	237
1.5	0.7	30	6	177
1	0.5	45	6	177
0.5	0.2	60	6	177

*No practice recommended.
From Peterson M, Peterson K: *Eat to compete: a guide to sports nutrition.* Chicago, Year Book Medical, 1988.

Successful hydration programs involve not only fluid intake but also fluid availability. Cool fluids infuse into the system more readily, so accessible liquids should be chilled or ice provided. Education of everyone involved with the activity, including parents and participants, is of paramount importance to ensure continued compliance. Knowledge of the common signs of dehydration—irritability, headache, nausea, dizziness, weakness, cramps, abdominal distress, and decreased performance—assist those involved with early recognition and intervention.[75]

RISK FACTORS FOR INJURY

Injury can be the result of a single macrotrauma or of repetitive microtrauma.[277] Seven risk factors for repetitive trauma, or "overuse," have been identified: (1) training errors; (2) musculotendinous imbalances of strength and/or flexibility; (3) anatomic malalignment of the lower extremity; (4) improper footwear; (5) faulty playing surface; (6) associated disease states of the lower extremity such as old injury or arthritis; and (7) growth factors.[249,275,398]

Training Error

Training error is frequently the cause of overuse injuries in children, as it is in adults. Dramatic increases in the total volume of activity, an increase in the rate of progression of training, or an attempt to participate at a level above the capacity of the athlete is a often identified as a mechanism of overuse injury.[4,277] The evolution of sports specialization has contributed to this phenomenon because more children are attempting to participate in several seasons of a single sport throughout the year. This results in few rest periods throughout a year and an increased focus on intense training. A sudden transition from casual, free play to 6 or 8 hours of intense participation daily, as may occur in a camp setting, has also contributed to the increased incidence of overuse injury in children.[185]

Muscle-Tendon Imbalance

Muscle-tendon imbalance can occur in strength, flexibility, or training. Until recently, little attention was paid to conditioning in children. This position may have been appropriate for free play activities but not for organized sport. The repetitive, often predictable, demands of a sport may result in imbalances of muscle and tendon unless the child is on a well-designed training plan. For example, an overhead athlete, such as a swimmer who does breast stroke, might develop a loose anterior capsule and a tight posterior capsule. This imbalance can lead to secondary shoulder impingement or excessive anterior shoulder laxity and even subluxation. Similarly, repetitive running can create strength and tightness in the quadriceps femoris and triceps surae muscles with relatively weaker hamstrings. This could be problematic if pace and hence stride length are increased.

Anatomic Malalignment

Anatomic malalignment, such as leg length difference or abnormal frontal and rotational plane alignments, can be a factor in the occurrence of injury. Anatomic malalignments may result in compensations for abnormally high forces created by the altered alignment under the demands of a sport. For example, femoral anteversion in a young dancer can cause compensatory excessive tibial external rotation and ankle pronation as substitutes for natural hip external rotation. Hyperlordosis of the spine or hyperextension of the knee creates abnormal loading on portions of the joint, leading to pain and increased risk of injury. Pes planus can increase the valgus moment at the knee, as well as allowing the weight of the body to land on a flexible foot. This malalignment can cause pain and abnormal wear on the medial knee joint and foot.

Improper Footwear and Playing Surface

Well-fitting shoes with a firm heel counter, slight heel lift, and flexible toe box are essential for the young athlete. Inadequate footwear that does not support the structures of the foot can lead to a number of foot and lower extremity problems. The shoe should compensate for changes in alignment and shock absorption. Likewise, improper playing surfaces can predispose the child to knee pain, shin splints, or stress fractures. These symptoms have been associated with playing on hard, banked surfaces or synthetic courts, as opposed to clay and hardwood surfaces.[282]

Associated Disease States

Associated disease has the potential to result in compensatory movement patterns during physical activity that may predispose athletes to overuse injuries. Conditions such as Legg-Calvé-Perthes disease (see Chapter 14) or juvenile idiopathic arthritis (see Chapter 7) may result in abnormal lower extremity alignment or abnormal movement patterns during dynamic activities, which may exacerbate joint pain or synovitis. Evaluation of dynamic movement patterns is an appropriate screening in these athletes to attempt to determine their risk for future injury.[292]

Growth Factors

The first aspect of growth that is a factor in overuse injuries is the articular cartilage (Fig. 15.2). Clinical and biomechanical evidence suggests that growing cartilage has low resistance to repetitive loading, resulting in microtrauma to either the

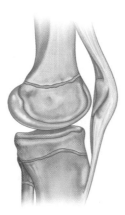

FIG. 15.2 Sites of susceptibility of the growth cartilage. (Redrawn from Micheli L: Overuse injuries in children's sports: the growth factor. *Orthop Clin North Am* 14(2):337-360, 1983.)

cartilage or the underlying growth plate. Damage may result in osteoarthritis or growth asymmetry.[275]

Growing articular cartilage is also less resistant to shear, particularly at the elbow, knee, and ankle. Repetitive shear has been implicated in osteochondritis dissecans of the capitellum in Little League pitchers and of the proximal and distal femur and talus in runners. Debate exists in the literature as to the etiology of osteochondritis dissecans; however, some authors postulate that a segment of subchondral bone becomes avascular and separates with its articular cartilage from the surrounding bone to become a loose body.[433] Shear stress has also been implicated in epiphyseal displacement.[433] The final site of growth cartilage weakness is the apophysis. The apophysis is a point of attachment of the tendon to the bone and represents an ossification center of the bone. Apophysitis is inflammation secondary to microavulsions at the bone-cartilage junction caused by repetitive motion and overuse at times of rapid growth. The apophysis will ultimately fuse as the child matures; however, until this time it is vulnerable to overuse injuries.[43] Increasing evidence suggests that traction apophysitis, such as Osgood-Schlatter disease, Sever disease, and irritation of the rectus femoris or sartorius muscle origins, is the result of degeneration of the growth center with tiny avulsion fractures and associated healing.[316,321]

The second element of growth involved in overuse injury is abnormal stress created by longitudinal growth. Long bone, longitudinal growth occurs initially in the bones, with secondary elongation of the soft tissues. During periods of rapid bone growth ("growth spurts"), the musculotendinous structures tighten and cause loss of flexibility. A coincidence of overuse injury and growth spurt has been noted.[275]

The biomechanical properties of bone also change with growth and maturation. As bone becomes less cartilaginous and stiffer, the resistance to impact decreases. Sudden overload may cause the bone to bow or buckle. The epiphysis, defined as the area of growth in the long bones, is more susceptible to injury and may shear or fracture. Examples of this process include avulsion fracture of the ACL, avulsion fracture of the ankle ligament, and growth plate fractures. Because fractures through the epiphysis can be difficult to visualize on radiographs, any injury to the epiphyseal area is considered a fracture and is treated as such in order to avoid potential growth disturbance.[250] Growth plate fractures are typically classified with a Salter-Harris

classification system. Salter-Harris I fractures represent a traction injury to the growth plate. More significant Salter-Harris II–V fractures involve additional portions of the bone and may represent more significant injuries that may affect growth.[364]

TYPES OF INJURIES

Although injuries in children have some similarity to those in adults, several are unique to the growing child. These specific injuries fall into three categories: (1) fractures, (2) joint injuries, and (3) muscle-tendon unit injuries.[152,275]

Fractures

A relatively new injury in children is the stress fracture, which usually results from repetitive microtrauma or poor training. Repetition causes cancellous bone fractures as opposed to cortical bone fatigue in adults.[90,249] These cancellous bone fractures are often imperceptible on radiographs until 6 to 8 weeks after the onset of pain. Clinical signs and symptoms indicative of a stress fracture can be confirmed by imaging tools, such as a bone scan or magnetic resonance imaging (MRI), to appropriately diagnose this condition. Stress fractures cause persistent, activity-related pain that can be reproduced by indirect force to the bone.

Growth plate or epiphyseal fractures are unique to the child. The cartilaginous growth plate is less resistant to shear or tensile-deforming force than either the ligament or bony cortex, so mechanical disruption frequently occurs through the plate itself, usually in the zone of hypertrophy.[249] This disruption can be caused by a single macrotrauma, such as jumping, or by repetitive microtrauma as in distance running. The potential for problems from epiphyseal fracture depends on the specific plate involved and on the extent of the injury. Physeal fractures are often classified according to a system proposed by Salter and Harris (Type I, fracture line within the physis; Type II, fracture line also extends to metaphysis; Type III, fracture line begins in physis and exits through epiphysis toward the joint; Type IV, involves a vertical split of the epiphysis, physis, and metaphysis; and Type V, involves crush injuries to the physeal plate).[119,364] The risk of growth disturbance following a physeal injury will vary depending on the nature of the injury and the individual's characteristics (i.e., injury during adolescence when growth is accelerated).[119] Shaft fractures are more common in the older child who is approaching adult status.[133]

Joint Injuries

Joint injuries in the young athlete include fractures (discussed above), ligamentous sprains, and other internal derangement. These injuries may result from a single discrete injury or from repetitive microtrauma. The diagnosis of ligament sprain must be made carefully in the child. During a growth spurt, ligaments may be stronger than the growth plate, so excessive bending or twisting forces cause the growth plate rather than the ligament to yield. Careful clinical examination and evaluation including physical examination (with special testing) and assessment of the mechanism of injury can assist in accurate differential diagnosis. Differential diagnosis can be further aided by imaging studies. The clinical assessment of ligamentous integrity can be complicated by the variability in anatomy and tendency for greater physiologic laxity, emphasizing the importance of side-to-side comparisons with ligamentous and soft tissue integrity examination. Often concomitant with ligament injuries are internal derangement of the joint, including meniscus (in the knee) and chondral injury. Although the true incidence of meniscus tears (knee) and chondral involvement in children is not known, there is a rise in the occurrence or recognition of these injuries in the pediatric and adolescent population.

Muscle-Tendon Unit Injuries

Another area at particular risk of injury in the growing child is the insertion of the musculotendinous unit into the bone through the apophyseal cartilage. Growth occurs at the apophyseal growth plate, where tendons and ligaments are attached. During growth spurts the increased tension on the attachments often leads to detachment of the structure at the apophysis (avulsion fracture). Tendonitis occurs much less frequently in the child than in the adult because the insertion becomes symptomatic before the tendon.[4]

Irritation of the insertional area of the musculotendinous unit, the enthesis, can cause pain and inflammation. This area is highly vascular and metabolically active. Pain and inflammation can cause inhibition of muscle activity with resultant weakness and loss of flexibility, potentially initiating a cycle of greater irritation and pain. In addition to experiencing acute injuries, children can overuse muscles, resulting in strain, just like adults. Children may also sustain injury or irritation to growth plates due to traction apophysitis from muscle attachment; such is the case with Osgood-Schlatter disease and Sinding-Larson-Johansson disease.

SITES OF INJURY

Mechanism, presentation, and management of injuries in children are often unique when compared to adult populations secondary to their developing anatomy and periods of rapid growth. The following sections will discuss the unique aspects of these various conditions in the pediatric and adolescent athlete.

Concussions

Concussion was defined at the Fourth International Conference on Concussion as "a complex pathophysiologic process affecting the brain, induced by traumatic biomechanical forces."[268] Generally, a concussion results from either compression, tensile, or shearing forces imposed on the brain and can be caused by a direct blow to the head, face, or neck or an impact to any body part that results in an impulsive force that is transmitted to the head.[268] It is important to recognize that a concussion may or may not result in a loss of consciousness.[268] Symptoms and signs from a concussion often emerge immediately following the injury; however, they may also evolve and develop over several hours, days, or even weeks.[82,268] Diagnosis of a concussion is typically indicated by new onset or worsening of at least one of the following criteria after a suspected head injury has occurred[254,268]:

  Any period of loss of or decreased level of consciousness
  A loss of memory for events immediately before or after the injury
  Any alteration in mental state at the time of injury such as confusion, disorientation, slowed thinking
  Signs or symptoms such as headache, slowed reaction times, dizziness, nausea, vomiting, sleep disturbances, irritability, emotional lability, feeling like in a fog, difficulty concentrating, visual disturbances, sensitivity to light or sound
Historically concussions have been viewed as relatively benign injuries. However, mounting evidence indicates that concussions can lead to multiple short-term impairments and potential long-term adverse outcomes such as cognitive declines, persistent motor control deficits, and actual structural changes in the brain (e.g., chronic traumatic encephalopathy).[35,103–105,252,267,268,271] Life-threatening complications from concussion include intracranial hemorrhage such as epidural and subdural hematoma. The leading cause of death from head injury is intracranial hemorrhage. Cantu and Mueller[73] reported that 86% of brain-injury deaths resulted from subdural hematoma. Symptoms of an epidural hematoma include initial preservation of consciousness with increasingly severe headache, lethargy, and focal neurologic signs. An acute subdural hematoma is the most common fatal head injury and should always be considered as a possible diagnosis in the athlete who loses and does not regain consciousness. A chronic subdural hematoma should be suspected in the athlete who is demonstrating abnormal behavior for days or weeks after a head injury. Signs may include progressive, worsening symptoms or new neurologic signs, persistent vomiting, deteriorating mental status, and the onset of seizures.[266,268] These conditions represent medical emergencies, and these patients should be immediately transported to emergency medical facilities.

Concussions Incidence

An estimated 1.6–3.8 million sport-related traumatic brain injuries occur in the United States each year,[228] a majority of which are mild traumatic brain injuries or concussions.[228] Pediatric patients make up a large portion of concussion injuries, with approximately 100,000 emergency department visits for concussion occurring for school-age children in the United States each year.[274,359] The actual incidence of concussions in youth is likely much higher because a large percentage of concussion injuries go unrecognized, unreported, or untreated.[359] Concussion rates differ by sport and gender, with boys experiencing more sports-related concussions overall, while girls have a higher concussion rate when comparing similar sports.[241,257,359] Football, ice hockey, lacrosse, and wrestling have been reported as sports with the highest risk for concussion for boys, and soccer, lacrosse, ice hockey, field hockey, and basketball are reportedly the highest-risk sports for girls.[257,359] Attempts to classify the severity of concussions have been controversial because these approaches are often dependent upon loss of consciousness and amnesia, both of which have been shown to be poor predictors of injury severity.[154]

As of February 2014, all 50 states and the District of Columbia have enacted legislation designed to help protect youth athletes. Most of these laws mandate that a child should not return to play the same day a suspected head injury has occurred and that a licensed health care provider must medically clear the athlete. Coinciding with an increase in the media attention surrounding concussive injuries and the enactment of the legislation, there has been a significant rise in health care utilization for concussive injuries as evidenced by the rates of pediatric concussion referrals to neurologists increasing by approximately 150% between 2008 and 2012.

Concussion Evaluation

Evaluation of a concussion is a multifactorial process, and a wide array of assessment tools are available to assist in the diagnosis and monitoring of concussive injuries. The initial assessment of the injury should occur on the field or at the time of injury if a potential head injury is suspected. There are a variety of sideline assessment tools that are now available such as the Sport

TABLE 15.6   Examples of Postconcussion Assessment Options and Strategies

	Musculoskeletal	Vestibular/Oculomotor	Cardiovascular
Balance Error Scoring System (BESS) Sensory organization test Force place assessments • Path length • Entropy • Stability index	Neck range of motion Neck strength Special tests for neck Posture assessment	Gaze stability Convergence Divergence Saccades Smooth pursuit Positional testing King-Devick test	Cycle ergometer exertional tests Treadmill exertional tests
Postural Control/Balance	**Musculoskeletal**	**Vestibular/Oculomotor**	**Cardiovascular**
Balance Error Scoring System (BESS) Sensory organization test Force place assessments • Path length • Entropy • Stability index	Neck range of motion Neck strength Special tests for neck Posture assessment	Gaze stability Convergence Divergence Saccades Smooth pursuit Positional testing King-Devick test	Cycle ergometer exertional tests Treadmill exertional tests

Concussion Assessment Tool (SCAT3) and the Child-SCAT3 (for ages 5 to 12 years).[81,368] The SCAT 3 and Child-SCAT3 are standardized tools for evaluating individuals with a suspected head injury that were designed for use by medical professionals. These tools provide specific, detailed instructions about how to conduct and record results for a series of background questions, the Glasgow coma scale, and cognitive and physical evaluation strategies.

Concussions are generally considered to represent a functional rather than a structural brain injury because in many cases conventional neuroimaging techniques such as computed tomography (CT) and MRI result in no abnormal findings.[359] However, various advanced neuroimaging techniques have demonstrated microstructural and functional brain changes in concussed individuals.[359] Even so, imaging is not often recommended for most patients with concussions as the cost and time to administer these tests do not typically result in changes in clinical management.[268,359]

It also recommended that a few days after injury patients be reassessed with neurocognitive screening techniques, symptom indices, and physical assessments. This is an area where the role of physical therapists in postconcussion care is evolving. Physical therapy evaluations for identification of postconcussion impairments in the postural control,[76-78,164,165] musculoskeletal,[373] vestibular/oculomotor,[377,415] and cardiovascular systems are becoming more common.[217,230-232] Much like the screening tools that are available for sideline assessments of concussions, a variety of options and strategies for screening for potential postconcussion impairments in patients in physical therapy clinics are also available (Table 15.6). Evaluation order and strategies may be individualized according to patient-specific symptoms, goals, and medical history.

Concussions Management and Recovery

Animal models suggest that there is a brief window of brain vulnerability following a concussion that appears to resolve gradually over 7–10 days.[82,359] It is unclear how well these findings generalize to the human population. Nevertheless, it is generally recognized that a typical recovery period for concussion is approximately 7–10 days for adults and about 2–4 weeks for children. Second impact syndrome is a potentially fatal condition that results from a second head injury being sustained before full resolution of an initial concussion. Young brains may be especially vulnerable to the rare but catastrophic

occurrence of second impact syndrome.[255,266] Consequently, current recommendations for initial management of concussions focus on rest until symptoms resolve or are back to baseline in a resting state.

Specific return-to-activity recommendations are controversial because the progression to activity should be individualized to each patient and focused on symptom and impairment recovery rather than days since the injury occurred. A gradual return to activity program is generally accepted as the safest way to help progress a patient back to preinjury activity levels (Table 15.7). If symptoms arise during this progression, modification should be made to allow the symptoms to resolve. Special consideration should be given to the individual who has suffered multiple concussions, and the potential disqualification for contact sports should be considered. In general, young athletes represent a unique population in the presence of concussions. The brain of a young athlete is still developing, and as a result the effect of a concussion in this population is still unknown.[82,112,166,171] General consensus in the literature does suggest that a more conservative approach to concussion management should be implemented in this younger population.[253] Therefore advancement through rehabilitation including time to return to play is often slower in this population. Future research needs to focus on better understanding the effects of concussion on a developing brain and developing more evidence-based guidelines related to management and return to activity following a concussion in a young athlete.

Approximately 10% to 30% of individuals who sustain a concussion will continue to experience persistent traumatic brain injury symptoms for months to years after the injury.[386] Individuals whose symptoms last for more than 4 weeks and fit the World Health Organization's diagnostic criteria are often diagnosed with postconcussion syndrome (PCS).[314,315] A rapidly emerging field of practice in physical therapy is the treatment of patients with PCS using physical therapy interventions. There is early evidence supporting such interventions as vestibular therapies, manual therapy, therapeutic exercise, and progressive aerobic training leading to growing recognition that physical therapy may facilitate recovery in patients with PCS.[8,9,28,145,146,372,373] At this time, specific evidence-based guidelines regarding physical therapy strategies for treating PCS are not currently available. Future research is needed to further develop an evidence base that can provide strong conclusions in these regards.

TABLE 15.7 Return to Activity Program

Rehabilitation Stage	Functional Exercise at Each Stage of Rehabilitation	Objective of Each Stage
No activity	Complete physical and cognitive rest	Recovery
Light aerobic exercise	Walking, swimming, or stationary cycling keeping intensity < 70% MPHR. No resistance training	Increase HR
Sport-specific exercise	Skating drills in ice hockey, running drills in soccer. No head impact activities	Add movement
Noncontact training drills	Progression to more complex training drills (e.g., passing drills in football and ice hockey). May start progressive resistance training	Exercise, coordination, cognitive load
Full-contact practice	Following medical clearance, participate in normal training activities	Restore confidence, assessment of functional skills by coaching staff
Return to play	Normal game play	

HR, heart rate; *MPHR*, .
(From McCrory P, et al.: Consensus statement on concussion in sport: the 3rd International Conference on Concussion in Sports Held in Zurich, November 2008. *J Athl Train* 44(4):434-448, 2009.)

Cervical Injuries

The incidence of central nervous system injury in children is low, varying from 1% to 5% of sports-related injuries, but these cases constitute 50% to 100% of the deaths from injury. Cervical spine injuries result in 30% to 50% of cases of childhood quadriplegia.[61] The rate of spinal cord injuries in children younger than age 11 years is low, but it escalates dramatically in the 15- to 18-year-old age bracket. The largest percentage of traumatic spinal cord injury in children ages 10–14 years old was due to sports injury,[86] with as many cervical spine injuries occurring in sports as seen in motor vehicle accidents in children between 8 and 15 years old.[235] Because the brain and spinal cord are largely incapable of regeneration, these injuries take on a singular importance.[72]

Participation in several sports carries a particularly high risk for head and neck injuries. Sports-related injuries account for 14% of all head trauma cases seen in pediatric emergency departments in the United States.[155] American football accounts for a large percentage of all concussion injuries in school sports, with as many as 9.6% of all injuries in football being diagnosed as concussions.[115] Although 69% of deaths between 1945 and 1999 were from brain injuries, the incidence of serious head injuries has decreased since the late 1980s.[73]

Severe spinal injuries may result in paralysis and total disability. A population-based study over 7 years identified 32 children younger than 15 years of age who sustained spinal fracture, dislocation, or severe ligamentous injury; sports were the cause of all injuries in children over the age of 10 years.[130] Rugby, a popular collision sport outside the United States, has head and neck injury rates similar to those of American football. Wrestling has the second highest injury rate of all high school sports, although the central nervous system injury rate is low. The rate of catastrophic wrestling injuries (cervical ligament injury, spinal cord contusion, severe head injury, or herniated disk) is 2.11 per year (1 per 100,000 participants) as a result of direct blows or falls.[52] Football, soccer, and basketball account for a large number of concussions secondary to collision, although exact incidence figures have not been reported. Diving accounts for 3% to 21% of all cervical spine injuries in young people.[49] Noguchi[303] noted that swimming and gymnastics accounted for 51% and 22.8%, respectively, of all spinal injuries in persons younger than 30 years of age.

Most neck injuries are caused by hyperflexion or hyperextension. Hyperflexion injuries, which are the most common, result from spearing (Fig. 15.3). Because of the undeveloped musculature in young athletes relative to adults and the commonly associated fracture, hyperflexion injury can be serious.

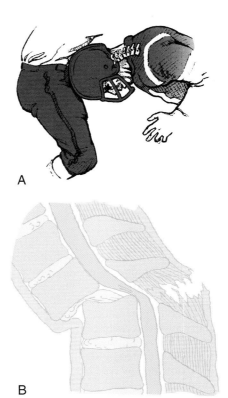

A

B

FIG. 15.3 Hyperflexion damage from head butting. ([A] From Birrer R, Brecher D: *Common sports injuries in youngsters.* Oradell, NJ, Medical Economics, 1987. [B] From Black JM, Hawks JH: *Medical-surgical nursing,* ed 8, St. Louis, 2009, Saunders.)

Hyperextension injuries often occur even in the absence of severe force because the anterior neck musculature is weaker than the posterior musculature. Common causes are face or head tackling (Fig. 15.4). Hyperextension injury with a rotatory component is the most common cause of nerve root damage.[48,394] Evaluation of these injuries should always include radiographs of the cervical spine. In the adolescent the second cervical vertebra is normally displaced posteriorly over the third secondary to hypermobility. This pseudosubluxation is normal and not the result of injury[72] but should be referred for assessment.

Another common injury is a "stinger" or "burner," which is a traction injury to the brachial plexus. It is caused by a forceful

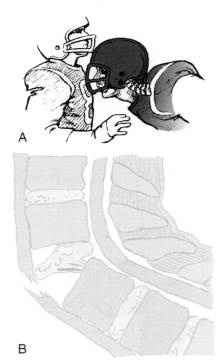

A

B

FIG. 15.4 Hyperextension injury from face blocking ([A] From Birrer R, Brecher D: *Common sports injuries in youngsters.* Oradell, NJ, Medical Economics, 1987. [B] From Black JM, Hawks JH: *Medical-surgical nursing,* ed 8, St. Louis, Saunders, 2009.)

blow to the head from the side creating lateral deviation of the head or from depression of the shoulder while the head and neck are fixed. Repeated injuries may cause weakness of the deltoid, biceps, and teres major muscles, which should be resolved with strengthening exercises. The use of a collar, a change in technique, and cervical/scapulothoracic strengthening are appropriate interventions to help resolve symptoms. If symptoms persist or if repeated injuries occur, restriction in ability to return to play is warranted.[93] Return to play in a collision or contact sport following any type of cervical injury should be closely monitored.[74,93]

Thoracic and Lumbar Spinal Injuries

Back injuries in children are different from those in adults and require careful evaluation.[219,420] Spinal injuries can occur in both the thoracic and the lumbar areas, although thoracic injuries are rare. Costovertebral injury secondary to compression of the rib cage may occur in sports such as football or from a forceful takedown in wrestling. Complaints include pain and muscle spasm along the associated rib with potential complaints of pain with thoracic rotation. Axial compression forces on a preflexed spine, as in sledding or tobogganing, can fracture the vertebrae, particularly at the vulnerable T12–L1 level. These injuries can cause pain but at times are asymptomatic.[48,394]

The most common injuries in the lumbar spine are spondylolysis and spondylolisthesis. One study of 3132 competitive athletes ages 15 to 27 years noted an incidence of spondylolysis of 12.5%.[360] Repeated and excessive hyperextension in football blocking, clean and jerk lift, diving, pole vaulting, wrestling, high jump, or gymnastic maneuvers can place excessive forces on the pars interarticularis and cause a stress fracture.

Spondylolisthesis is described as a fracture and slippage of one vertebra on another, usually L5 over S1 or L4 over L5. Loading of a bilateral spondylolysis, in which there is a defect in the bony connection of the posterior arch with the vertebral body, can cause a spondylolisthesis, as can traumatic or repetitive bilateral loading of a normal spine. The slippage is graded from 1 to 4, depending on the degree of slippage. Athletes with grade 2 or greater slippage should be counseled against participation in activities requiring excessive lumbar extension such as weight lifting, baseball, diving, gymnastics, or wrestling. Participation in basketball or football is permissible with use of a brace.[107,113,219,273] The growth spurt in the spine causes lumbar lordosis secondary to the enhanced anterior growth with posterior tethering by the heavy lumbodorsal fascia. This biomechanical situation increases the tendency of posterior element failure at the pars.[278] Athletes with spondylolysis are managed in a brace or, at minimum, with restricted activity until healing occurs. Physical therapy is indicated to maintain flexibility in the lumbosacral spine and the spinal and hip musculature and to improve trunk and abdominal muscle strength and core stability while braced. Surgery is indicated only in cases of unstable lesions or nerve root compression.[48,142,310]

The incidence of disk lesions in young athletes is unknown, but several studies have demonstrated that disk herniation can occur, with 95% of these cases occurring at L4/L5 or L5/S1. Although acute trauma may precede the diagnosis of disc herniation, degenerative changes of the vertebral bodies and intervertebral joints may be the contributing factors, with trauma being the acute precipitating incident.[139] Conservative management of this condition is often successful in the pediatric and adolescent population; however, if symptoms persist, surgical management may be necessary.[139]

Shoulder Injuries

Specific shoulder injuries can be predicted based on the biomechanics of the sport and the age of the athlete.[190,215] Participation in football, wrestling, and ice hockey may increase the likelihood of upper extremity fractures, subluxations, and dislocations. Sports with repeated overhead activities, such as volleyball, swimming, gymnastics, and baseball, are more likely to result in overuse injuries.[1,26,336] The hyperelasticity of juvenile joints, particularly the shoulder, makes them vulnerable to passive and dynamic instability patterns that can predispose the shoulder to injury.[190,323] The presence of disease processes or pathology that potentially increase this hyperelasticity, such as Ehlers-Danlos syndrome, can exacerbate this presentation.

Acromioclavicular (AC) sprains may occur in the immature athlete without clavicular fracture; however, it is more common in skeletally mature athletes. The most common mechanism is direct force from a fall or blow to the lateral aspect of the shoulder or a fall on an outstretched arm.[48,142,215,275] Grade I and II sprains are more common in the athlete whose skeleton is immature. Grade III sprains commonly rupture the dorsal clavicular periosteum, but the acromioclavicular and coracoclavicular ligaments remain intact.[215,323] There is some controversy regarding optimal management of AC joint separations. These lesions are often treated symptomatically with rest, ice, compression, and elevation (RICE) in a sling. Some cases may require surgical stabilization if conservative management fails.[55] Exercises are often necessary to increase scapulothoracic and glenohumeral mobility and strength after the sprain is healed.

Fractures are most common in the middle third of the clavicle from a direct blow. These can be actual fractures in the older child or greenstick fractures in the youngster. They are managed with a figure-of-eight strap or sling stabilization until healed.

The proximal humerus is an area of bone growth in children and is typically not as strong as the surrounding capsule and ligamentous structures. Therefore fractures are more common in children than in adults, who are more prone to dislocation. Epiphyseal displacements occur in the younger child, and metaphyseal fractures are more common in the older child or adolescent.[275] Once bony healing is identified, therapeutic intervention to normalize mobility and strength of the scapular, shoulder, and elbow muscles is frequently indicated.[323]

Little League shoulder, a relatively common injury in young pitchers and catchers, involves an injury of the proximal humeral growth plate secondary to rotatory torque. A skeletally immature athlete who complains of proximal shoulder pain in the absence of trauma should be suspected of having an epiphyseal injury until proved otherwise. The athlete should limit throwing and rotational activities until the pain subsides[190,215,323]; however, strengthening of the parascapular and core musculature is indicated to facilitate a smoother transition back to sports once the pain has subsided.

Frank anterior subluxation and dislocation of the glenohumeral joint are rare in children but common in adolescents. Because of the laxity of juvenile joints, a blow or forceful maneuver in abduction, external rotation, or extension can dislodge the head of the humerus.[48,142,323] This condition is common in contact sports, gymnastics, and overhead throwing sports. Patients with posterior glenohumeral instability respond better to conservative strengthening of appropriate musculature than those with anterior instability, although a program of scapular and shoulder muscle strengthening in a biomechanically correct range of motion should be attempted. Motion should be limited to ranges that prevent chronic subluxation. Surgery is more often an option with anterior or multidirectional instability but may occur in the case of posterior instability.[215,323] Debate exists in the literature regarding the most appropriate timing of arthroscopic stabilization following first-time shoulder dislocations in adolescent athletes.[108,221] Future research will need to identify if immediate surgical stabilization is indicated after first-time dislocation or if a trial of conservative management would be successful in some athletes.

Rotator cuff tears are not as common in the skeletally immature athlete as in the older athlete. They occur in throwing and racquet sports, as well as from direct contact blows in collision sports. These tears can be treated successfully with arthroscopic surgery and rehabilitation that includes strength and endurance training for all scapular and shoulder muscles, as well as training with correct biomechanical movements of the shoulder complex.[215]

Rotator cuff impingement syndrome (Fig. 15.5) is a frequent injury in athletes younger than 25 years of age. More than 50% of swimmers aged 12 to 18 years complain of shoulder pain.[48,142] Unlike adults who typically present with impingement resulting from a mechanical compression in the subacromial space (primary impingement), children often present with impingement symptoms caused by excessive laxity or mobility in the shoulder joint complex described as secondary impingement. This may be due to a laxity of the static stabilizers in the shoulder with an inability of the dynamic shoulder stabilizers to compensate appropriately. Others theorize altered arthrokinematics of the

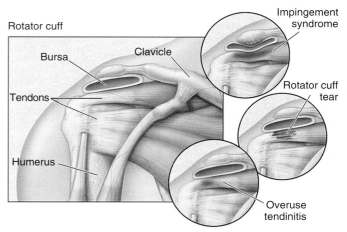

FIG. 15.5 Common causes of impingement. (By permission of Mayo Foundation for Medical Education and Research. All rights reserved.)

shoulder may be due to a contracture around the shoulder with loss of internal rotation at 90° of abduction and with increased external rotation in all positions of abduction. This might reflect a tightened posterior and a loosened anterior capsule, suggesting a tendency to translate anteriorly during functional movement patterns. Conservative physical therapy with a focus on improved strength and muscle activation of the dynamic shoulder-stabilizing musculature, along with normalization of mobility and dynamic movement patterns, has been successful in addressing the underlying instability.[215,275,323] All positions of impingement (anterior, lateral, or overhead) should be modified until the athlete is pain-free.

Elbow Injuries

Supracondylar fracture of the humerus is the second most common fracture in the skeletally immature client. Most of these fractures occur in the age group of 5 to 10 years. They are often the result of falling on an outstretched arm with significant forces into extension. Avulsion fractures of the medial epicondyle are also common in the population and are associated with elbow dislocations or throwing injuries. Anatomic reduction is indicated with internal fixation, when appropriate. Loss of motion is a common impairment following these injuries; therefore early protected range of motion to avoid loss of extension is critical.[152,215] Subsequent to healing, normalization of mobility and strength of the shoulder, elbow, and forearm are necessary for full function.

Repetitive microtrauma from pitching may result in epiphyseal injury of the radial head. Loss of extension and supination with a history of repetitive compressive loading of the radiocapitellar joint may indicate this injury. A radial head pathology is treated with rest.[101,190] Forceful distraction of the arm of a child younger than 7 years old can subluxate the radial head because of the poor development of the annular ligament, often referred to as "nursemaid's elbow."[418] Children who have sustained this injury often position the injured arm in flexion and pronation, dangling it at the side of the body.[48,142,215,394]

Elbow dislocation is seen in contact sports secondary to a fall on an abducted, extended arm. Early reduction will avoid neurovascular damage, and further evaluation and radiographs are necessary to assess the presence of associated fracture. Early protected mobility is necessary to preserve normal elbow motion.[48,142,215] Physical therapy to normalize elbow and forearm mobility and to improve strength at the elbow, forearm, and hand is appropriate.

Little League elbow commonly results from the extreme valgus stress placed on the epicondyles during the acceleration phase of pitching (Fig. 15.6). If this is not recognized and regular throwing continues, mild separation of the medial epicondyle with hypertrophy, irregularity, fragmentation, and avulsion can occur. The most serious damage occurs with the compressive loads experienced in the lateral joint between the radial head and the capitellum. This injury may occur in as many as 8% to 10% of young pitchers. This compressive mechanism can result in osteochondritis of the capitellum, avascular necrosis of the radial head, and loose bodies within the joint. Treatment is RICE and rest from throwing with an ultimate progression to rehabilitation to focus on restoration of full mobility and strength through the upper extremity.[48,142,152,310] Eventual alteration of throwing mechanics may be necessary.

Lateral epicondylitis, or tennis elbow, is seen in a variety of racquet sports as a result of repeated injury to the lateral epicondyle. Repetitive microtrauma to the wrist extensors, as often seen with faulty backhand strokes in tennis, can initiate the process. The resulting tensile overload in the wrist extensors as well as friction between the extensor muscles, the lateral epicondyle, and the radial head causes irritation, microtears in the extensor muscle origin, and adhesions between the annular ligament and the joint capsule. Using tightly strung racquets, racquets with small handles, and old tennis balls can aggravate the situation. Rehabilitation to decrease acute inflammation and chronic irritation, reduce adhesions, and strengthen the forearm and hand musculature is required. Alteration of technique and equipment, such as enlargement of the racquet grip area or reduction of string tension, is helpful.[142,152,190]

Wrist and Hand Injuries

The hand and wrist joint is an inherently complex anatomic structure. As a result, potentially serious injuries may be missed or underdiagnosed. Careful diagnosis using knowledge of anatomy, biomechanics, and pathomechanics of the wrist and hand is crucial.[48,152,215,394]

Fractures about the wrist follow an age-related pattern. In the young child a torus, or buckle fracture, of the distal radial epiphysis is common after a fall. Clinical signs include varying degrees of pain and tenderness, so careful radiologic examination is necessary. Simple splinting is adequate for healing.[48,215,310] Metaphyseal fractures of the distal radius and ulna are more common in the child. Often displaced, they require reduction with the use of anesthesia. In the younger adolescent, fractures through the growth plate are common, again from falls, and require operative reduction to minimize trauma to the growth plate.[215] Rehabilitation to regain normal forearm and wrist mobility as well as wrist and grip strength is desirable. Posttraumatic arthritis of the wrist and hand has been documented in active children. Management requires careful monitoring with nonoperative techniques to permit extensive remodeling, although occasionally surgery is necessary.[326] Stress injuries to the distal radial epiphysis, triangular fibrocartilage complex (TFCC) tears, as well as ligamentous injury in the carpal region have been noted in athletes such as gymnasts who bear weight on their hands. Complaints of wrist stiffness and pain with wrist dorsiflexion are common. Radiographs may demonstrate a widened epiphysis, cystic changes, and breaking of the distal metaphysis with distal radius injury. Carpal ligament and TFCC injuries often require MRI to confirm the diagnosis. Management of these conditions often consists of modification or avoidance of gymnastics with or without casting.[215] Rehabilitation and, at times, surgical management may be required.

Although fracture of most carpal bones is rare, fracture of the navicular or scaphoid bone is common in children from 12 to 15 years of age. This fracture results from a fall on the dorsiflexed hand of an outstretched arm. Although the fracture may not be initially visible on a radiograph, early diagnosis is important because of the high incidence of avascular necrosis and nonunion. If tenderness in the anatomic snuffbox occurs with a high degree of suspicion of fracture, use of a short-arm spica cast is the typical initial management.[48,142,153,394] Surgical management may be necessary in the cases of nonunion.

Because the hand and fingers are so essential in most sports, they absorb tremendous forces with sports participation, resulting in frequent injuries.[48,310,394] Dislocations are uncommon in the child's hand because as the child's developing bony anatomy is often more vulnerable than the ligamentous structure at this age. If dislocations do occur, it is usually in the older adolescent who is approaching skeletal maturity and in patterns similar to those in an adult. Thus the most common dislocation occurs

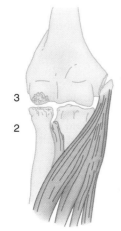
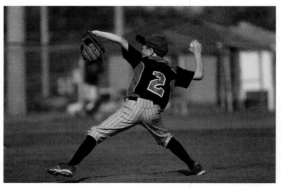

FIG. 15.6 Little Leaguer's elbow. Avulsion fracture of medial epicondyle *(1)*, compression fractures of the radial head *(2)*, and capitellum *(3)*. (*Left,* Redrawn from Connolly JF: *DePalma's management of fractures and dislocations,* Philadelphia, Saunders, 1981. *Right,* from iStock.com.)

at the carpometacarpal joint of the thumb, usually secondary to axial compression forces on the thumb tip in contact sports. Although reduction is easy, chronic instability can result. The thumb is put in a short-arm thumb spica, and participation in sports should be avoided for 6 weeks. Splint stabilization is advisable for the initial 6 weeks of reentry to play.[215]

Dorsal dislocation of the thumb metacarpophalangeal joint is the most common dislocation in the hand of a child. A fall or forceful contact hyperextends the metacarpophalangeal joint. If the proximal phalanx is parallel to the metacarpal, the volar plate has been avulsed and surgical reduction is necessary. Cast immobilization for 3 weeks with sports participation permitted is adequate for healing. Physical therapy may be indicated to normalize thumb mobility and strength following casting. Metacarpophalangeal dislocations in the fingers are rare except for those that affect the index finger. After this injury is reduced, splinting in flexion for 3 weeks with immediate mobilization after splint removal is the treatment of choice.[48,142,394]

Joint injuries are common in ball sports and skiing. The metacarpophalangeal joint of the thumb is the most commonly injured joint in skiers. The majority of these injuries in youth are bony gamekeeper's thumb in which the ulnar collateral ligament avulses a segment of bone, as compared with the purely ligamentous injury in adults. If the bony fragment lies close to its origin, good results are obtained with use of a short-arm thumb spica cast for 6 weeks, followed by exercises to normalize mobility and strength. Athletic participation may continue in some cases and can be facilitated by the use of a custom-molded splint to protect the healing tissues. If the radiograph is negative, integrity of the ulnar collateral ligament must be established by assessing radial deviation in extension and 30° of flexion. Deviation of greater than 30° indicates at least a partial tear. No firm end point in full extension or greater than 45° of deviation in flexion indicates full ligamentous tear with volar plate injury, which will require surgical repair.[48,215,394] Hand therapy is necessary to regain normal mobility, strength, and pinch.

"Jammed" fingers are common injuries in all age groups. Axial compression force to the fingertips causes distal interphalangeal flexion with proximal interphalangeal hyperextension. Reduction is easily accomplished by distal traction. Buddy taping will allow the athlete to return to play.[79,394] Caution should be exhibited, however, because fractures through the growth plate of the phalanx are common. These intra-articular, or neck, fractures have a great tendency to displace and then require open reduction with internal fixation.[275] In the absence of a fracture or dislocation, damage to the collateral ligaments can occur and is managed in similar fashion. Jamming at the distal interphalangeal joint can result in "mallet finger," or tearing of the terminal extensor tendon with or without a bony fragment. This injury is initially managed with use of a dorsal extension splint for 6 to 8 weeks. If active and passive extension ranges are equal at 6 weeks, active flexion can be initiated. If not, splinting is continued for another month. Participation may be permitted if a splint is in place.[48,142,215,394]

Pelvis and Hip Injuries

Pelvis and hip injuries account for 10% to 24% of injuries in the pediatric athlete, with high incidence in ballet, running, soccer, football, and hockey.[56] Because the hip and pelvis have complex ossification patterns and fuse late in childhood, the potential for injury is high. The acetabulum has three sections joined by triradiate cartilage. Likewise, three ossification centers exist on the femoral head: the capital femoral epiphysis, the greater trochanter, and the lesser trochanter. The circular vascularity of the femoral head and neck also creates risk for injury in the growing child.[318,376,422] Hip pain in the pediatric population is typically caused by skeletal (dislocation, avulsion, fracture), soft tissue, nontraumatic (slipped capital femoral epiphysis, Legg-Calvé-Perthes disease, developmental dysplasia) or neoplastic etiologies.[318,376,422]

Traumatic hip dislocations in children are most commonly posterior,[376] with clinical presentation of a limb that is flexed, adducted, and internally rotated. Prompt reduction of the dislocation is key to minimize risk of avascular necrosis.[376]

Fractures are uncommon but can occur in the epiphyseal plate, the femoral neck, or the subtrochanteric area. Fractures of the neck or subtrochanteric area can be the result of severe trauma, usually incurred during contact sports such as football and rugby. Often surgical reduction is required to obtain adequate reduction and promote proper healing.[376] Slipped capital femoral epiphysis (SCFE) is not caused by sports but must be suspected in any athlete with persistent hip or knee pain and a limp. SCFE typically occurs during the period of rapid growth in adolescence in either obese or very thin males, but it can occur in females as well. Surgical reduction with internal fixation is necessary (see Chapter 14).

The most common type of fracture in this region in the young athlete is an avulsion fracture. Avulsion fractures of the apophysis occur in 14% to 40% of athletes in sports[37,376] as a result of forceful contraction or excessive stretch of the muscle originating about the involved apophysis. The most common sites are the anterior-superior iliac spine (origin of the sartorius), the ischium (hamstring origin) (Fig. 15.7), the lesser trochanter (insertion of the iliopsoas), the anterior-inferior iliac spine (rectus femoris origin), and the iliac crest (abdominal insertion).[284] These injuries are classic in sprinting, jumping, soccer, football, and weight lifting. A majority of these injuries are managed nonoperatively with rest and activity modification, reducing tension in the involved area, followed by gradual increase of excursion to full mobility, progressive resistance exercise, and return to activity.[48,376] One less traumatic parallel of avulsion is iliac apophysitis, which usually affects adolescent track, field, or cross-country athletes or dancers. Repeated contraction of the tensor fasciae latae, rectus femoris, sartorius, gluteus medius, and oblique abdominal muscles causes nonspecific pain and tenderness over the iliac crest. Rest helps this problem,[48,142] but often exercises to increase strength and normalize two-joint muscle flexibility are required.

Stress fractures and osteitis pubis are being diagnosed more frequently as a result of repetitive microtrauma in runners or athletes who have suddenly increased their involvement in jumping or kicking activities. Persistent pain and tenderness in the groin with limited mobility and activity-related increases in pain could signal either of these conditions. Radiographs showing inflammation, demineralization, and sclerosis confirm the diagnosis of osteitis pubis, but a bone scan is necessary to diagnose a stress fracture. Stress fractures have been seen in the pelvis at the junction of the ischium and pubic ramus and in the femoral neck and shaft.[48] Relative rest, use of crutches, and restriction from percussive activities (running and jumping) are required for resolution of these disorders.

Snapping hip syndrome is an overuse problem noted in gymnasts, dancers, sprinters, and sports with a rotational component. The term *snapping hip syndrome* can refer either to irritation of the iliotibial band over the greater trochanter with

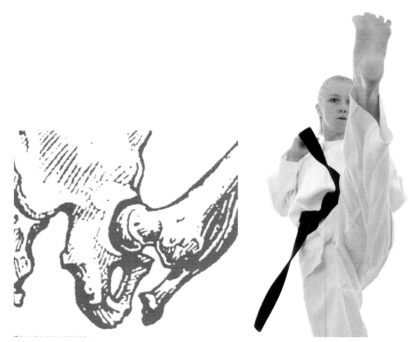

FIG. 15.7 Avulsion of the ischial tuberosity. (*Left,* from Birrer R, Brecher D: *Common sports injuries in youngsters.* Oradell, NJ, Medical Economics Books, 1987. *Right,* from iStock.com.)

hip motion or to tenosynovitis of the iliopsoas tendon near its femoral insertion. Usually, relative rest or activity modification, use of appropriate modalities, stretching, and improved muscle strength overcome these symptoms, with surgical intervention considered with failed conservative management.[191,275]

A serious condition seen in the young athlete age 5 to 12 years is avascular necrosis of the femoral head. Activity can irritate the synovium, leading to joint effusion and reduction of the blood supply to the femoral head. The initial complaint is nonspecific hip pain, but radiographs demonstrate periosteal rarefaction followed by sclerosis and irregular collapse of the femoral head. Bracing or surgery may be required, depending on the degree of progression of the problem.[142] (see Chapter 14).

Contusions are common, but the most frequent is the hip pointer. This iliac crest contusion, occurring typically in football or hockey, is caused by a driving blow by a helmet. The overlying muscle is damaged with a resultant subperiosteal hematoma. RICE and padding will resolve this problem with time.[142] Occasionally, use of ultrasound and soft tissue mobilization with stretching may be necessary.

Knee Injuries

As the largest joint in the body and one with minimal anatomic protection, the knee is the focal point of stress forces applied along the tibia and femur. The knee is the second most commonly injured body site in young individuals, and sports-related knee injuries are among the most economically costly sports injuries, commonly requiring surgical intervention and/or rehabilitation.[111,127,193,345,397] However, these data are likely an underestimation of the prevalence of knee injuries in the young population because overuse injuries account for as many as one half to one third of sports-related injury[248,335] and are often not registered in hospital or sport-specific settings.[200]

Fractures about the knee, although not frequent, are significant for their possible influences on growth.[401,434] Overall,

physeal fractures account for 30% of fractures in children less than 16 years old,[256] with distal femoral fractures accounting for 1% to 6% of all physeal fractures.[100,156,256] Acute fractures of the tibial tubercle are also relatively uncommon, with a reported incidence of 0.4% to 2.7%.[31,53,83,84,172,286,311] The mechanism of injury for fractures of the distal femoral physis is high-energy trauma, but older children and adolescents may sustain this type of fracture during lower-energy trauma, often sports related.[119] A fracture line that traverses through the physis and runs obliquely through the metaphysis (Saltar-Harris Type II[119]) is common during sports participation resulting from a valgus force producing medial physeal separation and is often concomitant with medial collateral ligament sprains.[119,246,276] In the proximal tibia, acute avulsion fractures are the most common occurring during athletic activity involving jumping or landing, either by a forceful quadriceps contraction against a fixed foot or by a forceful knee flexion against a tightly contracting quadriceps muscle.[138,237] There is a strong predominance of males with this injury.[119,138] Management of fractures in the distal femur or proximal tibia is dictated by the fracture type and displacement. Particular attention is given to restoration of joint alignment to minimize risk of growth disturbance.[119,138] Nondisplaced fractures can be managed with immobilization and protected weight bearing. Displaced and/or unstable fractures may be managed with either closed or open reduction, including percutaneous pin fixation, transphyseal pins, or internal fixation.[119,138] Displaced tibial tubercle fractures are typically managed with open reduction internal fixation to facilitate anatomic reduction and appropriate alignment and length of the extensor mechanism.[119,138] Rehabilitation will vary with regard to medical management and addresses primary and secondary impairments associated with the injury and management strategy, likely focusing on joint mobility/range of motion, muscle strengthening and activation, pain and effusion management, and functional movement progression.

Ligament injuries are becoming more common in the young athlete, with one study reporting medial collateral ligament injury in children as young as 4 years of age.[282] All ligament injuries should be assessed for coincident physis fractures. Medial collateral ligament tears in youth can include both the superficial and the capsular components of the ligament. Nonoperative treatment with splinting and avoidance of valgus stress has been successful in adolescents, so it may be possible to obtain equally good results in younger children.[142] Physical therapy to improve lower extremity strength and functional movement retraining is often indicated.

The incidence of ACL midsubstance tears in children has increased dramatically. The mechanism of injury is either noncontact, occurring during movements that involve deceleration or change of direction that results in valgus loading in combination with some anterior tibial shear.[181,197] This mechanism of injury may result in either an avulsion fracture at the tibial insertion or midsubstance tears of the ligament.[5,20] The fracture of the tibial spine usually occurs through the cancellous bone, demonstrating avulsion of the tibial spine on a radiograph. Diagnosis of midsubstance tears is done through clinical examination and MRI. Management of midsubstance ACL injuries relies on nonsurgical management or surgical reconstruction. Physical therapy is the focus of nonsurgical management, with an emphasis on acute injury management, strengthening and neuromuscular training, and functional progression for return to desired activity. In cases with recurrent instability, traditional reconstructive procedures are avoided in the adolescent under the age of 15 years because of fear of injury to the growth plate with the proximal tibial drill hole.[168,216] Instead, a modified ACL reconstruction will be performed to respect the still-open physes of the skeletally immature child, including partial transphyseal, physeal-sparing, and all epiphyseal-sparing techniques. These surgical procedures are utilized to provide mechanical stability to the knee and reduce the risk of secondary injury to the surrounding articular cartilage and meniscus during physical activity.[213] Postsurgical rehabilitation with a focus on joint projection, strengthening and neuromuscular development, and functional and return-to-play phases is key to optimize outcomes.

Juvenile osteochondritis dissecans is a focal lesion or injury of the subchondral bone region, with the risk of instability and disruption of the adjacent articular cartilage. The most common location is on the posterolateral aspect of the medial femoral condyle, where 70% of lesions occur.[163,214] There is increased incidence and prevalence in youth involved in sports activities, with boys being more affected than girls (5:3 ratio) and 25% of cases being bilateral with asymmetric lesion location.[188,214] The etiology of juvenile osteochondritis dissecans is still an enigma. Compression of the tibial spine against the medial femoral condyle, interruption of the vascularity, genetic predisposition, chronic inflammatory response, anatomic variations in the knee, and abnormal subchondral bone are all possible causes. The condition usually causes pain, recurrent swelling, and possibly catching in the knee. Pain is generally poorly localized and is exacerbated with activity. Physical examination may reveal tenderness over the anteromedial aspect of the knee with varying degrees of knee flexion. Because these lesions have a poor prognosis after skeletal maturity, every attempt should be made to gain healing before growth plate closure. In the child younger than 15 years of age, diminished activity to the point of not bearing weight is suggested. Drilling of the condyles with removal of fragments is recommended in children older than 15 years of age.[67] This procedure usually necessitates restriction of running, jumping, and other physical activity for a period of time, with concomitant intensive rehabilitation to regain strength, balance, and agility in the lower extremity.[142,370]

The challenge of meniscal injuries in the young athlete is accurate diagnosis.[287] Meniscus injuries are often concomitant with other acute knee injuries,[19,368] such as anterior cruciate ligament tears, chondral injuries, and tibial fractures. The preponderance of literature supports a management strategy that preserves as much of the meniscus as possible.[407] Rehabilitation management focuses on restoration of joint motion, strength, neuromuscular control, and endurance of the involved limb. If indicated, surgical management (repair versus debride) is dictated by tear location, chronicity of the tear, patient age, and other patient-specific factors. Postsurgical rehabilitation works to restore joint motion, strength, neuromuscular control, and endurance of the involved limb. Discoid lateral meniscus is a common abnormal meniscal variant in children.[224] Discoid lateral meniscus can create joint line tenderness, decreased joint mobility, effusion, and, most notably, a prominent snap in the lateral compartment as the knee is extended.[224] The complete type of discoid meniscus, producing symptoms in late adolescence, is distinguished by intact peripheral attachments. Good results are obtained with saucerization of the meniscus. The Wrisberg type of discoid meniscus, which is more common in the pediatric group, has an attachment only through the ligament of Wrisberg and can be resolved by cutting the ligament and removing the portions with no peripheral attachments.[224,304] Among the most common knee conditions in children are disorders involving the patella and patellofemoral joint.[41] Macrotrauma, repetitive microtrauma, and growth all can contribute to the disorders of the patellofemoral joint. Patellofemoral pain is the most frequent problem in the young athlete, with adolescent females being 2 to 10 times more likely than males to have patellofemoral pain.[51,124,143,144,356] Overuse of the extensor mechanism or extensor mechanism is a major cause of patellofemoral pain. Several other anatomic and biomechanical factors can increase stress in the patellofemoral joint and lead to pain (Fig. 15.8). Malalignment of the patellofemoral joint is the major cause of this pain. Several factors can cause or contribute to this malalignment. Anatomic factors such as patella alta, large Q angle, hip anteversion, flattened lateral femoral condyle, shallow femoral groove, or pes planus and hyperpronation can cause abnormal tracking of the patella during knee motion.[328] The malalignment of the patella in relation to the femoral groove can be the result of a more laterally positioned patella or a more internally rotated femur.[340] Biomechanical factors related to muscle strength (e.g., weak hip musculature) or altered movement strategies (e.g., dynamic knee valgus) can contribute to increased patellofemoral stress.[291,328] Nonoperative management is the standard of care for patellofemoral pain. Medical management may include nonsteroidal anti-inflammatory medications and bracing. A meta-analysis of randomized studies of physical therapy treatment in individuals with patellofemoral pain showed a positive effect for exercise on pain reduction,[175] with successful rehabilitation programs incorporating active stretching, lower extremity strengthening, balance, proprioception, and neuromuscular control activities with an emphasis on trunk, hip, and thigh musculature.[175]

Lateral patellar instability and subluxation/dislocation are common in young athletes, with an incidence of 107 per 100,000 in those 9 to 15 years old.[400] Injury occurs either by direct contact with the medial aspect of the knee, or indirect, noncontact mechanisms that relate to biomechanics and/or anatomic factors that result in a tendency for patellar lateralization. Sport-related movements, such as cutting or pivoting, that result in dynamic knee valgus place high strain on medial patellar restraints and are associated with lateral subluxation/dislocation.[400] Other factors such as pes planus or subtalar joint pronation are also thought to contribute to altered knee loading and to instability.[400] Other contributing factors include anatomic factors that reduce contact of the patella with the groove (e.g., trochlear dysplasia, patella alta, increased patellar tilt) and/or lateralize the pull of the quadriceps (e.g., increased quadriceps angle, high

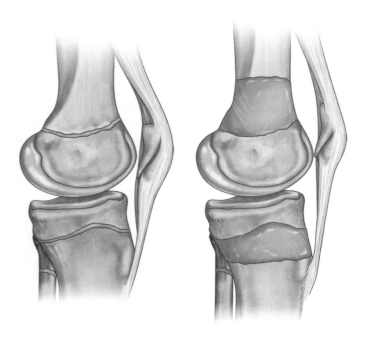

FIG. 15.8 Tension resulting from growth. Pain may occur at the patella (A), lower pole of the patella (B), or patellar tendon insertion on the tibia (C). (Redrawn from Micheli L: Overuse injuries in children's sports: the growth factor. *Orthop Clin North Am* 14(2):337-360, 1983.)

tibial tuberosity to trochlear groove).[109,400] The risk of recurrent instability is high, with studies reporting a 60% redislocation/subluxation rate for 11- to 14-year-olds and a 33% rate for 15- to 18-year-olds.[302,400] After primary dislocation, nonoperative management is considered, but early surgical intervention with a medial patellofemoral reconstruction procedure may also be considered, particularly if anatomic variations exist.[412] A medial patellofemoral reconstruction is often considered in those with recurrent instability. Rehabilitation management following acute dislocation focuses on pain/effusion management and activities that progress range of motion, strength, and neuromuscular control. Postoperative management will be dictated by the procedure performed but will include joint protection and pain/effusion management, as well as progressive range of motion, strengthening, and neuromuscular control activities.

Apophysitis, or irritation and inflammation of the secondary ossification centers where tendons attach, is common in the knee at the tibial tuberosity (Osgood-Schlatter disease) and inferior pole of the patella (Sinding-Larsen-Johansson syndrome) where localized pain and tenderness are clinical features of these conditions. Osgood-Schlatter disease (see Chapter 14) typically presents in boys age 12 to 15 years and girls age 8 to 12 years, is more common in boys than girls,[151,223,421] and is most often seen in sports involving repetitive running and/or jumping where there is a strong pull of the quadriceps muscles[106,151,380] (see Chapter 14). Sinding-Larsen-Johansson typically presents in adolescents between 10 to 14 years old but most often in males who participate in sports.[198] Relative rest, activity modification, ice/nonsteroidal anti-inflammatory medications, improving flexibility of surrounding muscles (particularly the quadriceps and rectus femoris muscles), and maintenance of quadriceps muscle strength or progressive quadriceps strengthening with pain-free exercise are treatment options.[48,389]

Ankle and Foot Injuries

As a result of their growing skeleton, children may suffer from foot and ankle problems not often seen in adults.[260] Injuries to the distal tibial and fibular growth plates are common in the young athlete. Gregg and Das[161] have classified growth plate injuries into a clinically useful system (Fig. 15.9). The

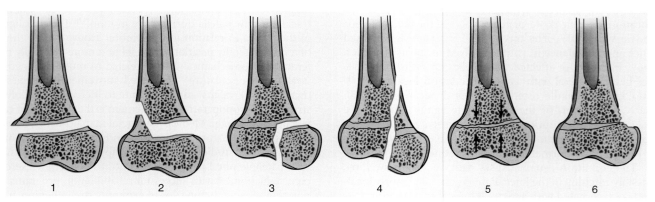

FIG. 15.9 Modified Salter-Harris classification of growth plate injuries: 1, Disruption entirely confined to the growth plate; distraction or slip injury. 2, Fracture line runs partially through the growth plate then extends through the metaphysis. 3, Fracture line runs partially through the growth plate then extends through the epiphysis. 4, Combined disruption of metaphysis, growth plate, and epiphysis. 5, Crush or compression injury of growth plate. 6, Abrasion, avulsion, or burn of the perichondrial ring of the growth plate. (From Marchiori D: *Clinical imaging: with skeletal, chest, & abdominal pattern differentials*, ed 3, St. Louis, Mosby, 2014.)

most common fractures to the ankle in the skeletally immature athlete are the Salter-Harris I and II injuries to the distal fibula. Although these fractures can occur with adduction and abduction injury to the distal tibia, they frequently occur alone as a result of inversion injury. The Ottawa rules for prediction of need for radiograph to rule out fracture have been validated in children.[239] The Ottawa rules state that an ankle series is indicated only for patients with pain in the malleolar zone and any of the following findings: (1) bone tenderness at the posterior edge of either the medial or lateral malleolus or (2) inability to bear weight immediately after injury and in the emergency room. The rules further state that a foot series is required only with midfoot pain and any of the following findings: (1) bone tenderness at the base of the fifth metatarsal, (2) bone tenderness at the navicular, or (3) inability to bear weight immediately and in the emergency room. Treatment with immobilization in a short leg cast for 2 to 6 weeks is suggested.[202] Physical therapy after casting to increase ankle and foot mobility and strength and to improve balance may be indicated. Increasing incidence of osteochondral defects of the talar dome may necessitate a review of surgical options for treatment of this condition.[403]

Type II injury of the distal tibia is a result of a variety of mechanisms, including supination and external rotation, supination and plantar flexion, and ankle pronation and eversion, to name a few. Common in football and soccer players, this injury is frequently associated with greenstick fracture of the distal fibula. Care must be taken to reduce these fractures and immobilize them in a long leg cast with knee flexion to prevent impaction of the tibial metaphysis into the growth plate. The results of this type of fracture are unpredictable; occasionally angulation or premature closure of the plate occurs.[142] The most common mechanism of injury in type III and IV fractures of the medial malleolus is ankle supination or inversion. Adduction injuries appear in approximately 15% of these injuries and are characterized by medial displacement of part or all of the distal tibial epiphysis. The affected children are usually young, so the incidence of growth disturbance is higher. Internal fixation with restoration of ankle joint congruity is critical.[236]

Because of the porosity of the bones of the foot in a child, stress fractures are common in the metatarsals in all jumping and distance-running activities. If suspected by local tenderness that is aggravated with activity, these injuries should be immobilized for 3 weeks. After immobilization, one can progressively and slowly increase activities to former levels over 3 more weeks.[142] Several types of ischemia can occur in the bones of the child's foot. Freiberg infarction, or avascular necrosis of the metatarsal epiphysis, occurs in those who walk or perform on their toes. Initial synovitis is followed by sclerosis, resorption, plate fracture and collapse, and bone reformation. It does not affect children younger than 12 years of age. Most commonly affected is the second metatarsal head. Treatment consists of cessation of toe-walking, wearing high-heeled shoes, and jumping. A negative-heel shoe is fitted. Kohler disease is seen in active boys age 3 to 7 years who have a tendency to cavus feet (see Chapter 14). Focal tenderness and swelling around the navicular bone are noted clinically. The radiograph reveals sclerosis and irregular rarefaction indicative of ischemia. Conservative treatment calls for use of a walking cast for 6 to 8 weeks followed by use of an arch support and limitation of activity for another 6 weeks.[282]

Although ankle sprains can occur in the young athlete, epiphyseal fractures are more common. Sprains occur in the older adolescent near the end of skeletal maturity. The common cause of injury is landing on the lateral border of a plantar-flexed foot (Fig. 15.10). Management is similar to that in adults. Surgery is indicated only in multiple sprains with gross instability limiting function or causing pain.

Sever disease, or apophysitis of the calcaneus, is comparable to Osgood-Schlatter syndrome in the knee (Fig. 15.11). It is seen most frequently in basketball and soccer players with complaint of heel pain on running. The usual age of occurrence is 8 to 13 years. Frequently, tight heel cords, a tendency toward in-toeing, and forefoot varus are noted. Treatment consists of heel cord stretching and initial use of a heel lift in well-constructed shoes (see Chapter 14).[142]

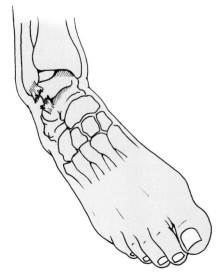
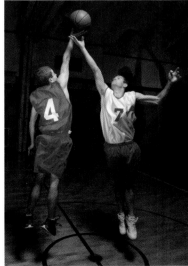

FIG. 15.10 Plantar flexion-inversion injury. (*Left,* from Manske RC: *Fundamental orthopedic management for the physical therapist assistant,* ed 4, St. Louis, Elsevier, 2016. *Right,* from iStock.com.)

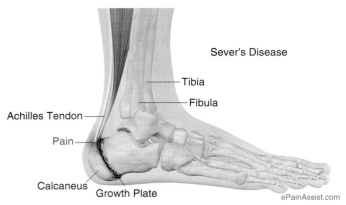

FIG. 15.11 Insertion of Sharpey's fibers from the Achilles tendon into the calcaneal apophysis. (From www.epainassist.com.)

FOREGROUND INFORMATION

REHABILITATION AND RETURN TO PLAY

In adults, rehabilitation following common sports injuries and subsequent medical treatment (i.e., ACL injury and reconstruction) is described in the literature. Commonly, rehabilitation guidelines that are accepted practice in adults are often applied to children and adolescents. However, rehabilitation in a child or adolescent requires age-appropriate modifications, specifically related to relevant anatomy, surgical procedures/modifications performed (if applicable), protection and preservation of future bone growth, as well as the unique psychosocial aspects of the pediatric or adolescent patient.

Children and adolescents require supervised rehabilitation programs that begin with first aid on the field of play. The goal of first aid is to contain the extent of injury and reduce any possibility of further harm. Following, or in conjunction with medical management of the injury, the long-term goal of rehabilitation is return to play in a safe manner with minimal risk of further injury. In healthy individuals, studies indicate that comprehensive training programs utilizing components of strength, balance, and core stability training, as well as biomechanical technique and plyometric training, induce changes in movement mechanics that are associated with reducing injury risk.[178,180,292] Similar principles are utilized when establishing a rehabilitation program for individuals following injury. Following injury, successful rehabilitation that advances toward unrestricted activity and sport participation requires a comprehensive, progressive, and criterion-based plan of physical therapy care.

A comprehensive rehabilitation program and individualized plan of care maximize outcomes. The physical therapy plan of care will vary based on the individual's unique characteristics and attributes within the context of his or her injury and relevant anatomy (e.g., open versus closed epiphyseal "growth" plates). Physical characteristics such as anatomic alignment, skeletal age, body mass, severity of impairments, and injury history are considered in rehabilitation planning.[348,426] Also considered are psychosocial attributes such as motivation, maturity level, patient/family goals, kinesthetic awareness, and demonstration of fear avoidance or kinesiophobic movement patterns. The young athlete's specific goals, as well as the magnitude of his or her impairments and functional limitations, will guide the specific interventions and pace of rehabilitation progression. For the young athlete, communication among the health care providers, as well as with the patient, family, coaches, and other involved personnel, will ensure effective collaboration with the recommended plan of care. Given the limited information available regarding injuries in young individuals, the rehabilitation specialist plays a large role in the education of the patient, patient's family, and the teaching and coaching staff involved with the young athlete.

Successful physical therapy management requires adherence to a systematic and criterion-based progression of interventions and considerations for the unique psychosocial and anatomic aspects of a young patient. This approach to rehabilitation will protect injured tissues, promote healing, maximize outcomes, and ultimately preserve long-term tissue and joint integrity.[348,426] A rehabilitation program that is developed and advanced based on criterion-based decision making, rather than time-based decision making, is advocated to ensure adequate tissue healing and adequate accommodation of the injured tissues to the forces associated with activity.[348,426] A thorough history and clinical examination are important to establish accurate differential diagnosis and to develop an individual plan of care based on severity of impairments and functional limitations.

Acute and Intermediate Phases of Rehabilitation

Protecting the injured tissue or joint during the early phases of healing is important for successful outcome. Adherence to necessary activity modifications may be a challenge for young, active patients. Patient and family education are important for effective cooperation with the plan of care. Resolution of impairments and progression toward functional activities are the goals of these phases of rehabilitation. Each patient's specific goals, as well as the magnitude of their impairments and functional limitations, will guide the specific interventions and pace of rehabilitation progression.

Advanced Stages of Rehabilitation

The long-term goal of rehabilitation is a safe transition and reintegration into sport following injury. The objective of the return-to-activity phase of rehabilitation is successful transition from advanced rehabilitation to safe participation in sports with minimal risk of injury. Criterion-based progression through the advanced stages of rehabilitation depends on achievement of clinical milestones, with consideration of the participation demands for the activity and position for which the individual desires to return (e.g., the amount of cutting/pivoting, amount of overhead throwing, amount of contact, and level of activity [elite versus recreational]). Advanced stages of rehabilitation should realize resolution of pain, effusion, range of motion, and joint-loading or weight-bearing restrictions. During the advanced stages of rehabilitation, the young athlete should be progressed through a functional program (based on activity- and position-specific demands) that optimizes strength and muscle performance in terms of intensity, frequency, and duration of activity.[293] Functional activities that progress neuromuscular control, including plyometric and technique training, should also be implemented.[293]

Return to Activity

Determination of timing for return to desired sports activities following injury should be based on objective measures during a comprehensive functional evaluation.[225,293] Patient reintegration into sport and activities is considered when there is demonstration of adequate tissue healing, resolution of impairments (such as pain, effusion, range of motion), adequate muscle strength and performance, and acceptable levels of functional performance necessary for the demands of the desired activity. Muscle strength should be objectively measured (via dynamometry), and the recommended criterion for return to activity is involved muscle strength that is 85% to 90% of the contralateral muscle.[203,225,285,306,358]

Patient-reported outcome tools and performance-based functional assessments are also utilized in physical therapy clinical decision making.[132] A number of region-specific patient-reported outcome measures are valid and reliable measures of function during activities of daily living, recreational activities, and sport activities, although most measures were developed based on adult patient populations. A recent study[371] demonstrated the internal consistency and validity of the International Knee Documentation Committee (IKDC) Subjective Knee Evaluation Form in young individuals, ages 6 to 18 years. Measures of general health assessment, such as the Pediatric Quality of Life Inventory 4.0 Generic Core Scales (PedsQL),[410,411] are valid, responsive, and reliable measures of health-related quality of life in children and adolescents (age 2 to 18 years). In addition to patient-reported measures of function, performance-based assessments are often used to determine readiness for return to sport and activity. Physical performance is often evaluated via jumping, hopping, or cutting tasks, depending on the demands of the activity of which the patient desires to return. Single-limb hop tests (such as the single hop, triple hop, crossover hop, and 6-meter timed hop[305]) are often used because of their convenience and reliability.[54,347] Recommended criteria for return to sport are performance of involved limb that is at least 85% to 90% of the uninvolved limb.[225] Additional performance measures may also be useful. Performance on the Star Excursion Balance Test has been associated with risk of lower extremity injury,[209,334] and a composite reach distance of > 94 is recommended to reduce injury risk.[209,334] Altered movement patterns and neuromuscular control have been associated with increased risk of injuries,[179] and movement and technique assessment during high-level activities are important for safe return to activity. The drop vertical jump task has been used repeatedly as an assessment tool of lower extremity biomechanics during a plyometric task.[120,136,179,294,313,317] The tuck jump exercise has been advocated as another clinician-friendly and reliable tool to identify lower extremity landing technique faults during a plyometric activity.[290,293]

For young athletes participating in overhead sports such as baseball, softball, and volleyball, a progressive return to overhead activity or throwing program is warranted following resolution of identified impairments and limitations. For overhead and throwing athletes, analyzing appropriate technique and addressing identified deviations are important to prevent further injury.[361,427] During the advanced and return-to-sport stages of rehabilitation, adherence to a progressive return to throwing or overhead activity program[22,427] will maximize performance and mitigate risk of further injury.

The clinical decision making for reintegration into sport activities utilizes a comprehensive and criterion-based approach that includes assessment of impairments as well as functional performance Box 15-2. A rehabilitation plan that culminates with a progressive reintegration of the young individual into the desired activity is advocated. A progressive approach toward unrestricted activity participation may be initiated with modification of activity participation, such as time of participation and demands of participation. Appropriate communication among the health care team and with the patient, family, and other involved persons (e.g., coaches) is important during the advanced stages of rehabilitation to ensure collaboration with the progressive plan of care.

BOX 15.2   Textbox for Intervention

Body Functions and Structures
- Static and dynamic stretching
- Open and closed kinetic chain strengthening
- Gait retraining
- Neuromuscular reeducation

Activities and Participation
- Functional return to activity progression

Other (e.g., Environment, QoL when applicable)
- Environmental integration to activity specific tasks

QoL, quality of life.

THE YOUNG ATHLETE WITH A PHYSICAL DISABILITY

The number of children with disabilities in the United States has continued to rise, with the greatest population living in lower socioeconomic status environments.[187] Children with disabilities benefit from physical activity similarly to their able-bodied or typically developing peers. Yet individuals with disabilities are less physically active and display higher risk for ailments associated with inactivity.[2,6,34,50,226,300,428] Children with intellectual impairments, especially those of low socioeconomic status, exhibit obesity rates among the highest in the nation.[2,134,300,355]

Despite increasing rates of participation in Paralympics and Special Olympics, individuals with disabilities still have limitations in accessing school and community resources.[2,21,34] According to a systematic review by Bloemen et al. in 2015, both positive and negative factors involving physical ability, sporting modification, and opinions toward wellness influence individuals' participation in physical activities (Table 15.8).[50,57,59,87,98,199,281,369,385] Many of these factors are similar to those affecting typically developing peers, yet medical impairments complicate normal requirements such as transportation and create a fear of trying a new activity. Health care providers are encouraged to promote healthy behaviors with patients, including strength, cardiovascular, and injury prevention training. Through collaboration with recreational therapists, occupational therapists, coaches, teachers, parents, and community advocates, therapists can best advocate for patients to safely participate in fitness, sports, and recreational training.

Both psychological and physiologic benefits of sports participation have been demonstrated in individuals with disabilities. Athletes with and without disabilities report improved social acceptance and enjoyment of participation in physical activities.[208] Fitness programs assist with cardiovascular fitness, mobility throughout the aging process, bone health, and muscle strength, and they decrease the risk of ailments of inactivity such as hypertension, fatigue, and difficulty performing daily activities.[114,355,357,414,425] Self-concept and self-acceptance were shown to be equal or greater in athletes as compared to nonathletes with disabilities.[174,363] According to a systematic review by Sahlin et al. in 2015, confidence, identity, competence, self-worth, life satisfaction, and community integration all increase through sports and recreational activities for individuals with neurologic pathologies.[363] Consistent with a systematic review performed in 2014, exercise can also help individuals with intellectual disabilities limit challenging behaviors associated with their cognitive impairments.[312] A variety of sports and recreational experiences promote social interactions, cognitive function, self-esteem, and skill acquisition through experience in the sport or recreational activity.[45,374]

TABLE 15.8 Personal, Environmental, and Other Factors Influencing the Physical Activity for People with a Disability

Barriers to Physical Activity	Facilitators to Physical Activity
Social Influence Physical activity and sports are not a priority at this time	**Social Influence** Parents are aware of the benefits of physical activity Parents desire their child to have a sense of normalcy, belonging to a group "like" them Physical activity assists with weight control, health
Health Conditions Presence of a cognitive impairment Concerns of pain, Injury Medical complications Current injury or disability Individual is currently in poor health Poor joint positioning or integrity	**Health Conditions** Physical activity assists in fundamental movement skills
Self-Efficacy Feeling insecure/lacking confidence Feeling an attractive sport is too difficult	**Self-Efficacy** Being able to independently negotiate barriers in the community Being able to adapt and teach others to help Feeling confident/gaining self-confidence Feeling competent in a sport Improving the ability to move without assistance from others
Attitude "Being active is not good for the body" Fear of increasing risk for injury Fear of injury, safety, or incontinence "I need to rest in my spare time"	**Intention** Desires to be active
Fitness Fatigue Lack of energy and endurance Lack of motor skills Poor physical condition Lack of skills	**Attitude** Motivation to be healthy Recognizing importance of physical activity Belief that symmetrical movement is beneficial Maintaining a healthy body
Motivation Poor motivation Preferences for sedentary behavior Physical activity/sports "are not fun"	**Socialization** Opportunity for social interaction Feeling accepted as part of a group
Age As individuals age, they report more fear and lack of motivation of participating in a new physical activity	**Abilities** Achieving fundamental movement skills
Time Lack of time Learning new skills is too time consuming Time to shower/change	**Other Personal Factors** Accepting disability Having perseverance Activities gives a sense of freedom
Other Personal Factors Awareness of differences from peers Resisting asking for help Feeling like an outsider/being ashamed Not accepting (extent of) disability Unsure how to use equipment Not knowing how to exercise Self-conscious/embarrassed Inconvenience of sweating	**Family** Family resilience Doing physical activity with parents Parental encouragement and motivation Parental support: getting them to places, helping with transfers, perseverance in exploring options, assertiveness (advocating for child), having a positive attitude Encouragement to be active
Family Reliant on parents for transport and entrance to facilities Lack of parental support Lack of time of parent to assist Parents not accepting extent of disability Parents concern for child's safety Parents feeling dissatisfaction with environment, fear of child "not fitting in," challenges with managing, and hesitating to ask for help from trainer(s) Low parental level of education	**Support From and Contact with People** Good teachers and instructors support Skilled helpers Motivation from PT teacher and friends Peer socialization Being accepted by peers and other parents Making friends Positive attitude of schoolmates, teachers, and other people Having someone who can provide support Having someone to do physical activity with
	Sports Activity type/sports they enjoy doing Chances to join competition Opportunities for sport/physical activity

TABLE 15.8 Personal, Environmental, and Other Factors Influencing the Physical Activity for People with a Disability—cont'd

Barriers to Physical Activity	Facilitators to Physical Activity
Support from and Contact with People Not being accepted or being bullied by peers Teachers and instructors giving negative comments Lack of role models Lack of physically active peers to play with Lack of professionals who know how to and can teach sport skills Professionals are not assisting child in physical activity People's misconception or unfriendly attitude "There's no one to do it with"	Sports facility: having good trainer, communication between trainers and coaches, training in small groups Advantages of wheelchair sorts: impact on child's confidence, community building, friendship, future aspirations, having necessary equipment, sport/club participation on weekend days
Sports Activity is too competitive Activity not adequately adapted Lacking necessary equipment/clothing Lack of opportunities (rules, regulation) Sports facility: teams are too big, there's a waiting list, not allowed to play matches, limited locations to exercise No space to exercise (with peers)	**Environment** Adaptive equipment Access to sport/physical activity in community Accessible community recreation facilities Accessible to suitable facilities
Environment Environment not adequately adapted Not suitable accessibility to facilities No showering/changing facilities	**School** Participation in PE classes at school
School Lack of professional training in physical education PE teachers only select students with better sport skills or performance Not suitable facilities at school Having a lot of homework	**Transport** Transport (living close to the city) Having transportation
Transport Lack of transportation	**Other Environmental Factors** Appropriate group activities Disability-adopted programs Opportunities away from home
Financial Support Financial restrictions High cost of sports/recreational activities	
Other Environmental Factors Stigma of disability Time commitment Inappropriate weather/too hot or cold	

Adapted from Bloemen MA, Backx FJ, Takken T, et al: Factors associated with physical activity in children and adolescents with a physical disability: a systematic review. *Dev Med Child Neurol* 57(2):137-148, 2015.

Between 11% and 61% of individuals with a lower extremity amputation participate in physical activity and/or sports.[58] The same pathologic process that caused the amputation may limit some individuals' ability to participate in activities after the amputation.[58] Yet improvements in strength, rehabilitation progressions, quality of life, aerobic and anaerobic fitness, as well as the body mass of individuals are all achieved through physical activity in individuals with amputations.[58] Once individuals start to participate in sport or recreational activity, there are improvements in the number of social contacts, their knowledge of sporting equipment, and motor skills, as well as a sense of acceptance of their disability.[58] Among children with limb deficiencies, athletic competence was one predictor of higher perceived physical appearance, lower levels of depression, and higher self-esteem.[363,409]

Individuals with Down syndrome are at a higher risk for inactivity, cardiac muscle atrophy, and obesity than those without disabilities or other diagnoses with intellectual impairments.[159,330,417] In a case series by Alesi et al., children with Down syndrome improved in both motor and intellectual scores after a 2-month training program that included cardiovascular warm-up, basic motor training, cognitive training games, and a breathing cool down.[7] Adolescents with Down syndrome displayed improved strength and agility after completing a 6-week fitness routine 3 days per week.[240] Therefore physical activity, cardiovascular fitness, strengthening, and motor training in a social environment are recommended for individuals with Down syndrome.[159,240]

Disability often causes a reduction of overall fitness relative to the general population.[129,162,333,346,354] According to Buffart et al., aerobic fitness in adolescents and young adults with spina bifida was 42% lower than in typically developing age-matched peers, with 39% of the participants with spina bifida classified as inactive and another 37% as extremely inactive.[63] Marques et al. attribute this lack of physical activity to feelings of a lack of competence in physical activity.[259] Similarly, individuals with cerebral palsy displayed an increased tendency toward sedentary behaviors, with lower bone density compared to typically developing individuals. The largest disparities are found in those with the greatest physical impairments and in those with a tendency toward sedentary behavior as they get older.[6,251]

Adaptive Sports

Legislative actions such as the United States of Public Law 94-142, the Rehabilitation Act of 1973, the Americans with Disabilities Act in 1991, and the National Park Service Director's Order #42 in 2000 have provided individuals with disabilities improved access to educational and community resources.[94,118,325,379] In 2013 the Department of Education issued a clarification regarding the Americans with Disabilities Act: that is, students must not only be provided equal access to educational opportunities but also to extracurricular activities.[353] This has increased the opportunities for individuals with disabilities to participate in sports and recreational activities and has advanced the possibilities for individuals with disabilities to obtain college scholarships and compete as NCAA athletes.[299]

Aside from the NCAA and local recreational opportunities, Special Olympics and Paralympics offer individuals with disabilities global recognition of their accomplishments through sports and recreational activities. Since the first Special Olympics world games in 1968, the number of competitors has more than doubled on the global stage. Special Olympics' mission is to provide year-round sports training and competitions for individuals with disabilities. Qualifications for Special Olympics include verification of a medical diagnosis of intellectual impairment. Athletes compete based on their skill sets for specific sporting activities. Some teams are unified, with individuals with and without disabilities competing on the same team. Paralympics, meaning parallel to the Olympics, began after World War II, with the first world games in 1948. Since that time, Paralympics has assessed individuals through classification processes of the individual's medical impairment in order to provide fair play. Originally, this was based on the medical diagnosis, but more recently it is based on an assessment of motion, strength, and coordination required for the specific sporting activity. Most United States Paralympic sports are managed through the same Olympic governing body as the Olympics.

Sports and recreational activities can be adapted either by the rules of the game or the equipment permitted in play. For example, runners with visual impairments are provided a guide runner to assist the athlete in safely completing the course. Size of the competition area, number of athletes, and additional personnel such as a sign language interpreter are other examples of modifications made to allow individuals to compete in the sport safely. Besides addressing strength, motion, and mobility impairments associated with physical disabilities, therapists can assist children and adults in appropriate adaptations to the physical activity in order to allow the individual to participate. Examples of such adaptations include providing a bicycle handlebar modification to allow an individual with a limb deficiency ample control of the bike, seen in Fig. 15.12A.[30] Paralympic adaptations are very specific and must be cleared with an official before use. Examples of this include a track and field throwing chair pictured in Fig. 15.12B, which may or may not have a seat back or hand pole depending on the thrower's

needs.[140,141,431] An important differentiation for therapists to note is between a handcycle, seen in Fig. 15.12C, which can only be used in cycling events, and a racing chair, pictured in Fig. 15.12D, which is appropriate only for running events. The biggest difference between these two chairs is that the handcycle has gears for the athlete to shift, allowing the athlete to have an easier push up and down hills, while the racing chair does not provide athletes this luxury.

Although Special Olympics and Paralympics offer individuals with physical and intellectual impairments opportunities to participate in sports and recreational activities, the incidence of obesity has continued to rise at a greater rate in individuals with disabilities than their peers without disabilities.[134,355] Education provided on the importance of physical activity and other health promotion interventions should be encouraged. This can include nutrition and promoting increased movement in more typical sedentary behaviors such as playing video games, cooking, and socializing through technological activities.[134,355,425] Fitness groups, off-season conditioning, cross training, active social gatherings, and wellness programs would benefit individuals with disabilities and assist in promoting activity.

Risk of Injury

The epidemiology of injuries of athletes with disabilities not only depends on the sport or activity the athlete is performing but also on the underlying pathology of the athlete's long-term impairment.[121,423] Generally speaking, wheelchair competitors have more upper extremity injuries, specifically injuries to the shoulder and spine, while ambulatory competitors have a higher incidence of lower extremity injuries, specifically injuries to the knee.[121,128,423] A systematic review by Webborn et al. in 2014 found that 5-a-side football had the greatest rate of injury at 22.4 injuries/1000 athlete-days and shooting had the least at 2.2 injuries/1000 athlete-days in summer Paralympic sports.[423] Skiing and sledge hockey had the greatest incidence of injury in winter Paralympic sports.[121,423] Ramirez et al. investigated injury rates of high school athletes with medical impairments including autism, emotional disturbances, and seizure disorders participating in basketball, softball, soccer, and field hockey.[344] They found the rate of injury in this population was 2.0 injuries/1000 athletic exposures, with abrasions and contusions accounting for over half of the injuries. The highest injury rate in this population was while playing soccer, recorded at 3.7/1000 athletic exposures.[344]

For athletes who compete in wheelchairs, shoulder pain may not only limit the individual in sport but also in mobility and activities of daily living.[99,121] In a survey of female wheelchair basketball players, over 90% of the 46 athletes reported experiencing shoulder pain since beginning wheelchair use, with 52% expressing current shoulder pain.[99] Nonambulatory athletes and individuals who do not regularly participate in physical activity are at high risk for low bone mineral density and fractures, which should be evaluated in the event of collision- or fall-related injuries.[80]

Head and neck injuries are of significant concern of contact wheelchair sports.[176,423] Out of 263 wheelchair basketball players, 6.1% reported sustaining a concussion in a single season, which is higher than the concussion rate in nondisabled basketball players. Most of those who did sustain a concussion did not report it, with female players sustaining concussions much more frequently than males.[424]

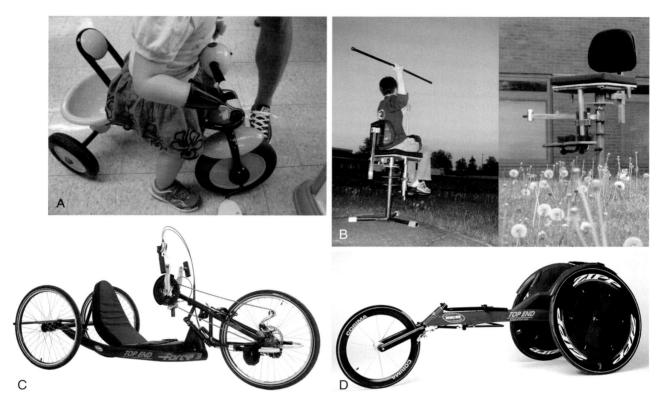

FIG. 15.12 Examples of appropriate adaptations to physical activities in order to allow individual participation. (A) Bicycle handlebar adaptation. (B) Track and field throwing chair. (C) Handcycle (for cycling events). (D) Racing chair (for track and field, road races). ([A] From Baker SA, Calhoun, VD: A custom bicycle handlebar adaptation for children with below elbow amputations. *J Hand Ther* 27(3):258-260, 2014. [B] From Chung C, Lin JT, Toro ML, et al.: Making assistive technology and rehabilitation engineering a sure bet/Uniform throwing chair for seated throwing sporting events. RESNA Annual Conference, June 26–30, 2010, Las Vegas, NV. Copyright © 2010 RESNA, Arlington, VA. [C–D] Courtesy Invacare Top End Wheelchair, Elyria, OH.)

Individuals with higher-level spinal cord injuries are at increased risk for heat intolerance. In cool conditions or at rest, trained individuals dissipate heat similarly to nondisabled trained athletes. However, due to the lack of thermoregulation and ability to dissipate heat through sweat below the level of injury, individuals with spinal cord injuries are at increased risk of heat-related injury.[341,354] It is recommended to keep athletes cool and shaded prior to competition and to provide ample cooling through cool misting stations, ice bags, or ice vests to limit heat illnesses.[220]

For athletes with spinal cord injuries at or above the sixth thoracic vertebra (T6), a life-threatening condition called autonomic dysreflexia should be monitored.[47,149,220] Autonomic dysreflexia arises when a noxious stimulus is not sensed due to a lack of sensation, and the sympathetic nervous system responds by increasing blood pressure and heart rate. It has been associated with increased performance, so is sometimes done as a method of performance enhancement, termed "boosting."[149] Boosting is performed before an event as a method of raising the blood pressure of the athlete to dangerous levels, placing the athlete at risk of stroke, heart attack, or even death. It is treated in Paralympic competitions as a doping method. Screenings before the events are performed at times to detect boosting, with a positive doping test noted when the systolic blood pressure is at or above 180 mm Hg.[47]

Overuse injuries such as tendinitis and muscle strains are common in athletes with disabilities and can be avoided through training modifications and conditioning.[23,121] The mechanism of the overuse is highly variable depending on the specific activity. For example, when comparing populations with reports of shoulder pain, scapular positioning and function may vary greatly in wheelchair basketball, amputee soccer, and disabled table tennis athletes.[15] Amputee soccer players competing on crutches had the best scapular positioning and function, likely due to differences in muscular demands and positioning of the shoulder.[23] Core stability, including scapular stabilizers and hip musculature, should be evaluated in combination with joint positioning and the athletic demands of the participant's sport.

Preparticipation Examination and Classification

Prior to initiating a physical activity program, all athletes should be screened by a physician for a medial release form in order to rule out neurologic, systemic, visual, auditory, or cardiovascular pathologies that would make it dangerous to participate in certain sports.[110] In order to qualify for Special Olympics, individuals must be at least 8 years of age and diagnosed with an intellectual impairment. Athletes are divided into teams or categories based on gender, age, and ability level.[192] In comparison, Paralympics classifies based on neurologic, visual, intellectual, or physical impairments with medical and technical classifiers evaluating the athlete's ability to participate in each sport. Minimal disability criteria qualify athletes to participate in Paralympics.[405]

Prior to participation, specific diagnoses may require additional screening. For individuals with Down syndrome, Special Olympics requires cervical radiographs to screen for atlantoaxial instability or other cervical spine instabilities prior to participation in certain sports, such as diving, high jump, equestrian, artistic gymnastics, football (soccer), power lifting, snowboarding, judo, skiing, and pentathlon.[192] The most recent recommendations from the American Academy of Pediatrics do not include routine radiographic screenings if a child is asymptomatic, unless it is required for specific Special Olympic sporting activities.[64] If a child becomes symptomatic, he or she is immediately referred to a pediatric neurosurgeon or pediatric orthopedic surgeon who has expertise in atlantoaxial instability to evaluate if a fusion is necessary.[64] Because individuals with Down syndrome often exhibit muscular hypotonia and joint hypermobility with poor stabilization, joint integrity should be evaluated for safety in positioning and participation in the sporting activity, including orthotics as needed.[3,70,247]

For individuals who compete with prosthetics, terminal overgrowth, bone spurs, socket fit, skin integrity, and abnormal sensations should be assessed in those with congenital limb deficiencies or acquired amputations.[62,238] Socket fit is critical for injury prevention for those competing with a prosthetic, especially when the prosthetic extends around bony prominences.[238] Socket modifications may be warranted as an individual prepares for increased physical activity.[238]

Athletes competing in a wheelchair should be screened for shoulder muscle imbalances in order to limit the risk of shoulder pathology through sports and recreational activities.[66,283] Similarly, athletes with a spinal cord injury should be assessed for motion, strength, and sensation to provide appropriate mobility and safety throughout participation in the sport.[71] For individuals with arthrogryposis or limited joint range of motion, joint integrity should be assessed prior to competition in sport.[44]

Sport-specific form should be assessed in both gross motor and fine motor movements of the sport with focus on limiting compensations. Equipment should be assessed for safety, size, fit, appropriate function for the athlete, and adherence to sporting rules and regulations.[140,141,408] Each athlete's needs are unique, so equipment that is adjustable is preferred over equipment that is fixed while an athlete is growing or learning a new skill.

Training Programs

When evaluating performance enhancement, a comprehensive assessment of strength, motion, nutritional analysis, body composition, and exercise capacity may best provide for the athlete. Testing should be impairment and sport specific with arm crank, wheelchair, or single-leg ergometry assessments provided as appropriate.[46,116,320]

Medical personnel in health facilities have traditionally provided fitness programs for individuals with disabilities.[425] However, people with disabilities benefit from sport-specific training, wellness, or conditioning programs just as do those without disabilities.[137] There are significant benefits to transitioning to more community-based fitness opportunities such as recreational sports, fitness clubs, or workout facilities including the promotion of self-efficacy in a sustainable workout routine.[425] It is recommended that fitness programs not only address mobility impairments but also promote healthy eating habits, strength training, cardiovascular fitness, and the

individual's community engagement.[2,34,137,158] If organized sport and recreational training programs are not available, after-school fitness programs are also a way to improve the health and wellness of children with disabilities.[173]

Several studies have evaluated the efficacy of these training programs in various groups with disabilities. Agility, aerobic capacity, strength, self-competence, functional movement, and quality of life all improved with an 8-month training program for ambulatory individuals with cerebral palsy.[413] Similarly, improvements in cardiovascular endurance and strength were found in a 10-week fitness program for children and adolescents with spina bifida.[18] In a study done by Baran et al., individuals with intellectual disabilities were able to improve in both fitness and sport-specific skills with the use of an 8-week training schedule of individuals training 3 times per week in soccer skills.[32] For youth with disabilities, task- or function-specific exercises that are fun and motivating yield greater results in functional outcomes.[201,207]

For older athletes, more traditional strength and conditioning tactics may yield greater gain. In a study of eight males with spinal cord injuries and eight male control subjects, both groups displayed similar improvements in strength and power with an 8-week heavy resistance training program, with improvements also noted in a 10-meter sprint.[404] Therefore as for able-bodied athletes who would not train the same for a 10-meter sprint or a 10,000-meter run, training programs should be individualized to the athlete's specific goals and sporting needs.

Biomechanical analyses of movement patterns are becoming more common in sports and recreational activities. Individuals with limb deficiencies have been specifically analyzed for running, swimming, and long jump. Runners and swimmers display decreased step length and stroke length on the involved side compared to the uninvolved side.[58] This is not associated with increased injury at this time, while runners with transfemoral amputations with low back pain display impaired frontal and transverse pelvic and lumbar motion.[374] Therefore not only are strength, power, anaerobic, aerobic, and sport-specific training appropriate, but biomechanical analysis of sport-specific movement patterns should also be evaluated with coaching provided as needed.

SUMMARY

Young athletes are not small adults. They have unique issues in sports participation that must be specifically addressed. Recognition of these unusual qualities is necessary for effective prevention and management of sports-related injuries.

Physical therapists should play a significant role in the total management of the child athlete. The broad-based and eclectic medical background of physical therapists makes them ideal professionals for the assessment and rehabilitation of sports injuries in athletes with full or altered physical capabilities. Depending on advanced experience or certification in sports physical therapy, athletic training, or exercise physiology, they may be the primary medical professionals to administer total management, from prevention to return to participation after injury.

A physical therapist is an important part of the comprehensive medical team that manages sports-related injuries in young athletes. Physical therapists may work with certified athletic trainers or exercise physiologists to provide comprehensive sports safety management. The certified trainer is appropriately skilled to assist with preparticipation screenings and to provide onsite coverage of practices and games with immediate triage and injury management. The exercise physiologist plays an integral part in preseason screening and in conditioning and training programs. The physical therapist can provide assessment and total rehabilitation of sports injuries and aid in phasing the athlete back to play with appropriate progression, supportive devices, or medical limitations. The certified trainer or the exercise physiologist often works with the physical therapist in the return-to-play planning and follow-up.

The goal of these programs is to promote the health and safety of the young athlete. All those involved should work in a manner appropriate to their education, skills, and practice statutes as members of a team, including coaches and parents, toward the goal of safe, rewarding, and successful participation in sport and recreation.

Case Scenarios on Expert Consult

Three case scenarios are presented:
  The post-concussion management of a 16-year-old elite swimmer.
  Management of a 10-year-old boy with osteochondritis dissecans at the knee.
  Postoperative management of anterior cruciate (ACL) reconstruction in a young female athlete.
  Video is also presented that addresses examination and includes both procedures and scoring protocols.

REFERENCES

1. Aagaard H, Jørgensen U: Injuries in elite volleyball, *Scand J Med Sci Sports* 6:228–232, 1996.
2. Abeysekara P, Turchi R, O'Neil M: Obesity and children with special healthcare needs: special considerations for a special population, *Curr Opin Pediatr* 26(4):508–515, 2014.
3. Abousamra O, Bayhan IA, Rogers KJ, Miller F: Hip instability in Down syndrome: a focus on acetabular retroversion, *J Pediatr Orthop*, 2015. [epub ahead of print].
4. Adirim TA, Cheng TL: Overview of injuries in the young athlete, *Sports Med* 33:75–81, 2003.
5. Aichroth PM, Patel DV, Zorrilla P: The natural history and treatment of rupture of the anterior cruciate ligament in children and adolescents: a prospective review, *J Bone Joint Surg Br* 84:38–41, 2002.
6. Al Wren T, Lee DC, Kay RM, Dorey FJ, Gilsanz V: Bone density and size in ambulatory children with cerebral palsy, *Dev Med Child Neurol* 53(2):137–141, 2011.
7. Alesi M, Battaglia G, Roccella M, Testa D, Palma A, Pepi A: Improvement of gross motor and cognitive abilities by an exercise training program: three case reports, *Neuropsychiatr Dis Treat* 10:479–485, 2014.
8. Alsalaheen BA, Mucha A, Morris LO, et al.: Vestibular rehabilitation for dizziness and balance disorders after concussion, *J Neurol Phys Ther* 34(2):87–93, 2010.
9. Alsalaheen BA, Whitney SL, Mucha A, Morris LO, Furman JM, Sparto PJ: Exercise prescription patterns in patients treated with vestibular rehabilitation after concussion, *Physiother Res Int* 18(2):100–108, 2013.
10. American Academy of Family Physicians: American Academy of Pediatrics, American College of Sports Med, American Medical Society for Sports Medicine, American Orthopaedic Society for Sports Medicine, American Osteopathic Academy of Sports Medicine: *PPE Preparticipation physical evaluation*, ed 4, Minneapolis, MN, 2010, McGraw-Hill.
11. American Academy of Pediatrics Committee on Sports Medicine and Fitness: Medical conditions affecting sports participation, *Pediatrics* 107:1205–1209, 2001. Available at URL: http://aappolicy.aappublications.org/cgi/reprint/pediatrics.
12. American Academy of Pediatrics: American Academy of Pediatrics. Organized athletics for preadolescent children, *Pediatrics* 84:583–584, 1989.
13. American Academy of Pediatrics: Climatic heat stress and the exercising child and adolescent. American Academy of Pediatrics. Committee on Sports Medicine and Fitness, *Pediatrics* 106:158–159, 2000.
14. American College of Sports Medicine: *Inter-Association Task Force on exertional heat illnesses consensus statement*, 2003.
15. American Medical Association: Ensuring the health of the adolescent athlete, *Arch Fam Med* 2:446–448, 1993.
16. American Medical Association: *Medical evaluation of the athlete: a guide*, Rev. ed, Chicago, 1976, American Medical Association.
17. Anderson SJ: Lower extremity injuries in youth sports, *Pediatr Clin North Am* 49:627–641, 2002.
18. Andrade CK, Kramer J, Garber M, Longmuir P: Changes in self-concept, cardiovascular endurance and muscular strength of children with spina bifida aged 8 to 13 years in response to a 10-week physical-activity programme: a pilot study, *Child Care Health Dev* 17(3):183–196, 1991.
19. Andrish JT: Meniscal injuries in children and adolescents: diagnosis and management, *J Am Acad Orthop Surg* 4(5):231–237, 1996.
20. Andrish JT: Anterior cruciate ligament injuries in the skeletally immature patient, *Am J Orthop* 30:103–110, 2001.
21. Antle BJ, Mills W, Steele C, Kalnins I, Rossen B: An exploratory study of parents' approaches to health promotion in families of adolescents with physical disabilities, *Child Care Health Dev* 34(2):185–193, 2008.
22. Axe MJ, Snyder-Mackler L, Konin JG, Strube MJ: Development of a distance-based interval throwing program for Little League-aged athletes, *Am J Sports Med* 24(5):594–602, 1996.
23. Aytar A, Zeybek A, Pekyavas NO, Tigli AA, Ergun N: Scapular resting position, shoulder pain and function in disabled athletes, *Prosthet Orthot Int* 39(5):390–396, 2014.
24. Bahrke MS, Yesalis CE, Brower KJ: Anabolic-androgenic steroid abuse and performance-enhancing drugs among adolescents, *Child Adolesc Psychiatr Clin North Am* 7:821–838, 1998.
25. Bailes JE, Cantu RC: Head injury in athletes, *Neurosurgery* 48:26–45, 2001.
26. Bak K: Nontraumatic glenohumeral instability and coracoacromial impingement in swimmers, *Scand J Med Sci Sports* 6(3):132–144, 1996.
27. Bak MJ, Doerr TD: Craniomaxillofacial fractures during recreational baseball and softball, *J Oral Maxillofac Surg* 62:1209–1212, 2004.
28. Baker JG, Freitas MS, Leddy JJ, Kozlowski KF, Willer BS: Return to full functioning after graded exercise assessment and progressive exercise treatment of postconcussion syndrome, *Rehabil Res Prac* 1–7, 2012.
29. Baker JS, Davies B: High intensity exercise assessment: relationships between laboratory and field measures of performance, *J Sci Med Sport* 5:341–347, 2002.
30. Baker SA, Calhoun VD: A custom bicycle handlebar adaptation for children with below elbow amputations, *J Hand Ther* 27(3):258–260, 2014.
31. Balmat P, Vichard P, Pem R: The treatment of avulsion fractures of the tibial tuberosity in adolescent athletes, *Sports Med* 9(5):311–316, 1990.
32. Baran F, Aktop A, Ozer D, Nalbant S, Aglamis E, Barak S, Hutzler Y: The effects of a Special Olympics Unified Sports Soccer training program on anthropometry, physical fitness and skilled performance in Special Olympics soccer athletes and non-disabled partners, *Res Dev Disabil* 34(1):695–709, 2013.
33. Bar-Or O: *Child and adolescent athlete*, vol. 6. Malden, MA, 1995, Blackwell.
34. Barr M, Shields N: Identifying the barriers and facilitators to participation in physical activity for children with Down syndrome, *J Intellect Disabil Res* 55(11):1020–1033, 2011.
35. Baugh CM, Stamm JM, Riley DO, et al.: Chronic traumatic encephalopathy: neurodegeneration following repetitive concussive and subconcussive brain trauma, *Brain Imaging Behav* 6(2):244–254, 2012.
36. Bauman M: Nutritional requirements for athletes. In Bernhardt DB, editor: *Sports physical therapy*, New York, 1986, Churchill Livingstone, pp 89–105.
37. Beaty JH: Hip, pelvis and thigh. In Sulliven JA, Anderson TE, editors: *Care of the young athletes*, Rosemont, IL, 2000, American Academy of Orthopaedic Surgeons, pp 3365–3376.
38. Bell DG, McLellan TM, Sabiston CM: Effect of ingesting caffeine and ephedrine on performance, *Med Sci Sports Exerc* 34:1399–1403, 2002.
39. Benson BW, Meeuwisse W: Ice hockey injuries, *Med Sport Sci* 49:86–119, 2005.

40. Benson LS, Waters PM, Meier SW, Visotsky JL, Williams CS: Pediatric hand injuries due to home exercycles, *J Pediatr Orthop* 20:34–39, 2000.

41. Bergstrom KA, Brandseth K, Fretheim S, Tvilde K, Ekeland A: Activity-related knee injuries and pain in athletic adolescents, *Knee Surg Sports Traumatol Arthrosc* 9:146–150, 2001.

42. Bernhardt DT, Gomez J, Johnson MD, et al.: Strength training by children and adolescents, *Pediatrics* 107:1470–1472, 2001.

43. Bernhardt DT, Landry GL: Sports injuries in young athletes, *Adv Pediatr* 42:465–500, 1995.

44. Bernstein RM: Arthrogryposis and amyoplasia, *J Am Acad Orthop Surg* 10(6):417–424, 2002.

45. Best JR: Effects of physical activity on children's executive function: contributions of experimental research on aerobic exercise, *Dev Rev* 30(4):331–551, 2010.

46. Bhambhani YN, Holland LJ, Steadward RD: Anaerobic threshold in wheelchair athletes with cerebral palsy: validity and reliability, *Arch Phys Med Rehabil* 74:305–311, 1993.

47. Bhambhani Y, Mactavish J, Warren S, et al.: Boosting in athletes with high-level spinal cord injury: knowledge, incidence and attitudes of athletes in Paralympic sport, *Disabil Rehabil* 32(26):2172–2190, 2010.

48. Birrer RB, Griesemer BA, Cataletto MB: *Pediatric sports medicine for primary care*, Philadelphia, 2002, Lippincott Williams Wilkins.

49. Blanksby BA, Wearne FK, Elliott BC, Blitvich JD: Aetiology and occurrence of diving injuries. A review of diving safety, *Sports Med* 23(4):228–246, 1997.

50. Bloemen MA, Backx FJ, Takken T, Wittink H, Benner J, Mollema J, de Groot JF: Factors associated with physical activity in children and adolescents with a physical disability: a systematic review, *Dev Med Child Neurol* 57(2):137–148, 2015.

51. Blond L, Hansen L: Patellofemoral pain syndrome in athletes: a 5.7-year retrospective follow-up study of 250 athletes, *Acta Orthop Belg* 64(4): 393–400, 1998.

52. Boden BP, Lin W, Young M, Mueller FO: Catastrophic injuries in wrestlers, *Am J Sports Med* 30:791–795, 2002.

53. Bolesta MJ, Fitch RD: Tibial tubercle avulsions, *J Pediatr Orthop* 6(2):186–192, 1986.

54. Bolgla LA, Keskula DR: Reliability of lower extremity functional performance tests, *J Orthop Sports Phys Ther* 26(3):138–142, 1997.

55. Bontempo NA, Mazzocca AD: Biomechanics and treatment of acromioclavicular and sternoclavicular joint injuries, *Br J Sports Med* 44(5): 361–369, 2010.

56. Boyd K, Peirce N, Batt M: Common hip injuries in sport, *Sports Med* 24(4):273–288, 1997.

57. Reference deleted in proofs.

58. Bragaru M, Dekker R, Geertzen JH, Dijkstra PU: Amputees and sports: a systematic review, *Sports Med* 41(9):721–740, 2011.

59. Reference deleted in proofs.

60. Brown RL, Koepplinger ME, Mehlman CT, Gittelman M, Garcia VF: All-terrain vehicle and bicycle crashes in children: epidemiology and comparison of injury severity, *J Pediatr Surg* 37:375–380, 2002.

61. Bruce DA, Schut L, Sutton LN: Brain and cervical spine injuries occurring during organized sports activities in children and adolescents, *Clin Sports Med* 1:495–514, 1982.

62. Bryant PR, Pandian G: Acquired limb deficiencies. 1. Acquired limb deficiencies in children and young adults, *Arch Phys Med Rehabil* 82(3 Suppl 1): S3–8, 2001.

63. Buffart LM, Roebroeck ME, Rol M, Stam HJ, van den Berg-Emons RJ: Triad of physical activity, aerobic fitness and obesity in adolescents and young adults with myelomeningocele, *J Rehabil Med* 40(1):70–75, 2008.

64. Bull MJ: Committee on Genetics: health supervision for children with Down syndrome, *Pediatrics* 128(2):393–406, 2011.

65. Bunc V: A simple method for estimating aerobic fitness, *Ergonomics* 37:159–165, 1994.

66. Burnham RS, May L, Nelson E, Steadward R, Reid DC: Shoulder pain in wheelchair athletes. The role of muscle imbalance, *Am J Sports Med* 21(2):238–242, 1993.

67. Cain EL, Clancy WG: Treatment algorithm for osteochondral injuries of the knee, *Clin Sports Med* 20:321–342, 2001.

68. Caine DJ, DiFiori J, Maffulli N: Physeal injuries in children's and youth sports. Reasons for concern? *Br J Sports Med* 40:749–760, 2006.

69. Caine D, Maffulli N, Caine C: Epidemiology of injury in child and adolescent sports: injury rates, risk factors and prevention, *Clin Sports Med* 27:19–50, 2008.

70. Caird MS, Wills BP, Dormans JP: Down syndrome in children: the role of the orthopaedic surgeon, *J Am Acad Orthop Surg* 14(11):610–619, 2006.

71. Cancel D, Capoor J: Patient safety in the rehabilitation of children with spinal cord injuries, spina bifida, neuromuscular disorders, and amputations, *Phys Med Rehabil Clin North Am* 23(2):401–422, 2012.

72. Cantu RC: Cervical spine injuries in the athlete, *Sem Neurol* 20:173–178, 2000.

73. Cantu RC, Mueller FO: Brain injury-related fatalities in American football, 1945-1999, *Neurosurgery* 52:846–852, 2003.

74. Cantu RC, Bailes JE, Wilberger Jr JE: Guidelines for return to contact or collision sport after a cervical spine injury, *Clin Sports Med* 17:137–146, 1998.

75. Casa DJ, Armstrong LE, Hillman SK, et al.: National Athletic Trainers' Association position statement: fluid replacement for athletes, *J Athl Train* 35:212–224, 2000.

76. Cavanaugh JT, Guskiewicz KM, Stergiou N: A nonlinear dynamic approach for evaluating postural control: new directions for the management of sport-related cerebral concussion, *Sports Med* 35(11):935–950, 2005.

77. Cavanaugh JT, Guskiewicz KM, Giuliani C, Marshall S, Mercer VS, Stergiou N: Recovery of postural control after cerebral concussion: new insights using approximate entropy, *J Athl Train* 41(3):305–313, 2006.

78. Cavanaugh JT, Guskiewicz KM, Giuliani C, Marshall S, Mercer V, Stergiou N: Detecting altered postural control after cerebral concussion in athletes with normal postural stability, *Br J Sports Med* 39(11):805–811, 2005.

79. Centers for Disease Control and Prevention: BMI for children and teens. Available at: URL: www.cdc.gov/nccdphp/dnpa/bmi/bmi-for-age.htm.

80. Chen CL, Lin KC, Wu CY, Ke JY, Wang CJ, Chen CY: Relationships of muscle strength and bone mineral density in ambulatory children with cerebral palsy, *Osteoporos Int* 23(2):715–721, 2012.

81. Child SCAT3, *Br J Sports Med* 47(5):263, 2013.

82. Choe MC, Babikian T, DiFiori J, Hovda DA, Giza CC: A pediatric perspective on concussion pathophysiology, *Curr Opin Pediatr* 24(6): 689–695, 2012.

83. Chow SP, Lam JJ, Leong JC: Fracture of the tibial tubercle in the adolescent, *J Bone Joint Surg Br* 72(2):231–234, 1990.

84. Christie MJ, Dvonch VM: Tibial tuberosity avulsion fracture in adolescents, *J Pediatr Orthop* 1(4):391–394, 1981.

85. Chun J, Haney S, DiFiori J: The relative contributions of the history and physical examination in the preparticipation evaluation of collegiate student-athletes, *Clin J Sport Med* 16(5):437–438, 2006.

86. Cirak B, Ziegfeld S, Knight VM, Chang D, Avellino AM, Paidas CN: Spinal injuries in children, *J Pediatr Surg* 39(4):607–612, 2004.

87. Reference deleted in proofs.

88. Clark N: Nutrition: pre-, intra-, and post-competition. In Cantu RC, Micheli LJ, editors: *ACSM's guidelines for the team physician*, Philadelphia, 1991, Lea Febiger, pp 58–65.

89. Clarkson PM: Nutrition for improved sports performance. Current issues on ergogenic aids, *Sports Med* 21:393–401, 1996.

90. Coady CM, Micheli LJ: Stress fractures in the pediatric athlete, *Clin Sports Med* 16:225–238, 1997.

91. Colletti TP: Sports preparticipation evaluation, *Physician Assist* 25(7): 31–41, 2001.

92. Collins MW, Lovell MR, Iverson GL, Cantu RC, Maroon JC, Field M: Cumulative effects of concussion in high school athletes, *Neurosurgery* 51:1175–1179, 2002.

93. Concannon LG, Harrast MA, Herring SA: Radiating upper limb pain in the contact sport athlete: an update on transient quadriparesis and stingers, *Curr Sports Med Rep* 11(1):28–34, 2012.

94. Congress: *Public Law* 94–142, 2015.

95. Conley KM, Bolin DJ, Carek PJ, Konin JG, Neal TL, Violette D: National Athletic Trainers' Association Position Statement: preparticipation physical examinations and disqualifying conditions, *J Athl Train* 49(1): 102–120, 2014.

96. Conn JM, Annest JL, Gilchrist J: Sports and recreation related injury episodes in the US population, 1997-1999, *Inj Prev* 9:117–123, 2003.

97. Cooper K: *Kid fitness*, New York, 1991, Bantam Books.

98. Reference deleted in proofs.

99. Curtis KA, Black K: Shoulder pain in female wheelchair basketball players, *J Orthop Sports Phys Ther* 29(4):225–231, 1999.

100. Czitrom AA, Salter RB, Willis RB: Fractures involving the distal epiphyseal plate of the femur, *Int Orthop* 4(4):269–277, 1981.

101. DaSilva MF, Williams JS, Fadale PD, Hulstyn MJ, Ehrlich MG: Pediatric throwing injuries about the elbow, *Am J Orthop* 27:90–96, 1998.

102. Day C, Stolz U, Mehan TJ, Smith GA, McKenzie LB: Diving-related injuries in children <20 years old treated in emergency departments in the United States: 1990-2006, *Pediatrics* 122(2):e388–e394, 2008.

103. De Beaumont L, Lassonde M, Leclerc S, Theoret H: Long-term and cumulative effects of sports concussion on motor cortex inhibition, *Neurosurgery* 61(2):329–336, 2007. discussion 336-327.

104. De Beaumont L, Mongeon D, Tremblay S, et al.: Persistent motor system abnormalities in formerly concussed athletes, *J Athl Train* 46(3): 234–240, 2011.

105. De Beaumont L, Theoret H, Mongeon D, et al.: Brain function decline in healthy retired athletes who sustained their last sports concussion in early adulthood, *Brain* 132(Pt 3):695–708, 2009.

106. de Lucena GL, dos Santos Gomes C, Guerra RO: Prevalence and associated factors of Osgood-Schlatter syndrome in a population-based sample of Brazilian adolescents, *Am J Sports Med* 39(2):415–420, 2011.

107. Debnath UK, Freeman BJ, Gregory P, de la Harpe D, Kerslake RW, Webb JK: Clinical outcome and return to sport after the surgical treatment of spondylolysis in young athletes, *J Bone Joint Surg Br* 85:244–249, 2003.

108. Deitch J, Mehlman CT, Foad SL, Obbehat A, Mallory M: Traumatic anterior shoulder dislocation in adolescents, *Am J Sports Med* 31(5):758–763, 2003.

109. Dejour H, Walch G, Nove-Josserand L, Guier C: Factors of patellar instability: an anatomic radiographic study, *Knee Surg Sports Traumatol Arthrosc* 2(1):19–26, 1994.

110. Deligiannis AP, Kouidi EJ, Koutlianos NA, et al.: Eighteen years' experience applying old and current strategies in the pre-participation cardiovascular screening of athletes, *Hellenic J Cardiol* 55(1):32–41, 2014.

111. deLoes M, Dahlstedt LJ, Thomee R: A 7-year study on risks and costs of knee injuries in male and female youth participants in 12 sports, *Scand J Med Sci Sports* 10:90–97, 2000.

112. DeMatteo C, Stazyk K, Singh SK, et al.: Development of a conservative protocol to return children and youth to activity following concussive injury, *Clin Pediatrics* 54(2):152–163, 2015.

113. d'Hemecourt PA, Gerbino 2 PG, Micheli LJ: Back injuries in the young athlete, *Clin Sports Med* 19:663–679, 2000.

114. Dodd KJ, Taylor NF, Damiano DL: A systematic review of the effectiveness of strength-training programs for people with cerebral palsy, *Arch Phys Med Rehabil* 83(8):1157–1164, 2002.

115. Dompier TP, Kerr ZY, Marshall SW, Hainline B, Snook EM, Hayden R, Simon JE: Incidence of concussion during practice and games in youth, high school, and collegiate American football players, *JAMA Pediatr* 169(7):659–665, 2015.

116. Draheim CC, Laurie NE, McCubbin JA, Perkins JL: Validity of a modified aerobic fitness test for adults with mental retardation, *Med Sci Sports Exerc* 31:1849–1854, 1999.

117. Drkulec JA, Letts M: Snowboarding injuries in children, *Can J Surg* 44:435–439, 2001.

118. EDUCATION, P. I. P: Creating equal opportunities for children and youth with disabilities to participate in physical education and extracurricular athletics, *Director*, 2011.

119. Edwards Jr PH, Grana WA: Physeal fractures about the knee, *J Am Acad Orthop Surg* 3(2):63–69, 1995.

120. Ekegren CL, Miller WC, Celebrini RG, Eng JJ, Macintyre DL: Reliability and validity of observational risk screening in evaluating dynamic knee valgus, *J Orthop Sports Phys Ther* 39(9):665–674, 2009.

121. Fagher K, Lexell J: Sports-related injuries in athletes with disabilities, *Scand J Med Sci in Sports* 24(5):e320–e331, 2014.

122. Faigenbaum AD, Kraemer WJ, Blimkie CJ, Jeffreys I, Micheli LJ, Nitka M, Rowland TW: Youth resistance training: updated position statement paper from the national strength and conditioning association, *J Strength Cond Res* 23(5 Suppl):S60–S79, 2009.

123. Faigenbaum AD, Milliken LA, Loud RL, Burak BT, Doherty CL, Westcott WL: Comparison of 1 and 2 days per week of strength training in children, *Res Q Exerc Sports* 73:416–424, 2002.

124. Fairbank JC, Pynsent PB, van Poortvliet JA, Phillips H: Mechanical factors in the incidence of knee pain in adolescents and young adults, *J Bone Joint Surg Br* 66(5):685–693, 1984.

125. Falk B, Dotan R: Physiologic and health aspects of exercise in hot and cold environments. In Hebestreit H, Bar-Or O, editors: *The young athlete*, Malden, MA, 2008, Blackwell Publishing. pp249–267.

126. Fehnel D, Johnson R: Anterior cruciate injuries in the skeletally immature athlete, *Sports Med* 29(1):51–63, 2000.

127. Ferguson RW, Green A, Hansen LM: Game changers: stats, stories and what communities are doing to protect young athletes, 2013. Available at: URL: http://www.safekids.org/research-report/game-changers-stats-stories-and-whatcommunities-are-doing-protect-young-athletes.

128. Ferrara MS, Peterson CL: Injuries to athletes with disabilities: identifying injury patterns, *Sports Med* 30(2):137–143, 2000.

129. Field SJ, Oates RK: Sports and recreation activities and opportunities for children with spina bifida and cystic fibrosis, *J Sci Med Sport* 4(1):71–76, 2001.

130. Finch GD, Barnes MJ: Major cervical spine injuries in children and adolescents, *J Pediatr Orthop* 18:811–814, 1998.

131. Finkelstein EA, Fiekbelkorn IC, Wang G: National medical spending attributable to overweight and obesity: how much and who's paying? *Health Aff (Millwood)* W3:219–226, 2003.

132. Fitzgerald GK, Lephart SM, Hwang JH, et al.: Hop tests as predictors of dynamic knee stability, *J Orthop Sports Phys Ther* 31(10):588–597, 2001.

133. Flynn JM, Skaggs DL, Sponseller PT, et al.: The surgical management of pediatric fractures of the lower extremity, *Instr Course Lect* 52:647–659, 2003.

134. Foley JT, Lloyd M, Vogl D, Temple VA: Obesity trends of 8-18 year old Special Olympians: 2005-2010, *Res Dev Disabil* 35(3):705–710, 2014.

135. *Food Guide Pyramid*, Washington, DC, 1992, US Department of Agriculture.

136. Ford KR, Myer GD, Hewett TE: Valgus knee motion during landing in high school female and male basketball players, *Med Sci Sports Exerc* 35(10):1745–1750, 2003.

137. Fowler EG, Kolobe TH, Damiano DL, et al.: Promotion of physical fitness and prevention of secondary conditions for children with cerebral palsy: section on pediatrics research summit proceedings, *Physical Therapy* 87(11):1495–1510, 2007.

138. Frey S, Hosalkar H, Cameron DB, Heath A, David Horn B, Ganley TJ: Tibial tuberosity fractures in adolescents, *J Child Orthop* 2(6):469–474, 2008.

139. Frino J, McCarthy RE, Sparks CY, McCullough FL: Trends in adolescent lumbar disk herniation, *J Pediatr Orthop* 26(5):579–581, 2006.

140. Frossard LA, O'Riordan A, Smeathers J: Performance of elite seated discus throwers in F30s classes: part I: does whole body positioning matter? *Prosthet Orthot Int* 37(3):183–191, 2013.

141. Frossard LA, O'Riordan A, Smeathers J: Performance of elite seated discus throwers in F30s classes: part II: does feet positioning matter? *Prosthet Orthot Int* 37(3):192–202, 2013.

142. Fu FH: *Sports injuries: mechanisms, prevention, and treatment*, ed 2, Philadelphia, 2001, Lippincott Williams Wilkins.

143. Fulkerson JP: Diagnosis and treatment of patients with patellofemoral pain, *Am J Sports Med* 30(3):447–456, 2002.

144. Fulkerson JP, Arendt EA: Anterior knee pain in females, *Clin Orthop Rel Res* 372:69–73, 2000.

145. Gagnon I, Galli C, Friedman D, Grilli L, Iverson GL: Active rehabilitation for children who are slow to recover following sport-related concussion, *Brain Inj* 23(12):956–964, 2009.

146. Gagnon I, Grilli L, Friedman D, Iverson GL: A pilot study of active rehabilitation for adolescents who are slow to recover from sport-related concussion, *Scand J Med Sci Sports* 26(3):299–306, 2016.

147. Gaillard B: *Handbook for the young athlete*, Palo Alto, CA, 1978, Bull Publishing.

148. Gassner R, Tuli T, Hachl O, Rudisch A, Ulmer H: Cranio-maxillofacial trauma: a 10 year review of 9,543 cases with 21,067 injuries, *J Cranio-maxillofac Surg* 31:51–61, 2003.

149. Gee CM, West CR, Krassioukov AV: Boosting in elite athletes with spinal cord injury: a critical review of physiology and testing procedures, *Sports Med* 45(8):1133–1142, 2015.

150. Gerstenbluth RE, Spirnak JP, Elder JS: Sports participation and high grade renal injuries in children, *J Urol* 168:2575–2578, 2002.

151. Gholve PA, Scher DM, Khakharia S, Widmann RF, Green DW: Osgood Schlatter syndrome, *Curr Opin Pediatr* 19(1):44–50, 2007.

152. Gill 4th TJ, Micheli LJ: The immature athlete: common injuries and overuse syndromes of the elbow and wrist, *Clin Sports Med* 15:401–423, 1996.

153. Gillon H: Scaphoid injuries in children, *Accid Emerg Nurs* 9:249–256, 2001.

154. Giza CC, Kutcher JS, Ashwal S, et al.: Summary of evidence-based guideline update: evaluation and management of concussion in sports: report of the Guideline Development Subcommittee of the American Academy of Neurology, *Neurology* 80(24):2250–2257, 2013.

155. Glass T, Ruddy RM, Alpern ER, et al.: Traumatic brain injuries and computed tomography use in pediatric sports participants, *Am J Emerg Med* 33(10):1458–1464, 2015.

156. Goldberg BA, Mansfield DS, Davino NA: Nonunion of a distal femoral epiphyseal fracture-separation, *Am J Orthop (Belle Mead NJ)* 25(11):773–777, 1996.

157. Goldberg B, Saraniti A, Witman P, Gavin M, Nicholas JA: Pre-participation sports assessment—an objective evaluation, *Pediatrics* 66(5):736–745, 1980.

158. Golubovic S, Maksimovic J, Golubovic B, Glumbic N: Effects of exercise on physical fitness in children with intellectual disability, *Res Dev Disabil* 33(2):608–614, 2012.

159. Gonzalez-Aguero A, Vicente-Rodriguez G, Moreno LA, Guerra-Balic M, Ara I, Casajus JA: Health-related physical fitness in children and adolescents with Down syndrome and response to training, *Scand J Med Sci Sports* 20(5):716–724, 2010.

160. Green GA: Drugs, athletes, and drug testing. In Sanders B, editor: *Sports physical therapy*, Norwalk, CT, 1990, Appleton Lange, pp 95–111.

161. Gregg JR, Das M: Foot and ankle problems in the preadolescent and adolescent athlete, *Clin Sports Med* 1:131–147, 1982.

162. Greydanus DE, Patel DR: Sports doping in the adolescent athlete: the hope, hype and hyperbole, *Pediatr Clin North Am* 49:829–855, 2002.

163. Grimm NL, Weiss JM, Kessler JI, Aoki SK: Osteochondritis dissecans of the knee: pathoanatomy, epidemiology, and diagnosis, *Clin Sports Med* 33(2):181–188, 2014.

164. Guskiewicz KM: Assessment of postural stability following sport-related concussion, *Curr Sports Med Rep* 2(1):24–30, 2003.

165. Guskiewicz KM: Balance assessment in the management of sport-related concussion, *Clin Sports Med* 30(1):89–102, 2011. ix.

166. Guskiewicz KM, Valovich McLeod TC: Pediatric sports-related concussion, *PM R* 3(4):353–364, 2011. quiz 364.

167. Guy JA, Micheli LJ: Strength training for children and adolescents, *J Am Acad Orthop Surg* 9:29–36, 2001.

168. Guzzanti V: The natural history and treatment of rupture of the anterior cruciate ligament in children and adolescents, *J Bone Joint Surg Br* 85:618–619, 2003.

169. Hagel B: Skiing and snowboarding injuries, *Med Sport Sci* 48:74–119, 2005.

170. Haller CA, Benowitz NL: Adverse cardiovascular and central nervous system events associated with dietary supplements containing ephedra alkaloids, *N Engl J Med* 343(25):1833–1888, 2000.

171. Halstead ME, Walter KD: American Academy of Pediatrics. Clinical report–sport-related concussion in children and adolescents, *Pediatrics* 126(3):597–615, 2010.

172. Hand WL, Hand CR, Dunn AW: Avulsion fractures of the tibial tubercle, *J Bone Joint Surg Am* 53(8):1579–1583, 1971.

173. Haney K, Messiah SE, Arheart KL, et al.: Park-based afterschool program to improve cardiovascular health and physical fitness in children with disabilities, *Disabil Health J* 7(3):335–342, 2014.

174. Hanson CS, Nabavi D, Yuen HK: The effect of sports on level of community integration as reported by persons with spinal cord injury, *Am J Occupat Ther* 55:332–338, 2001.

175. Harvie D, O'Leary T, Kumar S: A systematic review of randomized controlled trials on exercise parameters in the treatment of patellofemoral pain: what works? *J Multidisc Healthcare* 4:383–392, 2011.

176. Hawkeswood J, Finlayson H, O'Connor R, Anton H: A pilot survey on injury and safety concerns in international sledge hockey, *Int J Sports Phys Ther* 6(3):173–185, 2011.

177. Hayes JR, Groner JI: The increasing incidence of snowboard-related trauma, *J Pediatr Surg* 43(5):928–930, 2008.

178. Hewett TE, Ford KR, Myer GD: Anterior cruciate ligament injuries in female athletes: part 2: a meta-analysis of neuromuscular interventions aimed at injury prevention, *Am J Sports Med* 34(3):490–498, 2006.

179. Hewett TE, Myer GD, Ford KR: Reducing knee and anterior cruciate ligament injuries among female athletes: a systematic review of neuromuscular training interventions, *J Knee Surg* 18(1):82–88, 2005.

180. Hewett TE, Myer GD, Ford KR: Anterior cruciate ligament injuries in female athletes: part 1: mechanisms and risk factors, *Am J Sports Med* 34(2):299–311, 2006.

181. Hewett TE, Myer GD, Ford KR, et al.: Biomechanical measures of neuromuscular control and valgus loading of the knee predict anterior cruciate ligament injury risk in female athletes: a prospective study, *Am J Sports Med* 33(4):492–501, 2005.

182. Hewett TE, Pasque C, Heyl R, Wroble R: Wrestling injuries, *Med Sport Sci* 48:152–178, 2005.

183. Hewett TE, Zazulak BT, Myer GD: Effects of the menstrual cycle on anterior cruciate ligament injury risk: a systematic review, *Am J Sports Med* 35(4):659–668, 2007.

184. Hoeberigs JH, Debets-Eggen HB, Debets PM: Sports medical experiences from the International Flower Marathon for disabled wheelers, *Am J Sports Med* 18(4):418–421, 1990.

185. Hogan KA, Gross RH: Overuse injuries in pediatric athletes, *Orthop Clin North Am* 34(3):405–415, 2003.

186. Hosea TM, Carey OC, Harrer MF: The gender issue: epidemiology of ankle injuries in athletes who participate in basketball, *Clin Orthop* 372:45–49, 2000.

187. Houtrow AJ, Larson K, Olson LM, Newacheck PW, Halfon N: Changing trends of childhood disability, 2001-2011, *Pediatrics* 134(3):530–538, 2014.

188. Hughston JC, Hergenroeder PT, Courtenay BG: Osteochondritis dissecans of the femoral condyles, *J Bone Joint Surg Am* 66(9):1340–1348, 1984.

189. Hunter SC, Etchison WC, Halpern B, et al.: Standards and norms of fitness and flexibility in the high school athlete, *J Athl Train* 20:210–212, 1985.

190. Hutchinson MR, Ireland ML: Overuse and throwing injuries in the skeletally immature athlete, *Instr Course Lect* 52:25–36, 2003.

191. Ilizaliturri Jr VM, Villalobos Jr FE, Chaidez PA, Valero FS, Aguilera JM: Internal snapping hip syndrome: treatment by endoscopic release of the iliopsoas tendon, *Arthroscopy* 21(11):1375–1380, 2005.

192. Inc SO: *Special Olympics Sports Rules*, 2012.

193. Ingram JG, Fields SK, Yard EE, Comstock RD: Epidemiology of knee injuries among boys and girls in US high school athletics. *Am J Sports Med* 36(6):1116–1122.

194. *Invacare Top End Eliminator OSR Kneeling*, 2015.

195. *Invacare Top End Force 3 Handcycle*, 2015.

196. Iobst CA, Stanitski CL: Acute knee injuries, *Clin Sports Med* 19:621–635, 2000.

197. Ireland ML: Anterior cruciate ligament injury in female athletes: epidemiology, *J Athl Train* 34(2):150–154, 1999.

198. Iwamoto J, Takeda T, Sato Y, Matsumoto H: Radiographic abnormalities of the inferior pole of the patella in juvenile athletes, *Keio J Med* 58(1):50–53, 2009.

199. Jaarsma EA, Dijkstra PU, Geertzen JHB, Dekker R: Barriers to and facilitators of sports participation for people with physical disabilities: a systematic review, *Scand J Med Sci Sports* 24(6):871–881, 2014.

200. Junge T, Runge L, Juul-Kristensen B, Wedderkopp N: Risk factors for knee injuries in children 8-15 years: the CHAMPS-Study DK, *Med Sci Sports Exerc* 48(4):655–662, 2016.

201. Kanagasabai PS, Mulligan H, Mirfin-Veitch B, Hale LA: Association between motor functioning and leisure participation of children with physical disability: an integrative review, *Dev Med Child Neurol* 56(12):1147–1162, 2014.

202. Kay RM, Matthys GA: Pediatric ankle fractures: evaluation and treatment, *J Am Acad Orthop Surg* 9:268–278, 2001.

203. Keays SL, et al.: The relationship between knee strength and functional stability before and after anterior cruciate ligament reconstruction, *J Orthop Res* 21(2):231–237, 2003.

204. Kelleher CM, Metze SL, Dillon PA, Mychaliska GB, Keshen TH, Foglia RP: Unsafe at any speed–kids riding all-terrain vehicles, *J Pediatr Surg* 40(6):929–934, 2005. discussion 934-925.

205. Kerr IL: Mouth guards for the prevention of injuries in contact sports, *Sports Med* 5 415–427, 1986.

206. Kibler WB, Safran M: Tennis injuries, *Med Sport Sci* 48:120–137, 2005.

207. Kim JY, Kim JM, Ko EY: The effect of the action observation physical training on the upper extremity function in children with cerebral palsy, *J Exerc Rehabil* 10(3):176–183, 2014.

208. King G, Law M, Petrenchik T, Hurley P: Psychosocial determinants of out of school activity participation for children with and without physical disabilities, *Phys Occupat Ther Pediatr* 33(4):384–404, 2013.

209. Kinzey SJ, Armstrong CW: The reliability of the star-excursion test in assessing dynamic balance, *J Orthop Sports Phys Ther* 27(5):356–360, 1998.

210. Klish WJ: Childhood obesity: pathophysiology and treatment, *Acta Pediatrica Jpn* 37 1–6, 1995.

211. Knowles SB, Marshall SW, Guskiewicz KM: Issues in estimating risks and rates in sports injury research, *J Athl Train* 41(2):207–215, 2006.

212. Kocher MS, Garg S, Micheli LJ: Physeal sparing reconstruction of the anterior cruciate ligament in skeletally immature prepubescent children and adolescents, *J Bone Joint Surg* 87(11):2371–2379, 2005.

213. Kocher MS, Garg S, Micheli LJ: Physeal sparing reconstruction of the anterior cruciate ligament in skeletally immature prepubescent children and adolescents. Surgical technique, *J Bone Joint Surg Am* 88(Suppl 1 Pt 2): 283–293, 2006.

214. Kocher MS, Tucker R, Ganley TJ, Flynn JM: Management of osteochondritis dissecans of the knee: current concepts review, *Am J Sports Med* 34(7):1181–1191, 2006.

215. Kocher MS, Waters PM, Micheli LJ: Upper extremity injuries in the paediatric athlete, *Sports Med* 30:117–135, 2000.

216. Kouyoumjian A, Barber FA: Management of anterior cruciate ligament disruptions in skeletally immature patients, *Am J Orthop* 30:771–774, 2001.

217. Kozlowski KF, Graham J, Leddy JJ, Devinney-Boymel L, Willer BS: Exercise intolerance in individuals with postconcussion syndrome, *J Athl Train* 48(5):627–635, 2013.

218. Kraemer WJ, Voleck JS, French DN, et al.: The effects of L-Carnitine tartrate supplementation on hormonal responses to resistance exercise and recovery, *J Strength Cond Res* 17:455–462, 2003.

219. Kraft DE: Low back pain in the adolescent athlete, *Pediatr Clin North Am* 49:643–653, 2002.

220. Krassioukov A, West C: The role of autonomic function on sport performance in athletes with spinal cord injury, *PM R* 6(8 Suppl):S58–S65, 2014.

221. Kraus R, Pavlidis T, Heiss C, Kilian O, Schnettler R: Arthroscopic treatment of post-traumatic shoulder instability in children and adolescents, *Knee Surg Sports Traumotol Arthrosc* 18(12):1738–1741, 2010.

222. Kubiak R, Slongo T: Unpowered scooter injuries in children, *Acta Paediatr* 92:50–54, 2003.

223. Kujala UM, Kvist M, Heinonen O: Osgood-Schlatter's disease in adolescent athletes. Retrospective study of incidence and duration, *Am J Sports Med* 13(4):236–241, 1985.

224. Kushare I, Klingele K, Samora W: Discoid meniscus: diagnosis and management, *Orthop Clin North Am* 46(4):533–540, 2015.

225. Kvist J: Rehabilitation following anterior cruciate ligament injury: current recommendations for sports participation, *Sports Med* 34(4): 269–280, 2004.

226. Lai AM, Stanish WD, Stanish HI: The young athlete with physical challenges, *Clin Sports Med* 19:793–819, 2000.

227. Lambrick D, Westrupp N, Kaufmann S, Stoner L, Faulkner J: The effectiveness of a high-intensity games intervention on improving indices of health in young children, *J Sports Sci* 34(3):190–198, 2016.

228. Langlois JA, Rutland-Brown W, Wald MM: The epidemiology and impact of traumatic brain injury: a brief overview, *J Head Trauma Rehabil* 21(5):375–378, 2006.

229. Larsen GE, George JD, Alexander JL, Fellington GW, Aldana SG, Parcell AC: Prediction of maximum oxygen consumption from walking, jogging, or running, *Res Q Exerc Sp* 71:66–72, 2002.

230. Leddy JJ, Baker JG, Kozlowski K, Bisson L, Willer B: Reliability of a graded exercise test for assessing recovery from concussion, *Clin J Sport Med* 21(2):89–94, 2011.

231. Leddy JJ, Cox JL, Baker JG, Wack DS, Pendergast DR, Zivadinov R, Willer B: Exercise treatment for postconcussion syndrome: a pilot study of changes in functional magnetic resonance imaging activation, physiology, and symptoms, *J Head Trauma Rehabil* 28(4):241–249, 2013.

232. Leddy JJ, Kozlowski K, Donnelly JP, Pendergast DR, Epstein LH, Willer B: A preliminary study of subsymptom threshold exercise training for refractory post-concussion syndrome, *Clin J Sport Med* 20(1):21–27, 2010.

233. Lehnhard RA, Lehnhard HR, Young R, Butterfield SA: Monitoring injuries on a college soccer team: the effect of strength training, *J Strength Cond Res* 10:115–119, 1996.

234. Lenaway DD, Ambler AG, Beaudoin DE: The epidemiology of school-related injuries: new perspectives, *Am J Prevent Med* 8:193–198, 1992.

235. Leonard JR, Jaffe DM, Kuppermann N, Olsen CS, Leonard JC: Cervical spine injury patterns in children, *Pediatrics* 133(5):e1179–e1188, 2014.

236. Letts M, Davidson D, McCaffrey M: The adolescent pilon fracture: management and outcome, *J Pediatr Orthop* 21:20–26, 2001.

237. Levi JH, Coleman CR: Fracture of the tibial tubercle, *Am J Sports Med* 4(6):254–263, 1976.

238. Levy CE, Bryant PR, Spires MC, Duffy DA: Acquired limb deficiencies. 4. Troubleshooting, *Arch Phys Med Rehabil* 82(3 Suppl 1):S25–s30, 2001.

239. Libetta C, Burke D, Brennan P, Yassa J: Validation of the Ottawa ankle rules in children, *J Accid Emerg Med* 16:342–344, 1999.

240. Lin HC, Wuang YP: Strength and agility training in adolescents with Down syndrome: a randomized controlled trial, *Res Dev Disabil* 33(6):2236–2244, 2012.

241. Lincoln AE, Caswell SV, Almquist JL, Dunn RE, Norris JB, Hinton RY: Trends in concussion incidence in high school sports: a prospective 11-year study, *Am J Sports Med* 39(5):958–963, 2011.

242. Lipscomb AB, Anderson AF: Tears of the anterior cruciate ligament in adolescents, *J Bone Joint Surg Am* 68(1):19–28, 1986.

243. Lloyd RS, Faigenbaum AD, Stone MH, et al.: Position statement on youth resistance training: the 2014 International Consensus, *Br J Sports Med* 48(7):498–505, 2014.

244. Lombardo JA: Pre-participation physical evaluation, *Primary Care: clin Off Pract* 11(1):3–21, 1984.

245. Lombardo JA: Preparticipation examination. In Cantu RC, Micheli LJ, editors: *ACSM's guidelines for the team physician*, Philadelphia, 1991, Lea Febiger, pp 71–94.

246. Lombardo SJ, Harvey Jr JP: Fractures of the distal femoral epiphyses. Factors influencing prognosis: a review of thirty-four cases, *J Bone Joint Surg Am* 59(6):742–751, 1977.

247. Looper J, Benjamin D, Nolan M, Schumm L: What to measure when determining orthotic needs in children with Down syndrome: a pilot study, *Pediatr Phys Ther* 24(4):313–319, 2012.

248. Luke A, Lazaro RM, Bergeron MF, et al.: Sports-related injuries in youth athletes: is overscheduling a risk factor? *Clin J Sport Med* 21(4):307–314, 2011.

249. Maffulli N: Intensive training in young athletes, *Sports Med* 9:229–243, 1990.

250. Maffulli N, Bruns W: Injuries in young athletes, *Eur J Pediatr* 159:59–63, 2000.

251. Maher CA, Williams MT, Olds T, Lane AE: Physical and sedentary activity in adolescents with cerebral palsy, *Dev Med Child Neurol* 49(6): 450–457, 2007.

252. Makdissi M, Cantu RC, Johnston KM, McCrory P, Meeuwisse WH: The difficult concussion patient: what is the best approach to investigation and management of persistent (>10 days) postconcussive symptoms? *Br J Sports Med* 47(5):308–313, 2013.

253. Makdissi M, Davis G, Jordan B, Patricios J, Purcell L, Putukian M: Revisiting the modifiers: how should the evaluation and management of acute concussions differ in specific groups? *Br J Sports Med* 47(5):314–320, 2013.

254. Management of Concussion/m TBI: Working Group: VA/DoD clinical practice guideline for management of concussion/mild traumatic brain injury, *J Rehabil Res Dev* 46(6):CP1–68, 2009.

255. Mankovsky AB, Mendoza-Sagaon M, Cardinaux C, Hohlfeld J, Reinberg O: Evaluation of scooter-related injuries in children, *J Pediatr Surg* 37:755–759, 2002.

256. Mann DC, Rajmaira S: Distribution of physeal and nonphyseal fractures in 2,650 long-bone fractures in children aged 0-16 years, *J Pediatr Orthop* 10(6):713–716, 1990.

257. Marar M, McIlvain NM, Fields SK, Comstock RD: Epidemiology of concussions among United States high school athletes in 20 sports, *Am J Sports Med* 40(4):747–755, 2012.

258. Maron BJ, Thompson PD, Puffer JC, et al.: Cardiovascular preparticipation screening of competitive athletes. A statement for health professionals from the Sudden Death Committee (clinical cardiology) and Congenital Cardiac Defects Committee (cardiovascular disease in the young), American Heart Association, *Circulation* 94(4):850–856, 1996.

259. Marques A, Maldonado I, Peralta M, Santos S: Exploring psychosocial correlates of physical activity among children and adolescents with spina bifida, *Disabil Health J* 8(1):123–129, 2015.

260. Marsh JS, Daigneault JP: Ankle injuries in the pediatric population, *Curr Opin Pediatr* 12:52–60, 2000.

261. Maughan R: The athlete's diet: nutritional goals and dietary strategies, *Proc Nutr Soc* 61:87–96, 2002.

262. McArdle WD, Katch FI, Katch VL: *Exercise physiology: energy, nutrition, and human performance*, Philadelphia, 2001, Lippincott, Williams Wilkins.

263. McCarroll JR, Rettig AC, Shelbourne KD: Anterior cruciate ligament injuries in the young athlete with open physes, *Am J Sports Med* 16(1): 44–47, 1988.

264. McCrea M, Kelly J, Randolph C, et al.: Standardized assessment of concussion (SAC): on-site mental status evaluation of the athlete, *J Head Trauma Rehabil* 13(2):27–36, 1998.

265. McCrory P: Does second impact syndrome exist? *Clin J Sport Med* 11(3):144–149, 2001.

266. McCrory P, Davis G, Makdissi M: Second impact syndrome or cerebral swelling after sporting head injury, *Curr Sports Med Rep* 11(1):21–23, 2012.

267. McCrory P, Meeuwisse WH, Kutcher JS, Jordan BD, Gardner A: What is the evidence for chronic concussion-related changes in retired athletes: behavioural, pathological and clinical outcomes? *Br J Sports Med* 47(5):327–330, 2013.

268. McCrory P, Meeuwisse W, Aubry M, et al.: Consensus statement on concussion in sport-the 4th International Conference on Concussion in Sport Held in Zurich, November 2012, *Clin J Sport Med* 23(2):89–117, 2013.

269. McKeag D: Preseason physical examination for prevention of sports injuries, *Sports Med* 2:413–431, 1985.

270. McKeag DB: Preparticipation screening of the potential athlete, *Clin Sports Med* 8(3):373–397, 1989.

271. McKee AC, Cantu RC, Nowinski CJ, et al.: Chronic traumatic encephalopathy in athletes: progressive tauopathy after repetitive head injury, *J Neuropathol Exp Neurol* 68(7):709–735, 2009.

272. Reference deleted in proofs.

273. McTimoney CA, Micheli LJ: Current evaluation and management of spondylolysis and spondylolisthesis, *Curr Sports Med Rep* 2:41–46, 2003.

274. Meehan 3rd WP, Mannix R: Pediatric concussions in United States emergency departments in the years 2002 to 2006, *J Pediatr* 157(6):889–893, 2010.

275. Micheli LJ: Sports injuries in children and adolescents. Questions and controversies, *Clin Sports Med* 14:727–745, 1995.

276. Micheli LJ, Foster TE: Acute knee injuries in the immature athlete, *Instr Course Lect* 42:473–481, 1993.

277. Micheli LJ, Nielson JH: Overuse injuries in the young athlete: stress fractures. In Hebestreit H, Bar-or O, editors: *The young athlete*, Boston, 2008, Blackwell, pp 151–163.

278. Micheli LJ, Wood R: Back pain in young athletes. Significant differences from adults in causes and patterns, *Arch Pediatr Adolsc Med* 149:15–18, 1995.

279. Micheli LJ, Metzl JD, Canzio JD, Zurakowski D: Anterior cruciate ligament reconstructive surgery in adolescent soccer and basketball players, *Clin J Sport Med* 9(3):138–141, 1999.

280. Millar AL: Ergogenic aids. In Sanders B, editor: *Sports physical therapy*, Norwalk, CT, 1990, Appleton Lange, pp 79–93.

281. Reference deleted in proofs.

282. Mitchell LJ, Jenkins M: *Sports medicine bible for young athletes*, Naperville, IL, 2001, Sourcebooks, Inc.

283. Miyahara M, Sleivert GG, Gerrard DF: The relationship of strength and muscle balance to shoulder pain and impingement syndrome in elite quadriplegic wheelchair rugby players, *International Journal of Sports Med* 19(3):210–214, 1998.

284. Moeller JL: Pelvic and hip apophyseal avulsion injuries in young athletes, *Curr Sports Med Rep* 2:110–115, 2003.

285. Moller E, Forssblad M, Hansson L, et al.: Bracing versus nonbracing in rehabilitation after anterior cruciate ligament reconstruction: a randomized prospective study with 2-year follow-up, *Knee Surg Sports Traumotol Arthrosc* 9(2):102–108, 2001.

286. Mosier SM, Stanitski CL: Acute tibial tubercle avulsion fractures, *J Pediatr Orthop* 24(2):181–184, 2004.

287. Moti AW, Micheli LJ: Meniscal and articular cartilage injury in the skeletally immature knee, *Instr Course Lect* 52:683–690, 2003.

288. Mueller FO, Kucera K, Cox L: National Center for Catastrophic Injury Research. 31th Annual Report. Available at: URL: www.nccsir.unc.edu/files/2015/02/NCCSIR-31st-annual-all-sport-report-1982_2013.pdf.

289. Murphy N, Yanchar NL: Yet more pediatric injuries associated with all-terrain vehicles: should kids be using them? *J Trauma* 56(6):1185–1190, 2004.

290. Myer GD, Ford KR, Hewett TE: Tuck jump assessment for reducing anterior cruciate ligament risk, *Athl Ther Today* 13(5):39–44, 2008.

291. Myer GD, Ford KR, Barber Foss KD, et al.: The incidence and potential pathomechanics of patellofemoral pain in female athletes, *Clin Biomechan (Bristol, Avon)* 25(7):700–707, 2010.

292. Myer GD, Ford KR, Palumbo JP, Hewett TE: Neuromuscular training improves performance and lower-extremity biomechanics in female athletes, *J Strength Cond Res* 19(1):51–60, 2005.

293. Myer GD, Paterno MV, Ford KR, Quatman CE, Hewett TE: Rehabilitation after anterior cruciate ligament reconstruction: criteria-based progression through the return-to-sport phase, *J Orthop Sports Phys Ther* 36(6):385–402, 2006.

294. Myer GD, Ford KR, Brent JL, Hewett TE: Differential neuromuscular training effects on ACL injury risk factors in "high-risk" versus "low-risk" athletes, *BMC Musculoskel Dis* 8:39, 2007.

295. Nadler SF, Malanga GA, Feinberg JH, Rubanni M, Moley R, Foye P: Functional performance deficits in athletes with previous lower extremity injury, *Clin J Sport Med* 12:73–78, 2002.

296. Nalliah RP, Anderson IM, Lee MK, Rampa S, Allareddy V, Allareddy V: Epidemiology of hospital-based emergency department visits due to sports injuries, *Pediatr Emerg Care* 30(8):511–515, 2014.

297. Nathanson BH, Ribeiro K, Henneman PL: An analysis of US emergency department visits from falls from skiing, snowboarding, skateboarding, roller-skating, and using nonmotorized scooters, *Clin Pediatr (Phila)* 55(8):738–744, 2016.

298. National Safe Kids Campaign: Injury Facts. Available at: URL: www.safekids.org/.

299. NCAA: Boundless determination. Available at: URL: http://www.ncaa.org/champion/boundless-determination.

300. Neter JE, Schokker DF, de Jong E, Renders CM, Seidell JC, Visscher TL: The prevalence of overweight and obesity and its determinants in children with and without disabilities, *J Pediatr* 158(5):735–739, 2011.

301. Nguyen D, Letts M: In-line skating injuries in children: a ten year review, *J Pediatr Orthop* 21:613–618, 2001.

302. Nietosvaara Y, Aalto K, Kallio PE: Acute patellar dislocation in children: incidence and associated osteochondral fractures, *J Pediatr Orthop* 14(4):513–515, 1994.

303. Noguchi T: A survey of spinal cord injuries resulting from sport, *Paraplegia* 32:170–173, 2001.

304. Noyes FR, Barber-Westin SD: Arthroscopic repair of meniscal tears extending into the avascular zone in patients younger than twenty years of age, *Am J Sports Med* 30:589–600, 2002.

305. Noyes FR, Barber SD, Mangine RE: Abnormal lower limb symmetry determined by function hop tests after anterior cruciate ligament rupture, *Am J Sports Med* 19(5):513–518, 1991.

306. Noyes FR, Berrios-Torres S, Barber-Westin SD, et al.: Prevention of permanent arthrofibrosis after anterior cruciate ligament reconstruction alone or combined with associated procedures: a prospective study in 443 knees, *Knee Surg Sports Traumotol Arthrosc* 8(4):196–206, 2000.

307. Reference deleted in proofs.

308. Ogden CL, Carroll MD, Kit BK, Flegal KM: Prevalence of childhood and adult obesity in the United States, 2011-2012, *JAMA* 311(8):806–814, 2014.

309. Ogden CL, Flegal KM, Carroll MD, et al.: Relevance and trends in overweight among US children and adolescents 1999-2000, *JAMA* 288(14):1728–1732, 2002.

310. Ogden JA: *Skeletal injury in the child*, New York, 2000, Springer-Verlag.

311. Ogden JA, Tross RB, Murphy MJ: Fractures of the tibial tuberosity in adolescents, *J Bone Joint Surg Am* 62(2):205–215, 1980.

312. Ogg-Groenendaal M, Hermans H, Claessens B: A systematic review on the effect of exercise interventions on challenging behavior for people with intellectual disabilities, *Res Dev Disabil* 35(7):1507–1517, 2014.

313. Onate K, Cortes N, Welch C, Van Lunen BL: Expert versus novice interrater reliability and criterion validity of the landing error scoring system, *J Sports Rehabil* 19(1):41–56, 2010.

314. World Health Organization, 1992.

315. World Health Organization, 1993.

316. Outerbridge AR, Micheli LJ: Overuse injuries in young athletes, *Clin Sports Med* 14:503–516, 1995.

317. Padua DA, Marshall SW, Boling MC, Thigpen CA, Garrett Jr WE, Beutler AL: The Landing Error Scoring System (LESS) is a valid and reliable clinical assessment tool of jump-landing biomechanics: the JUMPACL study, *Am J Sports Med* 37(10):1996–2002, 2009.

318. Paletta Jr GA, Arish JT: Injuries about the hip and pelvis in the young athlete, *Clin Sports Med* 14:591–628, 1995.

319. Paralympic Games | Winter, Summer, Past, Future Paralympics. Available at: URL: http://www.paralympic.org/paralympic-games.

320. Pare G, Noreau L, Simard C: Prediction of maximal aerobic power from a submaximal exercise test performed by paraplegics on a wheelchair ergometer, *Paraplegia* 31(9):584–592, 1993.

321. Patel DR, Nelson TL: Sports injuries in adolescents, *Med Clin North Am* 84:983–1007, 2000.

322. Paterno MV, Schmitt LC, Ford KR, et al.: Biomechanical measures during landing and postural stability predict second anterior cruciate ligament injury after ACL reconstruction and return to sport, *Am J Sports Med* 38(10):1968–1978, 2010.

323. Paterson PD, Waters PM: Shoulder injuries in the childhood athlete, *Clin Sports Med* 19:681–692, 2000.

324. Pedraza J, Jadeleza JA: The preparticipation physical examination, *Prim Care* 40(4):791–799, vii. 2013.

325. Peel KA, Fagan C, Keener M, Shelton M: Director's Order #42: accessibility. doi: http://www.nps.gov/refdesk/DOrders/DOrder42.htm, 2000l.

326. Peljovich AE, Simmons BP: Traumatic arthritis of the hand and wrist in children, *Hand Clin* 16:673–684, 2000.

327. Pellman EJ, Viano DC, Withnall C, Shewchenko N, Bir CA, Halstead PD: Concussion in professional football: helmet testing to assess impact performance—part 11, *Neurosurgery* 58(1):78–96, 2006. discussion 78-96.

328. Petersen W, Ellermann A, Gosele-Koppenburg A, Best R, Rembitzki IV, Bruggemann GP, Liebau C: Patellofemoral pain syndrome, *Knee Surg Sports Traumotol Arthrosc* 22(10):2264–2274, 2014.

329. Peterson M, Peterson K: *Eat to compete: a guide to sports nutrition*, Chicago, 1988, Year Book Medical.

330. Phillips AC, Holland AJ: Assessment of objectively measured physical activity levels in individuals with intellectual disabilities with and without Down's syndrome, *PLoS One* 6(12):e28618, 2011.

331. Pieper P: Epidemiology and prevention of sports-related eye injuries. *J Emerg Nurs* 36(4):359–361.

332. Pieter W: Martial arts injuries, *Med Sport Sci* 48:59–73, 2005.

333. Pitetti KH, Rimmer JH, Fernhall B: Physical fitness and adults with mental retardation: an overview of current research and future directions, *Sports Med* 16:23–56, 1993.

334. Plisky PJ, Rauh MJ, Kaminski TW, Underwood FB: Star Excursion Balance Test as a predictor of lower extremity injury in high school basketball players, *J Orthop Sports Phys Ther* 36(12):911–919, 2006.

335. Pommering TL, Kluchurosky L: Overuse injuries in adolescents, *Adolesc Med State Art Rev* 18(1):95–120, ix. 2007.

336. Popchak A, Burnett T, Weber N, Boninger M: Factors related to injury in youth and adolescent baseball pitching, with an eye toward prevention, *Am J Phys Med Rehabil* 94(5):395–409, 2015.

337. Powell EC: Protecting children in the accident and emergency department, *Accid Emerg Nurs* 5:76–80, 1997.

338. Powell EC, Tanz RR: Cycling injuries treated in emergency departments: need for bicycle helmets among preschoolers, *Arch Pediatr Adolesc Med* 154:1096–1100, 2000.

339. Powell EC, Tanz RR: Tykes and bikes: injuries associated with bicycle-towed child trailers and bicycle-mounted child seats, *Arch Pediatr Adolesc Med* 154:351–353, 2000.

340. Powers CM: The influence of altered lower-extremity kinematics on patellofemoral joint dysfunction: a theoretical perspective, *J Orthop Sports Phys Ther* 33(11):639–646, 2003.

341. Price M: Thermoregulation during exercise in individuals with spinal cord injuries, *Sports Med* 36(10):863–879, 2006.

342. Prince JS, Laor T, Bean JA: MRI of anterior cruciate ligament injuries and associated findings in the pediatric knee: changes with skeletal maturation, *AJR Am J Roentgenol* 185(3):756–762, 2005.

343. Puffer JC: Organizational aspects. In Cantu RC, Micheli LJ, editors: *ACSM's guidelines for the team physician*, Philadelphia, 1991, Lea Febiger, pp 95–100.

344. Ramirez M, Yang J, Bourque L, Javien J, Kashani S, Limbos MA, Peek-Asa C: Sports injuries to high school athletes with disabilities, *Pediatrics* 123(2):690–696, 2009.

345. Rechel JA, Collins CL, Comstock RD: Epidemiology of injuries requiring surgery among high school athletes in the United States, 2005 to 2010, *J Trauma* 71(4):982–989, 2011.

346. Regan KJ, Banks GK, Beran RG: Therapeutic recreation programmes for children with epilepsy, *Seizure* 2(3):195–200, 1993.

347. Reid A, Birmingham TB, Stratford PN, et al.: Hop testing provides a reliable and valid outcome measure during rehabilitation after anterior cruciate ligament reconstruction, *Phys Ther* 87(3):337–349, 2007.

348. Reinold MM, Wilk KE, Macrina LC, et al.: Current concepts in the rehabilitation following articular cartilage repair procedures in the knee, *J Orthop Sports Phys Ther* 36:774–794, 2006.

349. Renstrom P, Ljungqvist A, Arendt E, et al.: Non-contact ACL injuries in female athletes: an International Olympic Committee current concepts statement, *Br J Sports Med* 42(6):394–412, 2008.

350. Rice SG: Medical conditions affecting sports participation, *Pediatrics* 121(4):841–848, 2008.

351. Rice SG, Congeni JA: Baseball and softball, *Pediatrics* 129(3):e842–e856, 2012.

352. Rifat SF, Ruffin 4th MT, Gorenflo DW: Disqualifying criteria in a preparticipation sports evaluation, *J Fam Pract* 41:42–50, 1995.

353. Rights, U. S. D. o. E. O. f. C: *Dear Colleague*, 2015.

354. Rimmer JH: Physical fitness levels of persons with cerebral palsy, *Dev Med Child Neurol* 43(3):208–212, 2001.

355. Rimmer JH, Rowland JL, Yamaki K: Obesity and secondary conditions in adolescents with disabilities: addressing the needs of an underserved population, *J Adolesc Health* 41(3):224–229, 2007.

356. Robinson RL, Nee RJ: Analysis of hip strength in females seeking physical therapy treatment for unilateral patellofemoral pain syndrome, *J Orthop Sports Phys Ther* 37(5):232–238, 2007.

357. Rogers A, Furler BL, Brinks S, Darrah J: A systematic review of the effectiveness of aerobic exercise interventions for children with cerebral palsy: an AACPDM evidence report. [1a (background)], *Dev Med Child Neurol* 50(11):808–814, 2008.

358. Roi GS, Creta D, Nanni G, et al.: Return to official Italian First Division soccer games within 90 days after anterior cruciate ligament reconstruction: a case report, *J Orthop Sports Phys Ther* 35(2):52–61, 2005. discussion, 61-66.

359. Rose SC, Weber KD, Collen JB, Heyer GL: The diagnosis and management of concussion in children and adolescents, *Pediatr Neurol* 53(2):108–118, 2015.

360. Rossi F, Dragoni S: Lumbar spondylolisthesis: occurrence in competitive athletes, *J Sports Med Fitness* 30:450–452, 1990.

361. Rudzki JR, Paletta Jr GA: Juvenile and adolescent elbow injuries in sports, *Clin Sports Med* 23(4):581–608, ix. 2004.

362. Sachtelben TR, Berg KE, Elias BA, Cheatham JP, Felix GL, Hofschire PJ: The effects of anabolic steroids on myocardial structure and cardiovascular fitness, *Med Sci Sports Exerc* 25:1240–1245, 1993.

363. Sahlin KB, Lexell J: Impact of organized sports on activity, participation, and quality of life in people with neurologic disabilities, *PM R* 10:1081–1088, 2015.

364. Salter RB, Harris WR: Injuries involving the epiphyseal plate, *J Bone Joint Surg* 45-A:587–622, 1963.

365. Samora 3rd WP, Palmer R, Klingele KE: Meniscal pathology associated with acute anterior cruciate ligament tears in patients with open physes, *J Pediatr Orthop* 31(3):272–276, 2011.

366. Sanders B, editor: *Sports physical therapy*, Norwalk, CT, 1990, Appleton Lange.

367. Sanders B, Blackburn TA, Boucher B: Preparticipation screening—the sports physical therapy perspective, *Int J Sports Phys Ther* 8(2):180–193, 2013.

368. Scat3: *Br J Sports Med* 47(5):259, 2013.

369. Reference deleted in proofs.

370. Schmitt LC, Byrnes R, Cherny C, et al.: Evidence-based clinical care guideline for management of osteochondritis dissecans of the knee, *Guideline* 037:1–16, 2009. http://www.cincinnatichildrens.org/svc/alpha/h/health-policy/otpt.htm.

371. Schmitt LC, Paterno MV, Huang S: Validity and internal consistency of the International Knee Documentation Committee Subjective Knee Form in Children and Adolescents, *Am J Sports Med* 38(223):2443–2447, 2010.

372. Schneider KJ, Iverson GL, Emery CA, McCrory P, Herring SA, Meeuwisse WH: The effects of rest and treatment following sport-related concussion: a systematic review of the literature, *Br J Sports Med* 47(5):304–307, 2013.

373. Schneider KJ, Meeuwisse WH, Nettel-Aguirre A, Barlow K, Boyd L, Kang J, Emery CA: Cervicovestibular rehabilitation in sport-related concussion: a randomised controlled trial, *Br J Sports Med* 48(17):1294–1298, 2014.

374. Schreuer N, Sachs D, Rosenblum S: Participation in leisure activities: differences between children with and without physical disabilities, *Res Dev Disabil* 35(1):223–233, 2014.

375. Schuller DE, Dankle SK, Martin M, Strauss RH: Auricular injury and the use of headgear in wrestlers, *Arch Otolaryngol Head Neck Surg* 115:714–717, 1993.

376. Scopp JM, Moorman 3rd CT: Acute athletic trauma to the hip and pelvis, *Orthop Clin North Am* 33(3):555–563, 2002.

377. Seidman DH, Burlingame J, Yousif LR, et al.: Evaluation of the King-Device test as a concussion screening tool in high school football players, *J Neurolol Sci* 365(1-2):97–101, 2015.

378. Selsby JT, Beckett KD, Kern M, Devor S: Swim performance following creatine supplementation in division III athletes, *J Strength Cond* 17(3):421–424, 2003.

379. Reference deleted in proofs

380. Seto CK, Statuta SM, Solari IL: Pediatric running injuries, *Clin Sports Med* 29(3):499–511, 2010.

381. Sharkey B: Training for sports. In Cantu RC, Micheli LJ, editors: *ACSM's guidelines for the team physician*, Philadelphia, 1991, Lea Febiger, pp 34–47.

382. Shea KG, Apel PJ, Pfeiffer RP: Anterior cruciate ligament injury in paediatric and adolescent patients: a review of basic science and clinical research, *Sports Med* 33(6):455–471, 2003.

383. Shea KG, Pfeiffer R, Wang JH, et al.: Anterior cruciate ligament injury in pediatric and adolescent soccer players: an analysis of insurance data, *J Pediatr Orthop* 24(6):623–628, 2004.

384. Sherrill C, Hinson M, Gench B, Kennedy SO, Low L: Self-concepts of disabled youth athletes, *Percept Mot Skills* 70:1093–1098, 1990.

385. Reference deleted in proofs.

386. Sigurdardottir S, Andelic N, Roe C, Jerstad T, Schanke AK: Post-concussion symptoms after traumatic brain injury at 3 and 12 months post-injury: a prospective study, *Brain Inj* 23(6):489–497, 2009.

387. Skokan EG, Junkins Jr EP, Kadish H: Serious winter sports injuries in children and adolescents requiring hospitalization, *Am J Emerg Med* 21:95–99, 2003.

388. Small E: The preparticipation physical evaluation. In Hebestreit H, Bar-or O, editors: *The young athlete*, Boston, 2008. Blackwell, pp 191–202.

389. Smith AD: The skeletally immature knee: what's new in overuse injuries, *Instr Course Lect* 52:691–697, 2003.

389a. Smith GE: Objective testing group certifies head protection, *Occup Health Safety* 57(3):18–20, 1988.

390. Smith J, Laskowski ER: The preparticipation physical examination: Mayo Clinic experience with 2,739 examinations, *Mayo Clinic Proc* 73:419–429, 1998.

391. Smith J, Wilder EP: Musculoskeletal rehabilitation and sports medicine, *Arch Phys Med Rehabil* 80:S68–S89, 1999.

392. Special Olympics: World and Regional Games Center. Available from: URL: http://www.specialolympics.org/Games/World_and_Regional_Games_Center.aspx.

393. Stanitski CL: Pediatric and adolescent sports injuries, *Clin Sports Med* 16:613–633, 1997.

394. Stanitski CL, Delee JC, Drez D: *Pediatric and adolescent sports medicine*, Philadelphia, 1994, WB Saunders.

395. Stracciolini A, Casciano R, Levey Friedman H, Stein CJ, Meehan 3rd WP, Micheli LJ: Pediatric sports injuries: a comparison of males versus females, *Am J Sports Med* 42(4):965–972, 2014.

396. Surgeon General: *Call to action to prevent and decrease overweight and obesity*, Washington, DC. Available at: URL: www.surgerongeneral.gov/topics/obesity, 2001.

397. Swenson DM, Collins CL, Best TM, Flanigan DC, Fields SK, Comstock RD: Epidemiology of knee injuries among U.S. high school athletes, 2005/2006-2010/2011, *Med Sci Sports and Exerc* 45(3):462–469, 2013.

398. Taimela S, Kujala UM, Osterman K: Intrinsic risk factors and athletic injuries, *Sports Med* 9:205–215, 1990.

399. Taylor BL, Attia MW: Sports-related injuries in children, *Acad Emerg Med* 7:1376–1382, 2000.

400. Team LPIM, Center CCsHM: Evidence-based clinical care guidelines for conservative management of lateral patellar dislocations and instability, *Guideline* 44:1–20, 2014. http://www.cincinnatichildrens.org/svc/alpha/h/health-policy/ev-based/Conservative Management of Lateral Patellar Dislocations and Instability.htm.

401. Tepper KB, Ireland ML: Fracture patterns and treatment in the skeletally immature knee, *Instr Course Lect* 52:667–676, 2003.

402. The National Federation of State High School Associations. Available at: URL: http://www.nfhs.org.

403. Tol JL, Struijs PA, Bossuyt PM, Verhagen RA, van Dijk CN: Treatment strategies in osteochondral defects of the talar dome: a systematic review, *Foot Ankle Int* 21:119–126, 2000.

404. Turbanski S, Schmidtbleicher D: Effects of heavy resistance training on strength and power in upper extremities in wheelchair athletes, *J Strength Cond Res* 24(1):8–16, 2010.

405. Tweedy SM, Beckman EM, Connick MJ: Paralympic classification: conceptual basis, current methods, and research update, *PM R* 6(Suppl 8): S11–17, 2014.

406. USDA/ARS Children's Nutrition Research Center at Baylor College of Medicine. Available at: URL: www.bcm.tmc.edu/cnrc/consumer/archives/percentDV.htm.

406a. US Department of Health and Human Services, Office for Civil Rights. Your rights under Section 504 of the Rehabilitation Act. Washington, D.C., 2006.

407. Vanderhave KL, Moravek JE, Sekiya JK, Wojtys EM: Meniscus tears in the young athlete: results of arthroscopic repair, *J Pediatr Orthop* 31(5):496–500, 2011.

408. Vanlandewijck YC, Verellen J, Tweedy S: Towards evidence-based classification in wheelchair sports: impact of seating position on wheelchair acceleration, *J Sports Sci* 29(10):1089–1096, 2011.

409. Varni JW, Setoguchi Y: Correlates of perceived physical appearance in children with congenital/acquired limb deficiencies, *J Dev Behav Pediatr* 12:171–176, 1991.

410. Varni JW, Seid M, Kurtin PS: PedsQL 4.0: reliability and validity of the Pediatric Quality of Life Inventory version 4.0 generic core scales in healthy and patient populations, *Med Care* 39(8):800–812, 2001.

411. Varni JW, Seid M, Rode CA: The PedsQL: measurement model for the pediatric quality of life inventory, *Med Care* 37(2):126–139, 1999.

412. Vavken P, Wimmer MD, Camathias C, Quidde J, Valderrabano V, Pagenstert G: Treating patella instability in skeletally immature patients, *Arthroscopy* 29(8):1410–1422, 2013.

413. Verschuren O, Ketelaar M, Gorter JW, Helders PJ, Uiterwaal CS, Takken T: Exercise training program in children and adolescents with cerebral palsy: a randomized controlled trial, *Arch Pediatr Adolesc Med* 161(11):1075–1081, 2007.

414. Verschuren O, Ketelaar M, Takken T, Helders PJ, Gorter JW: Exercise programs for children with cerebral palsy: a systematic review of the literature, *Am J Phys Med Rehabil* 87(5):404–417, 2008.

415. Vidal PG, Goodman AM, Colin A, Leddy JJ, Grady MF: Rehabilitation strategies for prolonged recovery in pediatric and adolescent concussion, *Pediatr Ann* 41(9):1–7, 2012.

416. Vinger PF: The mechanisms and prevention of sports eye injuries. Available at: URL: http://www.lexeye.com/pdf/section1.pdf.

417. Vis JC, de Bruin-Bon RH, Bouma BJ, Backx AP, Huisman SA, Imschoot L, Mulder BJ: 'The sedentary heart': physical inactivity is associated with cardiac atrophy in adults with an intellectual disability, *Int J Cardiol* 158(3):387–393, 2012.

418. Vitello S, Dvorkin R, Sattler S, Levy D, Ung L: Epidemiology of Nursemaid's Elbow, *West J Emerg Med* 15(4):554–557, 2014.

419. Wagner JC: Enhancement of athletic performance with drugs. An overview, *Sports Med* 12:250–265, 1991.

420. Waicus KM, Smith BW: Back injuries in the pediatric athlete, *Curr Sports Med Rep* 1:52–58, 2002.

421. Wall EJ: Osgood-Schlatter disease: practical treatment for a self-limiting condition, *Phys Sportsmed* 26(3):29–34, 1998.

422. Waters PM, Millis MB: Hip and pelvic injuries in the young athlete, *Clin Sports Med* 7:513–526, 1988.

423. Webborn N, Emery C: Descriptive epidemiology of Paralympic sports injuries, *PM R* 6(Suppl 8):S18–S22, 2014.

424. Wessels KK, Broglio SP, Sosnoff JJ: Concussions in wheelchair basketball, *Arch Phys Med Rehabil* 93(2):275–278, 2012.

425. Wiart L, Darrah J, Kelly M, Legg D: Community fitness programs: what is available for children and youth with motor disabilities and what do parents want? *Phys Occupat Ther Pediatr* 35(1):73–87, 2015.

426. Wilk KE, Briem K, Reinold MM, Devine KM, Dugas J, Andrews JR: Rehabilitation of articular lesions in the athlete's knee, *J Orthop Sports Phys Ther* 36(10):815–827, 2006.

427. Wilk KE, Reinold MM, Andrews JR: Rehabilitation of the thrower's elbow, *Clin Sports Med* 23(4):765–801, xii. 2004.

428. Wilson PE: Exercise and sports for children who have disabilities, *Phys Med Rehabil Clin North Am* 13(4):907–923, ix. 2002.

429. Reference deleted in proofs.

430. Winston FK, Weiss HB, Nance ML, Vivarelli O, Neill C, Strotmeyer S, Lawrence BA, Miller TR: Estimates of the incidence and costs associated with handlebar-related injuries in children, *Arch Pediatr Adolesc Med* 156:922–928, 2002.

431. Yasmingarcia: Uniform Throwing Chair for Seated Throwing Sporting Events. Available from: URL: http://aac-rerc.psu.edu/wordpressmu/RESNA-SDC/2010/05/13/uniform-throwing-chair-for-seated-throwing-sporting-events/.

432. Yesalis CE, Bahrke MS: Doping among adolescent athletes, *Baillieres Best Pract Res Clin Endocrinol Metab* 14:25–35, 2000.

433. Zanon G, Di Vico G, Marullo M: Osteochondritis dissecans of the knee, *Joints* 2(1):29–36, 2014.

434. Zoints LE: Fractures around the knee in children, *J Am Acad Orthop Surg* 10:345–355, 2002.

SUGGESTED READINGS

Background

American Academy of Pediatrics Committee on Sports Medicine and Fitness: Medical conditions affecting sports participation, *Pediatrics* 107: 1205–1209, 2001.

Bar-Or O: Child and adolescent athlete, vol. 6. Malden, MA, 1995, Blackwell.

Caine DJ, DiFiori J, Maffulli N: Physeal injuries in children's and youth sports. Reasons for concern? *Br J Sports Med* 40:749–760, 2006.

Caine D, Maffulli N, Caine C: Epidemiology of injury in child and adolescent sports: injury rates, risk factors and prevention, *Clin Sports Med* 27:19–50, 2008.

Conley KM, Bolin DJ, Carek PJ, Konin JG, Neal TL, Violette D: National Athletic Trainers' Association Position Statement: preparticipation physical examinations and disqualifying conditions, *J Athl Train* 49(1):102–120, 2014.

Giza CC, Kutcher JS, Ashwal S, et al.: Summary of evidence-based guideline update: evaluation and management of concussion in sports: report of the Guideline Development Subcommittee of the American Academy of Neurology, *Neurology* 80(24):2250–2257, 2013.

Foreground

Baran F, Aktop A, Ozer D, Nalbant S, Aglamis E, Barak S, Hutzler Y: The effects of a Special Olympics Unified Sports Soccer training program on anthropometry, physical fitness and skilled performance in Special Olympics soccer athletes and non-disabled partners, *Res Dev Disabil* 34(1):695–709, 2013.

DeMatteo C, Stazyk K, Singh SK, et al.: Development of a conservative protocol to return children and youth to activity following concussive injury, *Clin Pediatr* 54(2):152–163, 2015.

Faigenbaum AD, Kraemer WJ, Blimkie CJ, Jeffreys I, Micheli LJ, Nitka M, Rowland TW: Youth resistance training: updated position statement paper from the national strength and conditioning association, *J Strength Cond Res* 23(Suppl 5):S60–S79, 2009.

Fowler EG, Kolobe TH, Damiano DL, et al.: Promotion of physical fitness and prevention of secondary conditions for children with cerebral palsy: section on pediatrics research summit proceedings, *Phys Ther* 87(11):1495–1510, 2007.

Hewett TE, Myer GD, Ford KR, et al.: Biomechanical measures of neuromuscular control and valgus loading of the knee predict anterior cruciate ligament injury risk in female athletes: a prospective study, *Am J Sports Med* 33(4):492–501, 2005.

Kanagasabai PS, Mulligan H, Mirfin-Veitch B, Hale LA: Association between motor functioning and leisure participation of children with physical disability: an integrative review, *Dev Med Child Neurol* 56(12):1147–1162, 2014.

Kocher MS, Garg S, Micheli LJ: Physeal sparing reconstruction of the anterior cruciate ligament in skeletally immature prepubescent children and adolescents, *J Bone Joint Surg* 87(11):2371–2379, 2005.

Kocher MS, Tucker R, Ganley TJ, Flynn JM: Management of osteochondritis dissecans of the knee: current concepts review, *Am J Sports Med* 34(7):1181–1191, 2006.

Kozlowski KF, Graham J, Leddy JJ, Devinney-Boymel L, Willer BS: Exercise intolerance in individuals with postconcussion syndrome, *J Athl Train* 48(5):627–635, 2013.

Lloyd RS, Faigenbaum AD, Stone MH, et al.: Position statement on youth resistance training: the 2014 International Consensus, *Br J Sports Med* 48(7):498–505, 2014.

McCrory P, Meeuwisse W, Aubry M, et al.: Consensus statement on concussion in sport-the 4th International Conference on Concussion in Sport Held in Zurich, November 2012, *Clin J Sport Med* 23(2):89–117, 2013.

Paterno MV, Schmitt LC, Ford KR, et al.: Biomechanical measures during landing and postural stability predict second anterior cruciate ligament injury after ACL reconstruction and return to sport, *Am J Sports Med* 38(10):1968–1978, 2010.

Plisky PJ, Rauh MJ, Kaminski TW, Underwood FB: Star Excursion Balance Test as a predictor of lower extremity injury in high school basketball players, *J Orthop Sports Phys Ther* 36(12):911–919, 2006.

Shikako-Thomas K, Shevell M, Schmitz N, Lach L, Law M, Poulin C, Majnemer A: Determinants of participation in leisure activities among adolescents with cerebral palsy, *Res Dev Disabil* 34(9):2621–2634, 2013.

Vavken P, Wimmer MD, Camathias C, Quidde J, Valderrabano V, Pagenstert G: Treating patella instability in skeletally immature patients, *Arthroscopy* 29(8):1410–1422, 2013.

16

Pediatric Oncology

Victoria Marchese, Kristin M. Thomas, G. Stephen Morris

INTRODUCTION

The most common pediatric (children and adolescents 0–19 years of age) cancers are leukemia (specifically acute lymphocytic leukemia), lymphomas (Hodgkin's and non-Hodgkin's lymphoma), sarcomas, and central and peripheral nervous system tumors. The combined 5-year relative survival rate for all pediatric cancers has improved markedly since the 1980s, increasing from 61% for cases diagnosed between 1975 and 1977 to 83% for cases diagnosed during 2005 and 2011.[29] Although overall mortality has decreased, these rates vary widely depending on the type of cancer, age of the child, stage of disease at diagnosis, and presence of other comorbidities. For example, the 5-year survival rate for children with acute lymphoblastic leukemia (ALL) exceeds 90% and is 97% in children with Hodgkin's lymphoma, but it is only 71% and 72% in children with osteosarcoma and brain and central nervous system (CNS) tumors, respectively. (Note: All frequency, incidence, and prevalence numbers appearing in this chapter have a common reference: American Cancer Society: *Cancer Facts & Figures 2014*, Atlanta: American Cancer Society, 2014.)[1]

Pediatric cancers are treated with several therapeutic interventions (surgery, radiation, chemotherapy, and targeted therapy), either singly or in combination with one another. The increased survival rate of children with cancer is largely attributable to improvements in the efficacy of these interventions.[13,46,47] However, these interventions are increasingly recognized for the adverse effects that can result from their use, including functional impairments, cognitive changes, and morphologic alterations.[52,54,55,61,74] It is important for the physical therapist (PT) to recognize that these changes are superimposed on infants, children, and adolescents who are still growing and developing physically, mentally, and socially, which adds treatment complexities not typically seen in adults with cancer. It is also important for the PT to recognize that a child's cancer diagnosis significantly impacts the whole family. Treatment may require that the family travel away from home and remain absent for extended periods of time. Treatment and accompanying adverse effects may prevent the child from participating in age-appropriate play, school, sports, and family activities. Pediatric physical therapists and physical therapist assistants (PTAs) practice within this complex environment, making pediatric oncology a thoroughly unique specialty area within oncology rehabilitation specifically and physical therapy in general.

Increased survivorship in the pediatric cancer population has resulted in substantial growth in the number of adult survivors of childhood cancer, now estimated to be 350,000. Improved survival rates have revealed previously unknown late effects and comorbidities related to the disease, its treatment, or both. Specifically, research has shown that survivors of childhood cancer are at a greater risk for experiencing cognitive deficits, functional impairments, cardiovascular disease, pulmonary disease, and early onset frailty than their siblings.[30] Growth in the numbers of these survivors has highlighted their need for increased screening and regular follow-up care to identify potential impairments as early as possible and provide mitigating care. Screening and treatment guidelines have been developed for health care professionals, including PTs and PTAs, to guide the care and treatment of survivors and limit, as much as possible, late effects and additional impairment.[42] Specifically, the Children's Oncology Group Long-Term Follow-Up Guidelines for Survivors of Childhood, Adolescent, and Young Adult Cancer (COG LTFU Guidelines) assist in addressing the specialized and unique needs of survivors of childhood cancer.[11]

Since the 1990s, there has been an increased interest in the specialized practice area of pediatric oncology physical therapy. This is evidenced by an increase in the number of publications in the area of pediatric oncology rehabilitation, expansion in the number of centers providing pediatric cancer rehabilitation, and membership in the Oncology Section of the American Physical Therapy Association (APTA). PTs and PTAs are an essential part of the health care team that manages the care of children with cancer both during and after medical treatment. Pediatric PTs and PTAs play a key role in helping the children and their families manage the myriad of challenges they face, specifically related to functional mobility and participation in age-appropriate recreation. A pediatric PT and PTA provide patient and family education, treat acute or chronic impairments, and address gross motor delays and mobility limitations, all the while encouraging patient and family participation in daily life activities. Importantly, studies demonstrate that physical therapy interventions are effective and safe for children with cancer regardless of the stage of their disease or type of medical treatment received.[17,19,38,59,63]

Pediatric oncology physical therapy is a growing field, and to move the profession forward with new, cutting-edge tools and interventions, clinicians and researchers need to work together. Clinicians and researchers are encouraged to develop clinical pathways, practice guidelines, and models of care for infants, children, and adolescents who are being treated for a cancer diagnosis or are cancer survivors within and across all pediatric practice settings.

This chapter introduces the reader to the signs and symptoms of pediatric cancers, the most common medical interventions used to treat these diseases, the PT examination, and common therapeutic interventions.

BACKGROUND INFORMATION

COMMON PEDIATRIC CANCERS

In 2014, the American Cancer Society estimated that there were 15,780 new cancer cases in children (ages 0–14; 10,450) and adolescents (ages 15–19; 5330). Cancers of blood cells accounted for the majority of cancer cases in both children (41%) and adolescents (35%). Brain and CNS tumors accounted for 31% (children) and 10% (adolescents), respectively. Bone tumors occurred more frequently in adolescents (7%) than in children (4%).[1] The following discussion briefly describes the pathophysiology of these common pediatric cancers and some less common types of pediatric cancers seen in pediatric oncology physical therapy settings.

Leukemias

Leukemia is a form of cancer that begins in the blood-forming cells found in the bone marrow. This disease occurs when defective, nonfunctional white blood cells or leukocytes are produced in very large numbers. These defective leukocytes migrate from the bone marrow into the bloodstream, displacing the healthy leukocytes. Leukocytes play a central role in helping the body defend itself against infectious agents including viruses, bacteria, and fungi, and as the numbers of functional leukocytes in the blood decline, the body's ability to protect itself against these infectious agents also declines. This deterioration in immune function is reflected in several of the common symptoms of leukemia (Table 16.1).

Leukemia is categorized as either acute or chronic and by the type of cancerous cells (lymphoid or myeloid). Chronic lymphoblastic leukemia (CLL) or chronic myelogenous leukemia (CML) is less common in children. The two most common types of pediatric leukemia are acute lymphoblastic leukemia (ALL) and acute myeloid leukemia (AML). ALL is the most common, accounting for 80% of all pediatric leukemia cases and occurring most frequently in children between the ages of 2 and 5 years. ALL is considered acute because the proliferation of immature, nonfunctional leukocytes is rapid. If left untreated, death occurs quickly in these patients. Significant advances in the effectiveness of chemotherapeutic agents have increased the survival rate of patients with ALL to over 90%. However, treatment protocols for children with ALL often require a child to receive chemotherapy for 2 to 3 years and may result in multiple short- and long-term body function impairments, activity limitations, and participation restrictions.[18,20,30,36,53,60,71]

AML is the second most common pediatric leukemia and is also known as acute myelogenous leukemia, acute myelocytic leukemia, myeloblastic leukemia, granulocytic leukemia, or acute nonlymphocytic leukemia. This form of leukemia is characterized by the presence of defective and nonfunctional granulocytes (bacteria-destroying cells) or monocytes (macrophage-forming cells). As with ALL, AML compromises the body's immune system, increasing the patient's risk for infections. AML accounts for about 5% of all pediatric cancers and occurs most frequently during the first 2 years of life. Symptoms of AML are similar to those of ALL (see Table 16.1). AML is treated with chemotherapy, and the survival rate for pediatric patients with AML is approximately 63%, somewhat less favorable than that of children with ALL.

Lymphomas

Lymphomas, like leukemia, are cancers involving blood cells. In these particular diseases, the cancer occurs in lymphocytes, another subtype of mature white blood cells that play a major role in the body's immune function. Lymphocytes include B cells, which synthesize antibodies, and T cells, which activate phagocytes and inflammatory processes and can become cancerous. Because lymphocytes are found throughout the lymphatic system, lymphomas can occur in specific lymphatic structures including lymph nodes, spleen, bone marrow, and the thymus as well as within the lymphatic structures present in many organs including the brain, the gastrointestinal tract, and the liver.

Lymphomas are the third most common type of cancer found in children, accounting for approximately 10% to 12% of pediatric cancers. Signs and symptoms include pain-free swelling of lymph nodes (lymphadenopathy), which can occur anywhere in the body, fever, night sweats, and weight loss (see Table 16.1). Definitive diagnosis is made by examining a biopsy of lymph tissue for the presence of abnormal tissue architecture and lymphocytes.

There are two major types of lymphoma: Hodgkin's lymphoma (HL, 3% of childhood cancers) and non-Hodgkin's lymphoma (NHL). HL, which is the less common of these two lymphomas, is identified by the presence of abnormal B lymphocytes called Reed-Sternberg cells and typically begins in lymph nodes found in the chest, neck, and abdomen. HL is rare in children younger than 5 years, but the incidence rises rapidly in adolescents, accounting for 16% of the cancers in this age group. Treatment involves both chemotherapy and radiation. Current survival rates are about 97%.

NHL is a heterogeneous group of blood cancers that adversely impacts both B and T lymphocytes and includes all forms of lymphoma except HL. NHL occurs more frequently in children over the age of 3 years and presents with painless supraclavicular or cervical adenopathy, a nonproductive cough, fatigue, anorexia, and pruritus (see Table 16.1). Medical conditions or treatments that result in immune suppression, inherited immunodeficiency diseases, and HIV infection increase the risk for developing NHL. Chemotherapy, sometimes accompanied by radiation, is the main form of treatment for most forms of NHL and has resulted in a survival rate for children with NHL of approximately 87%.

TABLE 16.1	Signs and Symptoms of Common Pediatric Cancers
Type of Cancer	**Signs and Symptoms**
Leukemias	Enlarged lymph nodes (lymphadenopathy), enlarged liver or spleen (hepatosplenomegaly), fever, easy bleeding or bruising, night sweats, weight loss
Lymphomas	Painless enlargement of lymph node, night sweats, persistent fatigue, fever and chills, unexplained weight loss, anorexia, pruritus
Sarcomas (soft tissue and bone)	Intermittent pain that often worsens at night, swelling, decreased range of motion or altered gait pattern, swelling
Brain and central nervous system tumors	Headache, vomiting (especially in the morning); vision, speech, and hearing changes; worsening balance; unsteady gait; unusual sleepiness; weakness

Brain and Central Nervous System Tumors

Brain and spinal cord tumors are the second most common pediatric cancer, accounting for 21% of all pediatric cancer cases, and the third most common type of cancer found in adolescents. These tumors are classified by the type of cell or tissue in which they originate or by the tumor's location in the CNS. It is important to note that any tumor, including CNS tumors classified as benign, can cause significant adverse effects largely because the growth may cause compression of adjacent healthy, functioning tissue. The signs and symptoms of brain and CNS tumors depend on tumor location, the developmental stage of the child, the communication ability of the child, and the presence of increased intracranial pressure. Symptoms may include morning headaches, nausea and vomiting, vision loss, speech or hearing impairments, increased rate of loss of balance, occurrence of seizures, unusual sleepiness, and personality changes (see Table 16.1). Medical imaging plays a central role in diagnosing these tumors.

Three common categories of CNS tumors found in children and adolescents include astrocytomas, medulloblastomas, and ependymomas.

Astrocytomas

Astrocytomas are the most common CNS tumor found in children and adolescents, accounting for about 35% of CNS tumors in these age groups. These tumors arise in neural support cells known as astrocytes. These are neuroglial, star-shaped, non-neuronal cells that maintain brain homeostasis and the microarchitecture of the brain parenchyma, regulate the development of neuronal cells, and provide for brain tissue repair and protection. The pathogenicity of astrocytomas can range from low grade (less invasive) to high grade (more invasive). Because astrocytes are found throughout the CNS, tumors involving these cells also appear throughout the brain. Headaches, seizures, memory loss, and changes in behavior are the most common early symptoms of an astrocytoma (see Table 16.1). Treatment of astrocytomas, like that for all CNS tumors, depends on cancer type, grade, location, and size and other tumor-specific factors. Whenever possible, these tumors are first surgically resected, and then the patient is often treated with chemotherapy or radiation therapy.

Medulloblastomas

Medulloblastomas are a group of highly invasive embryonal tumors that are rare in adults but common in children, particularly those under 10 years of age. These tumors typically arise in the cerebellum but can spread throughout the central nervous system and account for about 18% of childhood cancers. Early symptoms include headaches, vomiting, and lethargy. More specific symptoms are dependent on the region of the brain invaded by the tumor.

Ependymomas

Ependymomas are tumors that arise from glial cells lining the ventricular system of the brain or the central canal of the spinal cord and can range in severity from low to high grade. These tumors account for about 5% of all childhood brain cancers. In addition to directly damaging brain tissue, these tumors can disrupt normal flow of the cerebral spinal fluid resulting in increased intracranial pressure and further CNS damage. Overall, the survival rate for these and other CNS tumors exceeds 70%; however, the survival rate for these tumors is variable, depending on tumor location, patient age at time of diagnosis, and responsiveness to treatment.

Embryonal Tumors

These are rapidly growing tumors that arise from embryonic tissues that fail to mature but continue to grow.

Neuroblastomas

This group of tumors includes neuroblastomas (accounting for 6%-10% of all childhood cancers), which are neuroendocrine tumors that arise from neuroblasts, or neuron precursor cells, and are found throughout the developing sympathetic nervous system.[64] This tumor begins most frequently in the adrenal gland but can begin in or spread to other areas including the neck, chest, abdomen, or pelvis. Neuroblastomas most commonly affect children under the age of 5 years, though they may occur in older children. Several disease characteristics are used to place children with a neuroblastoma into one of three risk groups— low, intermediate, and high—with prognosis becoming poorer and treatment more involved with increasing risk status.

Retinoblastomas

Retinoblastomas (2% of childhood cancers)[1] are tumors that originate in the retina, arising when immature retinoblasts mutate into cancerous cells. Retinoblastomas are most frequently diagnosed in children younger than 4 years of age, and 40% of these cases arise from a heritable gene defect located on chromosome 13.[5] Symptoms include a pupil that appears red or white instead of black, a crossed eye, vision changes, and an enlarged pupil. Retinoblastomas are commonly diagnosed during a baby's well-baby check, and treatment may include chemotherapy, radiation, and surgery.[12]

Wilms' Tumor or Nephroblastoma

Wilms' tumor or nephroblastoma (5% of childhood cancers) is the most common form of kidney cancer in children, with the majority of cases diagnosed in those younger than 5 years of age. These tumors tend to be unilateral and large when diagnosed. Symptoms typically include an asymptomatic, unilateral abdominal lump or mass, blood in the urine, fever, diarrhea, urogenital infections, and systemic symptoms including fever and malaise.[14] Treatment is dependent on the stage of the tumor but frequently involves both surgery and chemotherapy.

Bone Tumors and Soft Tissue Sarcomas

Sarcomas are solid tumors that arise in connective tissue (muscle, bone, cartilage, and fat) in the body. Pediatric sarcomas collectively account for 7% of all tumors found in children and adolescents. The most common childhood sarcomas include osteosarcoma (2% of childhood cancers), Ewing's sarcoma (1% of childhood cancers), and rhabdomyosarcoma (3% of childhood cancers).[1]

Osteosarcomas

Osteosarcomas are tumors found in bone that arise from the inappropriate growth and development of immature bone cells. The resulting bone tissue is weaker than normal bone tissue and more susceptible to fracture (Fig. 16.1). Osteosarcomas typically affect the distal femur or proximal tibia (metaphyseal area) with the next most common site being the proximal humerus. An osteosarcoma weakens the healthy bone increasing the risk for a pathologic fracture, which often is the first presenting sign. Long-term bone or

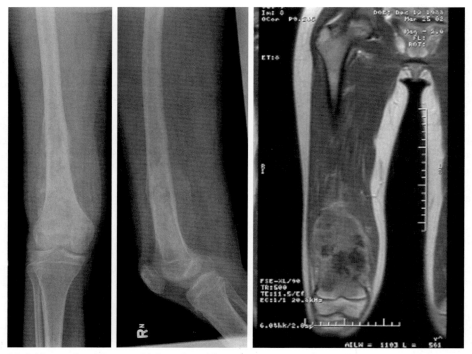

FIG. 16.1 X-ray of a 14-year-old female with osteosarcoma of the distal femur. (Courtesy Children's Hospital Colorado, Center for Cancer and Blood Disorders, Ortho-Oncology Program.)

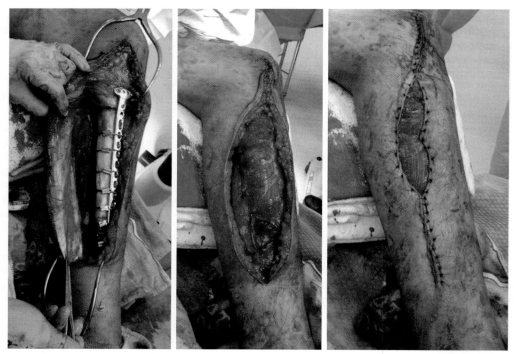

FIG. 16.2 Resection of tibial osteosarcoma with intercalary allograft reconstruction and gastrocnemius myoplasty. (Courtesy Children's Hospital Colorado, Center for Cancer and Blood Disorders, Ortho-Oncology Program.)

joint pain that worsens at night is symptomatic of osteosarcomas, and adolescents who are active in sports tend to complain about pain in the lower femur or right below the knee prior to the diagnosis of an osteosarcoma. If the osteosarcoma is large enough, it can visibly appear as a swelling (see Table 16.1). Treatment for osteosarcomas focuses on surgically removing the tumor using limb-sparing techniques with the aim to preserve as much of the bone and surrounding tissue as possible, thus preserving use of the affected limb (Figs. 16.2, 16.3, and 16.4). Occasionally the limb will be amputated if the neurovascular system is extensively involved.

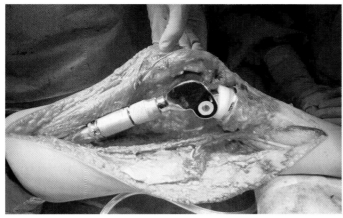

FIG. 16.3 Prosthetic reconstruction following proximal tibia osteosarcoma resection. (Courtesy Children's Hospital Colorado, Center for Cancer and Blood Disorders, Ortho-Oncology Program.)

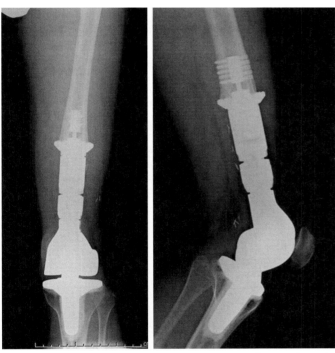

FIG. 16.4 X-ray of a prosthetic reconstruction of resection of a distal femur osteosarcoma. (Courtesy Children's Hospital Colorado, Center for Cancer and Blood Disorders, Ortho-Oncology Program.)

Rotationplasty (the Van Nes procedure) is an option in certain situations when the child would require an amputation but the surgeon and family choose to use the foot/ankle as the knee joint (for a more detailed discussion of this procedure, see Chapter 13) in order to assist with increasing functional mobility and giving the child a functional, neurovascularly intact knee joint, which greatly improves function and decreases energy expenditure with a prosthesis.[27] Chemotherapy may be administered before surgery to reduce the size of the tumor and is almost always administered following surgery. Radiation treatment is typically not effective in managing osteosarcoma.

Ewing's Sarcoma

Ewing's sarcoma is a malignant cancer found in both bone and in soft tissue. It is the second most common malignant bone tumor found in children and adolescents, and it occurs about equally in the bones of the extremities and bones in other parts of the body. Pain at the site of the tumor is typically the first symptom, sometimes with a mass or swelling present. Ewing's sarcoma may also arise in soft tissues. These tumors metastasize in about 25% of the cases, migrating to the lung, bone, and bone marrow. Metastases significantly reduce the chance of cure and survival.[10] Chemotherapy may be administered before surgery to reduce the size of the tumor and is almost always administered following surgery. Radiation treatment is typically not used to manage these tumors.[9]

Rhabdomyosarcoma

Rhabdomyosarcoma is a soft tissue sarcoma that arises from mesenchymal cells destined to become striated muscle cells. These tumors are found in children, adolescents, and young adults and can occur anywhere in the body. In children and adolescents, these tumors occur most frequently in the head and neck region and in urinary and reproductive organs. Treatment consists of surgery, chemotherapy, radiation therapy, or some combination of these interventions.

MEDICAL MANAGEMENT OF PEDIATRIC CANCERS

Once a child receives a diagnosis of cancer, decisions must be made regarding medical treatment. The medical treatment is dependent on the type of tumor present, its location, and the extent of the disease. Physicians use *staging* classification systems to describe the severity of a child's cancer, with larger stage numbers indicating greater disease severity. Staging classifications offer the medical team information on the size or extent or reach of the original tumor (i.e., whether or not the cancer has spread to other areas of the body). Oncologists use staging classifications to assist in determining the best treatment protocol to use for each patient. Understanding disease severity and treatment protocols allows the PT to better anticipate adverse effects of treatment and enables the PT to develop plans consistent with current and anticipated impairments and activity/limitation. Children are typically on treatment protocols that have been developed either at leading pediatric hospitals such as St. Jude Children's Research Hospital or from clinical trials undertaken by groups such as the Children's Oncology Group (COG) or a National Cancer Institute–supported clinical trials group. These protocols provide the medical team with a projected treatment and assessment time line for a specific medical treatment. Treatment options include surgery, radiation therapy, chemotherapy, and, more recently, alternative and complementary therapies. Some patients will require only one type of primary medical treatment intervention, but more typically a combination of treatments is required to successfully treat the disease.

The following section briefly describes these different medical treatment options.

Surgery

Surgery, in the context of cancer treatment, involves the resection or removal of a solid tumor (sarcomas, brain and CNS tumors, Wilms' tumors, etc.) along with sufficient amounts of the surrounding tissue to ensure that all tumor cells have been removed. For pediatric solid tumors, including CNS tumors and sarcomas, surgery remains the principal treatment strategy. However, some tumors may be too large to resect or may be located where surgical resection poses a significant risk for further injury to the tissue adjacent to tumor. Examples of the latter include brain stem gliomas or neuroblastomas that extend into the spinal cord. In these cases, alternative treatment options such as chemotherapy or radiation therapy may be used.

To ensure complete tumor resection and removal of all cancerous cells, surgeons resect the tumor along with a "clean" tissue margin (i.e., cancer-free, healthy tissue adjacent to the resected tumor). Clean margins suggest that all cancer cells have been removed. To further ensure that this is the case, chemotherapy and radiation therapy are frequently administered following a tumor resection. Radiation and chemotherapy may also be used prior to surgery in an effort to reduce the size of the tumor, making resection less difficult, and reducing surgical damage to surrounding, healthy tissue. In some cases surgery is used to debulk or resect as much of the tumor as possible, and chemotherapy and radiation therapy are then used to further shrink the remaining tumor. In cases of advanced or incurable cancers, surgery may be used to relieve side effects caused by a tumor, rather than to cure the disease itself. Many surgical procedures are used to treat pediatric cancers, and it is beyond the scope of this chapter to examine them. PTs treating pediatric patients with a surgical history for cancer treatment need to know where the tumor was located, what tissues (both cancerous and healthy) were resected, and what tissues were spared. Such understanding helps to identify impairments and possible impairments, thus providing guidance in developing physical therapy examination strategies and intervention plans.

Surgical interventions may play a tangential role in the diagnosis and treatment of some pediatric cancers. For example, tumor biopsies are often surgically acquired and subsequently used to stage and grade a tumor as well as determine its genetic makeup. Cerebrospinal fluid and bone marrow aspirates for analysis are typically collected surgically as well. Indwelling devices intended for long-term use such as implantable ports, central lines, Hickman catheters, or a peripherally inserted central venous catheter (PICC) line are often surgically implanted and then used to deliver drugs and collect blood samples. Medical shunts, such as a ventriculoperitoneal shunt, which drain cerebrospinal fluid from the brain into the abdominal cavity, are also surgically placed under either general or local anesthesia. Care must be taken not to dislodge these catheters during PT activities and to keep the area where they puncture the skin clean, dry, and protected from injury. Many pediatric patients receive anesthesia or light sedation prior to undergoing these procedures as well as imaging studies or radiation treatment. Following anesthesia, a child is at risk for a decrease in balance and postural control, thus increasing the risk of falling. Extra care should be taken if a PT session follows a procedure that requires anesthesia.

Radiation

Radiation has been a mainstay of cancer treatment for well over a century. This therapy exposes tumors to ionizing radiation, which damages the DNA of the irradiated cells, thus limiting the ability of these cells to successfully replicate. This treatment may be used to completely eradicate a tumor (curative), to reduce tumor size making resection less difficult or even

possible, or to prevent tumor recurrence. Radiation therapy can be delivered from either an external or an internal source; however, the majority of pediatric cancers are treated with radiation from an external source. Most doses of radiation required to successfully treat patients with cancer are too strong to be tolerated in a single dose. Rather, the total required radiation dose is usually *fractioned* or divided into smaller doses and delivered over a period of multiple days. Typical fraction schemes have the total dose divided into 30 equal units, delivered 5 times per week for 6 weeks; however, individual treatment doses can be increased or decreased depending on the patient response and the number of treatments received. Fractionation causes fewer toxic effects and often allows the patient to successfully receive needed amounts of radiation.

Radiation therapy may be used alone, or more frequently, in combination with surgery or chemotherapy. Regardless, radiation does not distinguish healthy tissue from cancerous tissue. As a result, healthy tissue can be damaged and destroyed by this intervention. Technological advances that allow more of the radiation beam to reach the tumor itself and less to strike healthy tissue has decreased collateral radiation damage. Despite these advances, radiation therapy often causes adverse side effects. These acute side effects include nausea and vomiting, diarrhea, hair loss, mucositis (inflammation of the mucus membranes lining the digestive tract), fatigue, and skin changes at the site irradiated (Table 16.2). Once treatment has been completed, these adverse effects typically diminish. Increased survivorship has led to the recognition that radiation used to treat pediatric cancers may cause adverse effects that do not

TABLE 16.2 Short-Term and Late Effects Associated With Receiving Radiation Therapy	
Short-Term Effect	**Late Effects**
Skin: redness, blistering, dry skin	Cardiac and vascular disease, metabolic impairment (low growth hormone), obesity, dyslipidemia
	Gurney JG, Ness KK, Sibley SD et al. Metabolic syndrome and growth hormone deficiency in adult survivors of childhood acute lymphoblastic leukemia. Cancer, 107(6): 1303-1312, 2006
Myelosuppression	Pulmonary fibrosis, restrictive lung disease
Fatigue	Osteoporosis, joint contractures, altered tooth development
Cognitive deficits	Cognitive deficits (impaired executive function), memory impairments
	Long-term decline in intelligence among adult survivors of childhood acute lymphoblastic leukemia treated with cranial radiation.
	Krull KR, Zhang N, Santucci A, Srivastava DK, Krasin MJ, Kun LE, Pui CH, Robison LL, Hudson MM, Armstrong GT. Blood. 2013 Jul 25;122(4):550-3. doi: 10.1182/blood-2013-03-487744. Epub 2013 Jun 6
Pain	Pain
Impaired digestive tract function (nausea, vomiting, mucositis diarrhea, difficulty swallowing)	Infertility
Hair loss	Increased risk for developing other cancers

Please note that this is not a complete list of adverse effects.

manifest themselves until years after the radiation therapy has been completed. Radiation is well recognized as causing fibrosis with resulting tissue injury; therefore, knowing the radiation field (area irradiated) allows a PT to anticipate, and ideally prevent, possible impairments to that area. For example, irradiation of the lungs in patients with mediastinal lymphoma can result in pulmonary fibrosis with accompanying respiratory defects; irradiation of the heart can cause fibrotic injury to the valves, coronary arteries, and myocardium, reducing cardiac function and increasing risk of cardiac disease; and radiation involving joints can result in fibrotic injury to the connective tissue components of the joint, thereby reducing joint range of motion and increasing the risk of osteoporosis in the involved bones. Cranial radiation can cause cognitive deficits during treatment, and these deficits may remain or reemerge after treatment has been completed. Abdominal and pelvic radiation can lead to kidney dysfunction and infertility in both males and females. A partial listing of these late effects is presented in Table 16.2.

Chemotherapy

Chemotherapy (CTX) refers to the use of drugs to either eradicate a tumor (curative) or to slow tumor growth, which may prolong life and reduce its immediate adverse effects (palliative). A large number of naturally occurring and synthesized compounds are used to treat pediatric cancer patients. These drugs (often simply referred to as "chemo") are perhaps best known for causing a number of adverse effects including nausea and vomiting, hair loss, and myelosuppression, a condition in which bone marrow activity is decreased, resulting in fewer red blood cells, white blood cells, and platelets. Chemotherapeutic agents can be administered as the primary treatment intervention. They can also be administered in conjunction with other primary therapies either before administration of the primary therapy, so-called neoadjuvant therapy, or after completion of the primary therapy, which is called adjuvant therapy. The purpose of delivering neoadjuvant therapy is to reduce the size of the tumor prior to delivery of the primary treatment (e.g., to shrink the tumor prior to surgical resection). Adjuvant therapy is provided in an effort to ensure that any cancer cells remaining after completion of primary therapy are killed, thus reducing the likelihood of recurrence. Chemotherapeutic agents act either by interrupting the cell cycle and hence cell division or by targeting specific proteins and disrupting metabolic processes that render the cells cancerous.

Traditional chemotherapeutic agents are cytotoxic (i.e., toxic to cells) and act by disrupting DNA structure, inhibiting DNA/RNA synthesis, or preventing cell division, thereby slowing or preventing tumor growth. Chemotherapy drugs are most effective against rapidly dividing cells, but they typically lack specificity for the cancer cells, thus they damage and kill rapidly dividing, healthy cells as well as cancer cells. There are a number of well-recognized acute adverse effects including damage to the bone marrow (causing myelosuppression, immune suppression, and increased frequency of bruising and bleeding), digestive tract (loss of appetite, nausea and vomiting, constipation/diarrhea, and mucositis), and hair follicles (alopecia) (Table 16.3). Children may experience a generalized myelosuppression resulting in decreased cell numbers of different blood cell types or may experience reductions in the number of specific types of blood cell types resulting in neutropenia (low number of neutrophils), thrombocytopenia (low platelet count), or anemia (low red blood cell count). When anemia is present, the patient may experience early fatigue, excessive tiredness, reduced endurance, headaches, and dizziness that may limit participation in the PT examination or treatment session. Leukopenia, a decrease in total number of white blood cells, is often used to identify the presence of an infection and as a signal of reduced infection-fighting ability. However, the cell numbers of neutrophils, the subpopulation of white blood cells most responsible for fighting infections, provide a better indicator of an individual's risk for developing an infection. The best estimate of neutrophil numbers is provided by the absolute neutrophil count (ANC), the product of the total white blood count and the contribution of neutrophils to the total blood cell count (%). Although an ANC value of 500 cells/mm^3 or lower signals an increased risk of infection, a decreasing ANC that includes this value is of more concern than a rising ANC that includes this value. It is important to remember that normal ranges for the different blood cell types vary by age and gender (Table 16.4).

Other adverse effects of chemotherapy can include hearing loss, peripheral neuropathy, neurocognitive changes, myopathy, and osteoporosis[3,4,9,56] (see Table 16.3). Platinum-based chemotherapeutic agents such as cisplatin are known to cause hearing loss, and all children taking this drug or class of drugs are at risk for permanent hearing loss, but those under 6 months of age are at particular risk. Children who are receiving cisplatin undergo routine hearing assessments from an audiologist. Both cisplatin and vincristine are known to cause peripheral neuropathy and loss of muscle strength (resulting in weakness). Functionally, these drugs impair gait, reduce endurance, and impair fine motor skills.[25] Glucocorticoid such as dexamethasone can cause a myopathy in proximal limb muscles and reduce blood flow to bones.[70] The resulting ischemic insult results in the death of bone cells or osteonecrosis, a condition associated with the loss of bone structure and rigidity, which increases the risk for the occurrence of pathologic fractures. Osteonecrosis can occur in the hips, knees, or ankles and may present with or without symptoms. In patients with ALL, it is more common in those aged 10 years or older.[33] There are limited data to support a relationship between joint pain and clinical symptoms of osteonecrosis such as decreased range of motion; therefore, PTs must be aware of the risk of osteonecrosis and avoid excessive high-impact activities during treatment sessions.[39] Children treated with vincristine often develop a chemo-induced peripheral neuropathy (CIPN), an adverse effect that typically presents with a loss of deep tendon reflexes, motor weakness (specifically decreased ankle dorsiflexion strength and handgrip strength), ankle dorsiflexion range of motion, paresthesias in hands and feet, and gait impairments (foot drop and increased hip flexion).[2,25] The onset of vincristine-induced CIPN can occur at any age, occur within a week of receiving the first dose of vincristine, or occur only after multiple doses have been received. The level of neuropathy can range from mild to moderate to severe, with the level of impairment paralleling the severity of the neuropathy.

Many chemotherapeutic agents cause cancer-related fatigue (CRF), a fatigue that is more severe, more distressing, and less likely to be relieved by rest than fatigue experienced by healthy people.[51] CRF is a complex, multidimensional problem arising from a number of factors including nutritional deficiencies, sleep disorders, depression and anxiety, anemia, and pain. Other acute, adverse effects of chemotherapy treatment include weight changes; skin changes; sores in the mouth, throat, and

TABLE 16.3   Chemotherapeutic Agents Used to Treat Specific Diseases With Resulting Short- and Late-Term Adverse Effects

Chemotherapeutic Agent	Diseases Treated	Short- and Late-Term Adverse Effects
L-asparaginase, Elspar	Leukemia, lymphoma	Drowsiness Nausea, vomiting, and cramping Allergic reaction: rash or increased breathing effort
Busulfan, Myleran	Leukemia	Fatigue, tiredness Decreased appetite Hair loss Nausea/vomiting Diarrhea Myelosuppression
Cisplatin (cisplatinum, Platinol, Platinol-AQ)	Osteosarcoma, HL, neuroblastoma, NHL, astrocytoma	Myelosuppression Allergic reaction: rash and increased breathing effort Nausea and vomiting that usually occurs for about 24 hours Tinnitus and hearing loss Fluctuations in blood electrolytes Kidney damage
Cyclophosphamide (cytoxan, Neosar)	HL, AML, Ewing's sarcoma, neuroblastoma,	Nausea, vomiting, and abdominal pain Decreased appetite Sore mouth and taste changes Diarrhea Hair loss (reversible) Bladder damage
Cytarabine (Ara-C, cytosine arabinoside, Cytosar-U)	Leukemia, lymphoma	Nausea, vomiting, and diarrhea Decreased appetite Decrease in blood cell counts Fever and flulike symptoms
Daunorubicin (Cerubidine), Doxorubicin (Adriamycin PFS, Adriamycin RDF, Rubex)	Lymphoma, AML	Nausea/vomiting Hair loss Red-colored urine (not bleeding but a drug effect) Myelosuppression Heart failure
Methotrexate (MTX)	Osteosarcoma, leukemia	Nausea/vomiting Decrease in blood cell counts Diarrhea Skin rashes Dizziness, headache, or drowsiness
Dexamethasone	ALL	Osteonecrosis, myopathy (typically proximal)
Vincristine (oncovin), vinblastine (Velban, Velbe)	Leukemia, HL, NHL, neuroblastoma, rhabdomyosarcoma	Weakness Loss of reflexes Nausea and vomiting Hair loss (reversible) Diarrhea or constipation, abdominal cramping Myelosuppression Peripheral neuropathy

AML, Acute myeloid leukemia; *HL,* Hodgkin's lymphoma; *NHL,* non-Hodgkin's lymphoma.

TABLE 16.4   Normal Ranges for Key Blood Parameters

Types of Cells	Purpose	Symptoms	Normal Ranges
White blood cells (leukocytes)	Fight infection	Leukopenia infections	4–11 k/ul
Neutrophil (absolute neutrophil count [ANC])	Fight infection	Leukopenia infections	1500–8000 cells/ml
Red blood cells (erythrocytes)	Transport of oxygen and nutrients	Anemia Pallor Fatigue Short of breath	3.8–6 million cells/ul
Hemoglobin	Transport of carbon dioxide and oxygen	See red blood cells	10–13 g/100 ml
Platelets (thrombocytes)	Helps blood to clot	Increased bruising Petechiae Bleeding from nose and gums	150,000–400,000 cells/mm³

Normal reference ranges for these cell counts may vary slightly between institutions.
From Garritan S, Jones P, Kornberg T, et al: Laboratory values in the intensive care unit, *Acute Care Perspect* 3:7-11, 1995.

TABLE 16.5 Diagnosis-Specific Body Structure/Function Impairments and Activity Limitations

Diagnosis	Body Function and Structure Impairments and Activity Limitations
Leukemia/lymphoma	Bone pain from buildup of blast cells in the bone marrow Decreased ankle dorsiflexion strength/ROM and handgrip strength, balance/postural control from vincristine peripheral neuropathy: pain, decreased hip, knee, ankle ROM from corticosteroid-induced osteonecrosis Decreased gross and fine motor skills Decreased mobility Decreased ability to carry or move objects Increased fatigue
Osteosarcoma/Ewing's sarcoma	Biomechanical changes to a limb causing increased energy expenditure for locomotion Neuropathic and nociceptive pain from tumor impingement, surgical pain, osteoporosis Decreased sensation from surgical nerve damage Decreased strength and ROM from slow wound healing, immobility, nerve damage, scar adhesions, CNS metastases Altered gait pattern/decreased ambulation Decreased stair climbing
Central and peripheral nervous system tumors	Pain from surgery, nerve impingement Decreased strength and ROM from tumor impingement, surgical pain, fear, immobility, inactivity Poor motor control, abnormal muscle tone

CNS, central nervous system; ROM, range of motion.

gums; and pain. Acute adverse effects vary from child to child, and most side effects are typically temporary, usually diminishing once chemotherapy has been completed. Symptoms of some adverse effects, however, including CIPN and CRF, may persist for months to years after the completion of chemotherapy.

Targeted therapies are a newer type of chemotherapy involving drugs that *target* molecular markers or cellular processes found exclusively or primarily in cancer cells thus allowing them to target cancer cells while sparing normal cells. This selectivity increases efficacy and decreases both short-term (myelosuppression, infection, and nausea, and vomiting), and long-term (neurocognitive impairment, infertility, cardiovascular morbidity and mortality, obesity, and second cancers) toxic effects.[6]

Table 16.3 lists common therapeutic agents used to treat pediatric and adolescent cancers and lists short-term and long-term adverse effects associated with these chemotherapeutic agents. PTs can use this information to guide their examination and assist in developing optimal interventions. Although the presence of these adverse effects may prevent delivering patient care, they more frequently require a modification of the interventions delivered (Table 16.5). For example, a PT treating a survivor of AML who received an anthracycline such as doxorubicin should carefully evaluate cardiac function, endurance, and fitness levels in this survivor, know the patient's blood cell counts, include exercise (reconditioning) as a treatment intervention, and carefully monitor the patient for the appearance of adverse cardiac signs and symptoms during each treatment session.

Chemotherapy drugs can be administered in a number of different ways. Standard intramuscular, intra-arterial, and intravenous delivery are sometimes used, but because these drugs are frequently given for extended periods, they are more frequently delivered via ports or central lines that provide long-term venous access. Because these lines puncture the skin, they can introduce bacteria into the bloodstream, resulting in sepsis. It is imperative that PTs treating patients with ports or central lines practice appropriate hand hygiene and clean toys and equipment before and after being used during an intervention session or examination. Some chemotherapy drugs may be delivered orally. Many chemotherapeutic agents used to treat brain tumors do not cross the blood–brain barrier and must be delivered through an intrathecal catheter. These catheters

are usually located in the lumbar spine or brain and are able to deliver drugs directly to the cerebral spinal fluid.

Chemotherapeutic agents are rarely given individually; rather they are typically given in combination with other chemotherapeutic agents. This multidrug strategy increases the likelihood that all cancer cells will be killed and reduces the chances of the cancer cells developing a resistance to these drugs. Because of cytotoxicity, these drugs are often given for a fixed period of time and then withheld for a period of time before restarting treatment. Such cycling allows the patient to recover from the deleterious effects of treatment. A course of chemotherapy treatment consists of a predetermined number of such cycles.

Chemotherapy has increased the long-term survivorship of pediatric cancer survivors. As these survivors have lived longer, it has become increasing obvious that they are at high risk for developing late adverse effects—impairments that can be linked to the chemotherapy regimen but emerge only years after completion of treatment. These late, chronic, adverse effects are common and can have potentially severe effects on the physical, cognitive, and psychosocial health of these survivors. These adverse health outcomes include pulmonary, cardiac, endocrine and reproductive dysfunction, osteoporosis, and neurocognitive/neurosensory loss.[25,30] In an effort to identify and screen for these late effects, long-term follow-up is now an established part of the posttreatment care of childhood cancer survivors.[66] For example, the Children's Oncology Group provides risk-based, exposure-related clinical practice guidelines for screening and managing late effects resulting from therapeutic treatment for pediatric malignancies.[34] Both the adolescent/young adult and the family need to be made aware of the risk of developing these late effects and understand the importance and need for ongoing screening and management of these late effects as well as preventive measures.

Bone Marrow Transplantation/Stem Cell Transplantation

Some pediatric patients with leukemia, HL, or NHL may not respond to available chemotherapy and thus become eligible for a stem cell (SC) transplant. SCs, once infused, repopulate the bone marrow and give rise to the array of mature blood cells found in the circulation. The transplant process first involves the elimination of all or nearly all blood cells and stem cells in the recipient, a process called the conditioning phase. This is accomplished by having the patient undergo whole body radiation therapy or a short-term, high-dose chemotherapy. Younger children do not receive whole body radiation due to the complex side effects of radiation to their growing bodies. The conditioning phase leaves the patient severely myelo- and immune suppressed. Immediately after completing this phase, the patient receives SCs by intravenous (IV) infusion. Transplanted SCs can be collected from three different sites including bone marrow, peripheral blood, or cord blood from the patient prior to treatment or from a donor. Stem cell transplants are characterized by the donor of the SCs. If the infused stem cells are harvested from the patient receiving them, the process is termed an *autologous* stem cell transplant; if the stem cells are harvested from another individual, it is termed an *allogeneic* transplant. Allogeneic transplants are also characterized by the quality of the relationship between the donor and the recipient. Those in which the donor and recipient are related and share common blood characteristics are referred to as matched transplants, and those from a nonrelative that matches the blood characteristics of the recipient are referred to as matched unrelated donors (MUDs).

Once infusion is completed, the stem cells migrate to the bone marrow, take up residence, establish a population of healthy stem cells, and begin producing functional, mature blood cells. During this time, called the *engraftment* period, the patient remains hospitalized (typically 28–35 days) and the SCs engraft, multiply, and cause a progressive increase in the number of functional blood cells found in the blood. Because the patients are often myelosuppressed and, as a result, severely immunocompromised, they receive medication prophylactically to prevent infections, including antivirals, antibiotics, and antifungals, as well as platelet infusions to limit bleeding and bruising, to prevent rejection (cyclosporine, methotrexate, tacrolimus, mycophenolate mofetil), and to manage adverse effects of these drugs and the transplant. An important milestone in this engraftment process occurs when the absolute neutrophil count is >500 cells/μL for at least 2 days in a row.[62,69] At this point, the patient is considered "neutrophil engrafted," a sign that the immune system is starting to recover. This process typically continues until the body can produce normal or nearly normal numbers of mature, functioning blood cells, which may take multiple months.

Patients who receive SC transplants are at risk for a disease called graft-versus-host disease (GVHD).[35,49,69] Cells that provide immunity to the recipient are eliminated during the conditioning phase and are subsequently replaced by the transplanted SCs. Immune protection now becomes a function of the blood cells arising from the transplanted SCs. This is a different scenario from that which occurs in a solid organ transplant, a situation where the recipient retains his or her own blood cells, giving the recipient the capacity to reject the transplanted organ. GVHD occurs when the transplanted stem cells give rise to blood cells, which recognize tissue of the recipient as foreign and reject those tissues. It occurs most frequently in patients receiving an allogeneic transplant and has a higher likelihood of occurring as the histocompatibility or tissue compatibility between donor and recipient decreases.[69] SC recipients can experience GVHD shortly after receiving the transplant, resulting in acute GVHD or aGVHD. The patient with aGVHD can experience a rash, itchy skin, skin discoloration, dry mouth, mouth ulcers, diarrhea and weight loss, joint contractures, and malabsorption. Antirejection drugs are given prophylactically during the engraftment period to prevent the occurrence of aGVHD, but when rejection does occur, the liver, skin, and gastrointestinal

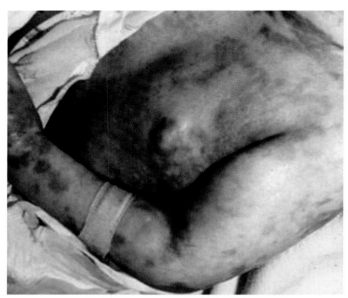

FIG. 16.5 Chronic graft versus host disease in a child following a stem cell transplant. (Courtesy Children's Hospital Colorado Pediatric Bone Marrow Transplant Program.)

tract are severely impacted. aGVHD is treated with high-dose glucocorticoid therapy, a treatment that has a number of adverse effects including infection, diabetes, sleep disorders, osteoporosis, hyperglycemia, and water retention.[35,49,69]

GVHD can also arise after completion of the acute phase of recovery from the transplant or simply persist after the transplant has engrafted, causing a disease known as chronic GVHD or chronic graft versus host disease (cGVHD), which typically occurs 1 year or more posttransplant. cGVHD lasts longer than acute graft versus host disease (aGVHD) and presents with similar symptoms (Fig. 16.5). Prednisone or other similar antiinflammatory or immunosuppressive medications are used to treat cGVHD.[35,49] Adverse effects of long-term glucocorticoid treatment have been previously noted.[70]

SC transplantation (stem cell rescue) is also used in the treatment of patients with high-risk neuroblastoma or medulloblastoma who have been treated with high doses of chemotherapy or radiation. Stem cells used in these patients are collected from the recipient's own bone marrow (autologous transplant) before chemo or radiation treatment begins and are then transplanted when needed. The transplantation procedure is similar to that described earlier. Although the risks are less than for those receiving allogeneic transplants, these patients remain at increased risk for infection. This SC rescue process allows for the use of higher doses of chemotherapeutic agents and radiation, ideally creating a greater likelihood of remission and cure.[23]

FOREGROUND INFORMATION

PHYSICAL THERAPY EXAMINATION

Children and adolescents who are undergoing cancer treatment, recovering from treatment, or are survivors may require PT services. These services are delivered in a number of different rehabilitation settings (acute care, in-patient rehabilitation hospital, out-patient, home, child care facilities, or school). Each cancer diagnosis presents with its own treatment protocols, systems involvement, and long-term effects, all of which influence the location and type of PT intervention provided. PTs treating these children must have the knowledge and skills necessary to perform a comprehensive physical therapy examination specific to the needs of the infant, child, and adolescent. Such knowledge and skills include typical age-appropriate gross/fine motor skills; musculoskeletal, neuromuscular, and cardiopulmonary development; understanding of the disease and medical protocols and short- and long term side effects of treatment; the essential role of the family–medical team relationship; and how to deliver these services in the context of family-centered care.[57,58] This information guides the PT in gathering an appropriate and detailed history, selecting correct assessment and outcome measures, developing a plan of care, and providing an evidence-based intervention program.[24,65,68]

History

The history section of the PT examination for a child with cancer will include all the typical key areas (past medical history, social history, home/school/child care environments, and family challenges/supports). PTs will want to take into consideration that children with cancer and their families have generally already shared their history with many health care professionals. Keeping this in mind, PTs should make every effort to gather information from the medical record and discussion with other health care professionals prior to talking with the child and family. Making this effort will help build mutual respect between the PT and the child and family and allow for more time during the initial physical therapy evaluation to focus on specific child/family needs. The PT will want to take note of the specific medical protocol the child is receiving with the medical management time lines for specific types of medications, surgeries, radiation, or other medical interventions. These protocols will help guide the physical therapy plan of care.

During the history-taking process, the PT should be aware of the child's blood cell counts. Children will have blood drawn regularly to determine the blood cell counts; however, these values can change daily and therefore the PT needs to know if the child is at risk for low blood cell counts and adapt evaluation appropriately. Cleaning all toys and mats prior to use and engaging in appropriate hand hygiene are the two most important ways to prevent the development and spread of infection. A child who is severely immunocompromised may need to be seen in an isolated area, and the therapist may need to wear a mask. In addition, if the child presents with low platelets, the PT will want to modify the examination so as not to put the child at risk for falls or apply resistance to an extremity to prevent bruising. If the red blood cell count is low, the child may present with fatigue and have decreased tolerance to physical activity.

Systems Review

Because children undergoing active treatment for cancer often have nausea, fatigue, and general malaise, the PT will want to quickly identify areas of concern during the initial evaluation. Due to the complex nature and involvement of multiple systems with the majority of oncologic diagnoses, the systems review is beneficial in prioritizing areas of impairments, activity limitations, and participation restrictions.[31,32] Areas of focus with this particular patient population typically include the following:

1. Musculoskeletal changes are observed easily through noticing asymmetries, decreased strength, and range of motion during standing, walking, or crawling.

> ### BOX 16.1 Recommended Measures for Children With Cancer
>
> **Body Functions and Structures**
> - Musculoskeletal: range of motion (goniometry), strength (handheld dynamometry)
> - Neuromuscular: pediatric modified Total Neuropathy Score (peds-mTNS)
> - Cardiopulmonary: endurance (heart rate, rate of perceived exertion)
>
> **Activities and Participation**
> - Timed up and down stairs
> - Timed up and go
> - Gross Motor Function Measure (GMFM)
> - Bruininks-Oseretsky Test of Motor Proficiency (BOT-2)
> - PedsQL
> - SF-36v2
> - Musculoskeletal Tumor Society (MSTS)
> - Toronto Extremity Salvage Scale (TESS)
>
> **Other**
> - Functional Mobility Assessment (FMA)

2. Neuromuscular symptoms such as pain, neuropathies, decreased sensation, proprioception, and auditory delays are often noted when the child avoids movement in a particular body part, refuses to bear weight on an extremity, does not respond to the PT's requests due to not hearing the instructions, or does not understand the instructions due to a neurocognitive delay.

3. Cardiopulmonary limitations are often identified by observing that the child uses a stroller or is excessively carried by the parents, or by noting increased work of breathing, nasal flaring, and changes in skin color during physical activity.

4. Integumentary changes such as bruising and pale complexion often indicate decreased platelets and red blood cells. Poor wound healing, edema, or open sores are common in children with cancer, thus the PT is advised to perform a thorough skin check as part of the physical exam.

Tests and Measures

Children with cancer will require a comprehensive, neuromuscular, musculoskeletal, cardiopulmonary, integumentary, developmental, and gait/functional mobility examination. The typical physical therapy test and measures are used for this population; additionally, a few tests and measures have been developed specifically for children with cancer (Box 16.1).

Neuromuscular

PTs assess muscle tone and spasticity using the Ashworth scale; pain with an age-appropriate scale (FLACC = face, legs, activity, consolability scale, FACES = Wong Baker FACES pain scale, visual analog scale); and sensation with light touch, sharp dull, and two-point discrimination. Visual and hearing examinations include eyes tracking in all directions and hearing quiet/loud sounds on the right and left sides.

The Pediatric modified Total Neuropathy Score (peds-mTNS) is an assessment scale used to measure CIPN in children with non-CNS cancers.[25,26] This tool assesses sensory symptoms, functional symptoms, autonomic symptoms, light touch sensation, pin sensibility, vibration sensibility, strength, and deep tendon reflexes. The ped-mTNS scores are reported to correlate with functional measures of balance and manual dexterity, and it is the most sensitive tool for assessing CIPN in this patient population.

Musculoskeletal

PTs determine range of motion (ROM) with a goniometer or inclinometer, strength by manual muscle testing or handheld dynamometer, function by visual observation during the performance of functional movements, and limb-length inequality by measuring leg lengths using a tape measure.

Children with a history of lower-extremity sarcoma (osteosarcoma or Ewing's sarcoma) require ongoing examination of their leg lengths. These growing children will typically have an expandable internal prosthesis (Repiphysis). The noninvasive expandable prosthesis allows expansion via external activation of a spring mechanism in the structure of the implant, allowing the leg to be lengthened without surgery through a fluoroscopic imaging procedure performed by the physician. The PT plays a role in this process by frequently measuring the child's leg length and notifying the physician when a limb length inequality is present.

Cardiovascular and Pulmonary

PTs use respiratory rate, heart rate, work of breathing (nasal flaring, accessory muscle breathing, belly breathing), physiologic cost index (PCI), rate of perceived exertion (RPE), and measures of endurance (2-, 3-, 6-, or 9-minute walk test, 30-second step test) to assess endurance and tolerance to activity in children with cancer.

PTs will want to assess fatigue with an age-appropriate assessment tool. The Parent Fatigue Scale (PFS) is often used for children 3 to 6 years of age. This scale consists of 17 items that ask the parents about their perceptions of the amount of fatigue experienced by their child in the past week on a 5-point Likert scale. The Childhood Fatigue Scale (CFS), a 14-item questionnaire, is used for children ages 7 to 12. The instrument is typically read to the child and the child is asked to rate how much the problem bothers him or her using a 5-point Likert scale ranging from "not at all" to "a lot." Scores range from 0 to 56 with higher scores reflecting greater amounts of experienced fatigue. The Fatigue Scale-Adolescent (FS-A), for adolescents 13 to 18 years of age, was specifically created to comprehensively measure cancer-related fatigue in adolescents who are receiving cancer treatment.[51] PTs can use the information obtained from these assessments to help develop intervention programs and evaluate the impact intervention programs have on cancer-related fatigue.[48]

Integumentary

PTs may assess edema with a tape measure, document wound size using pictures taken with a digital camera equipped with a grid scale, visually assess skin color, and determine bogginess and texture with manual palpation.

Gross Motor Development/Functional Mobility

PTs use the Timed Up and Go (TUG), Timed Up and Down Stairs (TUDS), Bayley Scales of Infant Development (BSID II), Peabody Developmental Motor Scales (PDMS-2), Gross Motor Function Measure (GMFM)[72], Bruininks-Oseretsky Test of Motor Proficiency (BOT-2),[73] and other common developmental tools to examine gross motor skills in children with cancer.

The Musculoskeletal Tumor Society (MSTS) is a tool used to identify the functional abilities of children following reconstructive surgery secondary to a tumor resection (osteosarcoma or Ewing's sarcoma). The MSTS examines factors pertaining to pain, physical function, emotional acceptance, use of supports (brace, cane, and crutches), walking ability, and quality of gait. This test involves patient observation by clinicians (nurse, physician, physical therapist) and patient report on pain, emotional acceptance, and support, and it is considered a subjective measure versus an objective measure of assessment.[27]

The Functional Mobility Assessment (FMA) was designed specifically for use with children and adolescents with a lower-extremity sarcoma and assesses six domains: (1) pain; (2) function using two specific measures, TUDS and TUG; (3) supports/assistive devices; (4) satisfaction with walking quality; (5) participation in work, school, sports; and (6) endurance as measured by results on the 9-minute run-walk test.[44] Heart rate (HR) and rate of perceived exertion (RPE) are both measured during the TUDS and TUG. Physiologic cost index, HR, and RPE are measured during the 9-minute run-walk. The FMA has norm-referenced values that allow health care professionals to compare the functional abilities of children, adolescents, and young adults with lower extremity sarcoma to age- and gender-matched healthy peers.[43] These comparisons assist the PT in identifying the need for physical therapy services, assisting the patient/family in setting goals, and initiating/progressing physical therapy intervention programs.

The Toronto Extremity Salvage Scale (TESS) is a self-administered questionnaire that allows patients to indicate the level of difficulty experienced in dressing, grooming, mobility, work, sports, and leisure. This tool measures patients' impressions of their level of physical disability. The 30 items are rated on a scale ranging from 1 (worst) to 5 (best).[27] Physical therapists use these types of measures to assist in identifying areas of importance to children with cancer or following the completion of cancer treatment.

Quality-of-Life Measures

SF-36v2 is a questionnaire consisting of 36 items combined into eight subscales that include physical functioning, role functioning (physical), pain, general health, vitality, social functioning, role functioning (emotional), and mental health. These subscales can be scored individually; aggregate physical component scales (PCSs) or mental health component scales (MCSs) can also be calculated as well as total Short Form-36 (SF-36) v2 score. PedsQL is a health-related, quality-of-life measure that incorporates a generic core and disease/symptom-specific modular approach for pediatric chronic health conditions.[38] Quality-of-life measures will guide the PT in focusing the intervention strategies. PTs will also want to explore factors that influence childhood cancer survivors' choice of occupation and choice to attend college to assist with guiding in enhancing physical activity to match career choices.[21,40,41]

PHYSICAL THERAPY INTERVENTION

Physical therapy intervention for children with cancer has been shown to be safe and effective in improving body structure and function impairments, activity limitations, and participation restrictions.[8,16,17,19,37,49,59,63,67] Due to the acute and long-term side effects of the cancer itself and the medical interventions used, physical therapists are essential members of the medical team and should be introduced into the medical plan of care starting at the initial diagnosis.

Numerous studies support the benefits of exercise and physical activity for children and adults with cancer.[15,17,28,37,50,75] The role of the health care team must extend beyond traditional recommendations of advising patients to be physically active. If children are medically stable, the PTs can recommend that they participate in physical activities during school such as gym class (modified if needed) and playing outside on the playground. If the children are in active medical treatment and do not feel as well, the PT can suggest physical activity such as encouraging parents to have their children walk, holding the child's hand versus carrying the child or pushing the child in a stroller. Parents are often concerned that their child will experience additional harm from overexertion or are hesitant to encourage them to participate in active play when their child is not feeling well. PTs provide patient and family education regarding safe physical activity and functional mobility that can be performed throughout treatment and should educate patients and their families on the importance of remaining as physically active as possible throughout the treatment process (Box 16.2). In addition physical activity is known to assist with decreasing cancer-related fatigue (CRF).[51]

PTs often are asked questions regarding when exercise and what exercise intensity is appropriate for children with myelosuppression. Currently available exercise guidelines for typically developing children recommend 60 minutes or more of physical activity per day at a moderate-to-vigorous intensity.[7] However, these guidelines are not often met by children with cancer. General recommendations for patient participation in exercise with depressed blood cell counts have been developed[1] and are shown in Table 16.6. Even when blood cell counts are low, there are still beneficial interventions the PT can provide, such as family education, pain management, supportive positioning, functional mobility, and addressing equipment needs. It is safe, effective, and important to encourage and provide opportunities for children with cancer to maintain their activity level and participation in age-appropriate recreation.

The PT bases the decision to progress a child's physical exercise, functional mobility, and intensity based on three primary factors: (1) the child's medical stability (cardiac, respiratory, hematologic, cognitive, surgical protocols), (2) the child's level of motivation, and (3) child and family goals. PTs have the responsibility to educate patients and families by letting them know that there will be good days and bad days (or weeks) but that in every situation it is important for the child to perform as much independent activity as is safe and possible. This will vary for each child, and one week it may mean walking to the bathroom with assistance, whereas in another week it may mean completing multiple flights of stairs or actively participating in sports and other age-appropriate activities (Fig. 16.6).[22] Due to the long treatment duration, PTs in the pediatric oncology setting have the unique opportunity to positively impact the child through many important stages of development and growth, all while maximizing functional mobility, independence, and participation.

Physical Therapy Intervention by Specific Cancer Diagnoses

Leukemia

Children with leukemia are likely to receive a PT referral at initial diagnosis due to decreased functional mobility because of severe bone pain from the buildup of cancer cells in the bone. Initiation of chemotherapy tends to lessen bone pain, but these children still frequently experience delays in gross motor function and functional mobility. The role of the PT during this period is to identify age-appropriate gross motor skills, employ therapeutic interventions that will help the child at least approach if not achieve these skills, encourage the child to achieve these skills, and involve the family in the pursuit of these goals. The PT educates the family on using toys and handling techniques to encourage the infant to crawl or the toddler to walk. The goal of the physical therapy intervention is to return the child to functional levels prior to a diagnosis of leukemia.

During medical treatment, children with leukemia are at risk for peripheral neuropathy impacting ankle dorsiflexion and handgrip ROM and strength. Research studies have found that daily ankle dorsiflexion stretching held for 30 seconds, 5 days a week, increased and prevented limitations in active ankle dorsiflexion.[38] In addition, performing lower-extremity

---

BOX 16.2   Recommended Interventions for Children With Cancer

Body Function and Structure
- Range-of-motion exercises
- Strengthening exercises
- Balance/coordination exercises

Activities and Participation
- Aerobic activity (walking, biking, swimming)
- Participation in sports and age-appropriate recreational groups (dance classes, taekwondo)
- Physical education classes

Communication Considerations for Physical Therapists
- Family and patient
- Other members of medical team (physicians, nurses, social work, child life, advanced care providers)
- Schoolteachers
- Primary care physician
- Other therapists from physical therapy or different disciplines

---

TABLE 16.6   Recommendations for Participation in Exercise Interventions With Below Normal Blood Cell Counts and Hemoglobin Levels

BLOOD PARAMETER	EXERTIONAL LEVEL		
	No Aerobic Exercise	Light Aerobic Exercises	Resistance Exercises[a]
White blood cells	<5 k cells/mm^3 and fever is present	>5 k cells/mm^3	>5 k cells/mm^3
Platelets	<20,000 cells/mm^3	20,000–50,000 cells/mm^3	>50,000 cells/mm^3
Hemoglobin	<8 g/dl	8–10 g/dl	>8 g/dl

Depending on the physical therapist's facility and individual protocols, these values may vary.
[a]Participation in resistance exercise interventions is recommended only if these levels are exceeded.
Garritan S, Jones P, Kornberg T, et al: Laboratory values in the intensive care unit, *Acute Care Perspect* 3:7-11, 1995.

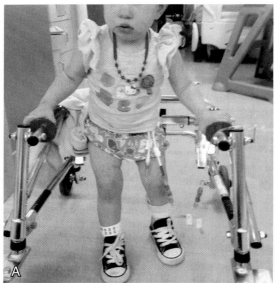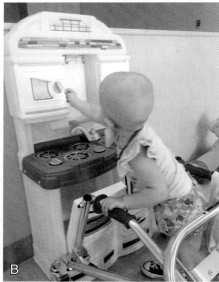

FIG. 16.6 A 20-month-old with an embryonal brain tumor ambulating (A) and playing (B) while using a posterior walker due to ataxia and weakness. (Courtesy Children's Hospital Colorado-Center for Cancer and Blood Disorders Physical Therapy Program.)

strengthening exercises such as mini-squats and step up and off a step for three sets of 10 repetitions, 3 days per week, improved lower-extremity strength.[38] PTs will also want to include a balance and coordination component to the intervention program to facilitate challenging ankle strategies and the use of vision and the vestibular systems when the somatosensory system is compromised to assist with preventing falls. When CIPN is significant and the child is not able to actively dorsiflex to neutral or is at risk for falls, the PT will recommend an ankle-foot orthosis and in severe cases the child may require forearm crutches. The primary goals of the stretching, strengthening, and balance/coordination exercises are to improve ROM, strength, and functional mobility while making the exercises fun and encouraging the child to incorporate the activities into the child's daily routines.

PT intervention that addresses aerobic endurance and fatigue is oftentimes challenging. PTs frequently recommend aerobic activity daily and should specify intensity and duration in their recommendations to ensure children are receiving the maximum benefit. PTs should encourage the child to select activities of interest, such as bike riding or dancing, to improve motivation and sustainability. PTs need to feel comfortable reassuring children and families that it is safe and important to work at a therapeutic intensity that is high enough to create positive changes in cardiovascular endurance, activity tolerance, and muscle strength. PTs may recommend heart rate monitors or measures such as rating of perceived exertion to encourage the appropriate exertional level for the individual child.

Osteonecrosis can occur in the hips, knees, or ankles and may present with or without symptoms in patients with leukemia[33,39]; therefore, PTs must be aware of the risk factors of osteonecrosis and avoid excessive high-impact activities during treatment sessions until osteonecrosis has been definitively ruled out by an MRI.[39,70] When a child does have osteonecrosis, the physician will often recommend non-weight-bearing or decreased weight-bearing periods; therefore, the PT will have to provide instruction on gait training with crutches. In addition,

PTs provide instructions on ROM exercises to improve or prevent limitations in active and passive ROM and limit strength losses caused by the weight-bearing status. Therapeutic interventions should focus on strengthening the muscles stabilizing the joint with the osteonecrosis to provide support and protection. The goal is to prevent or delay the need for surgical intervention. These exercises will help to increase blood flow to the area and decrease pain.

Children with leukemia who require a stem cell transplant will receive PT intervention during the engraftment period. Physical therapy is appropriate and should focus on using exercises and play to limit a loss of strength and endurance.[8,49] Due to the risk of thrombocytopenia and anemia, PT interventions during this phase of medical intervention will typically incorporate active ROM, body-supported (no weights) strengthening, and aerobic exercise according to the patient's tolerance. The PT session requires creative strategies because these children have to stay in their hospital rooms. Rehabilitation interventions must be delivered in the context of myelosuppression (practice good hand hygiene), fatigue (provide treatment when the patient's energy levels are highest), and nausea and vomiting (coordinate treatment in conjunction with the pharmacologic management of these symptoms).[8]

Lower-Extremity Sarcoma

Children and adolescents will receive physical therapy upon the initial diagnosis of upper- and lower-extremity sarcoma. PTs provide the child with crutch training consistent with the child's weight-bearing status on the involved lower extremity. Depending on the type of surgery (amputation, limb-sparing, rotation-plasty), the child might have non-weight-bearing or weight-bearing-to-tolerance orders. Children who have undergone limb-sparing procedures involving the femur typically begin knee ROM activities following surgery, but if the tumor involves the tibia, then the knee is typically immobilized for a period of time (according to the surgeon's preference, this phase usually lasts between 6 and 9 weeks), preventing such

ROM activities. Children with osteosarcomas receive intensive physical therapy to increase ROM, strength, and functional mobility. Temporary or permanent nerve damage may occur during limb-sparing surgery, therefore the PT may also provide the child with a modified ankle-foot orthosis to accommodate areas of wound healing.

ROM exercises are an important component of a physical therapy program for children and adolescents with lower-extremity sarcoma. ROM has been reported to correlate with functional mobility and quality of life in patients with lower-extremity sarcoma after limb-sparing surgery.[45]

Brain Tumor

Children with brain tumors, specifically medulloblastoma and less commonly astrocytoma or ependymoma, are at risk for posterior fossa syndrome following surgical resection of the tumor. These children may experience delays 1 to 5 days after surgery, causing apraxia of speech, dysarthria, mutism, irritability, ataxia, changes in muscle tone (hemiplegia, hypertonia), and poor motor coordination. Their skills will typically improve over many months, but some children have impairments for years. The PT will intervene to assist the family in positioning, use of assistive devices (orthotics, wheelchair, walker), and transfer training. The PT will work intensively with the child on functional mobility, balance, and coordination. During this time period, the PT's primary goal is to assist the child with positioning to prevent skin irritation, safety management to prevent falls, and family education. Because these are complex patients, the PT should strongly advocate for referrals to other health care providers including occupational therapists and speech language pathologists.

▌SUMMARY

This chapter has discussed multiple aspects of childhood cancers. Signs and symptoms are discussed. Specific cancer diagnoses and medical interventions including chemotherapy, radiation, and surgery are addressed. Survivorship is rising for many types of cancers, so children with these complex diagnoses often need and can benefit from physical therapy during the different stages of their treatment. They are at risk for complications such as musculoskeletal, neuromuscular, cardiopulmonary, integumentary impairments, and physical functional delays, which can be addressed by physical therapy. This chapter details specific physical therapy examinations and interventions used for children with cancer. The chapter also emphasizes working collaboratively with the other members of the medical team as well as how to include the family during therapy sessions, goal setting, and therapeutic education. The increased number of childhood cancer survivors has made it imperative that physical therapists be well educated and well prepared for this complex and rewarding specialty area.

Case Scenario on Expert Consult

The case scenario related to this chapter presents a 10-year-old girl with vincristine-induced peripheral neuropathy (VIPN) during treatment for high-risk acute lymphoblastic leukemia. It covers background information on peripheral neuropathy, the medical history, initial physical therapy examination and evaluation, and physical therapy intervention and management over the course of her treatment with a focus on family-centered care and evidence-based examination and decision making.

REFERENCES

1. American Cancer Society: *Cancer facts & figures 2014*, Atlanta, 2014, American Cancer Society.
2. Argyriou AA, Bruna J, Marmiroli P, et al.: Chemotherapy-induced peripheral neurotoxicity (CIPN): an update, *Crit Rev Oncol Hematol* 82:51–77, 2012.
3. Armstrong T, Almadrones L, Gilber MR: Chemotherapy-induced peripheral neuropathy, *Oncol Nurs Society* 32:305–311, 2005.
4. Arndt C, Hawkins D, Anderson JR, et al.: Age is a risk factor for chemotherapy-induced hepatopathy with vincristine, dactinomycin, and cyclophosphamide, *J Clin Oncol* 22:1894–1901, 2004.
5. Benavente CA, Dyer MA: Genetics and epigenetics of human retinoblastoma, *Annu Rev Pathol* 10:547–562, 2005.
6. Bernstein ML: Targeted therapy in pediatric and adolescent oncology, *Cancer* 117(Suppl 10):2268–2274, 2011.
7. Centers for Disease Control and Prevention: Division of nutrition, physical activity, and obesity. How much physical activity do children need? http://www.cdc.gov/physicalactivity/basics/children/.
8. Chamorro-viña C, et al.: Exercise during hematopoietic stem cell transplant hospitalization in children, *Med Sci Sports Exerc* 42:1045–1053, 2010.
9. Children's Oncology Group: In treatment. https://childrensoncologygroup.org/index.php/ewingsarcoma?id=184.
10. Children's Oncology Group: Just diagnosed. https://childrensoncologygroup.org/index.php/ewingsarcoma?id=183.
11. Children's Oncology Group: *Long-term follow-up guidelines for survivors of childhood, adolescent, and young adult cancers: version 4.0*, 2013.
12. Children's Oncology Group: Retinoblastomas. https://childrensoncologygroup.org/index.php/retinoblastoma.
13. Children's Oncology Group: What is cancer? https://childrensoncologygroup.org/index.php/home/64-medical-information/medical-information.
14. Children's Oncology Group: Wilms tumor and other kidney cancers. https://childrensoncologygroup.org/index.php/wilmstumorandotherkidneycancers.
15. Courneya KS, Friedenreich CM: Relationship between exercise during treatment and current quality of life among survivors of breast cancer, *J Psychosoc Oncol* 15:35–56, 1997.
16. Dimeo F, Bertz H, Finke J, et al.: An aerobic exercise program for patients with haematological malignancies after bone marrow transplantation, *Bone Marrow Transplant* 18:1157–1160, 1996.
17. Esbenshade AJ, Friedman DL, Smith WA, et al.: Feasibility and initial effectiveness of home exercise during maintenance therapy for childhood acute lymphoblastic leukemia, *Pediatr Phys Ther* 26:301–307, 2014.
18. Essig S, Li Q, Chen Y, et al.: Risk of late effects of treatment in children newly diagnosed with standard-risk acute lymphoblastic leukaemia: a report from the Childhood Cancer Survivor Study cohort, *Lancet Oncol* 15:841–851, 2014.
19. Farzin Gohar S, Price J, Comito M, et al.: Parent satisfaction of a physical therapy intervention program for children with acute lymphoblastic leukemia in the first six months of medical treatment, *Pediatr Blood Cancer* 56:799–804, 2011.
20. Florin TA, Fryer GE, Miyoshi T, et al.: Physical inactivity in adult survivors of childhood acute lymphoblastic leukemia: a report from the childhood cancer survivor study, *Cancer Epidemiol Biomarkers Prev* 16:1356–1363, 2007.
21. French AE, Tsangaris E, Barrera M, et al.: School attendance in childhood cancer survivors and their siblings, *J Pediatr* 162:160–265, 2013.
22. Garritan S, Jones P, Kornberg T, et al.: Laboratory values in the intensive care unit, *Acute Care Perspect* 3:7–11, 1995.
23. George RE, Li S, Medeiros-Nancarrow C, Neuberg D, et al.: High-risk neuroblastoma treated with tandem autologous peripheral-blood stem cell-supported transplantation: long-term survival update, *J Clin Oncol* 24:2891–2896, 2006.
24. Gilchrist LS, Galantino M, Wampler M, et al.: A framework for assessment in oncology rehabilitation, *Phys Ther* 89:286–306, 2009.
25. Gilchrist LS: Chemotherapy-induced peripheral neuropathy in pediatric cancer patients, *Semin Pediatr Neurol* 19:9–17, 2012.

26. Gilchrist LS, Marais L, Tanner L: Comparison of two chemotherapy-induced peripheral neuropathy measurement approaches in children, *Support Care Cancer* 22:359–366, 2014.

27. Ginsberg JP, Rai SN, Carlson CA, et al.: A comparative analysis of functional mobility in adolescents and young adults with lower-extremity sarcoma, *Pediatr Blood Cancer* 49:964–969, 2007.

28. Götte M, Kesting S, Winter C, et al.: Comparison of self-reported physical activity in children and adolescents before and during cancer treatment, *Pediatr Blood Cancer* 61:1023–1028, 2014.

29. Howlader N, Noone AM, Krapcho M, et al.: *SEER Cancer Statistics Review*, Bethesda, MD, 1975-2012, National Cancer Institute. http://seer.cancer.gov/csr/1975_2012/. Based on November 2014 SEER data submission, posted to the SEER website, April 2015.

30. Hudson MM, Ness KK, Gurney JG, et al.: Clinical ascertainment of health outcomes among adults treated for childhood cancer, *JAMA* 309:2371–2381, 2013.

31. International Classification of Functioning: *Disability, and Health (ICF): ICF full version*, Geneva, Switzerland, 2001, World Health Organization.

32. International Classification of Functioning: *Disability, and Health (ICF): children and youth version*, Geneva, Switzerland, 2007, World Health Organization.

33. Karimova EJ, Rai SN, Deng X, et al.: MRI of knee osteonecrosis in children with leukemia and lymphoma: part 1, observer agreement, *AJR Am J Roentgenol* 186:470–476, 2006.

34. Long-term follow-up guidelines for survivors of childhood, adolescent, and young adult cancers, *Children's oncology group version, 4.0*, 2013. www.survivorshipguidelines.org.

35. Mandanas R: Graft Versus Host Disease. Available at http://emedicine.medscape.com/article/429037-overview Accessed January 16, 2016.

36. Marchese VG, Chiarello LA, Lange BJ: Strength and functional mobility in children with acute lymphoblastic leukemia, *Med Pediatr Oncol* 40:230–232, 2003.

37. Marchese VG, Chiarello LA: Relationships between specific measures of body function, activity, and participation in children with acute lymphoblastic leukemia, *Rehabil Oncol* 22:5–9, 2004.

38. Marchese VG, Chiarello LA, Lange BJ: Effects of physical therapy intervention for children with acute lymphoblastic leukemia, *Pediatr Blood Cancer* 42:127–133, 2004.

39. Marchese VG, Connolly B, Able C, et al.: Relationships among severity of osteonecrosis, pain, range of motion, and functional mobility in children, adolescents, and young adults with acute lymphoblastic leukemia, *Phys Ther* 88:341–350, 2008.

40. Marchese VG, McEvoy CS, Brown H, et al.: Exploring factors that influence childhood cancer survivors' choice of occupation and choice to attend college, *Rehabil Oncol* 32:23–28, 2014.

41. Marchese VG, Miller M, Niethamer L, Koetteritz M: Factors affecting childhood cancer survivors' choice to attend a specific college: a pilot study, *Rehabil Oncol* 30:3, 2012.

42. Marchese VG, Morris GS, Gilchrist L, et al.: Screening for chemotherapy adverse late effects, *Top Geriatr Rehabil* 27:234–243, 2011.

43. Marchese VG, Oriel KN, Fry JA, et al.: Development of a normative sample for the functional mobility assessment, *Pediatr Phys Ther* 24:224–230, 2012.

44. Marchese VG, Rai SN, Carlson CA, et al.: Assessing functional mobility in survivors of lower-extremity sarcoma: reliability and validity of a new tool, *Pediatr Blood Cancer* 49:183–189, 2007.

45. Marchese VG, Spearing E, Callaway L, et al.: Relationships among range of motion, functional mobility, and quality of life in children and adolescents after limb-sparing surgery for lower-extremity sarcoma, *Pediatr Phys Ther* 18:238–244, 2006.

46. Mariotto AB, Rowland JH, Yabroff KR, et al.: Long-term survivors of childhood cancers in the United States, *Cancer Epidemiol Biomarkers Prev* 18:1033–1040, 2009.

47. Mattano LA, Devidas M, Nachman JB, et al.: Effect of alternate-week versus continuous dexamethasone scheduling on the risk of osteonecrosis in paediatric patients with acute lymphoblastic leukaemia: results from the CCG-1961 randomised cohort trial, *Lancet Oncol* 13:906–915, 2012.

48. Meeske KA, Siegel SE, Globe DR, et al.: Prevalence and correlates of fatigue in long-term survivors of childhood leukemia, *J Clin Oncol* 23:5501–5510, 2005.

49. Mello M, Tanaka C, Dulley FL: Effects of an exercise program on muscle performance in patients undergoing allogeneic bone marrow transplantation, *Bone Marrow Transplant* 32:723–728, 2003.

50. Mock V, Burke MB, Sheehan P, et al.: A nursing rehabilitation program for women with breast cancer receiving adjuvant chemotherapy, *Oncol Nurs Forum* 21:899–907, 1994.

51. NCCN Clinical Practice Guidelines in Oncology: *Cancer-related fatigue (version 1.2010 ed.)*, National Comprehensive Cancer Network, 2010.

52. Ness KK, Baker KS, Dengel DR, et al.: Body composition, muscle strength deficits and mobility limitations in adult survivors of childhood acute lymphoblastic leukemia, *Pediatr Blood Cancer* 49:975–981, 2007.

53. Ness KK, Hudson MM, Ginsberg JK, et al.: Physical performance limitation in the Childhood Cancer Survivor Study cohort, *J Clin Oncol* 27:2382–2389, 2009.

54. Ness KK, Armenian SH, Kadan-Lottick N, Gurney JG: Adverse effects of treatment in childhood acute lymphoblastic leukemia: general overview and implications for long-term cardiac health, *Expert Rev Hematol* 4:185–19711.

55. Ness KK, Hudson MM, Pui CH, et al.: Neuromuscular impairments in adult survivors of childhood acute lymphoblastic leukemia: associations with physical performance and chemotherapy doses, *Cancer* 118:828–838, 2012.

56. Ness KK, Jones KE, Smith WA, et al.: Chemotherapy-related neuropathic symptoms and functional impairment in adult survivors of extracranial solid tumors of childhood: results from the St. Jude Lifetime Cohort Study, *Arch Phys Med Rehabil* 94:1451–1457, 2013.

57. Ness KK, Leisenring WM, Huang S, et al.: Predictors of inactive lifestyle among adult survivors of childhood cancer: a report from the Childhood Cancer Survivor Study, *Cancer* 115:1984–1994, 2009.

58. Ness KK, Morris EB, Nolan VG, et al.: Physical performance limitation among adult survivors of childhood brain tumors, *Cancer* 116:3034–3044, 2010.

59. Ness KK, Esbenshade AJ, Friedman DL, et al.: Feasibility and initial effectiveness of home exercise during maintenance therapy for childhood acute lymphoblastic leukemia, *Pediatr Phys Ther* 26:301–307, 2014.

60. Nottage KA, Ness KK, Li C, et al.: Metabolic syndrome and cardiovascular risk among long term survivors of acute lymphoblastic leukaemia: from the St. Jude Lifetime Cohort, *Br J Haematol* 165:364–374, 2014.

61. Reilly JJ, Ventham JC, Callaway L, et al.: Reduced energy expenditure in preobese children treated for acute lymphoblastic leukemia, *Pediatr Res* 44:557–562, 1998.

62. Samuelson K: Standard of care: hematopoietic stem cell transplant (HSCT) in-patient phase, Department of Rehabilitation Services, *Brigham and Women's Hospital*, 2010.

63. San Juan AF, Fleck SJ, Chamorro-vina c, et al.: Effects of an intrahospital exercise program intervention for children with leukemia, *Med Sci Sport Exerc*13–21, 2007.

64. Schleiermacher G, Janoueix-Lerosey I, Delattre O: Recent insights into the biology of neuroblastoma, *Int J Cancer* 135:2249–2261, 2014.

65. Shin KY, Gillis TA, Fine SM: Cancer rehabilitation: general principles. In O'Young BJ, Young MA, Stiens SA, editors: *Physical medicine and rehabilitation secrets*, Philadelphia, 2002, Hanley & Belfus. VII:55, pp 325–333.

66. Skinner R, Wallace WH, Levitt GA, et al.: Long-term follow-up of people who have survived cancer during childhood, *Lancet Oncol* 7:489–498, 2006.

67. Silver JK, Gilchrist LS: Cancer rehabilitation with a focus on evidence based outpatient physical and occupational therapy intervention, *Am J Phys Med Rehabil* 90:S5–S15, 2011.

68. Steiner WA, Ryser L, Huber E, et al.: Use of the ICF model as a clinical problem solving tool in physical therapy and rehabilitation medicine, *Phys Ther* 82:1098–1107, 2002.

69. Styczynski J, Cheung Y-K, Garvin J, et al.: Outcomes of unrelated cord blood transplantation in pediatric recipients, *Bone Marrow Transplant* 34:129–136, 2004.

70. Tewinkel ML, Pieters R, Wind EJ, et al.: Management and treatment of osteonecrosis in children and adolescents with acute lymphoblastic leukemia, *Haematologica* 99:430–436, 2014.

71. Tonorezos ES, Snell PG, Moskowitz CS, et al.: Reduced cardiorespiratory fitness in adult survivors of childhood acute lymphoblastic leukemia, *Pediatr Blood Cancer* 60:1358–1364, 2013.

72. Wright MJ, Fairfield SM: Adaptation and psychometric properties of the gross motor function measure for children receiving treatment for acute lymphoblastic leukemia, *Rehabil Oncol* 25:14–20, 2007.

73. Wright MJ, Galea V, Barr RD: Proficiency of balance in children and youth who have had acute lymphoblastic leukemia, *Phys Ther* 85:782, 2005.

74. Wright MJ, Halton JM, Barr RD: Limitation of ankle range of motion in survivors of acute lymphoblastic leukemia: a cross-sectional study, *Med Pediatr Oncol* 32:279–282, 1998.

75. Young-McCaughan S, Sexton D: A retrospective investigation of the relationship between aerobic exercise and quality of life in women with breast cancer, *Oncol Nurs Forum* 18:751–757, 1991.

SUGGESTED READINGS

Background

Chemotherapy-related neuropathic symptoms and functional impairment in adult survivors of extracranial solid tumors of childhood: results from the St. Jude Lifetime Cohort Study, *Arch Phys Med Rehabil* 94:1451–1457, 2013.

Gilchrist LS: Chemotherapy-induced peripheral neuropathy in pediatric cancer patients, *Semin Pediatr Neurol* 19:9–17, 2012.

Ginsberg JP, Rai SN, Carlson CA, et al.: A comparative analysis of functional mobility in adolescents and young adults with lower-extremity sarcoma, *Pediatr Blood Cancer* 49:964–969, 2007.

Hudson MM, Ness KK, Gurney JG, et al.: Clinical ascertainment of health outcomes among adults treated for childhood cancer, *JAMA* 309:2371–2381, 2013.

Lavoie Smith EM, et al.: Patterns and severity of vincristine-induced peripheral neuropathy in children with acute lymphoblastic leukemia, *J Periph Nerv Syst* 2015:37–46, 2015.

Long-term follow-up guidelines for survivors of childhood, adolescent, and young adult cancers: Children's oncology group version, 4.0. 2013, www.survivorshipguidelines.org.

Meeske KA, Siegel SE, Globe DR, et al.: Prevalence and correlates of fatigue in long-term survivors of childhood leukemia, *J Clin Oncol* 23:5501–5510, 2005.

Foreground

Marchese VG, Chiarello LA, Lange BJ: Effects of physical therapy intervention for children with acute lymphoblastic leukemia, *Pediatr Blood Cancer* 42:127–133, 2004.

Marchese VG, Morris GS, Gilchrist L, et al.: Screening for chemotherapy adverse late effects, *Top Geriatr Rehabil* 27:234–243, 2011.

Marchese VG, Rai SN, Carlson CA, et al.: Assessing functional mobility in survivors of lower-extremity sarcoma: reliability and validity of a new tool, *Pediatr Blood Cancer* 49:183–189, 2007.

Mello M, Tanaka C, Dulley FL: Effects of an exercise program on muscle performance in patients undergoing allogeneic bone marrow transplantation, *Bone Marrow Transplant* 32:723–728, 2003.

Ness KK, Hudson MM, Ginsberg JK, et al.: Physical performance limitation in the Childhood Cancer Survivor Study cohort, *J Clin Oncol* 27:2382–2389, 2009.

San Juan AF, Fleck SJ, Chamorro-vina C, et al.: Effects of an intrahospital exercise program intervention for children with leukemia, *Med Sci Sports Exerc* 13–21, 2007.

Silver JK, Gilchrist LS: Cancer rehabilitation with a focus on evidence based outpatient physical and occupational therapy intervention, *Am J Phys Med Rehabil* 90:S5–S15, 2011.

Wright MJ, Fairfield SM: Adaptation and psychometric properties of the gross motor function measure for children receiving treatment for acute lymphoblastic leukemia, *Rehabil Oncol* 25:14–20, 2007.

17

Developmental Coordination Disorder

Lisa Rivard, Nancy Pollock, Jennifer Siemon, Cheryl Missiuna

Pediatric physical therapists evaluate and manage care for children presenting with a variety of motor challenges. They observe children's movement patterns and skills and ask key questions about children's motor abilities and development to differentiate among motor behaviors that are characteristic of particular conditions. This differentiation guides their selection of a course of intervention. Some of the children whom physical therapists observe are quite a "puzzle" to figure out. These children frequently trip over their feet and bump into others with clumsy, awkward movements. They may have an unusual gait pattern or a unique way of "fixing" or stabilizing their joints. Despite these differences, they are often observed to reach their motor milestones within normal age limits. Many of these children appear to have difficulty generalizing learned motor skills across settings or transferring skills to other contexts. Each child with motor difficulties such as these presents a little differently from the others, making it difficult to develop and apply a treatment approach. The children who are captured by this description are those who have developmental coordination disorder (DCD).[3]

Approximately 5% to 6% of school-age children have movement difficulties unrelated to specific neurologic conditions or cognitive impairment that limit their potential and affect their long-term academic achievement.[3] Recently, the prevalence rate for the most significantly impaired children in a UK birth cohort of 6990 children aged 7 to 8 years was close to 2% of the population.[107] These children struggle with everyday functional tasks such as handwriting,[9] dressing,[61,120] throwing and catching balls,[5,6] and learning to ride a bicycle.[114,128] They experience daily frustration with activities that are effortless for their peers, and, as a consequence of their motor problems, they may demonstrate additional difficulties, including poor perceived competence,[186,187] social isolation,[33,170] low self-worth,[57,153,155,187] anxiety,[54,132,171] and depressive symptoms,[57,108,125] even at early ages. These difficulties are characteristic features of DCD, a condition in which poorly developed fine and/or gross motor coordination has a substantial impact on motor skill performance with far-reaching consequences for daily life activities and scholastic achievement.[3] Although it was once believed that these difficulties would diminish with time and maturation, compelling evidence now suggests that DCD is a lifelong condition,[25,37,44,54] making this disorder one that warrants significant attention.

Physical therapists have a unique service to offer children with DCD and their families. Therapists' understanding of normal and abnormal motor control, motor learning, and motor development can be used to identify and evaluate the condition and to plan programs for children with DCD. Through education of children with DCD and their families, teachers, and others in the community, physical therapists can help children with DCD become more active and successful participants in their home, school, and community life.

The information presented in this chapter is intended to increase awareness, recognition, and understanding of children with DCD. The complex nature of DCD and its challenges for clinical management are described. The role of the physical therapist in managing children with this disorder and intervention approaches shown to be effective with children with DCD are explored. Evidence is presented to support the need for a multidisciplinary assessment and tailored, child- and family-centered intervention with collaborative consultation is emphasized. Three cases found on Expert Consult illustrate the heterogeneity of the disorder—a factor that greatly influences the decision-making process and strategies employed in the management of a child with DCD. Resources available for children with DCD and their families, as well as health professionals involved in their care, are provided on the Expert Consult website.

BACKGROUND INFORMATION

HISTORICAL BACKGROUND

A disorder of "clumsiness" whose key feature is poor motor coordination has been recognized and described for over a century. Much of our current understanding of DCD, however, has resulted from an explosion of research in the field over the past two decades.[115] DCD is a childhood disorder that is of interest to numerous professionals in the medical, rehabilitation, and education fields. Clinicians and researchers, each adopting various perspectives on the condition, have utilized diverse theoretical frameworks in their study of children with DCD. This wide-reaching interest in DCD has provided fertile ground for the development of knowledge about the condition. Historically, however, this diversity in perspectives also led to a lack of consensus, impacting the progression of research in the field. Different labels have been ascribed to children with DCD over the years, including the clumsy child syndrome,[69] the physically awkward child,[229] developmental dyspraxia[30] sensory integrative dysfunction,[7] disorder of attention, motor and perception (DAMP),[64] and minor coordination dysfunction,[233] each reflecting the perspectives of professionals who work with these children.[135] In 1994 an international consensus exercise was undertaken[163] and the term *DCD* was adopted to unify descriptions of children with significant motor incoordination. This decision, in part, was grounded in the recognition that DCD had become an officially recognized movement skills disorder.[3] In 2006, a second international consensus conference recommended maintaining use of the term *DCD*.[216] Although *DCD* is the term now most widely used in the literature, other terms have continued to persist, highlighting the diverse perspectives of researchers who study children with motor difficulties.

BACKGROUND INFORMATION

DEFINITION AND PREVALENCE

DCD is a chronic condition involving impairment in gross motor, postural, and/or fine motor performance that affects a child's ability to perform the skilled movements necessary for daily living, including the performance of academic and self-care tasks. By definition, DCD is not attributable to a known neurologic or medical disorder.[3] The manifestation of the disorder varies across children, with a spectrum of severity.

Research performed in many countries around the world has confirmed that large numbers of children are affected by this childhood motor disorder.[56,86,93,107,252] Attention is increasingly being paid to this disorder because of the impact of children's primary motor limitations on everyday life. The American Psychiatric Association (APA) estimates that DCD affects 5% to 6% of school-age children. Although it is commonly accepted that boys with DCD outnumber girls by a 2:1 ratio,[3] a recent population-based study of children with DCD would suggest that more equal numbers of boys and girls may be affected.[126] The prevalence of DCD appears to be substantially higher than average in preterm/low birth weight populations.[48,241,250] It has also been noted that, over time, preterm/low birth weight infants tend to exhibit poor coordination and many of the physical consequences associated with DCD such as decreased aerobic fitness, strength, and physical activity levels.[183]

Etiology and Pathophysiology

Although much has been learned regarding the body structure and function deficits of children with DCD and the potential sensory, motor control, and motor learning processes affected, the etiology of the disorder remains poorly understood.[227,256] Currently, no specific pathologic process or single neuroanatomic site has been definitively associated with DCD, but many behavioral studies, in particular studies on co-occurring conditions and possible subtypes of DCD, have led researchers to speculate as to the underlying mechanism(s) involved in DCD. Some researchers have postulated that diffuse, rather than distinct, areas of the brain may be affected, resulting in the variable expression of the disorder and the different profiles seen in children with DCD (including co-occurring conditions).[95] This would imply that the specific combination of co-occurring disorders depends on the location and severity of neurologic insult. This theory, however, does not take into account cases where developmental disorders occur alone.[227] Recent work conducted in the area of subtyping

has suggested that subcortical structures such as the thalamus may play a role.[223] Other researchers highlight the strong association between motor, attention, and perceptual processes and point to the possible role of neuroanatomic structures such as the cerebellum and basal ganglia.[64]

Research studies employing a dual-task paradigm indicate a lack of automatization of motor actions in children with DCD when attentional demands increase.[34,104] These findings implicate the cerebellum as a possible site of pathophysiology in children with DCD, given its known role in the automatization and learning of motor tasks.[26,102,191] The thinking behind the interference seen in dual-task paradigms is that performance of one task will be negatively affected by the second if both tasks need to make use of the same "pool" of resources, including visual and cognitive resources. Concurrent work examining motor adaptation, or the ability of children with DCD to adapt performance to changing environmental contexts, comes to a similar conclusion with respect to the potential role of the cerebellum in children with DCD. In these studies, children with motor difficulties show poor adaptation to gradual changes in environmental stimuli.[13,26] Given the rapid growth and vulnerability of the developing cerebellum to external events in the first year of life, theories regarding the possible link between cerebellar involvement and motor impairments are plausible.[66] Although the proposed link between motor coordination difficulties and the role of the cerebellum appears to be strong,[256] especially in situations of co-occurring conditions,[148,156] testing of causal models will be necessary to confirm these hypotheses.

Another avenue of research includes the investigation of motor imagery deficits in children with DCD. Understanding in this area has led to a proposal that impaired feed forward models could be a potential mechanism underlying DCD (efference-copy-deficit hypothesis).[246,249] In this theory, motor imagery deficits seen in children with DCD are related to difficulties in generating efference copies of motor commands through feed forward models, pointing to the possible involvement of the posterior parietal cortex.[246]

Recently, increasing interest in the possibility of impaired internal models can be seen in the DCD literature.[1,94] Internal models have been defined as neural representations of the visual-spatial coordinates of intended motor actions.[121] It has been hypothesized that children with motor impairment may have inadequate forward (predictive) modeling of movements and are unable to form, access, or update their internal models, which results in poor "online" error correction and ultimately affects motor learning over time.[209,248] It has been postulated that internal models may be located in the cerebellum or parieto-cerebellar network.[248,256] Findings from a recent metaanalysis of research conducted from 1997 to 2011 strongly suggest involvement of the cerebellum, given the pattern of deficits observed in DCD including poor predictive modeling and "online" correction, difficulties with rhythmic timing, executive function, posture and gait, catching and interceptive skills, as well as visual and tactile processing.[248] Parallel work investigating the role of "mirror neurons" (which are housed in the ventral premotor and posterior parietal cortices) has shed additional light on how motor representations are formed not only during the performance, but also in the observation, of movements.[121,181] Mirror neurons in the posterior parietal cortex may work in concert with internal models in the cerebellum through extensive neural projections between these two brain structures to code and update movement.[121]

Taken together, behavioral studies implicating different cortical and subcortical areas and the recent discovery and understanding of the role of mirror neurons suggest that a complex and shared interplay may occur between different neuroanatomic regions of the brain when learning, executing, and correcting movements. Research studies employing neuro-diagnostic technologies such as functional magnetic resonance imaging, diffusion tensor imaging, and electroencephalography are becoming more prevalent in the literature investigating possible mechanisms involved in DCD.[40,97,149] These experimental studies are demonstrating differences in brain activation patterns between children with and without DCD.[106,256] Combined with behavioral research, this work is beginning to shed more light on the specific neuroanatomic sites that may be involved in the pathophysiology of DCD.

In the end, why are there so many plausible theories regarding the origin of DCD and so many proposed sites of neurologic abnormality? The production of well-coordinated, smooth motor movements is a complex process requiring multiple levels of information processing, each of which requires different abilities such as sensory acuity, memory, decision making, attention, perception, as well as feedback and feed forward mechanisms. It is likely that children with DCD may have impairments in one or more of these functions and in related brain areas and that different groups of children may have abnormalities in different neural correlates.[66,87,256] Other possible influencing factors have already been alluded to earlier in this chapter. The heterogeneity of the disorder and the presence of co-occurring conditions give rise to different profiles of impairment, which may indeed have different underlying neural mechanisms.

DIAGNOSIS

DCD is present when (1) motor impairment and/or motor skill delay significantly impacts a child's ability to perform age-appropriate complex motor activities, (2) adequate opportunities for experience and practice have been provided, and (3) no other explanation can be offered for the motor impairment. In most states and provinces a diagnosis of DCD can be made only by a physician because it is critical to rule out any other underlying neurologic or medical reasons for the observed motor impairment. Four distinct criteria must be met for a diagnosis of DCD to be given, as outlined in the *Diagnostic and Statistical Manual of Mental Disorders* (Box 17.1)[3]: (1) The learning and performance of coordinated motor skills are not what would be expected based on a child's age and experiences/opportunities for motor skill development; (2) the motor difficulties have a significant impact on self-care activities, academic achievement, leisure, and play; (3) the difficulties begin early in development; and (4) the observed motor challenges are not better explained by intellectual or visual impairment or neurologic conditions that impact movement abilities.[3] In situations where more than one developmental or behavioral disorder is present (i.e., developmental coordination disorder with co-occurring attention deficit disorder, or autism spectrum disorder, etc.), it has been recommended that all diagnoses should be given.[11,216] Physical therapists have an important role to play in facilitating a diagnosis of DCD by providing physicians with an assessment of a child's motor coordination and the impact of motor challenges on everyday life activities. This will be discussed in greater detail later in this chapter.

> ### BOX 17.1 Diagnostic Criteria for Developmental Coordination Disorder (DCD)
>
> The acquisition and execution of coordinated motor skills is substantially below that expected given the individual's chronologic age and opportunity for skill learning and use. Difficulties are manifested as clumsiness (e.g., dropping or bumping into objects) as well as slowness and inaccuracy of performance of motor skills (e.g., catching an object, using scissors or cutlery, handwriting, riding a bike, or participating in sports).
>
> The motor skills deficit in Criterion A significantly and persistently interferes with activities of daily living appropriate to chronologic age (e.g., self-care and self-maintenance) and impacts academic/school productivity, prevocational and vocational activities, leisure, and play.
>
> Onset of symptoms is in the early developmental period.
>
> The motor skills deficits are not better explained by intellectual disability (intellectual developmental disorder) or visual impairment and are not attributable to a neurologic condition affecting movement (e.g., cerebral palsy, muscular dystrophy, degenerative disorder).

American Psychiatric Association: *Diagnostic and statistical manual of mental disorders* (5th ed.). Washington, DC, Author, 2013.

> ### BOX 17.2 Developmental Coordination Disorder (DCD): Differential Diagnosis
>
> Coordination difficulties are likely not DCD when a history of any of the following is reported:
> - Recent head injury or trauma
> - Deterioration in previously learned or acquired skills
> - Headaches, eye pain, blurred vision
> - Global developmental delays
> - Increased muscle tone, fluctuating tone, or significant hypotonia
> - Asymmetrical tone or strength
> - Musculoskeletal abnormality
> - Neurocutaneous lesion
> - Avoidance of eye contact, unwillingness to engage socially
> - Gowers' sign (difficulty rising to a standing position)
> - Ataxia, dysarthria
> - Absence of deep tendon reflexes
> - Dysmorphic features
> - Visual impairment (untreated)

From Missiuna C, Gaines R, Soucie H: Why every office needs a tennis ball: a new approach to assessing the clumsy child. *Can Med Assoc J 175*, 471-473, 2006.

DCD usually is not considered to be present if (1) recent head injury or trauma has occurred, (2) progressive deterioration in previously acquired skills is evident, or (3) increased or fluctuating muscle tone is present. DCD also would not be suspected routinely where there is a history of headaches or blurred vision, when evidence of asymmetrical tone or strength is observed, or when musculoskeletal abnormalities or Gowers' sign is present (Box 17.2).[70,130] If children do not show any of these signs but demonstrate uncoordinated movements and motor abilities below those expected for their age, they may have DCD, and it is important for these children to be seen by a physician. A medical practitioner can rule out other possible causes for poor coordination, including genetic causes (e.g., Down syndrome), neurologic disorders (e.g., cerebral palsy), degenerative conditions (e.g., muscular dystrophy, brain tumors), musculoskeletal abnormalities (e.g., Legg-Calvé-Perthes disease), sensory impairments (e.g., impaired visual acuity), cognitive impairment (e.g., developmental delay), pervasive developmental disorder (e.g., autism), and head injury (e.g., traumatic brain injury) (Box

BOX 17.3   **Developmental Coordination Disorder**

Medical and neurologic disorders that can be associated with motor incoordination must be excluded before a formal diagnosis of DCD is made. These include the following:
- Genetic disorders (e.g., Down syndrome)
- Neurologic disorders (e.g., cerebral palsy)
- Degenerative conditions (e.g., Duchenne muscular dystrophy, brain tumor)
- Musculoskeletal disorders (e.g., Legg-Calvé-Perthes disease)
- Physical impairments (e.g., impaired visual acuity)
- Cognitive impairments (e.g., developmental delay)
- Pervasive developmental disorders (e.g., autism)
- Injuries (e.g., traumatic brain injury)
- Environmental contaminants (e.g., lead, pesticides)

From Missiuna C, Gaines R, Soucie H: Why every office needs a tennis ball: a new approach to assessing the clumsy child. *Can Med Assoc J* 175:471-473, 2006.

17.3).[70,130] See respective chapters in this volume for further information on these other conditions.

CO-OCCURRING CONDITIONS

Strong associations have been demonstrated between DCD and attention deficit hyperactivity disorder (ADHD),[42,158,172,220] speech/articulation difficulties (specific language impairment [SLI]),[58,81,156,235] and language-based learning disabilities (LDs) (in particular, reading disability).[90] When a child has any of these conditions, the likelihood that DCD is also present is at least 50%. When criteria for more than one disorder are met, more than one diagnosis should be given.[3,216] It is recognized that the presence of co-occurring conditions may increase the probability of negative outcomes. In particular, children who have DCD in addition to ADHD have a significantly poorer outcome in terms of academic achievement and mental health than children with ADHD alone.[75,172,220] It is important to determine whether motor coordination problems are present and whether they are occurring in combination with another recognized condition. Knowledge of a child's complete profile (including associated conditions) will assist in the identification process and will help to determine intervention and management strategies. The frequently documented association between other developmental disorders and DCD underscores the need for a multidisciplinary assessment.

LONG-TERM PROGNOSIS

Longitudinal research clearly demonstrates that, without intervention, children with DCD do not "grow out of" the disorder. Strong evidence indicates that the motor problems of childhood persist into adolescence and adulthood.[25,37,44,54] In fact, children with DCD are at risk of developing serious negative physical, social, emotional, behavioral, and mental health consequences that are not limited to the presenting motor difficulties. Multiple studies have shown that, over time, children with DCD are more likely to demonstrate poor social, academic, and physical competence[186,232,255] social isolation,[33,210] academic and behavior problems,[172] poor self-esteem,[232] low self-efficacy,[49] victimization,[153] and higher rates of psychiatric and mental health problems.[125,172,204]

Children with DCD engage in less vigorous play and spend significantly more time away from the playground area than peers.[68,180] They spend more time alone on the playground and spend less time in formal and informal team play.[210] Many researchers have shown that they are less likely to be physically fit[180] or to participate voluntarily in motor activity,[231] predisposing them to an inactive lifestyle. Reduced physical activity participation[20,21] and the associated risks for long-term obesity[19,80,198] and poor cardiovascular health in children with DCD[50,51,91] are now being documented. Although this picture of the numerous consequences associated with motor impairment appears dire, the potential exists for positive trajectories and pathways of resilience.[138] The long-term outcome of the disorder is influenced not only by the severity of impairment and co-occurring conditions but also by the presence of supportive environments and the strengths of individuals with DCD, including coping mechanisms. It is possible to "tip the scale" in favor of more positive outcomes,[133] and physical therapists can be instrumental in preventing secondary impairments, which often become areas of greater focus as children mature.

The increased risk for children with DCD of secondary health issues and academic failure highlights the need to identify children with DCD as early as possible.[140] Early identification may facilitate the education of teachers and parents about how to make tasks easier and how to ensure that activities are matched to children's capabilities. In this way, children with DCD can be provided with optimally challenging situations that emphasize mastery and avoid multiple failed attempts.[141]

DESCRIBING CHILDREN WITH DCD

The International Classification of Functioning, Disability, and Health (ICF) provides a useful framework for understanding and describing the difficulties experienced by children with DCD.[251] In the ICF model, observable sensory/perceptual and motor impairments at the level of body structure and function can lead to difficulties with skill acquisition and task performance or activity limitations. These activity constraints, in turn, can place limitations on participation in the many aspects of daily life, conceptualized in the ICF framework as participation restrictions. In addition, personal and environmental factors are seen as important mediating factors at each of these levels (Table 17.1).

Body Structure and Function

Any description of children with DCD is influenced by the heterogeneity of the condition. The presentation of DCD is somewhat age dependent, is highly variable across children, and is complicated by the possible presence of co-occurring conditions. This variability in presentation has led investigators to examine multiple sensory and motor processes that contribute to the development of motor coordination. In a recent review of research into possible underlying mechanisms for DCD, primary impairments at the level of body structure and function have been proposed in the sensory, motor, and sensorimotor domains (Table 17.2).[227]

Primary Impairments

Sensory/perceptual deficits. Early research on children with DCD indicated deficiencies in kinesthetic processing and poor proprioceptive function.[110,197] Children with DCD have also been shown to have impairments in visual-spatial processing,

TABLE 17.1 Relationships Among Body Structures and Function, Activity, and Participation for a Child With Developmental Coordination Disorder (DCD)

Health Condition	Body Structure and Function	Activity Limitations	Participation Restrictions: Environmental Factors	Participation Restrictions: Personal Factors
Unknown/possibly heterogeneous nervous system insult (of prenatal, perinatal, or postnatal origin)	Neurologic "soft" signs Poor strength Poor coordination Jerky movements Poor visual perception Joint laxity Poor spatial organization Inadequate information processing Poor sequencing Poor feedback and feed forward motor control Poor memory	Awkward, slow gait Delayed and poor quality of fine and gross motor skills, such as hopping, jumping, ball skills, and writing Delayed oral-motor skills	Doors too heavy to open Physical education is competitive and skill oriented Time to dress and undress reduces participation in recess and readiness for home and community activities Slow and messy written communication in class limits academic performance	Depressed Quits trying to participate, unmotivated Low self-esteem Poor fitness Activities performed without concern for time restrictions Vocational anxiety

TABLE 17.2 Impairments of Body Structure and Function Identified in Children With Developmental Coordination Disorder (DCD)

Body Function	Reference
Visual-perceptual, visuospatial, and visuomotor impairment	Mon-Williams et al., 1999[143]; O'Brien et al., 1988[147]; Wilson and McKenzie, 1998[247]; Wilson et al., 2013[248]
Inefficient use of visual feedback in fast, goal-directed arm movements	van der Meulen et al., 1991[225]
Impaired visual memory	Dwyer and McKenzie, 1994[47]
More dependent on visuospatial rehearsal to memorize	Skorji and McKenzie, 1997[205]
Difficulty with visual and motor sequencing tasks requiring short- and long-term recall	Murphy and Gliner, 1988[144]
Impairments of size-constancy judgments, spatial position, and visual discrimination	Lord and Hulme, 1987[110]
Slow performance related to reliance on information feedback rather than feed forward programming	Missiuna et al., 2003[140]; Smyth, 1991[213]
Slow reaction time and movement time related to impaired response selection	Raynor, 1998[174]; Van Dellan and Geuze, 1988
Prolonged response latency related to the process of searching for and retrieving the correct responses with reliable timing	Henderson et al., 1992[77]
Poor timing, rhythm, and force control	Volman and Geuze, 1998[228]; Williams et al., 1992[240]
Impaired performance on kinesthetic acuity, linear positioning, and weight discrimination	Hoare and Larkin, 1991[84]
Prolonged burst of agonist activity and delayed onset of antagonist activity	Huh et al., 1998[85]
Reduced power and strength	Raynor, 2001[175]
Reduced ability to successfully inhibit an action	Mandich et al., 2002[116]

including difficulties determining object size and position, a limited ability to use visual rehearsal strategies,[43] and deficits with visual memory.[47] More recent research suggests that in children with DCD, visual feedback is managed differently and is processed more slowly than in typically developing children.[254] Several studies have confirmed that children with DCD demonstrate a heavy reliance on visual feedback to guide task performance.[52,77,124] This predominant use of vision to control movement is observed well beyond the age at which typically developing children would rely on vision.[124,205,212] As a result, children with DCD lack automation in movement patterns and remain at an early stage of motor learning for much longer.

Because both visual and kinesthetic perceptual deficits have been demonstrated in groups of children with DCD, it has been suggested that the deficit may not be confined to one specific sensory modality but may be multisensory in nature.[242] This seems plausible given that fluent, coordinated movements require multiple processes to plan, execute, and, when necessary, correct motor activity. Further, the motor impairments could be accounted for by impaired perception-action coupling

or poor integration of the senses,[202,211,254] including poor "mapping" of visual and proprioceptive information with the motor system.[143,184]

Research examining different profiles, or subtypes, of children with motor impairment has contributed to understanding in the area of possible sensory/perceptual deficits. Although studies have differed on the specific clusters of children identified and the individual characteristics of the subgroups,[44,83,112,142,223] there appears to be general agreement that there is a group of children who demonstrate a generalized, and often significant, perceptual deficit, including both visual and kinesthetic difficulties. Questions remain, however, because these specific perceptual deficits have not been shown to be present in all subgroups with motor impairment. This again serves to underscore the heterogeneity of the condition and suggests that different profiles of motor coordination problems may exist in children with DCD with varying sensory/perceptual impairments.

Motor deficits. Children with DCD move awkwardly and slowly, with a rigid, jerky movement quality.[5,94,238] They frequently bump into objects and people and have a tendency to trip and fall.[100] Poor balance, especially pronounced during single-leg stance, and difficulty maintaining postures are often noted (see video of Bill on Expert Consult for an example of a child with similar problems).[238] To compensate for balance instability, children with DCD may demonstrate many associated movements.[100] On physical examination, decreased muscle tone and neurologic soft signs can often be observed. This constellation of physical signs, combined with the possible sensory deficits outlined previously, has led many to hypothesize that the origins of the motor impairments seen in children with DCD may lie in faulty motor control and motor learning processes.

Motor control deficits. Children with DCD demonstrate inappropriate and ineffective neuromuscular strategies, both in muscular activation and in sequencing, using atypical postural control strategies,[82,84,229,238] including when balance is challenged.[239] An increased level of muscle co-contraction has also been described, with children with DCD demonstrating a much less effective method of muscular organization than peers, which did not improve with age.[151,175] Children with movement difficulties tend to "fix" or stabilize joints during task performance.[175,201] This deliberate joint stabilization leads to lack of movement fluency[140] and contributes to a stiff, awkward, and clumsy appearance[201]; it also increases the time it takes them to adapt to changes in their movement environment.[124] Fixing can be thought of as a strategy to control the multiple degrees of freedom of joints and muscles for efficient functioning. Children with DCD who "fix" joints during task performance are more likely to experience fatigue[150] and to demonstrate inconsistency in task performance.[124,201] Overall, the postural fixation and atypical muscular activation and sequencing seen in children with DCD result in less efficient movement patterns and reflect a less skilled stage of movement acquisition than is typical of age-matched peers.

When performing reaching tasks, children with DCD use different neuromuscular strategies than typically developing age-matched peers, contributing to slower and more variable movement and reaction times, as well as movement inaccuracy.[77,88,111,224,236,240] Evidence from subtyping and other research would suggest that, although some children with DCD exhibit problems primarily in execution and control of movements, others have difficulties related to motor planning processes.[61,209,213]

Children with DCD display gait differences that have also been suggested to be due to movement variability.[189] Decreased and variable force control and difficulties with temporal precision (both movement production and time perception) have also been noted in the motor control literature.[60,77,88,236,240]

As can be seen from extensive motor control research, in comparison with typically developing peers, children with DCD demonstrate variations in movement speed, timing, and force across a series of different tasks, resulting in qualitative differences in movement and motor control patterns. Difficulties with error detection and movement correction during the execution of motor skills are especially evident when motor tasks are complex and involve spatial uncertainty.

Motor learning deficits. In addition to poorly controlled movements, children with DCD exhibit limited movement repertoires, lacking both adaptability and flexibility in motor behavior.[103] This, along with the variability and inconsistency in motor performance, suggests difficulties in motor learning processes.[6]

Although children with DCD may achieve motor milestones within normal time limits, they have difficulty learning new motor skills.[76,124] They fail to see the similarities between motor tasks and thus are unable to transfer learned skills from one activity to a closely related activity. They also experience difficulty generalizing from one context or situation to another. Both of these processes reflect an early, more cognitive stage of motor learning (see Chapter 4 for more information on motor learning).[124,131,132] According to motor learning theory, as skills are learned, feedback requirements lessen and change, with proprioceptive and kinesthetic feedback relied on more than visual input.[53] Children with DCD continue to rely predominantly on visual information, as if they were still in the early stages of motor learning. As a result, the motor performance of children with DCD is sometimes more similar to that of younger children than to that of age peers.

Children with coordination difficulties have also been described as repeating tasks the same way over and over again, regardless of success with the task.[76,119] They appear to have difficulty understanding the demands of a task and its component parts, interpreting environmental cues, and selecting the best motor response for a task.[65] As a result, they do not effectively use the feedback originating from knowledge of past performance to prepare for upcoming actions (anticipatory preparation), and they have difficulty adapting to situational demands.[63,65,131] It has been postulated that children with DCD might attend to the wrong cues and not to the more salient aspects of available feedback.[65] Others have suggested that the problem might lie in the failure of children with DCD to use anticipatory control strategies for motor tasks[238]; as a result, they might have to rely heavily on a feedback or closed loop strategy to control movement.[184,209]

Secondary Impairments

Physical. Although slow, awkward movements are typical of children with DCD and are easy to casually observe (e.g., see video of Bill), what is less evident is the extra effort that motor skills seem to require and the struggle that children have in making adaptations and in "fine-tuning" movements.[28] Secondary impairments related to the primary motor coordination difficulties are of considerable concern and include lack of energy and fatigue, as well as decreased strength, power, and endurance.[175,180] Children with DCD complain of being tired more easily than peers and are often exhausted by the end of the day as they must exert more effort during motor-based activities at school and at home.[100] They can often be observed leaning against the wall or on other children when standing, or assuming a slouched posture when sitting (Fig. 17.1). Recent strong empirical evidence indicates a progressive decrease in strength and power in children with DCD over time, which is already apparent between the ages of 6 and 9 years.[175] Obesity in children with DCD and the relationship between motor difficulties and cardiovascular risk factors have begun to be studied in greater detail.[19,51] As will be discussed later in this chapter, these secondary sequelae are precursors for participation restrictions in sporting and/or leisure activities, reduced opportunities for social interaction, and diminished physical fitness across the life span. Secondary impairments in children with DCD may be preventable and are appropriate targets for physical therapy.

Social/Emotional/Behavioral. Often children with DCD demonstrate associated behavioral problems that become the focus of concern, especially in the classroom.[179] Children with DCD may be quiet and withdrawn at school, with avoidance of schoolwork and frequent "off-task" behaviors.[31,32,128]

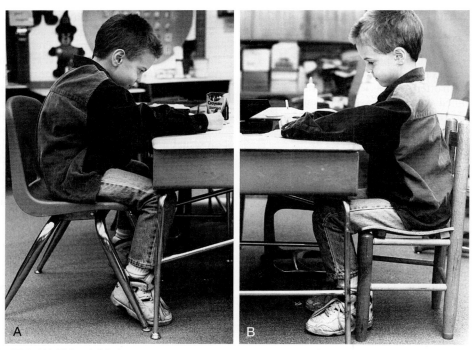

FIG. 17.1 (A) This child demonstrates poor posture that interferes with fine motor classroom activities. (B) A different desk and chair improve this child's posture and improve the precision of his fine motor activities.

Alternatively, children may act out in class, disrupting the teacher and/or others.[120] Learning new skills in physical education is a continuous challenge (e.g., see video of Bill), and children may try to avoid these classes with complaints of illness or problem behaviors. Avoidance of written work can result in "behaviors" such as needing to sharpen the pencil multiple times, talking and asking questions, attention seeking, and interference with other children. Low frustration tolerance, decreased motivation, and poor self-esteem are commonly observed.[204] Children with movement difficulties give up on tasks easily, which occasionally leads to angry, aggressive classroom behavior. Task initiation and task completion are often major issues, both at home and at school.[128]

Like the physical impairments outlined previously, these associated social, emotional, and behavioral difficulties can be significant but are not inevitable. All efforts should be made through early identification and management to prevent their occurrence.

Activity Limitations

How do the proposed body structure and function deficits manifest themselves in a practical sense? Children with DCD tend to have the greatest difficulty with skills that must be taught. In particular, skills requiring accuracy and refined eye-hand coordination and that require constant monitoring of feedback pose significant challenges for the child with DCD.[132,216] Children with DCD may experience difficulty with fine motor activities, gross motor activities, or both (see video of Bill).[113] These activity limitations are readily observable in the classroom, on the school playground, and at home.[31,128]

Fine Motor Activity Limitations

Self-care. The ability of children with DCD to perform self-care activities such as doing up snaps, zippers, and buttons,

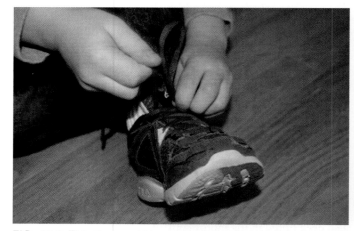

FIG. 17.2 This 8-year-old boy still cannot independently tie his shoes. His verbal cues were "loop around and go through." He forgot to "loop around" and forgot to make a second loop.

tying shoelaces, opening snack containers, and managing juice boxes is poorer than expected for their age. Tying shoelaces is an example of a skilled activity required at school by the time a student is in first grade. Children with impairments in sequencing skills cannot correctly sequence the steps in shoe tying, even though they may have practiced it many times before. When children with DCD make a mistake in one step of the sequence, they have to start over again rather than simply redo the last step. Or they might omit a different step in the sequence each time they try to tie shoes (Fig. 17.2). At home, parents notice difficulties when children are using cutlery, and there is a tendency to spill liquid from drinking glasses or when pouring from a container. Parents also describe problems

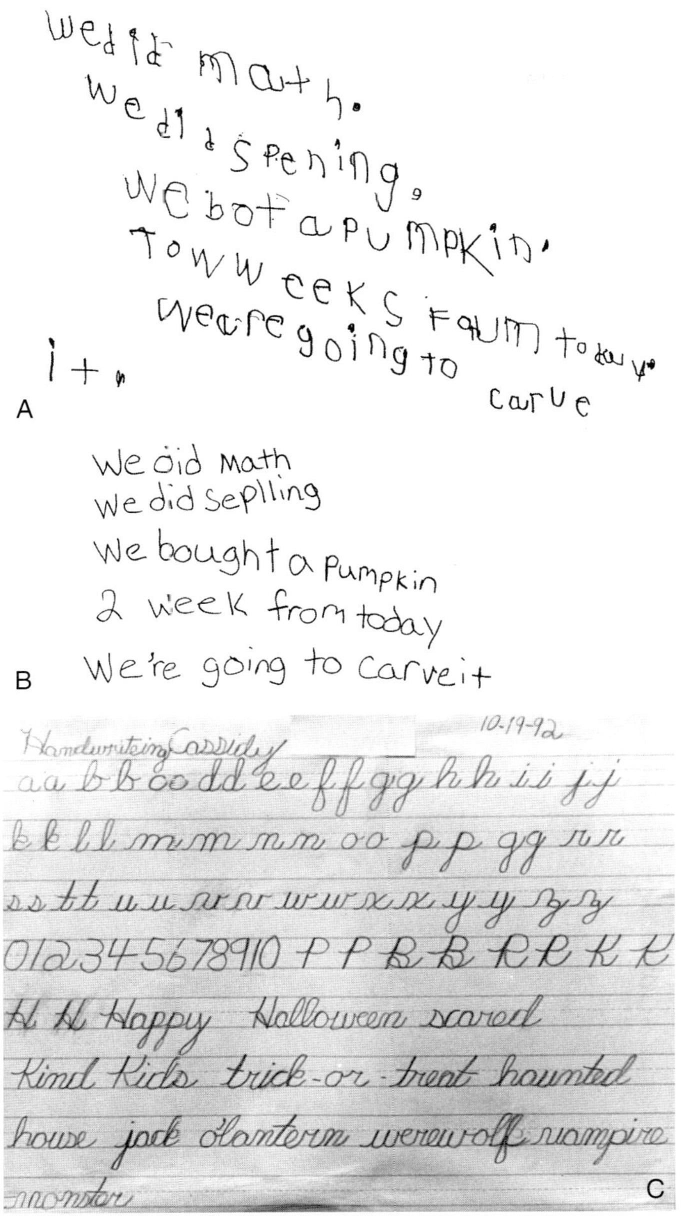

Handwriting samples (A, B, C)

A

Wedid math.
Wedid Spening,
We bot a pumpkin,
Toww eeks faum tokuy
weare going to
i+. carve

B

We did Math
We did seplling
We bought a pumpkin
2 week from today
We're going to carve it

C

Handwriting Cassidy 10-19-92

FIG. 17.3 (A) Handwriting sample of a third-grade child with developmental coordination disorder and a learning disability. (B) Handwriting sample obtained for comparison from a randomly selected third grade peer without motor difficulties. (C) Sample of cursive writing from another peer without motor difficulties demonstrates an even more advanced expectation of third grade students.

with grooming such as bathing, combing hair, and brushing teeth.[120,128,218] At school, children with movement difficulties are often the last to get snowsuits, jackets, and boots on or to get knapsacks organized to go home at the end of the day.

Academic. Classroom fine motor difficulties include problems with printing and handwriting (Fig. 17.3).[8,122] Written work is illegible and inconsistent in sizing and requires great effort.[188] Frequent erasures of work, inaccurate spacing of words, and unusual letter formation are evident.[100] Pencil/crayon grasps are awkward, and written work is not well aligned. Pencils may

be dropped frequently and pencil leads broken or paper torn as the result of excessive pressure on the page.[28,100] Because of this, teachers and parents often note that children with DCD have difficulty finishing academic tasks, including homework, on time. Children with these difficulties tend to rush through tasks or may be unusually slow (see video of Bill). Academic tasks that have a motor component require extra effort and attentional resources. Children with DCD can become fatigued and frustrated, as they work harder than children their age to complete the same activity. Teachers often describe a large discrepancy between oral and written work. Copying from the board and other fine motor tasks such as completing puzzles and turning door handles or washroom taps are also affected. Many children with DCD tend to avoid art projects and craft activities that require coloring, cutting, and pasting.[120,134]

Overall, children with DCD, in comparison with typically developing children of the same age, have been noted to require more support and assistance from those around them to complete motor-based self-care and academic tasks at home and at school.[129,218]

Gross Motor Activity Limitations

Lacking good balance and postural control, children with DCD often have difficulties with the flexibility and adaptability required for gross motor activities. They may show delays each time they learn a novel skill such as riding a push toy, learning to ride a tricycle or bicycle, and pumping a swing.[100,120,128] They demonstrate poorly coordinated running, skipping, hopping, and jumping and may have difficulty managing stairs, especially when they must maneuver around others (Fig. 17.4).[8,31] Coordination of eyes and hands at a whole body level is problematic, so children with DCD have difficulty with throwing, catching, and kicking a ball accurately.[4,5,26] Given current understanding about the etiology of DCD, difficulties with ball skills may result from challenges in a number of areas, including the ability to judge the amount of force required to throw/kick a ball to an intended distance, coordinating timing of limbs to intercept a ball, forward prediction of limb position when reaching for or striking a ball, and correction of limb trajectory as needed while in motion. As a result, performance on these tasks is often more like that of a younger child (see www.cmaj.ca/cgi/content/full/175/5/471, and click on "videos" in right-hand menu; also see video of Bill). Children with DCD have more difficulty with gross motor activities that require constant changes in body position or adaptation to changes in the environment, such as when playing baseball or tennis or jumping rope.[128] Activities that require the coordinated use of both sides of the body are difficult (e.g., stride jumps, swinging a bat, handling a hockey stick).[128]

The fine and gross motor activity limitations of children with DCD can be understood in the context of associated body structure and function deficits, according to the ICF model (Table 17.3). An appreciation of the link between underlying deficits and their expression in activities of daily living can be instrumental when planning effective and targeted interventions.

Participation Restrictions

In the context of the ICF framework, the fine and gross motor activity limitations seen in children with DCD in school and home environments can lead to participation restrictions that prevent them from having opportunities for optimal physical, social, and cognitive development.[114] When parents of children

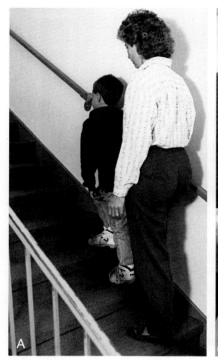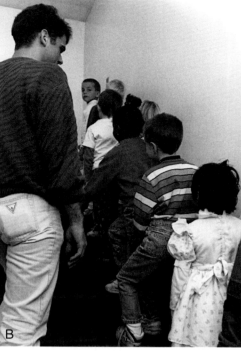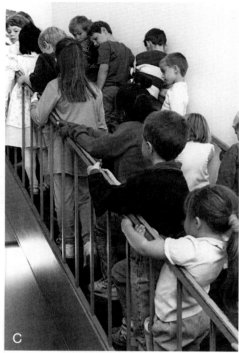

FIG. 17.4 (A) Managing stairs can be challenging for children with developmental coordination disorder because of difficulties with posture and balance. (B–C) Stair climbing is made more challenging when children with developmental coordination disorder must maneuver around others in a crowded environment.

TABLE 17.3   Examples of Activity Limitations and Related Body Structure and Function Deficits in Children With Developmental Coordination Disorder (DCD)

Activity Limitations	Related Body Structures and Functions
Self-Care Activities	
Eating:	Poor body awareness
Frequent spills, messy eating	Poor postural tone
Leaning on the table	Difficulties with in-hand manipulation
Poor use of cutlery when spreading/cutting	Difficulties judging force and distance, targeting
Dressing:	Poor use of dominant-assistant hands
Slow and disorganized	Poor body awareness and proprioception
Trouble with fasteners (buttons, zippers)	Lack of balance
Clothes twisted or on backward	Poor finger dexterity and strength
Shoes on wrong foot	Difficulties with touch perception, sequencing
Academic Activities	
Printing/handwriting:	Muscle tone and postural issues
Slow, poor legibility	Poor fine motor control
Awkward grasp	Overreliance on vision
Reduced volume of work	Use of attentional resources to maintain posture
Frequent erasures	Language and learning issues
Avoidance behaviors	Low muscle tone, fatigue
Sitting at a desk/in circle time:	Decreased postural control
Slumped posture	Poor body awareness
Holding head	Need for boundaries, increased sensory feedback
Leaning on others, lying down	Need to move to maintain muscle activity
Wiggling	
Falling out of chair	
Sports and Leisure Activities	
Ball-related activities:	Poor management of multiple degrees of freedom
Miss the ball, get hit by the ball	Timing issues
Slow to react	Difficulties correcting errors, poor generalization
Can't keep up	Difficulties attending to body position
Fatigue	Passivity response a coping mechanism
Passive—watch rather than play	Need to avoid failure, possibility of humiliation
Interact with adults rather than with peers	

with DCD are asked what their concerns are, they frequently identify restricted participation.[182,200] As a result of motor difficulties, children with DCD have reduced interest in physical activities and usually begin to withdraw from, and avoid, motor and sports activities at an early age.[21,180] Because of difficulties with self-care tasks at school, they are often slow to get to the playground for recess, restricting physical participation and further diminishing opportunities for physical and social interactions.

Complicating their physical challenges, children with motor difficulties often do not know how to play physical games, nor do they understand the rules of games,[100] limiting both physical and social participation with peers. They are often the last to "get picked" for teams and are not sought out to play with others.[120,231] As a result, these children can quickly become isolated from peer groups.[100] Difficulties in relating to peers have been noted in children with DCD.[100] This may be the result of not being chosen to participate in motor-based activities or because clumsy, less predictable movements may disrupt play with others.[120] Typically, children with DCD tend to watch more than play, preferring to wander the playground periphery or talk to teachers rather than engage in active play with others and socialize with peers[96]; this may be related to decreased self-confidence.[169] With fewer opportunities for social interaction, they often appear not to have learned the "intuitive" rules of social situations.[100]

Personal Factors

Children with DCD often self-impose restrictions on participation. They perceive themselves to be less competent than peers and have lower self-worth and greater anxiety.[154,204,255] When poor gross motor skills lead to inactivity and avoidance of physically challenging games, the child with DCD becomes less fit and further avoids physical activity. Avoidance of games requiring fine motor skill leads to decreased opportunities for practice, preventing ongoing academic skill development. Parents have reported that the more difficulty their children had with motor skills, the less willing they were to engage in physical activity.[160] Self-imposed isolation becomes a self-perpetuating cycle of poor skill development, limited skill practice, poor performance, and further isolation.[167]

Environmental Factors

With younger children, the environment tends to be more accepting of motor difficulties because of the wide range of normal variation. Early signs of incoordination may be viewed as part of normal developmental awkwardness or normal but slower maturation. As preschoolers become elementary school children, however, peers, parents, teachers, and/or communities may create unwarranted restrictions, artificial barriers, or rigid expectations.[170] If a physical education class or a community recreation program strictly adheres to performance criteria for group activities such as baseball, basketball, or dance class, a child with DCD can be prevented from participating with peers. If parents restrict their child's outdoor play to certain environments or to certain activities because they are afraid the child will get hurt, another barrier is established and peer relationships are potentially limited. If a family feels uncomfortable eating out at a restaurant or with relatives and friends because of a child's difficulty using utensils and messy eating[218] and restricts these opportunities to certain environments, social interactions will be unduly limited. Indoor manipulative play can pose just as much of a problem. When limitations

exist in fine motor skills, activities such as coloring, cutting, stacking objects, imaginative play with paper, handling small toys, or building blocks are very difficult. When children are not allowed to play with modified toys or when individualized expectations are not acceptable, a child's experiences can be artificially limited.

FOREGROUND INFORMATION

ROLE OF THE PHYSICAL THERAPIST

Physical therapists are skilled in the observation of gross motor task performance and can help to identify children whose poor motor performance leads to activity limitations and participation restrictions. Physical therapists can observe the lack of adaptive flexibility, the lack of premovement organization, and the "fixing" that is so characteristic of children with DCD in the early years.[140] These observations can facilitate early identification, which can help to prevent the development of secondary impairments. Physical therapists can provide education and guidance that will encourage the engagement of children with DCD in the typical activities of childhood, thereby reducing the risks of decreased physical health, as well as decreased self-esteem, self-efficacy, and social participation, that have been noted at an early age.[11,82]

Identification and Referral to Physical Therapy

The recognition of DCD will depend on the extent to which physical, social, and attitudinal factors have influenced motor skill acquisition. Although DCD must be considered at least theoretically to be present from birth, children differ with respect to the apparent age of onset because the developmental progression will vary depending upon the environmental and task demands placed upon the child in the early years. Because DCD is a disorder that has an impact on the development of movement skills, children with motor impairments often do not display the full extent of their functional difficulties until they are of school age. Limitations observed in the preschool years may be seen as "slow development" or temperamental differences. However, poor performance on everyday activities is tolerated less and less as children with DCD reach school age. Coordination difficulties may not be easy to observe until they reach the point at which they attempt to learn and perform skills that require adaptations in speed, timing, and grading of force. As has been mentioned, the presence of secondary impairments and co-occurring conditions can complicate the identification process.

Typically, children with motor difficulties are identified and referred to physical therapy via one of two principal routes—through the health care system or through the educational system. In the medical pathway, children with motor difficulties may have been investigated for possible musculoskeletal, orthopedic, or neurologic concerns. These may include concerns regarding ligament laxity, low tone, or an unusual gait pattern, or the results of regular monitoring after premature birth or low birth weight.[152] In the education system, referrals are usually made when poor motor performance affects academic functioning. Sources of initial identification within each of these pathways are varied and may include primary care physicians, community and developmental pediatricians, and hospital and infant programs, as well as classroom, physical education, and resource teachers, educational psychologists, and occupational therapists (OTs). Although some children are identified by the health care system, a significant number of the children referred to physical therapy for investigation of motor problems are referred through the educational route.

Although parents are often keenly aware early on of their child's activity limitations and participation restrictions,[2,182] classroom and special education teachers may be the initial source of referral to rehabilitation professionals when they notice poor skill development interfering with classroom work and overall academic performance.[217] Often, the structured demands of the classroom with expectations of increasingly precise motor skills and shorter time frames for performance stress a child with DCD to his or her limit. In fact, children with DCD are commonly underrecognized until academic failure begins to occur[70,122] and often are not identified before age 5.[122] In addition, teachers have many opportunities to compare the performance of children with poor motor coordination with that of more typically developing peers. At school age, poor written communication is frequently the first activity limitation that educators identify, so children with incoordination are most often referred to OTs for handwriting difficulties. This is often, however, just the "tip of the iceberg" because children commonly experience other challenges at school, on the playground, and at home. In the school setting, children with motor impairments may be referred to physical therapists for assistance with physical education programming and for safety concerns, as well as for strength and endurance issues. A physical therapist working in an educational setting has the advantage of screening children in natural environments while the children participate in everyday, functional activities. Immediate collaborative consultation with the classroom and/or physical education teacher can occur to gather information regarding the nature and extent of the motor concerns. After this, an appropriate physical therapy examination allows more comprehensive observation of function and functional difficulties in the classroom, at recess, and in physical education class. When children with possible DCD are referred and examined in a clinic setting, in-depth interviewing of parents and teachers regarding motor difficulties, as well as observation of functional activities, is needed to accurately identify concerns related to body structure and function and activity limitations.

Examination and Evaluation
History and Systems Review

Given the heterogeneous nature of DCD, it is important for a physical therapy examination to utilize multiple sources of information.[136] As part of the history, physical therapists should obtain information about motor development and medical background (pregnancy, delivery, and past and current health status); results of previous musculoskeletal and neuromuscular examinations; and a history of current functional status from the family and from school personnel. As part of the diagnostic process, physical therapists must differentiate the motor behaviors of children with DCD from those of other movement disorders. Children referred in the early years with poor coordination and/or motor delay may have disorders such as cerebral palsy, muscular dystrophy, global developmental delay, or DCD. Physical therapists must make evaluation hypotheses regarding the origin of the coordination difficulties. Some key questions may help therapists focus on differentiating among each of these patterns of motor behavior. In a young child, it would be important to ask and to observe during the systems review: (1) Is there evidence of increased or fluctuating tone? (observed alterations in muscle tone might be suggestive of

a condition such as cerebral palsy), (2) Are the delays more global in nature, rather than occurring in the motor domain alone—a situation in which global developmental delay might be suspected? (with a preschool- or school-aged child, questions might center around the history of the poor coordination), (3) Have the difficulties been present from an early age? (4) Are the motor concerns appearing to worsen over time? (5) Has there been a loss of previously acquired skills? (if so, this might be suggestive of a condition like muscular dystrophy). (See chapters in this volume on specific conditions noted here for further information on differential diagnosis.)

The following example suggests the process used in the examination of a young child who is demonstrating movement difficulties. A typical initial referral in a school-based service delivery environment might be made by a physical education teacher regarding a 5-year-old kindergarten student, Sarah, who is falling often. Initial hypotheses concerning why Sarah is falling more often than her peers might include the following: (1) She has mild cerebral palsy, spastic diplegia, or hemiplegia; (2) she has early symptoms of muscular dystrophy; (3) she has DCD; (4) she has characteristic symptoms of ADHD, and as a result she is impulsive and distracted to the extent that she bumps into people and objects; (5) her shoes are too big and she trips over the laces; or (6) she has a perceptual or visual impairment. Given the number of working hypotheses regarding the underlying cause of Sarah's difficulties, it will be important to conduct further physical examination and observation, with referral to additional health care professionals as warranted.

Direct observation of Sarah on the playground and during physical education class could rule out falling related to improperly fitting shoes (hypothesis 5) or significant impulsivity and distractibility possibly related to ADHD (hypothesis 4). Additional observation could identify a positive Gowers' sign and large calf muscles, suggesting further medical referral for possible muscular dystrophy (hypothesis 2). Observation of movement patterns during play may suggest typical symmetrical synergies of hip adduction and internal rotation with knee flexion and ankle plantar flexion (more suggestive of cerebral palsy, spastic diplegia; hypothesis 1), or unilateral shoulder retraction, internal rotation and adduction, elbow flexion with forearm pronation, wrist and finger flexion, and hip adduction and internal rotation with knee flexion and plantar flexion (indicative of cerebral palsy, hemiplegia; hypothesis 1). If none of these observations is made, the likelihood increases that Sarah has DCD (hypothesis 3).

Direct observation of functional activities in naturally occurring situations is an important part of the physical therapy examination. If the examination must be performed in a hospital or clinic setting, behavior might also need to be observed in a noisy, distracting, fast-paced environment such as a busy waiting room or a children's play area. Putting a coat on while surrounded by 25 other 7-year-old children, all struggling in a small space to get dressed and get outside for recess first, is much different from putting on a coat in a quiet room with one adult giving positive encouragement and will provide information on a child's ability to complete motor tasks in more usual settings.

Additional information obtained from parents (and where possible, teachers) is vital. A parent may describe her daughter as having a pattern of general incoordination with delayed speech, messy eating, and general clumsiness present from a young age but without a medical diagnosis related to a neurologic impairment (suggesting hypothesis 3). Suspicion that a child is demonstrating the characteristics of DCD would lead to questions about other developmental concerns as well (fine motor, self-care, leisure). It will be important to inquire whether or not difficulties are observed at home, such as struggling with buttons, using eating utensils, or tying shoelaces. Parents can provide information on the amount of effort required to complete motor tasks and whether their child participates in organized sports or other physical activities. The parent interview (combined with information from a teacher) can confirm the presence of a significant problem with academic achievement or activities of daily living—a key diagnostic finding in DCD.

Direct examination by the physical therapist might identify muscle hypertonicity that increases with faster movements (possible cerebral palsy; hypothesis 1). On the other hand, if direct examination suggests low muscle tone with shoulder, elbow, and knee hyperextension, DCD again becomes a valid hypothesis (3). If muscle testing reveals a weak gastrocnemius and pseudohypertrophy, the hypothesis of muscular dystrophy (2) would be supported. During direct examination the therapist may be able to relate the most striking activity limitations to difficulties in following directions when asked to perform a motor task or to poor attention to task. Children with DCD often cannot imitate body postures or follow two- or three-step motor commands. Frequent demonstration and actual physical assistance may be needed to accomplish items on standardized tests.

Tests and Measures

Initial screening. To identify children with motor challenges so that early and effective interventions can be implemented, the use of reliable and valid screening instruments is critical. To meet this need, several screening tools have been developed to elicit parent, teacher, and child perceptions of children's motor concerns.

Parent report. Parents know their children's developmental history, have observed functioning in multiple environments, and can provide important diagnostic information during screening for potential DCD.[56] The Developmental Coordination Disorder Questionnaire (DCDQ)[245] is a parent-report screening tool (at the ICF activity level) that measures the functional impact of a child's motor coordination difficulties. As a screening tool, the DCDQ can assist the clinician in determining the need to conduct a further, more in-depth evaluation of motor coordination. The DCDQ has recently been revised as the DCDQ'07.[243] Originally intended for use with parents of children 8 to 14 years of age, this 15-item tool has now been extended to include children 5 through 15 years old. Each item of the DCDQ describes tasks that are often of concern with children with motor impairment (e.g., catching a ball, riding a bicycle, writing), and parents are asked to compare their child's coordination to that of children the same age by choosing ratings on a 5-point scale. Percentiles are provided to assist the clinician in determining whether the child is demonstrating definite motor difficulties, is "suspect" for having motor difficulties, or is unlikely to have motor difficulties. The DCDQ is quick to complete and can provide valuable information to the family's physician regarding the impact of motor coordination difficulties on activities of daily life when a DCD diagnosis is being sought (i.e., Criterion B of the DSM-5).[3] Research performed on the original version of the DCDQ provides evidence of internal consistency of the test items, construct validity, and concurrent validity with both

the Movement Assessment Battery for Children (MABC) test of motor impairment[78] and the Bruininks-Oseretsky Test of Motor Proficiency (BOTMP),[15] as well as high sensitivity and specificity for identification of risk for DCD versus no DCD in populations of children in several different countries.[35,38,67,194] The new version of the DCDQ'07 was developed with a population-based sample from Alberta, Canada, and validated with typically developing children, as well as children with, or likely to have, coordination difficulties. The new DCDQ'07 was again noted to have high sensitivity and specificity, as well as construct and concurrent validity.[243] Findings from more recent studies of the criterion-related psychometric properties of the DCDQ have been conflicting.[22,109] This may relate, in part, to the fact that the DCDQ measures the functional impact of poor coordination, whereas several of the criterion standards to which the DCDQ has been compared measure difficulties in skill performance directly. The DCDQ'07 is available online at no charge (http://www.dcdq.ca/pdf/DCDQ_Administration_and_Scoring.pdf). The tool has been translated into many languages and validated for other cultural contexts.[27,96,145,173,222] In addition, the DCDQ has been modified for use with preschool children (The "Little" DCDQ)[177,244] and adults (Adult Developmental Coordination Disorder/Dyspraxia Checklist (ADC).[101] Evaluation of the psychometric properties of both of these modified versions is ongoing.[101,244]

Although teachers identify some children who have DCD, they have been shown to be inaccurate in some cases.[46,92,157] In one study of children 9 to 11 years of age, classroom teachers were able to identify only 25% and physical education teachers identified only 49% of the children with DCD.[157] This discrepancy is partially explained by the different environments on which the two types of teachers based their observations and may also be related to the fact that teachers may not be able to observe all functional tasks included in checklists. The popular teacher checklist (ICF activity level) used in this study, the Movement Assessment Battery for Children Checklist (MABC-C),[78] is also limited because it is somewhat lengthy, making it time consuming for teachers to complete. With regard to studies of the psychometric properties of this checklist, the results have been mixed. The MABC-C has been shown to demonstrate internal consistency, construct validity, and concurrent validity when measured against the MABC[78] test of motor impairment.[196] However, the checklist has been noted to have poor sensitivity, meaning that many of the children at risk for motor problems may not be identified.[92] The MABC checklist has recently been revised (MABC Checklist-2)[79] and includes fewer items, along with a new standardization sample of 395 children. Determination of the new checklist's psychometric properties will be important to determine whether the issues raised above have been addressed. Despite the limitations noted above, the MABC Checklist items may be useful to guide conversation and discussion with teachers when determining a child's functional difficulties.

Recently, the Children Activity Scale for Teachers (ChAS-T) has been developed for younger children 4 to 8 years of age.[188] In addition, the Motor Observation Scale for Teachers (MOQ-T) (previously known as the Groningen Motor Observation Scale) has been revised and new norms developed.[192] This checklist is intended for use with teachers of 5- to 11-year-old children. Only preliminary work has been conducted to examine the reliability and validity of these tools.[188,193] Until further validation studies have been done on these teacher checklists, caution should be exercised when relying only on the judgment of classroom or physical education teachers to identify children with DCD.

The Children's Self-Perceptions of Adequacy in, and Predilection for, Physical Activity Scale (CSAPPA)[72] is a brief 19-item child self-report measure of self-efficacy with regard to physical activity. It is intended for use with children aged 9 to 16 years. Specifically, the CSAPPA is a participation measure of children's perceptions of adequacy in performing, and desire to participate in, physical activity. It contains three subscales: perceived adequacy, predilection to physical activity, and enjoyment of physical education class. The CSAPPA uses a structured alternative choice format wherein children choose from two statements the one that best describes them (i.e., "some kids are among the last to be chosen for active games" versus "other kids are usually picked to play first") and then indicate whether the statement is true or very true for them. The tool has been shown to have high test-retest reliability, as well as predictive and construct validity.[72] The CSAPPA tool has been used in screening large groups of school-age children, primarily for research purposes, and scores on the CSAPPA have compared well with scores on a standardized test of general motor ability.[73] Several research studies suggest that the tool may be useful in the clinical setting for identification purposes.[20,23,73,74] Although it is possible to use only the subscales when screening for motor impairment, the use of additional sources of information on motor performance has been recommended to increase the specificity of the tool.[23]

Regardless of the type of screening tool used (parent, teacher, or child report), it should be noted that screening tools are just the first step in identifying potential DCD. Children identified through these tools as having possible motor impairment should undergo more detailed tests and measures intended for use with children with DCD to confirm motor difficulties (Criterion A).[216] When multiple measures are employed to confirm motor impairment (such as a checklist or questionnaire for initial screening followed by a test of motor ability), it should also be remembered that different tools may measure different constructs, including a child's capability (what the child can do, as measured by a standardized assessment) and the child's actual performance (what the child does do in everyday life and in multiple contexts or environments).[35] It is important to know a tool's strengths and limitations and to use a tool suited for the examination purpose. Each of these different tools can provide valuable information in understanding the complete picture of a child's difficulties.

Norm-Referenced Tests and Measures

One of the DSM-5 discriminating criteria for DCD is that motor coordination is markedly below expected levels for the child's chronologic age.[3] As such, a standardized, norm-referenced test must be used to determine whether a child experiencing motor difficulties is delayed compared to age-matched peers. Currently, there is no widely accepted standard to identify gross motor delay in children with DCD,[38,95,113,136] in part because of the heterogeneous nature of DCD and the frequent presence of co-morbidities. It is important to note that studies have reported inconsistencies in the numbers and types of children identified using different standardized tools specifically designed for children with DCD.[38] Without a gold standard to identify these children, researchers have often used more than one tool to confirm the DCD diagnosis in research study

samples.[252] It has been recommended that any examination of children with DCD should include information from a number of sources, including standardized tests, functional task analysis, and examination of tasks in natural environments.[38,136] The next sections describe a number of tests that are used with children with DCD. Further information on norm-referenced standardized tests can be found in Chapter 2.

A diagnosis of DCD is not recommended for children under 5 years of age.[11] However, it is important to identify children demonstrating early motor skill delays who are at risk for DCD and who may require ongoing monitoring, intervention, and reevaluation.[140] The Peabody Developmental Motor Scales–Second Edition (PDMS-2)[55] is a diagnostic and evaluative measure for children ages birth to 71 months and is an appropriate choice to monitor children at risk of DCD in this age group.

The Movement Assessment Battery for Children (MABC-2)[79] is a norm-referenced, multi-item test recommended for school-aged children suspected of DCD.[11] The MABC-2 (ICF activity level) contains three sections, and each section includes eight items for each of three age bands: 3 to 6 years, 7 to 10 years, and 11 to 16 years. Items are divided into manual dexterity (three items), aiming and catching (two items), and balance (three items) and include activities such as threading beads, putting pegs in a pegboard, catching and throwing a beanbag, balancing on one leg, jumping, hopping, and heel-to-toe walking. The total score is used to determine if performance is within normal ranges, if motor performance is borderline or at risk, if a motor impairment is present, and if the motor impairment is significant. When performance on the MABC-2 indicates risk for DCD, a child should be monitored and reevaluated for progression in the development of motor skills. If, during follow-up, progress continues to fall short of what is appropriate for their age and/or if movement quality is suspect, intervention may be warranted. When MABC-2 scores suggest that motor impairment is present, encouraging the family to follow up with their family physician to rule out other medical causes for the impairment and to seek a DCD diagnosis is important (see later sections in this chapter for long-term management of DCD), as is intervention. The form of intervention and setting in which it should take place will depend on a number of factors, including the severity of the impairment, the child and family goals, and the specific functional difficulties, but should in all cases include education and consultation with significant others in the child's life (see later sections in this chapter on intervention).

The original version of the MABC demonstrated good test-retest reliability and concurrent validity with the BOTMP.[38,39,78] In addition, numerous studies conducted worldwide have demonstrated that the MABC identifies children with DCD at the same prevalence rates as would be predicted,[185,207,252] and the body of evidence examining the use of the MABC has been steadily growing. After a literature review of 176 publications, Geuze and colleagues[62] concluded that the MABC is the best assessment tool for DCD in spite of the fact that it omits tasks related to handwriting—an important task to assess.[216] With regard to the newer MABC-2, two studies undertaken by the test developers demonstrate acceptable test-retest reliability (the tool was less reliable when the younger age band was used); information regarding other forms of reliability, however, is not available.[79] Although recent investigations of pilot versions of the lower and upper age bands of the updated MABC-2 provide some evidence of interrater, intrarater, and test-retest reliability, issues related to translation of the test items into other languages, cross-cultural examination, and use of single bands of the assessment tool in these studies have all been identified as issues influencing these results. To date, evidence of the new tool's construct and concurrent validity has not yet been firmly established.[14] Additional studies regarding these properties are emerging and include research on the concurrent validity of the MABC-2 with the MABC-C and the BOT-2, factor analytic validation, and further investigation of test-retest reliability.[199,208,226]

The MABC-2 has several advantages over other tools. The age bands for this instrument cover from 3-0 to 16-0 years, but testing time is short because the assessor presents only activities appropriate for that child's age. The original version has been shown to identify more children with coordination difficulties than the BOTMP[43] and appears to identify more readily those children who have additional learning or attention problems.[38] One of the key contributions of the MABC-2 is the inclusion of qualitative descriptors of motor behavior (i.e., impairment level descriptions) that the therapist can focus on during the administration of each test item. The MABC-2 also contains a behavioral checklist that can provide insight into the effects of motivation on test results and overall compliance with testing. Each of these unique features of the MABC-2 is of value to the clinician in identifying children with, or suspected of having, motor impairment. Although the MABC-2 demonstrates many clinical benefits, given that the psychometric properties of the MABC-2 have yet to be firmly established, therapists are encouraged to make use of several sources of information, including the MABC-2, in clinical decision making.[14]

Single-Item Activity Level Tests and Measures

Although initial tests of motor impairment can screen for, and confirm the presence of, significant motor difficulties, these tools do not provide a complete profile of a child's motor functioning,[89] an understanding of which is important for program planning and intervention.[234] In addition, the definition of DCD,[3] with its emphasis on the impact of motor coordination difficulties on daily life functioning, implies that a comprehensive evaluation of the child with DCD will include some examination of the child's ability to perform functional, everyday tasks in natural environments. Only a few assessment measures are available that include this functional and contextual emphasis, such as the Vineland Adaptive Behavior Scale, Second Edition (VABS).[214] Where secondary physical impairments are also present and significantly limit a child's activity and participation, it may be important to perform additional examinations at a body structure and function level (e.g., strength, physical fitness measures) to plan interventions to address these secondary issues specifically.[56] For more information on single-item activity level outcome measures, see Chapter 2.

FACILITATING A DIAGNOSIS OF DCD

It is not within the scope of practice of physical therapists to formally diagnose DCD. Nevertheless, physical therapists, through examination and evaluation of test results, are in an ideal position to recognize the motor and behavioral characteristics of potential DCD and can provide useful information to the child's physician regarding Criteria A and B of the diagnostic criteria.[3] Criterion A of the DSM-5 indicates that a significant delay in motor coordination must be present, which can be

difficult to determine in a physician's office.[3] Physical therapists can observe and test for motor delay and provide information to both the family and the physician. The DSM-5 Criterion B states that the motor impairment must interfere with academics, self-care, leisure, and play. The therapist can gather information from parents, teachers, and the child about what tasks are difficult for the child to perform and can relay this information to the physician.

Although health professionals may be hesitant to label the observed difficulties as DCD, a strong case can be made for the need to identify and recognize the disorder and for the role of the therapist in facilitating formal recognition of the motor difficulties.[138] DCD has a significant impact not only on the child but on the entire family.[133,134,218] Parental concerns are not often heard or acknowledged,[2,182] and parents are often frustrated with the health care and educational systems as they pursue answers to their concerns.[56] Significant family stress can occur regarding daily activities at home and around schoolwork. Parents not only are aware of the difficulties their child experiences from an early age[1,2,182] but are searching for answers and access to resources and are often relieved once they have a greater understanding of their children's difficulties. Recent research has shown that in pursuing answers to their concerns, parents are often involved with multiple education and/or health professionals before a diagnosis is made.[2,134]

Facilitating a diagnosis is critically important for the prevention of secondary consequences: in particular, self-esteem issues for the child. A diagnosis can help to initiate education, intervention, and accommodations for the child and allows parents to access resources. Equally important, the diagnosis can help to facilitate a long-term relationship with the family's primary care physician. This is critical for follow-up of potential secondary issues that may develop as the child matures and for identifying other developmental conditions that often coexist with DCD (e.g., expressive and receptive language difficulties, attention deficit disorder). Referral to other health care providers can then be made as appropriate. If DCD is suspected, the physical therapist should encourage the family to have the child seen by their primary care physician.

REFERRAL TO OTHER DISCIPLINES

As has already been discussed in this chapter, it should not be assumed that DCD is an isolated motor problem. An examination performed by any of the following individuals may be needed: (1) a family physician or neurologist when neuromuscular or musculoskeletal concerns are identified; (2) an occupational therapist when fine motor, self-help, or motor planning areas need further examination; (3) a speech and language pathologist when speech, oral-motor dysfunction, or possible cognitive-linguistic problems are observed; (4) a psychologist when intellectual or behavioral issues have surfaced; or (5) an adapted physical education teacher when more thorough gross motor skill training is needed.

INTERVENTION

Direct Intervention Approaches

According to the ICF model, physical therapy interventions can be directed toward remediating impairment, reducing activity limitations, and/or improving participation.[251] In the past, interventions used with children with DCD were aimed primarily at changing impairments of body structure and function by trying to improve either the child's sensory processing abilities (vision, kinesthesis) or the difficulties in individual motor components (balance, strength) that were believed to contribute to poor performance. These have been referred to as "bottom-up" interventions because they tend to address movement problems by emphasizing the building of foundational skills.[117] Examples of bottom-up interventions include perceptual-motor training, process-oriented approach, sensory integration (SI), and neurodevelopmental therapy (NDT). These interventions reflect more traditional theories of motor development and are based on the theoretical belief that, by changing these underlying deficits, task performance will be improved.[117] Some of these bottom-up interventions are still employed by therapists today when working with children with DCD, but several recent and comprehensive systematic reviews on the effectiveness of these approaches have found them to produce minimal change in functional outcomes and to offer no clear advantage of one approach over the other.[56,82,117,161,162,206] When gains are seen after the use of these approaches, the question has been posed as to whether they may be more a function of the skill of the therapists or application of general learning principles than of the treatment itself.[203,215] Physical therapists are challenged to rethink the importance of implementing intervention strategies for children with DCD that serve only to change primary impairments.

Dynamic systems theorists have proposed that improvement in functional tasks relies on many variables and tends to be environment-specific.[221] This way of thinking emphasizes that intervention must be contextually based, with intervention occurring in everyday situations and being of significance to the individual child. More recent interventions for children with DCD reflect these beliefs and now tend to emphasize the development of specific skills rather than underlying skill components alone. These have been referred to as "top-down" interventions,[117] which focus on motor learning principles in combination with other theories that emphasize the role of cognitive processes in the learning of new movement skills.[131] Top-down interventions include task-specific interventions and cognitive approaches. See Chapter 4 for more information on motor learning and task-specific intervention.

When selecting an intervention approach for children with DCD, physical therapists need to consider the motor learning difficulties that are particularly evident in this population such as the decreased ability to transfer and generalize skills and learn from past performance. It would seem reasonable from a motor learning perspective that giving feedback at the right stage of learning as well as opportunities to solve movement problems are instrumental guiding principles for interventions with children with movement difficulties.[131] It is likely that interventions that directly target the transfer and generalization of new skills and that emphasize motor learning will be the most successful. Many techniques to foster motor learning can be incorporated into intervention; these include providing verbal instructions, positioning, handling, and providing opportunities for visual or observational learning. Physically demonstrating or modeling movement sequences as well as helping children to learn strategies for managing feedback and organizing their bodies so they can attend to the most salient environmental cues may also be helpful, especially when intervening with young children. The use of frequent practice, practice in variable settings, and consistent provision of feedback should be key elements in any

intervention approach for children with DCD. It is important to create practice opportunities in a variety of environments so that each repetition of the action goal becomes a new problem-solving opportunity.[131]

Task-Specific Approaches

A growing body of research demonstrates the value of task-specific interventions.[159,176,203,206] Movement educators have found task-specific intervention to be a useful way to teach children with DCD specific gross motor skills[176]; they also emphasize its indirect effect in enhancing general participation in physical activity.[103]

Task-specific interventions have as their focus the direct teaching of functional skills in appropriate environments with the intended goal of reducing activity limitations and, by implication, increasing participation levels. Task-specific interventions are individualized approaches that attempt to increase the efficiency of movement by optimizing the way in which skills are performed, given the constraints within each of the several systems that interact during task performance—the child, the task itself, and the environment.[103] As children attempt to solve a movement problem, they may discover several ways to complete a motor task (Fig. 17.5). Children explore a variety of solutions to motor problems and are encouraged to experience the effects of using different aspects of their bodies or the environment. The therapist guides the child in choosing which of these different ways of performing represents the most efficient, optimal way for him individually and in a specific environment.

In task-specific interventions, the therapist is directive, providing verbal instructions, visual prompts, or physical assistance by guiding and directing movement so that children can appreciate the "feel" of efficient movement. Based on tasks that the child needs or wants to perform, the goal of task-specific instruction is to teach "culturally normative tasks in mechanically efficient ways" (p 238),[103] with the result that children will be less clumsy and will derive more enjoyment from the performance of tasks that were previously performed poorly.[176] Neuromotor task training[195] is one example of a task-oriented intervention that emphasizes components of motor learning such as verbal feedback and variable practice. Although there is good evidence that children learn the tasks that are taught through a task-oriented approach (and because they are culturally normative skills, this is important), there is not much evidence for transfer or generalization in this approach.[176] The latter are significant considerations when choosing an effective intervention for the child with DCD; more research is needed on how to best achieve these effects.

Cognitive Approaches

Like the task-oriented approaches described previously, interventions employing cognitive approaches also address activity and participation goals. Cognitive approaches, based on theoretical frameworks from cognitive and educational psychology as well as motor learning principles, use direct skill teaching but differ in their unique problem-solving framework that attempts to help children develop cognitive strategies, acquire tasks, and generalize from the learning of one skill to the next.[132] Cognitive approaches are based on the premise that children with DCD may be deficient in what has been termed "declarative knowledge" related to motor tasks: that is, they lack knowledge of how to approach a task, how to determine what is required for the task, and how to develop strategies to use when learning and

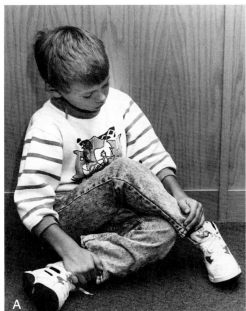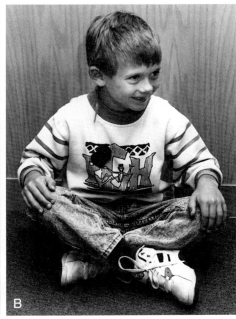

FIG. 17.5 (A) After many therapy sessions with verbal and physical prompts, this child is still unable to sit on the floor and cross his legs independently. (B) After being reminded of the verbal cues he needs to say to himself, he now successfully crosses his legs.

performing a motor task. Intervention approaches using cognition stress the importance of children learning to monitor performance and use self-evaluation. Mediation is used wherein children are guided to discover problems, generate solutions, and evaluate success independently.[141]

Evidence has been shown the effectiveness of a cognitive approach known as cognitive orientation to daily occupational performance (CO-OP).[165] This approach guides the child in discovering verbally based strategies that help him problem solve in new movement situations.[118,123,164,190] CO-OP emphasizes a child-centered approach with goals that are ecologically valid and performed in a realistic setting. Practice focuses on the child's ability to select, apply, evaluate, and monitor task-specific cognitive strategies with emphasis on facilitating transfer and generalization of the newly learned strategies (for a more in-depth review of the specific CO-OP protocol and the essential components of this approach, including the development of global and task-specific cognitive strategies, the reader is referred to Polatajko et al., 2001).[165] This cognitive approach was shown to be effective in a research clinic setting and, of note, demonstrated some generalization and transfer of skills in children with DCD.[164] Additional research studies have begun to investigate its suitability for use with younger children in clinical settings.[10,230]

The way in which cognitive intervention approaches are used by physical therapists will depend on the age of the child. For younger children, a participatory or consultative approach may be most effective. Using the principles of motor learning, it is important to provide appropriate feedback to children with DCD and to help them to focus on the salient aspects of a given activity by modeling and/or providing them with verbal guidance as they proceed through it. For older children, direct intervention with a more cognitive approach can be used to encourage them to think independently through motor problems. Whether a direct or consultative method of intervention

is used, increasing a child's self-efficacy should be a major aim of therapy. Finally, consultation with the child's family as outlined below will be critical to ensure that strategies learned through the cognitive approach can be transferred and generalized to home, school, and community settings to maximize participation.

Tools for Goal Setting and Measuring Intervention Effectiveness

Depending upon the target of intervention, several measures can be used to set collaborative goals and evaluate the efficacy of intervention. Whenever possible, goals should be child- and family-centered, as well as environmentally referenced to a problem related to participation in real-life situations.[56] The Canadian Occupational Performance Measure (COPM)[105] may be used as both a goal-setting and outcome measure and is therefore very appropriate for this population. This semistructured interview is used before intervention to have the child and/or family identify areas of functional difficulty (i.e., activity limitations or participation restrictions) and to rate the child's current performance of, and satisfaction with, each task. After intervention the rater is asked to reflect upon his performance and satisfaction for each targeted goal, and a change score can be generated. The COPM is best suited for use with children older than 8 or 9 years of age. With children younger than this, the Perceived Efficacy and Goal Setting System (PEGS)[166] may be a more appropriate goal-setting tool. In this pictorial measure, children reflect on and indicate their competence in performing 24 tasks that they need to do every day. They then identify any other activities that are difficult for them and select and prioritize tasks as goals for therapy. Using the PEGS, young children have been shown to be able to rate their competence at performing motor tasks and set goals for intervention.[137,139] The PEGS includes companion questionnaires that can be completed by caregivers and teachers. Research evidence indicates that children's goals often differ from those of parents and teachers, so the views of significant others may need to be solicited.[45,137]

Goal attainment scaling (GAS) is increasing in usage as a rehabilitation outcome measure with regard to the evaluation of individualized client outcomes and programs.[11,99] With GAS, five possible levels of specific functional attainment are developed for a child to create a criterion-referenced individualized measurement. To date, its use with children with DCD has been described mainly at a programmatic level. In this population, GAS that focuses on the levels of activity and/or participation, not on primary impairment, is warranted.

A measure that can be used to describe or evaluate activity and/or participation is the School Function Assessment (SFA).[36] The SFA has been used to describe the participation patterns of children with DCD,[253] but its use in a pre- to postintervention study of change has not been reported.

Parent/Child Instruction

An important, perhaps even primary, benefit of an evaluation for DCD is the follow-up consultation that allows the physical therapist the opportunity to discuss restrictions in activity and participation with the child, the parents, and school personnel.[43] Education and consultation with the family, school personnel, and the community lessen the impact of environmental and personal-contextual factors that may restrict participation.[56] Family members and school personnel are key players in identifying and improving outcomes for children with DCD. The physical therapist should always provide parents and school personnel with information about the disorder and its impact on functional activities and should provide additional resources regarding DCD tailored to the child's and family's needs, including print and web-based educational materials (see resources provided on Expert Consult website). After collaborative goal setting and intervention planning, written recommendations for home and school would also be helpful for families and school staff. When working toward the acquisition of specific skills, meaningful learning takes place over time and in multiple environments. Daily environmental modifications and task adaptations are critical for improved performance and motor learning for the child with DCD.[43]

Helping parents to understand their child's strengths and limitations is an important component of secondary prevention and risk management.[140] Family and cultural expectations can be inconsistent with a child's motor abilities. Expecting proficiency in competitive sports or dance or valuing perfect penmanship can lead to frustration and stress for everyone. Physical therapists can help families and children match interests and skills with expectations that lead to success. When parents are able to look at a play situation in their neighborhood or community recreation program and understand which motor skills are interfering with their child's ability to participate, the play situation can be adapted to maximize the child's participation and help prevent the imposition of societal limitations on full participation in community activities. Consultation with parents and teachers regarding promoting physical activity participation in children with DCD is addressed specifically in a later section in this chapter.

Coordination/Communication/Consultation

Communication with other disciplines is also an important component of physical therapy intervention for children with DCD.[56] DCD is a multifaceted disability, and more than one service provider may be involved with a child at any given time. If delays in speech and poor social language skills are associated with developmental incoordination, intervention by a speech/language pathologist may be appropriate. If oral-motor impairment is present, goals may be directed at improving articulation and fluency of speech.

OTs are able to contribute in a variety of ways when children are experiencing difficulties with self-care, academic performance, and social participation. Evaluations typically conducted by OTs will provide useful information about diagnostic Criterion B.[138] OTs are frequently asked to assist teachers in the evaluation and management of handwriting. OTs can also address classroom and home modifications that may remediate problems related to organization and spatial orientation in changing environments.[128]

Adapted physical education teachers can consult with regular physical education teachers to help modify the curriculum so that the child with DCD can participate and experience success. As has been discussed, children with DCD have a lower activity level than peers,[180] have decreased anaerobic power, and have decreased muscle strength.[175] For example, if a child cannot run fast enough or safely without falling, games such as baseball can be modified so that a designated runner is used or players are grouped into teams for all activities with one person hitting and one person running or one person catching and one person throwing. In addition, peer helpers can be identified to help the child with DCD practice basic motor skills such as hopping, jumping, or skipping.

If distractibility and attending to task are identified problems, a school psychologist can assist the physical therapist in managing disruptive or otherwise negative behaviors that interfere with learning motor skills. When concerns regarding distractibility and hyperactivity arise, a referral to a physician should be considered for evaluation of possible attention deficit disorder, or ADHD. Many children with ADHD but not DCD will appear clumsy. If they attend poorly, they will bump into and trip over objects in their environment. When ADHD is associated with DCD, the term DAMP (dysfunction of attention, motor control, and perception) has been used.[64] If behavioral and/or emotional problems such as poor self-esteem, depression, and anxiety become apparent, follow-up by the child's primary care physician is important. If the level of depression or anxiety is serious, psychiatric intervention, medication, and/or counseling might be needed. Physical and mental health complaints should be taken seriously, and previously unidentified medical conditions should be ruled out before other approaches to deal with the symptoms are implemented.

Recently, innovative service delivery models have begun to be explored, incorporating therapists in primary care settings (physician's office) as part of a multidisciplinary team. These service delivery models have the potential to increase awareness of DCD in the community, facilitating accurate and early identification and referral of children with DCD.[59] Other alternative service delivery models include those aimed at building capacity among families and educators, including through collaborative consultation and coaching in context (the "4 Cs," Partnering for Change) and focusing on graduated intensities of intervention,[127] as well as incorporating community level interventions.[24] These new methods of service delivery provide models to enhance collaboration among the many individuals involved in the management of children with DCD.

Consultation Regarding Physical Activity

Task-specific and cognitive approaches target intervention at the level of activity limitation. To increase participation levels, a key role for the physical therapist lies in early consultation with physical educators about strategies for the school environment and education for families about appropriate leisure activities that will likely be most successful for children with DCD.[56] These strategies emphasize participation without the risk of injury and are aimed at preventing the physical effects of inactivity.[8,140] In so doing, it may be possible to prevent many of the detrimental consequences that have been documented in children with DCD, including decreased physical activity,[180] participation,[21] strength,[175] and fitness,[180,198] as well as poor self-competence and self-esteem.[186,187,232] Although it may not be possible to change or "fix" the primary impairments of the child with DCD (such as low tone), the decrease in strength and fitness that can result from avoidance of physical activity is not inevitable and might be improved through promotion of an active lifestyle at home, at school, and in the community.[167]

Physical Education Class

Although teachers can often modify or adapt academic activities in which motor performance is not the primary focus, it may not be as easy to decrease the motor requirements in physical education class. Strategies can be used, however, to encourage children with DCD to make progress within their own range of abilities, to foster self-esteem, and to promote the value of physical activity for long-term fitness and health. As a general strategy, teachers can learn how to "MATCH" tasks to fit the needs of individual children with DCD to encourage maximal participation.[141] With the MATCH strategy, teachers are encouraged to Modify the task, Alter expectations, Teach strategies, Change the environment, and Help by understanding. (The reader is referred to the CanChild Centre for Childhood Disability website at http://www.canchild.ca for downloadable educator resources by grade level. These resources provide examples of different ways to adjust, i.e., MATCH, a task to improve fit with the abilities of a child with DCD.)

When physical activities are taught to children with DCD, emphasis should always be placed on encouraging fun, effort, and participation rather than proficiency. Noncompetitive games in which goals are measured against one's own performance and not that of other children may be helpful.[168] Another strategy is to divide the class into smaller groups when practicing skills because fewer obstacles will need to be avoided. When a new skill is taught to the class, children with DCD can be models while instructions are given so that they have an opportunity to experience the movement in addition to observing.[134] With ball skills, modifying the equipment will decrease the risk of injury and increase the likelihood of successful participation; beanbags, Nerf balls, and large balls can all be used effectively.

The School Playground

For outside play, introducing children with movement difficulties to playground equipment on an individual basis and teaching them how to use the equipment when in a relaxed environment will increase motivation to try independently. Children with DCD often avoid playground apparatus from an early age and have not had the experience of discovering how the equipment can be used.[231] The addition of moving objects (in this case, other children) increases the complexity of the environment significantly. Guiding them toward activities where they are more likely to have success (e.g., running or tag instead of ball games) will foster positive self-esteem and reward participation.

Sports and Leisure Activities

From what is now understood about the specific body structure and function impairments of children with DCD, it is possible to predict those types of functional tasks that are more likely to be problematic and to understand why certain sports and leisure activities may be more or less successful for them. It is important, first, to make the distinction between two types of motor behaviors. Early milestones such as sitting, crawling, and grasping (which are considered basic motor abilities) appear to develop relatively spontaneously in these children without any teaching (although milestones sometimes may be delayed and movement quality may not be optimal). Coordination difficulties appear to be much more evident when skills have to be purposefully learned. These skills include such things as catching or kicking a ball and playing baseball. Children with DCD experience particular difficulty with skills that require greater precision, continuous adaptability, and eye-hand coordination.[17,131] It is also important to appreciate the requirements of individual tasks. Some require constant monitoring of feedback during task performance, and others, once learned, do not require adaptations in response to environmental feedback. As one might expect, tasks with a heavy reliance on integrating feedback from the senses will be difficult for children with DCD.[131]

When recommending sporting and leisure activities for children with DCD, the type of task, as well as the degree of teaching involved, needs to be taken into account. Activities like swimming, skating, skiing, and cycling require some initial teaching of the skill and may pose a challenge for children with DCD during early learning of the skill because all novel skills are difficult for them and they do not generalize easily from previous learning.[178] Without encouragement and individualized attention, children with DCD may express dissatisfaction with these activities. Children with DCD, as well as parents, can be helped to understand that, because these sports contain a sequence of movements that are very repetitive and these activities do not require constant monitoring of feedback during performance, children with DCD can become very successful with these activities.[71,140] These are important "lifestyle" sports that individuals with DCD can continue to participate in throughout their lifetime (see the online PT DCD educational module at http://canchild.ca/elearning/dcd_pt_workshop/index.html for helpful tips on how to teach sports such as cycling applying evidence-based principles). In addition, because many of these sports tend to be taught through verbal guidance, they may be easier for children with DCD to learn. In contrast, activities such as hockey, baseball, football, and basketball (and other ball-related sporting activities) contain a high level of unpredictability. When the environment is changing or variable, the child not only has to learn the movement but also must continuously monitor the environment to adapt to change. Any time a player is required to hit or catch a baseball, contact a hockey stick to a puck, or move quickly around other players, changes must be made in the direction, force, speed, and distance of the movement. Even when the skill is learned, children must continue to adapt to changes in the environment and their place in it. Activities with a high degree of spatial and temporal uncertainty or unpredictability are likely to be challenging for the child with DCD.[74] The need for ongoing adaptation to changes in the environment is always a consideration; running on a smooth surface like a road or track, for example, will be much easier for a child with DCD than running on a forest trail.[140]

Parents of children with DCD have found that their child's involvement in organized sports is greatly enhanced if coaches are flexible about the child's role (e.g., having the child with DCD be the goalie).[134] Self-esteem is promoted through participation in organized sporting activities, and children appreciate when effort and personal mastery are emphasized.[29] Resources regarding ways to promote increased participation in community sports and leisure activities are available for parents, service providers, coaches, and community leaders on the CanChild website (http://www.canchild.ca).

TRANSITION TO ADULTHOOD AND LIFELONG MANAGEMENT OF DCD

High school classes, learning to drive a car, and vocational exploration present new challenges for the adolescent with DCD. It is now apparent that issues related to DCD are lifelong for many, if not all, individuals with DCD.[37] Physical therapy reexamination needs to include discussion of the prevention of secondary problems in adolescents with DCD. Identification of strategies to prevent impairments in body function from limiting activity or restricting participation can be one of the most important outcomes of physical therapy. Musculoskeletal or neuromuscular problems that would signal the need for future physical therapy care should be discussed because the changing environment and variables related to growth may place new demands on these systems. Preventive initiatives are needed because adults with DCD often have decreased strength, experience pain, and have poor aerobic capacity and endurance. Appropriate leisure activities that foster strength, endurance, and joint protection should be encouraged. The physical therapist can assist the individual with DCD to identify and participate in appropriate community fitness programs. Goals for lifelong leisure and recreational activity should be discussed with young adults. Activities should minimize competition and the need for quick motor responses. Swimming is likely to be more fun and more successful than playing tennis and therefore more likely to provide health benefits. Singing in a community choir may be a better choice than playing in a community basketball league. Riding a bike for exercise and enjoyment would be more appropriate than participating in a volleyball competition. Additional practical suggestions have been outlined in books for adolescents[100] and adults.[44]

Vocational choices are important decisions for individuals with DCD. Jobs that minimize the need for changing motoric and environmental expectations should be emphasized. Based on Henderson and Sugden's four-level categorization of motor skill difficulty, vocations that involve skills in which neither the individual nor the environment is moving or changing would be top choices.[78] Vocations in which the individual is moving and the environment is changing would be more challenging for the young adult with DCD (Table 17.4).

TABLE 17.4   Examples of Occupations Categorized by Motor Skill Difficulty

Individual	ENVIRONMENT	
	Stable	**Changing**
Stationary	Secondary school and college teaching Managerial occupations Psychologist Data processor Budget analyst	Air traffic controller Preschool and early elementary teaching Taxi driver in urban areas
Moving	Custodian Mail carrier Gardener Nurse Restaurant waiter	Fire fighter Physical education teacher Athlete in competitive sports

SUMMARY

DCD is a chronic condition affecting approximately 5% to 6% of the regular school-age population. A motor impairment disorder, its impacts are seen in academic underachievement and poor performance of everyday motor-based tasks. The exact etiology and pathophysiology are unknown, but DCD appears to have both motor production and motor learning components. Physical therapists have an important role to play both in identifying the impairments of body function and the activity limitations associated with DCD and in providing intervention to prevent or minimize the participation restrictions related to the person and the environment that might otherwise occur. DCD is a lifelong disability that presents challenges for adults, as well as for children and adolescents. Physical therapists function as members of the comprehensive team needed to manage the multiple ramifications of DCD and its many associated learning and medical problems.

Case Scenarios on Expert Consult

The cases scenarios related to this chapter describe several typical presentations of DCD. They are presented to demonstrate the variable nature of DCD and the different challenges that arise for physical therapy management.

ACKNOWLEDGMENTS

The authors are grateful to Doreen Bartlett, PhD, PT (Western University, London, Ontario, Canada), for her contributions to the ideas presented in this chapter and to Kathryn Steyer David for her work in previous editions of this chapter.

REFERENCES

1. Adams ILJ, Lust JM, Wilson PH, Steenbergen B: Compromised motor control in children with DCD: a deficit in the internal model? A systematic review, *Neurosci Biobehav Rev* 47:225–244, 2014.
2. Ahern K: Something is wrong with my child: a phenomenological account of a search for a diagnosis, *Early Ed Dev* 11:188–201, 2000.
3. American Psychiatric Association: *Diagnostic and statistical manual of mental disorders*, ed 5, Washington, DC, 2013, Author.

4. Asmussen MJ, Przysucha EP, Dounskaia N: Intersegmental dynamics shape joint coordination during catching in typically developing children but not in children with developmental coordination disorder, *J Neurophysiol* 111:1417–1428, 2014.

5. Astill S, Utley A: Two-handed catching in children with developmental coordination disorder, *Motor Control* 10:109–124, 2006.

6. Astill S, Utley A: Coupling of the reach and grasp phase during catching in children with developmental coordination disorder, *J Motor Behav* 40:315–323, 2008.

7. Ayres AJ: Types of sensory integrative dysfunction among disabled learners, *Am J Occup Ther* 26:13–18, 1972.

8. Barnhart RC, Davenport MJ, Epps SB, Nordquist VM: Developmental coordination disorder, *Phys Ther* 83:722–731, 2003.

9. Benbow M: Hand skills and handwriting. In Cermak S, Larkin D, editors: *Developmental coordination disorder*, Albany, NY, 2002, Delmar, pp 248–279.

10. Bernie C, Rodger S: Cognitive strategy use in school-aged children with developmental coordination disorder, *Phys Occup Ther Pediatr* 24:23–45, 2004.

11. Blank R, Smits-Engelsman B, Polatajko H, Wilson P: European Academy for Childhood Disability (EACD): recommendations on the definition, diagnosis and intervention of developmental coordination disorder (long version), *Dev Med Child Neurol* 54:54–93, 2011.

12. Reference deleted in proofs.

13. Brookes RL, Nicolson RI, Fawcett AJ: Prisms throw light on developmental disorders, *Neuropsychologia* 45:1921–1930, 2007.

14. Brown T, Lalor A: The Movement Assessment Battery for Children-Second edition (MABC-2): a review and critique, *Phys Occup Ther Pediatr* 29:86–103, 2009.

15. Bruininks RH: *Bruininks-Oseretsky Test of Motor Proficiency*, Circle Pines, MI, 1978, American Guidance Service.

16. Reference deleted in proofs.

17. Burton AW, Miller DE: *Movement skill assessment*, Champaign, IL, 1998, Human Kinetics.

18. Reference deleted in proofs.

19. Cairney J, Hay JA, Faught BE, Hawes R: Developmental coordination disorder and overweight and obesity in children aged 9-14 y, *Int J Obes (Lond)* 29:369–372, 2005.

20. Cairney J, Hay J, Faught B, et al.: Developmental coordination disorder, self-efficacy toward physical activity, and play: does gender matter? *Adapt Phys Activ Q* 22 67–82, 2005.

21. Cairney J, Hay JA, Faught BE, et al.: Developmental coordination disorder, generalized self-efficacy toward physical activity, and participation in organized and free play activities, *J Pediatr* 147:515–520, 2005.

22. Cairney J, Missiuna C, Veldhuizen S, Wilson B: Evaluation of the psychometric properties of the Developmental Coordination Disorder Questionnaire for Parents (DCD-Q): results from a community based study of school-aged children, *Hum Mov Sci* 27:932–940, 2008.

23. Cairney J, Veldhuizen S, Kurdyak P, et al.: Evaluating the CSAPPA subscales as potential screening instruments for developmental coordination disorder, *Arch Dis Child* 92:987–991, 2007.

24. Camden C, Leger F, Morel J, Missiuna C: A service delivery model for children with DCD based on principles of best practice, *Phys Occup Ther Pediatr early online*, 2014.

25. Cantell M, Kooistra L: Long-term outcomes of developmental coordination disorder. In Cermak S, Larkin D, editors: *Developmental coordination disorder*, Albany, NY, 2002, Delmar, pp 23–38.

26. Cantin N, Polatajko HJ, Thach WT, Jaglal S: Developmental coordination disorder: exploration of a cerebellar hypothesis, *Hum Mov Sci* 26:491–509, 2007.

27. Caravale B, Baldi S, Capone L, et al.: Psychometric properties of the Italian version of the Developmental Coordination Disorder Questionnaire (DCDQ-Italian), *Res Dev Disabil* 36:543–550, 2015.

28. Case-Smith J, Weintraub N: Hand function and developmental coordination disorder. In Cermak S, Larkin D, editors: *Developmental coordination disorder*, Albany, NY, 2002, Delmar, pp 157–171.

29. Causgrove Dunn J, Watkinson EJ: Considering motivation theory in the study of developmental coordination disorder. In Cermak S, Larkin D, editors: *Developmental coordination disorder*, Albany, NY, 2002, Delmar, pp 186–199.

30. Cermak S: Developmental dyspraxia, *Adv Psychol* 23:225–248, 1985.

31. Cermak S, Gubbay S, Larkin D: What is developmental coordination disorder? In Cermak S, Larkin D, editors: *Developmental coordination disorder*, Albany, NY, 2002, Delmar, pp 2–22.

32. Cermak S, Larkin D: Families as partners. In Cermak S, Larkin D, editors: *Developmental coordination disorder*, Albany, NY, 2002, Delmar, pp 200–208.

33. Chen HF, Cohn ES: Social participation for children with developmental coordination disorder: conceptual, evaluation and intervention considerations, *Phys Occup Ther Pediatr* 23:61–78, 2003.

34. Cherng RJ, Liang LY, Chen YJ, Chen JY: The effects of a motor and a cognitive concurrent task on walking in children with developmental coordination disorder, *Gait Posture* 29:204–207, 2009.

35. Civetta LR, Hillier SL: The Developmental Coordination Disorder Questionnaire and Movement Assessment Battery for Children as a diagnostic method in Australian children, *Pediatric Phys Ther* 20:39–46, 2008.

36. Coster W, Deeney T, Haltiwanger J, Haley S: *School function assessment*, San Antonio, TX, 1998, Psychological Corporation.

37. Cousins M, Smyth MM: Developmental coordination impairments in adulthood, *Hum Mov Sci* 22:433–459, 2003.

38. Crawford SG, Wilson BN, Dewey D: Identifying developmental coordination disorder: consistency between tests, *Phys Occup Ther Pediatr* 20:29–50, 2001.

39. Croce RV, Horvat M, McCarthy E: Reliability and concurrent validity of the Movement Assessment Battery for Children, *Percep Motor Skills* 93:275–280, 2001.

40. Debrabant J, Gheysen F, Caeyenberghs K, et al.: Neural underpinnings of impaired predicted motor timing in children with developmental coordination disorder, *Res Dev Disabil* 34:1478–1487, 2013.

41. Reference deleted in proofs.

42. Dewey D, Kaplan BJ, Crawford SG, Wilson BN: Developmental coordination disorder: associated problems in attention, learning, and psychosocial adjustment, *Hum Mov Sci* 21:905–918, 2002.

43. Dewey D, Wilson BN: Developmental coordination disorder: what is it? *Phys Occup Ther Pediatr* 20:5–27, 2001.

44. Drew S: *Developmental coordination disorder in adults*, West Sussex, UK, 2005, Whurr Publishers.

45. Dunford C, Missiuna C, Street E, Sibert J: Children's perceptions of the impact of developmental coordination disorder on activities of daily living, *Br J Occup Ther* 68:207–214, 2005.

46. Dunford C, Street E, O'Connell H, et al.: Are referrals to occupational therapy for developmental coordination disorder appropriate? *Arch Dis Child* 89:143–147, 2004.

47. Dwyer C, McKenzie BE: Impairment of visual memory in children who are clumsy, *Adapt Phys Activ Q* 11:179–189, 1994.

48. Edwards J, Berube M, Erlandson K, et al.: Developmental coordination disorder in school-aged children born very preterm and/or at very low birth weight: a systematic review, *J Dev Behav Pediatr* 32:678–687, 2011.

49. Engel-Yeger B, Hanna Kasis A: The relationship between developmental co-ordination disorders, child's perceived self-efficacy and preference to participate in daily activities, *Child Care Health Dev* 36:670–577, 2010.

50. Farhat F, Masmoudi K, Cairney J, et al.: Assessment of cardiorespiratory and neuromotor fitness in children with developmental coordination disorder, *Res Dev Disabil* 35:3554–3561, 2014.

51. Faught BE, Hay JA, Cairney J, Flouris A: Increased risk for coronary vascular disease in children with developmental coordination disorder, *J Adolesc Health* 37:376–380, 2005.

52. Ferguson GD, Duysens J, Smits-Engelsman BCM: Children with developmental coordination disorder are deficient in a visuo-manual tracking task requiring predictive control, *Neuroscience* 286:13–26, 2015.

53. Fitts PM, Posner MI: *Human performance*, Belmont, CA, 1967, Brooks/Cole Publishing.

54. Fitzpatrick DA, Watkinson EJ: The lived experience of physical awkwardness: adults' retrospective views, *Adapt Phys Activ Q* 20:279–297, 2003.

55. Folio MR, Fewell RR: *Peabody Developmental Motor Scales-2*, Austin, TX, 2000, Pro-Ed.

56. Forsyth K, Howden S, Maciver D, et al: Developmental co-ordination disorder: a review of evidence and models of practice employed by Allied Health Professionals in Scotland—summary of key findings. Available at: URL: http://www.healthcareimprovementscotland.org/our_work/reproductive,_maternal_child/programme_resources/dcd_review_response.aspx.

57. Francis M, Piek JP: The effects of perceived social support and self-worth on depressive symptomatology in children with and without developmental coordination disorder (DCD). *Presented at the 38th APS Annual Conference,* Perth, Western Australia, 2003.

58. Gaines R, Missiuna C: Early identification: are speech/language-impaired toddlers at increased risk for developmental coordination disorder? *Child Care Health Dev* 33:325–332, 2007.

59. Gaines R, Missiuna C, Egan M, McLean J: Interprofessional care in the management of a chronic childhood condition: developmental coordination disorder, *J Interprof Care* 22:552–555, 2008.

60. Geuze RH: Static balance and developmental coordination disorder, *Hum Mov Sci* 22:527–548, 2003.

61. Geuze RH: Motor impairment in DCD and activities of daily living. In Sugden D, Chambers M, editors: *Children with developmental coordination disorder,* London, England, 2005, Whurr Publishers, pp 19–46.

62. Geuze RH, Jongmans MJ, Schoemaker MM, Smits-Engelsman BCM: Clinical and research diagnostic criteria for developmental coordination disorder: a review and discussion, *Hum Mov Sci* 20:7–47, 2001.

63. Geuze RH, Kalverboer A: Inconsistency and adaptation in timing of clumsy children, *Journal of Hum Mov Sci* 13:421–432, 1987.

64. Gillberg C: Deficits in attention, motor control, and perception: a brief review, *Arch Dis Child* 88:904–910, 2003.

65. Goodgold-Edwards SA, Cermak SA: Integrating motor control and motor learning concepts with neuropsychological perspectives on apraxia and developmental dyspraxia, *Am J Occup Ther* 44:431–439, 1990.

66. Gramsbergen A: Clumsiness and disturbed cerebellar development: insights from animal experiments, *Neural Plast* 10:129–140, 2003.

67. Green D, Bishop T, Wilson B, et al.: Is questionnaire-based screening part of the solution to waiting lists for children with developmental coordination disorder? *Br J Occup Ther* 68:2–10, 2005.

68. Green D, Lingham R, Mattocks C, et al.: The risk of reduced physical activity in children with probable developmental coordination disorder, *Res Dev Disabil* 32:1332–1342, 2011.

69. Gubbay SS: *The clumsy child: a study of developmental apraxia and agnosic ataxia,* Philadelphia, 1975, Saunders.

70. Hamilton SS: Evaluation of clumsiness in children, *Am Fam Phys* 66:1435–1440, 2002.

71. Hands B, Larkin D: Physical fitness and developmental coordination disorder. In Cermak S, Larkin D, editors: *Developmental coordination disorder,* Albany, NY, 2002, Delmar, pp 172–184.

72. Hay J: Adequacy in and predilection for physical activity in children, *Clin J Sport Med* 2:192–201, 1992.

73. Hay JA, Hawes R, Faught BE: Evaluation of a screening instrument for developmental coordination disorder, *J Adolesc Health* 34:308–313, 2004.

74. Hay J, Missiuna C: Motor proficiency in children reporting low levels of participation in physical activity, *Can J Occup Ther* 65:64–71, 1998.

75. Hellgren L, Gillberg IC, Bagenholm A, Gillberg C: Children with deficits in attention, motor control and perception (DAMP) almost grown up: psychiatric and personality disorders at age 16 years, *J Child Psychol Psychiatry* 35:1255–1271, 1994.

76. Henderson SE, Henderson L: Toward an understanding of developmental coordination disorder, *Adapt Phys Activ Q* 19:12–31, 2002.

77. Henderson L, Rose P, Henderson S: Reaction time and movement time in children with developmental coordination disorder, *J Child Psychol Psychiatry* 33:895–905, 1992.

78. Henderson S, Sugden DA: *Movement Assessment Battery for Children,* San Antonio, TX, 1992, Psychological Corporation.

79. Henderson S, Sugden D: *The Movement Assessment Battery for Children-2,* London, 2007, Pearson Assessment.

80. Hendrix CG, Prins MR, Dekkers H: Developmental coordination disorder and overweight and obesity in children: a systematic review, *Obes Rev* 15:408–423, 2014.

81. Hill EL: Non-specific nature of specific language impairment: a review of the literature with regard to concomitant motor impairments, *Int J Lang Commun Disord* 36:149–171, 2001.

82. Hillier S: Intervention for children with developmental coordination disorder: a systematic review, *Internet J Allied Health Sci Pract* 5:1–11, 2007.

83. Hoare D: Subtypes of developmental coordination disorder, *Adapt Phys Activ Q* 11:158–169, 1994.

84. Hoare D, Larkin D: Kinaesthetic abilities of clumsy children, *Dev Med Child Neurol* 33:671–678, 1991.

85. Huh J, Williams H, Burke J: Development of bilateral motor control in children with developmental coordination disorders, *Dev Med Child Neurol* 40:474–484, 1998.

86. Iloeje SO: Developmental apraxia among Nigerian children in Enugu, Nigeria, *Dev Med Child Neurol* 29:502–507, 1987.

87. Ivry RB: Cerebellar involvement in clumsiness and other developmental disorders, *Neural Plast* 10:141–153, 2003.

88. Johnston LM, Burns YR, Brauer SG, Richardson CA: Differences in postural control and movement performance during goal directed reaching in children with developmental coordination disorder, *Hum Mov Sci* 21:583–601, 2002.

89. Johnston L, Watter P: Clinimetrics: movement assessment battery for children, *Aus J Physiother* 52:68, 2006.

90. Jongmans MJ, Smits-Engelsman BCM, Schoemaker MM: Consequences of comorbidity of developmental coordination disorders and learning disabilities for severity and pattern of perceptual-motor dysfunction, *J Learn Disabil* 36:528–537, 2003.

91. Joshi D, Missiuna C, Hanna S, et al.: Relationship between BMI, waist circumference, physical activity and probable developmental coordination disorder over time, *Hum Mov Sci* 40:237–247, 2015.

92. Junaid K, Harris S, Fulmer K, Carswell A: Teachers' use of the MABC checklist to identify children with motor coordination difficulties, *Pediatr Phys Ther* 12:158–163, 2000.

93. Kadesjö B, Gillberg C: Developmental coordination disorder in Swedish 7-year-old children, *J Am Acad Child Adolesc Psychiatry* 38:820–828, 1999.

94. Kagerer FA, Bo J, Contreras-Vidal JL, Clark JE: Visuomotor adaptation in children with developmental coordination disorder, *Motor Control* 8:450–460, 2004.

95. Kaplan BJ, Wilson BN, Dewey D, Crawford SG: DCD may not be a discrete disorder, *Hum Mov Sci* 17:471–490, 1998.

96. Kennedy-Behr A, Wilson BN, Rodger S, Mickan S: Cross-cultural adaptation of the developmental coordination disorder questionnaire 2007 for German-speaking countries: DCDQ-G, *Neuropediatrics* 44:245–251, 2013.

97. Kashiwagi M, Iwaki S, Narumi Y, et al.: Parietal dysfunction in developmental coordination disorder: a functional MRI study, *Brain Imaging* 20:1319–1324, 2009.

98. Reference deleted in proofs.

99. King G, McDougall J, Tucker M, et al.: An evaluation of functional, school-based therapy services for children with special needs, *Phys Occup Ther Pediatr* 19:5–29, 1999.

100. Kirby A: *Dyspraxia: the hidden handicap,* London, UK, 2001, Souvenir Press.

101. Kirby A, Edwards L, Sugden DA, Rosenblum S: The development and standardization of the adult developmental co-ordination disorders/dyspraxia checklist (ADC), *Res Dev Disabil* 31(1):131–139, 2010.

102. Konczak J, Timmann D: The effect of damage to the cerebellum on sensorimotor and cognitive function in children and adolescents, *Neurosci Biobehav Rev* 31:1101–1113, 2007.

103. Larkin D, Parker H: Task-specific intervention for children with developmental coordination disorder: a systems view. In Cermak S, Larkin D, editors: *Developmental coordination disorder,* Albany, NY, 2002, Delmar, pp 234–247.

104. Laufer Y, Ashkenazi T, Josman N: The effects of a concurrent cognitive task on the postural control of young children with and without developmental coordination disorder, *Gait Posture* 27:347–351, 2008.

105. Law M, Baptiste S, Carswell A, et al.: *Canadian Occupational Performance Measure,* ed 4, Ottawa, ON, 2005, CAOT Publications ACE.

106. Licari MK, Billington J, Reid SL, et al.: Cortical functioning in children with developmental coordination disorder: a motor overflow study, *Exp Brain Res* 233:1703–1710, 2015.

107. Lingam R, Hunt L, Golding J, et al.: Prevalence of developmental coordination disorder using the DSM-IV at 7 years of age: a UK population based study, *Pediatrics* 123:e693–e700, 2009.

108. Lingham R, Jongmans MJ, Ellis M, et al.: Mental health difficulties in children with developmental coordination disorder, *Pediatrics* 129: e882–e891, 2012.

109. Loh PR, Piek JP, Barrett NC: The use of the Developmental Coordination Disorder Questionnaire in Australian children, *Adapt Phys Activ Q* 26:38–53, 2009.

110. Lord R, Hulme C: Kinesthetic sensitivity of normal and clumsy children, *Dev Med Child Neurol* 29:720–725, 1987.

111. Mackenzie SJ, Getchell N, Deutsch K, et al.: Multi-limb coordination and rhythmic variability under varying sensory availability conditions in children with DCD, *Hum Mov Sci* 27:256–269, 2008.

112. MacNab JJ, Miller LT, Polatajko HJ: The search for subtypes of DCD: is cluster analysis the answer? *Hum Mov Sci* 20:49–72, 2001.

113. Maeland AF: Identification of children with motor coordination problems, *Adapt Phys Activ Q* 9:330–342, 1992.

114. Magalhaes LC, Cardoso AA, Misiuna C: Activities and participation in children with developmental coordination disorder: a systematic review, *Res Dev Disabil* 32:1309–1316, 2011.

115. Magalhaes L, Missiuna C, Wong S: Terminology used in research reports of developmental coordination disorder, *Dev Med Child Neurol* 48:937–941, 2006.

116. Mandich A, Buckolz E, Polatajko H: On the ability of children with developmental coordination disorder (DCD) to inhibit response initiation: the Simon effect, *Brain Cogn* 50:150–162, 2002.

117. Mandich AD, Polatajko HJ, MacNab JJ, Miller LT: Treatment of children with developmental coordination disorder: what is the evidence? *Phys Occup Ther Pediatr* 20:51–68, 2001.

118. Mandich AD, Polatajko HJ, Missiuna C, Miller LT: Cognitive strategies and motor performance in children with developmental coordination disorder, *Phys Occup Ther Pediatr* 20:125–143, 2001.

119. Marchiori GE, Wall AE, Bedingfield EW: Kinematic analysis of skill acquisition in physically awkward boys, *Adapt Phys Activ Q* 4:305–315, 1987.

120. May-Benson T, Ingolia P, Koomar J: Daily living skills and developmental coordination disorder. In Cermak S, Larkin D, editors: *Developmental coordination disorder*, Albany, NY, 2002, Delmar, pp 140–156.

121. Miall RC: Connecting mirror neurons and forward models, *NeuroReport* 14:2135–2137, 2003.

122. Miller LT, Missiuna CA, MacNab JJ, et al.: Clinical description of children with developmental coordination disorder, *Can J Occup Ther* 68:5–15, 2001.

123. Miller LT, Polatajko HJ, Missiuna C, et al.: A pilot trial of a cognitive treatment for children with developmental coordination disorder, *Hum Mov Sci* 20:183–210, 2001.

124. Missiuna C: Motor skill acquisition in children with developmental coordination disorder, *Adapt Phys Activ Q* 11:214–235, 1994.

125. Missiuna C, Cairney J, Pollock N, et al.: Psychological distress in children with developmental coordination disorder and attention-deficit hyperactivity disorder, *Res Dev Disabil* 35:1198–1207, 2014.

126. Missiuna C, Cairney J, Pollock N, et al.: A staged approach for identifying children with developmental coordination disorder from the population, *Res Dev Disabil* 32:549–559, 2011.

127. Missiuna C, Pollock N, Levac D, et al.: Partnering for Change: an innovative school-based occupational therapy service delivery model for children with developmental coordination disorder, *Can J Occup Ther* 79:41–50, 2012.

128. Missiuna C, Rivard L, Pollock N: Children with developmental coordination disorder: at home, at school, and in the community. (booklet). McMaster University, ON: CanChild (Online). Available at: URL: http://dcd.canchild.ca/en/EducationalMaterials/home.asp.

129. Missiuna C, Gaines BR, Pollock N: Recognizing and referring children at risk for developmental coordination disorder: role of the speech-language pathologist, *J Speech-Lang Pathol Audiol* 26:172–179, 2002.

130. Missiuna C, Gaines R, Soucie H: Why every office needs a tennis ball: a new approach to assessing the clumsy child, *Can Med Assoc J* 175: 471–473, 2006.

131. Missiuna C, Mandich A: Integrating motor learning theories into practice. In Cermak S, Larkin D, editors: *Developmental coordination disorder*, Albany, NY, 2002, Delmar, pp 221–233.

132. Missiuna C, Mandich AD, Polatajko HJ, Malloy-Miller T: Cognitive orientation to daily occupational performance (CO-OP): part I-theoretical foundations, *Phys Occup Ther Pediatr* 20:69–81, 2001.

133. Missiuna C, Moll S, King S, et al.: A trajectory of troubles: parents' impressions of the impact of developmental coordination disorder, *Phys Occup Ther Pediatr* 27:81–101, 2007.

134. Missiuna C, Moll S, Law M, et al.: Mysteries and mazes: parents' experiences of children with developmental coordination disorder, *Can J Occup Ther* 73:7–17, 2006.

135. Missiuna C, Polatajko H: Developmental dyspraxia by any other name: are they all just clumsy children? *Am J Occup Ther* 49:619–527, 1995.

136. Missiuna C, Pollock N: Beyond the norms: need for multiple sources of data in the assessment of children, *Phys Occup Ther Pediatr* 15:57–71, 1995.

137. Missiuna C, Pollock N: Perceived efficacy and goal setting in young children, *Can J Occup Ther* 67:101–109, 2000.

138. Missiuna C, Pollock N, Egan M, et al.: Enabling occupation through facilitating the diagnosis of developmental coordination disorder, *Can J Occup Ther* 75:26–34, 2008.

139. Missiuna C, Pollock N, Law M, et al.: Examination of the perceived efficacy and goal setting system (PEGS) with children with disabilities, their parents, and teachers, *Am J Occup Ther* 60:204–214, 2006.

140. Missiuna C, Rivard L, Bartlett D: Early identification and risk management of children with developmental coordination disorder, *Pediatric Phys Ther* 15:32–38, 2003.

141. Missiuna C, Rivard L, Pollock N: They're bright but can't write: developmental coordination disorder in school aged children, *Teaching Exceptional Children Plus 1*:Article 3, 2004.

142. Miyahara M: Subtypes of students with learning disabilities based upon gross motor functions, *Adapt Phys Activ Q* 11:368–382, 1994.

143. Mon-Williams MA, Wann JP, Pascal E: Visual-proprioceptive mapping in children with developmental coordination disorder, *Dev Med Child Neurol* 41:247–254, 1999.

144. Murphy J, Gliner J: Visual and motor sequencing in normal and clumsy children, *Occup Ther J* 8:89–103, 1988.

145. Nakai A, Miyachi T, Okada R, et al.: Evaluation of the Japanese version of the Developmental Coordination Disorder Questionnaire as a screening tool for clumsiness of Japanese children, *Res Dev Disabil* 32:1615–1622, 2011.

146. Reference deleted in proofs.

147. O'Brien V, Cermak S, Murray E: The relationship between visual-perceptual motor abilities and clumsiness in children with and without learning disabilities, *Am J Occup Ther* 42:359–363, 1988.

148. O'Hare A, Khalid S: The association of abnormal cerebellar function in children with developmental coordination disorder and reading difficulties, *Dyslexia* 8:234–248, 2002.

149. Pangelinan M, Hatfield B, Clark J: Differences in movement-related cortical activation patterns underlying motor performance in children with and without developmental coordination disorder, *J Neurophysiol* 109:3041–3050, 2013.

150. Reference deleted in proofs.

151. Parush S, Pindak V, Hahn-Markowitz J, Mazor-Karsenty T: Does fatigue influence children's handwriting performance? *Work* 11:307–313, 1998.

152. Peters JM, Henderson SE, Dookun D: Provision for children with developmental co-ordination disorder (DCD): audit of the service provider, *Child Care Health Dev* 30:463–479, 2004.

153. Piek JP, Barrett NC, Allen LS, et al.: The relationship between bullying and self-worth in children with movement coordination problems, *Br J Educ Psychol* 75:453–463, 2005.

154. Piek JP, Bradbury GS, Elsley SC, Tate L: Motor coordination and social-emotional behaviour in preschool-aged children, *Int J Disabil Dev Educ* 55:143–151, 2008.

155. Piek JP, Dworcan M, Barrett N, Coleman R: Determinants of self-worth in children with and without developmental coordination disorder, *Int J Disabil Dev Educ* 47:259–271, 2000.

156. Piek JP, Dyck MJ: Sensory-motor deficits in children with developmental coordination disorder, attention deficit hyperactivity disorder and autistic disorder, *Hum Mov Sci* 23:475–488, 2004.

157. Piek JP, Edwards K: The identification of children with developmental coordination disorder by class and physical education teachers, *Br J Educ Psychol* 67:55–67, 1997.

158. Pitcher TM, Piek JP, Hay DA: Fine and gross motor ability in males with ADHD, *Dev Med Child Neurol* 45:525–535, 2003.

159. Pless M, Carlsson M: Effects of motor skill intervention on developmental coordination disorder: a meta-analysis, *Adapt Phys Activ Q* 17:381–401, 2000.

160. Pless M, Carlsson M, Sundelin C, Persson K: Preschool children with developmental coordination disorder: a short-term follow-up of motor status at seven to eight years of age, *Acta Paediatr* 91:521–528, 2002.

161. Polatajko H, Cantin N: Attending to children with developmental coordination disorder: the approaches and the evidence, *Israel J Occup Ther* 14:E117–E150, 2005.

162. Polatajko HJ, Cantin N: Developmental coordination disorder (dyspraxia): an overview of the state of the art, *Sem Pediatr Neurol* 12:250–258, 2006.

163. Polatajko H, Fox M, Missiuna C: An international consensus on children with developmental coordination disorder, *Can J Occup Ther* 62:3–6, 1995.

164. Polatajko HJ, Mandich AD, Miller LT, MacNab JJ: Cognitive orientation to daily occupational performance (CO-OP): part II-the evidence, *Phys Occup Ther Pediatr* 20:83–106, 2001.

165. Polatajko HJ, Mandich AD, Missiuna C, et al.: Cognitive orientation to daily occupational performance (CO-OP): part III-the protocol in brief, *Phys Occup Ther Pediatr* 20:107–123, 2001.

166. Pollock N, Missiuna C: *The Perceived Efficacy and Goal-setting System*, ed 2, Hamilton, ON, 2015, CanChild Centre for Childhood Disability Research, McMaster University.

167. Poulsen AA, Ziviani JM: Can I play too? Physical activity engagement of children with developmental coordination disorders, *Can J Occup Ther* 71:100–107, 2004.

168. Poulsen AA, Ziviani JM, Cuskelly M: General self-concept and life satisfaction for boys with differing levels of physical coordination: the role of goal orientations and leisure participation, *Hum Mov Sci* 25:839–860, 2006.

169. Poulsen AA, Ziviani JM, Cuskelly M: Leisure time physical activity energy expenditure in boys with developmental coordination disorder: the role of peer relations self-concept perceptions, *OTJR (Thorofare N J)* 28:30, 2008.

170. Poulsen AA, Ziviani JM, Cuskelly M, Smith R: Boys with developmental coordination disorder: loneliness and team sports participation, *The Am J Occup Ther* 61:451–462, 2007.

171. Pratt ML, Hill EL: Anxiety profiles in children with and without developmental coordination disorder, *Res Dev Disabil* 32:1253–1259, 2011.

172. Rasmussen P, Gillberg C: Natural outcome of ADHD with developmental coordination disorder at age 22 years: a controlled, longitudinal, community-based study, *J Am Acad Child Adolesc Psychiatry* 39:1424–1431, 2000.

173. Ray-Kaeser S, Satink T, Andresen M, et al.: European-French cross-cultural adaptation of the Developmental Coordination Disorder Questionnaire and pretest in French-speaking Switzerland, *Phys Occup Ther Pediatr* 35:132–146, 2015.

174. Raynor AJ: Fractional reflex and reaction time in children with developmental coordination disorder, *Motor Control* 2:114–124, 1998.

175. Raynor AJ: Strength, power and co-activation in children with developmental coordination disorder, *Dev Med Child Neurol* 43:676–684, 2001.

176. Revie G, Larkin D: Task specific intervention for children with developmental coordination disorder: a systems view, *Adapt Phys Activ Q* 10:29–41, 1993.

177. Rihtman T, Wilson BN, Parush S: Development of the Little Developmental Coordination Disorder Questionnaire for preschoolers and preliminary evidence of its psychometric properties in Israel, *Res Dev Disabil* 32:1378–1387, 2011.

178. Rivard L, Missiuna C: Encouraging participation in physical activities for children with developmental coordination disorder. Available at: URL: http://dcd.canchild.ca/en/AboutDCD/resources/DCDPhysAct_Dec9Final.pdf.

179. Rivard LM, Missiuna C, Hanna S, Wishart L: Understanding teachers' perceptions of the motor difficulties of children with developmental coordination disorder (DCD), *Br J Educ Psycho!* 77:633–648, 2007.

180. Rivilis I, Hay J, Cairney J, et al.: Physical activity and fitness in children with developmental coordination disorder: a systematic review, *Res Dev Disabil* 32:894–910, 2011.

181. Rizzolatti G, Fogassi L, Gallese V: Mirrors of the mind, *Scientific American* 295:54–61, 2006.

182. Rodger S, Mandich A: Getting the run around: accessing services for children with developmental co-ordination disorder, *Child Care Health Dev* 31:449–457, 2005.

183. Rogers M, Fay TB, Whitfield MF, et al.: Aerobic capacity, strength, flexibility, and activity level in unimpaired extremely low birth weight (800 g) survivors at 17 years of age compared with term-born control subjects, *Pediatrics* 116, 2005.

184. Rosblad B: Visual perception in children with developmental coordination disorder. In Cermak S, Larkin D, editors: *Developmental coordination disorder*, Albany, NY, 2002, Delmar, pp 104–116.

185. Rosblad B, Gard L: The assessment of children with developmental coordination disorders in Sweden: a preliminary investigation of the suitability of the Movement ABC, *Hum Mov Sci* 17:711–719, 1998.

186. Rose B, Larkin D, Berger BG: Coordination and gender influences on the perceived competence of children, *Adapt Phys Activ Q* 12:210–221, 1997.

187. Rose E, Larkin D: Perceived competence, discrepancy scores and global self-worth, *Adapt Phys Activ Q* 19:127–140, 2002.

188. Rosenblum S: The development and standardization of the Children Activity Scales (ChAS-P/T) for the early identification of children with developmental coordination disorders, *Child Care Health Dev* 32:619–632, 2006.

189. Rosengren KS, Deconinck FJ, Diberardino 3rd LA, et al.: Differences in gait complexity and variability between children with and without developmental coordination disorder, *Gait Posture* 29:225–229, 2009.

190. Sangster CA, Beninger C, Polatajko HJ, Mandich A: Cognitive strategy generation in children with developmental coordination disorder, *Can J Occup Ther* 72:67–77, 2005.

191. Saywell N, Taylor D: The role of the cerebellum in procedural learning—are there implications for physiotherapists' clinical practice? *Physiother Theory Pract* 24:321–328, 2008.

192. Schoemaker MM: *Manual of the motor observation questionnaire for teachers*, Groningen, 2003, Internal Publication, Center for Human Movement Sciences (Dutch).

193. Schoemaker MM, Flapper BC, Reinders-Messelink HA, de Kloet A: Validity of the motor observation questionnaire for teachers as a screening instrument for children at risk for developmental coordination disorder, *Hum Mov Sci* 27:190–199, 2008.

194. Schoemaker MM, Flapper B, Verheij NP, et al.: Evaluation of the developmental coordination disorder questionnaire as a screening instrument, *Dev Med Child Neurol* 48:668–673, 2006.

195. Schoemaker MM, Niemeijer AS, Reynders K, Smits-Engelsman BC: Effectiveness of neuromotor task training for children with developmental coordination disorder: a pilot study, *Neural Plast* 10:155–163, 2003.

196. Schoemaker MM, Smits-Engelsman BC, Jongmans MJ: Psychometric properties of the M-ABC checklist as a screening instrument for children with a developmental co-ordination disorder, *Br J Educ Psychol* 73:425–441, 2003.

197. Schoemaker M, van der Wees M, Flapper B, et al.: Perceptual skills of children with developmental coordination disorder, *Hum Mov Sci* 20:111–133, 2001.

198. Schott N, Alof V, Hultsch D, Meermann D: Physical fitness in children with developmental coordination disorder, *Res Q Exer Sport* 78:438–450, 2007.

199. Schulz J, Henderson SE, Sugden DA, Barnett AL: Structural validity of the Movement-ABC-2 test: factor structure comparisons across three age groups, *Res Dev Disabil* 32:1361–1369, 2011.

200. Segal R, Mandich A, Polatajko H, Cook JV: Stigma and its management: a pilot study of parental perceptions of the experiences of children with developmental coordination disorder, *Am J Occup Ther* 56:422–428, 2002.

201. Sellers JS: Clumsiness: review of causes, treatments and outlook, *Phys Occup Ther Pediatr* 15:39–55, 1995.

202. Sigmundsson H, Hansen PC, Talcott JB: Do 'clumsy' children have visual deficits, *Behav Brain Res* 139:123–129, 2003.

203. Sigmundsson H, Pedersen AV, Whiting HT, Ingvaldsen RP: We can cure your child's clumsiness! A review of intervention methods, *Scand J Rehabil Med* 30:101–106, 1998.

204. Skinner RA, Piek JP: Psychosocial implications of poor motor coordination in children and adolescents, *Hum Mov Sci* 20:73–94, 2001.

205. Skorji V, McKenzie B: How do children who are clumsy remember modelled movements? *Dev Med Child Neurol* 39:404–408, 1997.

206. Smits-Engelsman BCM, Blank R, Van Der Kaay AC, et al.: Efficacy of interventions to improve motor performance in children with developmental coordination disorder: a combined systematic review and meta-analysis, *Dev Med Child Neurol* 55:229–237, 2013.

207. Smits-Engelsman BCM, Henderson SE, Michels CGJ: The assessment of children with developmental coordination disorder in the Netherlands: relationship between the Movement Assessment Battery for children and the Korperkoordinations Test Fur Kinder, *Hum Mov Sci* 17:699–709, 1998.

208. Smits-Engelsman BCM, Niemeijer A, Van Waelvelde H: Is the Movement Assessment Battery for Children - 2nd edition a reliable instrument to measure motor performance in 3 year old children? *Res Dev Disabil* 32:1370–1377, 2011.

209. Smits-Engelsman BCM, Wilson PH, Westenberg Y, Duysens J: Fine motor deficiencies in children with developmental coordination disorder and learning disabilities: an underlying open-loop control deficit, *Hum Mov Sci* 22:495–513, 2003.

210. Smyth MM, Anderson HI: Coping with clumsiness in the school playground: social and physical play in children with coordination impairments, *Br J Dev Psycholo* 18:389–413, 2000.

211. Smyth MM, Anderson HI, Churchill A: Visual information and the control of reaching in children: a comparison between children with and without development coordination disorder, *J Motor Behav* 33:306–320, 2001.

212. Smyth MM, Mason UC: Planning and execution of action in children with and without developmental coordination disorder, *J Child Psychol Psychiatry* 38:1023–1037, 1997.

213. Smyth TR: Abnormal clumsiness in children: a defect of motor programming? *Child Care Health Dev* 17:283–294, 1991.

214. Sparrow SS, Cicchetti DV, Balla DA: *Vineland adaptive behavior scales,* ed 2. Circle Pines, MN, 2005, American Guidance Service.

215. Sugden DA, Chambers ME: Intervention approaches and children with developmental coordination disorder, *Pediatr Rehabil* 2:139–147, 1998.

216. Sugden DA, Chambers M, Utley A: *Leeds consensus statement 2006.*

217. Sugden DA, Wright HC: *Motor coordination disorders in children,* Thousand Oaks, California, 1998, Sage Publication, Inc.

218. Summers J, Larkin D, Dewey D: Activities of daily living in children with developmental coordination disorder: dressing, personal hygiene, and eating skills, *Hum Mov Sci* 27:215–229, 2008.

219. Reference deleted in proofs.

220. Tervo RC, Azuma S, Fogas B, Fiechtner H: Children with ADHD and motor dysfunction compared with children with ADHD only, *Dev Med Child Neurol* 44:383–390, 2002.

221. Thelen E: Motor development: a new synthesis, *Am Psychol* 50:79–95, 1995.

222. Tseng M, Fu C, Wilson B, Hu F: Psychometric properties of a Chinese version of the Developmental Coordination Disorder Questionnaire in community-based children, *Res Dev Disabil* 31:33–45, 2010.

223. Vaivre-Douret L, Lalanne C, Ingster-Moati I, et al.: Subtypes of developmental coordination disorder: research on their nature and etiology, *Dev Neuropsychol* 36:614–643, 2011.

224. van der Meulen JH, Denier van der Gon JJ, Gielen CC, et al.: Visuomotor performance of normal and clumsy children: fast goal-directed arm movements with and without visual feedback, *Dev Med Child Neurol* 33:40–54, 1991.

225. van der Meulen JH, Denier van der Gon JJ, Gielen CC, et al.: Visuomotor performance of normal and clumsy children: arm-tracking with and without visual feedback, *Dev Med Child Neurol* 33:118–129, 1991.

226. van Waelvelde H, Peersman W, Debrabant J, Smits-Engelsman BCM: Factor analytical validation of the Movement Assessment Battery for Children-Second edition. *Paper presented at the DCD VIII Developmental Coordination Disorder International Conference,* 2009, June (Baltimore, MD).

227. Visser J: Developmental coordination disorder: a review of research on subtypes and comorbidities, *Hum Mov Sci* 22:479–493, 2003.

228. Volman M, Geuze RH: Relative phase stability of bimanual and visuomanual rhythmic coordination patterns in children with a developmental coordination disorder, *Hum Mov Sci* 17:541–572, 1998.

229. Wall AE, Reid G, Paton J: The syndrome of physical awkwardness. In Reid G, editor: *Problems in movement control,* Amsterdam, 1990, Elsevier Science, pp 284–316.

230. Ward A, Rodger S: The application of cognitive orientation to daily occupation performance (CO-OP) with children 5-7 years with developmental coordination disorder, *Br J Occup Ther* 67:256–264, 2004.

231. Watkinson EJ, Causgrove Dunn J, Cavaliere N, et al.: Engagement in playground activities as a criterion for diagnosing developmental coordination disorder, *Adapt Phys Activ Q* 18:18–34, 2001.

232. Watson L, Knott F: Self-esteem and coping in children with developmental coordination disorder, *Br J Occup Ther* 69:456–459, 2006.

233. Watter P: Physiotherapy management-minor coordination dysfunction. In Burns YR, MacDonald J, editors: *Physiotherapy and the growing child,* Toronto, Canada, 1996, Saunders, pp 415–432.

234. Watter P, Rodger S, Marinac J, et al.: Multidisciplinary assessment of children with developmental coordination disorder: using the ICF framework to inform assessment, *Phys Occup Ther Pediatr* 28:331–352, 2008.

235. Webster RI, Majnemer A, Platt RW, Shevell MI: Motor function at school age in children with a preschool diagnosis of developmental language impairment, *J Pediatr* 146:80–85, 2005.

236. Whitall J, Chang T-Y, Horn CL, et al.: Auditory-motor coupling of bilateral finger tapping in children with and without DCD compared to adults, *Hum Mov Sci* 27:914–931, 2008.

237. Reference deleted in proofs.

238. Williams H: Motor control in children with developmental coordination disorder. In Cermak S, Larkin D, editors: *Developmental coordination disorder,* Albany, NY, 2002, Delmar, pp 117–137.

239. Williams H, Woollacott M: Characteristics of neuromuscular responses underlying postural control in clumsy children, *Motor Dev Res Rev* 1:8–23, 1997.

240. Williams HG, Woollacott MH, Ivry R: Timing and motor control in clumsy children, *J Motor Behav* 24:165–172, 1992.

241. Williams J, Anderson P, Lee K: The prevalence of DCD in children born preterm: a systematic review. *Paper presented at the DCD VIII Developmental Coordination Disorder International Conference,* 2009, (Baltimore, MD).

242. Willoughby C, Polatajko HJ: Motor problems in children with developmental coordination disorder: review of the literature, *Am J Occup Ther* 49:787–794, 1995.

243. Wilson BN, Crawford SG, Green D, et al.: Psychometric properties of the revised Developmental Coordination Disorder Questionnaire, *Phys Occup Ther Pediatr* 29:184, 2009.

244. Wilson BN, Creighton D, Crawford SG, et al.: Psychometric properties of the Canadian Little Developmental Coordination Disorder Questionnaire for preschool children, *Phys Occup Ther Pediatr* 35:116–131, 2015.

245. Wilson BN, Kaplan BJ, Crawford SG, et al.: Reliability and validity of a parent questionnaire on childhood motor skills, *The Am J Occup Ther* 54:484–493, 2000.

246. Wilson PH, Maruff P, Ives S, Currie J: Abnormalities of motor and praxis imagery in children with DCD, *Hum Mov Sci* 20:135–159, 2001.

247. Wilson PH, McKenzie BE: Information processing deficits associated with developmental coordination disorder: a meta-analysis of research findings, *J Child Psychol Psychiatry* 39:829–840, 1998.

248. Wilson PH, Ruddock S, Smits-Engelsman B, et al.: Understanding performance deficits in developmental coordination disorder: a meta-analysis of recent research, *Dev Med Child Neurol* 55:217–228, 2013.

249. Wilson PH, Thomas PR, Maruff P: Motor imagery training ameliorates motor clumsiness in children, *J Child Neurol* 17:491–498, 2002.

250. Wocadlo C, Rieger I: Motor impairment and low achievement in very preterm children at eight years of age, *Early Hum Dev* 84:769–776, 2008.

251. World Health Organization: *The international classification of functioning, disability and health (ICF)*, Geneva, 2001, World Health Organization.

252. Wright HC, Sugden DA: A two-step procedure for the identification of children with developmental co-ordination disorder in Singapore, *Dev Med Child Neurol* 38:1099–1105, 1996.

253. Wynn K: *Exploring the participation of children with disabilities in school. Unpublished master's thesis*, Hamilton, Ontario, Canada, 2003, McMaster University.

254. Zoia S, Castiello U, Blason L, Scabar A: Reaching in children with and without developmental coordination disorder under normal and perturbed vision, *Dev Neuropsychol* 27:257–273, 2005.

255. Zwicker JG, Harris SR, Klassen AF: Quality of life domains affected in children with developmental coordination disorder, *Child Care Health Dev* 39:562–580, 2013.

256. Zwicker JG, Missiuna C, Boyd LA: Neural correlates of developmental coordination disorder: a review of hypotheses, *J Child Neurol* 24:1273–1281, 2009.

257. Reference deleted in proofs.

SUGGESTED READINGS

Background Information

Barnhart RC, Davenport MJ, Epps SB, Nordquist VM: Developmental coordination disorder, *Phys Ther* 83:722–731, 2003.

Blank R, Smits-Engelsman B, Polatajko H, Wilson P: European Academy for Childhood Disability (EACD): recommendations on the definition, diagnosis and intervention of developmental coordination disorder (long version), *Dev Med Child Neurol* 54:54–93, 2011.

Cantell M, Kooistra L: Long-term outcomes of developmental coordination disorder. In Cermak S, Larkin D, editors: *Developmental coordination disorder*, Albany, NY, 2002, Delmar, pp 23–38.

Wilson PH, Ruddock S, Smits-Engelsman B, et al.: Understanding performance deficits in developmental coordination disorder: a meta-analysis of recent research, *Dev Med Child Neurol* 55:217–228, 2013.

Foreground Information

Forsyth K, Howden S, Maciver D, et al.: Developmental co-ordination disorder: a review of evidence and models of practice employed by Allied Health Professionals in Scotland—summary of key findings. Available at: URL: http://www.healthcareimprovementscotland.org/our_work/reproductive,_maternal_child/programme_resources/dcd_review_response.aspx.

Magalhaes LC, Cardoso AA, Misiuna C: Activities and participation in children with developmental coordination disorder: a systematic review, *Res Dev Disabil* 32:1309–1316, 2011.

Mandich AD, Polatajko HJ, MacNab JJ, Miller LT: Treatment of children with developmental coordination disorder: what is the evidence? *Phys Occup Ther Pediatr* 20:51–68, 2001.

Mandich AD, Polatajko HJ, Missiuna C, Miller LT: Cognitive strategies and motor performance in children with developmental coordination disorder, *Phys Occup Ther Pediatr* 20:125–143, 2001.

Missiuna C, Pollock N, Levac D, et al.: Partnering for Change: an innovative school-based occupational therapy service delivery model for children with developmental coordination disorder, *Can J Occup Ther* 79:41–50, 2012.

Missiuna C, Rivard L, Pollock N: Children with developmental coordination disorder: at home, at school, and in the community. (booklet). McMaster University, ON: CanChild (Online). Available at: URL: http://dcd.canchild.ca/en/EducationalMaterials/home.asp.

Missiuna C, Rivard L, Bartlett D: Early identification and risk management of children with developmental coordination disorder, *Pediatr Phys Ther* 15:32–38, 2003.

Missiuna C, Rivard L, Pollock N: They're bright but can't write: developmental coordination disorder in school aged children. *Teaching Exceptional Children Plus* 1:Article 3, 2004.

Polatajko HJ, Cantin N: Developmental coordination disorder (dyspraxia): an overview of the state of the art, *Sem Pediatric Neurol* 12:250–258, 2006.

Smits-Engelsman BCM, Blank R, Van Der Kaay AC, et al.: Efficacy of interventions to improve motor performance in children with developmental coordination disorder: a combined systematic review and meta-analysis, *Dev Med Child Neurol* 55:229–237, 2013.

18

Children with Motor and Intellectual Disabilities

Mary Meiser, Melissa Maule, Irene McEwen, Maria Jones, Lorrie Sylvester

Children with intellectual disabilities often have secondary or associated delays in motor development and may have problems with motor learning and motor control. This is especially true of children whose intellectual functioning is moderately or severely limited. Some children's motor problems are minimal, requiring little, if any, physical therapy. Other children have cerebral palsy and other neurologic, musculoskeletal, and cardiopulmonary impairments that require considerable attention by physical therapists and other members of service delivery teams.

Many of the physical therapy examination and intervention methods used with children who have intellectual disabilities differ little from approaches used with any child who has similar motor characteristics, as described in other chapters of this volume. The learning characteristics of children with intellectual disabilities, however, can make it necessary to modify or supplement these approaches. These aspects of examination and intervention, along with current evidence-based and "best" practices for children with intellectual disabilities, are the foci of this chapter. The chapter will cover background information, including the definition, incidence, prevalence, origin, pathophysiology, and prevention of intellectual disabilities in children, and foreground information, including examination, determining outcomes and goals, and interventions to reduce impairments and activity limitations, prevent secondary complications, and promote participation. The chapter ends with consideration of the transition to adulthood.

BACKGROUND INFORMATION

DEFINITION OF INTELLECTUAL DISABILITIES

The definition of intellectual disabilities and the means by which children are identified as having intellectual disabilities are, and have been, highly controversial.[165] Much of the controversy surrounds the risk of inappropriately classifying children of cultural and linguistic minorities as having intellectual disabilities. The validity of this concern is supported by overrepresentation of children from cultural and linguistic minorities among children who have been identified as having intellectual disabilities and children placed in special education.[130,219]

Children with motor and sensory impairments also are at risk for being identified as having intellectual limitations when they do not or for being classified as having a greater degree of intellectual disability than actually exists. This is especially true if an examiner uses tests that require motor and spoken responses or has neither experience nor skill in examining children who require alternative input modes, such as manual signs, or alternative response modes, such as a voice output device.

In the United States, some organizations and educational and social service agencies still use the term *mental retardation* to refer to the condition of people with intellectual disabilities. The term *intellectual disability,* however, is being used increasingly, particularly since President Obama signed Rosa's Law (Public Law 111-256) in 2010,[156] which required changing references to "mental retardation" in health, education, and labor policy to "intellectual disability." The change has been gradual as laws and documents are revised.

The definition of intellectual disability has evolved over the years from a primary emphasis on intelligence test scores to an emphasis on individual functioning within natural environments. The American Association on Intellectual and Developmental Disabilities (AAIDD) proposed the most widely accepted definition, which has served as a basis for many other definitions, including those used by school districts for placement of students in special education.[164] AAIDD defines intellectual disability as being "characterized by significant limitations in both intellectual functioning and in adaptive behavior as expressed in conceptual, social, and practical adaptive skills originating before the age of 18" (p 1).[164]

This definition is based on the supports people need within authentic environments and natural routines, rather than on an intelligence quotient (IQ)–derived level of intellectual functioning, and incorporates the dimension of participation. Although an IQ of 70 to 75 or below still is required for a diagnosis of intellectual disability, the definition also includes adaptive skills, participation, interactions and social roles, health, and context consistent with the International Classification of Function, Disability, and Health (ICF).[216] Application of the definition depends on the following five assumptions:

1. Limitations in present functioning must be considered within the context of community environments typical of the individual's age, peers, and culture.
2. Valid assessment considers cultural and linguistic diversity as well as differences in communication, sensory, motor, and behavioral factors.
3. Within an individual, limitations often coexist with strengths.
4. An important purpose of describing limitations is to develop a profile of needed supports.
5. With appropriate personalized supports over a sustained period, the life functioning of the person with intellectual disability generally will improve.[164]

The assumptions emphasize the identification of the changing supports one needs over a lifetime to live successfully in the community, rather than simply on classification of the individual. Children identified as having intellectual disability who require supports to learn in school settings, for example, might not be labeled in adulthood when participating independently in home, work, and social roles.[164]

Other definitions of intellectual disability or mental retardation have coexisted with the AAIDD definition, including those used in the United States to qualify students for special education and for services for individuals with developmental disabilities. In the United States, Public Law 98-527, the Developmental Disabilities Act of 1984, authorized states to provide habilitation, medical, and social services for children and adults with intellectual disabilities and, in some states, for people with other disabilities. The term *developmental disabilities* was defined in the most recent version of the Developmental Disabilities Assistance and Bill of Rights Act of 2000 (Public Law 106-402) as "a severe, chronic disability that is attributable to a physical or mental disability that is likely to continue throughout the person's life and results in functional limitations in three or more areas of life activities" (Sec. 102[8][A]).[184] The only important difference between this definition and the AAIDD definition of intellectual disability is that the definition of developmental disability has no IQ requirement and the age of onset can be as high as 22 years.

Because of varying definitions of intellectual disability and eligibility criteria, confusion can exist both within and between states as to who is considered to have intellectual disability and who qualifies for which services. For this reason, physical therapists often need to seek information about programs in their own areas to determine the criteria for eligibility and who is qualified to classify a child as having an intellectual disability. Some programs provide wheelchairs, orthoses, and other equipment for children with intellectual disabilities; other programs pay for services such as physical therapy, respite care, and recreational activities.

For any child, a label of intellectual disability primarily is useful as a "passport" to early intervention, special education, and other educational, social, and medical programs. Such a label provides little, if any, insight into the strengths of the individual or the services needed and may limit a child's opportunities if the label causes others to have inappropriate or inadequate expectations of the child's capabilities.

INCIDENCE AND PREVALENCE OF INTELLECTUAL DISABILITIES

Reported estimates of the incidence and prevalence of intellectual disabilities vary widely. These differences are thought to be due to a number of factors, including variations in the definition; the methods employed; the sex, age, and communities of the samples; and the sociopolitical factors affecting the design and interpretation of the studies.[92] The US National Institute of Medicine[194] estimates that about 1% to 3% of the population have intellectual disabilities. Among students age 6 to 21 who received special education services under the Individuals with Disabilities Education Act (IDEA) in 2012, 7.3% were classified as having an intellectual disability and 2.2% were classified as having a multiple disability, which often includes an intellectual disability.[194] Mild intellectual disability is the most common (about 85% of those with intellectual disability). About 10% have moderate intellectual disability, 4% severe disability, and 4% profound disability.[104] Among children with cerebral palsy, approximately 50% have intellectual disability.[201]

ETIOLOGY AND PATHOPHYSIOLOGY OF INTELLECTUAL DISABILITIES

Multiple causes of intellectual disabilities exist, many of which have been identified and many of which have not. Shevell[169] reviewed retrospective and prospective studies and concluded that causes could be identified for approximately 50% of intellectual disabilities in children. Understanding the origin of a child's intellectual disability may assist physical therapists and others to better predict current or future needs for support and life planning and to identify other health-related problems that might be associated with a given diagnosis.[164]

More than 350 causes for intellectual disabilities have been identified that can be broadly categorized into prenatal, perinatal, and postnatal. Prenatal causes have been further classified as chromosomal disorders, genetic syndromes, inborn errors of metabolism, developmental disorders of brain formation, and environmental influences. Perinatal causes include intrauterine disorders and neonatal disorders. One meta-analysis of 15 studies that examined intellectual outcomes of children born prematurely provides evidence that prematurity alone may be associated with reduced scores on intellectual tests.[18] Pooled data demonstrated that test scores of children born at full gestation were significantly higher than scores of children born prematurely. Classifications of postnatal causes of intellectual disability include head injuries, infections, demyelinating disorders, degenerative disorders, seizure disorders, toxic-metabolic disorders, malnutrition, environmental deprivation, and hypoconnection syndrome.[164] Down syndrome, fetal alcohol syndrome, and fragile X syndrome are the most common causes of intellectual disability.[201]

Movement dysfunction is more often associated with some causes than with others, and in general, children with more severe intellectual disabilities are likely to have more severe motor delays and disabilities.[172] Years ago, Ellis[52] proposed that the relatively poor motor performance of people with intellectual disabilities is the result of their limited capacity to process information and the rapid decay of that information over time. Others have also proposed a relationship between intellectual and motor function, with cognitive processes affecting "attention, executive function, visuomotor skills, timing, and learning" (p e954).[172]

Prevention

Some forms of intellectual disability and associated disorders can now be prevented, such as those resulting from phenylketonuria, rubella, and lead poisoning. In addition, amniocentesis, ultrasound, and other techniques have enabled prenatal diagnosis of many conditions, which may help decrease morbidity, such as delivery of a child with myelodysplasia by cesarean section. Genetic counseling also can be offered.

Although the factors known to cause intellectual disabilities may be present in a given child, complex and powerful interactions between those factors and later environmental events can alter the actuality or the severity of intellectual limitations and associated impairments. In a review of research and theories on the development of intelligence, DiLalla[45] suggested that about half of a person's IQ may be influenced by environmental factors. Some infants, for example, who have severe medical problems during the postnatal course, with documented neuroanatomic pathology during this period, have few if any sequelae. On the other hand, children with no known pathology but who experience one or more environmental risk factors may eventually be classified as having intellectual disability. Two of the most common environmental causes of intellectual disability are early severe psychosocial deprivation and antenatal exposure to toxins, such as drugs or alcohol.[169]

In the United States the family-centered services directed by Part C of the IDEA[191], described in Chapters 28 and 29 of this volume, reflect a belief in the power of early social and physical environments to influence a child's development.[55] Part C regulations also imply confidence in the capability of physical therapists and other service providers to assist families in providing environments that both help to prevent unnecessary disability and promote the achievement of a child's potential.

PRIMARY IMPAIRMENT

The time at which impairments in intellectual functioning and movement become recognized varies widely, both within and between medical diagnoses. In some cases, prenatal or neonatal diagnosis can predict disabilities that may not yet be apparent, such as with children with Down syndrome or myelodysplasia. In other cases, a medical diagnosis will not be made until after impaired functioning is noted, perhaps not until months or years after birth.

Diagnosis/Problem Identification

Delay in achievement of developmental motor milestones or abnormal motor behaviors may be an early indication of intellectual disability that was present prenatally or perinatally. This is particularly true for children with severe intellectual disabilities. Some children, such as those with Rett syndrome or Tay-Sachs disease, will appear to develop normally for a period of time and then regress. In these cases, too, motor manifestations of the condition may be the first indication of a more global developmental problem.[50] Many children with autism, for example, have intellectual disabilities,[58] and studies have shown motor deficits in children with autism as early as during infancy.[138] Chapter 23 provides detailed information on autism.

Neuromotor Impairments of Children with Intellectual Disabilities

Children with intellectual disabilities are at high risk for motor impairments. One study, for example, found that 82% of children with mild intellectual disabilities scored below the 5th percentile on a test of motor coordination.[172] Although the study did not include children with greater than mild intellectual disabilities, children with more severely limited cognitive function are likely to have more severely limited motor skills.

The movement impairments of children with intellectual disabilities are as diverse as their primary and associated conditions. Many of the movement problems have their basis in central nervous system pathology that can lead to impairments in flexibility (too much or too little), force production, coordination, postural control, balance, endurance, and efficiency. Cardiopulmonary and musculoskeletal impairments also may contribute to movement problems, as well as cognitive processes that affect attention, executive function, timing, and learning.[172] Many children also have associated problems, such as vision and hearing disabilities, cerebral palsy, low levels of arousal, seizure disorders, and various other problems that can further negatively influence motor development, motor learning, and motor performance.

Although the type and degree of movement and related problems vary greatly, certain medical diagnoses are likely to be associated with specific constellations of neuromuscular, musculoskeletal, and cardiopulmonary impairments. Table 18.1 summarizes impairments that are common among children with selected diagnoses who often receive physical therapy. Box 18.1 summarizes common motor, cognitive, language, and medical characteristics of children with Down syndrome. A source of good information, including growth charts for children with Down syndrome, is the National Down Syndrome Society at http://www.ndss.org/. The National Association for Down Syndrome also has useful information at http://www.nads.org/.

Physical therapy examination of the movement impairments of children who have intellectual impairments is similar to that of other children who have problems addressed by physical therapists. Observation, criterion-referenced instruments, norm-referenced tests, and other formats are used, depending on the age of the child, the problem being assessed, and the purpose of the assessment.

Although the same examination methods[2,3,5,19,23,24] and tools may be used for children with and without intellectual impairments, recognizing that a child's intellectual impairment may affect performance of motor activities is important. This is especially the case when a child has to follow directions or perform motor tasks that have major intellectual components. Examination of infants and young children may be less affected by intellectual abilities than that of older children and adolescents, and intellectual disability may require more modification of methods to examine activity or participation than to measure impairments.

Relationship Between Environmental Exploration and Intellectual Abilities

Children who have motor impairments that restrict or prevent exploration of their environments may be at risk for secondary delays in domains that are not primarily affected, especially cognition, communication, and psychosocial development.[81] Campos and Bertenthal[31] suggested that independent mobility is an organizer of psychological changes in typically developing infants, especially developmental changes in social understanding, spatial cognition, and emotions. They also proposed theoretical links between independent mobility and the growth of brain structures, self-awareness, attachment to others, and ability to cope with the environment.

Relationships between mobility and spatial cognition have received considerable research attention. Several studies have demonstrated that locomotion, not age per se, is related to changes in such spatial intellectual tasks as recognition of cliffs[1] and slopes[3] and object permanence.[17] Results of individual studies were supported by a meta-analysis, which found that self-produced locomotion has an effect on spatial cognitive performance in typical children.[217] Self-produced locomotion also has been shown to influence social-communicative behaviors of infants[32] and to be linked to cognitive memory.[37] The proposed theoretical link between mobility and development of brain structures has been supported by studies demonstrating that experience shapes the brains of animals; for a review, see Kolb, Forgie, Gorny, and Rowntree.[90] Further research is needed to determine the relative contributions of innate mental capability and sensorimotor experiences on various aspects of intellectual development. It may be that the inborn intelligence

TABLE 18.1 Common Neuromuscular, Musculoskeletal, and Cardiopulmonary Impairments of Children with Intellectual Disabilities Caused by Selected Conditions[a]

Condition	Neuromuscular	Musculoskeletal	Cardiopulmonary
Angelman syndrome[197] Genetic mechanism with deletion of chromosome 15 as the most frequent cause; estimated prevalence 1 in 10,000 to 20,000. Up to 26% have no genetic cause and are diagnosed clinically.	Hypotonia and feeding problems within first 6 months followed by developmental delay. Tremulous movements, ataxia, hand flapping, and distinctive gait; microcephaly and seizure disorder	Facial abnormalities, flat occiput, strabismus, scoliosis, pronated or valgus at ankles	Vagal hypertonia resulting in cardiac rhythm disturbances
Cornelia deLange syndrome[119] Caused by mutations in the *NIPBL, SMC1A,* and *SMC3* genes; estimated to affect 1 in 10,000 to 30,000 newborn infants.	Spasticity, intention tremor, seizure disorder (10% to 20%), microcephaly	Severe growth retardation; decreased bone age, small stature, small hands and feet, short digits, proximal thumb placement, clinodactyly of fifth fingers, other arm and hand defects, limited elbow extension	Neonatal respiratory problems, congenital heart disease, recurrent upper respiratory infections
Cri du chat syndrome[40] A rare chromosomal disorder (1 in 50,000 live births) caused by loss of chromosomal material from region 5p (5p12).	Hypotonia in early childhood, sometimes hypertonia later	Facial and minor upper extremity anomalies, scoliosis	Congenital heart disease is common
Cytomegalovirus (prenatal)[62] One of the most common causes of prenatal infections in developed countries, with incidence estimated to be between 0.15% and 2.0%.	Cerebral palsy, seizure disorder, microcephaly (hearing problems)	Secondary to neuromuscular problems	Pulmonary valvular stenosis, mitral stenosis, atrial septal defect
Fetal alcohol syndrome[66] Caused by prenatal exposure to alcohol, the estimated prevalence of fetal alcohol syndrome is about 1%.	Fine motor and visual motor deficits, balance deficits	Minor facial abnormalities, joint anomalies with abnormal position or function, maxillary hypoplasia, poor growth	Heart defects
Fragile X syndrome[135] The most common form of inherited mental retardation, it is primarily caused by expansion of a sequence in the *FMR1* gene of the X chromosome.[135]	Poor coordination and motor planning, seizures	Connective tissue abnormalities, which may lead to congenital hip dislocation in infancy and later to scoliosis and pes planus	Mitral valve prolapse
Hurler syndrome[80] Autosomal recessive storage disorder with lack of lysosomal hydrolase α-l-iduronidase.	Hydrocephalus	Joint contractures, clawlike deformities of hands, short fingers, thoracolumbar kyphosis, shallow acetabular and glenoid fossae, irregularly shaped bones	Cardiac deformities, cardiac enlargement because right ventricular hypertension is common, death frequently due to cardiac failure
Lesch-Nyhan syndrome[98] Caused by a genetic deficiency of hypoxanthine-guanine phosphoribosyltransferase located on the X chromosome.	Hypotonia followed by spasticity and chorea, athetosis, or dystonia; compulsive self-injurious behavior	Secondary to neuromuscular problems	
Phenylketonuria (PKU)[178] Inherited metabolic disease, autosomal recessive disorder caused by mutation to the *PAH* gene. Treated with dietary means, enzyme therapy, and pharmaceutical supplementation. Occurs in 1 of 10,000 to 20,000 newborns. Neonates are screened for PKU. Progressive in untreated.	Tremors, microcephaly, epilepsy, hyperactivity	Reduced growth, eczema, distinct odor	
Prader-Willi syndrome[35] A chromosomal microdeletion disorder that occurs in 1 in 10,000 to 15,000 live births. It is the leading genetic cause of obesity.[35]	Severe hypotonia and feeding problems in infancy, excessive eating (usual onset 1-6 years) and obesity in childhood, poor fine and gross motor coordination, average age of sitting 12 months and walking 24 months	Small hands and feet, sometimes tapering fingers; scoliosis, kyphosis, or both are common; hip dysplasia in 10%; osteoporosis is frequent	Upper airway obstruction, sleep apnea, and oxygen desaturation are common
Rett syndrome[137] Definitive diagnosis is accomplished by mutation analysis on leukocyte DNA for the gene *MECP2*.	Deceleration in rate of head growth in infancy, gradual loss of acquired skills after 6 to 18 months of age, loss of purposeful hand skills, stereotypic hand movements (clapping, wringing, clenching), apraxia, teeth grinding, seizure disorder	Scoliosis/kyphosis, growth failure, bone demineralization	Breathing irregularities, such as hyperventilation and breath holding
Williams (elfin facies) syndrome[115] Caused by mutation or deletion of the *elastin* gene at 7q11.23; it occurs in 1 in 20,000 live births	Mild neurologic dysfunction, hypotonia, hyperreflexia, cerebellar dysfunction	Facial abnormalities, slow and abnormal growth, connective tissue abnormalities, radioulnar stenosis, spinal deformities, joint hyperextension when young, contractures when older	Supravalvar aortic stenosis, hypertension, peripheral pulmonic stenosis, and mitral valve prolapse

[a]Not all children with each condition exhibit all impairments.

BOX 18.1 Common Characteristics of Children with Down Syndrome

Motor Development

Hypotonia[199]
Hyperflexibility[199]
Problems with postural control and balance[199]
Delayed gross and fine motor development[131]
Gross motor development begins to level off after age 3 years[131]
Usually follow sequence of typical motor development[131]
Require more time to learn movements as complexity increases[131]
Atypical patterns of movement to maintain postural stability[199]
Reduced strength[199]
Better motor performance with visual than verbal instructions[109]
Perceptual-motor deficits in perception of complex visual motion cues[109]

Cognitive Development

Usually moderate to severe intellectual disability, although some have been reported to be within typical range[199]
Intelligence test scores progressively decrease with age[136]
Early onset (4th decade) of dementia is common[200,202]
Motivation may be low[199]

Language Development

Usually poor; below other areas of development and when compared with typical children or children with other causes for intellectual disabilities of the same mental age[199]
Impairment of verbal memory skills and other verbal processing abilities[202]
Language comprehension less impaired than expressive language[199]

Medical Problems[155]

Congenital heart disease (66%)
Vision deficit (60%)
Hearing impairments (60% to 80%)
Obesity (60%) and low levels of physical fitness
Skin conditions (50%)
Seizure disorder (6%)
Atlantoaxial instability (subclinical 14%; symptomatic 1%)
Hypothyroidism (subclinical 30% to 50%; overt 7%)
Periodontal disease

Other

Increased risk of early onset Alzheimer-type dementia[199]
Perhaps increased incidence of autism spectrum disorders[177]

---

of some children enables them to compensate for their motor limitations, thus making them less vulnerable to effects of sensorimotor deprivation than children whose intellectual capacities are more limited.

Learning in Children with Intellectual Impairments

By definition, *impaired learning* is what distinguishes children with intellectual impairments from other children. Although their motor problems often are similar to those of children without intellectual impairments and they respond to intervention based on the same physical therapy principles, the application of those principles must be sensitive to the children's learning characteristics and current theories on motor learning as explored in Chapter 4.

The degree and types of learning disabilities of children with intellectual limitations vary considerably, but several common learning characteristics have been identified. Compared with typically developing children, children with intellectual disabilities have been found (1) to be capable of learning fewer things; (2) to need a greater number of repetitions to learn; (3) to have greater difficulty generalizing skills; (4) to have greater difficulty maintaining skills that are not practiced regularly; (5) to have slower response times; and (6) to have a more limited repertoire of responses.[129] People with mild intellectual disabilities learn at about 50% to 66% the rate of people without intellectual disabilities, people with moderate intellectual disabilities at about 33% to 50% the rate, those with severe intellectual disabilities at about 24% to 33% the rate, and those with profound intellectual disabilities at about 25% the rate of people without intellectual disabilities.[201] Implications of these learning characteristics for physical therapy are described in later sections of this chapter.

Assessment of Intellectual Functioning

Determining if a child has an intellectual disability requires a standardized, norm-referenced measure of intelligence, which usually is administered by a psychologist or psychometrist. Even though most physical therapists do not administer intelligence tests, they are often able to promote an environment in which children with motor disabilities can perform optimally, such as by providing positioning to enhance a child's communication and eye and hand use[171] or by assisting the examiner to determine alternative response modes for use by children who have motor impairments.

Assessment of Infants

Physical therapists might be involved in the administration of tests designed to assess the intellectual abilities of infants because many of these tests focus on an infant's perceptual-motor development, such as accomplishment of motor developmental milestones or coordination of vision and hearing with body movement.[43] The Bayley Scales of Infant and Toddler Development[16] and the Test of Infant Motor Performance[30] discussed in Chapter 2 of this book are instruments that measure motor abilities and are often used to identify delay in infants.

Unfortunately, perceptual-motor–based infant evaluations are poor predictors of intellectual ability at later ages, with little, if any, relationship found between scores on infant tests and children's subsequent scores on intelligence tests for preschool or school-age children.[53] Hack and colleagues compared intellectual functioning of extremely low birth weight infants at 20 months corrected age and 8 years of age, using the Bayley Scales of Infant Development. They found that 80% of children born with extremely low birth weights, without neurosensory impairment, and with subnormal intellectual scores at 20 months demonstrated higher levels of intellectual functioning at 8 years.[70] The scores of children with extremely low birth weights and with neurosensory impairment were stable.[70] The limited stability of test scores in infants and young children is also influenced by other factors such as environment, experience, and rapid nature of developmental progress at early ages.[117]

Some tests of infant intellectual abilities attempt to measure infants' intellectual functioning through evaluation of their information-processing capacity rather than their perceptual-motor skills. These tests use infants' responses to novel and previously presented stimuli to assess their visual or auditory memory and their ability to discriminate among stimuli.[69] These tests are based on the tendency of infants, almost from birth, to respond for shorter periods of time to stimuli to which they have been previously exposed. Thus, if an infant has a longer response to a new stimulus than to one presented previously, memory for the familiar stimulus and discrimination of the two stimuli are demonstrated. Visual attention to stimuli is often assessed, as with the Fagan Test of Infant Intelligence (FTII),[54] but changes in physiologic status, like heart rate, respiration, and level of alertness can also be used to interpret response to stimuli.

One advantage of information-processing tests for infants is that they are essentially motor- and language-free, making them more appropriate for infants with motor and hearing impairments than many other tests.[53] Another advantage is that their predictive validity is much better than that of tests that focus on perceptual-motor behaviors; they may be most predictive when infants are tested at around 9 to 10 months corrected age.[69] These tests tap information-processing capacities similar to intelligence tests for older children. As noted by Sattler, cognitive development is highly changeable birth through age 5; after age 5, cognitive development can still change, but to lesser degrees.[162]

Assessment of Children

The Stanford-Binet Intelligence Scale V[152] for children ages 2 to 23, the Wechsler Intelligence Scale for Children V[84] for children ages 6 to 16.11, and the Differential Abilities Scale—Second Edition[51] for children ages 2.6 to 17.11 are common measures for assessing the intelligence of children.[162] Standardized administration of these and most other intelligence tests requires spoken and motor responses; however, these requirements seriously limit their usefulness with children who have communication and motor impairments.

A few intelligence tests have been developed that require children only to indicate a choice from among an array of alternatives. DeThorne and Schaefer provide an overview of intelligence testing that does not require an oral response in *A Guide to Child Nonverbal IQ Measures*.[44] Tests included meet five requirements: (1) used for testing of general cognitive functioning; (2) provides a standardized score of nonverbal ability; (3) developed or updated within the last 15 years; (4) suitable for preschool- or school-age children; and (5) developed for the population at large rather than specific groups. The Comprehensive Test of Nonverbal Intelligence,[73] the Pictorial Test of Intelligence,[60] and the Test of Nonverbal Intelligence[26] are tests that do not require manipulatives or verbal responses and, instead, require the student to indicate a pictorial response.

Raven's Progressive Matrices,[146] which requires selection of missing elements of abstract designs, and the Leiter International Performance Scale[153] are other non–language-based tests with minimal motor requirements. They may, however, suggest spuriously low intellectual abilities in children who have visual-perceptual deficits or visual impairments. It is also important to be aware that intelligence tests with limited motor and language requirements sample only a narrow range of abilities compared with more traditional tests of intelligence. Most intelligence tests have significant limitations in testing children who have lower levels of ability.[175] Current methods of testing inadequately address the needs of children with motor, visual, and/or communication impairments.[42] Capturing intelligence scores for these children continues to be elusive, requiring multiple assessment approaches to better gain a comprehensive and accurate picture of the child's strengths, needs, and performance abilities.

Assessment of Adaptive Behaviors

Although examiners often emphasize intelligence test scores in the diagnosis of intellectual disability, adaptive behaviors are also central in the assessment of intellectual functioning. The AAIDD defines adaptive behavior as the collection of conceptual, social, and practical skills necessary for daily function.[6] Assessment of adaptive behavior relies heavily on professional judgment, in both the selection of means to assess adaptive behaviors and in their interpretation. As with intelligence testing, psychologists and psychometrists typically administer tests of adaptive behavior when determining intellectual disability.

Instruments to measure adaptive behaviors have been developed that are of more recent vintage than many of the intelligence tests and are fewer in number. The AAMR Adaptive Behavior Scale-School (ABS-S:2)[75] is commonly used for older children to measure adaptive abilities. Results of a validity study of the ABS-S:2 indicated that the personal independence and social behavior scales of the tool demonstrated the largest difference between typical children and children with intellectual disabilities.[203] The Diagnostic Adaptive Behavior Scale (DABS) is under development by the AAIDD. The DABS measures three domains of adaptive behavior identified by the AAIIDD: Conceptual Skills, Social Skills, and Adaptive Skills.[7] Another test frequently used for older children is the Vineland Adaptive Behavior Scales, Second Edition (VABS-II).[176] The VABS-II is administered as a questionnaire or rating form that asks about activities of daily living, cognition, language, play, and social competency.

Physical therapists often can provide information about a child's adaptive behaviors, such as self-help and mobility skills, and may also be instrumental in providing assistive devices that can improve a child's adaptive skills. The Pediatric Evaluation of Disability Inventory (PEDI),[72] described in Chapter 2, is frequently used by physical therapists. The PEDI is a norm-referenced measure of adaptive behaviors in the areas of self-care in children age 6 months to 7.5 years with physical or combined physical and intellectual disabilities. The PEDI also can be used as a criterion-referenced test with older children whose function is below that of a typical 7-year-old.

Intellectual Referencing

Intellectual referencing is an assessment approach that has been used to determine whether children are eligible for services, especially for physical therapy, occupational therapy, and speech pathology, in public schools.[13,83] The approach is based on an assumption that children's potential for gains in motor and communication development is related to their intellectual abilities and that children whose intellectual abilities are lower than or equal to their motor or communication abilities would not benefit from services, so they are not eligible for them. Many children with intellectual disabilities could be declared ineligible for physical therapy services under such an assumption. Critics have been supported by at least one study that examined the association between IQ scores and progress in occupational therapy or physical therapy over the course of one school year.[13] Children were divided into two groups based on their IQ scores, and children received similar dosing of physical therapy for motor impairments with both groups showing significant change in their age-equivalence scores. There was not a significant correlation between IQ and change in motor test scores. The US Department of Education, Office of Special Education Programs (OSEP), declared intellectual referencing to be an unlawful means of determining whether a child should receive related services in public schools.[143] In the 2004 reauthorization of IDEA,[55] using cognitive referencing to identify severe discrepancies in ability was removed from federal policy.[120]

FOREGROUND INFORMATION

PHYSICAL THERAPY EXAMINATION

The complex problems of children with both intellectual and motor disabilities usually require a team approach for examination and for planning, implementation, and evaluation of intervention.[38,144] The team always will include the child's family or another caregiver, with other team members as required by the nature and severity of the child's problems, the child's age, and the service delivery setting. Many children need the services of two or more teams at the same time, such as a clinically based health care team and an early intervention or school team. Often, the health care team focuses on the child's body functions and structures, whereas the early intervention or school-based team is responsible for addressing activity limitations and ongoing efforts to promote the highest possible level of family and community participation. These teams, unfortunately, frequently function independently of each other,[68,125] creating overlaps and gaps in care while consuming considerable resources of time and money.[174,192] When the teams have mutual responsibilities and concerns, disagreements can occur, resulting in confusion for the family and an unnecessary expenditure of limited resources. Working toward family-centered care, understanding and appreciating the roles of each team, and integrating care across the care teams are important to achieve coordination of care for the child and family.[77,144] Regardless of team responsibility, the examination of a child with both intellectual and motor impairment should be guided by the ICF.[216]

History and Systems Review

As shown in Table 18.1, intellectual disability can be associated with a variety of causes and neuromuscular, musculoskeletal, and cardiopulmonary impairments. A child's history—obtained from family members, medical records, early intervention/education records, social service agencies, and any other relevant source—can help to identify systems on which to focus the systems review and examination. As with children without intellectual disabilities, the history also can identify activity and participation levels, prior interventions and outcomes, surgical procedures, family and child goals, and other information to help decide which tests and measures to use.

Tests and Measures: Activity

The norm- and criterion-referenced tools described in other chapters of this volume that are used to measure activity and participation among children with other types of disabilities can be used with many children with intellectual impairments. Depending on a test's properties, it can identify activity limitations and abilities, provide baseline data to measure change over time or change following intervention, predict future performance,[89] and/or help identify specific goals of intervention.

Norm-referenced tools, which compare a child's performance with the performance of other children of the same age, are primarily useful as discriminative measures to determine if a child's development is delayed and, if so, in what areas. The Peabody Developmental Motor Scales,[57] for example, frequently is used as part of an early intervention evaluation to determine if a child is eligible for services based on delays in gross and fine motor skills. The functional skills scale of the PEDI,[72] which measures mobility, self-care, and social function, is norm referenced for children from age 6 months to 7 years. The PEDI also can be used as a criterion-referenced test for older children whose function is below that of a typical 7-year-old. A newer computerized version of the PEDI, the PEDI-CAT, measures an additional domain of responsibility, which includes organizational skills, management of daily activities and health needs, as well as maintaining personal safety.[71]

The PEDI and other criterion-referenced tools, such as the Gross Motor Function Measure,[160] are useful as discriminative tests to identify a child's current performance of motor-related activities and also as evaluative tests to determine if change in performance occurs over time or following intervention. A few criterion-referenced tools, such as the Test of Infant Motor Performance[30] and the Gross Motor Function Classification System[132] are useful predictive measures that indicate what a child's future motor performance is likely to be. This information is particularly useful for intervention planning.

Tests and Measures: Participation

Examination of a child's participation often is best conducted in the environments in which the child actually participates or in environments in which children of similar age and social background participate.[108,144] Examination in natural environments is increasingly advocated to support the enablement model for all children who have disabilities, including children with intellectual disabilities, who have difficulty generalizing skills from one setting to another.[64] Because children function in multiple environments, episodic examination to address participation deficits or needs within a specific context may be necessary. Shummay-Cook and Woollacott note that motor-control challenges are best addressed through examination of both the task and the environment in which the task occurs.[170] An ecologic assessment can be a helpful way to examine a child's participation within the context of an identified goal. Table 18.2 shows an ecologic assessment for a young man whose goal is to shop independently for groceries at a neighborhood store.

If a child's and family's goals are related to participation, several tools are available to use as baseline and outcome measures. If a goal is for the child to participate in recreation and leisure activities outside of school, for example, the Children's Assessment of Participation and Enjoyment (CAPE) and Preferences for Activities of Children (PAC)[88] can provide useful information about participation of children and youth age 6 to 21. The CAPE measures the diversity, intensity, enjoyment, and context of the activities. The PAC measures preferences for involvement in activities. The Caregiver Assistance Scale of the PEDI[72] also measures participation related to mobility, self-care, and social function in the home environment. The School Function Assessment[41] measures participation, activities, and necessary task supports in the school environment of children in kindergarten through sixth grade.

Tests and Measures: Body Structures and Functions

Assessment of body structures and functions can help to identify reasons for activity and participation limitations. Methods for examination of body structures and functions of children described in other chapters of this volume are applicable to children with intellectual impairments. Modifications are often necessary, though, if a child has difficulty responding to verbal requests and directions. When determining pain levels, for

TABLE 18.2 Example of a Goal-Focused Ecologic Assessment

Name: Jeff
Goal: Grocery shopping independently
Environment: Dan's One-Stop

Steps Required	Jeff's Current Performance	Steps Can Acquire	Steps May Not Acquire	Compensatory Strategies	Intervention[a]
Go from home to Dan's and back using electric wheelchair.	Can open front door (outward), go down ramp, and drive to the corner. Cannot go down curb (no curb cut), cross street safely, or go up curb. Once on the sidewalk, can drive to Dan's. Cannot open door from outside. Can maneuver inside store and open door when leaving (outward). Cannot open door of home when returning.	Open doors of home and store when the door opens toward him. Go down curb. Ask for assistance and tell someone how to help him up a curb. Cross the street safely.	Go up a curb without assistance.	Curb cuts	Teach Jeff to open doors, go down curbs, and cross streets safely (PT, PCA). Talk with city about making curb cuts and with store and house manager about modifying doors (Jeff, CM). Program communication aid to request help with curbs and give instructions (mother, PT).
Select items in the store.	Does not always remember what he needs to get and cannot make or read a shopping list. Can get items that are at hand level, cannot shift weight or extend arm to reach low or high items.	Make and use shopping list. Improve ability to reach high and low items. Ask for assistance to get out-of-reach items.	Reach items that are very high or very low.	A reacher?	Teach Jeff To make and use a shopping list (OT, PCA), To use a reacher, if it seems feasible (OT, PCA), and To reach to higher and lower shelves (PT, PCA).
Carry items to checkout stand.	Cannot maneuver shopping cart. Items slide off lap, does not want to use tray.	Carry items in a bag or other container on lap or chair.	Push a grocery cart without endangering store and other people.	Bag or other container that is accessible to Jeff	Find container and teach Jeff to use it (OT and PCA).
Put items on counter.	Can put items on counter but is very slow, which annoys people in line behind him.	Put container on counter so clerk can remove items, or Ask for assistance.	Increase speed sufficiently, or Lift full container to counter.	None	Try to improve speed and lifting of container (PT, PCA), and Program communication aid and teach Jeff to ask for assistance (mother and PCA).
Pay for purchases.	Cannot get wallet out of pocket, cannot get money out of wallet. Does not recognize denominations of bills or coins, cannot pay correct amount or check change.	Get money out of suitable container. Recognize bills and coins. Give sufficient money to cover the purchase.	Get wallet out of pocket or money out of wallet. Determine if change is accurate.	Use an accessible container for money. Ask personal care assistant to compare bill and change occasionally.	Find accessible container for money, and teach Jeff to use it (OT, PCA). Teach Jeff to use money (OT, mother, PCA).
Carry purchases home.	Can carry small bag on lap, cannot carry large bag(s).	Carry purchases in container attached to chair.	Carry large or multiple bags on lap.	Alternate container (probably the same as in row 3, above).	Find appropriate container for purchases (OT, PCA).
Put purchases away.	Can open cupboards with flat surfaces or knobs, drawers with knobs, and the refrigerator. Cannot open high or low cupboards or drawers with flat surfaces. Can put purchases away in places he can open and reach.	Open all drawers he can reach. Put items away in higher and lower places.	Put items in very high or low places.	Make adaptations to allow Jeff to open kitchen drawers he can reach. Rearrange cupboards and drawers so items Jeff uses are accessible.	Discuss adaptations and rearrangement with house manager (OT). Improve Jeff's reach (also in row 2 above) (PT, PCA).

[a]*Note:* Those involved with each intervention are determined after the intervention is identified. At this time, Jeff has the assistance of his personal care assistant (PCA), case manager (CM), mother, occupational therapist (OT), and physical therapist (PT).
Format from Baumgart D, Brown L, Pumpian I, Nisbet J, Ford A, Sweet M, et al.: Principle of partial participation and individualized adaptations in educational programs for severely handicapped students. *J Assoc Severely Handicapped* 7:17-27, 1982.

example, the therapist might need to rely on the child's facial expressions or body movements, as well as caregiver input.[196] Similarly, a child with intellectual impairment may be unable to replicate standardized strength testing protocols. Instead, strength deficits might be identified by the child's inability to complete a functional skill, such as maintain a position against gravity or climb a step. For ambulatory children with

intellectual disabilities, a treadmill can be a reliable way to measure cardiorespiratory endurance, after allowing for practice.[128] In children with severe motor impairments, measurements of vital functions including heart rate and respiratory rate may be helpful in identifying endurance deficits. Use of the 9-point Beighton Hypermobility Score was found to be reliable and feasible in children with intellectual impairments, when provided prompting, guided movements and modification of the forward flexion testing position.[139] Examination of the integumentary system in children with intellectual and motor impairments is necessary because they may have several risk factors for skin breakdown including paralysis, immobility, insensate areas, poor nutrition, exposure to moisture from incontinence, shear from transfers, and use of accessory devices such as wheelchairs and splints.[105,148] *Smith's Recognizable Patterns of Human Malformation*[80] is a comprehensive resource of genetic abnormalities often with associated intellectual disability that can be useful for identifying body structure and function impairments that children with various conditions are likely to have that should be examined.

Tests and Measures: Contextual Factors

The AAIDD definition of *intellectual disability* requires consideration of function within context.[6] Similarly, the ICF views outcomes as resulting from interactions between health conditions and contextual factors. Contextual factors include both personal and environmental factors.[216] Environmental factors outside the child can profoundly affect child development, test scores, and intervention planning.[110] Brooks-Gunn and colleagues[23] found, for example, that differences between IQ test scores of African American and Caucasian children at age 5 years were nearly eliminated after adjustments were made for poverty and home environment.

Physical therapists often have less experience examining the social and attitudinal aspects of the environment than the physical aspects. Children rarely function alone in their environment, however, so social and attitudinal factors need to be considered. Young children are a part of their families, and older children spend their time in classrooms, in after-school activities, and in the community with their peers, family, and other community members. Acknowledgement of the complex relationship between the individual with a health condition and the environment has led to a shift toward greater emphasis on the environment in examination and intervention.[166]

In the ICF model, personal factors include those aspects of a person that are not part of the health condition, such as gender, race, coping styles, and those things that are intrinsically motivating.[216] Physical therapists need to consider such personal factors including motivation, self-efficacy, age-related interests, and engagement to effectively promote children's chosen activities and participation within the context of family, school, and community.[51] A tool that is helpful for identifying the level of supports that adolescents and adults with intellectual disabilities and other developmental disabilities need for quality participation in society is the Supports Intensity Scale (SIS).[5,185] The tool was normed with people age 16 to over 70 years and measures the supports needed in daily life activities and exceptional medical and behavioral support needs. A supplemental protection and advocacy scale also is included. The SIS-C, a version of the scale for children 5 to 15 years with intellectual disabilities, is currently being field tested.[8]

Determining Intervention Goals and Outcomes

Functional goals have been emphasized for many years in early intervention, special education, and physical therapy.[108,144,145] Functional skills have been defined as age-appropriate activities or tasks that someone else will have to do if the child does not[25] and should reflect the needs and interests of the child and family. Some children can learn to complete a task or activity,

whereas others will be capable of learning to carry out only a part of it. A child may, for example, be unable to transfer independently but can learn to unbuckle a seat belt and support weight in standing. Another child may be unable to put a DVD into a player but can learn to turn it on using a switch.

Outcomes of interventions to improve a child's abilities to participate in life must represent specific functional skills that the child will acquire. Team members cannot assume that interventions directed toward remediation of impairments, such as improving postural responses, range of motion, or strength, or toward reducing the degree of activity limitation indicated by failed items on a developmental test, will necessarily lead to meaningful outcomes.[108,144,145] This is especially true of children with intellectual disabilities who need many repetitions to learn, who forget easily, and who generalize poorly. These characteristics make it difficult or impossible for a child with intellectual disabilities to synthesize isolated activities or components of movement into meaningful skills.

Campbell[29] proposed a "top-down" approach to determining outcomes, in which the desired functional outcomes are determined first, then obstacles to their accomplishment are identified, and then intervention to overcome the obstacles is planned and implemented (Fig. 18.1). This process is similar to the decision-making process of the hypothesis-oriented algorithm for clinicians (HOAC II),[158] in which a person's goals for intervention are identified first, then the person is examined to generate a hypothesis about why the goals can or cannot be met at the present time.

Functional outcomes can be anything that is of high priority and meaningful to the child and family, is age appropriate, and is, or could be, a home, community, recreation-leisure, or vocational activity. Giangreco and colleagues[63] proposed five valued life outcomes for all children, including those with severe disabilities:

1. Having a safe, stable home in which to live now or in the future
2. Having access to a variety of places and engaging in meaningful activities
3. Having a social network of personally meaningful relationships
4. Having a level of personal choice and control that matches one's age
5. Being safe and healthy

Teams usually have the most difficulty determining meaningful outcomes for children with profound multiple disabilities, who often have extremely limited repertoires of behavior and movement. Even these children, however, can accomplish outcomes that require active behavioral changes, such as indicating a choice of food or activity or using body movements to activate switches. Such active outcomes lead to acquisition of skills that increase participation and are in contrast to passive activities that are done to the child, such as sensory stimulation, range of motion exercises, and positioning (often stated as something the child will "tolerate"). Passive activities may be part of the intervention to help a child accomplish a skill, but only the child's active behavior can increase true participation.

One helpful tool for assisting families to identify meaningful outcomes and to measure whether they have been accomplished is the Canadian Occupational Performance Measure (COPM).[94] The COPM was designed as an individualized measure of performance and satisfaction in self-care, productivity (work, household management, play/school), and leisure.

TOP-DOWN APPROACH

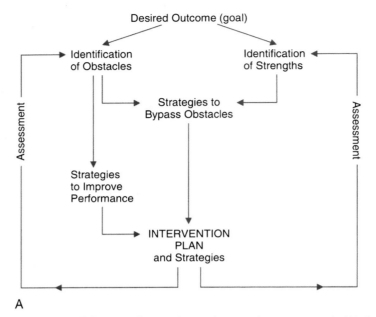

BOTTOM-UP APPROACH

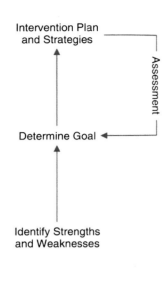

A

B

FIG. 18.1 Comparison of a top-down approach (A), in which assessments identify means to achieve desired outcomes, and a bottom-up approach (B), in which assessment results determine outcomes. (From Campbell PH: Evaluation and assessment in early intervention for infants and toddlers. *J Early Intervent* 15:42, 1991. Copyright ©1991 by Division for Early Childhood, the Council for Exceptional Children.)

Although the COPM was intended for occupational therapists, it is an equally useful tool for physical therapists. Another tool that is useful for children with receptive language at the 5-year level is the Perceived Efficacy and Goal Setting System (PEGS).[113] The PEGS uses a questionnaire format to help children rate their competence in everyday tasks and to select goals important to them.

When desired outcomes are determined first, they are discipline-free: that is, they describe the skills the child will accomplish without regard for discipline-related concerns. Only after team members identify the highest-priority outcomes do they decide which disciplines will be needed to help the child accomplish each one.[144] This team-oriented process for determining outcomes is not necessarily inconsistent with processes described in the HOAC II[158] or the *Guide to Physical Therapist Practice*[9] because both the HOAC II and the Guide describe primarily a unidisciplinary approach in which the physical therapist makes decisions in collaboration with the patient and perhaps the patient's family. When working with children whose complex problems require teams of professionals, the process must include other professionals as well.

INTERVENTION

During planning and implementation of intervention for children with intellectual disabilities, it is important to keep in mind what are widely regarded as best practices for working with children who have intellectual disabilities and other developmental disabilities. Some of these practices have been discussed previously and include families and children as full and equal team members, testing in natural environments[47] whenever

possible, and emphasizing functional outcomes with active participation by children.[108] Intervention based on environmental assessment and occurring in natural environments is far more likely to result in improved abilities to participate in everyday activities and in age-appropriate life roles than intervention that takes place in an isolated or clinical setting, is based on a normal development sequence, or focuses primarily on identification of impairments, such as range of motion, postural responses, or retention of reflexes.[24,86,108,144] Successful physical therapy services depend on more than developing intervention focused on the physical aspects of a task. Rather, successful intervention often depends on opportunities to practice within supportive social and attitudinal environments.

Other considerations that influence intervention for children with intellectual disabilities include interventions to limit impairments and promote activity and participation, use of teaching methods that are most likely to result in acquisition of skills by children with intellectual disabilities, and the role of physical therapists in promoting development in nonmotor domains.

Interventions for Impairments of Body Structures and Functions

Early identification of neuromuscular, musculoskeletal, and cardiopulmonary problems, at whatever age they occur, allows for intervention designed to limit the impairments, thus restricting the development of secondary impairments and activity limitations. Primary impairments are those associated with a condition at the time of diagnosis.[216] Secondary impairments are often the result of primary impairments, may develop over time, and can sometimes be avoided or reduced by intervention.[15] For example, children with Down syndrome are often

BOX 18.2   Physical Therapy for Children with Down Syndrome

Interventions for children with Down syndrome should be targeted to helping children achieve measurable goals identified with the parents and with the child when the child is old enough to have an opinion. Children's need for physical therapy and specific interventions changes as children age. Interventions are likely to be direct and more intensive for infants and toddlers and then involve more consultation than direct therapy as the child attends preschool and school.

Infants and Toddlers (Age Birth to 3 Years)

Early intervention services from the time the infant is medically stable to provide the parents with information about resources, the development of children with Down syndrome, and methods to promote their child's motor development and development of functional skill.[215]

Arrange access to parent-to-parent support.[116]

Attempt to prevent compensatory movements.

Consider treadmill training starting at about 10 months, which research has shown can reduce delay in walking and may promote developmental benefits of independent locomotion.[190]

When the child starts to stand, consider flexible supramalleolar orthoses to improve postural stability.[102]

Coordination and communication with other members of the early intervention team, such as speech/language pathologists, for strategies to promote communication development. Consider manual signs[202] or other forms of augmentative communication if the child is not communicating at age-appropriate levels.

Provide adaptive seating or other positioning devices to compensate for lack of postural control to facilitate reaching and hand function so the child can participate in learning activities.

Facilitate parent–child interactions.

Promote early perceptual-motor competencies such as eye gaze and joint attention to people, objects, and the environment.[200]

Coordinate and communicate with any day care or preschool providers.

Preschool

Coordinate and consult with preschool teachers about how to include the child in motor activities that will continue to promote motor development.

Consult with parents to involve child in active play, such as trike riding, swimming, etc.

Consider the need for orthoses to improve stability as necessary for development of higher-level motor skills.[102]

Consider manual signs or augmented assistive technology for communication.[202]

School Age

Prevention of problems associated with aging is important.[14]

Coordinate and consult with physical education teachers and parents to include the child in activities that promote fitness.

Promote regular physical activity including cardiovascular, flexibility, strengthening, balance, and agility.[49]

Minimize the risk of injury by structuring exercise of longer duration, greater frequency, and less intensity compared to that of typical peers.[49]

Refer to physician if child has symptoms of myelopathy (neck pain, head tilt, gait changes, weakness) due to increased risk of atlanto-axial subluxation.[4]

Choose a variety of activities that are enjoyable and motivating for the child.[49]

Teach and engage child in typical motor activities like bicycle riding.[189]

Consider a short-term exercise training program to improve strength and agility.[95]

Involve in organized programs that culminate in Special Olympics, Unified Sports, and inclusive events.

---

born with hypotonia and joint hypermobility.[199] The combination of these two factors can lead to joint instability, resulting in secondary musculoskeletal deformities including hip and patellar instability, scoliosis, and foot deformity.[61,112] Primary impairments in children with intellectual and motor impairments vary greatly and depend on the condition. Table 18.1 identifies impairments related to specific conditions and on consequences that often follow the natural history of these conditions. Pain,[126] diminished cardiopulmonary fitness,[128] obesity,[149] fatigue,[195] integumentary impairment,[105,150] impaired bone density,[87] and musculoskeletal deformity[127] are some of the many impairments that may occur secondary to the child's condition and may warrant physical therapy intervention.

Physical therapy intervention can potentially impact the development of secondary impairments as well as minimize the effect of the secondary impairment on activity, function, and participation. Continuing with the example of the child with Down syndrome, intervention designed to enhance postural control and force production may help promote accomplishment of motor milestones and decrease secondary impairments.[154] The use of foot orthoses can be helpful in improving stability and alignment for stance and gait,[102] reducing the risk of orthopedic problems. Box 18.2 provides recommendations for physical therapy for children with Down syndrome from infancy through school age.

Physical therapy intervention is often directed toward reducing the likelihood, severity, and impact of secondary impairments. Children with intellectual and motor disabilities can benefit from aerobic exercise interventions to increase cardiopulmonary fitness and endurance.[151] Strength training in children with intellectual and motor disabilities can improve functional mobility and muscular endurance.[159] Rowland and colleagues outlined strength protocols for children with Down syndrome, spina bifida, cerebral palsy, Duchenne muscular dystrophy, and autism.[159] Intervention also might focus on providing positioning equipment and supports as well as educating caregivers on the use of equipment, repositioning, and promoting alignment to help minimize pressure and positional causes of skin breakdown. The use of a standing frame has often been advocated as an intervention to help prevent osteoporosis in children with severe motor impairments. In one study a 6% increase in bone mineral density in the lumbar spine was observed with increased standing, but tibial bone density did not improve.[34] The use of a standing frame also can provide pressure relief, and standing can improve opportunities for socialization.[180] Additional information on intervention related to specific conditions and impairments is described in other chapters of this volume, including the effects of intervention on the musculoskeletal system (Chapter 5), management of spinal and orthopedic problems (Chapters 8 and 14), coordination impairment (Chapter 17), and impairments associated with cerebral palsy (Chapter 19).

Physical Therapy Interventions to Address Intellectual, Communication, and Psychosocial Limitations

If we assume that exploration and manipulation of the environment influence intellectual, communication, and social-emotional development, physical therapists play an obvious role in supporting the development of these nonmotor domains of children who have motor impairments. One means is through intervention strategies designed to improve motor performance, as described in Chapters 3 and 4 of this volume. Intervention specific to diagnoses that are often comorbid with intellectual disabilities is described in other chapters of this volume, including cerebral palsy (Chapter 19), myelodysplasia (Chapter 23), and autism (Chapter 24). Another potentially important strategy is to provide alternative means of mobility when children's motor impairments prevent exploration of the environment at an age when other children are crawling and walking.

Use of Power Mobility to Prevent Activity Limitations

Butler[27] asserted that self-produced locomotion can have such a powerful impact on development that functional means of mobility should be provided for all young children who have mobility restrictions, regardless of whether or not the child is expected to walk eventually. More recently, physical therapists and others are advocating for use of power mobility in very young children with severely delayed locomotor milestones and limited prognosis for independent ambulation.[81,97,100,157] Aided mobility is not seen as "giving up" on walking for young children but as providing critical assistance at a time when it is needed to promote age-appropriate activity and participation.

Several reports have demonstrated that very young children can learn to use power mobility devices by 7 to 11 months of age.[10,81,100,141] Use of power mobility is associated not only with increased mobility but also with improved social skills,[65,81] increased communication,[81,82,100] increased peer interaction,[142,213] and improved cognition.[81,100] Jones, McEwen, and Neas[82] studied the effects of power wheelchairs on the development of children who were 14–30 months of age at the beginning of the study and who used power wheelchairs for 1 year. The experimental group's *Battelle Developmental Inventory*[121] receptive communication, and their *Pediatric Evaluation of Disability Inventory*[72] mobility functional skills, mobility caregiver assistance, and self-case caregiver assistance scores improved more than the control group's scores from baseline to 1 year.

Although young children in these studies were believed to have normal intelligence, other studies have demonstrated that children with intellectual disabilities also can become independent users of power mobility devices.[20,124] Certain intellectual abilities probably are necessary to achieve independent power-aided mobility, but the specific abilities that are necessary and the means to assess them have not been determined. Because typically developing children learn to crawl and become independently mobile well before their first birthday and because children have become independently mobile using power mobility devices before age 2, children with intellectual disabilities who have adequate vision and the intellectual skills typical of an 18-month-old (or perhaps younger) are likely to be capable of learning to use powered means of mobility, given appropriate equipment, instruction, and opportunities. The rate of learning, however, varies, and the factors that influence the rate of learning require further study.[82] Tefft and colleagues[182] investigated intellectual predictors associated with young children who learn to use power mobility independently after six training sessions in a clinical setting. They found spatial relations and problem-solving abilities were better among children who learned to maneuver a chair than in those who did not. Children with poorer spatial relations and problem-solving abilities may be able to learn to use power mobility, but they also may require more frequent practice opportunities in their everyday settings and may take longer to achieve mobility independence.

When designing such practice opportunities, physical therapists should remember how frequently typically developing children practice and the miscues they make when learning to walk.[2]

Use of Assistive Positioning to Promote Environmental Interaction

Seating and other assistive positioning devices, as described in Chapter 33, also can influence interactions with physical and social environments through such variables as communication,[106] respiration,[96] self-care, fine motor function, and play.[148] Research suggests that positioning also can influence child communicative behaviors and opportunities for communication. After 1 month of age, infants looked at their mothers for longer periods of time when they were semireclined in supine on the couch than when held by the mother.[93] Similarly, children with profound intellectual disabilities and physical disabilities interacted with attentive teachers and classroom assistants for longer periods of time when they were in the supine position than when they were seated in wheelchairs or positioned in a sidelyer.[106] The reason for these findings is not known, although the environment might have been less distracting when children were in a supine position, or, in the case of children with disabilities who had inadequate head control, the supine position might have provided head support necessary to maintain eye contact and interact. Because a supine position may be socially isolating and physically detrimental, it should be monitored carefully and used only while the child is actively engaged in social interaction. Teachers were found to initiate interactions at higher rates when children were positioned in wheelchairs than when they were in sidelyers or supine on a mat.[106] Observations suggested that wheelchairs promoted interaction by placing students nearer the normal interaction level of adults, in contrast to being positioned on the floor.

Positioning might influence child interaction with the environment due to the impact of position on behavioral state or arousal. Low levels of arousal and behavioral states that interfere with attention to environmental stimuli are common among children with the most severe intellectual and motor disabilities.[67] Guess and colleagues[67] observed that children with multiple disabilities in upright positions demonstrated behavioral states that were more compatible with learning than when these children were placed in recumbent positions. When school-based therapists were surveyed, Taylor found that 90% of 386 respondents considered social interaction, self-esteem, and access to activities as benefits for a child utilizing a stander for upright positioning.[180] Although research concerning effects of positioning with children who have multiple disabilities is limited, it suggests that positioning may influence children's interactions with and participation within the environment through a variety of mechanisms. A systematic review of outcomes associated with adaptive seating found that although many studies linked positive effects of adapted seating on activity and participation of children with severe cerebral palsy, further investigation was needed to determine effects of adaptive seating on participation outcomes.[11]

Supporting Participation of Children with Intellectual and Motor Impairments

Many children with combined intellectual and motor disabilities will require extensive and pervasive supports as they grow up. Physical therapy services are likely to be intermittently provided across the life span and supports at all ages to mediate a child's adaptive behavior, health, context, and participation are important to consider.[212] Services frequently are initiated in infancy or early childhood, then support the child in the school environment, and eventually transition to support the individual in community, home, and work settings.

Provision of services in the least restrictive environments also is important to consider. The concept of least restrictive environments has its roots in the US Constitution, which affirms that the government shall intrude into peoples' lives in the least restrictive manner possible.[181] Since the 1960s, this concept has been incorporated into state and federal laws affecting services for people with intellectual disabilities, mandating that, to the extent possible, people with disabilities will go to school, live, and work in environments with people who do not have disabilities.

The definition of the *least restrictive environment* for people with intellectual disabilities has been moving steadily away from segregated services and toward full inclusion in community-based settings, as evidenced by closure of many institutions for people with intellectual disabilities and court-ordered inclusion of children with intellectual disabilities in general education classrooms. In 1992 a judge of the US Court for the District of New Jersey ordered a New Jersey school district to develop a plan to include an 8-year-old boy with Down syndrome in his neighborhood elementary school, with any needed supplementary aids and services. One of the court's findings was that "school districts ... must consider placing children with disabilities in regular classroom settings, with the use of supplementary aids and services ... before exploring other, more restrictive, alternatives."[179] The IDEA amendments of 2004 placed additional emphasis on the need for individualized education program (IEP) teams to consider whether a child's needs could be addressed in the general education classroom with supplementary aids and services.[55] Physical therapists are involved in the team considerations and decision-making process relative to a child's educational placement. Giangreco and colleagues[63] have written a helpful "how-to" manual for inclusion of children with severe disabilities in general education classrooms that addresses provision of physical therapy and other related services. Downing and associates[46] also provided practical and creative suggestions for including children with severe disabilities in typical classrooms.

Physical therapy services can assist in improving function in children with intellectual and motor disabilities as they transition between community settings and neighborhood schools. Collaboration and communication between school-based and habilitative service providers can be a powerful relationship in facilitating enhanced functional capacity and helping to ensure consistent and successful integration within community environments, such as religious, work, recreational, and social. As an example, after identifying child and family interests, the therapist might communicate with staff at a local YMCA, a scout leader, or a church youth group. Subsequently, the physical therapist might coordinate with the YMCA staff to establish a fitness program, with community transportation to schedule appropriate transportation to scout meetings, or with the church facility manager to facilitate ease of access to the youth club room. The physical therapist might provide specific education and training to community agency personnel in transfer, access, safety, and level of participation. Child-specific instruction might include skills needed for the YMCA fitness program, getting on/off the community transport van, or mobility within the church. Documentation by the team, including the physical therapist, of progress and problems encountered will

be important when evaluating the current plan of integrating the child into a specific community setting. Adjusting related procedures including community partner responsibilities, the need to consult with additional providers, frequency of physical therapy intervention, and the expected duration of services will all require consideration by all parties including the child and family, the community agency, and the physical therapist.

Teaching and Learning Considerations

Much of what physical therapists do to address activity limitations and participation restrictions involves teaching children to move more effectively and efficiently. Educational researchers have identified a number of teaching strategies that optimize the learning of students with intellectual disabilities and that might help physical therapists when designing and implementing intervention plans. Although most of these strategies were designed for educational programming, they can also be applied to motor learning. These strategies are closely related to current motor learning principles including antecedent verbal instruction and demonstration, providing feedback, allowing for error and consequences, and specificity of task in natural environment (see Chapter 4 on motor learning). Physical therapists should also communicate with other team members to identify opportunities for children to practice motor skills throughout their daily routine and should provide client and caregiver instruction so that these individuals are able to promote learning during those opportunities. Behavioral intervention is one of the areas in which physical therapists should take advantage of the expertise of other members of service delivery teams, such as teachers and psychologists. Physical therapy educational prerequisites and curricula rarely provide more than superficial information about behavioral strategies, and this limits the extent to which many physical therapists can use them effectively to promote the development of motor skills by children with intellectual disabilities.

Instruction in Natural Environments

Over 50 years ago, Mead, as cited in Dunst, et al. (2001),[48] observed that variations in natural environments and varied learning opportunities were related to differences in skill acquisition and generalization. Because students with intellectual disabilities may take a long time to learn a few things and because they have difficulty generalizing and maintaining skills, traditional curricula that build sequentially on fundamental nonfunctional skills have not generally led to meaningful gains.[46] Children are often unable to generalize such nonfunctional activities as putting pegs in pegboards, for example, to functional activities such as putting coins in a machine to get a soft drink. Practicing "prerequisite" skills, such as writing the letters of the alphabet, also often fails to result in such functional outcomes as the ability to sign one's name or select the correct restroom in a public place.

Children with severe motor impairments encounter similar difficulties when nonfunctional or presumed prerequisite skills are the focus of physical therapy. For instance, developing the skill of ascending and descending a set of therapy steps is vastly different from climbing a set of stairs at a library or other community setting due to contextual factors affecting the child's performance.[64,74] Contextual factors could include noise, visual distractions, other individuals, and inconsistencies in physical nature of stairs.[167] Little research supports generalization (carryover) of skills demonstrated during isolated physical therapy sessions to other settings or synthesis of presumed components and prerequisites of movement into measurable functional motor activities.[76]

When an emphasis is on acquisition of specific functional skills in natural environments, generalization is unnecessary or less difficult, and skills are likely to be maintained by natural reinforcers and ongoing occasions for practice.[85] If several people work with the child on the same skills using consistent methods, learning may be enhanced by providing more opportunities to learn (repetitions) and by varying the stimulus conditions under which the skill is practiced, thus promoting generalization. Providing client and caregiver education including strategies and daily opportunities to practice during routine, typical activities is critical to promote achievement of functional skills. These principles serve as a basis for integrated models of service delivery that have been advocated for a wide range of interventionists including physical therapists.[139] Although limited research has been conducted to support the effectiveness of teaching motor skills in natural environments, research in other areas, such as life skills, language, and social interaction, has suggested that such an approach would be valuable. [74,168]

Behavioral Programming Intervention

Behavioral programming is based on the assumption that behaviors are learned through interactions with social, physical, and biologic environments; by manipulating such environments, behaviors can be taught.[19] After a review of research on the effectiveness of motor skills instruction for children with neuromotor impairments, Horn[76] concluded that physical therapists and occupational therapists should develop procedures to incorporate behavioral techniques into their intervention programs. This recommendation was made based on the relative success of interventions using behavioral techniques compared with the neuromotor and sensory stimulation techniques that occupational therapists and physical therapists commonly use. By incorporating behavioral techniques into other intervention strategies, physical therapists not only may be able to increase the rate at which children with intellectual disabilities acquire motor skills and the number of skills they acquire but also may promote generalization and maintenance of motor behaviors.

Positive reinforcement. A child is positively reinforced by a stimulus if a behavior that preceded the stimulus increases.[134] Possible reinforcing stimuli are unlimited, ranging from tangible items, such as food and toys, to social reinforcers, such as attention or descriptive praise, and activity reinforcers, such as watching a video.[163] With children who have intellectual disabilities, especially severe or profound intellectual disabilities, common reinforcers such as praise, access to activities, and food often fail to lead to increases in behaviors, and identification of reinforcers can be a challenge.[79,173] Reinforcement has not been shown to result in acquisition of behaviors not previously in the child's repertoire. A combination of reinforcement with antecedent techniques and modification of consequences has, however, resulted in new behavioral responses.[173]

Antecedent techniques. The first step in shaping a new behavior is to prompt the desired behavior or an approximation by providing instructions, models, cues, or physical prompts.[173] Instructions can take a variety of forms, such as verbal or gestural instructions (e.g., "Reach for the toy") or verbal instructions paired with models, cues, or physical prompts (e.g., "Reach for the toy," paired with facilitation of movement at the shoulder). Modeling provides a demonstration of a behavior that the child

attempts to imitate. Cues direct a child's attention to a task that can result in the desired behavior, without a physical prompt. To cue the child to reach for the toy, the toy could be tapped on the table or held above the child to encourage the child to reach or to assume an erect posture or a standing position. Many of the techniques used by physical therapists provide physical prompts for motor behaviors.

For optimal learning to occur the type and amount of prompting must be matched to the skills of the child, with the least amount of help necessary being the most conducive to the child's learning.[173] Prompting should be faded as the child responds so that natural cues eventually provide the stimulus for response. A natural cue is the least intrusive prompt (e.g., the presence of a friend serving as a cue for a child to look up) and is the level of prompt required for independent behaviors. Physical prompts, often used by physical therapists, are the most intrusive.

Providing consequences. Once a behavior has been prompted, it can be improved or expanded through shaping or chaining techniques. Shaping and chaining can also be used to build new behaviors through reinforcement of behaviors that successively approximate the desired behavior.[173]

New behaviors can be shaped by reinforcing behaviors that are increasingly similar to the target behavior, such as reinforcing components of standing up from a chair, or chaining to link standing, walking, opening doors, and other behaviors necessary to accomplish a goal of walking to lunch. Backward chaining, in which the last step in the sequence is learned first, is often a useful technique because children receive the reward of task completion, often a natural reinforcer, throughout the process of learning the skill.[173]

Positive behavior support. Positive behavior support is another approach to intervention for children with developmental disabilities, including intellectual disabilities, who may lack knowledge, communication, or the social skills necessary to function effectively in their everyday environments. Lucyshyn and colleagues[99] hypothesized that children with these limitations may develop unwanted behaviors as a means of getting needs and wants met and for limiting aversive events. Positive behavior support interventions involve the use of methods to redesign children's social and attitudinal environments, and sometimes their physical environments, to enhance their ability to enjoy life with behaviors that are more acceptable to others. Intervention is aimed at replacing problem behaviors with more socially acceptable behaviors and making problem behaviors ineffective and undesirable.[33]

Positive behavior support shows promise as an intervention that encourages participation in everyday routines without limiting children's personal preferences. The interventionist begins by observing the child in the child's everyday environments to look for antecedents that may be triggering a problem behavior and identifying any environmental influences on the behavior.[33] The interventionist must work closely with family members or other primary care providers to develop hypotheses about causes of problem behaviors, learn what motivates the child, and develop a plan that is acceptable for the people in the environments in which the child spends time.[99] An effective plan redirects the child before the problem behavior occurs by adapting the task, the environment, or the demands.

Case studies have described the use of positive behavior support in a variety of everyday environments.[39,198] Vaughn and colleagues[198] utilized video task analysis of a child to identify the problem behavior and recurring antecedents, as well as the consequences, during a family routine that produced undesirable behavior. Hypotheses were developed as to the cause and function of the undesirable behavior and the identification of appropriate positive reinforcers. Interventions were put in place employing the positive reinforcers to decrease the disruptive behavior and enhance overall engagement in the family routine. Cole and Levinson[39] found that providing choice in aspects of unpleasant tasks (such as where to stand in line) reduced occurrence of problem behaviors in two children with developmental disabilities.

Bradshaw, Mitchell, and Leaf presented results from a randomized controlled study focusing on positive behavior support programs in schools over a 5-year period that showed reductions in suspensions and discipline referrals when positive behavior programs were carried out with fidelity.[21] This research and the case studies suggest that positive behavior support has promise to assist families, teachers, and other care providers in helping children with intellectual disabilities participate more successfully in everyday routines. As members of teams, physical therapists may participate in task analysis, developing an intervention plan and using the intervention while working with children. One important aspect of positive behavior support is promoting children's communication abilities so they can express desires and needs in behaviorally acceptable ways.

Promoting Children's Communication Development

When working with children who have intellectual disabilities, all team members are responsible for promoting development in areas often not considered part of their disciplinary domains. One of the most effective ways physical therapists can contribute to the overall development of children with intellectual disabilities is to assist efforts to improve communication abilities. At its most basic level, communication enables children to influence their social and physical environments to control what happens to them. All children, even those with the most profound multiple disabilities, can communicate.[118] Communication may be both aided and unaided and can be achieved in many forms including facial expression, body language, gestures, and both electronic and nonelectronic devices (see Chapter 33). The ability of children to control their environment and their interactions is key to prevention or reduction of these children's pervasive passivity or "learned helplessness," a condition that can result in difficulty with problem solving and mastering tasks.[218] Learned helplessness occurs when the child believes he or she is unable to accomplish a given skill and therefore is unwilling to try, relying on others. Learned helplessness can be the result of repeated failures, believing others are in control, or having others manage daily needs.[147] Providing environmental supports that give children the opportunity to make choices, solve simple problems, and promote self-regulation can help limit learned helplessness and promote self-determination.[133]

The importance of communication and the need for all team members to participate in communication development were recognized by creation of the National Joint Committee for the Communicative Needs of Persons with Severe Disabilities. Representatives of seven organizations, including the American Physical Therapy Association, served on the original joint committee and developed guidelines that cross traditional disciplinary boundaries and reflect a "shared commitment to promoting effective communication by persons with severe disabilities, thus providing a common ground on which the disciplines of the member organizations can unite their efforts to improve the quality of life of such persons" (p 1).[118] These guidelines, as well as the Communication Bill of Rights, were recently updated and continue to provide support to professionals and teams serving individuals with severe disabilities.[22] Physical therapists are responsible for promoting effective communication, not only through such traditional means as positioning and improving motor skills to enable access to communication aids but also through provision of environments that acknowledge and address the Communication Bill of Rights (Fig. 18.2) of children who have communication disabilities.[118]

Evaluation of Outcomes

Because children and young adults with intellectual disabilities, particularly those with severe disabilities, often progress slowly, using outcome measures that are responsive to small changes is important. This is necessary not only to determine if progress is being made but also to prevent expenditure of time and effort on intervention strategies that are not leading to meaningful improvement for the child and family. Three related methods that are especially useful for assessing outcomes of physical therapy for children with intellectual disabilities are (1) accomplishment of behavioral objectives and goal attainment scaling, (2) use of the Canadian Occupational Performance Measure,[94] and (3) single-subject research methods.

Use of Behavioral Objectives and Goal Attainment Scaling

Assessment of outcomes can be relatively straightforward if functional goals and behavioral objectives leading to them are identified before intervention. As described by Randall and McEwen,[145] the components of behavioral objectives should enable therapists to monitor a child's progress toward accomplishment of a goal, determine if it is necessary to modify an intervention, and determine when and if goals have been met. Once a goal, such as "David will go to the kitchen and make himself a peanut butter sandwich," has been identified, behavioral objectives leading to achievement of the goal can be developed by comparing David's abilities with the goal's requirements. Breaking goals into behavioral objectives helps team members determine if children with intellectual disabilities, who tend to change slowly, are making progress.

Behavioral objectives have five components: (1) Who will do (2) what, (3) under what condition, (4) how well, and (5) by when.[145] These five components permit a measurable evaluation of whether the objective is being met within the projected time frame. One of David's behavioral objectives, leading to the sandwich-making goal, might be to move himself from the living room to the kitchen, which could be written, "David will walk using his reverse walker from the living room to the kitchen in less than 2 minutes on four of five consecutive days after school by December 14, 20__." Assessing whether this objective, or part of it, is accomplished, regardless of the intervention methods used, should not be difficult.

To allow detection of smaller gains, objectives can be scaled using goal attainment scaling (GAS).[188] Starting with the behavioral objective that the child is expected to achieve, four additional objectives are determined: two that exceed the behavioral objective and two that fall below it. By identifying objectives above and below a child's anticipated achievement, a range of outcomes related to a general goal can be assessed. Information on goal attainment scaling can be found in Chapter 2, Tests and Measures. Table 18.3 shows an example of GAS with David's objective.

All persons, regardless of the extent or severity of their disabilities, have a basic right to affect, through communication, the conditions of their own existence. Beyond this general right, a number of specific communication rights should be ensured in all daily interactions and interventions involving persons who have severe disabilities. These basic communication rights are as follows:

1. The right to request desired objects, actions, events, and persons and to express personal preferences or feelings.
2. The right to be offered choices and alternatives.
3. The right to reject or refuse undesired objects, events, or actions, including the right to decline or reject all proffered choices.
4. The right to request, and be given, attention from and interaction with another person.
5. The right to request feedback or information about a state, an object, a person, or an event of interest.
6. The right to active treatment and intervention efforts to enable people with severe disabilities to communicate messages in whatever modes and as effectively and efficiently as their specific abilities will allow.
7. The right to have communication acts acknowledged and responded to, even when the intent of these acts cannot be fulfilled by the responder.
8. The right to have access at all times to any needed augmentative and alternative communication devices and other assistive devices and to have those devices in good working order.
9. The right to environmental contexts, interactions, and opportunities that expect and encourage persons with disabilities to participate as full communicative partners with other people, including peers.
10. The right to be informed about the people, things, and events in one's immediate environment.
11. The right to be communicated with in a manner that recognizes and acknowledges the inherent dignity of the person being addressed, including the right to be part of communication exchanges about individuals that are conducted in his or her presence.
12. The right to be communicated with in ways that are meaningful, understandable, and culturally and linguistically appropriate.

FIG. 18.2 Communication bill of rights. (From National Joint Committee for the Communication Needs of Persons With Severe Disabilities. (1992). Guidelines for meeting the communication needs of persons with severe disabilities [Guidelines]. Available from www.asha.org/policy or www.asha.org/njc.)

TABLE 18.3 Example of Goal Attainment Scaling

GOAL ATTAINMENT SCALING[156]

5-Point Scale based on the performance of the objective

OBJECTIVE: David will walk using his reverse walker from the living room to the kitchen in less than 2 minutes on four of five consecutive days after school by December 14, 20__.

Score	Objective
−2 Much less than expected	David will walk from the dining room to the kitchen in more than 3 minutes on four of five consecutive days after school by December 14, 20__.
−1 Somewhat less than expected	David will walk from the dining room to the kitchen in less than 3 minutes on four of five consecutive days after school by December 14, 20__.
0 Expected level of outcome	David will walk using his reverse walker from the living room to the kitchen in less than 2 minutes on four of five consecutive days after school by December 14, 20__.
+1 Somewhat more than expected	David will walk using his reverse walker from the living room to the kitchen in less than 1 minute on four of five consecutive days after school by December 14, 20__.
+2 Much more than expected	David will walk using his reverse walker from the living room to the kitchen in less than 30 seconds on four of five consecutive days after school by December 14, 20__.

Canadian Occupational Performance Measure

The COPM[94] was designed to help identify and measure individually meaningful goals for people in the areas of self-care, productivity (work, household management, and play/school), and leisure. More information on the COPM can be found in Chapter 2, Tests and Measures. In children with intellectual and motor impairments, gains in participation are often incremental and include partial completion of a task. The COPM can capture small changes in performance and resulting satisfaction of the child or family. As an example, a teen might identify participation in the cheer and pep squad as an important and meaningful goal. Rather than the ability to remember and perform intricate cheerleading maneuvers, meaningful participation gains and increased satisfaction might include the ability to sit with the pep squad in the bleachers, maintaining balance while using pom-poms. The COPM can measure the difference between how the teen perceives involvement in cheering on examination compared to the perception of participation following physical therapy intervention aimed at sitting on the bleachers, whether through improved sitting balance, if achievable, or with the use of adapted equipment.

Single-Subject Research Methods

Single-subject research methods are another useful means of assessing intervention outcomes in clinical, educational, and other service settings. These methods can be used to assess the outcomes for a single child or can assess effects of intervention across several children. Unlike case reports, single-subject research designs have controls that allow identification of cause–effect relationships among interventions and outcomes.[107] Several types of single-subject designs exist, including A-B, withdrawal, alternating treatment, and multiple baseline.[140]

Many examples of single-subject research exist in rehabilitation literature.[59,186,187] Meiser and McEwen,[111] for example, used an A-B-A single-subject design to compare the effect of ultralight and lightweight wheelchairs on the preference and propulsion of two young girls with myelodysplasia. Nearly all of the measured propulsion variables, including speed, distance, and effort, favored the ultralight wheelchairs, and the children and their mothers preferred them. A physical therapist in the home setting could use a similar design when choosing specialized equipment for the child at home. Likewise, school-based therapists could use a single-subject design to measure the impact of using a stander or gait trainer on the participation and social interaction of a child within the classroom. Textbooks and research articles are good resources for anyone interested in using single-subject research methods to measure outcomes of intervention. An excellent reference on single-subject methods is found in the text by Portney and Watkins.[140]

TRANSITION TO ADULTHOOD

Some people with intellectual disabilities, especially those with severe and profound multiple disabilities, may receive physical therapy, as a related service within special education, throughout their childhood years and during their transition to adulthood. Others will receive short episodes of physical therapy services as their abilities and needs change over time. The types of services provided, the intensity of services, and the model of service delivery should be individualized to the needs of the person. Therapists working in public schools are especially likely to be involved in the transition to adulthood because Part B of IDEA (2004) requires that transition planning begin by at least age 16 for all students with disabilities.[55] Transition services for students who have IEPs must promote movement from high school to meaningful community living, postsecondary education, training, and employment. The role of physical therapists, along with other IEP and interagency team members, should be to enable students to function meaningfully and as independently as possible in their current and possible future environments. See Chapter 32 in this volume for more information on postsecondary transition planning.

The transition to adulthood is difficult for many young people, regardless of their abilities or disabilities. Until recently, most young adults with intellectual and neuromotor impairments had few options available to them, and the greater their intellectual disabilities, the fewer options they had. Historically, employment options did not exist or were limited to sheltered workshops or activity centers. Although the decade between 2000 and 2010 revealed positive trends for young adults with disabilities for postsecondary employment, education, and independent living, students with intellectual and developmental disabilities were not expected to attend college and fewer than 10% achieved competitive employment.[123] Residential options usually included staying at home with aging parents or moving into a large residential facility, and few adults with intellectual and developmental disabilities expressed the desire or ability to live independently.[28,123] Young people also had few choices about how they spent their time, with whom they spent time, or where they could go. Thirty-five percent of youth with multiple disabilities reported no community engagement at all.[122]

In recent years, more employment and community life options have become available for people with severe intellectual disabilities, including those with the most severe multiple disabilities. To be able to take full advantage of these options, young people need to prepare for transition to adult life throughout their years in school and then should continue to receive support as the transition takes place and the new life begins. Physical therapy supports often can make a difference in the options available to young people with both intellectual and motor disabilities as they pursue successful transitions to adult life. Self-determination is often key to students' achieving their desired employment, educational, or adult living outcomes.

Self-Determination

Youth with disabilities often have difficulty achieving goals that their peers without disabilities achieve relatively easily, such as independent living, higher education, and employment. People with disabilities should have the same promise of self-determination as all people. Self-determination is defined by the Arc as having "opportunities, respectful support, and the authority to exert control in their lives, to self-direct their services to the extent they choose, and to advocate on their own behalf."[183] The Arc position statement is found in Box 18.3. Wehmeyer defined self-determination as "volitional actions that enable a person to improve their quality of life by acting with their own volitional intent."[206] Teaching and supporting self-determination have been found to improve school, employment, and community adult outcomes for youth with disabilities, including youth with intellectual disabilities.[204,207,211]

Self-determined people demonstrate four essential elements: autonomous behavior, self-regulated behavior, initiation and response to events, and self-realizing behavior.[206] These elements compose the *Self-Determined Learning Model of Instruction,*[205] which is a useful resource that has been validated in a variety of educational and employment settings.[103]

People exhibit self-determination by making everyday decisions and life decisions for themselves.[209] In a review of the self-determination literature, Malian and Nevin[101] found six curricula for teaching self-determination skills that have been field tested. Overall, the studies suggested that direct instruction in self-determination skills can lead to positive changes in the knowledge, attitudes, and behaviors associated with self-determination. Wehmeyer and Schwartz[210] examined the relationship between scores on a self-determination rating scale and outcomes of youth with intellectual or learning disabilities 1 year after leaving school. In their sample of 80 participants, students with higher scores on a self-determination rating scale were more likely to be employed and earn more per hour than students who achieved lower scores on the scale.

Wehmeyer and Bolding[208,209] also studied the relationship between environment and self-determination. In one study, they matched adults by intelligence, age, and gender to examine the relationship between living and working environments and self-determination. They found that those living or working in general community-based settings reported greater self-determination and autonomous function than matched peers living or working in segregated community-based settings or non–community-based segregated settings. This study suggested that environments and, in particular, inclusive community environments were important for greater self-determination and autonomy for people with intellectual disabilities. Wehmeyer and Bolding[209] also studied change in self-determination with changes in work or living environments. When 31 people moved from a restrictive environment (such as a nursing

---

BOX 18.3   **The Arc Position Statement on Self-Determination**

People with intellectual and/or developmental disabilities (I/DD)[a] have the same right to, and responsibilities that accompany, self-determination as everyone else. They must have opportunities, respectful support, and the authority to exert control in their lives, to self-direct their services to the extent they choose, and to advocate on their own behalf.

Issue

Many individuals with intellectual and/or developmental disabilities have not had the opportunity or the support to make choices and decisions about important aspects of their lives. Instead, they are often overprotected and involuntarily segregated, with others making decisions about key elements of their lives. Many individuals with I/DD have not had the experiences that would enable them to learn decision-making skills, take more personal control in their lives, and make choices. The lack of such learning opportunities has impeded people with I/DD from becoming participating, valued, and respected members of their communities, living lives of their own choosing.

Position

People with intellectual and/or developmental disabilities have the same right to self-determination as all people and must have the freedom, authority, and support to exercise control over their lives. To this end, they must:

In their personal lives have:

opportunities to advocate for themselves with the assurance that their desires, interests, and preferences will be respected and honored.

opportunities to acquire and use skills and knowledge which better enable them to exercise choice.

the right to take risks.

the right to choose their own allies.

the lead in decision-making about all aspects of their lives.

the option to self-direct their own supports and services and allocate available resources.

the choice and support necessary to hire, train, manage, and fire their own staff.

In their community lives have:

the right to receive the necessary support and assistance to vote.

opportunities to be supported to become active, valued members and leaders of community boards, advisory councils, and other organizations.

opportunities to take leadership roles in setting the policy direction for the self-determination movement.

the right to representation and meaningful involvement in policy-making at the federal, state, and local levels.

Adopted: Congress of Delegates, The Arc of the United States, 2011

[a]"People with intellectual and/or developmental disabilities" refers to those defined by AAIDD classification and DSM IV. In everyday language they are frequently referred to as people with cognitive, intellectual, and/or developmental disabilities although the professional and legal definitions of those terms both include others and exclude some defined by DSM IV.
From the Arc Position Statement on Self-Determination. Retrieved June 15, 2015 from http://www.thearc.org/who-we-are/position-statements/rights/self-determination.

---

home or sheltered workshop) to a less restrictive environment, self-determination increased when compared with premove test scores.

Physical therapists can help children with intellectual disabilities recognize what is important to them in their daily lives.[9] Providing physical therapy under this construct is best accomplished through a team approach that identifies priorities for the child and family and considers the environments in which the child does or will spend time. Self-determination is something that does not start in adolescence. It needs to begin early, with young children being offered opportunities to make choices in any way they are able to indicate preferences. Older children should be expected to be responsible for their choices, and young adults should be expected to thoughtfully decide what is best for them, and then others should support their choices.

Employment

Employment for individuals with intellectual and motor disabilities should include paid employment, including supported employment or self-employment, in integrated community settings.[184] Employment options in the United States for people with intellectual disabilities and multiple disabilities have expanded over the past several years, particularly in some parts of the country. This improvement was reflected in a 2013 report by the US Bureau of Labor Statistics,[193] which showed unemployment of people with intellectual and developmental disabilities (IDD) dropped from 15% in 2011 to 13% and the number of employed people with IDD rose from 4.9 million in 2011 to 5.1 million in 2013. Yet only 1 in 10 youth with developmental disabilities worked in integrated settings, and 5 in 10 were waiting for adult employment supports.[28,161,214]

Many places still primarily offer sheltered workshop and activity center alternatives, even as a first option out of high school,[28,114,161,214] but progress is being made nationwide as federal, state, and other public and private initiatives support development and expansion of employment opportunities for people with disabilities.[123] The Association of Supported Employment (APSE) supports *Employment First*, a concept that aims to facilitate full inclusion of people with the most significant disabilities into competitive work.[12] *Employment First* presumes that all people, regardless of disability, should have the opportunity to participate in community-based, competitive, integrated employment, with the appropriate supports in place, as a first and preferred employment option.

The Developmental Disabilities Act (2000)[184] described supported employment services as those that enable individuals with developmental disabilities to perform competitive work in integrated work settings when competitive employment has not traditionally occurred; when competitive employment has been interrupted or intermittent as a result of significant disability; or when intensive or extended supports are needed in order for a person to perform competitive work. Supported employment has helped to increase employment options for many people who have severe disabilities. Rather than working on prerequisite or prevocational skills in sheltered settings until they are "ready" for a job, people in supported employment learn real job skills, in competitive employment settings, with ongoing support from team members to learn and maintain the job.[56] The US Department of Health and Human Services described and verified supported employment as an evidence-based approach to enabling individuals with disabilities to achieve gainful employment.[192]

Even though supported employment received significant support from the Vocational Rehabilitation Act Amendments of 1986 (PL 99-506), which authorized new funds for states to provide supported employment services to people with severe disabilities, as yet few communities offer a supported employment alternative to sheltered workshops and day activity centers for those with the most severe disabilities. In 2000, Cimera reviewed 21 studies that investigated the economic value of supported employment. These studies overall continued to suggest that supported employment programs were cost effective from the perspective of the worker and the taxpayer. His review also found that supported employment was cost efficient for all individuals with disabilities, but those with more severe disabilities were less cost efficient than their peers with milder disabilities.[36]

Physical therapists can play a pivotal role in the successful employment of individuals who have both intellectual disabilities and limited motor skills. Physical therapists can assist employment specialists to assess an individual's abilities to perform job-related motor skills and to identify jobs that are compatible with those skills. They can also identify assistive technology and environmental modifications that may enable the person to perform a job that might not be possible otherwise. Physical therapists can include vocational planning assessment tools in their repertoire of skills and can also help develop training for job-related motor skills and for self-care and mobility during working hours.

SUMMARY

Regardless of their medical diagnoses, children with intellectual disabilities have learning characteristics that physical therapists need to consider for effective physical therapy management. Compared with typically developing children, children with intellectual disabilities have been shown, for example, to be able to learn fewer things, to need more repetitions for learning to occur, to have greater difficulty generalizing skills from one environment to another, to have greater difficulty maintaining skills that are not practiced regularly, to have slower response times, and to have a more limited repertoire of responses. Physical therapy intervention strategies that address these learning characteristics, which include motor learning principles, and that promote communication, inclusion, and self-determination can have an important role in the meaningful outcomes and participation of people with intellectual and motor disabilities. Although children with intellectual and motor impairments will likely need considerable support across their life spans, physical therapy services can often help expand the options for children and families, ease the child's transition into and participation in the community, and promote independence across environments in which people choose to live and work.

Case Scenario on Expert Consult

The case scenario related to this chapter illustrates assessment measures and modifications used to assess and establish a physical therapy plan of care for a child with an intellectual and motor impairment. Family concerns and participation in both assessment and intervention planning are included A video of a portion of the assessment accompanies the case.

REFERENCES

1. Adolph KE: Specificity of learning: why infants fall over a veritable cliff, *Psychol Sci* 11:290–295, 2000.
2. Adolph KE, Cole WG, Komati M, Garciaguirre JS, Badaly D, Lingeman JM, et al.: How do you learn to walk? Thousands of steps and dozens of falls per day, *Psychol Sci* 23:1387–1394, 2012.
3. Adolph KE, Joh AS, Eppler MA: Infants' perception of affordances of slopes under high- and low-friction conditions, *J Exp Psychol Hum Percept Perform* 36:797–811, 2010.
4. American Academy of Pediatrics: Clinical report-health supervision for children with Down syndrome, *Pediatrics* 128:393–406, 2011.
5. American Association on Intellectual and Developmental Disabilities: Supports Intensity Scale™ information, 2009.
6. American Association on Intellectual and Developmental Disabilities: Definition of intellectual disability, 2015. Available from: URL: http://aaidd.org/intellectual-disability/definition#.VX4tIEait28.
7. American Association on Intellectual and Developmental Disabilities: Diagnostic Adaptive Behavior Scale (DABS), 2016. Available from: URL: http://aaidd.org/intellectual-disability/diagnostic-adaptive-behavior-scale#.V9n5oYYrIdU.
8. American Association on Intellectual and Developmental Disabilities: Supports Intensity Scale for Children SIS-C, 2015. Available from: URL: http://aaidd.org/sis/for-children#.VX3LFkait28.
9. American Physical Therapy Association: Guide to physical therapist practice 3.0. Available from: URL: http://guidetoptpractice.apta.org/.
10. Anderson DI, Campos JJ, Anderson DE, Thomas TD, Witherington DC, Uchiyama I, Barbu-Roth MA: The flip side of perception-action coupling: locomotor experience and the ontogeny of visual-postural coupling, *Hum Mov Sci* 20:461–487, 2001.
11. Angsupaisal M, Maathuis CG, Hadders-Algra M: Adaptive seating systems in children with severe cerebral palsy across International Classification of Functioning, Disability and Health for Children and Youth version domains: a systematic review, *Dev Med Child Neurol* 57:919–930, 2015.
12. Association of People Supporting Employment, 2010. Available from: URL: http://www.apse.org/employment-first/statement/.
13. Baker BJ, Cole KN, Harris SR: Intellectual referencing as a method of OT/PT triage for young children, *Pediatr Phys Ther* 10:2–6, 1998.
14. Barnhart RC, Connolly B: Aging and Down syndrome: implications for physical therapy, *Phys Ther* 87:1399–1406, 2007.
15. Bartlett DJ, Palisano RJ: A multivariate model of determinants of motor change for children with cerebral palsy, *Phys Ther* 80:598–614, 2000.
16. Bayley N: *Bayley Scales of Infant and Toddler Development*, ed 3, San Antonio, TX, 2005, Pearson.
17. Bell MA, Fox NA: Individual differences in object permanence performance at 8 months: locomotor experience and brain electrical activity, *Dev Psychobiol* 31:287–297, 1998.
18. Bhutta AT, Cleves MA, Casey PH, Cradock MM, Anand KJS: Intellectual and behavioral outcomes of school-aged children who were born preterm, *JAMA* 288:728–737, 2002.
19. Bijou SW: A functional analysis of retarded development. In Ellis NR, editor: *International review of research in mental retardation*, vol. 1. New York, 1966, Academic Press, pp 1–19.
20. Bottos M, Bolcati C, Sciuto L, Ruggeri C, Feliciangeli A: Powered wheelchairs and independence in young children with tetraplegia, *Dev Med Child Neurol* 43:69–777, 2001.
21. Bradshaw C, Mitchell M, Leaf P: Examining the effects of schoolwide positive behavior interventions and supports on student outcomes: results from a randomized controlled effectiveness trial in elementary schools, *J Posit Behav Interv* 12(3):133–148, 2010.
22. Brady NC, Bruce S, Goldman A, Erickson K, Mineo B, Ogletree BT, et al.: Communication services and supports for individuals with severe disabilities: guidance for assessment, *Am J Intellect Dev Disabil* 121:121–138, 2016.
23. Brooks-Gunn J, Kelbanov PK, Duncan GJ: Ethnic differences in children's intelligence test scores: role of economic deprivation, home environment, and maternal characteristics, *Child Dev* 67:396–408, 1996.

24. Brown DA, Effgen SK, Palisano: Performance following ability-focused physical therapy interventions in individuals with severely limited physical and cognitive abilities, *Phys Ther* 78:934–950, 1998.

25. Brown L, Branston MB, Hamre-Nietupski S, Pumpian I, Certo N, Gruenewald L: A strategy for developing chronological age appropriate and functional curricular content for severely handicapped adolescents and young adults, *J Spec Ed* 12:81–90, 1979.

26. Brown L, Sherbenou RJ, Johnsen SK: *Test of nonverbal intelligence*, ed 4, Austin, 2010, Pro-Ed.

27. Butler C: Augmentative mobility: why do it? *Phys Med Rehabilitation Clin North Am* 2:801–815, 1991.

28. Cameto R, Levine P, Wagner M: *Transition planning for students with disabilities*, Menlo Park, CA, 2004, SRI International. Available from: URL: http://www.nlts2.org/reports/2004_11/index.html.

29. Campbell PH: Evaluation and assessment in early intervention for infants and toddlers, *J Early Interven* 15:36–45, 1991.

30. Campbell SK, Kolobe THA, Osten ET, Lenke M, Girolami GL: Construct validity of the Test of Infant Motor Performance, *Phys Ther* 75:585–596, 1995.

31. Campos JJ, Bertenthal BI: Locomotion and psychological development in infancy. In Jaffe KM, editor: *Childhood powered mobility: developmental, technical and clinical perspectives: proceedings of the RESNA First Northwest Regional Conference*, Washington, DC, 1987, RESNA, pp 11–42.

32. Campos JJ, Anderson DI, Barbu-Roth MA, Hubbard EM, Hertenstein MJ, Witherington D: Travel broadens the mind, *Infancy* 1:149–219, 2000.

33. Carr EG, Dunlap G, Horner RH, et al.: Positive behavior support: evolution of an applied science, *J Posit Behav Interv* 4:4–16, 2002.

34. Caulton J, Ward K, Alsop C, Dunn G, Adams J, Mughal M: A randomised controlled trial of standing programme on bone mineral density in non-ambulant children with cerebral palsy, *Arch Dis Child* 89:131–135, 2004.

35. Chen C, Visootsak J, Dills S, Graham Jr JM: Prader-Willi syndrome: an update and review for the primary pediatrician, *Clin Pediatr* 46:580–591, 2007.

36. Cimera RE: Cost efficiency of supported employment programs: a literature review, *J Voc Rehabil* 4:51–61, 2000.

37. Clearfield MW: The role of crawling and walking experience in infant spatial memory, *J Exp Child Psychol* 89:214–241, 2004.

38. Cloninger CK: Designing collaborative educational services. In Orelove FP, Sobsey D, Silberman RK, editors: *Educating children with multiple disabilities: a collaborative approach*, ed 4, Baltimore, 2004, Paul H. Brookes, pp 1–29.

39. Cole CL, Levinson TR: Effects of within activity choices on the challenging behavior of children with severe developmental disabilities, *J Posit Behav Interv* 4:29–37, 2002.

40. Cornish K, Bramble D: Cri du chat syndrome: genotype-phenotype correlations and recommendations for clinical management, *Dev Med Child Neurol* 44:494–497, 2002.

41. Coster W, Deeney T, Haltiwanger J, Haley S: *School Function Assessment (SFA)*, San Antonio, TX, 1998, Pearson.

42. Crisp C: The efficacy of intelligence testing in children with physical disabilities, visual impairments and/or the inability to speak, *Int J Spec Ed* 22:137–141, 2007.

43. Crowley JA, White-Waters K: Psychological assessment in pediatric rehabilitation. In Alexander MA, Matthews DJ, editors: *Pediatric rehabilitation: principles and practices*, ed 4, New York, 2009, Demos Medical, pp 21–52.

44. DeThorne LS, Schaefer BA: A guide to child nonverbal IQ measures, *Am J Speech Lang Pathol* 13:275–290, 2004.

45. DiLalla LF: Development of intelligence: current research and theories, *J School Psych* 38:3–7, 2000.

46. Downing J, Eichinger J, Demchak M: *Including students with severe disabilities in typical classrooms*, Baltimore, 2002, Paul H. Brookes.

47. Dunst CJ, Bruder MB, Trivette CM, Hamby D, Raab M, McLean M: Characteristics and consequences of everyday natural learning opportunities, *Top Early Child Spec Ed* 21:68–92, 2001.

48. Dunst CJ, Trivette CM, Humphries T, Raab M, Roper N: Contrasting approaches to natural learning environments, *Inf Young Child* 14:48–63, 2001.

49. Durstine JL, Painter P, Franklin BA, Morgan D, Pitetti KH, Roberts SO: Physical activity for the chronically ill and disabled, *Sports Med* 30:207–219, 2000.

50. Einspieler C, Kerr AM, Prechtl HF: Is the early development of girls with Rett disorder really normal? *Pediatr Res* 57:696–700, 2005.

51. Elliott CD: *Differential Ability Scales, 2nd edition: introductory and technical handbook*, San Antonio, TX, 2007, The Psychological Corporation.

52. Ellis NR: *Handbook of mental deficiency: psychological theory and research*, London, 1963, McGraw-Hill.

53. Fagan JF: A theory of intelligence as processing: implications for society, *Psych Pub Pol Law* 6:168–179, 2000.

54. Fagan JF, Shepherd PA: *The Fagan Test of Infant Intelligence Training Manual*, Cleveland, 1991, Infatest Corporation.

55. Federal Register, Part II, Department of Education: 34 CFR Parts 300 and 301 Assistance to States for the Education of Children With Disabilities and Pre-school Grants for Children With Disabilities, *Final Rule* 71(156), August 14, 2006.

56. Flexer RW, Simmons TJ, Luft P, Baer RM: *Transition planning for secondary students with disabilities*, Upper Saddle River, NJ, 2001, Merrill Prentice-Hall.

57. Folio MR, Fewell RR: *Peabody Developmental Motor Scales*, ed 2, Austin, TX, 2000, Pro-Ed.

58. Fombonne E: Epidemiological trends in rates of autism, *Mol Psychiatry* 7(Suppl 2):S4–S6, 2002.

59. Fragala MA, O'Neil ME, Russo KJ, Dumas HM: Impairment, disability, and satisfaction outcomes after lower-extremity botulinum toxin A injections for children with cerebral palsy, *Pediatr Phys Ther* 14:132–144, 2002.

60. French JL: *Pictorial Test of Intelligence-second edition*, Austin, 2001, Pro-Ed.

61. Galli M, Rigoldi C, Brunner R, Virji-Babul N, Giorgio A: Joint stiffness and gait pattern evaluation in children with Down syndrome, *Gait Posture* 28:502–506, 2008.

62. Gaytant MA, Rours GI, Steegers EA, Galama JM, Semmekrot BA: Congenital cytomegalovirus infection after recurrent infection: case reports and review of the literature, *Eur J Pediatr* 162:248–253, 2003.

63. Giangreco MF, Cloninger CH, Iverson VS: *Choosing options and accommodations for children: a guide to educational planning for students with disabilities*, ed 2, Baltimore, 1998, Paul H Brookes.

64. Goldstein DN, Cohn E, Coster W: Enhancing participation for children with disabilities: application of the ICF enablement framework to pediatric physical therapy practice, *Pediatr Phys Ther* 16:114–120, 2004.

65. Guerette P, Furumasu J, Tefft D: The positive effects of early powered mobility on children's psychosocial and play skills, *Assist Technol* 25:39–48, 2013.

66. Guerri C, Bazinet A, Riley EP: Fetal alcohol spectrum disorders and alterations in brain and behaviour, *Alcohol Alcohol* 44:108–114, 2009.

67. Guess D, Mulligan-Ault M, Roberts S, Struth J, Siegel-Causey E, Thompson B, et al.: Implications of biobehavioral states for the education and treatment of students with the most profoundly handicapping conditions, *J Assoc Persons Severe Handicaps* 13:163–174, 1988.

68. Gupta VB, O'Connor KG, Quezada-Gomez C: Care coordination services in pediatric practices, *Pediatrics* 113:1517–1521, 2004.

69. Guzzetta A, Mazzotti S, Tinelli F, Bancale A, Ferretti G, Battini R, et al.: Early assessment of visual information processing and neurological outcome in preterm infants, *Neuropediatrics* 37:278–285, 2006.

70. Hack M, Taylor HG, Drotar D, Schluter M, Cartar L, Wilson-Costello D, et al.: Poor predictive validity of the Bayley Scales of Infant Development for cognitive function of extremely low birth weight children of school age, *Pediatrics* 116:333–341, 2005.

71. Haley SM, Coster WJ, Dumas HM, Fragala-Pinkham MA, Moed R: *Pediatric evaluation of Disability Inventory-Computer Adaptive Test*, 2012. Available from: URL: http://pedicat.com/category/home/.

72. Haley SM, Coster WJ, Ludlow LH, Haltiwanger JT, Andrellos PJ: *Pediatric Evaluation of Disability inventory*, Boston, MA, 1992, Department of Rehabilitation Medicine, New England Medical Center.

73. Hammill DD, Pearson NA, Wiederholt JE: *Comprehensive Test of Non-verbal Intelligence*, ed 2, Austin, 2004, Pro-Ed.

74. Hanft BE, Pilkington KO: Therapy in natural environments: the means or end goal for early intervention, *Infant Young Child* 12:1–13, 2000.

75. Harrison PL, Oakland T: *Adaptive Behavior Assessment System® Second Edition (ABS-II)*, North Tonawanda, NY, 2004, MHS Inc.

76. Horn EM: Basic motor skills instruction for children with neuromotor delays: a critical review, *J Spec Ed* 25:168–197, 1991.

77. Idieshi RI, O'Neil ME, Chiarello LA, Nixon-Cave K: Perspectives of therapist's role in care coordination between medical and early intervention services, *Phys Occupat Ther Pediatr* 30:28–42, 2010.

78. Reference deleted in proofs.

79. Ivancic MT, Bailey JS: Current limits to reinforcer identification for some persons with profound multiple disabilities, *Res Dev Disabil* 17:77–92, 1996.

80. Jones KL, Jones MC, Casanelles MDC: *Smith's recognizable patterns of human malformation*, ed 7, Philadelphia, 2013, Elsevier Saunders.

81. Jones MA, McEwen IR, Hansen L: Use of power mobility for a young child with spinal muscular atrophy: a case report, *Phys Ther* 83:253–262, 2003.

82. Jones MA, McEwen IR, Neas BR: Effects of power wheelchairs on the development and function of young children with severe motor impairments, *Pediatr Phys Ther* 24:131–140, 2012.

83. Kaminker MK, Chiarello LA, O'Neil ME, Dichter CG: Decision making for physical therapy service delivery in schools: a nationwide survey of pediatric physical therapists, *Phys Ther* 84:919–933, 2004.

84. Kaplan E, Fein D, Kramer J, Delis D, Morris R: *Wechsler Intelligence Scale for Children®-Fourth Edition Integrated*, San Antonio, TX, 2004, Pearson Education.

85. Karnish K, Bruder MB, Rainforth B: A comparison of physical therapy in two school based treatment contexts, *Phys Occupat Ther Pediatr* 15:1–25, 1995.

86. Ketelaar M, Vermeer A, Hart H, van Petegem-van Beek E, Helders PJ: Effects of a functional motor program on motor abilities of children with cerebral palsy, *Phys Ther* 81:1534–1545, 2001.

87. Kilpinen-Loisa P, Paasio T, Soiva M, Ritanen UM, Lautala P, Palmu P, et al.: Low bone mass in patients with motor disability: prevalence and risk factors in 59 Finnish children, *Dev Med Child Neurol* 52:276–282, 2010.

88. King GA, Law M, King S, et al.: Measuring children's participation in recreation and leisure activities: construct validation of the CAPE and PAC, *Child Care Health Dev* 33:28–39, 2007.

89. Kirschner B, Guyatt G: A methodological framework for assessing health indices, *J Chronic Dis* 38:27–36, 1985.

90. Kolb B, Forgie M, Gibb R, Gorny G, Rowntree S: Age, experience and the changing brain, *Neurosci Biobehav Rev* 22:143–159, 1998.

91. Kolobe THA, Christy JB, Gannotti ME, Heathcock JC, Damiano DL, Taub E: Research Summit III Proceedings on dosing in children with an injured brain or cerebral palsy: executive summary, *Phys Ther* 94:907–920, 2014.

92. Larson SA, Lakin KC, Anderson L, Kwak N, Lee JH, Anderson D: Prevalence of mental retardation and developmental disabilities: estimates from the 1994/1995 national health interview survey disability supplements, *Am J Ment Retard* 106:231–252, 2001.

93. Lavelli M, Fogel A: Developmental changes in mother-infant face-to-face communication: birth to 3 months, *Dev Psychol* 2:288–305, 2002.

94. Law M, Baptiste S, Carswell A, McColl MA, Polatajko H, Pollock N: *Canadian Occupational Performance Measure*, ed 5, Toronto, 2014, Canadian Association of Occupational Therapists.

95. Linn HC, Wuang HP: Strength and agility training in adolescents with Down syndrome: a randomized controlled trial, *Res Dev Disabil* 33:2236–2244, 2012.

96. Littleton SR, Heriza CB, Mullens PA, Moerchen VA, Bjornson K: Effects of positioning on respiratory measures in individuals with cerebral palsy and severe scoliosis, *Pediatr Phys Ther* 23:159–169, 2011.

97. Livingstone R, Paleg G: Practice considerations for the introduction and use of power mobility for children, *Dev Med Child Neurol* 56:210–221, 2014.

98. Lopez JM: Is ZMP the toxic metabolite in Lesch-Nyhan disease? *Med Hypotheses* 71:657–663, 2008.

99. Lucyshyn JM, Horner RH, Dunlap G, Albin RW, Ben KR: Positive behavior support with families. In Lucyshyn JM, Dunlap G, Albin RW, editors: *Families and positive behavior support: addressing problem behavior in family contexts*, Baltimore, 2002, Paul H. Brookes, pp 3–43.

100. Lynch A, Ryu JC, Agrawal S, Galloway JC: Power mobility training for a 7-month-old infant with spina bifida, *Pediatr Phys Ther* 21(4):362–368, 2009.

101. Malian I, Nevin A: A review of self-determination literature: implications for practitioners, *Remedial Spec Ed* 23:68–74, 2002.

102. Martin K: Effects of supramalleolar orthoses on postural stability in children with Down syndrome, *Dev Med Child Neurol* 46:406–411, 2004.

103. Martin JE, Mithaug DE, Cox P, Peterson LY, Van Dycke JL, Cash ME: Increasing self-determination: teaching students to plan, work, evaluate, and ad-just, *Council Except Child* 69:431–447, 2003.

104. Maulik PK, Harbour CK: Epidemiology of intellectual disability. In Stone JH, Blouin M, editors: *International encyclopedia of rehabilitation*, 2010. Available from: URL: http://cirrie.buffalo.edu/encyclopedia/en/article/144/.

105. McCaskey MS, Kirk L, Gerdes C: Preventing skin breakdown in the immobile child in the homecare setting, *Home Health Nurse* 29:248–255, 2011.

106. McEwen IR: Assistive positioning as a control parameter of social-communicative interactions between students with profound multiple disabilities and classroom staff, *Phys Ther* 72:634–647, 1992.

107. McEwen IR, editor: *Writing case reports: a how-to manual for clinicians*, Alexandria, VA, 2001, American Physical Therapy Association.

108. McEwen IR, Shelden ML: Pediatric physical therapy in the 1990s: the demise of the educational versus medical dichotomy, *Phys Occupat Ther Pediatr* 15:33–45, 1995.

109. Meegan S, Maraj BK, Weeks D, Chua R: Gross motor skill acquisition in adolescents with Down syndrome, *Down Syndrome Res Pract* 9:75–80, 2006.

110. Meisels SJ, Atkins-Burnett S: The elements of early childhood assessment. In Shonkoff JP, Meisels SJ, editors: *Handbook of early childhood intervention*, ed 2, Cambridge, MA, 2000, Cambridge University Press, pp 231–257.

111. Meiser MJ, McEwen IR: Lightweight and ultralight wheelchairs: propulsion and preferences in two young children with spina bifida, *Pediatr Phys Ther* 19:245–253, 2007.

112. Mik G, Ghlove PA, Scher DM, Widmann RF, Green DW: Down syndrome: orthopedic issues, *Curr Opin Pediatr* 20:30–36, 2008.

113. Missiuna C, Polluck N, Law M: *Perceived efficacy and goal setting system (PEGS)*, Hamilton, Ontario, 2004, McMaster University. Available from: URL: http://www.canchild.ca/en/measures/pegs.asp.

114. Moon S, Simonsen ML, Neubert DA: Perceptions of supported employment providers: what students with developmental disabilities, families, and educators need to know for transition planning, *Ed Training Autism Dev Disabil* 46:94–105, 2011.

115. Morris CA, Mervis CB: Williams syndrome and related disorders, *Ann Rev Genom Human Genet* 1:261–284, 2000.

116. Muggli EE, Collins VR, Marraffa C: Going down a different road: first support and information needs of families with a baby with Down syndrome, *Med J Austral* 190:58–61, 2009.

117. Nagle RJ: Issues in preschool assessment. In Bracken BA, Nagle RJ, editors: *Psychoeducational assessment of preschool children*, ed 4, Mahwah, NJ, 2007, Lawrence Erlbaum Associates, pp 31–37.

118. National Joint Committee for the Communicative Needs of Persons with Severe Disabilities: Guidelines for meeting the communication needs of persons with severe disabilities, *ASHA* 34(Suppl 7):1–8, 1992.

119. National Library of Medicine: cornelia de Lange syndrome, 2007. Available from: URL: http://ghr.nlm.nih.gov/condition=corneliadelange syndrome.

120. Nelson NW: Developmental language disorders. In Patel DR, Grydanus DE, Omar HA, Merrick M, editors: *Neurodevelopmental disabilities*, New York, 2011, Springer, pp 178.

121. Newborg J: *Battelle Developmental Inventory*, ed 2, Itasca, IL, 2005, Riverside Publishing.

122. Newman L, Wagner M, Cameto R, Knokey AM: *The post-high school outcomes of youth with disabilities up to 4 years after high school: a report from the National Longitudinal Transition Study-2 (NLTS2) (NCSER 2009-3017)*, Menlo Park, CA, 2009, SRI International.

123. Newman L, Wagner M, Cameto R, Knokey AM, Shaver D: *Comparisons across time of the outcomes of youth with disabilities up to 4 years after high school. A report of findings from the National Longitudinal Transition Study-2 (NLTS2)*, Menlo Park, CA, 2010, SRI International. Available from: URL: www.nlts2.org/reports/2010_09/nlts2_report_2010_09 _complete.pdf.

124. Nilsson L: Training characteristics important for growing consciousness of joystick-use in people with profound cognitive disabilities, *Int J Ther Rehabil* 17:588–594, 2010.

125. Nolan K, Orlando M, Liptak GS: Care coordination services for children with special health care needs: are we family-centered yet? *Families Systems Health* 25:293–306, 2007.

126. Novak I, Hines M, Goldsmith S, Barclay R: Clinical prognostic messages from a systematic review on cerebral palsy, *Pediatrics* 130:e1285–e1312, 2012. Available from: URL: http://pediatrics.aappublications.org/content/130/5/e1285.short.

127. Odding E, Roebroeck ME, Stam HJ: The epidemiology of cerebral palsy: incidence, impairments, and risk factors, *Disabil Rehabil* 28:183–191, 2006.

128. Oppewal A, Hilgenkamp TI, van Wijick R, Evenhuis HM: Cardiorespiratory fitness in individuals with intellectual disability-a review, *Res Dev Disabil* 10:3301–3316, 2013.

129. Orelove FP, Sobsey D: Designing transdisciplinary services. In Orelove FP, Sobsey D, editors: *Educating children with multiple disabilities: a transdisciplinary approach*, ed 3, Baltimore, 1996, Paul H. Brookes, pp 1–33.

130. Oswald DP, Coutinho MJ, Nguyen N: Impact of sociodemographic characteristics on identification rates of minority students as having mental retardation, *Ment Retard* 39:351–367, 2001.

131. Palisano RJ, Walter SD, Russell DJ, Rosenbaum PL, Gémus M, Galuppi BE, Cunningham L: Gross motor function of children with Down syndrome: creation of motor growth curves, *Arch Phys Med Rehabil* 82:494–500, 2001.

132. Palisano R, Rosenbaum P, Russell D, Wood E, Galuppi B: Development and reliability of a system to classify gross motor function in children with cerebral palsy, *Dev Med Child Neurol* 39:214–223, 1997.

133. Palmer S, Summers JA: Building a foundation of self-determination in the early years of life, National Gateway to Self-Determination, 2012. Available from: URL: http://ngsd.org/sites/default/files/research_to _practice_sd_-_issue_4.pdf.

134. Parrish JM: Behavior management. In Batshaw ML, editor: *Children with disabilities*, ed 4, Baltimore, 1997, Paul H. Brookes, pp 657–686.

135. Penagarikano O, Mulle JG, Warren ST: The pathophysiology of fragile X syndrome, *Ann Rev Genom Human Genet* 8:109–129, 2007.

136. Pennington BF, Moon J, Edgin J, Stedron J, Nadel L: The neuropsychology of Down syndrome: evidence for hippocampal dysfunction, *Child Dev* 74:75–93, 2003.

137. Percy AK: Rett syndrome: current status and new vistas, *Neurolog Clin* 20:1125–1141, 2002.

138. Phagava H, Muratori F, Einspieler C, Maestro S, Apicella F, Guzzetta A, et al.: General movements in infants with autism spectrum disorders, *Georgian Med News* 156:100–105, 2008.

139. Pitteti K, Miller RA, Beets MW: Measuring joint hypermobility using the Beighton Scale in children with intellectual disability, *Pediatr Phys Ther* 127:143–150, 2015.

140. Portney LG, Watkins MP: *Foundations of clinical research: applications to practice*, ed 3, Upper Saddle River, NJ, 2009, Prentice Hall Health.

141. Ragonesi CB, Galloway JC: Short-term, early intensive power mobility training: case report of an infant at risk for cerebral palsy, *Pediatr Phys Ther* 24:141–148, 2012.

142. Ragonesi CB, Chen X, Agrawal S, Galloway JC: Power mobility and socialization in preschool: a case study of a child with cerebral palsy, *Pediatr Phys Ther* 22:322–329, 2010.

143. Rainforth B: *OSERS clarifies legality of related services eligibility criteria*, TASH Newsletter, 1991, p 8. April 1991.

144. Rainforth B, York-Barr J: *Collaborative teams for students with severe disabilities: integrating therapy and educational services*, ed 2, Baltimore, 1997, Paul H. Brookes.

145. Randall KE, McEwen IR: Writing patient-centered functional goals, *Phys Ther* 80:1197–1203, 2000.

146. Raven J, Raven JC, Court JH: *Standard Progressive Matrices—Parallel Form*, Oxford, England, 1998, Oxford Psychologists Press.

147. Richards SB, Brady MP, Taylor RL: *Cognitive and intellectual disabilities: historical perspectives, current practices, and future directions*, ed 2, New York, 2015, Routledge Taylor and Francis.

148. Rigby PJ, Ryan SE, Campbell KA: Effect of adaptive seating devices on activity performance of children with cerebral palsy, *Arch Phys Med Rehabil* 90:1389–1395, 2009.

149. Rimmer JH, Yamaki K, Davis Lowery BM, Wang E, Vogel LC: Obesity and obesity related secondary conditions in adolescents with intellectual/developmental disabilities, *J Intellect Disabil Res* 54:787–794, 2010.

150. Rodriguez-Key M, Alonzi A: Nutrition, skin integrity, and pressure ulcer healing in chronically ill children: an overview, *Ostomy Wound Manage* 53:56–66, 2007.

151. Rogers A, Furler B, Brinks S, Darrah J: A systematic review of aerobic exercise interventions for children with cerebral palsy: an AAPCDM evidence report, *Dev Med Child Neurol* 50:808–814, 2008.

152. Roid GH: *Stanford-Binet Intelligence Scales*, ed 5, Chicago, 2003, Riverside Publishing.

153. Roid GH, Miller L: *Lieter International Performance Scale—third edition*, Wood Dale, IL, 2013, Stoelting.

154. Roizen NJ: Down syndrome. In Batshaw ML, Roizen NR, Lotrecchiano G, editors: *Children with disabilities*, ed 7, Baltimore, 2013, Paul H. Brookes, pp 307–317.

155. Roizen NJ, Patterson D: Down's syndrome, *Lancet* 361:1281–1289, 2003.

156. Rosa's Law: pub L, pp 111–256. 2009. Available from: URL: https://www .govtrack.us/congress/bills/111/s2781.

157. Rosen L, Arva J, Furumasu J, Harris M, Lange ML, McCarthy E, Wonsettler T: RESNA position on the application of power wheelchairs for pediatric users, *Assist Technol* 21:218–225, 2009.

158. Rothstein JM, Echternach JL, Riddle DL: The hypothesis-oriented algorithm for clinicians II (HOAC II): a guide for patient management, *Phys Ther* 83:455–470, 2003.

159. Rowland JL, Fragala-Pinkham M, Miles C, O'Neil M: The scope of pediatric physical therapy practice in health promotion and fitness for youth with disabilities, *Pediatr Phys Ther* 27:2–15, 2015.

160. Russell DJ, Rosenbaum PL, Avery LM, Lane M: *Gross Motor Function Measure (GMFM 66 GMFM-88): user's manual*, London, 2002, MacKeith Press.

161. Sanford C, Newman L, Wagner M, Cameto R, Knokey AM, Shaver D: *The post-high school outcomes of young adults with disabilities up to 6 years after high school*, Key findings. From the National Longitudinal Transition Study-2 (NLTS2). NCSER 2011-3004. Menlo Park, CA, 2011, SRI International.

162. Sattler J: *Assessment of children: cognitive foundations*, ed 6, La Mesa, CA, 2008, Jerome M Sattler.

163. Sattler J, McGoey K: Functional behavior assessment. In Sattler J, editor: *Foundations of behavioral, social, and clinical assessment*, La Mesa, CA, 2014, Jerome M. Sattler, Publisher, Inc, pp 413–428.

164. Schalock RL, Borthwick-Duffy S, Bradley V, Buntinx WHE, Coulter DL, Craig EM, Yeager MH: *Intellectual disabilities: definition, classification, and system of supports*, ed 11, Washington, DC, 2010, American Association on Intellectual and Developmental Disabilities.

165. Schalock RL, Luckasson R, Shogren KA, et al.: The renaming of mental retardation: understanding the change to the term intellectual disability, *Intellect Dev Disabil* 45:116–124, 2007.

166. Schneidert M, Hurst R, Miller J, Üstün B: The role of environment in the International Classification of Functioning, Disability and Health (ICF), *Disabil Rehabil* 25:588–595, 2003.

167. Sekerak DM, Kirkpatrick DB, Nelson DC, Propes JH: Physical therapy in preschool classrooms: successful integration of therapy into classroom routines, *Pediatr Phys Ther* 15:93–104, 2003.

168. Shelden ML, Rush DD: The ten myths about providing early intervention services in natural environments, *Infants Young Child* 14:1–13, 2001.

169. Shevell M, Majnemer A, Platt RW, Webster R, Birnbaum R: Developmental and functional outcomes in children with global developmental delay or developmental language impairment, *Dev Med Child Neurol* 47:678–683, 2005.

170. Shumway-Cook A, Woollacott MH: *Motor control: translating research into clinical practice*, ed 3, Philadelphia, 2007, Lippincott Williams Wilkins.

171. Smith-Zuzovsky N, Exner CE: The effect of seated positioning quality on typical 6- and 7-year-old children's object manipulation skills, *Am J Occupat Ther* 58:380–388, 2004.

172. Smits-Engelsman B, Hill EL: The relationship between motor coordination and intelligence across the IQ range, *Pediatrics* 130:950–956, 2012.

173. Snell ME, Brown: Designing and implementing instructional programs. In Snell ME, Brown F, editors: *Instruction of students with severe disabilities*, ed 6, Upper Saddle River, NJ, 2006, Pearson, pp 111–169.

174. Sobo EJ: Mastering the health care system for children with special health care needs. In Sobo EJ, Kurtin PS, editors: *Optimizing care for young children with special health care needs: knowledge and strategies for navigating the system*, Baltimore, 2007, Paul H. Brookes, pp 115–134.

175. Sparrow SS, Davis SM: Recent advances in the assessment of intelligence and cognition, *J Child Psychol Psychiatry* 41:117–131, 2000.

176. Sparrow SS, Cichetti CV, Balla DA: *Vineland adaptive behavior scales*, ed 2, Upper Saddle River, NJ, 2005, Pearson Education.

177. Starr EM, Berument SK, Tomlins M, Papanikolaou K, Rutter M: Brief report: autism in individuals with Down syndrome, *J Autism Dev Disorders* 35:665–673, 2005.

178. Strisciuglio P, Concolino D: New strategies for the treatment of phenylketonuria (PKU), *Metabolites* 4:1007–1017, 2014.

179. TASH force strikes again: laski and Boyd win Oberti case in New Jersey: TASH Newsletter, November 1992, pp 1–2, 1992.

180. Taylor K: Factors affecting prescription and implementation of standing-frame programs by school-based physical therapists for children with impaired mobility, *Pediatr Phys Ther* 21:282–288, 2009.

181. Taylor SJ: Caught in the continuum: a critical analysis of the principle of the least restrictive environment, *Res Practice Persons Severe Disabil* 29:218–230, 2004.

182. Tefft D, Guerette P, Furumasu J: Intellectual predictors of young children's readiness for powered mobility, *Dev Med Child Neurol* 41:665–670, 1999.

183. The Arc: Arc Position Statement on Self-Determination, 2015. Available from: URL: http://www.thearc.org/who-we-are/position-statements/rights/self-determination.

184. The Developmental Disabilities Assistance and Bill of Rights Act (2000): PubL 106–402. Available from: URL: http://www.acl.gov/Programs/AIDD/DDA_BOR_ACT_2000.

185. Thompson JR, Bryant B, Campbell E, Craig M, Hughes C, Rotholz D, et al.: *Supports Intensity Scale*, Washington, DC, 2004, American Association on Mental Retardation.

186. Thorpe DE, Valvano J: The effects of knowledge of performance and intellectual strategies on motor skill learning in children with cerebral palsy, *Pediatr Phys Ther* 14:2–15, 2002.

187. Tunson J, Candler C: Behavioral states of children with severe disabilities in the multisensory environment, *Phys Occupat Ther Pediatr* 3:101–110, 2010.

188. Turner-Stokes L: Goal attainment scaling (GAS) in rehabilitation: a practical guide, *Clin Rehab* 23:362–370, 2009.

189. Ulrich DA, Burghardt AR, Lloyd M, Tiernan C, Hornyak JE: Physical activity benefits of learning to ride a two-wheel bicycle for children with Down syndrome: a randomized trial, *Phys Ther* 91:1463–1477, 2011.

190. Ulrich DA, Lloyd MC, Tiernan CW, Looper JE, Angulo-Barroso RM: Effects of intensity of treadmill training on developmental outcomes and stepping in infants with Down syndrome: a randomized trial, *Phys Ther* 88:114–122, 2008.

191. United States Department of Education: Thirty-sixth annual report to Congress on the implementation of the Individuals with Disabilities Education Act, Washington, DC, 2014, US Department of Education.

192. United States Department of Health and Human Services, Health Resources and Services Administration, Maternal and Child Health Bureau: The national survey of children with special healthcare needs chartbook 2005-2006, Rockville, MD, 2007, USDHHS.

193. United States Department of Labor, Bureau of Labor Statistics: Current Population Survey, 2014. Available from: URL: bls.gov/cps/tables.htm#charemp.

194. United States National Institute of Medicine: Intellectual disability, 2015. Available from: URL: http://www.nlm.nih.gov/medlineplus/ency/article/001523.htm.

195. Unnithan VB, Dowling JJ, Frost G, Bar-Or O: Role of co-contraction in the O2 cost of walking in children with cerebral palsy, *Med Sci Sports Exerc* 28:1498–1504, 1996.

196. Valkenburg AJ, van Dijk M, de Klein A, van den Anker JN, Tibboel D: Pain management in intellectually disabled children: assessment, treatment, and translational research, *Develop Disabil Res Rev* 16:248–257, 2010.

197. Van Buggenhout GJ, Fryns JP: Angelman syndrome, *Eur J Human Genet* 17:1367–1373, 2009.

198. Vaughn BJ, Wilson D, Dunlap G: Family-centered intervention to resolve problem behavior in a fast-food restaurant, *J Posit Behav Interv* 4:38–45, 2002.

199. Vicari S: Motor development and neuropsychological patterns in persons with Down syndrome, *Behav Genet* 36:355–364, 2006.

200. Virji-Babul N, Kerns K, Zhou E, Kapur A, Shiffrar M: Perceptual-motor deficits in children with Down syndrome: implications for intervention, *Down Syndrome Res Prac* 10:74–82, 2006.

201. Walker WO, Johnson CP: Cognitive and adaptive disabilities. In Wolraich ML, Drotar DD, Dworkin PH, Perrin EC, editors: *Developmental-behavioral pediatrics: evidence and practice*, Philadelphia, 2008, Mosby Elsevier, pp 405–443.

202. Wang P: In Wolraich ML, Drotar DD, Dworkin PH, Perrin EC, editors: *Developmental-behavioral pediatrics: evidence and practice*, Philadelphia, 2008, Mosby Elsevier, pp 317–336.

203. Watkins MW, Ravert CM, Crosby EG: Normative factor structure of the AAMR Adaptive Behavior Scale-School, ed 2, *J Psychoeducational Assess* 20:337–345, 2002.

204. Wehmeyer ML, Agran M, Hughes C, Martin J, Mithaug DE, Palmer S: *Promoting self-determination in students with intellectual and developmental disabilities*, New York, 2007, Guilford.

205. Wehmeyer ML, Palmer SB, Agran M, Mithaug DE, Martin JE: Promoting causal agency: the self-determined learning model of instruction, *Exceptional Child* 66:439–453, 2000.

206. Wehmeyer ML: Self-determination and individuals with severe disabilities: reexamining meanings and misinterpretations, *Res Fract Persons Severe Disabil* 30:113–120, 2005.

207. Wehmeyer ML, Abery B: Self-determination and choice, *Intellect Dev Disabil* 51:399–411, 2013.

208. Wehmeyer ML, Bolding N: Self-determination across living and working environments: a matched samples study of adults with mental retardation, *Ment Retard* 37:353–363, 1999.

209. Wehmeyer ML, Bolding N: Enhanced self-determination of adults with intellectual disability as an outcome of moving to community-based work or living environments, *J Intellect Disabil Res* 45:371–383, 2001.

210. Wehmeyer ML, Schwartz M: Self-determination and positive adult outcomes: a follow-up study of youth with mental retardation or learning disabilities, *Except Child* 63:245–255, 1997.

211. Wehmeyer ML, Abery B, Mithaug DE, Stancliffe RJ: *Theory in self-determination: foundations for educational practice*, Springfield, IL, 2003, Charles C Thomas.

212. Wehmeyer ML, Buntinx WHE, Lachapelle Y, Luckasson RA, Schalock RL, Verdugo MA, et al.: Perspectives: the intellectual disability construct and its relation to human functioning, *Intellect Dev Disabil* 46:311–318, 2008.

213. Wiart L, Darrah J, Hollis V, Cook A, May L: Mothers' perceptions of their children's use of powered mobility, *Phys Occupat Ther Pediatr* 24:3–21, 2004.

214. Wills J, Luecking R: *Making the connections: growing and supporting new organizations: intermediaries*, Washington, DC, 2004, National Collaborative on Workforce and Disability/Youth US Department of Education.

215. Winters PC: The goal and opportunity of physical therapy for children with Down syndrome, *Down Syndrome Quart* 6(2):1–5, 2001.

216. World Health Organization: *International Classification of Functioning, Disability, and Health (ICF)*, Geneva, 2001, WHO.

217. Yan JH, Thomas JR, Downing JH: Locomotion improves children's spatial search: a meta-analytic review, *Perceptual Motor Skills* 87:67–82, 1998.

218. Ylvisaker M, Feeney T: Executive functions, self-regulation, and learned optimism in paediatric rehabilitation: a review and implications for intervention, *Pediatr Rehabil* 5:51–70, 2001.

219. Zhang D, Katsiyannis A: Minority representation in special education: a persistent challenge, *RASE Rem Spec Ed* 23:180–187, 2002.

SUGGESTED READINGS

Background

Jones KL, Jones MC, Casanelles MDC: *Smith's recognizable patterns of human malformation*, ed 7, Philadelphia, 2013, Elsevier Saunders.

Linden DW, Paroli ET, Doron MW: *Preemies*, ed 2, New York, 2010, Gallery Books.

Riley EP, Infante MA, Warren KR: Fetal alcohol spectrum disorders: an overview, *Neuropsychol Rev* 21:73–80, 2011.

Schalock RL, Luckasson R, Shogren KA, Borthwick-Duffy S, Bradley V, Buntinx WH, et al.: The renaming of *mental retardation*: understanding the change to the term *intellectual disability*, *Intellect Dev Disabil* 45:116–124, 2007.

Foreground

American Association on Intellectual and Developmental Disabilities (AAIDD): Comprehensive website including education, policy, and publications about intellectual and developmental disabilities. Information available at aidd.org.

Downing JE, MacFarland S: Severe disabilities (education of individuals with severe disabilities: promising practices). In Stone JH, Blouin M, editors: *International encyclopedia of rehabilitation*, 2010. Available from: URL: http://cirrie.buffalo.edu/encyclopedia/en/article/114/.

Downing JE: *Including students with severe and multiple disabilities in typical classrooms*, ed 3, Baltimore, 2008, Paul H. Brookes.

Downing JE, Hanreddy A, Peckham-Hardin K: *Teaching communication skills to students with severe disabilities*, ed 3, Baltimore, 2015, Paul H. Brookes.

Levac D, Wishart L, Missiuna C, Wright V: The application of motor learning strategies within functionally based interventions with children with neuromotor conditions, *Pediatr Phys Ther* 21:345–355, 2009.

National Secondary Transition Technical Assistance Center: *Age appropriate transition assessment toolkit*, ed 3, University of North Carolina at Charlotte, 2013. Available from: URL: http://nsttac.org/content/age-appropriate-transition-assessment-toolkit-3rd-edition.

Novak I, McIntyre S, Morgan C, Campbell L, Dark L, Morton N, et al.: A systematic review of interventions for children with cerebral palsy: state of the evidence, *Dev Med Child Neurol* 55:885–910, 2013.

Palisano RJ, Walter SD, Russell DJ, Rosenbaum PL, Gémus M, Galuppi BE, Cunningham L, et al.: Gross motor function of children with Down syndrome: creation of motor growth curves, *Arch Phys Med Rehabil* 82:494–500, 2001.

Rosenbaum PL, Walter S, Hanna SE, Palisano RJ, Russell DJ, Raina P, et al.: Prognosis for gross motor function in cerebral palsy: creation of motor development curves, *JAMA* 288:1357–1363, 2002.

Washington State Department of Social and Health Services. Life skills inventory. *DSHS* 10-267. PDF available from: URL: http://www.iidc.indiana.edu/styles/iidc/defiles/INSTRC/Webinars/Life_skills_inventory.pdf.

Winders PC: *Gross motor skills for children with Down syndrome: a guide for parents and professionals*, ed 2, Bethesda, MD, 2014, Woodbine House.

19

Cerebral Palsy

Marilyn Wright, Robert J. Palisano

Physical therapists have an important role in the specialized interdisciplinary services to help children with cerebral palsy (CP) reach their full potential in their home, educational, and community environments. Children with cerebral palsy vary considerably not only in the nature of the movement disorder but also in their motor, communication, and cognitive abilities. Although the neurologic disturbance is static, there is risk of secondary musculoskeletal and neuromuscular impairments and environmental considerations change with age. As a consequence, goal setting and decisions on interventions are often complicated. This chapter provides background information on the etiology, diagnosis, prognosis, and characteristics of the movement disorders in children with CP, using the framework of the International Classification of Functioning Disability and Health. The Foreground Information section presents a framework for family–therapist collaboration for goal setting and intervention planning to achieve desired outcomes for activity and participation. Evidence-informed decision making is modeled. Comprehensive management is addressed during infancy, childhood, and adolescence. Topics include (1) communication and coordination with the child, family, health professionals, and educators; (2) the examination and evaluation process, including selecting tests and measures; (3) evidence-based interventions; and (4) supporting the child and family to engage in desired home and community activities. Physical therapists have great potential to influence the immediate and future lives of children with CP and their families.

BACKGROUND INFORMATION

"Cerebral palsy describes a group of permanent disorders of the development of movement and posture, causing activity limitations that are attributed to non-progressive disturbances that occurred in the developing fetal or infant brain" (p 9).[313] Although the brain lesion is static, secondary musculoskeletal impairments such as muscle/tendon contractures, bony torsion, hip displacement, and spinal deformity often contribute to activity limitations.[201,313] Factors that contribute to secondary impairments include physical growth, muscle spasticity and weakness, and the cumulative effect of biomechanical forces though joints.[313]

Motor impairments associated with CP are often accompanied by disturbances of cognition, behavior, communication, sensation, epilepsy, and perception.[313] Cognitive delays (IQ < 70) are present in 23% to 44% of children with CP, and behavioral issues have been recognized in 25%—a rate five times greater than that typically seen in children.

The prevalence of impaired speech (42%–81%), hearing (25%), and vision (62%–71%); seizure disorders (22%–40%); urinary incontinence (23%); and constipation (59%) is increased. Tactile sensory impairments, including problems with stereognosis, proprioception, and two-point discrimination, have been reported in 44% to 51% of children with CP. Visual-spatial and visual-perceptual problems are common—90% and 60%, respectively.[298] Rates of coexisting impairments vary with different subtypes. Children with more significant motor problems experience proportionately higher rates of associated impairments. The degrees of physical and cognitive disability are also related to lifetime costs.[203] Health care, social care, and productivity costs of people with CP contribute to significant societal financial burden.

CP is the most common childhood motor disability with a prevalence of 2 to 2.5 per 1000 live births. Oskoui et al.[272] performed a meta-analysis of 49 studies and reported an overall prevalence of 2.1 per 1000 live births. Prevalence was highest among children born before 28 weeks gestation (111.8 per 1000 live births) and children with a birth weight of 1000 to 1499 grams (59.2 per 1000 live births). Although the prevalence of CP is highest among children born preterm, they account for only 35% of children with CP. Life expectancy is associated with severity of motor, cognitive, and visual impairment. A 2-year-old with severe impairments has approximately a 40% chance of living to age 20, in contrast to a child with mild impairments, for whom the chance is 99%.[174] A decline in mortality of children with severe impairments has been noted since the 1990s, particularly for those with feeding problems, reflecting better management of feeding and swallowing difficulties and overall improvement in the care of medically fragile persons. People with CP have an increased incidence of mortality due to external causes such as drowning and being struck by motor vehicles.[348,349]

ETIOLOGY

There are multiple causes of CP, many of which are not fully understood. The exact cause for individual children is often not known. Originally CP was largely attributed to acute hypoxia during labor or birth; however, current evidence indicates that most lesions occur in the second half of gestation, an active period of brain development.[149]

Intrauterine pathology is attributed to environmental triggers such as bacterial and viral intrauterine infection, intrauterine growth restriction, antepartum hemorrhage, and tight nuchal cord, factors that are difficult to determine in retrospect.[228]

Evidence of genetic causes is emerging and may increase as technology improves.[228]

Advances in magnetic resonance imaging (MRI) have furthered understanding of the causes and timing of the pathogenesis of CP through visualization of physiologic and pathologic morphologic changes that occur during brain development.[200,201,261] The pathobiology of CP differs by nature, timing, and location of the brain insult.[201,261,262,321] Recognition of the impact of prenatal factors is increasing. Many perinatal complications occur secondary to preexisting central nervous system pathology. During the first and second trimesters of gestation, brain pathology is characterized by genetic or acquired impairments. From the late second trimester onward, disturbances are more often a result of infectious or hypoxic-ischemic mechanisms that result in lesions.[201] In infants born at term, CP most often results from prenatal influences.

Current evidence suggests that a multiplicity of risk factors contribute to CP rather than a single event. Single events such as uterine rupture, cord prolapse, or major placental abruption resulting in hypoxic insults to the brain account for a small proportion of cases.[261] Although birth asphyxia can result in CP, it is not a common antecedent. When it is the cause, hypoxic damage is typically bilateral and widespread, including the basal ganglia and gray and white matter, resulting in total body involvement with spastic and dyskinetic features. Additional factors such as inflammation can interact with asphyxia, multiplying the risk of CP.[261]

It has become increasingly clear that cerebral vascular events occurring within the first 28 days after birth are a significant cause of CP. The advent of neuroimaging has contributed significantly to further understanding in this area because neonates with strokes do not present clinically with hemiparesis. In contrast to the adult population, approximately one third of perinatal strokes are bilateral. Placental pathology such as thrombotic lesions may be an important factor.[261,262]

Infections such as toxoplasmosis, rubella, cytomegalovirus, herpes virus, hepatitis B, syphilis, human immunodeficiency virus, and streptococcus B can be transmitted from mother to infant, affecting the brain and resulting in CP. Placental inflammation (chorioamnionitis) has also been linked with adverse neurologic outcomes.[261,262] Children with CP have more congenital abnormalities, such as brain malformation, cleft lip or palate, and gut atresia, compared with children who do not have CP. This suggests further the significant contribution of prenatal factors to the origin of CP.[321] Maternal trauma resulting in direct fetal injury, placental abruption, or prenatal vascular insult can also cause CP. Possible mechanisms include reduced placental blood flow or placental embolization.[164] Maternal thyroid disease has been linked with cerebral palsy.[169]

Premature birth increases the risk of CP. In such cases, the underlying brain pathology is white matter injury in sensorimotor pathways. Prolonged rupture of the membranes predisposing to intrauterine infection is an important antecedent. Multiple gestation practices, increasingly common as a result of reproductive technology, can contribute to the risk for CP as a result of the tendency for premature birth or the death of a monozygotic fetus, causing malformation in a surviving infant due to vascular collapse.[261,262] The potentially complex medical course, including the use of postnatal steroids, adds to the risk of events that can disrupt development of the brain.

Infants with atypical intrauterine growth, either small or large for gestational age, are at increased risk for CP. Small birth weight can be associated with infection, preeclampsia, maternal vascular disease, or thrombophilia. Large babies may experience problematic deliveries. Maternal diabetes is a risk factor for macrosomia, but it is not a risk factor for CP. Excessively small or large babies are also at greater risk for perinatal stroke.[261]

Genetic factors can influence the risk of CP at a number of points along the causal pathway. Risk factors with a genetic component include preterm birth, placental abruption, preeclampsia, chorioamnionitis, and thrombophilias or the presence of certain genotypes such as apolipoprotein E.[206] Future research examining gene–gene and gene–environment interactions may provide important information.[261,262] A form of hereditary spastic paresis has also been identified.[96]

Reported rates of various brain pathologies vary. A study of a cohort of 154 children diagnosed with CP for whom MRI was available indicated the following proportions of brain scan findings: 16% normal, 31% periventricular white matter injury, 16% focal ischemic/hemorrhagic lesions, 14% diffuse encephalopathy, 12% brain malformations, 2% infections, and 8% unclassifiable.[304] Sixty-six percent of the children were born at term. Children with brain malformations were more likely to have been born at term and had more severe motor disabilities than other children with a CP diagnosis.

PROGRESS IN PREVENTION

Despite advances in neonatology and obstetrics, the prevalence of CP has not changed. Interventions such as cesarean section, earlier emergency delivery, and continuous electronic fetal monitoring during labor do not appear to address the cause of the brain disturbance for most children with CP. There is evidence of the effectiveness of antenatal magnesium sulphate therapy as a neuroprotective factor in women likely to give birth at less than 37 weeks' gestational age and therapeutic induced hypothermia (brain cooling). A Cochrane review[77] analyzed 37 randomized controlled trials involving 3571 women to determine the effect of antenatal magnesium sulphate therapy in women likely to give birth at less than 37 weeks' gestational age. The conclusion is that magnesium sulphate does not significantly delay birth or prevent preterm birth and has no apparent advantages for a range of neonatal and maternal outcomes. Antenatal magnesium sulphate, however, is effective in helping women who develop preeclampsia (high blood pressure and protein in the urine) and for helping to protect babies' brains. A Cochrane review[178] of 11 randomized controlled trials involving 1505 infants compared therapeutic hypothermia with standard care in term or late preterm infants with peripartum hypoxic ischemic encephalopathy. The conclusion is that therapeutic hypothermia initiated within 6 hours after birth for 48 to 72 hours reduces the combined outcome of mortality or major neurodevelopmental disability at 18 months of age. Nanomaterials such as dendrimers have been proposed as a means for targeted drug and gene delivery to cells responsible for neuroinflammation and injury.[14] Preclinical studies using several types of stem and adult cells have demonstrated some regenerative capacity; however, there are gaps in knowledge of the optimal source and type of cells, timing of treatment, and possible mechanisms of action.[113]

A social class gradient has been noted in the prevalence of CP, along with an association between birth weight and socio-economic status, suggesting that improvements in the education, health, and prenatal care of mothers at risk could improve outcomes. Avoidance of multiple fetus implantations during in vitro fertilization could decrease the incidence of CP due to multiple births.[262]

DIAGNOSIS

Neuroimaging findings and prenatal risk factors can assist in making a diagnosis of CP, but the sensitivity and specificity of single or combined risk factors, such as neonatal seizures, low birth weight, or maternal infection, in predicting CP have been disappointing.[287] As a result, CP remains a clinical diagnosis made when a child does not reach early motor milestones and exhibits abnormal muscle tone or qualitative differences in movement patterns.[309,310] Physical therapists can play an important role in the diagnosis of CP through their involvement in clinics for high-risk infants and early therapy intervention programs.[158] Assessment of asymmetry, involuntary movements, abnormal primitive reflexes, and the late development of postural responses can contribute to the clinical diagnosis.

Research on the General Movement Assessment suggests that the pathologic movement qualities characteristic of cerebral palsy can be reliably identified in the first few months of life with a sensitivity of 95% and specificity of 96%.[56,152] Prechtl and colleagues developed an assessment of general movement that characterizes the movement pattern in cerebral palsy as being one of "cramped synchrony," with a paucity of selective joint movements, especially in the rotational components.[55] Their work has also demonstrated that clinical examination of children with known signs of brain pathophysiologic impairment can identify the effects of such lesions on movement. These effects can then be qualitatively and quantitatively described longitudinally and used to predict recovery or nonrecovery from early disturbances in the neuromuscular system.

Predictive and discriminative infant neuromotor tests can augment clinical judgment to assist in prediction and identification of CP, respectively. The Alberta Infant Motor Scales (AIMS) assessment demonstrates good psychometric properties, especially between corrected ages 4 and 10 months, and has clinical utility in comparing an infant's development with that of other infants of the same age.[56] The Test of Infant Motor Performance (TIMP) and the NeuroSensory Motor Developmental Assessment (NSMDA) can be used before as well as after term.[57,70] Prechtl's Assessment of General Movements (GM) has the best combination of sensitivity and specificity for predicting CP in the early months, but the AIMS and the NSMDA are better predictors when the infants are older.[342]

Precise diagnosis can be difficult, especially early in development. No consensus has been reached on how early CP can be identified reliably,[56] although it has been postulated that an experienced physical therapist or pediatrician should be able to identify the signs of CP in all but the mildest cases by 6 months of age.[329] Nevertheless, variation in motor development must be considered and respected and a definitive diagnosis made cautiously in consideration of alternate explanations, while not withholding appropriate services.[59,310] It is important to differentiate between atypical motor trajectories that indicate CP and other situations such as recovery from early medical complications, including those associated with premature birth. For example, AIMS norms adjusted for gestational age at birth reflect variation in the gross motor trajectories of infants born preterm.[368] Physical therapists may also play a role in recognizing alternative diagnoses. Transient dystonia presents with similar but resolving neurologic signs of CP.[100,158,310,368]

Diagnosis should be confirmed by a pediatric physician specialist to rule out other causes of similar clinical signs such as brain tumors or metabolic disorders. Follow-up is necessary to ensure a nonprogressive nature. It is recommended that all children with CP have a brain MRI in cases of unknown origin. Metabolic workups should be considered in children who appear to have CP but have normal brain imaging, because genetic muscle disorders and mitochondrial disease may present similarly to CP.[200,304] Prenatal, perinatal, and postnatal medical complications that increase risk for cerebral palsy are addressed in Should state "Chapter 29, The Neonatal Intensive Care Unit".

CLASSIFICATION OF FUNCTIONAL ABILITIES

Children with CP demonstrate considerable variation in functional abilities. Four five-level classification systems have been validated for classifying gross motor function, manual ability, communication function, and eating and drinking ability of children and youth with cerebral palsy through age 18 years. Each system is based on the perspective that classification of children with CP on functional abilities and limitations should enhance communication among professionals and families with respect to (1) goal setting and intervention planning, (2) efficient utilization of medical and rehabilitation services, (3) assistive technology, and (4) comparing and generalizing research. The terms *functional related groups, severity of disability, case-mix complexity,* and *risk adjustment* refer to methods of grouping patients with the same diagnosis into subgroups for evaluating internal quality standards and comparative analysis of intervention outcomes. Because classification levels are based on performance in daily life, collaboration between parents, children/youth, and professionals is recommended to classify a child's levels of function. All four classification systems are available at no cost and have been translated into several languages. Collectively they provide an overview of a child's current functional abilities. It is important to recognize that the classification systems are *not* outcome measures and the goal of intervention *should not* be change in the child's classification level.

The *Gross Motor Function Classification System* (GMFCS) [281, 282] is available on the CanChild Centre website (www.canchild.ca).[58] Videos of young and older children functioning at each of the GMFCS levels are included on Expert Consult. The GMFCS was developed for children with cerebral palsy who are 12 years of age and younger and subsequently expanded to include a 12- to 18-year age band and revised to include environmental and personal considerations for the 6- to 12-year and 12- to 18-year bands. A summary of the descriptions for the 6- to 12-year age band is presented in Fig. 19.1. A classification is made by determining which of the five levels best represents the child's current abilities and limitations in gross motor function in home, school, and community settings. Classification is based on the child's self-initiated movement with emphasis on sitting and walking. The description for each level is broad and not intended to describe all aspects of the motor function of individual children. For each level, separate descriptions are

GMFCS E & R between 12ᵗʰ and 18ᵗʰ birthday: Descriptors and illustrations

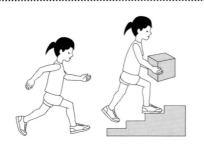

GMFCS Level I

Youth walk at home, school, outdoors and in the community. Youth are able to climb curbs and stairs without physical assistance or a railing. They perform gross motor skills such as running and jumping but speed, balance and coordination are limited.

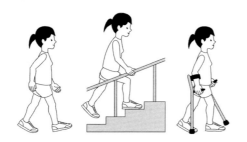

GMFCS Level II

Youth walk in most settings but environmental factors and personal choice influence mobility choices. At school or work they may require a hand held mobility device for safety and climb stairs holding onto a railing. Outdoors and in the community youth may use wheeled mobility when traveling long distances.

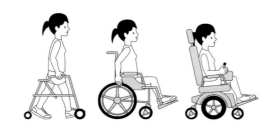

GMFCS Level III

Youth are capable of walking using a hand-held mobility device. Youth may climb stairs holding onto a railing with supervision or assistance. At school they may self-propel a manual wheelchair or use powered mobility. Outdoors and in the community youth are transported in a wheelchair or use powered mobility.

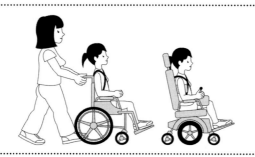

GMFCS Level IV

Youth use wheeled mobility in most settings. Physical assistance of 1-2 people is required for transfers. Indoors, youth may walk short distances with physical assistance, use wheeled mobility or a body support walker when positioned. They may operate a powered chair, otherwise are transported in a manual wheelchair.

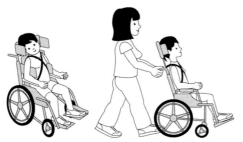

GMFCS Level V

Youth are transported in a manual wheelchair in all settings. Youth are limited in their ability to maintain antigravity head and trunk postures and control leg and arm movements. Self-mobility is severely limited, even with the use of assistive technology.

GMFCS descriptors: Palisano et al. (1997) Dev Med Child Neurol 39:214-23
CanChild: www.canchild.ca

Illustrations copyright © Kerr Graham, Bill Reid and Adrienne Harvey, The Royal Children's Hospital Melbourne   ERC151050

FIG. 19.1 The Gross Motor Function Classification System—Expanded and Revised for children ages 12 to 18 years of age. (CanChild Centre for Childhood Disability Research.)

provided for children in the following age bands: less than 2 years, 2 to 4 years, 4 to 6 years, and 6 to 12 years. Distinctions among levels of gross motor function are based on functional limitations, the need for handheld assistive mobility devices (walkers, crutches, canes), wheeled mobility, and, to a lesser extent, quality of movement. The scale is ordinal with no intent that the distances between levels be considered equal or that children with cerebral palsy are equally distributed among the five levels. Parents can apply the GMFCS reliably to their own children's functional status[127] and value being able to understand their child's level of function and what that means in terms of understanding future needs. Evidence of interrater reliability, stability, content, construct, and predictive validity has been reported.[239,281,282,286] Gorter et al.[141] found that classification of infants younger than 2 years of age is less precise than classification of older children and recommended reclassification at age 2 or older as more clinical information becomes available.

The *Manual Ability Classification System* (MACS)[109] is a five-level system to classify hand use of children with cerebral palsy, 4 to 18 years of age (www.macs.nu). Classification is based on the child's typical performance in handling objects during daily activities. Distinctions among the levels are based on the child's ability to handle objects and the amount of assistance or adaptation the child needs to complete tasks of daily living. Reliability and validity of the MACS have been demonstrated.[109,296] The authors of the MACS are in process of adapting and validating the MACS for children with CP below 4 years of age (Mini-MACS).

The *Communication Function Classification System* (CFCS)[167] is a five-level system to classify usual communication function of individuals with cerebral palsy (www.cfcs.us). A classification is based on everyday performance for all methods of communicating, including speech, gestures, eye gaze, facial expressions, and augmentative and alternative communication. Distinctions among the levels are based on the performance of sender and receiver roles, the pace of communication, and the type of conversational partner.

The *Eating and Drinking Abilities Classification System*[334] combines a five-level ordinal scale that describes the eating and drinking ability of people with CP, ages 3 to adulthood, and a three-level ordinal scale describing assistance required in bringing food and drink to mouth (www.EDACS.org). Distinctions between levels are based on ability to move food and drink in the mouth and coordinate breathing and swallowing. There is evidence of interobserver reliability between parents and speech and language therapists.[334]

Children with CP also are categorized by topographic distribution of impairments in body functions and structure and atypical movement. Topographic distributions include diplegia (lower limbs affected more than upper), hemiplegia or hemiparesis (upper and lower limbs on one side of the body), and quadriplegia or tetraplegia (all limbs). Although these designations focus on the limbs, involvement of the head and trunk muscles is typical. A more recent European classification designates spastic CP as bilateral or unilateral.[59] Lack of standardized definitions for topographic designations limits their reliability and validity.[142]

Movement differences are related to the location of brain damage. Types include spastic, dyskinetic, ataxic, and mixed.[59,330,331] Spastic CP results from involvement of the motor cortex or white matter projections to and from cortical sensorimotor areas of the brain. Spasticity and exaggerated reflexes result

in abnormal patterns of posture and movement. Dyskinesia reflects involvement of the basal ganglia. Dyskinetic features include atypical patterns of posture and involuntary, uncontrolled, recurring, and occasionally stereotyped movements of affected body parts. Dyskinetic CP may be classified further into subtypes: dystonic or athetotic. Dystonic movement is dominated by involuntary sustained or intermittent muscle contraction with repetitive movements and abnormal postures. Athetosis is characterized by slow, continuous, writhing movements that prevent maintenance of a stable posture. A cerebellar lesion produces ataxia—an inability to generate normal or expected voluntary movement trajectories that cannot be attributed to weakness or involuntary muscle activity about affected joints.[330] It results in general instability, abnormal patterns of posture, and lack of orderly, coordinated, rhythmic, and accurate movements.[59] In mixed CP, symptoms of spasticity and dyskinesia may be present.[59] The term should be used with an elaboration of the component motor disorders. Proportions of the various subtypes of CP vary with the reporting and sampling sources. Rates also change over time, as causes of CP are altered by advances in prevention and changing rates of prematurity and other medical problems associated with the diagnoses.

CHARACTERISTICS OF THE MOVEMENT DISORDERS IN CEREBRAL PALSY

The *International Classification of Functioning, Disability, and Health* (ICF) provides a common language and conceptual framework for describing complex interactions among body functions and structures, activities, and participation of individuals with CP in the context of personal and environmental factors. The ICF is applicable to clinical practice, research, teaching, and program evaluations.[129,332] A comprehensive core set and brief core sets grouped by age have been developed for children with CP to provide a systematic description of their functional profiles while considering the developmental trajectories of this population.[332]

Body Functions and Structures

Physical therapists address multiple body function and structure impairments in their comprehensive care of children with CP. Impairments can be primary or secondary. Primary impairments are an immediate result of the existing pathology, whereas secondary impairments such as contractures or skeletal malalignment develop over time as the result of other factors.[23] An understanding of these processes is integral to the prevention of unnecessary disability in children with CP. The following sections discuss the impairments addressed most often by physical therapists.

Muscle Tone and Extensibility

Tone is a clinical term used to describe the neural and mechanical properties of muscle. *Muscle tone* is defined as normal resting tension or resistance of muscle to passive movement or muscle lengthening.[59] It excludes resistance as a result of joint, ligament, or skeletal properties. Hypotonia is characterized by diminished resting muscle tone and decreased ability to generate voluntary muscle force. Hypertonia is an abnormal increase in resistance to an external force about a joint resulting from a number of factors, including neurally mediated reflex stiffness, passive muscle stiffness, and active muscle stiffness, all of which contribute to resistance of the muscle to stretch.[123] It is difficult to classify abnormal tone as a primary or secondary impairment because (1) it develops over time and with increasing attempts to overcome the force of gravity and gain mobility (except in those with severe impairment) and (2) the early neurally mediated abnormality of tone that is one of the signs leading to the diagnosis of CP is compounded over time by the addition of muscle stiffness and contracture. In children with CP, muscle tone has been found to increase up to 4 years of age and then decrease up to the age of 12.[151]

Spasticity is neural resistance to externally imposed movement, which increases with increasing speed of stretch and varies with the direction of joint movement. Resistance may rise rapidly above a threshold speed of passive movement or joint angle, resulting in a spastic catch that may represent the threshold for onset of the stretch reflex.[331] Spasticity may be associated with clonus, pathologic reflexes and particular patterns of posture and movement. Supraspinal and interneuronal mechanisms appear to be responsible for spasticity. Pathophysiologic mechanisms include reduced reciprocal inhibition of antagonist motoneuron pools, decreased presynaptic inhibition, and decreased nonreciprocal inhibition.[331,333]

Passive muscle stiffness is the sense of abnormally high tone or hypoextensibility of muscles resulting from abnormal mechanical properties. The muscle offers resistance to passive stretching at a shorter length than that expected in a normal muscle. In addition, if greater than normal amounts of force are required to produce a change in length, the muscle is said to have increased stiffness. This is represented as the passive tension curve for CP (p,CP) in contrast to the normal passive tension curve (p,N) in Fig. 19.2D, in response to moving the ankle from a position of plantar flexion to one of dorsiflexion. When it is not possible to manually stretch the muscle through a normal range using reasonable amounts of manual force, the muscle group is deemed to have a contracture. This is represented as *contracture*, the difference between the joint angle at which this extreme resistance is encountered in the CP muscle and that of the normal muscle. Fig. 19.2 shows hypothetical active force-length characteristics of spastic plantar flexors (a,CP; see Fig. 19.2B) and normal plantar flexors (a,N; see Fig. 19.2E)—that

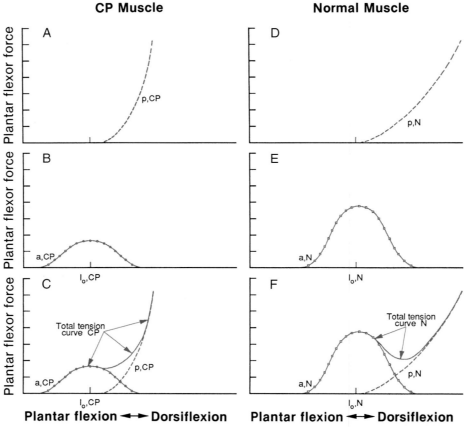

FIG. 19.2 Representation of force capabilities of ankle plantar flexor muscle at different joint angles in normal muscle (N) and spastic muscle (CP). A, Resistance to passive stretch of spastic muscle (p,CP) increasing with more dorsiflexion. B, The force of active contraction (a,CP) varying with the joint angle I_0 denoting resting length. C, The sum of passive and active effects in spastic muscle. D, Resistance to passive stretch in normal muscle (p,N). E, Force of active contraction in normal muscle (a,N). F, Total tension curve comprising the sum of passive and active effects in normal muscle. Note that (1) the slope (i.e., the stiffness) of p,CP in A is greater for the spastic muscle than for normal muscles (p,N) in D; (2) the maximal active force achieved by the spastic muscle (a,CP) in B is less than the maximal active force of normal muscle (a,N) in E; and (3) the maximal active force for spastic muscle (a,CP) shown in B occurs at a more plantarflexed position than that of the normal muscle (a,N) shown in E.

is, the force generated by the contractile elements of the muscle over the range of muscle lengths from a shortened position (plantarflexed) to a longer position (dorsiflexed). Note that the maximal force is lower for the CP muscle, and that the peak force occurs at a more plantarflexed position in the CP muscle than in the normal muscle. The sum of the combined effects of active force output and passive stiffness for the CP muscle is shown as total tension curve CP, and the corresponding curve for the normal muscle is shown as total tension curve N (Fig. 19.3). The complexity of the representation in Fig. 19.3 underscores the difficulty in determining the cause of increased tone through clinical methods such as passive manipulation of the limb and clinical assessment of muscle strength. The underlying mechanisms of these muscle extensibility alterations in CP are important in developing a rationale for interventions.[123]

Complex interactions among neurologic, mechanical, and biologic factors influence the structural integrity of muscle. This interplay between muscle innervation, altered loading, and impaired growth influences the development of contractile and noncontractile components of muscles in cerebral palsy.[143] The muscle structure has been characterized by alterations of sarcomere properties, muscle fiber size, type, variability, alignment, distribution, volume, and cell stiffness.[21,215] A proliferation and poor organization of extracellular materials with inferior mechanical properties have been noted in spastic muscle.[123] These abnormal collagen characteristics have been identified in the muscles of children with CP.[40]

Muscles grow and respond to the amount and type of activity during movement. Regular stretching of relaxed muscle under normal physiologic loading occurs in typically developing children. The muscles in children with CP may not relax during activity and may be subject to chronic muscle imbalance, abnormal posturing, and static positioning resulting from spasticity, weakness, and abnormal reflex activity. Muscle growth may not keep up with bone growth during periods of rapid linear growth, thereby contributing to hypoextensibility; conversely, some muscles may become overlengthened as the result of repeated mechanical stretch or orthopedic surgery.[405] Although patterns of tightness vary, the muscles most commonly at risk for contracture are the shoulder adductors;

the elbow, wrist, and finger flexors; the hip flexors and adductors; the knee flexors; and the ankle plantar flexors. A population-based study of adolescents with CP demonstrated that although those with lower gross motor function tended to have greater limitations in range of motion (ROM), variation within GMFCS levels could be seen. Some adolescents functioning at GMFCS level I had contractures; others functioning at level V did not.[401]

Muscle Strength

Considerable evidence suggests that children with CP are unable to generate normal voluntary force in a muscle or normal torque about a joint.[315,330] This impairment may be expressed as decreased moment of force output, a deficiency in power, or, when considered over time, a deficiency in work.[270] The term *strength* may refer to any of these measurable factors, and diminished force production capability is now understood to be a primary impairment in CP. Muscle weakness is consistent with low levels of electromyographic (EMG) activity and has been attributed to decreased neuronal drive, inappropriate co-activation of antagonistic muscle groups, secondary myopathy, and altered muscle tissue properties.[108,111,123,125,315,343] Additionally, muscle shortening and skeletal deformity can lead to changes in lever arm biomechanics, resulting in reduced output of muscle force in terms of torque.[269] Greater weakness has been reported in the distal musculature compared with the proximal musculature, for concentric versus eccentric contractions, and in faster versus slower speeds of movement.[85] Strength has been linked with activity capabilities such as walking speed and gross motor function.[84,269] Strength deficits can also contribute to bone deformity; for example, hip weakness is a postulated cause of hip deformity in ambulatory children and young adults.[240]

Skeletal Structure

Impairments such as weakness, spasticity, abnormal extensibility, and disturbed reflexes can result in excessive and abnormal biomechanical forces. Structures such as joint capsules, ligaments, and bones can become compromised. Torsion of long bones, joint instability, and premature degenerative changes in weight-bearing joints can occur. Alignment of the spine and extremities can be affected, particularly during times of physical growth. The prevalence of scoliosis in individuals with CP increases with age and GMFCS level and is greater than 60% in children with spastic quadriplegia.[10,216] Another concern is the lack of standing and ambulation on the growth and development of hip joint, putting children with CP at risk for subluxation and dislocation. Hip displacement can be painful and impact mobility, positioning, and activities of daily living.[391] A linear relationship exists between GMFCS and risk of hip instability. The overall prevalence of hip displacement (migration percentage greater than 30%) is 30%; however, children classified as GCMAS level V have a risk close to 90%.[403] Children with CP also have low bone mineral density and can be at risk for fragility fractures due to decreased weight bearing, the use of anticonvulsants, poor nutrition, and decreased exposure to sunlight.[115]

Selective Control

Normal movement is characterized by orderly phasing in and out of muscle activation, co-activation of muscles with similar biomechanical functions, and limited co-activation of antagonists during phasic or free movement. Children with CP have poor selective control of muscle activity. This is defined as

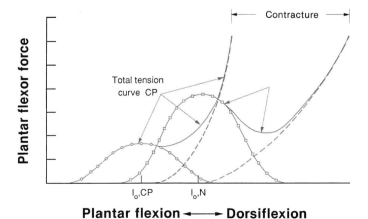

FIG. 19.3 Complete representation of force capabilities of ankle plantar flexor muscle at different joint angles in normal muscle (N) and spastic muscle (CP) shown in Fig. 19.2. a,CP = Force of active contraction of spastic muscle; l_o,CP = resting length of spastic muscle; l_o,N = resting length of normal muscle.

the impaired ability to isolate the activation of muscles in a selected pattern in response to demands of a voluntary posture or movement. Individuals with poor selective control exhibit reduced speed of movement, mirror movements, or abnormal reciprocal muscle activation.[124,330,333] They may be unable to move their hip, knee, and ankle joints independently of one another and exhibit coupled flexor and extensor patterns when attempting functional movement.[124] Deficiency in the control of selective movements is a major contributor to impaired motor function. For example, selective control of the lower extremity is related to the ability to extend the knee while flexing the hip and dorsiflexing the ankle at late swing and initial contact in gait.[124] Selective control is an important predictor of success for interventions such as dorsal rhizotomy[110] or orthopedic surgery.[124]

Postural Control

Postural control is the ability to control the body's position in space for stability or orientation, balancing the center of mass over the base of support.[101] (See Chapter 3, Motor Development and Control.) The sensory, motor, and musculoskeletal systems participate in coordinating postural activity through synergies and strategies. Children with CP have dysfunction in responding to postural challenges and have difficulty fine-tuning postural activity.[95] Reactive postural adjustments occur in response to unexpected external postural perturbations. Responses in children with CP vary with level of severity. Children with CP functioning at GMFCS levels I and II have some ability to produce direction-specific adjustments to counteract forces disturbing equilibrium through reactive control, whereas these abilities decrease with higher GMFCS levels and are largely absent in children with GMFCS level V.[45] Anticipatory postural adjustments are related to expected internal postural perturbations preceding the onset of voluntary movement. In healthy individuals, changes in posture are preceded by preparatory muscle contractions that stabilize the body and allow weight shifts in anticipation of movement, while keeping the center of mass within the stability limits of the body. Children with CP exhibit characteristic disorganization or adaptations, including cranial-caudal recruitment of postural muscles, excessive antagonistic co-activation, and reduced or absent capacity to adapt the degree of muscle contraction as appropriate to the specific task or situation.[45,95]

Pain

Acute and chronic pain can have a negative impact on accomplishment and satisfaction with daily activities, physical activity, mental health, social life, sleep, energy, and overall quality of life of people with CP.[23,104,356, 399] Pain can result from neuromuscular, orthopedic, or gastrointestinal impairments; overuse syndromes; and interventions such as surgery, bracing, and injections.[351] It can also be related to exercise, with stretching frequently being reported as painful.[351] Pain has been reported by 64% of girls and 50% of boys in adolescents with cerebral palsy, most frequently in the feet, ankles, knees, and lower backs of those functioning at all GMFCS levels as well as the lower back of those at levels I to IV and had a negative impact on daily activities.[104]

Fatigue

Fatigue of physiologic origin can results from high rates of energy expenditure. Possible underlying mechanisms in people with CP include decreased force production capacity and increased energy expenditure due excessive co-contraction and inefficient movement patterns.[49] Fatigue has the potential to impact participation in many aspects of life and can become more problematic with maturation as increased size and more demanding activities require greater physical exertion.

Activity and Participation

Physical therapists focus on motor activities and how they impact activity and participation in the domains of mobility, general tasks and demands, self-care, domestic life, and other life areas. Factors that contribute to variance in the motor abilities of children with CP are spasticity, quality of movement, postural stability, force production, range of motion, and endurance as well as distribution of involvement, adaptive behavior (GMFCS levels III-V only), and participation in community programs (GMFCS levels I-II only).[24]

Participation in children with disabilities is a complex phenomenon that allows them to pursue the learning of skills, to develop social engagement, and to find satisfaction in their lives.[175] Opportunities for children and adolescents with CP to participate in home, school, and community activities are increasing. Many have positive peer experiences.[176] This can be attributed to advances in technology and a legacy of striving for inclusion that has influenced social attitudes and policies regarding funding and environmental adaptation. Nevertheless, children and adolescents with CP experience restrictions in participation compared with children in the general population.[28,176,243] They may be overprotected, excluded from playing with peers, or bullied.[176] Adults with CP experience restrictions in participation. They can have challenges integrating socially, experiencing intimate and partner relationships, and securing paid employment.[305]

Many factors are associated with participation in life activities. Physical environment (Fig. 19.4), GMFCS level, hand function, toileting needs, pain, communication, cognition, attitudinal barriers, parental vigilance, and child motivation are important predictors[112,175,176,251] with walking ability being particularly significant.[112] Participation can vary significantly across countries even when other factors were controlled for. Denmark has higher rates of participation in all areas except relationships, most likely reflective of its policies and programs supporting the principle of equal access through public transportation, accessibility, assistive technology, and financial assistance. Such findings illustrate the impact of the social and legislative environment on the lives of people with disabilities.

RESEARCH EVIDENCE FOR INTERVENTIONS

Evidence-based practice is the standard for pediatric physical therapy. In the Foreground Information section of this chapter, research is applied to physical therapy management of infants, children, and adolescents with CP using the model of evidence-informed decision making described in Chapter 1. This section presents considerations for applying research to decision making for individual children.

The increase in the number of studies on interventions for children with CP has led to a proliferation of systematic reviews and meta-analyses. Systematic review is a retrospective appraisal of all research on an intervention in an effort to determine the overall effect. Meta-analysis refers to the use of

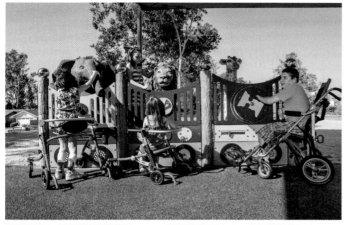

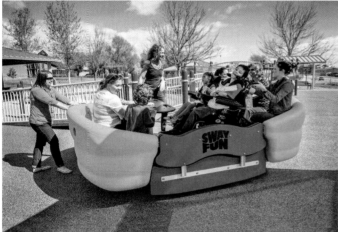

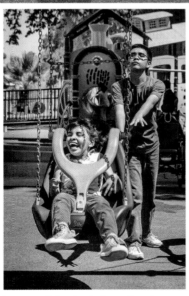

FIG. 19.4 Environmental adaptations to playgrounds can facilitate participation in normal childhood activities. (Courtesy Landscape Structures, Delano, MN.)

statistical methods to analyze the combined data from all studies to determine an overall effect. A current meta-analysis is a valuable resource for practitioners. A systematic review where results are analyzed descriptively requires more judgment in determining the overall effectiveness of an intervention.

Although systematic reviews are essential for evidence-informed decision making, the strength of evidence and effect size for physical therapy interventions for children with CP preclude prediction of outcomes for individual children. In other words, as will be presented in the Foreground Information section, research supports several interventions based on group data. The effect size for most interventions, however, is small to medium, indicating considerable overlap in outcomes between the children who received the intervention and the children in the comparison/control group. For this reason, the response of an individual child should not be inferred from group data.[80]

Also important is recognition that a systematic review is only as good as the quality of the research. Randomized controlled trials on the effects of interventions for children with CP are expensive and difficult to conduct. There is often variation in the ages and abilities of participants, the intensity of intervention, how the intervention is provided, and the outcomes measured. Sample size is often small and methodologic quality is variable. A concern when data are aggregated from studies with disparate features is applicability to evidence-informed decision making.

The caution urged when attempting to predict the response of an individual child from research evidence in many cases reflects the lack of knowledge of characteristics of children most likely to achieve the desired outcome, the age(s) when the intervention is most effective, the optimal intensity of intervention, and family and environmental factors associated with optimal outcomes. We encourage therapists to reflect on these considerations as part of the decision-making process.

FOREGROUND INFORMATION

EXAMINATION AND EVALUATION

Physical therapy examination of children with CP involves the identification of strengths and abilities, as well as participation restrictions, activity limitations, impairments of body structure and function, and environmental and personal factors as determined through interviews, observations, informal assessments, and objective measures.[192] Evaluation involves the integration of these findings with prognostic knowledge and consideration of contextual factors, which can be facilitators or barriers. It is important to differentiate among capacity (what someone can do in a standardized environment), capability (what someone can do in one's daily environment), and performance (what someone does do in daily life).[168] Capacity can exceed capability and capability can exceed performance. The gap between performance and capacity represents a therapy opportunity to enhance function and participation; however, an improvement in capacity may, but does not necessarily, translate into an improvement in capability or performance as personal factors such as age or motivation and physical or societal environmental factors impact change.[340] When motor skills are assessed, the use of equipment to carry out an activity should be taken into consideration. For example, wearing orthoses may substantially affect walking abilities.[320]

Ongoing assessments provide feedback for therapists, children, and their families that can be motivating, indicative of areas that need more attention, and helpful in determining prognosis; these assessments therefore guide ongoing shared and informed clinical decision making.[192] In addition to clinical practice, measurement is the foundation for research and can be used to enhance service delivery and allocation of health resources.[192]

The ICF provides a framework to guide the selection of measures. Selection should be consistent with the purpose of an examination: discrimination, prognosis, or evaluation. Measurement tools need to be psychometrically rigorous but also feasible for specific clinical or research situations. Cost, training, time to administer and score, amount of handling, and child and family acceptance must be considered.

An ever-increasing number of measurement tools are available. The concept of a toolbox of outcome measurements for children with cerebral palsy suggests a core set of outcome tools framed within the ICF.[397] Video and photographic recording of assessments can provide records for future comparison. Families can also use these techniques to share information about their child's functioning in environments outside the clinic setting. A selection of measures applicable to children and youth with CP will be reviewed (Box 19.1). A comprehensive compilation is available in Measures for Children with Developmental Disabilities—an ICF-CY Approach.[229]

Body Functions and Structures
Muscle Tone and Extensibility
No method of measuring muscle tone is universally accepted or has strong psychometric properties.[120] Choices depend on the purpose of measurement. It is important to consider both neurologic and passive mechanical components of tone and to measure accordingly. In the clinical setting, spasticity is assessed typically by measuring the resistance to passive movement imposed through available range. The modified Ashworth scale is an undifferentiated, ordinal measure of spasticity and extensibility. It has been shown to have variable levels of reliability for children with CP depending on muscle group and only fair

---

BOX 19.1 Selected Tests and Measures for Children and Youth with Cerebral Palsy

Body Functions and Structures
Modified Tardieu scale
Spinal Alignment Range of Motion Measure
Selective Control Assessment of the Lower Extremity
Accelerometers
Non-communicating Children's Pain Checklist/Pain Assessment Instrument for Cerebral Palsy

Activity and Participation
Timed distance tasks (walking or wheeled mobility)
Gait Laboratory Assessment/Video Assessment/Edinburgh Gait Score
Gross Motor Function Measure
Pediatric Evaluation of Disability Inventory
Activity Scale for Kids
Child Engagement in Daily Life
Assessment of Life Habits
Lifestyle Assessment Questionnaire for CP

Environment
Craig Hospital Inventory of Environmental Factors

Quality of Life
Pediatric Quality of Life Inventory (PedsQL), version 3.0, Cerebral Palsy Module
Caregiver Priorities and Child Health Index of Life with Disabilities
Cerebral Palsy Quality of Life Questionnaire for Children

---

to moderate interrater reliability for the plantar flexor muscles. It does not quantify spasticity exclusively as anatomic, and biomechanical factors such as intrinsic stiffness of the muscles can contribute to hypertonia in addition to a heightened, velocity-dependent stretch reflex response.

Measurements evaluating resistance at several speeds may be more useful for planning and evaluating interventions, particularly those that aim to reduce spasticity or manage contracture.[84,273] The modified Tardieu scale measures the point of resistance or "catch" to a rapid velocity stretch, giving an indication of the dynamic neural component of tone or the overactive stretch reflex and is sometimes referred to as "R1." Moving the limb slowly into a lengthened position indicates the mechanical component of tone or muscle length at rest, commonly known as passive ROM or "R2."[42] A large difference between the initial catch and the point of mechanical resistance indicates a large reflexive component to motion limitation, and a small difference suggests a more fixed muscle contracture.[42] The Tardieu scale has been found to be more reliable than the modified Ashworth scale, particularly for the plantar flexors, but wide intersessional variations between dynamic and static differences limit use as an outcome measure. Various biomechanical and neurophysiologic assessment tools such as dynamometers or electromyography, respectively, can also be used to quantify spasticity.[120] The Barry-Albright Dystonia Scale provides a tool for rating dystonia.[20] It is a 5-point ordinal scale based on severity of posturing and involuntary dystonic movements in eight body regions.

Goniometry is the most common measurement tool for ROM; however, measurement error necessitates caution when interpreting serial measurements to determine outcomes and or make clinical decisions.[87] Some researchers have suggested that a change of more than 15° to 20° between sessions is required to be 95% confident that a true change in ROM has occurred in many joints of children with CP.[191] Consistent positioning and procedures should be used for measuring and documenting ROM and skeletal alignment particularly for rotational movements and biarticular muscles. Relaxation of a child and consistency in therapists can also contribute to accuracy.

Visual estimation may be used for ease of measurement and has been shown to be correlated adequately to goniometry for assessing ankle dorsiflexion, hip extension, and the popliteal angle.[229] The Spinal Alignment Range of Motion Measure (SAROMM) is a discriminative tool that uses estimations of spinal alignment and ROM limitations to give a summary score. The SAROMM indicates whether the child has normal alignment and ROM; flexible deviation; or mild, moderate, or severe fixed limitations.[22] It is considered to be sufficiently reliable and valid for use with children with CP.

Strength/Endurance
Testing muscle strength in children with CP may be difficult because of age, cognitive level, spasticity, hyperactive reflexes, abnormal muscle and joint extensibility, or poor selective control. Isokinetic muscle strength testing is available in some settings, allowing for precise stabilization and quantification of strength at different speeds and for different types of contractions.[11] Clinically, muscle strength is more often measured isometrically by manual muscle testing using an ordinal 6-point scale, or with handheld dynamometry if a child can exert a maximal effort in a consistent manner.[84,125] A make test is more reliable than the break test for lower extremity muscles when

handheld dynamometry is used. It has been shown to have high within-session reliability and variable between-session reliability depending on muscle group, positioning, and stabilization.[76,376] As a result, changes in strength should be considered based on measurement error for particular muscle groups.

Strength can also be assessed in a functional context. Observation of activities such as moving between sitting and standing positions, or ascending and descending stairs, helps to assess both concentric and eccentric power. Counting the number of repetitions of a functional movement performed over a specific period of time can quantify functional muscle strength. Interrater reliability of 30-second repetitions of lateral step-ups, sit-to-stand, and standing through half kneeling is acceptable.[376] Muscle strength may differ depending on posture, joint angle, speed of movement, or presence of contracture. Ability to generate force may deteriorate as a result of early fatigue of muscles, reduced endurance, or an inability to generate a sufficiently rapid increase in force, and in some cases it may be important to measure both the ability to maintain force over time and the ability to generate a brief rapid force.

Endurance and efficiency of movement become increasingly important when children venture into the community on their own or with peers. Submaximal endurance can be evaluated by observing the ability to walk or propel a wheelchair for age-appropriate distances. The 10-meter, 1-minute, 6-minute, and 10-minute walk tests, 600-yard walk-run test, and 6-minute push test have been found to be reliable in children with CP.[65,357] Ambulation measured over longer distances more closely simulates community ambulation and therefore the ability to participate in community activities.[357] Shuttle run, wheeling, cycling, or ergometry tests have been validated as maximal exercise tests for children and adolescents with CP, and muscle power sprint running tests or Wingate tests can provide information about anaerobic muscle power.[372] Accelerometers can be used to measure physical activity levels of ambulatory children with CP.[177] Physiologic measures such as the energy expenditure index provide energy cost information in a clinically feasible manner, but these measures have limitations because heart rate may not be an accurate substitute for energy expenditure under all conditions.[125] They may be useful when two or more mobility options are compared for the same person. It is important to conduct exercise testing over time to track improvement or decline in exercise capacity.[372]

Selective Control and Postural Control

Examination of selective control of muscle activity, anticipatory regulation of postural muscle groups, and ability to learn unique movements may be broad—using measures of balance, coordination, and motor control—or specific—for example, using the selective motor control test to quantify active ankle dorsiflexion.[42] The Selective Control Assessment of the Lower Extremity (SCALE) is an objective tool used to quantify lower extremity selective voluntary motor control. It rates the ability to perform specific isolated movement patterns as normal, impaired, or unable and has been shown to be valid and reliable.[15,124,127]

Postural control is measured in many standardized and nonstandardized ways at impairment or activity levels.[101] Sway or response to perturbations can be assessed by disturbing the supporting surface or by perturbing the subject or environment. Visual observation; kinematic, kinetic, and center of pressure measures; or electromyography (EMG) can be used to assess responses. Analysis of EMG activity during perturbations

makes it possible to detect abnormal responses in the timing of muscle activity onset and duration, in the sequencing of agonists, and in the co-contraction of antagonists. Various balance tests such as the Automatic Reactions section of the Movement Assessment of Infants, the Pediatric Balance Scale, or the Early Clinical Assessment of Balance[233] can be used for children with CP. The Test of Infant Motor Performance (described in Chapter 29) includes assessment of primitive reflexes and automatic postural reactions.

Pain

Therapists should inquire about pain routinely, as people with CP may assume chronic pain to be the norm and not offer information spontaneously.[61] Self-report is optimal and can be verbal or through questionnaires or analog scales. Motor, cognitive, and communication problems can complicate but should not preclude the assessment of pain as behavioral cues or physiologic responses such as facial expression; vocalizations; or changes in cardiorespiratory status, sweating, movement, tone, affect, sleeping, and eating can indicate pain, despite the challenge of interpretation due to individual responses. The Non-communicating Children's Pain Checklist provides a standardized tool. The Pain Assessment Instrument for Cerebral Palsy is an instrument that allows self-report of pain and may indicate the range of potentially painful activities more accurately than proxy report.[38]

Activity and Participation

Pediatric physical therapists use a variety of tests to assess activity and participation. Some, such as the Test of Infant Motor Performance[254] (see video associated with Chapter 2 for an example of this test), the Alberta Infant Motor Scale,[89] the Movement Assessment of Infants,[63] and the Peabody Developmental Motor Scales[380] (see Chapter 2, Measurement) are not specific to CP. These are standardized measures normed on children with typical development to identify infants and children with delays in motor development or qualify children for services in early intervention and educational settings. For children with identified health conditions characterized by motor impairments and activity limitations, the value of such measures to plan interventions and document change is controversial. An alternative approach for measuring change over time or in response to an intervention in children with physical disabilities is to compare performance with expectations for children of the same age with a similar disability. This approach is dependent on disability-specific data.

The most widely used research and clinical tool for assessment of children with CP is the Gross Motor Function Measure (GMFM).[157] The GMFM is a reliable and valid criterion-referenced evaluative instrument designed to detect change in children with CP.[58,318] It has been validated on children 5 months to 16 years of age. The original GMFM has 88 items grouped in five dimensions: A: Lying and Rolling, B: Sitting, C: Crawling and Kneeling, D: Standing, and E: Walking, Running, and Jumping; these dimensions are scored on a generic 4-point ordinal scale. A gain of 5 to 7 percentage points is considered a medium positive, clinically important change for an individual child. The GMFM-66 is an interval-level version of the original GMFM developed and validated through Rasch analysis. Relative to the GMFM-88, the GMFM-66 demonstrates improved scoring, interpretation, and overall clinical and research utility; it requires fewer items to be tested and estimates the difficulty of items.[10] A computer program, the Gross Motor Ability Estimator (GMAE), converts scores to an interval scale, plots scores graphically or on an item map, and provides 95% confidence intervals. Item sets of the GMFM-66 (GMFM-66-IS) have been developed to further improve the efficiency of administration.[319] An algorithm with three decision items indicates which set to use. Another short form version uses a basal-ceiling approach (GMFM-66-B&C).[23]

A Challenge Module has been developed as an adjunct to the GMFM to target performance of higher-level gross motor skills in children functioning at GMFCS levels I and II. Items such as running around pylons are indicative of skills that facilitate participation in play and sports with peers.[138,392]

The Quality Function Measure (Quality FM) is an adaptation of the Gross Motor Performance Measure, a measure developed to rate qualitative aspects of motor skills. It is based on viewing video recordings to evaluate the quality of alignment, dissociated movement, coordination, stability, and weight shift in dimensions D: Standing and E: Walking, Running, and Jumping of the GMFM.[396] This reliable and valid tool assesses how well young people with CP move and what areas of function to target to enhance quality of motor control.

Walking is subject to more specific assessment, as it is a focus of many physical therapy interventions and is perceived by children and parents to impact quality of life.[182] *Gait analysis* is a broad term that refers to many different methods of measuring and studying primary and secondary walking deviations and compensatory patterns (Fig. 19.5). Three-dimensional instrumented gait analysis is promoted as an objective and accurate measurement tool that improves clinical decision making and allows critical evaluation of interventions aimed at better outcomes for children with CP, particularly around major decision making regarding orthopedic or selective dorsal rhizotomy surgery and as an outcome measure for these interventions.[223,259,303]

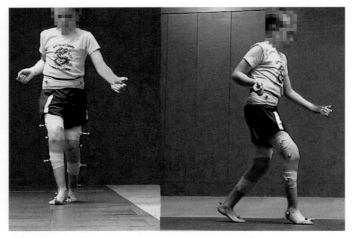

FIG. 19.5 Child taking part in gait analysis. Electromyography shows patterns of muscle activities and aids identification of the presence of co-contraction of muscle groups. Markers at joints allow computer calculation of joint movements; force platforms embedded in floor permit measurement of individual muscle group contributions to the work of walking. (From Chang FM, Rhodes JT, Flynn KM, Carollo JJ: The role of gait analysis in treating gait abnormalities in cerebral palsy, *Orthop Clin North Am* 41:489-506, 2010.)

A comprehensive gait analysis includes a clinical examination of physical impairments, including spasticity, ROM, bony deformity, strength, and selective control, coupled with a dynamic assessment of the biomechanical and physiologic aspects of walking. Findings from these measures are considered in relation to functional mobility performance outside the gait laboratory and in the context of a child's environment and participation in life activities. Visual observation can be used for subjective descriptions of stability and balance, speed and control, symmetry and movement patterns, weight transfer, foot placement, and the influence of assistive devices. The use of instrumentation to document and quantify temporal, spatial, kinematic, kinetic, and electromyographic information results in objective measures of multiple joints and limb segments simultaneously, providing complex data that could not be detected by visual inspection alone.[64,98] An understanding of power generation and absorption of muscle groups is of particular importance in assessing outcomes[406] (see Chapter 34, Development and Analysis of Gait and accompanying video on Expert Consult).

Although findings facilitate a wide range of clinical and research applications, clinical utility is controversial because of high costs and the questionable validity of laboratory results for representing daily function.[259] Proponents consider it to be the gold standard measure for clinical practice and research and believe computerized three-dimensional gait analysis is a requirement for the optimal treatment of problems related to ambulation in CP.[264] Others consider it to be an expensive tool that does not contribute sufficiently to warrant its use clinically.[71]

Video-based gait assessment is a simpler and less expensive alternative for basic description of key gait parameters that has been found to have moderate interrater reliability and validity based on three-dimensional gait analysis.[223] It can provide opportunities for frequent monitoring, to document change over time, the impact of treatments and interventions, and the impact of orthotics. It can be useful for very young children or those with behavioral or cognitive issues that could preclude fully instrumented gait analysis.[160] Observational gait scales have been developed to make video gait analysis more objective and reliable. The Edinburgh Gait Score was developed for people with CP and includes ratings of gait components in sagittal, coronal, and transverse planes of movement. It is the strongest tool psychometrically and correlates well with three-dimensional gait analysis.

Tests such as the Timed Up and Go, Timed Up and Down Stairs, and running tests provide measures of functional activities.[5] They may be useful in school or community settings because of their simplicity and are significant predictors of community mobility.[118]

The Activity Scale for Kids is a child or parent self-report measure for children with musculoskeletal disorders between the ages of 5 and 15 years and is robust psychometrically for children with CP. It has capacity and performance versions, which assess daily physical activities, including personal care, dressing, eating and drinking, play, locomotion, standing skills, climbing stairs, and transfers.[162,404]

The Pediatric Evaluation of Disability Inventory (PEDI) uses structured interviews to collect parental reports of functional skills in young children with disabilities.[379] The PEDI-CAT is a computerized version that selects items based on previous responses, thereby reducing the number of overall items. The

Functional Independence Measure for Children (WeeFIM), a pediatric version of the Functional Independence Measure, measures function as quantified by burden of care for children with developmental disabilities.[12] Chapter 2 provides more information on these tests. The Pediatric Outcomes Data Collection Instrument determines levels of various skills, including transfers and basic mobility, sports, and physical function, and it includes a participation component.[19]

Participation is a complex construct, but measures help to ensure that function in home, school, and community settings is recognized. They can help with goal setting, treatment planning, and overall patient care.[327] The Child Engagement in Daily Life is a parent-completed measure of frequency and enjoyment of participation in family and recreational activities and the degree a child participates in the self-care activities of feeding, dressing, bathing, and toileting for children 18 to 60 months of age.[66] The Assessment of Life Habits (LIFE-H) determines the daily life experiences of children.[248,263] It was developed from a theoretical framework aligned with the ICF and rates 11 domains of daily activities and social roles on levels of accomplishment, type of assistance, and level of satisfaction.

The Children's Assessment of Participation and Enjoyment (CAPE), a child-report instrument, captures diversity, intensity, location, and enjoyment of participation, including with whom the child participates, in formal and informal activities using five scales: recreational, active physical, social, skill-based and self-improvement, and educational. It does not incorporate assistance needed into the scoring system.[195] The Participation and Environment Measure for Children and Youth (PEM-CY) examines participation in home, school, and community settings and the environmental factors that support or hinder participation specific to these settings.[73] The Lifestyle Assessment Questionnaire for CP measures physical dependence, restriction of mobility, educational exclusion, clinical burden, economic burden, and restriction of social interaction. The contextual items provide information on the impact of disability on participation of the family unit.[227,248] The School Function Assessment may be used to assess participation, adaptations, assistance, and activity performance in educational settings, providing information about the environment as well as participation.[93,527]

Although the use of these standardized tools is important for diagnosis and quantification of outcomes, child and caregiver interviews remain important clinical tools for collecting useful and meaningful information about participation and environments. A family's recounting of their activities in a typical day and night, including accommodations made for their child with CP, is invaluable.[30,292,394] Information about the influence of personal and environmental attributes on enabling or creating barriers to function can be gathered through a description of daily activities. These range from specific factors internal to a child and family such as caregiver stress, family supports, and finances to broader factors such as community physical environments and societal attitudes toward children with disabilities.[30,385]

Health-Related Quality of Life

Measures of health-related quality of life (QOL) take into account various factors and values believed to be important by health care professionals, parents, and children themselves that contribute toward well-being and ability to fulfill certain life roles.[232,260,382] The Pediatric Quality of Life Inventory (PedsQL), version 3.0, Cerebral Palsy Module, measures health-related QOL dimensions specific to CP. It includes five dimensions: daily activities, movement and balance, pain and hurt, fatigue, and eating.[369] The Caregiver Priorities and Child Health Index of Life with Disabilities (CPCHILD) is a measure of health status and well-being of children with severe activity limitations.[260] The Cerebral Palsy Quality of Life Questionnaire for Children has self-report and parent proxy versions to assess seven domains of QOL, including social well-being and acceptance, feelings about functioning, participation and physical health, emotional well-being, access to services, pain and feeling about disability, and family health.[381] The Child Health Questionnaire is a health-related QOL measure that has been used in children with CP. Various health-related QOL measures such as the Short Form (SF)-36 have been used to study adults with CP.[179]

Individualized Outcomes

Individualized criterion-referenced measures are available to assist in formulating goals and measuring their attainment. The Canadian Occupational Performance Measure can be used to document and quantify goals that are relevant to a family and to determine whether they are achieved.[213] Goal Attainment Scaling can be used to evaluate whether specific individualized treatment goals or outcomes have been met.[97,279,344] These forms of assessment are highly responsive to clinically meaningful change in short time periods[192] and complement but do not replace standardized measures.

Evaluation of service delivery and environmental factors can provide valuable information to inform practice. The Measuring Processes of Care tool captures parental satisfaction with family-centered aspects of services. A 20-question version (MPOC-20) assesses five areas of care: enabling and partnership, providing general information, providing specific information about the child, providing coordinated and comprehensive care, and providing respectful and supportive care.[78] Giving Youth a Voice is an evolution of the MPOC designed to provide youth with disabilities an opportunity to give feedback.[132,337] The perceptions of service providers can be captured with the Measure of Processes of Care for Service Providers.[395] The Craig Hospital Inventory of Environmental factors (CHIEF) measures environmental barriers in school, work, and physical environments; policies; services and attitudes; and supports. The Supports and Services Inventory assesses the services families and children receive and their perception of the adequacy of services to meet their needs.

Physical therapy sessions can be described and evaluated in systematic, standardized, and reliable ways. Examples include determining the proportions of time spent facilitating movement versus challenging the production of motor behaviors in infant treatment or time spent in family involvement and education[35,103] or the Paediatric Rehabilitation Observational measure of Fidelity, which measures the degree to which interventions are delivered as intended.[102] These applications are used to increase research rigor and therefore better assess clinical effectiveness.

PROGNOSIS FOR GROSS MOTOR FUNCTION

Measurement findings coupled with knowledge of prognosis for gross motor function in children with CP can facilitate communication with families regarding outlook for gross motor function, facilitate collaborative and realistic goal setting, inform the selection of appropriate interventions, and evaluate intervention outcomes.[279] One of the first concerns for parents of children with CP is whether their child will walk. Walking ability varies by type of CP. Children with hemiplegic and ataxic CP are more likely to walk, whereas those with dyskinetic and bilateral CP are less likely to do so. Cognitive functioning, visual and hearing impairments, and epilepsy are also predictors of walking ability for all types of CP.[29] Independent sitting by 24 months remains the best predictor of ambulation for 15 meters or more with or without assistive devices by age 8 years.[383] If independent sitting is not achieved by age 3, there is very little chance of achieving functional independent walking. Some people with CP experience a decline in their walking abilities in adolescence or adulthood as a result of pain, fatigue, musculoskeletal deterioration, poor surgical outcome, weight and height gains, or fear of falling.[219]

Gross Motor Development Curves

The GMFM-66[318] and the GMFCS enabled researchers at the CanChild Centre for Developmental Disability Research to create gross motor development curves for children with cerebral palsy. Prospective longitudinal studies on a cohort of children with cerebral palsy randomly selected from an accessible population of 2108 children in the province of Ontario (Canada) were constructed. Children were stratified by age and GMFCS level. Each child's classification level at the start of the study was used to create five motor development curves. The first study[314] included 657 children who were administered the GMFM-66 an average of 4.3 times. The model that provided the best fit of GMFM-66 scores was nonlinear and included two parameters: the *rate parameter,* an estimate of how fast children approach their limit of gross motor function, and the *limit parameter,* an estimate of maximum potential for gross motor function.

A subsequent study was completed that followed 229 of the 343 older children in the original cohort for an additional 5 years during adolescence and early adulthood.[155] A consideration in deciding how to model the curves was the possibility that some youth might demonstrate a decline in gross motor function. To account for this possibility, a model was examined that included a third parameter to allow for a peak and decline in GMFM-66 scores, prior to a long-term limit. The data were modeled using both two and three parameters. The two-parameter model provided the best fit for children and youth in levels I and II, whereas the three-parameter model provided the best fit for children and youth in levels III, IV, and V. The gross motor development growth curves are presented in Fig. 19.6.

The gross motor development curves represent the average pattern of development for children and youth in each of the five classification levels. It should not be assumed, however, that the average patterns apply to all children with CP because there is large variability within levels. For all five curves, children progress faster to their maximum GMFM-66 score at younger ages and then demonstrate a leveling of scores (levels I and II) or a decline followed by a leveling (levels III-V). The predicted average maximum GMFM-66 score differs significantly for each level. On average, children in level I achieve a maximum score of 90, whereas children in level V achieve a score of 24 at age 6, which then declines to 17 age 21. Children and youth in levels III, IV, and V are predicted, on average, to demonstrate a decline in GMFM-66 score of 4.7 to 7.8 points. The gross motor development curves have important implications for evaluation

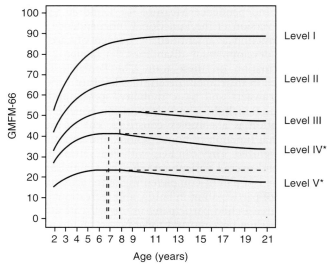

FIG. 19.6 Gross motor development curves for children and youth with cerebral palsy. (From Hanna SE, Rosenbaum PL, Bartlett DJ, et al.: Stability and decline in gross motor function among children and youth with cerebral palsy aged 2 to 21 years, *Dev Med Child Neurol* 51, 295-302, 2009.)

of interventions by providing evidence of the extent to which a particular intervention improves a child's gross motor function beyond what is predicted by the curves.

When sharing the gross motor curves with children, families, and other health care providers, therapists must clearly explain *what the curves do* and *do not measure.* The GMFM-66 measures activities, specifically what a child *can do* in a standard condition without shoes or orthotics. The activities measured are usually achieved by age 5 in children without motor impairments. The number of children below age 2 and the number above age 18 were low; therefore, the ends of the curves may not reflect actual development.

An example of the application of GMFCS, GMFM-66, and gross motor development curves to physical therapist examination, evaluation, and prognosis is provided in Box 19.2. The example is described in more detail by Palisano.[279] Prognosis for goals and outcomes such as wheeled mobility, ambulation with mobility aids or orthoses, movement efficiency, or performance of mobility during daily activities and routines *should not* be inferred from the motor development curve as these are not measured by the GMFM-66.

Reference percentile curves have been developed to provide further interpretation of GMFM-66 scores within GMFCS levels but should be used with caution and only as additional information becomes available to assist with the interpretation of change over time.[154] (Tabulated reference percentiles for the GMFM-66 are available at http://motorgrowth.canchild.ca/en/MotorGrowthCurves/percentiles.asp.)

The curves were based on data from children living in Canada; however, similar patterns of gross motor development were found in a Swedish study of 319 children between the ages of 1 and 15 years. Variability in GMFM-88 scores was noted among GMFCS levels, and most children reached a plateau at 6 to 7 years.[28] Such studies reflect descriptions of developmental trajectories as influenced by the intervention strategies available in developed countries.

BOX 19.2   Application of the Gross Motor Function Classification System (GMFCS), Gross Motor Function Measure (GMFM-66), and the Gross Motor Development Curves to Physical Therapist Examination, Evaluation, and Prognosis

Teresa Spataro is a 17-month-old twin born at 31 weeks' gestational age with a birth weight of 1570 g. She was recently diagnosed as having cerebral palsy and referred for physical therapy. During the initial interview, Mrs. Spataro identified the following needs and priorities: (1) information on when Teresa will walk, (2) concerns about leg stiffness, and (3) recommendations for what to do. Teresa crawls on hands and knees with leg reciprocation and is beginning to pull to stand and cruise. Using the GMFCS, the therapist classified Teresa's gross motor function at level II. The therapist uses the algorithm developed by Russell et al.[319] to identify the item set to administer (set B, which includes 29 items). Teresa achieved a GMFM-66 score of 44. As illustrated, her score is slightly above the average score predicted at 17 months of age for children in level II. Children with a GMFM-66 score of 56 have a 50% chance of walking 10 steps unsupported. On average, children at level II achieve a score of 56 at age 3 years. The therapist shared this evidence with Mr. and Mrs. Spataro when addressing their question, "When will Teresa walk?"

At age 4, Teresa continues to be classified at level II. She walks indoors and short distances outdoors. She has difficulty with initiation of walking, changing directions, and stopping. GMFM-66 item set C (39 items) was administered, and Teresa achieved a score of 60 on the GMFM-66. Hanna et al.[154] created percentiles for the GMFM-66 for children with cerebral palsy ages 2 to 12 years (not pictured). Teresa's score is at the 80th percentile. The therapist shares this information with Teresa and her parents. Teresa is proud saying she only has "a little cerebral palsy," and her parents express their delight at Teresa's progress in gross motor function.

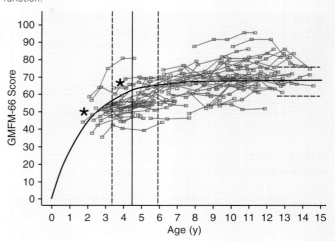

Probability Estimates for Methods of Mobility

Another type of data useful for decision making is performance of mobility in daily life. Performance of mobility or how children actually move at home, school, and in the community involves the interaction of the child and environment. Performance, therefore, is potentially influenced by several factors, including the child's physical capacity; the physical, social, and attitudinal features of the environment; and the child's (or family's) personal preference and choice. As part of the two longitudinal studies that led to creation of the motor development curves, parents of a population-based sample of 642 children reported their children's mobility at home, school, and outdoors at 6- or 12-month intervals for a mean of 5.2 times.[277] The data were analyzed to model the probabilities that children and youth with cerebral palsy walk (with or without mobility devices), use wheeled mobility (self-propelled or self-powered mobility), or use methods of mobility that require physical assistance (e.g., carried, takes steps with assistance, transported) as a function of age and environmental setting.

By age 3, almost all children in level I walked in all environmental settings, whereas only a small number of children and youth in level V moved without physical assistance of a person (powered mobility). Usual method of mobility varied by age and environmental setting for children and youth in levels II, III, and IV. Fig. 19.7 presents the estimated probabilities for children and youth in level III. At younger ages, there is a high probability that children are transported or carried outdoors. The probability of walking increases from age 4 and peaks at age 9 in the school setting (68%), age 11 in the outdoors setting (54%), and age 14 in the home setting (52%). The probability of walking at age 18 is about 50% in all three settings. At home, youth who do not walk as their usual method of mobility are more likely to move with physical assistance than use wheeled mobility. At school and outdoors, youth who do not walk as their usual method of mobility are almost as likely to use wheeled mobility as assisted mobility.

The probability estimates provide evidence that usual methods of mobility of children and youth with cerebral palsy are influenced by age and environmental setting. The probabilities are modeled from a population-based sample and, therefore, are likely to generalize to populations elsewhere whose resources and services are comparable to those in Ontario, Canada. The results have implications for long-term planning, clinical decision making, and family-centered services. Discussion of mobility options with children and families and involving children in decision making is recommended, with the understanding that the method of mobility that optimizes participation in one setting may not be the preferred method in another setting. Efficiency, safety, self-sufficiency, and environmental features such as distance and time requirements are important considerations when making decisions regarding goals and interventions for mobility. Therapists are encouraged to evaluate features of everyday environments when planning interventions to improve mobility.

Prognosis for overall functioning as an adult is dependent on many variables, and reports vary greatly. Mean values summarized from six studies showed that 31% of adults with CP lived independently, 12% were married, 24% achieved a tertiary/vocational level of education, and 28% had paid employment.[219] Positive prognostic factors for employment include mild physical involvement, good home support, education, vocational training, and good cognitive skills.[255] Increasing success rates in education and employment over the years have been attributed to advances in and access to technology such as power wheelchairs and computers, environmental access, and supportive legislation.

INTERVENTION

Framework for Evidence-Informed Decision Making

Planning effective physical therapy interventions for children and youth with CP is a complex process. Many approaches and treatments are available to address the physical therapy

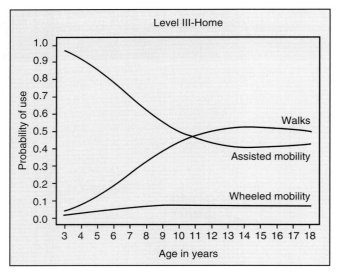

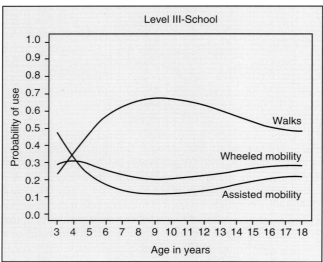

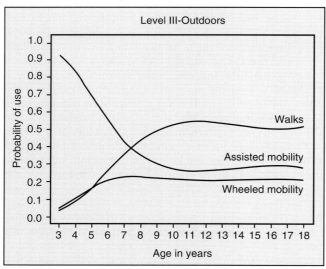

FIG. 19.7 Estimated probabilities of walking, wheeled mobility, and mobility with physical assistance as a function of age and environment for children and youth in GMFCS level III. (From Palisano RJ, Hanna SE, Rosenbaum PL, and Tieman B: Probability of walking, wheeled mobility, and assisted mobility for children and youth with cerebral palsy, *Dev Med Child Neurol* 52, 66-71, 2010.)

needs of a population that is heterogeneous in presentation of motor functioning, potential for change, and access to resources. In addition to these variances, characteristics of physical and social environments change as children get older and depend as well on what children want to do or need to do at their school and in the community. It can be challenging to determine what works best for whom and at what stage of life.[231] There is no singular right way to provide physical therapy interventions for children with cerebral palsy.[231] Evidence-informed decision making not only takes into consideration research evidence but also the therapist's clinical expertise and the values of a child and family, professionals, and society. These may overlap.

Family and Relationship-Centered Services

Family-centered care encompasses a set of values that improves parents' satisfaction with services and reduces parental stresses.[214] Therapists recognize that each family is unique and that parents know their child best. Therefore, they respect and encourage the family's roles and responsibilities as advocates for their child and are accepting of their autonomy in making choices.[16,196,279] Therapists strive to provide coordinated, collaborative, and comprehensive care in a respectful and supportive manner and are responsive to information needs, sharing general and specific information in a way that is most useful and meaningful to the family. Families value a therapist's honesty, commitment to their child, and belief that what they are doing is making a difference for their child.

Relationship-centered care recognizes that the formation and maintenance of relationships that value the perspectives of all players in the service delivery process are central to care and can be a source of satisfaction and positive experiences for all.[27,196] These include relationships between and among families, practitioners, organizations, and communities. Positive relationships result in mutually supportive interactions characterized by respect, trust, agreed-upon goals, and shared planning and decision making.

Collaboration in Setting Goals and Intervention Planning

Family–therapist collaboration in setting goals and deciding on how to achieve them can increase children's goal attainment, parental feelings of competency, and parental awareness of learning opportunities in daily activities. Goals should be meaningful to children and families in their everyday lives and are therefore determined based on a their concerns, needs, expectations, priorities, and values.[279,311] The process of goal setting is iterative. Goal attainment should be evaluated regularly in order to modify the intervention plan based on progress or lack thereof and the child and family's input.[367] The latter can be promoted by drawing attention to the gains the child is making, listening to parental concerns, and recognizing the personal values and strengths of the child, the family, and the community.[247] Parents value interventions that focus on short-term, realistic, small, and achievable goals.[202] If a family's goals are not realistic, therapists need to offer hope but be honest; sometimes they may serve as an outlet for a family's anger and fear.

Across the life span, physical therapy goals for people with CP encompass all components of the ICF: minimizing the impact of impairments, preventing secondary impairments and physical deterioration, maximizing motor function, and addressing environmental factors[273] with the overall aim of participation in age and developmentally appropriate home, leisure, educational, social, and employment activities and optimizing quality of life. Achievement of these goals includes the optimization of musculoskeletal function, enhancement of functional postures and movements, and attainment of fitness and overall health. Physical therapists must also be cognizant of environmental and personal factors that could be facilitators or barriers to activity and participation when planning interventions.

Physical therapy interventions for children with CP have evolved through research and knowledge of movement science, ecology, and family systems. Earlier assumptions based on neuromaturational theories suggesting that the development of movements and motor skills result from the neurologic maturation of the central nervous system have evolved. More recent theories describe motor development and coordination as emerging from the interaction of many subsystems in a task-specific context, suggesting a more active model of motor learning.[128] Motor control theory, dynamic systems theory,[88] neuronal group selection theory,[150] grounded cognition,[222] and motor learning strategies have provided newer conceptual frameworks for physical therapy interventions for children with CP.[103] For example, neurodevelopmental treatment (NDT) treatment, an approach that has evolved from the early work of the Bobaths, incorporates more recent principles and practices.[37,170] Physical therapists use goal-oriented, activity-focused, task-oriented, context-focused, child-focused, and ecologic interventions

that have emerged based on contemporary knowledge and research.[128] Application of contemporary theories of motor development and control are described in Chapter 3.

An approach to formulating an intervention plan to address goals is to (1) identify child, family, and environmental strengths specific to the goal; (2) identify aspects of the child, family, and environment that need to change to achieve goals; and (3) evaluate strengths and what needs to occur to achieve the goals.[278] Some goals may be achieved by focusing on personal attributes or modifying environmental factors. Personal factors might include the child's interest in and understanding of the goal and motivation to improve performance. A child's body functions and structures may need to be addressed to achieve other goals. It cannot be assumed that treatment of a specific impairment will lead to improvement in the ability to perform tasks in daily life.[273,400] Therapists use clinical reasoning skills to determine which intervention or combination of interventions is appropriate to achieve goals.

Treatments can be eclectic, including combinations of interventions for an individual child, while adhering to common principles. Despite the variety of approaches espoused and followed, any treatment plans and practice for children with cerebral palsy can be underpinned. We recommend an evidence-informed decision-making process for intervention planning that reflects child and family values, research evidence, and clinical expertise. General recommendations are included in Box 19.3.

How Much, How Often?

Decisions on the amount of physical therapy (how often, how long, over what period of time) are difficult and require consideration of many factors. To a large extent, decisions for both public funded services and services reimbursed by health insurance plans are constrained by policy, resources, and costs. Episodes of care focused on achievement of specific goals are an alternative to the traditional practice of regularly scheduled sessions for long periods of time. Short concentrated periods of intensive intervention during times of readiness have been advocated. Group sessions for children with similar goals have the potential to increase interest, motivation, and learning through peer modeling as well as reduce costs. The amount of direct therapy service may be less important than the total amount of practice and the opportunity for practice in natural environments. Similarly, the child's physical activity throughout the day and participation in community recreation and sports may be a consideration in the decision-making process.

Therapists must consider various ethical principles when providing services. Beneficence (doing what is best for the greatest number of people), non-maleficence (doing no or the least harm), and justice (doing what is fair and equitable, including moral and responsible use of family and institutional resources) must be considered when making decisions about service delivery at individual, programmatic, and institutional levels. Many of these issues involve some amount of physical therapy, which varies depending on the resources available, complementary programming, client goals, parental needs and desires, and the child's response to intervention. Optimal frequency is unknown, but periods of more intensive intervention have resulted in attainment of specific treatment goals at levels that were maintained when frequency was decreased, provided the skills were incorporated into daily

---

BOX 19.3   General Recommendations for Planning Interventions for Children and Youth With Cerebral Palsy

- Family-centered and relationship-focused services
- Address child and family priorities and information needs
- Effective communication and coordination with other service providers
- Goal-focused
  - Meaningful to and set collaboratively with child and family
  - Achievable
  - Revisited regularly
- Individualized intervention plans
- Attention to relationships among body functions and structures, activities and participation within the context of personal and environmental factors
- Management of health and co-morbidities
- Prevention of secondary impairment or functional deterioration
- Goal-related activities as follows:
  - Age and developmentally appropriate
  - Active rather than passive
  - Functional
  - Fun and motivating
  - Challenging
- Incorporate motor learning strategies
  - Problem solving
  - Task specificity
  - Active trial and error
  - High-frequency of practice
  - Self-correction, exploration
- Learning and practice in real-life environments
- Compensations, task modifications, or environmental adaptations to accommodate a child
- Life span approach

functional activities. Families and therapists must consider costs, accessibility, time, and the effect of the intervention on family dynamics. A regimen of short periods of intensive therapy separated by periods without therapy may allow for optimal motor gain and may be less demanding for the children and their families.[69,361]

The research on intervention intensity provides some guidance for developing service delivery models; however, the treatment frequencies in studies are often much higher than are realistically available in many situations. Intensive therapy, more than three times a week, compared to less intensive frequencies, may improve functional motor outcome as measured by the GMFM but with a modest effect size of questionable clinical significance, which must be considered in the context of fatigue—and can be tiring and stressful for children and families, with consequent low compliance and high costs for health care systems.[8] Many studies investigating the frequency of treatment or gross motor function have shown equal improvements between intervention provided and conventional therapy, and those with significant results in favor of intensive training tend to have a high risk of bias.[360]

One recommendation for children with CP who demonstrate continuous progress toward goals is one to two times per week or every other week; however, more intense frequencies or a less frequent consultative model will be appropriate in differing situations.[13] Families may need more intense input for specific circumstances such as pre-, peri-, and postsurgery. Periods of change and transition, such as school entry, are critical times, which may require extra support.[300] Episodes of more intensive frequencies are often alternated by periods of monitoring and consultation.

Models of service delivery, public health funding, private resources, and available family time can also impact decisions on amount of therapy.[277] Children with CP often receive therapy in more than one setting.[277] They often receive services at a treatment center and in a school setting, either with the same or a different therapist. Some families may purchase additional private services to augment or substitute for publicly funded services if these are deemed insufficient.[117] Ideally concurrent therapists can enter into cooperative relationships with each other; however, they may find themselves in situations of conflicting rehabilitation principles and practices. Collaboration and communication can help to avert such situations.[398]

Parents often consider complementary or alternative therapies for their children. The primary reason is to complement conventional approaches. Other reasons include a desire for more therapy, dissatisfaction with present therapy, the belief that their child could do better, and relief of symptoms.[173,328] Many complementary or alternative interventions lack research evidence.[265] Some families may pursue treatments even when shown to be ineffective. For example, some parents have had their children participate in hyperbaric oxygen programs, despite studies showing this treatment to be ineffective and associated with adverse effects.[234] Families may engage in treatments, such as massage, that do not achieve specific therapy goals but may improve feelings of well-being for children and their parents.[128] Alternative and complementary therapies are often expensive, and some professionals may not consider certain choices appropriate. If families choose to take an approach other than the one offered by a therapist, it is necessary to respect their choice. Therapists should not react defensively but rather should provide impartial, objective information about the therapies in question.

The following sections summarize interventions for children with CP at different ages. In addition to research evidence, child and family values and preferences, environmental strengths and potential barriers, and therapist practice knowledge are among the factors discussed when collaborating with families to make evidence-informed decisions.

INFANCY

Infants grow and develop in response to being loved and nurtured by parents and caregivers in a home environment. Despite being dependent in most aspects of life, infants interact with and develop an understanding of the people in their lives, their surroundings, and themselves. From the time of birth, a child with CP may not demonstrate the usual activities associated with infancy. As a result, parents of infants with CP may not receive some of the positive aspects of the nurturing experience and the satisfaction of observing the development of typical motor skills. Parents must cope with the impact of the diagnosis and the grieving process that accompanies the awareness that some of their hopes and expectations for their child may not be realized. They may be overwhelmed with the uncertainty that the future holds for them, their child, and their family. Many parents are also concerned with the immediate issues of providing basic infant care and may be challenged with the incorporation of the specialized care necessary for their child's optimal development while establishing relationships with health care professionals.

Physical Therapy Examination and Evaluation

Examination provides information on which to base prognosis, sometimes diagnosis, and establishes a baseline for the monitoring change through growth, maturation, and intervention. Therapists must determine the environment of an infant and the resources and the competencies and concerns of the family.

Various elements of movement and posture combine to produce gross motor skills. These skills include the ability to align one part of the body on another; to bear weight through different parts of the body; to shift weight; to move against gravity; to assume, maintain, and move into and out of different positions; and to perform graded, isolated, and variable movements with an appropriate degree of effort. When functional motor skills are examined, proficiency in incorporating these elements into purposeful and efficient movement must be evaluated. The effects of reflexes and postural reactions on positioning, handling, and movement should be considered. Standardized testing using the GMFM can be introduced in infancy and results shared as appropriate for an individual family's journey. Assessments of seating, feeding, or respiratory problems may be necessary for infants with problems in these areas. Growth is often affected in children with CP, as it is influenced by feeding, exercise, and energy efficiency.[205] Therefore therapists should be mindful of an infant's growth. When assessing infants, it is important to be aware of the influences of temperament, behavioral state regulation, and tolerance of handling on performance.

Physical Therapy Goals, Outcomes, and Intervention

A primary goal is to educate families about CP so they have the necessary information to make decisions related to physical therapy management of their child[103] (www.afcp.on.ca/guide.html).

Infancy is an important time to introduce the concepts of collaborative goal setting and ongoing communication. It may be difficult for families to contemplate specific goals while they are coping with a diagnosis of CP and are uncertain or even unrealistic about prognosis. Parents' goals may be overly optimistic during infancy. Therapists must be realistic about the prognosis and the efficacy of physical therapy while remaining positive, hopeful, and supportive.

Movement is an important component in the learning and interactions of infants. In babies who have CP, the nature and extent of their impairments affect their potential to develop and learn through movement, develop gross motor skills, and interact with their parents and their environment. Physical therapy focuses on facilitating parental caregiving and interactions and providing opportunities for optimal sensorimotor experiences and skills in enhanced environments. These allow infants to achieve their potential in developing relationships with others, developing play skills, and exploring their environment. Early intervention, within the first 2 years, is advocated to take advantage of the time when the brain is most plastic due to active sprouting and pruning in response to activity[236,245,365] despite there being no definitive support for its efficacy in changing outcomes.[54,342] Infants not diagnosed but at risk for CP should have access to early intervention. The observations of a physical therapist can facilitate making a diagnosis, and waiting for an absolute diagnosis of CP may preclude them from receiving intervention at a time of greater brain growth and plasticity.[103,245]

Everyday handling and positioning of infants by caregivers will influence development.[222] Activities such as prone positioning, promoting head control, weight bearing, encouraging sitting and standing, and midline hand activities provide enhanced perceptual-motor experiences to promote abilities including strength, postural control, hand activity, and social interaction.[222] Therapy should focus on the development of well-aligned postural stability coupled with smooth mobility to allow the emergence of motor skills such as exploration of one's and other's bodies, reaching during play, object interaction, and optimal transitional movements and postures. These skills allow infants to gain information about the interrelationships among their own bodies, objects, and people[222] and attain optimal mobility to facilitate play, language development, social interaction, and exploration of the environment.

Movements that include all planes of movement (anterior-posterior, then lateral, then rotational), selective control of body segments, weight shifting, weight bearing, and isolated and bimanual movements should be incorporated into gross motor exercises and activities. Abnormal postures and movements can make some infants challenging to handle and position. Physical therapists can promote ease and confidence in the handling and caring of infants with these problems. Parents are coached in positioning, carrying, feeding, and dressing techniques that promote comfort and symmetry, limit dysfunctional posturing and movement, facilitate postural stability and functional motor activity, and limit secondary impairments. They must learn how to be sensitive to their child's behavior and response to being handled.[103] The principles guiding these methods are to use a variety of movements and postures to promote a sensorimotor experience, to frequently include positions that promote the full lengthening of spastic or hypoextensible muscles, and to use positions that promote active, functional movement. The principles of central nervous system plasticity suggest that intensive, repetitive, task-specific intervention should be incorporated into practice. Even at a young age, focus on self-exploration, active trial and error, variability of practice, testing limits, and high frequency of practice are desirable components of treatment.[103,222] Some treatment approaches facilitate movements through handling, to guide self-generated movement, which is withdrawn as these children initiate them on their own, whereas others refrain from handling, allowing infants to learn through trial and error, using adaptive motor strategies and their own motor learning processes without concern about quality of movement.[103] Clinicians need to find a balance between hands-on and hands-off techniques.[231]

Some children will move through the typical developmental sequence of rolling, sitting, crawling, standing, and prewalking skills, whereas other children will be limited in their gross motor trajectories and require environmental adaptations. The stage at which this happens depends on the severity of the impairments; in some children, it may occur early in life.

Some infants will require environmental adaptation to achieve interaction with their bodies, object, or people. In children classified as level V on the GMFCS, slight gains in head control may be a goal, whereas a progression through the motor development sequence is expected for children classified as level I. Therapeutic interventions should not limit infants' spontaneous desires to move and play and explore their environments, because even very young children need to be able to assert themselves and manipulate their world.[55] Useful examples of various activities and strategies are noted by Dirk,[103] Lobo,[222] and Cameron et al.[54]

Ongoing support and encouragement are essential. Clearly written, illustrated, and updated home programs can be beneficial. Incorporating therapeutic activities into daily routines can ease the burden on home programs on families. Computer-generated programs or taking a video can be used to produce personalized, effective, and efficient information regarding activities, positioning, and exercises.

Equipment may facilitate activities when impairments otherwise prevent their development. For example, the sitting position promotes visual attending, upper extremity use, and social interaction. Infants with CP may be unable to sit independently, may sit statically only with precarious balance, or may not be able to be positioned in commercially available infant equipment. Customized seating or adaptations to regular infant seats may be necessary to allow function in other areas of development to progress. Infants who function at GMFCS levels IV and V should be provided with postural management programs for sleeping, sitting, and standing with postural support for sitting at 6 months of age and standing at 12 months.

The care of an infant exhibiting asymmetry, extensor posturing, and shoulder retraction illustrates these approaches. Such an infant should be carried, seated, and fed in a symmetrical position that does not allow axial hyperextension and keeps the hips and knees flexed; however, a variety of postures are necessary to allow elongation of all muscle groups and experiences in different positions. The therapist should work to ensure that no one position dominates daily activity. Positioning of or playing with the upper extremities to allow these infants to see their hands, practice midline play, reach for their feet, or suck on fingers or mouthing toys can promote sensorimotor awareness. Toys may need to be adapted to facilitate age-appropriate activities.

The frequency of intervention should be tailored to meet the needs of a family. Intensive therapy may help parents become comfortable with handling skills but may be challenging for parents to commit to, may be limited by resources, and does not necessarily demonstrate better motor outcomes compared with less frequent interventions.[365] Some settings may provide home-based early intervention programs that emphasize coaching parents in managing daily routines that include therapeutic input.

Role of Other Disciplines

At all ages, physical therapists work together with specialists from other disciplines to provide interprofessional care. Occupational therapists may be involved in upper extremity function, particularly as it relates to play and eye-hand coordination, as well as in sensory modulation/regulation. Speech and language therapists address early communication development. Various team members may address oral-motor and feeding issues. Community infant development workers may be involved in home-based programs to promote all areas of progress. Social workers may help parents through the grieving process, explain programs, and direct them to appropriate resources. Parent support groups or meetings with parents who have been through similar experiences may be helpful. A variety of medical and surgical specialists may be consulted, depending on individual needs.

PRESCHOOL PERIOD

During the preschool years, the development of locomotor, cognitive, communication, fine motor, self-care, and social abilities promotes functional independence in children. This developmental process is a dynamic one in which all of these areas constantly interact with one another. The children's environments remain oriented toward the parents, family, and home during this period, but they begin to interact with the outside world. Child care centers, babysitters, nursery schools, siblings, and playmates may become part of a preschooler's world.

For children with CP, limitations in motor activities may restrict participation in learning and socialization and limit independence. Parents become more aware of the extent and impact of their children's difficulties in all areas of development. These may include their child's ability to participate in and become integrated into preschool and community recreational activities, their child's development of cognitive and communication skills, and the long-term effect of their child's disability on future life and independence.

Physical Therapy Examination and Evaluation

Assessment of activity assumes a primary focus, but it is important to determine the interaction of impairment and activity and relation to participation. Through examination and evaluation, therapists document change and collaborate with families to ensure that goals and interventions address family priorities and concerns. Examination may focus on positioning and mobility for functional skills; however, therapists need to be cognizant of a child's communication, fine motor, self-care, sleep, and social functioning and how these interrelate with gross motor skills. The child's need for the caregiver assistance, adaptive equipment, and environmental modifications necessary to perform activities are important components of evaluation. Factors such as location of the examination, people present, and the child's

behavior, attention, and cooperation may affect the examination and evaluation process. Parents or other caregivers should be asked to comment on whether a child's performance is characteristic of his or her abilities.

Physical Therapy Goals, Outcomes, and Intervention

During the preschool years, a child's potential for attaining motor skills can be predicted with a greater degree of accuracy than during infancy, as the influences of impairments, activity limitations, and personal and environmental factors are more apparent. Families become more skilled at collaborative goal setting and comfortable communicating with service providers. Therapists can work with families to develop goals that are meaningful, realistic, noticeable, and measurable. The continued development of these skills empowers parents to make decisions, solve problems, and set priorities, as well as to become effective advocates for their children and themselves.

Physical therapy goals focus on promotion of control and alignment of postures and movements conducive to musculoskeletal development, fitness, gross motor, manual, and self-care activities, and participation. Muscles need to be extended to their limits on a regular basis to maintain range and used adequately and frequently to optimal strength; bones need compressive forces to stay strong; and the cardiovascular system needs to be challenged regularly at levels intense enough to maintain endurance and fitness.[86,125,388] During the preschool years, the focus of physical therapy is often on a child's ability to achieve independent mobility. Specific mobility goals will depend on the GMFCS level. Goals for children functioning at GMFCS levels IV and V may be achieved by using special equipment and adapted toys, rather than progressing through the normal developmental sequence.

In many cases, achievement of physical therapy goals serves as a building block for interventions by other disciplines to improve communication, self-care, social interaction, and problem solving. Therapists respect the priorities of children and families as well as other professionals when determining goals, as it may not be possible to work on all areas at once. Interventions should be goal directed, functional, motivating, and fun for the child.[82,189]

Home programs continue to be important for regular practice of activities to maximize potential and build confidence. These programs may also be carried out in other settings such as child care, preschool, or recreational sites. This can promote learning in a child's natural environment and lessen the burden on families as parents can struggle the stresses of balancing therapy programs and everyday life.[202]

Managing Primary Impairments and Preventing Secondary Impairments

Spasticity management may be introduced during the preschool years with the goals of preventing secondary impairments such as contractures and pain, ensuring comfort and ease of positioning and caregiving, improving functional movement, and reducing the need for orthopedic surgery. However, reducing spasticity will not necessarily improve motor function or participation, as only a single impairment in a multi-impairment condition is addressed.[400] Coexisting impairments such as weakness and selective motor control and contextual child and environment factors influence function.

Stretching has been shown to cause a short-term decrease in spasticity, but changes are minor and not sustained.[295]

Longer-lasting interventions are operative or pharmaceutical. Various oral, intramuscular, and intrathecal medications are used to reduce spasticity in people with cerebral palsy. A widely used method of spasticity intervention is the injection of small quantities of botulinum toxin A (Botox) into muscles to prevent the release of acetylcholine at the neuromuscular junction and impact activation for up to 4 months with peak effects observed 2 weeks after injection. The drug is expensive but covered often by insurance. Targeted muscles are those that have good ROM but exhibit spasticity that interferes with function and those most prone to developing contractures.[223] Evidence exists for injections of the calf muscles for equinus, the upper extremities, and the hip adductors for spasticity and pain control in children undergoing adductor-lengthening surgery.[25,116,225,339] Some studies of lower limb multilevel injections, including the iliopsoas, hamstrings, and rectus femoris muscles, have also demonstrated small improvements in gross motor functioning measured by the GMFM-66 and gait analysis.[98,324,333] Botox combined with therapy has been shown to be effective in improving positioning, ease of care, and comfort for nonambulatory children.[72] Botox addresses the impairment of spasticity and therefore outcomes are optimal when combined with interventions such as casting, orthotics, night splinting, positioning (prolonged stretch), and targeted motor training focus on coexisting impairments such as hypoextensibility and weakness in conjunction with functional motor activities.[97,223] Phenol injections may be used in conjunction with Botox to allow an increase in the number of injections at the maximal recommended dose.[139] Treatment algorithms can provide strategies to treat spasticity with Botox.[75] Studies following children who have received repeated injections of Botox over a period of a few years have had methodologic challenges and report varying results. Continued reduction in spasticity and improved ROM and gross motor function have been noted.[163]

Some have questioned whether Botox can prevent contractures and even question whether repeated injections may have a cumulative adverse effect on muscle growth in children with CP.[355] Longitudinal studies of the effects of Botox on muscle growth and morphology are needed. A systematic review of randomized controlled trials (RCTs) concluded that respiratory infection, bronchitis, pharyngitis, asthma, muscle weakness, urinary incontinence, seizures, fever, and unspecified pain have been related to the use of Botox in children with CP.[1] However, the rate of adverse effects has been determined to be no greater than those typically experienced by this population.[268] Discussion of potential advantages and disadvantages of options for spasticity management is recommended as part of the decision-making process.

The use of oral medications has been poorly studied, but they may be appropriate for some children.[106,370] Children must be assessed carefully for appropriateness and monitored closely for side effects. A pilot study showed that Artane in children with dystonic CP did not alter their dystonia or upper limb function but was associated with achieving therapeutic goals.[301] Baclofen, a synthetic agonist of gamma aminobutyric acid, has an inhibitory effect on presynaptic excitatory neurotransmitter release, reducing spasticity in individuals with CP.[294,370] Oral doses high enough to give the proper concentration in the cerebrospinal fluid can, however, cause side effects such as drowsiness. If this is a problem, baclofen can be administered intrathecally by a continuous infusion pump implanted in the abdomen that releases the drug at a slow, constant rate into the subarachnoid space once a child weighs 15 kilograms.[370] Intrathecal baclofen reduces spasticity most noticeably in the lower extremities. Improvements in function and ease of care and a reduced need for orthopedic surgery have been documented.[51] It is used most often in children with quadriplegic CP but has also been shown to improve the quality of gait and ability to perform gross motor activities in ambulatory children.[44,294] Complications related to catheter and pump malfunction, infection, leaks, or dosing have been reported. Some are associated with significant morbidity, but others are common and manageable in most cases.[199] Intrathecal baclofen has also been beneficial in treating patients with generalized dystonia, a difficult problem to manage. Levels of evidence are low but in addition to improved dystonia, subjective improvements have been reported in QOL, ease of care, speech, swallowing, posture, and upper and lower extremity functioning.[2,253]

Selective dorsal rhizotomy (SDR) is a neurosurgical procedure in which up to 60% to 70% of the sensory nerve rootlets for the lower extremities are cut selectively to reduce afferent drive to the reflex arc aiming to create a balance between the elimination of spasticity and preservation of adequate strength.[6,303] SDR is considered a safe procedure that offers significant and lasting functional gains to properly selected children. Selection criteria vary among institutions; however, it may be most effective for children functioning at GMFCS levels I to III, aged 3 to 8 years, with spastic diplegia, a history of prematurity, good selective control of muscles, lack of contracture or deformity, good cognitive abilities, motivation, parental support, and access to therapy.[148] Intensive postoperative physical therapy is necessary to address the resulting weakness (Fig. 19.8). Abnormalities in patterns of muscle activation may persist after SDR because of continuing problems with motor control and coordination. Long-term studies of 15 to 20 years have demonstrated lasting improvements in lower limb muscle tone, gait, gross motor function, and performance of activities of daily living; however, most children remain within their GMFCS level.[6]

All methods of spasticity management are considered to be optimized by therapy co-interventions. Therapy interventions include strengthening, stretch through exercise or prolonged

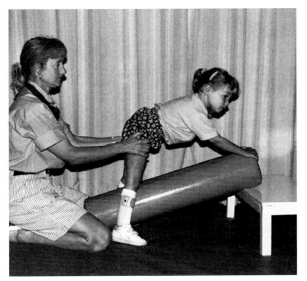

FIG. 19.8 Exercises after rhizotomy are frequently directed toward increasing force generation of extensor muscles.

positioning through splinting, orthotics, or casting, and interventions to improve gait and functional motor skills.[295] Physical therapy to optimize muscle strength involves the child performing activities that produce both concentric and eccentric muscle forces. These may include transitional movements against gravity, ball gymnastics, treadmill use, tricycle riding, scootering, and ascending and descending stairs.

Limitations in ROM can be observed in preschool children, particularly those in GMFCS levels IV and V. Considerable resources are directed toward maintaining or regaining muscle extensibility and joint mobility.[388] Ideally, range of motion is maintained through activities that involve active movements through full range of motion. A classic study by Tardieu found that plantar flexor contractures in children with CP were prevented if the muscles were stretched beyond a minimum threshold length for at least 6 hours during daily activity.[352] Threshold length was the length at which the muscle began to resist a stretch. However, the data prompting this statement are suggestive rather than conclusive. Stretching is unlikely to happen spontaneously in children with spastic CP who have limited active movement, particularly those at GMFCS levels IV and V. Knowledge is lacking on whether prolonged stretching and other interventions within the scope of physical therapy practice are effective in preventing muscle shortening in children with CP, particularly during periods of growth.

Consequently, combinations of approaches are often used, making it difficult to assess the usefulness of individual approaches.[33] Passive stretching programs are often recommended to maintain muscle length, but evidence of effectiveness and clinical relevance is limited and conflicting.[295,388] Some parents report that ROM exercises cause pain,[351] whereas others believe they relieve muscle cramps.[295]

Sustained low load passive stretching of longer duration has been shown to be more effective in increasing ROM and in reducing spasticity.[295] It can be achieved through casting, orthoses, or positioning. It is important to not position muscles at their fully lengthened state, as this can cause discomfort. A position just short of the initial catch has been advocated. This can be altered as muscle lengthening occurs. A single cast application or serial casting (the successive application of casts with progressive increases in the amount of stretch) has been used as a method of providing prolonged stretch to the calf muscles.[33,47] After serial casting of the foot and lower leg for equinus, often from 3 to 6 weeks, children with CP demonstrate decreased resistance to passive stretch and increased dorsiflexion end range.[47,362]

Peak strength will occur at longer muscle lengths. Substantial reduction in gains may occur following cast removal, suggesting the need to follow casting with orthoses.[362] Although it is clear that at least temporary mechanical changes result from casting, the precise nature of the changes and whether they involve an increase in the number of sarcomeres are unknown.[33] Casting has also been used for other muscle groups, such as the hamstrings and the upper extremity musculature. Research on the impact of casting on gait or motor function is inconsistent and lacks participation outcomes.[33,362] Clinically, casting has been observed to prevent surgery, but this has not been substantiated by research. Concern has been expressed that immobilization of growing muscle in a lengthened position can result in sarcomere loss and a reduction of the muscle belly girth with adaptation by lengthening of the tendon, exacerbating the altered morphology.[144]

Positioning, serial casting, and Botox injections are often used in combination to achieve optimal improvement.[33] Clinical reasoning suggests that Botox addresses spasticity and casting decreases contracture, but currently, no clear evidence indicates that casting, Botox, or the combination of both is superior to other options in the treatment of equinus. Analysis of research is complicated because of differing protocols and other methodologic problems. Ultimately, treatment choices should depend on research evidence combined with considerations such as availability, cost, convenience, family preference, and therapists' expertise and experience with the treatments and follow-up care.[33] Likewise, it is difficult to validate the effectiveness of interventions such as muscle strengthening and functional activities in conjunction with spasticity intervention, but the clinical value of these practices has been observed, and they are strongly advocated.[211]

The integrity of joints, particularly the hips, is a concern even at a young age. Early identification of subluxation can help prevent progression to dislocation, the complete lateral displacement of the femoral head from under the acetabulum through timely referral for orthopaedic assessment and management.[152,391,403] A program of surveillance based on GMFCS level and radiologic assessment of hip migration percentage, coupled with a clinical assessment of changes in ROM, muscle tone, spinal alignment, sitting tolerance, gait, pelvic obliquity, leg length discrepancy, or hip pain, is recommended. Clinical orthopedic assessment at diagnosis and an anteroposterior radiograph at 12 to 24 months of age or at diagnosis if older than 24 months and ongoing follow-up based on GMFCS level and clinical signs are recommended.[403]

Physical therapists provide education for families and may be involved in coordination of hip surveillance services.[134] They are often the first to recognize clinical warning signs of hip changes. Nonoperative interventions such as sleep positioning, seating, abduction bracing, and botulinum injections have not been shown to reduce the need for surgery or improve hip structure in a RCT,[391] but they may have value in positioning for comfort and function, maintaining muscle extensibility, and reducing early hip problems.[42,244] The impact of prophylactic interventions has been explored in a prospective study of groups of children receiving differing management.[152] Proactive practices—including early treatment of spasticity through rhizotomy, Botox injections, and intrathecal baclofen—and early detection and surgery to prevent dislocation were associated with improved ROM in nonambulatory children; a decrease in orthopedic surgery for contracture, rotational deformity, and foot deformity; and a reduction in salvage operations for dislocated hips, from 40% to 15%.

Lower extremity orthoses may be used to reduce primary impairment, prevent secondary impairment, and facilitate efficient and effective walking and other functional activities. Specific goals are to limit inappropriate joint movements and alignment due to spasticity or weakness; prevent contracture, hyperextensibility, and deformity; enhance postural control and balance; reduce the energy cost of walking; and provide postoperative protection of tissues.[247] In most studies, the use of ankle-foot orthoses (AFOs) compared with a barefoot condition has shown positive effects on gait kinematics and kinetics, including improvements in ground reaction forces, plantar flexion moments, stride length, foot clearance in swing, heel strike at initial contact, equinus during midstance, related hip and knee movement, temporal-spatial measures, and sometimes function measured by the walking, running, and jumping dimensions of the GMFM.[119,247,249] Research suggests that only orthoses that extend to the knee and have a rigid ankle, leaf spring, or hinged design with plantar flexion stop can prevent equinus deformities.[247,249] Little more than anecdotal observational evidence suggests that using orthoses to control movement into plantar flexion prevents muscle shortening and therefore joint contractures or deformity. Controlled trials are difficult to carry out, as contractures develop over many years. Despite these dynamic benefits, orthoses do not show clinically significant changes in the static bony alignment of the foot and ankle during weight bearing based on radiologic examination.[386] Results are variable depending on the specific gait problems of the child and the type of orthosis, demonstrating the need for individual assessment and prescription.

Many variations of AFOs are available. Decisions are made based on the biomechanical and functional needs of a child. Therapists and orthotists work together closely to decide on the optimal orthoses based on treatment goals. Solid AFOs are used if maximum restriction of ankle movement is desired. Children who would benefit from freedom of movement at the joint can use hinged AFOs, sometimes with stops to prevent movement into excessive plantar flexion. Hinged AFOs permit dorsiflexion, which allows stretching of the plantar flexor muscle group during walking, and have been found to promote a more normal and efficient gait pattern than rigid orthotics without a predisposition to crouch gait. Dynamic, energy storage and release, or posterior leaf spring orthoses, which are intended to prevent excessive equinus while mechanically augmenting push-off, have been found to reduce equinus in swing, permit ankle dorsiflexion in stance, and absorb more energy during midstance, but they actually reduce desirable power generation at push-off.[271] Foot orthoses, or supramalleolar orthoses, may be used for children with calcaneal valgus alignment or pronation but do not require the ankle stabilization of an AFO. Materials from a consensus conference on lower limb orthotic management of CP are available at www.ispoweb.org.[249]

Tape or elasticized garments have been used to assist children biomechanically and facilitate postural control function. Kinesio taping has been shown to improve dynamic activities, possibly through enhancement of the cutaneous receptors of the sensory system to improve proprioception resulting in improvement of voluntary control.[186] Garments made of spandex or neoprene can apply dynamic compression and are also hypothesized to provide somatic inputs, specifically proprioceptive and deep pressure, improving body awareness and muscle activation and therefore postural control.[226] In a perspective article, MacKenzie[226] stated that the limited research suggests an immediate benefit to motor function and quality of movements with some studies demonstrating short-term carryover. Skin tolerance may be an issue, and children and families sometimes find the garments uncomfortable and inconvenient for independent dressing and toileting.[122]

Children should have a variety of positions in which they can safely and comfortably function, travel, and sleep. Positioning needs vary greatly depending on GMFCS levels and personal and environmental factors.[323] Children functioning at GMFCS levels IV and V should have individually tailored postural management programs to prevent or ameliorate the secondary impairments of positional contractures and deformity, prevent skin breakdown, and facilitate function and participation.[134] Children with higher motor function may need some

alterations to seating to optimize postural control outcomes, hand function, self-care, and play.[5,323] At all ages, decreased ability to change body position during sleep can cause discomfort, pain, and respiratory problems, which can result in disrupted sleep for children with CP and their families.[399] Physical therapists may be involved in promoting safe, comfortable, and biomechanically optimal sleep positions. Orthoses, splints, and bed positioning systems have been used during sleep, but care must be taken to avoid overstretched muscles, disrupted sleep, or discomfort.[145]

Comfortable and safe sitting, standing, lying, and floor play positions are important for the preschooler's development. Children having difficulty with postural control may need adaptive seating systems. These can have a positive effect on children by improving communication, upper extremity function, feeding, toileting, independence, safety, social interaction, and contentment. These benefits translate into improvements in the lives of families through valuation of their children's well-being and the added benefits of expending less parental energy in caregiving and supervision. Adaptive seating should be individualized because of the wide variation in postural abilities and alignment. Specific suggestions are included in Chapter 33, Assistive Technology. Approved car seats and restraints are necessary for safe and comfortable vehicular transportation.[224] Positioning can also contribute to pulmonary health. Children with limited movement are at risk for chest complications because of chest wall biomechanics, feeding difficulties, immobility, and poor coughing abilities. Adaptive seating or orthoses have been shown to improve pulmonary functioning, but research is very limited.[18]

Weight bearing is thought to reduce or prevent secondary impairments. Optimally, standing involves movement and activity to provide intermittent loading and muscle strain. Maintenance of lower extremity weight bearing may allow continued ability to participate in standing transfers and reduce the need for lifting when children are older. Standers are often used, starting when children are as young as 9 to 10 months and are not able to bear weight effectively on their own. Dosing recommendations based on limited research and clinical expertise include the following: 45 to 60 minutes a day to maintain or increase hip, knee, and ankle range of motion; 60 to 90 minutes a day to affect bone mineral density; 60 minutes a day in 30° to 60° of total hip abduction to influence hip stability; and 30 to 45 minutes for short-term decrease in spasticity.[275] There may also be benefits to bowel bladder function, alertness, circulation, or interactions with peers.[275] It is important to determine the actual weight being borne through the lower extremities when in a stander. This has been shown to vary from 23% to 102%, with a mean of 68% body weight.[166]

Lifelong management of pain should begin in early childhood. As noted, seating, positioning, and spasticity management can provide immediate comfort and long-term pain management through the prevention of secondary impairments such as skeletal malalignment. Therapists should ensure physical therapy interventions are as pain-free as possible but in situations when discomfort cannot be avoided, such as postoperative mobilization, the development of a positive therapeutic relationship can influence children's ability to cope with uncomfortable therapeutic procedures. Behavioral approaches such as distraction, imagery, breathing, or relaxation along with empathy, praise, and breaks can be helpful.[351]

Promotion of Activity

Complex relationships exist among the impairments of spasticity, strength, sensation, ROM, selective motor control, and cognition impacting the ability to analyze movement and provide instruction to improve performance.[358] These problems, as well as the lack of opportunity to experience motor skills in variable settings, contribute to the ability to learn movement strategies and therefore gross motor function and achievement of tasks in mobility, self-care, and social function. A child with CP may have to use different or additional cognitive strategies when planning and performing motor skills.

Physical therapy to promote activity is often intensive during the preschool years. Therapists need to recognize when it is realistic to work on a child's impairments to achieve success in an activity and when it is necessary to adapt a task or the environment. Intervention often involves components of both; however, children functioning at GMFCS levels I and II may need very little adaptation, whereas children functioning at level V may require considerable adaptation and environmental modifications. Components of the dynamic systems theory, motor control theory, and motor learning principles and strategies should be integrated into activity-oriented treatment (see Chapters 3 and 4).

Motor learning comprises a set of processes associated with practice or experience that leads to relatively permanent changes in the ability to produce skilled action (see Chapter 4). Children with CP can be constrained in their ability to learn movement strategies due to impairments of muscle tone, strength sensory processing, perceptual-motor skills, and cognition, as well as the lack of opportunity to perform motor skills in variable settings. They have difficulty analyzing their own movement and utilizing feedback to improve performance.[358] Motor memory is frequently impaired.[107] As a consequence, children with CP may use different or additional cognitive strategies when planning and performing motor skills. Limited research exists on the cognitive aspects of motor learning in children with neurologic disability, and more research is needed.[358]

Motor learning principles advocate the encouragement of movement exploration and child-initiated solutions to motor tasks, adaptation to changes in the environment, and repetitive practicing of goal-related functional tasks that are meaningful to the child.[189] Ample and variable practice in home, school, and community settings is important. Feedback is important in the process of learning skilled movement. Information is received intrinsically through a child's sensory receptors and extrinsically from external sources. Knowledge of results contributes information about movement outcome, and an understanding of performance supplies feedback about the nature of the movement. Trial and error can form the basis for selecting efficient movement patterns.[45] Feed forward mechanisms must also be considered, as movement skills have a cognitive component. In some instances, cognitive strategies may be able to compensate for the inherent motor limitations. Children with CP may understand concrete instructions much more readily than abstract ones. Transfer between tasks may be limited, particularly in children with cognitive impairments, so practice of a targeted skill is recommended.[366] Integration of skills into functional and cognitively directed tasks may promote carryover.

Therapists should focus on time periods when the child demonstrates prerequisite abilities (readiness) associated with a particular task and engage the child in goal setting and intervention planning.[329] Therapy should be challenging and interesting

to maintain motivation. Embedding activities into daily routines supports the principles of motor learning.[278] For example, kicking a soccer ball is a more functional and fun method of developing balance skills than practicing while standing on one foot. A task can be achieved through many different means based on the child's unique movement capabilities, provided the action is safe and will not cause secondary impairments over time.[366] Ketelaar and colleagues found that children receiving interventions based on these principles demonstrated greater improvement in both capability and performance of self-care and mobility activities in daily situations when compared with children receiving intervention designed to normalize movement quality.[189]

Although the body of literature on many aspects of therapy for children with CP is growing, optimal strategies and interventions are not known. Consequently it is important to analyze the child, task, and environment to identify what needs to occur to achieve the goal. Practice-based, goal-directed interventions such as constraint-induced therapy (restraining the unaffected limb of children with unilateral CP while encouraging high-repetition active arm and hand movements of the more involved extremity) or bimanual training (using motor learning principles to promote use of the more affected arm and hand as an assist) have evidence of improving arm function and hand movement quality and effectiveness associated with cortical reorganization as measured by functional magnetic resonance imaging and magnetoencephalography.[265,327,350] Functional relevance, cognitive engagement, massed practice, high intensity of training, age-appropriate activities, peer engagement, and the incorporation of home programs are aspects of successful programs.[3,86,327,360] See Chapter 4 for more information.

Physical therapists may be involved in a variety of roles related to health and well-being. Children with CP are at risk for a wide range of feeding, hydration, and nutritional problems due to problems with oral-motor control and swallowing, drooling, aspiration, impaired self-feeding, and difficulties in expressing hunger or food preferences.[9,205] Feeding problems coupled with impaired movement can impact growth, particularly in children with GMFCS levels III, IV, and V. Poor growth is associated with poorer health, increased use of health care resources, decreased social participation, and missed school days and may impact a family's ability to take part in usual activities and feel they are able to adequately nurture their child.[9,205,346] Gastroesophageal reflux and aspiration can also occur. Oral-motor programs, proper positioning, and parent education and support are important aspects of comprehensive care. Lack of physical activity can contribute to chronic constipation. In some cases, gastrostomy and antireflux procedures are recommended. Growth curves have been developed for children with complex medical conditions.[9,205,346]

Conversely, increasing rates of obesity in children, including those with CP, are a matter of concern. The overall prevalence of overweight or risk of overweight in children with CP is over 29% and is relatively greater in those who are ambulatory.[172] Concerns associated with obesity, such as muscle loss, pain, pressure sores, and mobility limitations, can be amplified for people with cerebral palsy.[238] Interventions with positive outcomes include encouraging physical activity with techniques such as motivational strategies that allow self-direction of goal setting and activity choice, self-monitoring, positive reinforcement, incremental increases in workload, and engaging in strength training for longer than 15 minutes. Targeting body weight is more challenging.[238] Child behavior, personality, and family recreational styles predict variation in leisure and recreational participation.[193] Physical therapists can be involved in the early promotion of healthy behaviors including participation in physical activity and healthy eating.

Children with limited mobility or feeding problems may have poor pulmonary function and respiratory muscle weakness.[207] Problems including poor clearance of secretions, aspiration, and susceptibility to pneumonia may necessitate chest physical therapy, suctioning, and other techniques to maintain optimal respiratory function.

Failure to develop an appropriate toileting routine during the preschool years can result in participation restrictions and negative reactions from peers. Development of bladder control in children with CP may be delayed in comparison with typically developing children, but most become continent. Cognitive abilities and a diagnosis of quadriplegia can negatively influence the development of control.[307] Therapists may need to recommend appropriate adaptive equipment.

Mobility

Walking is a preoccupation of parents at the time of diagnosis, a frequent goal of families, a predictor of participation, and a skill that can deteriorate over time. As a result, walking is a major focus of clinical practice and research in children with CP in the preschool years and beyond. Walking is not always a realistic or optimal method of mobility. Alternative means of mobility are essential for some children and are chosen by some children and adults for efficiency in certain environments.[359]

The GMFCS and the Gross Motor Development Curves provide evidence-based information to assist in identifying realistic mobility goals.[314] If the prognosis for walking is good, intervention will include promotion of preparatory ambulation skills, such as effective and well-aligned weight bearing, selective control of movement, and weight shifting needed for gait and balance. Body-weight-support harnesses with treadmill training may provide a learning opportunity for the task of walking.[230] Ambulatory aids, such as walkers, crutches, or canes, may be used, either temporarily while a child is progressing to more advanced gait skills or as long-term aids for independent mobility. The use of posterior walkers has been found to encourage a more upright posture during gait, promote better gait characteristics, and decrease energy expenditure compared with the use of anterior walkers (Fig. 19.9).[289] Children functioning at GMFCS level IV can use wheeled walking devices that support the trunk and pelvis to provide the benefits of upright positioning, the ability to take steps, and a limited degree of mobility. Although there is limited evidence of therapeutic impact, these devices provide opportunities for participation with others and exploration of environments.[276]

Children 3 to 5 years of age are becoming aware of the concept of achievement. Walking may be a coveted skill, but it should not become an all-consuming goal, particularly if it may not be attainable or sustainable at older ages. Adults who are nonambulatory remember walking as the most important goal set for them by their parents and therapists, resulting in feelings of failure from an early age and loss of faith in rehabilitation professionals.[135,190]

The provision of alternative methods of functional, independent mobility is recommended when ambulation is not possible or is inefficient. This need may be met with an adapted tricycle (Fig. 19.10), a manual wheelchair, or a power mobility device,

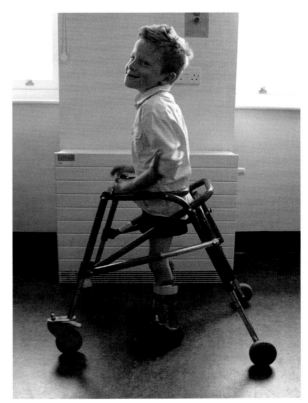

FIG. 19.9 Child using a posterior walker, reported to promote upright posture and higher walking speeds than an anterior walker. (From Lissauer T, Clayden G. *Illustrated textbook of paediatrics,* ed 4. St. Louis, 2011, Elsevier.)

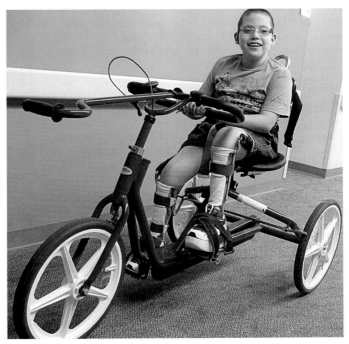

FIG. 19.10 An adapted tricycle may meet a child's needs for mobility. (Courtesy Texas Children's Hospital, Houston.)

sometimes with special controls. The University of Delaware's GoBabyGo! program (http://www.udel.edu/gobabygo/program) has developed guidelines to motorize and adapt toy ride-on cars for young children with disabilities.[171] These devices enable children with CP to explore their environment, achieve a sense of independence and competence, and experience increased participation in family, school, and community life. Power mobility may also promote the overall development of self-initiated behaviors and the acquisition of spatial concepts. The lack of self-propelled locomotion can result in apathy, withdrawal, passivity, and dependent behavior that can persist into later life.

Powered mobility is often a sensitive topic for families of young children with CP. Therapists are encouraged to raise the possibility and encourage the family members to share their thoughts. It is important to respect family preferences. Some families may prolong the use of strollers to delay wheelchair use due to acceptance or assumed stigma.[135] Parents initially may be hesitant about introducing power mobility to young children, fearing that it signifies giving up on walking. The topic can be revisited at a later time. Power mobility does not preclude goals for supported walking or walking using a mobility device such as a walker but provides the child with a method of self-mobility for exploration and experiential learning. For children who will continue to be wholly dependent on power mobility for independence, it provides mobility at an appropriate age and gives families an indication of the implications of power mobility for housing, schooling, and transportation needs.

If power mobility is being considered, fine motor control, cognitive skills, visual and auditory abilities, behavior, environmental accessibility, transportation, and financial resources must all be taken into account. Consensus regarding clinical practice suggests that children can begin augmented mobility as early as 8 months of age, when children typically begin to crawl, and can begin to learn how to maneuver a power mobility device before they are 14 months of age. Those able to use a joystick or other steering device can demonstrate control as young as 18 to 24 months of age.[220] Some children with significant cognitive or sensory impairments can learn to use power mobility devices with appropriate practice and environmental support. For more information, see Chapter 33, Assistive Technology.

Play

Play, the primary productive activity of children, should be intrinsically motivating and pleasurable. The benefits of play include helping children discover the effects they can have on objects and people in their environment; development of social skills; and enhanced development of perceptual, conceptual, intellectual, and language skills. Children with CP are often constrained in their playfulness even when they have the capacity to be playful. They receive more support in play at home than in community or school environments.[302] Limitations in the play of children with physical disabilities due to physical impairments, time limitations, and social and environmental barriers may affect the experiential learning derived from play and may result in decreased independence, motivation, imagination, creativity, assertiveness, social skills, and self-esteem.[34] Therapy should provide and demonstrate play opportunities and provide input on dealing with social and environmental barriers to play (Fig. 19.11).

Appropriate toys and play methods should be suggested to parents and caregivers. If children are physically unable to play

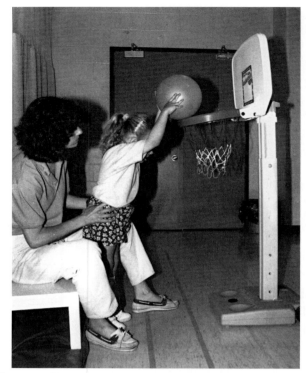

FIG. 19.11 Therapeutic exercise programs can include highly motivating play activities. Throwing a basketball may be more motivating than trunk extension exercises.

with regular toys, a variety of adaptations, such as switch access, can make their toys usable.[208] Environmental control equipment also can be introduced to preschoolers.

It is important to not overprotect children with CP. Parents should be encouraged to let their children enjoy typical play activities, such as rolling down hills and getting dirty in the mud. Therapists must ensure that therapy and home programs promote, rather than interfere with, normal play experiences. Early integration of children into community recreational activities can introduce a child and family to the benefits of a healthy active lifestyle and social opportunities.

Family Involvement

Planning of interventions should consider the child within the context of the family. Therapists should be sensitive to the family's stresses, dynamics, child-rearing practices, coping mechanisms, privacy, values, and cultural variations and be flexible in their approach and programming. Family–therapist collaboration is crucial for integrating goals into learning opportunities during daily activities and routines. Home programs are important for optimal therapy results because strengthening, extensibility, and motor learning require more input than can be provided in treatment sessions. Parents use the guidance and support that they gain from home programs to build confidence about how to help their child.[267]

Therapists need to be sensitive to the well-being of families and must find a balance between providing home programs that the family cannot realistically be expected to carry out, especially programs that do not promote positive parent–child interactions. Asking a family to spend 15 minutes on a treatment activity means 15 minutes will be lost from another activity.[30] Obstacles may include constraints on time, energy, skills, or resources, and negative effects on the parent–child relationship. Factors that have a positive influence on the participation of parents in home programs include collaborative decision making regarding the content and intensity of programs, recognition of the needs of individual families, and use of activities that are integrated easily into daily routines and are not stressful for the child or the caregiver.[267] Siblings can have a role in care and play.[103] Their education about CP and ways in which they can help their brother or sister can contribute toward achieving more independence.[74] Sibling well-being must also be considered.

Role of Other Disciplines

Occupational therapists work closely with preschool children to develop independence in activities such as dressing, feeding, toileting, and playing. Speech and language therapists promote use of efficient methods of communication. Psychologists assess cognitive skills and consult with other professionals on the interaction of intellectual abilities with other areas of development. Social workers and behavior therapists provide ongoing support to families because the stresses involved in parenting a child with a disability persist but change. Team assessment and intervention are imperative for addressing issues such as feeding problems, augmentative communication, and transition to school. Orthopedic surgeons monitor musculoskeletal development.

SCHOOL-AGE AND ADOLESCENT PERIOD

During the school-age and adolescent years, children typically participate in school and community life while remaining dependent on their families and living in their parental homes. They refine and maintain the basic functional skills they have learned, develop independence in life skills activities that will enable them to cope effectively with the demands of daily living, interact with peers, and transition to adult life. These years, particularly those spent in high school, can be difficult for children with CP.[255] Youth become increasingly aware of the reality, extent, and impact of their disabilities on themselves, their families, and their relationships with peers. As they strive to contend with the normal stresses of growing up, particularly those of adolescence, they must also cope with being different, acknowledge the potential obstacles to attaining independence, and work to overcome them.

Participation in life activities has been shown to be more challenging as children reach adolescence.[175] Problems encountered during adolescence include mobility limitations, poor endurance in performing routine activities, and continued difficulty and slowness with self-care and hygiene skills at a time when privacy is becoming increasingly important. Adolescents may not have sufficient opportunities to develop socially and sexually or achieve age-appropriate levels of independence from the family. Dating is often delayed and less frequent than for other teenagers.[389] Environmental factors may contribute to reduced access to community and school facilities, limiting opportunities for participation in social, cultural, recreational, and athletic activities.

Parents may be anxious about the effects of their child's disabilities on their participation in age-appropriate endeavors and their future as an adult.[153] They continue to be naturally attentive but have to avoid being hypervigilant or overprotective and must begin to allow their child to take risks and become independent in the outside world.[255] In some cases, financial concerns regarding the need for special equipment, transportation, and home renovations must be addressed. Parents of children who are dependent in activities of daily living (ADLs) and transfers may suffer from physical stresses, such as back problems.

Physical Therapy Examination and Evaluation

Identification of risk for secondary impairment is an important part of the examination. Gross motor assessments may be less frequent as children naturally plateau in this area,[155] but they are still important for monitoring change resulting from interventions such as spasticity management, surgery, the use of orthoses, or periods of intensive therapy or deterioration. Assessment in a child's natural environment may provide valuable information for differentiating between capacity and performance and determining necessary accommodations to allow participation. For example, the walking speed, endurance, and agility necessary for negotiating school hallways with other children, noise, and obstacles may differ from those assessed in a gait laboratory or a structured timed distance test. The mean velocity of typical 7-year-old children leading a line of students in a school hallway is 4 feet/second.[92] Information such as this can provide guidelines for the walking abilities necessary for participation in school mobility and for determination of treatment goals.

Privacy of individuals of all ages should be respected, but this is particularly important during these years, when children are becoming more aware of their bodies and their sexuality. They should be appropriately dressed when attending therapy sessions and clinics, particularly if they will be seen by unfamiliar people or photographed or a video taken. If it is necessary for children to remove their clothing, a reason should be given for doing so and their permission requested.

Physical Therapy Goals, Outcomes, and Interventions

Goals shift during these years to reflect lifestyle and potential for change. Most children with CP achieve their gross motor ceiling capacity at around 5 years of age.[59,155,314] Some children and adolescents may improve their motor function or skills. For example, a systematic review on exercise interventions to improve postural control in children with CP by Dewar et al. (2014) concluded that moderate-level evidence supports the effectiveness of gross motor task training, hippotherapy, treadmill training with no body support, trunk-targeted training, and reactive balance training. However, emphasis tends to focus on prevention of secondary impairments, maintenance of achieved level of motor function, participation in age-appropriate pursuits, and exploration of compensations and environmental accommodations. Potential challenges include contracture, pain, increasing size, puberty, cumulative physical overuse, fatigue, and a more demanding and competitive lifestyle.[23]

School-age children and adolescents should be active participants in conversations regarding goals and programming if they are cognitively able. They should be encouraged to take increasing responsibility for their own health, nutrition, fitness, personal care, finances, and decision making so that they are prepared to assume these responsibilities in adulthood. Therapists should strive to foster self-esteem, self-efficacy, and assertiveness in children and adolescents by emphasizing their abilities, encouraging activities in which they can excel, and helping them to acknowledge their difficulties with a view toward identifying appropriate compensations such as use of attendant care. In the case of children with more severe involvement, goals may be oriented toward minimizing impairments to facilitate caregiving and comfort. To the extent possible children and adolescents should be knowledgeable of their health condition and learning to self-manage. When motor capacity is limited, self-management involves instruction of others to provide assistance.

Secondary impairments must be anticipated and avoided if possible. Maintenance of muscle extensibility, strength, joint integrity, and fitness is important in preventing secondary impairments. Children and youth need to develop problem-solving strategies to overcome environmental and societal barriers to become as independent and active as possible in home, school, recreational, social, and community life. Education about their disability is an important but often lacking component of assuming self-management.[305] This may occur because the initial education of families occurs when a child is young, and continued provision of age-appropriate information to the child is often inadequate.

Mobility is important for overall health, well-being, and independence. Adolescents may be capable of employing methods of mobility used at younger ages, but environmental and personal factors may influence performance.[312] It is vital to identify underlying causes of excessive energy use, to develop effective strategies to reduce energy-wasteful movements, and to implement physical fitness interventions through community exercise and sport programs. These goals are important for children across the spectrum of GMFCS levels but will be achieved in different ways.[125]

Reducing Primary Impairment and Preventing Secondary Impairment

Progressive resistance training has become a common intervention for children and adolescents with CP, as it has been shown that the effort associated with training is not associated with the exacerbation of spasticity or pain.[136] Elastic bands, free weights, isokinetic equipment, and functional movements have been used, and programs have taken place in home, clinic, or community settings. Many studies have shown that resistance training in the lower limbs of children and adolescents increases isotonic, isokinetic, isometric, and functional strength but has a lesser effect on functional activity and participation.[128,136,353] However, some studies have reported concurrent improvements in activity as measured by gross motor function, gait parameters such as stride length and kinematics, and perception of body image.[128,288,363]

A review of methodologies suggests that protocols may not have implemented evidence-based guidelines for resistance training.[371] Protocol suggestions for school-aged children and adolescents with CP are discussed by Vershuren et al.,[371] Park and Kim,[288] and Gillett et al.[136] and include the following: (1) single-joint training when muscles are very weak or compensations are evident with multijoint muscles; (2) rest intervals greater than 1 minute (perhaps up to 3 minutes); (3) interventions of sufficient length (12 weeks), three times a week, and 40- to 50-minute sessions; and (4) consideration of National Strength and Conditioning Association Guidelines for Children for other parameters.

Youth with CP should exercise in positions that are comfortable and allow optimal selective control of targeted muscle groups. Changes in prepubescent youth are due to neural factors

such as improvements in motor skills, increases in motor unit recruitment and firing rate, and changes in coordination more than muscle hypertrophy.[371] Strengthening should be included in regular exercise or physical activity regimens to maintain optimal musculoskeletal function throughout the life span.[125] Strength training is more likely to enhance motor functioning in younger children but may counteract deterioration in youth, thus statistically nonsignificant results may be clinically worthwhile. Protocols involving high-velocity training, plyometric training, or the addition of anaerobic training may be promising.[136,183]

Electrical stimulation, mental imagery, and biofeedback may be helpful for children who have problems contracting their muscles voluntarily.[371] Various methods of neuromuscular electrical stimulation have been used as an adjunct to the treatment of CP in attempts to reduce spasticity, increase strength and muscle extensibility, promote the initial learning of selective control, and improve functional activities such as gait.[68,402] Therapeutic electrical stimulation, low intensities that do not produce a muscle contraction over an extended period of time, has not been shown to have a clinical effect.[79] Functional electrical stimulation, stimulation at high intensities for short durations during practice of an activity, has been shown to have favorable effects on gait parameters when applied to the plantar flexors alone or in combination with dorsiflexors. Protocols should be individualized for patients after careful analysis of movement, and application should be closely monitored. Treatment effects have been observed when stimulation is applied for 30 to 60 minutes per day for at least 6 to 8 weeks.[402] Some studies have shown that functional electrical stimulation is no more effective than activity training alone but might be useful for children who have problems initiating movements due to cognitive or selective control problems.[68]

Spasticity management is still important in this age group. Botulinum toxin continues to be effective and is often combined with serial casting if contractures are present, to provide more marked and long-lasting effects.[99] Contractures are prevalent in this age group, particularly in more severely affected patients.[401] The interventions described in the preschool section are appropriate, but it is important for therapists to ascertain which structures are causing restriction in movement. Joint hypomobility resulting from capsular or ligamentous tightness can be treated with joint mobilization.[46,159]

Continued surveillance of hip joint integrity is necessary even after skeletal maturity for adolescents with risk factors such as scoliosis, leg length discrepancy, or changes in gait or sitting.[403] Although spasticity management and positioning programs may delay or reduce the need for orthopedic surgery, some children benefit from surgical intervention to address progressive contractures or bone deformity and to address problems with gait, posture, hygiene, and pain. Children may become progressively flexed in their gait and may develop a crouch gait pattern, which can be worsened by their pubertal growth spurt. This pattern is characterized by excessive ankle dorsiflexion, knee flexion, and hip flexion and may be accompanied by excessive femoral anteversion, hip subluxation, patella alta, excessive external tibial torsion, calcaneal valgus, and knee pain. Possible surgical procedures include muscle/tendon lengthenings and transfers, tenotomies, osteotomies, and joint stabilization procedures.

Single-event multilevel surgery, including procedures for the hip, knee, and ankle, allows biomechanical alignment and can take place at all joints simultaneously. Children and families have to deal with only one hospital admission and one period of rehabilitation. Research on the long-term effects of orthopedic surgery is limited due to ethical issues with conducting randomized control trials, a lack of stratification by GMFCS, and inconsistent reporting of the timing of evaluations, procedures, adverse events, postoperative care, and rehabilitation protocols. However, multilevel orthopedic surgery has been shown to improve range of motion, torsion, kinematic and kinetic gait parameters including summary measures, and energy efficiency but only small changes in overall gross motor function and a less predictable effect on quality of life.[235]

More complex surgeries that include procedures such as femoral extension osteotomies and patellar tendon advancements are resulting in promising improvements in knee function and gains in community function.[347] Orthopedic priorities for children functioning at GMFCS level V are the ability to sit comfortably with a stable straight spine over a level pelvis with flexible located hips and plantigrade, braceable feet. The ability to participate in standing transfers is a goal for those functioning at GMFCS level IV. [235]

Physical therapists play important roles in surgical decision making and the management of preoperative and postoperative care. Therapists, surgeons, and families are collaborators in surgical choices based on assessments of gait and other gross motor activities, equipment tolerance, pain, ROM, strength, selective motor control, spasticity, and respiratory function. Child and family goals, resources, motivation, and priorities, as well as surgeon experience, must be considered. As children get older, they should be active participants in making decisions about their care. Their interests, priorities, and concerns about interruptions in their lives as a result of hospitalizations, immobilizations, recovery periods, and commitment to postoperative rehabilitation should be respected.

Preoperatively, therapists can educate the family about postoperative needs such as positioning, lifting, transferring, transportation, respiratory care, feeding, sleeping, and pain management and the potential need for extra help at home. Botox and other forms of spasticity management may be considered to reduce postoperative discomfort.[25] Strengthening and respiratory exercises for preoperative conditioning may be beneficial. Home adaptations and equipment may be put in place in collaboration with occupational therapists, who may provide consultation regarding toileting and bathing needs.

Positioning during the immediate postoperative period is important for comfort and muscle extensibility. Caregiver body mechanics are important when dealing with children who are compromised as the result of casts, movement restrictions, and pain. Postoperative rehabilitation contributes to optimal surgical outcomes, which may continue to improve 12 to 24 months following surgery and may be maintained for many years. Muscle strength, particularly that of the hamstrings, can decrease significantly after surgery.[335] A goal is motor control of lengthened and transferred muscle in the context of functional motor tasks. Specific exercises will vary according to immobilization and weight-bearing and movement restrictions, but extensibility and strengthening exercises to promote functional motor skills will serve as the basis of training programs.[26,335] Hydrotherapy may be beneficial. Re-evaluation of orthotic management, walking aids, and seating may be necessary to maintain alignment, protect surgical correction, and facilitate functional movement.

Spasticity, abnormal extensibility of muscles, muscular imbalance, and weakness can result in scoliosis, which, in turn, can affect positioning, respiratory status, pain, and skin integrity and therefore can be a difficult problem, particularly in the children with spastic quadriplegia.[216] Various types of orthoses can be used in the management of spinal deformity. Evidence does not indicate that bracing prevents the progression of scoliosis in children with CP and may not be tolerated well; however, it may provide benefit by stabilizing trunk posture.[216,249] Surgical correction of severe spinal deformities may be necessary. Despite concerns of morbidity and even mortality, caregivers are satisfied typically with outcomes (see Chapter 8, Spinal Conditions).[216]

Osteopenia with an increased rate of fracture in moderately to severely involved children with CP has been associated with limited ambulation, previous fractures, the use of anticonvulsants, feeding problems, and lower body fat mass.[208] Physical activity that involves weight bearing and bisphosphonate therapy has been shown to have positive effects on bone mineral density in children and adolescents with CP.[115]

Activity and Participation

Attainment of new gross motor skills levels off during these years; however, improvements may be possible, even in children with severe physical and cognitive limitations, if goals are realistic and appropriate behavioral, communication, and motor learning techniques are used.[48] It has been considered that neuroplasticity can continue into the adolescent years or even across the life span but needs to be taken advantage of using optimal types and intensities of treatment.[393] Regardless of the lack of potential for large gains in gross motor skills, therapy programs are necessary to maintain optimal levels of functioning and prevent unnecessary deterioration. Intervention principles such as family-centered service remain the same, but goals, tasks, and motivators may adjust to be age appropriate.

Youth with CP value mobility for independence and participation. Walking in CP is not a dichotomous outcome.[135] As discussed in the section on prognosis for gross motor function, children and youth may have more than one method of mobility depending on varying situations and related to energy expenditure, the activity, the environment, and personal preferences, particularly as children become larger and need to travel greater distances to participate in their social and educational activities.[135,283] Youth who are functioning at GMFCS levels II to IV often choose to use manual or powered wheeled mobility for safety, practicality, or social appropriateness in school or community settings even if they can walk.[283,359] The use of mobility devices may require environmental modifications, such as entrance ramps or washroom renovations, for accessibility. Driver training offers the freedom to travel independently for those capable of driving a car. When driving is not feasible, instruction in the use of public or special transportation should be provided. Dependence on special transportation programs or parents limits the ability to be spontaneous in attending community activities.[283]

Walking may continue to be considered a symbol of normalcy but may become an activity for exercise or to fulfill the expectations of others rather than function.[135] Treadmill training with partial-body-weight-support harnesses can provide safe, task-specific gait training, providing multiple repetitions and active participation for children functioning at GMFCS levels III, IV, and V.[230,257] Studies have small sample sizes but have demonstrated clinically relevant improvements in walking skills, gait velocity, and endurance, as well as improved standing transfers, in children who do not walk by themselves. To date, the quantity and quality of these studies are insufficient to conclude that partial-body-weight-support treadmill training results in significant improvements for children with CP.[83,257,391] Programs with higher intensities and extended durations have resulted in better outcomes. Robotic-assisted treadmill training using a driven gait orthosis requires less personal effort, allowing high-dose, high-repetition walking practice at increased speeds and longer distances during treatment sessions, and possibly enhancing neural reorganization.[242] This intervention shows promise as a therapeutic option to improve walking velocity and gross motor function in children functioning at GMFCS levels I, II, III, and IV.[241] Treadmills also are useful for increasing endurance and strength and can be used without harnesses in higher-functioning children.

School-age children have usually developed abstract thinking and sufficient cognitive ability to use biofeedback, electronic feedback about muscle activity to teach voluntary control. Research is limited; however, it has been found to improve active ROM, strength, and control of movement such as dorsiflexion in a study of children with CP.[105] Carryover is often limited, generalization to real-life situations is not readily demonstrated, and treatment can be time consuming. Biofeedback has been incorporated into robotic technologies.

Readily available technologies such as smart phones, tablets, and computers and a multitude of games and apps provide youth with disabilities access to the many options of activities and social media typically used by peers. Virtual reality technology has provided opportunities for active, repetitive sensory and motor sensory practice that are relatively low cost, commercially available, enjoyable, motivating, socially acceptable, and safe for children of all GMFCS levels. They can improve balance and enhance visual-perceptual processing, postural control, and functional activities.[114] Active video games that require participants to engage in physical activity can lead to moderate-intensity exercise levels with the potential to promote physical fitness and decrease sedentary behavior and therefore enhance cardiovascular fitness.[114]

Habitual physical activity levels in children and youth with CP have been reported to be 13% to 53% lower than their peers and approximately 30% lower than recommended guidelines.[60] Impairments in strength, muscle tone, balance, coordination, and fatigue can contribute to low levels of participation in physical activity, which can in turn result in obesity, poorer cardiorespiratory fitness, lower physical work capacity, and higher oxygen costs.[125,373] Bidirectional associations can result. Energy expenditure for walking can be up to three times as great as that of typically developing children, with significant differences across GMFCS levels.[184,375]

Physical therapists can play an important role in the promotion of health lifestyle practices. Personal or environmental factors can be facilitators or barriers to physical activity. Therapists need to be aware of and should address contextual factors including self-efficacy, knowledge on why and how to exercise, pain management, family support, availability of time, availability and awareness of appropriate equipment or programs, facility accessibility, transportation, finances, trained recreation staff, and people's conceptions about their abilities and conditions.[185,194,256,373]

Physical activity behaviors in childhood and adolescence are important, as they can establish lifestyle habits that continue into adulthood.[336] Research has shown that exercise interventions can increase habitual physical activity in children and youth with CP, but maintenance can be difficult.[17] Aerobic training studies have shown overall positive effects on children with CP, but few report on the impact on daily activity and participation level.[129] The training intensity may be insufficient or the duration of training is too short to show results in these areas.[129]

Strategies include education about the benefits of fitness activities, goal setting, a mix of structured and unstructured programs, feedback, positive role modeling, and providing support to families to find suitable activities and navigate barriers to participation.[17,317] Physical activity recommendations can be grounded in guidelines for the general population that children and youth participate in an accumulated minimum of 60 minutes of moderate to vigorous physical activity daily including aerobic and muscle and bone strengthening activities and FITTE (frequency, intensity, type, time, and enjoyment) principles.[317] Evidence of the impact of physical activity on body functions (strength, flexibility, aerobic and anaerobic capacity, cognition, daily activity, participation, self-competence, and QOL) is promising.[126,374,375] Qualitative finding such as the ability to play outside longer and walk for longer periods have been reported.[140] Activities can include circuit training; trampoline, running, jumping, treadmill, and cycling activities; and swimming. Physical activity should be incorporated into home, school, and community environments. Programs offered in school settings can contribute to adherence and feasibility. Community fitness programs have been shown to improve muscle strength and perception of physical appearance; participants feel confident and motivated enough to take responsibility for continuing in fitness programs.[91] Online programs have shown success.[17]

Youth with CP have twice the recommended amounts of daily sedentary time.[60] The negative health impacts of sedentary time must be considered; however, the definition of sedentary activity may not be appropriate for people with CP. For example, although long periods of time may be spent in sitting, impairments such as atypical muscle tone, co-contraction, and poor balance may actually lessen the sedentary nature of being seated.[177] Finding ways to limit the total time spent being sedentary and ensuring that prolonged periods of sedentary time are broken up with bursts of movement and light activity, such as sitting exercises or even wiggling in a wheelchair, may lessen the risks of too much sedentary time.[177,373]

Recreational and sports activities provide excellent opportunities for exercise, fun, and social interaction.[345] These include horseback riding,[94] swimming, bicycling,[292] skiing,[345] sailing, canoeing, camping, kayaking, fishing, bungee jumping, yoga, skiing, and tai chi (Fig. 19.12). Adapted games provide exercise, athletic competition, participation in team experiences, and social opportunities (www.medicalhomeinfo.org/health/recreation.html).

All athletes are at risk for sports-related injuries, but relatively minor injuries can incapacitate people with CP. They should be encouraged to be responsible for their bodies during sports activities by completing appropriate conditioning, warm-up, and cool-down routines; following comprehensive injury-prevention programs, which include strengthening, flexibility, and aerobic and anaerobic training activities and protection

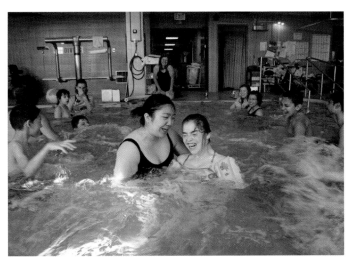

FIG. 19.12 Participating in an aquatic class can provide fitness and social opportunities.

of long-term joint integrity; and using appropriate protective and orthotic equipment. Knee injuries commonly involve the patellofemoral joint secondary to spasticity of muscle groups surrounding the joint. Deformities of the ankle and foot, including equinus, equinovarus, and valgus deformities, can lead to an increased risk for injury.[198] Injuries should be taken seriously and treated promptly. For more information, see Chapter 15, Sports Injuries in Children.

School and Community

Tremendous progress has been made in the inclusion of children with physical disabilities into the educational system and community activities. Although many experiences are very successful, some children experience isolation, marginalization, social or physical exclusion, bullying, or constant adult presence.[176] Physical therapists are involved in school-based therapy programs to support student access to and participation in all school activities. These may include positioning, mobility in and between classrooms and during recess, physical education, noncurricular social activities, and field trips. Facilities and resources such as support personnel, equipment, building accessibility, and computer technology may be necessary to meet the educational, physical, and self-care needs of children in the school system. Therapists develop and maintain collaborative partnerships with school personnel. They may interpret the impact of medical conditions; instruct assistants and teachers in positioning, lifting, and transferring children and carrying out exercise programs; and adapt activities through modification and accommodation.[212] Therapists may also be involved in transportation, evacuation, and other safety issues. Therapists working in school settings must be sensitive to the physical and scheduling constraints of the educational environment and must be willing to compromise to meet the educational priorities of students. Therapy may range from consultation and monitoring for students thought to have reached their maximal level of functioning to active therapy for children who have specific goals. When children are seen primarily through the educational system, efforts must be made to keep the family involved in all aspects of care and treatment. Therapists may be involved in the coordination of services among family members, school professionals, health services,

and community agencies and influential in empowering students as they become capable of being involved in decision making.[212] See Chapter 31, The Educational Environment, for in-depth information on the role of the physical therapist in the US educational system.

Therapists can also be involved in educating students about cerebral palsy to reduce teasing and bullying and to increase acceptance of children with disabilities. Children with knowledge about and social contact with individuals with disabilities have more positive attitudes toward peers with disabilities and are more likely to have empathy for, and feel less anxious about, interacting with people with disabilities.[7]

Children and adolescents learn about their bodies, their sexuality, and appropriate interactions with other people. Children and adults with disabilities can suffer abuse, including sexual exploitation, which may result in physical, social, emotional, and behavioral consequences.[341] Some abusers have relationships specifically related to the victim's disability. These people may include personal care attendants, transportation providers, residential care staff, and other disabled individuals. Physical therapists must know how to detect the signs of abuse, be sensitive and receptive to clients who may choose to confide in them, and know the proper procedures to follow if they suspect abuse. They must work with other professionals to promote assertiveness and positive self-esteem in their clients.

All people involved with youth with CP must educate them in being streetwise. Their physical and sometimes cognitive limitations can make them particularly vulnerable to crime. They should be taught to avoid unsafe situations and warned about protecting valuables. Purses or knapsacks slung over a wheelchair handle can be easy to grab. Self-defense courses specifically designed for people with disabilities may be available.

Health care professionals must realize that although parents have been coping with their child's needs for a number of years, parent education is still important because the child and the child's needs are constantly changing. Parents of children with CP may experience physical and psychological health problems and need to be encouraged to take good care of themselves. Reported health issues include back problems, stomach/intestinal ulcers, migraine headaches, arthritis, emotional problems, pain, and chronic physical conditions.[43] Continued attention to education in lifting and transferring is necessary to prevent injury to caregivers whose children are growing larger and heavier as they, themselves, are aging.

Role of Other Disciplines

Occupational therapists may be involved in promoting independence in activities of daily living and work closely with physical therapists in managing upper extremity function.[67] Interdisciplinary life skills training can focus on self-care, community living, and interpersonal relationships. Prevocational training and related activities, such as money management and employment searching, may be beneficial. Psychologists or social workers may be involved in various aspects of adolescent life such as social and sexuality issues.

TRANSITION TO ADULTHOOD

Adults strive to be independently functioning and self-sufficient, employed individuals who have satisfying social and emotional lives and contribute to society. They endeavor to live independently in the community, alone or with others.

They have romantic relationships and sexual experiences, enjoy social outings, often marry, and sometimes have children. Adolescents with CP have the same dreams and aspirations for adult life as all young people.[196] The extent to which these goals can be realized depends on factors such as independence in self-care activities and mobility, level of cognition, communication skills, and available resources and support. A review of adults with CP without intellectual disability showed 60% to 80% completed high school, 14% to 25% completed college, up to 61% were living independently in the community, 25% to 55% were competitively employed, and 14% to 28% were involved in long-term relationships with partners or had established families.[121]

Many adults with CP continue to live with their families or in group homes or institutions.[219] At a time when most parents are experiencing freedom from caregiving responsibilities, many parents of youth with CP continue to have these obligations.[153] Their concerns focus on how their child can function as an independent adult, how they can continue to care for their child as they themselves age, and who will care for the child when they are unable to do so. Parents of children who have the potential to live independently must deal with the anxieties of letting go.[142] Many may also be coping with a decrease in the number of relatively organized and available programs and equipment resources that are available for younger children. Continuity of care may be lacking, and it may be difficult to find medical professionals with experience in managing the health care of people with disabilities.

The transition to adult lifestyle and services is complex. Planning and problem solving should take place throughout adolescence. Successful transition has been characterized by self-determination, enhanced knowledge of self and community, problem-solving and decision-making skills, identification of support systems, and supportive environments, including transition clinics.[31] During the transition there should be a gradual shift in responsibilities from parents to the young person, as developmentally appropriate, to develop capacity in self-management.[142] This can start with having adolescents see health care professionals by themselves. Areas of transition to be addressed include vocational or postsecondary education, living arrangements, personal management, leisure time, recreational and social activities, and financial planning. The latter involves education about governmental benefits, guardianship, conservatorship, wills, and trusts. Primary and preventive health care services must be organized. These include provision of therapy when needed, medical consultation, primary care, and equipment needs and maintenance. Internet resources from institutions provide guides to assist adolescents and families in navigating the transition to adulthood. These include Bloorview Kids Rehab (www.bloorview.ca/programsandservices/programserviceaz/growingupready) and Ministry of Children and Family Development in British Columbia (www.mcf.gov.bc.ca/spec_needs/pdf/your_future_now.pdf).

In-depth information is presented in Chapter 32, Transition to Adulthood for Youth with Physical Disabilities.

Role of Physical Therapy

Pediatric physical therapists work together with the individual, the family, and the health care team to provide comprehensive planning to facilitate the transition to managing the challenges of adulthood. Major physical therapy goals during this period of transition are aimed at maximizing the capability to maintain function, prevent deterioration, and achieve optimal independent living. Ideally, the medical, therapeutic, and educational outcomes achieved throughout childhood have prepared youth with CP for success in these areas. Therapists need to encourage problem solving in adolescents who have the potential to live on their own, as they will need to be self-sufficient in managing their health condition.

Adults with CP must deal with the normal effects of aging in addition to their preexisting impairments.[274] They may experience early onset of frailty, chronic pain, fatigue, osteoarthritis, osteoporosis, cardiometabolic disease, sarcopenia, and decreased extensibility and endurance.[291] These can contribute to falls and a decline in mobility and independence and impact employment, social integration, and participation in exercise and other leisure activities.[291] Among adults with CP who are able to walk, 25% are estimated to have reduced abilities compared to when they were younger, more so in those with less capacity to walk, bilateral rather than unilateral motor impairment, older age, and higher levels of pain or fatigue.[246] Gait decline may be characterized by the need for more assistance to walk, greater perceived effort, a reduction in walking distance, speed or environments managed, the ability to climb stairs, or the emergence or increase of features such as onset of pain, breathlessness, or fatigue.[246] Deterioration in function, mobility, and participation in daily life has been attributed to pain, physical fatigue, obesity, and losses of muscle strength, balance, and cardiovascular fitness.[291] Adults with CP who report preservation of mobility accredit this to regular physical activity participation and maintenance of balance, strength, and overall fitness.[291]

Fatigue is a major concern for some youth and adults with CP, particularly with walking long distances, suggesting an association with overuse.[49] Fatigue is associated with pain, lack of physical activity, general health problems, deterioration of physical skills, emotional issues, and low life satisfaction. Physical therapists can encourage youth to be aware of their own bodies, adapt activities to allow continued participation in various aspects of their lives, and counsel regarding the positive and negative effects of activity on pain and fatigue, the use of adaptive equipment, and pacing.[50]

Strength training can improve walking ability and may prevent a decline in mobility.[4] Strength training for adults with CP has been found to increase strength of targeted muscles by 27% compared to a control group but with no improvements in measures of mobility.[353]

Prevention of overuse syndromes, early joint degeneration, progression of contractures, osteoporosis, poor endurance, and pathologic fractures is important. Cervical and back pain, nerve entrapment syndromes, or tendinitis can occur as a result of excessive and repetitive physical stresses.[131] A survey of adults found that 67% reported one or more areas of pain, with lower extremity and back pain most common; 53% had pain of moderate to severe intensity.

Adherence to exercise programs of stretching, strengthening, and aerobics may be poor, and access to therapy programs may decrease in the adult years. Therapists should encourage the use of community and recreational programs that provide the necessary opportunities to promote fitness and focus on healthy lifestyles. Poor exercise habits may start during adolescence, if not earlier, and can result in a cycle of poor fitness and endurance.[131]

Young adults with CP may experience a wide variation in physical problems with intimacy including spasticity, stiffness, movement, fatigue, weakness, and impaired manual ability.[390] Health professionals may be able to provide counseling and necessary information on adaptations for sexual activities.

Overall, adults with CP need to find a balance between alleviating unnecessary energy costs in daily living and staying fit to achieve optimal health and functioning.[81] Preventive strategies that may minimize the long-term effects of neuromuscular dysfunction include choosing exercises that minimize excessive joint stress, using additional mobility aids or devices such as orthoses, and opting for surgery when appropriate. Changes to the environment may be necessary to maintain optimal independence.[274] Technological advances provide many options for adults with CP. These include computers for written communication, artificial speech devices, environmental controls, and power mobility. For more information, see Chapter 33: Assistive Technology.

In many parts of the world, society is becoming more conscious of the rights and needs of individuals with limitations. This recognition has had a positive effect on environmental factors that influence participation. Human rights legislation exists to accommodate people with disabilities and to prevent discrimination in areas such as employment, accessibility, the legal system, and education. Government programs and services are available to people with disabilities. Theaters, restaurants, libraries, museums, government buildings, educational facilities, shopping areas, parks, campground facilities, and parking lots are often accessible through the provision of ramps, appropriate washroom facilities, and other modifications. Air and rail travel are also becoming more available to people with special mobility needs. Some travel organizations cater to people with disabilities. Therapists should be aware of the facilities and resources available to people with physical disabilities. In some situations, funding for assistive devices, living allowances, and housing and tax exemptions helps prevent undue hardship. Therapists also should be cognizant of the political policies and issues affecting the lives of those with disabilities and should advocate for advancement of equal access to community and governmental resources.

GLOBAL ISSUES

Resources and services for children with CP vary throughout the world. Physical therapists use many different approaches or combinations of approaches, depending on the facilities available, the child's and the family's needs, the therapist's training and background, and the diversity of client values, beliefs, and priorities. Many of the interventions and technologies discussed in this chapter are practiced in high-resource countries, where services, although variable in their extent, quality, and funding, are generally available and accessible. However, much of the world's population lives in low-resource, underserved areas, particularly in developing nations or in remote areas of developed nations. In many countries, children with disabilities are not able to realize basic rights and are subject to policies of institutionalization rather than receiving community-based and family-focused care.[299] They may be deprived of opportunities to participate in society, may be denied access to education, and may suffer from stigma. Nevertheless many of the principles and equipment ideas developed elsewhere can be adapted to various situations. Using indigenous materials to fabricate effective and affordable equipment, recycling used equipment, and training local personnel or fostering exchange programs can help to provide resources to underserved areas.

It is important to be sensitive to local customs, cultures, and environmental situations when adapting programs for different settings. Often the direct application of a certain method is impractical or inappropriate because of economic, geographic, or cultural differences. Throughout the world, increasing emphasis is being placed on community-based rehabilitation, which promotes interventions that are practical and functional for specific settings, lifestyles, and cultures.

PROFESSIONAL ISSUES

Many potential facilitators and barriers to the practice of efficacious, effective, and efficient physical therapy are known. Therapists who provide services to children with CP and their families should be aware that the work can be physically and emotionally demanding. They must practice appropriate lifting and handling techniques and should maintain a suitable level of fitness if they are treating patients actively. Working with children and their families can be both fulfilling and emotionally stressful. Therapists may be challenged by ethical issues, unrealistic expectations and demands, limited resources, and the pressures of dealing with families during periods of grieving and times of crisis.

Therapists are encouraged to collaborate with families and focus on family and environment strengths and solutions to challenges. Therapists also have a role in advocating for public policy and resources to enable individuals with CP to have good health and full participation in desired roles throughout life. Professionals must acknowledge their own needs and reactions and feel comfortable seeking assistance and support from others.

The lifelong physical therapy needs of children with CP and their families are often influenced and constrained by service availability, accessibility, costs, and policy. These parameters can affect wait times for services and may have an impact on service frequency. The psychosocial well-being of families may be affected by long wait periods for therapy.[117] Therapists are often faced with the stressful challenges of providing equitable services within their facility or practice while justifying differences in services among facilities or clients. Intensity of services, including decisions regarding how often, how long, and the duration of an episode, varies considerably among families, therapists, administrators, policy makers, and insurers.[280] Family and fiscal resources challenge therapists to create strategies to provide equitable and appropriate services for all children in their care. Alternatives to continuous therapy include consultation, monitoring, or providing blocks of treatment, while taking into consideration periods of readiness for change. Determining whether children are at a stage of acquiring, improving, maintaining, or generalizing skill, and assessing motivation, supports, and environments, can help indicate optimal times to provide services. Small or large group programs and recreation and sports opportunities can provide alternatives to direct individual therapy.[280]

Best practice encompasses the best research evidence available, clinical expertise, and needs and values.[326] These must be considered in the context of a child, the family, and the health care system resources. Physical therapists are encouraged to reflect on these considerations and collaborate with the family to make individualized decisions for each child. Therapists must critically appraise available and appropriate knowledge, including accessing recent literature, using the Internet, attending educational sessions, and sharing practice-generated knowledge with colleagues and families to promote optimal decision making. Organizations need to support these strategies.[21,188]

◼ SUMMARY

Physical therapists play an important role on the team of professionals who provide services to children with CP and their families. Therapists offer choices and advice and provide interventions to optimize the development of functional abilities, enable participation in all aspects of life, and prevent secondary impairments. The support given during infancy, childhood, and adolescence can have an impact on functioning and quality of life in adulthood. The ICF framework, systems to classify functional abilities, improved prognostic information, psychometrically strong yet clinically feasible tests and measures, established and innovative interventions, progressive advances in assistive technology, and increasing knowledge of the lived experiences, priorities, and preferences of individuals with CP combine to make the practice of physical therapy for children and adolescents with CP challenging but exciting. The "F-words" paper by Rosenbaum and Gorter[308] exemplifies many of these concepts: *fitness, function, family, fun, friends,* and the addition of *future,* suggesting an emphasis on promoting health promotion by enhancing fitness, activities, and accomplishments that are meaningful to the child and family; encouraging friendships while having fun; and aiming for a future that embodies dreams and desires.[308] In our experience, families are particularly interested in planning for the future. The term *anticipatory guidance* refers to collaborating with families to prepare children for new roles and changing environments such as the transition from early intervention to primary school and the transition from secondary education to adulthood.

Case Scenarios on Expert Consult

The case scenarios related to this chapter present two patients (Noelle and Nicole) with accompanying videos. They illustrate some of the management principles discussed in this chapter. Nicole's story recounts her life over the five editions of *Physical Therapy for Children*, from infancy to adulthood.

ACKNOWLEDGMENTS

Acknowledgments are extended to the children, adolescents, and their families involved in the case studies for their time and valuable perspectives. We also would like to acknowledge the clinical expertise of our colleagues. The literature provides us with research evidence, but best practice would not be possible without our day-to-day learning from each other.

REFERENCES

1. Albavera-Hernandez C, et al.: Safety of botulinum toxin type A among children with spasticity secondary to cerebral palsy: a systematic review of randomized clinical trials, *Clin Rehab* 23:394–407, 2009.
2. Albright AL, et al.: Intrathecal baclofen for generalized dystonia, *Dev Med Child Neurol* 43:652–657, 2001.
3. Anderson JC, et al.: Intensive upper extremity training for children with hemiplegia: from science to practice, *Pediatr Neurol* 20:100–105, 2013.
4. Andersson C, et al.: Adults with cerebral palsy: walking ability after progressive strength training, *Dev Med Child Neurol* 45:220–228, 2003.
5. Angsupaisal M, et al.: Adaptive seating systems in children with severe cerebral palsy across International Classification of Functioning, Disability and Health for Children and Youth version domains: a systematic review, *Dev Med Child Neurol* 57:919–931, 2015.
6. Aquilina K, Graham D, Wimalasundera N: Selective dorsal rhizotomy: an old treatment re-emerging, *Arch Dis Child* 100:798–802, 2015.
7. Armstrong M, et al.: Children's with people with disabilities and their attitudes towards disability: a cross-sectional study, *Disabil Rehabil* 14:1–10, 2015.
8. Arpino C, et al.: Efficacy of intensive versus nonintensive physiotherapy in children with cerebral palsy: a meta-analysis, *Int J Rehab Res* 33:165–171, 2010.
9. Arvedson JC: Feeding children with cerebral palsy and swallowing difficulties, *Eur J Clin Nutr* 67(Suppl 2):S9–S12, 2013.
10. Avery LM, et al.: Rasch analysis of the Gross Motor Function Measure: validating the assumptions of the Rasch model to create an interval-level measure, *Arch Phys Med Rehab* 84:697–705, 2003.
11. Ayalon M, et al.: Reliability of isokinetic strength measurements of the knee in children with cerebral palsy, *Dev Med Child Neurol* 42:398–402, 2000.
12. Bagley AM, et al.: Outcome assessments in children with cerebral palsy, part II. Discriminatory ability of outcomes tools, *Dev Med Child Neurol* 49:181–186, 2007.
13. Bailes AF, et al.: Development of guidelines for determining frequency of therapy services in a pediatric medical setting, *Pediatr Phys Ther* 20:194–198, 2008.
14. Balakrishnan B, et al.: Nanomedicine in cerebral palsy, *Int J Nanomed* 8:4183–4195
15. Balzer J, et al.: Construct validity and reliability of the Selective Control Assessment of the Lower Extremity in children with cerebral palsy, *Dev Med Child Neurol* 58:167–172, 2016.
16. Bamm EL, Rosenbaum P: Family-centered theory: origins, development, barriers, and supports to implementation in rehabilitation medicine, *Arch Phys Med Rehabil* 89:1618–1624, 2008.
17. Bania T, et al.: Habitual physical activity can be increased in people with cerebral palsy: a systematic review, *Clin Rehab* 25:303–315, 2011.
18. Barks L: Therapeutic positioning, wheelchair seating, and pulmonary function of children with cerebral palsy: a research synthesis, *Rehabilitation Nursing* 29:146–153, 2004.
19. Barnes D, et al.: Pediatric outcomes data collection instrument scores in ambulatory children with cerebral palsy: an analysis by age groups and severity level, *J Pediatr Orthop* 28:97–102, 2008.
20. Barry MJ, et al.: Reliability and responsiveness of the Barry-Albright Dystonia Scale, *Dev Med Child Neurol* 41:404–411, 1999.
21. Barrett RS, Lichtwark GA: Gross morphology and structure in spastic cerebral palsy: a systematic review, *Dev Med Child Neurol* 52:798–804, 2010.
22. Bartlett D, Purdy B: Testing of the spinal alignment and range of motion measure: a discriminative measure of posture and flexibility for children with cerebral palsy, *Dev Med Child Neurol* 47:739–743, 2005.
23. Bartlett DJ, et al.: Correlates of decline in gross motor capacity in adolescents with cerebral palsy in Gross Motor Function Classification System levels III to V: an exploratory study, *Dev Med Child Neurol* 52:e155–e160, 2010.
24. Bartlett DJ, et al.: Determinants of gross motor function of young children with cerebral palsy: a prospective cohort study, *Dev Med Child Neurol* 56:275–282, 2014.
25. Barwood S, et al.: Analgesic effects of botulinum toxin A: a randomised placebo trial, *Dev Med Child Neurol* 42:116–121, 2000.
26. BC Children's Hospital: http://www.bcchildrens.ca/NR/rdonlyres/37804B05-9233-463F-B352-AF91DC0611E4/63909/SEMLSclinicalpathway.pdf.
27. Beach MC, Inui T: Relationship-centered care research network: relationship-centered care: a constructive reframing, *J Gen Intern Med* 21:S1, S3–S8, 2006.
28. Beckung E, et al.: The natural history of gross motor development in children with cerebral palsy aged 1 to 15 years, *Dev Med Child Neurol* 49:751–756, 2002.

29. Beckung E, et al.: Probability of walking in children with cerebral palsy in Europe, *Pediatrics* 121:e187–e192, 2008.

30. Bernheimer LP, Weisner TS: "Let me just tell you what I do all day …" The family story at the center of intervention research and practice, *Infants Young Child* 20:192–201, 2007.

31. Binks JA, et al.: What do we really know about the transition to adult-centered health care? A focus on cerebral palsy and spina bifida, *Arch Phys Med Rehabil* 88:1064–1073, 2007.

32. Reference deleted in proofs.

33. Blackmore AM, et al.: A systematic review of the effects of casting on equinus in children with cerebral palsy: an evidence report of the AACPDM, *Dev Med Child Neurol* 49:781–790, 2007.

34. Blanche EI: Doing with—not doing to: play and the child with cerebral palsy. In Parham LD, Fazio LS, editors: *Play in occupational therapy for children*, St. Louis, 1997, Mosby, pp 202–218.

35. Blauw-Hospers CH, et al.: Development of a quantitative tool to assess the contents of physical therapy for infants, *Pediatr Phys Ther* 22:189–197, 2010.

36. Reference deleted in proofs.

37. Bly L: A historical and current view of the basis of NDT, *Pediatr Phys Ther* 3:131–135, 1991.

38. Boldingh EJ, et al.: Assessing pain in patients with severe cerebral palsy: development, reliability, and validity of a pain assessment instrument for cerebral palsy, *Arch Phys Med Rehabil* 85:758–766, 2004.

39. Reference deleted in proofs.

40. Booth CM, et al.: Collagen accumulation in muscles of children with cerebral palsy and correlation with severity of spasticity, *Dev Med Child Neurol* 43:314–320, 2001.

41. Reference deleted in proofs.

42. Boyd R, Graham HK: Objective clinical measures in the use of botulinum toxin A in the management of cerebral palsy, *Eur J Neurol* 6(Suppl 4): 23–36, 1999.

43. Brehaut JC, et al.: The health of primary caregivers of children with cerebral palsy: how does it compare with that of other Canadian caregivers? *Pediatrics* 114:e182–e191, 2004.

44. Brochard S, Remy, et al.: Intrathecal baclofen infusion for ambulant children with cerebral palsy, *Pediatr Neurol* 40:265–270, 2009.

45. Brogren Carlberg E, Hadders-Algra M: Postural dysfunction in children with cerebral palsy: some implications for therapeutic guidance, *Neural Plasticity* 12:221–228, 2005.

46. Brooks-Scott S: *Mobilization for the neurologically involved child*, Tucson, AZ, 1995, Therapy Skill Builders.

47. Brouwer B, et al.: Serial casting in idiopathic toe-walkers and children with spastic cerebral palsy, *J Pediatr Orthoped* 20:221–225, 2000.

48. Brown DA, et al.: Performance following ability-focused physical therapy intervention in individuals with severely limited physical and cognitive abilities, *Phys Ther* 78:934–950, 1998.

49. Brunton LK, Rice CL: Fatigue in cerebral palsy, *Dev Neurorehabil* 15:54–62, 2012.

50. Brunton LK, Bartlett DJ: The bodily experience of cerebral palsy: a journey to self-awareness, *Disabil Rehabil* 35:1981–1990, 2013.

51. Butler C, Campbell S: Evidence of the effects of intrathecal baclofen for spastic and dystonic cerebral palsy. AACPCM Treatment Outcomes Committee Review Panel, *Dev Med Child Neurol* 42:634–645, 2000.

52. Reference deleted in proofs.

53. Reference deleted in proofs.

54. Cameron EC, et al.: The effects of an early physical therapy intervention for very preterm, very low birth weight infants: a randomized controlled clinical trial, *Pediatr Phys Ther* 17:107–119, 2005.

55. Campbell SK: Therapy programs for children that last a lifetime, *Phys Occup Ther Pediatr* 17:1–15, 1997.

56. Campbell SK, Barbosa V: The challenge of early diagnosis, *Dev Med Child Neurol* 45(Suppl 94):5–6, 2003.

57. Campbell SK, Hedeker D: Validity of the Test of Infant Motor Performance for discriminating among infants with varying risk for poor motor outcome, *J Pediatr* 139:546–551, 2001.

58. CanChild Centre for Childhood Disability Research. Retrieved from: http://www.canchild.ca.

59. Cans C: Surveillance of cerebral palsy in Europe: a collaboration of cerebral palsy surveys and registers, *Dev Med Child Neurol* 42:816–824, 2000.

60. Carlon SL, et al.: Differences in habitual physical activity levels of young people with cerebral palsy and their typically developing peers: a systematic review, *Disabil Rehabil* 35:647–655, 2013.

61. Castle K, et al.: Being in pain: a phenomenological study of young people with cerebral palsy, *Dev Med Child Neurol* 49:445–449, 2007.

62. Reference deleted in proofs.

63. Chandler LS, et al.: *Movement assessment of infants: a manual*, Rolling Bay, WA, 1980, Infant Movement Research.

64. Chang FM, et al.: Effectiveness of instrumented gait analysis in children with cerebral palsy: comparison of outcomes, *J Pediatr Orthop* 26: 612–616, 2006.

65. Chen F, et al.: The use of the 600 yard walk-run test to assess walking endurance and speed in children with CP, *Pediatr Phys Ther* 18:86, 2006.

66. Chiarello LA, et al.: Child engagement in daily life: a measure of participation for young children with cerebral palsy, *Disabil Rehabil* 36: 1804–1816, 2014.

67. Chin TYP, et al.: Management of the upper limb in cerebral palsy, *J Pediatr Orthop B* 14:389–404, 2005.

68. Chiu H, Ada L: Effect of functional electrical stimulation on activity in children with cerebral palsy: a systematic review, *Pediatr Phys Ther* 26:283–288, 2014.

69. Christiansen AS, Lange C: Intermittent versus continuous physiotherapy in children with cerebral palsy, *Dev Med Child Neurol* 50:290–293, 2008.

70. Cioni G, et al.: Comparison between observation of spontaneous movements and neurological examination in preterm infants, *J Pediatr* 130:704–711, 1997.

71. Cook RE, et al.: Gait analysis alters decision-making in cerebral palsy, *J Pediatr Orthop* 23:292–295, 2003.

72. Copeland L, et al.: Botulinum toxin A for nonambulatory children with cerebral palsy: a double blind randomized controlled trial, *J Pediatr* 165:140–146, 2014.

73. Coster W, et al.: Psychometric evaluation of the Participation and Environment Measure for Children and Youth (PEM-CY), *Dev Med Child Neurol* 53:1030–1037, 2012.

74. Craft MJ, et al.: Siblings as change agents for promoting the functional status of children with cerebral palsy, *Dev Med Child Neurol* 32:1049–1057, 1990.

75. Criswell SR, et al.: The use of botulinum toxin therapy for lower-extremity spasticity in children with cerebral palsy, *Neurosurg Focus* 21:e1, 2006.

76. Crompton J, et al.: Hand-held dynamometry for muscle strength measurement in children with cerebral palsy, *Dev Med Child Neurol* 49:106–111, 2007.

77. Crowther CA, et al.: Magnesium sulphate for preventing preterm birth in threatened preterm labour, *Cochrane Database Syst Rev* 8:CD001060, 2014.

78. Cunningham BJ, Rosenbaum PL: Measure of processes of care: a review of 20 years of research, *Dev Med Child Neurol* 56:445–452, 2014.

79. Dali C, et al.: Threshold electrical stimulation (TES) in ambulant children with CP: a randomized double-blind placebo-controlled clinical trial, *Dev Med Child Neurol* 44:364–369, 2002.

80. Damiano DL: Meaningfulness of mean group results for determining the optimal motor rehabilitation program for an individual child with cerebral palsy, *Dev Med Child Neurol* 56:1141–1146, 2014.

81. Damiano DL: Strength, endurance, and fitness in cerebral palsy, *Dev Med Child Neurol* 45(Suppl 94):8–10, 2003.

82. Damiano DL: Activity, activity, activity: rethinking our physical therapy approach to cerebral palsy, *Phys Ther* 86:1535–1540, 2006.

83. Damiano DL, DeJong SL: A systematic review of the effectiveness of treadmill training and body weight support in pediatric rehabilitation, *J Neurol Phys Ther* 33:27–44, 2009.

84. Damiano DL, et al.: Should we be testing and training muscle strength in cerebral palsy? *Dev Med Child Neurol* 44:68–72, 2002.

85. Damiano DL, et al.: Deficits in eccentric versus concentric torque in children with spastic cerebral palsy, *Med Sci Sports Exercise* 33:117–122, 2001.

86. Damiano DL: Is addressing impairments the shortest path to improving function? *Phys Occup Ther Pediatr* 28:327–330, 2008.

87. Darrah J, et al.: Stability of serial range-of-motion measurements of the lower extremities in children with cerebral palsy: can we do better? *Phys Ther* 94:987–994, 2014.

88. Darrah J, Bartlett D: Dynamic systems theory and management of children with cerebral palsy: unresolved issues, *Infants Young Child* 8:52–59, 1995.

89. Darrah J, et al.: Assessment of gross motor skills of at-risk infants: predictive validity of the Alberta Infant Motor Scale, *Dev Med Child Neurol* 40:495–491, 1998.

90. Reference deleted in proofs.

91. Darrah J, et al.: Evaluation of a community fitness program for adolescents with cerebral palsy, *Pediatr Phys Ther* 11:18–23, 1999.

92. David KS, Sullivan M: Expectations for walking speeds: standards for students in elementary schools, *Pediatr Phys Ther* 17:120–127, 2005.

93. Davies PL, et al.: Validity and reliability of the School Function Assessment in elementary school students with disabilities, *Phys Occup Ther Pediatr* 24:23–43, 2004.

94. Davis E, et al.: A randomized controlled trial of the impact of therapeutic horse riding on the quality of life, health, and function of children with cerebral palsy, *Dev Med Child Neurol* 51:111–119, 2009.

95. De Graaf-Peters VB, et al.: Development of postural control in typically developing children and children with cerebral palsy: possibilities for intervention? *Neurosci Biobehav Rev* 31:1191–1200, 2007.

96. Depienne C, et al.: Hereditary spastic paraplegia: an update, *Curr Opin Neurol* 20:674–680, 2007.

97. Desloovere L, et al.: The effect of different physiotherapy interventions in post-BTX-A treatment of children with cerebral palsy, *Eur J Paediatr Neurol* 16:20–28, 2011.

98. Desloovere K, et al.: Do dynamic and static clinical measurements correlate with gait analysis parameters in children with cerebral palsy? *Gait Posture* 24:302–313, 2006.

99. Desloovere K, et al.: A randomized study of combined botulinum toxin type A and casting in the ambulant child with cerebral palsy using objective outcome measures, *Eur J Neurol* 8:75–87, 2001.

100. DeVries AM, deGroot L: Transient dystonia revisited: a comparative study of preterm and term children at 2½ years of age, *Dev Med Child Neurol* 44:415–421, 2002.

101. Dewar R, et al.: Exercise interventions improve postural control in children with cerebral palsy: a systematic review, *Dev Med Child Neurol* 57:504–520, 2015.

102. Di Rezze B, et al.: Development of a generic fidelity measure for rehabilitation intervention for children with physical disabilities, *Dev Med Child Neurol* 55:737–744, 2013.

103. Dirks T, et al.: Differences between the family-centres "COPCA" program and traditional infant physical therapy based on neurodevelopmental treatment principles, *Phys Ther* 91:1303–1322, 2011.

104. Dorlap S, Bartlett DJ: The prevalence, distribution, effect of pain among adolescents with cerebral palsy, *Pediatr Phys Ther* 22:26–33, 2010.

105. Dursun E, et al.: Effects of biofeedback treatment on gait in children with cerebral palsy, *Disabil Rehabil* 26:116–120, 2004.

106. Edgar TS: Oral pharmacotherapy of childhood movement disorders, *J Child Neurol* 18(Suppl 1):S40–S49, 2003.

107. Ehrsson HH, et al.: Brain regions controlling nonsynergistic versus synergistic movement of the digits: a functional magnetic resonance imaging study, *J Neurosci* 22:5074–5080, 2002.

108. Elder GC, et al.: Contributing factors to muscle weakness in children with cerebral palsy, *Dev Med Child Neurol* 45:542–550, 2003.

109. Eliasson A-C, et al.: The Manual Ability Classification System (MACS) for children with cerebral palsy: scale development and evidence of validity and reliability, *Dev Med Child Neurol* 48:549–554, 2006.

110. Engsberg JR, et al.: Predicting functional change from preintervention measures in selective dorsal rhizotomy, *J Neurosurg* 106(Suppl 4): 282–287, 2007.

111. Engsberg JR, et al.: Ankle spasticity and strength in children with spastic diplegia cerebral palsy, *Dev Med Child Neurol* 42:42–47, 2000.

112. Fauconnier J, et al.: Participation in life situations of 8-12 year old children with cerebral palsy: cross sectional European study, *BMJ* 338:b1458, 2009.

113. Faulkner SD, et al.: -The potential for stem cells in cerebral palsy-piecing together the puzzle, *Sem Pediatr Neurol* 20:146–153, 2013.

114. Fehlings D, et al.: Interactive computer play as "motor therapy" for individuals with cerebral palsy, *Sem Pediatr Neurol* 20:127–138, 2013

115. Fehlings D, et al.: Informing evidence-based clinical practice guidelines for children with cerebral palsy at risk of osteoporosis: a systematic review, *Dev Med Child Neurol* 54:106–116, 2011.

116. Fehlings D, et al.: An evaluation of botulinum: a toxin injections to improve upper extremity in children with hemiplegia cerebral palsy, *J Pediatr* 137:331–337, 2000.

117. Felman DE, et al.: Is waiting for rehabilitation services associated with changes in function and quality of life in children with physical disabilities? *Phys Occup Ther Pediatr* 28:291–304, 2008.

118. Ferland C, et al.: Locomotor tests predict community mobility in children and youth with cerebral palsy, *Adapt Phys Activ Q* 29:266–277, 2012.

119. Figueiredo EM, et al.: Efficacy of ankle-foot orthoses on gait of children with cerebral palsy: systematic review of literature, *Pediatr Phys Ther* 20:207–223, 2012.

120. Flamand VH, et al.: Psychometric evidence of spasticity measurement tools in cerebral palsy children and adolescents: a systematic review, *J Rehabil Med* 45:14–23, 2013.

121. Frisch D, Msall ME: Health, functioning, and participation of adolescents and adults with cerebral palsy: a review of outcomes research, *Dev Disabil Res Rev* 18:84–94, 2013.

122. Flanagan A, et al.: Evaluation of short-term intensive orthotic garment use in children with cerebral palsy, *Pediatr Phys Ther* 21:201–204, 2009.

123. Foran JRH, et al.: Structural and mechanical alterations in spastic skeletal muscle, *Dev Med Child Neurol* 47:713–717, 2005.

124. Fowler EG, Goldberg EJ: The effect of lower extremity selective voluntary motor control on interjoint coordination during gait in children with spastic diplegic cerebral palsy, *Gait Posture* 29:102–107, 2009.

125. Fowler EG, et al.: Promotion of physical fitness and prevention of secondary conditions for children with cerebral palsy: section on Pediatrics Research Summit Proceedings, *Phys Ther* 87:1495–1510, 2007.

126. Fowler EG, et al.: Pediatric endurance and limb strengthening (PEDALS) for children with cerebral palsy using stationary cycling: a randomized control trial, *Phys Ther* 90:367–381, 2010.

127. Fowler EG, et al.: Selective control assessment of the lower extremity (SCALE): development, validation and interrater reliability of a clinical tool for patients with cerebral palsy, *Dev Med Child Neurol* 51:607–614, 2009.

128. Franki I, et al.: The evidence-base for conceptual approaches in children with cerebral palsy: a systematic review using the international classification of functioning, disability and health as a framework, *J Rehabil Med* 44:396–405, 2012.

129. Franki I, et al.: The evidence-base for basic physical therapy techniques targeting lower limb function in children with cerebral palsy: a systematic review using the International Classification of Functioning, Disability and Health as a framework, *J Rehabil Med* 44:385–395, 2012.

130. Reference deleted in proofs.

131. Gajdosik CG, Cicirello N: Secondary conditions of the musculoskeletal system in adolescents and adults with cerebral palsy, *Phys Occup Ther Pediatr* 21:4967, 2001.

132. Gan D, et al.: Giving Youth a Voice (GYC): a measure of youth's perceptions of the client-centeredness of rehabilitation services, *Can J Occup Ther* 75:96–109, 2008.

133. Reference deleted in proofs.

134. Gericke T: Postural management for children with cerebral palsy: consensus statement, *Dev Med Child Neurol* 48:244, 2006.

135. Gibson BE, et al.: Children's and parents' beliefs regarding the value of walking: rehabilitation implications for children with cerebral palsy, *Child Care Health Dev* 38:61–69, 2011.

136. Gillet JG, et al.: FAST CP: protocol of a randomized controlled trial of the efficacy of a 12-week combined Functional Anaerobic and Strength Training programme on muscle properties and mechanical gait deficiencies in adolescents and young adults with spastic-type cerebral palsy, *BMJ Open* 5:e008059, 2015.

137. Reference deleted in proofs.

138. Glazebrook CM, Wright FV: Measuring advanced motor skills in children with cerebral palsy: further development of the Challenge module, *Pediatr Phys Ther* 26:201–213, 2014.

139. Gooch JL, Patton CP: Combining botulinum toxin and phenol to manage spasticity in children, *Arch Phys Med Rehabil* 85:1121–1124, 2004.

140. Gorter H, et al.: Changes in endurance and walking ability through functional training in children with cerebral palsy, *Phys Ther* 21:31–37, 2009.

141. Gorter JW, et al.: Use of the GMFCS in infants with CP: the need for reclassification at age 2 years or older, *Dev Med Child Neurol* 50:46–52, 2008.

142. Gorter JW, et al.: Limb distribution, motor impairment, and functional classification of cerebral palsy, *Dev Med Child Neurol* 46:461–467, 2004.

143. Gough M, Shortland AP: Could muscle deformity in children with spastic cerebral palsy be related to an impairment of muscle growth and altered adaptation? *Dev Med Child Neurol* 54:495–499, 2012.

144. Gough M: Serial casting in cerebral palsy: panacea, placebo, or peril? *Dev Med Child Neurol* 49:725, 2007.

145. Gough M: Continuous postural management and the prevention of deformity in children with cerebral palsy: an appraisal, *Dev Med Child Neurol* 51:105–110, 2009.

146. Reference deleted in proofs.

147. Reference deleted in proofs.

148. Grunt S, et al.: Selection criteria for selective dorsal rhizotomy in children with spastic cerebral palsy: a systematic review of the literature, *Dev Med Child Neurol* 56:302–312, 2014.

149. Hadders-Algra M: Early diagnosis and early intervention in cerebral palsy, *Front Neurol* 5:1–13, 2014.

150. Hadders-Algra M: The neuronal group selection theory: promising principles for understanding and treating developmental motor disorders, *Dev Med Child Neurol* 42:707–715, 2000.

151. Hagglund D, Wagner P: Development of spasticity with age in a total population of children with cerebral palsy, *BMC Musculoskelet Disord* 9:150, 2008.

152. Hagglund G, et al.: Prevention of severe contracture might replace multilevel surgery in cerebral palsy: results of a population-based health care programme and new techniques to reduce spasticity, *J Pediatr Orthop B* 14:269–273, 2005.

153. Hallum A: Disability and the transition to adulthood: issues for the disabled child, the family, and the pediatrician, *Curr Prob Pediatr* 25:12–50, 1995.

154. Hanna SE, et al.: Reference curves for the Gross Motor Function Measure: percentiles for clinical description and tracking over time among children with cerebral palsy, *Phys Ther* 88:596–607, 2008.

155. Hanna SE, et al.: Stability and decline in gross motor function among children and youth with cerebral palsy aged 2 to 21 years, *Dev Med Child Neurol* 51:295–302, 2009.

156. Reference deleted in proofs.

157. Hanna SE, et al.: Measurement practices in pediatric rehabilitation: a survey of physical therapists, occupational therapists, and speech-language pathologists in Ontario, *Phys Occup Ther Pediatr* 27:25–42, 2007.

158. Harris SR: Listening to patients' voices: what can we learn? *Physiother Can* 39–47, 2006.

159. Harris SR, Lundgren BD: Joint mobilization for children with central nervous system disorders: indications and precautions, *Phys Ther* 71:890–896, 1991.

160. Harvey A, Gorter JW: Video gait analysis for ambulatory children with cerebral palsy: why, when, where and how, *Gait Posture* 33:501–503, 2011.

161. Reference deleted in proofs.

162. Harvey A, et al.: A systematic review of measures of activity limitation for children with cerebral palsy, *Dev Med Child Neurol* 50:190–198, 2008.

163. Hawamdeh ZM, et al.: Long-term effect of botulinum toxin (A) in the management of calf spasticity in children with diplegic cerebral palsy, *Europa Medicophysica* 43:311–318, 2007.

164. Hayes B, et al.: Cerebral palsy after maternal trauma in pregnancy, *Dev Med Child Neurol* 49:700–706, 2007.

165. Refernce deleted in proofs.

166. Herman D, et al.: Quantifying weight-bearing by children with cerebral palsy while in passive standers, *Pediatr Phys Ther* 19:283–287, 2007.

167. Hidecker MJC, et al.: Development of the communication function classification system (CFCS) for individuals with cerebral palsy, *Dev Med Child Neurol* 51(Suppl 2):48, 2009.

168. Holsbeeke L, et al.: Capacity, capability, and performance: different constructs or three of a kind? *Arch Phys Med Rehabil* 90:849–855, 2009.

169. Hong T, Paneth N: Maternal and infant thyroid disorders and cerebral palsy, *Sem Perinatol* 32:438–445, 2008.

170. Howle J: *Neuro-developmental treatment approach: theoretical foundations and principles of clinical practice*, Laguna Beach, CA, 2003, North American Neuro-developmental Treatment Association.

171. Huang H, et al.: Modified toy cars for mobility and socialization: case report of a child with cerebral palsy, *Pediatr Phys Ther* 26:76–84, 2014.

172. Hurvitz EA, et al.: Body mass index measures in children with cerebral palsy related to gross motor function classification: a clinic based study, *Am J Phys Med Rehabil* 87:395–403, 2008.

173. Hurvitz EA, et al.: Complementary and alternative medicine use in families of children with cerebral palsy, *Dev Med Child Neurol* 45:364–370, 2003.

174. Hutton JL, Pharoah POD: Life expectancy in severe cerebral palsy, *Arch Dis Child* 91:254–258, 2006.

175. Imms C, et al.: Diversity of participation in children with cerebral palsy, *Dev Med Child Neurol* 50:363–369, 2008.

176. Imms C: Children with cerebral palsy participate: a review of the literature, *Disabil Rehabil* 30:1867–1884, 2008.

177. Innes J, Darrah J: Sedentary behavior: implications for children with cerebral palsy, *Pediatr Phys Ther* 25:402–408, 2013.

178. Jacobs SE, et al.: Cooling for newborns with hypoxic ischaemic encephalopathy, *Cochrane Database Syst Rev* 1: CD003311, 2013.

179. Jahnsen R, et al.: Fatigue in adults with cerebral palsy in Norway compared with the general population, *Dev Med Child Neurol* 45:296–303, 2003.

180. Reference deleted in proofs.

181. Reference deleted in proof.

182. Jaspers E, et al.: Lower limb functioning and its impact on quality of life in ambulatory children with cerebral palsy, *Eur J Paediatr Neurol* 17:561–567, 2013.

183. Johnson BA, et al.: Plyometric training: effectiveness and optimal duration for children with unilateral cerebral palsy, *Pediatr Phys Ther* 26:169–179, 2014.

184. Johnston TE, et al.: Energy cost of walking in children with cerebral palsy: relation to the Gross Motor Function Classification System, *Dev Med Child Neurol* 46:34–38, 2004.

185. Kang M, et al.: Exercise barrier severity and perseverance of active youth with physical disabilities, *Rehabil Psychol* 52:170–176, 2007.

186. Kara OK, et al.: The effects of Kinesio Taping on body functions and activity in unilateral spastic cerebral palsy: a single-blind randomized controlled trail, *Dev Med Child Neurol* 57:81–88, 2014.

187. Refernce deleted in proof.

188. Ketelaar M, et al.: The challenge of moving evidence-based measures into clinical practice: lessons in knowledge translation, *Phys Occup Ther Pediatr* 28:191–206, 2008.

189. Ketelaar M, et al.: Effects of a functional therapy program on motor abilities of children with cerebral palsy, *Phys Ther* 81:1534–1545, 2001.

190. Kibele A: Occupational therapy's role in improving the quality of life for persons with cerebral palsy, *Am J Occup Ther* 43:371–377, 1989.

191. Kilgour G, et al.: Intrarater reliability of lower limb sagittal range-of-motion measures in children with spastic cerebral diplegia, *Dev Med Child Neurol* 45:391–399, 2003.

192. King G, et al.: Understanding paediatric rehabilitation therapists' lack of use of outcome measures, *Disabil Rehabil* 33:2262–2671, 2011.

193. King G, et al.: Predictors of the leisure and recreation participation of children with physical disabilities: a structural equation modeling analysis, *Child Health Care* 35:209–234, 2006.

194. King G, et al.: A conceptual model of the factors affecting the recreation and leisure participation of children with disabilities, *Phys Occup Ther Pediatr* 23:63–90, 2003.

195. King GA, Law, et al.: Measuring children's participation in recreation and leisure activities: construct validation of the CAPE and PAC, *Child Care Health Dev* 33:28–39, 2007.

196. King S, et al.: Family-centered service for children with cerebral palsy and their families: a review of the literature, *Sem Pediatr Neurol* 11:78–86, 2004.

197. Reference deleted in proof.

198. Klenck C, Gebke K: Practical management: common medical problems in disabled athletes, *Clin J Sport Med* 17:55–60, 2007.

199. Kolaski K, Logan LR: A review of the complication of intrathecal baclofen in patients with cerebral palsy, *Neurorehabilitation* 22:383–395, 2007.

200. Korzeniewski SJ, et al.: A systematic review of neuroimaging for cerebral palsy, *J Child Neurol* 23:216–227, 2009.

201. Kragloh-Mann I, et al.: The role of magnetic resonance imaging in elucidating the pathogenesis of cerebral palsy: a systematic review, *Dev Med Child Neurol* 49:144–151, 2007.

202. Kruijsen-Terpstra AJA, et al.: Parents' experiences with physical and occupational therapy for their young child with cerebral palsy: a mixed studies review, *Child Care Health Dev* 40:787–796, 2013.

203. Kruse M, et al.: Lifetime costs of cerebral palsy, *Dev Med Child Neurol* 51:622–629, 2009.

204. Reference deleted in proofs.

205. Kuperminc MN, et al.: Nutritional management of children with cerebral palsy: a practical guide, *Eur J Clin Nutr* 67(Suppl 2):S21–S23, 2013.

206. Kuroda MM, et al.: Association of apolipoprotein E genotype and cerebral palsy in children, *Pediatrics* 119:303–313, 2007.

207. Kwon YH, Lee HY: Differences of respiratory function according to level of the gross motor function classification system in children with cerebral palsy, *J Phys Ther Sci* 26:389–391, 2014.

208. Lagone J, et al.: Technology solutions for young children with developmental concerns, *Infants Young Child* 11:65–78, 1999.

209. Reference deleted in proofs.

210. Reference deleted in proofs.

211. Lannin N, et al.: AACPDM systematic review of the effectiveness of therapy for children with cerebral palsy after botulinum toxin A injections, *Dev Med Child Neurol* 48:533–539, 2006.

212. Laverdure PA, Rose DS: Providing educationally relevant occupational and physical therapy services, *Phys Occup Ther Pediatr* 32:347–354, 2012.

213. Law M, et al.: The Canadian Occupational Performance Measure: an outcome measure for occupational therapy, *Can J Occup Ther* 57:82–87, 1990.

214. Law M, et al.: Factors affecting family-centered service delivery for children with disabilities, *Child Care Health Dev* 29:357–366, 2003.

215. Leiber RL, et al.: Structural and functional changes in spastic skeletal muscle, *Muscle Nerve* 29:615–627, 2004.

216. Legg J, et al.: Surgical correction of scoliosis in children with spastic cerebral palsy: benefits, adverse effects, and patient selection, *Evid Based Spine Care J* 5:38–51, 2014.

217. Reference deleted in proofs.

218. Reference deleted in proofs.

219. Liptak GS: Health and well being of adults with cerebral palsy, *Curr Opin Neurol* 21:136–142, 2008.

220. Livingstone R, Paleg G: Practice considerations for the introduction and use of mobility for children, *Dev Med Child Neurol* 56:210–222, 2014.

221. Reference deleted in proofs.

222. Lobo MA, et al.: Grounding early intervention: physical therapy cannot just be about motor skills anymore, *Phys Ther* 93:94–103, 2013.

223. Love SC, et al.: Botulinum toxin assessment, intervention an after-care for lower limb spasticity in children with cerebral palsy: international consensus statement, *Eur J Neurol* 17(Suppl 2):9–37, 2010.

224. Lovette B: Safe transportation for children with special needs, *J Pediatr Health Care* 22:323–328, 2008.

225. Lundy CT, et al.: Botulinum toxin type A injections can be an effective treatment for pain in children with hip spasms and cerebral palsy, *Dev Med Child Neurol* 51:705–711, 2009.

226. MacKenzie C, McIlwain S: Evidence-based management of postural control in a child with cerebral palsy, *Physiother Can* 67:245–247, 2015.

227. Mackie PC, et al.: The lifestyle assessment questionnaire: an instrument to measure the impact of disability on the lives of children with cerebral palsy and their families, *Child Care Health Dev* 24:473–486, 1998.

228. MacLennan AH, et al.: Cerebral palsy: causes, pathways, and the role of genetic variants, *Am J Obstet Gynecol* 213:779–788, 2015.

229. Majnemer A, editor: *Measures for children with developmental disabilities: an ICF-CY approach. Clinics in Developmental Medicine No. 194-195*, London, 2012, Mac Keith Press.

230. Mattern-Baxter K: Effects of partial body weight supported treadmill training on children with cerebral palsy, *Pediatr Phys Ther* 21:12–22, 2009.

231. Mayston M: From 'one size fits all' to tailor-made physical intervention for cerebral palsy, *Dev Med Child Neurol* 53:969–970, 2011.

232. McCarthy ML, et al.: Comparing reliability and validity of pediatric instruments for measuring health and well-being of children with spastic cerebral palsy, *Dev Med Child Neurol* 44:468–476, 2002.

233. McCoy SW, et al.: Development and validity of the early clinical assessment of balance for young children with cerebral palsy, *Dev Neurorehabil* 17:375–383, 2014.

234. McDonagh MS, et al.: Systematic review of hyperbaric oygen therapy for cerebral palsy: the state of the evidence, *Dev Med Child Neurol* 49: 942–947, 2007.

235. McGinley JL, et al.: Single-event multilevel surgery for children with cerebral palsy: a systematic review, *Dev Med Child Neurol* 54:117–128, 2012.

236. McIntyre S, et al.: Cerebral palsy—don't delay, *Dev Disabil Res Rev* 17:114–129, 2011.

237. Reference deleted in proofs.

238. McPherson AC, et al.: Obesity prevention for children with physical disabilities: a scoping review of physical activity an nutrition interventions, *Disabil Rehabil* 36:1573–1587, 2014.

239. Mergler S, et al.: Epidemiology of low bone mineral density and fractures in children with severe cerebral palsy: a systematic review, *Dev Med Child Neurol* 51:773–778, 2009.

240. Metaxiotis D, et al.: Hip deformities in walking patients with cerebral palsy, *Gait Posture* 11:86–91, 2000.

241. Meyer-Heim A, van Hedel HJ: Robot-assisted and computer enhanced therapies for children with cerebral palsy: current state and clinical implementation, *Sem Pediatr Neurol* 20:139–145, 2013.

242. Meyer-Heim A, et al.: Improvement of walking abilities after robotic-assisted locomotion training in children with cerebral palsy, *Arch Dis Child* 94:615–620, 2009.

243. Michelsen SI, et al.: Frequency of participation of 8-12-year-old children with cerebral palsy: a multi-centre cross-sectional European study, *Eur J Paediatr Neurol* 13:165–177, 2008.

244. Molenaers G, et al.: The effects of quantitative gait assessment and botulinum toxin A on musculoskeletal surgery in children with cerebral palsy, *J Bone Joint Surg Am* 88-A:161–169, 2006.

245. Morgan C, et al.: Enriched environments and motor outcomes in cerebral palsy: systematic review and meta-analysis, *Pediatrics* 132e: e737–e746, 2013.

246. Morgan P, McGinley J: Gait function and decline in adults with cerebral palsy: a systematic review, *Disabil Rehabil* 36:1–9, 2014.

247. Morris C: A review of the efficacy of lower-limb orthoses used for cerebral palsy, *Dev Med Child Neurol* 44:205–211, 2002.

248. Morris C: Child or family assessed measures of activity performance and participation for children with cerebral palsy: a structured review, *Child Care Health Dev* 31:397–407, 2005.

249. Morris C: Aiming to improve the health care of people with cerebral palsy worldwide: a report of an International Society for Prosthetics and Orthotics conference, *Dev Med Child Neurol* 51:689, 2000.

250. Reference deleted in proofs.

251. Morris C, et al.: Do the abilities of children with cerebral palsy explain their activities and participation? *Dev Med Child Neurol* 48:954–961, 2006.

252. Reference deleted in proofs.

253. Motta F, et al.: Effect of intrathecal baclofen on dystonia in children with cerebral palsy and the use of functional scales, *J Pediatr Orthoped* 28:213–217, 2008.

254. Murney ME, et al.: The ecological relevance of the Test of Motor Performance elicited scale items, *Phys Ther* 78:479–489, 1998.

255. Murphy KP, et al.: Employment and social issues in adults with cerebral palsy, *Arch Phys Med Rehabil* 81:807–811, 2000.

256. Murphy NA, Carbone PS: Promoting the participation of children with disabilities in sports, recreation, and physical activities, *Pediatrics* 121:1057–1061, 2008.

257. Mutlu A, et al. Treadmill training with partial body-weight support in children with cerebral palsy: a systematic review, *Dev Med Child Neurol* 51:268–275, 2009.

258. Reference deleted in proofs.

259. Narayanan UG: The role of gait analysis in the orthopedic management of ambulatory cerebral palsy, *Curr Opin Pediatr* 19:38–43, 2007.

260. Narayanan UG, et al.: Initial development and validation of the Caregiver Priorities and Child Health Index of Life with Disabilities (CPCHILD), *Dev Med Child Neurol* 48:804–812, 2006.

261. Nelson KB: Causative factors in cerebral palsy, *Clin Obstet Gynecol* 51:749–762, 2008.

262. Nelson K, Chang T: Is cerebral palsy preventable? *Curr Opin Neurol* 21:129–135, 2008.

263. Noreau L, et al.: Measuring participation in children with disabilities using the Assessment of Life Habits, *Dev Med Child Neurol* 49:666–671, 2007.

264. Novacheck TF, Gage JR: Orthopedic management of spasticity in cerebral palsy, *Child Nerv Syst* 23:1015–1031, 2007.

265. Novak I, et al.: A systematic review of interventions for children with cerebral palsy: state of the evidence, *Dev Med Child Neurol* 55:885–910, 2013.

266. Reference deleted in proofs.

267. Novak I: Parent experience of implementing effective home programs, *Phys Occup Ther Pediatr* 31:198–213, 2011.

268. O'Flaherty S, et al.: Botulinum toxin A adverse events and health status in children with cerebral palsy in all GMFCS levels, *Dev Med Child Neurol* 53:125–130 2011.

269. Nystrom EM, Beckung E: Walking ability is related to muscle strength in children with cerebral palsy, *Gait Posture* 28:366–371, 2008.

270. Olney SJ, et al.: Work and power in hemiplegic cerebral palsy gait, *Phys Ther* 70:431–438, 1990.

271. Oonpuu S, et al.: An evaluation of the posterior leaf spring orthosis using joint kinematics and kinetics, *J Pediatr Orthoped* 16:378–384, 1996.

272. Oskoui M, et al.: An update on the prevalence of cerebral palsy: a systematic review and meta-analysis, *Dev Med Child Neurol* 55:509–519, 2013.

273. Ostensjo S, et al.: Motor impairment in young children with cerebral palsy: relationship to gross motor function and everyday activities, *Dev Med Child Neurol* 46:580–589, 2004.

274. Overeynder JC, Turk MA: Cerebral palsy and aging: a framework for promoting the health of older persons with cerebral palsy, *Topics Geriatr Rehabil* 13:19–24, 1998.

275. Paleg GS, et al. Systematic review and evidence-based clinical recommendations for dosing of pediatric supported standing programs, *Pediatr Phys Ther* 25:232–247, 2013.

276. Paleg G, Livingstone R: Outcomes of gait trainer use in home and school settings for children with motor impairments: a systematic review, *Clin Rehab* 29:1077–1091, 2015.

277. Palisano RJ, et al.: Probability of walking, wheeled, and assisted mobility in children and adolescents with cerebral palsy, *Dev Med Child Neurol* 52:66–71, 2010.

278. Palisano RJ, et al.: Amount and focus of physical therapy and occupational therapy for young children with cerebral palsy, *Phys Occup Ther Pediatr* 32:368–382, 2012.

279. Palisano RJ: A collaborative model of service delivery for children with movement disorders: a framework for evidence-based decision making, *Phys Ther* 86:1295–1305, 2006.

280. Palisano RJ, Marr S: Intensity of therapy services: what are the considerations? *Phys Occup Ther Pediatr* 29:107–112, 2009.

281. Palisano RJ, et al.: Content validity of the expanded and revised Gross Motor Function Classification System, *Dev Med Child Neurol* 50:744–750, 2008.

282. Palisano RJ, et al.: Development and reliability of a system to classify gross motor function in children with cerebral palsy, *Dev Med Child Neurol* 39:214–223, 1997.

283. Palisano RJ: Mobility experiences of adolescents with cerebral palsy, *Phys Occup Ther Pediatr* 29:133–153, 2009.

284. Palisano RJ, et al.: Stability of the Gross Motor Function Classification System, *Dev Med Child Neurol* 48:424–428, 2006.

285. Reference deleted in proofs.

286. Palisano RJ, et al.: Validation of a model of motor development for children with cerebral palsy, *Phys Ther* 80:974–985, 2000.

287. Palmer FB: Strategies for the early diagnosis of cerebral palsy, *J Pediatr* 145:S8–S11, 2004.

288. Park EY, Kim WH: Meta-analysis of the effect of strengthening interventions in individuals with cerebral palsy, *Res Dev Disabil* 35:239–249, 2014.

289. Park ES, et al.: Comparison of anterior and posterior walkers with respect to gait parameters and energy expenditure in children with spastic diplegic cerebral palsy, *Yonsei Med J* 42:180–184, 2001.

290. Reference deleted in proofs.

291. Peterson MD, et al.: Chronic disease risk among adults with cerebral palsy: the role of premature sarcopenia, obesity and sedentary behaviour, *Obesity Rev* 14:171–182, 2013.

292. Pickering DM, et al.: Adapted bikes: what children and young people with cerebral palsy told us about their participation in adapted dynamic cycling, *Disabil Rehabil Assist Technol* 81:30–37, 2013.

293. Reference deleted in proofs.

294. Pin TW, et al.: Use of intrathecal baclofen therapy in ambulant children and adolescents with spasticity and dystonia of cerebral origin: a systematic review, *Dev Med Child Neurol* 53:885–895, 2011.

295. Pin T, et al.: The effectiveness of passive stretching in children with cerebral palsy, *Dev Med Child Neurol* 48:855–862, 2006.

296. Plasschaert VF, et al.: Classification of manual abilities in children with cerebral palsy under 5 years of age: how reliable is the manual ability classification system? *Clin Rehab* 23:164–170, 2009.

297. Reference deleted in proofs.

298. Pueyo R, et al.: Neuropsychologic impairment in bilateral cerebral palsy, *Pediatr Neurol* 40:19–26, 2009.

299. Puras D: Developmental disabilities: challenged for research practices and policies in the 21st century, *Dev Med Child Neurol* 51:415, 2009.

300. Reid A, et al.: "If I knew then what I know now": parents' reflections on raising a child with cerebral palsy, *Phys Occup Ther Pediatr* 31:169–183, 2011.

301. Rice J, Waugh M: Pilot study on trihexyphenidyl in the treatment of dystonia in children with cerebral palsy, *J Child Neurol* 24:176–182, 2009.

302. Rigby P, Gaik S: Stability of playfulness across environmental settings: a pilot study, *Phys Occup Ther Pediatr* 27:27–43, 2007.

303. Roberts A, et al.: Gait analysis to guide a selective dorsal rhizotomy program, *Gait Posture* 42:16–22, 2015.

304. Robinson MN, et al.: Magnetic resonance imaging findings in a population-based cohort of children with cerebral palsy, *Dev Med Child Neurol* 50:39–45, 2008.

305. Roebroeck ME, et al.: Adult outcomes and lifespan issues for people with childhood-onset physical disability, *Dev Med Child Neurol* 51:670–678, 2009.

306. Reference deleted in proofs.

307. Roijen LE, et al.: Development of bladder control in children and adolescents with cerebral palsy, *Child Neurol* 43:103–107, 2001.

308. Rosenbaum P, Gorter JW: The "F-words" in childhood disability: I swear this is how we should think! *Child Care Health Dev* 38:457–463, 2011.

309. Rosenbaum PL: Cerebral palsy: what parents and doctors want to know, *BMJ* 326:970–974, 2003.

310. Rosenbaum P: Variation and abnormality: recognizing the differences, *J Pediatr* 149:593–594, 2006.

311. Rosenbaum P, et al.: Family-centered service: a conceptual framework and research review, *Phys Occup Ther Pediatr* 18:1–20, 1998.

312. Rosenbaum PL, et al.: Development of the Gross Motor Classification System for cerebral palsy, *Dev Med Child Neurol* 50:249–253, 2008.

313. Rosenbaum P, et al.: A report: the definition and classification of cerebral palsy, *Dev Med Child Neurol Suppl* 109:8–14, 2007.

314. Rosenbaum PL, et al.: Prognosis for gross motor function in cerebral palsy: creation of motor development curves, *JAMA* 288:1357–1363, 2007.

315. Ross SA, Engsberg JR: Relation between spasticity and strength in individuals with spastic diplegic cerebral palsy, *Dev Med Child Neurol* 44:148–157, 2002.

316. Reference deleted in proofs.

317. Rowland JL, et al.: The scope of pediatric physical therapy practice in health promotion and fitness for youth with disabilities, *Pediatr Phy Ther* 27:2–15, 2015.

318. Russell DJ, et al.: *Gross Motor Function Measure (GMFM-66 & GMFM-88) user's manual. Clinics in Developmental Medicine*, ed 2, London, 2013, Mac Keith Press.

319. Russell DJ, et al.: Development and validation of item sets to improve efficiency of administration of the Gross Motor Function Measure (GMFM-66) in children with cerebral palsy, *Dev Med Child Neurol* 52:e48–e54, 2010.

320. Russell DJ, Gorter JW: Assessing functional differences in gross motor skills in children with cerebral palsy who use an ambulatory aid or orthoses: can the GMFM-88 help? *Dev Med Child Neurol* 47:462–467, 2005.

321. Russman BS, Ashwal S: Evaluation of the child with cerebral palsy, *Sem Pediatr Neurol* 11:47–57, 2004.

322. Reference deleted in proofs.

323. Ryan SE: An overview of systematic reviews of adaptive seating interventions for children with cerebral palsy: where do we go from here? *Disabil Rehabil Assist Technol* 7:104–111, 2012.

324. Ryll U, et al.: Effects of leg muscle botulinum toxin A injections on walking in children with spasticity-related cerebral palsy: a systematic review, *Dev Med Child Neurol* 53:210–216, 2011.

325. Reference deleted in proofs.

326. Sackett DL, et al.: *Evidence-based medicine: how to practice and teach EBM*, ed 2, Edinburgh, 2000, Churchill Livingstone.

327. Sakzewski L, et al.: Clinimetric properties of participation measure for 5- to 13-year-old children with cerebral palsy: a systematic review, *Dev Med Child Neurol* 49:232–240, 2007.

328. Samdup DZ, et al.: The use of complementary and alternative medicine in children with chronic medical conditions, *Am J Phys Med Rehabil* 85:842–846, 2006.

329. Samson JF, et al.: Muscle power development in preterm infants with periventricular flaring or leukomalacia in relation to outcome at 18 months, *Dev Med Child Neurol* 44:734–740, 2002.

330. Sanger TD, et al.: Definitions and classification of negative motor signs in childhood, *Pediatrics* 118:2159–2167, 2006.

331. Sanger TD, et al.: Classification and definition of disorders causing hypertonia in childhood, *Pediatrics* 111:e89–e97, 2003.

332. Schiariti V, et al.: International Classification of Functioning, Disability, and Health Core Sets for children and youth with cerebral palsy: a consensus meeting, *Dev Med Child Neurol* 57:149–158, 2015.

333. Scholtes VAB, et al.: Clinical assessment of spasticity in children with cerebral palsy: a critical review of available literature, *Dev Med Child Neurol* 48:64–73, 2006.

334. Sellers D, et al.: Development and reliability of a system to classify the eating and drinking ability of people with cerebral palsy, *Dev Med Child Neurol* 56:245–251, 2014.

335. Seniorou M, et al.: Recovery of muscle strength following multi-level orthopedic surgery in diplegic cerebral palsy, *Gait Posture* 26:475–481, 2007.

336. Shortland AP, et al.: Architecture of the medial gastrocnemius in children with spastic diplegia, *Dev Med Child Neurol* 44:158–163, 2002.

337. Siebes RC, et al.: Validation of the Dutch Giving Youth a Voice Questionnaire (GYV-20): a measure of the client-centeredness of rehabilitation services from an adolescent perspective, *Disabil Rehabil* 29:373–380, 2007.

338. Reference deleted in proofs.

339. Simpson DM, et al.: Assessment: botulinum neurotoxin for the treatment of spasticity (an evidence-based review): report of the Therapeutics and Technology Assessment Subcommittee of the American Academy of Neurology, *Neurology* 70:1691–1698, 2008.

340. Smits D, et al.: How do changes in motor capacity, motor capability, and motor performance relate in children and adolescents with cerebral palsy? *Arch Phys Med Rehabil* 95:1577–1584, 2014.

341. Sobsey D, Doe T: Patterns of sexual abuse and assault, *Sex Disabil* 9:243–259, 1991.

342. Spittle AJ, et al.: A systematic review of the clinimetric properties of neuromotor assessments for preterm infants during the first year of life, *Dev Med Child Neurol* 50:254–266, 2008.

343. Stackhouse SK, et al.: Voluntary muscle activation, contractile properties, and fatigability in children with and without cerebral palsy, *Muscle Nerve* 31:594–601, 2005.

344. Steenbeek D, et al.: Goal attainment scaling in pediatric rehabilitation: a critical review of the literature, *Dev Med Child Neurol* 49:550–556, 2007.

345. Sterba JA: Adaptive downhill skiing in children with cerebral palsy: effect on gross motor function, *Pediatr Phys Ther* 18:289–296, 2006.

346. Stevensen RD, et al.: Growth and health in children with moderate-to-severe cerebral palsy, *Pediatrics* 118:1010–1018, 2006.

347. Stout J, et al.: Distal femoral extension osteotomy and patellar tendon advancement to treat persistent crouch gait in cerebral palsy, *J Bone Joint Surg Am* 90:2470–2484, 2008.

348. Strauss D, et al.: Life expectancy in cerebral palsy: an update, *Dev Med Child Neurol* 50:487–493, 2008.

349. Strauss D, et al.: Survival in cerebral palsy in the last 20 years: signs of improvement? *Dev Med Child Neurol* 49:86–92, 2007.

350. Sutcliffe TL, et al.: Cortical reorganization after modified constraint-induced movement therapy in pediatric hemiplegic cerebral palsy, *J Child Neurol* 22:1281–1287, 2007.

351. Swiggum M, et al.: Pain in children with cerebral palsy: implications for pediatric physical therapy, *Pediatr Phys Ther* 22:86–92, 2010.

352. Tardieu C, et al.: For how long must the soleus muscle be stretched each day to prevent contracture? *Dev Med Child Neurol* 30:3–10, 1998.

353. Taylor NF, et al.: Progressive resistance training and mobility-related function in young people with cerebral palsy: a randomized controlled trial, *Dev Med Child Neurol* 55:806–812, 2013.

354. Reference deleted in proofs.

355. Tedroff K, et al.: Long-term effects of botulinum toxin A in children with cerebral palsy, *Dev Med Child Neurol* 51:120–127, 2009.

356. Tervo RC, et al.: Parental report of pain and associated limitations in ambulatory children with cerebral palsy, *Arch Phys Med Rehabil* 87:928–934, 2006.

357. Thompson P, et al.: Test-retest reliability of the 10-metre fast walk test and 6-minute walk test in ambulatory school-aged children with cerebral palsy, *Dev Med Child Neurol* 50:370–376, 2008.

358. Thorpe DE, Valvano J: The effects of knowledge of performance and cognitive strategies on motor skill learning in children with cerebral palsy, *Pediatr Phys Ther* 14:2–15, 2002.

359. Tieman BL, et al.: Variability in mobility of children with cerebral palsy in GMFCS levels II-IV, *Pediatr Phys Ther* 19:180–187, 2007.

360. Tinderholt Myrhaug H, et al.: Intensive training of motor function and functional skills among young children with cerebral palsy: a systematic review and meta-analysis, *BMC Pediatr* 14:292, 2014.

361. Trahan J, Malouin F: Intermittent intensive physiotherapy in children with cerebral palsy: a pilot study, *Dev Med Child Neurol* 44:233–239, 2002.

362. Tustin K, Patel A: A critical evaluation of the updated evidence for casting for equinus deformity in children with cerebral palsy, *Physiother Res Int*, 2015. http://dx.doi.org/10.1002/pri.1646.

363. Unger M, et al.: Strength training in adolescents learners with cerebral palsy: a randomized controlled trial, *Clin Rehab* 20:469–477, 2006.

364. Reference deleted in proofs.

365. Ustad T, et al.: Effects of intensive physiotherapy in infants newly diagnosed with cerebral palsy, *Pediatr Phys Ther* 21:140–149, 2009.

366. Valvano J: Activity-focused motor interventions for children with neurological conditions, *Phys Occup Ther Pediatr* 24:79–107, 2004.

367. Van den Broeck C, et al.: The effect of individually defined physiotherapy in children with cerebral palsy, *Eur J Paediatr Neurol* 14:519–525, 2010.

368. Van Haastert IC, et al.: Early gross motor development of preterm infants according to the Alberta Infant Motor Scale, *J Pediatr* 149:617–622, 2006.

369. Varni JW, et al.: The PedsQL in pediatric cerebral palsy: reliability, validity, and sensitivity of the Generic Core Scales and Cerebral Palsy Module, *Dev Med Child Neurol* 48:442–449, 2006.

370. Verrotti A, et al.: Pharmacotherapy of spasticity in children with cerebral palsy, *Pediatr Neurol* 34:1–6, 2006.

371. Verschuren O, et al.: Muscle strengthening in children with cerebral palsy: considerations for future resistance training protocols, *Phys Ther* 91:1130–1139, 2011.

372. Verschuren O, Balemans ACJ: Update of the core set of exercise, *Pediatr Phys Ther* 27:187–189, 2015.

373. Verschuren O, et al.: Health-enhancing physical activity in children with cerebral palsy: more of the same is not enough, *Phys Ther* 94:297–305, 2014.

374. Verschuren O, et al.: Exercise training program in children and adolescents with cerebral palsy: a randomized controlled trial, *Arch Pediatr Adolesc Med* 161:1075–1081, 2007.

375. Verschuren O, et al.: Exercise programs for children with cerebral palsy: a systematic review of the literature, *Am J Phys Med Rehabil* 87:404–417, 2008.

376. Verschuren O, et al.: Reliability of hand-held dynamometry and functional strength tests for the lower extremity in children with cerebral palsy, *Disabil Rehabil* 30:1358–1366, 2007.

377. Reference deleted in proofs.

378. Reference deleted in proofs.

379. Vos-Vromans DC, et al.: Responsiveness of evaluative measures for children with cerebral palsy: the Gross Motor Function Measure and the Pediatric Evaluation of Disability Inventory, *Disabil Rehabil* 27:1245–1252, 2005.

380. Wang HH, et al.: Reliability, sensitivity to change, and responsiveness of the Peabody Developmental Motor Scales second edition for children with cerebral palsy, *Phys Ther* 86:1351–1359, 2006.

381. Waters E, et al : Psychometric properties of the quality of life questionnaire for children with CP, *Dev Med Child Neurol* 49:49–55, 2007.

382. Waters E, et al : Quality of life instruments for children and adolescents with neurodisabilities: how to choose the appropriate instrument, *Dev Med Child Neurol* 51:660–669, 2009.

383. Watt J, et al.: Early prognosis for ambulation of neonatal intensive care survivors with cerebral palsy, *Dev Med Child Neurol* 31:766–773, 1989.

384. Reference deleted in proofs.

385. Welsh B, et al.: How might districts identify local barriers to participation for children with cerebral palsy? *Public Health* 120:167–175, 2006.

386. Westberry DE, et al.: Impact of ankle-foot orthoses on static foot alignment in children with cerebral palsy, *J Bone Joint Surg Am* 89:806–813, 2007.

387. Reference deleted in proofs.

388. Wiart L, et al.: Stretching with children with cerebral palsy: what do we know and where are we going? *Pediatr Phys Ther* 20:173–178, 2008.

389. Wiegeriak DJ, et al.: Social, intimate and sexual relationships of adolescents with cerebral palsy compared with able-bodies age-mates, *J Rehabil Med* 40:112–118, 2006.

390. Wiegerink D, et al.: Sexuality of young adults with cerebral palsy: experienced limitations and needs, *Sex Disabil* 29:119–128, 2011.

391. Willoughby K, et al.: The impact of botulinum toxin A and abduction bracing on long-term hip development in children with cerebral palsy, *Dev Med Child Neurol* 54:743–747, 2012.

392. Wilson A, et al.: Development and pilot testing of the challenge module: a proposed adjunct to the Gross Motor Function Measure for high-functioning children with cerebral palsy, *Phys Occup Ther Pediatr* 31:135–149, 2011.

393. Wittenberg GF: Neural plasticity and treatment across the lifespan for motor deficits in cerebral palsy, *Dev Med Child Neurol* 51(Suppl 4):130–133, 2009.

394. Woods JJ, Lindeman DP: Gathering and giving information with families, *Infants Young Child* 21:272–284, 2008.

395. Woodside JM, et al.: Family-centered service: developing and validating a self-assessment tool for paediatric service providers, *J Child Health Care* 30:237–252, 2001.

396. Wright FV, et al.: The Quality Function Measure: reliability and discriminant validity of a new measure of quality of gross motor movement in ambulatory children with cerebral palsy, *Dev Med Child Neurol* 56:770–778, 2014.

397. Wright FV, Majnemer A: The concept of a toolbox of outcome measures for children with cerebral palsy: why, what, and how to use? *J Child Neurol* 29:1055–1065, 2014.

398. Wright MJ, et al: *Ethics in childhood neurodisability: cases, principles and clinical practice*, London, in press, Mac Keith Press.

399. Wright MJ, et al.: Sleep issues in families of children with physical disabilities, *Phys Occup Ther Pediatr* 26:55–72, 2003.

400. Wright FV, et al.: How do changes in body functions and structures, activity, and participation relate in children with cerebral palsy? *Dev Med Child Neurol* 50:283–289, 2008.

401. Wright M, Bartlett DJ: Distribution of contractures and spinal malalignments in adolescents with cerebral palsy, *Dev Neurorehabil* 13:46–52, 2010.

402. Wright PA, et al.: Neuromuscular electrical stimulation for children with cerebral palsy: a review, *Arch Dis Child* 97:364–371, 2012.

403. Wynter M, et al.: Australian hip surveillance guideline for children with cerebral palsy: 5-year review, *Dev Med Child Neurol* 57:808–820, 2015.

404. Young NL, et al.: Measurement properties of the Activity Scales for Kids, *J Clin Epidemiol* 53:125–137, 2000.

405. Ziv I, et al.: Muscle growth in normal and spastic mice, *Dev Med Child Neurol* 26:94–99, 1984.

406. Zwick EB, et al.: Propulsive function during gait in diplegic children: evaluation after surgery for gait improvement, *J Pediatr Orthop Br* 10:226–233, 2001.

SUGGESTED READINGS

Bania T, Dodd KJ, Taylor N: Habitual physical activity can be increased in people with cerebral palsy: a systematic review, *Clin Rehab* 25:303–315, 2011.

Bloemen MAT, Backx FJG, Takken T, et al.: Factors associated with physical activity in children and adolescents with a physical disability: a systematic review, *Dev Med Child Neurol* 57:137–148, 2015.

Cahill-Rowley K, Rose J: Etiology of impaired selective motor control: emerging evidence and its implications for research and treatment in cerebral palsy, *Dev Med Child Neurol* 56:522–528, 2013.

Dewar R, Love S, Johnston LM: Exercise interventions improve postural control in children with cerebral palsy: a systematic review, *Dev Med Child Neurol* 57:504–520, 2015.

Gannoti ME, Christy JB, Heathcock JC, Kolobe THA: A path model for evaluating dosing parameters for children with cerebral palsy, *Phys Ther* 94:411–421, 2014.

Gibson BE, Teachman G, Wright V, et al.: Children's and parents' beliefs regarding the value of walking: rehabilitation implications for children with cerebral palsy, *Child Care Health Dev* 38:61–69, 2011.

Hadders-Algra M: Early diagnosis and early intervention in cerebral palsy, *Front Neurol* 5:1–13, 2014.

Livingstone R, Paleg G: Practice considerations for the introduction and use of mobility for children, *Dev Med Child Neurol* 56:210–222, 2014.

Park EY, Kim WH: Meta-analysis of the effect of strengthening interventions in individuals with cerebral palsy, *Res Dev Disabil* 35:239–249, 2014.

Penner M, Xie WY, Binepal N, et al.: Characteristics of pain in children and youth with cerebral palsy, *Pediatrics* 132:e407–e413, 2013.

Rosenbaum P, Gorter JW: The "F-words" in childhood disability: I swear this is how we should think! *Child Care Health Dev* 38:457–463, 2011.

Sakzewski L, Ziviani J, Boyd RN: Efficacy of upper limb therapies for unilateral cerebral palsy: a meta-analysis, *Pediatr Phys Ther* 26:28–37, 2014.

Verschuren O, Darrah J, Novak I, et al.: Health-enhancing physical activity in children with cerebral palsy: more of the same is not enough, *Phys Ther* 94:297–305, 2014.

Vos RC, Becher JG, Ketalaar M, et al.: Developmental trajectories of daily activities in children and adolescents with cerebral palsy, *Pediatrics* 132:e915–e923, 2013.

20

Brachial Plexus Injury

Susan V. Duff, Darl Vander Linden

This chapter focuses on perinatal brachial plexus injury (PBPI), yet the concepts presented apply to resultant impairments, activity limitations, and participation restrictions caused by brachial plexus injury in children at any age. Therapists may work with infants and children with PBPI in a variety of settings, including early intervention programs, acute care hospitals, and specialty clinics. Therapists may also be involved with this population after microsurgical repair to the brachial plexus in infants or after shoulder reconstruction in toddlers and older children. This chapter reviews the etiology and pathophysiology, examination, procedural interventions, family education, and medical management of children with PBPI.

BACKGROUND INFORMATION

ETIOLOGY AND INCIDENCE

A traction injury to the brachial plexus (Fig. 20.1) can occur during a difficult delivery.[28] During a vaginal delivery, forceful traction and rotation of the head during a vertex presentation to deliver the shoulder tends to injure the C5 and C6 roots or the associated nerves. Traction on the newborn's shoulder during delivery of the head in a breech delivery can injure the cervical roots or nerves, fracture the clavicle or humerus, or cause a subluxation of the shoulder. The likelihood of injury to the brachial plexus drops from 0.2% to 0.02% during delivery by cesarean section.[28] Associated damage to the phrenic nerve at C4 is less common but will cause ipsilateral hemiparesis of the diaphragm. Congenital anomalies such as a cervical rib, abnormal thoracic vertebrae, or a shortened scalenus anticus muscle can also cause pressure on the lower plexus.[62]

The incidence of PBPI has been reported to range from 0.38 to 5.1 per 1000.[14,21,34,78] Risk factors that can contribute to PBPI include shoulder dystocia (catching of the shoulder), birth weight greater than the 90th percentile (4500–5000 g), prolonged maternal labor, maternal gestational diabetes, and breech delivery.[1,19,29,51,78] In a prospective study of 62 infants with PBPI of whom 17 had permanent impairment, 16 of the 17 infants had birth weights over 3500 g and only 1 of the 17 had a birth weight less than 3500 g. Twelve of 13 infants (92%) diagnosed with PBPI at birth who weighed less than 3500 g had full recovery of function, but only 67% of infants (33 of 49) who weighed more than 3500 g had full recovery.[78]

PATHOPHYSIOLOGY

Damage to the nerve structure can occur at the level of the nerve rootlets attached to the spinal cord, at the anterior or posterior rootlets (distal to where the rootlets coalesce to form the mixed nerve root that exits the vertebral canal), or in the spinal nerve itself.[79] Roots, trunks, divisions, cords, and peripheral nerves can all suffer neurotmesis (complete rupture), axonotmesis (disruption of axons while the endoneurium remains intact), or neurapraxia (temporary nerve conduction block with intact axons).[65,79] Partial or complete rupture may evolve into a neuroma and a mass of fibrous tissue as disorganized neurons on the proximal end attempt to reach the distal end.

Recovery is usually limited after ruptures and often requires microsurgical repair. Prognosis after axonotmesis is better as the neurons reconnect more successfully through the intact endoneurium. Axon regrowth reportedly proceeds at approximately 1 mm per day.[65] Given this timeline, recovery in most infants with PBPI can take up to 4 to 6 months in the upper arm and 7 to 9 months in the lower arm.[65] Continued recovery can occur for up to 2 years in the upper arm and 4 years in the lower arm.[22] Early recovery after neurapraxia occurs as edema resolves and is usually quick and complete, sometimes within days or weeks.[34] Among infants and children with PBPI, a combination of these types of lesions is common. Furthermore, axon regrowth in young children may be quicker due to neuroplasticity and the shorter growth distance, which may explain the variability of the return of motor function in individual muscles.

NATURAL HISTORY AND PROGNOSIS

The natural history and recovery of PBPI are difficult to determine because few studies have followed children over a long period of time and authors have primarily used outcome measures of impairment and not of activity and participation. In early studies, a recovery rate of 80% to over 90% was reported.[10,50] As a result, a favorable prognosis has been perceived for the majority of infants with PBPI. More recent studies, however, have reported recovery rates of 66% to 73%.[34,54] Thus, close to 35% of infants and children do not fully recover. In a systematic review designed to describe the natural history of PBPI, Pondaag and colleagues[60] examined the literature on PBPI outcomes. The inclusion criteria were (1) a prospective design, (2) all children with PBPI from a demographic area be followed, (3) a minimum follow-up of 3 years with < 10% loss to follow-up, and (4) use of a well-defined outcome measure with a reproducible scoring system and no surgical intervention. Of the 103 identified articles, none met even three of the four criteria defined for the systematic review, but 27 of the 103 met two criteria. Based on the findings, the authors concluded that the excellent prognosis often cited for PBPI was not based on sound scientific evidence.[60]

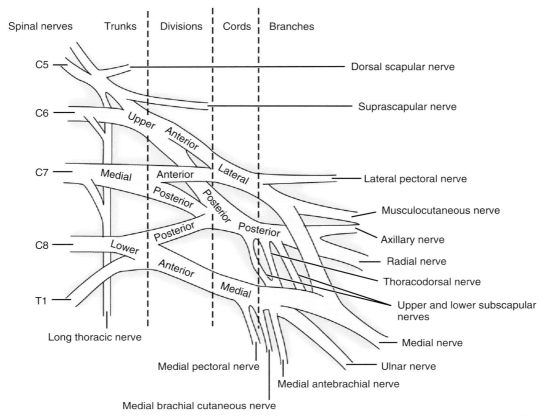

FIG. 20.1 The brachial plexus. Injury can occur at any point along the nerves as they branch off the spinal cord and weave into the brachial plexus. (Redrawn from Waters PM: Obstetric brachial plexus palsy, *J Am Acad Orthop Surg* 5:205-214, 1997.)

Estimates of spontaneous recovery from PBPI are difficult to establish because many children have neurapraxic lesions that resolve within a few days or weeks so these children are not included in many follow-up studies. Hoeksma and colleagues[34] found, in fact, that 34% of infants (19 of 56) diagnosed with PBPI at birth had full recovery by 3 weeks of age. However, they also found that 32% (18 of 56) had "late" recovery by 1 year of age, and 19 of 56 (34%) did not have full recovery of muscle strength when assessed at a mean age of 3 years. The authors indicated that if the criteria for a "good" outcome as described by Michelow and colleagues[50] of "more than ½ of normal range of shoulder and elbow motion" had been used with their cohort of 56 children, 93% would have had a "good" outcome.[33] DiTaranto and colleagues[13] followed 91 infants in Argentina who did not have access to neurosurgical intervention for at least 2 years. They reported that although 69% had full recovery, 18% of infants had minimal recovery and 13% had global PBPI with flaccid and insensate arms.

The differences reported in the natural history and outcomes for children with PBPI make it difficult for parents and professionals to accurately predict to what extent children will recover postinjury. Studies have begun to use outcome measures standardized for infants and children with PBPI such as the Active Movement Scale[10] and the Modified Mallet Scale.[2] Although more recent reports have specifically defined outcomes based on strength of specific muscle groups,[34,35] few studies report outcomes in terms of activity limitations and participation restrictions in children, adolescents, and adults.

CHANGES IN BODY STRUCTURE AND FUNCTION

Injury Classification and General Impairments

Injury can occur at any level of the brachial plexus, but the most common injury is to the upper plexus (C5 and C6) resulting in a condition referred to as Erb's palsy.[28] Strombeck and colleagues reported that of 247 children followed for PBPI, 52% had C5-C6 involvement and an additional 34% had C5-C7 involvement.[63] As a result of injury to the fibers from the upper plexus, the child's shoulder is usually held in extension, internal rotation, and adduction; the elbow is extended; the forearm is pronated; and the wrist and fingers are flexed in the *waiter's tip* position (Fig. 20.2). Paralysis or decreased activation of the rhomboids, levator scapulae, serratus anterior, subscapularis, deltoid, supraspinatus, infraspinatus, teres minor, biceps, brachialis, brachioradialis, supinator, and long extensors of the wrist, fingers, and thumb can be expected. Grasp is left intact, but sensation may be diminished or lost. Elbow and finger extension are compromised if C7 is also involved and are referred to as an extended Erb's palsy.

Global palsy involves injury to the upper and lower plexus (C5-T1) resulting in paralysis or decreased activation of all muscles of the affected arm with loss of or diminished sensation.[28] Strombeck and colleagues reported that 13% of the children with PBPI in their follow-up study had involvement of the C5-T1 roots.[63] Involvement is usually unilateral but has been reported to be bilateral in a low percentage of children.[71] The pattern of motor loss does not always fit the classic definitions,

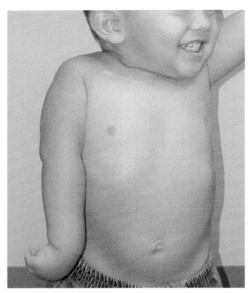

FIG. 20.2 Child with Erb's palsy, a C5-C6 brachial plexus injury, resulting in the *waiter's tip* position of the UE, which is typically observed with this type of injury. (From Shenaq SM, Bullocks JM, Dhillon G: Management of infant brachial plexus injuries, *Clin Plast Surg* 32:79-98, 2005.)

indicating incomplete or mixed upper and lower types of injury. Horner's syndrome, as a result of T1 root avulsion, or the sympathetic ganglion, can cause deficient sweating, recession of the eyeball, abnormal pupillary contraction, myosis, ptosis, and irises of different colors.[14]

Klumpke's palsy by definition involves only the lower roots or spinal nerves C8-T1.[37] In a 1995 review, Al-Qattan and colleagues found Klumpke's palsy in only 20 of 3508 cases of PBPI reported in the papers they reviewed, for an incidence of only 0.6%.[3] When pure Klumpke's palsy is present, the child's shoulder and elbow movements are not impaired, but the resting position of the forearm is typically in supination with paralysis of the wrist flexor and extensor muscles and the intrinsic muscles of the wrist and hand.

Positional torticollis can develop as a result of the infant's head being habitually positioned away from the affected arm, or it may be present from the same trauma that caused the PBPI.[31] In addition, some infants develop plagiocephaly from prolonged positioning. See Chapter 9 for more information regarding examination of and interventions for torticollis and plagiocephaly.

During the period of neural regeneration following PBPI, infants and toddlers use muscle substitutions that are the most advantageous given the strength of the available innervated muscles. For example, internal rotation at the shoulder, combined with forearm pronation and wrist flexion, is often used to obtain objects. Neglect of the affected extremity may occur due to diminished sensibility or the comparative ease with which the opposite arm and hand can accomplish a task. Some infants also demonstrate self-mutilation of the limb such as biting if there is diminished sensation.[45] Patterns of substitution, neglect, or abuse are reinforced with repetition. The problems that arise from these repetitive patterns include soft tissue and muscle contractures, muscle atrophy, and abnormal bone growth. The contractures most likely to develop are scapular

protraction; shoulder extension, adduction, and internal rotation; and elbow flexion. Contractures into forearm pronation as well as wrist and finger flexion may occur in those with severe injury or Klumpke's palsy. These patterns will obviously vary depending on the denervation pattern.

Shoulder Impairment

As the infant develops, persistent muscle imbalance and habitual posturing contribute to common anatomic changes in the shoulder. These changes can include flattening of the humeral head, an abnormally short clavicle, humeral head hypoplasia, posterior subluxation of the humeral head, an irregular glenoid fossa, ligamentous pathology, and muscle tightness.[24,33,39] These deficits correlate with a loss of passive and active shoulder external rotation (ER) along with other changes in shoulder biomechanics.[14,39] The mean glenohumeral-to-scapulothoracic (GH-to-ST) ratio in typically developing children is reportedly 1.3 to 1 in children 6.7 ± 1.5 years[12] and 1.43 to 1 in children 9.12 ± 1.51 years.[27] Duff and colleagues[15] examined the GH-to-ST ratio in children 7.81 ± 2.93 years who sustained PBPI yet had not undergone microsurgery or shoulder reconstruction. During active abduction in the scapular plane, the authors found a mean loss in the GH-to-ST ratio (0.6 to 1) in the affected arm of children with limited arm elevation (< 75°). This first group of children tended to rely on scapular upward rotation versus GH joint elevation to raise the affected arm. Children who could raise the affected arm 75° and above displayed a mean GH-to-ST ratio of 1.7 to 1 during shoulder range of 15° to 75°. Thus, the GH joint of the second group made a greater contribution to arm elevation in the affected arm.

ACTIVITY AND PARTICIPATION LIMITATIONS

Activity limitations will vary greatly, depending on the extent of the initial pathology, neurologic regeneration, and residual impairments. The primary activity limitations in children with PBPI relate to reach-to-grasp skills and the performance of tasks that require bilateral arm use such as catching a large ball or lifting a large object. Activities of daily living (ADLs) that require bilateral upper extremity (UE) use will be compromised. These activities would include donning and removing shirts and pants, tying shoes, and securing fasteners. Studies that examine the nature and extent of activity limitations such as dressing and eating or participation restrictions are emerging.[32]

Typical developmental activities may be compromised as a result of PBPI. Transitions from prone or supine to sitting could habitually be done from one side, thereby asymmetrically strengthening one side of the trunk or delaying development of balance reactions. The developmental milestone of creeping on all fours may not occur or may be adapted because the child may not be able to safely bear weight on the affected arm or may not be able to extend the wrist sufficiently. The child may also scoot around while sitting or progress directly to walking at the appropriate age.

Neglect of the affected limb during activity and self-abusive behavior such as biting can occur because of diminished sensory awareness.[46] Injuries such as burns, insect bites, and abrasions may go unnoticed if sensibility is severely compromised. Shoulder pain and neuritis in adults are complications that can interfere not only with the function of the affected arm but also with other aspects of the individual's social or vocational activities.

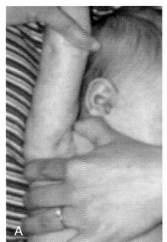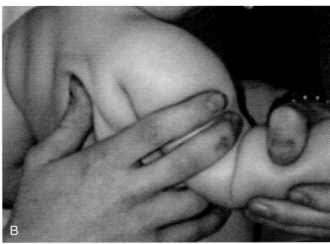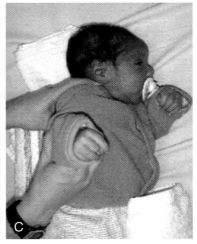

FIG. 20.3 Stabilization of the scapula during passive ROM: A, Lateral stabilization during humeral elevation. B, Medial and superior stabilization during humeral external rotation. C, Medial and superior stabilization during humeral external rotation in sidelying. (Images courtesy of SV Duff. From Duff SV, DeMatteo C: Clinical assessment of the infant and child following perinatal brachial plexus injury, *J Hand Therapy* 28:126-134, 2016.)

FOREGROUND INFORMATION

THERAPEUTIC EXAMINATION

Clinical examination of the neonate with PBPI may be requested before discharge from the hospital. Infants and children may also be referred to therapy in the days, weeks, months, or years after the initial injury. An examination of active and passive range of motion (ROM), posture, pain, sensory status, and visual skills is key in establishing a baseline of early function and capability.[4] Screening the developmental status of the infant or child will ensure that other pathologic conditions are not missed. In the infant, frequent reexamination documents motor and sensory recovery as neural regeneration occurs. These data aid in program planning, whether it be therapeutic exercise, positioning, splinting, determining eligibility for surgery, or establishing readiness for discharge from intervention.

Impairments
Imaging: Electromyography
Neonatally, radiographs are taken to assess for clavicular or humeral fractures.[79] Infants not showing evidence of recovery may initially undergo imaging between 1 and 6 months of age, yet the exact timing of testing varies. Imaging is frequently done to examine the integrity of the nerve roots and neural structure as well as the integrity of the glenohumeral joint. Imaging in the form of magnetic resonance imaging (MRI), electrodiagnostic studies, computed tomography (CT), CT with metrizamide (CT-myelogram), and ultrasound can be used diagnostically and to aid in surgical planning.[2,47,69] CT myelography and MRI are the most frequent modes used to examine nerve structures.[79] Noninvasive ultrasound of the glenohumeral joint[72] between 3 and 6 months of age is reportedly useful to diagnose posterior subluxation of the humeral head.[61] Imaging studies are often repeated in older infants and children to examine glenohumeral joint structure before shoulder reconstruction. However, imaging does not replace the careful physical examination of the clinical and functional consequences of neurologic damage and neural regeneration.

Electromyography (EMG), although of little prognostic value, can determine the extent of involvement and is often recommended as a preoperative baseline.[64,69,70] Repeated EMG testing can alert the clinician to muscles that are undergoing reinnervation before obvious motor changes occur. Findings from diagnostic EMG have been used to assess the extent and severity of the lesion, but they may not correlate well with findings upon surgical exploration.[30] Reinnervation after microsurgery can be identified by EMG immediately after surgery or in the following weeks and months, before clinical signs of motor return are present. This information may alter therapeutic goals and intervention strategies, and it may change a patient's prognosis significantly.

Range of Motion
At any age, passive ROM measurements of the affected arm and cervical area are performed and compared with the contralateral side. Initially, movements should be performed with great care because the child's joints can be unstable[38] and the child may be experiencing pain or diminished/absent sensibility in the affected limb. It is critical to establish baseline passive ROM with goniometry before examining muscle strength. It is also essential that during passive assessment of the GH joint the scapula is stabilized,[16,24] as shown in Fig. 20.3A-C. Gharbaoui and colleagues[24] published a review of the anatomic changes in the GH joint and shoulder in children with perinatal brachial plexus palsy. The authors recommend measuring five shoulder motions: (1) scapulohumeral (SH) angle in abduction, (2) SH angle in adduction, (3) SH angle in horizontal adduction, (4) GH internal rotation (IR) arc of motion in 90° abduction and 90° elbow flexion, and (5) GH ER arc of motion in 90° abduction and 90° elbow flexion. The reader is referred to this article for a full description and photos of the measurement positions and goniometry placement.

Muscle Strength and Motor Function
In the infant, clinicians can observe limb movement or palpate muscle contractions when testing a variety of responses

TABLE 20.1 Active Movement Scale

15 Active Motions*	Grade
Gravity Minimized	
No contraction	0
Isometric contraction, no motion	1
Motion ≤ ½ available passive range	2
Motion > ½ available passive range	3
Full motion	4
Against Gravity	
Motion ≤ ½ available passive range	5
Motion > ½ available passive range	6
Full motion	7

*Shoulder (abduction, adduction, flexion, external rotation, internal rotation), elbow (flexion, extension), forearm (supination, pronation), wrist (flexion, extension), thumb (flexion, extension). Full active range of motion with gravity minimized (grade 4) must be achieved before active range against gravity is scored (grades 5 to 7).
From Clarke HM, Curtis GC: An approach to obstetrical brachial plexus injuries, Hand Clin 11:567, 1995.

and reflexes/reactions such as visual tracking, asymmetrical neck righting reflex, the Moro reflex, the Galant reflex, or the hand-placing reaction.[16] Arm and head movement can be observed during wakeful play periods as a child tries to bring the hand to the mouth or reach for a toy. Care should be taken to document whether movements are made with gravity minimized or against gravity. Asymmetry of abdominal and thoracic movement may indicate phrenic nerve paralysis.

A muscle grading system, titled the Active Movement Scale (AMS) has been developed specifically for infants and children with PBPI to capture subtle but significant changes in active movement of the arm (Table 20.1).[10] This measure has been shown to have adequate interrater reliability and validity to accurately measure motor function of the UE in infants younger than 1 year of age.[11] Curtis and colleagues also provided a review of other measures of impairment that have been used for children with PBPI including the British Medical Research Council (BMRC) system of manual muscle testing and the modified BMRC that uses a 4-point scale (M0 to M3) to measure muscle activity.[11]

Older children can be examined using standard manual muscle tests and dynamometers to obtain an objective measure of muscle strength (see Chapters 2 and 5 for more information on strength testing in children). Patterns of movement, atypical substitution patterns, and posturing of the arm as a result of muscle imbalance and diminished or absent sensation should be documented. The Mallet classification of UE function can be used for children older than 3 to 4 years of age and has been shown to be reliable when used with children with PBPI.[6, 44] The Modified Mallet (Fig. 20.4)[2] expands on the original Mallet scale with the addition of a sixth item, IR with elbow flexion to the abdomen from a position of 90° shoulder abduction.

The impairments present in PBPI do not include spasticity. As a result, any spasticity identified during the examination would suggest an upper motor neuron lesion warranting further diagnostic evaluation by the child's primary physician or neurologist.

Sensation

Narakas[53] developed the Sensory Grading System for children with PBPI. A grade of S0 is regarded as no reaction to painful or other stimuli; S1 is reaction to painful stimuli, none to touch; S2 is reaction to touch, not to light touch; and S3 is regarded as normal sensation. Diminished or absent sensation does not necessarily correspond to the extent of motor impairment;[18] therefore, care should be taken not to ignore this component of the examination in children with milder involvement.

As neural regeneration proceeds, sensory loss may change to hyperesthesia before progressing through diminished or normal sensation.[53] Infants or older children may experience pain or discomfort in reaction to sensory stimulation and touch. This change should be documented and may indicate progression of neural regeneration. More definitive sensory testing to touch pressure, light touch, and two-point discrimination is possible in older children, and specific areas of diminished sensibility can be mapped. Sensation may take as long as 2 years to recover.[53]

Pain

Light palpation to the affected neck and upper shoulder may induce a pain response such as grimacing in an infant or child with PBPI. Active movement as elicited with visual tracking can provide further information on the influence pain may have on neck motion and visual scanning. These behavioral cues can be used to rate pain on the Face, Legs, Activity, Cry, Consolability (FLACC) scale. The FLACC rates pain on a score of 0 to 2 based on behavioral cues from five categories: face, legs, activity, cry, and consolability.[49] Many clinical sites have adopted the resultant 0-to-10 FLACC scale to objectively measure pain in infants. The Wong-Faces pain rating scale[77] is recommend to assess pain in older children.

Activity and Participation

Developmental tests of gross and fine motor performance can be used to establish and track any delays caused by the UE impairment and dysfunction in infants and toddlers. Although no research exists on its use in PBPI, the Test of Infant Motor Performance (TIMP) may be useful for infants younger than 4 months of age postterm to document changes in motor function because it has nine activities that are scored independently for each side of the body.[9] Another useful gross motor assessment standardized for use with children 0 to 18 months of age is the Alberta Infant Motor Scale (AIMS).[59] Gross screens can be conducted to assess the ability the older child has to perform functional activities such as bringing the hand to mouth for eating, bringing the hand to the head for brushing hair, and sufficiently holding select tools (e.g., toothbrush) for their intended use. Taking a video of these activities would allow comparison with follow-up testing.

For older children, anecdotal information about activity limitations and participation such as difficulty with ADLs, carrying a tray at school for lunch, or playing a recorder should be documented.[66] Fortunately, specific measures of activity and participation for use with children with PBPI have been developed.[32,41] The Brachial Plexus Outcome Measure (BPOM) and the BPOM Activity Scale were designed for children 4 to 19 years of age. The BPOM tests the quality of UE movement during completion of 11 activities aimed at measuring the key deficient functional movement patterns in children with brachial plexus palsy. Performance is graded on a 5-point ordinal scale based on task completion and visible movement quality. The Assisting Hand Assessment (AHA)[41] and the Mini-AHA[25] assess the bimanual skills of children with unilateral cerebral

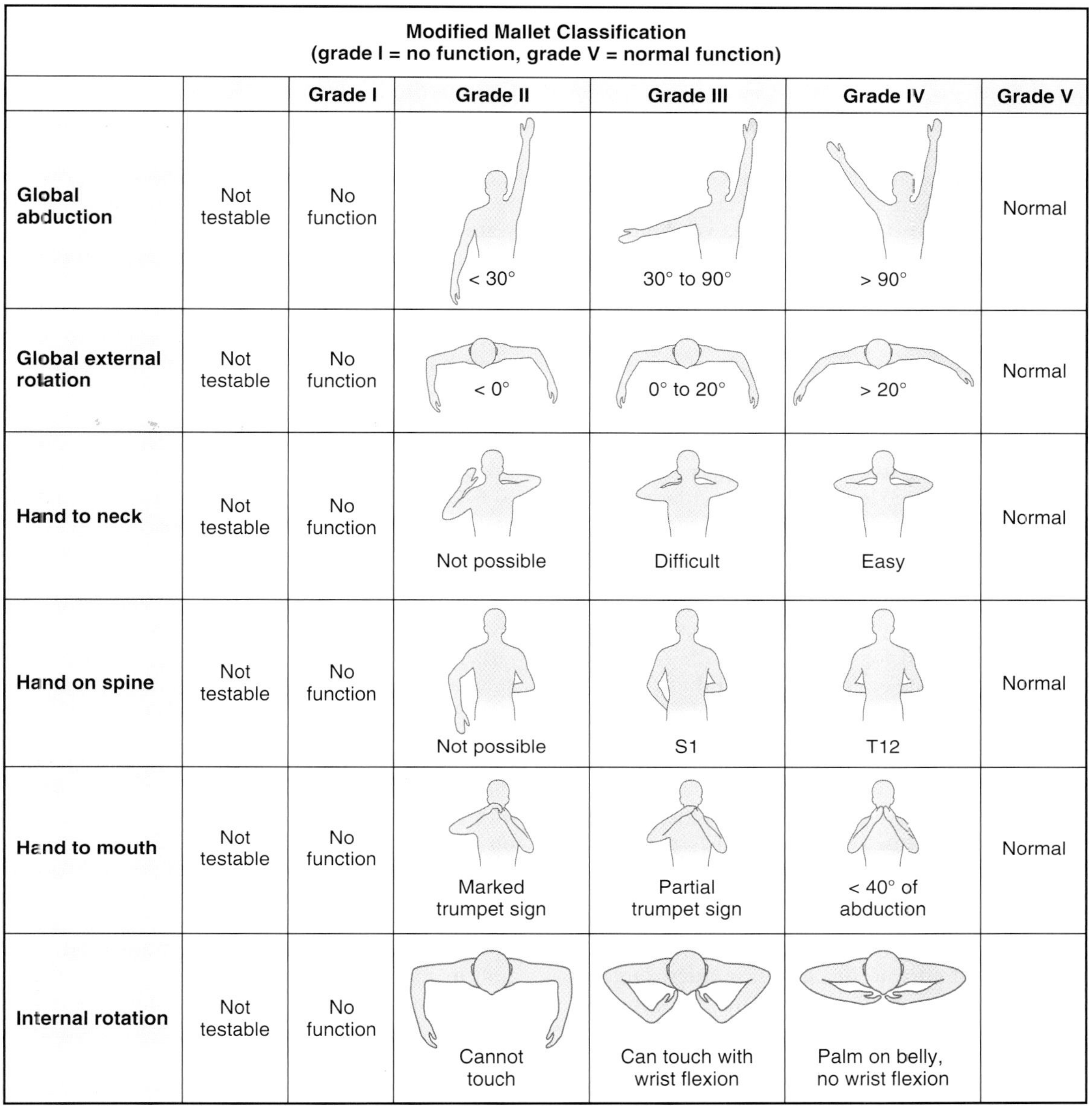

Modified Mallet Classification (grade I = no function, grade V = normal function)						
		Grade I	Grade II	Grade III	Grade IV	Grade V
Global abduction	Not testable	No function	< 30°	30° to 90°	> 90°	Normal
Global external rotation	Not testable	No function	< 0°	0° to 20°	> 20°	Normal
Hand to neck	Not testable	No function	Not possible	Difficult	Easy	Normal
Hand on spine	Not testable	No function	Not possible	S1	T12	Normal
Hand to mouth	Not testable	No function	Marked trumpet sign	Partial trumpet sign	< 40° of abduction	Normal
Internal rotation	Not testable	No function	Cannot touch	Can touch with wrist flexion	Palm on belly, no wrist flexion	

FIG. 20.4 Modified Mallet's classification of function in brachial plexus palsy. Grade 0 (not shown) is no movement in the desired plane, and grade V (not shown) is full movement. (From Skirven TM, Osterman AL, Fedorczyk JM, et al.: *Rehabilitation of the hand and upper extremity*, ed 6, Philadelphia, 2011, Mosby.)

palsy or who sustained brachial plexus injury. The AHA is standardized for children 18 months to 12 years and the Mini-AHA for children 8 to 18 months of age. The AHA, Mini-AHA, and the BPOM are criterion-referenced tools designed to measure how effectively children with unilateral dysfunction actually use the affected hand and arm during bimanual tasks within a play session. These assessment tools could be used to measure change over time or following therapeutic or surgical intervention.

SURGICAL MANAGEMENT

Neurosurgery

For infants who are not displaying sufficient recovery of spontaneous or intentional affected arm motion, microsurgery is recommended. Microsurgical techniques used in the treatment

of PBPI include nerve transfers, nerve grafting, neuroma dissection and removal, neurolysis (decompression and removal of scar tissue), and direct end-to-end anastomosis of the nerve ends.[42,68] The technique chosen depends on the anatomic findings and surgical background of the physician.

Indications and Timing of Neurosurgery

It is typically recommended that microsurgical repair of the brachial plexus be done between 3 and 8 months of age for optimal results with select clinical sites opting for surgery at an earlier age (e.g., 3 months).[7,26] For infants who present with complete paralysis and Horner's syndrome, surgery is highly recommended by 3 months of age.[30] Lack of biceps function and elbow flexion are frequently used to determine which infants with incomplete neural recovery are candidates for surgery.[22,23]

Interestingly, Hoeksma and colleagues found that available shoulder ER and forearm supination were more useful determinants of the need for surgical intervention than elbow flexion.[34] Fisher and colleagues[20] also reported that lack of active elbow flexion is not as useful in determining candidates for surgery as total AMS scores are. Hence, diminished or absent active ER and forearm supination as well as total AMS score may be the most useful criteria for determining if an infant should have microsurgical repair secondary to a brachial plexus lesion.

Outcomes of Neurosurgery

The results from brachial plexus microsurgery are far better in infants than in adults due to the reduced distance, better potential for neural regeneration, and the potential for central adaptation.[68]

Interestingly, Terzis and Kokkalis[67] found that a group of infants who underwent microsurgery before 3 months had better shoulder function than those who had surgery between 4 and 6 months and demonstrated less need for secondary reconstruction. However, some authors have demonstrated that late nerve reconstruction can result in improved shoulder function and have recommended this option to extend the window for surgery past 3 to 8 months.[26]

During the immediate postoperative period after microsurgery, the limb is immobilized for about 3 weeks.[42] After this period, the rehabilitation strategies of passive ROM and muscle activation are initiated. It is important to remember that the timing of muscle activation will be variable based on the type of microsurgical procedure that was done. Children who receive nerve transfers should achieve muscle activation months sooner than children who undergo nerve grafting.[43] It is recommended that the therapist communicate closely with the surgeon to determine the best plan of intervention for each child.

Strombeck and colleagues[63] reported that for children with global palsy (C5-T1), those who had microsurgery displayed significant improvements in active shoulder motion when compared to children who did not have microsurgery. In a long-term follow-up of the same group of children who had microsurgery,[64] the integrity of the EMG findings from the deltoid muscle was noted to deteriorate over time, even in those children with full recovery. However, sensibility was less affected. More recently, Lin and colleagues[42] reported that neurosurgical repair that included resection and grafting (n = 92) as opposed to neurolysis only (n = 16) had better movement outcomes based on the AMS. A multicenter retrospective review was conducted to examine the outcome from ulnar or median nerve fascicle transfers to increase elbow flexion and supination.[43] Reportedly, postoperatively 27/31 subjects achieved full elbow flexion and 24/31 achieved elbow flexion against gravity.

In a systematic review of outcomes for children with PBPI who underwent neurosurgery, McNeely and Drake[46] found most studies to be case-series designs without control groups (level III evidence). Although the findings were generally favorable, the authors determined that there was no conclusive evidence of a benefit of microsurgery over conservative management in the medical treatment of children with PBPI. Because most of the studies related to timing and outcomes of microsurgery from a case-series design, it would seem essential that randomized controlled trials (RCTs) examining the outcome of microsurgery in this population be conducted. It would be interesting to compare early versus late surgery, as both have been shown to be beneficial. Ideally, the RCTs should use standardized, reliable, and valid outcome measures in each of the three domains of impairment, activity, and participation.

Orthopedic Surgery

The main goal of orthopedic surgery is to provide the necessary active and passive ROM to enable the patient's hand to reach the head and mouth for meaningful ADLs. Hand and wrist reconstruction may be delayed until spontaneous recovery has plateaued and the child can fully participate in postoperative hand therapy. However, shoulder reconstruction is frequently done much earlier.

Persistent muscle imbalances and soft tissue contractures in children who do not experience complete return after PBPI contribute to progressive GH joint dysplasia.[24,33,75] Prolonged weakness of the shoulder external rotators with overpull of the internal rotators often leads to glenoid retroversion, flattening of the humeral head, and progressive posterior subluxation of the humeral head.[24,75] The GH joint deformity is present in up to 67% of children with PBPI[30,45] and is frequently associated with a shoulder IR contracture. Hoeksma and colleagues found that even mild contractures are strongly associated with shoulder deformity.[33]

Common shoulder surgeries include extraarticular tendon transfers of the latissimus dorsi and teres major to the rotator cuff, musculotendinous lengthenings of the pectoralis major or subscapularis, reductions of GH joint dislocations, and osteotomies.[74,75] In one study, 23 children with GH deformity had transfers of the latissimus dorsi and the teres major tendons to the rotator cuff for weakness in ER, as well as lengthening of the pectoralis major or subscapularis. For these children at a mean follow-up of 31 months, active ER improved significantly on the Mallet[44] (preop score of 2 and postop score of 4) and on the AMS (preop score of 3 and postop score of 6). Tendon transfers reportedly improve shoulder motion,[37] and whereas some studies documented the presence of GH remodeling postoperatively,[75] other postoperative studies did not find a reduction in humeral head subluxation and GH joint alignment.[40] Derotational osteotomies are done to place the arm and hand in more functional positions for use if shoulder impairments persist > 5 to 7 years of age.[76]

Parents pursuing orthopedic surgery for their child should become knowledgeable of the most current research on the technique and outcome of procedures being considered. Transferring a muscle can be expected to result in the loss of one muscle strength grade; therefore, the muscle chosen for transfer should be as strong as possible before surgery. Also, clearly identified functional goals should be established before any surgery. For an excellent review of the evaluation and management of shoulder problems in infants and children with PBPI, parents and therapists are referred to Pearl[58] or Gharbaoui et al.[24]

The rehabilitation goals after shoulder reconstruction resemble those that were outlined previously but also vary depending on the orthopedic procedure. Immediately after most shoulder procedures, stabilization with an orthotic brace or spica cast is employed for 4 to 6 weeks.[76] After the stabilization period the child is often weaned off a brace during the day but may continue to wear one at night, depending on the treatment plan of the surgeon.

Active motion and strengthening can usually begin after the brace or cast is removed.[76] After tendon transfers, place and hold isometric strategies aid the child in activating the tendon/muscle unit in a new functional role. Isotonic exercises can follow isometrics and when cleared resistive work can begin. Joint releases and muscle-lengthening procedures require diligence with regard to maintenance of the full passive range of motion (PROM) achieved and active motion in the improved range. Strengthening exercises and the performance of functional tasks in the new range are encouraged when tolerated. As the child progresses, rehabilitation strategies that maximize performance and function will be encouraged. Assessment of postsurgical and rehabilitation outcome is ongoing to allow the program to be adjusted as needed.

REHABILITATION GOALS

The ideal outcome for the neonate who sustains a PBPI is complete return of motor control and sensation with no activity limitations or participation restrictions. It is recommended that therapy begin immediately in early infancy, but further research is needed to examine the best modes of treatment to obtain a beneficial effect. The therapy goals during the first few months after diagnosis are to support spontaneous recovery, minimize pain, prevent secondary impairments (e.g., muscle or joint contracture), promote typical movement patterns, and foster overall development. Depending on the extent of the impairment and dysfunction, increasing PROM, strength, and sensory awareness while minimizing pain during functional tasks remains the goal in the first 2 years of life. Neural regeneration and restoration of motor control may be augmented through surgical procedures. Most spontaneous recovery occurs by 9 months of age, but continued recovery may occur up to 2 years after the injury.[22]

Children with PBPI need ongoing monitoring of ROM, sensibility, pain, functional status, and development. At some point in the infant or toddler phase, it may become apparent that significant neural regeneration is no longer occurring, even after microsurgery. Goals would need to be revised for children who lose range or plateau in their recovery over several months. Even with the most diligent implementation of a home program, full FROM can be difficult to maintain when muscle imbalance is present. If GH joint limitations are present, the child may be a candidate for shoulder reconstruction.

The desired outcomes during the toddler-to-childhood phase would be that the child develop age-appropriate self-care skills such as dressing and grooming using either extremity and participate in age-appropriate movement activities and school programs. Goals would include maintaining or increasing PROM and strength in motion critical to specific activities that the child has difficulty with or is invested in performing. For example, the child may need to increase shoulder elevation and elbow extension strength in the affected arm to shoot a basketball.

THERAPEUTIC PROCEDURAL INTERVENTIONS AND FAMILY EDUCATION

During infancy, a therapist may perform a consultation before discharge from the hospital. Once cleared for assessment and treatment, the clinician can perform baseline examinations described earlier in this chapter. A home program is developed for parents featuring passive ROM to the neck and UE joints at risk for contracture. Positioning strategies and therapeutic play activities useful to maintain ROM and activate or strengthen weak muscles are also emphasized. In addition, precautions regarding regions of pain, sensory loss, or diminished sensibility are reviewed. For older children, the provision of DVDs has been shown to improve compliance with the home program.[52] Anecdotally, videos or photos taken with a cell phone have also been used to reinforce home programs for infants and children of any age. Intuitively, therapeutic treatment and home programs seem beneficial for this population whether they progress without surgery or require surgical intervention. However, high-quality evidence in support of various intervention strategies is warranted.

Active Movement

The objective of the rehabilitation program is to facilitate the highest functional outcome possible for the infant or child, particularly in regard to prehensile skills as they relate to meaningful, developmentally appropriate activities. Simple strategies often work best. For example, while being held on a parent's lap, placement of a finger into the palm of a young infant's hand while the elbow/forearm is supported in flexion/neutral supination often encourages activation of the grasp reflex or an intentional grasp. This action can potentially foster activation of weak arm muscles such as the biceps. The use of positioning strategies in clinic and home programs is vital early in rehabilitation.

Strategic positioning in sidelying, prone, and supine positions can aid the activation of weak muscles in young infants. Lying on the affected side (with the head supported in neutral) encourages isolated elbow flexion, whereas lying on the unaffected side encourages shoulder motion. Given the high risk for muscle and GH joint contracture, it is important to prevent sustained shoulder IR of the affected arm (as feasible) when sidelying on the unaffected side. When prone, the infant who does not yet prop on the elbows can stretch the GH joint into ER and horizontal abduction while resting in this position. Alternatively, chest support provided with a rolled-up receiving blanket can allow the infant to prone prop on the elbows when this is developmentally appropriate and tolerated by the affected shoulder. This supported weight-bearing position can encourage activation of the shoulder musculature and neck/trunk extensors. When the infant is placed in the supine position, it is important to place the elbows and hands of the both arms higher than the shoulders to prevent posturing into shoulder extension and to allow greater ease of arm movement against gravity.

During reaching activities, careful attention to the scapula is critical because paralysis of the rhomboids and contracture of muscles that link the humerus to the scapula interfere with the normal 6:1 humeral-scapular rhythm in the first 30° of shoulder movement.[36] The scapula can be manually stabilized as the shoulder is assisted in active elevation while the child reaches for toys. Alternatively, strategically setting up the environment to allow active shoulder movement with gravity minimized can allow for recruitment of weaker muscles and prevent atypical movements from occurring. For young infants the sidelying position allows for shoulder flexion with gravity minimized. For older infants and children, kinesiotaping[73] may be one method to foster scapular stabilization from any position. The published case study by Walsh[73] reported that kinesiotaping and exercise seemed to facilitate muscular support to position the humeral head in the glenoid fossa. Despite the positive outcomes from this case study, further research on the specific benefits of kinesiotaping and exercise for scapular stabilization is warranted.

In clinic and home programs, one must be creative to provide opportunities for activation of weak muscles during prehensile and functional tasks that minimize gravity and prevent substitution patterns. The number of motor behaviors and tasks that need emphasis in this population of children are endless and include hand-to-mouth tasks, hand-to-hand transfer of objects, weight shifting in prone prop and quadruped, tailor sitting with hands propped anteriorly or posteriorly, transitional movements, creeping, and reach-to-grasp behaviors. Simple place and hold isometric exercises are an efficient way to initiate muscle activation in weak musculature. Manual guidance to aid in the accomplishment of tasks is also useful but can be replaced with environmental set-up to ease task completion and encourage self-generated movement as muscle strength improves. Fig. 20.5A illustrates a nonfunctional position that an infant with a classic C5-C6 injury may assume. Fig. 20.5B demonstrates how manually guiding the shoulder into flexion and ER allows the infant to experience a more typical, functional movement pattern and obtain more appropriate sensory information through an open palm. This action can be followed by task practice without manual guidance by setting up the environment to allow the production of self-generated motion and reinforce motor learning. Because active shoulder ER and forearm supination are often weak or absent in children with C5-C6 injuries, toys should be presented strategically in different areas of the workspace to encourage variable muscle activation patterns and different prehensile skills. Intervention strategies designed to augment muscle activation of weak muscles through visual-auditory biofeedback are emerging and showing promise as rehabilitation strategies.[17]

In any position, gravity or toys held in the hand can provide resistance as muscles gain strength for prehensile behaviors. At times, the unaffected arm may need to be gently restrained when encouraging the child to use the affected arm. Tactile stimulation or facilitation of the weak muscles with gentle joint compression in weight bearing, biofeedback, or electrical stimulation can also encourage activation of weak muscles.

Typical posture and developmental activities may be compromised as a result of PBPI. Transitional movement to a seated position may always be done from one (i.e., the unaffected) side, and as a result, posture of the trunk may be asymmetrical and balance reactions may be delayed on the affected side. To address reliance on the unaffected side, movement into sitting and other transitional movements can be practiced from the affected side using manual guidance and facilitation as needed. When sitting is achieved, challenging protective reactions to the affected side can facilitate shoulder abduction.

Typical bilateral UE use will likely be delayed and often needs to be emphasized. Opportunities for the child to experience and practice symmetrical two-handed activities such as tossing and catching large balls can be encouraged as well as the performance of asymmetrical tasks that require stabilization with one hand manipulating the other. Intervention strategies provided in the context of purposeful tasks versus the performance of exercises are also motivating for children. For example, strengthening of the shoulder flexors could be done by asking the child to lift 10 toy people up and into a dollhouse (purposeful) instead of performing 10 repetitions of shoulder flexion (exercise). In the older child who has not experienced full return of motor function, adaptations and devices to assist in ADLs and recreational activities should be made available for the child's consideration. Swimming programs are often recommended at this time because they engage both UEs and are often enjoyable for children.

The use of botulinum toxin has been found to improve active motion in muscles antagonistic to those injected with the toxin.[5] Arad and colleagues[5] examined the short- and long-term outcome after Botox injections to the shoulder internal rotators and triceps musculature to improve shoulder ER and elbow flexion/supination in children who had not undergone microsurgery. The study included children who first received an injection at a mean age of 30 to 36 months of age. Based on AMS scores the authors found that shoulder ER significantly improved after 1 month yet decreased by 1 year of age. Elbow flexion/supination did not initially improve, but after 1 year a significant improvement was noted based on AMS scores. Only the elbow/forearm motions were sustained over time. The authors caution that it is important to determine whether the cause of the muscle imbalance is differential muscle weakness or co-contraction.

Range of Motion

Passive ROM and stretching can be done in isolation, during positioning, or in the context of typical developmental activities

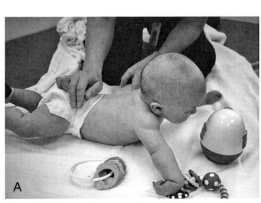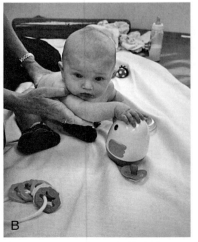

FIG. 20.5 A, Infant with C5-C6 brachial plexus injury trying to prop and reach. B, Infant assisted to reach and grasp with manual guidance.

by parents and clinicians. Goniometric measures of UE PROM should be performed weekly or biweekly and the clinic/home program adjusted based on the findings. Maintaining ROM is important, as up to 65% of children with incomplete recovery of PBPI have been found to have limited ROM at the shoulder.[35] Stretching should never cause pain and should always be gentle. Although passive ROM is encouraged, overstretching can be harmful to joints and joint capsules that are already unstable. Placing the child's arm in optimal positions is a time-efficient way to stretch soft tissue restrictions because this can be done during feeding, carrying, or positioning in a car seat. As the child's arm relaxes during sleep, even more passive range can be attempted.

Prevention of scapulohumeral adhesions is an important goal of therapeutic intervention. The infant or child can do passive shoulder ROM in isolation as tolerated. As mentioned previously, stabilization of the scapula is critical, as shown in Fig. 20.3A-C. Again, the reader is encouraged to review the article by Gharbaoui and colleagues,[24] which introduces five critical stretches that should be used with children to prevent GH joint contractures or encourage an increase in passive ROM.

During reaching tasks, the scapula can be stabilized or restrained to stretch muscles that link the scapula to the humerus during the first 30° of abduction. As mentioned previously, Kinesiotape can be used to foster scapular stabilization during tasks performed at home.[73] Beyond 30°, the scapula must rotate along with humeral ER to avoid harmful impingement of soft tissues on the acromion process, thus, rotation should be encouraged. For a visual demonstration of scapulohumeral rhythm, the reader is encouraged to search for appropriate videos online by using the search term *scapulohumeral rhythm.*

Sensory Awareness

Diminished sensibility can lead to neglect or even self-abuse of the affected arm.[45] Parents must be cautioned about the risk of injury to body areas where sensation is compromised and should watch for any signs of self-mutilation such as biting an insensate area. Enlisting the participation of the affected limb in play activities such as holding a bottle allows the child to perceive the extremity as being a purposeful part of the body. Sensory perception can be enhanced by placing objects of different textures and temperatures in the hand, playing games such as finding toys under sudsy water or in rice with the affected hand, or in the case of older children having them name familiar objects placed in their hand while blindfolded. Parents themselves should be encouraged not to neglect the arm but to caress and play with it as usual while holding or guiding it through movement patterns that need reinforcement.

Orthotics

Intermittent use of orthotics for the wrist and fingers may sometimes be indicated. Wrist orthoses may preserve the integrity of the wrist and finger tendons/muscles until motor function returns. Resting night orthoses can help prevent wrist and finger/thumb contractures by providing a low-load prolonged stretch to the tissues. A dorsal or volar wrist orthotic can maintain the wrist in neutral or partial extension yet free the fingers to grasp and release toys. To prevent shoulder adduction and IR contractures, a "statue of liberty" orthotic or an abduction orthotic has been suggested. However, the child may not tolerate this position for long periods or may not tolerate it at all.

A semi-stretchable strap (e.g., Fabrifoam) that wraps around the hand/forearm and extends from the palm to above the elbow can be used to foster forearm supination. For young infants this strap can be ½-inch wide, and for older infants and children it can be ¾- to 1-inch wide. This type of strap is often worn during waking hours as tolerated with frequent breaks to induce a bias of forearm supination during activities. If the strap does not sufficiently position the forearm, a plastic supination orthotic can be fabricated to use with an additional wide supination strap instead.

Restraining casts, splints, or slings can be used on the unaffected extremity to successfully encourage use of the affected arm and hand as a form of forced use.[8] If shaping activities for the affected arm and hand are employed while the restraint is on the unaffected arm, the approach would be regarded as constraint-induced movement therapy (CIMT). In the case study reported by Berggren and Baker,[8] the child had to use his affected arm to bring a toy to his mouth or self-feed when elbow flexion was restrained on the unaffected side. It is recommended that the restraint be used for brief periods only during the day with frustration levels monitored carefully. It is important to remember that some children will not tolerate any form of restraint, particularly if it is unrealistic that the affected arm can perform functional activities with some independence.

Electrical Stimulation

As introduced previously, Berggren and Baker[8] published a retrospective case report of an infant/toddler who sustained a right global PBPI and presented with Horner's syndrome. At 6 weeks of age he received sensory electrical stimulation (ES) (100 μs pulse duration) at submotor threshold until motor recovery was noted. At 3 months of age he underwent microsurgical repair of the brachial plexus. At 11 months of age, reciprocal ES (150 μs pulse duration with trace [1/5] level of contraction) was initiated to foster efficient motor recruitment and active movement. CIMT was employed over four separate time periods during his first 2 years of life. The outcome based on scores from the AMS, Modified Mallet, and the AHA changed after intervention with significant increases in AHA scores after episodes of CIMT. Okafor and colleagues[55] reported from a small study (eight children per group) that ES paired with conventional physical therapy improved active shoulder abduction and elbow flexion when compared with conventional therapy after 6 weeks. Further research is recommended on the use of ES as an adjunct to increase muscle activation in this population of infants and children.

OUTCOMES

The information available on long-term outcomes in adults with a history of PBPI suggests that disability in daily activities can be lifelong and frequently associated with orthopedic disorders and pain. Strombeck and colleagues[64] evaluated long-term changes in function in a group of 70 participants aged 7 to 20 years. Of this group, 43% had improvements in shoulder function, whereas about 50% had decreased active elbow extension at follow-up. Interestingly, 75% of participants perceived they had no difficulty with ADLs. In another study of 36 adults aged 21 to 72 years with PBPI, Partridge and Edwards[57] found that 60% had painful arthritic joints and 27% had scoliosis. In this group, 80% reported trouble with dressing, 55%

with bathing, and 66% with cooking. Furthermore, 33 of 36 participants surveyed (91%) reported experiencing pain, with 28 of those 33 reporting that their pain was "getting worse." Outcomes research using health-related quality-of-life and participation measures would be extremely helpful for therapists and parents to aid long-term planning for children with PBPI.

PREVENTION

Although the risk factors are known, the positive predictive values for identifying PBPI before birth are lower than 15%.[56] Despite this observation, the goal of prevention continues, thus, risk factors continue to be investigated.[19,47,48] Modified delivery practices such as cesarean section should be considered when there are multiple risk factors for an infant to present with shoulder dystocia during the birth process.

SUMMARY

A unilateral traction injury secondary to shoulder dystocia is the most common cause of PBPI.[29] Infants with PBPI present with impairments of flaccidity or reduced muscle activity that are readily apparent at birth. Therapists and parents can employ strategies to foster early activation of partially denervated muscles and an increase in sensory awareness. It is essential that methods are used to maintain muscle extensibility and joint ROM while reinforcing motor recovery, function, and the acquisition of age-appropriate developmental behaviors. Microsurgery may be considered if substantial spontaneous recovery is not apparent by the age of 3 to 6 months. 28 Shoulder reconstruction can be pursued in a timely manner for cases presenting with GH joint dysplasia. Long-term outcome studies suggest that PBPI affects ADLs and causes disability in adulthood with minimal effects on social participation. As intervention strategies expand, perhaps disability can be reduced and therefore better partner with the positive aspects of social participation.

Case Scenario on Expert Consult

The case related to this chapter presents a child with PBPI, and a video illustrates the outcomes for a child who underwent microsurgical intervention as an infant.

REFERENCES

1. Åberg K, Norman M, Ekéus C: Preterm birth by vacuum extraction and neonatal outcome: a population-based cohort study, *BMC Pregnancy Childbirth* 14:42, 2014.
2. Abzug JM, Kozin SH: Evaluation and management of brachial plexus birth palsy, *Orthop Clin N Am* 45:225–232, 2014.
3. Al-Qattan NM, Clarke HM, Curtis CG: Klumpke's birth palsy: does it really exist? *J Hand Surg Br* 20B:19–23, 1995.
4. American Physical Therapy Association: *Guide to physical therapist practice*, ed 2, American Physical Therapy Association, 2001. 81:9-744.
5. Arad E, Stephens D, Curtis CG, et al.: Botulinum toxin for the treatment of motor imbalance in obstetrical brachial plexus palsy, *Plast Reconstr Surg* 131:1307–1315, 2013.
6. Bae DS, Waters PM, Zurakowski D: Reliability of three classification systems measuring active motion in brachial plexus birth palsy, *J Bone Joint Surg* 85A:1733–1738, 2003.
7. Bain JR, DeMatteo C, Gjertsen D, et al.: Navigating the gray zone: a guideline for surgical decision making in obstetrical brachial plexus injuries, *J Neurosurg Pediatr* 3:173–180, 2009.
8. Berggren J, Baker LL: Targeted strategies using electrical stimulation and constraint induced movement therapy for muscle activation and active movement in neonatal brachial plexus palsy: a case review, *J Hand Ther* 28:217–220, 2015.
9. Campbell SK, Wright BD, Linacre JM: Development of a functional movement scale for infants, *J Applied Measure* 3:191–204, 2002.
10. Clarke HM, Curtis CG: An approach to obstetrical brachial plexus injuries, *Hand Clin* 11:563–580, 1995.
11. Curtis C, Stephens D, Clarke HM, et al.: The active movement scale: an evaluative tool for infants with obstetrical brachial plexus injury, *J Hand Surg Am* 27A:470–478, 2002.
12. Dayanidhi S, Orlin M, Kozin S, et al.: Scapular kinematics during humeral elevation in adults and children, *Clin Biomech* 20:600–606, 2005.
13. DiTaranto P, Campagna L, Price AE: Outcome following nonoperative treatment of brachial plexus birth injuries, *J Child Neurol* 19:87–90, 2004.
14. Dodds SD, Wolfe SW: Perinatal brachial plexus palsy, *Curr Opin Pediatr* 12:40–47, 2000.
15. Duff SV, Dayanidhi S, Kozin SH: Asymmetrical shoulder kinematics in children with brachial plexus birth injury, *Clin Biomech [Bristol, Avon]* 22:630–638, 2007.
16. Duff SV, DeMatteo C: Clinical assessment of the infant and child following perinatal brachial plexus injury, *J Hand Ther* 28:126–133, 2015.
17. Duff SV, Sargent B, Kutch JJ, et al.: Self-generated feedback to increase muscle activation in infancy, *Poster presentation at the Combined Sections Meeting of the American Physical Therapy Association*, February 2015.
18. Eng GD, Koch B, Smokvina MD: Brachial plexus palsy in neonates and children, *Arch Phys Med Rehabil* 59:458–464, 1978.
19. Executive summary: neonatal brachial plexus palsy. Report of the American College of Obstetricians and Gynecologists' Task Force on Neonatal Brachial Plexus Palsy, *Obstet Gynecol* 123:902–904, 2014.
20. Fisher DM, Borschel GH, Curtis C, et al.: Evaluation of elbow flexion as a predictor of outcome in obstetrical brachial plexus palsy, *Plast Reconstruct Surg* 120:1585–1590, 2007.
21. Foad SL, Mehlman CT, Ying J: The epidemiology of neonatal brachial plexus palsy in the United States, *J Bone Joint Surg Am* 90:1258–1264, 2008.
22. Gilbert A: Long-term evaluation of brachial plexus surgery in obstetrical palsy, *Hand Clin* 11:583–593, 1995.
23. Gilbert A, Tassin JL: [Surgical repair of the brachial plexus in obstetrical paralysis], *Chirurgie* 110:70–75, 1984.
24. Gharbaoui IS, Gogola GR, Aaron DH, et al.: Perspectives on glenohumeral joint contractures and shoulder dysfunction in children with perinatal brachial plexus palsy, *J Hand Ther* 28:176–183, 2015.
25. Greaves S, Imms C, Dodd K, Krumlinde-Sundholm L: Development of Mini-Assisting Hand Assessment: validation of the play session and item generation, *Dev Med Child Neurol* 55:1030–1037, 2013.
26. Grossman AL, Ditaranto P, Yaylali I, et al.: Shoulder function following late neurolysis and bypass grafting for upper brachial plexus birth injuries, *J Hand Surg Br* 29B:356–358, 2004.
27. Habechian FA, Fornasari GG, Sacramento LS, et al.: Differences in scapular kinematics and scapulohumeral rhythm during elevation and lowering of the arm between typical children and healthy adults, *J Electromyogr Kinesiol* 24:78–83, 2014.
28. Hale HB, Bae DS, Waters PM: Current concepts in the management of brachial plexus birth palsy, *J Hand Surg* 35A:322–331, 2010.
29. Hansen A, Chauhan SP: Shoulder dystocia: definitions and incidence, *Sem Perinatol* 38:184–188, 2014.
30. Haerle M, Gilbert A: Management of complete obstetrical brachial plexus lesions, *J Pediatr Ortho* 24:194–200, 2004.
31. Hervey-Jumper SL, Justice D, Vanaman MM, et al.: Torticollis associated with neonatal brachial plexus palsy, *Pediatr Neurol* 45:305–310, 2011.
32. Ho ES, Curtis CG, Clarke HM: The brachial plexus outcome measure: development, internal consistency, and construct validity, *J Hand Ther* 25:406–416, 2012.

33. Hoeksma AF, ter Steeg AM, Dijkstra P, et al.: Shoulder contracture and osseous deformity in obstetrical brachial plexus injuries, *J Bone Joint Surg Am* 85A:316–322, 2003.

34. Hoeksma AF, ter Steeg AM, Nelissen RG, et al.: Neurological recovery in obstetric brachial plexus injuries: an historical cohort study, *Dev Med Child Neurol* 46:76–83, 2004.

35. Hoeksma AF, Wolf H, Oei SL: Obstetrical brachial plexus injuries: incidence, natural course and shoulder contracture, *Clin Rehabil* 14:523–526, 2000.

36. Inman VT, Saunders JDM: Observations on the function of the clavicle, *Calif Med* 65:158, 1946.

37. Jennette RJ, Tarby TJ, Krauss RL: Erb's palsy contrasted with Klumpke's and total palsy: different mechanisms involved, *Am J Obstet Gynecol* 186:1216–1220, 2002.

38. Justice D, Rasmussen L, DiPietro M, et al.: Prevalence of posterior shoulder subluxation in children with neonatal brachial plexus palsy after early full passive range of motion exercises, *PMR*1–8, 2015, http://dx.doi.org/10.1016/j.pmrj.2015.05.013. Accessed September 1, 2015.

39. Kozin SH: The evaluation and treatment of children with brachial plexus palsy, *J Hand Surg* 36A:1360–1369, 2011.

40. Kozin SH, Chafetz RS, Shaffer A, et al.: Magnetic resonance imaging and clinical findings before and after tendon transfers about the shoulder in children with residual brachial plexus palsy: a 3-year follow-up study, *J Pediatr Orthop* 30:154–160, 2010.

41. Krumlinde-Sundholm L, Holmefur M, Kottorp A, Eliasson A-C: The Assisting Hand Assessment: current evidence of validity, reliability, and responsiveness to change, *Dev Med Child Neurol* 49:259–264, 2007.

42. Lin JC, Schwenker-Colizza A, Curtis CG: Final results of grafting versus neurolysis in obstetrical brachial plexus palsy, *Plastic Reconstruct Surg* 123:939–948, 2009.

43. Little KJ, Zlotolow DA, Soldado F, et al.: Early functional recovery of elbow flexion and supination following median and/or ulnar nerve fascicle transfer in upper neonatal brachial plexus palsy, *J Bone Joint Surg Am* 96:215–221, 2014.

44. Mallet J: Primaute du traitement de l'epaule—methode d'expresion des resultants, *Rev Chir Orthop* 58S:166–168, 1972.

45. McCann ME, Waters P, Goumnerova LC: Self-mutilation in young children following brachial plexus birth injury, *Pain* 110:123–129, 2004.

46. McNeely PD, Drake JM: A systematic review of brachial plexus surgery for birth-related brachial plexus injury, *Pediatr Neurosurg* 38:57–62, 2003.

47. Medina LS, Yaylali I, Zurakowski D, et al.: Diagnostic performance of MRI and MR myelography in infants with a brachial plexus birth palsy, *Pediatr Radiol* 36:1295–1299, 2006.

48. Mehta H, Sokol RJ: Shoulder dystocia: risk factors, predictability, and preventability, *Sem Perinatol* 38:189–193, 2014.

49. Merkel S, Voepel-Lewis T, Malviya S: Pain assessment in infants and young children: FLACC scale, *Am J Nurse* 10255–10258, 2002.

50. Michelow BJ, Clarke HM, Curtis CG, et al.: The natural history of brachial plexus palsy, *Plast Reconstruct Surg* 93:675–680, 1994.

51. Mollberg M, Hagberg H, Bager B, et al.: High birthweight and shoulder dystocia: the strongest risk factors for obstetrical brachial plexus palsy in a Swedish population-based study, *Acta Obstet Gynecol Scand* 84:654–659, 2005.

52. Murphy KM, Rasmussen L, Hervey-Jumper SL, et al.: An assessment of the compliance and utility of a home exercise DVD for caregivers of children and adolescents with brachial plexus palsy: a pilot study, *PMR* 4:190–197, 2011.

53. Narakas AO: Obstetrical brachial plexus injuries. In Lamb DW, editor: *The hand and upper limb, the paralyzed hand*, vol. 2. Edinburgh, Scotland, 1987, Churchill Livingstone, p 116.

54. Noetzel MJ, Park TS, Robinson S, et al.: Prospective study of recovery following neonatal brachial plexus injury, *J Child Neurol* 16:488–492, 2001.

55. Okafor UA, Akinbo SR, Sokunbi OG, et al.: Comparison of electrical stimulation and conventional physiotherapy in functional rehabilitation in Erb's palsy, *Nigerian Quarter J Hosp Med* 18:202–205, 2008.

56. Ouzounian J: Risk factors for neonatal brachial plexus palsy, *Sem Perinatol* 38:219–221, 2014.

57. Partridge C, Edwards S: Obstetric brachial plexus palsy: increasing disability and exacerbation of symptoms with age, *Physiother Res Int* 9:157–163, 2004.

58. Pearl M: Shoulder problems in children with brachial plexus birth palsy: evaluation and management, *J Am Acad Ortho Surg* 17:242–254, 2009.

59. Piper MC, Darrah J: *Motor assessment of the developing infant*, Philadelphia, 1994, WB Saunders.

60. Pondaag W, Malessy MJ, van Dijk JG, et al.: Natural history of obstetric brachial plexus palsy: a systematic review, *Dev Med Child Neurol* 46:138–144, 2004.

61. Pöyhiä TH, Lamminen AE, Peltonen JI, et al.: Brachial plexus birth injury: US screening for glenohumeral joint instability, *Radiology* 254:253–260, 2010.

62. Shepherd RB: Brachial plexus injury. In Campbell SK, editor: *Pediatric neurologic physical therapy*, ed 2, New York, 1991, Churchill Livingstone, pp 101–130.

63. Strombeck C, Krumlinde-Sundholm L, Forssberg H: Functional outcome at 5 years in children with obstetrical brachial plexus palsy with and without microsurgical reconstruction, *Dev Med Child Neurol* 42:148–157, 2000.

64. Strombeck C, Krumlinde-Sundholm L, Remalh S, et al.: Long-term follow-up of children with obstetric brachial plexus I; functional aspects, *Dev Med Child Neurol* 49:198–203, 2007.

65. Sunderland S: Nerves and nerve injuries. In Green DP, Hotchkiss RN, Pederson WD, et al., editors: *Green's operative hand surgery*, ed 4, New York, 1999, Churchill Livingstone, pp 750–779.

66. Sundholm LK, Eliasson AC, Forssberg H: Obstetric brachial plexus injuries: assessment protocol and functional outcome at age 5 years, *Dev Med Child Neurol* 40:4–11, 1998.

67. Terzis JK, Kokkalis ZT: Primary and secondary shoulder reconstruction in obstetric brachial plexus palsy, *Injury* 39S:S5–S14, 2008.

68. Tse R, Kozin SH, Malessy MJ, Clark HM: International Federation of Societies for Surgery of the Hand Committee Report: the role of nerve transfers in the treatment of neonatal brachial plexus palsy, *J Hand Surg Am* 40:1246–1259, 2015.

69. Vanderhave KL, Bovid K, Alpert H, et al.: Utility of electrodiagnostic testing and computed tomography myelography in the preoperative evaluation of neonatal brachial plexus palsy, *J Neurosurg Pediatr* 9:283–289, 2012.

70. van Dijk JG, Pondaag W, Buitenhuis SM, et al.: Needle electromyography at 1 month predicts paralysis of elbow flexion at 3 months in obstetric brachial plexus lesions, *Dev Med Child Neurol* 54:753–758, 2012.

71. van Ouwerkerk WJR, van der Sluijs JA, Nollet T, et al.: Management of obstetric brachial plexus lesions: state of the art and future developments, *Childs Nerv Syst* 16:638–644, 2000.

72. Vathana T, Vathana T, Rust S, et al.: Intraobserver and interobserver reliability of two ultrasound measures of humeral head position in infants with neonatal brachial plexus palsy, *J Bone Joint Surg Am* 89:1710–1715, 2007.

73. Walsh SF: Treatment of a brachial plexus injury using kinesiotape and exercise, *Physiother Theory Pract* 26:490–496, 2010.

74. Waters PM: Comparison of the natural history, the outcome of microsurgical repair, and the outcome of operative reconstruction in brachial plexus birth palsy, *J Bone Joint Surg Am* 81:649–659, 1999.

75. Waters PM, Bae DS: The early effects of tendon transfers and open capsulorrhaphy on glenohumeral deformity in brachial plexus birth palsy, *J Bone Joint Surg Am* 90:2171–2179, 2008.

76. Waters PM, Bae DS: The early effects of tendon transfers and open capsulorrhaphy on glenohumeral deformity in brachial plexus birth palsy. Surgical technique, *J Bone Joint Surg Am* 91(Suppl 2):213–222, 2009.

77. Wong D: *Reference manual for the Wong-Baker FACES pain rating scale*, Duarte, CA, 1995, Mayday Pain Resource Center.

78. Wolf H, Hoeksma AF, Oei SL, et al.: Obstetric brachial plexus injury: risk factors related to recovery, *Eur J Obstet Gyn R B* 88:133–138, 2000.

79. Yang LJ: Neonatal brachial plexus palsy: management and prognostic factors, *Sem Perinatol* 38:222–234, 2014.

SUGGESTED READINGS

Bae DS, Waters PM, Zurakowski D: Reliability of three classification systems measuring active motion in brachial plexus birth palsy, *J Bone Joint Surg* 85A:1733–1738, 2003.

Bain JR, DeMatteo C, Gjertsen D, et al.: Navigating the gray zone: a guideline for surgical decision making in obstetrical brachial plexus injuries, *J Neurosurg Pediatr* 3:173–180, 2009.

Clarke HM, Curtis CG: An approach to obstetrical brachial plexus injuries, *Hand Clin* 11:563–580, 1995.

Duff SV, DeMatteo C: Clinical assessment of the infant and child following perinatal brachial plexus injury, *J Hand Ther* 28:126–133, 2015.

Ho ES, Curtis CG, Clarke HM: The brachial plexus outcome measure: development, internal consistency, and construct validity, *J Hand Ther* 25:406–416, 2012.

Krumlinde-Sundholm L, Holmefur M, Kottorp A, Eliasson A-C: The Assisting Hand Assessment: current evidence of validity, reliability, and responsiveness to change, *Dev Med Child Neurol* 49:259–264, 2007.

Mollberg M, Hagber H, Bager B, et al.: High birthweight and shoulder dystocia: the strongest risk factors for obstetrical brachial plexus palsy in a Swedish population-based study, *Acta Obstet Gynecol Scand* 84:654–659, 2005.

Vanderhave KL, Bovid K, Alpert H, et al.: Utility of electrodiagnostic testing and computed tomography myelography in the preoperative evaluation of neonatal brachial plexus palsy, *J Neurosurg Pediatr* 9:283–289, 2012.

van Dijk JG, Pondaag W, Buitenhuis SM, et al.: Needle electromyography at 1 month predicts paralysis of elbow flexion at 3 months in obstetric brachial plexus lesions, *Dev Med Child Neurol* 54:753–758, 2012.

Waters PM, Bae DS: The early effects of tendon transfers and open capsulorrhaphy on glenohumeral deformity in brachial plexus birth palsy, *J Bone Joint Surg Am* 90:2171–2179, 2008.

Yang LJ-S: Neonatal brachial plexus palsy: management and prognostic factors, *Sem Perinatol* 38:222–234, 2014.

21

Spinal Cord Injury

Christina Calhoun Thielen, Therese Johnston, Christin Krey

Acquired lesions of the spinal cord occur far less commonly in children than in adults, but the unique aspects of growth and development can make treatment of the child with spinal cord injury (SCI) a challenge for pediatric physical therapists. The rehabilitation process may take years because the young child requires time to achieve adequate strength, adult body proportions, developmental milestones, and cognitive skills for maximal independence. The child who is not skeletally mature may develop orthopedic problems during growth, which may result in altered function. Direct intervention, monitoring skill acquisition, education, and assessing equipment needs are important roles for the physical therapist.

This chapter describes the pathophysiology, resulting neurologic changes, changes in body functions and structures, and their impact on activity and participation of children with SCI. Examination, prognosis, goals, and outcomes and physical therapy intervention for the child with SCI are discussed.

BACKGROUND INFORMATION

Epidemiology

Spinal cord injuries account for a small number of all injuries sustained by children; however, the consequences of SCI can be devastating. The overall incidence of pediatric SCI in the United States is approximately 1.99 cases per 100,000 children and adolescents.[141] Additionally, approximately 5% of the SCIs sustained each year occur in children 15 and younger, although this estimate is likely below the actual percentage due to limited availability of data.[33] From birth to 5 years of age, the ratio of males to females affected by SCI is fairly equal. With increasing age, the ratio of males to females increases to approximately 4:1.[32,33,41,141] Motor vehicle crashes (MVCs), sports, falls, and violence are the leading causes of traumatic SCI; however, this varies as a function of age (Table 21.1).[32-34,41,141,143] MVCs are the most prevalent cause in all age groups, but violence, sports, and falls increase as the cause with increasing age. Injuries sustained due to sports are greatest in the 13- to 15-year-old age group.[14,32,34,41] Child abuse accounts for some cases of SCI, but the frequency of abuse as a cause is unknown.[34]

When an MVC is the cause of injury, a high cervical lesion usually occurs in children younger than 4 years of age, with continued risk for cervical level injuries through age 8.[41,43] Lap belt injuries tend to occur in children between 5 to 8 years of age. Lap belt injuries frequently occur when a child transitions too early from a car seat to sitting in a passenger seat, causing the lap portion of a lap/shoulder seat belt to ride high on the abdomen. Spinal injury from a lap belt in an MVC is typically at the thoracolumbar junction, and significant retroperitoneal injury also occurs.[59,120] Teens injured as a result of an MVC typically sustain cervical level injuries.

Whether a child sustains an injury leading to tetraplegia verses paraplegia and the severity (complete versus incomplete) varies with age.[32,41] If a child is injured prior to the age of 12, about two thirds are paraplegic and a complete injury is sustained. In the adolescent population, approximately half of those injured are paraplegic and slightly more than half sustain a complete injury. It is difficult to classify an injury in a child age 4 or younger due to the reliability of the examination used to classify SCI; therefore, limited data are available for the 0 to 4 age group.[105] This topic will be discussed in more detail later in the chapter.

Nontraumatic causes of SCI in children include tumor (predominantly intramedullary tumors[152]), transverse myelitis, epidural abscess, arteriovenous malformation, multiple sclerosis, and spinal cord infarction due to thromboembolic disorders. Developmental anomalies of the cervical vertebrae can place the spinal cord at increased risk of injury. These anomalies include instability of the atlantoaxial joint, as seen in Down syndrome, juvenile rheumatoid arthritis, os odontoideum (a congenital failure of fusion of the odontoid process to the C2 vertebral body), and dysplasia of the base of the skull or upper cervical vertebrae, as seen in achondroplasia.

The long-term survival rates of children with an SCIs range from 83% of normal life expectancy with an incomplete injury to 50% with a high cervical injury without ventilator dependency,[127] with primary mortality resulting from respiratory complications.[3] Mortality overall seems to follow a different pattern than for individuals with adult-onset SCI as well as the general population of comparable age.[3] A small-scale study suggests that recovery of neurologic function occurs more frequently in pediatric patients than in adults and that recovery can be identified for a longer period of time after injury.[148]

PREVENTION

Proper use of vehicle restraints, water safety instruction, and preparticipation sports physical examinations are important measures for preventing traumatic SCI in children. Lap seat belts must be placed across the pelvis, not across the waist, and shoulder harnesses should cross the clavicle, not the neck, to avoid lumbar or cervical spine injury in the event of a collision. Children should use a booster seat until the lap belt and shoulder harness fit correctly. This typically occurs when the child is about 4 feet 9 inches tall, 8 to 12 years old, or 80 pounds. Once a child is old enough and tall enough to transition to a standard seat, both a lap and shoulder belt should be used and the child restrained in the rear seat until at least 13 years of age. According to the National Highway Transportation and Safety

TABLE 21.1	Causes of Pediatric Spinal Cord Injury Related to Age					
Age (years)	Vehicular	Violence	Sports	Falls	Medical/Surgical	Other
0–5	65%	9%	0.2%	6.5%	12%	8%
6–12	52%	22%	11%	6.5%	5%	5%
13–15	41%	19%	28%	8%	3%	1.5%
16–21	49%	22%	18%	8%	0.6%	2%

Adapted from Vogel LC, Betz RR, Mulcahey MJ: Spinal cord injuries in children and adolescents. In Verhaagen J, McDonald JW III, editors: *Handbook of clinical neurology,* vol 109, Amsterdam, 2012, Elsevier, Chapter 8, pp 131-148.

Administration (NHTSA), American Academy of Pediatrics, and federal law, infants and toddlers should remain in a rear-facing-only seat or rear-facing convertible car seat until at least 2 years of age or until they reach the highest weight or height determined by the car seat manufacturer. Car seat manufacturers have been producing car seats rated to a higher weight in the rear-facing position, as it has been suggested that remaining in the rear-facing position for as long as possible is preferred. Once a child has outgrown a rear-facing weight or height limit, a forward-facing car seat with a harness should be used as long as possible, again to the highest weight and height allowed by the car seat's manufacturer. This again is reflected in the manufacturing of combination car seats with harnesses rated to higher weights. It should also be noted that proper car seat installation as well as proper harness snugness and retainer clip placement is imperative to properly restrain an infant, toddler, or child in an appropriate vehicle safety system (http://www.safercar.gov-/parents/CarSeats/Car-Seat-Safety.htm).

Organizations such as Safe Kids Worldwide (www.safekids.org) and the Center for Childhood Injury Prevention Studies (CChIPS) carry missions to reduce accidental childhood injury through research, public policy, and education and awareness. By determining preventable risks to children, programs are developed to educate adults and children about how and why injuries happen and how they can be prevented. Many health care facilities and schools utilize the programs developed by these organizations to raise awareness and educate the public. Some of these programs include tips on how to prevent injuries and be safe in motor vehicles with restraints, as pedestrians, and during sports, as well as instructions on water safety (https://injury.research.chop.edu/center-child-injury-prevention-studies-cchip).

Because children with Down syndrome have some risk of atlantoaxial instability, the American Academy of Pediatrics[36] recommends screening radiographs to assess cervical spine stability for this population of children between the ages of 3 and 5 years. This radiographic screening is most helpful for children who may participate in sports or who are symptomatic. The Committee on Genetics[135] also recommends that children with achondroplasia be encouraged to participate in activities such as biking or swimming but to avoid gymnastics and contact sports because of the potential for neck or back injury.

ADVANCES IN RECOVERY

Researchers in spinal cord regeneration are focusing on neuroprotection, neuroplasticity, neuroregeneration, and cellular transplant therapy. Many have tried pharmacologic interventions to halt the chain of secondary events producing neural damage and to protect compromised but viable cells. Antioxidants, free radical scavengers, opiate antagonists, vitamins, thyrotropin-releasing hormone, and calcium channel

blockers are a few of the agents that have been tested.[119] The only current practice is the administration of methylprednisolone (corticosteroids) in the acute phase to decrease cord edema and limit cell death. High doses, administered within the first 8 hours and continued for 24 to 48 hours, have been shown to slightly enhance motor recovery in humans.[17-19,62,83] Data are lacking on the effects of methylprednisolone in the pediatric population. There have been no pediatric-specific studies, and past studies have had a minimal number of subjects in the 13- to 19-years-of-age category.[19] Currently, the use of the steroid overall is being questioned,[66,67,110,128] and it is even proposed to cause acute myopathy when administered.[119]

After a professional football player was injured while tackling during a game, a treatment of modest hypothermia gained attention.[24] This technique of slowly cooling the body's core temperature to 92°F for a period of time and then slowly rewarming potentially minimizes metabolic demands and edema within an injured spinal cord. Results are promising in terms of safety and have shown improvements in neurologic outcomes.[42] This neuroprotective therapy is still being studied in clinical trials.

A major focus in the SCI community most recently has been on stem cell transplants. Various sources have been used, such as olfactory epithelial cells, bone marrow stromal cells, and, most recently, human embryonic stem cells. Several physicians outside the United States[45,122] have injected humans with these cells, but none of these regimens were conducted through rigorous research, and reported results are mixed. It is a slow process to bring new pharmacotherapies into clinical practice, owing to the necessary steps of animal trials, followed by preliminary and then larger-scale trials in humans. Human trials must be placebo controlled and have a sufficient period of follow-up to assess the efficacy of the treatment. Because SCI is not common, clinical trials usually require collaboration among many medical centers. Approval to move these adult-based studies into the pediatric population is extremely difficult secondary to reluctance to approve studies by human subjects review boards and the Food and Drug Administration (FDA) in an attempt to protect this vulnerable population. It is not clear whether the young, immature spinal cord responds exactly the same way to injury as a mature spinal cord. Therefore, additional studies are being conducted in young animals to evaluate the sequelae of events after injury.

It is important to realize that patients and their families have been and will continue to be tempted by unproved therapies, often at considerable personal financial expense. Therapists can help them to evaluate the evidence regarding potential therapies. Any purported cure should be subjected to randomized clinical trials before being offered to hopeful but vulnerable patients. It is reasonable for patients and therapists to hold out hope for a cure for SCI. It is often just this hope that motivates patients and caregivers to be meticulous about preventing secondary complications.

PATHOPHYSIOLOGY

As mentioned earlier, the site or level at which SCI occurs is often related to the cause of injury and the child's age. Many of the nontraumatic causes (tumors, stenosis) of SCI occur in the thoracic spinal cord and result in incomplete injuries.[98] By contrast, vertebral dysplasias place the upper cervical spinal cord or lower brain stem at risk. Birth trauma as a result of traction and angulation of the spine in a breech delivery most commonly causes SCI at the cervicothoracic junction. In the child younger than 8 to 10 years old, the cervical spine has greater mobility than it does in adults because of ligamentous laxity, shallow angulation of the facets, incomplete ossification of vertebrae, and relative underdevelopment of the neck muscles for the size of the head.[151] Young children are therefore more likely to experience injury at the upper cervical spine than are adults,[15] and SCI may occur without any signs of bone damage by radiography, a finding referred to as SCI without radiographic abnormality, or SCIWORA.[16] Studies have reported the incidence of SCIWORA to be anywhere between 6% and 38% in skeletally immature children.[21,34] In children, 55% of cases of traumatic SCIs result in tetraplegia as a result of injury between the first cervical and first thoracic root levels, and 45% result in paraplegia from injury below the first thoracic level.[112]

Most cases of traumatic SCI are caused by a blunt, nonpenetrating injury to the spinal cord in which the cord is not lacerated or transected, and in the majority of cases, some white matter tracts remain intact across the lesion. The direct effect of the trauma is immediate disruption of neural transmission in the gray and white matter of the spinal cord at and below the injury site, resulting in spinal shock. Reactive physiologic events evolve over a period of hours and induce secondary injury to the spinal cord.[78] The exact sequence of events between transfer of kinetic energy to the cord and subsequent neuronal death is unknown. Animal models have shown that ischemia, hemorrhage, edema, calcium influx into cells, and generation of free radicals contribute to cell membrane degradation and death of neurons.[62] In gray matter, neurons that die are not replaced. In white matter, axonal segments distal to the injury degenerate and synapses no longer function. Although axonal sprouting does occur to a limited degree in the central nervous system (CNS), it appears to be functionally insignificant, and most of the recovery observed in patients with incomplete lesions is probably due to resolution of neurapraxic injury. Case reports of neurologic improvement years after SCI are rare but provide hope that therapies can be developed to enhance function in the remaining spinal cord tissue.[96]

The zone of injury within the spinal cord is usually large enough to cause a transition in neurologic function from normal to abnormal or from normal to absent over several spinal root levels. Soon after SCI, the level of injury may appear to move cephalad as the secondary or indirect injury processes set in. Later, the level of injury may move caudally as these factors resolve, as sprouting develops (either within the spinal cord or peripherally to denervated muscles), or as hypertrophy of weak muscles occurs. The extent of injury may diminish for as long as 1 year, and it is obvious that until the natural history of SCI and recovery is delineated, experimental treatments may be inappropriately credited with enhancing recovery.

There are several distinct patterns of neuroanatomic incomplete syndromes that have distinct clinical representations.

Anterior cord syndrome is usually due to damage of the anterior spinal artery causing infarction to the spinal cord. This injury produces variable motor paralysis, with reduced sensation of pain and temperature but with preserved dorsal column function. Prognosis for return of function is poor. Hemorrhage in the *central part of the cervical spinal cord* produces flaccid weakness of the arms and strong but spastic legs, with preservation of bladder and bowel function. As a result, ambulation is a potential goal for this population, but hand function may be impaired depending on the level of injury. *Posterior cord lesions* are rare and produce selective loss of proprioception with preserved motor function. Ambulation remains unlikely because of loss of proprioception. A *Brown-Séquard lesion* results in ipsilateral paralysis and proprioceptive loss and contralateral loss of pain and temperature sensation. Brown-Séquard is primarily seen with penetrating trauma to one side of the spinal cord, such as in a stab wound. Prognosis for ambulation as well as bladder and bowel control is good. Injury to the lumbosacral nerve roots results in *cauda equina syndrome,* with lower extremity weakness and areflexia of the legs and bladder. Cauda equina lesions are essentially lesions of the peripheral nerve or lower motoneuron and may show recovery over several years owing to resolution of neurapraxia or to regrowth of damaged axons, as well as to peripheral sprouting.

MEDICAL DIAGNOSIS, ACUTE MANAGEMENT, AND STABILIZATION

Emergent Stabilization (In the Field)

Initial management of a child with SCI is focused on stabilization of the spine to prevent further damage to the intact but injured spinal cord. The spine is immobilized during transport and throughout all assessments and procedures. Modified spine boards should be utilized with infants and toddlers to allow for proper neutral alignment of the cervical spine. Because of their larger head-to-torso ratio, their neck will be flexed on a regular spine board, potentially causing further injury. Modifications include either creating an occipital cutout or elevating the torso on an additional pad (preferred) to allow the cervical spine to be positioned neutrally[12,13,63] (Fig. 21.1).

Diagnostic Studies

At the hospital, a thorough neurologic examination is performed to determine the motor and sensory level of SCI and the completeness of injury. Spinal shock is usually present, although occasionally it has resolved by the time the patient is treated in the emergency department. In spinal shock, the muscles are flaccid below the SCI and all cutaneous and deep tendon reflexes are absent. This state persists for hours to weeks and is said to be over when sacral reflexes, including the bulbocavernous and anal reflexes, are present.

Further evaluation is undertaken with plain radiographs of the whole spine from the first cervical to the sacral vertebrae to identify any fractures, facet subluxations, or dislocations. Full radiographic evaluation is imperative as multiple, noncontiguous fractures occur in 30% of children.[14] Anteroposterior (AP) and lateral radiographs of the entire spine are needed to rule this out.[14] Computed tomography (CT) and magnetic resonance imaging (MRI) are used to diagnose root impingement, the presence of bone fragments in the spinal canal, cord compression, and spinal cord hemorrhage. Because of the high incidence of SCIWORA, particularly in children younger than

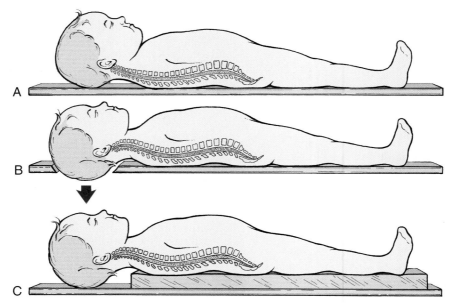

FIG. 21.1 Emergent stabilization. A, the enlarged occiput causes child to flex the head forward. Note improved spinal alignment with pediatric spine board modifications cut out (B) or elevation of torso (C), which is preferred. (From Mencio GA, Swiontkowski MF: *Green's skeletal trauma in children,* ed 5, Philadelphia, 2015, Elsevier.)

10 years of age, an MRI is indicated for all children who have sustained an SCI and can show problems that are not seen on plain radiographs.[14]

Surgical Stabilization

Whether immediate surgical intervention to correct bone injury and decompress the spinal cord is effective in reducing paralysis is unknown because the numerous surgical procedures have never been subjected to randomized clinical trials. The main goal of surgery is to prevent later deformity, pain, or loss of neurologic function. Surgery may not be necessary if spinal alignment can be achieved with traction and maintained with an orthosis. Tonged cervical traction in children under 12 years of age, however, has increased risks as compared with its use in adults. Therefore, halo traction may be safer and preferred,[12] even in axis (C2) fractures.[88] A variant in the use of halo traction is an increase in the number of pins used, while decreasing the amount of torque on each pin. If a halo cannot be applied, a Minerva-type cervicothoracolumbosacral orthosis (CTLSO) would be an option (Fig. 21.2). External halo orthoses[88] have also traditionally been used in conjunction with internal posterior wiring in children with atlantoaxial and occipital-cervical instability. However, investigation has identified successful rigid internal fixation for children requiring C1-C2 and occipital-cervical stabilization.[6]

Surgery is indicated if there is a penetrating injury, if traction has failed to reduce a dislocation, if nerve root impingement exists, if the spine is highly unstable and at risk of further damaging the cord, or if bone fragments are compressing the cauda equina.[50] Regardless of whether surgery is performed, if bone injury has occurred patients usually wear an external orthosis until bone fusion is complete, often for 3 or more months. There is, however, regional variation in practice among orthopedic surgeons in the use of spinal orthoses after spinal fusion. For some lower lumbar (L4 or L5) injuries, the surgeon may

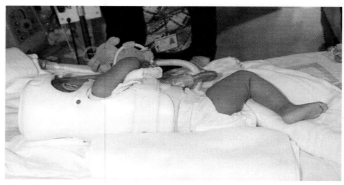

FIG. 21.2 Infant wearing CTLSO for acute stabilization secondary to C1-2 injury.

have the child wear an orthosis with a thigh piece, which permits only limited hip flexion (e.g., to only 60°). This is done to reduce torque on the immature fusion mass that could occur from pull of the hamstrings on the pelvis in a position of hip flexion.

Underlying Injuries and Comorbidities

Traumatic brain injury is one of the most commonly associated comorbidities and has been reported to occur in 38% of patients with SCI.[21] Traumatic brain injury, which can occur with any type of loss of consciousness, is important to recognize at initial examination as it can significantly affect the rehabilitation process and warrant additional therapies such as speech pathology and neuropsychologic testing (see Chapter 22 on acquired brain injuries for further information).

Another comorbidity that can be easily overlooked, particularly in someone with a cervical-level SCI, is injury to the brachial plexus. Brachial plexus injury should be considered if the mechanism of injury included any type of distraction to the shoulder or impingement or fracture of the clavicle in the presence of asymmetrical weakness in the upper extremities.

MEDICAL COMPLICATIONS, LONG-TERM MEDICAL MANAGEMENT, AND PREVENTION OF SECONDARY IMPAIRMENTS

A child's participation in SCI rehabilitation may be affected by a number of medical complications. Each of the following complications must be addressed by the entire rehabilitation team, physicians, nurses, therapists, and caregivers in order to achieve optimum outcomes.

Autonomic Dysreflexia

Autonomic dysreflexia (AD) is a massive reflex sympathetic discharge that occurs after an SCI of T6 or above in response to noxious stimuli below the level of injury, causing a sudden increase in blood pressure (BP > 15 mm Hg over baseline systolic).[97] If left untreated, the hypertensive crisis can cause stroke, seizures, or even death. Clinical features include headache, flushing, sweating, pilomotor activity, bradycardia or tachycardia, and hypertension. School-age children and adolescents are capable of reporting headaches, but younger children may have difficulty verbalizing symptoms and may have more nonspecific symptoms because of their maturing central and peripheral nervous systems. As a result, autonomic dysreflexia is often overlooked in these youngsters. Infants and children who are unusually sleepy, irritable, or crying may be experiencing an AD episode and should have their vital signs checked. Knowledge of baseline BPs are imperative, as infants, toddlers, and children up to 13 years of age have different normal values for BP.[137] Additionally, patients with SCI typically have lower resting BP (i.e., 90/60).[97]

The primary causes of an AD episode/noxious stimulus below the level of injury are an overdistended bladder and the need for catheterization or a kinked catheter in the instance of an indwelling system; an overdistended bowel and the need to complete a bowel program; and excessive pressure to the skin below the level of injury caused by a wrinkle in clothing, compression hose, or shoes that are too tight/small.

Treatment of AD includes monitoring BP, pulse, and temperature (at least every 5 minutes); elevation of the patient's head (unless contraindicated); removal of compression stockings and abdominal binders; and loosening of tight clothes/shoes. Next the clinician performs bladder management steps and, if BP does not decrease, completes a bowel regimen. It is important to continuously check vital signs for reduction in BP and return to normal as the various management techniques are completed. If none of the above methods resolve the dysreflexic episode, pharmacologic intervention by a physician or nurse practitioner may be warranted.

Respiratory Dysfunction

Respiratory insufficiency may occur with lesions of the cervical and thoracic spinal cord and is a prominent cause of morbidity and mortality in the population with SCI.[3] Dysfunction ranges anywhere from complete diaphragm paralysis and the requirement of mechanical ventilation (C1-C3 and occasionally C4 depending on age/size of child) to diminished vital capacity or weakened forced expiration during coughing as a result of absent/weakened accessory breathing muscles (lower cervical

and thoracic level injuries). Respiratory/breathing exercises are all too often overlooked as part of physical therapy rehabilitation but must be included. Respiratory exercises can occur during any part of treatment sessions, including during mat mobility and sitting balance activities. *Quad coughing* techniques are to be taught to the child and caregivers in order to assist with forced expiration when a cough alone is ineffective in clearing secretions. A quad cough is forced compression of the abdomen with a hand in an inward and upward fashion during expiration.

Deep Vein Thrombosis

Paralyzed and dependent lower extremities can develop edema and deep vein thromboses (DVTs). Although common in adults with SCI, deep vein thrombosis occurs less frequently in children with SCI (5%)[136] but does have a significant occurrence rate in 14- to 19-year-old adolescents.[136] A DVT prophylactic protocol of either insertion of an inferior vena cava filter (typically in older adolescents) or pharmacologic treatment is typically initiated during acute care hospitalization and completed during acute inpatient rehabilitation.

Hypercalcemia/Bone Density/Muscle Atrophy

Almost unique to children is the problem of immobilization hypercalcemia.[91] During the first 12 to 18 months after SCI, approximately 40% of bone mineral density is lost via calcium excreted in the urine. Children are more likely to have rapid bone turnover, resulting in a larger load of calcium than the kidneys can excrete. This produces elevated serum calcium level, or hypercalcemia. Nonspecific symptoms include lethargy, nausea, altered mood, and anorexia. Remobilization is an important aspect of treatment in persons without SCI (e.g., the child with a femur fracture), but it is not known if this is effective in reducing hypercalcemia after SCI. The mainstays of treating immobilization hypercalcemia are primarily medical through hydration for improved excretion of the excessive calcium in urine and administration of etidronate (Didronel) and calcitonin (Miacalcin) to avoid excessive calcification in unwanted areas, such as joints (heterotopic ossification) or kidneys (renal stones).

Pathologic fractures, which occur at an increased rate in persons with bone mineral densities below 40% of normal, are a potential complication of osteopenia. Deposition of new bone in periarticular soft tissue can also occur in paralyzed extremities. This heterotopic ossification can be asymptomatic, or it may interfere with range of motion (ROM) around a joint or even cause ankylosis. The most commonly affected joints are hips, knees, shoulders, and elbows. Muscle atrophy begins early and occurs at a rapid rate during acute immobilization through 24 weeks postinjury when it begins to plateau at approximately 15% loss of lean muscle mass below the level of injury.[57]

Orthostatic Hypotension

Orthostatic hypotension, a position-related drop in BP, is a common side effect with SCI. There is a decrease in the venous return of blood from the lower extremities as a result of muscle paralysis, which decreases cardiac output and arterial pressure, causing a quick drop in BP. As a result, the person's BP cannot adjust quickly enough during positional changes such as supine to sit, sit-to-stand, or coming out of a tilted position in a power wheelchair. Treatment for orthostatic hypotension can include gradient compression stockings, an abdominal binder, utilization of a wheelchair with a reclining back (particularly during acute care mobilization), tilt table, or pharmacologic intervention.

Early physical therapy sessions may address the goal of maintaining a stable BP when transitioning out of bed or while in the wheelchair. The patient's BP should be monitored throughout the treatment session.

Thermoregulatory Dysfunction

Persons with SCIs have an impaired ability to regulate body temperature resulting from the loss of hypothalamic thermoregulatory control and interruption of afferent pathways from peripheral temperature receptors below the level of injury. With injuries above T6, there is the complete loss of shivering and sweating and no peripheral circulatory adjustment below the level of injury. Education provided to children and caregivers must include the increased risk of hypothermia and frostbite in cold weather, as well as heat exhaustion and heat stroke in hot weather. Children with SCI should avoid excessive sun exposure and maintain adequate hydration.

Syringomyelia

Delayed cavitation (syringomyelia) within the damaged spinal cord can occur in patients with complete or incomplete lesions. The occurrence of a cystic cavitation, or syrinx, appears to be common after SCI and it may progressively enlarge, resulting in further loss of neurologic function months to years after SCI.[145] Signs and symptoms that may herald the presence of a syrinx include loss of motor function, ascending sensory level, increased spasticity or sweating, and a new onset of pain or dysesthesia.

Spasticity and Pain

Spasticity is a frequent occurrence after SCI and usually evolves over a period of 1 to 2 years. Although initially the patient is flaccid, hypertonus gradually appears, and in the first 3 to 6 months after SCI hyperreflexia, clonus and flexor spasms develop. Later, extensor spasms usually predominate. Evolution of spasticity after CNS insult is common and is seen in other conditions such as cerebral palsy and stroke. In SCI, the immediate effects of loss of supraspinal inhibition and the later-developing effects of denervation supersensitivity and sprouting by afferent and collateral neurons probably all contribute to the development of spasticity, but the sequence of events behind the evolution of clinical manifestations of spasticity is not known.

Spasticity can be controlled pharmacologically with oral medications, such as baclofen, intramuscular injections, such as Botox, or nerve block injections, such as phenol. Therapeutic interventions to control spasticity include passive ROM, passive and functional electrical stimulation (FES)–assisted cycling, and static standing. Many patients feel a certain amount of spasticity is helpful during transfers, bed mobility, or even some activities of daily living, so pharmacologic or other therapeutic interventions are usually withheld unless the spasticity is severe enough to limit function.

Neurogenic, or neuropathic, pain can occur after SCI at, above, or below the level of injury. Children and adolescents describe neurogenic pain as a burning pain, which anecdotally precedes the return of function or sensation at the dermatologic level(s) where pain is experienced. This type of pain can be unbearable but can be pharmacologically controlled with gabapentin (Neurontin) or pregabalin (Lyrica).

Skin Breakdown and Pressure Ulcers

Pressure ulcers occur as a result of improper positioning, both in bed as well as in a wheelchair, or inadequate pressure relief, which can limit the ability to sit. Pressure ulcers may also occur because of the improper fit of spinal orthoses, upper and lower extremity splints, and braces for ambulation. It is important to remember that skin breakdown is also caused by friction, shear, and moisture. All too often skin breakdown on the buttocks occurs from shearing across the wheel of the wheelchair during transfers and moisture secondary to improper bladder management or continuation of wearing a diaper beyond the age when the child should be dry between catheterizations.

Young children may not exhibit skin breakdown in the typical sense (from poor wheelchair or bed positioning) as seen with adolescents and adults because they are under direct care and guidance of their caregiver; however, young children typically have complete disregard for any body area that is insensate. They often will drag their lower extremities on the ground while crawling, or they may even bite insensate fingertips to the point of self-injury. As children grow older, it is often difficult for them to understand the importance of routine pressure-relief activities, particularly in the adolescent population with their tendency to test boundaries with caregivers. Patients and caregivers must also pay special attention to hot items on insensate skin to avoid burns (e.g., on the thighs from food that has been in the microwave such as popcorn or the heat generated by a laptop computer).

Pressure-relief techniques must also be taught. During acute care hospitalization and rehabilitation, the child/adolescent is turned every 2 hours and frequently is utilizing a specialty low air loss mattress. Children using power mobility can perform pressure-relieving techniques through powered seating, such as tilt and recline. Those using manual wheelchairs can perform wheelchair push-ups or lean laterally and anteriorly. The recommended frequency of pressure-relieving techniques varies between 15 to 30 minutes and should last 1 minute to allow return of blood flow to compressed tissue.[38] Children often utilize a watch with a timer to provide an audio reminder to complete weight-shift/pressure-relief measures at designated times.

Orthopedic Management

Contractures can arise as a result of static positioning, spasticity, or heterotopic bone formation and may interfere with positioning or voluntary movement. As a result, passive ROMs or the prolonged stretches, which an upright stander can provide, are imperative to use as treatments. Tightness is most typically seen in the hip flexor, hamstring, adductor, and ankle plantar flexor muscles. Of note is the fact that children and adolescents with flaccid paralysis may develop "pseudo hip flexion contractures," in which the iliotibial band is actually the tight muscle rather than the iliopsoas and rectus femoris muscles.

Hip subluxation (Fig. 21.3) and dislocation are common in children who have onset of SCI before age 10, with an incidence up to 66% in children under 4 years of age.[93] Management to prevent subluxation/dislocation includes stretching of hip adductor and flexor muscles; proper bed positioning in an abducted position with either a wedge or pillow; and wheelchair seating positioning that encourages proper femoral alignment, such as a medial thigh build-up or pommel. Prevention is important, because although typically nonpainful, hip dislocation can lead to pelvic obliquity and other postural changes that will place the child at greater risk of skin breakdown as well as

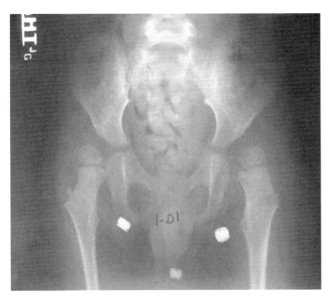

FIG. 21.3 Hip instability.

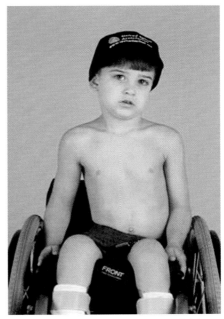

FIG. 21.4 Neuromuscular scoliosis.

exacerbate a neuromuscular scoliosis.[93] Treatment can include surgical plating and pinning to restore joint alignment.

Pathologic fractures can occur to osteopenic extremities as a result of disregard of lower extremities during transfers, falls, or forceful ROM exercises. The osteopenia has been found to be greatest at the hip and knee as compared to children their age without a disability.[84]

Neuromuscular scoliosis occurs in virtually all children with SCI (up to 98% has been reported[13]), particularly in patients injured before their adolescent growth spurt, and can affect the comfort of seating and respiratory function. Sixty-seven percent progress to the point of requiring spinal fusion.[13] Although it is important to provide proper pelvic alignment and trunk support in wheelchairs, external support devices in wheelchairs do not seem to ultimately prevent the development of scoliosis (Fig. 21.4).[14]

Prophylactic bracing is a controversial topic in therapy because the wear of a thoracolumbosacral orthosis (TLSO) will most likely inhibit independent activities, mobility, and reachable workspace while worn.[30,130] The argument, however, is that wearing the brace prophylactically can prevent (curves < 10°) or even delay (curves < 20°) spine fusion. If surgery can be delayed until these children have achieved nearly all of their trunk growth, bracing is considered successful. Once a curve nears or surpasses 20°, however, bracing may be futile.[99] Typical brace prescription can range from "while out of bed" for less significant curves to 23 hours a day, for which aggressive brace wear can delay progression when close to the 20° cutoff, particularly during growth spurts.[99] Brace wear compliance is always a question, as many children and teens tend to return for follow-up and leave the brace at home. Surgery for neuromuscular scoliosis becomes indicated once the degree of curve causes respiratory compromise or significant pelvic obliquity that increases the risk of ischial pressure ulcers.

FOREGROUND INFORMATION

PHYSICAL THERAPY EXAMINATION

The physical therapy examination of the child with spinal cord injury is influenced by many factors, including the age of the child presently as well as age at injury, the development and maturation of the child, any concomitant injuries such as a traumatic brain injury or cognitive delay, and the family's understanding of SCI. Physical therapists examine children with SCI in the acute care, rehabilitation, outpatient, home, and school settings. What is examined in each setting will depend on the age of the child, the child's abilities and needs, and the setting itself.

Key History and Systems Review Information

The physical therapist must have an understanding of the child's history, comorbidities, and restrictions. Children with SCI are at risk for secondary conditions such as skin integrity issues, pain, cardiovascular issues and disease, pulmonary and respiratory issues, and musculoskeletal issues. These issues should be screened for during the examination. Box 21.1 lists questions that should be included in the examination history and systems review. Depending on the child's age, these questions may be answered by the parents/caregiver or the child.

Tests for Impairments of Body Structure and Function

Quantification of changes in body structure and function in the young child is often unreliable because young children are unable to cooperate consistently with formal testing. Passive ROM measurement is possibly an exception, but intrarater and interrater reliability in children with SCI have not been established. In children without SCI and in children with myelodysplasia, manual muscle testing is generally unreliable if the child is younger than 5 years of age.[95,101] In young children, strength testing is often estimated by encouraging and observing movement. Ideally, the therapist places the child in various positions and encourages him or her to reach for toys with a single extremity. This allows examination of gravity-eliminated and antigravity movements, as well as comparison of left and right extremities. Resistance can be provided with small wrap weights (0.25 lb) or the weight of handheld toys. In reality, the best choice may be for the physical therapist to observe

BOX 21.1 **History and Systems Review Questions**

Date, cause, level, ASIA, AIS classification if known
Concomitant injuries
Current medications
Medical, surgical, and rehabilitative management
Neurologic change
Pain and response to pain
Current functional performance: what the child is capable of doing versus
    what the child typically does, how function has changed with growth
    and development
History of orthostatic hypotension and autonomic dysreflexia
Secondary conditions such as scoliosis, hip subluxation, or new medical
    diagnosis
Current equipment and issues or problems with the equipment
Environmental barriers
Social support
Level of participation at home, school, and in the community
Modes of transportation
Psychological status
Changes since last examination
Current goals
Questions the child or parent may have

TABLE 21.2 **Key Muscles for Motor Level Classification**

C5	Elbow flexors (biceps, brachialis)
C6	Wrist extensors (extensor carpi radialis longus and brevis)
C7	Elbow extensors (triceps)
C8	Finger flexors to the middle finger (flexor digitorum profundus)
T1	Small finger abductors (abductor digiti minimi manus)
L2	Hip flexors (iliopsoas)
L3	Knee extensors (quadriceps)
L4	Ankle dorsiflexors (tibialis anterior)
L5	Long toe extensors (extensor hallucis longus)
S1	Ankle plantar flexors (gastrocnemius, soleus)

From American Spinal Injury Association: *International standards for neurological and functional classification of spinal cord injury*, Chicago, 2000, revised 2002, American Spinal Injury Association.

spontaneous play and record descriptions of available movements. Ruling out substitutions can be challenging. Muscle strength is recorded as 0 through 5, as with adults (rarely with the finer + or − gradations). Scores of 4 and 5 are subjective measures, particularly in growing children, but with experience the therapist can become an increasingly more accurate evaluator. While examining muscle strength and function, spasticity and spasms should be noted. The physical therapist also facilitates the child's basic postural responses, such as positive support of the lower extremities or protective extension of the upper extremities. Postural alignment should be assessed as well as balance in sitting and standing if applicable.

International Standards for Neurological Classification of Spinal Cord Injury or American Spinal Injury Association Examination

Professionals should use a common terminology when describing the motor or sensory levels of SCI in children or adults. Most widely used are the International Standards for Neurological Classification of Spinal Cord Injury (ISNCSCI), which are published by the American Spinal Injury Association (ASIA).[2,80] The ISNCSCI standards were developed by consensus of a multidisciplinary group of clinical experts and have been revised periodically since initial publication in 1982. The ISNCSCI standards, more commonly referred to as the ASIA Examination, define right and left motor levels, right and left sensory levels, the neurologic level, the severity of injury (i.e., complete versus incomplete), and a classification called the ASIA Impairment Scale (AIS). The ISNCSCI standards have been used as the primary indicators to predict recovery of neurologic function,[20,89,92,150] and the exams have been used to determine inclusion for entry into drug and device trials that pertain to SCI,[19,60,96,114,125,133,134] including outcomes of activity-based rehabilitation, a program of intensive cycling, assisted treadmill training, and swimming.[96]

Precise description of the motor and sensory loss after SCI is important for two reasons. First, it helps predict the likelihood of further neurologic recovery in both complete and incomplete syndromes. For instance, in motor complete C5 tetraplegia, most if not all patients gain one full motor level, achieving grade 3 wrist extensor movement (a C6 muscle) during the first 8 months after injury.[44] Researchers have also determined that in SCI above T11, preservation of pinprick sensation has predictive value for return of motor function and independent ambulation, probably because of the proximity of the ascending pain fibers and descending motor fibers in the spinal cord.[114] The second reason for the importance of a precise definition of the level of SCI is that it helps predict the ultimate level of independence a patient can expect to achieve in the areas of mobility, self-care, and even communication. Patients with incomplete SCI may exceed the expectations for any given level of injury. Such expectations for independence must also be tempered by consideration of the child's age, which influences developmental expectations. It can take years for preschoolers to reach the expected level of independence, or they may fall short of expectations if complications, particularly orthopedic problems, arise. Environmental and personal factors also play an important role in determining the child's participation in home life, education, community activities, and social relationships.

Defining the Level of Spinal Cord Injury

The ASIA standards accept the widely used system of muscle grading: 0 = absence, total paralysis; 1 = trace, palpable, or visible contraction; 2 = poor, active movement through full ROM with gravity eliminated; 3 = fair, active movement through full ROM against gravity; 4 = good, active movement through full ROM against moderate resistance; and 5 = normal, active movement through full ROM against full resistance. Motor levels may differ for right and left sides of the body. The key muscles for determining motor level are listed in Table 21.2. Because all muscles have innervation from more than one root level, the presence of innervation by one root level and the absence by the next lower level result in a weakened muscle. The ASIA-defined motor level is the most caudal root level in which muscle strength is grade 3 or more and the next most rostral muscle a grade 5. By convention, if a muscle has grade 3 strength and the next most rostral muscle is grade 5, the grade 3 muscle is considered to have full innervation by the higher root level, for which it is named. For example, for a patient with a grade 2 C8 key muscle, grade 3 C7 key muscle, grade 4 C6 key muscle, and grade 5 C5 key muscle, the motor level as defined by ASIA is C6. One disadvantage to using only the ASIA key muscles to define a level of function is the omission of examination of hip extensor, hip abductor, and knee flexor muscles. These L5 and S1 muscles play an important role in activities such as transfers, ambulation, and stair climbing. Strength grades of the key muscles can be added together for both sides of the body to create a composite ASIA motor score. This score has been used in research studies assessing the efficacy of pharmacologic treatment of SCI.[7,17-19,45,79,83,122] It can also be used to predict function and need for assistance.[121,123,150]

The sensory level may not correspond exactly to the motor level. Determining the sensory level is especially helpful in injuries above C5 or to the thoracic spinal cord, where there are no key muscles to define the level of SCI. Rather than relying on dermatome charts, which vary from one text to another, the ASIA standards rely on the presence of normal light touch and sharp/dull discrimination (pinprick) sensation at a key point in each of the 28 dermatomes on the right and left sides of the body (Fig. 21.5A, and Table 21.2). Proprioception should also be assessed below the level of injury in patients with incomplete SCI to determine the integrity of dorsal column function.

Classification

A complete injury, or AIS A classification, is defined as the total absence of motor or sensory function in the lowest sacral segments (Fig. 21.5B). There may be some preservation of sensation or motor levels below the level of injury. This is defined as a *zone of partial preservation*, a term used only with complete injuries.

A patient is said to have an incomplete SCI, AIS B, C, or D classification, only if motor or sensory function is present in the lowest sacral segment, implying voluntary control of the external anal sphincter, sensation at the mucocutaneous junction, or both. Further delineation between incomplete classifications occurs based on the extent of preservation of sensory or motor function below the level of injury.

An addition has been the Autonomic Standards Assessment Form (Fig. 21.5C), which highlights autonomic function/dysfunction and can be used to complement the ISNCSCI standards.

Application to the Pediatric Population

Historically, the ISNCSCI standards or ASIA examination has routinely been the clinical tool used for assessing pediatric patients with SCI. It is considered the gold standard assessment for assessing prognosis and outcomes, yet the actual utility in the pediatric population was not assessed until recently. Research suggests that the ISNCSCI exams may have poor utility overall in children under 4 years of age, as they were unable to complete the exam.[105] Additionally, the results suggest poor cooperation of children age 10 and under in terms of anxiety during the pinprick portion of the discrimination exam. Results also showed low precision in confidence intervals for total motor scores in children up to the age of 15, bringing into question the reliability of the motor examination.[105]

Additional questions revolve around the clinical validity of the anorectal exam in classifying children with SCI, particularly children who were injured prior to being potty trained who have never had to conceptualize holding in a bowel movement (which is the verbiage typically used during the anal contraction portion of the exam).[147] Preteens and teenagers may also have difficulty with the anorectal portion of the examination because of privacy concerns.

The WeeSTeP, a complement to InSTeP, is an electronic training module developed to outline pediatric considerations for the current ISNCSCI standards (www.asialearningcenter.org). Some modifications include altering the method of approaching child, conducting sensory testing in a nonthreatening manner, altering vocabulary used to make it more child friendly, and giving the child sense of control during test. Alternatives also include an observational motor assessment or infant motor scale to a certain age. Most important, however, is explaining to the parents/caregivers the current standards, how classification may not be able to be ascertained due to the child's age, and that repeated testing during various points of follow-up will be used in an attempt to identify neurologic change until the child is old enough to reliably complete the ISNCSCI standards (or until a pediatric version becomes available to use as a clinical tool).

Depending on experience and the policy of the facility, a physical therapist may be the clinician completing the ISNCSCI standards examination. In the case of the pediatric patient, it would be the examiner's responsibility to educate the parent and possibly the patient on the purpose of the examination, how it may be modified for the child, as well as the outcome. Based on the age of the child and the examination results, the physical therapist may be able to determine the SCI characteristics such as severity and level of injury.

Tests for Activity and Participation

The physical therapist must establish a thorough baseline report of the child's abilities and activity and determine whether activity limitations and participation restrictions are due to the child's age, primary neurologic changes in body structure and function, secondary conditions such as contractures, pain, decreased endurance, the need to wear a spinal orthosis, or other causes. The Functional Independence Measure (FIM) (for adolescents), Functional Independence Measure for Children (WeeFIM),[1,113] Pediatric Evaluation of Disability Inventory (PEDI),[61,111] Pediatric Quality of Life (PedsQL), and Canadian Occupational Performance Measure (COPM) have all been used to describe function and measure outcomes for children with SCI; however, none fully identifies changes with recovery and rehabilitation in children with SCI.

The FIM and WeeFIM are measures used in acute rehabilitation across many diagnoses to determine the "burden of care." These measures, when used with patients with SCI, may not be sensitive enough to detect change associated with return of function, and some areas tested have ceiling and floor effects. Additionally, a change in FIM or WeeFIM score may be based more on lack of injury severity rather than length of inpatient rehabilitation.[56] For example, in comparing a child with a complete cervical injury to a child with an incomplete thoracic injury, each of whom had a 4-week inpatient rehabilitation stay, the child with the incomplete thoracic injury may show a much larger change in FIM or WeeFIM scores. This change is more related to the fact that, based on level of injury, the amount of functional change is inherently greater as measured by the FIM or WeeFIM, rather than reflecting the effectiveness or amount of rehabilitation received.

Overall, no one measure or test has been deemed the most effective and efficient for children and adolescents with SCIs. One option may be the Spinal Cord Independence Measure (SCIM) III, developed in 1994, which measures performance of daily activities in patients with spinal cord lesions. It has

INTERNATIONAL STANDARDS FOR NEUROLOGICAL CLASSIFICATION OF SPINAL CORD INJURY (ISNCSCI)

ASIA · ISCOS

Patient Name _____ Date/Time of Exam _____
Examiner Name _____ Signature _____

RIGHT — MOTOR KEY MUSCLES — SENSORY KEY SENSORY POINTS: Light Touch (LTR), Pin Prick (PPR)

C2, C3, C4

UER (Upper Extremity Right)
Elbow flexors C5
Wrist extensors C6
Elbow extensors C7
Finger flexors C8
Finger abductors (little finger) T1

Comments (Non-key Muscle? Reason for NT? Pain?):

T2, T3, T4, T5, T6, T7, T8, T9, T10, T11, T12, L1

LER (Lower Extremity Right)
Hip flexors L2
Knee extensors L3
Ankle dorsiflexors L4
Long toe extensors L5
Ankle plantar flexors S1

S2, S3, S4-5

(VAC) Voluntary anal contraction (Yes/No)

RIGHT TOTALS (MAXIMUM) (50) (56) (56)

LEFT — SENSORY KEY SENSORY POINTS: Light Touch (LTL), Pin Prick (PPL) — MOTOR KEY MUSCLES

C2, C3, C4

C5 Elbow flexors
C6 Wrist extensors
C7 Elbow extensors
C8 Finger flexors
T1 Finger abductors (little finger)

UEL (Upper Extremity Left)

MOTOR (SCORING ON REVERSE SIDE)
0 = total paralysis
1 = palpable or visible contraction
2 = active movement, gravity eliminated
3 = active movement, against gravity
4 = active movement, against some resistance
5 = active movement, against full resistance
5* = normal corrected for pain/disuse
NT = not testable

SENSORY (SCORING ON REVERSE SIDE)
0 = absent   2 = normal
1 = altered   NT = not testable

T2, T3, T4, T5, T6, T7, T8, T9, T10, T11, T12, L1

L2 Hip flexors
L3 Knee extensors
L4 Ankle dorsiflexors
L5 Long toe extensors
S1 Ankle plantar flexors

LEL (Lower Extremity Left)

S2, S3, S4-5

(DAP) Deep anal pressure (Yes/No)

LEFT TOTALS (56) (56) (50) (MAXIMUM)

• Key Sensory Points
Palm / Dorsum

MOTOR SUBSCORES
UER ___ + UEL ___ = UEMS TOTAL ___   LER ___ + LEL ___ = LEMS TOTAL ___
MAX (25) (25) (50)   MAX (25) (25) (50)

SENSORY SUBSCORES
LTR ___ + LTL ___ = LT TOTAL ___   PPR ___ + PPL ___ = PP TOTAL ___
MAX (56) (56) (112)   MAX (56) (56) (112)

NEUROLOGICAL LEVELS Steps 1-5 for classification as on reverse
1. SENSORY (R) (L)
2. MOTOR (R) (L)

3. NEUROLOGICAL LEVEL OF INJURY (NLI)

4. COMPLETE OR INCOMPLETE? Incomplete = Any sensory or motor function in S4-5
5. ASIA IMPAIRMENT SCALE (AIS)

(In complete injuries only) **ZONE OF PARTIAL PRESERVATION** Most caudal level with any innervation
SENSORY (R) (L)
MOTOR (R) (L)

A — This form may be copied freely but should not be altered without permission from the American Spinal Injury Association. REV 11/15

Muscle Function Grading

0 = total paralysis
1 = palpable or visible contraction
2 = active movement, full range of motion (ROM) with gravity eliminated
3 = active movement, full ROM against gravity
4 = active movement, full ROM against gravity and moderate resistance in a muscle specific position
5 = (normal) active movement, full ROM against gravity and full resistance in a functional muscle position expected from an otherwise unimpaired person
5* = (normal) active movement, full ROM against gravity and sufficient resistance to be considered normal if identified inhibiting factors (i.e. pain, disuse) were not present
NT = not testable (i.e. due to immobilization, severe pain such that the patient cannot be graded, amputation of limb, or contracture of > 50% of the normal range of motion)

Sensory Grading

0 = Absent
1 = Altered, either decreased/impaired sensation or hypersensitivity
2 = Normal
NT = Not testable

When to Test Non-Key Muscles:

In a patient with an apparent AIS B classification, non-key muscle functions more than 3 levels below the motor level on each side should be tested to most accurately classify the injury (differentiate between AIS B and C).

Movement	Root level
Shoulder: Flexion, extension, abduction, adduction, internal and external rotation / Elbow: Supination	C5
Elbow: Pronation / Wrist: Flexion	C6
Finger: Flexion at proximal joint, extension / Thumb: Flexion, extension and abduction in plane of thumb	C7
Finger: Flexion at MCP joint / Thumb: Opposition, adduction and abduction perpendicular to palm	C8
Finger: Abduction of the index finger	T1
Hip: Adduction	L2
Hip: External rotation	L3
Hip: Extension, abduction, internal rotation / Knee: Flexion / Ankle: Inversion and eversion / Toe: MP and IP extension	L4
Hallux and Toe: DIP and PIP flexion and abduction	L5
Hallux: Adduction	S1

ASIA Impairment Scale (AIS)

A = Complete. No sensory or motor function is preserved in the sacral segments S4-5.

B = Sensory Incomplete. Sensory but not motor function is preserved below the neurological level and includes the sacral segments S4-5 (light touch or pin prick at S4-5 or deep anal pressure) AND no motor function is preserved more than three levels below the motor level on either side of the body.

C = Motor Incomplete. Motor function is preserved at the most caudal sacral segments for voluntary contraction (VAC) OR the patient meets the criteria for sensory incomplete status (sensory function preserved at the most caudal sacral segments (S4-S5) by LT, PP or DAP), and has some sparing of motor function more than three levels below the ipsilateral motor level on either side of the body. (This includes key or non-key muscle functions to determine motor incomplete status.) For AIS C–less than half of key muscle functions below the single NLI have a muscle grade >3.

D = Motor Incomplete. Motor incomplete status as defined above, with at least half (half or more) of key muscle functions below the NLI have a muscle grade ≥ 3.

E = Normal. If sensation and motor function as tested with the ISNCSCI are graded as normal in all segments, and the patient had prior deficits, then the AIS grade is E. Someone without an initial SCI does not receive an AIS grade.

Using ND: To document the sensory, motor and NLI levels, the ASIA Impairment Scale grade, and/or the zone of partial preservation (ZPP) whey they are unable to be determined based on the examination results.

Steps in Classification

The following order is recommended for determining the classification of individuals with SCI.

1. Determine sensory levels for right and left sides.
The sensory level is the most caudal, intact dermatome for both pin prick and light touch sensation.

2. Determine motor levels for right and left sides.
Defined by the lowest key muscle function that has a grade of at least 3 (on supine testing), providing the key muscle functions represented by segments above that level are judged to be intact (graded as ≥ 5).
Note: in regions where there is no myotome to test, the motor level is presumed to be the same as the sensory level, if testable motor function above that level is also normal.

3. Determine the neurological level of injury (NLI).
This refers to the most caudal segment of the cord with intact sensation and antigravity (3 or more) muscle function strength, provided that there is normal (intact) sensory and motor function rostrally respectively.
The NLI is the most cephalad of the sensory and motor levels determined in steps 1 and 2.

4. Determine whether the injury is Complete or Incomplete.
(i.e. absence or presence of sacral sparing)
If voluntary anal contraction = **No** AND all S4-5 sensory scores = **0** AND deep anal pressure = **No**, then injury is **Complete**.
Otherwise, injury is **Incomplete**.

5. Determine ASIA Impairment Scale (AIS) Grade:

Is injury **Complete?** If YES, AIS=A and can record
NO ↓ ZPP (lowest dermatome or myotome on each side with some preservation)

Is injury Motor Complete? If YES, AIS=B
NO ↓ (No=voluntary anal contraction OR motor function more than three levels below the motor level on a given side, if the patient has sensory incomplete classification)

Are at least half (half or more) of the key muscles below the neurological level of injury graded 3 or better?
NO ↓   YES ↓
AIS=C   AIS=D

If sensation and motor function are normal in all segments, AIS=E
Note: AIS E is used in follow-up testing when an individual with a documented SCI has recovered normal function. If at initial testing no deficits are found, the individual is neurologically intact; the ASIA Impairment Scale does not apply.

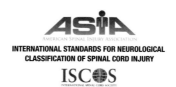

INTERNATIONAL STANDARDS FOR NEUROLOGICAL CLASSIFICATION OF SPINAL CORD INJURY

AMERICAN SPINAL INJURY ASSOCIATION

INTERNATIONAL SPINAL CORD SOCIETY

B

FIG. 21.5 A, Scoring sheet with key sensory testing areas by dermatome for ASIA Examination. Dot in each dermatome indicates exact location within dermatome to complete sensory testing. B, Muscle grading, impairment scale, and steps in classification.

Autonomic Standards Assessment Form

Autonomic Diagnosis: (Supraconal ☐, Conal ☐, Cauda Equina ☐)

Patient Name: _____

General Autonomic Function

System/Organ	Findings	Abnormal conditions	Check mark
Autonomic control of the heart	Normal		
	Abnormal	Bradycardia	
		Tachycardia	
		Other dysrhythmias	
	Unknown		
	Unable to assess		
Autonomic control of blood pressure	Normal		
	Abnormal	Resting systolic blood pressure below 90 mmHg	
		Orthostatic hypotension	
		Autonomic dysreflexia	
	Unknown		
	Unable to assess		
Autonomic control of sweating	Normal		
	Abnormal	Hyperhydrosis above lesion	
		Hyperhydrosis below lesion	
		Hypohydrosis below lesion	
	Unknown		
	Unable to assess		
Temperature regulations	Normal		
	Abnormal	Hyperthermia	
		Hypothermia	
	Unknown		
	Unable to assess		
Autonomic and Somatic Control of Bronchopulmonary System	Normal		
	Abnormal	Unable to voluntarily breathe requiring full ventilatory support	
		Impaired voluntary breathing requiring partial vent support	
		Voluntary respiration impaired does not require vent support	
	Unknown		
	Unable to assess		

C

Lower Urinary Tract, Bowel and Sexual Function

System/Organ		Score
Lower Urinary Tract		
Awareness of the need to empty the bladder		
Ability to prevent leakage (continence)		
Bladder emptying method (specify)_____		
Bowel		
Sensation of need for a bowel movement		
Ability to Prevent Stool Leakage (continence)		
Voluntary sphincter contraction		
Sexual Function		
Genital arousal (erection or lubrication)	Psychogenic	
	Reflex	
Orgasm		
Ejaculation (male only)		
Sensation of Menses (female only)		

2=Normal function, 1=Reduced or Altered Neurological Function
0=Complete loss of control, NT=Unable to assess due to preexisting or concomitant problems

Date of Injury_____ Date of Assessment _____

This form may be freely copied and reproduced but not modfied.
This assessment should use the terminology found in the International
SCI Data Sets (ASIA and ISCoS - http://www.iscos.org.uk)

Examiner _____

Appendix II

INTERNATIONAL SPINAL CORD INJURY DATA SETS[4]

Urodynamic Basic Data Set Form

Date performed:_____ ☐ Unknown

Bladder sensation during filling cystometry:
☐ Normal ☐ Increased ☐ Reduced ☐ Absent
☐ Non-specific ☐ Unknown

Detrusor function
☐ Normal ☐ Neurogenic detrusor overactivity
☐ Underactive detrusor ☐ Acontractile detrusor
☐ Unknown

Compliance during filling cystometry:
Low (< 10 mL/cm H_2O) ☐ Yes ☐ No ☐ Unknown

Urethral function during voiding:
☐ Normal ☐ Detrusor sphincter dyssynergia
☐ Non-relaxing urethral sphincter obstruction
☐ Not applicable ☐ Unknown

Detrusor leak point pressure_____cm H_2O
☐ Not applicable ☐ Unknown

Maximum detrusor pressure_____cm H_2O
☐ Not applicable ☐ Unknown

Cystometric bladder capacity_____mL
☐ Not applicable ☐ Unknown

Post void residual volume_____mL
☐ Not applicable ☐ Unknown

FIG. 21.5, cont'd C, Autonomic standards assessment, newly added assessment sheet to complement muscle and sensory testing of ASIA examination. (Adapted from American Spinal Injury Association: *International standards for neurological classification of spinal cord injury*, revised 2011, Atlanta, GA, Revised 2011, ASIA., Updated 2015.)

been shown to have strong construct validity (.8–1.4, $p < .05$), interrater reliability (SCIM III kappa .64–.84; ICC > .94), and sensitivity to change (SCIM II, 2001)[26-28] in adults even when compared to the FIM.[27] Evaluating the utility and psychometric properties of the SCIM-III in children with SCI is currently underway. Another option may be Computerized Adaptive Testing (CAT), which employs an algorithm and adapts the number of questions to each specific individual based on previous answers given to achieve the desired precision of scores for all children on a standard metric.[47] Work on development of parent- and child-report CAT specifically for children with SCI has been completed,[22,103,104] and clinical deployment is under way. These SCI-specific CATs, which evaluate general mobility, wheeled mobility, self-care, school, chores, and leisure functions as well as participation, can be used to monitor the child longitudinally or determine change due to an intervention.

It is also critical to systematically test the child's ability to reach in a variety of positions, roll, position in bed, come to sitting, balance in sitting, scoot, crawl, transfer to and from a variety of surfaces, come to kneel, stand, and ambulate. Some or all of these may not be possible, so the type and amount of assistance needed are recorded, or the therapist may simply record the movement as "unable." In general, when assessing function, the dependent, maximal, moderate, and minimal assistance, supervision, and independent scale is used (Table 21.3); however, it is often further qualified based on developmental appropriateness. For example, a child may be able to physically push his or her wheelchair across the street; however, children do not do this independently because the average young child does not move across the street without supervision. Additionally, children may be able to complete a task independently but on a typical basis their parent does it for them (i.e., getting dressed in the morning). Both can be noted and monitored over time.

The examination of the infant, young child, or adolescent with SCI will require modification based on chronologic as well as developmental age. As previously mentioned, determination of motor and sensory levels in infants and young children is challenging and may require multiple examinations to determine what movement is voluntary and what is reflexively mediated. The therapist can determine activity limitations by comparing the infant's motor skills such as head control,

rolling, sitting balance, transitional movements, crawling, and standing with expected developmental milestones. Very young children with SCI require careful follow-up over time to ensure that they meet functional goals and are not infantilized by caregivers.

PHYSICAL THERAPY INTERVENTION

Rehabilitation and Habilitation

Research in the adult population has shown that timely referral of patients with SCI to comprehensive, multidisciplinary SCI centers is more cost effective, with improved patient outcomes, reduced hospital and long-term nursing care charges, and an improved prospect for long-term patient earnings, compared with unspecialized care for SCI patients.[25]

The acute rehabilitation and long-term treatment of children with SCI require a comprehensive interdisciplinary approach involving both hospital and school-based personnel. Team members typically include physical therapists, physicians, nurses, a dietitian, occupational and speech therapists, therapeutic recreation specialists, a social worker, an orthotist, a clinical psychologist, teachers, the child, and the family.

Physical therapists often work alongside a pediatric physiatrist, who typically provides medical management and serves as a team leader. In some centers, however, an orthopedist, a neurologist, or a pediatrician may fill this role. The lead physician may also request consultation by other physicians such as an orthopedic surgeon or neurosurgeon to monitor spine stability and alignment, a urologist to monitor urinary tract function, and a pulmonologist for ventilator management.

Physical therapists develop age-appropriate ROM, strengthening, and SCI education programs. They address functional mobility, including bed mobility, transfers, sitting balance, ambulation, and basic and advanced wheelchair skills. The physical therapist makes recommendations on lower extremity orthoses and plays a primary role in the ordering of a wheelchair. Goals must be set according to usual expectations for age. Greater independence with varying degrees of transfers and mobility will be expected the older the child.

Continuum of Care

Like the physical therapy examination, the interventions may differ in each setting based on the age, abilities, and needs of the child. In general, in the acute care setting, the physical therapy focus is on education, prevention of secondary complications, and discharge planning. During inpatient rehabilitation, physical therapy interventions include trialing, choosing appropriate equipment, and functional activities such as engaging in developmentally appropriate and continued education. With development and increasing age, returning to the inpatient rehabilitation setting for "brush up rehab" is an option. Learning new skills or advancing skills as developmentally appropriate can also occur in the outpatient setting. Home care services may be warranted if the focus is to allow for independence in the home setting, whereas school-based interventions will address the needs of the child while functioning at school.

Education

Physical therapists should include parents as active participants during both the examination and intervention phases. Parent goals often focus on wanting the child "to walk again." However, parents must become experts in all aspects of their

TABLE 21.3	Levels of Assistance for Functional Assessment
Terminology	**Definition**
Independence	Able to complete the activity safely and timely without assistance of another person and without the use of aids or devices
Modified independence	Able to complete the activity safely without assistance but requires aids or devices or takes extra time to complete
Supervision	Able to complete the activity without physical assistance but another person is present for safety or to provide support if needed
Minimal assistance	A small amount of assistance is required; typically the patient does 75% or more of the task
Moderate assistance	A greater amount of assistance is required, typically the patient does 50%–74% of the task
Maximal assistance	The patient does 25%–49% of the task
Dependent/unable to do	The patient does less than 25% of the task

child's mobility and use of adaptive equipment. Parent education and training should be an ongoing process that begins soon after the initial examination and supports success with day or overnight outings. Physical therapy goals for this population focus on education, as the family must be thoroughly trained in all aspects of the child's mobility and care. Children must also be trained to instruct others in their care, including use and maintenance of the wheelchair, mechanical lift, environmental control unit (ECU), computer access, and any other equipment.

Outcomes

The therapist and SCI team must assist the family and child in establishing realistic outcomes. One must consider the child's level of injury (Tables 21.4 and 21.5), the completeness of injury, the age of the child, and the family's expectations for the child. Parents should be included in treatment sessions whenever possible. Although many children work better in therapy sessions in the absence of parents, parents should be regularly included to see the new skills their child can independently accomplish and the emerging skills that require assistance.

Every parent and caregiver want the child with an SCI to walk again. Ambulation is feasible and can be tried with certain portions of this population; however, the goals for ambulation must be realistic.[23] In many cases, ambulation does not replace the use of a wheelchair, especially with braced ambulation, as it is both time and energy consuming. Studies have looked at the relationship between results of the ISNCSCI examination and ambulatory ability.[29,123,150] One pediatric study determined that the total lower extremity motor score can predict ambulatory potential, including the use of ambulation as a primary mode of mobility.[29] Two

adult-based studies found that the total lower extremity motor score is directly related to the potential for an individual with SCI to ambulate. If the total lower extremity motor score is less than or equal to 20, an individual's ambulatory ability is typically limited to household situations, in contrast to those with scores greater than or equal to 30, who are often community ambulators.[150] Additionally, the greater the total lower extremity motor score, the greater the individual's walking speed and endurance.[123]

Guidelines have been developed based on developmental level and neurologic impairment to aid in decision making regarding mobility and appropriate clinical goals.[23,37] A stander is recommended for patients with injuries at T1 and higher and either a stander or bracing for injuries below T1. For those with levels of injury at T1 and below, ambulation may be achieved via various types of bracing depending on level of injury and lower extremity muscle strength. With higher-level injuries, ambulation is more of a therapeutic/exercise goal rather than a true functional goal. The cost of bracing and assistive devices must be balanced against the practicality of ambulation and the willingness of the patient and family to follow through with ambulation after discharge/ training sessions. The most common reasons for discontinuing use of the braces are the excessive energy costs and the need for assistance to don and remove them for ambulation.[146] Periodic reexamination of the child's physical abilities and outcomes as an outpatient can be used to determine whether ambulation with braces is a reasonable goal. Many patients become less interested over time in ambulation requiring extensive bracing as the permanence of the injury becomes more apparent. Those who remain interested may have specific needs for standing or limited walking that increase the likelihood of long-term use of the orthoses.[146]

TABLE 21.4 Mobility in Complete Tetraplegia, Expected Function, and Necessary Equipment for Level of Injury

Functional Skill	C1-C4	C5	C6	C7-T1
Bed mobility	D	A, Even with electrical bed	I, May use equipment; electrical bed helpful	I, Electrical bed helpful
Transfers	D, May need mechanical lift	D, May need mechanical lift	Some I with or without sliding board	I, May need sliding board
Wheelchair	I, PWC, head, chin, mouth, or tongue control	I, PWC, hand control with splint	I, MWC, may use adapted rims; likely to use PWC in community	I, MWC
Pressure relief	D, Bed, MWC I, Power tilt PWC	D, Bed, MWC I, Power tilt PWC	I, Leaning to side	I, Push-up on open hands
Transportation	U, Driving; van with lift needed	I, Upper extremity controls; van with lift needed	I, Hand controls A, Load MWC	I, Hand controls I, Load MWC

A, assistance required; *D*, dependent; *I*, independent; *MWC*, manual wheelchair; *PWC*, power wheelchair; *U*, unable.
Adapted from Massagli TL, Jaffe KM: Pediatric spinal cord injury, treatment and outcome, *Pediatrician* 17:244-254, 1990.

TABLE 21.5 Mobility in Complete Paraplegia, Expected Function, and Necessary Equipment for Level of Injury

Functional Skill	T2-T10	T11-L2	L3-S2
Manual wheelchair	I, Indoors and in community	I, Indoors and in community	May not need MWC except long distances, recreation
Ambulation	SBA, Exercise only; need KAFOs or RGOs and forearm crutches or walker; not practical for T2-T6	I, Indoors with KAFOs or RGOs and forearm crutches; some can do stairs with railing	I, Indoors and community with AFOs; may need forearm crutches or cane
Driving	I, Hand controls I, Load MWC	I, Hand controls I, Load MWC	Can drive automatic transmission; may prefer hand controls

AFOs, ankle-foot orthoses; *I*, independent; *KAFOs*, knee-ankle-foot orthoses; *MWC*, manual wheelchair; *RGOs*, reciprocating gait orthoses; *SBA*, standby assistance.
Adapted from Massagli TL, Jaffe KM: Pediatric spinal cord injury, treatment and outcome, *Pediatrician* 17:244-254, 1990.

Physical therapy intervention sessions will be structured around the child's motivation for play. Within that framework, the therapist designs activities that encourage strengthening, balance, reaching, rolling, sitting, transitions, and mobility in various combinations.

Sitting balance is often one of the major goals of therapy. Balance is impaired by altered strength and sensation and often by the presence of a spinal orthosis. Conversely, a child with tetraplegia or high paraplegia may benefit from a soft orthosis to facilitate sitting, leaving hands free for other activities (Fig. 21.6). The seated child is encouraged to progress from therapist support to self-support at a tabletop or on a mat and to independent sitting if this is a realistic goal given the level and completeness of injury. These goals may be achieved by engaging the child in play activities.

All innervated musculature must be strengthened, including muscles that have normal grade 5 strength because these will be used to compensate for weakened or paralyzed muscles. Maintaining full ROM, particularly at specific joints, is imperative. For example, full ROM at the shoulders must be maintained for ease of dressing. Historically, patients with tetraplegia who have wrist extension but no hand function were provided with a stretching program that allowed them to develop mild finger flexor tightness to provide for a tenodesis grasp during wrist extension. Current recommendations, however, are to maintain a supple hand and to even splint with metacarpophalangeal flexion and interphalangeal extension ("intrinsic plus" position) to maintain this ROM. The change in practice is due to the evolution of upper extremity reconstructive surgery for the population with tetraplegia, which can augment wrist extension, grasp, lateral pinch, and finger extension.[102] Stretching the hamstrings to allow 100° to 110° of hip flexion is necessary for dressing and self-care. It is important to have excessively flexible hamstrings to prevent overstretching of the low back. Ankle ROM must be maintained at neutral for proper placement on the wheelchair footrest.

A small number of children with tetraplegia have upper cervical injuries (C1-C3) that necessitate mechanical ventilation (see Chapter 25). Physical therapy for these children and for those with C4 tetraplegia has a more narrowed focus because the child is dependent in bed mobility, transfers, and sitting balance (see Table 21.2). Spasticity tends to be more problematic with this population, although daily passive ROM can reduce tone and facilitate positioning.

Bed Mobility and Transfer Techniques

Depending on the level of injury and personal preference for the patient, several strategies can be used when teaching mobility and transfer techniques. It can be challenging for both the physical therapist and patient. The International Network of Spinal Cord Injury Physiotherapists website (www.scipt.org) is a valuable resource, as it contains videos of patients at various levels performing bed mobility, transfers, wheelchair mobility, and gait techniques. Extended detail can also be found in SCI rehabilitation textbooks.[51,131]

Bed mobility and transferring techniques for children and adolescents are similar to those used for adults. Successful mobility focuses on maximizing biomechanics, using momentum, and understanding the head-hips relationship. The head-hips relationship, or the concept of moving your head and upper trunk *opposite* to the direction you are moving and looking away from where you are moving in order to unweight the pelvis for transfers or mat mobility, is not intuitive for a child. Mastery of this concept, however, will open up much more opportunity for mobility.

For children with paraplegia and lower level tetraplegia (C6 and below), transfer training may initially include the use of a transfer (sliding) board. Calling it a transfer board is preferred so that children do not think they can slide on the board, as doing so can shear the skin. Push-up blocks can also be helpful when first learning transfers (Fig. 21.7). As upper extremity strength and balance increase, the child may be able to transfer

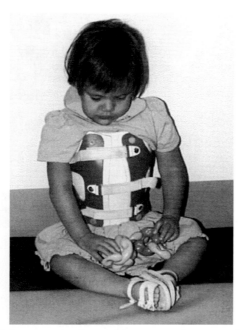

FIG. 21.6 A soft orthosis provides external support, improving sitting balance and allowing this child with a high thoracic spinal cord injury to use both hands in play.

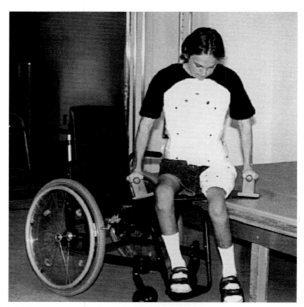

FIG. 21.7 Teen wearing a thoracolumbosacral orthosis with a thigh piece that restricts hip flexion uses a sliding board and push-up blocks to begin learning transfers.

without a transfer board. Types of transfers learned should include those for level and nonlevel surfaces, as well as floor to wheelchair and wheelchair to floor. Older children should also learn how to transfer in and out of a vehicle. Young children can be physically capable in transferring themselves; however, they may require a caregiver's assistance from a safety standpoint as they may totally disregard their legs, putting themselves at risk for a lower extremity fracture. Rather than taking a lateral approach to the surface they wish to transfer to, young children may take more of an anterior approach and scoot forward/backward with their legs in either a long or ring-sit position. Children and adolescents with C5 and above tetraplegia are dependent for transfers and require either a caregiver to lift them or the use of a mechanical lift. In either situation, all caregivers must be educated in proper technique, and the child must be able to verbalize the steps that need to be taken for a safe transfer.

Wheeled Mobility

If community ambulation is not an expected outcome, the child needs a wheelchair for mobility. Guidelines for appropriate mobility have been developed for children with SCI to assist the therapist and team.[23] Young children with an SCI at or above C6 need a power wheelchair for independent mobility. Some young children with lower levels of cervical SCI, or even high thoracic injuries, may be able to propel a manual wheelchair for only limited distances on smooth, level surfaces owing to lack of upper body strength and endurance. For these children to be exposed to a broader range of environments, such as preschool playgrounds or uneven or steep terrain around the family home, prescription of a power wheelchair is justifiable to promote age-appropriate functional mobility. A child as young as 18 to 24 months may be trained to use a power wheelchair but requires adult supervision for safety.[82,100,119a] An environmental control unit (ECU) and a complex power wheelchair are needed for independent mobility when a joystick is not appropriate due to a higher level of injury. The joystick is replaced with head, tongue, or sip-and-puff controls and the power tilt

must allow for ventilator placement. In addition, a manual tilt-in-space wheelchair is necessary to provide these children with a substitute when the power chair needs repairs. The manual wheelchair is also useful for transport in places where the larger, heavier power chair is impractical. Many families do not have a home with hallways or doors large enough to accommodate a power wheelchair, so power mobility may be used primarily in community and school settings and the manual wheelchair is used in the home.

Power-assist wheels are motorized wheels that can be added onto or are already a part of a manual wheelchair. These allow the user to provide some propulsion forces, and the motors enhance their propulsion to allow them to be functional. This type of wheel is most applicable for patients with C6-T1 level injuries or where upper body endurance is lacking. Power-assist wheels do add weight to the wheelchair, but the trade-off is that there is still a manual wheelchair that can typically be transported in the trunk of a car, rather than a power chair that requires an adapted van or lift. One case series[35] demonstrates positive outcomes of independent propulsion over terrain and ascending ramps in children, ages 7 to 11, with SCI or dysfunction affecting upper extremity strength.

For children/adolescents for whom manual wheelchair propulsion is going to be the primary means of independent mobility, extra attention must be paid to the configuration of the wheelchair in addition to the weight of the chair (Fig. 21.8). Focus is frequently placed on ultra-lightweight materials; however, setup is just as important, if not more so. Proper setup details include overall width and depth of the chair, axle placement, seat-to-floor height, wheel and rim size, caster size, and back type and height. Variances in setup can now be quantified through the use of the SmartWheel (Fig. 21.9), which measures propulsive forces, speed, and cadence.

The Paralyzed Veterans Association (PVA) has also published guidelines on proper wheelchair setup in the adult population[39,82] to preserve the joints of the upper extremity, and because literature is lacking in the pediatric population,[23,82] these may be considered, as best practice is in

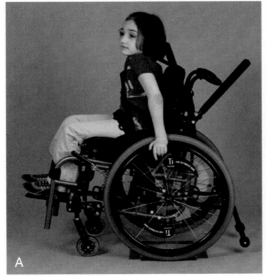
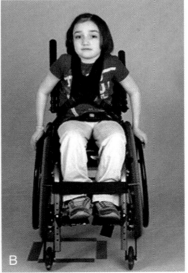

FIG. 21.8 A-B, Manual wheelchair setup.

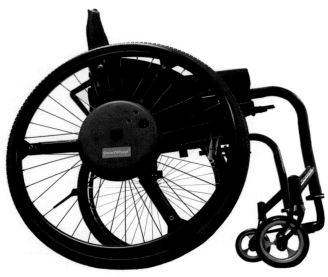

FIG. 21.9 SmartWheel. (Courtesy of Out Front, Mesa, Arizona.)

the pediatric population. Overuse injuries at the shoulder (rotator cuff impingement, capsular injury) and the wrist (carpal tunnel syndrome) are seen in a large percentage of the adult population.[39] It is likely that these same injuries will occur in pediatrics, as they are pushing wheelchairs for more years, and presumably with more force, because the chair can weigh more than the child. Additionally, the tendency is to add backpacks on the back of the chair, only to increase the overall amount of weight the child needs to propel. Finally, oftentimes the wheelchairs provided are larger than needed with the anticipation that the child will grow and the chair needs to "grow" with the child, particularly because insurers will only pay for a new chair approximately every 5 years. Manufacturers have designed chairs that can change seat width and depth, but often proper setup is sacrificed. Other manufacturers have a trade-in program or "growth kit" option to allow for a more appropriately sized and setup frame to be delivered when needed.

The seating components of either a power or manual wheelchair are prescribed with skin protection and spinal alignment in mind (see Chapter 33 for additional information). A level pelvis decreases the amount of pressure placed over individual ischial tuberosities of the sacrum, thereby improving overall pressure distribution. A solid seat and back are preferred to sling upholstery in this age group. Many types of wheelchair cushions are available, but none is universally effective for maintaining skin integrity in all persons with SCI, and individual assessment is required to minimize ulcerative forces (pressure, shear, friction and moisture).

Wheelchair positioning and fit can also limit the development of secondary peripheral neuropathies. Too frequently, peroneal nerve neuropathies are seen as a result of the lateral lower leg, just distal to the head of the fibula, resting against the front end or leg rest of the wheelchair. Additionally, some children and teens use an upper extremity to "hook" around a back cane of a wheelchair for either pressure relief or to assist with balance. Excessive pressure in the antecubital fossa over time may cause median nerve neuropathy.

Wheelchair evaluations can occur in all settings, but often the first time is in the rehabilitation setting. During this time it is best to trial as many wheelchair frames and seating systems as possible to determine what is clinically most appropriate and what the child and parents like best. If no change in neurologic status and function is expected, the wheelchair must be ordered as soon as possible, although because it is unlikely that the new wheelchair will arrive before discharge, a rental wheelchair may be necessary. As the child grows, wheelchair evaluations may occur at the rehabilitation hospital, at an outpatient facility, or in school. All wheelchairs and ECUs should be chosen by the rehabilitation team, child, and family in consultation with a knowledgeable vendor (see Chapter 33). The therapist should be aware of available funding for wheelchairs and other durable medical equipment. There may be limitations in coverage, and the therapist can assist the family in prioritizing equipment needs.

The physical therapist will address a variety of skills. There is no set time to initiate these mobility skills, and the appropriate timing depends on the child's age currently and age at injury, their abilities, and the environments in which they typically interact. Some of these skills include propulsion over even and uneven terrain, negotiation of obstacles, ascending and descending ramps and curbs, assuming a wheelie, falls, and stairs (www.scipt.org).

Ambulation

For those with absent or limited active hip flexion, a hip-knee-ankle-foot orthosis (HKAFO) may be prescribed. The hip joint can be locked for a swing-through gait pattern and unlocked to use active hip flexion for a reciprocal gait. Another option is an reciprocating gait orthose (RGO), which has a cable system that allows for passive reciprocating gait, but the child must be adept at weight shifting and trunk extension. Children who have at least three-fifths strength in the quadriceps muscles or stronger hip flexors can achieve ambulation with KAFOs. The swing-through gait pattern is more efficient than other gait patterns. Many adults who have RGOs or knee-ankle-foot orthoses (KAFOs) prescribed do not use them at all in the long term, and the majority of the remaining patients use them only for standing or exercise. Children with lower-level injuries, L3 and below, and some incomplete injuries may achieve independent ambulation with ankle-foot orthoses (AFOs). Ambulation typically also requires an upper extremity assistive device, particularly for those using H/KAFOs and RGOs. Gait training may be initiated in parallel bars and advance to use of an appropriate assistive device (typically front wheeled walkers or Loftstrand crutches) as the child improves in standing balance. Parastance, where the hips and lower trunk are in excessive extension and balance is achieved by resting on the y-ligaments in the hip, must be achieved in order for those ambulating with H/KAFOs to be successful. Donning and doffing, and general orthoses management, must be taught and practiced with both the child and caregivers. Controlled sit-to-stand transitions must also be practiced.

Preschool-age children (5 years and younger) are more likely to pursue ambulation, perform a higher level of ambulation, and ambulate for a longer number of years as compared to older children and adolescents.[146] Once these younger children enter the preteen and adolescent period, however, ambulation is typically abandoned for wheeled mobility beyond an indoor home or school level in order to keep up with peers.[146]

For children who wish to be upright for physiologic and psychological benefits but do not necessarily wish to ambulate,

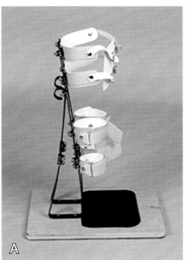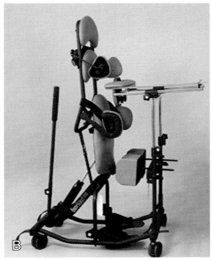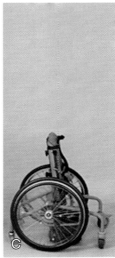

FIG. 21.10 A-C, Options for static and mobile standing.

various devices are available. A standing frame (Fig. 21.10B) can be used for static standing, but there are also parapodiums (Fig. 21.10A) or swivel standers, which have a footplate that, in combination with an assistive device, allows a child to swivel the trunk for very short distance mobility. Mobile standers (Fig. 21.10C) are also available in which a child can assume a standing position while propelling with large, wheelchair-like wheels (see the video that accompanying Chapter 21).

Locomotor training (LT) is an activity-based therapy that typically consists of step training via a body-weight-supported (BWS) system, initially on a treadmill often followed by overground gait training. BWS systems are commercially available; some are developed specifically for use overtop a treadmill, whereas others use a track from a ceiling allowing for more movement. The term *activity-based therapy* is used to describe an intervention that results in neuromuscular activation below the level of spinal cord lesion to promote recovery of motor function, thus demonstrating the neuroplasticity of the spinal cord.[8-10] A reported goal of LT is to stimulate the locomotor central pattern generators (CPGs) in the spinal cord.[52] It is believed that reflexive movements of ambulation can be restored by stimulating these CPGs through the repetitive motion.[52] One case study in which LT was performed as part of a young child's acute inpatient rehabilitation demonstrated the return of isolated volitional contractions of lower extremity muscles and significant gains in functional mobility.[117] Research continues in this area, but early results are promising and suggest the potential value of incorporating LT into physical therapy intervention.[10]

Ambulation may also be achieved by using a robotically assisted walking device. These systems allow users to stand and ambulate by wearing an exoskeleton "suit" that provides motorized assistance to leg musculature. There are specific criteria for their use. Most require the user to be able to shift weight in order to activate the motor and therefore take a step. These robotic systems are geared toward adults, as another criterion for use is based on weight and height. There are systems designed for use with a physical therapist in the medical setting as well as devices for personal use.

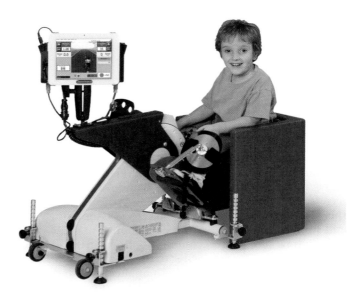

FIG. 21.11 A 5-year-old child with Spina Bifida using the RT300-SLP FES cycle. (Courtesy Restorative-Therapies, Inc., Baltimore, Maryland.)

Functional Electrical Stimulation for Children

Cycling with FES has gained increased popularity as an activity-based rehabilitation strategy to encourage neuroplasticity and health gains for people with SCI. FES during cycling can be performed at home, and cycles appropriately sized for children are now available (Fig. 21.11). The cycles are FDA approved for children ages 4 years and older; however, the primary limiting factor is the child's size. Typically the bilateral quadriceps, hamstrings, and gluteal muscles are stimulated at the appropriate times during the revolution of the cycle. This intervention has been applied to people with SCI with and without lower extremity sensation. For children with sensation, the FES can be gradually applied and limited in intensity in order to not exceed the child's tolerance. Exercise protocols in the literature commonly involve cycling for 30 to 60 minutes three to five times per week at cadences of 40 to 50 revolutions per minute (rpm).[54] The ideal protocol, however, is not known, especially for children. The only published literature with children applied FES cycling for 60 minutes, three times per week, at a cadence of 40 to 50 rpm.[77]

Outcomes reported for FES cycling with adults include improvements in bone mineral density,[11,31,40] strength in stimulated muscles,[77] muscle size,[40,55,64] oxygen uptake,[40,65,77] cardiac output,[49,65] stroke volume,[49] and decreased adiposity.[64,124] In children, the literature is more limited with changes reported in bone mineral density,[77] oxygen uptake,[75,77] muscle volume,[77] stimulated muscle strength,[77] as well as decreased resting heart rate.[77] In addition, FES cycling has been shown not to increase the degree of hip subluxation after 6 months of cycling.[75]

Most clinically available applications for FES in pediatric SCI use electrodes placed on the skin surface. For all FES applications, a critical portion of the evaluation is the determination of the ability to stimulate the muscle.[106,134] With a lower motor neuron injury, muscle cannot be adequately stimulated and FES is therefore not appropriate.[72] For example, a child with a C5 SCI is likely to have lower motor neuron damage to C6 due to concomitant damage to the alpha motor neuron or nerve root at C6, and thus stimulation for wrist extension may be problematic. A thorough evaluation using electrical stimulation will provide information as to what muscles are appropriate for FES applications.

FES walking options using surface stimulation for standing and walking are known as neuroprostheses. These systems use the peroneal withdrawal reflex to mimic a step, allowing the leg to advance.[81] The commercially available system is only approved for use when skeletally mature; however, the peroneal withdrawal reflex can be obtained using a portable neuromuscular electrical stimulation (NMES) unit and a trigger if desired for children with incomplete SCI who have some ability to maintain stability during stance. For this technique, an electrode is placed near the fibular head and stimulation intensity is set high enough to cause the leg to withdraw into flexion. Another option during gait for a child with an incomplete SCI is to use a portable NMES unit to create dorsiflexion.[116] For both applications during gait, a switch can be placed into the shoe to control the timing of the FES. Surface systems are commercially available for specific applications such as foot drop or hand function and are available in pediatric sizes. To provide these applications without a commercially available surface system, a more generic neuromuscular electrical stimulation NMES device can be used, and the ability to use a trigger or switch to turn on the stimulation is important for FES applications. Common stimulation parameters for FES include pulse duration sufficient to create a muscle contraction (200 to 400 usec) and a low frequency, measured in pulses per second (pps) (20 to 30 pps) to minimize fatigue. On and off times will be determined by the activity itself, and ramp time can be set for comfort or to minimize spasticity as long as it does not impact the timing of the activity (i.e., during gait when on times are very short).[77]

Implanted devices have been used in pediatric clinical and research applications including facilitation of grasp, standing and walking, bladder and bowel function,[132] and phrenic or diaphragmatic pacing.[48,126] Phrenic and diaphragmatic pacing systems are FDA approved for use in children. With this device, bilateral phrenic nerve electrodes are placed thoracoscopically and after a period of conditioning can provide full-time ventilatory support without a mechanical ventilator.[48] A report of nine children implanted with the phrenic pacemaker showed that eight were able to meet their pacing goals.[126]

Coordination/Communication/Consultation

While hospitalized, the child and adolescent must practice mobility skills outside the structured therapy sessions. For instance, nurses should be updated on progress in mobility skills so that the child can be encouraged to incorporate these abilities into play activities or getting to meals.

Community and school reentry activities are often the combined responsibility of physical therapists, occupational therapists, and therapeutic recreation specialists. Children must become familiar with common architectural barriers such as curbs, heavy doors, and high shelves and learn how to negotiate them or ask for help. Caregivers need to be trained in the type and amount of assistance to provide and cautioned against being overly helpful. Teenagers should be encouraged to problem solve the management of architectural barriers and ask for assistance if safety is jeopardized. Discharge planning and long-term management should address mobility issues in the child's home, school, and community. Whenever possible, a home evaluation should be conducted early in the child's hospital stay. If home modifications are necessary for wheelchair accessibility or safety, the family needs time to gather financial resources and complete modifications. Physical therapists may be asked to consult regarding modifications being made to the home. The US Department of Housing and Urban Development has resources available and has published guidelines on making homes more accessible.[118,139] These modifications can be evaluated during weekend passes. Public schools employ physical therapists and occupational therapists who can provide accessibility information while the child is still hospitalized. Upon school entry, the child can be assisted with accommodations under the provisions of Section 504 of the Vocational Rehabilitation Act of 1973.[140] The therapist plays a major role as a consultant to the school administration, faculty, family, and student regarding accessibility issues and needed modifications to architectural barriers or curriculum. For children living great distances from the hospital, physical therapists in the school can provide a local perspective and become a resource to the family.

Another area of concern in community reentry is safe transportation. The physical therapist can assist the family with evaluating safe transportation for the child. If a van will be used, wheelchair tie-downs will be necessary. If the child has a lower thoracic injury with adequate balance and can sit in a vehicle seat, an appropriate car seat or booster seat may be needed. For teenagers, friends may need to be trained in car transfers so that the patient can stay socially active. The teenager returning to driving needs to be independent with transfers and with loading and unloading the wheelchair.

Exercise and Fitness

Cardiovascular fitness is a major health concern in the SCI population. Adults with tetraplegia have a 16% increased risk of cardiovascular diseases as compared to the general population, whereas those with paraplegia have a 70% greater risk of coronary artery disease (a subset of the cardiovascular diseases).[107]

Greater risk (44%) of cardiovascular diseases is also seen with complete versus incomplete SCI. The prevalence of cardiovascular disease in the SCI population is difficult to estimate because of the presence of silent ischemia that may go undetected, but cardiovascular disease has been reported to be the leading cause of death for people with SCI of greater than 30 years in duration. These data suggest that interventions are desperately needed to decrease the incidence of cardiovascular disease in the SCI population.[107]

People with SCI tend to lead sedentary lifestyles, which further increases their risk for coronary heart disease (CHD).[68] The level of inactivity seen in the SCI population poses a serious health risk because of the accompanying secondary health complications of CHD, obesity, and diabetes.[58,115] Voluntary exercise, however, is difficult for many people with SCI based on the extent of the paralysis, lack of proper exercise equipment, and lack of trained professionals to provide guidance. Although people with paraplegia have more capability to exercise, they are not more fit than people with tetraplegia who have fewer exercise options.[108] In addition, 25% of healthy young people with SCI lack the fitness levels to perform important daily activities.[108] Given the significant impact that SCI has on cardiovascular health, compounded with the lack of availability and need for exercise in this population, there is a dire need for exercise interventions.

Regular exercise can decrease the extent of the metabolic, skeletal, and muscle complications for people with SCI.[73,108,109] Some options for exercise include upper extremity ergometry, FES-assisted activity, swimming, and adapted sports.[68,107] Strong level 1 evidence exists for the ability of upper extremity exercise to improve cardiovascular fitness and oxygen uptake.[149] Central effects (heart and lungs) of exercise reported with people with SCI include increases in peak oxygen uptake up to 65%, as well as improvements in stroke volume of approximately 16%.[115] In addition, regular exercise can have a positive impact on lipid profiles[107,149] and glucose homeostasis.[149] The evidence suggests that more intense exercise than currently being performed may be needed to have an impact on lipids post SCI and that effects are possible with both arm exercise and FES cycling.[149]

Little research has been done on health and fitness in children with SCI, but with the increasing prevalence of obesity among children as a whole, intervening early with children with SCI may help to develop healthy habits that persist into adulthood. Some evidence suggests that 10- to 21-year-old children with SCI have an increased incidence of metabolic syndrome (present in 11 out of 20 children),[109] decreased lean tissue mass compared to overweight and control subjects,[87] increased fat mass (by 22.9% with paraplegia and 25.9% with tetraplegia),[94] and decreased aerobic capacity compared to controls.[149] In addition, children 5 to 13 years of age have been shown to have decreased aerobic capacity.[74] Exercise interventions targeting some of these deficits have been limited.[86] Liusuwal and colleagues[87] studied the outcomes of a 16-week program targeting nutrition, exercise (aerobic and resistance training), and lifestyle change and reported increases in lean body tissue and in power and efficiency during an upper extremity ergometry test. Johnston and colleagues[76] studied the effects of 6 months of FES cycling and reported increases in peak oxygen uptake during an upper extremity ergometry test. These studies suggest that exercise can have a positive impact on the health of children with SCI; however, more research is needed to determine optimal ways to address the health concerns for people with SCI.

Sports and Recreation

Therapists should encourage regular aerobic exercise in children and young adults with SCI to help them develop lifelong habits that promote health, particularly because of their general tendency toward lower-intensity, more sedentary leisure activities.[71] With childhood obesity and type 2 diabetes rates on the rise in the pediatric population, those with SCIs are at greater risk. A majority of children and teens are not involving themselves in organized activities such as sports, clubs, or those offered by youth centers.[71] Therapeutic recreation specialists facilitate participation in an adaptive physical education program, community-based recreational programs for people with disabilities, or competitive wheelchair sports. Offering specific recreation programs during inpatient rehabilitation or camps after discharge can significantly contribute to overall rehabilitation and quality-of-life outcomes.

PSYCHOSOCIAL ASPECTS

A team member skilled in mental health should monitor the child's adaptation to disability and be available to help the child verbally process the injury and rehabilitation. This could be a skilled social worker, but if a behavior management program using reinforcers is needed, a clinical psychologist should be consulted. In rare cases, the child may truly be clinically depressed, and a psychiatrist can be consulted if a medication trial is contemplated. As described by Fordyce,[53] acquisition of an SCI accompanied by pain, medical complications, altered cosmesis, and body image and the new and challenging rehabilitation procedures can be expected to have a significant impact on the patient's affect, self-esteem, and behavior. The child's adjustment to SCI does not necessarily follow predictable stages of crisis response such as shock, denial, depression, and adaptation. Adjustment to SCI probably occurs over several years. The verbal or attitudinal expressions of children with a new SCI are less predictive of outcome than are their behaviors. Physical therapists can facilitate adjustment by actively engaging the child in acquiring the skills needed to maximize independence. Therapists must include parents and caregivers when teaching these skills to children and adolescents, and they must not forget the importance for adolescents of incorporating peers. The psychologist or psychiatrist may also need to confront issues of premorbid risk-taking behavior or even substance abuse. Psychologists, nurses, and pediatric physiatrists collaborate in discussing sexuality and changes in sexual functioning with teenagers who have had SCI. Sexuality is often a difficult topic to approach with teens and their caregivers. If a teen is not ready to verbalize questions or concerns related to sexuality, there are a number of online resources from adult spinal cord injury model systems that may provide additional assistance, such as University of Alabama at Birmingham (www.spinalcord.uab.edu).

A concern commonly expressed by teenagers is that of not being able to trust their bodies. The altered motor and sensory processes and potential changes in bowel and bladder function can make their bodies feel foreign to them. In addition, teenagers are accustomed to privacy and independence in their lives. Both the injury and subsequent reliance on a hospital environment, adaptive equipment, and caregivers can disrupt any sense of control. The rehabilitation team should respect privacy and encourage participation in scheduling therapy, nursing care, and free time.

QUALITY OF LIFE

Physical therapists can have a positive impact on quality-of-life issues a child may face as a result of SCI. Chronic pain has been determined to be one of the most common[69] and limiting factors in terms of quality of life following SCI, resulting in decreased perceived mental and physical health, as well as decreased activity levels[142] (although activity does not seem to decrease as significantly as in the adult population[70]). Musculoskeletal pain is most prevalent in the shoulder, elbow, and wrist. Visceral pain is also frequently identified, particularly originating from the genitourinary tract, as is neuropathic pain.[69]

Depression can hinder quality of life and life satisfaction as it limits community participation and self-inclusion in activities. Adults with pediatric-onset SCI experience depression to varying degrees, which is related to medical complications, perceived mental-health quality of life, occupation, and the severity of their injuries (complete versus incomplete).[5]

By being aware of these potential issues, physical therapists can monitor for them and make referrals to appropriate providers as necessary. By constantly monitoring developmental changes and a child's participation, age-appropriate habilitation and rehabilitation can be addressed as needed.

FOLLOW-UP AND TRANSITION TO ADULTHOOD

The key to ensuring maximal participation in young children with SCI is to provide ongoing examination of impairments and activity and to regularly update expected outcomes that are appropriate. At least two mechanisms are available to accomplish this objective. Children who are discharged from rehabilitation centers are routinely seen in follow-up visits two or more times each year. These reassessments include medical follow-up to reexamine the level and completeness of injury, to evaluate changes in bladder and bowel function and skin integrity, to monitor the spine and hip for development of scoliosis and hip subluxation/dislocation, respectively, to determine the need for medications to treat spasticity or bladder or bowel incontinence, and developmental appropriateness.

Reexamination by the physical therapist is an important part of these follow-up visits. Any changes should be noted, including changes in ROM, strength, sensation, and spasticity. For children, age-appropriate habilitative skills can be taught (i.e., self-catheterization, skin checks, advanced wheelchair skills, and transfers). The wheelchair should be reassessed and adapted as needed to accommodate the child's growth and to ensure that any modifications enhance positioning and propulsion independence.

The physical therapy reexaminations at the rehabilitation facility follow a consultative model. The ongoing progress toward age-appropriate outcomes may occur in a hospital-based outpatient therapy program, but it is more typically accomplished through therapy services offered in the outpatient physical therapy setting, early intervention programs, or in publicly funded schools. Therapists in these programs ideally are in contact with the rehabilitation centers on a regular basis to update progress and goals and to identify new concerns and equipment needs.

Although the majority of young school-age children with SCI receive direct physical therapy and occupational therapy services in school, few adolescents receive such services.[90] The therapist works from a consultative model, using the faculty and student to carry out programs and recommendations.

Issues may include supporting the teen to continue with regular pressure releases, stretching and impairment-based home activities, and progressing mobility skills to community distances. The physical therapist and occupational therapist should also consult with the faculty and student regarding an appropriate physical education program; modification of classroom and desk setup; and accessibility to lockers, bathroom, and lunchroom. In reality, many adolescents with SCI have no physical education program, face problems of accessibility at school, and report that breakdown of wheelchairs (both power and manual) contributes to absences at school.[90] Although completion of education is supported by accommodations and modifications, such supports are more often implemented to enhance the child's participation in classroom activities and are not geared toward competitive performance and productivity. Therapists should assist adolescents in achieving independence with assistive technology for mobility, communication, and environmental control. Skills development in directing and managing human assistants may also be needed.[46] Few adolescents with SCI receive educational or vocational counseling beyond the selection of classes each term.[90] Such students may qualify for transition planning under the Individuals with Disabilities Education Act, Public Law 105-17.[138] School physical therapists might participate in a transition program by assessing functional mobility skills in the community or work-study setting. When teenagers with SCI become 18 years of age, they are eligible in the United States for state vocational counseling services. Such services are often important sources of funding for vocation-related education or even equipment. The importance of facilitating education and employment is underscored by research showing that the life satisfaction of adults with pediatric-onset SCI is associated with education, income, satisfaction with employment, and social opportunities but not with level of, age at, or duration of SCI.[144]

For teenagers, follow-up visits should also include discussions related to sexuality and reproduction.[85] Fertility in women is not impaired by SCI, but sexual response and orgasm may be. Pregnant women with SCI should be managed at high-risk medical centers to avoid respiratory and urinary tract complications, detect threatened preterm births, and prevent autonomic dysreflexia during delivery. Although the majority of males with SCI can have erections, these are often fleeting and not adequate for vaginal penetration. Few men with SCI have ejaculations, and sperm quality decreases over time for reasons that are not entirely clear. New techniques for retrieval of sperm and for artificial insemination have helped some men with SCI to father children. In addition to this physiologic information, it is important to include issues of intimacy and relationships in candid discussions of sexuality.

Successful transition to adulthood is a goal of all children/adolescents with SCI. The rehabilitation team plays an important role in fostering success. Transition into a spinal cord injury model system (www.mscisdisseminationcenter.org) is ideal to continue specialized care; however, travel to these facilities may not be feasible. Continued care from a specialized center will not only provide optimum medical care but will also support the services required for seeking education, vocational development, and independent living. Many adults with pediatric-onset SCI do complete an education level equivalent to noninjured peers; however, employment rate, income, rate of independent living, and marital status do not correlate with noninjured peers.[4] See Chapter 32 for more information.

SUMMARY

Physical therapy for the child with SCI can, at first glance, appear straightforward. Preserving ROM and promoting strength and endurance are the cornerstones for the functional achievement predicted by the level of injury. Yet predicting realistic long-term outcomes and attaining them require respect for the broader and more complex picture. The physical therapist must consider the cause of the injury (progressive versus stable), the completeness of the injury (preserved motor function, sensory function), and the potential for, or presence of, secondary complications (scoliosis, skin breakdown, contractures). The therapist must also be sensitive to the child's age, personal and environmental factors, and the child's ability to meet age-appropriate expectations in the home, school, and community. Unlike adults with SCI, who may be very close to expected levels of independence at discharge from inpatient rehabilitation, children often require years of outpatient therapy to achieve optimal outcomes. Thus, it becomes imperative to provide the child and the family with a team approach incorporating multiple disciplines and settings to maximize the child's potential for functional independence and participation in life roles.

Case Scenarios on Expert Consult

The cases related to this chapter present three case scenarios (Stacey, Alex, and Adam) with additional videos. They illustrate some of the management principles discussed in this chapter.

REFERENCES

1. Allen DD, et al.: Motor scores on the Functional Independence Measure after pediatric spinal cord injury, *Spinal Cord* 47:213–217, 2009.
2. American Spinal Injury Association: *International standards for neurological and functional classification of spinal cord injury*, Chicago, 2000, American Spinal Injury Association.
3. Anderson CJ, DeVivo M: Mortality in pediatric spinal cord injury. Paper abstract #10, *J Spinal Cord Med* 27:S113, 2004.
4. Anderson CJ, et al.: Overview of adult outcomes in pediatric-onset spinal cord injuries, implications for transition to adulthood, *J Spinal Cord Med* 27 S98–S106, 2004.
5. Anderson CJ, et al.: Depression in adults who sustained spinal cord injuries as children or adolescents, *J Spinal Cord Med* 30:S76–S82, 2007.
6. Anderson R, et al.: Untitled selection of rigid internal fixation construct for stabilization at the craniovertebral junction in pediatric patients, *J Spinal Cord Med* 30(Suppl):S193–S194, 2007. [abstract].
7. Baptiste DC, Fehlings MG: Pharmacological approaches to repair the injured spinal cord, *J Neurotrauma* 23:318–334, 2006.
8. Behrman AL, Harkema SJ: Locomotor training after human spinal cord injury: a series of case studies, *Phys Ther* 80:688–700, 2000.
9. Behrman AL, Harkema SJ: Physical rehabilitation as an agent for recovery after spinal cord injury, *Phys Med Rehabil Clin N Am* 18:183–202, 2007.
10. Behrman AL, et al.: Restorative rehabilitation entails a paradigm shift in pediatric incomplete spinal cord injury in adolescence: an illustrative case series, *J Pediatr Rehabil Med* 5:245–259, 2012.
11. Belanger M, et al.: Electrical stimulation: can it increase muscle strength and reverse osteopenia in spinal cord injured individuals? *Arch Phys Med Rehabil* 81:1090–1098, 2008.
12. Betz RR, Mulcahey MJ: Pediatric spinal cord injury. In Vaccaro AR, et al., editors: *Principles and practice of spine surgery*, Philadelphia, 2003, Mosby.
13. Betz RR, et al.: Sagittal analysis of patients with spinal cord injury: a radiographic analysis and implications for treatment. Poster presentation abstract #36, *J Spinal Cord Med* 27:S135, 2004.
14. Bilston LE, Brown J: Pediatric spinal injury type and severity are age and mechanism dependent, *Spine* 32:2339–2347, 2007.
15. Bohn D, et al.: Cervical spine injuries in children, *J Trauma* 30:463–469, 1990.
16. Bosch PP, et al.: Pediatric spinal cord injury without radiographic abnormality (SCIWORA): the absence of occult instability and lack of indication for bracing, *Spine* 27:2788–2800, 2002.
17. Bracken MB, et al.: A randomized, controlled trial of methylprednisolone or naloxone in the treatment of acute spinal cord injury: results of the second national acute spinal cord injury study, *N Eng J Med* 332:1405–1411, 1990.
18. Bracken MB, et al.: Efficacy of methylprednisolone in acute spinal cord injury, *JAMA* 251:45–52, 1984.
19. Bracken MB, et al.: Methylprednisolone for 24 or 48 hours or tirilazad mesylate for 48 hours in the treatment of acute spinal cord injury: results of the Third National Acute Spinal Cord Injury Randomized Controlled Trial. National Acute Spinal Cord Injury Study, *JAMA* 277:1597–1604, 1997.
20. Brown PJ, et al.: The 72-h examination as a predictor of recovery in motor complete quadriplegia, *Arch Phys Med Rehabil* 72:546–548, 1991.
21. Brown RL, et al.: Cervical spine injuries in children: a review of 103 patients treated consecutively at a level 1 pediatric trauma center, *J Pediatr Surg* 36:1107–1114, 2001.
22. Calhoun CL, et al.: Development of items designed to evaluate activity performance and participation in children and adolescents with spinal cord injury, *Int J Pediatr* 854904, 2009.
23. Calhoun CL, et al.: Recommendations for mobility in children with spinal cord injury, *Top Spinal Cord Inj Rehabil* 19:142–151, 2013.
24. Cappuccino A: Moderate hypothermia as treatment for spinal cord injury, *Orthopedics* 31:243, 2008.
25. Cardenas DD, et al.: A bibliography of cost-effectiveness practices in physical medicine and rehabilitation, American Academy of Physical Medicine & Rehabilitation white paper, *Arch Phys Med Rehabil* 82:711–719, 2001.
26. Catz A, Itzkovich M: Spinal Cord Independence Measure: comprehensive ability rating scale for the spinal cord lesion patient, *J Rehabil Res Dev* 44:65–68, 2007.
27. Catz A, et al.: SCIM: Spinal Cord Independence Measure: a new disability scale for patients with spinal cord lesions, *Spinal Cord* 35:850–856, 1997.
28. Catz A, et al.: The Spinal Cord Independence Measure (SCIM), sensitivity to functional changes in subgroups of spinal cord lesion patient, *Spinal Cord* 39:97–100, 2001.
29. Chafetz RS, et al.: Relationship between neurological injury and patterns of upright mobility in children with spinal cord injury, *Top Spinal Cord Inj Rehabil* 19:31–41, 2013.
30. Chafetz RS, et al.: Impact of prophylactic thoracolumbosacral orthosis bracing on functional activities and activities of daily living in the pediatric spinal cord injury population, *J Spinal Cord Med* 30:S178–S183, 2007.
31. Chen SC, et al.: Increases in bone mineral density after functional electrical stimulation cycling exercises in spinal cord injured patients, *Disabil Rehabil* 27:1337–1341, 2005.
32. Chen Y, DeVivo MJ: Epidemiology. In Vogel LC, et al., editors: *Spinal cord injury in the child and young adult*, London, 2014, Mac Keith Press, pp 15–27.
33. Chen Y, et al.: Causes of spinal cord injury, *Top Spinal Cord Inj Rehabil* 19:1–8, 2013.
34. Cirak B, et al.: Spinal injuries in children, *J Pediatr Surg* 39:607–612, 2004.
35. Clayton GH, et al.: The use of push-rim power-assist wheels in three pediatric patients. Poster presentation abstract #13, *J Spinal Cord Med* 27:S126, 2004.
36. Committee on Genetics: American Academy of Pediatrics: health supervision for children with Down syndrome, *Pediatrics* 107:442–449, 2001.
37. Consortium for Spinal Cord Medicine: *Outcomes following traumatic SCI: clinical practice guidelines for healthcare professionals*, Washington, DC, 1999, Paralyzed Veterans of America.
38. Consortium for Spinal Cord Medicine: Clinical practice guideline: *Pressure ulcer prevention and treatment following spinal cord injury: a clinical practice guideline for health care professionals*, ed 2, Washington, DC, 2014, Paralyzed Veterans of America.

39. Consortium of Spinal Cord Medicine: Clinical practice guideline: *Preservation of upper limb function following spinal cord injury: a clinical practice guideline for healthcare professionals*, Washington, DC, 2002, Paralyzed Veterans of America.

40. Davis GM, et al.: Cardiorespiratory, metabolic, and biomechanical responses during functional electrical stimulation leg exercise: health and fitness benefits, *Artif Organs* 32:625–629, 2008.

41. DeVivo MJ, Vogel LC: Epidemiology of spinal cord injury in children and adolescents, *J Spinal Cord Med* 27:S4–S10, 2004.

42. Dididze M, et al.: Systemic hypothermia in acute cervical spinal cord injury: a case-controlled study, *Spinal Cord* 51:395–400, 2013.

43. Di Martino A, et al.: Pediatric spinal cord injury, *Neurosurg Q* 14:84–197, 2004.

44. Ditunno JF, et al.: Recovery of upper-extremity strength in complete and incomplete tetraplegia: a multicenter study, *Arch Phys Med Rehabil* 81:389–393, 2000.

45. Dobkin BH, et al.: Cellular transplants in China: observational study from the largest human experiment in chronic spinal cord injury, *Neurorehabil Neural Repair* 20:5–13, 2006.

46. Dudgeon BJ, et al.: Educational participation of children with spinal cord injury, *Am J Occup Ther* 51:553–561, 1997.

47. Dumas HM, et al.: Self-report measures of physical function for children with spinal cord injury: a review of current tools and an option for the future, *Dev Neurorehabil* 12:113–118, 2009.

48. Elefteriades JA, et al.: Long-term follow-up of pacing of the conditioned diaphragm in quadriplegia, *Pacing Clin Electrophysiol* 25:897–906, 2002.

49. Faghri PD, et al.: Functional electrical stimulation leg cycle ergometer exercise: training effects on cardiorespiratory responses of spinal cord injured subjects at rest and during submaximal exercise, *Arch Phys Med Rehabil* 73:1085–1093, 1992.

50. Fehlings MG, et al.: The role and timing of decompression in acute spinal cord injury, *Spine* 26:S101–S110, 2001.

51. Field-Fote EC: *Spinal cord injury rehabilitation*, Philadelphia, 2009, F.A. Davis.

52. Field-Fote EC, Behrman A: Locomotor training after incomplete spinal cord injury, neural mechanisms and functional outcomes. In Field-Fote EC, editor: *Spinal cord injury rehabilitation*, Philadelphia, 2009, F.A. Davis.

53. Fordyce WE: Behavioral methods in medical rehabilitation, *Neurosci Biobehav Rev* 5:391–396, 1981.

54. Fornusek C, Davis GM: Cardiovascular and metabolic responses during functional electric stimulation cycling at different cadences, *Arch Phys Med Rehabil* 89:719–725, 2008.

55. Frotzler A, et al.: High-volume FES-cycling partially reverses bone loss in people with chronic spinal cord injury, *Bone* 43:169–176, 2008.

56. Garcia RA, et al.: Functional improvement after pediatric spinal cord injury, *Am J Phys Med Rehabil* 81:458–463, 2002.

57. Giangregorio L, McCartney N: Bone loss and muscle atrophy in spinal cord injury, epidemiology, fracture prediction, and rehabilitation strategies, *J Spinal Cord Med* 29:489–500, 2006.

58. Ginis KA, Hicks AL: Considerations for the development of a physical activity guide for Canadians with physical disabilities, *Can J Public Health* 98(Suppl 2):S135–S147, 2007.

59. Glassman SD, et al.: Seatbelt injuries in children, *J Trauma* 33:882–886, 1992.

60. Glenn WW, et al.: Twenty years of experience in phrenic nerve stimulation to pace the diaphragm, *Pacing Clin Electrophysiol* 9:780–784, 1986.

61. Haley SM, et al.: *Pediatric evaluation of disability inventory*, Boston, 1992, New England Medical Center.

62. Hall ED: Pharmacological treatment of acute spinal cord injury: how do we build on past success? *J Spinal Cord Med* 24:142–146, 2001.

63. Herzenberg JE, et al.: Emergency transport and positioning of young children who have an injury to the cervical spine, *J Bone Joint Surg* 71A:15–22, 1989.

64. Hjeltnes N, et al.: Improved body composition after 8 wk of electrically stimulated leg cycling in tetraplegic patients, *Am J Physiol* 273:R1072–R1079, 1997.

65. Hooker SP, et al.: Physiologic effects of electrical stimulation leg cycle exercise training in spinal cord injured persons, *Arch Phys Med Rehabil* 73:470–476, 1992.

66. Hugenholtz H: Methylprednisolone for acute spinal cord injury: not a standard of care, *Can Med Assoc J* 168, 2003.

67. Hurlbert RJ: The role of steroids in acute spinal cord injury: an evidence-based analysis [review], *Spine* 26(Suppl 24):S39–S46, 2001.

68. Jacobs PL, Nash MS: Modes, benefits, and risks of voluntary and electrically induced exercise in persons with spinal cord injury, *J Spinal Cord Med* 24:10–18, 2001 (and exercise and fitness).

69. Janm FK, Wilson PE: A survey of chronic pain in the pediatric spinal cord injury population, *J Spinal Cord Med* 27:S50–S53, 2004.

70. Johnson KA, Klaas SJ: The changing nature of play: implications for pediatric spinal cord injury, *J Spinal Cord Med* 30:S71–S75, 2007.

71. Johnson KA, et al.: Leisure characteristics of the pediatric spinal cord injury population, *J Spinal Cord Med* 27:S107–S109, 2004.

72. Johnston TE, et al.: Patterns of lower extremity innervation in pediatric spinal cord injury, *Spinal Cord* 43:476–482, 2005.

73. Johnston TE, McDonald CM: Health and fitness in pediatric spinal cord injury: medical issues and the role of exercise, *J Pediatr Rehabil Med* 6:35–44, 2013.

74. Johnston TE, et al.: Exercise testing using upper extremity ergometry in pediatric spinal cord injury, *Pediatr Phys Ther* 20:146–151, 2008.

75. Johnston TE, et al.: A randomized controlled trial on the effects of cycling with and without electrical stimulation on cardiorespiratory and vascular health in children with spinal cord injury, *Arch Phys Med Rehabil* 90:1379, 2009.

76. Johnston TE, et al.: A randomized controlled trial on the effects of cycling with and without electrical stimulation on cardiorespiratory and vascular health in children with spinal cord injury, *Arch Phys Med Rehabil*. In press.

77. Johnston TE, et al.: Outcomes of a home cycling program using functional electrical stimulation or passive motion for children with spinal cord injury: a case series, *J Spinal Cord Med* 31:215–221, 2008.

78. Kakulas BA: A review of the neuropathology of human spinal cord injury with emphasis on special features, *J Spinal Cord Med* 22:119–124, 1999.

79. Kigerl K, Popovich P: Drug evaluation, ProCord: a potential cell-based therapy for spinal cord injury, *IDrugs* 9:354–360, 2006. [abstract].

80. Kirshblum SC, et al.: International standards for neurological classification of spinal cord injury, *J Spinal Cord Med* 34:535–554, 2011.

81. Klose KJ, et al.: Evaluation of a training program for persons with SCI paraplegia using the Parastep 1 ambulation system, Part 1. Ambulation performance and anthropometric measures, *Arch Phys Med Rehabil* 78:789–793, 1997.

82. Krey CH, Calhoun CL: Utilizing research in wheelchair and seating selection and configuration for children with injury/dysfunction of the spinal cord, *J Spinal Cord Med* 27(Suppl 1):S29–S37, 2004.

83. Lammertse DP: Invited review: update on pharmaceutical trials in acute spinal cord injury, *J Spinal Cord Med* 27:319–325, 2004.

84. Lauer RT, et al.: Bone mineral density of the hip and knee in children with spinal cord injury, *J Spinal Cord Med* 30:S10–S14, 2007.

85. Lisenmeyer TA: Sexual function and infertility following spinal cord injury, *Phys Med Rehabil Clin N Am* 11:141–156, 2000.

86. Liusuwan RA, et al.: Behavioral intervention, exercise, and nutrition education to improve health and fitness (BENEfit) in adolescents with mobility impairment due to spinal cord dysfunction, *J Spinal Cord Med* 30(Suppl 1):S119–S126, 2007.

87. Liusuwan RA, et al.: Body composition and resting energy expenditure in patients aged 11 to 21 years with spinal cord dysfunction compared to controls: comparisons and relationships among the groups, *J Spinal Cord Med* 30(Suppl 1):S105–S111, 2007.

88. Mandabach M, et al.: Pediatric axis fractures: early halo immobilization, management and outcome, *Pediatr Neurosurg* 19:225–232, 1993.

89. Mange KC, et al.: Recovery of strength at the zone of injury in motor complete and motor incomplete cervical spinal cord injured patients, *Arch Phys Med Rehabil* 71:562–565, 1990.

90. Massagli TL, et al.: Educational performance and vocational participation after spinal cord injury in childhood, *Arch Phys Med Rehabil* 77:995–999, 1996.

91. Massagli TL, Reyes MR: Hypercalcemia and spinal cord injury. http://emedicine.medscape.com/article/322109, 2008.

92. Maynard FM, et al.: Neurological prognosis after traumatic quadriplegia, *J Neurosurg* 50:611–616, 1979.

93. McCarthy JJ, et al.: Incidence and degree of hip subluxation/dislocation in children with spinal cord injury, *J Spinal Cord Med* 27:S80–S83, 2004.

94. McDonald CM, et al.: Body mass index and body composition measures by dual x-ray absorptiometry in patients aged 10 to 21 years with spinal cord injury, *J Spinal Cord Med* 30(Suppl 1):S97–S104, 2007.

95. McDonald CM, et al.: Assessment of muscle strength in children with meningomyelocele: accuracy and stability of measurements over time, *Arch Phys Med Rehabil* 67:855–861, 1986.

96. McDonald JW, et al.: Late recovery following spinal cord injury: case report and review of the literature, *J Neurosurg* 97:252–265, 2002.

97. McGinnis KB, et al.: Recognition and management of autonomic dysreflexia in pediatric spinal cord injury, *J Spinal Cord Med* 27:S61–S74, 2004.

98. McKinley WO, et al.: Nontraumatic spinal cord injury, incidence, epidemiology, and functional outcome, *Arch Phys Med Rehabil* 80:619–623, 1999. [abstract].

99. Mehta S, et al.: Effect of bracing on paralytic scoliosis secondary to spinal cord injury, *J Spinal Cord Med* 27:S88–S92, 2004.

100. Meyer A: Pediatric mobility issues, *Rehabil Management* 21:20–23, 2008.

101. Molnar GE, Alexander MA: History and examination. In Molnar GE, editor: *Pediatric rehabilitation*, ed 3, Philadelphia, 1999, Hanley & Belfus, pp 1–12.

102. Mulcahey MJ: An overview of the upper extremity in pediatric spinal cord injury, *Top Spinal Cord Inj Rehabil* 3:48–55, 1997.

103. Mulcahey MJ, et al.: Children's reports of activity and participation after sustaining a spinal cord injury: a cognitive interviewing study, *Dev Neurorehabil* 12:191–200, 2009.

104. Mulcahey MJ, et al.: Children's and parent's perspectives about activity performance and participation after spinal cord injury: initial development of a patient reported outcome measure, *Am J Occup Ther* 64:605–613, 2010.

105. Mulcahey MJ, et al.: The International Standards for Neurological Classification of Spinal Cord Injury: reliability of data when applied to children and youths, *Spinal Cord* 45:1–8, 2008.

106. Mulcahey MJ, et al.: Evaluation of the lower motor neuron integrity of upper extremity muscles in high level spinal cord injury, *Spinal Cord* 37:585–591, 1999.

107. Myers J, et al.: Cardiovascular disease in spinal cord injury, An overview of prevalence, risk, evaluation, and management, *Am J Phys Med Rehabil* 86:142–152, 2007.

108. Nash MS: Exercise as a health-promoting activity following spinal cord injury, *J Neurol Phys Ther* 29:87–103, 106, 2005.

109. Nelson MD, et al.: Metabolic syndrome in adolescents with spinal cord dysfunction, *J Spinal Cord Med* 30(Suppl 1):S127–S139, 2007.

110. Nesathurai S: Steroids and spinal cord injury: revisiting the NASCIS 2 and 3 trials, *J Trauma* 45:1088–1093, 1998.

111. Nichols DS, Case-Smith J: Reliability and validity of the Pediatric Evaluation of Disability Inventory, *Pediatr Phys Ther* 8:15–24, 1996.

112. Nobunaga AI, et al.: Recent demographic and injury trends in people served by the Model Spinal Cord Injury Care Systems, *Arch Phys Med Rehabil* 80:1372–1382, 1999.

113. Ottenbacher KJ, et al.: The stability and equivalence reliability of the Functional Independence Measure for children (WeeFIM), *Dev Med Child Neurol* 38:907–916, 1996.

114. Peckham PH, et al.: Efficacy of an implanted neuroprosthesis for resorting hand grasp in tetraplegia: a multicenter study, *Arch Phys Med Rehabil* 82:1380–1388, 2001.

115. Phillips WT, et al.: Effect of spinal cord injury on the heart and cardiovascular fitness, *Curr Probl Cardiol* 23:641–716, 1998.

116. Pierce SR, et al.: Comparison of percutaneous and surface functional electrical stimulation during gait in a child with hemiplegic cerebral palsy, *Am J Phys Med Rehabil* 83:798–805, 2004.

117. Prosser LA: Locomotor training within an inpatient rehabilitation program after pediatric incomplete spinal cord injury, *Phys Ther* 87:1224–1232, 2007.

118. Residential Remodeling and Universal Design: Making homes more comfortable and accessible. Prepared by NAHB Research Center, Inc. US Department of Housing and Urban Development, May 1996.

119. Rhoney DH, et al.: New pharmacological approaches to acute spinal cord injury, *Pharmacotherapy* 16:382–392, 1996.

119a. Rosen L, Arva J, Furumasu J, Harris M, Lange M, McCarthy E et al.: RESNA position on the application of power wheelchairs for pediatric users, *Assist Technol* 21:218–226, 2009.

120. Rumball K, Jarvis J: Seat-belt injuries of the spine in young children, *J Bone Joint Surg (Br)* 74:571–574, 1992.

121. Saboe LA, et al.: Early predictors of functional independence 2 years after spinal cord injury, *Arch Phys Med Rehabil* 78:644–650, 1997.

122. Samdani AF: Commentary: spinal cord regeneration, injury modulation, repair strategies, and clinical trials: the Howard H. Steel Conference Precourse, *J Spinal Cord Med* 30(S1):S3–S4, 2007.

123. Scivoletto G, et al.: Clinical factors that affect walking level and performance in chronic spinal cord lesion patients, *Spine (Phila Pa 1976)* 33:259–264, 2008.

124. Scremin AM, et al.: Increasing muscle mass in spinal cord injured persons with a functional electrical stimulation exercise program, *Arch Phys Med Rehabil* 80:1531–1536, 1999.

125. Sharkey PC, et al.: Electrophrenic respiration in patients with high quadriplegia, *Neurosurgery* 24:529–535, 1989.

126. Shaul DB, et al.: Thoracoscopic placement of phrenic nerve electrodes for diaphragmatic pacing in children, *J Pediatr Surg* 37:974–978, 2002.

127. Shavelle RM, et al.: Long-term survival after childhood spinal cord injury, *J Spinal Cord Med* 30:S48–S54, 2007.

128. Short DJ, et al.: High dose methylprednisolone in the management of acute spinal cord injury: a systematic review from a clinical perspective, *Spinal Cord* 38:278–286, 2000.

129. Reference deleted in proofs.

130. Sison-Williamson M, et al.: Effect of thoracolumbosacral orthoses on reachable workspace volumes in children with spinal cord injury, *J Spinal Cord Med* 30:S184–S191, 2007.

131. Sisto SA, et al.: *Spinal cord injuries, management and rehabilitation*, St. Louis, MO, 2009, Mosby.

132. Spoltore T, et al.: Innovative programs for children and adolescents with spinal cord injury, *Orthoped Nurs* 19:55–62, 2000.

133. Stein RB, et al.: Electrical systems for improving locomotion after spinal cord injury: an assessment, *Arch Phys Med Rehabil* 74:954–959, 1993.

134. Triolo RJ, et al.: Application of functional electrical stimulation to children with spinal cord injuries: candidate for selection for upper and lower extremity research, *Paraplegia* 32:824–843, 1994.

135. Trotter TL, et al.: Health supervision for children with achondroplasia, *Pediatrics* 116:771–783, 2005.

136. Ugalde V, et al.: Incidence of venous thromboembolism in patients with acute spinal cord injury by age. Paper abstract #6, *J Spinal Cord Med* 27:S112, 2004.

137. Urbina E, et al.: Ambulatory blood pressure monitoring in children and adolescents, recommendations for standard assessment: a scientific statement from the American Heart Association Atherosclerosis, Hypertension, and Obesity in Youth Committee of the Council on Cardiovascular Disease in the Young and the Council for High Blood Pressure Research, *Hypertension* 52:433–451, 2008.

138. US Department of Education: 105th Congress, *Public Law* 105–117, 1997.

139. US Department of Housing and Urban Development: adaptable housing: a technical manual for implementing adaptable dwelling unit specifications. Publication # HUD-1124-PDR, Barrier Free Environments, Inc.

140. US Equal Employment Opportunity Commission: The Rehabilitation Act of 1973, sec, 504. 1973.

141. Vitale MG, et al.: Epidemiology of pediatric spinal cord injury in the United States, 1997 and 2000, *J Spinal Cord Med* 30:S196, 2006.

142. Vogel LC, et al.: Pain and its impact in adults with pediatric onset spinal cord injury, *J Spinal Cord Med* 30:S193, 2007.

143. Vogel LC, et al.: Spinal cord injuries in children and adolescents. In Verhaagen J, McDonald III JW, editors: *Handbook of clinical neurology*, vol. 109. Amsterdam, 2012, Elsevier, pp 131–148. Chapter 8.

144. Vogel LC, et al.: Long-term outcomes and life satisfaction of adults who had pediatric spinal cord injuries, *Arch Phys Med Rehabil* 79:1496–1503, 1998.

145. Vogel LC, et al.: Adults with pediatric-onset spinal cord injury, part 2, musculoskeletal and neurological complications, *J Spinal Cord Med* 25:117–123, 200.

146. Vogel LC, et al.: Ambulation in children and youth with spinal cord injuries, *J Spinal Cord Med* 30:S158–S164, 2007.

147. Vogel LC, et al.: Intra-rater agreement of the anorectal exam and classification of injury severity in children with spinal cord injury, *Spinal Cord* 47:687–691, 2009.

148. Wang MY, et al.: High rates of neurological improvement following severe traumatic pediatric spinal cord injury, *Spine* 29:1493–1497, 2004.

149. Warburton DER, et al.: Cardiovascular health and exercise following spinal cord. In Eng JJ, et al., editors: *Spinal cord injury rehabilitation evidence*, Vancouver, 2006, British Columbia, 7, 1–7, 28.

150. Waters RL, et al.: Prediction of ambulatory performance based on motor scores derived from standards of the American Spinal Injury Association, *Arch Phys Med Rehabil* 75:756–760, 1994.

151. Wilberger JE: *Spinal cord injuries in children*, New York, 1986, Futura.

152. Wilson PE, et al.: Pediatric spinal cord tumors and masses, *J Spinal Cord Med* 30:S15–S20, 2007.

SUGGESTED READINGS

Calhoun CL, et al.: Recommendations for mobility in children with spinal cord injury, *Top Spinal Cord Inj Rehabil* 19:142–151, 2013.

Chen Y, et al.: Causes of spinal cord injury, *Top Spinal Cord Inj Rehabil* 19:1–8, 2013.

Consortium of Spinal Cord Medicine: *Clinical practice guideline. Preservation of upper limb function following spinal cord injury: a clinical practice guideline for healthcare professionals*, Washington, DC, 2002, Paralyzed Veterans of America.

Consortium for Spinal Cord Medicine: *Clinical practice guideline. Pressure ulcer prevention and treatment following spinal cord injury: a clinical practice guideline for healthcare professionals*, ed 2, Washington, DC, 2014, Paralyzed Veterans of America.

Consortium for Spinal Cord Medicine: *Outcomes following traumatic SCI: clinical practice guidelines for healthcare professionals*. Washington, DC, 1999, Paralyzed Veterans of America.

Field-Fote EC: *Spinal cord injury rehabilitation*, Philadelphia, 2009, F.A. Davis.

Harvey LA, Somers MF, Glinsky JV: Physiotherapy management. In Chhabra JS, editor: *ISCoS textbook on comprehensive management of spinal cord injuries*, New Dehli, India, 2015, Wolters Kluwer, pp 514–537. Chapter 34.

Johnston TE, McDonald CM: Health and fitness in pediatric spinal cord injury: medical issues and the role of exercise, *J Pediatr Rehabil Med* 6:35–44, 2013.

Kirshblum SC, et al.: International standards for neurological classification of spinal cord injury, *J Spinal Cord Med* 34:535–554, 2011.

McCarthy JJ, et al.: Incidence and degree of hip subluxation/dislocation in children with spinal cord injury, *J Spinal Cord Med* 27:S80–S83, 2004.

McGinnis KB, et al.: Recognition and management of autonomic dysreflexia in pediatric spinal cord injury, *J Spinal Cord Med* 27:S61–S74, 2004.

Mehta S, et al.: Effect of bracing on paralytic scoliosis secondary to spinal cord injury, *J Spinal Cord Med* 27:S88–S92, 2004.

Mulcahey MJ, et al.: The International Standards for Neurological Classification of Spinal Cord Injury: reliability of data when applied to children and youths, *Spinal Cord* 45:1–8, 2007.

Sisto SA, et al.: *Spinal cord injuries, management and rehabilitation*, St. Louis, MO, 2009, Mosby.

Vogel LC, et al.: Spinal cord Injuries in children and adolescents. In Verhaagen J, McDonald III JW, editors: *Handbook of clinical neurology, vol. 109.* Amsterdam, 2012, Elsevier, pp 131–148. Chapter 8.

Vogel LC, et al.: Ambulation in children and youth with spinal cord injuries, *J Spinal Cord Med* 30:S158–S164, 2007.

22

Acquired Brain Injuries: Trauma, Near-Drowning, and Tumors

Michal Katz-Leurer, Hemda Rotem

Acquired brain injury (ABI) in children is a highly stressful event for the child and the family. Damage occurring at a time of development extensively affects the child's abilities to do what children usually do: play, learn, establish friendships, and gradually develop to become independent young adults. The injury commonly causes a variety of physical, emotional, cognitive, and behavioral impairments. Suddenly, the child's expectations from life and the parents' aspirations for their child may be dramatically changed. These unique emotional, social, and developmental needs of the child and family demand a holistic and inclusive approach by a multidisciplinary team, both as a team and by each member of the team as an expert in a unique specialty. This chapter focuses on the role of the physical therapist and the elements of patient/client management: examination, diagnosis, prognosis, and intervention strategies, with emphasis on the child with ABI and the parents and family as they progress through the rehabilitation process.

ABI is a general categorization that describes any injury to the brain that occurs after birth and may be the result of trauma (e.g., head injury after traffic accidents, falls), anoxia (e.g., near-drowning), or a nontraumatic event (e.g., stroke, brain tumor, infection). ABI is the most common cause of morbidity and mortality in children and in young adults.[35] ABI might cause a variety of disorders involving motor dysfunction, cognitive impairment, behavioral disturbance, emotional difficulties, and abnormal function of the autonomic nervous system. Even a mild injury might result in a serious disability that interferes with the child's daily functioning and activities for the rest of his or her life.

Different theories have been put forth regarding the recovery and adaptation processes of brain function following a brain injury. One theory suggests that intact areas of the brain that are anatomically linked to the damaged site might be functionally depressed. Because return of activity occurs in these functionally depressed areas, recovery of function might also occur.[110] Another theory suggests that recovery and adaptation of brain function might occur as the original brain area responsible for that function recovers or through the adaptation of noninjured brain regions that normally contribute indirectly to that function. Furthermore, recovery of function occurs as a result of behavioral substitution in which new strategies are learned to compensate for the behavioral deficit.[110]

These theories serve as the foundation for a variety of interventions physical therapists use for children with ABI, ranging from preventive treatment with the expectation for brain function recovery at one end of the spectrum to a structured motor training program to facilitate compensation processes of brain function at the other. The latter is the source of many innovative treatment strategies for patients with brain damage. Advances in basic science have demonstrated morphologic changes in neural structures within the motor cortex during the process of motor skill acquisition, resulting in behavioral changes in motor performance.[91] The use of functional neuroimaging techniques may help researchers and clinicians to clarify the effect of treatment on neural reorganization and to identify the sequence and timing of interventions that will optimally and efficiently improve function. Although the outcome of the injury depends largely on the nature and severity of the injury itself, appropriate and timely treatment may play a vital role in determining the level of recovery.[73]

The first part of this chapter describes the epidemiology, pathology, and prognosis of ABI among children and adolescents. Examples of three common causes of brain injury among children—trauma, near-drowning as an example of an anoxic event, and brain tumor—are described in detail. The second part focuses on foreground information related to physical therapy examination and intervention throughout the rehabilitation process.

BACKGROUND INFORMATION

TRAUMATIC BRAIN INJURY

Epidemiology

Traumatic brain injury (TBI) is the most common cause of acquired disability in childhood, with an incidence death rate of 4.5, a hospitalization rate for nonfatal TBI of 63, and an emergency department visit rate of 731 cases, all per 100,000 children aged 0 to 14 years per year in the United States.[65] The most frequent causes of injury are motor vehicle accidents and falls, the latter being the primary cause among younger, preschool children; adolescents and young adults are more commonly injured in motor vehicle accidents. The incidence is higher in boys and highest in boys between the ages of 15 and 20 years, followed by children between the ages of 6 and 10 years.[56] Other demographic and socio-environmental factors associated with an increased risk of TBI include poverty, crowded neighborhoods, family instability, history of alcohol or drug abuse, and learning disability.[61] Preexisting behavioral characteristics such as impulsivity and hyperactivity, as well as attention deficit disorder, have been associated with an increased risk of accidental injury[15]; the *shaken baby syndrome* resulting from vigorous shaking of an infant or small child by the shoulders, arms, or legs can also be a cause of brain injury.[12] Preventive efforts are essential and should include educational programs for children, adolescents, and parents. The effectiveness of preventive activities regarding risky behavior and the use of protective equipment have been described. For example, awareness about head injury in children not wearing helmets during bicycle riding arose during the early 1980s, when it was noted that only approximately 15% of riders younger than 15 years of age wore helmets. Societal interest resulted in the implementation of helmet laws that reduced the incidence of pediatric TBI. The results of a case-control study in Seattle in 1989 indicated that the use of bicycle helmets reduced the risk of bicycle-related head injury by 74% to 85%.[105]

Pathology

Brain damage due to TBI is typically divided into primary and secondary damage. *Primary damage* is related to the forces that occur at the time of initial impact; *secondary* damage occurs as the result of processes evoked in response to the initial trauma.

Primary Brain Damage

Primary brain damage can be classified according to the mechanism of injury, including acceleration-deceleration injury, crush injury, and penetration injury. *Acceleration-deceleration* injuries occur when the force applied is translational (Fig. 22.1) or rotational (Fig. 22.2) and commonly results from motor vehicle accidents; the head hits an immobile object or a mobile object hits the immobile head. Such injuries can lead to lesions that might be microscopic or combined with a focal macroscopic lesion with a predilection for the midbrain, pons, corpus callosum, and white matter of the cerebral hemispheres.[80] Acceleration-deceleration injuries, particularly the rotational component, produce differential displacement of adjacent brain tissue layers. This shearing force has its greatest effect in areas where the density differences of the tissues are greatest. Therefore approximately two thirds of lesions of this type—that is, diffuse axon injury (DAI)—occur at the gray-white matter interface.[92] The child's brain has a higher water content (88%) than the adult brain (77%), meaning that the brain is softer and more prone to acceleration-deceleration injury. *Contusion or crush injuries* are usually frontal or temporal. These injuries result from relatively low-velocity impact such as blows to the head or falls. Skull fractures may be associated, which is significant only when underlying compression of the brain or hemorrhage occurs. Or multiple small intracerebral hemorrhages and occasionally more extensive bleeding may be observed. *Penetration injuries* constitute a minority of pediatric TBI and are classified as nonmissile penetrating injuries and missile penetrating injuries. Children are prone to nonmissile penetrating injuries that result from a fall or from a home or playground accident. These injuries often involve nails, pencils, and sharp sticks, which, in most cases, cause focal damage. Missile injuries caused by gunshots or air pellet rifles lead to substantive intracranial damage.

Secondary Brain Damage

Secondary brain damage usually results from hypoxia or ischemia, which can be caused by *intracranial factors* or *extracranial factors* such as hypoxemia or hypotension (systolic blood pressure <90/mm Hg).[14] The main *intracranial causes* of secondary injuries are hemorrhage and brain swelling. Intracranial hemorrhage is due to laceration of blood vessels within the brain or on its surface, resulting in an epidural, subdural, or subarachnoid hematoma, according to the site. Displacement of the brain can occur as the result of a rise in intracranial pressure due to edema or can be caused by a mass lesion. Diffuse swelling is more common in infants and children than in adults. It has been suggested that the relatively compliant skull and membranous suture properties of the infant skull allow a significant cranial shape change and a more diffuse pattern of brain distortion

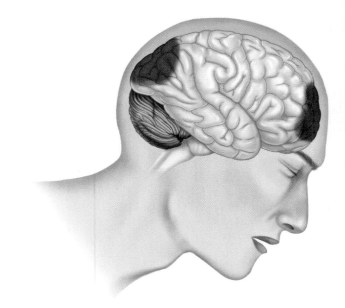

FIG. 22.1 Mechanism of translation injury.

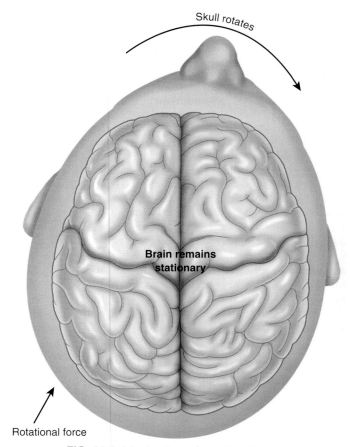

FIG. 22.2 Mechanism of rotational injury.

than is seen in adults after TBI. Experimental studies have suggested that the edema setting in early after injury might be related to enhanced diffusion of excitotoxic neurotransmitters in the immature brain, to an enhanced inflammatory response in the developing brain, or to enhanced blood-brain barrier permeability after central nervous system (CNS) injury in the immature versus the adult brain.[60]

Further brain damage may occur as the result of complications such as infection, hydrocephalus, hygroma, or convulsions. Infection of the brain may occur after an open fracture or cerebrospinal fluid (CSF) rhinorrhea, or it may be iatrogenic, caused by intracranial monitoring or surgery.[4] A hygroma develops as the result of localized CSF collection or resolution of a hematoma. Posttraumatic seizures typically are divided into three types, depending on their time of onset as related to the trauma. Seizures that occur within minutes are referred to as immediate seizures, early seizures occur within 1 week of the trauma, and late seizures occur beyond the first week of injury. A child who suffers two or more late seizures is diagnosed as having posttraumatic epilepsy.

Prognosis

Studies designed to identify prognostic factors for survival and function after TBI have resulted in an overall conclusion that no single factor adequately predicts outcome from an injury as complex and heterogeneous as TBI. Nevertheless, the severity of the brain injury seems to be directly associated with the outcome.[61]

The most commonly used parameters for determining brain damage severity are the Glasgow Coma Scale, coma duration, and posttraumatic amnesia. The Glasgow Coma Scale (GCS) is a widely accepted method of initially evaluating and characterizing trauma patients with head injuries.[114] The scale has been adapted for infants and young children as the Pediatric Coma Scale.[101] The GCS assesses the level of coma by ranking three aspects of function: motor response, verbal performance, and eye opening. The best response for each is noted on a scale from 1 to 5. The sum of the scores (3 to 15 points) is used as an indication of the depth of the coma and the severity of injury. A GCS score of 13 to 15 points is considered mild, a GCS score of 9 to 12 points is considered moderate, and a GCS score of 3 to 8 points is considered severe. A limitation of the GCS is that it is a time-dependent assessment tool designed to evaluate injury severity within the first 48 hours after the trauma.

Coma duration classifies injury severity as mild (coma lasting less than 20 minutes), moderate (coma lasting 20 minutes to 6 hours), severe (coma lasting 6 to 24 hours), and very severe (coma for longer than 24 hours).[6] Depth and duration of impaired consciousness are negatively associated with functional outcome. Coma duration may be a better predictor of motor and cognitive recovery than coma depth measured with the GCS. The longer the duration of the coma, particularly a duration of coma of longer than 4 weeks, the less likely is a good recovery.[49] Nevertheless it has been noted that coma duration as brief as 1 hour may lead to attention deficits, behavioral disturbances, and irritability.[98]

Posttraumatic amnesia (PTA) is defined as a period of variable length after trauma, during which the patient is confused and disoriented; retrograde amnesia is defined as an inability to remember and recall new information. The longer the duration of PTA, the worse is the outcome. It is unlikely that a person will have an outcome of severe disability if the duration of PTA is less than 2 months. Conversely, it is unlikely that a person will have a good recovery if the duration of PTA extends beyond 3 months.[49]

Of all children who sustain TBI, 95% survive.[61] Among those with severe TBI, that percentage drops to 65%. The highest mortality rate is seen in children younger than 2 years of age, with a decline in mortality rate until age 12 years, and then a second peak at age 15 years.[56] Death is seldom due to

the primary damage but is more often the result of secondary intracranial or extracranial complications of brain damage or other related injuries.

NEAR-DROWNING

Hypoxic injury refers to any injury caused by tissue oxygen deficiency and includes drowning and near-drowning, inhalation of a foreign body, hanging and strangulation, suffocation and asphyxia, apnea, and others.[42] Although near-drowning is unique in some aspects, it can serve as a model for understanding many of the pathophysiologic, therapeutic, and prognostic aspects of all types of hypoxic injury in the pediatric population.[118]

Epidemiology

Drowning, defined as death within 24 hours of a submersion incident, and near-drowning, defined as survival for at least 24 hours following a submersion incident, represent significant causes of morbidity and mortality in children.[130] In the United States in 2013, 2% of all deaths were due to drowning among children age 0-14 years. Males were more likely to die of drowning than were females in all age groups; boys 1 to 4 years of age had the highest rate of drowning (2.5 per 100,000), followed by boys 15 to 19 years of age (3.25 per 100,000). http://www.cdc.gov-/nchs/data/nvsr/nvsr64/nvsr64_02.pdf. Efficient preventive procedures include adult supervision of young children in bathtubs and pools and well-maintained four-sided pool fencing that prevents direct entry to the pool from the house or yard.[111]

Pathology

Submersion of a child usually leads to panic and a struggle to surface. In attempting to breathe, the child may aspirate water (wet drowning), or laryngospasm may occur without aspiration (dry drowning).[119] The most significant factors causing morbidity and mortality from near-drowning are hypoxemia and a decrease in oxygen delivery to vital tissues. Sustained hypoxemia causes neuronal injury and finally leads to circulatory collapse, myocardial damage, and dysfunction of multiple organ systems, with further ischemic brain damage. During the first few minutes, the brain is deprived of oxygen (hypoxic injury). As the cardiovascular system fails, cerebral blood flow decreases and ischemic injury occurs. The vulnerability of the brain tissue to hypoxic-ischemic injury varies in the white matter and the gray matter. Areas of greatest susceptibility to ischemic injury are usually in vascular end zones, in the hippocampus, insular cortex, and basal ganglia. Even within the hippocampus itself, vulnerability to hypoxic-ischemic damage varies.[62] More severe hypoxia-ischemia leads to more extensive and global cortical damage.

Prognosis

CNS damage and its outcomes determine survival and long-term morbidity. About one third of all children who survive will have significant neurologic damage caused by hypoxic-ischemic encephalopathy.[21] The prognosis for those who are severely injured may be difficult to determine in the first hours after the hypoxic-ischemic event, although prolonged cardiopulmonary resuscitation, fixed and dilated pupils, and a GCS of 3 suggest a poor outcome.[42] Attention to the adequacy of oxygenation with optimal ventilator strategies to minimize brain and lung injury, provide cardiovascular support, and avoid iatrogenic complications may minimize secondary brain damage.[42]

BRAIN TUMORS

Epidemiology

Brain tumors are the most common form of solid tumors in children and the second most common form of pediatric cancer overall.[36] The annual incidence of brain tumors in the United States is about 38 cases per million children. Brain tumors occasionally are congenital, occur most frequently in children ages 1 to 10 years, and are slightly more common in boys than in girls.[36]

Pathology

Brain tumors may be benign or malignant, primary or metastatic. The term *benign* may imply that a complete cure is possible, but it can be life threatening if it is large or if it results in increased intracranial pressure, cerebral edema, or brain herniation, especially if it is located in a critical area of the brain for maintaining vital functions, such as the pons or medulla. Malignant brain tumors, which make up 80% of brain tumors among children, are life threatening. Primary brain tumors are those that originate directly from cells in the brain and rarely spread outside of the CNS. Metastatic brain tumors originate from tissues outside the brain.

Tumors can cause symptoms directly, by penetration or compression of an area of the brain, or indirectly, by causing an increase in intracranial pressure. Most common symptoms include headache, nausea, vomiting, irritability, balance disturbances, ataxia, seizures, hemiparesis, and visual problems.[67]

Young children have a relatively high incidence of cerebellum and brain stem tumors.[37] The tumors are classified according to their cellular characteristics and location (Fig. 22.3). The most common entities throughout childhood and adolescence are astrocytoma and medulloblastoma, which occur predominantly in the cerebellum. Early signs are those of increased intracranial pressure, as well as cerebellar signs such as ataxia.

Metastases may occur throughout the meninges and may involve sites outside the brain. Ependymoma is a primary brain tumor that may occur in the posterior fossa and the cerebral hemispheres. Initial signs and symptoms include those related to increased intracranial pressure in the posterior fossa, seizures, and focal cerebellar deficits.[67] Craniopharyngiomas are histologically benign and occur primarily at the midline of the suprasellar region. Visual disturbances, headaches, and vomiting, as well as endocrine disturbances, are the primary symptoms. Initial signs of brain stem gliomas include progressive cranial nerve dysfunction and gait disorders.

Prognosis

Treatment of brain tumors usually includes surgical resection, radiation therapy, and chemotherapy. Radiation therapy must be used cautiously in young children because of late-onset effects on cognition and learning. Chemotherapy effectiveness is often limited owing to difficulty in crossing the blood-brain barrier. Shunt placement may be necessary to relieve hydrocephalus resulting from blockage of CSF flow by the tumor. The survival rate has been growing continuously, but in general, it depends on the grade of the malignancy and age. The prognosis is better the older the child is at onset and, for example, the prognosis is better for astrocytomas than for medulloblastomas.[100] The astrocytomas arise from astrocytes, cells that play a role in nutrition and various cleanup functions within the central nervous system, and are usually more slow-growing tumors and are therefore considered treatable. However, medulloblastomoas, which are primitive neuroectodermal tumors usually located in the cerebellum, are fast growing and highly malignant.[67] A rough estimate of the 5-year survival rate for malignant brain tumors in children is about 70%.[36] In spite of generally encouraging prognostic data, many long-term survivors continue to have major neuropsychological or cognitive deficits.[83]

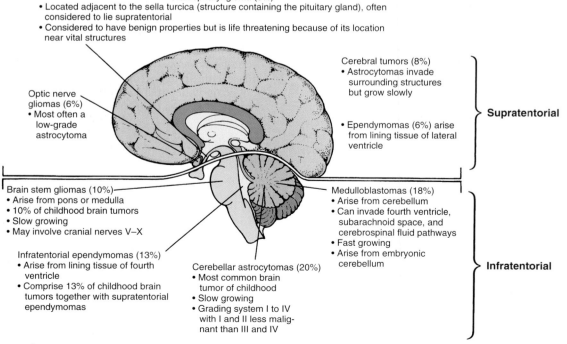

FIG. 22.3 Common sites of pediatric brain tumors. *PNET,* primitive neuroectodermal tumor. (From James SR, Nelson K, Ashwill J: *Nursing care of children: principles and practice,* ed 4, St. Louis, 2013, Saunders.)

ACQUIRED BRAIN INJURY: DIAGNOSTIC TECHNIQUES

Imaging techniques can provide specific and accurate information on the structure of the brain, its metabolic activity, and its functional activity. The techniques assist in making a diagnosis and planning a treatment strategy, and they may provide insight as to the prognosis.

Imaging techniques that provide information about brain structure include magnetic resonance imaging (MRI), x-ray (least informative), computed tomography (CT), and angiography.[57] MRI is based on signals produced by tissue protons when placed in a magnetic field. MRI is sensitive in detecting hemorrhage or hypoxic-ischemic damage, and it can often discriminate between benign and malignant masses and other changes in tissue density. CT illustrates thin slices through the brain based on x-rays. This technique can be used to distinguish among many soft tissues and can indicate the location, density, and the presence of a tumor or edema. CT is particularly effective in identifying foreign bodies and bone abnormalities. MRI has greater tissue contrast resolution than does CT; it does not use ionizing radiation and has not been shown to produce side effects. On the other hand, CT is less expensive, faster, and safer, because an MRI scan requires the child to lie still for an extended period of time, often under sedation. Angiography is used primarily to diagnose and to map vascularization. It is particularly helpful in providing information on blood supply to the brain.[7]

Imaging techniques that provide information about cellular metabolic activity and thereby assist with functional mapping of the brain include functional magnetic resonance imaging (fMRI), positron emission tomography (PET), and magnetic resonance spectroscopy (MRS). The advantage of these techniques is their superior resolution with reference to spatial relationships that define areas of activated brain tissue. fMRI takes a rapid succession of scans that can detect small changes in the level of oxygen consumption and blood flow taking place in areas of the brain that are activated during a test protocol. PET detects the differing levels of glucose uptake that occur in brain tissue. Brain tumors, for example, have a higher level of glucose uptake than normal brain tissue, whereas necrotic tissue has little to no glucose uptake. MRS is another imaging technique that detects metabolic changes; it is noninvasive and does not require contrast agents or labeled tracers.[103]

Techniques that provide information about brain functional activity include electroencephalography (EEG) and evoked potential tests (EPTs)—sensory, motor, or cognitive. Advantages of these techniques are their superior resolution in relation to time. The EEG is a recording of ongoing electrical brain activity, which presents frequency, amplitude, and organization of the waveform at rest and as a response to stimuli. EPT is an electrical potential recorded from the brain after presentation of a stimulus, as opposed to spontaneous potentials as detected by EEG. Sensory EPTs are recorded from the brain after stimulation of sense organs, for example, visual (elicited by a flashing light), auditory (elicited by a click or tone stimulus presented through earphones), or tactile- or somatosensory-evoked potentials (elicited by touch or electrical stimulation of a sensory or mixed nerve in the periphery). In motor-evoked potentials, an area of the brain is stimulated electrically, and the response is recorded in the peripheral musculature.[74] The appropriate choice of tests depends on the suspected pathology, and tests are often repeated to monitor the progress of treatment.

FOREGROUND INFORMATION

PHYSICAL THERAPY MANAGEMENT FOR A CHILD WITH ACQUIRED BRAIN INJURY

Physical therapy for a child with brain injury is a unique and challenging process. The varied clinical presentation and the unpredictable and varied recovery processes obligate the therapist to carry out frequent reevaluation and, as a consequence, modification of the plan of care. Additionally, evaluation and intervention are impacted by the age of the child and the ongoing maturation and refinement of cognitive and functional abilities. In addition, the management of a child with ABI should be based on identifying levels of activity and participation that the child and family wish to assume or reassume after the injury. Only then can the therapist design a plan of care that includes the interventions needed to address the physiologic mechanisms of recovery and adaptation at both impairment and activity skill levels.

Behavioral and Cognitive Disorders

Often the clinical situation is complicated in that not only does neuronal injury directly interfere with motor function, but damage to the cognitive processes *associated* with motor performance and learning has been reported. In the period after the injury, children present with a variety of organic, behavioral, and cognitive disorders, as well as with individual emotional reactions to injury and disability, which might influence their ability to participate in examination and intervention activities. Common situations include the following:

- Low tolerance to frustration, poor social judgment, aggression, and impulsivity are frequent phenomena among children with ABI.[129] Attention deficits might include inability to concentrate, increased distractibility, or even perseveration. Children tend to experience global attention difficulties, which often persist beyond the acute recovery phase and may affect performance and learning capabilities.
- Memory disorders in children with brain injury are varied. Memory is assessed with respect to the child's ability to learn new material. *Explicit* memory, which is memory for facts and events, is mediated by medial temporal cerebral areas that include the hippocampus and the diencephalic nuclei.[109] *Implicit* memory is the ability to develop skills and habits. Motor skill learning is a form of implicit learning in which changes in motor performance with practice can accrue without conscious awareness of all the movement-related abilities that are being learned. Areas associated with implicit learning include the sensory, motor, and prefrontal cerebral cortices, the basal ganglia, and cerebellar areas, which include the neural network for movement.[109] Explicit and implicit learning systems are functionally and neuroanatomically distinct. For example, it is possible that children will present with cognitive deficits that interfere with their ability to have explicit recall but may not interfere with their ability to learn new motor skills.
- Language skill impairment, expressive or receptive, might be due to temporal lobe lesions and can obstruct the child's ability to follow instructions.[129] Expressive disorders impair the child's ability to communicate with others, leading to frustration and aggravation.

TABLE 22.1 **Rancho Pediatric Levels of Consciousness**

Rancho Pediatric Level	Infants: 6 Months to 2 Years	Preschool: 2 to 5 Years	School Age: 5 Years and Older
I	Interacts with environment Shows active interest in toys; manipulates or examines before mounting or discarding Watches other children at play, may move toward them purposefully Initiates social contact with adults; enjoys socializing Shows active interest in bottle Reaches for or moves toward person or object	Oriented to self and surroundings Provides accurate information about self Knows he or she is away from home Knows where toys, clothes, and the like are kept Actively participates in treatment program Recognizes own room, knows way to bathroom, nursing station, and so on Is potty trained Initiates social contact with adults, enjoys socializing	Oriented to time and place Provides accurate detailed information about self and present situation Knows way to and from daily activities Knows sequence of daily routine Knows way around unit, recognizes own room Finds own bed; knows where personal belongings are kept Is bowel and bladder trained
II	Demonstrates awareness of environment Responds to name Recognizes mother and other family members Enjoys imitative vocal play Giggles or smiles when talked to or played with Fussing is quieted by soft voice or touch	Is responsive to environment Follows simple commands Refuses to follow command by shaking head or saying no Imitates examiner's gestures or facial expressions Response to name Recognizes mother and other family members Enjoys imitative vocal play	Is responsive to environment Follows simple verbal or gestured requests Initiates purposeful activity Actively participates in therapy program Refuses to follow request by shaking head or saying no Imitates examiner's gestures or facial expressions
III	Gives localized response to sensory stimuli Blinks when strong light crosses field of vision Follows moving object passed within visual field Turns toward or away from loud sound Gives localized response to painful stimuli		
IV	Gives generalized response to sensory stimuli Gives generalized startle to loud sound Responds to repeated auditory stimulation with increased or decreased activity Gives generalized reflex response to painful stimuli		
V	No response to stimuli Complete absence of observable change in visual, auditory, or painful stimuli		

Adapted from Professional Staff Association of Rancho Los Amigos Hospital, Inc: *Rehabilitation of the head injured child and adult: pediatric levels of consciousness, selected problems*, Downey, CA, 1982, Rancho Los Amigos Medical Center, Pediatric Brain Injury Service and Los Amigos Research and Education Institute, Inc.

- Visuospatial and perceptual impairments may affect the child's perception of the environment—for example, the ability to distinguish a given shape from its surroundings.[129] A child may not be able to put on an orthosis and thereby becomes dependent in functional mobility, even though the child is able to ambulate independently once the orthosis is on. Areas associated with these impairments involve the temporal or occipital lobes of the cerebral cortex.

These cognitive and psychological impairments are frequently present to various degrees and often interfere with the child's ability to participate in examination and intervention activities. Although the neuropsychologist formally performs specific testing of these areas, the physical therapist needs to grossly determine the child's level of cognitive ability in order to enhance the effectiveness of the examination and ongoing intervention. The Rancho Levels of Cognitive Functioning (RLCF) is a simple ordinal scale that uses behavioral observation to categorize the child's cognitive functioning level and classifies the level of pediatric consciousness by three age groups: infants (6 months to 2 years), preschool-aged children (2 to 5 years), and school-aged children (5 years and older). The levels of each scale range from V (no response to stimuli) to I (oriented). Behavioral expectations at each level are variable, depending on the age group (Table 22.1). Cognitive function of children 12 years of age and older can be assessed using the RLCF for adults. This scale is reversed in order compared with

pediatric forms and delineates adult cognitive functioning into eight levels (Table 22.2).

Table 22.3 provides a basic frame for examination and evaluation that would be appropriate at various stages of cognitive functional recovery of a child with ABI. The next section describes assessments of impairment and functional activity appropriate for the child with ABI.

Physical Therapy Examination

Most children with ABI change their environmental settings during the rehabilitation process from the acute care unit to the inpatient rehabilitation ward, outpatient therapy departments, community services, and educational settings. A systematic examination and evaluation should be performed upon entry into each new setting.

History

The examination process should include a review of the medical record and history. Medical record information may include medical history before the injury, cause of injury, earliest GCS, imaging reports specifying locations and extent of injury, other injuries, procedures and surgeries performed, medications, complications, and previous therapy progress reports. Consultations with other rehabilitation personnel and education professionals enable every team member to have a greater understanding of the child's needs and abilities.

TABLE 22.2   Rancho Levels of Cognitive Functioning

Rancho Adult Level

I	No response	Completely unresponsive to any stimuli
II	Generalized response	Inconsistent and nonpurposeful response to stimuli
III	Localized response	Specific yet inconsistent response to stimuli; response is related to type of stimuli (turning head toward sound)
IV	Confused–agitated	Heightened state of activity. Demonstrates bizarre and nonpurposeful behaviors relative to the environment
V	Confused–inappropriate	Inconsistently follows simple commands. Shows gross attention to environment but is easily distractible and lacks ability to focus attention on specific task. Memory is severely impaired, new information is difficult to learn
VI	Confused–appropriate	Goal direction behavior appropriate, responds to environment. Can consistently follow simple commands and demonstrates carryover of relearned tasks. Dependent on external cues for direction. Shows little carryover to independent performance of newly learned tasks
VII	Automatic–appropriate	Appears appropriate and oriented to self and environment. Participates in automatic daily routines. Recent memory is impaired, resulting in shallow recall of activities and decreased rate of learning new information
VIII	Purposeful–appropriate	Recalls and integrates past and recent events. Adapts responses to environment. Demonstrates carryover of new learning and does not require supervision once an activity is learned. Deficits remain in the areas of abstract reasoning, tolerance to stress, and judgment in emergencies

Adapted from Malkmus D, Booth B, Kodimer C: *Rehabilitation of head injured adult: comprehensive cognitive management,* Downey, CA, 1980, Los Amigos Research and Education Institute, Inc.

TABLE 22.3   Examination Strategy Based on Rancho Levels of Cognitive Functioning Categories

Rancho Adult Level	Rancho Pediatric Level	Global Description	Examination Strategies
I–III	V–III	None to early response	Testing should focus on passive manipulation and observation of spontaneous or stimulus-induced movements.
IV–V	II	Agitated, confused	Testing should focus on observation of spontaneous and simple instructed tasks.
VI–VIII	I	Higher-level response	Testing should focus on more complex, two or more staged functional and nonfunctional instructed tasks.

Data to be collected from the family as part of the examination procedure include information regarding developmental history, including learning ability, behavior, and cognitive level. Talking with the parents and family enables the therapist to more fully understand the family's perception of the extent of the injuries and their impact on the previous level of function, and it allows the family to express expectations and goals. During these discussions, the therapist builds up a picture of the child's personality before the injury, the child's favorite music or television programs, specific heroes for the younger children, special hobbies, leisure activities, and information on friends and siblings. This information may enable the therapist to incorporate familiar, attractive, and motivating components into the treatment sessions and to plan for participation in home and community activities.

Systems Review

The physiotherapist should obtain information regarding medical status, medications, cardiac, respiration, musculoskeletal or abdominal status, and injuries prior to performing physical assessments and testing.

Brain injury can cause revealed and concealed dysfunction. An example of more concealed impairment is the neuroendocrine, pituitary dysfunction, which is frequently observed post brain injury. Diabetes insipidus may present with diagnosis in the acute phase post injury; nevertheless the loss of other pituitary hormones may not be diagnosed for months or years. The appearance of the syndrome of growth hormone deficiency, characterized by decreases in strength, aerobic capacity, and the sense of well-being, has to be considered, especially in those with associated facial fractures, cranial nerve injuries, and dysautonomia.[18]

Tests and Measures

In the next stage, the therapist selects appropriate tests and measures in an effort to diagnose impairments, activity limitations, and participation restrictions, and to define appropriate short- and long-term treatment goals in the design of a plan of care. It should be emphasized that many of the described tests have not yet been validated or assessed for reliability in children with ABI. One must consider that children who have experienced trauma or near-drowning might sustain other injuries that impair their ability to perform a test according to its guidelines and that may affect the test's outcomes. Such problems must be noted as limitations when test results are evaluated.

Impairments of body structure and function

Passive range of motion. Limitations to range of motion (ROM) might be associated with one or more factors, such as prolonged bed rest, immobilization, pain, peripheral nerve injury, spasticity, side effects of medical treatment, and skeletal injury due to periarticular new bone formation (PNBF), also known as heterotopic ossification (HO).[22] PNBF is a localized and progressive formation of pathologic bone that develops in the soft tissues adjacent to large joints (hips, elbows, shoulders, and knees). The risk that a child with TBI will develop PNBF is about 20%, and this risk increases with severity of the injury, length of immobilization, duration of coma, and presence of spasticity or fracture, especially if the fracture involves an open reduction with internal fixation or joint dislocation.[41] Assessing the ROM in a child who is unable to follow commands might be problematic, as the child may resist the movement and cry in response to pain. Observations of spontaneous movements and performance of gentle passive ROM exercises will enlighten the therapist regarding joint limitations.

Diagnosis of periarticular new bone formation. Decreased passive range of motion and a painful joint might be the first clinical signs of PNBF. The serum alkaline phosphatase level test, which reflects osteoblastic activity, is useful for obtaining an early diagnosis, especially in patients who cannot report pain. Although radiographs offer a feasible method for recognizing a neurogenic heterotopic ossification, it may take up to 6 weeks for ossification to be evident. Ultrasonography (US) can be used in the early diagnosis of HO, although bone scans such as MRI and CT are considered the most sensitive methods for the early detection of ossification.[112]

Spasticity is characterized by muscles that are perceived as stiff, in which velocity-dependent resistance to passive movement produces increased muscle tone; spasticity is assessed by the Modified Ashworth Scale,[13] which is a simple, quick, but subjective tool with questionable reliability.[23]

Active range of motion/muscle strength. Muscle atrophy and weakness typically result after prolonged bed rest or sedentary behavior. For example, bed rest for 30 days can result in an 18% to 20% reduction in knee extensor peak torque.[11] Peripheral or spinal nerve damage due to trauma or chemotherapy can cause a reduction in muscle strength. Manual muscle testing (MMT) demands careful attention and the ability of the examinee to follow simple commands—not suitable requirements for the confused child. At this stage, the therapist must evaluate strength simply by observation. Movement should be observed in varied situations with gravity eliminated, as well as against gravity in lying, sitting, and standing, statically and dynamically, and with variable task demands. When a child can follow simple commands such as standing from sitting or lifting weights (e.g., plantar flexor muscle strength might be assessed by asking children to raise their heels in standing),[77] then this simple procedure might provide information about the functional strength of the muscle groups. Among children with TBI older than 7 years who can follow simple instructions, lower extremity muscle strength can be reliably tested using a standardized measurement protocol and a handheld dynamometer[55]; hand strength may be measured objectively in children 5 years and older with quantitative analyses of precision-grip forces.[34] See Chapter 2 for more information on strength testing.

Sensory testing. *Sensory testing* in children with ABI is challenging. Children may have cognitive deficits that impair their ability to accurately respond to sensory input. Their young age may also lead to difficulty in perceiving and expressing sensations. Sensory stimuli should be introduced selectively with careful observation to determine the response. Responses are noted as being generalized, with a full-body response, or localized. Localized responses are more appropriate, with the response being specific to the system that is being stimulated.

Activity level tests and measures

Motor performance. Status and change in motor performance might be identified by using a multi-item activity level test of motor performance such as the Gross Motor Function Measure (GMFM), designed and validated to measure change in gross motor function over time in children with cerebral palsy (CP).[107] The maximum performance detectable is that of a typical 5-year-old child (see Chapters 2 and 19 for more information on the GMFM). It is important to note that this measure has not been validated for children with ABI, even though it may provide the therapist with objective information for identifying the child's abilities and may assist in planning intervention and evaluating the child's progress in motor function.

Several norm-referenced, multi-item standardized tests are available to compare a child with ABI to a reference group such as the child's same-aged peers. These tools are used to determine whether the child performs at, below, or above expectations for age on motor skills. These include the Alberta Infant Motor Scale (AIMS) for children from birth to 18 months[96]; the Bayley Scales of Infant Development III, appropriate for children from birth to 42 months of age[9]; the Peabody Developmental Motor Scales (PDMS),[99] appropriate for children from birth to 83 months of age; and the Bruininks-Oseretsky Test of Motor Proficiency (BOTMP), with age standards for children from 4.5 to 21 years of age (see Chapter 2 for further psychometric information on these tests).[27]

Upper limb motor performance can also be compared to age-matched peers using the PDMS fine motor scale or the BOTMP. Fine motor coordination can be evaluated using the Purdue Pegboard Test, in which the child places pegs into board holes in three 30-second test sessions as fast as possible; the numbers of pegs from these trials are then averaged and compared with age standards.[1] The Developmental Hand Function Test measures the time required to complete seven standardized timed subtests: writing, page turning, small object manipulation, simulated feeding with a spoon, stacking checkers, lifting light objects, and lifting heavy objects.[46]

Ataxia is primarily a disorder of balance and control in the timing of coordinated movement. Oscillations during movement, along with an increase in oscillations as the task increases in difficulty, can be detected during functional activities and documented by clinical observation. Ataxia might express itself in the limbs and be observed in tasks such as active reaching or in the trunk, and then it is evident in upright postures with increasing antigravity demands. Common causes of ataxia are injuries to the cerebellum or to sensory structures. Sensory ataxia worsens when the child's eyes are closed.[8]

Postural control and balance. Several studies have reported long-lasting deficits in the motor proficiency of children with TBI, leading to significant balance impairment and functional disability.[54,63] Postural orientation problems may result from sensory impairment such as hemianopsia or impaired proprioception or tactile sensation or may be due to other CNS deficits, including the inability to coordinate sensory inputs from the vestibular, visual, and somatosensory systems. Postural responses may be affected by neurologic impairment or biomechanical constraint. The effect of perceptual deficits on a child's postural control may vary with age and postural development. Younger children have a greater reliance on visual input; the adult-like patterns might be present at the age of 7 years and older.[123] With an increase in active movement and in the use of antigravity positions, impairments in equilibrium and righting reactions may be observed. These reactions can be tested in a variety of positions and activities. Completion, symmetry, and speed of the reactions constitute qualitative information that should be noted when testing. Structured assessment of postural control and balance can be performed only in children who can respond accurately to at least simple instructions. The Pediatric Clinical Test of Sensory Interaction for Balance, for children 4 to 9 years,[102] and the Clinical Test of Sensory Interaction for Balance, for children 8 years and older,[108] require the child to maintain standing balance under six sensory conditions that assist in the identification of impairments in motor responses in variable sensory environments. Tests that assess balance in relation to gross motor skills include the pediatric balance scale, which contains 14 tasks including sitting and standing unsupported, lifting an object from the floor in standing, and turning 360°.[33] The Functional Reach Test has excellent within-session test-retest reliability for children with TBI,[53,89] The Timed Up and Go[125] exhibits good within-session test-retest reliability values for children with ABI.[53] (See Chapter 2 for more detail about the FRT and TUG for children.) The balance subtest of the Bruininks-Oseretsky Test of Motor Proficiency (BOTMP) is a static and dynamic balance assessment. It focuses primarily on the assessment of the child's anticipatory postural control.[27]

Gait. The walking items of motor assessments can be used as a measure of gait function (see Chapter 2 for further detail on gait tests and measures). For children who ambulate and achieve the highest scores on these items, it is often useful to include an assessment of other gait parameters such as walking speed, distance, and temporal and spatial assessments. Broad-based gait, prolonged time of double limb support, and increased step length variability have been observed in children with TBI.[54] The electronic walkway may provide the therapist with a reliable and valid (i.e., as demonstrated by concurrent assessment with a three-dimensional motion analysis system) measure for assessing walking improvement in children who showed a ceiling effect in the functional gait measures.[122] The timed walking tests and the shuttle walk-run assessment have good test-retest reliability with normative data available; the last has been designed specifically for the patient after TBI.[121]

Cardiorespiratory Status and Fitness. Autonomic instability is common following an ABI, often presenting with signs and symptoms of hyperstimulation of the sympathetic nervous system (including tachycardia, rhythm disturbances, and decreased heart rate variability). The prevalence of these symptoms decreases with neurologic recovery.[58] Respiratory or pulmonary complications noted after ABI include those directly related to the trauma, such as pneumothorax, hemothorax, and flail chest, and those directly related to the drowning event. A number of pulmonary complications may occur that are related, at least in part, to subsequent neurologic dysfunction, including respiratory failure, aspiration pneumonia, neurogenic pulmonary edema, and tracheal-airway complications.[124] Cardiorespiratory status should be screened during the systems review by measuring baseline heart rate, respiratory rate, blood pressure, and oxygen saturation; it is then reevaluated during and after activities. This is particularly important at the initial therapy session in a child with impaired consciousness or after prolonged bed rest, as responses to muscle stretch, pain, or position change may be abnormal. Once the child achieves ambulation, endurance limitations and difficulties in performance may become evident. It has been noted that peak exercise capacity and cardiorespiratory fitness of patients with moderate to severe brain injury are significantly lower compared with the capacity of normal healthy adults of a similar age.[86] Heart rate monitoring as an indicator of exercise intensity is important during endurance training; in addition, a rating of perceived exertion scale such as the OMNI Walk/Run scale can be used. Rossi and Sullivan described a functional fitness battery for children and adolescents with TBI aged 8 to 17 years.[32] The battery includes items assessing flexibility, strength, cardiorespiratory endurance, agility, power, balance, speed, and coordination.[106]

Participation level tests and measures. The Pediatric Evaluation of Disability Inventory (PEDI)[38] and the WeeFIM[117] (see Chapter 2) are standardized criterion-referenced indicators of status and change in functional skills such as mobility and self-care. The PEDI yields normative and scale scores that can be used to compare the child's performance over time. The PEDI focuses on the function of specific tasks and also rates caregiver assistance and modification. It has demonstrated good sensitivity to both global and item-specific changes in children with ABI.[115] About 11 points on a 0 to 100 scaled score is considered to be a minimal clinically important difference for change on any of the PEDI scaled scores.[43] The WeeFIM was designed for use with children 6 months to 7 years of age; the FIM might be used for children 7 years of age and older.[117]

The child and parents can collaborate with health care professionals in setting clear and important functional goals by using individualized outcome measures, which reflect the opinions, preferences, and concerns of child and the child's parents.[26] The Canadian Occupational Performance Measure (COPM) is an individualized child- and family-focused tool that is used to measure a change in goals that are meaningful to the child. The COPM is carried out as an interview and is structured around the areas of self-care, leisure, and productivity. The child and family identify areas of difficulty, prioritize these difficulties, then rate the child's performance and satisfaction in those areas identified as most important to the child. The Goal Attainment Scale (GAS) is a criterion-referenced measure of treatment-induced change. The GAS allows children and their parents to set clear functional goals together with their therapists. It is a 5-point scale, constructed before an intervention period, with 0 representing the expected level of functioning after a predefined period. If a patient achieves more than is expected, a score of 1 or 2 is given, depending on the level of achievement. If the patient's progress is less than expected, a score of 1 or 2 is given.

Two self-report measures of a child's participation in recreation and leisure activities are the Children's Assessment of Participation and Enjoyment (CAPE) and its companion measure, Preferences for Activities of Children (PAC). The CAPE is a 55-item measure of five dimensions of participation: diversity, intensity, with whom, where, and enjoyment, providing three levels of scoring: (1) overall participation scores, (2) domain scores reflecting participation in formal and informal activities, and (3) scores reflecting participation in five types of activities: recreational, active physical, social, skill-based, and self-improvement activities. The PAC is a parallel measure of preference for activities, which can be scored on the same three levels.[5,59]

Outcomes and Intervention Strategies

Based on the data gathered during the examination, and in collaboration with the child, family, and other team members, the physical therapist needs to formulate appropriate discipline-specific outcomes and then decide which intervention strategies are most appropriate for the specific child. The therapist needs to consider all injuries present: the time elapsed since the brain damage event, the rate of recovery, prior interventions, the age of the child, and the child's consciousness and cognitive state. A detailed description of this process is presented in the case scenario found on Expert Consult. General concepts related to global treatment goals

TABLE 22.4 Intervention Strategy Related to Rancho Levels of Cognitive Functioning Level

Rancho Adult Level	Rancho Pediatric Level	Global Description	Global Treatment Goals and Strategies
I–III	V–III	None to early response	Prevent musculoskeletal complications Sensory stimulation Family education
IV–V	II	Agitated, confused	Directed activity Increase child's motivation for activity Family education
VI–VIII	I	Higher-level response	Practice progressively challenging tasks Reduce environmental restrictions Increase physical conditioning

and treatment strategies can be outlined using the child's RLCF grade as a framework (Table 22.4). Next we provide information on some of the typical intervention needs of children at each level of cognitive functioning.

Intervention

Physical therapists employ numerous therapeutic strategies to address issues of motor control. Traditional approaches commonly used to facilitate motor and postural control—such as neuro-developmental Treatment (NDT), proprioceptive neuromuscular facilitation (PNF), and the Brunnstrom approach—were derived from the concept that proprioceptive afferent sensory stimulation can be used to modify abnormal tone and facilitate movement patterns and that recovery from brain damage occurs in a predictable sequence that corresponds to normal development.[72] Another treatment approach may be to target the impairment, as in, for example, muscle strengthening. More contemporary, task-specific training is based on the hypothesis that the most effective form of motor reeducation and learning occurs when performance during practice matches performance during retention and transfer (see Chapter 4 on motor learning).

Unfortunately, clinical trials that specifically examine treatment efficacy in children with ABI are sparse. Evidence from work done on children with cerebral palsy and on adults post stroke might provide a basis for the design of future trials targeting children with ABI to identify the interventions that optimally and efficiently improve function. A systematic review of physical therapy interventions for patients post stroke reveals a greater benefit from task-oriented specific training than from impairment-focused intervention, and almost no evidence suggests improved functional outcome to support the use of traditional approaches.[90,114] Nevertheless, traditional approaches continue to influence practice today. Proximal control and midline alignment, isolated joint movement and selective control as a sign of recovery, and the use of developmental postures to enhance outcome for functional tasks are all components of therapy sessions.

Nonresponse to Early Response Stage

A child with severe cognitive impairment functioning at RLCF adult level I–III, pediatric level V–III is unable to follow commands. The primary focus of physical therapy intervention is to prevent complications associated with prolonged immobilization while creating an environment conducive to recovery. Procedural interventions and patient-related instruction include the following:

- Prevention of musculoskeletal complications
- Multisensory stimulation
- Family education

Prevention of musculoskeletal complications. The main treatment strategies to achieve this goal include positioning in bed, passive movement, splints or serial casting, and assisted sitting and standing.

Positioning. Positioning includes prevention of contractures and minimization of asymmetry. The supine position should be avoided if possible because this position stimulates dystonic posturing or reflex hyperactivity. The child is positioned in a sidelying or semiprone position. A pillow placed between the slightly flexed legs prevents the child from adducting. The upper limb may be positioned on a pillow with the shoulder girdle protracted and the elbow extended. Attention to skin integrity, especially over bony prominence, is important.

The standard practice is to elevate the head above the level of the heart as part of an effort to reduce intracranial pressure by facilitating venous outflow without compromising cerebral perfusion pressure and cardiac output.[88]

Passive range-of-motion exercise. It is unclear whether or not passive ROM exercise has any effect on preventing the development of contractures, unless the muscle at risk is stretched for at least 30 minutes every day.[3,126] In addition, passive ROM exercise may have harmful effects on soft tissue; movements performed too vigorously or in too large a range may cause microtears in muscle, resulting in bleeding into the muscle and subsequent risk for development of PNBF.[79,84] In paralyzed or very weak muscle, exercises performed at the end of the range might overstretch the periarticular connective tissue, and if performed too quickly they may cause an increase in spasticity.[2] Therefore passive ROM exercises should be performed only if no other way of moving the child's joints is known. These exercises should be done slowly, with care taken to avoid overstretching at the end of the range. While doing the exercise, the therapist (or parent) should verbally describe to the child what is being done. An alternative is continuous passive motion (CPM) by an external motorized device, which enables a joint to be moved passively throughout an arc of motion and assists in attaining and increasing ROM. When CPM is used, the range and arc of motion should be carefully determined and reassessed periodically.

Periarticular new bone formation treatment. Prevention should start with early joint mobilization. The role of physical therapy is somewhat controversial. There are those who believe that aggressive ROM may increase bone formation.[62] Nonsteroidal anti-inflammatory drugs (NSAIDs) have demonstrated good results in preventing heterotopic ossification. The role of bisphosphonates in prevention is to inhibit the mineralization of organic osteoid, and they may have long-term effects on the prevention of significant HO years after they are discontinued. It has to be remembered, however, that post TBI there are frequently other musculoskeletal injuries and, therefore, the use of agents that inhibit new bone may impair fracture healing.[112]

Radiation therapy (RT) is another treatment used in managing patients with HO, and it is thought to work by preventing the differentiation of mesenchymal progenitor cells into HO-forming osteoblasts. The surgical management of HO aims to improve mobility and decrease the complications of immobility such as pressure ulcers, intractable pain, and impingement of important neurovascular structures. In addition, surgery allows the patient or the caretaker to improve mobility and ease of care.[45,112]

Serial casting or positional splints. Serial casting and splints have been found to prevent and correct muscle contractures in the short term[85] and to increase ROM in the elbow and ankle joints in adults with brain injury.[66] Few studies among adults with brain injury reported an improvement in spasticity.[20,40] Whereas splints are used early, mainly for prevention, serial casting is used once a developing contracture is evident. When a two-joint muscle is casted, a lengthened position is easily achieved if the cast is applied while the muscle is not lengthened over both joints (i.e., by first addressing one joint with the other flexed and then extending the cast). Casts should be well padded and particularly well molded. Casts should be changed regularly so that skin status can be assessed and further correction gradually achieved with each change. A little overcorrection is useful to allow for loss of correction and the need to repeat the casting.[70,71]

Although casting and splits are frequently used, there are no well-structured protocols for how long a splint or cast should be applied.[28,68,69,78] In addition, the available literature presents better results for children with CP when splints are combined with other therapy such as goal-directed training, bimanual therapy, constraint-induced movement therapy, or botulinum toxin A injections.[30,64]

Passive sitting and standing. As soon as the vital signs are stable, particularly blood pressure and pulse rate, periods of sitting and standing with external constraints are implemented. The standing position on a tilt table loads bones and cartilage,[24] stretches soft tissues, stimulates internal functions such as bowel movement and bladder emptying, and promotes lung expansion and as a result improves ventilation.[17] The child needs to be stood up slowly while blood pressure changes are monitored. Passive standing for at least 45 to 60 minutes, five times a week, should be part of the daily routine until the child achieves the ability to stand unsupported.[95,116]

Multisensory stimulation. The therapist typically stimulates the five senses directly, and the child's responses are assessed with the intent of advancing the stimulation as the complexity of the response increases. The efficacy of a prolonged sensory stimulation program is controversial. Cochrane's review of sensory stimulation in individuals with TBI in a comatose or vegetative state revealed that most of the literature in this particular area of cognitive-physical rehabilitation is mainly at the level of case studies or case series and as such does not provide strong evidence of its efficacy in raising the level of consciousness.[76]

Family education. Family members are encouraged to participate in intervention sessions as much as possible to facilitate carryover of treatment and practice. In the early stages, the child is dependent in all functional mobility and self-care

activities. The parent should therefore be instructed on how to safely and effectively perform all caregiving functions (i.e., dressing, grooming, bathing, and feeding), as well as on how to perform bed mobility activities and transfers into and out of bed to the wheelchair. The caregiver may also contribute to carrying out interventions such as contracture prevention and maintenance of optimal skin integrity.

Vegetative State and Minimal Conscious State

The vegetative state in a child with RLCF adult level I, pediatric level V, is defined as the absence of an adequate response to the outside world and absence of any evidence of reception or projection of information in the presence of a sleep-wake cycle.[47] Children may have periods of restlessness with open eyes and movement, but responsiveness is limited to primitive postural and reflex movements of the limbs. Children in a minimal conscious state have limited self-awareness, but they do feel pain and have sleep-wake cycles. The vegetative and minimal conscious states are directly due to primary brain pathology and are not an extension of coma. Coma is a transient state, characterized by an inability to obey commands, utter recognizable words, or open the eyes with the absence of sleep-wake cycles.[97] The vegetative state and the minimal conscious state may be masked by the state of coma, thus hindering diagnosis.

Spasticity and muscle contractures are two common features associated with the vegetative and minimal conscious states. For a child in these states, maintaining ROM is important for hygiene and nursing. Pharmacologic intervention and neurosurgical procedures to reduce muscle spasticity and improve ROM must be followed by physical therapy. Intervention to maintain passive ROM as described previously was found to be effective in a few studies among adults with TBI.[128] Botulinum toxin type A combined with a cast or splint and intensive physical therapy resulted in improvement on the modified Ashworth scale and in ROM.[120]

Agitation/Confused Stage

A child functioning at RLCF adult levels IV and V, pediatric level II, may follow simple commands but would have impaired judgment and problem-solving ability, thereby necessitating constant supervision to prevent injury. The therapist's aim is to encourage successful performance through adaptive task practice.

The main procedural interventions and patient-related instructional strategies to achieve treatments goals include the following:
- Directed activity
- Increasing the child's motivation for activity
- Family education

Directed activity and *increasing child motivation* may be achieved through the following components of intervention:
- Simple task training
- Modification of tasks to ensure success
- Building a structured environment
- Carrying out many short-interval treatments

Simple task training. Functional activities might be learned using procedural memory and implicit learning through repetition of tasks with appropriate orientation to time, self, and place. At this stage, the child exhibits frequent errors and variable performance. Practice and feedback are two of the more important training variables that can affect motor performance and learning. Children are mainly dependent on

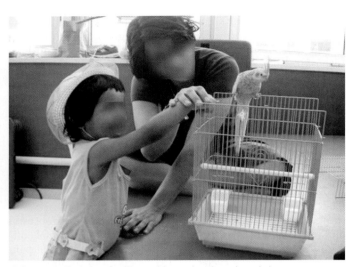

FIG. 22.4 Training facilitated by animal-assisted therapy.

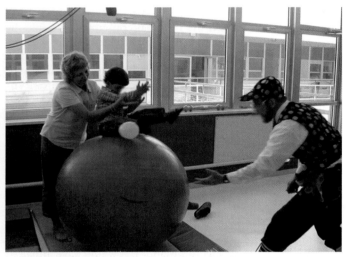

FIG. 22.5 Training facilitated by the "Clown Doctors."

visual and verbal cues to organize their movements. At this early stage of learning, therapists serve as important sources of augmented verbal, visual, or tactile feedback that provides information on outcome and error. Some children with TBI simply fail to act without extensive cueing. A highly structured, consistent, and reinforcing environment is required to ensure active participation in training. Adequate session training time is needed for the child to work on each task and improve performance. When errors decrease, other forms of feedback such as kinesthetic information will be used for error detection and correction.

Modification of the task to ensure success. Often, the physical therapist needs to be creative to keep the child focused on treatment and to increase the child's motivation. The therapist ensures that the activities practiced are relevant to the child's needs but at the same time motivate the child to participate (Figs. 22.4 and 22.5). Too much input or a request for difficult or complex movements may result in frustration and agitation at this stage of recovery.

Building a structured environment. A calm environment with structured stimuli may enhance the child's ability to follow

commands for a short time. The therapist should observe the child's behavior in different settings and with different people and should identify the environmental variables that affect the child's behavior either positively or negatively. Negative factors should be eliminated and replaced with those that reinforce desired behavior. This procedure is dynamic, and the therapist needs to reevaluate the effects of environmental modification on progress and modify intervention to facilitate further improvement.

Carrying out many short-interval treatments. At this stage, the child's tolerance of and attention span during treatment is short. Multiple short treatment sessions are preferred to maximize the child's alertness and attention to the demands of therapy.

Family education. At this stage, the caregiver is usually with the child all day long. The child has impaired judgment and a short attention span and as such needs close supervision. A consistent schedule of daily activities and therapy is most effective. Collaborating with the caregiver on how best to implement intervention strategies as part of the daily routine is extremely important. The expectation is that practicing repetitive tasks during this stage will gradually improve motor performance as the child reacquires motor skills that may be independent of any verbal recollection of the task training.

It is often noted that the child may at times become bored and even frustrated during the rehabilitation period. At such times, innovations such as an outing appropriate to the child's condition might be a good solution. A visit to a park with younger children while practicing intervention-related activities in the playground enables children to enjoy themselves while the therapist achieves treatment goals. Observation of the child in a natural environment might lead to the formulation of additional treatment goals. In addition, parents may pick up clues on working toward treatment goals during free-time play activities.

Higher-level response stage. At this level (RLCF pediatric level I or RLCF adult levels VI–VIII), less confusion is noted than in the previous stage, as are an improvement in short-term memory, more appropriate and focused behavior, and increased interaction with others and the environment. Limitations of insight, abstract reasoning, and problem solving, however, can still exist. Although the child is relatively independent at this level, complexities in activities of daily living and therapy may require focus on the tasks and skills needed to facilitate community reintegration. The focus is on helping the child to acquire skills that will lead to meeting self-care, social, and educational goals. Muscle strengthening and endurance activities are implemented if needed. The main procedural intervention strategies to achieve treatment goals include the following:

- Practice progressively challenging tasks.
- Reduce environmental restrictions.
- Increase physical conditioning.

Practice progressively challenging tasks. The therapist should provide opportunities for the child to actively participate and practice meaningful and motivating activities (Figs. 22.6 and 22.7). Functional, relevant, and varied skills should be practiced in an effective manner and in a variety of environmental circumstances. It is common, however, for children to show improvement in the practiced tasks but not be able to transfer the skills to other contexts.[87] Determining the number of repetitions needed to learn a new task, the ability of the child to do the same task the following day, and

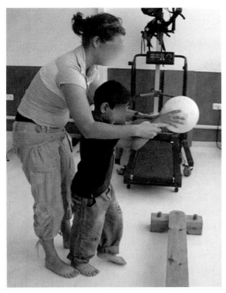

FIG. 22.6 Ball exercise.

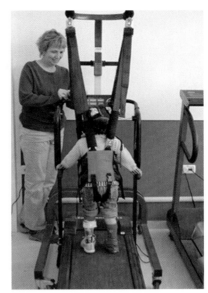

FIG. 22.8 Treadmill walking with suspension.

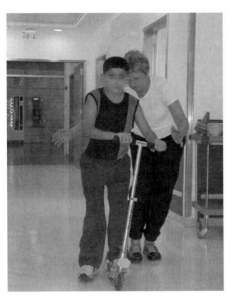

FIG. 22.7 Riding on a scooter.

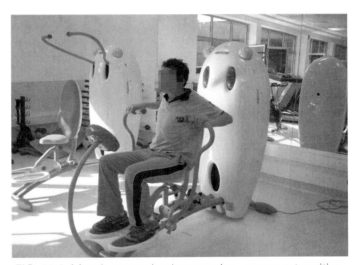

FIG. 22.9 Muscle strengthening exercise—upper extremities.

the ability to do the same task in different contexts provides additional clues to the child's learning capabilities.[81,87]

More recently introduced therapies include the constraint-induced technique and the use of treadmill training with and without body-weight support (Fig. 22.8). These treatment strategies have come about as the result of basic research in neuroplasticity and neurorecovery. The feasibility of such interventions has been assessed in adults with brain damage and in children with CP. The strength of the evidence that exists in relation to the efficacy of treadmill training with body-weight support in children with CP is generally weak,[25] and this approach has not yet been found to be preferable to regular gait therapy in improving functional parameters in adults with ABI.[16] Evidence suggests that children with hemiplegia due to CP may benefit from constraint-induced movement therapy to improve hand function.[113,127] For children with severe ABI, participation in constraint-induced movement therapy

may be problematic given the required practice intensity and the frustration that constraint may induce over time. A multiple case study of children with ABI noted that it is possible to implement constraint-induced movement protocols only if the whole team, including parents, totally adhere to the treatment regimen.[48]

Reduce environmental restrictions. The therapist may modify the task or the environment to adjust the difficulty of the functional activity. For example, ambulation can be practiced progressively first indoors and then outdoors and then on different surfaces and so on.

Increase physical conditioning. Weakness is a common impairment in children with ABI.[29] An adolescent might participate in a standard muscle-strengthening program, with repetitions and duration as needed, or perhaps the adolescent would prefer to participate in gym activities with peers (Figs. 22.9 and 22.10). For a younger child, the therapist has to choose appropriate developmental activities that will facilitate muscle strengthening (e.g., play activities combined with stair climbing).

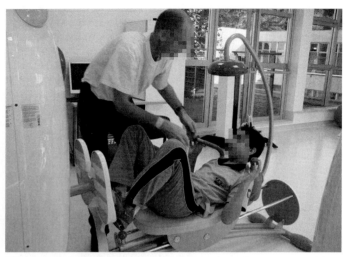

FIG. 22.10 Muscle strengthening exercise—lower extremities.

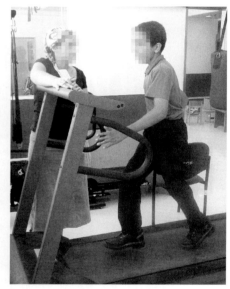

FIG. 22.11 Aerobic exercise on the treadmill.

Cardiorespiratory fitness may be reduced by impaired motor abilities, due to prolonged bed rest and inactivity, or due to lesions that affect the autonomic nervous system. Among children with TBI, the mean heart rate at rest was found to be significantly higher and heart rate variability significantly lower as compared with healthy controls.[52] Only a few studies have investigated the outcome of challenging the cardiovascular system of the child with ABI, making it difficult for clinicians to make an evidence-based decision concerning the applicability of a fitness program for a child. Responsiveness and tolerance of adult patients at the subacute stage following moderate to severe brain injury to aerobic training have been demonstrated.[10,44] Evidence suggests that this is a safe, well-accepted, and feasible intervention (Fig. 22.11). In the light of insufficient data for children, the therapist must monitor and adhere to acceptable physiologic parameters during endurance therapy sessions.[94]

BACK AT HOME

Once the child is discharged from the rehabilitation setting, outpatient services should continue as necessary to maximize independence at home, at school, and in the community. High cognitive functions of decision making, judgment, and problem solving usually have not fully recovered, and activities that demand these skills usually require close supervision to ensure safety.

At this time, parents, siblings, and the child all try to adapt to a new family constellation. Many aspects of family life, from emotional to financial, might be influenced directly as a result of the injury or its consequences. Siblings frequently experience adverse effects. About half of the families reported that siblings exhibited behavioral problems such as withdrawal from their injured sibling, symptoms such as increased fearfulness, or, on the other hand, became overly involved in family issues.[82] Approximately one third of families reported deterioration in their financial status after the child's injury.[93] Parents need help and guidance to rebuild the family framework, and they need time to reinforce continued development of the child and the child's siblings while getting on with their own lives.

An outpatient treatment program in combination with a home-based program might be proposed to the family because the rehabilitation process might need to continue throughout childhood, and intervention provided in the educational system may be inadequate for addressing medical, as opposed to educational, needs. A home-based program was found to be effective for children with ABI[50,51] and included the advantage of reducing travel time. In adults with TBI, home-based exercise programs were found to improve cardiorespiratory fitness.[39] In addition, home-based activities that educate children to perform exercise as a part of their daily routine might have a long-lasting advantage in preventing secondary impairments such as weight gain, contractures, and pain.[104]

Few studies have examined the effects of repetitive practice of weight-bearing exercises that share similar characteristics to those found in typical functional activities involving the lower limbs (support, balance, and force).[75] For example, sit-to-stand and step-up exercises are mechanically demanding functional activities that children perform many times during their daily routine. Both require muscle strength to raise the body mass, and both require the ability to transfer the center of mass from a larger to a relatively smaller base of support, thereby challenging the muscular system as well as the equilibrium system. As such, these exercises have the potential to train aspects of motor performance such as balance, strength, and endurance. It was found that a short task-oriented exercise program of sit-to-stand and step-up exercises for children with severe ABI carried out at home resulted in increased functional balance performance[50] and walking performance,[51] which were maintained even after the training had ended.

Because adherence to an exercise program is crucial for its success, simple adjustments to increase compliance were found to be effective. For example, a phone call once a week to the child and parent encouraged them to continue with the program, as did providing each child and family with written information about the program, a detailed explanation and practice run on how to perform each task, and a diary in which the child is requested to keep a record of the number of sets performed each day. All of these tactics have the potential to increase compliance and adherence to the program to well over 50%.[31,50]

For school-aged children, involvement in sports and physical leisure time activities should be encouraged. These have the potential to increase self-esteem and acceptance by peers. Bicycle riding, horseback riding, and other challenging sports activities for children with special needs are recommended and are available in many areas.

ASSISTIVE DEVICES

Nonambulatory children need appropriate assistive technology, and proper use of this technology can be one of the most important aspects of therapeutic intervention. The process of selecting the right equipment requires considerations regarding availability, cost, source of funding, portability, stability, ease of adjustment, ease of modification, construction materials, and aesthetics. Equipment must be reevaluated more frequently than when used by adults because of the functional changes and growth that occur in children.

For preschool children, exploring the environment is crucial for development. For children who cannot ambulate, a device such as a tricycle is a fun alternative to a wheelchair. Many options for adapted equipment are commercially available. When choosing the equipment, one should consider the environment in which the child functions and the needs of caregivers. Another factor to consider is the family's lifestyle and typical activities. For teenagers, who are often greatly concerned about their physical appearance and social acceptance by their peers, the prescribed equipment and devices should be as cosmetic and minimal as possible.

Case Scenario on Expert Consult

The case scenario related to this chapter presents a detailed look at a 6-year-old boy with a severe traumatic brain injury. A video accompanies the case. An additional video is provided that illustrates the course of physical therapy management for a 10-month-old child who was affected by a brain tumor.

REFERENCES

1. Aaron DH, Jansen CW: Development of the Functional Dexterity Test (FDT): construction, validity, reliability, and normative data, *J Hand Ther* 16:12, 2003.
2. Ada L, et al.: Care of the unconscious head-injury patient. In Ada L, Canning C, editors: *Key issues in neurological physiotherapy*, Oxford, 1990, Butterworth Heinemann, pp 249–286.
3. Ada L, et al.: Thirty minutes of positioning reduces the development of shoulder external rotation contracture after stroke: a randomized controlled trial, *Arch Phys Med Rehabil* 86:230–234, 2005.
4. Adamo MA, et al.: Decompressive craniectomy and postoperative complication management in infants and toddlers with severe traumatic brain injuries, *J Neurosurg Pediatr* 3:334–339, 2009.
5. Anaby D, et al.: Predictors of change in participation rates following acquired brain injury: results of a longitudinal study, *Dev Med Child Neurol* 54:339–346, 2012.
6. Asikainen I, et al.: Predicting late outcome for patients with traumatic brain injury referred to a rehabilitation programme: a study of 508 Finnish patients 5 years or more after injury, *Brain Inj* 12:95–107, 1998.
7. Baridd J, et al.: Static neuro-imaging in the evaluation of TBI. In Zasler N, et al., editors: *Brain injury medicine*, New York, 2007, Demos Medical Publishing.
8. Bastian AJ: Mechanisms of ataxia, *Phys Ther* 77:672–675, 1997.
9. Bayley N: *Bayley Scales of Infant Development II*, San Antonio, 1993, Psychological Corporation.
10. Bhambhani Y, et al.: Effects of circuit training on body composition and peak cardiorespiratory responses in patients with moderate to severe traumatic brain injury, *Arch Phys Med Rehabil* 86:268–276, 2005.
11. Bloomfield SA: Changes in musculoskeletal structure and function with prolonged bed rest, *Med Sci Sports Exerc* 29:197–206, 1997.
12. Blumenthal I: Shaken baby syndrome, *Postgrad Med J* 78:732–735, 2002.
13. Bohannon RW, Smith MB: Interrater reliability of a modified Ashworth scale of muscle spasticity, *Phys Ther* 67:206–207, 1987.
14. Bouma GJ, Muizelaar JP: Cerebral blood flow in severe clinical head injury, *New Horiz* 3:384–394, 1995.
15. Brehaut JC, et al.: Childhood behavior disorders and injuries among children and youth: a population-based study, *Pediatrics* 111:262–269, 2003.
16. Brown TH, et al.: Body weight-supported treadmill training versus conventional gait training for people with chronic traumatic brain injury, *J Head Trauma Rehabil* 20:402–415, 2005.
17. Chang AT, et al.: Standing with the assistance of a tilt table improves minute ventilation in chronic critically ill patients, *Arch Phys Med Rehabil* 85:1972–1976, 2004.
18. Casano-Sancho P, et al.: Pituitary dysfunction after traumatic brain injury in children: is there a need for ongoing endocrine assessment? *Clin Endocrinol (Oxf)* 79:853–858, 2013.
19. Centers for Disease Control, National Center for Injury Prevention and Control: WISQARS. Retrieved from: http://www.cdc.gov/ncipc/wisqars, 2002.
20. Childers MK, et al.: Inhibitory casting decreases a vibratory inhibition index of the H-reflex in the spastic upper limb, *Arch Phys Med Rehabil* 80:714–716, 1999.
21. Christensen DW, et al.: Outcome and acute care hospital costs after warm water near drowning in children, *Pediatrics* 99:715–721, 1997.
22. Citta-Pietrolungo TJ, et al.: Early detection of heterotopic ossification in young patients with traumatic brain injury, *Arch Phys Med Rehabil* 73:258–262, 1992.
23. Clopton N, et al.: Interrater and intrarater reliability of the Modified Ashworth Scale in children with hypertonia, *Pediatr Phys Ther* 17:268–274, 2005.
24. Damcott M, et al.: Effects of passive versus dynamic loading interventions on bone health in children who are nonambulatory, *Pediatr Phys Ther* 25:248–255, 2013.
25. Damiano DL, DeJong SL: A systematic review of the effectiveness of treadmill training and body weight support in pediatric rehabilitation, *J Neurol Phys Ther* 33:27–44, 2009.
26. de Kloet AJ, et al.: Gaming supports youth with acquired brain injury? A pilot study, *Brain Inj* 26:1021–1029, 2012.
27. Deitz JC, et al.: Review of the Bruininks-Oseretsky Test of Motor Proficiency, Second Edition (BOT-2), *Phys Occup Ther Pediatr* 27:87–102, 2007.
28. Elliott CM, et al.: Lycra arm splints in conjunction with goal-directed training can improve movement in children with cerebral palsy, *NeuroRehabilitation* 1:47–54, 2011.
29. Foran JR, et al.: Structural and mechanical alterations in spastic skeletal muscle, *Dev Med Child Neurol* 47:713–717, 2005. review.
30. Reference deleted in proofs.
31. Fragala-Pinkham MA, et al.: A fitness program for children with disabilities, *Phys Ther* 85:1182–1200, 2005.
32. Reference deleted in proofs.
33. Franjoine MR, et al.: Pediatric Balance Scale: a modified version of the Berg Balance Scale for the school-age child with mild to moderate motor impairment, *Pediatr Phys Ther* 15:114–128, 2003.
34. Gölge M, et al.: Recovery of the precision grip in children after traumatic brain injury, *Arch Phys Med Rehabil* 85:1435–1444, 2004.
35. Greenwald BD, et al.: Congenital and acquired brain injury. I. Brain injury: epidemiology and pathophysiology, *Arch Phys Med Rehabil* 84:S3–S7, 2003.

36. Gurney JG, et al.: Brain and other central nervous system tumors: rates, trends, and epidemiology, *Curr Opin Oncol* 13:160–166, 2001.

37. Gurney JG, et al.: *CNS and miscellaneous intracranial and intraspinal neoplasms. SEER pediatric monograph*, Washington, DC, 1999, National Cancer Institute.

38. Reference deleted in proofs.

39. Hassett LM, et al.: Efficacy of a fitness centre-based exercise programme compared with a home-based exercise programme in traumatic brain injury: a randomized controlled trial, *J Rehabil Med* 41:247–255, 2009.

40. Hill J: The effects of casting on upper extremity motor disorders after brain injury, *Am J Occup Ther* 48:219–224, 1994.

41. Hurvitz EA, et al.: Risk factors for heterotopic ossification in children and adolescents with severe traumatic brain injury, *Arch Phys Med Rehabil* 73:459–462, 1992.

42. Ibsen LM, Koch I: Submersion and asphyxial injury, *Crit Care Med* 30:402–408, 2002.

43. Reference deleted in proofs.

44. Jackson D, et al.: Can brain-injured patients participate in an aerobic exercise programme during early inpatient rehabilitation? *Clin Rehabil* 15:535–544, 2001.

45. Jang SH, et al.: Radiation therapy for heterotopic ossification in a patient with traumatic brain injury, *Yonsei Med J* 41:536–539, 2000.

46. Jebsen RH, et al.: An objective and standardized test of hand function, *Arch Phys Med Rehabil* 50:311–319, 1969.

47. Jennett B, Plum F: Persistent vegetative state after brain damage: a syndrome in search of a name, *Lancet* 1:734–737, 1972.

48. Karman N, et al.: Constraint-induced movement therapy for hemiplegic children with acquired brain injuries, *J Head Trauma Rehabil* 18: 259–267, 2003.

49. Katz DI, Alexander MP: Traumatic brain injury: predicting course of recovery and outcome for patients admitted to rehabilitation, *Arch Neurol* 51:661–670, 1994.

50. Katz-Leurer M, et al.: Effects of home-based treatment in acquired brain injury children using a task-oriented exercise program, *Physiotherapy* 94:71–77, 2008.

51. Katz-Leurer M, et al.: The effects of a "home-based" task-oriented exercise programme on motor and balance performance in children with spastic cerebral palsy and severe traumatic brain injury, *Clin Rehabil* 23:714–724, 2009.

52. Katz-Leurer M, et al.: Heart rate and heart rate variability at rest and during exercise in boys who suffered a severe traumatic brain injury and typically-developed controls, *Brain Inj* 24:110–114, 2010.

53. Katz-Leurer M, et al.: Functional balance tests for children with traumatic brain injury: within-session reliability, *Pediatr Phys Ther* 20:254–258, 2008.

54. Katz-Leurer M, et al.: Relationship between balance abilities and gait characteristics in children with post-traumatic brain injury, *Brain Inj* 22:153–159, 2008.

55. Katz-Leurer M, et al.: Hand-held dynamometry in children with traumatic brain injury: within-session reliability, *Pediatr Phys Ther* 20:259–263, 2008.

56. Keenan HT, Bratton SL: Epidemiology and outcomes of pediatric traumatic brain injury, *Dev Neurosci* 28:256–263, 2006.

57. Kemp AM, et al.: What neuroimaging should be performed in children in whom inflicted brain injury (iBI) is suspected? A systematic review, *Clin Radiol* 64:473–483, 2009.

58. Keren O, et al.: Heart rate variability (HRV) of patients with traumatic brain injury (TBI) during the post-insult sub-acute period, *Brain Inj* 19:605–611, 2005.

59. King G, et al.: *Children's Assessment of Participation and Enjoyment (CAPE) and Preferences for Activities of Children (PAC)*, San Antonio, TX, 2004, Harcourt Assessment.

60. Kochanek PM: Pediatric traumatic brain injury: quo vadis? *Dev Neurosci* 28:244–255, 2006.

61. Kraus JF: Epidemiological features of brain injury in children: occurrence, children at risk, causes and manner of injury, severity, and outcomes. In Broman SH, Michel ME, editors: *Traumatic head injury in children*, New York, 1995, Oxford University Press, pp 22–39.

62. Kreisman NR, et al.: Regional differences in hypoxic depolarization and swelling in hippocampal slices, *J Neurophysiol* 83:1031–1038, 2000.

63. Kuhtz-Buschbeck JP, et al.: Sensorimotor recovery in children after traumatic brain injury: analyses of gait, gross motor, and fine motor skills, *Dev Med Child Neurol* 45:821–828, 2003.

64. Lai JM, et al.: Dynamic splinting after treatment with botulinum toxin type-A: a randomized controlled pilot study, *Adv Ther* 26:241–248, 2009.

65. Langlois JA, et al.: The incidence of traumatic brain injury among children in the United States: differences by race, *J Head Trauma Rehabil* 20:229–238, 2005.

66. Lannin NA, et al.: Effects of splinting on wrist contracture after stroke: a randomized controlled trial, *Stroke* 38:111–116, 2007.

67. Laws ER, Thapar K: Brain tumors, *CA Cancer J Clin* 43:263–271, 1993.

68. Law M, et al.: Neurodevelopmental therapy and upper extremity inhibitive casting for children with cerebral palsy, *Dev Med Child Neurol* 33:379–387, 1991.

69. Law M, et al.: A comparison of intensive neurodevelopmental therapy plus casting and a regular occupational therapy program for children with cerebral palsy, *Dev Med Child Neurol* 10:664–670, 1997.

70. Leong B: Critical review of passive muscle stretch: implications for the treatment of children in vegetative and minimally conscious states, *Brain Inj* 16:169–183, 2002.

71. Leong B: The vegetative and minimally conscious states in children: spasticity, muscle contracture and issues for physiotherapy treatment, *Brain Inj* 16:217–230, 2002.

72. Lettinga AT: Diversity in neurological physiotherapy: a content analysis of the Brunnstrom/Bobath controversy, *Adv Physiol* 4:23–36, 2002.

73. Levin M, et al.: What do motor "recovery" and "compensation" mean in patients following stroke? *Neurorehabil Neural Repair* 23:313–319, 2009.

74. Lew H, et al.: Electrophysiologic assessment technique: evoked potentials and electroencephalography. In Zasler M, et al., editors: *Brain injury medicine*, New York, 2007, Demos Medical Publishing, pp 150–157.

75. Liao HF, et al.: Effectiveness of loaded sit-to-stand resistance exercise for children with mild spastic diplegia: a randomized clinical trial, *Arch Phys Med Rehabil* 88:25–31, 2007.

76. Lombardi F, et al.: Sensory stimulation for brain injured individuals in coma or vegetative state, *Cochrane Database Syst Rev*, 2002. CD001427.

77. Lunsford BR, Perry J: The standing heel-rise test for ankle plantar flexion: criterion for normal, *Phys Ther* 75:694–698, 1995.

78. McNee AE, et al.: The effect of serial casting on gait in children with cerebral palsy: preliminary results from a crossover trial, *Gait Posture* 25:463–468, 2007.

79. Melamed E, et al.: Periarticular new bone formation following traumatic brain injury, *Harefuah* 139:368–371, 2000.

80. Meythaler JM, et al.: Current concepts: diffuse axonal injury-associated traumatic brain injury, *Arch Phys Med Rehabil* 82:1461–1471, 2001.

81. Monfils MH, et al.: In search of the motor engram: motor map plasticity as a mechanism for encoding motor experience, *Neuroscientist* 11:471–483, 2005.

82. Montgomery V, et al.: The effect of severe traumatic brain injury on the family, *J Trauma* 52:1121–1124, 2002.

83. Moore BD, et al.: Neuropsychological outcome of children diagnosed with brain tumor during infancy, *Childs Nerv Syst* 14:504, 1998.

84. Morley J, et al.: Does traumatic brain injury results in accelerated fracture healing? *Injury* 36:363–368, 2005. review.

85. Mortenson PA, Eng JJ: The use of casts in the management of joint mobility and hypertonia following brain injury in adults: a systematic review, *Phys Ther* 83:648–658, 2003.

86. Mossberg KA, et al.: Aerobic capacity after traumatic brain injury: comparison with a nondisabled cohort, *Arch Phys Med Rehabil* 88:315–320, 2007.

87. Neistadt ME: Perceptual retraining for adults with diffuse brain injury, *Am J Occup Ther* 48:225–233, 1994.

88. Ng I, et al.: Effects of head posture on cerebral hemodynamics: its influences on intracranial pressure, cerebral perfusion pressure, and cerebral oxygenation, *Neurosurgery* 54:593–597, 2004.

89. Reference deleted in proofs.

90. Novak I, et al.: A systematic review of interventions for children with cerebral palsy: state of the evidence, *Dev Med Child Neurol* 55:885–910, 2013.

91. Nudo RJ, et al.: Neural substrates for the effects of rehabilitation training on motor recovery after ischemic infarct, *Science* 171:1791–1794, 1996.

92. Ommaya AK, et al.: Biomechanics and neuropathology of adult and paediatric head injury, *Br J Neurosurg* 16:220–242, 2002.

93. Osberg JS, et al.: Pediatric trauma: impact on work and family finances, *Pediatrics* 98:890–897, 1996.

94. Peel C: The cardiopulmonary system and movement dysfunction, *Phys Ther* 76:448–455, 1996.

95. Paleg GS, et al.: Systematic review and evidence-based clinical recommendations for dosing of pediatric supported standing programs, *Pediatr Phys Ther* 25:232–247, 2013.

96. Piper MC, et al.: Construction and validation of the Alberta Infant Motor Scale (AIMS), *Can J Public Health* 83:S46–S50, 1992.

97. Plum F: Coma and related global disturbances of the human conscious state, *Cerebral Cortex* 9:25–42, 1991.

98. Ponsford J, et al.: Impact of early intervention on outcome after mild traumatic brain injury in children, *Pediatrics* 108:1297–1303, 2001.

99. Provost B, et al.: Concurrent validity of the Bayley Scales of Infant Development II Motor Scale and the Peabody Developmental Motor Scales-2 in children with developmental delays, *Pediatr Phys Ther* 16:149–156, 2004.

100. Reference deleted in proofs.

101. Reilly PL, et al.: Assessing the conscious level in infants and young children: a pediatric version of the Glasgow Coma Scale, *Childs Nerv Syst* 4:30–33, 1988.

102. Richardson PK, et al.: Performance of preschoolers on the Pediatric Clinical Test of Sensory Interaction for Balance, *Am J Occup Ther* 46:793–800, 1992.

103. Ricker J, Arenth P: Functional neuro-imaging in TBI. In Zasler N, et al., editors: *Brain injury medicine*, New York, 2007, Demos Medical Publishing, pp 130–149.

104. Rimmer JH, et al.: Physical activity participation among persons with disabilities: barriers and facilitators, *Am J Prev Med* 26:419–425, 2004.

105. Rodgers GB: *Bicycle and bicycle helmet use patterns in the United States: a description and analysis of national survey data*, Washington, DC, 1993, US Consumer Product Safety Commission.

106. Rossi C, Sullivan SJ: Motor fitness in children and adolescents with traumatic brain injury, *Arch Phys Med Rehabil* 77:1062–1065, 1996.

107. Russell D, et al.: *Gross motor function manual*, Hamilton, Ontario, 1993, McMaster University.

108. Shumway-Cook A, Horak FB: Assessing the influence of sensory interaction of balance: suggestion from the field, *Phys Ther* 66:1548–1550, 1986.

109. Squire LR, Zola SM: Structure and function of declarative and non-declarative memory systems, *Proc Natl Acad Sci U S A* 93:13515–13522, 1996.

110. Stein DG: Concepts of CNS plasticity and their implication for understanding recovery after brain damage. In Zasler N, et al., editors: *Brain injury medicine*, New York, 2007, Demos Medical Publishing.

111. Stevenson MR, et al.: Childhood drowning: barriers surrounding private swimming pools, *Pediatrics* 111:e115–e119, 2003.

112. Sullivan MP, et al.: Heterotopic ossification after central nervous system trauma: a current review, *Bone Joint Res* 2:51–57, 2013.

113. Taub E, et al.: Efficacy of constraint-induced movement therapy for children with cerebral palsy with asymmetric motor impairment, *Pediatrics* 113:305–312, 2004.

114. Teasdale G, Jennett B: Assessment of coma and impaired consciousness: a practical scale, *Lancet* 13:81–84, 1974.

115. Tokcan G, et al.: Item-specific functional recovery in children and youth with acquired brain injury, *Pediatr Phys Ther* 15:16–22, 2003.

116. Tremblay F, et al.: Effects of prolonged muscle stretch on reflex and voluntary activations in children with spastic cerebral palsy, *Scand J Rehabil Med* 22:171–180, 1990.

117. *Uniform Data System for Medical Rehabilitation*, 2000. http://www.udsmr.org/WebModules/WeeFIM/Wee_About.aspx.

118. Reference deleted in proofs.

119. Van Peppen R, et al.: The impact of physical therapy on functional outcomes after stroke: what's the evidence? *Clin Rehabil* 18:833–862, 2004.

120. van Rhijn J, et al.: Botulinum toxin type A in the treatment of children and adolescents with an acquired brain injury, *Brain Inj* 19:331–335, 2005.

121. Vitale AE, et al.: Reliability for a walk/run test to estimate aerobic capacity in a brain-injured population, *Brain Inj* 11:67–76, 1997.

122. Webster KE, et al.: Validity of the GAITRite walkway system for the measurement of averaged and individual step parameters of gait, *Gait Posture* 22:317–321, 2005.

123. Westcott SL, et al.: Evaluation of postural stability in children: current theories and assessment tools, *Phys Ther* 77:629–645, 1997.

124. Wiercisiewski DR, McDeavitt JT: Pulmonary complications in traumatic brain injury, *Head Trauma Rehabil* 13:28–35, 1998.

125. Reference deleted in proofs.

126. Williams PE: Use of intermittent stretch in the prevention of serial sarcomere loss in immobilised muscle, *Ann Rheumat Dis* 49:316–317, 1990.

127. Willis JK, et al.: Forced use treatment of childhood hemiparesis, *Pediatrics* 110:94–96, 2002.

128. Yablon SA, et al.: Botulinum toxin in severe upper extremity spasticity among patients with traumatic brain injury: an open-labeled trial, *Neurology* 47:939–944, 1996.

129. Ylvisaker M, Feeney T: Pediatric brain injury: social, behavioral, and communication disability, *Phys Med Rehabil Clin N Am* 18:133–144, 2007.

130. Zuckerman GB, et al.: Predictors of death and neurologic impairment in pediatric submersion injuries: the Pediatric Risk of Mortality Score, *Arch Pediatr Adolesc Med* 152:134–140, 1998.

SUGGESTED READINGS

Anaby D, Law M, Hanna S, et al.: Predictors of change in participation rates following acquired brain injury: results of a longitudinal study, *Develop Med Child Neurol* 54:339–346, 2012.

Casano-Sancho P, Suárez L, Ibáñez L, et al.: Pituitary dysfunction after traumatic brain injury in children: is there a need for ongoing endocrine assessment? *Clin Endocrinol (Oxf)* 79:853–858, 2013.

Hassett LM, Moseley AM, Tate RL, et al.: Efficacy of a fitness centre-based exercise programme compared with a home-based exercise programme in traumatic brain injury: a randomized controlled trial, *J Rehab Med* 41:247–255, 2009.

Katz-Leurer M, Rotem H, Keren O, et al.: Heart rate and heart rate variability at rest and during exercise in boys who suffered a severe traumatic brain injury and typically developed controls, *Brain Injury* 24:110–114, 2010.

Keenan HT, Bratton SL: Epidemiology and outcomes of pediatric traumatic brain injury, *Develop Neurosci* 28:256–263, 2006.

Paleg GS, Smith BA, Glickman LB: Systematic review and evidence-based clinical recommendations for dosing of pediatric supported standing programs, *Pediatric Phys Ther* 25:232–247, 2013.

Ricker J, Arenth P: Functional neuro-imaging in TBI. In Zasler N, Katz DI, Zafonte RD, editors: *Brain injury medicine*, New York, 2007, Demos Medical Publishing.

Stein DG: Concepts of CNS plasticity and their implication for understanding recovery after brain damage. In Zasler N, Katz DI, Zafonte RD, editors: *Brain injury medicine*, New York, 2007, Demos Medical Publishing.

Sullivan MP, Torres SJ, Mehta S, et al.: Heterotopic ossification after central nervous system trauma: a current review, *Bone Joint Research* 2(3):51–57, 2013.

Ylvisaker M, Feeney T: Pediatric brain injury: social, behavioral, and communication disability, *Phys Med Rehabil Clin North Am* 18:133–144, 2007.

23

Myelodysplasia

Kathleen Hinderer, Steven Hinderer, William O. Walker, Jr., David Shurtleff

Children and adolescents with myelodysplasia, perhaps more than most diagnostic groups of children with disabilities, challenge pediatric physical therapists to use and integrate many facets of their knowledge and skills. The multiple body systems affected by this congenital malformation make intervention for these patients more complex than the congenital spinal cord defect alone might imply. Awareness of the many possible manifestations of this condition, knowledge of methods to examine and detect their presence, and the ability to evaluate the relative contribution of each manifestation to current activity limitations are important. This knowledge, combined with the ability to anticipate future needs and potential problems, empowers the physical therapist to select interventions that will optimize function and prevent the development of secondary impairments. Conversely, lack of awareness of these issues is not without consequences, as significant secondary permanent impairments can result when clinicians are not aware of or do not recognize early signs and symptoms of preventable complications related to myelodysplasia.

The objectives of this chapter are to familiarize the physical therapist with the numerous manifestations of myelodysplasia; describe its impact on body systems and functional skills; provide developmental expectations and prognosis based on the level of involvement; outline the roles of the various disciplines involved in team management; discuss methods of examination, evaluation, and diagnosis; and highlight intervention strategies for specific problems.

BACKGROUND INFORMATION

TYPES OF MYELODYSPLASIA

Dorland's Medical Dictionary defines myelodysplasia as "defective development of any part (especially the lower segments) of the spinal cord." The various types of myelodysplasia are illustrated in Fig. 23.1. Spina bifida is a commonly used term referring to various forms of myelodysplasia. Spina bifida is classified into aperta (visible or open) lesions and occulta (hidden or not visible) lesions.[101] The degree of motor and sensory loss from these lesions can range from no loss to severe impairment. Regardless of initial level of neurologic impairment, individuals with any of these lesions are at risk for further loss of function over time. Paralysis may occur later in life as a complication of abnormal tissue growth (dysplasia) causing pressure on nerves (e.g., lipomatous or dermoid tissue). Lack of proper growth of associated connective tissues around the malformed spinal cord can also cause ischemia and progressive neurologic impairment by tethering of the cord.

Spina bifida aperta is commonly thought of as myelomeningocele (MM), which is an open spinal cord defect that usually protrudes dorsally. MMs are not skin covered and are usually associated with spinal nerve paralysis (see Fig. 23.1C–D). Meninges and nerves can also protrude anteriorly or laterally, making them not visible externally but still associated with nerve paralysis. Some individuals with MM do not have associated paralysis.

Meningoceles are also classified as spina bifida aperta. They are skin covered and are initially associated with no paralysis (see Fig. 23.1B). Meningoceles contain only membranes or nonfunctional nerves that end in the sac wall.[101] Other skin-covered lesions, however, can be associated with paralysis.

The next most common form of myelodysplasia is a lipoma of the spinal cord. Lipomas are classified as spina bifida occulta, but most are visible. They may be large or small and manifest as distinct, subcutaneous masses of fat, frequently associated with abnormal pigmentation of the skin, hirsutism, skin appendages, and dimples above the gluteal cleft. A lipomatous or fibrous tract descends ventrally from the subcutaneous lipoma to varying extents into the subdural space adjacent to the spinal cord. Lipomas of the spinal cord are therefore classified based on the location of the tract. They can be (1) lipomyelomeningocele with paralysis, (2) lipomeningoceles with no paralysis, (3) lipomas of the filum terminale usually with no paralysis, and (4) lipomas of the cauda equina or conus medullaris with or without paralysis at birth. If paralysis is absent at birth, it is acquired over time, and if present at birth, it will worsen with time. Some lipomas involving the spinal cord are not associated with an extension to subcutaneous fat. Lipomas of the spinal cord may or may not be associated with bifid vertebrae (true spina bifida occulta).

Diastematomyelia is a fibrous, cartilaginous, or bony band or spicule separating the spinal cord into hemicords, each surrounded by a dural sac. It can occur as an isolated defect along with vertebral anomalies or in conjunction with either MM or lipomyelomeningocele. Depending on the associated involvement of the spinal cord and meninges, diastematomyelia may be associated with paralysis initially, or progressive weakness can develop later in occulta lesions as a result of cord tethering.

The least common of the myelodysplasias are separate or septated cysts. These myelocystoceles are separate from the central canal of the spinal cord and from the subarachnoid space. They occur in the low lumbar and sacral area and are skin covered. They may or may not be associated with nerve impairment or lipomas of the spinal cord. When a myelocystocele is associated with a primitive gut and an open abdomen, it is classified as an exstrophy of the cloaca. When the bony elements of the sacrum are missing or abnormal, such myelocystic lesions are termed *sacral agenesis*.

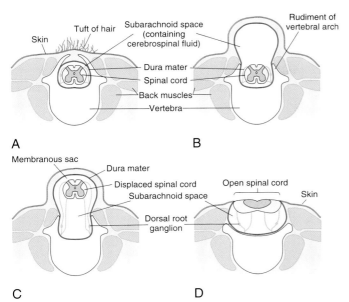

FIG. 23.1 Diagrammatic sketches illustrating various types of spina bifida and commonly associated malformations of the nervous system. (A) Spina bifida occulta. About 10% of people have this vertebral defect in L5 and/or S1. It usually causes no back problems. (B) Spina bifida with meningocele. (C) Spina bifida with meningomyelocele. (D) Spina bifida with myeloschisis. The types illustrated in B through D are often referred to collectively as spina bifida cystica because of the cystic sac that is associated with them. (From Hagen-Ansert SL: *Textbook of diagnostic sonography.* 7th ed. St Louis: Mosby, 2012.)

PATHOEMBRYOLOGY

Embryologically, myelodysplastic lesions can be related to two different processes of nervous system formation: abnormal neurulation or canalization. Neurulation is the folding of ectoderm (primitive skin and associated structures) on each side of the notochord (primitive spinal cord) to form a tube that extends from the hindbrain to the second sacral vertebra. Meningoceles can therefore occur both over the skull and along the spinal column. Encephaloceles (containing brain if along the midline of the skull) and MMs, which can occur along the spinal canal from the C1 to S2 vertebrae, result from a failure of complete entubulation with associated abnormal mesodermal (primitive connective tissue, muscle, and nervous tissue) development. Abnormal mesodermal development produces epidermal sinus tracts, lipomas, and diastematomyelia, as well as unfused posterior vertebral laminae (i.e., true spina bifida occulta).[101] Neurulation occurs early in development, before day 28 of gestation.

The spinal cord distal to the S2 vertebra develops by canalization. Groups of cells in the dorsal, central midline of the mesoderm, distal to the S2 vertebra, become nerve cells. These cells clump together into masses, which develop cystic structures that join to form many canals. The canals ultimately fuse into one tubular structure that joins with the distal end of the spinal cord, which was developing from the neurulation process described previously. Failure of proper canalization, with subsequent retrogressive development of this region, embryologically explains the occurrence of skin-covered meningoceles, lipomas of the spinal cord, and MMs, all of which most frequently develop caudal to the L3 vertebra.[101]

The much better formed, essentially normal, central nervous system (CNS) observed in lesions associated with abnormal canalization and the frequency of CNS malformations (e.g., Arnold-Chiari type II, mental impairment, cranial nerve palsies, and hydrocephalus) associated with neurulation can be explained by the way that neurulation takes place. The neural crests first fuse at approximately the C1 vertebra, and closure of the neural tube progresses simultaneously in cephalad and caudal directions. The same embryologic neurulation processes are simultaneously forming the CNS from the tectal plate to the midlumbar area. It is therefore logical that an influence sufficient to interfere with neurulation along the spinal canal would also interfere with development of the cephalad end, producing CNS malformations above the spinal cord level, which are commonly exhibited in this population.[101] Because canalization occurs by different embryologic processes at a different time period than neurulation, any factor interfering with canalization will not necessarily affect neurulation, so the CNS usually forms normally above the midlumbar area (Fig. 23.2).

ETIOLOGY

The cause of canalization disorders is unknown. This discussion therefore focuses on disorders of neurulation and, in particular, on MM. These causes may also apply to other MMs that can result from defective neurulation (anencephaly, encephalocele, meningocele, and lipomyelomeningocele, all with or without diastematomyelia). For brevity, we refer to all these lesions throughout this chapter as MM for myelomeningocele and its associated malformations.[181]

Genetics

MMs as a group are multifactorial, arising from a complex combination of genetic and environmental factors. MM is often associated with genetic abnormalities, including chromosomal aberrations (Trisomy 13, 18, and 21) and other classic "syndromes"/single gene disorders. Each child born with MM, therefore, warrants a careful physical examination by a pediatrician because the "syndrome" is usually more important than the spinal lesion for defining prognosis. The recurrence risk for siblings in the United States is 2% to 3%.[181]

The prevalence estimates of MM among children and adolescents vary according to region, race/ethnicity, and gender, which suggests possible variations in prevalence at birth or inequities in survival rates.[84] The occurrence of MM varies among races and regions of the world. African blacks have the lowest incidence at 1 in 10,000. Celts (Eastern Irish, Western Scots, and all Welsh) have had a birth incidence recorded as high as 1 in 80. One can conclude from these data that either there are many genetic causes for MM or that there are many genetically determined responses to one or more teratogens.[181] However, with the advent of antenatal diagnosis and elective termination of pregnancy (TOP), the prevalence of MM at birth is no longer reliable as an estimate of incidence.[169]

Teratogens

Teratogens can cause MM. Excess maternal alcohol intake can produce a classic fetal alcohol syndrome with MM. Ingestion of valproic acid or carbamazepine (anticonvulsant medications) during pregnancy are also associated with an increased

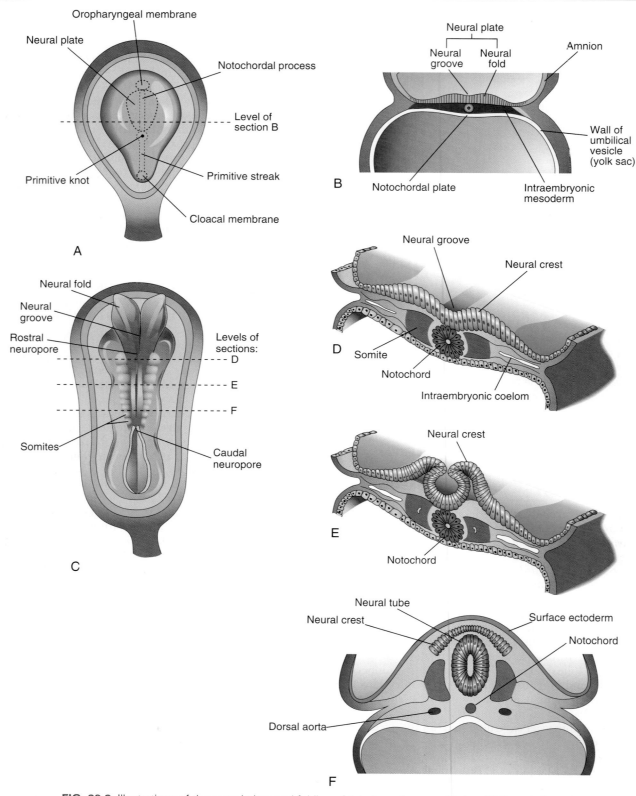

FIG. 23.2 Illustrations of the neural plate and folding of it to form the neural tube. (A) Dorsal view of an embryo of approximately 17 days, exposed by removing the amnion. (B) Transverse section of the embryo showing the neural plate and early development of the neural groove and neural folds. (C) Dorsal view of an embryo of approximately 22 days. The neural folds have fused opposite the fourth to sixth somites but are open at both ends. (D–F) Transverse sections of this embryo at the levels shown in C illustrating formation of the neural tube and its detachment from the surface ectoderm. Note that some neuroectodermal cells are not included in the neural tube but remain between it and the surface ectoderm as the neural crest. (From Moore KL, Persaud TVN, Torchia MG: *Before we are born: essentials of embryology and birth defects.* 9th ed. Philadelphia: Elsevier, 2016.)

birth incidence of MM. Many other possible teratogens have been studied, but inadequate descriptions of the pathology of the lesions and the relative infrequency of their occurrence have resulted in inconclusive observations. Maternal pregestational insulin-dependent diabetes is associated with a 2- to 10-fold increase, and maternal pregestational obesity (BMI > 29) is associated with a 1.5- to 3.5-fold increase in the occurrence of MM.[132] More studies combining detailed family histories, pathologic anatomy, and detailed physical examinations must be conducted to determine the relative contribution of teratogens to MM formation.[181]

Nutritional Deficiencies

A significant decrease in the incidence of MM births and abortions was observed for MM diagnosed prenatally in the United Kingdom during a placebo-controlled trial of prenatal folic acid administration for women who had given birth to a previous baby with a MM.[134] Other reports suggested that European and United Kingdom studies regarding the benefit of supplementation of folic acid could be applied to other culturally and genetically diverse populations where there are different racial and regional differences in the birth incidence of MM.[16,35,59,150] Early data from the United States did not include pregnancies terminated because of in utero diagnosis of MM and, therefore, led to controversy.[17,128,130,165]

MM stands out as one of the few birth defects for which a primary prevention strategy (folic acid [FA] fortification of food) is available. It has been a highly effective intervention compared with dietary improvement or supplementation because fortification made FA accessible to all women of childbearing age without requiring behavior change. In 1998, the United States was the first country to require mandatory FA fortification of standardized enriched cereal grain products, infant formulas, medical foods, and foods for special dietary use. MM prevalence decreased by 31% after fortification, from 5.04 per 10,000 during 1995 to 1996 to 3.49 at the end of 2006. Unfortunately, this decrease is not uniform across ethnic groups. The reasons for the disparity between declines in the prevalence of MM since FA fortification are unknown. However, no European countries, including the United Kingdom, had implemented mandatory food fortification as of June 2013.[209]

Current Centers for Disease Control recommendations advise women to take folic acid in an effort to reduce both the recurrence in families with[134] and the occurrence in families without a member with MM.[16,33] Women with a first-degree relative with MM or with history of having an open MM in a previous child or fetus should be advised to take 4 mg per day, and women without a positive history should be advised to take 0.4 mg per day. Both should begin the folic acid at least 3 months before conception. Folic acid is believed to be harmless in this age group because the only possible concern is the masking of pernicious anemia resulting from cobalamin deficiency. Both observational and intervention studies, including randomized, controlled trials, showed that adequate consumption of FA periconceptionally can prevent 50% to 70% of MM. Taking folic acid does not eliminate the occurrence of open neural tube defects and has no known effect on the occurrence of closed MM. How FA acts to prevent MM in some individuals and does not appear to have any prevention ability in others remains an important but unanswered question.

INCIDENCE AND PREVALENCE

Superimposed on a general worldwide decrease in the birth incidence of MM are a number of influences to cause both a reduction in birth incidence and increased prevalence resulting from improved survival. Better nutrition applies to many areas of the industrialized world. Wider availability of amniocentesis, maternal serum alpha-fetoprotein screening, and more refined resolution of diagnostic ultrasonography for fetal examination have given parents an option to terminate pregnancies because their fetus has MM.[7,111] Measurement of maternal serum alpha-fetoprotein is now part of the triple test (alpha-fetoprotein, human chorionic gonadotropin, and estradiol) and the quad screen (alpha-fetoprotein, human chorionic gonadotropin, estradiol, inhibin A). Alpha-fetoprotein levels are reported as multiples of the median (MoM); concerning results for an open MM are levels greater than 2.5 MoM.

Diagnosis now occurs frequently at 18 weeks' gestation allowing time for parents to deliberate.[192] It is estimated that internationally approximately 23% of pregnancies where a prenatal diagnosis of a MM is made are voluntarily terminated.[139] TOP is the most common outcome of pregnancy after prenatal diagnosis of anencephaly and MM.[84] One systematic review showed an overall frequency of TOP after prenatal diagnosis to be 83% for anencephaly (range, 59% to 100%) and 63% for MM (range, 31% to 97%). TOP for MM was more common when the prenatal diagnosis occurred at less than 24 weeks' gestation (86 vs. 27%), with defects of greater severity, and in Europe versus North America (66 vs. 50%).[84] Conversely, prenatal diagnosis has allowed other parents to select cesarean section prior to rupture of the amniotic membranes and onset of labor, avoiding trauma to the neural sac from vaginal delivery. The outcome of cesarean delivery compared to vaginal delivery has been children with less paralysis and with minimal risk for CNS infection, both of which were previously a cause for increased morbidity and early death.[182] Improved medical care has resulted in increased survival and, secondarily, an increased prevalence of MM. Incidence at birth in the United States has been reported to range from 0.4 to 0.9 per 1000 births, depending on the reporting source.[181] Prevalence per 1000 births in the United States is reported to be 4.17 for Hispanic, 3.22 for non-Hispanic white, and 2.64 for non-Hispanic black mothers.

PERINATAL MANAGEMENT

Since the late 1980s, the intervention for MM has changed from a postnatal crisis of horrendous magnitude to a prenatal option of either pregnancy termination or improved pregnancy outcome by prelabor cesarean section birth. This advance has been made possible by widespread use of maternal serum alpha-fetoprotein screening as part of the triple screen or quad screen.[111] Unfortunately, this type of screening will not detect skin-covered neural defects such as meningoceles, lipomyelomeningoceles, or other rare lesions covered by skin.

Technical improvements in ultrasonography allow for the identification of anatomic variations/markers to diagnose MM. It is believed that ultrasonography is a reliable method to identify MM by the end of the first trimester of gestation. These markers are more specific for open spinal defects and represent the consequence of the associated Chiari II malformation.

Common cranial ultrasonographic signs described in MM include[34]:

1. The lemon sign (scalloping/overlapping of the frontal bones): the cross-section view of the brain appears lemon shaped rather than oval and is predictive of MM. Seen in 80% of cases.
2. Small cerebellum (transcerebellar diameter < 10th percentile)
3. Effacement of the cisterna magna (width < 2 mm on axial scan of posterior fossa)
4. The banana sign (small cerebellum hemispheres curling anteriorly and obliteration of the cisterna magna as a result of downward displacement of the hindbrain structures). Seen in 93% of cases.
5. Ventriculomegaly (atrial width: severe: > 14 mm; borderline: > 10 mm)
6. Funneling of the posterior fossa (clivus-supraocciput angle < 72 degrees)

Their sequence has not been established; investigators disagree whether cerebellar signs precede cerebral signs or vice versa. These ultrasonographic signs are more accurate in defining the cranial malformations associated with MM than in detecting abnormalities of the spine. As discussed in the section on pathoembryology, these ultrasonographic signs are pertinent to MM cephalad to the S2 vertebra (i.e., neurulation defects) but not to canalization defects, which are usually not associated with cranial malformations responsible for the Arnold-Chiari type II malformation,[176] the cause of the "lemon" and "banana" signs. Some spinal dysraphic states and dorsal lumbosacral masses consistent with canalization defects such as myelocystocele or lipomyelomeningocele can be identified with ultrasonography. Other anomalies consistent with syndromes or organ malformations that are incompatible with survival beyond intrauterine life (e.g., anencephaly) can also be detected.

A third modality for prenatal diagnosis, amniotic fluid analysis, is critical in the evaluation of a fetus with a MM. Up to 10% of fetuses with a MM detected in the first half of the second trimester or before have an associated chromosome error, usually trisomy 13 or 18.[108] Chromosome analysis of amniotic cells is therefore essential to the parental decision-making process regarding abortion of the pregnancy. From the same amniotic fluid specimen obtained for chromosome analysis, the acetylcholinesterase level can be determined. This test is more accurate than determination of the amniotic fluid level of alpha-fetoprotein used previously because the former is positive only in a fetus with an open MM.[111] The presence of a dorsal spine lesion and a negative result of an acetylcholinesterase test suggest a skin-covered meningocele or other skin-covered MM, which is an indication for normal vaginal delivery. A MM lesion containing nerves protruding dorsal to the plane of the back, in the presence of fetal knee or ankle function observed on ultrasonography, warrants prelabor cesarean section, sterile delivery, and closure of the open-back lesion to preserve nerve function.[108]

Prenatal diagnosis also allowed the introduction of repair of the MM sac in utero. While the goal of previous fetal interventions in other conditions was to prevent fetal/neonatal demise, the goal of fetal meningomyelocele (fMMC) repair was to improve long-term outcome in a condition that already had an effective postnatal treatment. Tulipan and associates[197] reported a decreased need for a cerebrospinal fluid shunt and claimed improvement in the Chiari II malformation, as evidenced solely by improved appearance on magnetic resonance imaging (MRI) when intrauterine repairs were performed. Bannister[9] cautioned that the MRI appearance was not as important as function. The claims of Tulipan and associates,[197] however, were not substantiated by the results of cases treated at other centers. Differences in selection criteria and the lack of comparison populations undergoing postnatal repair led the National Institute of Child Health and Human Development to initiate the Management of Myelomeningocele Study (MoMS) (2003–2010) at three centers with prior intrauterine surgery experience. MoMS showed the efficacy of fMMC in a specific homogeneous population under ideal circumstances; these results may not be generalizable outside the eligibility criteria set forth in MoMS. As a result, it is not clear that fMMC is effective in real patients in typical settings. The initial MoMS results were published in 2011,[1] when the majority of the participants were 12–30 months of age. They reported important benefits in children who underwent prenatal closure/repair compared with infants repaired postnatally:

1. Decreased need for postnatal ventriculoperitoneal shunt placement (40% vs. 82%, $P < .001$)
2. Significant reversal of severe hindbrain herniation (22% vs. 6%, $P < .001$)
3. Greater likelihood to walk without devices (42% vs. 21%, $P < .01$)
4. Motor function 2 or more levels better than expected by anatomic level (32% vs. 12%, $P < .005$).

However, MoMS also showed that fMMC surgery increased several risks in children who underwent prenatal closure/repair compared with infants repaired postnatally:

1. Increased risk of spontaneous rupture of membranes (46% vs. 8%, $P < .001$)
2. Increased risk of oligohydramnios (21% vs. 4%, $P < .001$)
3. Increased risk of preterm delivery (79% vs. 15%, $P < .001$); 13% of the fetal surgery group were born before 30 weeks of gestation

Urologic outcomes are a particular area in which the benefits of fMMC repair remain unclear. All of these questions will require further evaluation and extended follow-up. This is a primary goal of the MoMS II study that will evaluate participants between 5 and 8 years of age.

IMPAIRMENTS

The discussions of pathoembryology and diagnosis describe the potential involvement of the brain and brain stem in addition to the spinal cord in individuals with MM. The multifocal involvement of the CNS results in several possible complex problems, making the care of these individuals more challenging than and substantially different from that of children with traumatic spinal cord injuries. The broad spectrum of problems encountered with MM requires a multidisciplinary team approach in a comprehensive care outpatient clinic setting. This section describes the variety of impairments that can occur with MM. In addition, general examination and intervention issues related to each impairment are discussed. Impairment, for the purpose of this discussion, is defined as a change in body structure and function, whereas activity limitation is the inability to perform tasks as a consequence of impairments. Activity limitations and participation restrictions encountered at specific age levels, along with age-specific examination, evaluation, and intervention issues, are discussed in subsequent sections of this chapter.

Musculoskeletal Deformities

Spinal and lower limb deformities and joint contractures occur frequently in children with MM. Orthopedic deformities and joint contractures negatively affect positioning, body image, weight bearing (both in sitting and standing), activities of daily living (ADLs), energy expenditure, and mobility from infancy through adulthood. Several factors contribute to abnormal posture, limb deformity, and joint contractures, including muscle imbalance secondary to neurologic dysfunction, progressive neurologic dysfunction, intrauterine positioning, coexisting congenital malformations, arthrogryposis, habitually assumed postures after birth, reduced or absent active joint motion, and deformities after fractures.[115,175] The upper limbs can also be involved as a result of spasticity or poor postural habits. The upper limb region most likely to have restricted motion is the shoulder girdle due to overuse of the arms for weight bearing and poor postural habits.

Postural stability is essential to effectively perform functional tasks. Symmetric alignment is important to minimize joint stress and deforming forces and to permit muscles to function at their optimal length. Uncorrected postural deficits can result in joint contractures and deformities, stretch weakness, and musculoskeletal pain. Deficits that may appear insignificant during childhood often become magnified once an individual has adult body proportions, resulting in activity limitations and discomfort (e.g., low back pain resulting from an increased lumbar lordosis and hip flexion contractures). Consequently, limb, neck, and trunk range of motion (ROM), muscle extensibility, and joint alignment should be monitored throughout the life span so that appropriate interventions can be implemented as indicated.

Typical postural problems include forward head, rounded shoulders, kyphosis, scoliosis, excessive lordosis, anterior pelvic tilt, rotational deformities of the hip or tibia (in-toeing, out-toeing, or windswept positions), flexed hips and knees, and pronated feet. It is important to observe posture and postural control after a given position has been maintained for a period of time to determine the effects of fatigue. Static and dynamic balance should be observed in sitting, four-point positioning, kneeling, half-kneeling, and standing, as well as during transitions between these positions. Symmetry and weight distribution should also be noted. In addition, typical sleeping and sitting positions should be identified to determine if habitual positioning is contributing to postural or joint deformities (e.g., "frog-leg" position in prone or supine, W-sitting, ring sitting, heel sitting, cross-legged sitting, and crouch standing). These habitual positions should be avoided because they may produce deforming forces and altered musculotendon length that result in the development of secondary impairments such as the progression of orthopedic deformities, joint contractures, and strength deficits. Photographs or videos of sitting and standing postures are often useful to document current status and to provide a visual baseline for future reference.

Postural deviations and contractures that are typical for individual lesion levels are summarized as follows. Individuals with high-level lesions (thoracic to L2) often have hip flexion, abduction, and external rotation contractures; knee flexion contractures; and ankle plantar flexion contractures. The lumbar spine is typically lordotic. Individuals with mid- to low-lumbar (L3–L5) lesion levels often have hip and knee flexion contractures, an increased lumbar lordosis, genu and calcaneal valgus malalignment, and a pronated position of the foot when bearing weight. They often walk with a pronounced crouched gait and bear weight primarily on their calcaneus. Individuals with sacral level lesions often have mild hip and knee flexion contractures and an increased lumbar lordosis, and the ankle and foot can either be in varus or valgus, combined with a pronated or supinated forefoot. They may walk with a mild crouch gait and may bear weight primarily on their calcaneus unless plantar flexor muscles are at least grade 3/5.

Crouch standing is a typical postural deviation that is observed across lesion levels and is characterized by persistent hip and knee flexion and an increased lumbar lordosis. The crouch posture often occurs because of muscle weakness (e.g., insufficient soleus muscle strength to maintain the tibia vertical) and orthopedic deformities (e.g., calcaneal valgus, which results in obligatory tibial internal rotation and knee flexion). Hip and knee flexion contractures often occur secondarily, in response to adaptive shortening of muscles from prolonged positioning in the crouch-standing posture. Altered postures, such as crouch standing, negatively affect both the task requirements (by increasing the muscle torque required to maintain the position) and the torque-generating capacity of the musculoskeletal system.[66] Such increased demands placed on the musculoskeletal system when standing and walking in a crouched posture may negatively impact function and result in secondary impairments.[5,25,66,107,136,137,177,198,206] It is important that appropriate intervention be implemented to ameliorate crouch standing so that the excessive physical demands and stress placed on the musculoskeletal system are reduced and the development of secondary impairments is minimized.

Scoliosis occurs in about 50% of children with MM and can be congenital or acquired; the congenital form is usually related to underlying vertebral anomalies and the curve is often inflexible, whereas the acquired type is usually caused by muscle imbalance and the curve is flexible until skeletal maturity is reached,[115] at which point little further progression is usually observed.[175] Scoliosis is more frequently observed in higher lesion level groups (thoracic 90%; midlumbar 40%; low lumbar 10%) and becomes more prevalent and increasingly severe with age in all groups.[115]

Other spinal deformities that can occur in conjunction with or separate from scoliosis are kyphosis and lordosis deformities (Fig. 23.3). Congenital kyphosis occurs in 10% to 15% of infants with MM.[131,196] Paralytic kyphosis is acquired in approximately one third by early adolescence,[25] progressing at a rate of 7% to 8% per year.[11] Kyphosis can occur in the lumbar spine with reversal of the lumbar lordosis, or the kyphosis can be more diffusely distributed over the entire spine. Hyperlordosis of the lumbar spine is another commonly observed deformity. Like scoliosis, both kyphosis and lordosis are more commonly observed in children with higher spinal lesions and the curves tend to progress with age.[115] Severe kyphosis and scoliosis can limit chest wall expansion with consequent restriction of lung ventilation and frequent respiratory infections. The resulting restrictive lung condition can limit exercise tolerance and can be life threatening in extreme cases.[115] Poor sitting posture, muscle imbalance, and recurrent skin ulcerations are additional problems encountered.[25]

The goal of treatment of spinal deformities is to maintain a balanced trunk and pelvis.[86] Orthotic intervention, usually with a bivalved Silastic thoracolumbosacral orthosis (TLSO), is helpful in maintaining improved trunk position for functional

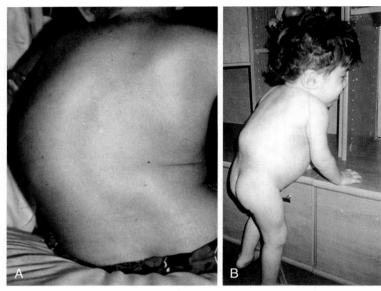

FIG. 23.3 Spinal deformities. (A) Collapsing type of lordoscoliosis. (B) Kyphotic spinal deformity. ([A] From Zitelli BJ, McIntire SC, Nowalk AJ: *Zitelli and Davis' atlas of pediatric physical diagnosis.* 6th ed. Philadelphia: Saunders, 2016. [B] From Hoyt CS, Taylor D: *Pediatric ophthalmology and strabismus.* 4th ed. Edinburgh: Saunders, 2013.)

activities but does not prevent progression of acquired spinal deformity.[115] For children with progressive spinal deformities, orthotic intervention is continued until the child reaches a sufficient age to allow surgical fusion of the spine to prevent further progression of these deformities. Long spinal fusions before the skeletal age of 10 result in greater loss of trunk height because of ablation of the growth plates of vertebral bodies included in the fusion mass.[115] In addition, surgery at too young a skeletal age is associated with an increased frequency of instrumentation failure as a result of fragile bones and skin breakdown over the bulky spinal instrumentation.[115] The ideal minimum age for spinal fusion is 10 to 11 years old in girls and 12 to 13 years old in boys.[115] In general, children with MM reach puberty and their growth spurt earlier than their able-bodied peers, so only minimal truncal shortening occurs as a consequence of long spinal fusion when it is performed at the appropriate age. With the introduction of growing constructs such as the vertically expanding prosthetic titanium rib systems and growing rods, children with severe scoliosis at younger ages can undergo a spine stabilization procedure without sacrificing the final truncal height.

It is important to note that a history of recurrent urinary tract infections or poor nutrition increases the risk of perioperative infections with spinal instrumentation procedures for children with MM.[64]

Hip joints also are prone to deformity in children with MM. Fixed flexion deformities often require surgical intervention because they interfere with ambulation and orthotic fit. Correction after surgery should be maintained by encouraging standing and walking.[41,125] Children with high lumbar lesions (L1, L2) have unopposed flexion and adduction forces that gradually push the femoral head superiorly and posteriorly. The resulting contractures and secondary bony deformities of the proximal femur and acetabulum can lead to subluxation or dislocation (Fig. 23.4A and B) in nearly one third to one half of children with MM.[41]

In children with hip subluxation or dislocation, long-term follow-up studies have indicated that reduction of the hips is not a prerequisite for ambulation.[168] Mayfield[115] stated that a level pelvis and good ROM are more important for function than hip reduction. Furthermore, he stated that the presence of the femoral head in the acetabulum does not necessarily improve ROM at the hip or the ability to ambulate. In addition, unlike in children with cerebral palsy, it does not appear to affect the amount of orthotic support required, hip pain, or gait deviation.[159] The indications for hip surgery in children with MM continue to be controversial; however, a basic principle practiced at many centers is to operate only on children with a lesion level at or below L3, when quadriceps muscle function is present, because these children are more likely to be functional ambulators into adulthood.[115,175] Fixed pelvic obliquity caused by unilateral subluxation or dislocation interferes with sitting or standing posture, contributes to scoliosis, and makes skin care unmanageable. It is another indication for surgical relocation of the hip, regardless of lesion level or ambulatory potential, along with painful hip dysplasia in ambulators.[189]

Shurtleff[175] evaluated the frequency of all types of hip contractures in large numbers of children with various spinal lesion levels. He noted that contractures measured in infancy tended to decrease in severity until approximately age 3 to 4 years, then increased to much higher values by adolescence. The initial decrease in severity of hip contractures can potentially be explained as a normal physiologic phenomenon resulting from intrauterine positioning. The increase in severity of contractures by adolescence, however, is of special concern to physical therapists. Mild contractures of minimal functional significance in young children can increase dramatically during later childhood and adolescence, necessitating persistent intervention and follow-up by the therapist to prevent significant functional loss. Consequently, physical therapists should be proactive in preventing the progression of contractures. Thoracic and high lumbar (L1, L2) groups of children have a higher incidence and

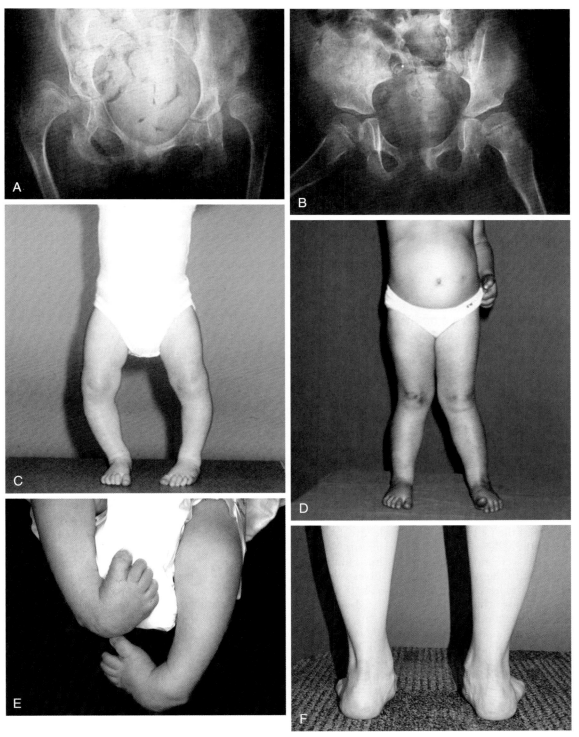

FIG. 23.4 Lower limb deformities. (A) Hip dislocation. (B) Hip dysplasia and subluxation. (C) Genu varus. (D) Genu valgus. (E) Equinovarus. (F) Calcaneal valgus. ([C–D] From Macnicol MF: Paediatric knee problems. *Orthop Trauma* 4[5]:369-380, 2010. [E] From Herring JA: *Tachdjian's pediatric orthopaedics: from the Texas Scottish Rite Hospital for Children.* 5th ed. Philadelphia: Saunders, 2014. [F] From Sahrmann S: *Movement system impairment syndromes of the extremities, cervical and thoracic spines.* St. Louis: Mosby, 2011.)

greater severity of contractures owing to unopposed iliopsoas muscle function, regardless of whether or not they were participating in a standing program.[103] Shurtleff[175] reported progressively declining frequency and severity of contractures in groups of children with lesions at L3, L4 to L5, and sacral levels, respectively. An unexpected finding from Shurtleff's study was that only a certain percentage of children in each lesion level group had hip contractures, subluxation, or both. These relative percentages were not altered by surgical procedures on the hip and stayed constant across age groups. No clear reasons were discerned why certain individuals were susceptible to contractures, whereas others with similar neurologic function were not.

The knee joints of children with MM frequently have contractures or deformities. These include both flexion and extension contractures; the former more commonly occur in children who primarily use a wheelchair for mobility,[103] and the latter often occur after periods of immobility from fractures, decubitus ulcers, or surgical procedures. Varus and valgus deformities (see Fig. 23.4C–D) are also observed. Flexion deformities may make walking difficult or impossible, and extension deformities may complicate sitting. If either flexion or extension deformities are significant, they may need to be ameliorated via surgical release.[189] Wright and associates[208] reported that 60% of individuals with fixed flexion contractures less than 20° and a lesion level higher than L3 were still biped ambulators in late adolescence, as compared to fewer than 5% of individuals with fixed flexion contractures greater than 20°. They also concluded that muscle imbalance and spasticity do not appear to be major causative factors; rather, the lack of normal joint movement may lead to joint stiffness. As described earlier for the hip joints, Shurtleff[175] studied the frequency of knee contractures and deformities in children with different lesion levels. An initial decrease from the contractures measured in infants was also noted at the knees, with the lowest prevalence occurring at age 4 to 5 years for patients with L3 or higher lesions and at age 2 to 3 years for children with lesions below L3. The frequency and severity of contractures increased in all groups from early childhood into adolescence. Knee joint contractures occurred in 65% to 70% of the thoracic and high lumbar groups by age 6 to 8, 20% to 25% of the L4 to L5 group by age 9 to 12, and sporadically among the children with sacral level lesions. Valgus and varus deformities were most frequently observed in the L3 and above groups, with a slight increase during adolescence.

Deformities of the ankles and feet can occur in both ambulatory and nonambulatory children and are most common in children with lesion levels at L5 and above.[175] Partial innervation and consequent muscle imbalance determine the type of deformity that occurs. Even with surgical correction, these deformities will recur unless the deforming forces are removed. Progressive ankle and foot deformities can also be observed in conjunction with the development of spasticity and motor strength loss associated with tethering of the spinal cord. Children with "skip" lesions (see the section on motor paralysis) are particularly prone to progressive foot deformities.[175]

A variety of foot and ankle deformities can occur (see Fig. 23.4E–F), including ankle equinovarus (clubfeet), forefoot varus or valgus, forefoot supination or pronation, calcaneal varus or valgus, pes cavus and planus, and claw-toe deformities. The most frequent contracture observed is of the ankle plantar flexor muscles. The frequency of foot deformities has been reported to vary from 20% to 50% between lesion level groups[175] and has been reported to be as high as 90% for

high-level paralysis and 60% to 70% for lower-level paralysis.[24,52,189] Although some deformities are more frequently associated with certain neurosegmental levels (e.g., clubfeet in thoracic and high lumbar lesions, claw-toes in sacral lesions), all types of ankle and foot deformities are observed in children at every lesion level. Congenital clubfeet are common, and surgery is indicated once the child is developmentally ready to stand.[25] Other foot deformities may develop over time as a result of muscle imbalance. Dias[40] noted that ankle valgus occurs in the presence of fibular shortening, the latter being highly correlated with paralysis of the soleus muscle. Surgical treatment of a valgus ankle is indicated when the deformity cannot be functionally alleviated with orthotics. The presence of ankle and foot deformities can greatly affect sitting and standing posture, balance, mobility, foot ulcerations, and shoe fit, regardless of lesion level. Weight-bearing forces often result in ankle and foot deformities. Even partial weight bearing on wheelchair footrests in poor alignment over time can result in deformities and foot ulcerations. Consequently, achieving a plantigrade position of the feet is a priority, regardless of ambulatory status. Surgical procedures are often necessary and are effective.[189] Orthoses and assistive devices should be adjusted properly to maintain neutral subtalar alignment and a plantigrade foot position.

Torsional deformities are common. Excessive foot progression angles and windswept positions of the lower limbs are often present (Fig. 23.5) as a result of hip anteversion, hip retroversion, or tibial torsion. These torsional deformities negatively affect sitting and standing balance, weight distribution, and walking. See Cusick and Stuberg[32] for factors that contribute to torsional deformities in individuals with developmental disabilities, examination procedures, normative values, and intervention suggestions.

Joint alignment and evidence of abnormal joint stress are often most apparent during dynamic activities such as walking or wheelchair propulsion. Joint stresses are often magnified when walking on uneven surfaces, stairs, or curbs. Observing wear patterns on shoes and orthoses can provide additional clues to abnormal stress and malalignment. If joint deformities are supple, they may respond to stretching, combined with orthoses or positioning splints to maintain alignment. Fixed deformities may respond to serial casting (e.g., foot deformities) but will often require surgical intervention (e.g., scoliosis, unilateral hip dislocation, or tibial torsion). If muscle imbalance is severe and the deforming forces are not effectively counteracted by stretching, strengthening, or positioning, muscle transfers may be indicated (e.g., partial transfer of the anterior tibialis muscle to the calcaneus to achieve a plantigrade foot position by balancing the unopposed dorsiflexion force in a child with L5 motor function).

There are several reasons for maintaining joint ROM. Limited ROM can interfere with ADLs, bed mobility, and transfers. Bed mobility is more efficient and self-care is easier for individuals who have maintained their flexibility.[68] Restricted ROM, combined with muscle weakness, can result in poor postural habits and gait deviations. Adequate ROM must be maintained to perform ADLs such as bathing and toileting. Restricted joint motion can result in overlengthening of weak muscles, not permitting them to function in the optimal range of the length-tension curve. Limited ROM may result in discomfort, especially when lying down (e.g., tight hip flexors pulling on the lumbar spine). Severe contractures also can negatively affect body image. Contractures that may seem insignificant

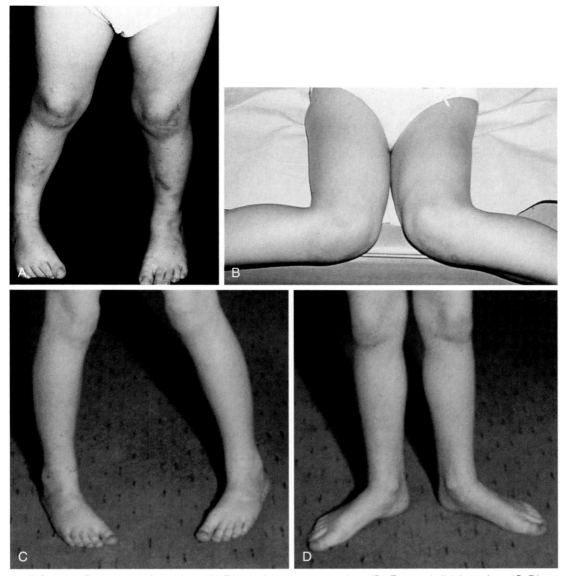

FIG. 23.5 Torsional deformities. (A) Femoral neck anteversion. (B) External tibial torsion. (C–D) Internal tibial torsion. ([A–B] From Zitelli BJ, McIntire SC, Nowalk AJ: *Zitelli and Davis' atlas of pediatric physical diagnosis.* 6th ed. Philadelphia: Saunders, 2016. [C–D] From Coughlin MJ, Saltzman CL, Anderson RB: *Mann's surgery of the foot and ankle.* 9th ed, Philadelphia: Saunders, 2014.)

during childhood may become functionally limiting once the individual has adult-sized body proportions (e.g., knee extension contractures can interfere with the ability to maneuver in a wheelchair). In extreme cases, difficulty in managing paralyzed limbs because of joint contractures can put individuals at risk for skin breakdown and possibly amputations because of the increased incidence of injury.[68] The impact of limited ROM on functional performance should be considered before deciding whether intervention is indicated.

ROM and positioning of paralytic limbs should be done carefully, without excessive force, to avoid fractures.[163] Caution should also be exercised when adducting the hips to avoid hip dislocation. The prone hip extension test[188] for measuring hip extension is the method of choice in this population because of interference of spinal and pelvic deformities and lower limb spasticity with the traditional Thomas test method.[13] Ankle

ROM should always be measured with the ankle joint in subtalar neutral so that measurements are comparable across time and therapists.

The long-term effects of surgical interventions and weight bearing on insensate joints are becoming evident as individuals with MM reach adulthood.[25] Secondary impairments of knee joint deterioration and arthritis occur with increased frequency in older individuals.[107] Nagankatti and associates[137] reported a prevalence of 1 per 100 cases of Charcot arthroplasty in the MM population.

There are several ways to minimize musculoskeletal stress and reduce the incidence of acquired orthopedic deformities. Improving traction of the hands by providing biking gloves for community wheelchair mobility reduces the grip forces required for wheelchair propulsion. Wheelchair seat positions influence propulsion effectiveness and the amount of stress on upper limb joints and muscles.[114] For ambulators, shoes with nonskid soles improve foot traction. Symmetric neutral joint alignment should be maintained in both sitting and standing via appropriate orthotics or seating devices. It is important to avoid shifting weight to one leg when standing and to avoid crossing the legs when sitting. Extreme ROM should be avoided, especially when bearing weight. Crutch and walker handgrips should be angled to avoid hyperextension of the wrists, and weight should be distributed across a broad, cushioned area. Orthoses should provide total contact to minimize the risk of development of pressure areas. Excessive pressure on tendons and the palms of the hand should be avoided to reduce the risk of developing carpal tunnel syndrome. Overhead reaching and work activities should be minimized by adapting the home, school, and work environments. In addition, long-distance mobility options should be provided to reduce joint stresses. When sitting, weight bearing should be symmetric, pelvic tilt should be neutral with a slight lumbar lordosis, the hips and knees should be at 90°, and the feet should be flat on the floor. Good lumbar support should be provided. Inclining the seat backward 15° minimizes stress on the lumbar spine and helps keep the pelvis seated back in the chair.[28] Tilting the desk or tabletop upward improves the position of the upper trunk, head, and shoulders.

Osteoporosis

The incidence of fractures is reported to be 11% to 30% in children with MM.[44,113,193] This high rate of fractures is believed to be secondary to reduced bone mineral density from limited ambulation and muscle weakness caused by the MM.[112]

Decreased bone mineral density, thought to be secondary to hypotonic or flaccid musculature combined with decreased loading of long bones from altered mobility, is frequently observed in children with MM and often results in osteoporotic fractures. In a comprehensive review of studies evaluating pediatric supported standing programs, Paleg[148] concluded: "Standing programs 5 days per week positively affect bone mineral density (60 to 90 min/d); hip stability (60 min/d in 30° to 60° of total bilateral hip abduction); range of motion of hip, knee, and ankle (45 to 60 min/d); and spasticity (30 to 45 min/d)." These issues must be studied further in the MM population, however. Bone responses in children with flaccid paralysis may be quite different. Rosenstein and associates[157] examined this issue in the MM population and reported that bone mineral density was 38% to 44% higher in household or community ambulators compared with nonfunctional ambulators (exercise-only ambulators or nonambulators). Salvaggio and associates[160] reported that walking ability was a highly significant determinant of bone density in prepubertal children with MM. Because the effects of lesion level were not controlled in either of these studies, however, the potential contribution of muscle activity versus weight-bearing status to the differences in bone mineral density cannot be determined. In addition, neither study addressed the issue of reduction of the incidence of osteoporotic fractures.

Studying the frequency of fractures is a more direct and clinically significant method of examining the benefits of standing programs. Shurtleff[175] asked the question, "Are fractures less common among those patients in standing or ambulatory programs than among similarly paralyzed sedentary peers?" Asher and Olson[6] showed no correlation between fractures and the use of wheelchairs. DeSouza and Carroll[39] reported no fractures in 7 nonambulators and 38 fractures in 16 ambulators. Their data implied that exposure to forces that can produce fractures (i.e., upright mobility) is the important risk factor for fractures, rather than the level of flaccid paralysis, as would be expected. Liptak and associates[103] found no difference in the frequency of fractures between a group of children who were wheelchair users and a comparable group of children who ambulated with orthoses. Clinically, the use of standing frames, parapodiums, or hip-knee-ankle-foot orthoses (HKAFOs) in children with high lumbar and thoracic lesions does not appear warranted for the purpose of fracture prevention. For children with lower lumbar and sacral lesion levels, for whom upright positioning and mobility are important functional skills, undue restriction of physical activity for fear of a fracture is not indicated. The fact that passive weight bearing does not decrease the risk of fractures in these children makes sense if one considers that bone density is more likely maintained by torque generated from volitional muscle activity. Active muscle contraction generates forces through the long bones that are several times greater than the forces from passive weight bearing.

Fractures often present subacutely because of lack of sensation, with swelling and warmth at the fracture site and a low-grade fever often being the only symptoms. Fractures frequently occur after surgery, immobilization in a cast, or as a sequela to foot arthrodesis. Because of the correlation between the duration of casting and the incidence of fracturing, immobilization in a cast is kept to a minimum and fractures are contained in soft immobilization for alignment.[25] Weight bearing is resumed as soon as possible to avoid the risk of additional fractures.[86]

Motor Paralysis

The inherently obvious manifestation of MM is the paraplegia resulting from the spinal cord malformation. Upper limb weakness can also occur in this population, regardless of lesion level, and is often a sign of progressive neurologic dysfunction. Knowledge of the motor lesion level is useful for predicting associated abnormalities and for prognostication of functional outcome. A detailed discussion regarding developmental and functional expectations for each motor lesion level is provided later in the section on outcomes and their determinants. Strategies for assessing strength and planning intervention programs to enhance motor function are provided in the section on age-specific examination and physical therapy intervention strategies.

The motor level is defined as the lowest intact, functional neuromuscular segment. For example, an L4 level indicates that the fourth lumbar nerve and the myotome it innervates are functioning, whereas segments below L4 are not intact. Table 23.1 provides the International Myelodysplasia Study Group (IMSG) criteria for assigning motor levels from manual muscle strength test results.[80] The IMSG criteria have been shown to best reflect the innervation patterns of individuals with MM as opposed to other spinal segment classification systems. MM spinal lesions can be asymmetric when motor or sensory functions of the right and left sides of the body are compared. Consequently, motor function should be classified individually for the right and left sides.

Neuromuscular involvement of individuals with MM may manifest in one of three ways: (1) lesions resembling complete cord transection, (2) incomplete lesions, and (3) skip lesions.[175] Lesions resembling complete cord transection manifest as normal function down to a particular level, below which there is flaccid paralysis, loss of sensation, and absent reflexes.

Incomplete lesions have a mixed manifestation of spasticity and volitional control. Skip lesions are also observed, where more caudal segments are functioning despite the presence of one or more nonfunctional segments interposed between the intact more cephalad spinal segments. Individual skip motor lesions manifest either with isolated function of muscles noted below the last functional level of the lesion or with inadequate strength of muscle groups that have innervation higher than the lowest functioning group.[149] Consequently, it is important to evaluate muscles with lower innervation than the last functional level to determine whether a skip lesion exists. The presence of spasticity and reflexes should also be carefully documented.

McDonald and associates[119] demonstrated that muscle strength grades for the gluteus medius and medial hamstring muscles correlate more highly with strength grades of the hip adductors, hip flexors, and knee extensors than lower limb anterior compartment muscles that have been previously described as being innervated by the L4, L5, and sacral nerve roots. These data potentially explain the clinical observation that individuals with MM often have functional strength in the gluteus medius and medial hamstrings despite having weak or nonactive lower limb anterior compartment muscles. It was concluded from this study that it is more useful clinically to group individuals with MM by the strength of specific muscle groups, as outlined in Table 23.1, rather than by traditional neurosegmental levels.

Sensory Deficits

Sensory deficits are not clear-cut in this population because sensory levels often do not correlate with motor levels and there may be skip areas that lack sensation. Because skip areas can occur within a given dermatome, it is important to test all dermatomes and multiple sites within a given dermatome to have an accurate baseline examination. Deficits should be recorded on a dermatome chart with areas of absent and decreased sensation color-coded for the various sensory modalities (e.g., light touch, pinprick, vibration, and thermal). Proprioception and kinesthetic sense should also be evaluated in both the upper and lower extremities.

Based on the results of a study conducted on 30 adults with MM, testing with both light touch and pinprick stimuli is not necessary in this population because there is little discriminating value for detecting insensate areas.[70] In contrast, vibratory stimuli could be felt one dermatome below light touch and pinprick sensation. Based on these results, vibration sensation should be evaluated in addition to either light touch or pinprick sensation.

It is important for individuals with MM to be aware of their sensory deficits and to be taught techniques to compensate by substituting other sensory modalities (e.g., vision). The impact of decreased sensation on safety should be emphasized, especially when checking temperature (e.g., bath water or when sitting near a fireplace) and when barefoot. Skin inspection and pressure relief techniques should be taught early so that they are incorporated into the daily routine. The importance of pressure relief cushions and sitting push-ups for pressure relief should be emphasized. Proper intervention of lower limbs and joint protection techniques should be taught when learning how to perform ADLs such as transfers.

The impact of sensory deficits on functional performance should be kept in mind when teaching functional tasks. Individuals with MM may rely heavily on vision to compensate for sensory deficits.[166] They may lack the kinesthetic acuity that

TABLE 23.1   International Myelodysplasia Study Group Criteria for Assigning Motor Levels

Motor Level	Criteria for Assigning Motor Levels
T10 or above T11	Determined by sensory level or palpation of abdominal muscles.
T12	Some pelvic control is present in sitting or supine (this may come from the abdominals or paraspinal muscles). Hip hiking from the quadratus lumborum may also be present.
L1	Weak iliopsoas muscle function is present (grade 2).
L1-L2	Exceeds criteria for L1 but does not meet L2 criteria.[a]
L2	Iliopsoas, sartorius, and the hip adductors all must be grade 3 or better.
L3	Meets or exceeds the criteria for L2 plus the quadriceps are grade 3 or better.
L3-L4	Exceeds criteria for L3 but does not meet L4 criteria.
L4	Meets or exceeds the criteria for L3 and the medial hamstrings or the tibialis anterior is grade 3 or better. A weak peroneus tertius may also be seen.
-	Exceeds criteria for L4 but does not meet L5 criteria.
L5	Meets or exceeds the criteria for L4 and has lateral hamstring strength of grade 3 or better plus one of the following: gluteus medius grade 2 or better, peroneus tertius grade 4 or better, or tibialis posterior grade 3 or better.
L5-S1	Exceeds criteria for L5 but does not meet S1 criteria.
S1	Meets or exceeds the criteria for L5 plus at least two of the following: gastrocnemius/soleus grade 2 or better, gluteus medius grade 3 or better, or gluteus maximus grade 2 or better (can pucker the buttocks).
S1-S2	Exceeds criteria for S1 but does not meet S2 criteria.
S2	Meets or exceeds the criteria for S1, the gastrocnemius/soleus must be grade 3 or better, and gluteus medius and maximus are grade 4 or better.
S2-S3	All of the lower limb muscle groups are of normal strength (may be grade 4 in one or two groups). Also includes normal-appearing infants who are too young to be bowel and bladder trained (see "no loss").
"No loss"	Meets all of the criteria for S2-S3 and has no bowel or bladder dysfunction.

[a]When description states "meets criteria ...," strength of muscles listed for preceding levels should be increasing respectively.
Adapted with permission from Patient Data Management System. Myelodysplasia Study Data Collection Criteria and Instructions, 1994. (Available from D. B. Shurtleff, MD, Professor, Department of Pediatrics, University of Washington, Seattle, WA 98195.)

permits subconscious completion of many repetitive motor tasks. Consequently, visual attention may not be available to be directed at other factors in the environment.[4] Adding small amounts of weight to the ankles or a walker may enhance proprioceptive awareness and facilitate gait training. Use of patellar tendon-bearing orthoses (Fig. 23.6) instead of traditional ankle-foot orthoses (AFOs) may also facilitate foot placement for individuals with innervation through L3 because the orthosis contacts the skin in an area of intact sensation.

Hydrocephalus

Hydrocephalus is excessive accumulation of cerebrospinal fluid (CSF) in the ventricles of the brain. Approximately 25% or more of children with MM are born with hydrocephalus. An additional 60% develop it after surgical closure of their back lesion.[153] If left untreated, the continued expansion of the ventricles can cause loss of cerebral cortex with additional cognitive

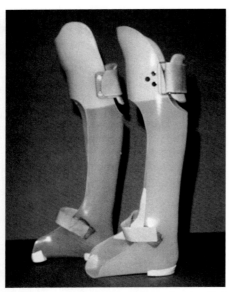

FIG. 23.6 Ground-reaction ankle-foot orthosis. Polypropylene patellar tendon-bearing ground-reaction ankle-foot orthoses molded with the foot in a subtalar neutral position. Note the zero heel posts and posts under the first metatarsal heads.

BOX 23.1 Early Warning Signs and Symptoms of Shunt Dysfunction

Changes in speech
Fever and malaise
Recurring headache
Decreased activity level
Decreased school performance
Onset of or increased strabismus
Changes in appetite and weight
Incontinence begins or worsens
Onset or worsening of scoliosis
Onset of or increased spasticity
Personality change (irritability)
Decreased or static grip strength
Difficult to arouse in the morning
Decreased visuomotor coordination
Decreased visual acuity or diplopia
Decreased visuoperceptual coordination
Onset or increased frequency of seizures

Adapted with permission from Shurtleff DB, Stuntz JT, Hayden P: Hydrocephalus. In Shurtleff DB, editor: *Myelodysplasias and exstrophies: significance, prevention, and treatment.* Orlando, FL: Grune & Stratton, 1986.

and functional impairment. Cerebellar hypoplasia with caudal displacement of the hindbrain through the foramen magnum, known as the Arnold-Chiari type II malformation, is usually associated with hydrocephalus.

The hydrocephalus will occasionally arrest spontaneously; however, 80% to 90% of children with hydrocephalus will require a CSF shunt.[181] A ventriculoperitoneal catheter shunts excess CSF from the lateral ventricles of the brain to the peritoneal space, where the CSF is resorbed. Because a shunt is a foreign body, it can be a nidus for infection or can become obstructed, requiring neurosurgical intervention. Repeated or prolonged shunt dysfunction and infections often lead to additional functional and cognitive decline of the child. Shunt dysfunction is often gradual, with subtle symptoms. Therapists should be familiar with these symptoms to facilitate early detection and appropriate referral to a physician for further evaluation. Box 23.1 provides a list of early symptoms and signs of shunt obstruction. Of particular interest are the findings of Kilburn and associates,[90] which suggest that static or declining grip strength measurements are potentially an early indicator of neurologic dysfunction such as shunt malfunction or symptomatic Arnold-Chiari malformation. Hydrocephalus persists throughout life with consequent need of ongoing follow-up by a physician who is familiar with the medical complications associated with MM.

Cognitive Dysfunction

Early closure of spinal lesions with antibiotic intervention to prevent meningitis and improved CSF shunt intervention have increased the expected cognitive function of children born with MM. However, an increasing body of work supports the concept that specific intellectual deficiencies in individuals with MM can be attributed to structural brain defects. A higher level of spinal lesion has been used as a marker for more severe anomalous brain development. Intelligence scores have traditionally been reported as higher in lumbar and sacral lesion level groups

than in thoracic lesion level groups.[166] However, recent studies comparing lesion level and measures of intelligence, academic skills, and adaptive behavior are not consistent in their findings.

Dise and Lohr[43] demonstrated the need for individual analysis of "higher-order" cognitive functions, including conceptual reasoning, problem solving, mental flexibility, and efficiency of thinking for individuals with MM, regardless of lesion level or general intelligence level. They argued that such neuropsychological deficits likely underlie the "motivational" and academic difficulties observed in this population, especially for those with an average IQ. The impairments in areas such as language, mathematics, and executive functioning persist throughout life.

The current neuropsychological focus is on a MM phenotype that is the product of multiple complex processes rather than a dichotomous (visual vs. auditory perception; verbal vs. nonverbal learning disability) approach. The result of these multiple complex processes is the recognition of a more variable cognitive phenotype. Particularly important are deficits in assembled processing (the ability to assemble, construct, and integrate information across various content domains) and relatively intact associative processing (the ability to activate or categorize information; data driven).[38] About 25% of school-aged children with spina bifida have a mathematical learning disability; children with spina bifida have difficulties with specific aspects of executive functioning: problem solving, planning and goal-directed behavior, focused attention, ability to shift attention, response inhibition, and working memory.[87]

Structural brain abnormalities in MM are important determinants of the neuropsychological profile. Three core deficits have been described in the neuropsychological assessment of individuals with MM and have been associated with specific brain structural anomalies:

deficits in timing related to the volume of the cerebellum;

deficits in attention related to the status of the midbrain, posterior cortex, and corpus callosum;

deficits in movement related to spinal cord dysfunction and cerebellar dysmorphologies that affect sensory motor timing and motor regulation.

The majority of children without hydrocephalus or with uncomplicated hydrocephalus (no infections or cerebral hemorrhage) will have intellect falling within the broad range of normal scores on intelligence testing. The distribution of scores tends to be skewed toward the upper and lower ends of normal, however, with fewer children scoring in the middle of the curve and a greater proportion scoring at the lower end of the range.[166] The intellectual performance of children who have had significant CNS infections is lower than those who have not had infection.[173] Verbal subtest scores usually exceed performance subtest scores.[166] The poorer scores on performance subtests, however, may not represent true differences in verbal versus nonverbal reasoning skills. Instead, these differences can potentially be explained by upper limb dyscoordination (discussed later) and by memory deficits.[166] Dyscoordination and memory deficits are manifested as distractibility on subtests assessing acquired knowledge (e.g., arithmetic), integrated right-left hemisphere function (e.g., picture arrangement, block design, and coding), speed of motor response (e.g., coding), and memory (e.g., digit span, coding, and arithmetic). Further controlled studies must be conducted to determine the source or sources of discrepant verbal versus performance intelligence scores observed in individuals with MM.

The "cocktail party personality" is a cognitively associated behavioral disorder that occurs in some individuals with hydrocephalus, regardless of age or intelligence level.[78] These individuals are articulate and verbose, superficially appearing to have high verbal skills. Close examination of the content of their speech, however, shows frequent and inappropriate use of clichés and jargon. Individual words are often misused. Despite the initial appearance of being capable, these individuals are often impaired, their performance in daily life is below what they superficially appear capable of,[78] and they lack social skills.[183] They often have difficulties with behavioral regulation. Difficulties include identifying the rules, maintaining goal-directed activities during play, performance in unstructured social situations, and a failure to benefit from feedback or instruction about their behavior. Children with spina bifida have a higher incidence of attention deficit/hyperactivity disorder (ADHD) than the general population and typically show problems with inattention rather than with impulsivity and hyperactivity on objective and subjective measures of attention, even when controlling for differences in intellectual functioning. It is important for the physical therapist to directly observe skills that these children report that they can perform and to confirm regular performance of the task at home with parents and care providers to determine if information provided by the patient is accurate.

Language Dysfunction

Although language was once viewed as an asset, children with MM and hydrocephalus demonstrate a profile of both intact and impaired language skills. Their strengths are in the formal, fixed structures of grammar and single words or phrases (vocabulary) and "stored" meanings. Their weaknesses include deficits in discourse, characterized by a high frequency of irrelevant utterances and poorer performance with abstract rather than concrete language. Their communication can be difficult to process and is uneconomic and unclear. These language weaknesses adversely affect their success in social discourse settings. Culatta and Young[31] administered the Preschool Language

Assessment Instrument (PLAI) at four levels of abstraction to children with MM and comparable language-age control children. Children with MM performed comparably to control subjects on concrete tasks of the PLAI, but they produced more "no response" and irrelevant responses than control participants on abstract tasks.

Latex Allergy

A range of up to 73% of children with MM have been reported to have latex allergies[167,210] compared to 1% to 5% of control groups. Unfortunately, 2% of latex consists of major IgE-sensitizing proteins that are ubiquitous in our culture, and some children with MM have life-threatening anaphylaxis when exposed to them. Latex-containing materials are almost never present in operating rooms or in products used elsewhere in the hospital; however, latex is still present throughout the general community. The IgE proteins in latex may be present in wheelchair seats and tires, foam rubber lining on splints and braces, elastic on diapers and clothes, pacifiers, balls, examination gloves used for bladder and bowel programs, and many other everyday objects. While almost all children's hospitals have latex precaution policies, it is important for therapists in schools and clinics in the community to be aware of the need for children with MM to avoid exposure to latex products.

Upper Limb Dyscoordination

Children with MM frequently display upper limb dyscoordination, especially those with hydrocephalus.[166] The dyscoordination can potentially be explained by three possible causes: (1) cerebellar ataxia most likely related to the Arnold-Chiari type II malformation; (2) motor cortex or pyramidal tract damage secondary to hydrocephalus; or (3) motor learning deficits resulting from the use of upper limbs for balance and support rather than manipulation and exploration. These children perform poorly on timed fine motor skill tasks.[166] Their movements can be described as halting and deliberate, rather than the expected smooth, continuous motion of able-bodied children. It often appears that there is a heavy reliance on visual feedback instead of kinesthetic sense. Consequently, even with extensive training, these children often have difficulty integrating frequently used fine motor movements at a subconscious level.[166] Practicing fine motor tasks has been found to be beneficial, however, and often carries over into functional tasks.[49] These coordination deficits have been described by some authors as apparent motor apraxias or motor learning deficits.[26,97] Given the frequent occurrence of upper limb dyscoordination in these children, true apraxias are probably less common than these studies indicate.

An additional factor that may contribute to upper limb dyscoordination is delayed development of hand dominance.[166] A large number of children with MM have mixed hand dominance or are left-handed, suggestive of possible left hemisphere damage.[166] Brunt[26] indicated that delayed hand dominance may contribute to deficits in bilateral upper limb function integration, resulting in further difficulty with fine motor tasks.

Visuoperceptual Deficits

Studies assessing visual perception have not clearly determined whether deficits in children with MM are common, as has been described in the literature.[126,161,195] Tests that require good hand-eye coordination, such as the Frostig Developmental

Test of Visual Perception, may artificially lower scores of children with MM as a result of the upper limb dyscoordination described earlier. When upper limb motor function has been removed as a factor in testing by using the Motor Free Visual Perception Test, children with MM have performed at age-appropriate levels.[166] Consequently, results of visuoperceptual tests must be interpreted carefully, in conjunction with other examinations, before a diagnosis of a visuoperception deficit is made.

Cranial Nerve Palsies

The Arnold-Chiari malformation, along with hydrocephalus or dysplasia of the brain stem, may result in cranial nerve deficits. Ocular muscle palsies can occur,[176] such as involvement of cranial nerve VI (abducens) with consequent lateral rectus eye muscle weakness and esotropia on the involved side. Correction with patching of the eye, prescription lenses, or minor outpatient surgery is necessary to prevent amblyopia and for cosmesis.[153] Gaston[55] studied 322 children with MM for 6 years to monitor them for ophthalmic complications. Forty-two percent of these children had a manifest squint, 29% had an oculomotor nerve palsy or musculoparetic nystagmus, 14% had papilledema, and 17% had optic nerve atrophy. Only 27% of those surveyed had definite normal vision. Seventy percent of proven episodes of raised intracranial pressure (ICP) from CSF shunt malfunction had positive ophthalmologic evidence of the ICP. Shunt surgery is the first priority but may not restore normal ocular motility and visual function, requiring further compensatory interventions.

Cranial nerves IX (glossopharyngeal) and X (vagus) can also be affected with pharyngeal and laryngeal dysfunction (croupy, hoarse cry) and swallowing difficulties.[176] Apneic episodes and bradycardia may occur with a severely symptomatic Arnold-Chiari type II malformation and can potentially be life threatening. These severe symptoms usually appear within the first few weeks of life but can occur at any time.[153] The survival rate is only about 40% in these severe cases.[174] Those infants who do survive, however, have been noted to have gradual improvement in cranial nerve function. Neurosurgical posterior fossa decompression and high cervical laminectomies do not seem to substantially improve the outcome.[57,174] In contrast, surgical decompression of the Arnold-Chiari malformation has been shown to be beneficial for the intervention of progressive upper and lower limb spasticity.[57]

Spasticity

The muscle tone of infants and children with MM can range from flaccid to normal to spastic. Stack and Baber[187] found that some upper motoneuron signs were present in approximately two thirds of children with MM whom they examined; however, only about 9% had true spastic paraparesis. The remainder of this group had predominantly a lower motor neuron presentation with scattered upper motor neuron signs (e.g., flexor withdrawal reflex). In the group of children without upper motor neuron signs, most had totally flaccid paralysis below the segmental level of their spinal lesion, but a small percentage had normal tone. In contrast, Mazur and Menelaus[117] stated that approximately 25% of individuals with MM exhibit lower extremity spasticity because of associated CNS abnormalities. As with other CNS conditions, spasticity and abnormal reflexes can affect function, positioning, or comfort in individuals with MM.

Progressive Neurologic Dysfunction

Minor improvements in strength or development of sensation, although rare, can occur even as late as the fourth decade of life. More important, however, is the deterioration from neurologic changes that are due to treatable complications. These changes that can occur in the upper or lower extremities or trunk include loss of sensation, loss of strength, pain at the site of the sac repair, pain radiating along a dermatome, initial onset or worsening of spasticity, development or rapid progression of scoliosis, development of a lower limb deformity not explained by previously documented muscle imbalance, or change in bowel or bladder sphincter control. Such changes can be due to CSF shunt obstruction, hydromyelia (syringohydromyelia, syrinx), growth of a dermoid or lipoma at the site of repair, subarachnoid cysts of the cord, or spinal cord tethering and can be detected via MRI. Cord tethering occurs from scarring of the neural placode or spinal cord to the overlying dura or skin with resultant traction on neural structures.[180] One third of children with MM will require surgery for a tethered spinal cord. The tethered cord syndrome may also result from other congenital anomalies, including thickening of the filum terminale and diastematomyelia.[154] An acquired cause of progressive spinal cord dysfunction that has been reported is severe herniation of intervertebral disks into the spinal canal, causing compression of the cord.[177] Lais and associates[96] stated that slow deterioration of neurologic function is not uncommon.

Progressive deterioration of spinal cord function resulting from any of these causes can be arrested by neurosurgical interventions. Deterioration of the gait pattern is frequently the first complaint by patients or their parents. Because physical therapists see these patients more frequently than physicians or surgeons, the therapist is often the first to observe these changes and should be alert to the need for immediate referral to a neurosurgeon. Owing to this risk of progressive loss of function, it is essential that individuals with MM be closely monitored throughout their life span.

Seizures

Seizures have been reported to occur in 10% to 30% of children and adolescents with MM.[168] The etiologies of seizure activity include associated brain malformation, CSF shunt malfunction or infection, and residual brain damage from shunt infection or malfunction. Anticonvulsant medications, which are necessary for prophylaxis against seizures, unfortunately can also accentuate any cognitive deficits or dyscoordination already present.[54,155] Untreated seizures, however, can lead to permanent cognitive or neurologic functional loss, or even death.

Neurogenic Bowel

Fewer than 5% of children with MM develop voluntary control of their urinary or anal sphincter.[153] Abnormal or absent function of spinal segments S2 through S4, which provide the innervation to these organs, is the primary reason for the incontinence. The anal sphincter can be flaccid, hypotonic, or spastic, causing different manifestations of dysfunction during defecation. Anorectal sensation is also often impaired, preventing the individual from receiving sensory input of an imminent bowel movement so that he or she can take appropriate action. In addition to incontinence, constipation and impaction can also occur. Fortunately, conscientious attention to individually designed bowel programs can have effective results, minimizing problems of incontinence and constipation.[92,153,201,202] The presence of a bulbocavernosus or anal cutaneous reflex (indicating that lower motor neuron innervation of the sphincter is present) is highly predictive of success with a bowel training program.[92] King and associates[92] also reported that instituting bowel training before age 7 years correlates with improved outcomes by means of better compliance. When stool incontinence is interfering with a child's school and social activities, the physical therapist may want to become involved to help address the problem. Incontinence often affects feelings of self-image and competence, which in turn can affect performance in other activities pertinent to the therapist's intervention program.

Neurogenic Bladder

Just as the nerves to control defecation are impaired, so are the nerves that produce bladder control. Eighty-five percent of patients with MM have an underlying neurogenic bladder.[53] A variety of different types of dysfunctions can occur, depending on the relative tonicity of the detrusor muscle in the bladder wall and the outlet sphincters of the bladder. Bladder intervention strategies are directed toward the point or points of dysfunction. The goal is infection-free social continence with preservation of renal function. Retrograde flow of urine from the bladder up the ureters to the kidneys, termed *vesicoureteral reflux,* can occur without symptoms or signs being evident until the later stages of irreversible renal failure. Inadequate emptying of the bladder with residual urine retention within the bladder provides an optimal culture medium for bacteria, causing recurrent urinary tract infections and possible generalized sepsis. Adequate bladder intervention is therefore an essential component of health maintenance and normal longevity of people with MM, in addition to being an important social issue.

The bladder dysfunction can begin in utero (5% to 10% of newborns with MM show evidence of hydronephrosis and reflux). This is typically due to dyssynergy between the detrusor muscle of the bladder and the external urethral sphincter (i.e., the bladder contracts but the sphincter does not relax to allow the flow of urine out of the urethra). This results in high bladder pressures and vesicoureteral reflux. It is now standard practice for all newborns with MM to undergo an extensive urologic workup in the neonatal period. Early implementation of intermittent catheterization in infancy helps to prevent later problems with detrusor muscle function from overstretching the bladder wall.[14]

For most individuals, effective bladder intervention is achieved with clean intermittent catheterization on a regularly timed schedule for voiding. A small catheter is inserted into the bladder through the urethra until urine begins to flow. After the bladder is empty or urine stops flowing, the catheter is withdrawn, cleansed with soap and water, and stored for future use. It has been shown that the clean method of catheterization, as opposed to sterile technique, is sufficient for prevention of urinary tract infections.[153] The risk of injury to the urethra or bladder from clean intermittent catheterization is sufficiently low to allow young children to be taught to catheterize themselves. Mastery of the technique is usually achieved by age 6 to 8 years depending on the severity of the involvement.[179] Supplementation of clean intermittent catheterization with medication is frequently recommended to decrease bladder storage pressure and improve urinary continence and achieve intervention goals by altering spastic detrusor muscle function (e.g., oxybutynin [Ditropan], tolterodine [Detrol]), spastic sphincter function (phenoxybenzamine), or hypotonic

sphincter function (ephedrine, pseudoephedrine, phenylpropanolamine). Medications may be delivered orally, transdermally, and via intravesicular injection. Botulinum toxin A is a relatively new addition to the therapeutic armamentarium for these patients, and onabotulinumtoxinA (Botox) has recently received US Food and Drug Administration approval for use in patients with neurogenic bladder conditions. Overnight catheter drainage has also been effectively used in a select group of patients with small, poorly compliant neurogenic bladders to decrease the risk of upper urinary tract deterioration. It is recommended that individuals with MM have regular follow-up with a urologist every 6 months until age 2, and yearly thereafter, throughout the life span.[91]

The physical therapist must be aware of the method used for urine drainage as it relates to wheelchair positioning, transfer techniques, and orthoses so that assistive devices do not interfere with effective performance of urine drainage techniques. It is important to allow adequate time for patients with MM to attend to bowel and bladder needs before and after examination and therapy sessions so that they are comfortable and continent during physical activities. Discomfort from a distended bladder or rectum may impair performance. Patients are often not assertive in requesting necessary time for personal care, and therapists should encourage them to do so to avoid embarrassing accidents.

Sexual function is also impacted, especially by diminished or absent sensation of the genitalia. For males, a transposition of the ilioinguinal nerve to the dorsal nerve of the penis can provide sensation for sexual activity.[144] The procedure has helped to contribute to the quality of life and overall adjustment to adulthood for adolescents and young men who have undergone the procedure.

Skin Breakdown

Decubitus ulcers and other types of skin breakdown have previously been shown to occur in 85% to 95% of all children with MM by the time they reach young adulthood.[172] Okamoto and associates[141] performed an extensive study of skin breakdown on 524 patients with MM who were 1 to 20 years old. Perineal decubiti and breakdown over the apex of the spinal kyphotic curve (gibbus) occurred in 82% of children with thoracic level lesions, 62% of those with high lumbar level lesions, and 50% to 53% of those with lower level lesions. Lower limb skin breakdown was approximately equivalent in all lesion level groups (30% to 46%). Although the sites and causes of skin breakdown varied among lesion level groups, the overall frequency was the same. The prevalence of skin breakdown at any one time was 20% to 25% for the population sampled. Several etiologies for skin breakdown were ascertained. In 42% of the children, tissue ischemia from excessive pressure was the cause. In 23% a cast or orthotic device produced the breakdown. In another 23% urine and stool soiling produced skin maceration. Friction and shear accounted for another 10%; burns accounted for 1%; and 1% of causes were not recorded or were unknown. Other authors have described additional causes of skin breakdown.[172] These include excessive weight bearing over bony prominences of the pelvis as a result of spinal deformity, obesity, lower limb autonomic dysfunction with vascular insufficiency or venous stasis, and tenuous tissue postoperatively over bony prominences. One might expect at least modest improvement in the prevalence of skin breakdown for children with MM owing to improved wheelchair cushion technologies and seating options;

however, no recent studies have been performed to assess the breadth or severity of this problem.

Age is an important factor in the etiology of skin breakdown. Shurtleff[172] showed that young children who are not toilet trained have the greatest problem with breakdown from skin soiling (ammonia burns). Young active children with MM have the greatest frequency of friction burns on knees and feet from scooting along rugs, hot water scalds, and pressure ulcers from orthoses or casts. Older children, adolescents, and young adults develop skin breakdown over lower limb bony prominences (even if they did not have ulcers when they were younger) from the increased pressure of a larger body habitus, asymmetric weight bearing resulting from deformities, abrasions of the buttocks or lower limbs resulting from poor transfer skills, improperly fitted orthoses, and lower limb vascular problems. Strategies for prevention taught by the physical therapist therefore should be directed to the likely causes of skin breakdown for the age of the individual. Helping the child develop an awareness of his insensate extremities is important during the early years in order to later develop independence with personal care. Mobley and associates[133] found that preschoolers with MM exhibited altered self-perception as evidenced by their drawing fewer trunks, legs, and feet on self-portraits than their able-bodied peers.

Pressure sores can result in a delay or loss of ambulation.[42] Skin breakdown of the insensate foot is often a cause of decreased ability to ambulate. Predictors of skin breakdown resulting from excessive pressure during ambulation or while resting feet on wheelchair footrests are foot rigidity, nonplantigrade position, and surgical arthrodesis.[116] Clawing of the toes may be another contributing factor that also affects shoe wear. To avoid foot ulcerations, physical therapists should examine and document foot deformity, level of sensation, and pressure areas. The insensate foot can be protected with appropriate footwear, orthotics, or surgery. Total contact casting can be useful in healing ulcers.[25]

Obesity

Obesity is a common and difficult multifactorial problem occurring in children with MM that complicates orthotic and wheelchair fitting and can affect independence and proficiency with transfers, mobility, and self-care activities. For children who are ambulatory, a greater expenditure of energy is required to participate in physical play activities, so it is likely that less time will be spent engaged in physical play and that more sedentary activities (e.g., watching television) will be adopted. Children with mobility limitations, whether they are ambulatory or wheelchair mobile, may not be well accepted by able-bodied peers when they attempt to participate in physically challenging play, or they may feel conspicuous because they have difficulty keeping up. The likelihood of participation under these circumstances is diminished. As obesity develops, this further complicates participation and negatively affects self-image, creating an undesirable cycle perpetuating weight gain. In addition, children with MM probably are at a disadvantage physiologically. Studies evaluating the caloric intake required for children with MM[173] have shown that the intake should be lower than for able-bodied obese peers. This is probably not just a function of the decreased activity level of children with MM. Decreased muscle mass of large lower limb muscle groups diminishes the ability to burn calories (i.e., the basal metabolic rate of children with MM is probably lower than normal). This is consistent with the observation that children with high lumbar and thoracic lesions have greater problems with obesity. Decreased muscle mass coupled with lower extremity inactivity reduces the daily caloric needs such that a young adult who uses a wheelchair as his primary means of mobility will need fewer than 1500 calories a day to maintain his current weight.[109] Liusuwan and associates[105] showed that in a population of children ages 11 to 21, children with MM, when compared to a control group, have significantly less lean body mass measured using dual energy x-ray absorptiometry as well as significantly lower resting energy expenditure measured with an open-circuit indirect calorimeter.

An easy and readily available mechanism to screen for obesity in the general population is height-weight ratios; however, arm span–weight ratios are more appropriate for monitoring individuals with MM. Shurtleff[173] noted that height-weight ratios are not useful in children with MM because of their short stature, decreased linear length secondary to spine or lower limb deformities, and decreased growth of paretic limbs. He recommended monitoring individuals with MM by measuring serial subscapular skinfold thickness, linear length measured along the axis of long bones to take into consideration hip and knee joint contractures, arm span measured with a spanner, and weight measured on a platform scale (subtracting the weight of the wheelchair or adaptive aids). Results should be recorded on National Center for Health Statistics percentile charts.[61] Arm span measurements should be adjusted using correction factors to avoid underestimating body fat content: 0.9 arm span for children with no leg muscle mass (thoracic and high-lumbar levels), 0.95 arm span for those with partial loss of muscle mass (mid- and low-lumbar lesions), and 1.0 arm span for children with minimal or no muscle mass loss. Del Gado and associates[37] reported that in comparison to a control group, 32 children with MM had significantly lower stature, higher weights, and greater subcutaneous fat deposits in their trunks, the latter being associated with cardiovascular disease risk factors.

Weight control is not just a function of decreased caloric intake for children with MM, however, and must involve a regular exercise program. The challenge of the physical therapist is to find age-appropriate physical activities for their clients that are fun and at which they can succeed; in this way, physical activity is positively reinforced and a lifelong pattern of engaging in such activities is developed. Liusuwan and associates[104] piloted a program combining behavioral intervention, exercise, and nutrition education that showed promise as a method for improving health and fitness of adolescents with spinal cord dysfunction.

FOREGROUND INFORMATION

AGE-SPECIFIC EXAMINATION AND PHYSICAL THERAPY INTERVENTION

There are issues of particular importance for specific age groups with MM. Intervention should be provided to keep pace with the normal timing of development.[18,171] Throughout the life span, it is important to keep in mind the overall picture of the needs of the patient and family. The medical problems and the number of health care professionals involved in the care of individuals with MM can be overwhelming. Many members of other disciplines, in addition to the physical therapist, may also be making requests of the family's time. Each professional should prioritize his or her goals relative to those of other disciplines and coordinate planning so that the demands placed on the patient and the family are realistic. It is best to work as a team with the family and other disciplines to integrate appropriate intervention programs into the patient's daily routine. In addition, if conflicting information is provided to parents, they often become confused and may lack appropriate information to set realistic goals for their children and adolescents (e.g., goals for mobility, self-care, employment, and independent living). Consequently, multidisciplinary team collaboration with the family is important to establish appropriate goals and expectations.

The following sections focus on special considerations throughout the life span. Four age groups are discussed: infancy, preschool age, school age, and adolescence. Participation restrictions that are typically present, as well as the causes and impact of activity limitations on expected life roles, are discussed for each of the four age groups. Examination and evaluation of body structure and function, activity limitations, and participation restrictions, along with recommendations for ongoing monitoring, typical physical therapy goals, intervention, and strategies to prevent secondary impairments and activity limitations, are also discussed. In addition, typical secondary participation restrictions and activity limitations encountered during adolescence and their impact on the transition to adulthood are discussed in the section on adolescence and transition to adulthood. The information presented in this latter section has important implications for preventive intervention during childhood and adolescence to minimize the incidence of acquired impairments and activity limitations that often surface later in life.

It is important to keep in mind that the interaction of a multitude of impairments may affect an individual's functional performance, yet only a few key impairments are discussed for each age group. The reader is referred to the previous section on impairments for a more thorough discussion of other factors. Similarly, only key examination and intervention strategies that are specific to a given age category are discussed in each section. Common goals across the life span are to prevent joint contractures, correct existing deformities, prevent or minimize the effects of sensory and motor deficiency, and optimize mobility within natural environments.[117]

Infancy

Typical Participation Restrictions: Causes and Implications

The multiple impairments and overwhelming medical needs of a newborn with MM may interfere with parent-infant interaction. Parents are often afraid to handle their infant with MM, and the opportunities for handling and interacting with their child may be further limited by medical complications. Parents and extended family members may be cautious in handling the infant, resulting in decreased stimulation. Naturally occurring opportunities for early environmental stimulation, observation, exploration, and social interaction also may be limited as a result of somatosensory and motor deficits, hypotonia, and visual deficits. Family and infant interaction may be further impeded by the additional parental duties required (e.g., bowel and bladder intervention), frequent medical visits, and hospitalizations for complications.

The achievement of fine motor and gross motor developmental milestones is usually delayed during infancy because of multiple impairments, including joint contractures and deformities, motor and sensory deficits, hypotonia, upper limb dyscoordination, CNS dysfunction, visual and perceptual disorders, and cognitive deficits. The lack of normal infant movements, combined with impaired sensation, decreases kinesthetic awareness and inhibits perceptuomotor development. Independence with early ADLs such as holding a bottle or finger feeding is also negatively affected by impairments resulting from MM, especially swallowing disorders, upper limb dyscoordination, and visuoperceptual deficits.

Examination of Impairments

As discussed in Chapter 5, therapists must be aware of normal physiologic flexion of the hips and knees when assessing newborns. Limitations of up to 35° are present in normal newborns. These contractures may be more pronounced at birth in the infant with MM after prolonged intrauterine positioning of the relatively inactive fetus. Physiologic flexion spontaneously reduces in able-bodied infants from the effects of gravity and spontaneous lower limb movements. Physiologic flexion of infants with MM typically does not spontaneously reduce because of decreased or absent spontaneous lower limb activity secondary to muscle weakness. Consequently, contractures may develop even in children with sacral level function if they lack full strength of the gluteal muscles.

Two primary orthopedic concerns during this period are to identify and manage dislocated hips and foot deformities. Early orthopedic intervention of these deformities results in improved potential for standing balance and more timely achievement of motor milestones such as sitting and walking.[115,124] Achieving a plantigrade foot position is important regardless of ambulatory prognosis. Plantigrade alignment is optimal for shoe fit, positioning and weight distribution in sitting, and stability when bearing weight for standing pivot transfers or ambulation.

When assessing muscle tone in infants, either the Harris Infant Neuromotor Test[63] (HINT) or the Movement Assessment of Infants[29] is a useful tool. Hypotonia is typical in infants with MM, even if sacral level function is present.[207] Poor head control, delayed neck and trunk righting, automatic reactions, and low trunk and lower limb muscle tone are typical. A mixture of hypotonia and spasticity may be present in the limbs. It is important to distinguish between voluntary and reflexive movements when assessing muscle function.

One of the key physical therapy considerations in managing the newborn with MM is to establish a reliable baseline of muscle function. This baseline is important for predicting future function and for monitoring status. In addition, it is important to identify muscle imbalance around joints and existing joint contractures that are unlikely to reduce spontaneously.

In the newborn, muscle function is assessed before and after surgical closure of the back to determine the extent of motor paralysis. Sidelying is usually the position of choice for testing the newborn to avoid injury to the exposed neural tissue.[163] The state of alertness must be considered and documented when testing newborns or infants. Repeated examinations may need to be conducted at different times of the day to observe the infant's muscle activity in various behavioral states. Optimal performance cannot be elicited if the infant is in a sleepy state. Muscle activity is best observed when the infant is alert, hungry, or crying. Several techniques can be used to arouse the drowsy infant, including assessing limb ROM, rocking vertically to stimulate the vestibular system, and providing tactile and auditory stimulation.[69,163] Ideally, the infant's spontaneous activity should be observed in supine, prone, and sidelying positions before the examiner starts handling the infant. Handling the infant may suppress spontaneous activity. Movement can often be elicited through sounds, visual tracking, reaching for toys, tickling, placing limbs in antigravity positions to elicit holding responses, and moving limbs to end-range positions to see if the infant will move out of the position.[69] For older infants, muscle activity can be observed, palpated, and resisted in developmental positions. If leg movements in myotomes caudal to the MM occur concurrently with performance of general movements in infants, functional neural conduction through the MM is implicated.[184]

Therapists often do not record specific strength grades for infants and young children. Instead, either a dichotomous scale (present or absent) or a 3-point ordinal scale (apparently normal, weak, or absent) is often advocated.[135,146,163] This 3-point scale, however, lacks sensitivity and predictive validity.[135] In contrast, specific manual muscle test strength scores (grades 0 to 5) have been found to provide useful information for infants and young children with MM and are predictive of later function.[120] Consequently, when strength is assessed manually, we recommend using the full manual muscle testing scale, regardless of age. The estimated quality of the examination should also be recorded, indicating the examiner's degree of confidence in the results based on the child's level of cooperation. Neck and trunk musculature should be graded as "normal for age" if the child is able to perform developmentally appropriate activities.[88]

Testing sensation in infants and young children presents special challenges. Complete testing of multiple sensory modalities is not possible until the child has acquired sufficient cognitive and language abilities to accurately respond to testing.[163] Parents can often provide useful information to help focus on probable insensate areas. It is best to test the child in a quiet state. Testing with a pin or other sharp object should begin at the lowest level of sacral innervation and progress to more proximally innervated dermatomes until a noxious response is noted (e.g., crying or facial grimace).

Teulier and associates[194] used a motorized treadmill to evaluate stepping responses of infants with MM from 1 to 12 months of age. Treadmill practice elicited steps and increased motor activity. Holding infants with MM on a moving treadmill resulted in 17% more motor activity of their entire body during the year than holding them on a nonmoving treadmill. Infants with MM stepped less than typically developing infants (14.4 versus 40.8 steps/minute), however, and they were less likely to produce alternating steps than typically developing infants at any age level. Responses were affected by lesion level but varied markedly among infants because of other confounding factors such as shunt revisions, medications, joint and ligament structures, and family support resources. Infants with the highest lesion levels (L1–3) exhibited a very low step rate over time, which the authors proposed was due to marked delays in muscle strength and limb control, rather than an innate lack of capacity as three of four infants in this group developed the ability to walk with walkers by 44 months of age. In contrast to interlimb stepping patterns, the within-limb step parameters of infants with MM were quite similar to typically developing infants. The authors plan to study the potential for treadmill practice to produce positive outcomes for infants with MM such as increasing muscle and cardiovascular strength, bone density, and neuromotor control required for upright locomotion.

Ongoing Monitoring

During the first year of life, it is important to monitor joint alignment, muscle imbalance, and the development of contractures. Typical lower limb contractures that develop are hip and knee flexion contractures combined with external rotation at the hips. Children with weak or absent hip musculature often lie in a "frog-legged" position with the hips flexed and externally rotated and the knees flexed. Consequently, these muscle groups are typically in a shortened position. It is important to closely monitor ROM and muscle extensibility during periods of rapid growth. Soft tissue growth typically lags behind skeletal changes, resulting in decreased extensibility. Stretching exercises should be initiated early on, if indicated, when contractures are relatively flexible and respond well to intervention. If orthoses or night-positioning splints are used to correct orthopedic deformities, the fit of these devices should be monitored to prevent skin breakdown.

Changes in muscle tone and muscle function are observed with progressive neurologic dysfunction. Baseline measurements, therefore, are essential, and these parameters should be closely monitored. Therapists should also watch for behavioral changes, decreases in performance, and other subtle signs of shunt malfunction (see Box 23.1) or seizure disorders. Motor development must also be observed to determine whether an infant is keeping pace with normal developmental expectations. Abnormalities in any of these areas should be reported to the child's primary care physician.

Typical Physical Therapy Goals and Strategies

During the newborn period, physical therapists must be sensitive to the feelings and needs of parents and other extended family members who are learning to cope with the overwhelming problems of a child with MM. Parents go through a period of tremendous adjustment. They are required to meet the demands of a normal infant, plus deal with the extensive medical and surgical needs of their newborn and adjust to the long-term implications of their child's multiple impairments. Not all instructions may be assimilated at any one time given the large amount of information to which parents are asked to attend. Often instructions must be reviewed and reinforced during subsequent visits. Written instructions should be provided to augment verbal explanations.

If ROM is limited, parents should be instructed in positioning techniques. It is optimal to maintain ROM by means of positioning because little additional time is required of the family. If contractures do not resolve with positioning, or if contractures are not supple, parents should also be instructed in stretching exercises and soft tissue mobilization techniques. It is usually most efficient to perform stretching exercises and soft tissue mobilization techniques in conjunction with diaper changes.

For infants who exhibit hypotonia, parents should be instructed in handling techniques to facilitate head and trunk control. Techniques advocated for children with hypotonic cerebral palsy[21] are often beneficial. Parents should be encouraged to provide sitting opportunities for the infant to facilitate the development of head and trunk control. Additional head and trunk support are often required in high chairs, strollers, and car seats. If motor development is significantly delayed and requires intervention, optimal handling techniques and treatment methods to improve posture and motor control discussed in the Infancy section in Chapter 19 in this text are potentially applicable to this population as well. Therapeutic interventions and adaptive equipment should ideally be planned to keep pace with the normal timing of development so that the child is provided with typical developmental experiences. During the latter half of the first year, preparatory activities for mobility are indicated. Emphasis should be placed on balance, trunk control, and facilitating an upright posture as the child progresses through the developmental sequence.

Prevention of Secondary Impairments and Activity Limitations

Parents should be instructed in proper positioning, ROM, and handling techniques with the lower limbs in neutral alignment to prevent the development of contractures. If the hips are dislocated or subluxed, parents should be instructed in proper positioning, double diapering, and the use of a night-positioning orthosis, if indicated.[158,162] If surgery is indicated to relocate hip dislocations (see previous section on orthopedic deformities), it is generally performed after 6 months of age. Foot deformities are generally treated through serial casting or positioning splints.

Parents should also be instructed to inspect insensate skin areas during diaper changes and dressing for signs of pressure or injury. Parents need to understand the importance of skin inspection and that insensate areas should be inspected on a daily basis throughout the life span.

Toddler and Preschool Years

Typical Participation Restrictions: Causes and Implications

The achievement of fine motor and gross motor developmental milestones continues to be delayed. Mobility is typically impaired in this population owing to orthopedic, motor, and sensory deficits. As the child nears the end of the first year of life, it is important to provide opportunities for environmental exploration. If the child does not have an efficient, effective mode of independent mobility by the end of the first year, provision of a mobility device is indicated.

Environmental exploration is essential for the development of initiative and independence. Limited early mobility may result in a lack of curiosity and initiative and may negatively affect other aspects of development.[15,27,175] If a toddler does not have an effective means of independently exploring and interacting with the environment, he or she may learn to be passively dependent. The negative influence of limited early mobility on personality and behavior development can persist throughout life. Passive-dependent behavior is a commonly observed personality trait of adolescents and adults with MM.

Limited mobility also negatively affects socialization, especially interaction with other children. If a stroller is used as the primary mode of community mobility beyond the normal age of weaning a child from a stroller, other children will view the child with MM as a "baby." Play opportunities are also limited if a child does not have an effective means of mobility.

Independence with ADLs is often impaired in this population because of fine and gross motor impairments, upper limb dyscoordination, and CNS dysfunction. Children who are not independent with ADLs may miss out on normal childhood experiences (e.g., play time) while waiting for others to assist them with basic skills. Their self-esteem may also be negatively affected if other children tease them regarding their dependency.

It is important that parents, child care personnel, and preschool teachers be aware of other motor deficits that are often exhibited in this population, such as poor eye-hand coordination. The potential impact of these deficits on functional performance in handwriting and the acquisition of ADL skills such as feeding and dressing should be realized so that reasonable goals can be established and the use of appropriate adaptive equipment implemented.

Examination and Evaluation of Impairments and Activity Limitations

By the end of the first year, ROM is expected to be within normal limits. If limited ROM persists, it is important to distinguish between fixed and supple contractures, determine muscle extensibility, and evaluate orthopedic deformities to determine whether they are fixed or flexible.

To assess strength, functional muscle testing techniques are advocated for children 2 to 5 years old because they may not cooperate with traditional test procedures.[69,146] Functional activities that are helpful in determining the strength of key lower limb muscle groups include gait observations, heel- and toe-walking, climbing up and down a step, one-legged stand, toe touching, squat to stand, bridging, bicycling while supine, the Landau position, prone kicking, the wheelbarrow position, sit-ups, pull to sit, and sitting and standing push-ups. It is often possible for young children to cooperate with isolated muscle actions by having them push against a puppet to show how strong they are. To elicit the cooperation of older preschoolers (3- to 4-year-olds), it is often helpful to name the muscle and describe its "job" (the muscle action). The children think that the muscle names are humorous, maintaining their attention. Asking children to have the muscle do its "job" makes strength testing more understandable.[65] We have found it possible to obtain objective, reliable measures of strength from children as young as 4 years of age using handheld myometry techniques.[69] The degree of confidence regarding whether the child's optimal performance was elicited should be recorded.

Once the child is 2 years of age, light touch and position sense can usually be assessed by eliciting tickling responses or having the child respond to the touch of a puppet. Other sensory modalities can ordinarily be accurately tested once the child is 5 to 7 years old. The accuracy of responses often must be double-checked because of short attention span and response perseveration. Two sensory testing techniques minimize perseveration of responses. The first is to randomly alternate between testing light touch and pinprick and have the child identify the type of sensation. The second is to have the child point to the spot that was touched and correctly state when no area was touched.

Fine and gross motor development should be measured using appropriate standardized tests such as those discussed in Chapter 2 of this text. Examination of ADLs should focus on what the individual actually does on a daily basis, in addition to what she or he is capable of doing. If independence with ADLs is limited, appropriate adaptations and interventions should be implemented to foster independence. The Functional Activities Assessment[142,185,186] provides specific ADL performance data for MM (Fig. 23.7). Items may be scored by direct observation or by parent report. Assistive devices required to perform a given task are also documented. The "Can" and "Does" scoring format permits the examiner to record what the child can do versus what the child actually does on a regular basis. In addition, if the child is directly observed performing the task, the degree of independence and the time to complete the task are recorded.

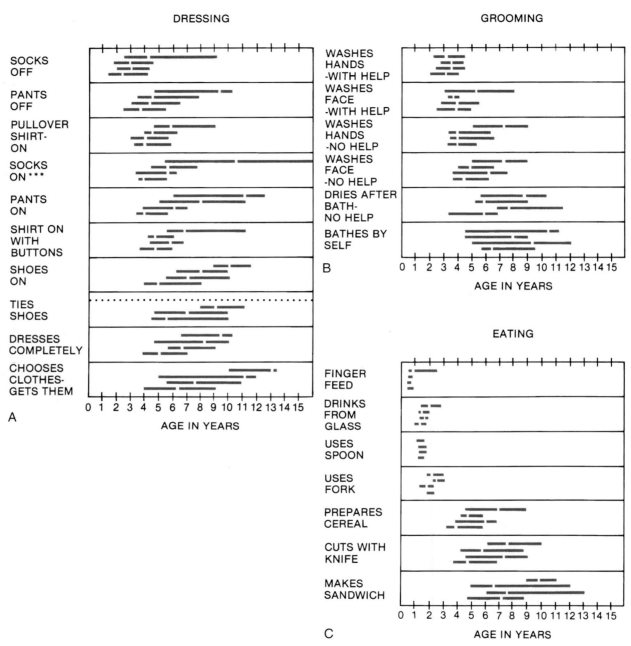

FIG. 23.7 Functional activities assessment. The age at which 20%, 50%, and 80% of a group of 173 children with MM learned dressing (A), grooming (B), and eating (C) skills is indicated by the beginning of, space between (white space), and end of the black bars, respectively. Triple asterisks indicate that this group never achieved an 80% learning proportion. Dotted line indicates activity was attempted with this group. The bars in each category represent, from top to bottom, (1) thoracic and L1–L2; (2) L3 and mixed lesions, L2–L4; (3) L4–L5; and (4) sacral-level groups. All data were recorded as the child achieved the skill during the 2.5-year period of the study, within 4 months of entering the study, or when the caretaker entered a specific date of achievement in the child's diary. These charts were created from data published by Okamoto and associates[142] and Sousa and associates.[186] (From Shurtleff DB, editor: *Myelodysplasias and exstrophies: significance, prevention, and treatment.* Orlando, FL: Grune & Stratton, 1986.)

Ongoing Monitoring

Joint alignment, muscle imbalance, contractures, posture, and signs of progressive neurologic dysfunction should continue to be monitored. Contractures that seem insignificant during childhood may become functionally limiting once the individual has adult-sized body proportions. For example, knee extension contractures can interfere with the ability to maneuver in a wheelchair.

Typical Physical Therapy Goals and Strategies

Joint alignment, contractures, muscle strength, and postural alignment should continue to be treated as necessary. Proper positioning in sleeping and sitting should continue. If stretching or strengthening exercises are indicated, it is often helpful to involve other family members in the exercise program so that the child does not feel singled out. For ambulatory candidates with weak hip and knee musculature, strengthening activities may be beneficial if the child is cooperative. In addition to traditional posture exercises,[88] many play activities promote strengthening and the development of good posture.[48] The use of therapy ball techniques to strengthen postural muscles is also beneficial. Muscle reeducation techniques, such as functional electrical stimulation and biofeedback, are useful to teach muscles to function in new ROM after stretching exercises. Electrical stimulation has also been found to be beneficial in increasing strength and enhancing functional performance in this population.[85]

During the preschool years, the focus is on improving the independence, efficiency, and effectiveness of ADLs and mobility. Development of independence with dressing and feeding should be encouraged. Appropriate guidance should be provided so that parents have age-appropriate expectations. It is important for young children to actively participate in skin inspection, bowel and bladder intervention, donning and removing orthoses, wheelchair intervention, and other ADL tasks. Teaching these skills early on and actively involving the child facilitates independence and incorporation of these activities into the daily routine. As a result, these extra responsibilities required of the child with MM become as natural as other ADLs such as brushing teeth. Waiting to introduce tasks until the child is older often is met with resistance, especially when the child observes that siblings do not have the same requirements.

By kindergarten age, children without disabilities are able to dress and toilet themselves (with the exception of some fasteners), eat independently, and be mobile.[49] These skills must be emphasized at an early age in children with MM so that they achieve independence by the time they begin school. A wide range of age of achievement of independence with ADLs is evident in this population when examining the normative data provided on the Functional Activities Assessment (see Fig. 23.7). This wide variability in age of achieving skills within a given motor level suggests that a significant percentage of children are delayed in ADL skill acquisition because of attitudes and expectations. Fay and associates[49] suggested that these delays may be partially caused by low parental expectations and protective attitudes, perceptions that it is faster for the parent to perform the task, and parental difficulty accepting the reality of the child's activity limitations. Showing parents the ADL normative data for children with MM and promoting positive parental expectations of independence are beneficial. It is important for parents to positively reinforce the child's attempts to be independent so that she or he is motivated to

achieve. It is also important to help the parents understand how incontinence retards their child's normal sexual exploration, learning, and social inhibitions that normal preschool children learn. Alternative opportunities should be offered to children with MM.[22]

Skin inspection and pressure relief techniques should be taught early so that they are incorporated into the daily routine. Proper intervention of lower limbs and joint protection techniques should be taught to avoid injury of insensate areas when learning how to perform ADLs such as transfers. The impact of sensory deficits on functional performance should be kept in mind during gait training and when teaching other functional tasks.

Provision of an effective means of independent mobility is essential for young children. Consequently, if a child does not begin maneuvering effectively within the environment by 1 year of age, alternative means of mobility must be considered to achieve independent home and short-distance community mobility.[27,175] Mobility options should be explored and implemented as frequently as is needed so that the child is able to actively participate in normal childhood activities. Various mobility options are available from manual devices such as a caster cart to electric wheelchairs. Electric wheelchair use has been found to be feasible and beneficial for children as young as 24 months of age.[27] If a wheelchair is indicated, it is important to present this option to the parents in a positive way. Based on our clinical experience, the use of a wheelchair does not preclude walking. In fact, children who use wheelchairs at an early age generally are more interested in mobility, independence, and environmental exploration. Consequently, they tend to be more independent in all forms of mobility later in life. For example, Ryan and associates[159] recommended introducing a wheelchair as early as 18 months to enable children to keep up with their peers, boost self-confidence, facilitate independence, and increase activity levels. A more recent case report[110] suggests that it is potentially feasible to train infants as young as 7 months old to safely operate a power mobility device.

Preparatory activities for mobility are indicated for 1- to 2-year-olds. Emphasis should be placed on balance, trunk control, and facilitating an upright posture. For ambulatory candidates, once the child begins to pull to stand, the need for orthoses to improve weight-bearing alignment should be considered. It is important to anticipate future ambulatory needs when recommending orthoses to maximize their utility.

For children with high-level lesions (thoracic to L3), preparatory activities for wheelchair mobility should be emphasized (e.g., sitting balance, arm strengthening, transfer training, wheelchair propulsion, and electrical switch operation if indicated). The focus of wheelchair training for toddlers and preschoolers with high-level lesions should include mobility, environmental exploration, safety, and transfer skills. Household distance ambulation using a parapodium, HKAFO, knee-ankle-foot orthosis (KAFO), or reciprocating gait orthosis (RGO) may be attempted, but energy expenditure is very high. Consequently, wheelchairs are generally used for community mobility of children with thoracic to L3 motor function, particularly once body proportions increase.

Effective biped ambulation is feasible for toddlers and preschoolers with L4 and below motor function. They will require wheelchair skills as older children, however, to participate in sports and prolonged activities. It is essential to maintain adequate ROM and to emphasize an upright posture so that weight-bearing forces are properly distributed and muscles can function at their optimal length. Therapeutic activities that promote trunk control and balance are beneficial. Children with lumbar level lesions will require upper limb support for walking. In general, a reverse-facing walker is best when the child is learning to walk because it allows the child to be upright and minimizes upper limb weight bearing. Reverse-facing walkers have been found to promote better postural alignment than anterior-facing walkers.[106] At the point an upright gait is established, the child can be advanced to forearm crutches.

If children with sacral level motor function require upper limb support to begin walking, a reverse-facing walker is also usually best to minimize upper limb weight bearing. Alternatively, forearm crutches can be used if the child is able to walk upright while manipulating the crutches. Children with L5 and S1 level lesions often abandon their upper limb aids when they are young and their center of mass is low to the ground. Upper limb aids may still be indicated for endurance and to decrease trunk sway when walking long distances, for balance when walking on rough terrain, or to minimize the stress on weight-bearing lower limb joints. The need for upper limb aids should be reevaluated when the child is older and body proportions and environmental demands have changed.

The use of positive reinforcement is often recommended for this population to enhance cooperation with examination procedures and intervention programs. In general, food is not an appropriate form of reinforcement because obesity is often a concern. Verbal reinforcement is preferred at this age.

Prevention of Secondary Impairments and Activity Limitations

Individuals are at risk for joint contractures when there is muscle imbalance around joints, when a substantial portion of the day is spent sitting, when there is a prolonged period of immobilization or bed rest, following surgery, and during periods of rapid growth when soft tissue growth may lag behind skeletal changes. It is important to closely monitor individuals with MM during these periods so that intervention can be initiated early on, if needed, when contractures are still flexible and respond well to intervention. Early detection and intervention of contractures can prevent fixed deformities and stretch weakness of overlengthened muscles. Similarly, the importance of skin inspection of insensate areas, use of pressure relief cushions, and sitting push-ups for pressure relief should be emphasized at an early age so that these preventive measures become routine. Daily monitoring of insensate areas can be taught at an early age by jointly inspecting the skin and verbalizing that there are no red areas. Body image can be promoted by playing games that involve touching and finding body parts.

Habitual postural positions that contribute to deforming forces should be discouraged. It is essential to emphasize an upright posture when a child is learning to walk. If children are permitted to stand and walk in a crouched posture, habits become established and it is difficult to teach a more upright posture because of the development of secondary impairments (e.g., joint contractures and stretch weakness of excessively lengthened muscles). Therapists should closely observe joint alignment and posture when a child is standing. Postural deviations that look insignificant when a child is young are often magnified once body proportions increase.

School Age
Typical Participation Restrictions: Causes and Implications

Independence with ADLs often continues to be impaired in this age group. Children who are not independent with ADLs may miss out on normal childhood experiences (e.g., playtime or recess) while waiting for parents or teachers to assist them with basic skills. Their self-esteem may continue to be negatively affected if other children tease them regarding their dependency.

Mobility limitations are magnified once a child begins school because of the increased community mobility distances and skills required. Advanced mobility skills are needed because of environmental barriers such as curbs, ramps, uneven terrain, and steps. Ineffective or inefficient community mobility can further reinforce dependent behaviors if other children carry his or her schoolbooks and lunch tray or push the wheelchair.

The negative effects of limited mobility and physical limitations on socialization become more apparent at this age. Play and recreational opportunities are restricted if a child does not have an effective method of mobility. Often children with MM are excluded from recess or physical education class. Consequently, they miss out on opportunities for social interaction. Even if they are included in these activities, often their involvement is peripheral (e.g., serving as the score keeper during physical education class). Mobility limitations, dependency with ADLs, difficulties with toileting, and the difficulty of managing adaptive equipment often interfere with other aspects of peer interaction, such as going over to friends' houses to play or spending the night with friends.

Finally, it is important that parents and teachers be aware of perceptuomotor, visuoperceptual, and sensory deficits. The potential impact of these deficits on writing speed, legibility, and accuracy; the efficiency and effectiveness of performing ADL skills; problem solving; and cognitive abilities should be realized so that reasonable goals can be established and the use of appropriate adaptive equipment can be implemented. Multiple hospitalizations or medical complications can also negatively affect school performance.

Examination and Evaluation of Impairments and Activity Limitations

As with younger children, joint alignment, strength, muscle imbalance, contractures, muscle extensibility, and posture should continue to be monitored. Other parameters that should be assessed include sensation, coordination, fine motor skills, ADLs, mobility, gait, body awareness, and functional skills.

Reliable, sensitive, objective measures of strength can be obtained in school-age children.[65] We recommend that objective methods of strength examination, such as handheld myometry, be used to serially monitor strength of individuals with MM who are old enough to cooperate (typically age 4 or older). Stationary isokinetic or strain gauge devices can also provide objective measures of strength, but these devices are not available in the typical clinic or school setting.

Independence with ADLs should be assessed. In addition to the basic ADL skills evaluated in the Functional Activities Assessment, the school-age child's ability to carry items and assist with basic household chores should be evaluated. The physical therapist also assesses the adequacy of clearance, duration, frequency, and reliability of performance of wheelchair push-ups. A nurse usually evaluates bowel and bladder function and the degree of continence. It is important that the physical therapist understand these and degree of independence with bowel and bladder function, however, because positioning, adaptive equipment, and mobility issues can often restrict independence with bowel and bladder intervention programs.

The home, school, and community environments should be accessible so that individuals with MM can participate fully in all activities. The Americans with Disabilities Act of 1990 mandates access to all buildings, programs, and services used by the general public in the United States. Even partial exclusion from a school program can have lasting negative effects on a student's social and emotional development.[8] Providing accessibility to the entirety of school, home, and community activities lets individuals with MM know that they have the same opportunities and rights of access as everyone else. Limited access broadcasts a message of exclusion and estrangement. Both physical and social barriers to participation must be addressed. For a more thorough discussion of evaluating environmental accessibility in the school setting, see Baker and Rogosky-Grassi.[8] Community accessibility should also be evaluated. Ideally, the patient should have access to the community school, church, grocery and drug stores, post office, bank, cleaners, stores and shopping malls, library, restaurants, theaters, sports arenas, hospital, physician's office, work environment, and public transportation. Streets, sidewalks, crosswalks, and parking lots should also be accessible.

Ongoing Monitoring

Joint alignment, muscle imbalance, contractures, posture, and signs of progressive neurologic dysfunction should continue to be monitored. As school-age children mature, they should become more responsible for daily inspection of insensate skin areas when they are bathing and dressing. Appropriate performance of pressure relief strategies should also be monitored. Areas of skin breakdown should be noted so that appropriate adjustments in equipment and preventive behaviors can be implemented or reviewed.

School-age children should be observed closely during periods of rapid growth because they are at risk for loss of function as a result of cord tethering. Parents and teachers should be made aware of signs of progressive CNS complications so that they know when to refer the child to a primary care physician.

Typical Physical Therapy Goals and Strategies

The stretching and strengthening strategies discussed for the two previous age groups also apply to the school-age child. Improving the flexibility of low back extensor, hip flexor, hamstring, and shoulder girdle musculature should be emphasized. When possible, stretching and strengthening exercises should also be incorporated into the physical education program. It is important that children with MM participate in physical education classes and sports activities in a meaningful way. As noted earlier, if children dependent on braces and crutches learn wheelchair skills and use at an early age, they will not be depressed and perceive wheelchair use as a failure when they arrive at adolescence.

Proper positioning while sleeping and sitting should continue. In the classroom, seating should provide stability and symmetric alignment. Feet should be flat on the floor or on wheelchair footrests. The seat and desk height should be adjusted to fit the child's body proportions. The desktop should be tilted up to improve neck and upper trunk alignment. Appropriate cushioning should be provided. The child's chair should be positioned in the room so that the teacher and blackboard can easily be viewed while maintaining neutral alignment, without having to turn in the chair.

If a child has not achieved independence with a given ADL task by the age at which 50% of the normative group achieved independence on the Functional Activities Assessment, the child's performance should be assessed to determine if adaptive equipment is required or if further interventions are indicated. Goals for ADL performance should include efficiency in addition to independence. If the child is not as efficient as the primary caretaker, the caretaker will most likely perform the task. The target goal, therefore, is for the child to be able to perform the task as efficiently as the primary caretaker. Showing parents the ADL normative data for children with MM and promoting positive parental expectations of independence are beneficial (see Fig. 23.7). It is important for parents to positively reinforce the child's attempts to be independent so that he or she is motivated to achieve. Pressure relief techniques should be incorporated into the daily routine. Joint protection measures should also be implemented early on to prevent the development of future degenerative changes.

Once children with MM begin school, it is important that they have an independent, efficient, and effective means of mobility for home and long community distances. Alternative means of mobility may need to be considered for long distances to ensure that children with MM are able to keep up with their peers and still have energy left to attend to classroom activities. Various mobility options should be evaluated according to the criteria outlined in Box 23.2 to determine the most effective means of mobility for a given environment. Community-level wheelchair and ambulation skills should be taught, emphasizing efficiency and safety. Community, home, and school environments should be assessed to determine if there are architectural barriers that interfere with daily activities. It is essential for normal social development to permit accessibility to all school, home, and community activities, including recess, physical education, and field trips.[8]

A functional environment should be created at home and school by removing obstacles and adapting the environment to facilitate efficient and independent function. Adaptive equipment and effective mobility devices should be provided to maximize function. Community mobility skills may need to be practiced to facilitate independent function. Endurance training may also be indicated to ensure that the individual has sufficient endurance and efficiency to function effectively in all activities.

Recreation and physical fitness are important for physical, psychological, and social reasons. Psychosocial benefits of participation in recreational activities include enhancing confidence and self-esteem, increasing socialization, improving group participation skills, providing a means of exercising in a more normal way, and increasing interest and motivation in maintaining flexibility, strengthening, and endurance. In contrast, perceived physical restrictions result in a sedentary lifestyle, potentially predisposing these individuals to problems with obesity and degenerative diseases. It is important to stimulate a lifelong interest in fitness and recreation. In addition, community resources, feasibility of transportation, and the family's lifestyle must be taken into account.

Recreation activities must be carefully selected to ensure that they are beneficial and feasible yet enjoyable so they will be continued on a regular basis. Ideally, recreation activities should

---

BOX 23.2 Feasibility of Wheelchair and Biped Ambulation: Criteria for Evaluation

Household Distances

Endurance
Adequate to go between rooms in house?
Adequate to get to yard and car?

Efficiency
Record heart rate and calculate energy expenditure.
Record normal and fast household walking speeds.
Is fast pace adequate for emergency situations?
Is normal pace practical for everyday activities?

Effectiveness
Independent with all transfers?
Able to carry, reach, lift, and climb?
Able to perform activities of daily living?
Able to go forward, backward, sideways, and turn?

Safety
Has good stability and balance?
Observes joint and skin protection?
Able to maneuver around obstacles?
Safe on smooth surfaces and rugs?
Safe when turning?

Accessibility
Maneuvers in and out of house independently?
Necessary household rooms accessible?
Emergency exit routes accessible?

Community Distances

Endurance
Sufficient at a functional speed for average community distances (e.g., going to school, store, medical appointments, and social activities)?
Adequate for play and recreational activities (e.g., playground, park, beach, theater, sports arenas, sports participation)?
Adequate for long-distance community distances (e.g., shopping mall, zoo, concert, sporting events, hiking)?

Efficiency
Record heart rate and calculate energy expenditure.
Record normal and fast walking paces.
Adequate speed to cross intersections?
Is typical pace practical for community distances?

Effectiveness
Independent with all transfers?
Able to maneuver in all directions?
Able to climb and step over obstacles?
Able to carry packages and groceries?
Able to reach and lift items from shelves?

Safety
Has good stability and balance?
Observes joint and skin protection?
Safe on wet or slippery surfaces?
Able to maneuver around obstacles?
Able to maneuver in congested areas?
Safe on uneven terrain, curbs, inclines, and steps?

Accessibility
Maneuvers in and out of car and bus independently?
Necessary community buildings accessible?

---

incorporate forms of aerobic exercise along with socialization. It is important for individuals with MM to be involved in regular aerobic exercise to maintain their physical fitness and effectively control their weight. Recreational and physical fitness goals include maintaining and improving flexibility, strength, endurance, aerobic capacity, cardiovascular fitness, and coordination and controlling weight. Low-impact aerobics are preferred to minimize stress on joints. Aerobic exercise videos have been developed for individuals with disabilities. Swimming is an ideal sport for this population because they are often able to be competitive with their able-bodied peers and there is minimal stress on joints (www.brighthub.com/education/special/articles/44574.aspx). Other low-impact activities include cycling, rowing, cross-country skiing, roller and ice skating, and aerobic dance (www.cureourchildren.org/sports.htm).

Verbal reinforcement or implementation of a token economy system to earn special privileges is preferred at this age to enhance cooperation with examination procedures and intervention programs. As mentioned above, food is not an appropriate form of reinforcement.

Prevention of Secondary Impairments and Activity Limitations

Deficits that may appear insignificant during childhood often become magnified once an individual has adult body proportions, resulting in activity limitations and discomfort (e.g., low back pain resulting from an increased lumbar lordosis and hip flexion contractures). Joint protection is also important, beginning in early childhood. Joint trauma from excessive stress is cumulative over the life span. Children do not typically complain of pain, and children with MM may not be able to reliably detect pain in insensate areas. Consequently, sources of excess joint stress must be identified by carefully observing children while they perform ADLs and transfers, walk, and propel their wheelchair. Permitting school-age children to assume responsibility for daily skin inspection checks with supervision prepares them for independence in adolescence.[151] One method of teaching careful skin inspection involves letting the child locate a small colored adhesive dot that is placed randomly on insensate skin.

Children and their parents should be involved as much as possible in the decision-making process and intervention for their disability. The rationale for assistive devices and therapeutic interventions should be explained so that they agree with intervention plans and become knowledgeable regarding acquisition of medical care and services, rather than being passive recipients.

Adolescence and Transition to Adulthood
Typical Participation Restrictions: Causes and Implications
If normal stages for early childhood development have not been successfully accomplished, adolescence can present a crisis. The preparation of individuals with MM for a successful transition into adult life must be based on developmental concerns and timely issues from infancy through all stages of development to young-adult life.[151] Adolescence brings expanded domains of travel for individuals with MM. School buildings become larger, with more

environmental barriers for people with physical disabilities. To keep up with peers, community mobility must include mobility skills to travel long distances quickly and efficiently between classrooms, out to athletic fields as a participant or spectator, around shopping malls, and into crowded movie theaters, dances, and nightclubs. Independent adult living also requires mobility and balance skills that permit completion of advanced ADL tasks such as cooking, cleaning, clothes washing, shopping, yard work, house and equipment maintenance, driving, riding on public transportation, and going to work. Children who have gotten by with slow, inefficient ambulation skills using cumbersome adaptive equipment or who have had basic wheelchair mobility on level surfaces but suddenly cannot handle ramps, hills, curbs, and uneven ground find themselves lagging behind their peers. Nearly all of the adults in a study of 30 individuals with MM[72] required referral to a physical therapist to address advanced mobility or equipment issues. It has been the observation of the authors that many adolescents and young adults do not have sufficient mobility skills to succeed independently in the community and must play catch-up to achieve their functional potential. The price paid for this delayed development of functional community mobility and lack of independence is social incompetence, dependence for advanced living skills, and unemployability, all of which must subsequently be addressed once mobility skills are improved. It is also important to train for competence and self-reliance. Blum and associates[18] reported that young people with MM who perceived that they were overprotected had less happiness, lower self-esteem, higher anxiety, lower self-perceived popularity, and greater self-consciousness.

Changes in functional mobility skills often occur concurrently with the rapid changes of adolescence. Individuals who have previously been ambulatory often become more reliant on a wheelchair. Dudgeon and associates[45] reported that adolescents with MM often exhibit changes in ambulation that are not explained by progressive complications. They suggested that these changes reflect adaptation of mobility to new environmental and social demands that require different speed, accessibility, and energy demands than those encountered in childhood. If orthotic stabilization of the hip, knee, or both is required, it is unlikely that adolescents with MM will maintain community ambulation; instead, most become nonambulators.[45] Brinker and associates[23] reported a decline in the ability to walk in 11 of 35 adults with sacral level MM (19 to 51 years old). Of the 34 adults who were initially community ambulators, 5 had become household ambulators, 2 were nonfunctional ambulators, and 4 were nonambulators. The one adult who had been a household ambulator became a nonambulator. The most common reasons for their declining ambulatory status were foot ulcerations, infections, and amputations. Wheelchair transfer skills have also been observed to decline during the transition from adolescence to adulthood. In a study of 30 adults with MM who had thoracic through sacral level motor function, the mobility status for 43% had declined since previous examinations performed during adolescence.[72] Several potential factors can play a role in this decreased function.

Changes in body proportions and body composition occur throughout the growing years, but the rate of these changes is accelerated dramatically during adolescence.[69] Increases in limb length affect the torque generated by muscles because of altered muscle length and resistance force moment arms. In addition, increases in height raise the location of the center of mass higher off the ground, making upright balance more difficult and energy expenditure greater to perform mobility tasks. Changes in body composition also alter the biomechanics of movement and affect performance. The relative percentage of force-generating muscle to fat and bone tissue changes the ratio of force-producing tissue to the load of the limbs. The development of obesity often occurs during adolescence and can further accentuate these changes. Banta[10] stated that body mass increases by the cube or volume whereas strength increases only by the square or cross-sectional area. The inevitable result during the adolescent growth spurt is that walking efficiency declines as the energy demands increase. Furthermore, during the adolescent growth spurt, the rate of skeletal growth exceeds the increase in muscle mass; the latter catches up after skeletal growth slows in late adolescence. Decreased flexibility of the trunk and two-joint limb muscles is often observed as part of this process. Normal adolescents frequently become clumsy during this period of adjustment while learning how to coordinate their longer limb lengths and increased muscle mass. Adolescents with MM already have a mechanical disadvantage and are consequently more susceptible to dyscoordination and decreased flexibility. It is likely that these developmental changes contribute to the decline in mobility that often occurs in adolescents with MM.

Progression of the neurologic deficit is another potential cause for decline in mobility function, and adolescents are particularly at risk during rapid periods of growth. Forty percent of the participants in our adult follow-up study[72] had lower limb strength loss compared with previous strength examinations as adolescents. Twenty-seven percent had a reduction in lower limb sensory perception. The greatest motor and sensory losses occurred in the group with lesions at L5 and below—the individuals with the most function to lose. In addition, 10% of study participants demonstrated upper limb strength loss. Progressive neurologic loss, therefore, appears to be an important factor in the changes in mobility status of many individuals during the transition from adolescence to adulthood.

Immobilization for intervention of secondary complications of MM can also contribute to decreased mobility skills. Decubiti, fractures, and orthopedic surgeries such as spinal fusions often require extended periods of immobilization with consequent disuse weakness, decreased endurance, and contracture development, all of which can decrease performance of mobility and transfer tasks.

Prolonged periods of bed rest are often necessary to heal decubitus ulcers to avoid bearing weight on pressure areas. Adolescents often have an increased incidence of decubiti compared with younger children. This is due to their increased body mass causing greater pressure over bony prominences around the buttocks and because of the development of adult sweat patterns in these areas. Fifty-six percent of the adults evaluated in our study[72] had a history of skin breakdown since their last examination as adolescents; nearly 17% had breakdown present at the time of the examination. An alarming number of these people had little insight into the causes or methods for preventing skin breakdown despite their previous care in a large multidisciplinary pediatric clinic. Even more disturbing was the fact that three individuals (10%) had sustained lower limb amputations since adolescence (two bilateral, one unilateral) as a result of nonhealing ulcers that had progressed to osteomyelitis. Clearly, functional mobility is affected by decubitus ulcers and especially by limb loss.

Musculoskeletal problems can also affect the mobility of adolescents. Progression of spinal deformities often occurs during the growth spurt or in conjunction with one of the neurologic complications previously discussed. Sitting and standing balance can be affected by these spinal changes, leading to decreased mobility and transfer skills. Spinal orthoses prescribed to maintain optimal postural alignment also limit trunk ROM and hip flexion, interfering with wheelchair transfers and moving from sitting to standing. Surgical fusion of the spine to correct deformity and prevent its further progression can lead to immobilization with its consequent effects on mobility described earlier. Lower limb fractures secondary to osteoporosis can also necessitate immobilization with increased risk of functional loss.

Adolescents often begin to develop degenerative changes of weight-bearing joints and overuse syndromes as a result of the excessive loading of these joints necessitated by their neurologic deficit. Joint pain, ligamentous instability, or tendinitis can further limit mobility capabilities. Fifty percent of the adult study participants[72] complained of joint pain, and 100% had joint or spinal deformities noted at the time of their examination.

Several other issues become important for the physical therapist to be cognizant of during adolescence. Independence with self-care and other daily activities is essential for normal socialization and for preparing individuals to lead normal adult lives. Bowel and bladder continence and independent intervention of bowel and bladder emptying are essential for social acceptance by peers and are even more critical at this stage because of the impact on dating, sexuality, higher education, employment, and independent living. Design and fit of wheelchair equipment, mobility aids, and orthoses affect independence with these tasks. Cosmesis is also a consideration with regard to equipment selection because body image and appearance become increasingly important issues during adolescence. Improper design or fit of equipment can significantly limit normal development in these areas.

Examination and Evaluation of Impairments and Activity Limitations

Based on the discussion of participation restrictions and their causes, the physical therapist should assess several impairments. Emphasis of specific impairments should be based on the known or suspected concurrent medical problems.

Joint ROM and muscle extensibility of two-joint muscles (especially hip and knee flexors) and trunk muscles should be assessed. Neck and low back motions are often restricted, particularly in adolescents and adults, because of muscle imbalance and poor postural habits. Joint swelling, ligamentous instability, crepitus, and pain with or without joint motion should be documented. If these conditions are progressive or severe enough to interfere with function, the patient should be referred to a physician for further evaluation and intervention. The distribution of degenerative joint changes should be noted with regard to performance of mobility tasks and obesity to determine the contribution of abnormal joint stresses to joint pain and dysfunction.

Muscle strength should continue to be monitored for all major upper and lower limb muscle groups. When progressive neurologic dysfunction is suspected, coordination testing and serial grip strength measurements can also be helpful. Posture and trunk balance in sitting and standing (for ambulators) should be assessed. Real or apparent leg length discrepancy may be present in individuals with foot and ankle deformities, lower limb contractures, unilateral or bilateral hip dislocation, or pelvic obliquity related to spinal curves.

Thorough examination of bed mobility, floor mobility, wheelchair mobility and transfers, and appropriateness and fit of wheelchair equipment is essential for wheelchair users. Endurance and effectiveness of mobility should be assessed to determine whether the individual's current mode of mobility is practical for community-level function. Box 23.2 provides further detail regarding important areas to assess. When orthoses are needed to maintain proper alignment or to facilitate efficient ambulation, the physical therapist must assess their appropriateness and fit. Boxes 23.3 and 23.4 provide further information regarding lower limb orthoses used in this population.

Ongoing Monitoring

Given the multitude of potential problems that can occur during adolescence and adulthood, comprehensive examinations should continue on at least a yearly basis, and potentially more frequently when problems are suspected or known to be present. Without regular reexamination, these individuals often fall through the cracks and endure permanent loss of

---

BOX 23.3   Indicators for Lower Limb Orthoses

Foot Orthoses and Supramalleolar Orthoses

Advantages
Permits full active dorsiflexion and plantar flexion
Maintains the subtalar joint in neutral alignment
Provides medial and lateral ankle stability

Motor Function
S1 to "no loss"
Must have adequate toe clearance and sufficient gastrocnemius/soleus strength to provide adequate push-off and decelerate forward movement of tibia

Indications
Unequal weight distribution, resulting in skin breakdown, foot deformities, or abnormal shoe wear
Medial and lateral ankle instability, resulting in balance problems, especially difficulty traversing uneven terrain
Poor alignment of the subtalar joint, forefoot, or rearfoot

Ankle-Foot Orthoses (Standard AFOs and Ground-Reaction Force AFOs)

Advantages
In general, the ground-reaction force (see Fig. 23.6) is advantageous for this population. The proximal trim line can be extended medially to control genu valgus. The ground-reaction force AFO also facilitates push-off and knee extension during the stance phase and improves static standing balance. The ground-reaction force AFO has a patellar tendon-bearing design. This design distributes pressure across a broad area, preventing skin breakdown and lower leg deformities, which are common when traditional AFO anterior straps have been worn for an extended period of time. If traditional AFOs are used in this population, the anterior straps must be well padded.

Motor Function
L4 to S1
Weak or absent ankle musculature
Knee extensors at least grade 4

BOX 23.3   Indicators for Lower Limb Orthoses—cont'd

Indications

Medial and lateral instability of knee or ankle
Insufficient knee extension moment (ground-reaction force AFO)
Lack of or ineffective push-off
Inadequate toe clearance
Crouched gait pattern

Knee-Ankle-Foot Orthoses

Advantages

If unable to maintain upright posture because of joint contractures or muscle weakness, or if the knee joints are unstable, KAFOs are indicated.

If the knee joint is primarily required for medial and lateral stability so the knee joint is unlocked, or if there is potential to progress to ambulation with the knee joints unlocked, it is best to incorporate the ground-reaction force AFO component into the KAFO design to provide the advantages listed earlier in the AFO section.

Motor Function

L3 to L4
Weak knee musculature
Absent ankle musculature

Indications

Medial and lateral instability of knee
Weak quadriceps (grade 4 or less)

Reciprocating Gait Orthoses or Hip-Knee-Ankle-Foot Orthoses

Advantages

The reciprocating gait orthosis (RGO) cable system facilitates hip extension during stance phase and hip flexion during swing phase by coupling flexion of one hip with extension of the opposite hip.

Release of both cables permits hip flexion when sitting.

The RGO reduces the energy required for ambulation compared with walking with traditional KAFOs.

Motor Function

L1 to L3 (some centers also advocate for thoracic level)
Weak hip flexion is required to effectively operate the cables.

Indications

Unable to maintain an upright posture with the hip joints extended
RGO is indicated to facilitate hip extension and swing phase.

Thoracic-Hip-Knee-Ankle-Foot Orthoses, Parapodiums, or Verlos

Advantages

Upright positioning for high-level lesions
Generally for exercise walking only

Motor Function

Thoracic to L2. Walking is usually nonfunctional for these high-level lesions because of the high energy expenditure required and the slow, cumbersome walking pace.

Indications

Limited distance mobility
Upright positioning
"Exercise" walking

BOX 23.4   Lower Limb Orthotic Specifications, Objectives, and Examination Criteria

Orthotic Specifications

Shoe Heel Height

A low heel (¼ to ½ inch) may improve balance by shifting the center of gravity forward in a person with a calcaneal weight-bearing position.

A low heel (¼ to ½ inch) may decrease knee hyperextension by shifting the center of gravity forward.

A high heel shifts the center of gravity too far forward and causes balance problems in a person with weak plantar flexors.

A high heel may result in increased hip and knee flexion, combined with an increased lordosis or swayback posture.

Ankle Angle

Ideally molded or set in 5° plantar flexion with a rigid anterior and posterior stop to reduce energy requirements and to increase the knee extension moment as long as toe clearance is adequate and the knee does not hyperextend. If foot clearance is a problem, set angle more acutely, no higher than neutral, at the minimum angle required to clear the foot during swing phase. Plastic orthoses must enclose the malleoli to effectively resist dorsiflexion and provide a rigid anterior stop.[100]

Do not set ankle angle more acutely than a neutral angle unless trying to control a knee hyperextension problem because the energy expenditure will increase.

Keel

Generally, keel should be rigid to the distal aspect of the metatarsal heads (to decrease energy expenditure by providing a longer lever). The plastic should extend to the end of the toes to maintain proper toe alignment, but it must be pulled thin distal to the metatarsal heads to provide a flexible toe break. If a flexible toe break is not provided, the knee extension moment may be excessive, resulting in knee hyperextension. The alternative is to trim the plastic at the metatarsal heads, but the toes are not adequately supported in this latter case.

Extending a rigid keel out to the end of the toes may be indicated to increase the extension moment at the knee. Do not extend the rigid lever arm to the end of the toes if it results in knee hyperextension or difficulty with balance (especially on stairs).

Plantar Aspect

Posting may be required to accommodate the hindfoot and rearfoot position so that the subtalar joint is maintained in a neutral position, yet a plantigrade position is achieved.[200]

Posting helps distribute the weight across the plantar aspect and prevents varus or valgus.

Straps

All straps should be well padded.

An instep strap angled at 45° helps hold the heel in place and prevents pistoning and friction.

KAFOs should have a three-point pressure distribution.

A combined suprapatellar and infrapatellar strap distributes the pressure best. A spider kneecap pad can also be used but results in greater shear forces through the knee joint.

An infrapatellar strap often deforms the lower leg when worn for a prolonged period of time because the pressure is not well distributed. The patellar tendon-bearing orthotic trim line is preferred in this population because the pressure is better distributed.

Orthotic Fabrication Objectives

Increase Medial and Lateral Stability

Mold in subtalar neutral position.[93,200]

Continued

BOX 23.4   Lower Limb Orthotic Specifications, Objectives, and Examination Criteria—cont'd

Proximal trim line should be sufficiently proximal and anterior to provide adequate leverage to control the ankle and to distribute pressure evenly.

Increase base of support and equalize weight-bearing forces by means of external posting.

Valgus or Pronated Foot

Post medially under first metatarsal head and medial aspect of calcaneus.

Flare posting medially to increase the base of support and to prevent deviation into valgus.

Varus or Supinated Foot

Post medially under first metatarsal head to accommodate supinated position of forefoot and equalize pressure distribution.

Zero posting under calcaneus (with lateral flare if needed) to prevent deviation into supination at heel strike.

Orthoses must sit level in shoes, and the shoes should be fastened securely so they do not slide on orthoses.

Decrease Energy Expenditure

Ankle angle ideally molded or set at 5° plantar flexion with rigid anterior stop (see ankle angle, earlier).

Distal trim line at metatarsal heads to provide a long rigid lever arm.

Provide adequate toe clearance and simulate push-off.

Plantar flexion stop, ideally set at 5° of plantar flexion if able to adequately clear toe without increasing knee flexion during swing phase (see ankle angle, earlier).

Generally a rigid dorsiflexion stop is required unless the patient has sufficient plantar flexor strength to control forward movement of tibia during stance phase.

Increase Knee Extension Moment

Ground-reaction force, patellar tendon-bearing orthosis.

Solid ankle, cushioned heel, or wedge heel anteriorly to move ground-reaction force forward at heel strike.

Rigid dorsiflexion stop set in 5° plantar flexion (see ankle angle, earlier).

Keel rigid to distal aspect of metatarsal heads to provide a long rigid lever and yet still permit a flexible toe break (see keel, earlier). An even greater extension moment can be provided by extending the rigid lever to the end of the toes. This is usually contraindicated, however, because it results in difficulties with balance (especially on stairs).

Prevent Knee Hyperextension

Prevent knee hyperextension by increasing knee flexion moment.

Flare heel posteriorly to move ground-reaction force behind knee joint axis at heel strike to produce a flexion moment.

Ankle set at neutral angle with rigid dorsiflexion and plantar flexion stop (if this does not adequately prevent knee hyperextension, the angle may need to be set more acutely, into dorsiflexion). The more acute the angle, however, the greater the energy expenditure.[93]

A low heel (¼ to ½ inch) may decrease knee hyperextension by shifting the center of gravity forward.

Keel rigid to the distal aspect of the metatarsal heads to provide a long rigid lever to decrease energy expenditure. Plastic must be pulled thin beyond this point, however, to provide a flexible toe break (do not extend the rigid keel to the end of the toes because this will increase the knee extension moment at push-off).

If knee hyperextension cannot be adequately controlled with previously described modifications, use KAFOs with knee extension stops.

Improve Pressure Distribution

Use total contact orthoses.

All straps should be well padded.

Bony prominences should be padded (e.g., mallecli, prominent naviculi, patellar tendon region).

Posting to equalize pressure distribution on foot and minimize pressure on malleoli and naviculi.

Patellar tendon-bearing orthosis distributes pressure better than a proximal strap.

KAFOs: the combination of a suprapatellar and infrapatellar strap distributes pressure most effectively.

Improve Balance

Adding a low heel (¼ to ½ inch) may improve balance by shifting the center of gravity forward in a person with a calcaneal weight-bearing position.

A high heel shifts the center of gravity too far forward and causes balance problems, particularly in a person with weak or absent plantar flexors.

Orthotic Examination Criteria

Check for pressure areas.

Heel must seat well in orthosis.

Check for rigid keel and flexible toe break.

Check knee alignment and congruency of knee joint axis.

All straps and bony prominences should be well padded.

Check medial and lateral alignment, and make sure the orthosis is posted properly with subtalar joint in neutral.

Check angle at ankle (anterior/posterior and medial/lateral).

Check anterior and posterior stops to make sure they adequately control motion, facilitate push-off, and permit toe clearance during swing phase.

Insert orthosis in shoe to check alignment. If molded properly, the orthosis should be able to balance and stand without support on a flat surface.

---

function that was avoidable. An unfortunate example was one of the adult study participants with a diagnosis of lipomeningocele and a neurosegmental classification of "no loss" as an adolescent. His lesion level was reclassified at an L5 level at the time of our study. His loss of neurologic function was caused by a recurrent lipoma on his spine that went undetected and was not surgically removed until permanent neurologic loss had occurred. This individual thought that because his original lesion was removed as an infant with preservation of his spinal cord function, he had no risk of future problems; therefore he did not seek medical care until neurologic loss was irreversible. Early detection of progressive muscle strength loss, scoliosis, progression of spasticity, or contractures by the physical therapist with timely referral to a physician familiar with the potential complications associated with MM, along with aggressive physical therapy to reverse lost function (see section on prevention of secondary impairments and activity limitations), can prevent this scenario. This patient's story underscores the need for all individuals with MM to be followed throughout life, even if there are seemingly no current problems or their lesion has been classified as "no loss" after surgical closure.

Typical Physical Therapy Goals and Strategies

Functional goals for adolescents and adults are based on a number of factors that have been discussed in preceding sections of this chapter. The section on outcomes and their determinants provides guidelines for outcome expectations based on neurologic system function. In general, the goal for all but the most severely involved patients is to achieve independent basic and community mobility skills. The physical therapist must, therefore, be aware of all environments, distances, and barriers the individual is required to negotiate to adequately prepare the patient for all eventualities. Instruction in advanced community skills, along with endurance training, is often indicated. Physical and occupational therapists often need to be involved with driver's education programs and with the provision of adaptive equipment required for driving.

Goodwyn[56] expanded the Functional Activities Assessment format to include adolescent skills required for independent living. The items were selected from existing adult-oriented skill achievement tests, and normative data were studied in this population. The Assessment of Motor and Process Skills (AMPS) was also studied in a group of individuals ranging in age from 6 to 73 years old (mean = 21.3 years) and was found to be a valid assessment of ADL performance.[94] The AMPS assesses motor and process skills in terms of efficiency, effort, safety, and level of independence. The Kohlman Evaluation of Living Skills[122] is also a useful screening tool for determining independence with adult living skills such as self-care, safety, health maintenance, money management, transportation, telephone use, and work and leisure activities. For adolescents and adults, the ability to lift and carry items such as a hot dish, grocery bags, a laundry basket, and heavy household items is also important to assess. It is particularly important to observe safety issues and the use of proper body mechanics for advanced living skills. In addition, the maximum carrying distance should be determined and contrasted with functional demands. If independence and effectiveness with ADLs are limited, appropriate adaptations and interventions should be made to foster independence. Environmental adaptations or assistive devices required to perform functional tasks should be determined and specifically selected for application to social, educational, vocational, and work capacity requirements of the adolescent and adult. Vocational counseling and planning should begin early during the high school years. A social worker may need to assist the family with the transition to independent living because a mutually dependent relationship is often fostered by the intense lifelong involvement of parents and siblings in assisting the individual with MM. Recreation therapy may be used to assist with shopping for and purchasing personal items, use of public transportation, and developing appropriate adult leisure activities. Occupational therapy is useful to address advanced living skills such as cooking, cleaning, laundry, money management, and driver's training for appropriate candidates. A social worker can assist with locating accessible housing and obtaining appropriate support services for physical tasks that are too difficult for the patient. Depending on the practice setting, however, it may be necessary for the physical therapist to manage these areas. The expectation for individuals with MM who have intelligence in the normal range and sufficient motor function to care for themselves is the ability to thrive as an independent adult in our society. See Chapter 32 for more information on transition to adulthood.

Prevention of Secondary Impairments and Activity Limitations

The physical therapist plays an important role in anticipating the potential for functional loss when one of the medical complications of MM previously described increases the risk of secondary impairments. For example, when an adolescent undergoes a surgical procedure that requires extended bed rest, maintenance of muscle extensibility, joint ROM, and strength at the bedside followed by resumption of physical mobility tasks as soon as possible postoperatively can prevent long-term or permanent decline in mobility skills. Unfortunately, care providers are often not aware of these issues, and intervention is not instituted until it is too late to recover lost function. The physical therapist must serve as an advocate for the patient under these circumstances. Regular skin inspection continues to be important to monitor skin integrity. Another mechanism for preventing secondary impairments is education of patients and their parents regarding the fit, specifications, condition, and maintenance of their adaptive equipment. They should know how to monitor skin tolerance and the fit of adaptive equipment. They should also understand the rationale for equipment and design features that are recommended. Knowledgeable consumers can detect and report potential problems before they result in complications such as decubiti. They need to be aware of the potential consequences of poorly fitted equipment so that they can advocate for quality equipment. The majority of adults in our follow-up study had improperly fitted equipment or lacked equipment that was essential for optimal function. These adults were also unaware of proper equipment maintenance techniques.[72] As a result, many of them were functioning well below their capabilities and had skin breakdown, back pain, or joint pain as a result of poorly fitted orthoses or improper wheelchair design and seating.

OUTCOMES AND THEIR DETERMINANTS

Survival, disability, health, and lifestyles were investigated in a complete cohort of adults with MM in Cambridge, England.[77,138] Outcomes were investigated at age 35 for 117 individuals who were born between 1963 and 1971. Sixty-three (54%) had died, primarily the most severely affected. The mean age of the survivors was 35 years (range 32 to 38), and 39 of the 54 survivors had an IQ above 80. Sixteen could walk for community distances (50 meters or more) with or without aids. These 16 individuals all had a sensory lesion level at or below L3. Thirty had pressure sores, 30 were overweight, and only 11 were fully continent. In terms of independent living status, 22 survivors lived independently in the community, 12 lived in sheltered accommodations where help was available if required, and 20 needed daily assistance. Twenty of the survivors drove cars and another nine had given up driving. Thirteen were employed, with five of them being in wheelchairs. Seven females and two males had had a total of 13 children (none with visible MM). Hunt and colleagues[76] also reported that shunt revisions, particularly after the age of 2, were associated with poor long-term achievement in this same group of adult survivors with MM. Achievement was operationally defined according to their independent living status, employment, and use of a car. McDonnell and McCann[121] in a commentary to Hunt and associates' article reported more optimistic outcomes in terms of mobility and employment for shunt-treated survivors of MM in Belfast, Northern Ireland. Hunt[75] reported that only 50% of adults were capable of living independently based on a sample of 69, of whom 68% had normal intelligence. In a sample of 18 patients 16 to 47 years old in Japan, Oi and associates[140] reported that patients with spina bifida occulta (spinal lipoma) have a risk of neurologic deterioration whether or not they have undergone radical preventive surgery in infancy. This deterioration is primarily related to lower spinal functions, such as ambulation and bowel and bladder control, that likely result from tethered cord, reexpansion of the residual lipoma, or syringomyelia. In contrast, these authors reported psychological problems in patients with spina bifida aperta. Padua and associates[147] reported that adolescents with MM who have relatively mild activity limitations (i.e., they are able to walk and run) but who have urologic problems need psychological support to a greater extent than adolescents with severe activity limitations and limited independence. There are many factors that contribute to the observed outcomes.

The motor function present is an important factor for predicting outcomes. Common characteristics of each lesion level are described in this section. The functional motor level does not always correspond to the anatomic lesion level because of individual variations in nerve root innervation of muscles. The information presented here is intended to serve as general guidelines for expectations at a given level of motor function. Many factors besides muscle strength influence an individual's functional potential and result in variations of performance within a given lesion level group. These factors include age, body proportions, weight, sensation, orthopedic deformities, joint contractures, spasticity, upper limb function, and cognition. The relative contribution of these factors is highly individual, and a thorough examination and follow-up of each child is necessary to maximize potential capabilities.

Thoracic Level

Individuals with thoracic level muscle function have innervation of neck, upper limb, shoulder girdle, and trunk musculature, but no volitional lower limb movements are present. Banta[10] stated that at the thoracic level the orthopedic goals are to maintain a straight spine, level pelvis, and symmetric lower limbs. Neck, upper limb, and shoulder girdle muscle groups are innervated by the C1 to T4 spinal nerves; back extensors by the C2 to L4 spinal nerves; intercostals by the thoracic nerves; and abdominals by T5 to L1. Consequently, individuals with motor function at or above T10 have strong upper limbs and upper thoracic and neck motions, but their lower trunk musculature is weak. They have difficulty with unsupported sitting balance and may have decreased respiratory function. Sliding boards may be required to perform wheelchair transfers because of the combination of poor trunk control and upper limb dyscoordination.

Individuals with motor function at T12 have strong trunk musculature and good sitting balance and may have weak hip hiking by means of the quadratus lumborum (innervated by T12 to L3). Ambulation may be attempted for exercise at this level using a parapodium; however, it is generally not an effective means of mobility.[103] A wheelchair is required for functional household and community mobility.

Children with thoracic level lesions also tend to have greater involvement of other areas of the CNS, with corresponding cognitive deficits. Consequently, even though many of these people achieve independence with basic self-care skills and mobility by late childhood, they often require a supervised living situation throughout life. They are rarely competitively employed but often participate in sheltered workshop settings or perform volunteer work.[72]

High Lumbar (L1–L2) Level

Individuals with high lumbar motor function have weak hip movements. The iliopsoas muscle is supplied by nerve roots L1 through L4, with its primary innervation at L2 and L3. The sartorius muscle is supplied by L2 and L3 and the adductors by L2 through L4. With L1 motor function, weak hip flexion may be present, and with L2 motor function the hip flexors, adductors,

and rotators are grade 3 or better. According to Schafer and Dias,[162] unopposed hip flexion and adduction contractures are often present at the L2 motor level, and this muscle imbalance often results in dislocated hips. Short-distance household ambulation is possible with high lumbar innervation (L1 and L2) when body proportions are small, using KAFOs or RGOs and upper limb support. These children generally use a wheelchair for community distances. By the second decade of life, a wheelchair is typically the sole means of mobility commensurate with increased energy requirements and enlarged body proportions.[72,175]

The prognosis of children with high lumbar lesions for function and independent living as adults is similar to that of the thoracic group described earlier.[72] More individuals in this group, however, achieve independent living status (approximately 50%), but they are rarely able to maintain competitive employment as adults.

L3 Level

Individuals with L3 muscle function have strong hip flexion and adduction, weak hip rotation, and at least antigravity knee extension. The quadriceps muscle group is innervated by nerve roots L2 through L4. Children with grade 3 quadriceps strength usually require KAFOs and forearm crutches to ambulate for household and short community distances and a wheelchair for long community distances. By adulthood, most individuals with L3 level lesions are primarily wheelchair mobile.[72,178,190]

Approximately 60% of individuals with lesions at this level achieve independent living status as adults.[68] Despite their higher level of independence, only a small percentage (about 20%) actively participate in full-time competitive employment.[72]

L4 Level

At the L4 motor level, antigravity knee flexion and grade 4 ankle dorsiflexion with inversion may be present. The medial hamstrings are innervated by nerve roots L4 through S2, and the anterior tibialis is innervated primarily by L4 and L5, with some innervation from S1. An individual is considered to have L4 motor function if the medial hamstrings or anterior tibialis is at least grade 3. Calcaneal foot deformities are common at this motor level as a result of the unopposed action of the tibialis anterior muscle.[162] Knee extension is usually strong, and these individuals are generally functional ambulators with AFOs and forearm crutches. When first learning to walk, however, KAFOs, a walker, or both may be required. A wheelchair is often needed for long distances.

In the adult follow-up study that we conducted, only 20% of individuals with L4 motor function continued to ambulate as adults.[72] Many individuals stopped ambulation after their adolescent growth spurt. Others were unable to maintain ambulation because of ankle and knee valgus joint deformities and elbow and wrist pain resulting from years of weight bearing in poor alignment. To increase the likelihood of maintaining biped ambulation for individuals with L4 motor function throughout adulthood, upright posture should be emphasized when ambulating to minimize the weight-bearing stress on upper limb joints. Orthoses must be aligned properly and posted to support the ankle in a subtalar neutral position. If the ankle joint is malaligned, the knee joint position is adversely affected. It is essential to maintain the knee and ankle in neutral alignment when weight bearing. A flexed and valgus position should not be permitted. Ounpuu and associates[143] demonstrated that 30%

of the mechanical work occurs at the ankle during normal gait, underscoring the importance of controlling the ankle in order to provide proper alignment of the body to the ground reaction force. Often a patellar tendon-bearing, ground-reaction force orthotic design is optimal to protect the knee and increase the knee extension moment. The proximal medial trim line can be extended higher to provide additional medial knee support, if needed, to reduce a genu valgus deformity (see Fig. 23.4). Knee musculature should be strengthened to help maintain the knee in neutral alignment when weight bearing. Every effort should be made to progress ambulation to using AFOs and forearm crutches to allow short-distance ambulation to easily be combined with long-distance wheelchair mobility. Crutches can be transported on the wheelchair, and AFOs are optimal because, unlike KAFOs, they do not interfere with dressing or toileting and do not cause skin breakdown when sitting. The prognosis for independent living and employment is similar to that for the group with L3 lesions.

L5 Level

According to the IMSG criteria, classification of an L5 motor level is based on the presence of lateral hamstring muscles with at least grade 3 strength, and either grade 2 gluteus minimus and medius muscles (L4–S1), grade 3 posterior tibialis muscles (L5–S1), or grade 4 peroneus tertius muscles (L4–S1). Therefore an individual with an L5 motor level has at least antigravity knee flexion and weak hip extension using the hamstrings and may have weak hip abduction, as well as weak plantar flexion with inversion, strong dorsiflexion with eversion, or both. Weak toe movements may also be present. Hindfoot valgus deformities or calcaneal foot deformities are common as a result of muscle imbalance. Individuals with motor function through L5 are able to ambulate without orthoses yet require them to correct foot alignment and substitute for lack of push-off. A gluteal lurch is typically evident unless upper limb support is used. Bilateral upper limb support is usually recommended for community distances to decrease energy expenditure, decrease gluteal lurch and trunk sway, maintain symmetric alignment, protect lower limb joints, and improve safety. The need for upper limb support often becomes more apparent with increased height following growth spurts. Traversing uneven terrain is often difficult. A wheelchair may be required when there is a rapid change in body proportions (e.g., pregnancy) or for long distances on rough terrain. A bike is also useful for long community distances.

Approximately 80% of individuals with lesions at L5 and below achieve independent living status as adults.[72] About 30% are employed full time and an additional 20% part time, well below the average employment rate of the general adult population.

S1 Level

With muscle function present through S1, at least two of the following additional muscle actions are present: gastrocnemius/soleus (grade 2), gluteus medius (grade 3), or gluteus maximus (grade 2). Individuals with S1 motor function have improved hip stability and can walk without orthoses or upper limb support. A weak push-off is evident when running or climbing stairs. A mild to moderate gluteal lurch is often present. Vankoski and associates[199] documented the benefits of crutch use for this lesion level, which resulted in improved pelvis and hip kinematics during gait. Gait deviations and activity limitations are often more pronounced after the adolescent growth spurt. The toe musculature is generally strong. Foot deformities are less common at this level, but foot orthoses or AFOs may be required to improve lower limb alignment and permit muscle groups to function at a more optimal length. Medial and lateral stability at the ankle are required for adequate function of the plantar flexor muscles during push-off.[98]

S2, S2–S3, and "No Loss" Levels

Motor function is classified at the S2 level if the plantar flexor muscles are at least grade 3 and the gluteals grade 4. The only obvious gait abnormality present at this level is generally a decreased push-off and stride length when walking rapidly or running as a result of the decreased strength of the plantar flexor muscles. If all lower limb muscle groups have grade 5 strength except for one or two groups with grade 4 strength, the motor level is classified as S2–S3 according to the IMSG criteria. The term "no loss" is used if the bowel and bladder function normally and lower limb strength is judged to be normal through manual muscle testing. Functional deficits may be present, however, for individuals classified as having no loss. Foot orthoses are often used to maintain the ankle in the subtalar neutral position and optimize ankle muscle function by maintaining optimal muscle length.

EXAMINATION, EVALUATION, AND DIRECT INTERVENTIONS FOR MUSCULOSKELETAL ISSUES, MOBILITY, AND FUNCTIONAL SKILLS

There are three primary reasons for evaluating the individual with MM: (1) to define an individual's current status so that appropriate program planning can occur, (2) to identify the potential for developing secondary impairments so that preventive measures can be implemented, and (3) to monitor changes in status that could indicate progressive neurologic dysfunction. Because of the complexity of problems associated with MM, numerous dimensions of disability must be assessed by various disciplines. The physical therapist provides essential information to other team members for program planning and to monitor status. Careful documentation is important for communication among team members and for serial comparisons over time. General examination and intervention strategies will be discussed in this section. Considerations that are specific to certain age categories are discussed in the section on age-specific examination and physical therapy interventions.

Examination Strategies

The tests and measures typically used by physical therapists include ROM, muscle extensibility, joint alignment or orthopedic deformities, muscle tone, muscle strength and endurance, sensation, posture, motor development, ADLs, mobility skills, equipment needs, and environmental accessibility. It is important to follow standardized procedures, when available, that have good reliability and validity to permit comparison within and between individuals.[71,185,186] (Refer to Fig. 23.7 Functional Activities Assessment for ADL performance ranges of children with MM). If more than one measurement method exists (e.g., hip extension ROM), the specific method employed should be documented and used consistently. Comprehensive examinations should be conducted at regular intervals throughout the life span on all individuals with MM. In addition, to avoid potential biases it is recommended that therapists remain blind to previous results of the more subjective measures (e.g., manual muscle testing scores or gait deviations) until the examination is complete. Videos and photographs are often useful adjuncts to clinical examination of gait, joint deformities, and posture. These visual records provide an excellent baseline for comparison purposes if deterioration in status is suspected. It is beneficial to conduct examination of activities that are influenced by environmental or endurance factors (e.g., wheelchair mobility, gait, or ADLs) in more natural settings.

The IMSG recommends a comprehensive, multidisciplinary assessment for all individuals with MM, regardless of functional level, because they all are at risk for progressive neurologic dysfunction, as discussed earlier. The following examination intervals are recommended: newborn preoperatively, newborn postoperatively, 6 months, 12 months, 18 months, 24 months, and annually thereafter, continuing through adulthood.[174] Annual examinations are suggested to occur around an individual's birth date so that they are not forgotten. ROM, muscle extensibility, strength, endurance, coordination, and functional parameters should be monitored more closely during periods of rapid growth, when individuals with MM are at increased risk for loss of function. Family members and caregivers should be educated regarding symptoms of neurologic loss to help with monitoring. Preintervention and postintervention measurements should be obtained for individuals undergoing surgery or other therapeutic procedures. More frequent evaluation of specific goal attainment is indicated for individuals receiving ongoing therapeutic intervention. Mobility and independence with ADLs should be assessed when body proportions or environmental demands change to determine if the individual has the strength, endurance, coordination, and adaptive equipment required to function effectively.

Individuals with MM should be examined on at least a yearly basis by multiple disciplines at a comprehensive care center. It is important, however, for comprehensive care centers and local school and intervention settings to coordinate their examinations, goals, and intervention programs to avoid duplication of effort and to ensure appropriate prioritization of intervention goals. The use of the PDMS facilitates communication and coordination of services between team members. The School Needs Identification and Action Forms[158] also provide a useful format for identifying impairments, academic and activity limitations, and the remedial action recommended. The areas assessed by the school needs forms include health-related services required, physical intervention instructions, accessibility, safety and fire drills, preparation for school entry, educational rights and related services, academic difficulties, psychological evaluation, perceptuomotor deficits, visuoperceptual deficits, self-help skills, social acceptance, social and emotional issues, parent and school relationships, transitional services, and other needs. The School Function Assessment (SFA) measures needs and abilities during school-related functional tasks for kindergarten through sixth-grade students.[30] The SFA consists of three sections: (1) participation in a variety of school activity settings, (2) task supports required (physical and cognitive/behavioral assistance and adaptations), and (3) activity performance in school-related functional activities (e.g., using materials, following rules, and communicating needs). The School Function Assessment Technical Report available at www.pearsonassessments.com/NR/rdonlyres/D50E4125-86EE-43BE-8

001-2A4001B603DF/0/SFA_TR_Web.pdf describes the standardization sample of 676 students, including 363 students with special needs from 112 sites in 40 US states and Puerto Rico.

Intervention Strategies

Once primary and secondary impairments, activity limitations, and participation restrictions are identified through a comprehensive examination and evaluation, the functional significance must be determined to plan appropriate intervention strategies. Intervention of an impairment is indicated if it currently interferes with function or if the deficit can progress to a point where it may negatively affect future function. Intervention is also indicated if the efficiency, effectiveness, or safety of performance can be improved. Strength, endurance, and efficiency of performing tasks should be emphasized. Weight-bearing joints must be protected to prevent early onset of osteoarthritis and pain and to prolong mobility. In addition, the most efficient and effective means of mobility for a given environment should be determined. Goal setting for intervention must consider the impact of the multiple impairments discussed earlier on functional performance expectations. The cognitive, social, and behavioral issues discussed in the impairments section should also be considered.

Fay and associates[49] recommended three specific intervention approaches for developmental delays in this population. The first is developmental programming in which children are encouraged by parents, teachers, and therapists with a "high dose" of normal developmental activities in "at-risk" areas. The philosophy behind this approach is that supplemental early emphasis and practice in potential problem areas will minimize later deficits. These early intervention programs are often initiated for children with MM before measurable delays are identified. The second approach, remediation, is implemented once problem areas are clearly identified. This approach consists of repeating a set of graded tasks in the domain of concern. Improved performance through practice theoretically carries over into functional activities. The third approach is teaching compensatory skills. Compensation is often implemented when the other two approaches have not produced sufficient results or when the child is older or more severely impaired. This intervention approach involves identifying and developing strategies to help the child become as independent as possible or providing adaptive equipment to compensate for underlying problems and minimize disability in daily life.

Specific Examination and Intervention Strategies

Specific examination and intervention strategies as they pertain to strength, mobility, gait, and equipment issues are highlighted in this section because of the magnitude of the impact of these factors on function in this population, regardless of age or lesion level. Suggestions for impairment-specific parameters (e.g., ROM, orthopedic deformities, and sensation) were discussed in the section on impairments. Developmental issues were discussed in the section on age-specific examination and physical therapy interventions.

Strength

Upper limb, neck, and trunk musculature should be screened for weakness. If evidence of weakness exists, a more specific examination of strength should be conducted. For individuals with thoracic or high lumbar level involvement, it is important to palpate trunk musculature to determine which portions of muscle groups are functioning. Dynamometer values of grip and pinch strength should also be obtained. Kilburn and associates[90] suggested that grip strength measurement can be a sensitive gauge of progressive neurologic dysfunction. Level[102] provided a standardized protocol for obtaining grip strength measurements and normative values for children.

Specific testing of isolated motions of lower limb muscles is essential to determine if individual muscles are functioning. Standardized test protocols should be used.[73,82,88] It is essential to detect changes in strength in this population as soon as possible because loss of strength can be a sign of progressive neurologic dysfunction. As a result, we recommend using quantitative strength measurements in conjunction with traditional manual muscle testing techniques. It is also important to distinguish between reflexive and voluntary movements. Reflexive movements should be documented, but they should not be considered when determining motor lesion levels.

Manual muscle testing is the most common method used to assess strength in this population because of its adaptability in a typical clinic setting. Manual muscle testing is the method of choice for screening muscle strength to determine the presence of volitional activity in specific muscles and to determine whether an individual muscle's function varies throughout the ROM. There are several limitations to relying only on manual muscle testing scores for serially monitoring strength, as discussed in Chapter 5.

Manual muscle testing has limited interrater and test-retest reliability.[65] Manual muscle test scores must change more than one full grade to reliably indicate that a true change in strength has occurred.[62] In addition, manual muscle testing has poor concurrent validity compared with more quantitative measures. Several studies have demonstrated that deficits in strength exceeding 50% are not detected by manual muscle testing.[2,3,20,58,127] Agre and colleagues[2] examined this issue in 33 adolescents with MM. Individuals who had been classified as having "no motor deficits" by means of manual muscle testing actually had strength deficits compared with normative data. These deficits were 40% for the hip extensor and 60% for the knee extensor muscles. The lack of concurrent validity of manual muscle testing compared with quantitative measurements demonstrates that the sensitivity of manual muscle testing in detecting weakness is limited and is inadequate for detecting early strength loss in individuals with MM.

The predictive validity of manual muscle testing has been examined in two studies on children with MM. Murdoch[135] examined the predictive validity of neonatal manual muscle testing examinations using a truncated 3-point scale. The correlation between muscle power of the newborn and subsequent mobility of the child at age 3 to 8 years was "very poor." In contrast, McDonald and associates[119] examined the predictive validity of manual muscle testing for individual muscle groups on 825 children with MM using the complete 0- to 5-point grading scale. Predictive validity of manual muscle testing generally increased from birth to age 5. The probability that a given manual muscle test score precisely predicted future scores varied with age and the particular muscle group tested. These probabilities ranged from 23% to 68% for newborns and from 54% to 87% for older children. The probability that a single test score predicted future strength within ±1 manual muscle test grade, however, was considerably higher, ranging from 70% to 86% for newborns and from 87% to 97% for older children.

These results indicate that manual muscle testing is useful for predicting future muscle function within one manual muscle test grade. Strength test results obtained in infancy using the complete manual muscle test scale, therefore, appear to provide useful information for prognosis and for planning the course of intervention.

The limited reliability and concurrent validity of manual muscle testing indicates that it is not the method of choice for monitoring changes in strength over time. In contrast, strength testing using handheld instruments has been found to be a reliable and sensitive method for assessing strength in children and adolescents with MM. Intraclass interrater and test-retest correlation coefficients using this technique ranged from 0.73 to 0.99.[47,65] Other authors report good to high levels of reliability when testing the strength of other populations of children and adolescents with handheld instrumentation.[51,67,69,74,79,123,191] Several portable, handheld instruments are available for use in conjunction with manual muscle testing.[69] The advantages of these tools over nonportable instruments are that they are easily applied in typical clinic settings and can be used with standard manual muscle testing techniques to obtain objective force readings from most muscle groups.

It is best to obtain three myometry trials and report the average score because the mean is more stable over time and between raters.[60,65] Torque values should be reported (force times lever arm length) to permit comparison over time, regardless of changing body proportions, at least until skeletal maturity has been attained. Torque values also permit direct comparison of force production capabilities between individuals with different body proportions. Standardized testing techniques must be implemented when assessing strength with handheld instruments to ensure the consistency of measurements. Many factors influence test results and must be controlled for when testing, including test positions, instructions and commands provided, use of reinforcement and feedback, application of resistance, the type of contraction, and the examiner's body mechanics. For more information regarding techniques used in testing with handheld instruments, see Hinderer and Hinderer.[69]

Several factors should be considered when testing the muscle strength of children with MM, including age, developmental level, cognitive level, ability to follow directions, attention span, motivation, motor planning skills, sensation, and proprioception. The examiner must carefully watch for muscle substitutions. This is particularly challenging in the MM population because of altered angles of pull from orthopedic deformities. It is often difficult for multijoint muscles such as the hamstrings to initiate motions. Any differences in function between end-range and midrange positions should be noted. Special considerations when testing infants and young children are discussed in the section on age-specific examination and physical therapy interventions.

As discussed in the impairments section, several CNS complications can account for loss of muscle function in this population, necessitating serial strength testing for early detection. There are many factors that can result in normal variations in strength, however, that should also be considered when interpreting test results. These factors include changes in body proportions, hormonal influences, motor learning, illness, injury, surgery, immobilization, physical or psychological fatigue, the prior state of activity, seasonal variations, temporal factors, motivation, cooperation, and comprehension. Discussion of the specific influences of these factors is beyond the scope of this chapter. For further information regarding the impact of these factors on force production, see Hinderer and Hinderer.[69] Because of the multiple factors that can influence force production, it is important to repeat the testing at more frequent intervals, if strength loss is suspected, to determine whether consistent test results are obtained. Several variables should be considered when interpreting muscle test results, including the reliability and standard error of measurement of the testing method used, the concurrent and predictive validity of test results, and factors that can account for fluctuations in strength.[69]

Static strength measurements should be correlated with functional measures to observe the effects of fatigue and to determine the effect of reduced strength and limited endurance on function. Individuals with neurogenic muscle weakness may have a higher degree of variability in force production as a result of the lower threshold of fatigue and slower rate of recovery of weak musculature. Local muscle endurance appears to be deficient in some neuromuscular diseases.[12,129] Although this issue has not been specifically tested in the MM population, these results suggest that force production may be more variable in weak muscle groups of individuals with MM.

If function is present but weakness exists in muscle groups that are important for postural stability, ADLs, mobility, or balance of muscle forces around joints, strengthening exercises are indicated. The specific muscle groups to emphasize vary depending on the lesion level and functional requirements. In general, strong upper limb muscle groups are required for performing transfers, for wheelchair propulsion, and when using assistive devices to walk. Increasing the strength of trunk musculature improves sitting balance and postural stability. Increasing the strength of key lower limb muscle groups that are critical for ambulation can improve gait and can possibly minimize the need for orthoses and assistive devices. For example, increasing the quadriceps and hamstrings strength in an individual with L4 motor function may enable progression of ambulation from using KAFOs to using AFOs (see the case scenario found on Expert Consult).

Muscle groups should be strengthened within functional ROM. In addition to traditional strengthening exercises, many play activities promote strengthening.[48] Muscle reeducation techniques such as functional electrical stimulation and biofeedback are useful to teach muscles to function in new parts of the ROM. Electrical stimulation has also been found to be beneficial to increase strength and enhance functional performance in this population.[85] Strengthening programs should be implemented during periods when an individual is at risk for loss of muscle strength and endurance (e.g., after recent surgery, immobilization, illness, or bed rest) and during periods of rapid growth when individuals often lose function as a result of changes in body proportions.

Endurance activities are also important for weight control and to enhance aerobic capacity. Individuals with MM must have adequate endurance to meet the challenges of community mobility. Low-impact aerobic activities to minimize joint stress are preferable. In general, jumping activities should be avoided because joint stress is increased as a result of the inadequate deceleration provided by weak lower limb muscles. Indications for endurance training and instruction in energy conservation techniques include decreased aerobic capacity, high energy cost of mobility, and limited endurance.

Mobility

Ineffective mobility is a hallmark of MM. Effective mobility is defined as any efficient and effective means of moving about in space that enables the individual to easily traverse and explore the environment, grow and develop, and independently pursue an education, vocation, or avocation.[175] Mobility options provided should meet these criteria for all environments encountered by the individual so that lifestyle is not limited by endurance and difficulty traversing uneven terrain.

Changes in body proportions can significantly affect mobility. Mobility options, orthoses, and assistive device requirements that are ideal at one time may not be effective once body proportions, environmental demands, or both change. Consequently, the appropriateness of adaptive equipment and mobility options must be reevaluated throughout the life span. Health care providers should emphasize this point to patients to help prevent the feeling of failure if alternative mobility options are required in the future. Too often, individuals with MM grow up being praised for walking instead of using a wheelchair or for walking without assistive devices, depending on their lesion level. This emphasis gives the impression that normal biped ambulation is the only socially acceptable form of mobility. Several of the adults in our follow-up study reported that it was difficult to accept the use of a wheelchair or other assistive devices as they grew up because they felt that they were a failure or that they would disappoint their parents and health care providers.[72] It is important to emphasize that wheelchairs and other assistive devices are aids for effective mobility and that their use does not represent a failure of biped ambulation.

Bed mobility, floor mobility, wheelchair mobility, ambulation, and transfers should be assessed and compared with the requirements for independent function. Criteria for assessing mobility parameters are endurance, efficiency, effectiveness, safety, degree of independence, and accessibility. Objective information regarding these parameters is often helpful to convince children and their parents that alternative methods of mobility should be considered. Efficiency can be estimated by measuring the time required to complete a task. Energy expenditure can be estimated by measuring heart rate (HR). Regression equations have been determined for this population to equate heart rate with the energy expenditure required for a given task.[205] The regression equations for energy expenditure and efficiency of this population are as follows:

$$\text{Energy cost (ml O}_2/\text{kg min)} = 0.073 \, (\text{HR}) + 6.119$$

$$\text{Energy efficiency (ml O}_2/\text{kg meter)} = 0.006 \, (\text{HR}) - 0.313$$

Criteria for determining the most practical and effective mode of mobility for household and community distances are provided in Box 23.2. Standardized tests that are useful for assessing mobility in the population with lower level lesions are discussed in Chapter 2. In addition, the Timed Test of Patient Mobility[83] is beneficial for assessing the efficiency of mobility because the time required to perform bed mobility, transfers, wheelchair mobility, and gait mobility tasks is documented. Normative data are available for comparison purposes.[83] We suggest augmenting the efficiency time score of the Timed Test of Patient Mobility with a rating scale for the level of independence, safety, practicality, and assistive devices required for each task.[72] Other tests that are specific to function in wheelchairs include the Functional Task Performance Wheelchair Assessment of positioning, reaching, and driving tasks[36] and the Seated Postural Control Measure for sitting posture and functional movements.[50]

Gait

Delays in achieving ambulation can be expected for all children with MM, including those with sacral level lesions, and children with high level lesions may cease walking after a period of 3 to 4 years of biped ambulation.[203] Thorough examination and documentation of gait status are essential to monitor functional motor status and to watch for signs of progressive neurologic dysfunction. Patients or their parents typically notice changes in gait patterns and walking endurance before they notice increased muscle weakness. Careful gait observation is also needed to determine the most appropriate orthoses and assistive devices. Examination of orthoses and assistive devices for wear patterns helps determine if they are being used on a regular basis or just to perform in the clinic setting. Gait should be assessed in a natural environment on a variety of walking surfaces. Patients should be observed walking for typical household and community distances to determine the effects of fatigue. The 10-meter walk test for gait velocity and the 6-minute walk test for endurance are standardized tests that are useful for assessing upright mobility in clients with MM. More information about these tests is provided in Chapter 2 of this text-book.

All too often, decisions regarding gait problems and the need for orthoses and assistive devices are made by observing short-distance ambulation on a smooth clinic floor. Performance in the home or community environment may be vastly different from in a clinic situation, especially when walking around a number of obstacles, when in congested areas, when traversing uneven terrain, or with inclement weather. The impact of these factors must be considered when making recommendations.

Requirements for orthoses and ambulatory aids should be documented. Gait deviations should be closely observed and recorded. If possible, gait deviations and efficiency parameters both with and without orthoses and assistive devices should be observed. Typical gait parameters assessed include arm swing, trunk position and sway, pelvic tilt and rotations, compensated or uncompensated Trendelenburg position, excessive hip flexion and rotation, excessive knee flexion or hyperextension, toe clearance, foot position, push-off effectiveness, and foot progression angle.

Observational gait analysis is the technique used most commonly to assess gait in clinical settings.[95] Video analysis augments clinical observations by allowing the evaluator to observe gait multiple times at slow speeds and by providing a permanent record that is invaluable for comparison purposes if deterioration of functional status is suspected. The interrater reliability of observational analysis through videos, however, has been reported to be low to moderate.[46,95] Footprint analysis is a low-cost method of obtaining objective information regarding velocity, cadence, foot progression angle, base of support, toe clearance, stride length, and step length.[170] More sophisticated methods of objective gait analysis are described by Stout in Chapter 34, Development and Analysis of Gait (on Expert Consult).

Criteria for the effectiveness, efficiency, and safety of household and community ambulation are provided in Box 23.2. Efficiency and practicality of ambulation can be estimated by monitoring heart rate, normal and fast walking velocity, and maximum walking distance. Other time-distance variables (e.g., step and stride length, cadence, and cycle time) provide useful information regarding symmetry, stability, and function. These variables can be used for comparison purposes if they are normalized (adjusted) for stature.[156]

Time-distance variables provide information about gait symmetry by comparing right-left differences in step lengths and stance-to-swing phase ratios. Examining cadence and the percentage of time spent in the stance phase versus the swing phase provides information regarding the stability of gait. For instance, a high cadence or an imbalance in the stance versus swing phase duration may indicate instability. Parameters such as walking velocity and cadence provide information regarding the functional practicality of gait. If the velocity is too low or step rate is too high, the individual may not be able to meet environmental demands.

It is essential to normalize time-distance variables for stature to compare these parameters serially over time for a given individual or to compare between individuals of different stature (e.g., comparing with normative data). These parameters are normalized by dividing by leg length. An alternative but less precise method of normalizing time-distance parameters is to divide by height because overall height is closely correlated to individual limb lengths. If these parameters are not normalized for stature, conclusions regarding differences in function may be confounded by changes in body proportions over time.

Indications for lower limb orthoses are provided in Box 23.3. Specifications and their effect on gait are outlined in Box 23.4. Indications for gait training include when a child is first learning to walk; when there is potential for progression to a new type of orthosis or upper limb aid; for progression to a more efficient gait pattern (e.g., from a four-point to a two-point alternative gait); when there is potential for improving gait (e.g., crouched gait pattern, excessive foot progression angle); to improve safety and confidence with advanced walking activities (e.g., walking on inclines, rough terrain, steps; learning to fall safely and stand up independently from floor; carrying and lifting objects); and to improve the efficiency and safety of gait, transfers, and intervention of aids.

Strength of the quadriceps muscles has been suggested by some authors to be the best predictor of ambulatory potential in children with MM[164,205]; others indicate that iliopsoas muscle strength is better.[118] McDonald and associates[118] examined the relationship between the patterns of strength and mobility in 291 children with MM who had received at least three serial standardized strength examinations after age 5 and who were classified for their mobility status as community ambulators, partial (household) ambulators, and nonambulators. Iliopsoas muscle strength was found to be the best predictor of ambulation. The quadriceps, anterior tibialis, and gluteal muscles also were determined to have significant importance for ambulation in these children. Grade 0 to 3 iliopsoas strength was always associated with partial or complete reliance on a wheelchair. Patients with grade 4 to 5 iliopsoas and quadriceps muscle strength were almost all community ambulators, and no members of this group were completely wheelchair dependent. Children with grade 4 to 5 gluteal and anterior tibialis muscle strength were all classified as community ambulators and did not require the use of an assistive device or orthosis.

Key muscle groups for community ambulation, listed in order of importance, are the iliopsoas, gluteus medius and maximus, quadriceps, anterior tibialis, and hamstring muscles.[12] Specific strength of these muscles accounted for 86% of the variance in mobility status. Gluteus medius muscle strength was found to be the best predictor of requirements for aids or orthoses. In individuals with gluteus medius strength grade 2 to 3, 72.2% required aids, orthoses, or both. If activity in this muscle was absent or trace, 95.7% required aids, orthoses, or both. In contrast, if gluteus medius strength was grade 4 to 5, only 11.2% required aids, orthoses, or both. Mazur and Menelaus[117] reported that 98% of all individuals with quadriceps strength of grade 4 to 5 were at least household ambulators, with 82% being community ambulators. In contrast, for individuals with quadriceps strength of grade 3 or less, 88% were exclusive wheelchair users.

Agre and associates[2] reported that maximum walking velocity was correlated with hip and knee extensor muscle strength. They compared the energy expenditure and efficiency of ambulation in children with MM versus able-bodied peers and found that children with MM used almost twice as much energy when walking and had a 41% lower ambulation velocity. They also reported that mobility in a wheelchair was considerably more efficient than walking, approximating normal gait in terms of energy requirements. In addition, individuals classified as having "no loss" by means of manual muscle testing had a decreased walking velocity and increased energy expenditure compared with able-bodied peers.

Equipment

A wide variety of adaptive equipment typically is required for individuals with MM. Equipment needs vary considerably with level of lesion and age. Therapists must be aware of the available options and be able to select the most appropriate type of equipment for a given situation. In addition, it is important to educate parents and patients regarding the fit and appropriateness of adaptive equipment so that they can be knowledgeable consumers. It is beyond the scope of this chapter to discuss specific equipment items. See Baker and Rogosky-Grassi,[8] Knutson and Clark,[93] and Pomatto[152] for further information regarding adaptive equipment and orthoses for this population. Indications for lower limb orthotics are provided in Box 23.3. Design specifications, objectives, and considerations when assessing the components and fit of orthoses are included in Box 23.4.

Examinations of adaptive equipment and orthotics should be conducted on at least a yearly basis. Examinations should occur more often during periods of rapid growth; when environmental demands change (e.g., changing school or work settings); when there are changes in lifestyle, goals, or vocation; or when there is a change in status that may affect motor control or mobility.

■ SUMMARY

Few populations challenge the skill and knowledge domains of the physical therapist as extensively as individuals with MM. This discussion has highlighted the multitude and complexity of problems encountered by children and adolescents with MM. Each lesion level group has general functional expectations that help direct physical therapy goals from an early age. Although MM is a congenital-onset problem requiring intervention by the physical therapist during infancy and childhood, most of the impairments and functional deficits described in this chapter occur throughout the life span. Individuals with MM

should be followed on a regular basis, even as adults, in multidisciplinary specialty clinics by care providers familiar with this population. Because the physical therapist has extended contact with these individuals from infancy through adolescence, the therapist plays an important role in screening and triaging for potential problems, in addition to more traditional physical therapy roles. The challenges and rewards of working with this population are therefore extraordinary.

Case Scenarios on Expert Consult

The cases related to this chapter present two case scenarios (Sally and Megan), along with an additional case scenario presented on video (Megan). Each of the cases illustrates several of the management principles discussed in this chapter.

REFERENCES

1. Adzick N: Fetal surgery for spina bifida: past, present, future, *Semin Pediatr Surg* 22:10–17, 2013.
2. Agre JC, Findley TW, McNally MC, et al.: Physical activity capacity in children with myelomeningocele, *Arch Phys Med Rehabil* 68:372–377, 1987.
3. Aitkens S, Lord J, Bernauer E, et al.: Relationship of manual muscle testing to objective strength measurements, *Muscle Nerve* 12:173–177, 1989.
4. Andersen EM, Plewis I: Impairment of motor skill in children with spina bifida cystica and hydrocephalus: an exploratory study, *Br J Psychol* 68:61–70, 1977.
5. Andersson C, Mattsson E: Adults with cerebral palsy: a survey describing problems, needs, and resources, with special emphasis on locomotion, *Dev Med Child Neurol* 43:76–82, 2001.
6. Asher M, Olson J: Factors affecting the ambulatory status of patients with spina bifida cystica, *J Bone Joint Surg Am* 65:350–356, 1983.
7. Babcook CJ: Ultrasound evaluation of prenatal and neonatal spina bifida, *Neurosurg Clin North Am* 6:203–218, 1995.
8. Baker SB, Rogosky-Grassi MA: Access to the school. In Kelly FL, Reigel DH, editors: In *Teaching the student with spina bifida*, Baltimore, 1992, Paul H. Brookes, pp 31–70.
9. Bannister CM: The case for and against intrauterine surgery for myelomeningocele, *Eur J Obst Gynecol Reproduct Biol* 92:109–113, 2000.
10. Banta JV: Bracing for ambulation: basic principles, brace alternatives by motor level and predictive long-term goals. In Matsumoto S, Sato H, editors: *Spina bifida*, New York, 1999, Springer Verlag, pp 307–311.
11. Banta J, Hamada J: Natural history of the kyphotic deformity in myelomeningocele, *J Bone Joint Surg* 58A:279, 1976.
12. Bar-Or O: Pathophysiological factors which limit the exercise capacity of the sick child, *Med Sci Sports Exerc* 18:276–282, 1986.
13. Bartlett MD, Wolf LS, Shurtleff DB, Staheli LT: Hip flexion contractures: a comparison of measurement methods, *Arch Phys Med Rehabil* 66:620–625, 1985.
14. Bauer SB: Neurogenic bladder: etiology and assessment, *Pediatr Nephrol* 23:541–551, 2008.
15. Becker RD: Recent developments in child psychiatry: I. The restrictive emotional and cognitive environment reconsidered: a redefinition of the concept of therapeutic restraint, *Isr Ann Psychiatr Relat Discip* 12:239–258, 1975.
16. Berry RJ, Li Z, Erickson JD, et al.: Prevention of neural-tube defects with folic acid in China, *New Engl J Med* 341:1485–1491, 1999.
17. Birth Defects and Genetic Diseases Branch of Birth Defects and Developmental Disabilities Office: National Center for Environmental Disease and Injury: use of folic acid prevention of spina bifida and other neural tube defects, 1983-1991, *MMWR Morb Mortal Wkly Rep* 40:1–4, 1991.
18. Bleck EE, Nagel DA: *Physically handicapped children: a medical atlas for teachers*, Orlando, FL, 1982, Grune Stratton.
19. Reference deleted in proofs.
20. Bohannon RW: Manual muscle test scores and dynamometer test scores of knee extension strength, *Arch Phys Med Rehabil* 67:390–392, 1986.

21. Bower E, editor: *Finnie's handling the young child with cerebral palsy at home*, Burlington, MA, 2009, Butterworth- Heinemann.

22. Brazelton TB: Touchpoints: *your child's emotional and behavioral development*, Reading, MA, 1992, Perseus Books.

23. Brinker M, Rosenfeld S, Feiwell E, et al.: Myelomeningocele at the sacral level: long-term outcomes in adults, *J Bone Joint Surg* 76A:1293–1300, 1994.

24. Broughton NS, Graham G, Menelaus MB: The high incidence of foot deformity in patients with high-level spina bifida, *J Bone Joint Surg* 76B:548–550, 1994.

25. Brown JP: Orthopedic care of children with spina bifida: you've come a long way, baby! *Orthop Nurs* 20:51–58, 2001.

26. Brunt D: Characteristics of upper limb movements in a sample of meningomyelocele children, *Percept Mot Skills* 51:431–437, 1980.

27. Butler C, Okamoto GA, McKay TM: Motorized wheelchair driving by disabled children, *Arch Phys Med Rehabil* 65:95–97, 1984.

28. Chaffin DB, Andersson GBJ, Martin BJ: *Occupational biomechanics*, ed 3, New York, 1999, John Wiley Sons.

29. Chandler LS, Andrews MS, Swanson MW: *Movement assessment of infants: a manual*, Rolling Bay, WA, 1980, Authors.

30. Coster W, Deeney TA, Haltiwanger JT, Haley SM: *School function assessment*, Boston, 1998, Boston University.

31. Culatta B, Young C: Linguistic performance as a function of abstract task demands in children with spina bifida, *Dev Med Child Neurol* 34(5):434–440, 1992.

32. Cusick BD, Stuberg WA: Assessment of lower extremity alignment in the transverse plane: implications for management of children with neuromotor dysfunction, *Phys Ther* 72:3–15, 1992.

33. Czeizel AE, Dudas I: Prevention of first occurrence of neural tube defects by periconceptual vitamin supplementation, *New Engl J Med* 327:131–137, 1992.

34. D'Addario V, Rossi AC, Pinto V, et al.: Comparison of six sonographic signs in the prenatal diagnosis of spina bifida, *J Perinat Med* 36(4):330–334, 2008.

35. De Villarreal LM, Perez JZ, Vasquez PA, et al.: Decline of neural tube defects after a folic acid campaign in Neuvo Leon, Mexico, *Teratology* 66:249–256, 2002.

36. Deitz JC, Jaffe KM, Wolf LS, et al.: Pediatric power wheelchairs: evaluation of function in the home and school environments, *Assist Technol* 3:24–31, 1991.

37. Del Gado R, Del Gaizo D, Brescia D, et al.: Obesity and overweight in a group of patients with myelomeningocele. In Matsumoto S, Sato H, editors: *Spina bifida*, New York, 1999, Springer Verlag, pp 474–475.

38. Dennis M, Barnes MA: The cognitive phenotype of spina bifida meningomyelocele, *Dev Disabil Res Rev* 16(1):31–39, 2010.

39. DeSouza L, Carroll N: Ambulation of the braced myelomeningocele patient, *J Bone Joint Surg Am* 58:1112–1118, 1976.

40. Dias L: Management of ankle and hindfoot valgus in spina bifida. In Matsumoto S, Sato H, editors: *Spina bifida*, New York, 1999, Springer Verlag, pp 374–377.

41. Dias L: The management of hip pathology in spina bifida. In Matsumoto SS, Sato HH, editors: *Spina bifida*, New York, 1999, Springer Verlag, pp 321–322.

42. Diaz Llopis I, Bea Munoz M, Martinez Agullo E, et al.: Ambulation in patients with myelomeningocele: a study of 1500 patients, *Paraplegia* 31:28–32, 1993.

43. Dise JE, Lohr ME: Examination of deficits in conceptual reasoning abilities associated with spina bifida, *Am J Phys Med Rehabil* 77:247–251, 1998.

44. Dosa NP, Eckrich M, Katz DA, et al.: Incidence, prevalence, and characteristics of fractures in children, adolescents, and adults with spina bifida, *J Spinal Cord Med* 30(Suppl 1):S5–S9, 2007.

45. Dudgeon BJ, Jaffe KM, Shurtleff DB: Variations in midlumbar myelomeningocele: implications for ambulation, *Pediatr Phys Ther* 3:57–62, 1991.

46. Eastlack ME, Arvidson J, Snyder-Mackler L, et al.: Interrater reliability of videotaped observational gait-analysis assessments, *Phys Ther* 71:465–472, 1991.

47. Effgen SK, Brown DA: Long-term stability of hand-held dynamometric measurements in children who have myelomeningocele, *Phys Ther* 72:458–465, 1992.

48. Embrey D, Endicott J, Glenn T, Jaeger DL: Developing better postural tone in grade school children, *Clinical Management in Phys Ther* 3:6–10, 1983.

49. Fay G, Shurtleff DB, Shurtleff H, Wolf L: Approaches to facilitate independent self-care and academic success. In Shurtleff DB, editor: *Myelodysplasias and exstrophies: significance, prevention, and treatment*, Orlando, FL, 1986, Grune Stratton, pp 373–398.

50. Fife SE, Roxborough LA, Armstrong RW, et al.: Development of a clinical measure of postural control for assessment of adaptive seating in children with neuromotor disabilities, *Phys Ther* 71:981–993, 1991.

51. Florence JM, Pandya S, King W, et al.: Strength assessment: comparison of methods in children with Duchenne muscular dystrophy (Abstract), *Phys Ther* 68:866, 1988.

52. Frawley PA, Broughton NS, Menelaus MB: Incidence and type of hindfoot deformities in patients with low-level spina bifida, *J Pediatr Orthop* 18:312–313, 1998.

53. Frimberger D, Cheng E, Kropp BP: The current management of the neurogenic bladder in children with spina bifida, *Pediatr Clin North Am* 59(4):757–767, 2012.

54. Gadow K: *Children on medication*, San Diego, CA, 1986, College Hill Press.

55. Gaston H: Ophthalmic complications of spina bifida and hydrocephalus, *Eye* 5:279–290, 1991.

56. Goodwyn MA: *Biomedical psychological factors predicting success with activities of daily living and academic pursuits*. Unpublished doctoral dissertation, Seattle, 1990, University of Washington.

57. Griebel ML, Oakes WJ, Worley G: The Chiari malformation associated with myelomeningocele. In Rekate HL, editor: *Comprehensive management of spina bifida*, Boca Raton, FL, 1991, CRC Press, pp 67–92.

58. Griffin JW, McClure MH, Bertorini TE: Sequential isokinetic and manual muscle testing in patients with neuromuscular disease: pilot study, *Phys Ther* 66:32–35, 1986.

59. Gucciardi E, Pietrusiak MA, Reynolds DL, Rouleau J: Incidence of neural tube defects in Ontario, 1986-1999, *CMAJ* 167:237–240, 2002.

60. Hack SN, Norton BJ, Zahalak GI: A quantitative muscle tester for clinical use (Abstract), *Phys Ther* 61:673, 1981.

61. Hamill PV, Drizd TA, Johnson CL, et al.: Physical growth: National Center for Health Statistics percentiles, *Am J Clin Nutr* 32:607–629, 1979.

62. Harms-Ringdahl K: *Muscle strength*, Edinburgh, 1993, Churchill Livingstone.

63. Harris SR, Megans AM, Daniels LE: *Harris Infant Neuromotor Test (HINT)*, Test User's Manual Version 1.0 Clinical Edition. Chicago, IL, 2010, Infant Motor Performance Scales, LLC, p 2009.

64. Hatlen T, Song K, Shurtleff D, Duguay S: Contributory factors to postoperative spinal fusion complications for children with myelomeningocele, *Spine* 35:1294–1299, 2010.

65. Hinderer KA: *Reliability of the myometer in muscle testing children and adolescents with myelodysplasia*, Unpublished master's thesis, Seattle, 1988, University of Washington.

66. Hinderer KA: *The relationship between musculoskeletal system capacity and task requirements in simulated crouch standing*, Doctoral dissertation, Ann Arbor, MI, 2003, University of Michigan.

67. Hinderer KA, Gutierrez T: Myometry measurements of children using isometric and eccentric methods of muscle testing (Abstract), *Phys Ther* 68:817, 1988.

68. Hinderer KA, Hinderer SR: Mobility and transfer efficiency of adults with myelodysplasia (Abstract), *Arch Phys Med Rehabil* 69:712, 1988.

69. Hinderer KA, Hinderer SR: Muscle strength development and assessment in children and adolescents. In Harms-Ringdahl KK, editor: *International perspectives in physical therapy: muscle strength*, Vol. 8. London, 1993, Churchill Livingstone, pp 93–140.

70. Hinderer SR, Hinderer KA: Sensory examination of individuals with myelodysplasia (Abstract), *Arch Phys Med Rehabil* 71:769–770, 1990.

71. Hinderer SR, Hinderer KA: Principles and applications of measurement. In Frontera WR, editor: *DeLisa's Rehabilitation medicine: principles and practices*, ed 5, Philadelphia, 2010, Lippincott-Williams Wilkins, pp 221–242.

72. Hinderer SR, Hinderer KA, Dunne K, Shurtleff DB: Medical and functional status of adults with spina bifida (Abstract), *Dev Med Child Neurol* 30(Suppl 57):28, 1988.

73. Hislop HJ, Montgomery J: *Daniels and Worthingham's muscle testing*, ed 7, Philadelphia, 2002, WB Saunders.

74. Hosking GP, Bhat US, Dubowitz V, Edwards RHT: Measurements of muscle strength and performance in children with normal and diseased muscle, *Arch Dis Child* 51:957–963, 1976.

75. Hunt GM: Open spina bifida: outcome for complete cohort treated unselectively and followed into adulthood, *Dev Med Child Neurol* 32:108–118, 1990.

76. Hunt GM, Oakeshott P, Kerry S: Link between the CSF shunt and achievement in adults with spina bifida, *J Neurol Nerosurg Psychiatry* 67:591–595, 1999.

77. Hunt G, Oakeshott P: Outcome in people with open spina bifida at age 35: prospective community based cohort study, *Br Med J* 326:1365–1366, 2003.

78. Hurley AD: Conducting psychological assessments. In Rowley-Kelly FL, Reigel DH, editors: *Teaching the student with spina bifida*, Baltimore, 1992, Paul H. Brookes, pp 107–124.

79. Hyde S, Goddard C, Scott O: The myometer: the development of a clinical tool, *Physiotherapy* 69:424–427, 1983.

80. IMSG: International Myelodysplasia Study Group Database Coordination: *Department of Pediatrics*, Seattle, 1993, University of Washington.

81. Reference deleted in proofs.

82. Janda V: *Muscle function testing*, Boston, 1983, Butterworths.

83. Jebsen RH, Trieschman RB, Mikulic MA, et al.: Measurement of time in a standardized test of patient mobility, *Arch Phys Med Rehabil* 51:170–175, 1970.

84. Johnson C, Honein MA, Dana Flanders W, et al.: Pregnancy termination following prenatal diagnosis of anencephaly or spina bifida: a systematic review of the literature, *Birth Defects Res A Clin Mol Teratol* 94:857–863, 2012.

85. Karmel-Ross K, Cooperman DR, Van Doren CL: The effect of electrical stimulation on quadriceps femoris muscle torque in children with spina bifida, *Phys Ther* 72:723–731, 1992.

86. Karol L: Orthopedic management in myelomeningocele, *Neurosurg Clin North Am* 6:259–268, 1995.

87. Kelly NC, Ammerman RT, Rausch JR, et al.: Executive functioning and psychological adjustment in children and youth with spina bifida, *Child Neuropsychol* 18(5):417–431, 2012.

88. Kendall FP, McCreary EK, Provance PG: *Muscles: testing and function*, ed 4, Baltimore, 1999, Williams Wilkins.

89. Reference deleted in proofs.

90. Kilburn J, Saffer A, Barnes L, et al.: *The Vigorimeter as an early predictor of central neurologic malformation in myelodysplastic children*, Seattle, 1985, Paper presented at the meeting of the American Academy for Cerebral Palsy and Developmental Medicine.

91. Kimura DK, Mayo M, Shurtleff DB: Urinary tract management. In Shurtleff DB, editor: *Myelodysplasias and exstrophies: significance, prevention, and treatment*, Orlando, FL, 1986, Grune Stratton, pp 243–266.

92. King JC, Currie DM, Wright E: Bowel training in spina bifida: importance of education, patient compliance, age, and anal reflexes, *Arch Phys Med Rehabil* 75:243–247, 1994.

93. Knutson LM, Clark DE: Orthotic devices for ambulation in children with cerebral palsy and myelomeningocele, *Phys Ther* 71:947–960, 1991.

94. Kottorp A, Bernspang B, Fisher AG: Validity of a performance assessment of activities of daily living for people with developmental disabilities, *J Intellect Disabil Res* 47(8):597–605, 2003.

95. Krebs DE, Edelstein JE, Fishman S: Reliability of observational kinematic gait analysis, *Phys Ther* 65:1027–1033, 1985.

96. Lais A, Kasabian NG, Dryo FM, et al.: The neurosurgical implications of continuous neurological surveillance of children with myelodysplasia, *J Urol* 150:1879–1883, 1993.

97. Land LC: Study of the sensory integration of children with myelomeningocele. In McLaurin RL, editor: *Myelomeningocele*, Orlando, FL, 1977, Grune Stratton, pp 115–140.

98. Lehmann JF, Condon SM, de Lateur BJ, Price R: Gait abnormalities in peroneal nerve paralysis and their corrections by orthoses: a biomechanical study, *Arch Phys Med Rehabil* 67:380–386, 1986.

99. Reference deleted in proofs.

100. Lehmann JF, Esselman PC, Ko MJ, et al.: Plastic ankle-foot orthoses: evaluation of function, *Arch Phys Med Rehabil* 64:402–404, 1983.

101. Lemire RJ, Loeser JD, Leech RW, Alvord ED, editors: *Normal and abnormal development of the human nervous system*, Hagerstown, MD, 1975, Harper Row.

102. Level MB: *Spherical grip strength of children*, Unpublished master's thesis. Seattle, 1984, University of Washington.

103. Liptak GS, Shurtleff DB, Bloss JW, et al.: Mobility aids for children with high-level myelomeningocele: parapodium versus wheelchair, *Dev Med Child Neurol* 34:787–796, 1992.

104. Liusuwan RA, Widman LM, Abresch RT, et al.: Behavioral intervention, exercise, and nutrition education to improve health and fitness (BENEfit) in adolescents with mobility impairment due to spinal cord dysfunction, *J Spinal Cord Med* 30:S119–S126, 2007.

105. Liusuwan RA, Widman LM, Abresch RT, et al.: Body composition and resting energy expenditure in patients aged 11 to 21 years with spinal cord dysfunction compared to controls: comparisons and relationships among the groups, *J Spinal Cord Med* 30:S105–S111, 2007.

106. Logan L, Byers-Hinkley K, Ciccone CD: Anterior versus posterior walkers: a gait analysis study, *Dev Med Child Neurol* 32:1044–1048, 1990.

107. Lollar D: *Preventing secondary conditions associated with spina bifida or cerebral palsy. Proceedings and Recommendations of a Symposium* (pp. 54–64, Washington, DC, 1994, Spina Bifida Association of America.

108. Luthy DA, Wardinsky T, Shurtleff DB, et al.: Cesarean section before the onset of labor and subsequent motor function in infants with myelomeningocele diagnosed antenatally, *New Engl J Med* 324:662–666, 1991.

109. Lutkenhoff M, Oppenheimer S: *Spinabilities: a young person's guide to spina bifida*, Bethesda, MD, 1997, Woodbine House.

110. Lynch A, Ryu J, Agrawal S, Galloway JC: Power mobility training for a 7-month old infant with spina bifida, *Pediatr Phys Ther* 21:362–368, 2009.

111. Main DM, Mennuti MT: Neural tube defects: issues in prenatal diagnosis and counseling, *Obstet Gynecol* 67:1–16, 1986.

112. Marreiros H, Loff C, Calado E: Osteoporosis in paediatric patients with spina bifida, *J Spinal Cord Med* 35(1):9–21, 2012.

113. Marreiros H, Monteiro L, Loff C, et al.: Fractures in children and adolescents with spina bifida: the experience of a Portuguese tertiary-care hospital, *Dev Med Child Neurol* 52(8):754–759, 2010.

114. Masse LC, Lamontagne M, O'Riain MD: Biomedical analysis of wheelchair propulsion for various seating positions, *J Rehabil Res Dev* 29:12–28, 1992.

115. Mayfield JK: Comprehensive orthopedic management in myelomeningocele. In Rekate HL, editor: *Comprehensive management of spina bifida*, Boca Raton, FL, 1991, CRC Press, pp 113–164.

116. Maynard J, Weiner J, Burke S: Neuropathic foot ulceration in patients with myelodysplasia, *J Pediatr Orthop* 12:786–788, 1992.

117. Mazur JM, Menelaus MB: Neurologic status of spina bifida patients and the orthopedic surgeon, *Clin Orthop Rel Res* 264:54–63, 1991.

118. McDonald CM, Jaffe KM, Mosca VS, Shurtleff DB: Ambulatory outcome of children with myelomeningocele: effect of lower-extremity muscle strength, *Dev Med Child Neurol* 33:482–490, 1991.

119. McDonald CM, Jaffe KM, Shurtleff DB, Menelaus MB: Modifications to the traditional description of neurosegmental innervation in myelomeningocele, *Dev Med Child Neurol* 33:473–481, 1991.

120. McDonald CM, Jaffe K, Shurtleff DB: Assessment of muscle strength in children with meningomyelocele: accuracy and stability of measurements over time, *Arch Phys Med Rehabil* 67:855–861, 1986.

121. McDonnell GV, McCann JP: Link between the CSF shunt and achievement in adults with spina bifida, *J Neurol Neurosurg Psychiatry* 68:800, 2000.

122. McGourty LK: Kohlman Evaluation of Living Skills (KELS). In Hemphill BJ, editor: *Mental health assessment in occupational therapy*, Thorofare, NJ, 1988, Black, pp 131–146.

123. Mendell JR, Florence J: Manual muscle testing, *Muscle Nerve* 13 (Suppl):16–20, 1990.

124. Menelaus MB: Orthopedic management of children with myelomeningocele: a plea for realistic goals, *Dev Med Child Neurol* 18(Suppl 37):3–11, 1976.

125. Menelaus MD: The hip: current treatment. In Matsumoto S, Sato H, editors: *Spina bifida*, New York, 1999, Springer Verlag, pp 338–340.

126. Miller E, Sethi L: The effect of hydrocephalus on perception, *Dev Med Child Neurol* 13(Suppl 25):77–81, 1971.

127. Miller LC, Michael AF, Baxter TL, Kim Y: Quantitative muscle testing in childhood dermatomyositis, *Arch Phys Med Rehabil* 69:610–613, 1988.

128. Mills JL, Rhoads GG, Simpson JL, et al.: The absence of a relation between the periconceptual use of vitamins and neural tube defects, *New Engl J Med* 321:430–435, 1989.

129. Milner-Brown HS, Miller RG: Increased muscular fatigue in patients with neurogenic muscle weakness: quantification and pathophysiology, *Arch Phys Med Rehabil* 70:361–366, 1989.

130. Milunsky A, Jick H, Jick SS, et al.: Multivitamin/folic acid supplementation in early pregnancy reduces the prevalence of neural tube defects, *JAMA* 262:2847–2852, 1989.

131. Mintz L, Sarwark J, Dias L, Schafer M: The natural history of congenital kyphosis in myelomeningocele, *Spine* 16(Suppl 5):348–350, 1991.

132. Mitchell L: Epidemiology of neural tube defects, *Am J Med Genet C Semin Med Genet* 135C:88–94, 2005.

133. Mobley C, Harless L, Miller K: Self perceptions of preschool children with spina bifida, *J Pediatr Nurs* 1:217–224, 1996.

134. MRC Vitamin Study Research Group: Prevention of neural tube defects: results of the Medical Research Council vitamin study, *Lancet* 338:131–137, 1991.

135. Murdoch A: How valuable is muscle charting? A study of the relationship between neonatal assessment of muscle power and later mobility in children with spina bifida defects, *Physiotherapy* 66:221–223, 1980.

136. Murphy KP, Molnar GE, Lankasky K: Medical and functional status of adults with cerebral palsy, *Dev Med Child Neurol* 37:1075–1084, 1995.

137. Nagankatti D, Banta J, Thomson J: Charcot arthropathy in spina bifida, *J Pediatr Orthop* 20:82–87, 2000.

138. Oakeshott P, Reid F, Poulton A, et al.: Neurologic level at birth predicts survival to the mid-40s and urological deaths in open spina bifida: a complete prospective cohort study, *Dev Med Child Neurol* 57(7):634–638, 2015.

139. Oi S: Current status of prenatal management of fetal spina bifida in the world: worldwide cooperative survey on the medico-ethical issue, *Child Nerv Syst* 19:596–599, 2003.

140. Oi S, Sato O, Matsumoto S: Neurologic and medico-social problems of spina bifida patients in adolescence and adulthood, *Child Nerv Syst* 12:181–187, 1996.

141. Okamoto GA, Lamers JV, Shurtleff DB: Skin breakdown in patients with myelomeningocele, *Arch Phys Med Rehabil* 64:20–23, 1983.

142. Okamoto GA, Sousa J, Telzrow RW, et al.: Toileting skills in children with myelomeningocele: rates of learning, *Arch Phys Med Rehabil* 65(4):182–185, 1984.

143. Ounpuu S, Davis RB, Banta JV, DeLuce PA: *The effects of orthotics on gait in children with low-level myelomeningocele*, Chicago, IL, 1992, Proceedings of the North American Congress on Biomechanics, pp 323–324.

144. Overgoor MLE, Kon M, Cohen-Kettenis PT, et al.: Neurologic bypass for sensory innervations of the penis in patients with spina bifida, *J Urol* 176:1086–1090, 2006.

145. Reference deleted in proofs.

146. Pact V, Sirotkin-Roses M, Beatus J: *The muscle testing handbook*, Boston, 1984, Little, Brown.

147. Padua L, Rendeli C, Rabini A, et al.: Health-related quality of life and disability in young patients with spina bifida, *Arch Phys Med Rehabil* 83:1384–1388, 2002.

148. Paleg GS, Smith BA, Glickman LB: Systematic review and evidence-based clinical recommendations for dosing of pediatric supported standing programs, *Pediatr Phys Ther* 25(3):232–247, 2013.

149. *Patient Data Management System: Myelodysplasia Study Data Collection Criteria and Instructions*, 1994.

150. Persad VL, Van den Hof MC, Dube JM, Zimmer P: Incidence of open neural tube defects in Nova Scotia after folic acid fortification, *CMAJ* 167:241–245, 2002.

151. Peterson P, Rauen K, Brown J, Cole J: Spina bifida: the transition into adulthood begins in infancy, *Rehabil Nurs* 19:229–238, 1994.

152. Pomatto RC: The use of orthotics in the treatment of myelomeningocele. In Rekate HL, editor: *Comprehensive management of spina bifida*, Boca Raton, FL, 1991, CRC Press, pp 165–183.

153. Reigel DH: Spina bifida from infancy through the school years. In Kelly FL, Reigel DH, editors: *Teaching the student with spina bifida*, Baltimore, 1992, Paul H. Brookes, pp 3–30.

154. Rekate HL: Neurosurgical management of the newborn with spina bifida. In Rekate HL, editor: *Comprehensive management of spina bifida*, Boca Raton, FL, 1991, CRC Press, pp 1–28.

155. Reynolds EH: Mental effects of antiepileptic medication: a review, *Epilepsia* 24(Suppl 2):S85–S95, 1983.

156. Rose SA, Ounpuu S, DeLuca PA: Strategies for the assessment of pediatric gait in the clinical setting, *Phys Ther* 71:961–980, 1991.

157. Rosenstein BD, Greene WB, Herrington RT, Blum AS: Bone density in myelomeningocele: the effects of ambulatory status and other factors, *Dev Med Child Neurol* 29:486–494, 1987.

158. Rowley-Kelly FL, Kunkle PM: Developing a school outreach program. In Rowley-Kelly FL, Reigel DH, editors: *Teaching the student with spina bifida*, Baltimore, 1992, Paul H. Brookes, pp 395–436.

159. Ryan KD, Pioski C, Emans JB: Myelodysplasia—the musculoskeletal problem: habilitation from infancy to adulthood, *Phys Ther* 71:935–946, 1991.

160. Salvaggio E, Mauti G, Ranieri P, et al.: Ability in walking is a predictor of bone mineral density and body composition in prepubertal children with myelomeningocele. In Matsumoto S, Sato H, editors: *Spina bifida*, New York, 1999, Springer Verlag, pp 298–301.

161. Sand PL, Taylor N, Rawlings M, Chitnis S: Performance of children with spina bifida manifest on the Frostig Developmental Test of Visual Perception, *Percept Mot Skills* 37:539–546, 1973.

162. Schafer MF, Dias LS: *Myelomeningocele: orthopaedic treatment*, Baltimore, Williams Wilkins 13.

163. Schneider JW, Krosschell K, Gabriel KL: Congenital spinal cord injury. In Umphred DA, editor: *Neurologic rehabilitation*, ed 4, St. Louis, 2001, Mosby, pp 454–483.

164. Schopler SA, Menelaus MB: Significance of strength of the quadriceps muscles in children with myelomeningocele, *J Pediatr Orthop* 7:507–512, 1987.

165. Seller MJ, Nevin NC: Periconceptual vitamin supplementation and the prevention of neural tube defects in south-east England and Northern Ireland, *J Med Genet* 21:325–330, 1984.

166. Shaffer J, Wolfe L, Friedrich W, et al.: Developmental expectations: intelligence and fine motor skills. In Shurtleff DB, editor: *Myelodysplasias and exstrophies: significance, prevention, and treatment*, Orlando, FL, 1986, Grune Stratton, pp 359–372.

167. Shapiro E, Kelly KJ, Setlock MA, et al.: Complications of latex allergy, *Dia Pediatr Urol* 15:1–5, 1992.

168. Sherk H, Uppal G, Lane G, Melchionni J: Treatment versus nontreatment of hip dislocations in ambulatory patients with myelomeningocele, *Dev Med Child Neurol* 33:491–494, 1991.

169. Shin M, Besser LM, Siffel C, et al.: Prevalence of spina bifida among children and adolescents in 10 regions in the United States, *Pediatrics* 126:274–927, 2010.

170. Shores M: Footprint analysis in gait documentation, *Phys Ther* 60:1163–1167, 1980.

171. Shurtleff DB: Timing of learning in the myelomeningocele patient, *Phys Ther* 46(2):136–148, 1966.

172. Shurtleff DB: Decubitus formation and skin breakdown. In Shurtleff DB, editor: *Myelodysplasias and exstrophies: significance, prevention, and treatment*, Orlando, FL, 1986, Grune Stratton, pp 299–312.

173. Shurtleff DB: Dietary management. (1986b). In Shurtleff DB, editor: *Myelodysplasias and exstrophies: significance, prevention, and treatment*, Orlando, FL, 1986, Grune Stratton, pp 285–298.

174. Shurtleff DB: Health care delivery. In Shurtleff DB, editor: *Myelodysplasias and exstrophies: significance, prevention, and treatment*, Orlando, FL, 1986, Grune Stratton, pp 449–514.

175. Shurtleff DB: (1986d). Mobility. In Shurtleff DB, editor: *Myelodysplasias and exstrophies: significance, prevention, and treatment*, Orlando, FL, 1986, Grune Stratton, pp 313–356.

176. Shurtleff DB: Selection process for the care of congenitally malformed infants. In Shurtleff DB, editor: *Myelodysplasias and exstrophies: significance, prevention, and treatment*, Orlando, FL, 1986, Grune Stratton, pp 89–116.

177. Shurtleff DB, Dunne K: Adults and adolescents with myelomeningocele. In Shurtleff DB, editor: *Myelodysplasias and exstrophies: significance, prevention, and treatment*, Orlando, FL, 1986, Grune Stratton, pp 433–448.

178. Shurtleff DB, Lamers J: Clinical considerations in the treatment of myelodysplasia. In Crandal DB, Brazier MAB, editors: *Prevention of neural tube defects: the role of alpha-fetoprotein*, New York, 1978, Academic Press, pp 103–122.

179. Shurtleff DB, Mayo M: Toilet training: the Seattle experience and conclusions. In Shurtleff DB, editor: *Myelodysplasias and exstrophies: significance, prevention, and treatment*, Orlando, FL, 1986, Grune Stratton, pp 267–284.

180. Shurtleff DB, Duguay S, Duguay G, et al.: Epidemiology of tethered cord with meningomyelocele, *Eur J Pediatr Surg* 7(Suppl 1):7–11, 1997.

181. Shurtleff DB, Lemire RJ, Warkany J: Embryology, etiology and epidemiology. In Shurtleff DB, editor: *Myelodysplasias and exstrophies: significance, prevention, and treatment*, Orlando, FL, 1986, Grune Stratton, pp 39–64.

182. Shurtleff DB, Luthy DA, Benededetti TJ, Mack LA: Meningomyelocele: management in utero and post partum. Neural tube defects, *CIBA Found Symp* 181:270–286, 1994.

183. Simeonsson RJ, Huntington GS, McMillen JS, et al.: Development factors, health, and psychosocial adjustment of children and youths with spina bifida. In Matsumoto S, Sato SH, editors: *Spina bifida*, New York, 1999, Springer Verlag, pp 543–551.

184. Sival DA, Brouwer OF, Bruggink JLM, et al.: Movement analysis in neonates with spina bifida aperta, *Early Hum Dev* 82:227–234, 2006.

185. Sousa JC, Gordon LH, Shurtleff DB: Assessing the development of daily living skills in patients with spina bifida, *Dev Med Child Neurol* 18(Suppl 37):134–142, 1976.

186. Sousa JC, Telzrow RW, Holm RA, et al.: Developmental guidelines for children with myelodysplasia, *Phys Ther* 63:21–29, 1983.

187. Stack GD, Baber GC: The neurological involvement of the lower limbs in myelomeningocele, *Dev Med Child Neurol* 9:732, 1967.

188. Staheli LT: Prone hip extension test: method of measuring hip flexion deformity, *Clin Orthop* 123:12–15, 1977.

189. Staheli LT: *Practice of pediatric orthopedics*, Philadelphia, 2001, Lippincott Williams Wilkins.

190. Stillwell A, Menelaus MB: Walking ability in mature patients with spina bifida, *J Pediatr Orthop* 3:184–190, 1983.

191. Stuberg WA, Metcalf WK: Reliability of quantitative muscle testing in healthy children and in children with Duchenne muscular dystrophy using a hand-held dynamometer, *Phys Ther* 68:977–982, 1988.

192. Sutton LN: Fetal surgery for neural tube defects, *Best Pract Res Clin Obstet Gynaecol* 22:175–188, 2008.

193. Szalay EA, Cheema A: Children with spina bifida are at risk for low bone density, *Clin Orthop Relat Res* 469(5):1253–1257, 2011.

194. Teulier C, Smith BA, Kubo M, et al.: Stepping responses of infants with myelomeningocele when supported on a motorized treadmill, *Phys Ther* 89(1):60–72, 2009.

195. Tew B, Laurence KM: The effects of hydrocephalus on intelligence, visual perception, and school attainments, *Dev Med Child Neurol* 17(Suppl 35):129–134, 1975.

196. Torode I, Godette G: Surgical correction of congenital kyphosis in myelomeningocele, *J Pediatr Orthop* 15:202–205, 1995.

197. Tulipan N, Sutton LN, Cohen BM: The effect of intrauterine myelomeningocele repair on the incidence of shunt-dependent hydrocephalus, *Pediatr Neurosurg* 38:27–33, 2003.

198. Turk MA, Weber RJ: Adults with congenital and childhood onset disability disorders. In DeLisa JB, Gans BM, editors: *Rehabilitation medicine: principles and practice*, ed 3, Philadelphia, 1998, Lippincott-Raven, pp 953–962.

199. Vankoski S, Moore C, Satler K, et al.: The influence of forearm crutches on pelvic and hip kinematic parameters in childhood community ambulators with low-level myelomeningocele-Don't throw away the crutches, *Dev Med Child Neurol* 37(Suppl 75):5–6, 1995.

200. Weber D, Agro M: *Clinical aspects of lower extremity orthotics*, Winnipeg, Manitoba, 1993, Canadian Association of Prosthetists and Orthotists.

201. Wicks K, Shurtleff DB: (1986a). An introduction to toilet training. In Shurtleff DB, editor: *Myelodysplasias and exstrophies: significance, prevention, and treatment*, Orlando, FL, 1986, Grune Stratton, pp 203–219.

202. Wicks K, Shurtleff DB: (1986b). Stool management. In Shurtleff DB, editor: *Myelodysplasias and exstrophies: significance, prevention, and treatment*, Orlando, FL, 1986, Grune Stratton, pp 221–242.

203. Williams EN, Broughton NS, Menelaus MB: Age-related walking in children with spina bifida, *Dev Med Child Neurol* 41:446–449, 1999.

204. Reference deleted in proofs.

205. Williams LV, Anderson AD, Campbell J, et al.: Energy cost of walking and of wheelchair propulsion by children with myelodysplasia: comparison with normal children, *Dev Med Child Neurol* 25:617–624, 1983.

206. Winter DA: Knee flexion during stance as a determinant of inefficient walking, *Phys Ther* 63:331–333, 1983.

207. Wolf LS, McLaughlin JF: Early motor development in infants with myelomeningocele, *Pediatr Phys Ther* 4:12–17, 1992.

208. Wright J, Menelaus M, Broughton N, Shurtleff D: Natural history of knee contractures in myelomeningocele, *J Pediatr Orthop* 11:725–730, 1991.

209. Yi Y, Lindemann M, Colligs A, et al.: Economic burden of neural tube defects and impact of prevention with folic acid: a literature review, *Eur J Pediatr* 170(11):1391–1400, 2011.

210. Zsolt S, Seidl R, Bernert G, et al.: Latex sensitization in spina bifida appears disease-associated, *J Pediatr* 134:344–348, 1999.

24

Children With Autism Spectrum Disorder

Toby Long, Jamie M. Holloway

INTRODUCTION

Autism spectrum disorder (ASD) is a developmental disability that results in significant social, communication, and behavioral challenges. Data from the Centers for Disease Control and Prevention (CDC) suggest that, although an experienced professional can identify ASD by the time a child is age 2, ASD is often not diagnosed until a child is age 4 or later.[23] The cause of ASD is unknown, but suspected genetic and environmental risk factors are associated with the diagnosis. The CDC currently estimates that 1 in 68 children are diagnosed with autism.[23] Blumberg et al.,[17] however, surveyed parents regarding the ASD diagnosis, and their results indicate that the prevalence may be as high as 1 in 50. Boys are four times more likely to be diagnosed with ASD than girls.[6,22]

This chapter describes the characteristics of ASD, the diagnostic process, program planning, and evidence-based decision making for children with ASD. The chapter also emphasizes the role of the physical therapist in a comprehensive interdisciplinary team–based approach to the intervention of children and youth with ASD.

BACKGROUND INFORMATION

ETIOLOGY AND PATHOPHYSIOLOGY OF AUTISM SPECTRUM DISORDER

There is no one etiology for autism. Autism is considered a neurologically based condition, probably due to a genetic predisposition and environmental interactions. In addition to the increased incidence of children in families being diagnosed with ASD, there are also several genetic disorders associated with ASD. These include tuberous sclerosis, fragile X syndrome, chromosome 15 deletion syndromes such as Prader-Willi syndrome and Angelman syndrome, Down syndrome, moebius, and CHARGE syndrome (of the eye, heart defects, atresia of the choanae, retardation of growth and development, and ear abnormalities and deafness).[56]

Family studies have also provided information on the genetic basis for ASD. Hallmayer et al.[53] found that in a sample of 192 sets of twins in California, 77% of the identical twin boys and 31% of the fraternal twin boys had ASD. Chawarska and colleagues from the Baby Siblings Research Consortium (BSRC)[24] found that as young as 18 months of age, siblings of children diagnosed with ASD have distinct patterns of behavior that may predict the diagnosis of autism at 36 months of age. The BSRC study indicates that siblings of children with autism are 14.7 times more likely than siblings of children without autism to be diagnosed with autism at 36 months of age. The study found patterns of behavior at 18 months of age that identified the amount of risk to be diagnosed with ASD at age 36 months.

Children at 18 months of age who showed poorly modulated eye contact to initiate, terminate, or regulate social interactions; the absence of giving objects to others to share; and limited use of emotional or descriptive communicative gestures other than pointing were three times more likely to be diagnosed with ASD at 36 months. Other children who showed impaired eye contact and the inability to spontaneously engage in pretend play were almost two times more likely to be diagnosed with ASD. A third group of siblings in this study demonstrated repetitive and stereotyped behaviors and rarely or never engaged in sharing behaviors, typical eye contact, and other appropriate communication behaviors. Despite being what the authors considered to be borderline at 18 months, children in this group were three times more likely to be diagnosed with ASD at 36 months than were peers who did not have siblings with ASD.

Evidence of a variety of neurologic abnormalities has been found in people with ASD. Studies suggest that *underconnectivity* in the brain leads to decreased communication between brain regions and resultant impairments.[49,61,86] Libero[71] also found significantly decreased cortical thickness, white matter connectivity, and neurochemical concentrations in the brains of adults with ASD. Evidence of inflammation in the glia of the brains of people with ASD has also been found.[52] These brain abnormalities may be associated with the motor deficits seen in children with ASD. For example, Bailey et al.[8] showed a decrease in the number of Purkinje cells in the vermis and hemispheres in the cerebellum. This may contribute to the poor coordination seen in children with ASD.[44]

Other neurologic evidence suggests that the function of mirror neurons might be altered in children with ASD. Mirror neurons are activated when people perform a task as well as when they observe a task.[41] Mirror neurons are thought to be involved in the recognition of motor tasks. Studies have suggested that the dysfunction in this system might also explain the social and cognitive impairments observed in children with ASD.[97]

Although environmental factors may interact with genes to contribute to the expression of autistic symptoms, there is little indication of what these specific environmental factors may be.[56]

DIAGNOSTIC CRITERIA ACROSS AUTISM SPECTRUM DISORDER

A diagnosis of ASD is made based on criteria listed in the *Diagnostic and Statistical Manual,* Fifth Edition (DSM-5).[34] The DSM-5 combines the criteria for autistic disorder, Asperger disorder, childhood disintegrative disorder, and pervasive developmental disorder not otherwise specified (PDD-NOS) under

the umbrella of autism. The diagnosis is based on symptoms that do the following:
- Cause functional impairment
- Are present in early childhood
- Are not better described by another condition

The criteria define the severity of ASD based on the level of support the child needs to communicate, problem solve, use movement, and use behavior above what would be expected for his or her age. The severity also reflects the impact of co-occurring conditions such as an intellectual disability or attention deficit disorder.

There are three categories of symptoms:
- Social reciprocity
- Communication intent
- Repetitive behaviors

These three categories of symptoms fall under two types of ASD:
- Social communication/interaction
- Restricted and repetitive behaviors

For a child to be diagnosed with the *social communication/ interaction* type of ASD, three behaviors must be present. The child must have difficulty establishing/maintaining back and forth interactions, maintaining relationships, and communicating nonverbally. For a child to be diagnosed with the *restricted/ repetitive behaviors* type of ASD, two of four behaviors must be present. The child must display stereotyped, repetitive speech, movements, or object play; excessive adherence to routines or rituals; highly restrictive, abnormal interests; or hyper/hyperoactivity to sensory input or unusual interest in sensory input. Box 24.1 delineates the criteria as defined by the DSM-5.

Several additional features associated with ASD have been identified.[6] These include the following:
- Motor deficits such as unusual gait, clumsiness, or toe-walking
- Self-injurious behavior such as head banging or biting
- Anxiety or depression

- A large gap between intellectual ability and adaptive/self-care skills
- Significant delays or impairments in performing routine daily caregiving tasks, even if the child does not have an intellectual disability

Motor skill performance has previously been thought of as a strength for children with autism. Research, however, indicates that this area may be a strength only in comparison to other areas of difficulty or deficits. Several studies synthesized by Downey and Rapport[33] have found that children with ASD score lower on tests of fine and gross motor skill development when compared to children without autism. Current literature also shows difficulties with coordination and postural control in children with ASD.[33] Green et al.[50] found that 79% of their sample of children with ASD had motor impairments based on the *Movement Assessment Battery of Children–2,* and the scores of 10% more of their sample were in the borderline range. More recently, children with ASD demonstrated greater overall motor impairment in comparison to children who are typically developing or have a diagnosis of attention deficient disorder (ADHD).[2] Children with ASD are also likely to have more difficulty maintaining balance and catching a ball, findings that are consistent with previous reports.[2,50]

Associated Conditions

Children with autism may also have a variety of related conditions. ASD commonly co-occurs with other developmental, psychiatric, neurologic, chromosomal, and genetic diagnoses (Table 24.1). The co-occurrence of one or more non-ASD developmental diagnoses such as intellectual disability, learning disabilities, or sensory processing disorders is 83%.[70] The co-occurrence of one or more psychiatric diagnoses such as anxiety or depression is 10%.[70] It is critical for the interdisciplinary team determining the diagnosis of ASD to differentiate autism from other possible diagnoses and share with families all conditions that may be contributing to a child's behavior and characteristics. Table 24.1 describes associated conditions often seen in children with ASD.

GENERAL/MEDICAL DIAGNOSTIC PROCESS

Screening

Early identification and intervention are critical for children with autism.[128] Research indicates that early intervention positively effects developmental and functional outcome of children with ASD.[100] Screening tools are helpful to determine if a family should explore further evaluation. Studies show that routine screening increases the rates of referral to appropriate intervention services and supports.[31,51] Several tools have been developed to screen for ASD in young children. Caution should be taken when using these tools because they were developed using previous diagnostic criteria and may not accurately screen for ASD under current DSM-5 criteria. There has been little research assessing the accuracy of these screening tools against the DSM-5 criteria. However, as clinical tools to determine if referral for further testing is necessary, they still are useful. General developmental screening tools, such as the *Ages and Stages Questionnaires–3*[113] or the *Denver Developmental Screening Tool,*[48] are also used to determine if a child has generalized developmental delays. Table 24.2 describes commonly used tools developed specifically for screening children for ASD. The American Academy of Pediatrics[60] recommends screening for autism during well child checks at 18 and 24 months of age for all children, with earlier screening recommended if a specific

---

BOX 24.1 DSM-5 Criteria for the Diagnosis of Autism Spectrum Disorder

- Deficits in social communication and social interaction across multiple contexts
  - Deficits may be in social-emotional reciprocity
  - Deficits in nonverbal communication
  - Deficits in developing, maintaining, and understanding relationships
- Restricted repetitive patterns of behavior, interest, or activities; the individual must demonstrate two of the following four criteria
  - Stereotyped or repetitive motor movement, use of objects, or speech (lining up toys, echolalia, etc.)
  - Insistence on sameness, inflexible adherence to routines, or ritualized patterns of verbal or nonverbal behavior (difficulties with transitions, greeting rituals, etc.)
  - Highly restricted, fixated interests that are abnormal in intensity or focus (perseverative interests, strong attachment to or preoccupation with unusual objects, etc.)
  - Hyper- or hyporeactivity to sensory input or unusual interest in sensory aspects of the environment (adverse responses to sounds or textures, apparent indifference to pain/temperature, etc.)
- Symptoms must be present from early developmental period
- Symptoms must cause clinically significant impairment in social, occupational, or other important areas of current functioning
- Disturbances are not better explained by intellectual disability or global developmental delay

From Autism spectrum disorder. In American Psychiatric Association: *Diagnostic and statistical manual of mental disorders,* ed 5, Washington, DC, 2013, American Psychiatric Association.

TABLE 24.1	Co-occurring Conditions Associated With Autism Spectrum Disorder
Condition	**Characteristics/Prevalence**
Attention deficit hyperactivity disorder	*Children with developmentally inappropriate inattention, impulsiveness, and hyperactivity* 41%–95%[4]
Communication disorders	*Difficulty making intentions known through talking or other forms of expression (gestures, signs, assistive technology) or understanding the spoken or written word*[3] Speech disorders: Difficulty formulating sounds Language disorders: Difficulty understanding Pragmatics: Functional and socially appropriate communication Processing disorders: Deficit of CNS processing information Production disorder: Inability to produce sounds. Includes fluency disorders such as stuttering 63.4%[70]
Epilepsy	*The occurrence of two unprovoked seizures of any type* 16%–44%[69]
Gastrointestinal disorders	*The most common gastrointestinal symptoms reported are constipation, diarrhea, reflux, food regurgitation, food selectivity, food intolerance, or allergy* 42%[129]
Intellectual disability	*Children with below average intelligence (< 70) and adaptive* skills 18.3%[70]
Learning disabilities	*Children with at least average intelligence who have difficulty or an inability to acquire and use the academic skills of oral language, reading, written language, and math (DSM-5)* 6.3%[70]
Motor planning disorders or dyspraxia	*Difficulty planning, coordinating, initiating movements and actions* Praxis or motor planning requires: —Ideation (generating the idea of a movement), —Motor planning (organizing the action), and —Execution (actually performing the movement) Etiology may be due to underlying sensory processing disorders or CNS inefficiency or injury Evidence indicates that dyspraxia may be a core component of autism spectrum disorder (ASD) Characteristics Difficulties with eye movements, walking, hopping, skipping Tend to bump into objects Difficulty with fine motor skills May be sensitive to touch In older children dyspraxia may contribute to: —Difficulty coordinating more sophisticated motor skills needed to play sports —Speech difficulties —Writing difficulties —Difficulty developing social relationships 34%[134]
Obesity	*Body mass index > 95th %* 31.8% of adolescents[93]
Psychiatric disorders (mood disorders, anxiety, depression, obsessive-compulsive disorder, schizophrenia)	*Patterns of psychological or behavioral symptoms that interfere with the way a person behaves, interacts with others, and functions in daily life; anxiety is the most common and schizophrenia the least in children with ASD* 10%[70]
Sensory processing disorders	*Inability to organize, process sensory input from the body (visual, auditory, taste, olfactory, tactile, vestibular) and environment* Three categories have been described [9,10,84,123] —Under-responsive —Over-responsive —Sensation seeking 15.7%[70]
Sleep disorders	*Difficulty with sleep initiation or maintenance* 50%–80%[64]
Tic disorders	0.5%[70]
Toe-walking	20.6%[12]

concern arises from the parent or pediatrician or if the child has a sibling with ASD. Physical therapists working with young children may also be involved in screening for ASD to make appropriate referral to an interdisciplinary team for diagnostic evaluation if concerns are noted. Based on screening results, recommendations for a comprehensive diagnostic examination will be made to determine eligibility and to develop a comprehensive program plan if necessary.

Diagnostic Evaluation

A diagnostic evaluation should be completed to determine an appropriate diagnosis if a screening indicates that a child may have ASD. Research shows that an accurate diagnosis can be made by 24 months of age.[31] Best practice guidelines recommend diagnostic evaluations be conducted by an interdisciplinary team. Team members may include a psychologist, psychiatrist, developmental pediatrician, neurologist, physical therapist, occupational therapist,

Tool	Age	Format	Sensitivity/Specificity[a]	Comments	Availability	References
Modified Checklist for Autism Spectrum Disorder in Toddlers (M-CHAT)	16–48 months	Parent-completed questionnaire	0.85/0.93	Free online Higher specificity than sensitivity	First Signs http://www.firstsigns.org/downloads/m-chat.PDF	References 98, 109
Pervasive Developmental Disorders Screening Test-II (PDDST-II)	18–48 months	Parent-completed questionnaire	0.92/0.91	Must be purchased and distributed to parent	Pearson Clinical Assessments Ordering Department P.O. Box 599700 San Antonio, Texas 78259 800.627.7271 http://www.pearsonclinical.com/psychology/products/100000132/pervasive-developmental-disorders-screening-test-ii-pddst-ii-html.	Reference 79
Screening Tool for Autism Spectrum Disorder in Two-Year-Olds (STAT)	24–36 months	Interactive format with the clinician	0.92/0.85	High sensitivity Clinician administered Lengthy Training required	Vanderbilt University http://stat.vueinnovations.com/products	References 115, 135
Social Communication Questionnaire (SCQ)	> 4 years old	Parent-completed questionnaire	0.85–0.96/0.67–0.80	Must be purchased	Western Psychological Services 625 Alaska Avenue Torrance, CA 90503-5124 800.648.8857 http://www.wpspublish.com/store/p/2954/social-communication-questionnaire-scq	Reference 18

TABLE 24.2   Comparison of Selected Screening Tools for Autism Spectrum Disorder

From Long T, Brady R: *Contemporary practices in early intervention for children birth through five: a distance learning curriculum,* Washington, DC, 2012, Georgetown University. Available at teachingei.org.
[a]Based on reported research.

speech-language pathologist, and sometimes a special educator. Physical therapists who are involved in the diagnostic evaluation process will conduct a comprehensive physical therapy examination of a child's sensory-motor abilities and behaviors and make recommendations for services. Physical therapists may also be involved in the administration of specific tools used to aid in the diagnosis of ASD if they have received specialized training in these tools.

The comprehensive interdisciplinary evaluation examines all areas of development including communication, speech, language, fine, gross, and perceptual motor skills, self-help skills, social-emotional, and cognitive skills. A diagnosis is made based on criteria in the DSM-5 described previously. Some tools also exist to help clinicians gather information specific to the diagnosis of ASD based on salient characteristics. As indicated under screening, these diagnostic tools were also developed prior to the publication of the DSM-5, thus caution should be used when interpreting the information in relationship to the DSM-5 diagnostic criteria. Table 24.3 provides salient information on the three most popular diagnostic tools administered by trained members of interdisciplinary teams that evaluate and serve individuals with ASD and their families. Box 24.2 delineates specific information about the *Childhood Autism Rating Scale,* Second Edition,[106] a commonly used tool to differentiate children with ASD from those with severe cognitive disabilities. All members of the team are eligible to be trained in the use of these tools, including physical therapists.

FOREGROUND INFORMATION

PHYSICAL THERAPY EXAMINATION

History

A comprehensive physical therapy examination includes obtaining a thorough history through chart review, family interviews, and interviews with other caregivers such as child care providers or teachers. Critical medical history may include history of seizures, allergies, medications, immunizations, and any significant hospitalization. Specific to children with ASD, information such as involvement in and outcomes of past therapeutic history, early intervention services, and community-based activities should be obtained. Children with ASD often participate in alternative programs such as special diets. Documenting these programs and what effects these may have had is important.

Systems Review

The physical therapy examination begins with an anatomic and physiologic review of systems. Any issues or concerns identified during systems review warrant further testing during examination of body structures and function, activity, and participation. Children with ASD often have co-occurring conditions in a variety of physiologic and psychological systems (see Table 24.1). Because ASD is a complex, multisystem condition, the physical therapy examination is most often one component of a multidisciplinary evaluation. Information specific to cognition, communication, social skills, and the like will be examined by other team members; however, the physical therapist should be aware of the child's communication and interaction style and skill level to interact effectively with him or her, thus the physical therapist should review current information in these areas. The physical therapy examination will include specific examination of the musculoskeletal, neuromuscular, and sensory-motor systems, but a brief assessment of these systems should begin during the systems review to identify initial concerns related to these systems. Older children with physical activity limitations or who are obese may identify issues in these areas that warrant further cardiovascular/pulmonary system examination assessing endurance and speed for example. A brief assessment of the integumentary system is also important

TABLE 24.3 Tools Used for the Diagnosis of Autism Spectrum Disorder

Tool	Description	Population	Format	Availability	References
Autism Diagnostic Interview-Revised (ADI-R)	Gathers information in three domains: language/communication, reciprocal social interactions, and restricted, repetitive, and stereotyped behaviors and interests	Children and adults with mental age above 2.0 years	Parent interview format that takes about 1.5 to 2.5 hours to complete	http://www .wpspublish .com/	Rutter, Le Couteur, and Lord 2003
Autism Diagnostic Observation Schedule-Revised (ADOS-2)	Consists of five modules Select module based on expressive language level and chronologic age Modules 1 through 4 provide cutoff scores that fall into classifications of autism spectrum disorder, or nonspectrum Module 1: Children 31 months and older who do not consistently use phrase speech Module 2: Children of any age who use phrase speech, but are not verbally fluent Module 3: Children who are verbally fluent and young adolescents Module 4: Older adolescents and adults who are verbally fluent The Toddler module provides "ranges of concern" to help inform clinical impressions but avoid formal classification. Children between 12 and 30 months of age who do not consistently use three or more word phrases to communicate (phrase speech)	People aged 12 months through adulthood	Direct observation of child taking about 40–60 minutes to administer	www.pearson-clinical.com	Lord, Rutter, and DiLavore et al., 2012
Childhood Autism Rating Scale 2nd Ed (CARS-2)	Rates behaviors of children to determine severity of symptoms 4-point response scale based on the frequency, intensity, peculiarity, and duration of the behavior Discriminates between children with ASD and those with severe cognitive disabilities Standard Version Rating Scale (ST) and a High-Functioning Rating Scale (HF) each contain 15 items (see Table 24.5) The test also includes a questionnaire for parents and caregivers to assess early development; social, emotional, and communication skills; repetitive behaviors; play and routines; and unusual sensory interests (see Table 24.5)	People 2 years of age through adulthood	Direct observation	http://www .wpspublish .com/	Schopler et al., 2010

BOX 24.2 CARS-2 Functional Areas of Assessment

- Relating to people
- Imitation (ST); social-emotional understanding (HF)
- Emotional response (ST); emotional expression and regulation of emotions (HF)
- Body use
- Object use (ST); object use in play (HF)
- Adaptation to change (ST); adaptation to change/restricted interests (HF)
- Visual response
- Listening response
- Taste, smell, and touch response and use
- Fear or nervousness (ST); fear or anxiety (HF)
- Verbal communication
- Nonverbal communication
- Activity level (ST); thinking/cognitive integration skills (HF)
- Level and consistency of intellectual response
- General impressions

HF, High-Functioning Rating Scale (HF); *ST,* Standard Version Rating Scale.

to evaluate the integrity of the child's skin and inquire about the child's history of self-injurious behavior or falls. Important findings from the review of systems will determine specific tests and measures to be performed during the physical therapy examination. Physical therapists should review, through family interview or chart review, systems such as the gastrointestinal, hearing, and vision.

Tests and Measures

Impairment

Impairments in body structure and function may impact a child's activities and participation. Measures of strength, range of motion, muscle tone, and balance described elsewhere in this text can also be used with children with ASD.

Measurement of sensory processing is an important factor in the physical therapy examination for children with autism. Sensory processing differences have been well documented in people with ASD. Prevalence rates range from 40% to > 90%.[101] Tomchek, Huebner, and Dunn[123] have provided background information on these differences documented in the basic science literature, clinical literature, and in first-person accounts. Sensory processing difficulties have been associated with social communication challenges,[130] social participation,[96] and social adaptive behaviors.[14]

The *Sensory Profile 2 (SP-2)*[36] is one of a family of tools developed to determine how people process sensory information in everyday situations. The SP-2 is a parent-report tool on children from birth through 14 years 11 months that measures sensory processing through six sensory systems: auditory, visual, touch, movement, body position, and oral. Scores are used to develop a sensory pattern for the child. The tool also includes a planning report to link findings to participation in a variety of settings such as home and school.

Research using the Sensory Profile[35,36] has identified sensory processing dysfunction in children with autism and differentiating patterns of sensory processing in children with ASD in comparison to typically developing peers.[123] Tomchek, Huebner, and Dunn[124] conducted a large-scale study (n = 400) identifying six sensory processing factors using a short form of the Sensory Profile, which may impact development, learning, and social interaction. These include low energy/weak, tactile/movement sensitivity, taste/smell sensitivity, auditory/visual sensitivity, sensory seeking/distractibility, and hyporesponsitivity. These factors are consistent with findings from smaller-scale studies conducted since the 1990s[35,81,82] indicating that deficits in these areas limit a child's attention, contribute to distractibility, and influence arousal, all necessary components for learning. Physical therapists' knowledge in the sensory processing area and their expertise in evaluating this area are unique contributions to the team's ability to describe the child comprehensively, explain performance, and develop comprehensive, responsive, functional program plans.

Activity and Participation

Examination of a child's strengths and limitations in activities and participation during daily routines is an important part of physical therapy examination. When possible, the examination should occur during the child's natural routines to obtain a true picture of the child's abilities. The examination should focus on activities most relevant to the child and family's needs.

Tools are available to assist the physical therapist (PT) in determining developmental skill level.[13,19,46] There are also tools that assess underlying components of movement or motor skills that may be helpful for children with dyspraxia, a characteristic seen in many children with ASD.[101] Tools such as the *Test of Gross Motor Development–3;*[125] the *Movement Assessment Battery for Children–2;*[54] and the *Miller Function and Participation Scales*[83] may be helpful for children with less severe forms of ASD. As discussed earlier, Ament et al.[2] demonstrated that findings from the *Movement Assessment Battery for Children–2 (MABC-2)* differentiated children with ASD from those with ADHD and typically developing children, thus the MABC-2 may be a particularly helpful tool for physical therapists. The MABC-2 is designed to differentiate skills that require visual, temporal, and spatial characteristics of an action such as ball catching.

Emphasis on examining a child's participation has become increasingly important, and tools have become available to guide this component of a comprehensive physical therapy exam. The *Children's Assessment of Participation and Enjoyment (CAPE)* and the *Preferences for Activities of Children (PAC)*[63] are designed to measure the participation of children ages 6 to 21. These tools are self-report measures of the child's participation in recreation and leisure activities outside of required school activities. The *CAPE* measures formal and informal activities of recreational, active physical, social, skill-based, and self-improvement domains. The *PAC* has an additional dimension to examine the child's preferences. The *Preschool Activity Card Sort (PACS)*[15] was developed to examine participation for children between the ages of 3 and 6 years old. The PACS is administered through parent interview. Domains of the PACS include domestic life, self-care, mobility, education, interpersonal interactions and relationships, and community, social, and civic measurements.

McWilliam and colleagues[80] have developed a family of routines-based tools that help providers determine a young child's engagement and independence in participating in a variety of functional activities. These routines-based interviews are especially helpful for team-based decision making and outcome determination in early intervention or early childhood programming. The *School Function Assessment (SFA)*[28] is another tool that teams find helpful for determining a child's activity limitations and participation. The SFA helps school-based teams determine how participatory early elementary-aged children are in completing nonacademic skills required in classrooms and school wide. Skills include classroom activities such as computer use, mobility around the school environment, and participation in the cafeteria. See Chapter 2 for a full description of these and other tools that therapists may find helpful for assessing activity limitations and participation. Also, *Selected Assessment Tools for the Evaluation of Children with Autism Spectrum Disorder in School Based Practice*, developed by the Academy of Pediatric Physical Therapy of the American Physical Therapy Association, describes a variety of tools across domains that the PT may find helpful.

Assessment of gait is another important component of the examination, as toe-walking and other gait abnormalities are common in children with ASD. Over 20% of children with ASD walk on their tiptoes.[12] A study by Esposito et al.[42] found that toddlers with ASD showed more asymmetry in gait compared to toddlers with developmental delay and toddlers who were typically developing. Gait abnormalities such as toe-walking can lead to decreased range of motion in the ankle joint, thus, it is important to address this issue as early as possible.

Determining the child's level of independence and participation in adaptive skills such as self-care is also important. Research suggests that higher adaptive functioning is associated with positive outcomes in adults with ASD.[43] The *Pediatric Evaluation of Disability Inventory-Computer Adapted Test (PEDI-CAT)* as described in Chapter 2 is commonly used to measure capability and performance of skills in the self-care, mobility, and social function in children from birth to 21 years of age. The authors have adapted the PEDI-CAT to meet the unique characteristics of children with autism.[65] Research indicates that the PEDI-CAT (ASD) is a reliable tool that parents find easy to use. The *Vineland Adaptive Behavior Scales, Second Edition (VABS-II)*[111] measures adaptive behavior from birth through adulthood. Domains on the VABS-II include communication, daily living skills, socialization, motor skills, and an optional maladaptive behaviors index. The VABS-II is administered via parent or teacher interview. Using the daily activities, social/cognitive and responsibility domains of the PEDI-CAT (ASD), Kramer, Lilenquist, and Coster[65] found that those constructs are similar to the VABS-II in children with autism, providing validity for its use with this population. The authors also found that parents preferred the PEDI-CAT (ASD) to the VABS-II as they found the computer version easier to use, quicker, more efficient, and more strength based.

Environmental Considerations

The International Classification of Functioning, Disability and Health (ICF) model views disability and functioning as the outcome of the interaction between the health condition and contextual factors.[133] Contextual factors include external environmental factors and internal personal factors. Environmental factors include limiting and enabling factors that are external to the individual such as social attitudes, legal policies, and architectural characteristics. The physical therapist may not be able to directly control or change the environmental factors; however, understanding the child's functioning within the context of the environment is important for establishing appropriate intervention strategies. Consideration of the environmental stimuli that are present is important when working with children with ASD. For example, a child with ASD might prefer an environment with low noise and minimal visual distractions, whereas another child may prefer a loud, busy environment. Personal factors are those that are internal to the individual, including age, coping style, and past experience. An understanding of personal factors that motivate an individual can provide an important context for meaningful interventions for the child. This is especially important when working with children with ASD who have very narrow interests. The Sensory Profile 2 is a helpful tool for linking environmental factors to a child's behavior. Although it may be challenging to achieve change in certain characteristics of a child with ASD (for example, tactile sensitivity), removing tags from clothing or avoiding certain materials may decrease the child's negative behaviors that are a preferred response to tactile stimulation.

Evaluation/Interpretation–Clinical Decision Making Regarding Need for Physical Therapy Services

Using the examination information and that obtained from team members, the physical therapist, in collaboration with the team, will design an appropriate, meaningful, functional intervention plan. The evidence-informed decision-making process considers the strengths and needs of the child and family, research evidence on intervention strategies and procedures, clinical expertise, and the home and community environment. Current practice indicates that children should be served in the natural environment by those practitioners with the skills and knowledge to best help the child and family meet their outcomes.[38,120]

Determining Outcomes and Goals

The comprehensive physical therapy examination process includes collecting information specifically to help the program planning process. Program planning includes determining outcomes and goals that promote a child's functional activity and participation, limit impairments, or prevent further disability. Depending on the physical therapy practice environment (early intervention, school based, inpatient, outpatient, etc.) these outcomes may be developed within a team process or independently. In addition to tools described previously such as the routines-based interviews, the CAPE/PAC, SFA, and so on, the *Canadian Occupational Performance Measure*,[68] goal attainment scaling,[105] and the top-down approach are useful for program planning.

The top-down approach described in Chapter 18 is very helpful for identifying possible barriers to the accomplishment of specific tasks for children with complex diagnoses such as ASD. This approach is consistent with a family-centered, team-based practice that is supported for children with disabilities, especially those being served by the part B and part C components of the Individuals with Disabilities Education Act (IDEA).

The approach helps providers to link specific impairments or activity limitations to a desired outcome, easing the measurement and documentation of change toward reaching functional outcomes.

As discussed previously, decisions regarding which professionals will provide intervention to the child and how often are based on the outcomes determined by the team.

PHYSICAL THERAPY INTERVENTION

Coordination, Communication, Documentation

Physical therapists must coordinate their services with other service providers to ensure that children with ASD are receiving comprehensive services delivered in a manner that reinforces goals and outcomes across providers, builds on the child's strengths, and assists the child to bypass barriers in performing functional and meaningful skills and activities. PTs are responsible for communicating their examination findings to other team members, explaining perspective and findings, and developing with the team a comprehensive integrated service plan. Physical therapists may be required to document their services in a variety of ways depending on the payment and regulatory systems. For example, under the Infants and Toddlers Program of IDEA, physical therapists will need to document their services through the Individualized Family Service Plan (IFSP) process. They may also have to document their services as required by a third-party payment system such as Medicaid. Physical therapists often voice concern about inefficiency, duplication of documentation, and the changing requirements for documentation as children age due to the variety of regulatory and payment systems serving children with complex developmental disorders such as autism spectrum disorder.

Patient/Caregiver Instruction

Pediatric physical therapy requires ongoing collaboration with family members and other caregivers. Evidence indicates that children develop new skills, learn tasks, and participate effectively when intervention is intensive and embedded into the context of daily routines and activities. Parent and caregiver instruction should focus on strategies to promote a child's participation in daily routines and activities.

Procedural Interventions

Contemporary practice supports a team-based approach to intervention planning and service delivery that promotes active participation of children with ASD in the community. As with all children with disabilities or developmental delays, intervention for children with ASD should be evidence based and represent contemporary best practices. These practices include those that are (1) team based, in which the family is an equal, contributing member of the team; (2) delivered in what is considered the natural context for learning the skills desired; (3) based on the interests of the child; and (4) lead to mastery.[25] Information about interventions for children with ASD can be found readily in professional literature as well as in popular media.

Families receive a variety of mixed messages in regard to intervention effectiveness. Professionals should be aware that parents, who ultimately choose interventions for their children, more often base those decisions from nonmedical professionals and lay publications.[85] It is critical that professionals present intervention choices to families based on objective, evidence-based information and help families sort through the plethora of information presented. This is particularly relevant for interventions considered complementary and alternative medicine (CAM). It is estimated that between 52% and 95% of children with ASD have used CAM.[1] Physical therapists should discuss nonjudgmentally with families the evidence for the effects of various types of CAM. A thorough summary of common CAM used by families with children with ASD has been provided by Akins, Anguskustsiri, and Hansen.[1] A unique aspect to this review, which may be particularly helpful for physical therapists, is categorization of each intervention as being safe or unsafe, and it provides an evidence-based recommendation to discourage or monitor its use.

Guiding Principles of Effective Intervention

Many interventions and programs exist for children with autism. The appendix describes a variety of programs commonly used for children with ASD. Although research is emerging to support some approaches, it is apparent that no single approach works for every child with ASD. A 2003 review of the literature on ASD-specific interventions, however, revealed six common characteristics or threads among programs that have been deemed effective for children with ASD.[57] The literature continues to support these characteristics[62,89]:

- *Early intervention.* Research supports the importance of earliest possible intervention. Children who receive intervention early tend to make changes across all domains.[128]
- *Family involvement.* Because families are the consistent and stable influence in a child's life, it is imperative that families are involved in the intervention. Family involvement includes teaching parents strategies to promote development or desired behaviors. Family involvement during an individualized family support plan (IFSP) and individualized education program (IEP) development is mandated by the Individuals with Disabilities Education Act (IDEA) and research indicates that children whose families are a part of the intervention program meet outcomes faster.[37]
- *Individualized programming.* Given that no single approach appears to benefit all children with ASD, it is recommended that interventions are individualized to meet the needs of the child with ASD and his or her family and team. Individualized programming involves consideration of the family's preferences and child expectations (for example, classroom expectations) when determining the intervention methods used and outcomes to be met. Incorporating the child's preferences and interests into the program and focusing on the child's strengths are also important factors for individualized programming.
- *Systematic intervention.* Systematic intervention refers to the systematic collection of data to identify developmental outcomes and carefully outline intervention procedures for serving children as well as evaluating the effectiveness of the procedures. Systematic intervention targets the promotion of meaningful skills and the collection of specific data to determine change over time.[55,104]
- *Structured/predictable environments.* Environments are considered structured when the activities, schedule, and environment are clear to the child, teacher, therapist, and family. Young children, including those with ASD, have been shown

to prefer and thrive in structured, predictable environments.[27]
- *Functional approach to behavior.* Current research recommends using positive behavior support to identify the function of a problem behavior and teach new skills to replace the challenging behavior with a new socially appropriate skill or communication method.[30]

Evidence of Effectiveness

Two major research studies have examined the effectiveness of interventions for children with ASD. The National Standards Project,[87] in an update of its 2009 systematic review of the effectiveness research, categorized and described interventions used for children with ASD that were found to be effective for improving behavior, communication, social skills, and other skills (i.e., motor) important for participation. Teams providing services to children with ASD should be aware of these reviews to assist families in making intervention decisions. Many intervention components are described in these reviews that, although not considered traditional physical therapy techniques, are certainly strategies used within a comprehensive treatment session—for example, modeling, practice, prompting, schedules, parent training, and natural environments. Additionally, a strategy often used by physical therapists serving children with ASD, sensory integration, is categorized as an unestablished treatment. The following categories are used for describing levels of evidence:

- *Established:* These interventions have sufficient evidence to confidently determine that they produce beneficial treatment effects.
- *Emerging:* One or more studies have suggested that these interventions will produce beneficial treatment effects, but further study on effectiveness is needed.
- *Unestablished:* There is little or no evidence to support the use of these intervention strategies (Table 24.4).

The National Professional Development Center on ASD[29] reviewed the literature and found 27 intervention strategies met its criteria for evidence-based practice. This review also described strategies that are effectively incorporated into a physical therapy session. For example, in addition to the strategies described by the National Standards Project, the National Professional Development Center on ASD described task analysis, extinction, visual supports, and reinforcement as evidence based.

It is clear from these reviews that service providers should focus their attention on the components of the models rather than the model in its entirety. Physical therapists incorporate these interventions within a comprehensive physical therapy session. For example, within a preschool program a PT may lead a small motor group intervention session that promotes the acquisition of developmental motor skills. To be most effective, the PT would incorporate strategies such as modeling, extinction, peer teaching, prompting, and time delay, thereby supporting what Bhat, Landa, and Galloway[16] described as multisystem physical therapy intervention for children with ASD. Research, however, has examined the effects of specific motor interventions used to improve developmental and functional skills as well as behavior. The next section discusses two types of motor-based interventions often used by physical therapists in a comprehensive intervention approach for children with autism.

TABLE 24.4   Interventions for Children Under 22 Years of Age With Autism Spectrum Disorder (National Standards Project, 2015)

Established (n = 14)	Emerging (n = 18)	Unestablished (n = 13)
• Behavioral interventions (discrete trial training, joint attention training, reinforcement, practice, modeling, etc.) • Cognitive-behavioral intervention package • Comprehensive behavioral treatment for young children: intensive services based on principles of applied behavioral analysis • Language production training • Modeling (live or video) • Naturalistic teaching strategies: natural environment, context specific • Peer training • Parent training • Pivotal response training • Schedules • Scripting • Self-management • Social skills package: turn-taking, recognizing facial expressions, initiating interactions, etc. • Story-based intervention	• Augmentative/alternative communication devices • Developmental relationship-based treatment • Exercise • Exposure package • Functional communication training • Imitation-based intervention • Initiation training • Language training (production and understanding) • Massage therapy • Multicomponent package • Music therapy • Picture exchange communication system • Reductive package • Sign instruction • Social communication intervention • Structured teaching • Technology-based intervention • Theory of mind training	• Animal-assisted therapy • Auditory integration training • Concept mapping • Developmental, individual difference, relationship based/floor time • Facilitated communication • Gluten-free/casein-free diet • Movement-based intervention • SENSE Theatre intervention • Sensory intervention package • Shock therapy • Social behavioral learning strategy • Social cognition intervention • Social thinking intervention

From National Autism Center: Findings and conclusions: National Standards Project, Phase 2. Retrieved on May 2, 2015, from http://www.nationalautismcenter.org/national-standards-project/phase-2/.

Motor Specific Interventions

Exercise and physical activity. Children with autism demonstrate delays in motor skill development, impairments in motor skill performance, and recent reports indicate increasing rates of obesity[114] in addition to sensory processing difficulties, poor social skills, difficulty communicating, and behavioral challenges. Like children with other types of developmental disabilities, children with ASD participate in more sedentary activities or individual physical activities (i.e., swimming), limiting the social components of group or team-based activities.[110] Research on the effectiveness of exercise and physical activity is limited and has focused primarily on changes in behavioral or social interactions. Lang et al.[67] conducted a systematic review of 18 research studies that incorporated exercise as a treatment for children with ASD (ages 4 to 20 years). Findings indicate that exercise was effective in decreasing stereotypic behaviors, aggression, off-task behavior, and elopement and an increase in on-task behavior and improvement in motor skill acquisition. Various exercise programs were used such as weight training, aerobic exercise, bike riding, and jogging. Although promising, these results must be interpreted with caution as the number of participants across the 18 studies was low (n = 64), most of the research designs were single-subject or within-subject designs, and the programs combined exercise with other behavioral interventions such as reinforcement, prompting, and modeling, all which have been shown to be effective practices. Sowa and Meulenbroek's meta-analysis of the effects of exercise for children and adults indicated similar findings.[110] Additionally, they found that individual rather than group interventions were more successful. Again, in a one-to-one situation, other behavioral strategies may have affected the outcomes.

Because of the lack of information on the effect of exercise on cardiovascular and musculoskeletal fitness and weight management, Srinivasan, Pescatello, and Bhat[114] recommended that this is a rich opportunity for physical therapists to increase involvement. As exercise specialists, physical therapists are in the ideal position to ensure that exercise and physical activity are included in a comprehensive intervention program. It is necessary to systematically collect data and use specific measures to assess physical fitness.

One exercise that shows promise for children with autism is swimming. Physical therapists have used aquatics as a therapeutic strategy for many years, thus they are in an ideal position to design programs and determine the effectiveness of aquatic programs for children with ASD.

Although limited, research on the effectiveness of swimming on children with ASD appears promising. Pan conducted a series of experiments testing the effectiveness of swimming on improving aquatic skills,[92] physical fitness,[91,92] and social behaviors[91] in young children with ASD. The findings from his most recent study, which involved 23 children with ASD and their typically developing siblings, indicate that children with ASD and their siblings without ASD improved on a variety of parameters following a 14-week aquatic program. As compared to other studies that incorporated swimming into the methodology, this program focused on the principles of motor learning and physical fitness. All groups demonstrated improvement in swimming skills as well as physical fitness as tested by strength, flexibility, and endurance. There was no positive effect on body composition as assessed by body mass index nor were the results long lasting, however. As previously recommended, this study incorporated a goal-directed, structured curriculum that taught skills in a progressive fashion. Additionally, the program's dosage was at a level from which change was more likely to occur: frequent (twice weekly), intense (60-minute sessions), and long duration (14-week time period.) Because the positive changes were not sustained, it is recommended that providers help children adopt a healthy active lifestyle rather than only providing limited program-specific interventions. Physical therapists are ideally positioned to support families in adopting lifestyle changes and advocating for a variety of community-based opportunities to help families and children maintain active lifestyles throughout the life span.

Sensory processing intervention. As discussed previously, many children with ASD demonstrate sensitivity to sensory input and have been identified with sensory processing dysfunction,[123] dyspraxia,[76] and incoordination.[47] A variety of strategies have been used with the intention of improving sensory-based impairments with limited, if any, effectiveness.[21,99] These ineffective strategies include (1) weighted vests and other compression garments used to provide proprioceptive input and calming to increase attention, concentration, and focus; (2) brushing and sensory diets[131] to increase tolerance to tactile input, increase focus, and improve organization; (3) fidget and fiddle toys to help sustain attention and concentration; and (4) Auditory Integration and Therapeutic Listening programs.[108]

Although sensory impairment remediation focused interventions have not been shown to be effective, Dunn and colleagues[37] have indicated that sensory-based symptomatology that prevents functional behaviors can be effectively addressed through management strategies such as adapting tasks, environments, and routines. Based on Dunn's model of sensory processing,[35] Dunn and colleagues improved parental competence and child outcomes through contextually based interventions that focused on managing the detrimental effects of sensory processing symptoms in young children with ASD.[37] Parents were provided coaching within the naturally occurring context that they identified as problematic. Contexts were primarily the home and the community. Therapists used the findings from the family-completed Sensory Profile 2[36] to determine sensory strengths or barriers to accomplishment of the functional skill desired. The therapists coached families to identify strengths-based solutions to promote outcome attainment rather than telling the family what to do. This study illustrates that using information from tools like the Sensory Profile 2 to help families identify solutions to family-identified outcomes may be an effective strategy to produce functional change.

Outcome Measures and Clinical Decision Making Regarding Response to Physical Therapy Intervention

After intervention strategies are selected and implemented, providers must continue to collect data and monitor the child's progress toward achieving the outcomes. Physical therapists conduct ongoing assessment to determine if any changes or modifications need to be made to their intervention plan. Data collection plans should consider the following:

- Use data to monitor progress and troubleshoot intervention approaches.
- Link assessment results to intervention by using them to guide and plan what skills to promote.
- Consider several intervention methods while remembering that no single approach will be right for every child. Some children may benefit from a combination of methods.
- Provide data indicating the effectiveness of the interventions used.
- Observe and record data consistently. Consider different approaches when the data indicate that the child is not progressing or succeeding.
- Collect information regarding the family's perspective on the child's success. Ask the family members how they see the child progressing.

Measuring effectiveness of intervention using goal attainment scaling (as described in Chapter 2) may be helpful when working with children who have complex needs. Schaaf, Benevides, Kelly, and Mailloux-Maggio[105] found that goal attainment scaling was useful for linking changes in function/participation to changes in sensory processing as a result of a sensory integration–based therapeutic program for children with ASD. Using goal attainment scaling, the Canadian Occupational Performance Measure, and the Parent Sense of Competence as outcome measures, Dunn and colleagues[37] found that a sensory processing–based family coaching intervention improved parent competence and children's participation in everyday activities.

Determining Intervention Dosage: Type, Intensity, and Frequency

Providers and families often have questions and concerns about the type, frequency, and intensity of services delivered. The type, frequency, and intensity of intervention should be individualized to meet the needs of the child and family. Five evidence-based factors have been identified to assist providers and families as they determine services for children with ASD[26]:

1. *Intensity.* Intensity refers to the amount of service provided and is often conceptualized by families and providers as number of hours of direct service. Research suggests that true intensity may be better measured by the child's level of *engagement* in everyday routines and activities as engagement is a powerful predictor of developmental growth.[80,116] Rather than thinking about the number of hours on a program plan (IFSP, IEP, PT Plan of Care) the team should consider whether or not the strategies and services are sufficient to influence the child's engagement across all daily routines and meet the outcomes or goals established.

2. *Fidelity of intervention delivery.* When selecting an evidence-based intervention, the team should examine what experience the provider has with the approach and whether or not the provider has a method to determine if the intervention is being correctly implemented and a plan if the outcomes are not achieved. Providers may need additional training, support, and supervision to reach the fidelity of a specific method.

3. *Social validity of outcomes.* Social validity refers to the degree in which there is an impact on the child's social participation in life when a particular outcome has been met. For example, teaching a toddler to walk up three steps in the clinic only to turn around at the top to come back down would have low social validity compared to teaching the same toddler to walk up the carpeted stairs at home to get to a playroom. In the latter case, the child's new knowledge can directly control the environment and meet immediate needs. Therefore, this activity would have high social validity.[7,88]

4. *Comprehensiveness of intervention.* Research on intervention for children with ASD suggests that progress in one developmental domain has minimal impact on other domains.[75,118] These findings have been widely replicated and strongly support a comprehensive program plan design that addresses all relevant domains of performance for the child and family.[77]

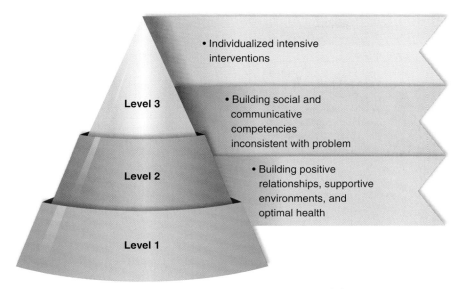

FIG. 24.1 Three-tiered intervention model.

5. *Data-based decision making.* An important component to effective intervention is to collect and monitor data to inform decision-making strategies and optimize the delivery of effective services.[59]

In addition to considering the preceding five factors, there are further considerations that impact the decisions regarding type, frequency, and intensity of services, which include the following:

- Outcomes identified by the team
- Child's age
- Total hours of engagement the family currently implements
- Developmental profile of the child
- Learning characteristics of the child
- Child's previous involvement in intervention
- Family's availability for level of service including daily routines of the child and family
- Quality and quantity of concerning behaviors

Members of the team collaborating with the family decide the type of service and the frequency and intensity of the service necessary to meet the team-developed outcomes. The team will include a variety of people depending on the age of the child and the system delivering the services, but no matter the system, the family is a team member and the family's opinions are equal to those of other team members. Team decision making requires that all members share information, and decisions are reached through consensus based on what will best meet the outcomes and expectations deemed beneficial to the child, not based on any one member's opinions, desires, or administrative constraints. The roles of team members may vary depending on the system. Ultimately, the decision regarding frequency and intensity should be based on whatever is necessary to help the child achieve the identified outcomes. It is imperative that teams identify relevant outcomes and objectively monitor the progress.

The Academy of Pediatric Physical Therapy of the American Physical Therapy Association has three key documents that may be helpful in determining the dosage of physical therapy across a variety of intervention environments school-based services, acute care, outpatient; (Academy of Pediatric Physical

Therapy, 2014, 2013, 2012). Although these documents are not written specifically for children with ASD, therapists may find them helpful for decision making. Physical therapists collaborating with family members and other team members use these documents, the five evidence-based factors, and the individual family and child characteristics to design program plans and implement therapeutic strategies at a level of intensity, frequency, and duration to influence the attainment of outcomes. The dosage of therapeutic input will change over time due to the changing capacities of the child, the child and family's involvement in services and support in addition to physical therapy, and the family's constraints. Outcome-driven, family-centered physical therapy balances the shifting needs, concerns, and priorities of the family and child.

Tiered Levels of Intervention

A tiered intervention model (Fig. 24.1) for children with ASD to support developmental, functional, and social skill acquisition and to limit the impact of atypical or problematic behaviors is promoted[26,104]:

- Level 1 describes general experiences and supports that are reasonable for any child with ASD, regardless of the child's abilities.
- Level 2 involves strategies designed to enhance a child's behavioral competences and prevent problem behaviors. Level 2 is used when strategies from level 1 are insufficient to meet the child's needs.
- Level 3 strategies are used when problem behaviors have developed to the point that they have become obstacles to learning and healthy social emotional development. Level 3 consists of procedures that are most readily associated with problem behavior interventions. Table 24.5 provides a detailed explanation of the three tiers as depicted in Fig. 24.1.

The three-tiered model shows that an early emphasis on prevention has the potential to influence a child's development of more positive social behaviors and prevent the occurrence of severe problem behaviors. Additionally, the model implies that a strong foundation of level 1 and level 2 strategies will reduce the need for more labor-intensive interventions at level 3.

TABLE 24.5   Description of Tiered Levels of Intervention

Level	Description	Examples
1	• Development of positive relationships between caregivers and child • Provision of a safe, comprehensive, stimulating, and responsive environment • Procedures to ensure that the child's physical health is sound • Activities that promote the acquisition of functional movement skills	• An engaging game is initiated by adult with child and then stopped to allow the child to look or gesture to indicate the game should continue • Creating opportunities for children to walk on a variety of surfaces, play with a variety of sizes or textures of balls, or play games that require a child to start and stop quickly, hold postures, etc.
2	• Procedures designed to enhance a young child's behavioral competencies and help prevent display of problem behaviors	• Appropriate engagement strategy such as incorporating motor activities into the intervention strategies used to promote communication and language or building on the child's strengths in the motor area to promote social skills • Pivotal response training (PRT) • Incidental teaching
3	• Procedures used to improve impairments, bypass activity limitations, or to eliminate problematic behaviors	• Positive behavior support • Specific teaching of motor skills using individualized behavior management strategies • Providing sensory-motor intervention to diminish negative effects of sensory input

Lifelong Implications and the Role of Physical Therapy
Transition to Adulthood
The transition from adolescence to adulthood can be difficult for people with ASD. Unlike early intervention or school system services, adult systems often do not utilize a service coordination model, making it difficult for families to become aware of available programs and to synchronize services between programs. Young adults with ASD were 3 to 14 times more likely to be socially isolated than young adults with an intellectual disability, emotional disturbance, or learning disability.[90] Physical therapists working with adolescents with ASD should talk with the teenager and family about plans for education or employment after high school graduation and refer them to appropriate resources to help achieve their goals. Early involvement with transition and employment programs is key to a successful transition.[78]

▮ SUMMARY

Many opportunities exist for physical therapists to help children with ASD achieve optimal outcomes throughout the life span. Physical therapists should be aware of the signs of ASD and refer the family for diagnostic evaluation as necessary. In addition, incorporating appropriate behavior strategies and current evidence-based interventions for children with ASD into physical therapy interventions is imperative to meet outcomes.

Case Scenario on Expert Consult

The case related to this chapter presents Micah, a 30-month-old child, and illustrates some of the management principles discussed in this chapter.

Behavioral
Applied Behavior Analysis (ABA)
ABA-based interventions have been shown to improve a wide variety of skills across all areas of development. Tasks are broken down into discrete trials and then coupled with reinforcement to build positive behaviors. ABA is usually administered with low adult–child ratios and can be done at home, in a classroom, or in the community. Intervention is usually intense (25–40 hours a week) and consists of individualized targeting of skills. Parents are trained to become active co-teachers. Strong evidence exists to support the use of ABA-based interventions in children over the age of 3.[112,127]

Differential Reinforcement
A form of ABA, this approach is used to increase the occurrence of desired, functional behaviors using rewards. Interfering behaviors decrease because they are not reinforced. Evidence exists to support the use of differential reinforcement in children over 4 years of age.[66]

Discrete Trial Training (DTT)
DTT is a one-on-one approach that is used to teach skills that are best taught in steps. Positive praise or rewards are used to reinforce the behavior or desired skill. Practitioners collect data to determine progress and challenges, skill acquisition, and generalization of skills. Evidence suggests that DTT is beneficial for children between 2 to 9 years of age.[45]

Schedules
Schedules can assist with managing challenging behavior by providing a visual learning strategy as well as making a routine more predictable. Schedules may consist of photographs, line drawings, three-dimensional objects, or icons. This method is flexible and may consist of a schedule for an entire day or for a specific event. They may also be used in a single place such as the classroom or may travel with a child between places within the community. Schedules are an established intervention for children ages 3 to 14.[87]

Self-Management
Self-management interventions teach children with ASD to regulate their behavior by recording when the target behavior does or does not occur. The child with ASD independently seeks or delivers reinforcers. Self-management may involve the use of checklists, visual prompts, tokens, or wrist counters. Self-management is an established intervention for children 3 to 18 years old. Studies have shown improvements in interpersonal skills and self-regulation.[87]

Communication
Augmentative and Alternative Communication (AAC)
A variety of AAC approaches are used to improve the social and communication skills of individuals with autism. Approaches such as the use of gestures, sign language, and facial expressions are classified as unaided AAC. The use of pictures, symbols, or written cues and the use of tools such as speech-generating devices are classified as aided AAC. Research suggests that speech-generating devices have been used to teach requesting skills.[126] AAC is considered an emerging intervention for children 3 to 9 years of age with ASD.[87]

Continued

Communication–cont'd
Hanen Program

The Hanen Program for Parents of Children with Autism Spectrum Disorders, also known as *More Than Words,* is a program for families of children with ASD who are under the age of 5. The program focuses on teaching families to become the primary facilitator of their child's communication and language development. Families using this approach maximize the child's opportunities to develop communication skills through everyday situations. Preliminary studies have shown that the More Than Words program may enhance early language skills, positively impact parent–child interactions, and increase social interaction.[119]

Picture Exchange System (PECS)

The PECS is one type of unaided AAC. This approach consists of using pictures as a means for individuals with autism to communicate. PECS is considered an emerging intervention for children 0 to 9 years of age.[87]

Educational
Learning Experiences and Alternative Program for Preschoolers and Their Parents (LEAP)

LEAP is an inclusive educational program where children with autism are included with peers who are typically developing. The model teaches the child's peers to facilitate the social and communicative behaviors of children with autism. ABA, peer-mediated instruction, incidental teaching, self-maintenance training, and parent training strategies are all incorporated into the LEAP model.[117]

Naturalistic Teaching Strategies

Naturalistic teaching strategies teach functional skills in the environment using child-directed interactions. Interventions may include modeling how to play, providing choices, encouraging conversation, or providing a stimulating environment. Naturalistic teaching is an established intervention for ASD. It has been shown to improve communication, interpersonal skills, learning readiness, and play skills.[87]

Pivotal Response Training (PRT)

PRT is an educational intervention designed to target "pivotal" behavioral areas. These areas include motivation to engage in social communication, self-management, and responsiveness to multiple cues. PRT also focuses on family involvement and intervention in the natural environment. PRT is an established intervention for children with ASD ages 3 to 9. It has been shown to improve communication, interpersonal skills, and play skills.[87]

Social Communication Emotional Regulation Transactional Supports (SCERTS)

SCERTS is a multidisciplinary, comprehensive educational model used to improve function in children with ASD. The model is used to increase participation in developmentally appropriate activities within a variety of settings by achieving "authentic progress." Authentic progress is defined as "the ability to learn and spontaneously apply functional and relevant skills in a variety of settings and with a variety of partners." The SCERTS model can be also combined with other approaches.[94]

Treatment and Education of Autistic and Related Communication-Handicapped Children (TEACCH)

TEACCH is a comprehensive educational program designed to help children develop key life skills used for independent living. TEACCH is based on the idea that all individuals with ASD have similar neuropsychological deficits as well as strengths. The model uses "structured teaching," based on understanding the learning characteristics of children with ASD and the use of visual supports to promote independence. TEACCH can be done in all settings, including the home and classroom.[121]

Relationship Based
Developmental, Individual Difference, Relationship-Based Model (DIR)

The DIRFloortime model focuses on building healthy foundations for social, emotional, and intellectual capacities rather than focusing on skills and isolated behaviors. Parents, educators, and clinicians work together to conduct a comprehensive assessment and to develop an intervention program specific to the strengths and challenges of the child with ASD. The *d*evelopmental part of the model focuses on six developmental milestones (self-regulation and interest in the world; intimacy, engagement, and falling in love; two-way communication; complex communication; emotional ideas; and emotional and logical thinking) that are necessary for healthy emotional and intellectual growth. The *i*ndividual differences section examines the biologic challenges that are unique to the child. These may include processing issues that are interfering with the child's ability to learn. The *r*elationship part of the DIR model refers to learning how to develop relationships with caregivers, peers, educators, and therapists whose affect-based interactions are tailored to the child's individual differences and developmental capacities.[32]

Early Start Denver Model (ESDM)

The Early Start Denver Model focuses on increasing the child's social-emotional, cognitive, and language skills. This approach combines behavioral and relationship-based intervention with a developmental, play-based approach that is individualized and standardized. Intervention is provided in the home by trained therapists and takes place within naturally occurring routines. Parents and caregivers are involved in all aspects of this treatment approach.[40]

Joint Attention Intervention

Joint attention interventions teach a child to respond to the nonverbal social communication of others or to initiate joint attention interactions. This may include showing items to another person, following eye gaze, or pointing to objects. Joint attention intervention is an established treatment approach to ASD for children 0 to 5 years of age. Studies have shown benefits in the areas of communication and interpersonal skills.[87]

Modeling

Modeling is a type of intervention in which an adult or peer demonstrates a target behavior for an individual with ASD and encourages the individual to imitate it. This approach is often combined with other strategies such as prompting and reinforcement. This intervention may involve live or video modeling. Modeling is an established intervention for children 3 to 18 years of age with ASD. Studies have shown improvements in communication, cognitive skills, interpersonal skills, self-regulation, and personal responsibility. Decreases in problem behaviors have also been noted in research.[87]

Play and Language for Autistic Youngsters (PLAY Project)

The PLAY project is based on the principles of the DIR model and aims to help parents become their child's best PLAY partner. The program is designed to be used with children 18 months or older. PLAY is administered at least 25 hours per week and uses a one-on-one approach.[122]

Relationship Development Intervention (RDI)

RDI is a cognitive-developmental approach in which the parents or caregivers are trained to provide daily opportunities for successful functioning. The approach is taught to families by trained consultants, beginning with 6 days of intensive training and followed by weekly or biweekly meetings with reevaluation at 6 months. RDI is most appropriate for children younger than 9 years of age without intellectual disabilities.[95]

Sensory-Motor

Alert

The Alert program focuses on teaching children to recognize their body's state of alertness and how it can be regulated to be appropriate for the current situation and environment. Children learn how to self-regulate their state of arousal while parents and teachers learn how to promote these behaviors. The Alert program can be used for children of all ages with sensory processing disorders and is often done in conjunction with sensory diet.[132]

Sensory Diet

A sensory diet is an individualized activity plan designed to provide the specific sensory input a child needs during the day. The goal of a sensory diet is to help children to tolerate different sensations, regulate their alertness, increase attention span, limit sensory seeking behaviors, and handle transitions with less stress by reorganizing the nervous system.[11]

Sensory Integration

Sensory integration intervention focuses on creating an environment that challenges children to use all of their senses effectively. The goal of sensory integration therapy is to address overstimulation or understimulation from the environment. Some studies suggest sensory integration intervention may improve play performance, enhance social interaction, and decrease sensitivity.[11] Sensory integration is considered an unestablished intervention because research findings have been inconsistent or do not apply to children with ASD.[87]

Pharmacologic Interventions

These interventions are generally used in children with ASD to control or improve attention, obsessive-compulsive behaviors, tantrums, irritability, self-injury, or aggression. There are varying levels of evidence for the use and effectiveness of medications for children with ASD. Decisions to use medications are made by the family in consultation with the primary care provider, and they may be used in combination with other interventions. Interventions include the following categories of medications: anticonvulsants, antidepressants, antipsychotics, and stimulants.

Dietary Interventions

Dietary interventions for ASD include the Defeat Autism Now (DAN) protocol gluten- and casein-free diets, and omega-3 fatty acids. There is little evidence that these dietary interventions are effective in promoting skills or positively impacting behavior or symptoms for children with ASD. Families may ask questions about or have an interest in trying these interventions. It is important to have an open discussion about the use of these interventions, the minimal evidence to support them, and the benefits, risks, and costs that may be associated with their use for their individual child. Families should consult their health care providers before beginning any dietary intervention.

REFERENCES

1. Akins RS, et al.: Complementary and alternative medicine in autism: an evidence-based approach to negotiating safe and efficacious interventions with families, *Neurotherapeutics* 7:307–319, 2010.
2. Ament K, et al.: Evidence for specificity of motor impairments in catching and balance in children with autism, *J Autism Dev Disord* 45:742–751, 2015.
3. American Speech and Hearing Association, *Ad Hoc Committee on Service Delivery in the Schools: definitions of communication disorders and variations*, 1993. Available from: http://www.asha.org/policy/RP1993-00208.htm.
4. Antshel K, Hier B: Attention deficit hyperactivity disorder (ADHD) in children with autism spectrum disorders. In *Comprehensive guide to autism*, New York, 2014, Springer, pp 1013–1029.
5. Reference deleted in proofs.
6. Autism spectrum disorder. In *Diagnostic and statistical manual of mental disorders*, ed 5, Washington, DC, 2013, American Psychiatric Association, pp 50–51.
7. Bagnato SJ, et al.: Authentic assessment as "best practice" for early childhood intervention: national Consumer Social Validity Research, *Topics Early Child Spec Educ* 34:116–127, 2014.
8. Bailey A, et al.: A clinicopathological study of autism, *Brain* 121(Pt 5): 889–905, 1998.
9. Baranek GT, et al.: Sensory experiences questionnaire: discriminating sensory features in young children with autism, developmental delays, and typical development, *J Child Psychol Psychiatry* 4:591–601, 2006.
10. Baranek GT: Autism during infancy: a retrospective video analysis of sensory-motor and social behaviors at 9-12 months of age, *J Autism Dev Disord* 29:213–224, 1999.
11. Baranek GT, et al.: Efficacy of sensory and motor interventions for children with autism, *J Autism Dev Disord* 32:397–422, 2002.
12. Barrow W, et al.: Persistent toe walking in autism, *J Child Neurol* 26:619–621, 2011.
13. Bayley N: *Bayley scales of infant and toddler development III*, San Antonio, TX, 2006, Psychological Corporation.
14. Ben-Sasson A, et al.: A meta-analysis of sensory modulation symptoms in individuals with autism spectrum disorders, *J Autism Dev Disord* 39:1–11, 2009.
15. Berg C, LaVesser P: The preschool activity card sort, *OTJR: Occupation, Participation, Health* 26:143–151, 2006.
16. Bhat AN, et al.: Current perspectives on motor functioning in infants, children, and adults with autism spectrum disorders, *Phys Ther* 91: 1116–1129, 2011.
17. Blumberg SJ, et al.: Changes in prevalence of parent-reported autism spectrum disorder in school-aged US children: 2007 to 2011-2012, *Natl Health Stat Report* 65:1–12, 2013.
18. Bolte S, et al.: The social communication questionnaire (SCQ) as a screener for autism spectrum disorders: additional evidence and cross-cultural validity, *J Am Acad Child Adolesc Psychiatry* 47:719–720, 2008.
19. Bruininks R, Bruininks B: *Bruininks-Oseretsky test of motor proficiency*, ed 2, Minneapolis, MN, 2005, NCS Pearson.
20. Reference deleted in proofs.
21. Case-Smith J, et al.: A systematic review of sensory processing interventions for children with autism spectrum disorders, *Autism* 19:133–148, 2015.
22. Centers for Disease Control and Prevention: facts about AUTISMs, 2012. Retrieved on May 3, 2015, from: http://www.cdc.gov/ncbddd/autism/facts.html.
23. Centers for Disease Control: *Prevalence of autism spectrum disorder among children aged 8 years: Autism and Developmental Disabilities Monitoring Network, 11 Sites, United States, 2010, Surveill Summ*, 2014, pp 1–21.
24. Chawarska K, et al.: 18-month predictors of later outcomes in younger siblings of children with autism spectrum disorder: a baby siblings research consortium study, *J Am Acad Child Adolesc Psychiatry* 53: 1317–1327, 2014.
25. Childress DC, et al.: Infants and toddlers with autism spectrum disorder. In Raver SA, Childress DC, editors: *Family centered early intervention*, Baltimore, MD, 2015, Brookes Publishing, pp 190–210.
26. Connecticut Birth to Three System: *Autism spectrum disorder intervention guidance for service providers*. Retrieved May 3, 2015, from: http://www.birth23.org/files/SGsPlus/SG1-ASDSpectrum, 2011. DisoderAutism.pdf.
27. Corsello CM: Early intervention in autism, *Infants Young Child* 18:74–85, 2005.
28. Coster W, et al.: *School function assessment*, San Antonio, TX, 1988, Pearson.
29. Cox AW, et al.: National Professional Development Center on ASD: an emerging national educational strategy, *Autism Services Across America*, 2013, pp 249–266.
30. Crosland K, Dunlap G: Effective strategies for the inclusion of children with autism in general education classrooms, *Behav Modif* 36:251–269, 2012.

31. Daniels AM, et al.: Approaches to enhancing the early detection of autism spectrum disorders: a systematic review of the literature, *J Am Acad Child Adolesc Psychiatry* 53:141–152, 2014.

32. DIR and the DIRFLoortime Approach. Retrieved May 3, 2015, from: http://www.icdl.com/DIR.

33. Downey R, Rapport MK: Motor activity in children with autism: a review of the current literature, *Pediatr Phys Ther* 24:2–20, 2012.

34. DSM-5 Autism Spectrum Disorder Fact Sheet: retrieved on June 8, 2013, from: http://www.dsm5.org/Documents/Autism Spectrum Disorder Fact%20Sheet.pdf.

35. Dunn W: The impact of sensory processing abilities on the daily lives of young children and their families: a conceptual model, *Infants Young Child* 9:23–35, 1997.

36. Dunn W: *Sensory profile 2*, San Antonio, TX, 2014, Pearson Clinical.

37. Dunn W, et al.: Impact of a contextual intervention on child participation and parent competence among children with autism spectrum disorders: a pretest-posttest repeated-measures design, *Am J Occup Ther* 66:520–528, 2012.

38. Dunst CJ, et al.: Family capacity-building in early childhood intervention: do context and setting matter? *School Community J* 24:37–48, 2014.

39. Reference deleted in proofs.

40. Early Start Lab. Retrieved on May 3, 2015, from: http://www.ucdmc .ucdavis.edu/mindinstitute/research/esdm/.

41. Enticott PG, et al.: Mirror neuron activity associated with social impairments but not age in autism spectrum disorder, *Biol Psychiatry* 71:427–433, 2012.

42. Esposito G, et al.: Analysis of unsupported gait in toddlers with autism, *Brain Dev* 33:367–373, 2011.

43. Farley MA, et al.: Twenty-year outcome for individuals with autism and average or near-average cognitive abilities, *Autism Res* 2:109–118, 2009.

44. Fatemi SH, et al.: Consensus paper: pathological role of the cerebellum in autism, *Cerebellum* 11:777–807, 2012.

45. Fleury VP: Discrete trial teaching (DTT) fact sheet. Chapel Hill: the University of North Carolina, Frank Porter Graham Child Development Institute, The National Professional Development Center on Autism Spectrum Disorders. Retrieved May 12, 2015, from: http://autismpdc .fpg.unc.edu/sites/autismpdc.fpg.unc.edu/files/DTT_factsheet.pdf.

46. Folio MR, Fewell RR: *Peabody developmental motor scales*, ed 2, Austin, TX, 2000, Pro-Ed.

47. Fournier K, et al.: Motor coordination in autism spectrum disorders: a synthesis and meta-analysis, *J Autism Dev Disord* 40:1227–1240, 2010.

48. Frankenburg WK, et al.: *Denver II*, Denver, CO, 1990, Denver Developmental Materials.

49. Gotts S, et al.: Fractionation of social brain circuits in autism spectrum disorders, *Brain* 135:2711–2725, 2012.

50. Green D, et al.: Impairment in movement skills of children with autistic spectrum disorders, *Dev Med Child Neurol* 51:311–316, 2009.

51. Guevara J, et al.: Effectiveness of developmental screening in an urban setting, *Pediatrics* 131:30–37, 2013.

52. Gupta S, et al.: Transcriptome analysis reveals dysregulation of innate immune response genes and neuronal activity-dependent genes in autism, *Nat Commun* 5:1–8, 2014.

53. Hallmayer J, et al.: Genetic heritability and shared environmental factors among twin pairs with autism, *Arch Gen Psychiatry* 68:1095–1102, 2011.

54. Henderson SE, et al.: In *Movement assessment battery for children*, ed 2, San Antonio, TX, 2007, Pearson Clinical, 2007.

55. Hurth J, et al.: Areas of agreement about effective practices among programs serving young children with autism spectrum disorders, *Infants Young Child* 12:17–26, 1999.

56. Hyman S, Levy S: Autism spectrum disorders. In Batshaw M, et al., editors: *Children with disabilities*, ed 7, Baltimore, MD, 2013, Paul H. Brookes, pp 345–367.

57. Iovannone R, et al.: Effective educational practices for students with autism spectrum disorders, *Focus Autism Other Dev Disabl* 18:150–165, 2003.

58. Reference deleted in proofs.

59. Jimenez BA, et al.: Data-based decisions guidelines for teachers of students with severe intellectual and developmental disabilities, *Educ Train Autism Dev Disabil* 407–413, 2012.

60. Johnson CP, et al.: Identification and evaluation of children with autism spectrum disorders, *Pediatrics* 120:1183–1215, 2007.

61. Just MA, et al.: Autism as a neural systems disorder: a theory of frontal-posterior underconnectivity, *Neurosci Biobehav Rev* 36:1292–1313, 2012.

62. Kasari C, Smith T: Interventions in schools for children with autism spectrum disorder: methods and recommendations, *Autism* 17:254–267, 2013.

63. King G, et al.: *Children's Assessment of Participation and Enjoyment (CAPE) and Preferences for Activities of Children (PAC)*, San Antonio, TX, 2004, Harcourt Assessment.

64. Kotagal S, Broomall E: Sleep in children with autism spectrum disorder, *Pediatr Neurol* 47:242–251, 2012.

65. Kramer JM, et al.: Validity, reliability, and usability of the Pediatric Evaluation of Disability Inventory-Computer Adaptive Test for autism spectrum disorders, *Dev Med Child Neurol* 58:255–261, 2016.

66. Kucharczyk S: *Differential reinforcement of alternative, incompatible, or other behavior (DRA/I/O) fact sheet*, Chapel Hill, NC, 2013, The University of North Carolina. Frank Porter Graham Child Development Institute, The National Professional Development Center on Autism Spectrum Disorders. Retrieved May 12, 2015, from: http://autismpdc.fpg.unc .edu/sites/autismpdc.fpg.unc.edu/files/Differential_Reinforcement _factsheet.pdf.

67. Lang R, et al.: Physical exercise and individuals with autism spectrum disorders: a systematic review, *Res Autism Spectr Disord* 4:565–576, 2010.

68. Law M, et al.: *Canadian occupational performance measure*, ed 4, Toronto, 2005, Canadian Association of Occupational Therapists.

69. Lee BH, et al.: Autism spectrum disorder and epilepsy: disorders with a shared biology, *Epilepsy Behav* 47:191–201, 2015.

70. Levy SE, et al.: Autism spectrum disorder and co-occurring developmental, psychiatric, and medical conditions among children in multiple populations of the United States, *J Dev Behav Pediatr* 31:267–275, 2010.

71. Libero LE, et al.: Multimodal neuroimaging based classification of autism spectrum disorder using anatomical, neurochemical, and white matter correlates, *Cortex* 66:46–59, 2015.

72. Long T, Brady R: *Contemporary practices in early intervention for children birth through five: a distance learning curriculum*, Washington, DC, 2012, Georgetown University. Available at: teachingei.org.

73. Reference deleted in proofs.

74. Reference deleted in proofs.

75. Lovaas OI: Behavioral treatment and normal education and intellectual functioning in young autistic children, *J Consult Clin Psychol* 53:3–9, 1987.

76. MacNeil LK, Mostofsky SH: Specificity of dyspraxia in children with autism, *Neuropsychology* 26:165–171, 2012.

77. Magiati I, et al.: Patterns of change in children with autism spectrum disorders who received community based comprehensive interventions in their pre-school years: a seven year follow-up study, *Res Autism Spectr Disord* 5:1016–1027, 2011.

78. McDonough JT, Revell G: Accessing employment supports in the adult system for transitioning youth with autism spectrum disorders, *J Vocat Rehabil* 32:89–100, 2010.

79. McQuistin A, Zieren C: Clinical experiences with the PDDST-II, *J Autism Spectrum Disord Devel Disord* 36:577–578, 2006.

80. McWilliam RA, et al.: The routines-based interview: a method for assessing needs and developing IFSPs, *Infants Young Child* 22:224–233, 2009.

81. Miller LJ, Lane SJ: Toward a consensus in terminology in sensory integration theory and practice: part 1: taxonomy of neurophysiological processes, *Sensory Integration Special Interest Sect Q* 23:1–4, 2000.

82. Miller LJ, Summers C: Clinical applications in sensory modulation dysfunction: assessment and intervention considerations, *Understanding the nature of sensory integration with diverse populations* 247–274, 2001.

83. Miller LJ: *Miller function and participation scales*, San Antonio, TX, 2006, Pearson Clinical.

84. Miller LJ, et al.: Concept evolution in sensory integration: a proposed nosology for diagnosis, *Am J Occup Ther* 61:135–140, 2007.

85. Miller VA, et al.: Factors related to parents' choices of treatments for their children with autism spectrum disorders, *Res Autism Spectr Disord* 6:87–95, 2012.

86. Nair A, et al.: Impaired thalamocortical connectivity in autism spectrum disorder: a study of functional and anatomical connectivity, *Brain* 136:1942–1955, 2013.

87. National Autism Center: Findings and conclusions: national Standards Project, Phase 2. Retrieved on May 2, 2015, from: http://www.nationalautismcenter.org/national-standards-project/phase-2/.

88. Noyes-Grosser DM, et al.: Conceptualizing child and family outcomes of early intervention services for children with ASD and their families, *J Early Interv* 35:332–354, 2013.

89. Odom S, et al.: Moving beyond the intensive behavior treatment versus eclectic dichotomy evidence-based and individualized programs for learners with ASD, *Behav Modif* 36:270–297, 2012.

90. Orsmond GI, et al.: Social participation among young adults with an autism spectrum disorder, *J Autism Spectr Disord Dev Disord* 43:2710–2719, 2013.

91. Pan CY: Effects of water exercise swimming program on aquatic skills and social behaviors in children with autism spectrum disorders, *Autism* 14:9–28, 2010.

92. Pan CY: The efficacy of an aquatic program on physical fitness and aquatic skills in children with and without autism spectrum disorders, *Res Autism Spectr Disord* 5:657–665, 2011.

93. Phillips KL, et al.: Prevalence and impact of unhealthy weight in a national sample of US adolescents with autism and other learning and behavioral disabilities, *Matern Child Health J* 18:1964–1975, 2014.

94. Prizant BM, et al.: *The SCERTS model and evidence-based practice*, 2010. Retrieved on May 2, 2015, from: http://www.scerts.com/docs/scerts_ebp%20090810%20v1.pdf.

95. RDI Connect: Retrieved on May 3, 2015, from: http://www.rdiconnect.com/.

96. Reynolds S, et al.: Sensory processing, physiological stress, and sleep behaviors in children with and without autism spectrum disorders, *OTJR: Occupation, Participation Health* 32:246–257, 2012.

97. Rizzolatti G, Fabbri-Destro M: Mirror neurons: from discovery to autism, *Exp Brain Res* 200:223–237, 2010.

98. Robins DL, et al.: The modified checklist for autism spectrum disorder in toddlers: an initial study investigating the early detection of ASD and pervasive developmental disorders, *J Autism Spectr Disord Dev Disord* 31:131–144, 2001.

99. Rodger S, Polatajko HJ: Occupational therapy for children with autism. In *Comprehensive guide to autism*, New York, 2014, Springer, pp 2297–2314.

100. Rogers SJ, et al.: Autism treatment in the first year of life: a pilot study of infant start, a parent-implemented intervention for symptomatic infants, *J Autism Spectr Disord Dev Disord* 44:2981–2995, 2014.

101. Roley SS, et al.: Sensory integration and praxis patterns in children with autism, *Am J Occup Ther* 69, 6901220010p1–6901220010p8, 2015.

102. Reference deleted in proofs.

103. Rutter M, et al.: *Autism spectrum disorder diagnostic interview—revised*, Torrance, CA, 2003, Western Psychological Services.

104. Sansosti FJ: Teaching social skills to children with autism spectrum disorders using tiers of support: a guide for school-based professionals, *Psychol in Schools* 47:257–281, 2010.

105. Schaaf RC, et al.: Occupational therapy and sensory integration for children with autism: a feasibility, safety, acceptability and fidelity study, Department of Occupational Therapy Faculty Papers, paper 13, 2012. http://jdc.jefferson.edu/otfp/13.

106. Schopler E, et al.: *Childhood autism spectrum disorder rating scale*, ed 2, Torrance, CA, 2010, Western Psychological Services.

107. Reference deleted in proofs.

108. Sinha Y, et al.: Auditory integration training and other sound therapies for autism spectrum disorders, *Cochrane Database Syst Rev*, 2004. CD003681.

109. Snow AV, Lecavalier L: Sensitivity and specificity of the modified checklist for autism spectrum disorder in toddlers and the social communication questionnaire in preschoolers suspected of having pervasive developmental disorders, *Autism* 12:627–644, 2008.

110. Sowa M, Meulenbroek R: Effects of physical exercise on autism spectrum disorders: a meta-analysis, *Res Autism Spectr Disord* 6:46–57, 2012.

111. Sparrow SS, et al.: *Vineland adaptive behavior scales*, ed 2, Upper Saddle River, NJ, 2005, Pearson Education.

112. Spreckley M, Boyd R: The efficacy of applied behavioral intervention in preschool children with autism for improving cognitive, language, and adaptive behavior: a systematic review and meta-analysis, *J Pediatr* 154:338–344, 2009.

113. Squires J, et al.: *Ages & Stages Questionnaires®*, (ASQ-3™), ed 3, Baltimore, MD, 2009, Brookes Publishing.

114. Srinivasan SM, et al.: Current perspectives on physical activity and exercise recommendations for children and adolescents with autism spectrum disorders, *Phys Ther* 94:875–889, 2014.

115. Stone WL, et al.: Use of the screening tool for autism spectrum disorder in two year olds for children under 24 months: an exploratory study, *Autism* 12:557–573, 2008.

116. Strain P, Schwartz I: Positive behavior support and early intervention for young children with autism: case studies on the efficacy of proactive treatment of problem behavior. In Sailor W, et al., editors: *Handbook of positive behavior support*, New York, 2009, Springer, pp 107–123.

117. Strain P: Empirically-based social skill intervention, *Behav Disord* 27:30–36, 2001.

118. Strain PS, Hoyson M: On the need for longitudinal, intensive social skill intervention: LEAP follow-up outcomes for children with autism spectrum disorder as a case-in-point, *Topics Early Child Spec Educ* 20:116–122, 2000.

119. Sussman F: More than words research summary. Retrieved May 3, 2015, from: http://www.hanen.org/SiteAssets/Helpful-Info/Research-Summary/More-Than-Words-Research-Summary.aspx.

120. Swanson J, et al.: Strengthening family capacity to provide young children everyday natural learning opportunities, *J Early Child Res* 9:66, 2011.

121. TEACCH Autism Spectrum Disorder Program. Retrieved on May 3, 2015, from: http://www.teacch.com/.

122. The PLAY Project. Retrieved on May 3, 2015, from: www.playproject.org.

123. Tomcheck SD, Dunn W: Sensory processing in children with and without autism: a comparative study using the short sensory profile, *Am J Occup Ther* 61:190–200, 2007.

124. Tomchek SD, et al.: Patterns of sensory processing in children with an autism spectrum disorder, *Res Autism Spectr Disord* 8:1214–1224, 2014.

125. Ulrich D, Webster EK: *Test of gross motor development*, ed 3, Austin, TX, 2015, Pro-Ed.

126. Van der Meer LAJ, Rispoli M: Communication interventions involving speech-generating devices for children with autism: a review of the literature, *Dev Neurorehabil* 13:294–306, 2010.

127. Virues-Ortega J: Applied behavioral analytic intervention for autism in early childhood: meta-analysis, meta-regression and dose response meta-analysis of multiple outcomes, *Clin Psychol Rev* 30:387–399, 2010.

128. Volkmar FR: Editorial: the importance of early intervention, *J Autism Dev Disord* 44:2979–2980, 2014.

129. Wang LW, et al.: The prevalence of gastrointestinal problems in children across the United States with autism spectrum disorders from families with multiple affected members, *J Dev Behav Pediatr* 32:351–360, 2011.

130. Watson LR, et al.: Behavioral and physiological responses to child-directed speech as predictors of communication outcomes in children with autism spectrum disorders, *J Speech Language Hearing Res* 53:1052–1064, 2010.

131. Wilbarger P, Wilbarger JL: *Sensory defensiveness in children ages 2-12: an intervention guide for parents and other caretakers*, Santa Barbara, CA, 1991, Avanti Educational Programs.

132. Williams MS, Shellenberger S: How does your engine run? The Alert Program™ for Self-Regulation, *Autism-Asperger's Digest Magazine* 14, 2000.

133. World Health Organization: *Towards a common language for functioning, disability, and health ICF*, Geneva, Switzerland, 2002, Author.

134. Xue M, et al.: Prevalence of motor impairment in autism spectrum disorders, *Brain Deve* 29:565–570, 2007.

135. Zwaigenbaum L: The screening tool for autism in two year olds can identify children at risk of autism, *Evid Based Ment Health* 8:69, 2005.

SUGGESTED READINGS

Background

Autism spectrum disorder: In *Diagnostic and statistical manual of mental disorders*, ed 5, Washington, DC, 2013, American Psychiatric Association, pp 50–51.

Centers for Disease Control: Prevalence of autism spectrum disorder among children aged 8 years: Autism and Developmental Disabilities Monitoring Network, 11 Sites, United States, 2010, *Surveill Summ*, 2014, pp 1–21.

Chawarska K, et al.: 18-month predictors of later outcomes in younger siblings of children with autism spectrum disorder: a Baby Siblings Research Consortium Study, *Child Adolesc Psychiatry* 53:1317–1327, 2014.

Cox AW, et al.: National Professional Development Center on ASD: an emerging national educational strategy, Autism Services Across America, 2013, pp 249–266.

Hyman S, Levy S: Autism spectrum disorders. In Batshaw M, et al.: *Children with disabilities*, ed 7, Baltimore, MD, 2013, Paul H. Brookes, pp 345–367.

Levy SE, et al.: Autism spectrum disorder and co-occurring developmental, psychiatric, and medical conditions among children in multiple populations of the United States, *J Dev Behav Pediatr* 31:267–275, 2010.

Foreground

Ament K, et al.: Evidence for specificity of motor impairments in catching and balance in children with autism, *J Autism Dev Disord* 45:742–751, 2015.

Bhat AN, et al.: Current perspectives on motor functioning in infants, children, and adults with autism spectrum disorders, *Phys Ther* 91:1116–1129, 2011.

Case-Smith J, et al.: A systematic review of sensory processing interventions for children with autism spectrum disorders,, *Autism* 19:133–148, 2015.

Downey R, Rapport MK: Motor activity in children with autism: a review of the current literature, *Pediatr Phys Ther* 24:2–20, 2012.

Lang R, et al.: Physical exercise and individuals with autism spectrum disorders: a systematic review, *Res Autism Spectr Disord* 4:565–576, 2010.

Odom S, et al.: Moving beyond the intensive behavior treatment versus eclectic dichotomy evidence-based and individualized programs for learners with ASD, *Behav Modif* 36:270–297, 2012.

Pan CY: The efficacy of an aquatic program on physical fitness and aquatic skills in children with and without autism spectrum disorders, *Res Autism Spectr Disord* 5:657–665, 2011.

Rush DD, Shelden MLL: *The early childhood coaching handbook*, Baltimore, MD, 2011, Brookes Publishing.

Shelden M, Rush D: *The early intervention teaming handbook: the primary service provider approach*, Baltimore, MD, 2013, Brookes Publishing.

Sowa M, Meulenbroek R: Effects of physical exercise on autism spectrum disorders: a meta-analysis, *Res Autism Spectr Disord* 6:46–57, 2012.

Srinivasan SM, et al.: Current perspectives on physical activity and exercise recommendations for children and adolescents with autism spectrum disorders, *Physical Ther* 94:875–889, 2014.

Tomchek SD, et al.: Patterns of sensory processing in children with an autism spectrum disorder, *Res Autism Spectr Disord* 8:1214–1224.

Volkmar FR: Editorial: the importance of early intervention, *J Autism Dev Disord* 44:2979–2980, 2014.

25

Children Requiring Long-Term Mechanical Ventilation

Helene M. Dumas, M. Kathleen Kelly

Advances in medicine and biomedical technologies have improved the survival of children with complex health care needs, in particular those who require prolonged mechanical ventilation. Mechanical ventilation (MV) is a life-sustaining form of medical technology that either substitutes for or assists a child's respiratory efforts. Children require MV as a treatment modality because of underlying disease processes resulting in respiratory insufficiency. By definition, an individual is considered to be a *long-term* ventilator user if MV is required for more than 21 days.[90] Although the degree of support and care varies from child to child, each child dependent on long-term MV requires high-cost care that demands sophisticated equipment and round-the-clock monitoring.

The child with ventilator dependence represents a unique challenge for all health care professionals, as providers have moved beyond the goal of increasing survival rates and are now identifying evidence-informed practices that result in optimal quality-of-life outcomes. For the child dependent on long-term MV, goals include minimizing impairments, reducing the incidence of activity limitations, and maximizing participation in home, school, and the community.[52] The role of the pediatric physical therapist is an important one in addressing these aims. Children dependent on MV may be seen by physical therapists in a hospital-based setting such as a neonatal or pediatric intensive care unit (NICU or PICU), in a tertiary care hospital, or in a postacute care rehabilitation facility. Children dependent on MV may also be seen by a physical therapist in the community in a public or private school, a medical day care, a home- or center-based early intervention program, or at home.

This chapter presents a framework for physical therapist examination, intervention, and outcomes for children dependent on long-term MV. The pathophysiologic processes associated with chronic respiratory failure are described, as are the common modes of ventilatory support.

INCIDENCE

Although children dependent on long-term MV are a small percentage of the overall group of children with medical complexity, the number continues to increase as a result of continuing advances in medical care and improved technology.[49,60,88]

From 2000 to 2006, there was a 55% increase in the number of hospital discharges for children dependent on mechanical ventilation.[4] Estimates indicate that in the state of Utah, the number of children using MV at home increased by 33% from 1996 to 2004.[26] In Indiana, the incidence of children with chronic respiratory failure secondary to bronchopulmonary dysplasia (BPD) and dependent on MV at home was 1.23 per 100,000 live births in 1984 and increased to 4.77 per 100,000 live births in 2010. In Massachusetts, the number of children dependent on MV has increased nearly threefold from an estimated 70 children in 1990 to 197 in 2005.[27] In 2012, it was estimated that 8000 children in the United States are dependent on MV and live at home.[8] This steadily growing prevalence has also been established outside the United States.[31,49,60,70,88]

The introduction of safe and portable respiratory equipment for home care use and the presumption of an overall reduced cost of care have added to the positive expectations of care for children at home on a ventilator in various geographic regions.[15,20] Geographic differences in the prevalence of children with ventilator dependence may exist, however, as a result of differing medical practices, parental expectations of long-term survival, and the expectation of being able to care for a child on a ventilator at home.[3,13,15,26,27,88] Unfortunately, no central tracking system exists for documenting ventilator use, outcomes of care, or care settings for children dependent on long-term MV.[27]

The highest percentage of children requiring MV is no longer due to the chronic lung disease associated with premature birth but rather is the result of congenital and neurologic disorders and neuromuscular diseases.[13,27,31,69] This shift is of particular importance to physical therapists because children with congenital, neurologic, and neuromuscular diagnoses are common diagnostic groups referred to physical therapists, and it is thus increasingly more likely that physical therapists will encounter a child who is dependent on MV. In a study of children requiring MV and admitted to one of six inpatient postacute hospitals in the northeastern United States, 83% received rehabilitation services during their hospitalization, and 50% of those children discharged using ventilators required rehabilitation services following discharge from the hospital.[59]

CHRONIC RESPIRATORY FAILURE

The need for long-term MV is due to ongoing impaired respiratory function. Adequate respiratory function requires the effective exchange of oxygen and carbon dioxide with an organ for gas exchange (the lungs), a "pump" mechanism (the rib cage, diaphragm, and external intercostals for inspiration and the rectus abdominis, internal intercostals, and accessory muscles for nonpassive expiration), and the neural control centers for breathing (involuntary-medulla and pons and voluntary-cerebral cortex). Under normal conditions, an individual's respiratory function adapts to satisfy the increased metabolic needs that occur during exercise, hyperthermia, or other demands, but when these systems are unable to deliver oxygen and remove carbon dioxide from the pulmonary circulation, respiratory failure ensues and gas exchange is impaired.[55,66,85]

Chronic respiratory failure and dependence on technology characterize the health condition of children requiring long-term ventilator assistance rather than the medical or rehabilitation diagnosis. Acute respiratory failure may develop in minutes or hours, whereas chronic respiratory failure develops over several days or weeks (Box 25.1). Chronic respiratory failure is the result of an uncorrectable imbalance in the respiratory system in which a failure of the exchange of oxygen and carbon dioxide occurs within the alveoli, along with failure of the muscles required to expand the lungs or failure of the brain centers controlling respiration. In this situation, ventilatory muscle power and central respiratory drive are inadequate to overcome the respiratory load. Regardless of the etiology, there is a need to balance the medical, developmental, and psychological needs of these children.[66,67,85]

Generally, the causes of chronic respiratory insufficiency in children have been grouped into the following categories: (1) conditions that cause *central dysregulation of breathing* (e.g., ischemic encephalopathy, traumatic brain injury, spinal cord injury), (2) conditions that affect the *lungs, lung parenchyma, and airway* (e.g., BPD, tracheobronchomalacia), and (3) diseases/disorders of the chest wall and thorax that affect the *respiratory pump* (e.g., spinal muscular atrophy, scoliosis).[55,56,74,85] See Table 25.1.

Central Dysregulation of Breathing

Central dysregulation of breathing is characterized by disorders affecting the central respiratory centers (i.e., brain stem or cervical spinal cord) that control the depth and frequency of involuntary breathing. Appropriate rhythmic depth and frequency of breathing maintain homeostatic levels of oxygen, carbon dioxide, and hydrogen ions in arterial blood. Voluntary control of breathing is under control from the cerebral cortex (i.e., speaking, breath holding); these voluntary pathways bypass the respiratory centers in the medulla and directly affect the respiratory motor neurons that are located in the spinal cord.

BOX 25.1 Signs of Chronic Respiratory Failure

Clinical Signs
Decreased inspiratory breath sounds
Use of accessory muscles/chest wall retractions
Altered depth and pattern of respiration (deep, shallow, apnea, irregular)
Weak cough
Nasal flaring
Wheezing/expiratory grunting/prolonged expiration
Retained airway secretions/incompetent swallowing/weak or absent gag reflex (neurologic, neuromuscular, and skeletal conditions)
Cyanosis
Tachycardia
Hypertension
Bradycardia
Hypotension
Cardiac arrest
Fatigue/decreased level of activity
Poor weight gain
Excessive sweating
Changes in mental status
Retained airway secretions
Restlessness/irritability
Headache
Papilledema
Seizures
Coma

Physiologic/Laboratory Findings
Hypoxemia (acute or chronic): $PaO_2 < 65$ mm Hg
Hypercapnia (acute or chronic): $PaCO_2 > 45$ mm Hg
O_2 saturation <95% breathing room air (metabolic or respiratory)

Mechanical ventilation: Beyond the ICU quick reference guide. (July 2009). Retrieved from: <http://www.chestnet.org/education/cs/mech_vent/qrg/p14.php>.
Vo P, Kharasch VS: Respiratory Failure. Pediatrics in Review 35: 476-486, 2014.
From Sarnaik A, Clark JA, Sarnaikk AA: Respiratory distress and failure. In Kliegman RM, Stanton BMD, St. Geme J, et al., editors: Nelson textbook of pediatrics, ed 20, Philadelphia: Elsevier, 2016.
From Noah ZL, Budek CE: Chronic severe respiratory insufficiency. In Kliegman RM, Stanton BMD, St. Geme J, et al., editors: Nelson textbook of pediatrics, ed 20, Philadelphia: Elsevier, 2016.
From Panitch HB: Children dependent on respiratory technology. Wilmott RW, Bush A, Boat TF, et al., editors: Kendig and Chernick's disorders of the respiratory tract in children, ed 8, Philadelphia: Saunders, 2012.

TABLE 25.1 Common Pathophysiologic Mechanisms Leading to Chronic Respiratory Failure

Lungs, Lung Parenchyma, and Airway	Central Dysregulation of Breathing	Diseases/Disorders of the Chest Wall and Thorax (Pump Failure)
Bronchopulmonary dysplasia	Congenital central hypoventilation syndrome	Congenital myopathies
Respiratory distress syndrome	Infectious disease of the brain/brain stem	Muscular dystrophies
Chronic lung disease of infancy	Brain tumor	Phrenic nerve trauma
Tracheobronchomalacia	Arnold-Chiari malformation	Diaphragmatic dysfunction
Tracheomegaly	Traumatic brain injury	Botulism
Tracheoesophageal fistula	Spinal cord injury	Dwarfism
Subglottic stenosis	Intracranial hemorrhage	Scoliosis
Laryngeal atresia	Hypoxic encephalopathy	Guillain-Barré syndrome
Bronchial atresia		

Congenital central hypoventilation syndrome (CCHS) (previously known as Ondine's curse) is a rare disorder that presents shortly after birth or early in infancy. CCHS is characterized by failure of the central autonomic control of ventilation in the absence of primary pulmonary or neuromuscular disease or in the absence of a brain stem lesion. CCHS is due to a defect in the *PHOX2B* homeobox gene, the product of which is a transcription factor important for regulation of neural crest cell migration.[5,42] Symptoms of this disorder are generally noted in the neonatal period when the infant experiences hypoventilation and apneic episodes during sleep. CCHS is known to be associated with genetic or oncologic conditions such as Hirschsprung's disease[41] and neuroblastoma. Although the incidence of CCHS is low, this group of patients faces a lifelong dependence on MV, almost exclusively with positive-pressure ventilators or diaphragmatic pacemakers. Early treatment is essential to minimize the neurologic effects of hypoxia.[42] CCHS is fatal if untreated.[78]

Disorders of the brain stem that affect respiration typically result from trauma, infectious disease processes, brain stem tumors, or complications of Chiari malformations.[82] In these instances, chronic respiratory failure may be transient or long term and may present as apnea or other forms of sleep-disordered breathing. Traumatic injuries or acquired disorders of the spinal cord can also result in chronic respiratory failure, leading to dependence on MV. The prognosis for dependence on MV depends on the level of the lesion, the extent of nerve damage, and the nature of the lesion.[14] Following injuries involving the upper cervical or cervicothoracic area, respiration is often compromised because of phrenic and intercostal nerve root damage affecting the function of the diaphragmatic and accessory muscles of respiration. Patients with cervical-level injuries usually require MV throughout the day and night or, occasionally, only at night. The rate and extent of recovery of respiratory sufficiency and motor function after a spinal cord injury are contributing factors to quality-of-life outcomes.[75]

Lungs, Lung Parenchyma, and Airway

A common cause of primary lung failure is respiratory distress syndrome (RDS), in which primary lung or airway disease compromises pulmonary gas exchange. Respiratory distress syndrome, associated with preterm birth, pulmonary immaturity, and deficiency of surfactant, is a common cause of ventilator dependence in infants, as well as a major cause of neonatal death. Because of anatomic and physiologic immaturities, infants are predisposed to respiratory dysfunction such as atelectasis, airway obstruction, increased pulmonary vascular resistance, and pulmonary edema. As well, they are predisposed to diaphragmatic fatigue and instability in the neural control of breathing. Treatment of neonatal respiratory distress includes antenatal steroids, surfactant replacement therapy, oxygen therapy, and high-frequency ventilators used in the early neonatal period.[7,47,62,86,91]

Smaller and more immature infants requiring prolonged MV are at risk for ventilator-induced lung injury resulting in BPD and chronic lung disease of infancy (CLDI). BPD, first described by Northway et al. in 1967, is diagnosed when an infant is 28 days of chronologic age, continues to require supplemental oxygen, and has an abnormal clinical examination and chest radiograph. CLDI is diagnosed at 36 weeks of postmenstrual age if the clinical examination and chest radiographs continue to be abnormal and the need for oxygen is still present; BPD accounts for the majority of cases of CLDI.

A newer and milder form of BPD has emerged as a result of surfactant administration and improved critical care practices

that are more lung protective.[68] The classification of BPD is based on several factors, and disease severity is categorized as *mild, moderate,* or *severe* based on the need for supplemental oxygen or positive-pressure ventilation at 36 weeks of postmenstrual age for infants born before 32 weeks or 56 days of postnatal age for infants born at 32 weeks or after. This new phenotype is characterized by impaired/disrupted alveolar development, rather than the airway damage and fibrosis seen in the classical form of BPD.[47] Although no breakthroughs have occurred in the prevention of BPD, long-term outcomes have improved, and disease severity has been reduced as a result of improvements in medical and pharmacologic treatment, including the use of surfactant and lung protective ventilatory strategies such as high flow oxygen and noninvasive positive-pressure ventilation.[62,6] Although many infants "recover" from BPD and eventually achieve respiratory function independent of assisted ventilation or supplemental oxygen therapy, a small proportion require long-term ventilation. The reader is referred to Chapter 29 for information on early management of RDS, BPD, and CLDI.

Chronic respiratory failure may also result from congenital or acquired airway anomalies. These can include tracheal anomalies such as tracheomalacia, tracheomegaly, and tracheal atresia; abnormalities of the bronchi such as bronchial atresia, bronchial stenosis, and bronchomalacia; laryngeal atresia; tracheal and esophageal fistulas; and subglottic stenosis. All of these conditions can prevent alveolar ventilation and increase the respiratory workload, necessitating the need for MV support.[66]

Respiratory Pump Failure

Respiratory compromise can also occur with failure of the respiratory pump. Inadequate pump output can result from decreased respiratory muscle capacity due to weakened or fatigued respiratory muscles or from a workload that exceeds the capabilities of the pump. In either case the imbalance results in an inadequate generation of force and an inability to sustain ventilator requirements.

Congenital muscle disorders that affect respiratory muscles are a common cause of respiratory pump failure. Children with congenital myopathies typically manifest symptoms of respiratory failure early in the course of the disease, whereas those with muscular dystrophies typically do not present with respiratory compromise until late childhood or early adolescence. The degree of muscle weakness varies based on the type and nature of the disorder. In either case, MV may be warranted to compensate for the significantly reduced respiratory muscle function.[2,22,66] Muscular dystrophy and spinal muscular atrophy are presented in Chapter 12.

Pump failure can also result from congenital anomalies of the thorax and rib cage. In these conditions, reduced chest wall compliance or structural abnormalities restrict lung and chest expansion. Thoracic abnormalities are often associated with a variety of syndromes such as asphyxiating thoracic dystrophy, arthrogryposis (Chapter 10), osteogenesis imperfecta (Chapter 11), and dwarfism, as well as scoliosis (Chapter 8).[38,48,84]

MECHANICAL VENTILATION

Although the underlying disease processes and severity of respiratory failure differ considerably among individuals, MV is the final common treatment approach for individuals with chronic respiratory failure. MV is designed to assist with or substitute for respiratory function (i.e., moving air into and out of the lungs) in order to give the respiratory muscles a rest until the disease process resolves or lessens.

The decision to institute MV is often made as a lifesaving measure, and MV is increasingly used to preserve physiologic function and improve quality of life. In many instances involving infants and children, the clinical decision is to take advantage of the growth and maturational potential of the lungs and to maximize the child's overall developmental potential. Thus, the desired outcome for many children is medical stability with adequate growth and healing of the lungs and then the eventual withdrawal of assisted ventilation.[66,84,90]

Decisions on the type and parameters of MV are individualized and based on limited research evidence and, to some extent, on the experience of the medical team. The optimal ventilator settings for each patient are determined by the patient's metabolic requirements, respiratory drive, and pulmonary mechanics. The type of MV and the various parameters chosen depend on the child's age, the underlying disease process that precipitated ventilatory failure, available equipment, available research evidence, provider experience with specific types of machines, and site of care (e.g., PICU, home environment) (Table 25.2). In general, ventilators are adjusted to maintain an oxygen saturation > 95% and a CO_2 tension within the range of 35 to 45 mm Hg while the child is awake or asleep.[66,67,85]

Since the beginning of the modern era of MV in the 1950s, ventilators have continued to undergo significant technologic advances. Specifically, pediatric MV has undergone continual changes that reflect increased knowledge, understanding, and appreciation of the developing cardiorespiratory system. Currently, ventilation approaches utilize protective strategies to avoid atelectrauma and lung overdistention through the use of maximal alveolar pressures, minimal positive end-expiratory pressure, and permissive hypercapnia. Contemporary knowledge of respiratory physiology and a more detailed understanding of the pathophysiologic mechanisms underlying diseases of the respiratory system continue to drive research and development in this area. Although it is beyond the scope and intent of this chapter to detail available technical information on MV, a brief overview of MV will be provided.

Positive-pressure ventilation (PPV) is the most commonly used assisted ventilation strategy and can be delivered using noninvasive approaches as well as invasive methods. Most often, PPV is delivered invasively via an endotracheal (for the short term in the tertiary care hospital) or tracheostomy tube (for long-term management) with pressurized gas delivered into the airways and ventilator circuit during inspiration until the ventilator breath is terminated. As the airway pressure drops to zero, elastic recoil of the chest accomplishes passive exhalation by pushing the tidal volume out. Positive-pressure ventilators can be broadly classified as pressure limited or volume limited, the description indicating the method used to switch from the inspiratory phase to the expiratory phase. For a volume-cycled ventilator, the signal to terminate the inspiratory activity of the ventilator is a preset *volume*. For pressure-cycled ventilators, a preset *pressure* limit is used. The modes within each of those classes are categorized according to the type of inspiratory support (Box 25.2).

There has been an increasing use of partial ventilator assistance strategies to avoid the complications related to controlled MV.[73] Ideally, the desirable mode of ventilation is one with optimal synchrony and patient-ventilator interface, along

TABLE 25.2   Selection Criteria for Mechanical Ventilation

Parameter	Findings
Clinical	
Respiratory[a]	Apnea; decreased breath sounds; rigorous chest wall movement; weakening ventilatory effort
Cardiac	Asystole; peripheral collapse; severe bradycardia or tachycardia
Cerebral	Coma; lack of response to physical stimuli; uncontrolled restlessness; anxious facial expression
General	Limpness; loss of ability to cry
Laboratory[b]	
$PaCO_2$	Newborn: > 60–65 mm Hg
	Older child: > 55–60 mm Hg
	Rapidly rising > 5 mm Hg
PaO_2	Newborn: < 40–50 mm Hg
	Older child: < 50–60 mm Hg

[a]More than one episode of apnea with bradycardia or an episode of cardiac arrest is an adequate indication for initiating mechanical ventilation (MV), even in the absence of blood gas data.
[b]Laboratory values less extreme than those indicated must be supplemented by clinical evidence of severity to warrant initiating MV.
From Laghi F, Tobin M: Indications for mechanical ventilation. In M. Tobin, editor: *Principles and practice of mechanical ventilation*, ed 2, New York: McGraw Hill, 2006; Venkataraman ST: Mechanical ventilation and respiratory care. In Fuhrman BP, Zimmerman JJ, editors: *Pediatric critical care*, ed 4, Philadelphia: Saunders, 2011.

with the use of lung-protective strategies. With the advent of microprocessor technology, newer models of ventilators are able to offer greater flexibility with respect to modes of oxygen delivery.

Although long-term MV has decreased mortality rates for infants and children, complications can impact overall health, growth and development, and quality of life. Long-term invasive PPV requires a tracheostomy, which increases the complexities of care (Fig. 25.1).[35,64] Complications due to tracheotomy such as tracheitis, accidental decannulation, tracheal ulceration, or granuloma development are common. Tracheostomy placement or complications require routine surgical surveillance or surgical intervention (bronchoscopy).[36] An artificial airway also interferes with speech and nutrition. Secondary illnesses that have been reported include ventilator-associated pneumonia[79] and respiratory syncytial virus infection.[87]

Despite the benefits of PPV, there is risk of secondary lung injury. Numerous complications can occur with invasive PPV (Box 25.3), making it essential that individuals who work with children requiring long-term MV understand normal and pathologic respiratory physiology, anatomic and physiologic changes of the developing respiratory system, and how the machine interfaces with the patient's physiology.

Positive-pressure ventilatory support may also be accomplished noninvasively. Positive pressure via facemask can be accomplished using continuous positive airway pressure (CPAP) or bilevel positive airway pressure (BiPAP). CPAP applies continuous distending pressure to the alveoli throughout the respiratory cycle, keeping the alveoli partially inflated so that they may expand more easily with each cycle. CPAP may be delivered nasally, thus minimizing discomfort. BiPAP uses

BOX 25.2 Types of Positive-Pressure Ventilations

Noninvasive Positive-Pressure Ventilation
Modes of Application
- CPAP: single level of airway pressure applied throughout the respiratory cycle
- BiPAP: provides airway pressure during inspiration and an expiratory pressure to maintain lung expansion during expiration

Invasive Positive-Pressure Ventilation
Types of Ventilation
Pressure limited ventilation: inspiration ends after delivery of a set inspiratory pressure; tidal volume variable

Modes
- Pressure-controlled MV: minute ventilation determined by set respiratory rate and inspiratory pressure; patient does not initiate additional minute ventilation
- Pressure-limited assist-controlled MV: minimum minute ventilation set and patient can trigger additional pressure-limited breaths
- Pressure-limited synchronized intermittent MV (SIMV): ventilator breaths are synchronized with patient's spontaneous inspiratory efforts
- Pressure-support ventilation: patient-triggered breath with preset positive pressure, thus uses patient's own inspiratory timing and tidal volume; *often used in weaning*
- Volume limited ventilation: inspiration ends after delivery of a set tidal volume

Modes
- Controlled MV: preset tidal volume and respiratory rate delivered; patient does not initiate any ventilation
- Assist-controlled MV: preset minute ventilation; patient can trigger additional breaths, which have a set tidal volume
- Intermittent mandatory ventilation (IMV): allows patient to breathe in between mandatory ventilator breaths
- Synchronized intermittent MV (SIMV): allows the mandatory breaths to be triggered by the patient's spontaneous breaths

Siegel TA: Mechanical Ventilation and Non-invasive Ventilatory Support. In Marx JA, Hockberger RS, Walls RM, editors: *Rosen's Emergency Medicine*, ed 8, Philadelphia: Saunders, 2014.
Venkataraman ST: Mechanical Ventilation and Respiratory Care. In Fuhrman BP, Zimmerman JJ: *Pediatric Critical Care*, ed 4, Philadelphia: Saunders, 2011.
Hyzy RC: *Modes of Mechanical Ventilation*. UpToDate http://www.uptodate.com/contents/modes-of-mechanical-ventilation?source=search_result&search=modes+of+mechanical+venatilation&selectedTitle=17~150#H29, 2015.
Vo P, Kharasch VS: Respiratory failure. Pediatrics in Review 35: 476-486, 2014.

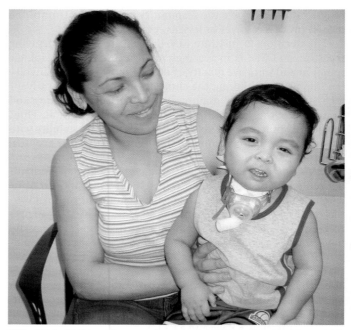

FIG. 25.1 Child with a tracheostomy. (From Hockenberry MJ, Wilson D: *Wong's nursing care of infants and children,* ed 10, St. Louis, 2015, Mosby.)

Another strategy for noninvasive MV is the use of negative-pressure ventilation (NPV). NPV provides a pressure gradient, which is established by creating a negative pressure around the person's entire body (from the neck down) during inspiration, causing air to enter the lungs. The typical interface used with this type of ventilation is a customized chest shell, a wrap/poncho, or a tank ventilator (Fig. 25.2). A major advantage of NPV is that it avoids or delays the need for a tracheostomy, thereby reducing the risk of infection. Another advantage of NPV is that ventilation is not interrupted when secretions are suctioned. NPV has been used most successfully for patients with normal lung mechanics and hypoventilation, as seen in patients with neuromuscular disease and pulmonary disease requiring periodic or nocturnal ventilatory support. There are limitations in use of NPV with infants and young children. Airway occlusion may occur during sleep. The chest shell or wrap is not effective for children who require high respiratory rates, tidal volumes, or distending pressures; thus NPV is not commonly used.[49,66,88]

Weaning From a Ventilator

The transition from mechanical ventilation to unassisted breathing is a complex process. Weaning a child from the support of a mechanical ventilator is highly individualized, is accomplished in response to recovery from respiratory insufficiency, and may not be a goal for some children. The primary consideration is whether a child is capable of maintaining adequate alveolar ventilation while breathing spontaneously. This requires adequate central nervous system regulation, respiratory muscle capacity to support the work required for breathing, and that the lungs and airway are not severely compromised by disease. Although weaning from MV may be a goal for many children, no standard protocol exists for the discontinuation of long-term ventilator support.

cycling variations between two CPAP levels, allowing spontaneous breathing during every ventilatory phase and has been used effectively to wean children from long-term MV.

In addition to the obvious advantage of avoiding a tracheostomy, noninvasive forms of PPV reduce the risk of acquired infection and allow patients to be more mobile.[37] Difficulties with noninvasive ventilation in children, however, such as poor mask fit, inadequate ventilation because of leaks, and eye irritation and nasal dryness due to high flow, have been reported. In addition, the use of noninvasive ventilation is limited in patients with congenital facial anomalies, which may preclude a tight-fitting mask, and with conditions that have the potential for infection, such as facial trauma or burns.[37]

BOX 25.3   Complications Associated With Mechanical Ventilation

Respiratory

Tracheal lesions (erosion, edema, stenosis, granuloma, obstruction, perforation)
Accidental endotracheal tube displacement or actual extubation
Air leaks (pneumothorax, pneumomediastinum, interstitial emphysema)
Infection (tracheitis, pneumonitis)
Trapping of gas (hyperinflation)
Excessive secretions (atelectasis)
Oxygen hazards (depression of ventilation, bronchopulmonary dysplasia)
Pulmonary hemorrhage

Circulatory

Impairment of venous return (decreased cardiac output and systemic hypotension)
Oxygen toxicity (retinopathy of prematurity, cerebral vasoconstriction)
Septicemia
Intracranial hemorrhage
Hyperventilation (decreased cerebral blood flow)

Gastrointestinal

Gastrointestinal hypomotility
Stress ulcer

Metabolic

Increased work of breathing ("fighting the ventilator")
Alkalosis (potassium depletion, excessive bicarbonate therapy)

Renal and Fluid Balance

Antidiuresis
Excess water in inspired gas

Equipment Malfunction

Power source failure
Improper humidification (overheating of inspired gas, inspiratory line condensation)
Improper tubing connections (kinked line, disconnection)
Ventilation malfunction (leaks, valve dysfunction)

From Zielinska MS, et al: Mechanical ventilation in children: problems and issues. Adv Clin Exp Med 23:843–848, 2014; Slutsky AS, Ranieri VM: Ventilator-induced lung injury. N Engl J Med 369:2126–2136, 2013; Venkataraman ST: Mechanical ventilation and respiratory care. In Fuhrman BP, Zimmerman JJ, editors: Pediatric critical care, ed 4, Saunders, 2012.

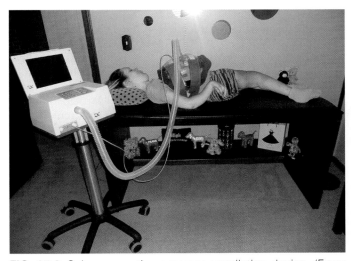

FIG. 25.2 Cuirass negative pressure ventilation device. (From McDonald CM, Joyce NC: Neuromuscular disease management and rehabilitation, part II: specialty care and therapeutics. *Phys Med Rehabil Clin N Am* 23:xiii-xvii, 2012.)

In critical care, the process of endotracheal tube extubation and ventilator weaning is often done by trial and error, whereby time off the ventilator is variable, dependent on when hypercapnia and hypoxia develop. In addition to the increased length of time for the weaning process, weaning strategies for children in a postacute setting are inherently different from those used in the neonatal or pediatric ICU because of differences between the use of a short-term endotracheal tube and a more permanent stable airway with a tracheostomy. Proposed criteria for weaning readiness in the postacute pediatric hospital setting include the following: (1) no escalation in ventilator support within 2 days before weaning; (2) stable chest radiograph; (3) blood $PaCO_2$ level not more than 10% above baseline; (4) blood pH within normal range; (5) supplemental FiO_2 of 0.6 or lower; (6) stable blood pressure over the previous 5 to 7 days; (7) heart rate no greater than 95% maximal normal for age; (8) tolerance of adequate nutrition; (9) absence of active infection, acute pain, or

other medical problems that might negatively affect the weaning process; and (10) reported understanding by the family/guardian and all health care providers of the desirability of weaning. In pediatric pulmonary rehabilitation, children may be weaned completely off MV, advanced to portable equipment, progressed to milder levels of ventilation (i.e., reduced pressure support), or weaned to a less invasive mode of support (i.e., CPAP).[58]

Despite the expected financial, clinical, and psychosocial advantages of weaning children with ventilator dependency in a postacute inpatient setting, only a few studies have reported outcomes on cohorts of children with long-term NV dependence undergoing weaning programs. In a single-site study, successful ventilator weaning was achieved during 30% of admission-discharge episodes, with diagnosis (prematurity with BPD) and age (younger) being the strongest predictors of weaning success. Nearly half of children admitted to a prospective multisite study over a 1-year enrollment period who were dependent on MV 24 hours per day at admission no longer required MV at discharge from inpatient rehabilitation. In addition, four children required only 12 or fewer hours per day of ventilator support at discharge.[59] Even though respiratory function is not monitored as closely, reports have described children's dependence on MV being minimized while they are cared for at home. Programs report that up to 57% of children are weaned from MV while at home.[26,57]

Weaning can be an arduous task, both physiologically and psychologically, and must be done with caution. The weaning prognosis can be enhanced by improvements in cardiorespiratory strength and endurance, adequate nutrition, and overall health; however, both muscular and respiratory fatigue should be avoided during this time. The timing and prognosis for weaning are important for physical therapists to understand so that physical therapist management may be directed appropriately. It is imperative for the physical therapist to coordinate and communicate with the medical team as to the amount of physical exertion that can be tolerated safely. During a time of weaning, the child's schedule of activities may need to be altered. In addition, the observations and ongoing clinical assessments made by the physical therapist may be influential in ventilator weaning. Ventilator settings are often influenced by the child's physical capacity such as strength, endurance, and developmental/functional skills. When these findings are communicated to the medical care team, weaning may be progressed, halted, or interrupted. Conversely, unpublished clinical observations by the authors indicate that when children are being actively weaned from the ventilator, physical therapy participation may be limited. Infants may sleep more, and older children often do not tolerate the same level of physical activity, until they accommodate to the increased demands of reduced ventilator settings on their respiratory system.

CONTINUUM OF CARE

Children who require mechanical ventilation may be seen by a physical therapist anywhere along the health care continuum. Infants in a neonatal intensive care unit may be placed on MV because of lung or airway anomalies, neurologic disorders affecting respiration, or disorders of the respiratory pump.[83] Children in a pediatric ICU may be placed on MV for postsurgical indications; as the result of recent trauma, illness, or organ failure; or because of a history of chronic respiratory failure. Only a small percentage of these children, however, will require long-term MV.[81]

For children who require MV for an extended period, the locus of inpatient care has shifted from acute care hospital neonatal and pediatric ICUs to postacute rehabilitation units or hospitals, where children can spend longer periods of time at a lower financial cost. In the rehabilitation unit or hospital, children may be weaned from their oxygen or ventilators or weaned to a less invasive mode of ventilation.[31,59] The more developmentally appropriate environment and rehabilitation services are intended to optimize weaning from a ventilator to a less restrictive mode of respiratory support for safe discharge home. Parent–child interaction, parent education, and growth and development can be promoted along with medical stability.[59] This is an important consideration for referring children to rehabilitation programs and for setting realistic expectations for referral sources, children and families, clinical staff, and payers. Whether fully weaned, weaned to fewer hours per day of MV, or weaned to a less invasive mode of ventilation, the ultimate goal is to discharge children home.

Children dependent on MV can be cared for at home and can participate in community activities when medically stable on a ventilator suitable for nonhospital use and with appropriate caregiver support.[57] Technological advances in design, efficiency, and portability have contributed to an increase in the use of MV outside the hospital environment. This option is dependent on many factors but primarily on a stable airway, an oxygen requirement typically less than 40%, a $PaCO_2$ level not more than 10% above baseline, and an adequate nutritional intake to maintain growth and development.[58] Home ventilation minimizes nosocomial infections and improves children's psychosocial development, social integration, and quality of life.[13,15,63,67,69]

Barriers to discharge from the hospital include the inability to recruit qualified home nursing staff inadequate or delayed funding of home care resources, unsuitable housing, delays in obtaining the appropriate equipment, and a limited number of capable family caregivers. It is imperative that the family or designated caregivers be involved in, and capable of learning, all aspects of the child's care. This care includes not only managing the ventilator and other monitoring equipment but also being able to recognize signs of medical distress and provide emergency medical procedures. The high degree of medical and technological expertise required by parents or caregivers can be a tremendous drain on a family.[19,67,116]

The transition to home carries with it other circumstances that can increase stress such as financial burden and significant changes in a family's routine, lifestyle, and relationships. The shift in responsibility for medical care from health care professionals to a family results in a myriad of issues that require psychological, social, ethical, financial, and policy solutions.[12,13,19,46,116] In many cases, the primary caregiver has to leave the workforce to care for the child at home.[51] Also, for children using MV at home, hospital readmissions are common.[11,34,87] Burdens of a hospital readmission for the child and family may include separation from family, coping with the illness itself, and financial concerns such as loss of income and the cost of the hospital admission. Children and families also face the possibility of a breakdown in their established network of community service providers caused by the interruption in service.[19] Although these added burdens do not necessarily outweigh the tremendous benefits of children being raised at home and integrated into their communities, they can be overwhelming and can have an impact on the quality of life of the child and family.[12,19,46,67]

As the degree and complexity of impairment, activity limitations, and participation restrictions increase, quality of life usually decreases—especially when financial, psychosocial, and emotional supports dwindle. With this in mind, one of the most important roles of health care providers is to work closely with family members as a child is being considered for discharge from the hospital and while at home. Physical therapists are encouraged to collaborate with families to identify their information needs and share intervention options in ways that enable informed decision making about caring for their children at home.[30,43,67] It is essential that the child's therapy program be integrated into the family's daily routine and not be the focus of a family's daily schedule.[43,51]

PHYSICAL THERAPIST MANAGEMENT

Physical therapy may be provided for children dependent on long-term MV who have or may develop impairments, activity limitations, and participation restrictions related to congenital or acquired conditions of the musculoskeletal, neuromuscular, cardiovascular, pulmonary, or integumentary systems. As noted previously, children who require long-term mechanical ventilation are a diverse and heterogeneous group. Despite differences in the underlying cause of respiratory insufficiency, children may have similar activity limitations and participation restrictions. The video accompanying this chapter illustrates some of the physical therapist interventions used with a 22-month-old girl with a diagnosis of Moebius syndrome, central respiratory dysfunction, and long-term mechanical ventilator dependence.

Children dependent on long-term MV may have limitations in self-care, mobility, cognitive, communication,[32] or oral feeding activities. Limitations in self-care and mobility activities may increase with fatigue, due to reduced cardiorespiratory endurance or limited access to environmental surroundings because of tubing length and the ventilator itself. The lack of frequent and variable practice opportunities makes skill acquisition particularly difficult, and thus the repertoire of skills in a variety of developmental domains is limited (see Chapter 4 for additional details on motor learning). As a point of illustration, the acquisition of independent mobility in children who are typically developing allows them to acquire information about their world and develop perceptions upon which they can act. Thus, development of cognitive skills such as object permanence is facilitated through motoric competencies. This interweaving of developmental domains and their interdependence is a well-known phenomenon, so the impact of limitations in the amount and type of mobility and lack of environmental affordances can be substantial.

A case report described the achievement of independent ambulation while a child was using CPAP.[16] An 18-month-old child with chronic lung disease of infancy and tracheobronchomalacia was provided with a CPAP device that allowed compressed air to be delivered via tracheostomy tube with extended tubing. It was hypothesized that the shorter, heavier tubing of the traditional CPAP device had severely restricted the child's mobility, but the application of the new CPAP device afforded the child the space to move up to 10 meters, and thus, psychomotor development was stimulated. Unfortunately, no studies documenting the relationship of physical therapist intervention, ventilator weaning, and motor/mobility outcomes are available for children dependent on long-term MV.

In addition to the aforementioned impairments and activity limitations, the additive effects of secondary complications such as recurrent hypoxic episodes, recurrent infections, poor weight gain, and poor physical growth can directly result in any number of secondary impairments and subsequent activity limitations. For example, because of the often prolonged periods of immobility or restricted activity early in the course of their disease, children may demonstrate impairments such as sensory defensiveness, generalized weakness, and soft tissue or muscular tightness. Likewise, if the child has hypoxic or ischemic episodes, neurologic damage may additionally limit motor skill acquisition and fluency. Infants with BPD and extremely low birth weight with a history of MV have an increased risk of being diagnosed with cerebral palsy, attention deficit disorder, and developmental coordination disorder (DCD).[92]

Due to children's impairments, reliance on external equipment requiring a power source and back-up safety materials (e.g., Ambu bag, extra tracheostomy tube), and the need for a trained adult caregiver, participation in activities outside the home may be difficult and appropriate recreation and leisure activities may be hard to find. Reports of participation in an ice skating program[23] and in a hospital-based fitness program are available.[24] Summer outdoor overnight camps for children dependent on MV are offered in multiple states throughout the United States.[39]

A multidisciplinary team approach is essential in the management of children with long-term MV and should be the standard of practice, regardless of the physical therapist's practice setting. For optimal patient management, the physical therapist who works with infants, children, and adolescents dependent on MV should have a thorough understanding of cardiorespiratory physiology and the implications of a compromise to that system in addition to an understanding of typical and atypical motor skill development. Physical therapists should be aware of the pathophysiology of chronic respiratory failure, the physiologic conditions requiring MV, the parameters of ventilator machinery, the varied types of MV, and the use of physiologic monitoring devices (Table 25.3). Types and

TABLE 25.3	Commonly Encountered Noninvasive Monitoring Devices[a]
Equipment	Physiologic Parameters Monitored
Cardiorespiratory monitors	Heart rate and respiratory rate
Pulse oximeter[b]	Transcutaneous arterial oxygen saturation to monitor hypoxemia
Ventilator alarms	Various modes chosen for the individual case, as well as airway pressures, gas concentrations, and expiratory tidal volumes
Transcutaneous PaO$_2$ and PaCO$_2$	Partial pressure of oxygen and carbon dioxide in the arterial blood
Oxygen analyzers on the ventilator	Oxygen supply in the ventilator circuit
Sphygmomanometer	Blood pressure

[a]These are some noninvasive devices that one may use to monitor response to activity and general status. Before any examination or treatment session, the therapist should be familiar with all of the equipment used for the child.
[b]Pulse oximeters are not useful for discriminating hyperoxia because the blood is fully saturated at PaO$_2$ of 150 mm Hg.

settings of ventilators will vary according to the child's age and diagnosis, site of care, availability of equipment, and providers' knowledge and experience with specific types of ventilators. Although the infant or child may be medically stable, the presence of an artificial airway creates a critical situation because it may become dislodged or occluded. In addition, the infant or young child may not communicate well; thus it is up to the therapist to interpret any signs of impending or actual distress.

Examination

Before any examination or intervention session, the therapist should confer with the child's primary caregiver to determine the child's current medical status, in addition to his or her baseline physiologic parameters. Depending on the nature and severity of the predisposing condition, cardiorespiratory parameters may vary from what is considered to be typical for the child's age (Table 25.4). It is always prudent to establish safe physiologic parameters within which to work. Typically, heart rate, respiratory rate, and oxygen saturation are monitored electronically while the child is on the ventilator.

Physical therapists should familiarize themselves with the type of mechanical ventilator being used by the child. The therapist should understand whether the ventilator is doing all the work of breathing for the child or whether it is assisting the child with the number or depth of breaths. Physical therapists should be knowledgeable of the clinical signs that indicate that the child needs respiratory assistance and the alarm systems of the ventilator, monitors that record oxygen saturation levels, heart and respiratory rates, and the emergency response procedures of the care setting. Therapists should be competent observing the child for signs of respiratory distress, skin color changes indicative of hypoxia, and changes in respiratory rate, breathing pattern, symmetry of chest expansion, posture, and general comfort. Signs of respiratory distress such as retractions, nasal flaring, expiratory grunting, and stridor may not be evident when a child is on a mechanical ventilator. For more information specific to the assessment of the cardiorespiratory system, the reader is referred elsewhere.[53]

As with any child referred for physical therapy services, the therapist must first complete a comprehensive examination that includes a history, a systems review, and specific tests

TABLE 25.4 Normal Ranges of Physiologic Values[a]

Parameter	Newborn/Infant (< 1 year)	Older Infant and Child (> 1 year)
Respiratory rate (breaths/minute)	24–40 40–70 (preterm infant)	20–30 (1–3 years) 20–24 (4–9 years) 14–20 (> 10 years)
Heart rate (beats/minute)	100–160 120–170 (preterm infant)	70–120 (1–10 years) 60–100 (> 10 years)
Blood pressure-systolic (mm Hg)	60–90 55–75 (preterm infant)	80–130 (1–3 years) 90–140 (> 3 years)
Blood pressure-diastolic (mm Hg)	30–60 35–45 (preterm infant)	45–90 (< 3 years) 50–80 (> 3 years)
PaO_2 (mm Hg)	60–90	80–100
$PaCO_2$ (mm Hg)	30–35	30–35 (< 2 years) 35–45 (> 2 years)
Arterial oxygen saturation (%)	87–89 (low) 94–95 (high) 90–95 (preterm infant)	95–100

[a]These measures represent "normal" physiologic values; in the case of infants and children with varying pathophysiologic processes, the "normal" values may be different.

From Bernstein D: History and physical examination. In Kliegman RM, Stanton BMD, St. Geme J, et al., editors: Nelson textbook of pediatrics, ed 20, Philadelphia: Elsevier 2016; Marx J, Hockberger R, editors: Rosen's emergency medicine: concepts and clinical practice, ed 8, Philadelphia: Saunders, 2014.

and measures. Because of varying ages, diagnoses, prognoses, and intervention settings for children dependent on MV, tests and measures must be aimed at quantifying a child's aerobic capacity and endurance, motor function, musculoskeletal performance (flexibility, strength, posture), and general adaptive behaviors that are age appropriate and most relevant to the child and family goals and the clinical setting.

The neuromuscular/musculoskeletal examination should provide information about the child's general neurologic and musculoskeletal status and includes assessment of active control of movement and strength, flexibility, sensation, and posture. Examination procedures will vary, depending on the age and cognitive level of the child, and areas of emphasis may be different, depending on the diagnosis, the care setting, and child and family goals. An important component is the measurement of neuromotor development and motor control as children on long-term MV are at great risk for global developmental delays that may or may not have a pathophysiologic component.

An examination of the child's functional activity level should include age-appropriate activities of daily living, general mobility skills, communication skills, and an assessment of the child's role within the family and within the relevant environment. The functional assessment provides an indication of how well the child is integrated into his environment, family, and, if applicable, community. A performance-based assessment or a patient-reported measure may be appropriate. A performance-based standardized developmental assessment or functional assessment tool can be used to quantify achievement of motor milestones or changes in functional mobility skills. No specific tool has been recommended for children dependent on ventilators, and only a few of the currently available tools have been reported to be used in populations in which children were ventilator dependent. When choosing an assessment, therapists

should consider the child's age, as well as the care setting, prognosis, diagnosis, and intended outcomes (e.g., developmental milestones such as rolling, functional skills such as transfers, factors influencing quality of life such as accessing transportation to school), while remembering that standardized developmental assessments seldom take into account factors related to endurance for exercise. See Chapter 2 for information on physical therapy tests and measures.

A reexamination will include performing selected tests and measures to evaluate progress in response to parent/caregiver questions or concerns, physical therapist intervention, growth and development, and medical recovery. Reexamination is indicated at times of new clinical findings or failure to respond to physical therapist intervention, or as dictated by the care setting.[29] For children dependent on MV, a change in type of ventilator or ventilator settings, or a decrease in the number of hours of ventilator support per day, may warrant a reexamination of aerobic capacity and endurance for motor tasks or the appropriateness of adaptive equipment.

Evaluation and Diagnosis

Information gathered during the physical therapy examination should be used for the therapist's evaluation and determination of a physical therapy diagnosis. Results of the examination should be synthesized to determine the child's impairments, activity limitations, and participation restrictions, as well as to identify strengths and resources available to minimize disability. Ideally, a multidimensional approach to the use of tests and measures should be employed and the results correlated to relevant activity limitations and participation restrictions interfering with the child's quality of life. For example, the child with chronic lung disease and mechanical ventilator dependence secondary to BPD may have coexisting neurologic impairments, gastrointestinal abnormalities, and growth disturbance. The physical therapy diagnosis therefore might include developmental delay, aerobic capacity and endurance limitations, and a decreased repertoire of movement patterns. On the other hand, children with the neurologic diagnosis of congenital central hypoventilation syndrome may be otherwise medically stable and at risk for developmental delay only if they are hospitalized for a prolonged time. Thus, at this stage of clinical decision making, diagnostic determinations will vary depending on the age of the child, the severity and chronicity of the lung disease, and the coexisting diagnoses.

Prognosis and Plan of Care

The physical therapy prognosis for a child who is dependent on long-term MV may be difficult to establish. The prognosis is the determination of the predicted maximal level of improvement and the estimate of how long it will take the child to achieve that improvement. As this population of children is diverse in its medical diagnoses and age range, the literature base on which to base a prognosis for the reduction of impairments, improvement of function, and facilitation of participation in home and community life is limited.

Decisions regarding the mode, intensity, and frequency of activity need to be made in conjunction with other members of the child's medical team and modified as the disease process changes. The physical therapist must recognize the potential for adverse physiologic stress when implementing any intervention and the potential impact on the child's prognosis. The amount and type of motor activities must be individualized and graded to the child's level of tolerance so that risks associated with the physiologically immature or unstable systems are not magnified.

One of the ultimate goals for pediatric physical therapists, however, should be to promote the concept of lifelong health and fitness. Barring any medical contraindication, physical activity in children who are dependent on a ventilator should be encouraged and incorporated into the plan of care. The long-term benefits of physical activity and lifelong fitness include mental health benefits such as improved self-esteem and confidence.[61]

Physical Therapist Intervention

The multiple medical, emotional, educational, and rehabilitative needs of the child with ventilator dependence are beyond the expertise of a single provider and thus require the care and coordination of an interdisciplinary team. This team will include a primary care physician and multiple specialty physicians. Therapists working with a child dependent on long-term MV should routinely communicate with the child, family, other daily caregivers (e.g., nurse, home health aide), and the child's primary physician. Therapists should also communicate with other medical specialists such as the pulmonologist, physiatrist, orthopedist, and neurologist about the child's therapy goals and physical response to intervention.

Members of the child's team in the home setting may expand to include a case manager, a respiratory equipment provider, and a durable medical equipment vendor. Additionally, team members in a school setting may include teachers, classroom aides, the school nurse, and transportation personnel (bus driver and monitor[s]). In many states, it is typical for a child with a tracheostomy on a ventilator outside the hospital to have a nurse with him or her at all times. Sharing of successful strategies for communication and motivation, as well as carry-over of all rehabilitation goals among physical, occupational, and speech therapists, can facilitate a successful therapist–client relationship and can enhance a consistent approach to the needs of the child and family. Short-term and long-term goals developed by the team should be formulated in conjunction with the family, while the ultimate goal of maximizing function from a physical, cognitive, social-emotional, and family dynamics perspective is kept in mind.

No one intervention strategy or intensity is unanimously embraced by physical therapists for any diagnostic group. Similarly, in the case of children with long-term ventilator dependence, physical therapy varies widely because of differing philosophies of management and the wide range of problem areas that might be identified. Thus, the intent of this section is not to recommend specific interventions but to present a conceptual framework from which one can organize an appropriate plan of care and to emphasize considerations unique to this group of children. Specific interventions are listed and detailed in the Guide to Physical Therapist Practice.[29] Table 25.5 summarizes key consideration for physical therapy intervention for children dependent on MV. Before continuing, readers unfamiliar with children requiring long-term mechanical ventilation might want to first view the video accompanying this chapter on Expert Consult that illustrates physical therapist intervention with a 22-month-old girl who is ventilator dependent.

Infants and children who are typically developing are capable of using a variable repertoire of motor skills to explore and learn. Motor development in childhood presumes a smooth

TABLE 25.5	**Considerations for Physical Therapy Interventions**
Type of Intervention	**Procedures**
Airway clearance techniques	Breathing strategies for airway clearance Manual/mechanical techniques for airway clearance Positioning Postural drainage
Assistive technology	Splints, casts, prosthetics, and orthotics Activity of daily living and bathroom technologies (e.g., adaptive commodes, shower benches) Mobility technologies: strollers, standers, and wheelchairs Seating and positioning equipment Transfer technologies (e.g., mechanical lifts)
Biophysical agents	Biofeedback Taping Electrical stimulation Hydrotherapy
Integumentary repair and protection techniques	Debridement Dressing selection Orthotic, protective, and supportive device recommendations and modifications Topical agents
Manual therapy techniques	Manual traction Massage Mobilization/manipulation Passive range of motion
Motor function training	Balance training Gait training Manual and power wheelchair training Perceptual training Postural stabilization and training Task-specific performance training Vestibular training
Therapeutic exercise	Aerobic capacity/endurance conditioning or reconditioning Aquatic therapy Developmental activities Flexibility exercises Gait and locomotor training Relaxation techniques Training for strength, power, and endurance
Patient or client instruction	Activity tolerance, vital sign monitoring, and clinical signs indicating the need for emergency intervention Diagnosis/prognosis Indications for ventilator use and impact of ventilator on motor and mobility skills Positioning, orthotic and equipment use Mobility strategies-home, school, and community transportation options Resources for leisure and recreation activities

interaction of the cardiopulmonary and musculoskeletal systems, as well as the necessary cognitive requirements. In the case of a child with chronic respiratory insufficiency, compromised physiologic stability may limit the seemingly endless exploration and practice in which children typically engage. In children with a chronic illness, a reduced capacity for activity or exercise can be a direct or indirect result of their underlying pathophysiologic process. For example, Smith et al.[78] reported on a large cohort of school-aged children born very preterm and noted significant impairment in exercise capacity despite evidence of only mild small-airway obstruction and gas trapping. Regardless of the cause, a vicious circle of inactivity may ensue—inactivity with reluctance to move and explore resulting in decreased endurance and fitness and further inactivity.

Another consideration is that children with long-term MV may associate movement with negative experiences such as fatigue, hypoxia, and pain, which limits their motivation to be active. A major goal of the physical therapist in the management of children who are dependent on ventilators should be secondary prevention—that is, to prevent deprivation of sensory and motor experiences because of inactivity and the various sequelae that result from that deprivation. Regardless of the child's medical diagnosis, intervention should be aimed at providing a variety of opportunities for movement challenges and for exploration, as well as increasing their function and capacity for exercise. Depending on whether the child has a specific motor impairment, these goals may be accomplished with or without the use of assistive devices. For example, in the case of a child with BPD who also had an intraventricular hemorrhage, adaptive equipment may be needed for positioning because of poor antigravity trunk control or for ambulation because of lower extremity weakness and spasticity. Alternatively, the child with congenital central hypoventilation syndrome and no impairments in motor control may be independent in all motor skills but may exhibit exercise intolerance.

Patient or Client Instruction

The pediatric health care environment embraces family-centered care,[40] recognizing that family members are the most important people in a child's life. The role of the family in shaping the child's environment to be the most conducive for growth and development is crucial. Importantly, from a practical point of view, the child's life depends on parents' knowledge of the intensive care needed to maintain the child's health and safety when dependent on long-term MV.

Physical therapists can provide the child, family, and other team members with information about the child's diagnosis, indications for ventilator use, and the functional abilities of the child. Therapists can also provide consultation on positioning, orthotic and equipment use, activity tolerance, vital sign monitoring, clinical signs indicating the need for emergency intervention, mobility strategies within the home and school environments, transportation options, resources for leisure and recreation activities, and psychosocial factors affecting intervention.

Airway Clearance Techniques

Although therapists often focus on strengthening the muscles of respiration and core trunk muscles, maintaining mobility of the rib cage, spine, and shoulder girdle is important to promote any nonassisted ventilation. Physical therapists select, prescribe, and implement airway clearance techniques that may include breathing strategies for airway clearance, manual/mechanical techniques for airway clearance, positioning, and pulmonary postural drainage. Although the goals of physical therapists are to enhance exercise performance; reduce risk factors and complications; enhance or maintain physical performance; improve cough; improve oxygenation and ventilation; or prevent or remediate impairments in body functions and structures, activity limitations, or participation restrictions, they may also teach a child and family airway clearance techniques and positioning for pulmonary drainage.

Assistive Technology

Appropriate assistive technology can minimize caregiver dependence and help children to attain functional skills and mobility unattainable on their own. Assistive technology may also be used to decrease pain, minimize the chance of secondary impairments due to the underlying disease process or immobility, and promote function and participation. Examples of assistive technologies to improve safety, function, and independence include splints, casts, prosthetics, and orthotics; transfer technologies (e.g., transfer boards, mechanical lifts/hoists); activity of daily living and bathroom technologies (e.g., adaptive commodes, shower benches); and strollers, standers, and wheelchairs.

Orthoses may be needed to manage joint contractures, maintain joint flexibility, or provide proper alignment of the trunk, feet, legs, and hands or arms. Of particular importance for children who require a trunk orthosis in order to maintain an upright posture or manage a scoliosis is an orthosis that is fabricated to allow the rib cage to expand fully and accommodate a gastrostomy tube.

Seating, positioning, and mobility equipment options are extensive (e.g., custom-molded seating, upper extremity support trays for wheelchairs, prone standers, manual or power wheelchairs). Young children may require specialized adapted strollers with ventilator-carrying capability. Older children may require manual or power wheelchairs adequately outfitted to transport a ventilator. The ventilator and other equipment must be safely secured to the seating system (Fig. 25.3). If the child is ambulatory, a portable ventilator may be transported in a backpack that the child or the care provider can carry.

All systems of transport should meet the Federal Motor Vehicle Safety Standard for car seats and bus transport. This includes securing the ventilator on the seat next to the child. In addition, when transporting a ventilator, in the authors' experience it is common for the child to have a spare tracheostomy tube, Ambu bag, oxygen tank, or portable suction unit with sterile catheters, as well as an external battery for the ventilator.

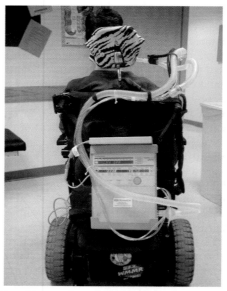

FIG. 25.3 Portable ventilator is placed on the back of the wheelchair. (From Panitch HB: Diurnal hypercapnia in patients with neuromuscular disease, *Paediatr Respir Rev* 11:3-8, 2010.)

Although physical therapists are not the ones who prescribe assistive technology to promote communication for children without speech and those with learning challenges, they may be consulted regarding the design and access of these devices.

Biophysical Agents

Biophysical agents—modalities that use various forms of energy primarily to increase muscle force, tissue perfusion, healing or tissue extensibility, or decrease pain or inflammation—may be used in conjunction with other physical therapist interventions.[29] There is, however, no evidence supporting or refuting the efficacy of such agents with children dependent on long-term MV. Examples of biophysical agents used with children with neuromuscular diagnoses that may also be applicable for a child with a neuromuscular diagnosis and long-term MV dependence include biofeedback, taping, electrical stimulation, hydrotherapy, and mechanical devices (e.g., standing frame).

Integumentary Repair and Protection Techniques

Methods and techniques may include debridement, dressing selection, orthotic selection, protective and supportive device recommendations and modifications, biophysical agents, and topical agents.[29] Often because of the multiple medical providers involved with a child who has ventilator dependence, another member of the health care team may be the one to employ several of these techniques. Of particular concern for children with long-term MV is the skin around the tracheostomy, which is at high risk for breakdown due to the moisture and tubing and requires vigilant monitoring.

Manual Therapy Techniques

Manual therapy techniques include skilled movements of joints and soft tissue intended to improve tissue extensibility; increase range of motion; induce relaxation; mobilize joints; and reduce pain, swelling, inflammation.[29] Techniques may include manual traction, massage, mobilization/manipulation, and passive range of motion. The child's dependence on a ventilator does not in itself prohibit the use of these techniques if indicated.

Motor Function Training

Motor function training is the systematic performance or execution of planned physical movements, postures, or activities. Motor function training may include balance training, both static and dynamic; gait training; manual and power wheelchair training; perceptual training; task-specific performance training; vestibular training; and postural stabilization and training.[29] Physical therapists commonly use motor function training activities for children with neuromuscular diagnoses; thus, these methods may be applicable for the plan of care for children with long-term MV dependence.

Therapeutic Exercise

Therapeutic exercise may include the following: aerobic capacity/endurance conditioning or reconditioning; developmental activities training; aquatic therapy; flexibility exercises; gait and locomotor training; relaxation techniques; and training for strength, power, and endurance for head, neck, limb, pelvic-floor, trunk, and ventilator muscles (active, active-assistive, and resistive exercises). This broad group of activities is intended to improve strength, flexibility, muscular and cardiorespiratory endurance, balance, coordination, posture, and motor function or development.

Simply stated, the "normal" response to exercise is an increase in heart rate, followed by a return to baseline. Ventilation also increases linearly with the metabolic rate until approximately 60% of oxygen consumption, at which time it increases more rapidly (see Chapter 6 for a summary of the cardiorespiratory and musculoskeletal components of exercise and fitness). These relationships, as well as the other physiologic processes that support adequate ventilation and perfusion during exercise, are altered in conditions of lung disease. Whereas exercise is normally cardiac limited, in individuals with chronic lung disease, exercise may be ventilator limited as a result of deficient exercise capacity and gas exchange or poor pulmonary mechanics. The optimal level of physical activity for children with chronic lung disease, however, is not related to disease severity.[80] Response to exercise and capacity for improvement, therefore, are evaluated for each child.

The beneficial effects of exercise have been documented in certain populations with respiratory conditions such as individuals with cystic fibrosis[50] (see Chapter 26) and asthma (see Chapter 27).[21] No group design study has examined active exercise and strength training for children who require MV. Strength training has been found to be useful for children with neurologic and neuromuscular disorders.[25] As with any health condition, exercise limitations and restrictions should be determined before the start of an exercise program, and with all exercise, children should be supervised closely to avoid musculoskeletal injury, excessive heart and respiratory rate, and dislodgement of tubing.

In infants and children dependent on MV, physical activity can be viewed as exercise and a means of improving endurance and tolerance for movement. There is a paucity of research on the effect of developmental interventions on cardiopulmonary function and exercise tolerance. In one study investigating physical therapist intervention activities and cardiorespiratory response for young children with chronic respiratory insufficiency, sitting activities were the most frequently applied and prone activities were used the least.[18] Ventilator dependence often dictates limited movement and mobility if the child must remain close to a nonmobile ventilator. For example, time spent in a prone position is often limited and may occur only during physical therapy. Exercise and activity in a prone position are useful for strengthening the neck and shoulder girdle musculature and for developing righting reactions. Rotational movements and crossing the midline of the body are important for many functional activities but are often constrained by the child's ventilator tubing. For children of all ages, upright positioning in sitting or standing is important for physiologic function and bone density and should be encouraged when developmentally and medically appropriate. Activities such as pulling to stand and cruising may occur in a crib if a young child is in the hospital with limited opportunities for playtime on the floor.[17]

SUMMARY

Children dependent on long-term MV have complex medical conditions including prematurity and chronic lung disease, cardiac conditions, congenital anomalies, and, most commonly, neuromuscular and neurologic conditions. The prevalence of infants and children dependent on MV continues to increase due to medical and technological advancements. Children requiring long-term MV are at high risk for secondary illness, recurring hospitalizations, global developmental delays, tracheostomy-related complications, and equipment failure.

Minimizing a child's dependence on MV has important benefits for the quality of life of both the child and the family. This includes a reduction in hospital stays, improved physical and mental health, and more opportunities for social participation. There is limited evidence on how often successful weaning from a ventilator is achieved.

Physical therapists have an important role in fostering the health and development of infants, children, and youth with chronic respiratory failure and supporting families. Once the decision is made to begin artificial ventilation, prevention and treatment of associated complications are primary goals of medical and rehabilitation management. Although the type and intensity of intervention varies, desired outcomes of physical therapy include maximizing children's mobility, self-care, and participation. Some physical therapist interventions are medically related, such as percussion and postural drainage. A major focus of physical therapist interventions is to integrate goals into everyday activities and support the family in managing the child's health and developmental needs. The ecologic validity of intervention increases if goals are made a part of daily activities and routines.

Physical therapists are encouraged to participate in clinical research to contribute to the evidence supporting management of children who require long-term ventilation. Research is needed to determine effective program planning, program improvements, and appropriate resource utilization, and to set outcome expectations for infants, toddlers, and children dependent on long-term MV. Additional research questions may involve the impact of rehabilitation interventions on the weaning process and the impact of rehabilitation interventions on quality-of-life outcomes for children and their families.

Case Scenario on Expert Consult

Two case scenarios on the Expert Consult website illustrate the physical therapy management of children who require long-term mechanical ventilation. The first case is a video of a 22-month-old child with Mobius syndrome and central respiratory dysfunction. The second case describes a 24-month-old child with chronic lung disease using the *Guide to Physical Therapist Practice* and the International Classification of Functioning, Disability and Health as frameworks.

The case scenario related to this chapter illustrates the physical therapy management of a child requiring long-term MV who has several comorbidities.

REFERENCES

1. Reference deleted in proofs.
2. Allen J: Pulmonary complications of neuromuscular disease: a respiratory mechanics perspective, *Paediatr Respir Rev* 11:18–23, 2010.
3. Bach JR, et al.: Long-term survival in Werdnig-Hoffmann disease, *Am J Phys Med Rehabil* 86:339–345, 2007.
4. Benneyworth BD, et al.: Inpatient health care utilization for children dependent on long-term mechanical ventilation, *Pediatrics* 127:e1533–e1541, 2011.
5. Berry-Kravis EM, et al.: Congenital central hypoventilation syndrome: PHOX2B mutations and phenotype, *Am J Respir Crit Care Med* 174:1139–1144, 2006.
6. Bertrand P, et al.: Home ventilatory assistance in Chilean children: 12 years' experience, *Arch Bronconeumol* 42:165–170, 2006.
7. Bhandari V, Gruen JR: The genetics of bronchopulmonary dysplasia, *Semin Perinatol* 30:185–191, 2006.
8. Boroughs D, Dougherty JA: Decreasing accidental mortality of ventilator-dependent children at home: a call to action, *Home Healthc Nurse* 30:103–111, 2012.
9. Reference deleted in proofs.
10. Reference deleted in proofs.
11. Carrozzi L, Make B: Chronic respiratory failure as a global issue. In Ambrosino N, Goldstein R, editors: *Ventilatory support for chronic respiratory failure: lung biology in health and disease*, vol. 225. New York, 2008, Informa Healthcare, pp 27–38.
12. Cockett A: Technology dependence and children: a review of the evidence, *Nurs Child Young People* 24:32–35, 2012.
13. Com G, et al.: Outcomes of children treated with tracheostomy and positive-pressure ventilation at home, *Clin Pediatr (Phila)* 52:54–61, 2013.
14. Como JJ, et al.: Characterizing the need for mechanical ventilation following cervical spinal cord injury with neurologic deficit, *J Trauma* 59:912–916, 2005.
15. Cristea AI, et al.: Outcomes of children with severe bronchopulmonary dysplasia who were ventilator dependent at home, *Pediatrics* 132:e727–e734, 2013.
16. Dieperink W, et al.: Walking with continuous positive airway pressure, *Eur Respir J* 27:853–855, 2006.
17. Dudek-Shriber L, Zelazny S: The effect of prone positioning on the quality and acquisition of developmental milestones in four-month old infants, *Pediatr Phys Ther* 19:48–55, 2007.
18. Dumas HM, et al.: Cardiorespiratory response during physical therapist intervention for infants and young children with chronic respiratory insufficiency, *Pediatr Phys Ther* 25:178–185, 2013.
19. Dybwik K, et al.: Fighting the system: families caring for ventilator-dependent children and adults with complex health care needs at home, *BMC Health Serv Res* 11:156, 2011.
20. Edwards EA, et al.: Paediatric home ventilatory support: the Auckland experience, *J Paediatr Child Health* 41:652–658, 2005.
21. Fanelli A, et al.: Exercise training on disease control and quality of life in asthmatic children, *MedSci Sports Exerc* 39:1474–1480, 2007.
22. Fauroux B, Khirani S: Neuromuscular disease and respiratory physiology in children: putting lung function into perspective, *Respirology* 19:782–791, 2014.
23. Fragala-Pinkham MA, et al.: Evaluation of an adaptive ice skating programme for children with disabilities, *Dev Neurorehabil* 12:215–223, 2009.
24. Fragala-Pinkham MA, et al.: A fitness program for children with disabilities, *Phys Ther* 85:1182–1200, 2005.
25. Fragala-Pinkham MA, et al.: Evaluation of a community-based group fitness program for children with disabilities, *Pediatr Phys Ther* 18:159–167, 2006.
26. Gowans M, et al.: The population prevalence of children receiving invasive home ventilation in Utah, *Pediatr Pulmonol* 42:231–236, 2007.
27. Graham RJ, et al.: Chronic ventilator need in the community: a 2005 pediatric census of Massachusetts, *Pediatrics* 119:e1280–e1287, 2007.
28. Reference deleted in proofs.
29. Guide to pysical therapist practice 3.0, Alexandria, VA, 2014, American Physical Therapy Association. Available at: http://guidetoptpractice.apta.org/. Accessed August 5, 2015.
30. Hefner JL, Tsai WC: Ventilator-dependent children and the health services system: unmet needs and coordination of care, *Ann Am Thorac Soc* 10:482–489, 2013.
31. Hsia SH, Lin JJ, Huang IA, Wu CT: Outcome of long-term mechanical ventilation support in children, *Pediatr Neonatol* 53:304–308, 2012.
32. Hull EM, et al.: Tracheostomy speaking valves for children: tolerance and clinical benefits, *Pediatr Rehabil* 8:214–219, 2005.
33. Reference deleted in proofs.
34. Jurgens V, et al.: Hospital readmission in children with complex chronic conditions discharged from subacute care, *Hosp Pediatr* 4:153–158, 2014.
35. Kendirli T, et al.: Mechanical ventilation in children, *Turk J Pediatr* 48:323–327, 2007.

36. Kharasch VS, et al.: Bronchoscopy findings in children and young adults with tracheostomy due to congenital anomalies and neurological impairment, *J Pediatr Rehabil Med* 1:137–143, 2008.

37. Kissoon N, Adderley R: Noninvasive ventilation in infants and children, *Minerva Pediatr* 60:211–218, 2008.

38. Koumbourlis AC: Chest wall abnormalities and their clinical significance in childhood, *Paediatr Respir Rev* 15:246–255, 2014.

39. Krcmar S: Room to breathe, RT: for decision makers in respiratory care, Overland Park, Kansas. *Allied Media*, LLC 2006.

40. Kuo DZ, et al.: Family-centered care: current applications and future directions in pediatric health care, *Matern Child Health J* 16:297–305, 2012.

41. Lai D, Schroer B: Haddad syndromes: a case of an infant with central congenital hypoventilation syndrome and Hirschsprung disease, *J Child Neurol* 23:341–343, 2008.

42. Lesser DJ, et al.: Congenital hypoventilation syndromes, *Sem Respir Crit Care Med* 30:339–347, 2009.

43. Lindahl B, Lindblad BM: Family members' experiences of everyday life when a child is dependent on a ventilator: a metasynthesis study, *J Fam Nurs* 17:241–269, 2011.

44. Reference deleted in proofs.

45. Reference deleted in proofs.

46. Mah JK, et al.: Parental stress and quality of life in children with neuromuscular disease, *Pediatr Neurol* 39:102–107, 2008.

47. Maitre NL, R, et al.: Respiratory consequences of prematurity: evolution of a diagnosis and development of a comprehensive approach, *J Perinatol* 35:321, 2015.

48. Mayer OH: Chest wall hypoplasia: principles and treatment, *Paediatr Respir Rev* 16:30–34, 2015.

49. McDougall CM, et al.: Long-term ventilation in children: longitudinal trends and outcomes, *Arch Dis Child* 98:660–665, 2013.

50. McIlwane M: Chest physical therapy, breathing techniques and exercise in children with CF, *Paediatr Respir Rev* 8:8–16, 2007.

51. Meltzer LJ, et al.: The relationship between home nursing coverage, sleep and daytime functioning in parents of ventilator-assisted children, *J Pediatr Nurs* 25:250–257, 2010.

52. Mesman GR, et al.: The impact of technology dependence on children and their families, *J Pediatr Health Care* 27:451–459, 2013.

53. Moffat M, Frownfelter D: *Cardiovascular/pulmonary essentials: applying the preferred physical therapist practice patterns*, Thorofare, NJ, 2007, Slack.

54. Reference deleted in proofs.

55. Nitu Mara E, Eigen H: Respiratory failure, *Pediatr Rev* 30:470–478, 2009.

56. Noah ZL, Budek CE: Chronic severe respiratory insufficiency. In Marx JA, Hockberger RS, Walls RM, editors: *Rosen's emergency medicine*, ed 8, 2014, Philadelphia: Saunders (imprint of Elsevier).

57. Noyes J: Health and quality of life of ventilator-dependent children, *J Adv Nurs* 56:392–403, 2006.

58. O'Brien JE, et al.: Weaning children from mechanical ventilation in a post-acute setting, *Pediatr Rehabil* 9:365–372, 2006.

59. O'Brien JE, et al.: Ventilator weaning outcomes in chronic respiratory failure in children, *Int J Rehabil Res* 30:171–174, 2007.

60. Oktem S, et al.: Home ventilation for children with chronic respiratory failure in Istanbul, *Respiration* 76:76–81, 2007.

61. O'Neil ME, et al.: Community-based programs for children and youth: our experiences in design, implementation, and evaluation, *Phys Occup Ther Pediatr* 32:111–119, 2012.

62. O'Reilly M, et al.: Impact of preterm birth and bronchopulmonary dysplasia on the developing lung: long-term consequences for respiratory health, *Clin Exp Pharmacol Physiol* 40:765–773, 2013.

63. Ottonello G, et al.: Home mechanical ventilation in children: retrospective survey of a pediatric population, *Pediatr Int* 49:801–805, 2007.

64. Overman AE, et al.: Tracheostomy for infants requiring prolonged mechanical ventilation: 10 years' experience, *Pediatr* 131:e1491–e1496, 2013.

65. Reference deleted in proofs.

66. Panitch HB: Children dependent on respiratory technology. In Wilmott RW, et al., editors: *Kendig & Chernick's disorders of the respiratory tract in children*, 2012, Philadelphia: Elsevier.

67. Peterson-Carmichael SL, Cheifetz IM: The chronically critically ill patient: pediatric considerations, *Respir Care* 57:993–1002, 2012.

68. Philip AGS: Bronchopulmonary dysplasia: then and now, *Neonatology* 102:1–8, 2012.

69. Preutthipan A: Home mechanical ventilation in children, *Indian J Pediatr* 82:852–859, 2015.

70. Racca F, et al.: Invasive and non-invasive long-term mechanical ventilation in Italian children, *Minerva Anestesiologica* 77:892–901, 2011.

71. Reference deleted in proofs.

72. Reference deleted in proofs.

73. Rsovac S, et al.: Complications of mechanical ventilation in pediatric patients in Serbia, *Adv Clin Exp Med* 23:1, 57–61, 2014.

74. Sarnaik AP, et al.: Chapter 71. In Marx JA, et al., editors: *Rosen's emergency medicine*, ed 8, 2014, Philadelphia: Saunders (imprint of Elsevier).

75. Sharma H, et al.: Treatments to restore respiratory function after spinal cord injury and their implications for regeneration, plasticity and adaptation, *Exp Neurol* 235:18–25, 2012.

76. Reference deleted in proofs.

77. Reference deleted in proofs.

78. Smith LJ, et al.: Reduced exercise capacity in children born very preterm, *Pediatrics* 122:e287–e293, 2008.

79. Srinivasan R, et al.: A prospective study of ventilator-associated pneumonia in children, *Pediatrics* 123:1108–1115, 2009.

80. Sritippayawan S, et al.: Optimal level of physical activity in children with chronic lung disease, *Acta Paediatrica* 97:1582–1587, 2008.

81. Traiber C, et al.: Profile and consequences of children requiring prolonged mechanical ventilation in three Brazilian pediatric intensive care units, *Pediatr Crit Care Med* 10:375–380, 2009.

82. Van den Broek MJ, et al.: Chiari type I malformation causing central apnoeas in a 4-month-old boy, *Eur J Pediatr Neurol* 13:463–465, 2008.

83. van Kaam AH, et al.: Ventilation practices in the neonatal intensive care unit: a cross-sectional study, *J Pediatr* 157:767–771, 2010.

84. Venkataraman ST: Mechanical ventilation and respiratory care. In Fuhrman BP, Zimmerman JJ, editors: *Pediatric critical care*, ed 4, Philadelphia: Elsevier, 2012.

85. Vo P, Kharasch VS: Respiratory failure, *Pediatr Rev* 35:476–486, 2014.

86. vom Hove M, et al.: Pulmonary outcome in former preterm, very low birth weight children with bronchopulmonary dysplasia: a case-control follow-up at school age, *J Pediatr* 164:40–45, 2014. e4.

87. von Renesse A, et al.: Respiratory syncytial virus infection in children admitted to hospital but ventilated mechanically for other reasons, *J Med Virol* 81:160–166, 2009.

88. Wallis C, et al.: Children on long-term ventilatory support: 10 years of progress, *Arch Dis Child* 96:998–1002, 2011.

89. Reference deleted in proofs.

90. White AC: Long-term mechanical ventilation: management strategies, *Respir Care* 57:889–899, 2012.

91. Wilmott RW: Long-term respiratory impairment with the new Bpd, *J Pediatr* 164:1–3, 2014.

92. Wocadlo C, Rieger I: Motor impairment and low achievement in very preterm children at eight years of age, *Early Human Dev* 84:769–776, 2008.

93. Reference deleted in proofs

94. Reference deleted in proofs.

26

Cystic Fibrosis

Jennifer L. Agnew, Blythe Owen

The increasing life expectancy of individuals with cystic fibrosis (CF) and continuing advances in treatment have contributed to an expanded role of the physical therapist as a member of a multidisciplinary health care team. In this chapter, background information is presented on pathophysiology, etiology, diagnosis, and medical management of CF that is critical for setting goals, developing, and modifying the physical therapy plan of care. The role of the physical therapist in promoting self-management of respiratory function and physical activity beginning at a young age and progressing through childhood, adolescence, and adulthood is discussed. Supporting families and children's self-efficacy are essential components of intervention to promote well-being and quality of life.

BACKGROUND INFORMATION

CF was identified in 1928, when Andersen published a paper describing the clinical course of a number of children who had died of pulmonary and digestive problems. She labeled the disorder "cystic fibrosis of the pancreas."[5] This disease thereafter was classified as a disorder of exocrine gland function, influencing the respiratory system, pancreas, reproductive organs, and sweat glands. At times the first presenting sign has been the subjective report, "My child tastes salty to kiss"; the "sweat test" often confirms the diagnosis. Subsequent study and interest led to a clearer understanding of the disease and a coordinated approach to treating the associated impairments. Over time the disorder that had so intrigued Andersen has come to be known as cystic fibrosis, and research has continued, yielding vast knowledge about this chronic illness.

Classified as a hereditary disease, CF is inherited through an autosomal recessive pattern in which two copies of the gene responsible for CF are passed on to an affected individual. Both parents of a child diagnosed with CF must be carriers of at least one copy of a mutation at the gene locus responsible for CF. Those persons with one copy of the CF gene are termed *heterozygote carriers* and are not diagnostically positive for CF. In 1989 a major scientific breakthrough occurred with discovery of the precise locus on chromosome 7 of the gene responsible for CF.[169] The pathology of the physical manifestations of CF has since been determined.

Although cystic fibrosis was once referred to the most commonly inherited life-shortening illness in the Caucasian population, advances in its management have improved the quality of life and prognosis for life expectancy.[55] In the United States, 45% of the approximately 30,000 individuals diagnosed with CF are over the age of 18; therefore CF is no longer thought of as exclusively a childhood disease. The median predicted age of survival for individuals with CF is currently 41.1 years in the United States.[151,198] An increasing number of people with CF are reaching the fifth decade of life; the median age of survival in Canada is 50.9 years.[46] Surgical advances in lung transplantation offer hope of prolonging life for people with chronic pulmonary disabilities.

CF is diagnosed in 1 in 3500 children born to white American parents, and statistical analysis of this incidence yields a best estimate of the rate of heterozygote carriers as about 5% of the population in areas of the world where significant white populations have settled.[19,147] The incidence of CF in black and Asian peoples is considerably lower than that in whites: approximately 1 in 17,000 births in the black population and an estimated 1 in 90,000 births in Asian societies.[19] Several reports have documented the incidence of CF in the South Asian population, estimated to be 1 in 10,000 to 1 in 40,750.[125] Recent research and carrier screening are producing more precise statistical estimates of the incidence of individuals who are heterozygote CF carriers, suggesting that previous rates were underestimated.[210] Prenatal diagnosis of CF is now possible, as is screening for carrier status, which is discussed in detail later in this chapter.

The gene responsible for CF was identified in 1989 by an international team of researchers led by Drs. Tsui, Collins, and Riordan.[93] This discovery was an extraordinary achievement in molecular genetics and has led to subsequent research advances in the understanding of genetic and pathologic components of CF worldwide. Approximately 2000 distinct mutations within the CF gene have been identified in many ethnic groups, although fewer than 10 mutations occur with a frequency greater than 1%.[182] The trinucleotide deletion, delta-F508, is the most common mutation associated with clinical CF, occurring in 66% of patients worldwide.[166] This mutation results in loss of the amino acid phenylalanine from the product protein, which ultimately affects its production, regulation, and/or function. The specific genetic mutation can now be used to predict the severity of lung disease and the prognosis in terms of survival.[43,124]

Specialized health care is most often provided through regional CF centers. Comprehensive treatment programs for CF were established over 55 years ago[59] and are the primary mode of delivery of specialized health care. CF centers changed the practice of focusing on the treatment of ongoing disease to taking a proactive approach of early intervention, maintenance of health, and preservation of lung function.[198] CF centers can offer their clients the services of respirologists, gastroenterologists, physical therapists, respiratory therapists, pharmacists, dietitians, genetic counselors, social workers, psychologists, exercise physiologists, and specialty care nursing personnel. The multidisciplinary team is dedicated to the delivery of the most effective and palatable treatments and promoting the optimal level of well-being for patients with CF and their families. CF centers worldwide work collaboratively in sharing their clinical expertise and their knowledge base to develop new treatment possibilities and to renew hopes for an ultimate cure for CF. Definitions of key terms used in the chapter are provided in Box 26.1.

PATHOPHYSIOLOGY

The CF gene defect leads to absent or malfunctioning of the cystic fibrosis transmembrane conductance regulator (CFTR) protein, which results in abnormal chloride conductance on the epithelial cell. The main organ systems affected are the respiratory system and the gastrointestinal system, although the reproductive system, sinuses, and sweat glands are also impaired. Blockage of exocrine glands prevents the delivery of their product to target tissues and organs and creates clinical abnormalities in these body systems.

In the lung, abnormal CFTR protein leads to depletion of the airway surface liquid layer (ASL) due to obstruction of mucus secreting exocrine glands and hyperviscous secretions, which can lead to ciliary collapse and decreased mucociliary transport. The accumulation of hyperviscous secretions leads to progressive airway obstruction, secondary infection by opportunistic bacteria, inflammation, and subsequent bronchiectasis and irreversible airway damage. This vicious cycle can be complicated by bronchoconstriction of the airways and chronic lung hyperinflation. Deconditioning of the respiratory muscles and malnutrition also affect the functional limitations of the respiratory system.[166]

Obstruction of the small airways in CF and subsequent air trapping and atelectasis result in ventilation and perfusion mismatch, which leads to hypoxemia. Long-standing hypoxemia may result in pulmonary artery hypertension and cor pulmonale or right ventricular failure. Large airway bronchiectasis combined with small airway obstruction reduces vital capacity and tidal volume and results in decreased volumes of airflow at the alveolar level. Consequently, progressively increasing arterial carbon dioxide concentration ($PaCO_2$) occurs, which may lead to hypercapnic respiratory failure. Respiratory failure accounts for 95% of the mortality rate in CF.[143]

In the gastrointestinal tract, viscous secretions begin to obstruct the pancreatic duct in utero, and periductal inflammation and fibrosis cause the loss of pancreatic exocrine function. The resulting maldigestion of fats and proteins results in steatorrhea and the excretion of excessive quantities of fat in the stools.[60] The stools are described as bulky, frequent, and "greasy" and as having a strongly offensive odor. Infants with CF can display evidence of protein-calorie malnutrition with a protruding abdomen, muscle wasting, and initial diagnosis of failure to thrive despite reports from parents of hearty appetites.[111] Compensating for loss of pancreatic function remains a critical feature of management throughout the life span.

Another pathologic finding that presents in 10% to 20% of individuals with CF is meconium ileus, which is demonstrated in neonates.[133] The combination of abnormal pancreatic function and hyperviscous secretions of the intestinal glands creates an altered viscosity of the meconium, which causes an obstruction at the distal ileum, thus preventing passage of meconium in the first neonatal days.[111] Distal intestinal obstruction syndrome (DIOS) is seen in some older patients, associated with abnormal intestinal secretions and increased adherence of mucus in the intestines.[35]

Hepatobiliary disease has been reported with greater frequency among patients with pancreatic insufficiency. CF-related liver disease occurs in up to 30% of people with CF, but it is a significant clinical problem only in the minority of individuals (cirrhosis, portal hypertension). Patients with CF and pancreatic sufficiency have an increased risk of developing acute pancreatitis.[62] CF-related diabetes mellitus (CFRD) is a systemic complication whose prevalence increases with age. CFRD occurs in 2% of children, 19% of adolescents, and 40% to 50% of adults. Incidence and prevalence are higher in females age 30 to 39, but otherwise, no gender difference is noted.[128]

In the reproductive system, obstruction of the vas deferens causes infertility in 98% of males with CF.[35] Older studies reported that the fertility rate for females with CF was 20% to 30% of normal, but more recent data have suggested that the reproductive tract is normal in most women with CF. Therefore females with CF who have good weight and lung function can expect to have normal hormone levels that contribute to regular ovulation and menstruation. The only mechanical barrier present in females with CF is the cervical mucous plug.[61]

In the upper respiratory tract, chronic pansinusitis occurs in 99% of individuals with CF and contributes to the infection of the lower respiratory tract by acting as a reservoir of infection. Sinusitis may cause persistent headache and nasal polyps occur in 6% to 40% of patients and can recur after initial resection.[35] Hypertrophic pulmonary osteoarthropathy is often associated with advanced severity of pulmonary disease and is most noticeable in the clinical finding of "clubbing," or rounded hypertrophic changes in the terminal phalanges of the fingers and toes.[110] Osteopenia is present in up to 85% of adult patients, and osteoporosis in 10% to 34%. In children, the reported prevalence is not consistent because of comparisons with different control populations and corrections for bone size in growing children.[180]

BOX 26.1 Definitions of Key Terms

Airway Clearance: Cardiopulmonary techniques used to open up the airways and to loosen, unstick, collect, and mobilize secretions from the peripheral airways to the central airway to promote mucus transport in the lungs.

Cystic Fibrosis: Autosomal recessive disorder that results from the 2 CFTR mutations.

Cystic Fibrosis Transmembrane Conductance Regulator (CFTR): A protein channel that transports negatively charged chloride ions across the membrane of exocrine cells, resulting in the movement of water and other ions across the epithelial cell membrane. In the lung the balance of ions and water hydrate the airway surface liquid layer to support ciliary stability and functioning and ultimately to promote mucociliary transport.

Exercise Testing: An objective exercise assessment used to evaluate physical limitations and aerobic capacity, in which the results can be used to make recommendations for an individualized exercise program.

Forced Expiratory Volume in 1 sec (FEV_1): The amount of air that is forcefully expired in 1 second during spirometry.

Inhalation Therapy: The administration of aerosolized medications with proper breathing technique.

Pulmonary Function Tests: A group of tests that assess how well the lungs are working; determine how much air the lungs can hold, how well air moves in and out of the lungs, and how efficient gas exchange is.

Sweat Chloride Test: Clinical diagnostic test used to detect elevated chloride levels in sweat and help make a diagnosis of cystic fibrosis.

ETIOLOGY

The cause of CF is traced to the abnormal gene product, CFTR protein, which seems to be most abundantly expressed in the apical membrane surface of epithelial cells of the respiratory, gastrointestinal, and reproductive systems and in the sweat glands. Normal epithelial cells secrete fluid by allowing chloride ions (negatively charged) to pass through the luminal membrane of the cell. Because this membrane is permeable to sodium ions (positively charged), they passively follow; increased levels of sodium chloride then stimulate fluid secretion. Fluid levels in the airways must be maintained at a sufficient level to provide for normal mucociliary transport. There are 6 different classes of CFTR mutations: i) defective synthesis of the protein; ii) defective protein processing and trafficking; iii) defective CFTR channel gating; iv) defective protein channel conductance; v) reduced synthesis of CFTR; vi) high CFTR protein turnover at the cell surface.[22,53] The consequence is an electrolyte abnormality (chloride impermeability and sodium hyperpermeability) that leads to excessive amounts of fluid being removed from the airway lumen, resulting in reduced airway surface liquid (ASL) volume and underhydrated mucus. These impairments, in turn, lead to impaired mucociliary clearance and retention of mucus in the lower airways.[21,111] Abnormal expression or regulation of the CFTR protein in airway epithelial cells is the primary cause of the respiratory manifestations of CF.

DIAGNOSIS

Early diagnosis, including prenatal determination of the presence of the CF gene mutation, has enabled researchers to follow the expression and progression of the disease from birth in many patients. Impairment of the respiratory system may not manifest immediately, and at birth the lungs often appear normal on radiologic examination. A history of respiratory illness such as repeated respiratory tract infections, recurrent bronchiolitis, or even pneumonia is often reported, but in 80% of newly diagnosed cases, no family history of CF is known.[111] Chest CT scans can detect infection and inflammation that are present in a significant proportion of infants with CF at 3 months of age, and it has been shown that these early structural changes are progressive. Dilation and hypertrophy of mucus-secreting goblet cells begin early in life, leading to subsequent impaired mucociliary clearance, obstructive mucous plugs, air trapping, atelectasis, and bronchiectasis, which all reflect abnormal ventilation and perfusion. Data from CT scans have been correlated with survival and health-related quality of life; it can also be used to identify children at risk for worse pulmonary outcomes and may help to guide treatment.[192]

A diagnosis of CF is made if the patient has one or more clinical features of the disease, a history of CF in a sibling, or a positive newborn screening test, plus laboratory evidence of an abnormality in the CFTR gene or protein. Acceptable evidence of a CFTR abnormality includes biologic evidence of channel dysfunction (i.e., abnormal sweat chloride concentration or nasal potential difference) or identification of a CF disease-causing mutation in each copy of the CFTR gene (i.e., on each chromosome).[64] An elevated level of sodium chloride in the sweat has been the principal diagnostic indicator for CF for more than 50 years.[70] A positive sweat test occurs if the chloride concentration is greater than 60 mmol/L or is within the intermediate range (30–59 mmol/L for infants younger than 6 months of age and 40–59 mmol/L for older individuals).[147]

In a few centers with specialized laboratory and trained personnel, another diagnostic test, nasal potential difference (PD), is possible. This test measures the electrical charge (potential difference) across the epithelial surface (mucous membrane) of the nose. In normal subjects, a small charge of −5 to −30 mV is present, whereas subjects with CF demonstrate values between −40 and −80 mV.[143] The degree of CFTR dysfunction as measured by the nasal PD correlates with the number and severity of CFTR gene mutations.[192]

Screening tests for prospective parents who are known carriers (with prior offspring with CF or with CF themselves) are now possible and raise a number of ethical issues when CF is suggested prenatally. Genetic counseling therefore is available at CF centers. Analysis of the blood of known heterozygote parents and of tissue from the fetus obtained through amniocentesis or chorionic villus sampling can determine the presence of the CF gene mutation common to the family history.

Newborn screening is being performed increasingly in many states and provinces within North America and around the world. A sample of blood is taken, and the IRT/DNA test is a two-stage test that is used to screen for CF. The first stage of the test looks for high levels of an enzyme called IRT (immunoreactive trypsinogen) in the blood sample from the baby's foot. If the amount of IRT is above a certain level, a DNA test is performed on the same blood sample. The DNA test looks for the most common genetic mutations associated with CF. A positive finding indicates that the child is at increased risk of CF and a sweat test must be performed to confirm the diagnosis. Without the onset of newborn screening, children with CF were not diagnosed with the disease until they became symptomatic with respiratory signs or failure to thrive. Several studies have shown that newborn screening for CF leads to improved nutritional outcomes, which in turn lead to improved pulmonary outcomes later in life.[147]

The diagnosis of CF may even be discovered in adulthood because these patients usually present with milder lung disease and pancreatic sufficiency. Their diagnosis is often delayed because of the belief that CF is a pediatric disease and the finding that some adults have normal to borderline sweat test results. The criteria for making a diagnosis are the same for adults and children.[213]

MEDICAL MANAGEMENT

Individuals with CF should be followed periodically at CF clinics (usually every 3–4 months, although this can vary) by a multidisciplinary team; this practice has contributed to increasing life expectancy.[55] To determine the plan of care for each individual, the clinical team evaluates the radiologic assessment, pulmonary function testing (PFT), sputum cultures, nutritional status and patterns of weight loss, blood analysis, exercise testing, and subjective reports of treatment adherence. All of these findings help the team address the changing therapeutic needs of patients with CF and initiate treatment regimens with the aim of preventing or slowing development of functional limitations. Increased frequency of monitoring and increased use of appropriate medications have been associated with an improvement in forced expired volume in 1 second (FEV$_1$: see section on measuring pulmonary function) in CF centers.[89]

Morbidity in individuals with CF is primarily related to deteriorating pulmonary status. The treatment of CF lung disease aims to decrease airway obstruction due to chronic bronchorrhea (abnormal mucous secretions) and the progressive inflammation that occurs secondary to chronic bacterial infection.[112] Irreversible airway damage is caused by bacteria that infect the respiratory tract at an early age (which may be difficult to eradicate) and the associated aggressive host inflammatory response. The development of antibiotic resistance after multiple antibiotic courses leads to chronic persistent infection. In infants and younger children, *Staphylococcus aureus* and *Haemophilus influenzae* predominate, although the most common CF pathogen is *Pseudomonas aeruginosa*. It has been suggested that inhaled *P. aeruginosa* has a high affinity for CF airways, which may explain the high prevalence of this organism in patients with CF. Some bacteria such as *P. aeruginosa* and *Burkholderia cepacia* complex can also produce biofilms that protect themselves, explaining the persistence of bacterial infection in the majority of CF patients despite attempts at eradication.[52] Chronic *Pseudomonas* infection is associated with a reduction in lung function and a poorer prognosis.[134]

Antibiotic therapy appears to have significantly influenced the effects of the chronic endobronchial infection that typifies CF and has been a mainstay of treatment regimens for over 60 years.[55] Optimally, the choice of antibiotics should be based on the results of sputum culture and sensitivity tests.[19] Sputum cultures show infection by a number of organisms in a common pattern that changes with severity of disease and with the age of the patient. Opportunistic bacteria, such as *P. aeruginosa, S. aureus, H. influenzae, B. cepacia* complex, *Stenotrophomonas maltophilia,* and *Achromobacter xylosoxidans,* are the organisms most frequently seen. Combinations of infectious organisms are common, particularly when disease severity and age of the patient advance. Some evidence suggests that early and vigorous use of antibiotics produce better results than delaying their administration until symptoms are well developed or advanced.[19]

Inhaled antibiotics, such as tobramycin and colistin, are beneficial in suppressing bacterial pulmonary infection because aerosolized medications can be delivered in higher doses directly to the airways while minimizing systemic exposure and toxicity. Ramsey and colleagues showed that inhaled preservative-free tobramycin twice a day resulted in a significant increase in FEV_1 and a 36% reduction in the use of intravenous antibiotics for pulmonary exacerbations.[4,164] In the Early Intervention TOBI Eradication (ELITE) trial, a 1-month course of inhaled TOBI (preservative-free tobramycin solution) monotherapy achieved an eradication rate > 90%. Approximately 70% of patients remained culture-negative for > 800 days after the short-course eradication protocol. Inhaled antipseudomonal antibiotics have been associated with improved quality of life, decreased risk of pulmonary exacerbation, improved pulmonary function, and decreased mortality.[65]

Delaying the onset of chronic *P. aeruginosa* and the development of a mucoid strain may help to preserve lung function over the longer term.[167] Intravenous antibiotics such as ceftazidime and other aminoglycosides are used to target *Pseudomonas* infections in hospitalized patients when oral or inhaled antibiotics do not improve their respiratory symptoms related to a pulmonary exacerbation. The combination of IV antibiotics with intensified airway clearance was shown to improve lung function more than with IV antibiotics alone.[17] Nebulized aztreonam (Cayston) is a relatively new inhaled antibiotic that has been shown to improve lung function and respiratory symptoms such as decreased cough, sputum, and wheezing in patients with CF. The drug is prescribed three times daily and must be taken with a special nebulizer system, the e-flow device that is a type of vibrating mesh technology.[2]

B. cepacia complex is made of 9 different species (e.g., *B. cenocepacia, B. multivorans*) and is an opportunistic pathogen in individuals with CF and other compromised hosts.[111] *B. cepacia* complex is recognized as a particularly virulent pathogen because of its high level of intrinsic antibiotic resistance, its tenacity to persist in the lungs, and its association with more advanced pulmonary disease. Synergy studies combining antibiotics may help identify a more effective antimicrobial therapy.[24] *B. cepacia* complex is highly transmissible from person to person, which has led to initiation of segregation practices and attempts to control cross-contamination of equipment in many centers. Infection with *B. cepacia* complex can cause a rapid decline in pulmonary function and can increase mortality fourfold in individuals with CF, due to the possibility of a sepsislike condition.[35]

An organism that can be present in the airways without causing infection is *Aspergillus fumigatus,* though an intense allergic response to this fungus, allergic bronchopulmonary aspergillosis (ABPA), is seen in up to 15% of patients with CF. Clinical manifestations of ABPA include wheezing, pulmonary infiltrates, and central bronchiectasis.[147] Non-tuberculous mycobacterium, such as *Mycobacterium abscessus* complex and *Mycobacterium avium* complex, is the most emerging threat to individuals with CF. It was previously regarded as a relatively benign environmental bacteria and now has been recognized as an opportunistic pathogen that can affect morbidity and mortality in CF.[162]

Although several of the virulent products of bacterial infection cause airway inflammation and progressive epithelial destruction and therefore contribute significantly to the severity of the pulmonary impairment in CF,[111] it has also been reported that inflammation can precede infection, as was observed in bronchoalveolar lavage (BAL) studies in infants.[96] Anti-inflammatory corticosteroids may slow progressive pulmonary deterioration but are associated with numerous side effects when used on a long-term basis and require careful consideration before use.[111] They may be used in a small percentage of patients for specific indications such as fungal infection and ABPA.[19]

Influenza, rubella, and pertussis infections are particularly harmful to individuals with CF and can trigger a downward spiral of lung function. Early immunization is highly recommended, and a routine yearly influenza vaccine should be addressed in the regular clinic routine.[19]

The use of inhaled hypertonic saline has been suggested as an inexpensive treatment option to improve mucociliary clearance and pulmonary function in patients with CF. Hypertonic saline is associated with bronchospasm, so patients should be pretreated with bronchodilators. Recent studies suggest that hypertonic saline (7%) may increase the airway surface layer (ASL) to facilitate mucociliary clearance, thereby producing a short-term improvement in lung function in older children and adults.[202] Most studies have included patients with moderate to severe lung disease. In children with CF under the age of 6, there was no difference in the rate of pulmonary exacerbations between inhaled hypertonic and isotonic saline, although it has been shown to be tolerated in this age group.[63,170]

Another mucolytic agent, recombinant human DNase (dornase alfa), thins mucus by cleaving the DNA released by dead neutrophils that are responsible for the tenacity of the mucus in the airways. Daily inhalation of aerosolized DNase can reverse early air trapping and ventilation inhomogeneity, decrease markers of inflammation in sputum, reduce pulmonary exacerbation risk, and improve or slow down the decline of pulmonary function.[65]

Malnutrition is a key feature of CF because defective CFTR in the pancreatic epithelium results in obstruction of the pancreatic duct. CF patients become pancreatic insufficient when more than 95% of total pancreatic exocrine function is lost. These patients develop nutrient malabsorption and are at risk for vitamin and mineral deficiencies.[4] Nutrition and lung function are linked such that poor nutritional status and poor somatic growth affect the ability to repair lung disease. Similarly, pulmonary disease affects growth through appetite suppression and increased energy expenditure. Special attention to a properly balanced, high-calorie diet with supplementary pancreatic enzymes and vitamins requires acceptance and compliance in patients. During acute episodes of respiratory exacerbations, the anorexia that accompanies the frequent racking cough, the increase in mucus production, and the increased work of breathing pose a challenge to provision of adequate nutritional intake. Levels of resting energy expenditure have been shown to be in excess of 150% of normal in patients with CF with more progressive pulmonary disease or malnutrition.[111] Oral nutritional supplements are available, but if patients fail to improve their weight, a gastrostomy feeding tube may be inserted for additional nutritional supplementation.[4]

Cystic fibrosis–related diabetes (CFRD) can develop in CF patients, with the average age of onset between 18 and 21 years. Annual screening for CFRD with an oral glucose tolerance test starts at age 10. Hyperglycemia during times of stress, such as pulmonary exacerbations or while on steroids, can occur.[4] Female patients with CFRD have a poorer survival than male patients.[147] Intermittent CFRD can be treated with insulin, with the goal of normalizing glucose levels.

In patients with CF the airway lumen is compromised not only by secretions but also by airway edema, smooth muscle hypertrophy, and bronchoconstriction. Inhaled steroids, although never proven effective in CF in controlled clinical trials, may reduce airway edema. Bronchodilators such as β-adrenergic agonists or theophylline, intended to relax airway smooth muscle, are routinely administered, although not all patients respond to them in direct testing. Some patients may have paradoxical decreases in pulmonary function likely due to extensively damaged airways, which normally are held open by muscle tone.[55] When used immediately before exercise or pulmonary physical therapy, bronchodilators may help prevent induced bronchospasm in some people and therefore are often prescribed as an important adjunct to physical therapy.[111]

Many medications employed in the treatment of CF require nebulization. As a result, the performance characteristics of the nebulizer must be considered when a method of delivery for inhaled medications is selected. Studies comparing the efficiency of different aerosol delivery systems found a significant difference among systems in terms of particle size, total delivery of fluid, and time taken to deliver the medication.[38,107] Less drug wastage, reduced treatment time, and more specific matching of the delivery system to the breathing pattern of the individual are possible.[38]

Effective clearance of mucus-obstructed airways benefits the pulmonary system by allowing for improved ventilation and gas exchange and by limiting the tissue damage associated with recurrent infection. Today's airway clearance techniques are based on the physiologic strategy of opening up the airways and getting air behind the secretions, mobilizing and collecting secretions from the peripheral airways, transporting them toward the central airways, and finally evacuating the secretions.[102] Physical therapy techniques to promote airway clearance include postural drainage and percussion, positioning, expiratory vibrations, positive expiratory pressure (PEP) therapy, oscillating PEP therapy, high-frequency chest wall oscillations (HFCWO), directed breathing techniques such as the active cycle of breathing technique (ACBT), and autogenic drainage and are all combined with huffing and coughing. Exercise, thoracic mobility, and postural realignment exercises are often prescribed to maximize pulmonary fitness.

More research is needed to scientifically support the efficacy of the use of pulmonary physical therapy modalities in CF. Most studies assess only short-term effects on airway clearance by measuring qualities of sputum (i.e., volume, weight, and viscosity) or rates of clearance of radiolabeled aerosol from the lung. Although some modalities yield short-term improvements in these markers, few measure long-term and clinically important end points like health-related quality of life or rates of exacerbation, hospitalization, and mortality. Cochrane reviews demonstrate the need for more adequate controls, randomized design and sampling, larger sample sizes, and use of valid outcome measures.[119,131] The ethics of performing long-term randomized trials that withhold airway clearance from patients with CF is problematic because this treatment is considered to be the standard of care and has an established short-term benefit in increasing expectorated sputum volume and enhancing mucus clearance. In addition to airway clearance, exercise should be included in the management of CF. In a study at the Hospital for Sick Children in Toronto that evaluated the effects of a 3-year home exercise program, it was found that pulmonary function declined more slowly in the exercise group than in the control group, suggesting a benefit for patients with CF participating in regular aerobic exercise.[175]

Increased understanding of how CFTR dysfunction causes lung disease has resulted in new therapies that target the basic defect. CFTR replacement therapy involves the use of gene transfer therapy. This approach has been limited by the selection of an appropriate vector because of adverse side effects, transfection efficiency, and short-lived gene expression. Another treatment alternative is CFTR pharmacotherapy, which affects the trafficking, expression, or functioning of CFTR, depending on the class mutation. Most recently, a tremendous breakthrough in the disease-modifying therapy ivacaftor (Kalydeco), an oral pharmacologic potentiator that restores the function of defective CFTR at the cell surface caused by the class III mutation G551D, demonstrated improvements in lung function, weight, quality of life, and sweat chloride levels and a reduction in the frequency of pulmonary exacerbations in randomized placebo-controlled trials. This drug is approved in Canada and the United States in children older than 2 years old with the specific CFTR mutation. Moreover, ivacaftor is currently being investigated in phase 3 trials as a combination therapy with lumacaftor in patients older than 12 years of age with two F508 CFTR mutations. This novel approach involves a two-step strategy: lumacaftor brings the defective CFTR to the cell surface,

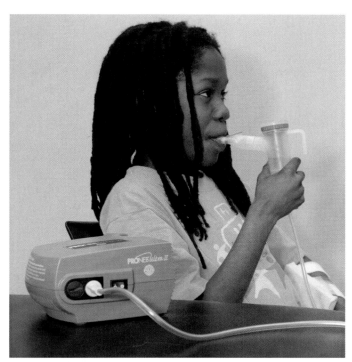

FIG. 26.1 A teenager is performing inhalation therapy via a reusable breath-enhanced nebulizer with a mouthpiece.

and ivacaftor supports the activity of the protein to restore salt and water balance for less viscous secretions.[53] Inhaled osmotic agents are being developed because they are thought to increase the airway fluid layer (Fig. 26.1). These exciting therapies are being developed to treat the early and root causes of CF, which will improve outcomes and potentially reduce the burden of care.[166] The unprecedented volume of current research and the emergence of new, successful therapies for CF dictate a need for conscientious practitioners to remain educated and receptive to adjusting their management plans and critical pathways for care of patients with CF.

LUNG TRANSPLANTATION

Organ transplantation is now a treatment option in many different terminal illnesses, including CF. Advances in surgical technique and postoperative care with improved immunosuppressive therapies have given some patients with CF a new lease on life. (See Chapter 28 for a more detailed discussion of the involvement of physical therapy in postsurgical care.)

In North America, both heart-lung and double-lung transplants have been performed on patients with CF with end-stage pulmonary disease. The Toronto Lung Transplant Group performed the world's first successful double-lung transplant in 1987.[155] Cystic fibrosis has gradually become a leading indication for lung transplantation and accounts for 54% of pediatric lung recipients in North America and 73% in Europe[14] while in adults, 17% of international lung recipients are due to CF.[216] Survival rates in pediatric lung transplantation are similar to those reported in adults, with a median survival of 4.9 years versus 5.4 years, respectively, in recipients undergoing transplantation between January 1990 and June 2011.[14]

Living-donor lobar lung transplantation has been performed since 1993, but because it involves recruitment of two donors

and the surgical procedure carries inherent risks to the donors, it is not without its problems. The impact of this technique on survival statistics appears comparable with that of other approaches, but long-term analysis is needed.[184] Complications most often arise from infections or graft rejection in the early post-transplant period. In children, development of bronchiolitis obliterans syndrome is an indicator of chronic rejection and a leading cause of death after lung transplantation.[14] The problem with malabsorption in patients with CF dictates difficulties with the therapeutic regimen for adequate immunosuppression after transplantation. Individual transplant centers should direct and monitor the immunosuppressive regimen because close monitoring of serum levels and adjustment of doses are vital to successful post-transplant management.[212]

Guidelines for listing a patient with CF for lung transplantation include FEV_1 30% of predicted or rapidly declining lung function (increased frequency and duration of hospitalizations for pulmonary exacerbations, increasing antibiotic resistance of infectious bacteria, and increasing oxygen requirements, hypercapnia, and pulmonary hypertension). Patients also should have a history of compliance with medical treatment, an acceptable psychosocial profile, and functional vital organs.[99,212] A referral for transplant (and acceptance onto the waiting list) must be made early enough to allow for a substantial wait for a suitable donor and creates a need for the development of a preoperative program of physical conditioning for these patients, which is a component of the lung transplantation program in many centers. These conditioning programs are designed to optimize the patient's functional ability and exercise tolerance and to help maintain emotional well-being during the long wait for a transplant.[45] Recently, a study found that pediatric lung transplant candidates that are ambulatory prior to transplant and able to walk greater than 229–305 m during a 6-MWT have better outcomes postoperatively.[215] The inclusion of a home-based or hospital-attended semiindividualized exercise program following lung transplantation in children demonstrated improved health-related fitness.[57] Physical therapists play a primary role in the development and implementation of both preoperative and postoperative exercise programs.

Double-lung transplantation is now most often performed by bilateral anterolateral thoracotomies using bilateral submammary incisions, as first described in 1990.[149] The lungs are transplanted as sequential single-lung grafts. The lung with the worst pulmonary function is replaced first, while oxygenation and ventilation are maintained by the native lung. Replacement of the second lung can then proceed with the newly implanted lung supporting the patient. Use of this technique has reduced to 30% to 35% the number of patients requiring anticoagulation and cardiopulmonary bypass during surgery. This surgical innovation has also reduced the degree of complications from perioperative bleeding, which can be a significant problem for patients with CF because of the presence of inflammatory adhesions within the pleural space.[209]

Single-lung transplants are not performed on patients with CF because the remaining native lung continues to be ventilated after transplantation, and its overexpansion will compress the transplanted lung.[110] Contamination of the native lung could also spread infection to the transplanted lung.

Impairments in Pulmonary Function and Digestive Absorption

Mucous plugging and bronchiolitis in the patient's airways cause ventilation-perfusion abnormalities, and the subsequent hypoxemia worsens as severity of the obstruction increases.[110] Further declines in arterial oxygenation can occur during sleep, so blood gases may have to be monitored throughout the night to assess the need for nocturnal supplementary oxygen.[132] Increased oxygen demands during exercise can be a contributing factor to hypoxemia in individuals with CF. Although arterial blood gas measures are considered the "gold standard" in blood gas analysis,[218] they are not commonly used in patients with CF because of their invasive nature. Other noninvasive techniques are preferred, such as pulse oximetry, which measures the level of oxygen saturation in the blood. This assessment tool can be used to evaluate the suitability of supplemental oxygen during exercise performance.

Other changes in blood gas readings forewarn of serious advanced pathology. Hypercapnia in CF indicates advanced pulmonary disease and carries a poor prognosis. In a study of survival patterns of patients with CF who demonstrated hypercapnia, it was found that death usually occurred within 1 year of the development of chronic hypercapnia[201] without interventions such as noninvasive ventilation or lung transplantation.

Chest radiographs can provide detailed evidence of the progressive nature of pulmonary disease in CF (Fig. 26.2). In the initial stages of pulmonary involvement, the chest radiograph may reveal signs of hyperinflation and peribronchial thickening. As the disease progresses, bronchiectasis can become apparent, particularly in the upper lobes, and pulmonary infiltrates appear as nodular shadows on radiographs. With severe pulmonary disease the hyperexpanded lungs can precipitate flattening of the diaphragm, thoracic kyphosis, and bowing of the sternum—all detectable on radiography.[110] Confirmation of the development of a pneumothorax can also be provided by examining the chest radiographs. When pulmonary disease is advanced, pulmonary artery hypertrophy may be noticed on radiography as a sign of the pulmonary hypertension associated with cor pulmonale.[110]

Cultures from sputum of a patient with CF identify the variety of bacteria that have infected the lower respiratory tract. Sensitivity studies can then be performed to identify effective antibiotic therapies.[143] CF centers perform regular sputum bacteriologic tests to ensure adequate antibiotic coverage for their patients and to help monitor the state of bacterial infection.[112]

The physical examination provides valuable information on pulmonary function. Examination of the chest includes inspection, palpation, percussion, and auscultation. Inspection can reveal postural abnormalities (Fig. 26.3), modifications of breathing pattern (Fig. 26.4), or signs of respiratory distress. Evidence of a chronic productive cough is desirable. Examination of the comparative dimensions of the chest in the anterior-posterior and transverse planes is important because barrel chest deformity is common to obstructive lung diseases.[86] Inspection of the fingers and toes may reveal bluish nail beds and clubbing of the digits, which reflect a change in the amount of soft tissue at the nail bed associated with lung disease. Palpation of the chest wall for excursion and for tactile fremitus may reveal atelectasis, pneumothorax, or large airway secretions. The resonance pattern of the chest is examined by percussion. Audible changes in the resonance pattern are an indication of abnormally dense areas of the lungs.[86] Age of the patient may limit the reliability and clinical usefulness of components of the physical examination. In infants, measurement of chest wall expansion may be difficult and percussion may not be appropriate.[44]

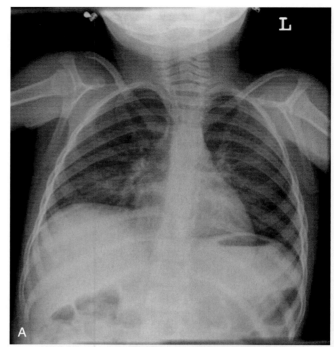

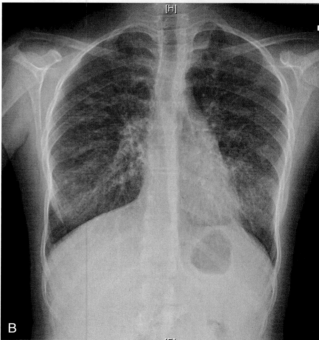

FIG. 26.2 Two chest radiographs of the same individual showing marked deterioration over the course of 10 years. (A) At age 4, there is already evidence of bilateral perihilar peribronchial thickening and patchy infiltrates in the right middle lobe, suggestive of mucous plugging. (B) Diffuse bilateral bronchiectasis associated with cystic fibrosis with hyperinflation and bilateral areas of consolidation.

Auscultation of the chest contributes information on the quality of airflow and evidence of obstruction in different areas of the lungs. Reduced ventilation is suggested by decreased breath sounds or the presence of inspiratory crackles (also called *rales*). If crackles are heard throughout the ventilation

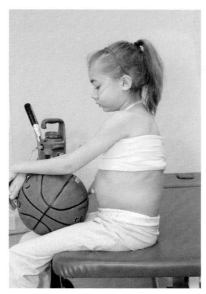

FIG. 26.3 An example of postural changes in an individual: elevation of the shoulders, protracted scapulae, and increased anterior-posterior diameter of the chest. Note the intercostal indrawing.

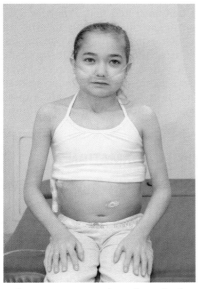

FIG. 26.4 Use of accessory muscles of respiration, tracheal tug, and supraclavicular indrawing is apparent on physical inspection. Note the gastrostomy tube and the port-a-catheter line.

cycle, this suggests impaired secretion clearance. Diffuse airway obstruction may cause polyphonic wheezing. The examiner must be aware that chronically hyperinflated lungs tend to mask or make it difficult to hear adventitious sounds on auscultation.[86] Familiarization with a patient's lung sounds is important because a change may signal a change in pulmonary function that might otherwise have gone undetected.

Individuals with CF must make a concerted effort to consume adequate calories to meet the increased work of breathing and altered digestive absorption. Individuals with CF who are pancreatic insufficient require oral supplementary enzymes

to absorb adequate nutrients from their diet. Pancreatic function is determined by a number of methods including fecal fat assessment, pancreatic substrate assays, and direct collection of pancreatic secretions by duodenal intubation.[111] Individuals with CF whose pancreatic function is sufficient are able to maintain fat absorption and have less pulmonary dysfunction than individuals who have pancreatic insufficiency.[42] Because pulmonary function is strongly associated with adequate nutrition and weight gain, the goal of treatment is prevention of the cascade of wasting precipitated by reduced lung function, increased energy expenditure, decreased intake due to poor appetite, and increased losses due to malabsorption.

Other factors that are associated with a preferred prognosis include single-organ involvement at diagnosis, absent or single-organism sputum colonization, and a normal chest radiograph 1 year after diagnosis. Multiple organ involvement, abnormal chest radiographs at diagnosis, colonization of multiple organisms in the sputum, a falloff from typical growth, and recurrent hemoptysis are all factors associated with a poor prognosis. There also appears to be a gender bias in severity of disease expression, with males having a better prognosis than females.[112]

Pulmonary Function Testing

Pulmonary function tests (PFTs) are used to evaluate lung function and are administered by pulmonary function technicians. PFTs are indicated to determine the presence or absence of lung disease, to quantify the effects of a known lung disease on lung function, and to determine the beneficial or negative effects of various types of therapy.

PFTs consist of a number of different tests, and the type of test ordered depends on the question to be answered. The most common question for patients with CF is, "What is the degree of obstruction?" This parameter is easily measured with spirometry, which measures forced vital capacity (FVC), FEV_1, and airflow rates (forced expired flow between 25% and 75% of the vital capacity) during different phases of expiration, yielding an indication of the amount of bronchial obstruction present. The measure of FEV_1 chronicles the early portion of expiration and is often reported as a ratio of FVC. In a healthy individual, FEV_1/FVC is 0.70 to 0.80 indicating that 70% to 80% of the FVC is expired in the first seconds of a forced exhalation.[78] A decrease in this ratio reflects an obstructed expiratory airflow.

Early detection of abnormalities in lung function in CF is critical because these initial changes involve the small airways. Miller suggests that forced expiratory flow (FEF) 25%–75% is more sensitive than FEV_1 or FEV_1/FVC in detecting changes in small airway obstruction.[127] Timed volumes at high lung volumes (e.g., FEV_1) may remain within typical limits because the contribution of the small airways to overall resistance is low.[91] FEV_1 therefore is not a sensitive test in early lung disease but indicates obstruction of the central bronchi and becomes markedly abnormal as disease progresses.[111] (A video demonstrating administration of pulmonary function testing is included on Expert Consult.)

Another form of PFTs is plethysmography, in which the patient breathes through a mouthpiece to measure changes in air pressure within a sealed chamber (body box) while the volume of air remains constant. The volumes that can be measured include functional residual capacity (FRC), total lung capacity (TLC), and residual volume (RV), which can also be assessed by gas dilution methods.[172] Both of these techniques can further evaluate severity of lung disease by determining the degree of gas trapping that occurs in an obstructive disease such as CF.

The US National Institutes of Health's comparative review of 307 cases of CF reported that PFT scores showed a common pattern: progressive decline in flow rates and vital capacity (VC) and an increase in the RV/TLC ratio, correlating with clinically gauged worsening of disease.[58] As pulmonary disease becomes progressively more severe, deteriorating PFT scores can be used to help predict life expectancy. In one study, patients with poor arterial gases and an FEV_1 of less than 30% of predicted value had 2-year mortality rates of greater than 50%.[94] Individuals with CF demonstrate a characteristic decline in mid-expiratory flow rate ($FEF_{25\%-75\%}$); noting the rate of this decline becomes an important prognostic indicator.[77] Steadily worsening PFT scores correlate with declining clinical conditions and are used as an indicator in assessment for lung transplantation.[95] FEV_1 has been shown to be the strongest predictor of mortality in CF and has been the primary outcome measure in many clinical trials[206]; however, it may not be sensitive enough to detect changes in lung function because most patients with CF have normal FEV_1 until adolescence.

Although PFTs are informative and invaluable for early detection in advance of lung disease, these tests are not always easily performed. Patients must be cooperative, must be able to follow specific instructions, and must give maximum effort. Children younger than age 6 years usually cannot perform the standard test of forced expiration in 1 second in a reliable manner. Recent reports document that children between 3 and 6 years can successfully undergo spirometry[139]; however, there is a large learning curve and extra time may have to be scheduled into their clinic appointment. Another study examining children age 2 to 5 years found that modifying the FEV_1 test to $FEV_{0.75}$ gave a reliable measure of pulmonary function for young children.[10] Various techniques are being developed to measure pulmonary function in infants, such as the raised-volume rapid thoracoabdominal compression (RVRTC) technique and fractional lung volumes. Revised techniques of rapid thoracic compression following increasing lung volumes near TLC and multiple breath washouts have also been investigated. Infant PFTs require sedation, special equipment, and trained personnel, which currently are available in only a few centers.[206]

In older children and adults, many other factors, such as sputum retention, poor nutrition, and fatigue, can influence the individual's performance during spirometry. Notably, many children with CF show performance scores on repeat tests that have a significantly greater range of variability than scores of typical test subjects.[41] The body plethysmography test can help to more accurately assess lung function by measuring the patient's lung volumes (FRC, TLC, and RV). Some claustrophobia may be experienced by patients undergoing testing in the "body box," and plethysmography may not be appropriate for all young children.

The lung-clearance index (LCI) is a more sensitive test than spirometry at the early stages of disease because it correlates with structural changes on computed tomography imaging and has been shown to be predictive of later lung function abnormalities.[186] The test consists of multiple-breath washout of a nonabsorbable gas (sulfur hexafluoride, nitrogen gas) to measure ventilation inhomogeneity caused by airways narrowing from inflammation or partial obstruction by mucus. The technique is easy to perform, requiring only tidal breathing; no additional coordination or forced maneuvers are needed,

TABLE 26.1   Selected Tests and Measures Used and/or Interpreted by Physical Therapists

Test/Measure	Performed by
Exercise testing: cycle ergometer, stationary bike, treadmill	Exercise physiologist
Pulmonary function test (PFT): Spirometry, LCI	PFT technician
Exercise field tests (6 MWT, 12 MWT, shuttle test, 3 MST)	Physical therapist
15-Count breathlessness score	Physical therapist
RPE (rate of perceived exertion) using modified Borg scale	
Radiologic tests	Technician
Pulse oximetry	Physical therapist
Heart rate	Physical therapist
Respiratory rate	Physical therapist
Sputum: quantity, color, viscosity, odor	Physical therapist
Manual muscle testing	Physical therapist
Postural screening and range of motion (ROM)	Physical therapist
Breathing patterns	Physical therapist

LCI, lung clearance index; *MST*, Minute Shuttle Test; *MWT*, Minute Walk Test.

making it possible to use the technique in infancy and during preschool ages to generate repeatable and reproducible results. A small study demonstrated that abnormal LCI values could be present in younger children with CF who have apparently normal FEV_1.[196] One disadvantage is that the inhaled gas does not reach regions of the lung that are completely obstructed and therefore may underestimate disease severity.[51] Recently, the measurement technique was standardized and was shown to provide good short- and medium-term repeatability as well as being responsive to interventions such as intravenous antibiotics, hypertonic saline, and DNase.[192]

FOREGROUND INFORMATION

PHYSICAL THERAPY EXAMINATION, EVALUATION, AND INTERVENTION

The role of the physical therapist in serving children and families is described during infancy, preschool and school age, adolescence, and transition to adulthood. Readers are encouraged to navigate the website of the Cystic Fibrosis Foundation (http://www.cff.org) to become familiar with the available resources. Selected tests and measures and interventions for children with CF are provided in Tables 26.1 and 26.2.

Infancy

Newborn screening for CF is currently carried out in many countries around the world, including the United States and in most provinces of Canada. The current method of screening suggests that many but not all newborns with CF can be identified. Studies have suggested that through newborn screening, nutritional deficits are detected and that early intervention may be useful to protect against loss of lung function.[19] A shorter prediagnostic period is associated with less negative feelings and increased confidence in the medical profession among parents of children with CF.[126]

A diagnosis of CF for their child can mean many things to parents. At the most basic level, it means they have a child with

TABLE 26.2 Summary of Physical Therapy Interventions for Children With Cystic Fibrosis

Intervention	Example
Airway clearance techniques	Modified postural drainage and percussions, positive expiratory pressure, oscillating positive expiratory pressure, active cycle of breathing technique, autogenic drainage
Postural exercises	Chin and shoulder retraction
Mobility exercises	Side trunk flexion, chest expansion
Stretches	Pectoral stretch over ball
Strengthening	Core muscles, large muscle groups
Aerobic training	Swimming, running
Inhalation therapies	Compressor, nebulizer education on administering medications
Energy conservation	Positioning for shortness of breath, pacing, timing of activities
Efficient breathing pattern training	Diaphragmatic pursed lip breathing
Urinary incontinence training	Core and pelvic floor muscle strengthening *The Knack* (contraction of the pelvic floor muscles before and during events that increase pressure on the pelvic floor)

"special needs," and those needs can be seen to influence the family dynamics.[106] The child's family members are forced to familiarize themselves with CF and with the psychological and practical demands inherent in this diagnosis. Addressing family information needs including what to expect for their child is critical. Intervention often must be implemented immediately upon diagnosis, and the family needs assistance in making the necessary adjustments and provisions to ensure adherence with the recommended therapeutic regimen.

Supporting Families

Sensitivity and equanimity while interacting with families of infants diagnosed with CF are important for effective communication because this is a very stressful time for all involved. Active listening, asking for feedback after information is shared, and clarification are strategies used by physical therapists to minimize miscommunication; what the family or professional may "hear" can differ from what is actually said.[26] Families seem to want information that acknowledges the seriousness of the disease while emphasizing the likelihood of a happy and fulfilling family life. Flexibility promotes better integration of the child's treatment into the family's routines. Parents may have many concerns and a host of questions and can be especially confused by all the uncertainty that typifies the disease. Because the progression of CF is so variable from case to case, ongoing examination of the child is the only way to ensure that treatments are individualized to meet child and family needs. This means that family members must have continued association with the CF center and appreciate their role as integral members of the caregiving team.

Children with a chronic condition have been shown to have increased risk of psychosocial dysfunction with low self-esteem, poor school attendance, and family factors all playing a significant role in their ability to adjust.[193] Because parental overprotection is strongly linked to the existence of psychosocial maladjustment in children,[85] the parents of a child with CF must be alerted to the dangers of unnecessarily shielding their child from aspects of normal life. In infancy, this may take the form of overdressing the child to guard against drafts or neglecting to

allow the child to participate in exploratory play. Physical therapists should reassure parents that infants with CF have the same interests and learn through social interactions, movement, and play similar to other infants. Parents are encouraged to position and play with their infant following developmental milestones to encourage chest mobility, leg strengthening, and endurance training.

In a large study across nine countries, 17% of patients with CF reported depression, which was two times that reported in community populations; 37% of mothers and 31% of fathers reported clinically elevated depression, which were three times the rate in the community samples. The authors conclude that assessing and treating mental health issues in patients and families coping with a serious, chronic illness should be performed.[161] The physical therapist can help to identify individuals with CF and their families who appear to be struggling and refer them to the psychologist or psychiatrist on the team so issues can be addressed early. Excellent reference materials are available in most CF centers. Teaching manuals designed to supplement the information imparted by the CF center staff are often distributed to families and can be made available to other interested caregivers such as child care workers or school teachers.

Management of Impairments in Pulmonary Function

In the neonate the most common symptoms of CF are meconium ileus, malabsorption of nutrients, and failure to thrive, all of which are associated with involvement of the gastrointestinal tract.[171] Overt pulmonary involvement is not apparent in the neonatal period because the lungs are morphologically normal at birth.[80,110] Within a few months, however, some infants with CF develop signs of impaired respiratory function, manifesting symptoms suggesting bronchiolitis. Pronounced wheeze, an indication of hyperactive airways, is sometimes apparent, and chest radiographs can reveal evidence of hyperinflation. Obstruction of airflow may be related to airway inflammation, mucosal edema, copious mucus secretion retention, and increased airway tone.[189] The bronchioles are the main site of airflow obstruction in infancy. Studies using bronchoalveolar lavage revealed that every infant with CF, whether symptomatic or not, has small airway obstruction in the form of bronchial mucous casts.[211] Pulmonary function cannot be measured in the conventional way (e.g., spirometry) in infants; therefore researchers have had to modify standard methods by using the raised-volume rapid thoracoabdominal compression technique (RVRTC). $FEV_{0.5}$ was measured and was found to be significantly lower in infants with CF shortly after diagnosis (median age of 28 weeks) and 6 months later on retest.[165]

Infants with CF demonstrate decreased lung compliance and a less homogeneous distribution of ventilation when compared with typical control subjects.[191] Tepper and colleagues found these changes in both symptomatic and asymptomatic infants.[190] Abnormalities in flow-volume curves[71] and low values of maximal expiratory flow[83] indicate that limitations to airflow in infancy are associated with bronchoconstriction.[80] Infants with CF have indeed displayed altered bronchial tone after the administration of a bronchodilator, as revealed by the fact that airflow rates showed significant increases not seen in a control group.[83] Methacholine challenge testing also revealed heightened airway responsiveness.[1]

The PFTs used for infants in research are not feasible or practical in most clinics or CF centers. Examination of pulmonary involvement in infancy is usually limited to observation of chest and breathing patterns, history of respiratory symptoms, and chest radiographs. Carefully observing for signs of respiratory distress, such as nasal flaring, expiratory grunting, retractions of the chest wall, tachypnea, pallor, or cyanosis, produces an indication of respiratory status. Interpretation of auscultation of an infant or young child is more challenging because of easily transmitted sounds from close structures underlying the thin chest wall,[44] but careful auscultation is necessary to ascertain if there is any evidence of wheezing. Changes visible on radiography are the most reliable indication of early pulmonary involvement because it has been demonstrated that airflow obstruction may precede the presence of overt respiratory symptoms. Historical accounts of respiratory illness must also be carefully considered.

The rate of deterioration of pulmonary function in individuals with CF may be slowed by early initiation of treatment. Bronchoalveolar lavage findings in infants with CF show the presence of infection and inflammation within the airways as early as 4 weeks postpartum even before clinical manifestations, which can damage the respiratory epithelium resulting in an impairment of mucociliary transport and secretion retention. The airways of infants with CF have also been shown to be morphologically abnormal with greater diameter and thicker walls.[108] The change in respiratory patterns and mechanics suggests that early therapeutic intervention might actually delay the onset of overt symptoms of respiratory impairment, but the value of initiating pulmonary treatment before development of symptoms remains controversial, although various theoretical arguments for initiating therapy as soon as possible can be presented. The time before onset of structural changes provides an opportunity for intervention and prevention of onset of progressive airway damage.[23] Adherence may be improved if airway clearance therapy is incorporated into the child's daily routine; prevention of respiratory impairment should be emphasized early in the treatment plan.[211] Parents of infants with CF can also develop sensitive observational skills needed to detect changes in their infant's status and to liaise with the team appropriately.[102]

A study was conducted to evaluate the combined effects of a bronchodilator and cardiopulmonary physical therapy on infants newly diagnosed with CF, addressing the controversy surrounding treatment for asymptomatic children.[80] Baseline, preintervention measurements of the mechanics and energetics of breathing were obtained for all subjects. Twenty minutes after the inhalation of a bronchodilator, cardiopulmonary physical therapy was given to the subjects, consisting of 20 minutes of chest percussions and vibrations applied in five different postural drainage positions. Immediately after the physical therapy session, repeat pulmonary function measurements were taken. Most of the infants (10 of 13) demonstrated decreases from baseline values in pulmonary resistance, with subsequent decreases in the work of breathing, after administration of the bronchodilator and physical therapy.[80] The investigators postulated that the bronchodilator relieved subclinical bronchospasm and aided the reduction of mucosal edema, and physical therapy assisted the mucociliary system by effectively mobilizing secretions and improving the patency of the airways.[80] When serial PFTs are possible, objective measures of the progression of impairment and the effects of specific treatments may provide evidence of the effects of early intervention.[80]

Prevention of obstructive mucous plugging is the initial goal of pulmonary physical therapy. Historically, in infants with CF

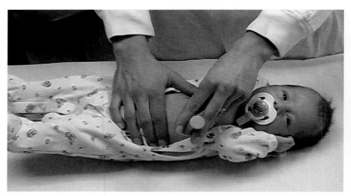

FIG. 26.5 Modified postural drainage and percussion on an infant performed by a parent using a palm cup.

the primary modalities used in airway clearance were postural drainage, percussion, and vibration, which all use gravity-assisted positions to drain secretions while using a cupped hand to percuss. More recently, assisted autogenic drainage, baby PEP mask, and mobility exercises have been recognized as alternatives to airway clearance in infants.[87]

In obstructive airway diseases such as CF, the effectiveness of the antireflux mechanism at the esophagogastric junction is reduced.[145] Increases in intraabdominal pressure associated with coughing also promote gastroesophageal reflux.[176] The effectiveness of the antireflux barrier is further reduced in infants because of the anatomy of their chest. Their chests are more cylindrically shaped with a more cartilaginous rib cage, making the ribs more horizontally aligned while flattening the diaphragm and increasing the sternocostal angle.[102] Of newly diagnosed infants with CF, 35% had symptomatic gastroesophageal reflux in one study,[197] and 24-hour esophageal monitoring revealed abnormalities in 10 successive infants newly diagnosed with CF in another.[48] There are suggestions that reflux can worsen lung disease in CF and cause upper respiratory symptoms.[214] A 5-year comparative study by Button and colleagues compared the standard 30° head-down tilt position versus the modified position (no tip) in 20 infants with CF who were asymptomatic.[29] The investigators found that infants positioned in the modified position had significantly fewer days with upper respiratory tract symptom, shorter courses of antibiotics during the first year of life, better chest x-ray scores at 2.5 years of age, and better pulmonary function at 5 years compared with children who received postural drainage with their heads-down tilt. Therefore it is recommended that the modified postural drainage position be used for postural drainage.

Timing physical therapy around feeding schedules may also be necessary to reduce the risk of gastroesophageal reflux. Postural drainage positions are easily achieved by placing the infant in the desired position on the caregiver's lap. Holding the small child in this way also seems to offer the child an extra measure of security. Adapting hand position (by "tenting" the middle finger) or using a rubber palm cup suits the application of percussion on a tiny chest wall (Fig. 26.5). The applied force of percussion should vary with the size and condition of the infant, and conscientious monitoring of the infant's response guides the amount of vigor used in percussion. Timing of manual vibrations to coincide with the expirations of an infant is difficult because of the infant's rapid respiratory rate, and this technique may be very challenging to teach to parents. (A video demonstrating modified postural drainage and percussion is included on Expert Consult.)

Use of a PEP mask has been compared with postural drainage in infants with CF. Constantini and colleagues studied 26 newborns with CF over 12 months using PEP and postural drainage as airway clearance techniques.[39] The use of PEP was associated with less severe gastroesophageal reflux when compared with postural drainage. No significant difference in the effectiveness of airway clearance was noted; however, patients and parents preferred PEP. Assisted autogenic drainage is an alternative airway clearance technique for infants or individuals who are unable to cooperate.[195] The goal of this technique is to prolong expiration toward residual volume and increase the expiratory flow, which can enhance mucus transport toward the larger airways. The placement of the therapist's hands on the individual chest wall provides pressure and gradually restricts the inspiratory level.[87] Ongoing communication, education, and instruction with the family are important. Periodically asking the parent or caregiver to demonstrate treatment positions and manual technique allows the therapist to reinforce proper technique and identify problems with proper application. Instructing parents to play breathing games with their infants and toddlers is a first step in learning to perform diaphragmatic breathing and huffing. Breathing exercises can promote use of collateral ventilation and can introduce concepts of techniques that will be used at older ages. In some CF centers, the physical therapist is also responsible for ordering, demonstrating, and arranging equipment necessary for the aerosol delivery of medications. Instruction on the care and use of these nebulizers is vitally important to ensure correct delivery of prescribed medications.

Adherence to a therapeutic regimen requires commitment on the part of the caregiver. The demands of caring for a child with CF can seem extreme when considering the extra attention to nutritional issues, medications, and physical therapy. Signs of excessive stress or evidence that the family is having difficulty in coping with the caregiving requirements may become obvious. Referral to a social worker or a psychologist might help identify the family in crisis and aid the family in developing strategies to enable adjustment to the various challenges that lie ahead of them as they nurture their child with CF.

Preschool and School Age

More than 75% of children with CF are now diagnosed before their second birthday.[151] When there is a positive family history of CF, parents are familiar with the disease, but in many cases, there is no prior knowledge of the disorder and the diagnosis can be startling. Initial shock may be followed by disbelief, anger, or grief.[106] The age of the child when diagnosed affects parental reaction to some extent. The older the child, the greater the likelihood that the parents may experience extreme shock at the time of diagnosis.[25] Sensitivity to the anguish experienced by the family must be shown.

The clinical status of children with CF is highly variable. Some toddlers may have already experienced pulmonary complications and been hospitalized repeatedly, whereas others exhibit little or no detrimental impact on their respiratory function. The effects of protein-calorie deficits due to malabsorption may be manifest in stunted development such as small stature or a lower than average weight-to-height ratio; therefore a difference in appearance from their healthy siblings or friends may be perceptible.

Self-Efficacy and Participation

Young children need to develop the ability to function socially outside the family circle. Demands of school and new friendships dictate a lessening of parental attachments and a capacity for some measure of independence.[106] This type of autonomy may be difficult to achieve for the child with CF. If parents perceive that their child is fragile with exceptionally vulnerable health, they may become overprotective. Cappelli and colleagues found a strong correlation between parental overprotection and psychological maladjustment in the child.[31] Encouraging children with CF to participate in a variety of social and physical activities could prove beneficial for their physical and emotional health. The physical therapist should stress the importance of incorporating an active lifestyle into the family dynamic.

Assisting children to gain a sense of self-efficacy is an important goal. A key factor of lifelong adherence to necessary treatment is incorporating a sense of self-efficacy (the confidence that one has the ability to perform a behavior). Adherence is promoted through interaction with a credible role model, encouragement to perform tasks of self-management, and development of competency. Individual care plans are developed with each child, and a self-care manual is provided to the families to act as a guide. Initiating teaching when the child is young and regularly reinforcing education with both parents and children may counteract the negative correlation between adherence and aging.[7] Better adherence to CF therapies is more likely in children whose parents strongly believe that the treatments are necessary.[72] In a study evaluating the association between adherence to pulmonary medications and health care use, low adherence was a significant predicator of subsequent health care use and costs.[160]

Examination and Evaluation

Examination and evaluation in the young child include history, physical examination, chest radiographs, blood gases, oximetry, and sputum bacteriology. The pulmonary function of younger children can be assessed by the lung clearance index (LCI) if the equipment is available and in children who are able to execute the necessary voluntary maneuver spirometry.

Examination by the physical therapist should include thorough history taking, a physical examination including posture when applicable, and some type of exercise tolerance testing. A minority of young children with CF may have chronic cough, hypoxemia, and decreased compliance of the lungs,[191] leading to restrictions in maximal oxygen consumption, an increase in the work of breathing, and an increase in resting energy expenditure.[181] These factors all compromise exercise tolerance.

Exercise testing is an objective method by which the physical therapist can quantify the patient's disease severity and functional ability.[163] Individuals with CF often will not be aware of the extent of their physical limitations owing to the slow progression of their disease.[33] An exercise test can detect mild pulmonary dysfunction, which may go undetected during investigations at rest, and will also help reveal how individuals cope with work despite their disability. (A video demonstrating exercising testing is included on Expert Consult.)

When an exercise test protocol is chosen, the purpose of the test and the age and disease severity of the subject should be carefully considered. Choosing the appropriate exercise test depends on the specific question being asked. For example, to assess activity limitations in aerobic performance, the exercise test should be progressive and should stress the subject's cardio-respiratory system to a symptom-limited maximum. The test should also be reproducible and capable of providing meaningful results.[81]

Cycle ergometers are often used for testing exercise capacity in children with pulmonary disease.[34,138] An accurate prediction of oxygen consumption can be obtained because the mechanical efficiency for pedaling a cycle is independent of body weight and therefore is almost identical for all individuals.[33] Although the treadmill test generally yields higher oxygen consumption values, the cycle ergometer offers the advantages of being relatively inexpensive, portable, and safe. Because cycling is a familiar exercise for many people, it is less likely to cause apprehension. As with the treadmill test, cycle ergometry is reproducible. In addition, the subject is relatively stationary, and therefore vital signs are more easily monitored. Most ergometers have adjustable seat heights suitable for children, and it is important to be able to adjust handlebars and pedal crank length.

Several progressive exercise protocols are used on the cycle ergometer to determine maximum oxygen consumption or individual peak work capacity (Fig. 26.6; see Chapter 6). Cerny and colleagues examined subjects with CF matched to a control group without CF to monitor cardiopulmonary response to incrementally increased workloads with cycle ergometry.[34] Workloads were increased every 2 minutes until the subject could not continue. The study demonstrated that subjects with typical development needed an increased workload of 0.32 W/kg on average for an increase in heart rate of 10 beats per minute. Subjects with CF required workload increases ranging from 0.15 to 0.35 W/kg, depending on the severity of their disease, to demonstrate the same change in heart rate. Cerny and colleagues concluded that the limiting factor in exercise tolerance was severity of pulmonary involvement and not cardiovascular limitation.[34]

If the child is too small to successfully use a cycle ergometer, a treadmill can be used because only the ability to walk is required. The child should be monitored closely to maintain a sense of confidence during the test. Elevation and speed are adjusted according to the size and skill of the subject and should be selected to allow even the subject with severe dysfunction

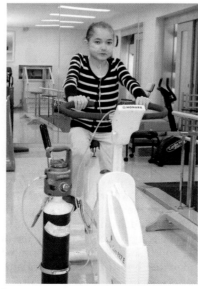

FIG. 26.6 Exercise testing with a young patient on oxygen.

to exercise at two to three levels of difficulty.[33] Two protocols frequently used for children with CF are the Godfrey protocol for cycle tests and the Bruce protocol for treadmill testing.[163]

For individuals with severe lung disease, field walking tests such as 6- or 12-minute walks[27] or the shuttle walking test[177] may be preferred. The reliability and validity of the 6-minute walk test[76] and the shuttle test[179] with children with CF have been demonstrated, and normative values for children who are healthy have been published.[163] Walking tests are simple, inexpensive, and can be performed by individuals of all ages and abilities with little risk of injury.[156] Because they are highly reproducible, walking tests correspond closely to the demands of everyday activity. Another quick and portable test that may prove useful in a clinical setting is the 3-minute step test, which showed similar results as the 6-minute walk test when outcome measures were oxygen saturation, maximum pulse rate, and the Modified Borg Dyspnea Scale.[11] Narang and colleagues, however, found that when the 3-minute step test was compared with the cycle ergometer, the 3-minute step test provided limited information related to exercise performance in a group with mild lung disease.[135] They suggest that a more suitable test for this group must be given at a higher intensity and must equate better to typical levels of physical activity.

Subjects performing an exercise test must be closely monitored and special attention must be given to signs of increased work of breathing that are disproportionate to what is expected.[33] Subjective measures of the perceived level of respiratory labor with a dyspnea scale such as Borg's Scale of Ratings of Perceived Exertion[16] can be taken before, during, and after the exercise test. Borg's scale is a good indicator of physiologic and psychological strain and allows individuals to interpret the intensity of their exercise according to subjective impressions.[148] For more information on quantifying increased work of breathing, a 15-count breathlessness scale is an objective measure that can be used with the Borg scale or a visual analog scale.[157]

Maximal work capacity is limited by ventilation in individuals with pulmonary disease.[33] Deficiencies in gas exchange and poor pulmonary mechanics compound the effects of decreased exercise capacity.[34] The limitation to exercise caused by pulmonary restrictions is further evidenced by failure to reach predicted peak heart rates in exercise test subjects with CF, suggesting that exercise capacity is not limited by cardiovascular factors.[30]

A complete physical examination should assist in revealing the individual's level of fitness, thus aiding the physical therapist in choosing the most appropriate exercise testing protocol. By assessing an individual's response to exercise, physical limitations, exercise-related symptoms, and aerobic capacity can be measured. The results of an exercise test can be used to design an individualized exercise program to improve one's exercise capacity and fitness level while encouraging individuals with CF to be physically active throughout their lives.

Management of Impairments in Respiratory Function

Individuals with CF demonstrate wide variance in the severity of illness because the disease progresses in individuals at different rates, but some amount of chronic airflow obstruction is often already present in childhood. The small peripheral airways are the site of most of these early pulmonary changes, and patchy atelectasis and ventilation-perfusion abnormalities lead to increases in functional dead space and discernible hypoxemia.[110]

The goals of physical therapy for the young child encompass improvement of exercise tolerance with continued attention to secretion clearance techniques. Correction and maintenance of proper postural alignment are also stressed. Goals of intervention are determined with the child and his or her family and take into account the developmental stage of the child and the family's priorities and concerns. The intervention plan must accommodate the child's learning style and avoid prescriptive tasks that are beyond the child's capabilities to promote self-efficacy and adherence. Collaboration with caregivers is essential when planning the home program. Children with a chronic illness should be encouraged to assume a degree of responsibility for their own treatment. Feeling some level of control over one's own health fosters self-esteem and helps subdue anxiety.[92]

Although the practice of postural drainage and percussion has long been used in the treatment of CF, it has been criticized as being too time consuming and difficult to perform independently. Adherence to a daily physical therapy regimen is reported as lower than with all other aspects of treatment.[150] Evidence of effectiveness might promote adherence, but research that has examined the effects of postural drainage and percussion is difficult to interpret because of the wide variety of outcome measures, including different PFTs, volume of secretions produced, and participants' subjective impressions.[185] It is also problematic to compare studies done on children at different stages of the disease and/or characteristics. Identifying the independent variable is sometimes troublesome because of the diverse combinations of techniques used; for example, percussion is rarely performed independently of postural drainage and coughing, making it difficult to determine the effect of each procedure. Recent reviews suggest the need for studies comparing treatment versus no treatment, but the ethical considerations of withholding treatment have prevented researchers from conducting this type of research.[82]

In a study by Lorin and Denning, the short-term effect of postural drainage and percussion physical therapy for patients with CF, compared with cough alone, was production of more sputum.[109] Other studies support the effectiveness of postural drainage and percussion in increasing amounts of sputum expectorated by subjects when excess secretion production is already a feature of the patient's condition.[13,114] The amount of sputum produced may be quantified by volume or weight, but caution must be used when interpreting the findings from this type of measurement. Because many individuals may swallow a portion of their sputum, the output can underestimate the true volume produced. The amount of saliva that contaminates the product is difficult to determine, and this has resulted in measurement of the dry weight of sputum in some studies. Measurement of dry weight is not practical in most clinical settings. In addition, the amount of sputum produced does not indicate where it originated.

Alternative methods for mobilizing secretions and stimulating cough have been suggested, usually involving directed breathing techniques. These include huffing, PEP, oscillating PEP (Flutter and Acapella), autogenic drainage, and active cycle of breathing (formerly known as forced expiratory technique, or FET). The rationale for use of huffing, a type of forced expiration with a similar mechanism to coughing, was suggested by a study that bronchoscopically demonstrated that maintenance of an open glottis throughout the maneuver stabilized the collapsible airway walls of subjects with chronic airflow obstruction.[84] The glottis normally closes in the compression phase of a cough, translating high compressive pressures on the tracheobronchial tree that may cause bronchiolar collapse.[185] Uncontrolled coughing is often nonproductive and exhausting.

The concept of the equal pressure point (EPP) in which the intraluminal pressure and the extraluminal pressure are equal, helps to explain how huffing is effective in clearing secretions. During a huff, the intraluminal pressure decreases from the peripheral airways toward the mouth thereby manipulating the position of the EPP to control the degree of compression of the airway. To perform huffing, the subject is asked to take either a low-, mid-, or large-volume (depending on the location of the secretions) inspiration and then, without allowing the glottis to close, to render a strong contraction of the abdominal muscles to aid in forceful expiration. Maintaining an open glottis can be compared with vocalizing "ha" or "ho."[185] Huffing is an uncomplicated breathing technique that can be easily taught to young children, and performing huffs can introduce the child to the concept of controlled or directed breathing techniques. (A video demonstrating huffing is included on Expert Consult.)

Forced expiratory technique (FET) employs forceful expirations combined with an open glottis as in huffing, interspersed with controlled breathing at mid to low lung volumes. A 3-year study conducted by Reisman et al. compared the treatment effects of FETs versus postural drainage and percussion physical therapy in subjects with mild to moderate pulmonary involvement and found that subjects who performed only FETs had significantly greater rates of decline in measures of FEV_1, midexpiratory flow rates ($FEF_{25\%-75\%}$), and lower Shwachmann CXR scores compared to subjects performing postural drainage and percussion.[168]

To clarify how to properly use FET, which always includes finer breathing control techniques and thoracic expansion exercises, Pryor and associates reclassified it as an active cycle of breathing techniques.[158] The three components are combined in a set cycle: relaxation and breathing control and three to four thoracic expansion exercises repeated twice, then relaxation and breathing control followed by one or two forced expirations. The number of breaths within a cycle can be modified to suit the individual's need. When secretions reach the larger, proximal airways, they may be cleared by a huff or a cough at high lung volume. Postural drainage positions may augment the effect, but the sitting position may be used if a gravity-assisted position is contraindicated.[205]

PEP (Fig. 26.7) as a means of secretion mobilization for individuals with CF has been proposed. Introduced for use in this

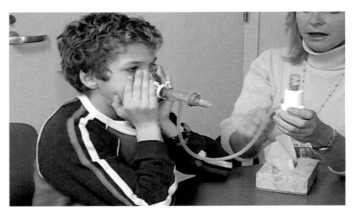

FIG. 26.7 An adolescent doing his routine PEP therapy technique with the physiotherapist.

population in the 1980s in Denmark, PEP has been shown to be as effective as traditional cardiopulmonary physical therapy both for chronic (baseline) stages of CF[69,118,140] and during an acute exacerbation of pulmonary complications.[119,141] This flow-regulated technique aims to temporarily increase functional residual capacity (FRC) to allow the tidal volume to be above the opening volume of obstructed alveoli.[28] The transmural pressure generated by maintaining positive pressure throughout the expiration phase is thought to allow airflow to reach some obstructed alveoli through use of collateral airway channels. Airways are "splinted open" through the maintenance of PEP, thereby facilitating movement of peripheral secretions toward central airways.[103] The PEP technique usually consists of diaphragmatic and pursed lipped breathing followed by 10–15 slightly larger than tidal volume breaths into the mouthpiece or mask after which huffing and coughing are performed. These steps are repeated 5–6 times, for a total of 15–20 minutes of airway clearance. (A video demonstrating a cycle of PEP therapy is included on Expert Consult.)

A 1-year randomized study that compared postural drainage and percussion with PEP in children and adolescents showed an improvement in lung function in the PEP group, while the postural drainage and percussion group deteriorated.[118] A 2-year study of[66] subjects found that PEP therapy is a valid alternative to postural drainage and percussions.[69] In another long-term study, pulmonary function scores improved in subjects using PEP versus postural drainage and percussions, which indicated that PEP was preferred by subjects, thereby increasing adherence.[118] The physiologic basis for the efficacy of low PEP and high PEP was shown to improve gas mixing in individuals with CF, and these improvements are associated with increased lung function, sputum expectoration, and arterial blood oxyhemoglobin saturation.[49] Contraindications for PEP include undrained pneumothorax and frank hemoptysis.[28]

Oscillating PEP is another effective alternative to other forms of airway clearance techniques.[131] Oscillating PEP (Flutter device, Acapella, RC Cornet) was developed to generate a controlled oscillating positive pressure and interruptions to airflow during expiration through a handheld device (Fig. 26.8). The Flutter was developed in Europe in the late 1980s, and the device consists of a steel ball in a plastic cone with perforated cover and a plastic mouthpiece. The effect of this device is angle dependent and the position of the ball determines the frequency of vibrations (range: 6–26 Hz). The range of PEP generated with the Flutter is 18–35 cm H_2O. The Acapella, developed in the United States in the 21st century, uses a counterweighted plug and magnet to create airflow oscillation.[28] Compared to the Flutter, the Acapella is not angle dependent and has an adjustable dial to modify the amount of PEP and oscillations provided depending on the individual. Oscillating PEP has been shown to be as effective as other commonly practiced airway clearance techniques.[131] A long-term comparative study in children found that using Flutter in isolation from other airway clearance techniques did not prove as effective as PEP in maintaining pulmonary function and that it was more costly because of the increased number of hospitalizations and antibiotic use.[123] The Flutter technique has been altered since this study. Newbold and colleagues reported no significant difference between PEP and Flutter in terms of pulmonary function and health-related quality of life in adult patients using the now-recommended technique.[136] One study comparing Acapella versus Flutter found that they had similar performance

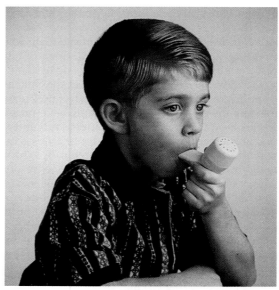

FIG. 26.8 A child performing his daily airway clearance using the Flutter device. (From Hockenberry MJ, Wilson D: *Wong's nursing care of infants and children*. 10th ed. St. Louis: Mosby, 2015.)

characteristics. Investigators suggested that Acapella may have some advantages over Flutter because it is not position dependent and can be used at very low expiratory flows.[199] Main and colleagues compared the RC Cornet, a type of oscillatory PEP, to the use of PEP alone and showed that neither PEP nor Cornet was associated with significant changes in lung function over a 6- or 12-month period.[113]

BubblePEP is another form of oscillating PEP that can be used in young children. It can be made at home using a container of water with a height of 5–10 cm of water and 5-mm diameter tubing to create 10- to 20-cm H_2O pressure. The bubbles created in the water by expiring through the tubing create oscillations into the airways. Food coloring or bubble solution can be added to make the activity fun for younger children. This apparatus is not a closed system and will cause only transient increases in FRC. Appropriate cleaning of devices or BubblePEP apparatuses should be performed routinely to prevent growth of microorganisms. Contraindications to oscillating PEP are frank hemoptysis and an undrained pneumothorax, and precautions should be taken in individuals with increased intracranial pressure, hemodynamic instability, recent facial or oral surgery, acute sinusitis, or middle ear pathology.[28]

High-frequency chest wall oscillation (HFCWO) consists of an inflatable fitted vest attached to a pump that generates high-frequency oscillations applied to the external chest wall. It is proposed that HFCWO enhances mucociliary transport in three ways: by altering the rheologic properties of mucus, by creating a coughlike expiratory flow bias that shears mucus from the airway walls and encourages its movement upward, and by enhancing ciliary beat frequency.[79] Short-term studies have found that HFCWO and postural drainage and percussion are comparable for airway clearance,[73,188,203] but caution must be used when comparing these studies because a number of manufacturers producing this device use different protocols.[153] Recently, a 12-month long-term multicenter randomized controlled study of HFCWO versus PEP mask in 107 children and adults older than 6 years old with CF across Canada was conducted. The study found that the number of pulmonary exacerbations (PE) requiring antibiotics and the time to the first pulmonary exacerbation were significantly higher in the HFCWO group than the PEP group.[120] The number of PEs and the time to PEs have been associated with greater lung function decline and higher morbidity and mortality and have been shown to be a more sensitive measure of improvement in studies.[204] McIlwaine et al. report that the results of their study do not support the use of HFCWO as the primary means of airway clearance in patients with CF.

Intrapulmonary percussive vibration (IPV) is a form of physiotherapy that is administered through the mouth to the airways to mobilize secretions centrally while increasing resting lung volumes. The goal of IPV is to integrate percussion and oscillatory vibration to mobilize retained secretions, high-density aerosol delivery to hydrate mucus, and PEP to recruit alveolar lung units.[28] IPV has been compared with other airway clearance techniques in individuals with CF though more long-term studies are warranted.

Physical Activity

Physical activity is an integral part of managing cystic fibrosis from a musculoskeletal point of view as well as cardiorespiratory perspective. Exercise is known to stimulate the respiratory system by changing breathing patterns, expiratory flows, and ventilation distribution while mobilizing secretions at the same time. A 30-month study of the effects of discontinuing other airway clearance modalities in favor of participation in aerobic exercise activities demonstrated no significant declines in clinical status, radiographic results, or PFT outcomes.[6] In an acute exacerbation, exercise proved as effective as postural drainage and percussion for the study subjects when pulmonary function was reviewed. The group assigned to "exercise" continued to receive one bronchial hygiene treatment session by a physical therapist daily, whereas the postural drainage and percussion physical therapy group received three of these sessions per day. Cerny concluded that hospitalized patients could substitute exercise for part of the standard in-hospital care.[32] It has also been shown that nasal epithelial sodium channels are inhibited during exercise in patients with CF, which may help to hydrate mucus and improve mucociliary clearance.[194]

Benefits of an exercise program extend beyond increases in peak oxygen consumption, increased maximal work capacity, improved mucus expectoration, and improved expiratory flow rates.[144,217] Exercise also improves general fitness, self-esteem, and measures of quality of life. Exercise is socially acceptable and helps to normalize the patient's life rather than adding a therapy that accentuates differences from peers. Fitness level also has implications as a prognostic indicator. An improved survival rate is found in individuals with CF who demonstrate higher levels of aerobic fitness. Although this may simply reflect less severe illness, the ability to maintain aerobic fitness appears to have value in improving longevity.[138] In a habitual physical activity study of 187 (99 females) patients age 7 to 25 years, subjects were divided into high- and low-activity groups and were followed over a 6-year period. Those in the low activity group had a significantly steeper rate of decline in FEV_1 compared with those in the high-activity group. The authors conclude that higher activity levels are clearly associated with a slower rate of decline of FEV_1.[208] Selvadurai and colleagues discovered that prepubescent activity levels were similar between genders in

patients with CF and between patients with CF and controls.[178] After puberty, girls with similar severity of CF were significantly less active than boys. In another habitual physical activity study, Nixon found that children with CF engage in less vigorous physical activities than their non-CF peers despite having good lung function. Therefore it was concluded that individuals with CF should be encouraged to engage in more vigorous activities to promote aerobic fitness that may ultimately have an impact on survival.[137]

Low activity levels are also related to low bone mineral density and vice versa. It is important to encourage children with CF to optimize nutrition and to participate in regular physical activity to maximize the potential to acquire bone mass in childhood.[207] Prevention and treatment of CF-related bone disease must address the myriad of risk factors. These factors include decreased absorption of fat-soluble vitamins and poor nutritional status due to pancreatic insufficiency, altered sex hormone production, chronic lung infection with increased levels of bone active cytokines, physical inactivity, and glucocorticoid therapy. Chronic pulmonary inflammation leads to increased serum cytokine levels, which are thought to increase bone resorption and decrease bone formation. Decreased quantity and quality of bone mineral density can lead to pathologic fractures and kyphosis in late childhood. Kyphosis contributes to diminished stature, pain and debilitation, rib and vertebral fractures, and chest wall deformities that reduce lung function, inhibit effective cough, hinder airways clearance, and ultimately accelerate the course of CF. The prevalence of bone disease appears to increase with the severity of lung disease and malnutrition. Cross-sectional studies have reported a higher incidence of fractures in individuals with CF.[8] Postural exercises aimed at preserving good mobility of the thorax, back, and shoulders are recommended to prevent thoracic kyphosis while maintaining the functionality of bodily structures and improving self-image and body awareness. It is helpful to teach individuals how to distinguish between acceptable shortness of breath and abnormal dyspnea and how to modify exercise intensity in response to symptoms.[104]

Young children with CF should be encouraged to use the treatments that best suit their requirements for adequate secretion clearance and prevention of deterioration of clinical status. Attitudes toward adherence with treatment can greatly influence the effectiveness of any therapeutic regimen, and the challenge for the physical therapist is to design an intervention strategy that is useful for both efficacy and practicality. Factors that should be considered in designing a therapy program include disease presentation and severity; patient's age; motivation and ability to concentrate; physician, caregiver, and child goals; research evidence; training considerations; work required; need for assistance or equipment; and costs. Children who learn to adopt their physical therapy as an aspect of daily living, as opposed to a burden or punishment, are more likely to adhere with the intervention plan.

Adolescence

Adolescence is a time of rapid transformation in many areas of development. Sexual maturation comes about as a result of major changes in circulating hormones occurring around the time of maturity of the skeletal system, typically when the child is about 11 or 12 years old. These hormonal secretions cause a "growth spurt" in the adolescent.[74] "Delay of maturity" occurs when there has been slowed or prolonged skeletal maturation.

This is often the cause of delayed puberty in adolescents with CF.[58] Arrested sexual development, combined with a smaller than average physical build, can intensify feelings of isolation from healthy peers. Osteopenia (low bone mass) is a possible complication of CF that may be linked to nutritional factors, delayed puberty, reduced exercise or weight-bearing activities, treatment with corticosteroids, and chronic infection.[40] The prevention of osteoporosis and the risk of fracture in patients with signs of osteopenia must be considered when developing a therapy program. The need for increasing independence can conflict with the demands of daily medical care, making adherence with the routine seem arduous. Adolescents with CF who look and feel different from the perceived "norm" may rebel against continuation of time-consuming treatments that reinforce their sense of being dissimilar or abnormal.[20]

Management of Impairments in Respiratory Function

Adherence with the routine of daily postural drainage and percussion sessions is poor in the adolescent population.[150] One challenge with this population is to promote self-efficacy with alternative methods of treatment. The use of PEP, active cycle of breathing technique, or a program of regular exercise may help to promote independence and has already been discussed. Autogenic drainage (AD) is another treatment modality involving self-controlled breathing techniques.

Autogenic drainage requires no equipment or special environment to execute and relies on the user's ability to control both inspiratory and expiratory airflow to generate maximum airflow within the different generations of bronchi.[36] Three separate phases of the technique are believed to "unstick" mucus in the peripheral airways, "collect" the mucus in the middle airways, and "evacuate" it from the central airways according to the volume level of controlled breaths.[117] Mobilization of airway secretions by autogenic drainage does not rely on the gravity assistance needed for postural drainage and can be performed in a sitting position.

Research on the effectiveness of AD is scarce.[130] A study comparing AD with postural drainage and percussion physical therapy and PEP in patients with CF[122] and a 2-year comparison trial of AD and postural drainage and percussion physical therapy found no significant differences between treatment groups when clinical status and PFT scores were used as outcome measures.[50] Learning the technique of AD poses difficulties for both the adolescent and the instructor. The technique requires concentration and the ability to use proprioceptive and sensory cues to localize secretions in the various levels of bronchi. A hands-on approach is essential, with a minimum of environmental distractions. Frequent training sessions and reviews are necessary. This type of concentrated self-directed activity usually is not achievable by children younger than age 12.

Maintenance of proper posture is important for individuals with CF to provide efficient breathing mechanics. Changes in the length-tension relationships of the respiratory musculature may occur with increases in FRC creating a mechanical disadvantage that contributes to increased work of breathing and muscle fatigue.[33] Several postural changes are found in adolescents with CF to varying degrees, associated with chronically hyperinflated lungs, including increased anterior-posterior diameter of the chest, shoulder elevation, and forward protraction and abdominal flexion. Thoracic kyphosis predisposes individuals to back pain with up to 94% of adults with CF reporting chronic back pain.[105]

The physical therapist examines posture and evaluates whether deviations are reversible or amenable to treatment. Exercises to promote improved posture include a strengthening program for the supporting muscles of the back and spine, stretching of shortened musculature, and increasing awareness of postural alignment. Weight-bearing exercises should be included to promote bone formation. An innovative way to keep adolescents active that can address the above issues is "ball therapy" (Fig. 26.9). Ball therapy can also be used to promote aerobic fitness, balance, coordination, and relaxation.[183] Projecting a good appearance is usually very important to adolescents, and informing the teenager with CF of the benefits of a good postural maintenance and weight-bearing program may provide the incentive necessary to ensure adherence to recommendations for exercises.

More recently, Schneidermann and colleagues found that despite natural progression of CF lung disease, increased habitual physical activity of 17 min/day is feasible and is associated with a slower rate of decline in FEV_1 at 1.63% per year, which is lower than the documented average decline in lung function. This study highlights the opportunity to have a positive impact on lung function decline, by promoting a physically active lifestyle throughout childhood, to encourage the maintenance of activity and enhance the carryover into adulthood.[174] A retrospective pilot study in the United Kingdom analyzed data for a 5-year period and compared 24 CF patients identified as partaking in an exercise group or no record of exercise. Despite no difference in FEV_1 between the two groups, the exercise group required significantly shorter days of IV antibiotics, suggesting that more intensive treatment was required to maintain lung function in the group that did not exercise regularly.[115]

A secondary effect of strength training with weights may be an improvement in self-confidence in the adolescent because training has been shown to be beneficial in promoting weight gain.[187] As pulmonary function declines, nutritional status is a consideration that requires a great deal of focus. Reduced anaerobic performance in individuals with CF is predominantly due to poor nutritional status.[97] The dietitian can identify situations in which intervention is necessary and may be a valuable ally in reinforcing the message that exercise can promote weight gain when appropriately managed. A liaison with the dietitian can ensure coordination of dietary and physical therapy recommendations.

Urinary incontinence is an underreported problem in individuals with CF due to embarrassment,[129,146] although it occurs in 5% to 16% of males and in 30% to 68% of females. Girls with CF as young as 9–11 years of age may experience urinary incontinence, which is exacerbated by the repeated physical strain of coughing, airway clearance, worsening lung disease, and various types of physical exercise.[2] Addressing this issue should become part of routine management and should be followed up regularly. Strategies that focus on the contraction of the pelvic floor muscles ("the Knack"), strengthening and endurance training of the lower abdominal core muscles, and optimal positioning during airway clearance all help to decrease stress on the pelvic floor muscles.

Transition to Adulthood

When CF was first described in 1938, fewer than half of the patients survived their first year,[54] but CF is no longer a purely pediatric disease. The currently reported median age of survival is 41.1 years, although many patients live well into their fifth

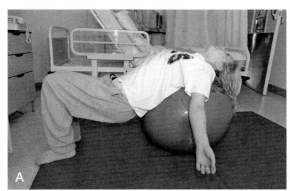
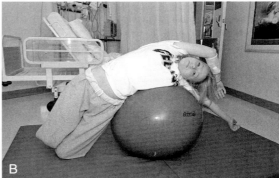
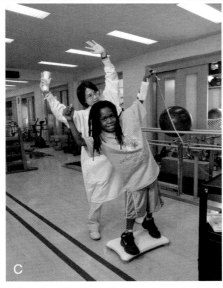

FIG. 26.9 (A–B) Therapy ball stretches to promote proper posture and thoracic mobility. (C) Using modern forms of technology, Nintendo Wii Fit System, for exercise.

decade of life.[198] Although many of the issues physical therapists are concerned with in the pediatric patient are similar for adults, some special differences should be considered. Standard programs of transition from a pediatric to an adult center should include all team members to ensure continuity of the patient's care.[64] Continuity of care enhances the effectiveness of care and minimizes uncertainty and distress for young individuals and their families. Transition from the pediatric to the adult CF team is an important milestone for patients and must be handled sensitively. Transfer is more easily achieved when the pediatric and adult clinics work closely together.[101]

The psychosocial issues in adulthood are distinct because the normal progression of psychological maturation brings new concerns with each developmental stage.[54] Greater clinical awareness, early treatment, and more effective management of CF have all contributed to improvement in prognosis.[154] Choices regarding education, employment (medical insurance), marriage, and family will have to be made. These choices are more complex than usual for the adult with CF, who not only has to consider present health status but also must attempt to predict and prepare for future health status.

Consideration should be given to medical insurance coverage, flexible work hours, and sick time when choosing employment.[213] Physically demanding occupations may not be appropriate for the adult with CF with pulmonary limitations;

therefore careful consideration of the physical demands of any task must be undertaken. Jobs involving constant exposure to dust, chemical fumes, or smoke should be avoided.[54,143] Adults with CF will face few restrictions on choice of employment; however, infection control issues should be well thought out when choosing a career in health care.[213] Treatment complexity and high treatment burden are highest among adults and pose a challenge to patient self-management and adherence.[173] Physical therapists should help to accommodate the adult's busy lifestyle and incorporate strategies for fitting treatment into work schedules. Methods that are more convenient and promote independence, such as the PEP mask, Flutter, or AD, may be more agreeable to the adult at work or school.

Because many adults with CF witness death among their peers, deterioration of their own health may have heightened significance for them. The adult who as an adolescent chose to be nonadherent with a physical therapy regimen may decide to initiate one again. Generally, individuals with CF have a strong positive outlook and are able to fully enjoy many of the typical pleasures of adulthood despite having to contend with unusual difficulties.[143] Patients' attitudes and outlook on life can have a tremendous influence on the medical progression of CF and are considered in prognostic scores.[54]

In general, cardiac status is related to severity of pulmonary involvement: the more severe the pulmonary adaptation to hypoxemia, the worse the pulmonary hypertension and right-sided heart strain. With comparable degrees of pulmonary disease, adults, especially those with mild lung disease, have more severe echocardiographic abnormalities than children. This may reflect the accumulative effects of episodes of mild hypoxemia and nocturnal oxygen desaturation that occur in even minimally affected individuals.[54]

Management of Impairments in Pulmonary Function

The progressive nature of CF may predispose many adults to have more symptoms and activity limitations than they had as children[143]; thus it is essential that the physical therapist works closely with the individual to adapt the intervention plan accordingly. Minor hemoptysis or blood streaking occurs in up to 60% of adults with CF[58]; in most cases, the cause is an increase in bronchial infection that has irritated a blood vessel.[142,144] Bleeding within the lungs can worsen infection by providing a more hospitable environment for bacteria; thus routine airway clearance can be continued if increased hemoptysis does not occur. Webber and Pryor believe that physical therapy should be continued with blood streaking.[205] Strategies that emphasize huffing and breathing control may be less likely to increase the amount of bleeding than the frequent uncontrolled coughing that may occur with completely stopping airway clearance.

Massive hemoptysis, which is also strongly related to advancing age,[54] is defined as rupture of a bronchial blood vessel into the airways, producing greater than 240 ml of blood in 24 hours or recurrent bleeding greater than 100 ml/d over several days. The average incidence of massive hemoptysis is 1 in 115 patients per year, and approximately 4.1% of all patients with CF will suffer this complication during their lifetime, with a median age of 23 years.[66] This complication warrants hospitalization and possible blood transfusion.[106] The CF Foundation Pulmonary Therapies Committee recommends that an individual's usual airway clearance technique can be continued in the presence of scant hemoptysis but that with massive hemoptysis airway clearance therapies should be ceased until the active bleeding stops.[67]

Spontaneous pneumothorax occurs 1 in 167 patients with CF per year, and approximately 3.4% of all patients will suffer from this complication during their lifetime with a median onset age of 21 years.[66] A common cause of pneumothorax is the spontaneous rupture of apical bullae, which develop as the result of increased air trapping and microabscess formation in the diseased lung.[110] Cardiopulmonary physical therapy is contraindicated in the presence of an untreated, progressing, or tension pneumothorax; however, treatment can continue with a small, stable pneumothorax and with a pneumothorax that has resolved through treatment with a thoracotomy and insertion of a chest tube for vacuum drainage of air.[56] Percussion must not be performed directly over the chest tube site owing to the danger of displacement, but percussion may be safely performed elsewhere on the thorax as tolerated. The PEP mask is a relative contraindication because theoretically it could make the pneumothorax worse as a result of repetitive increased pressure generated in the airways. In the event of a large or unstable pneumothorax, it is recommended that certain airway clearance therapies be stopped, including PEP, oscillating PEP, and IPV.[67] In summary, if a particular technique appears to make the situation worse, it should be discontinued and other modalities using breathing techniques may be beneficial at this time.

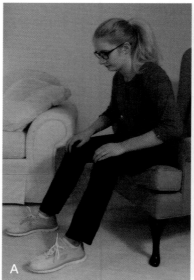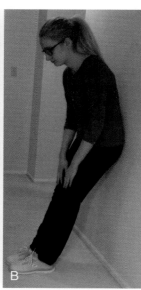

FIG. 26.10 (A–B) Positioning for energy conservation, promoting relaxation and ease of breathing.

Episodes of hypertrophic pulmonary osteoarthropathy also increase in prevalence with advancing age.[54] Digital clubbing can become more noticeable in people whose pulmonary disease is severe.[143] Standard anti-inflammatory agents are used to treat the joint pain associated with hypertrophic pulmonary osteoarthropathy.[152] Physical therapists have a role in helping to relieve pain while maintaining joint range of motion (ROM). A home treatment program consisting of stretching, muscle strengthening, and ROM exercises for the specific joints involved can be easily added to the individual's existing exercise program.

When pulmonary disease becomes so disabling that the individual is having difficulty performing activities of daily living, physical therapy goals should encompass these needs. The patient may have to be instructed on energy conservation techniques such as diaphragmatic pursed-lip breathing and assuming positions that relieve breathlessness. These positions should promote comfort and relaxation and should encourage mobility of the thorax and support of the spinal column. They should also include hip flexion to relax the abdominal musculature and aid in increasing intraabdominal pressure for coughing.[56] Examples of energy conservation positions are shown in Fig. 26.10. Retraining of the respiratory pattern using pursed-lip breathing in conjunction with diaphragmatic excursion has shown temporary benefits in increased tidal volume, decreased respiratory rate, reduction in $PaCO_2$ levels, and improved PaO_2 levels, as well as subjective benefits reported by patients. It may be that pursed-lip breathing improves confidence and decreases anxiety by providing some temporary control over oxygenation.[37]

Oxygen needs with exercise may have to be assessed at this time. Continuation of an active lifestyle should be promoted for all individuals with CF to optimize physical condition and maintain an optimistic outlook. If the individual is considering lung transplantation as an option, physical therapists must involve the individual in a formalized exercise program. The Toronto Lung Transplant Program at the Toronto General Hospital has a well-established rehabilitation program. Exercise capacity is determined by using a 6-minute walk test and ear oximetry, or the Modified Bruce Protocol on the treadmill.[45] The purpose of assessing a patient's exercise capacity is to determine if the severity of disability warrants consideration for transplant. A 6-minute walk test result of less than 400 meters was found to be a significant indicator for a patient to be listed for transplantation.[90] Individuals can also be monitored at regular intervals with these tests to gauge potential deterioration in their functional status. Once accepted into the lung transplantation program, most centers require attendance at a formal rehabilitation program[75] featuring aerobics, muscle strengthening, stretching, and light calisthenics.

Expected physical therapy outcomes for the adult with CF include optimizing functional ability, physical exercise tolerance, and emotional well-being. For individuals awaiting a lung transplant, improvement in overall function should enable them to handle the surgery and immediate postoperative period with less difficulty.[45] Arnold and associates found that 13 patients with end-stage CF showed improvement in their functional exercise capacity by participating in pulmonary rehabilitation while awaiting double-lung transplantation.[9] Pulmonary rehabilitation entailed treadmill walking and lower extremity ergometry three to five times per week, initiated at the time of listing for double-lung transplant. Six-minute walks were performed biweekly to assess changes in functional exercise capacity and workload on the treadmill and bicycle ergometer was recorded. Six-minute walk distances and treadmill and bicycle workloads all increased significantly. Conclusions from this data confirm the possibility of improving functional exercise capacity in patients with end-stage CF awaiting double-lung transplantation, despite severe limitations in pulmonary function.

Noninvasive ventilation, most commonly biphasic positive airway pressure (BiPAP), may benefit CF patients who are experiencing respiratory failure and awaiting lung transplantation. Although nocturnal oxygen therapy has not been shown to improve long-term prognosis, nighttime BiPAP reduces hypoxia, hypercarbia, and work of breathing and may enhance airway clearance and reduce pulmonary hypertension.[200]

Physical therapists have a role in serving individuals in the terminal stages of their disease. Intervention at this stage includes the provision of comfort measures and must be directed by the patient's wishes. Treatment sessions may have to decrease in duration and be offered with increased frequency throughout the day. Adaptations to postural drainage positions may have to be adopted so treatment can be tolerated. As the work of coughing becomes too tiring or painful, other modalities such as splinting and huffing can be reviewed. Pain control measures and relaxation and anxiety-reducing techniques, such as massage, may be the primary need of the dying patient. Simply listening to the concerns of these patients can be therapeutic. The value of a compassionate ear should not be underestimated. Physical therapists treating patients who are terminally ill should be careful to incorporate the families' needs, respecting the fact that this is an emotionally volatile time for all involved.

SUMMARY

Physical therapists have an important role in promoting self-management of respiratory function and physical activity of children and youth with CF beginning at a young age. Supporting families and children's self-efficacy are important to promote well-being and quality of life. The multisystem involvement and chronicity of CF requires physical therapists to keep abreast of medical management and continually interact with a team of professionals to communicate and coordinate care. Collaboration with a multidisciplinary health care team is stimulating and fosters creative and fulfilling practice of physical therapy. New advances suggest exciting possibilities for the future care of people with CF. Physical therapists serving children and youth with CF are encouraged to continually adapt their interventions based on current knowledge and research.

Case Scenario on Expert Consult

The case scenario related to this chapter follows a child with cystic fibrosis from diagnosis at 2 months of age to 16 years of age. Changes in his health condition and the role of the physical therapist at different ages are described.

REFERENCES

1. Ackerman V, Montgomery G, Eigen H, Tepper R: Assessment of airway responsiveness in infants with cystic fibrosis, *Am Rev Resp Dis* 144:344–346, 1991.
2. Agent P, Parrott H: Inhaled therapy in cystic fibrosis: agents, devices and regimens, *Breathe* 11(2):111–118, 2015.
3. Reference deleted in proofs.
4. Amin R, Ratjen F: Cystic fibrosis: a review of pulmonary and nutritional therapies, *Adv Pediatr* 55:99–121, 2008.
5. Andersen DH: Cystic fibrosis of the pancreas and its relation to celiac disease: a clinical and pathologic study, *Am J Dis Child* 56:344–395, 1938.
6. Andreasson B, Jonson B, Kornfalt R, et al.: Long-term effects of physical exercise on working capacity and pulmonary function in cystic fibrosis, *Acta Paediatr Scand* 76:70–75, 1987.
7. Arias Llorente RP, Bousono Garcia C, Diaz Mattin JJ: Treatment compliance in children and adults with cystic fibrosis, *J Cyst Fibros* 7(5):359–367, 2008.
8. Aris RM, Merkel PA, Bachrach LK, et al.: Consensus statement: guide to bone health and disease in cystic fibrosis, *J Clin Endocrinol Metabol* 90:1888–1896, 2005.
9. Arnold CD, Westerman JH, Downs AM, Egan TM: Benefits of an aerobic exercise program in C.F. patients waiting for double lung transplant, *Pediatr Pulmonol* (Suppl 6):287, 1991.
10. Aurora P, Stocks J, Oliver C, et al.: Quality control for spirometry in preschool children with and without lung disease, *Am J Resp Crit Care Med* 169:1152–1159, 2004.
11. Balfour-Lynn IM, Prasad SA, Laverty A, et al.: A step in the right direction: assessing exercise tolerance in cystic fibrosis, *Pediatr Pulmonol* 25:223–225, 1998.
12. Reference deleted in proofs.
13. Bateman JRM, Newton SP, Daunt KM, et al.: Regional lung clearance of excessive bronchial secretions during chest physiotherapy in patients with stable chronic bronchial obstruction, *Lancet* 1:294–297, 1979.
14. Benden C, Edwards LB, Kucheryavaya AY, et al.: The Registry of the International Society for Heart and Lung Transplantation: sixteenth Official Pediatric Lung and Heart-Lung Transplantation Report-Focus Theme: age, *J Heart Lung Transplant* 32(10):989–997, 2013.
15. Reference deleted in proofs.
16. Borg GAV: Psychophysical bases of perceived exertion, *Med Sci Sport Exerc* 14:377–381, 1982.
17. Bosworth DG, Nielson DW: Effectiveness of home versus hospital care in the routine treatment of cystic fibrosis, *Pediatr Pulmonol* 24:42–47, 1997.
18. Reference deleted in proofs.
19. Boucher RC, Knowles MR, Yankaskas JR: Cystic fibrosis. In Murray J, Nadel J, editors: *Textbook of respiratory medicine,* ed 3, vol. 2. Toronto, 2000, WB Saunders, pp 1291–1323.

20. Boyle IR, di Sant'Agnese PA, Sack S: Emotional adjustment of adolescents and young adults with cystic fibrosis, *J Pediatr* 88:318–326, 1976.

21. Brennan G, Brennan AL, Geddes DM: Bringing new treatments to the bedside in cystic fibrosis, *Pediatr Pulmonol* 37:87–98, 2004.

22. Brodlie M, Haq IJ, Roberts K, Elborn JS: Targeted therapies to improve CFTR function in cystic fibrosis, *Genome Med* 7:101, 2015.

23. Brody AS: Early morphological changes in the lungs of asymptomatic infants and young children with cystic fibrosis, *J Pediatr* 144:145–146, 2004.

24. Burns JL: Treatment of cepacia: in search of the magic bullet, *Pediatr Pulmonol* (Suppl 14):90–91, 1997.

25. Burton L: *The family life of sick children: a study of families coping with chronic childhood disease*, London, 1975, Routledge Kegan Paul.

26. Bush A: Giving the bad news-your child has cystic fibrosis, *Pediatr Pulmonol* (Suppl 14):206–208, 1997.

27. Butland RJA, Pang J, Gross ER, et al.: Two, six and 12-minute walking test in respiratory disease, *Br Med J* 284:1607–1608, 1982.

28. Button BM, Button B: Structure and function of the mucus clearance system of the lung, *Cold Spring Harb Perspect Med* 3(8):a009720, 2013. http://doi.org/10.1101/cshperspect.a009720.

29. Button BM, Heine R, Catto-Smith A, et al.: Chest physiotherapy in infants with cystic fibrosis: to tip or not? A five-year study, *Pediatr Pulmonol* 35:208–213, 2003.

30. Canny GJ, Levison H: Exercise response and rehabilitation in cystic fibrosis, *Sports Med* 4:143–152, 1987.

31. Cappelli M, McGrath PJ, MacDonald NE, et al.: Parental care and overprotection of children with cystic fibrosis, *Br J Med Psychol* 62:281–289, 1989.

32. Cerny FJ: Relative effects of bronchial drainage and exercise for in-hospital care of patients with cystic fibrosis, *Phys Ther* 69:633–639, 1989.

33. Cerny FJ, Darbee J: Exercise testing and exercise conditioning for children with lung dysfunction. In Irwin S, Tecklin JS, editors: *Cardiopulmonary physical*, St. Louis, 1990, Mosby, pp 461–475.

34. Cerny FJ, Pullano TP, Cropp GJA: Cardiorespiratory adaptations to exercise in cystic fibrosis, *Am Rev Resp Dis* 126:217–220, 1982.

35. Chernick V, Boat T, Wilmott R, Bush A: *Kendig's disorders of the respiratory tract in children*, ed 7, Philadelphia, 2006, Saunders, pp 848–900.

36. Chevaillier J: Autogenic drainage. In Lawson D, editor: *Cystic fibrosis: horizons*, New York, 1984, Wiley, p 235.

37. Ciesla N: Postural drainage, positioning and breathing exercises. In Mackenzie CF, editor: *Chest physiotherapy in the intensive care unit*, Baltimore, 1989, Williams Wilkins, pp 93–133.

38. Coates AL, MacNeish CF, Lands LC, et al.: Comparison of the availability of tobramycin for inhalation from vented vs. unvented nebulizers, *Chest* 113:951–956, 1998.

39. Constantini D, Brivio A, et al.: PEP-mask versus postural drainage in CF infants: a long-term comparative trial, *Pediatr Pulmonol* (Suppl 22):308, 2001. A400.

40. Conway SP: Impact of lung inflammation on bone metabolism in adolescents with cystic fibrosis, *Paediatr Respir Rev* 2:324–331, 2001.

41. Cooper PJ, Robertson CF, Hudson IL, Phelan PD: Variability of pulmonary function tests in cystic fibrosis, *Pediatr Pulmonol* 8:16–22, 1990.

42. Corey M, Gaskin K, Durie P, et al.: Improved prognosis in C.F. patients with normal fat absorption, *J Pediatr Gastroenterol Nutrit* 3(Suppl 1):99–105, 1984.

43. Corvol H, Blackman SM3, Boëlle PY, et al.: Genome-wide association meta-analysis identifies five modifier loci of lung disease severity in cystic fibrosis, *Nat Commun* 6:8382–8382, 2015. http://dx.doi.org/10.1038/ncomms9382.

44. Crane L: Physical therapy for the neonate with respiratory disease. In Irwin S, Tecklin JS, editors: *Cardiopulmonary physical therapy*, St. Louis, 1990, Mosby, pp 389–416.

45. Craven JL, Bright J, Dear CL: Psychiatric, psychosocial, and rehabilitative aspects of lung transplantation, *Clins Chest Med* 11:247–257, 1990.

46. Cystic Fibrosis Canada: *The Canadian Cystic Fibrosis Registry: annual Report*, Toronto, 2013, Cystic Fibrosis Canada. Available at: URL: http://www.cysticfibrosis.ca/wp-content/uploads/2015/02/Canadian-CF-Registry-2013-FINAL.pdf.

47. Reference deleted in proofs.

48. Dab I, Malfroot A: Gastroesophageal reflux: a primary defect in cystic fibrosis, *Scand J Gastroenterol* (Suppl 143):125–131, 1988.

49. Darbee JC, Ohtake PJ, Grant BJ, Cerny FJ: Physiologic evidence for the efficacy of positive expiratory pressure as an airway clearance technique in patients with cystic fibrosis, *Phys Ther* 84:524–537, 2004.

50. Davidson AGF, McIlwaine PM, Wong LTK, Pirie GE: Long-term comparative trial of conventional percussion and drainage physiotherapy versus autogenic drainage in cystic fibrosis, *Pediatr Pulmonol* (Suppl 8):298, 1992.

51. Davies JC, Alton E: Monitoring respiratory disease severity in cystic fibrosis, *Respir Care* 54:606–617, 2009.

52. Davies JC, Bilton D: Bugs, biofilms, and resistance in cystic fibrosis, *Respir Care* 54:628–638, 2009.

53. Davies JC, Ebdon A, Orchard C: Recent advances in the management of cystic fibrosis, *Arch Dis Child* 99:1033–1036, 2014.

54. Davis PB: Cystic fibrosis in adults. In Lloyd-Still JD, editor: *Textbook of cystic fibrosis*, Stoneham, MA, 1983, Wright, pp 351–370.

55. Davis PB: Cystic fibrosis since 1938, *Am J Resp Crit Care Med* 73:475–482, 2006.

56. DeCesare JA, Graybill CA: Physical therapy for the child with respiratory dysfunction. In Irwin S, Tecklin JS, editors: *Cardiopulmonary physical therapy*, St. Louis, 1990, Mosby, pp 417–460.

57. Deliva R, Hassall A, Manlhiot C, et al.: Effects of an acute, outpatient physiotherapy exercise program following pediatric heart or lung transplantation, *Pediatr Transplant* 16(8):879–886, 2012.

58. di Sant'Agnese PA, Davis PB: Cystic fibrosis in adults: 75 cases and a review of 232 cases in the literature, *Am J Med* 66:121–132, 1979.

59. Doershuk CF, Matthews LW, Tucker AS: A five-year clinical evaluation of a therapeutic program for patients with cystic fibrosis, *J Pediatr* 65:1112–1113, 1964.

60. Durie PR, Gaskin KJ, Corey M, et al.: Pancreatic function testing in cystic fibrosis, *J Pediatr Gastroenterol Nutrit* 3(Suppl 1):S89–S98, 1984.

61. Edenborough FP: Women with cystic fibrosis and their potential for reproduction, *Thorax* 56:649–655, 2001.

62. Elborn J: How can we prevent multi-system complications of cystic fibrosis? *Pediatr Pulmonol* 28:303–311, 2007.

63. Emer PR, Molloy K, Pohl K, McElvaney NG: Hypertonic saline in treatment of pulmonary disease in cystic fibrosis, *ScientificWorldJournal*, 2012. http://dx.doi.org/10.1100/2012/465230.

64. Farrell PM, Rosenstein BJ, White TB, et al.: Guidelines for diagnosis of cystic fibrosis in newborns through older adults: cystic fibrosis foundation consensus report, *J Pediatr* 153:s4–s14, 2008.

65. Flume P, Van Devanter DR: State of progress in treating cystic fibrosis respiratory disease, *Medicine* 18:88, 2012.

66. Flume P: Pulmonary complications of cystic fibrosis, *Respir Care* 54(5):618–627, 2009.

67. Flume P, Mogayzel PJ, Robinson KA, et al.: Cystic fibrosis pulmonary guidelines, *Am J Respir Crit Care Med* 180(9):802–808, 2009.

68. Reference deleted in proofs.

69. Gaskin L, Shin J, Reisman JJ, et al.: Long term trial of conventional postural drainage and percussion vs. positive expiratory pressure, *Pediatr Pulmonol* (Suppl 15):345a, 1998.

70. Gibson LE, Cooke RE: A test for concentration of electrolytes in sweat in cystic fibrosis of the pancreas utilizing pilocarpine by iontophoresis, *Pediatrics* 23:545–549, 1959.

71. Godfrey S, Bar-Yishay E, Arad I, et al.: Flow-volume curves in infants with lung disease, *Pediatrics* 72:517–522, 1983.

72. Goodfellow NA, Hawwa AF, Reid AJ, et al.: Adherence to treatment in children and adolescents with CF: a cross-sectional, multi-method study investigating the influence of beliefs about treatment and parental depressive symptoms, *BMC Pulm Med* 15:43, 2015. http://dx.doi.org/10.1186/s12890-015-0038-7.

73. Grece CA: Effectiveness of high frequency chest compression: a 3-year retrospective study, *Pediatr Pulmonol* (Suppl 20):302, 2000.

74. Green OC: Endocrinological complications associated with cystic fibrosis. In Lloyd-Still JD, editor: *Textbook of cystic fibrosis*, Stoneham, MA, 1983, Wright, pp 329–349.

75. Grossman RF: Lung transplantation, *Med Clin North Am* 24:4572–4579, 1988.

76. Gulmans VAM, van Veldhoven NHMJ, de Meer K, Helders PJM: The six-minute walking test in children with cystic fibrosis: reliability and validity, *Pediatr Pulmonol* 22:85–89, 1996.

77. Gurit D, Corey M, Francis PJ, et al.: Perspectives in cystic fibrosis, *Pediatr Clin North Am* 26:603–615, 1979.

78. Hancox B, Whyte K: *Pocket guide to lung function tests*, ed 2, New York, 2006, McGraw-Hill.

79. Hansen LG, Warwick WJ, Hansen KL: Mucus transport mechanisms in relation to the effect of high frequency chest compression (HFCC) on mucus clearance, *Pediatr Pulmonol* 17:113–118, 1994.

80. Hardy KA, Wolfson MR, Schidlow DV, Shaffer TH: Mechanics and energetics of breathing in newly diagnosed infants with cystic fibrosis: effect of combined bronchodilator and chest physical therapy, *Pediatr Pulmonol* 6:103–108, 1989.

81. Hebestreit H, Arets H, Aurora P, et al.: Statement on exercise testing in cystic fibrosis, *Respiration* 90(4), 2015 http://dx.doi.org/10.1159/000439057.

82. Hess DR: The evidence for secretion clearance techniques, *Respir Care* 46:1276–1293, 2001.

83. Hiatt P, Eigen H, Yu P, Tepper RS: Bronchodilator response in infants and young children with cystic fibrosis, *Am Rev Resp Dis* 137:119–122, 1988.

84. Hietpas B, Roth R, Jensen W: Huff coughing and airway patency, *Respir Care* 24:710–713, 1979.

85. Holmbeck GN, Johnson SZ, Wills KE, et al.: Observed and perceived parental overprotection in relation to psychosocial adjustment in pre-adolescents with a physical disability: the mediational role of behavioral autonomy, *J Consult Clin Psychol* 70(1):96–110, 2002.

86. Humberstone N: Respiratory assessment and treatment. In Irwin S, Tecklin JS, editors: *Cardiopulmonary physical therapy*, St. Louis, 1990, Mosby, pp 283–322.

87. International Physiotherapy Group for Cystic Fibrosis: Canada, International Physiotherapy Group. 2009. Available at: URL: http://www.cfww.org/docs/ipg-cf/bluebook/bluebooklet2009websiteversion.pdf.

88. Reference deleted in proofs.

89. Johnson C, Butler SM, Konstan MW, et al.: Factors influencing outcomes in cystic fibrosis, *Chest* 123:20–27, 2003.

90. Kadikar A, Maurer J, Kesten S: The six-minute walk test: a guide to assessment for lung transplantation, *J Heart Lung Transplant* 16:313–319, 1997.

91. Kattan M: Pediatric pulmonary function testing. In Miller A, editor: *Pulmonary function tests: a guide for the student and house officer*, Philadelphia, 1987, WB Saunders, pp 199–212.

92. Kellerman J, Zeltzer L, Ellenberg L: Psychological effects of illness in adolescence: anxiety, self-esteem and perception of control, *J Pediatr* 97:126–131, 1980.

93. Kerem BS, Rommens JR, Buchanan JA, et al.: Identification of the cystic fibrosis gene: gene analysis, *Science* 245:1073–1080, 1989.

94. Kerem E, Reisman J, Corey M, et al.: Prediction of mortality in patients with cystic fibrosis, *N Eng J Med* 326:1187–1191, 1992.

95. Khaghani A, Madden B, Hodson M, Yacoub M: Heart-lung transplantation for cystic fibrosis, *Pediatr Pulmonol* (Suppl 6):128–129, 1991.

96. Khan TZ, Wagener JS, Bost T, et al.: Early pulmonary inflammation in infants with cystic fibrosis, *Am J Resp Crit Care Med* 151:1075–1082, 1995.

97. Klijn PH, Terherggen-Largo SW, van der Ent CK, et al.: Anaerobic exercise in pediatric cystic fibrosis, *Pediatr Pulmonol* 36:223–229, 2003.

98. Reference deleted in proofs.

99. Kreider M, Kotloff RM: Selection of candidates for lung transplantation, *Proc of the Am Thoracic Soc* 6:20–27, 2009.

100. Reference deleted in proofs.

101. Landau LI: Cystic fibrosis: transition from paediatric to adult physician's care, *Thorax* 50:1031–1032, 1995.

102. Lannefors L, Button BM, McIlwaine M: Physiotherapy in infants and young children with cystic fibrosis: current practice and future developments, *J R Soc Med* 97(Suppl 44):8–25, 2004.

103. Lannefors L: Different ways of using positive expiratory pressure to loosen and mobilize secretions, *Pediatr Pulmonol* (Suppl 8):136–137, 1992.

104. Lannefors L, Dennersten U, Gursli S. Stanghelle J: In Johan Sundberg C, editor: *Chapter 22: Cystic Fibrosis in Physical Activity in the Prevention and Treatment of Disease*, Sweden, 2010, Swedish National Institute of Public Health, Professional Associations for Physical Activity. http://www.fyss.se/wp-content/uploads/2011/02/fyss_2010_english.pdf.

105. Lee A, Holdsworth M, Holland A, Button B: The immediate effect of musculoskeletal physiotherapy techniques and massage on pain and ease of breathing in adults with cystic fibrosis, *J Cyst Fibros* 8:79–81, 2009.

106. Lloyd-Still DM, Lloyd-Still JD: The patient, the family and the community. In Lloyd-Still JD, editor: *Textbook of cystic fibrosis*, Stoneham, MA, 1983, Wright, pp 443–446.

107. Loffert DT, Ikle D, Nelson HS: A comparison of commercial jet nebulizers, *Chest* 106:1788–1792, 1994.

108. Long FR, Williams RS, Castile RG: Structural airway abnormalities in infants and young children with cystic fibrosis, *J Pediatr* 144:154–161, 2004.

109. Lorin MI, Denning CR: Evaluation of postural drainage by measurement of sputum volume and consistency, *Am J Phys Med Rehabil* 50:215–219, 1971.

110. MacLusky IB, Levison H: Cystic fibrosis. In Chernick VI, editor: *Kendig's disorders of the respiratory tract in children*, vol. 5. Philadelphia, 1990, WB Saunders, pp 692–730.

111. MacLusky IB, Levison H: Cystic fibrosis. In Chernick VI, editor: *Kendig's disorders of the respiratory tract in children*, vol. 6. Philadelphia, 1998, WB Saunders, pp 838–882.

112. MacLusky IB, Canny GJ, Levison H: Cystic fibrosis: an update, *Paediatr Rev Commun* 1:343–384, 1987.

113. Main E, Tannenbaum E, Stanojevic S, Scrase E, Prasad A: The effects of positive expiratory pressure (PEP) or oscillatory positive pressure (RC Cornet) on FEV1 and lung clearance index over a twelve month period in children with CF, *Pediatr Pulmonol* (Suppl 29):351, 2006.

114. Mazzacco MC, Owens GR, Kirilloff LH, Rogers RM: Chest percussion and postural drainage in patients with chronic bronchiectasis, *Chest* 88:360–363, 1985.

115. McAuley K, Green S, Major E, Daniels T: Does exercise participation affect FEV1 and the number of IV antibiotic days over 5 years in adults with CF? *J Cystic Fibro* 14(Suppl 1):S27, 2015.

116. Reference deleted in proofs.

117. McCool FD, Rosen MJ: Nonpharmacologic airway clearance therapies: ACCP evidence-based clinical practice guidelines, *Chest* 129(Suppl 1):250S–259S, 2006.

118. McIlwaine, et al.: Long-term comparative trial of conventional postural drainage and percussion versus positive expiratory pressure physiotherapy in the treatment of cystic fibrosis, *J Paediatr* 131(4):570–574, 1997.

119. McIlwaine M, Button B, Dwan K: Positive expiratory pressure physiotherapy for airway clearance in people with cystic fibrosis, *Cochrane Database Syst Rev* 17;6:CD003147, 2015.

120. McIlwaine MP, Alarie N, Davidson GF, et al.: Long-term multicentre randomised controlled study of high frequency chest wall oscillation versus positive expiratory pressure mask in cystic fibrosis, *Thorax* 68(8):746–751, 2013. http://dx.doi.org/10.1136/thoraxjnl-2012-202915.

121. Reference deleted in proofs.

122. McIlwaine PM, Davidson AGF, Wong LTK: Comparison of positive expiratory pressure and autogenic drainage with conventional percussion and drainage therapy in the treatment of cystic fibrosis, *Pediatr Pulmonol* 4(Suppl 2):132a, 1988.

123. McIlwaine PM, Wong LT, Peacock D, Davidson AG: Long-term comparative trial of positive expiratory pressure versus oscillating positive expiratory pressure (flutter) physiotherapy in the treatment of cystic fibrosis, *J Pediatr* 138:845–850, 2001.

124. McKone EF, Velentgas P, Swenson A, Goss CH: Association of sweat chloride concentration at time of diagnosis and CFTR genotype with mortality and cystic fibrosis phenotype. *J Cystic Fibro* 14(5):580–58, 2015.

125. Mei-Zahav M, Durie P, Zielenski J, et al.: The prevalence and clinical characteristics of cystic fibrosis in South Asian Canadian immigrants, *Arch Dis Child* 90:675–679, 2005.

126. Merelle ME, Huisman J, Alderden-van der Vecht A, et al.: Early versus late diagnosis: psychological impact on parents of children with cystic fibrosis, *Pediatrics* 111(2):346–350, 2003.

127. Miller A: Spirometry and maximum expiratory flow-volume curves. In Miller A, editor: *Pulmonary function tests: a guide for the student and house officer*, Philadelphia, 1987, WB Saunders, pp 15–32.

128. Moran A, Dunitz J, Nathan B, et al.: Cystic fibrosis related diabetes: current trends in prevalence, incidence and mortality, *Diabetes Care* 32:1626–1631, 2009.

129. Moran F, Bradley JM, Boyle L, Elborn JS: Incontinence in adult females with cystic fibrosis: a Northern Ireland survey, *Int J Clin Pract* 57:182–183, 2003.

130. Morgan K, Osterling K, Gilbert R, Dechman G: Effects of autogenic drainage on sputum recovery and pulmonary function in people with cystic fibrosis: a systematic review, *Physiother Can* 67(4):319–326, 2015.

131. Morrison L, Agnew J: Oscillating devices for airway clearance in people with cystic fibrosis, *Cochrane Database Syst Rev* CD006842, 2014. http://dx.doi.org/10.1002/14651858.CD006842.pub3.

132. Muller N, Frances P, Gurwitz D, et al.: Mechanisms of hemoglobin desaturation during rapid-eye movement sleep in normal subjects and in patients with cystic fibrosis, *Am Rev Resp Dis* 119:338, 1980.

133. Munck A, Gerardin M, Alberti C, et al.: Clinical outcome of cystic fibrosis present with or without meconium ileus: a matched cohort study, *J Pediatr Surg* 41:1556–1560, 2006.

134. Murray TS, Egan M, Kazmierczak BI: *Pseudomonas aeruginosa* chronic colonization in cystic fibrosis patients, *Curr Opin Pediatr* 19(1):83–88, 2007.

135. Narang I, Pike S, Rosenthal M, et al.: Three-minute step test to assess exercise capacity in children with cystic fibrosis with mild lung disease, *Pediatr Pulmonol* 35:108–113, 2003.

136. Newbold E, Tullis E, Corey M, et al.: The Flutter device versus the PEP mask in the treatment of adults with cystic fibrosis, *Physiother Can* 57:199–207, 2005.

137. Nixon PA, Orenstein DM, Kelsey SF: Habitual physical activity in children and adolescents with cystic fibrosis, *Med Sci Sport Exerc* 33:30–35, 2001.

138. Nixon PA, Orenstein DM, Kelsey SF, Doershuk CF: The prognostic value of exercise testing in patients with cystic fibrosis, *N Eng J Med* 327:1785–1788, 1992.

139. Nystad W, Samuelsen SO, Nafstad P, et al.: Feasibility of measuring lung function in preschool children, *Thorax* 57:1021–1027, 2002.

140. Oberwaldner B, Evans JC, Zach MS: Forced expirations against a variable resistance: a new chest physiotherapy method in cystic fibrosis, *Pediatr Pulmonol* 2:358–367, 1986.

141. Oberwaldner B, Theissl B, Rucker A, Zach MS: Chest physiotherapy in hospitalized patients with cystic fibrosis: a study of lung function effects and sputum production, *Eur Respir J* 4:152–158, 1991.

142. Orenstein DM: *Cystic fibrosis: a guide for patient and family*, ed 2, Philadelphia, 1997, Lippincott-Raven.

143. Orenstein DM: *Cystic fibrosis: a guide for patient and family*, ed 3, New York, 2003, Lippincott-Raven.

144. Orenstein DM, Franklin BA, Doershuk CF, et al.: Exercise conditioning and cardiopulmonary fitness in cystic fibrosis, *Chest* 80:292–298, 1981.

145. Orenstein SR, Orenstein DM: Gastroesophageal reflux and respiratory disease in children, *J Pediatr* 112:847–858, 1988.

146. Orr A, McVean RJ, Webb AK, Dodd ME: Questionnaire survey of urinary incontinence in women with cystic fibrosis, *Br Med J* 322:1521, 2001.

147. O'Sullivan B, Friedman S: Cystic fibrosis, *Lancet* 373:1891–1904, 2009.

148. Paley CA: A way forward for determining optimal aerobic exercise intensity? *Physiotherapy* 83:620–624, 1997.

149. Pasque MK, Cooper JD, Kaiser LR, et al.: Improved technique for bilateral lung transplantation: rationale and initial clinical experience, *Ann Thorac Surg* 49:785–791, 1990.

150. Passero MA, Remor B, Solomon J: Patient-reported compliance with cystic fibrosis therapy, *Clin Pediatrics* 20:264–268, 1981.

151. Pettit RS, Fellner C: CFTR modulators for the treatment of cystic fibrosis, *P T* 39(7):500–511, 2014.

152. Phillips BM, David TJ: Pathogenesis and management of arthropathy in cystic fibrosis, *J R Soc Med* 79(Suppl 12):44–49, 1986.

153. Phillips GE, Pike SE, Jaffe A, Bush A: Comparison of active cycle of breathing and high-frequency oscillation jacket in children with cystic fibrosis, *Pediatr Pulmonol* 37:71–75, 2004.

154. Pinkerton P, Trauer T, Duncan F, et al.: Cystic fibrosis in adult life: a study of coping patterns, *Lancet* 2:761–763, 1985.

155. Pizer HF: *Organ transplants: a patient's guide*, Cambridge, MA, 1991, Harvard University Press.

156. Porcari JP, Ebbeling CB, Ward A, et al.: Walking for exercise testing and training, *Sports Med* 8:189–200, 1989.

157. Prasad SA, Randall SD, Balfour-Lynn IM: Fifteen-count breathlessness score: an objective measure for children, *Pediatr Pulmonol* 30:56–62, 2000.

158. Pryor JA: The forced expiratory technique. In Pryor J, editor: *Respiratory care*, London, 1991, Churchill Livingstone, pp 79–100.

159. Reference deleted in proofs.

160. Quittner AL, Zhang J, Marynchenko M, et al.: Pulmonary medication adherence and health-care use in cystic fibrosis, *Chest* 146(1):142–151, 2014. http://dx.doi.org/10.1378/chest.13-1926.

161. Quittner AL, Goldbeck L, Abbott J, et al.: Prevalence of depression and anxiety in patients with cystic fibrosis and parent caregivers: results of The International Depression Epidemiological Study across nine countries, *Thorax* 69:1090–1097, 2014.

162. Qvist T, Pressler T, Høiby N, Katzenstein TL: Shifting paradigms of nontuberculous mycobacteria in cystic fibrosis, *Respir Res* 15(1):41, 2014.

163. Radtke R, Stevens D, Benden C, Williams C: Clinical exercise testing in children and adolescents with cystic fibrosis, *Pediatr Phys Ther* 21(3):275–281, 2009.

164. Ramsey BW, Pepe MS, Quan JM, et al.: Intermittent administration of inhaled tobramycin in patients with cystic fibrosis. Cystic Fibrosis Inhaled Tobramycin Study Group, *N Engl J Med* 340:23–30, 1999.

165. Ranganathan SC, Stocks J, Dezateux C, et al.: The London Collaborative Cystic Fibrosis Group. The evolution of airway function in early childhood following clinical diagnosis of cystic fibrosis, *Am J Resp Crit Care Med* 169:928–933, 2004.

166. Ratjen FA: Cystic fibrosis: pathogenesis and future treatment strategies, *Respir Care* 54:595–602, 2009.

167. Ratjen F, Munck A, Kho P: Short and long-term efficacy of inhaled tobramycin in early *P. aeruginosa* infection: the ELITE study, *Pediatr Pulmonol* (Suppl 31):319–320, 2008.

168. Reisman JJ, Rivington-Law B, Corey M, Marcotte J, et al.: Role of conventional physiotherapy in cystic fibrosis, *J Pediatr* 113:632–636, 1988.

169. Riordan JR, Rommens JM, Kerem BS, et al.: Identification of the cystic fibrosis gene: cloning and characterization of complementary DNA, *Science* 245:1066–1073, 1989.

170. Rosenfeld M, Ratjen F, Brunback L, et al.: Inhaled hypertonic saline in infants and children younger than 6 years with cystic fibrosis: the ISIS randomized controlled trial, *JAMA* 307(21):2269–2277, 2012.

171. Rosenstein B, Langbaum T: Diagnosis. In Taussig LM, editor: *Cystic fibrosis*, New York, 1984, Thieme-Stratton, pp 85–115.

172. Ruppel G: *Manual of pulmonary function testing*, ed 7, St. Louis, 1998, Mosby.

173. Sawicki GS, Ren CL, Konstan MW, et al.: Treatment complexity in cystic fibrosis: trends over time and associations with site-specific outcomes, *J Cystic Fibro* 12(5):461–467, 2013.

174. Schneiderman JE, Wilkes DL, Atenafu EG, et al.: Longitudinal relationship between physical activity and lung health in patients with cystic fibrosis, *Eur Respir J* 43(3):817–823, 2014.

175. Schneiderman-Walker J, Pollock S, Corey M, et al.: A randomized controlled trial of a 3-year home exercise program in cystic fibrosis, *J Pediatr* 136:304–310, 2000.

176. Scott RB, O'Loughlin EV, Gall DG: Gastroesophageal reflux in patients with cystic fibrosis, *J Pediatr* 106:223–227, 1985.

177. Scott SM, Walters DA, Singh SJ, et al.: A progressive shuttle walking test of functional capacity in patients with chronic airflow limitation, *Thorax* 45:781a, 1990.

178. Selvadurai HC, Blimkie J, Cooper PJ, et al.: Gender differences in habitual activity in children with cystic fibrosis, *Arch Dis Child* 89:928–933, 2005.

179. Selvadurai HC, Cooper PJ, Meyers N, et al.: Validation of shuttle tests in children with cystic fibrosis, *Pediatr Pulmonol* 35:133–138, 2003.

180. Sermet-Gaudelus I, Castanet M, Retsch-Bogart G, Aris R: Update on cystic fibrosis-related bone disease: a special focus on children, *Pediatr Respir Rev* 10:134–142, 2009.

181. Shepherd R, Vasques-Velasquez L, Prentice A, et al.: Increased energy expenditure in young children with cystic fibrosis, *Lancet* 2:1300–1303, 1988.

182. Sosnay PR, Siklosi KR, Van Goor F, et al.: Defining the disease liability of variants in the cystic fibrosis transmembrane conductance regulator gene, *Nat Genet* 45(10):1160–1167, 2013.

183. Spalding A, Kelly L, Santopietro J, Posner-Mayor J: *Kid on the ball: Swiss balls in a complete fitness program*, Windsor, 1999, Human Kinetics.

184. Starnes VA, Bowdish ME, Woo MS, et al.: A decade of living lobar lung transplantation: recipient outcomes, *J Thorac Cardiovasc Surg* 127:114–122, 2004.

185. Starr JA: Manual techniques of chest physical therapy and airway clearance techniques. In Zadai CC, editor: *Pulmonary management in physical therapy*, New York, 1992, Churchill Livingstone, pp 99–133.

186. Subbarao PJ, Stanojevic S, Brown M, et al.: Clearance Index as an outcome measure for clinical trials in young children with cystic fibrosis, *Am J Respir Crit Care Med* 188:456–460, 2013.

187. Swisher AK, Hebestreit H, Mejia-Dopwns A, et al.: Exercise and habitual physical activity for people with cystic fibrosis: expert consensus, evidence-based guide for advising patients, *Cardiopul Phys Ther J* 26(4):85–98, 2015.

188. Tecklin JS, Clayton RG, Scanlin TF: High frequency chest wall oscillation vs. traditional chest physical therapy in CF: a large, 1-year, controlled study, *Pediatr Pulmonol* (Suppl 20):304, 2000.

189. Tepper RS: Assessment of pulmonary function in infants with cystic fibrosis, *Pediatr Pulmonol* (Suppl 8):165–166, 1992.

190. Tepper RS, Hiatt PW, Eigen H, Smith J: Total respiratory compliance in asymptomatic infants with cystic fibrosis, *Am Rev Resp Dis* 135:1075–1079, 1987.

191. Tepper RS, Hiatt P, Eigen H, et al.: Infants with cystic fibrosis: pulmonary function at diagnosis, *Pediatr Pulmonol* 5:15–18, 1988.

192. Tiddens H, Puderbach M, Venegas J, et al.: Novel outcome measures for clinical trials in cystic fibrosis, *Pediatr Pulmonol* 50(3):302–315, 2015.

193. Turkel S, Pao M: Late consequences of pediatric chronic illness, *Psychiatr Clin North Am* 30(4):819–835, 2007.

194. van de Weert-van Leeuwan, Arets H, van der Ent CK, Beekman JM: Infection, inflammation and exercise in cystic fibrosis, *Respir Rese* 14:32, 2013.

195. Van Ginderdeuren F, Malfroot A, Dab I: Influence of 'assisted autogenic drainage (AAD),' 'bouncing' and 'AAD combined with bouncing' on gastro-oesophageal reflux (GOR) in infants, *J Cyst Fibros Book of abstracts* 112, 2001.

196. Vermeulen F, Proesmans M, De Boeck K: Longitudinal changes in lung clearance index in children with CF, *J Cystic Fibr* 14(Supp):S48, 2015.

197. Vinocur CD, Marmon L, Schidlow DV, Weintraub WH: Gastroesophageal reflux in the infant with cystic fibrosis, *Am J Surg* 149:182–186, 1985.

198. Volsko TA: Cystic fibrosis and the respiratory therapist: a 50-year perspective, *Respir Care* 54:587–593, 2009.

199. Volsko TA, DiFiore JM, Chatburn RL: Performance comparison of two oscillating positive expiratory pressure devices: Acapella versus Flutter, *Respir Care* 48:124–130, 2003.

200. Wagener JS, Headley AA: Cystic fibrosis: current trends in respiratory care, *Respir Care* 48:234–244, 2003.

201. Wagener JS, Taussig LM, Burrows B, et al.: Comparison of lung function survival patterns between cystic fibrosis and emphysema or chronic bronchitis patients. In Sturgess JM, editor: *Perspectives in cystic fibrosis*, Mississauga, Canada, 1980, Imperial Press, pp 236–245.

202. Wark P, McDonald VM: Nebulized hypertonic saline for cystic fibrosis, *Cochrane Database Syst Rev* 2:CD001506, 2009.

203. Warwick WJ, Hansen LG: The long term effect of high frequency chest compression therapy on pulmonary complications of cystic fibrosis, *Pediatr Pulmonol* 11:265–271, 1991.

204. Waters V, Stanojevic S, Atenafu EG, et al.: Effect of pulmonary exacerbations on long term function decline in cystic fibrosis, *Eur Respir J* 40(1):61–66, 2012.

205. Webber BA, Pryor JA: *Physiotherapy for respiratory and cardiac problems*, ed 2, New York, 1998, Churchill Livingstone.

206. Weiser G, Kerem E: Early intervention in CF: how to monitor the effect, *Pediatr Pulmonol* 42:1002–1007, 2007.

207. Wilkes DL, Schneiderman-Walker J, Atenafu E, et al.: Bone mineral density and habitual physical activity in cystic fibrosis, *Pediatr Pulmonol* (Suppl 31):436, 2008.

208. Wilkes DL, Schneiderman-Walker J, Corey M, et al.: Long-term effect of habitual physical activity on lung function in patients with cystic fibrosis, *Pediatr Pulmonol* (Suppl 30):358, 2007.

209. Winton T: Double lung transplantation for cystic fibrosis: operative technique and early post-operative care, *Pediatr Pulmonol* (Suppl 8):208–209, 1992.

210. Witt DR, Blumberg B, Schaefer C, et al.: Cystic fibrosis carrier screening in a prenatal population, *Pediatr Pulmonol* (Suppl 8):235, 1992.

211. Wood RE: Why commence conventional chest physiotherapy for CF at diagnosis? *Pediatr Pulmonol* (Suppl 9):89–90, 1993.

212. Yankaskas JR, Mallory, GB, and the Consensus Committee: Lung transplantation in cystic fibrosis: consensus conference statement, *Chest* 113(1):217–226, 1998. 1998.

213. Yankaskas JR, Marshall BC, Sufian B, et al.: Cystic fibrosis adult care: consensus conference report, *Chest* 125:1S–39S, 2004.

214. Yellon RF: The spectrum of reflux-associated otolaryngologic problems in infants and children, *Am J Med* 103:125–129, 1997.

215. Yimlamai D, Freiberger DA, Gould A, et al.: Pretransplant six-minute walk test predicts peri- and post-operative outcomes after pediatric lung transplantation, *Pediatr Transplant* 17(1):34–40, 2013.

216. Yusen RD, Christie JD, Edwards LB, et al.: The Registry of the International Society for Heart and Lung Transplantation: thirtieth Adult Lung and Heart-Lung Transplant Report-2013; Focus theme: age, *J Heart Lung Transplant* 32(10), 2013.

217. Zach MS, Purrer B, Oberwaldner B: Effect of swimming on forced expiration and sputum clearance in cystic fibrosis, *Lancet* 2:1201–1203, 1981.

218. Zadai CC: Comprehensive physical therapy evaluation: identifying potential pulmonary limitations. In Zadai CC, editor: *Pulmonary management in physical therapy*, New York, 1992, Churchill Livingstone, pp 55–78.

SUGGESTED READINGS

Bush A, Bilton D, Hodson M: Physiotherapy. In Bush A, Bilton D, Hodson M, editors: *Hodson and Geddes' cystic fibrosis*, ed 4, London, 2015. CRC Press.

Button BM, Button B: Structure and function of the mucus clearance system of the lung, *Cold Spring Harb Perspect Med* 3(8):a009720 2013. http://doi.org/10.1101/cshperspect.a009720.

Cystic Fibrosis Foundation. Available at: URL: https://www.cff.org/.

International Physiotherapy Group for Cystic Fibrosis: *Canada:* International Physiotherapy Group, 2009. Available at: URL: http://www.cfww.org/docs/ipg-cf/bluebook/bluebooklet2009websiteversion.pdf.

Lannefors L, Button BM, McIlwaine M: Physiotherapy in infants and young children with cystic fibrosis: current practice and future developments, *J R Soc Med* 97(Suppl 44):8–25, 2004.

Ratjen FA: Cystic fibrosis: pathogenesis and future treatment strategies, *Respir Care* 54:595–602, 2009.

Schneiderman JE, Wilkes DL, Atenafu EG, et al.: Longitudinal relationship between physical activity and lung health in patients with cystic fibrosis, *Eur Respir J* 43(3):817–823, 2014.

Swisher AK, Hebestreit H, Mejia-Downs A, et al.: Exercise and habitual physical activity for people with cystic fibrosis: expert consensus, evidence-based guide for advising patients, *Cardiopul Phys Ther J* 26(4):85–98, 2015.

Tiddens H, Puderbach M, Venegas J, et al.: Novel outcome measures for clinical trials in cystic fibrosis, *Pediatr Pulmonol* 50(3):302–315, 2015.

Volsko TA: Cystic fibrosis and the respiratory therapist: a 50-year perspective, *Respir Care* 54:587–593, 2009.

27

Asthma: Multisystem Implications

Mary Massery

Asthma is a common childhood health condition that can result in activity limitations and participation restrictions that impact quality of life. Asthma is characterized by airway inflammation, airway obstruction, and bronchial hyperresponsiveness to stimuli. The pathophysiology is complex with multiple system interactions making each child's presentation of asthma unique. The purpose of this chapter is to: (1) describe pathophysiology from infancy to adulthood, (2) discuss the primary and secondary impairments of asthma and their impact on children's long-term health and development, and (3) present medical and physical therapy management. The physical therapist needs to be knowledgeable of pathophysiology, primary and secondary impairments, and pharmacologic management to understand how asthma affects a child's ability to participate in physical activities and what role the therapist can play in optimizing the child's health, motor development, and physical activity. An extensive longitudinal case scenario on Expert Consult illustrates physical therapy management.

BACKGROUND INFORMATION

PREVALENCE

According to the Centers for Disease Control (CDC), nearly one in 10 children in the United States has a diagnosis of asthma.[2,11] The percentage nearly doubles among children born preterm.[5] A full listing of national asthma facts and figures can be found on the CDC website (http://www.cdc.gov/asthma/faqs.htm).

PATHOPHYSIOLOGY

According to the National Institutes of Health (NIH), asthma is defined as a pulmonary disease with recurring symptoms that are variable in presentation and show three significant characteristics: (1) airway inflammation, (2) airway obstruction that is often reversible either spontaneously or with pharmacologic intervention, and (3) bronchial hyperresponsiveness to stimuli.[40] Asthma is a disease of both the large and the small airways with recurrent episodes of shortness of breath, wheezing, chest tightness, and coughing.[40] Extrinsic or allergic (atopic) stimuli include but are not limited to pollen, mold, animal dander, cigarette smoke, foods, drugs, dust, and other environmental factors. Intrinsic or nonallergenic stimuli include but are not limited to viral infections, inhalation of irritating substances, exercise, and emotional stress (Fig. 27.1). An individual may be sensitive to either type of stimuli or to both types. The hyperresponsiveness to stimuli in turn causes an inflammatory response. Inflammation has been

identified as a central component of asthma and is likely the primary contributor to airway remodeling leading to chronic inflammation.[40] This structural change may make the airways less responsive over time to medications.

Genetics plays a role but does not account for all types and severities of asthma. The physical, environmental, neurogenic, chemical, and pharmacologic factors that are associated with asthma vary among individuals. They stimulate or trigger the immune system (i.e., mast cells, eosinophils, neutrophils, T lymphocytes, macrophages, epithelial cells) to release chemical mediators, which in turn cause constriction of the bronchial muscles, increased mucus production, and swelling of the mucous membranes. The most recent NIH guidelines, developed by a panel of asthma experts, point to two major environmental factors that significantly increase the risk of developing asthma: airborne allergens and respiratory viral infections (especially respiratory syncytial virus [RSV]).[40] Recent findings confirm and explain the increased risk of developing asthma when exposed to RSV in infancy.[6] Other environmental factors such as secondhand smoke increase the risk of asthma and influence the severity of the disease. For example, 6- to 11-year-old children with asthma who were exposed regularly to secondhand smoke showed greater adverse health and participation outcomes than their asthma peers not exposed to smoke.[1]

PRIMARY IMPAIRMENT

Diagnosis

The diagnosis of asthma is made on the basis of history, physical examination, auscultation and palpation, and pulmonary function tests (PFTs), especially in response to a methacholine challenge.[4] Wheezing and rhonchi may be detected by auscultation even when the child does not show difficulty breathing. Breathing is often reported as being worse at night or early in the morning. Hyperexpansion of the thorax, increased accessory muscle breathing, postural changes, increased nasal secretions, mucosal swelling, nasal polyps, "allergic shiners" (darkened areas under the eyes), and evidence of an allergic skin condition may be noted on physical examination.

During an acute asthma attack, the child may show an increased respiratory rate, expiratory grunting, intercostal muscle retractions and nasal flaring, an alteration in the inspiration-expiration ratio, and coughing. In severe cases, a bluish color of the lips and nails may be noted (oxygen desaturation). Other conditions mimic asthmatic symptoms, such as vocal cord dysfunction, airway hyperreactivity, other small airway diseases, dysfunctional breathing, nonobstructive dyspnea, and hyperventilation condition. These "copy-cat" conditions

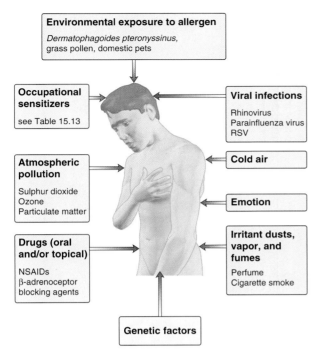

FIG. 27.1 Causes and triggers of asthma. (From Kumar P, Clarke ML: *Kumar and Clark's clinical medicine*. 8th ed. Edinburgh: Saunders, 2012.)

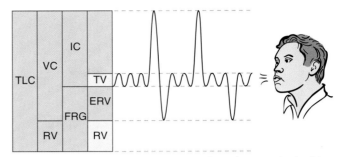

FIG. 27.2 A spirogram (pulmonary function testing). (From Frownfelter DL, Dean E: *Cardiovascular and pulmonary physical therapy: evidence to practice*. St. Louis: Mosby, 2012.)

should be ruled out during a differential diagnosis process to avoid making the wrong diagnosis.[3,27,33]

Classification and Guidelines for Treatment

A classification system and guidelines for stepwise treatment of asthma were developed by an expert panel to streamline communication among medical professionals and researchers and were published by the NIH in 2007.[40] The classification system lists childhood asthma by age (0–4 years old, 5–11 years old, 12 years old and older) and by clinical symptoms. The disease is classified as (1) intermittent, or persistent; (2) mild persistent; (3) moderate persistent; or (4) severe persistent. The summary of the report and recommendations for each age range can be found online at: http://www.nhlbi.nih.gov/health-pro/guidelines/current/asthma-guidelines/summary-report-2007. The severity classification table for children 12 years old and older is presented as an example of this classification system (Table 27.1). The classification system facilitates more consistent communication between practitioners and researchers. Desired goals of classification include improved treatment choices and more accurate documentation of patient outcomes by disease severity. Taken together, it is hoped that a national classification and treatment guideline will lead to better management of this chronic condition. New panels of experts are organized to report and compile the latest findings in the management of asthma approximately every 10 years.[32]

Pulmonary Function Tests (PFTs)

PFTs are a group of tests that measure lung function. Test values are compared with predicted values based on age, sex, and height.[12] PFTs are performed for patients with asthma to determine the location and degree of the respiratory impairment as well as the reversibility of bronchoconstriction following

administration of a bronchodilator (methacholine challenge) (Fig. 27.2).[29] PFT measurements are typically used to reveal one or more of the following: (1) decreased forced vital capacity (FVC), (2) decreased forced expiration during the first second of FVC (FEV_1), (3) decreased forced expiratory volume compared with forced vital capacity (FEV/FVC), (4) decreased peak expiratory flow rate (PEFR) because of airway obstruction in large or small airways, (5) forced expiratory flow (FEF) during 25% to 75% of FVC (FEF 25% to 75%) because of airway obstruction in the small airways, (6) increased residual volume (RV), and (7) increased functional residual capacity (FRC) because of air trapping.[40] Asthma is an obstructive lung disease, meaning the inflamed airways trap the air in the distal segments making it hard for the patient to exhale; thus his or her expiratory flows such as FEV_1 and PEFR are likely to be low. However, the swelling and mucus may also restrict the patient's ability to inhale (restrictive lung condition); thus FVC may be low as well. The physician will determine which tests are the most sensitive measures to indicate sickness/wellness for each individual patient.

School-age children and youth with asthma often monitor their pulmonary status at home by daily or weekly testing of their PEFR with a peak flow meter to assist the physician in adjusting medication. A peak flow meter is not a substitute for a formal PFT, but it can help to monitor the child's condition at home.[40] PFTs are generally not reliable for children under the age of 5 years old because they require cooperation and consistent maximal effort.[40] Children under the age of 5–6 years old are monitored on the basis of clinical signs and symptoms.[10] Asthma guidelines for pediatricians are constantly being updated.[26,57] Check the current literature for updates.

Impairments in Body Functions and Structures

Asthma is a pulmonary disease with recurring symptoms; thus the diagnosis is not typically made until the child is 3 to 5 years of age when numerous episodes of pulmonary problems have been demonstrated and are consistent with symptoms of asthma.[40] Initially, a child may be diagnosed with "reactive airway disease."[30] Over time, the physician will determine if the diagnosis of asthma is appropriate. The young child diagnosed with asthma may present with a multiple of risk factors that interact to cause asthma and influence disease severity: family history of asthma or atopic (allergy) predispositions, prematurity, lung abnormalities, exposure to secondhand smoke or other environmental pollutants, history of episodes of wheezy bronchitis, croup, recurrent upper respiratory tract infections, chronic bronchitis, recurrent pneumonia, respiratory distress syndrome, difficulty sleeping, bronchopulmonary dysplasia,

TABLE 27.1 NIH Classification of Asthma Severity

Pediatric asthma severity is classified according to 3 age groups: 0 to 4 years, 5 to 11 years, and 12 years old or older. This example is for the older child; youths 12 years old or older.

Assessing severity and initiating treatment for patients who are not currently taking long-term control medications

Components of Severity		Classification of Asthma Severity ≥12 years of age			
		Intermittent	Persistent		
			Mild	Moderate	Severe
Impairment	Symptoms	≤2 days/week	>2 days/week but not daily	Daily	Throughout the day
Normal FEV$_1$/FVC: 8–19 yr 85% 20–39 yr 80% 40–59 yr 75% 60–80 yr 70%	Nighttime awakenings	≤2x/month	3–4x/month	>1x/week but not nightly	Often 7x/week
	Short-acting beta$_2$-agonist use for symptom control (not prevention of EIB)	≤2 days/week	>2 days/week but not daily, and not more than 1x on any day	Daily	Several times per day
	Interference with normal activity	None	Minor limitation	Some limitation	Extremely limited
	Lung function	• Normal FEV$_1$ between exacerbations • FEV$_1$ >80% predicted • FEV$_1$/FVC normal	• FEV$_1$ >80% predicted • FEV$_1$/FVC normal	• FEV$_1$ >60% but <80% predicted • FEV$_1$/FVC reduced 5%	• FEV$_1$ <60% predicted • FEV$_1$/FVC reduced >5%
Risk	Exacerbations requiring oral systemic corticosteroids	0–1/year (see note)	≥2/year (see note) Consider severity and interval since last exacerbation. Frequency and severity may fluctuate over time for patients in any severity category. Relative annual risk of exacerbations may be related to FEV$_1$.		
Recommended Step for Initiating Treatment (See "Stepwise Approach for Managing Asthma" for treatment steps.)		Step 1	Step 2	Step 3	Step 4 or 5 and consider short course of oral systemic corticosteroids
				In 2–6 weeks, evaluate level of asthma control that is achieved and adjust therapy accordingly.	

Key: EIB, exercise-induced bronchospasm; FEV1, forced expiratory volume in 1 second; FVC, forced vital capacity; ICU, intensive care unit

Notes:
- The stepwise approach is meant to assist, not replace, the clinical decisionmaking required to meet individual patient needs.
- Level of severity is determined by assessment of both impairment and risk. Assess impairment domain by patient's/caregiver's recall of previous 2–4 weeks and spirometry. Assign severity to the most severe category in which any feature occurs.
- At present, there are inadequate data to correspond frequencies of exacerbations with different levels of asthma severity. In general, more frequent and intense exacerbations (e.g., requiring urgent, unscheduled care, hospitalization, or ICU admission) indicate greater underlying disease severity. For treatment purposes, patients who had ≥2 exacerbations requiring oral systemic corticosteroids in the past year may be considered the same as patients who have persistent asthma, even in the absence of impairment levels consistent with persistent asthma.

From NIH: *Expert panel report 3: guidelines for the diagnosis and management of asthma: National Institutes of Health: National Heart, Lung, and Blood Institute. Expert Panel Report 3*, p. 43.

respiratory syncytial virus (RSV) infection, gastroesophageal reflux (GERD), sleep dysfunction, rapid weight gain in infancy, obesity later in childhood, chronic dehydration, and low vitamin D levels.[16,31,41,42,45,48,51,55,58] Research has recently focused on early life events and exposures that appear to increase the risk of asthma or the risk of disease severity. Significant co-morbidities that contribute to a higher risk of asthma and are easily screened for by pediatric physical therapists are highlighted.

Gastroesophageal reflux disease: GERD occurs when stomach acid is involuntarily refluxed up into the esophagus and sometimes into the upper airway, causing chemically induced damage to the tissues.[7,13] Reflux can cause hyperirritation to the upper airway, triggering the onset of asthma or contributing to the severity of asthma. Children with asthma work harder to breathe at rest and with exertion. They pull the air in (inhalation) with greater muscular effort to overcome airway restrictions, and some have to push their air out with abdominal muscles (exhalation) to overcome obstructed airways. This increases the pressure differential across the lower esophageal sphincter, increasing risk for developing reflux. There are conflicting results on whether GERD causes asthma or whether it just contributes to disease severity.[15,30,52,54] There is agreement that children with suspected asthma should be screened for GERD.[42]

Sleep: Disrupted or poor sleep patterns are common symptoms of asthma[41,51] that have been linked to GERD as well.[13] What is not understood is which came first: the GERD, the disrupted sleep, or the asthma? Sleep-disordered breathing was found to be significantly more prevalent in individuals with asthma (26%) than age-matched controls (11%), as was habitual snoring (36%, 16%, respectively).[20] Sleep dysfunction is an important part of the child's asthma profile and should be ruled out as a significant contributor to disease severity.[9,36,45,51] In children, chronic sleep-disordered breathing is positively correlated with problems in neuropsychological development and adverse brain development, which makes it absolutely critical to rule out a sleep disorder for this high-risk population.[24,35] Because of relationships between the quality of sleep and the increased risk for poor health (such as asthma) and impaired cognitive performance, physical therapists should routinely inquire about a child's sleep pattern to screen for a possible sleep disorder.

Infant rapid weight gain: It is known children born preterm are at increased risk of developing asthma,[30,55] but there is mounting evidence that rapid weight gain by infants born preterm, especially in the first 3–4 months, is also associated with higher risk of asthma as a school-aged child.[48] In a study of > 800 preterm infants, rapid body weight gain in the first year of life was independently associated with an increased risk of developing asthma, whereas increased longitudinal growth in the same period was not associated with an increased risk of asthma.[5] The higher risk for asthma with fast weight gain as an infant was also noted in a large study of more than 25,000 infants born full-term who were followed to school age.[58] With the current preponderance of evidence on the adverse pulmonary health outcomes of early weight gain, practitioners should be compelled to instruct parents about this modifiable risk factor for asthma. Physical therapists need to be aware of this risk as well.

Viral infections: Viral infections, especially severe RSV infection in infancy, is highly associated with a later diagnosis of asthma.[55] Two recent studies found inflammatory markers that

begin to explain this increased risk.[6,46] It is hoped that understanding the physiology of the inflammatory response will lead to improved treatments that lower the risk of developing asthma later in childhood. In the meantime, physical therapists should carefully watch children with a history of infant RSV infections for signs of asthma.

Prognosis

By adolescence, asthmatic symptoms often decrease. However, even if adolescents are symptom free, they often have impairments in respiratory growth and development. Their lungs are smaller compared with healthy peers, and they are more likely to demonstrate decreased lung function.[25,50] Infants born preterm with respiratory problems are even more likely to have lung and airway restrictions later in childhood and young adulthood.[6,22,25,38] It is speculated that children born preterm who develop asthma are at higher risk for developing emphysema-like conditions in middle age.[4,21,50] This remains an hypothesis, however, because survivors of extreme prematurity have not yet reached middle age. For these reasons, pediatric physical therapists are encouraged to screen and educate children and families about the ongoing risk of developing asthma and other chronic lung diseases all the way into adulthood.

Medical Management

Asthma is not a curable disease, so the medical treatment plan is focused on short-term relief and long-term management to control or prevent symptoms as best as possible.[40] The NIH has been the leader in developing and disseminating national guidelines on asthma based on the best available evidence and a consensus of asthma experts.[40] To see the full, current guidelines go to: http://www.nhlbi.nih.gov/health-pro/guidelines/current/asthma-guidelines/summary-report-2007. Short-term goals focus on managing acute airway obstruction (bronchoconstriction). Long-term management addresses the triggers that cause the bronchial hyperresponsiveness and the underlying inflammatory response.

Short term: The frequency, duration, and severity of asthma attacks can be highly variable even for the same individual. Symptoms are usually reversible and can be prevented or modified to some degree when individual-specific triggers are identified. Acute treatment is aimed at reversing the bronchoconstriction; thus bronchodilator medications are the drugs of choice. Bronchodilators, such as the generic albuterol, are short-acting beta2-agonists (SABAs).[40] Bronchodilators relax the smooth muscles of the airway, providing immediate relief of the constriction, usually within 5 minutes. Relief may last for 3–6 hours. SABAs are inhaled via a metered dose inhaler (MDI) or through a nebulizer treatment (Fig. 27.3). SABAs do not control asthma, but they are typically used to manage acute asthma attacks or purposely taken before a known trigger such as exercise (exercise-induced asthma). The most common adverse side effects are rapid heart rate, headaches, nausea, and anxiety. The physician takes the child's individual response to SABAs into account when developing an asthma plan of care. Typically, when SABAs are used more than 2×/week, the plan of care is adjusted to focus on long-term control rather than quick acute relief.[40]

If an asthma attack is severe and does not respond to bronchodilator medications, the child may develop status asthmaticus.[40] This is a life-threatening emergency. Physical therapists should stop treatment immediately and seek medical attention

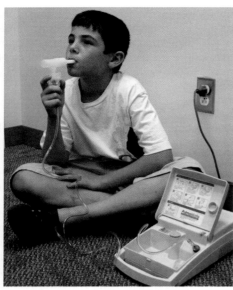

FIG. 27.3 Nebulized aerosol treatment with a mouthpiece. (Courtesy Texas Children's Hospital, Houston. From Hockenberry MJ, Wilson D: *Wong's nursing care of infants and children*. 10th ed. St, Louis: Mosby, 2015.)

by the hospital emergency team (in-patient setting) or by calling for an ambulance (community setting).

Long term: The goals of long-term asthma management are to prevent chronic and troublesome symptoms, to maintain pulmonary function and physical activity level, to prevent recurrent exacerbations, to minimize the need for emergency room visits or hospitalizations, to provide optimal pharmacotherapy, and to meet the patient's and family's expectations and satisfaction.[40] To achieve all of the goals, no two medical care plans will be exactly the same. Each written action plan should address disease severity, disease control, and responsiveness to treatment and should be considered a fluid document that changes with the child over time.[40]

NIH guidelines have specific treatment plan suggestions based on the disease severity: intermittent asthma, or persistent asthma (mild, moderate, or severe) (see Table 27.1). In addition to managing asthma itself, it is critical to manage the co-morbidities that influence disease severity such as allergens, environmental factors (e.g., smoke, pollutants), exercise response (exercise-induced asthma), GERD, sleep dysfunction, rhinitis, sinusitis, obesity, stress, depression, nutrition, etc.[40] Factors that can be easily modified such as allergies, secondhand smoke, initiating exercise safely to avoid EIA response, and weight gain should be addressed immediately. After assessing the child's response to the initial program and assessing the risk of exacerbations, the action plan should be appropriately modified. This plan should be shared with school and other personnel who are involved with the child on a regular basis. The child's or family's knowledge, understanding, and willingness to follow through (adherence) with the program are essential for successful long-term management of asthma.[18,40] Researchers have repeatedly found poorer health outcomes for children with poor adherence to their asthma treatment plans and are continually looking for methods to improve adherence.[44,49]

Medications: The current NIH Publication on the Guidelines for Asthma describes a terraced approach to pharmacologic management for long-term control of asthma.[40] Recommendations for dosing medication are based on severity and age (0 to 4 years, 5 to 11 years, and 12 years and older) because evidence indicates that children respond differently to asthma medications than adults. Long-term control starts with managing the inflammatory component of asthma. Inhaled corticosteroids continue to be the drug of choice across all age groups for long-term management of inflammation.[40] Cromolyn sodium and nedocromil medications are used to stabilize the mast cell response and may be useful in managing exercise-induced asthma symptoms and allergen triggers.[40] Other medications include immunomodulators, leukotriene modifiers, long-acting beta2-agonists, and methylxanthines. These medications are more likely to be prescribed if the child's symptoms are not well controlled using an inhaled corticosteroid. Most children take a combination of medications, each adjusted to meet their asthma management goals. Physical therapists need to understand the pharmacologic management of their patients with asthma.

Although the medications used in the management of asthma are necessary, the side effects may have an unintended impact on daily life. For example, oral corticosteroids may cause an increased appetite and weight gain, fluid retention, increased bruising, and mild elevation of blood pressure.[40] Other side effects reported from asthma medications include nervousness, headache, trembling, heart palpitations, dizziness or light-headedness, dryness or irritation of the mouth and throat, heartburn, nausea, bad taste in the mouth, restlessness, difficulty concentrating, and insomnia.[40] Thus for children with asthma, adverse motor, cognitive, or emotional behaviors could be related to their medication and should be ruled out as a factor for such behaviors. For example, concentration difficulties could be misdiagnosed as a primary attention deficit disorder; anxiety consequences could be misdiagnosed as primary psychological disorder; overeating could be misdiagnosed as a primary eating disorder; and dizziness and trembling consequences could be misdiagnosed as primary motor impairments to balance and fine motor performance and ultimately to the child's participation level.

New drugs are constantly being researched and developed; thus, any listing of medications is relevant only within a limited time frame. The overall goal of long-term asthma management is to find the medication or combination of medications that will stop the inflammatory process at an earlier point or prevent the presentation of asthma altogether. As the understanding of the pathophysiology and genetics of asthma increases, new medications with more specific but fewer side effects will likely be developed. Medications to address coexisting conditions such as allergies and GERD will also contribute to the effective management asthma. Physical therapists should communicate with the child's physician about current medications and the implications for optimal physical activity and endurance.

SECONDARY IMPAIRMENTS

Quality of Life

Asthma is a chronic condition that is managed, not cured. Thus the diagnosis of asthma affects the life of the entire family and not just the child.[57] Numerous quality-of-life studies show extensive effects on family life.[8,14,56] For example, adolescents with asthma don't thrive as well as their nonasthmatic peers.[39]

This poor outcome is exacerbated when parents aren't coping well with the child's asthma.[39] Other family decisions reflect the parents' concerns for their child's health. For example, parents may restrict their child's participation in normal childhood activities out of fear of asthma exacerbations or social retributions.[56] In fact, it is not only the child who suffers from restricted participation. Parents are forced to miss days of work just like the child is forced to miss days of school; taken together they reduce the quality of life for the entire family.[47]

Growing up with this chronic childhood disease undoubtedly influences quality of life and choices made by individuals with asthma across the life span.[17] In fact, a recent study shows that 88% of adults with moderate to severe asthma report that their asthma is not well controlled, which negatively affects their burden of care and life choices.[59] When developing a plan of care for children with asthma, physical therapists are encouraged to engage the child and family in conversation about health and wellness, suggesting how the child can safely participate in his or her preferred physical and social activities. The therapist's recommendations should support the importance of adherence to medical management and encourage the child's self-management.

Growth and Development

Children with asthma are often shorter than their peers. Prolonged use of high-dose inhaled corticosteroids has been shown to reduce height compared to peers without asthma.[53] Recognition of the potential for reduced height as an adult is taken into consideration when developing a plan of care, but control of the child's asthma is paramount. Some modifications include recognition that bone mineral density (BMD) levels were better maintained with inhaled corticosteroids rather than with frequent bursts of oral corticosteroids.[19] Thus physicians may alter their choice of medication or delivery to control asthma while trying to minimize adverse secondary effects. Current recommendations call for the lowest dose of inhaled corticosteroids that will control the asthma symptoms but minimize the adverse effect on the child's musculoskeletal development to optimize adult lung growth and height growth and to maximize BMD.[19] Vitamin D is being explored as an asthma supplement to counteract the adverse effects of inhaled corticosteroids on height and BMD. Early results are promising, but more long-term studies are needed.[16]

Financial Impact on the Family and Society

According to the CDC, asthma is associated with the high related costs of care, reportedly topping $56 billion a year: http://www.cdc.gov/asthma/impacts_nation/asthmafactsheet.pdf. Children with moderate to severe asthma had higher costs, and those with exacerbations had the highest care costs.[28] Thus having a child with asthma not only increases the family's focus on the child's medical needs but also consumes the family's and the community's financial resources.

FOREGROUND INFORMATION

PHYSICAL THERAPY MANAGEMENT

Physical therapists are traditionally involved in exercise programs for children with asthma, and studies have shown the efficacy of such programs in improving endurance and decreasing

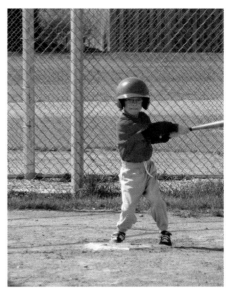

FIG. 27.4 Seven-year-old boy with asthma playing baseball. This is representative of an exercise that the child enjoys doing.

asthmatic symptoms.[43] The specifics of exercise testing and the development of a fitness program are covered in Chapter 6 and will not be covered here. Endurance programs such as treadmill training, which are also common, will not be covered either because this author prefers to find ways to improve fitness and endurance through participation in typical childhood activities rather than in contrived activities, circumstances permitting. If physical fitness is seen as an "exercise duty," it is this author's experience that the child and family are less likely to follow through, seeing physical exercise as a chore rather than an opportunity for growth. Interventions that improve adherence to the child's asthma program are associated with improved health outcomes; thus finding exercises or activities that a child likes to do is well matched with those desired outcomes (Fig. 27.4).[44]

The child with asthma may need more than a nudge and emotional support to engage in age-appropriate physical activities. Few studies address possible secondary physical restrictions due to asthma (or other childhood chronic pulmonary diseases), such as adverse musculoskeletal changes/alignments and neuromotor strategies for breathing or trunk control that could limit the child's functional potential.[34,37] In the *Guide to Physical Therapist Practice*, physical therapy is defined as a "profession with ... widespread clinical applications in the restoration, maintenance and promotion of optimal physical function."[23] Thus if physical function and activity limitations are identified as occurring secondary to asthma, physical therapy would be the appropriate service to restore, maintain, and promote optimal physical functioning and address activity limitations.

Physical therapy examination and evaluation and considerations for physical therapy interventions will be discussed in an in-depth case longitudinal scenario presented on Expert Consult. The case involves "Jonathan," who was referred to physical therapy at age 9 because his exercise-induced asthma limited his ability to participate in competitive soccer. In addition, a congenital chest wall deformity (pectus excavatum) was exacerbated by his asthma and further limited his inspiratory capacity and posture. The case scenario is intended to: (1) inform the physical therapist of the process of a differential diagnosis for the potential physical and activity limitations that may occur in children with asthma and (2) present intervention strategies and procedures to enable children with asthma to play and participate in age-appropriate physical activities with peers, rather than participating in adult-supervised exercise programs. This is an especially important consideration for children with exercise-induced asthma because it is a common reason for decreased participation in school-age activities. Long-term outcomes from these interventions are presented.

SUMMARY

This chapter presented the pathophysiology and current medical management strategies associated with childhood asthma. Asthma has three primary traits: airway inflammation, airway obstruction, and bronchial hyperresponsiveness to stimuli. The pathophysiology is complex and interactive; thus physical therapy and medical plans of care must be developed specific to each patient. The child and family's adherence to the medical management of asthma is critical to positive long-term outcomes. A detailed longitudinal case scenario on Expert Consult illustrates physical therapist diagnosis and management from a multisystem and multidiscipline perspective. Therapists are encouraged to screen for impairments in cardiopulmonary, neuromuscular, musculoskeletal, integumentary, and gastrointestinal systems that contribute to activity limitations and participation restrictions that cannot be fully explained by asthma alone. The individualized physical therapy program presented in the case scenario along with the short-term and long-term outcomes serve as a template for setting goals and planning interventions for children with asthma.

Case Scenario on Expert Consult

The case scenario related to this chapter demonstrates the process of a differential physical therapy diagnosis for potential physical and activity limitations secondary to asthma. There is a special focus on the potential long-term outcomes of physical therapy procedural interventions on the maturation and physical performance of a child with asthma.

REFERENCES

1. Akinbami LJ, Kit BK, Simon AE: Impact of environmental tobacco smoke on children with asthma, United States, 2003-2010, *Acad Pediatr* 13(6):508–516, 2013.
2. Akinbami LJ, Moorman JE, Simon AE, Schoendorf KC: Trends in racial disparities for asthma outcomes among children 0 to 17 years, 2001-2010, *J Allergy Clin Immunol* 134(3):547–553, 2014. e545.
3. Balkissoon R, Kenn K: Asthma: vocal cord dysfunction (VCD) and other dysfunctional breathing disorders, *Semin Respir Crit Care Med* 33(6):595–605, 2012.
4. Baraldi E, Carraro S, Filippone M: Bronchopulmonary dysplasia: definitions and long-term respiratory outcome, *Early Hum Dev* 85(Suppl 10):S1–S3, 2009.
5. Belfort MB, Cohen RT, Rhein LM, McCormick MC: Preterm infant growth and asthma at age 8 years, *Arch Dis Child Fetal Neonatal Ed* 101:F230–F234, 2016.
6. Bertrand P, Lay MK, Piedimonte G, et al.: Elevated IL-3 and IL-12p40 levels in the lower airway of infants with RSV-induced bronchiolitis correlate with recurrent wheezing, *Cytokine* 76(2):417–423, 2015.
7. Bhatia J, Parish A: GERD or not GERD: the fussy infant, *J Perinatol* 29(Suppl 2):S7–S11, 2009.
8. Bravata DM, Gienger AL, Holty JE, et al.: Quality improvement strategies for children with asthma: a systematic review, *Arch Pediatr Adolesc Med* 163(6):572–581, 2009.
9. Brockmann PE, Bertrand P, Castro-Rodriguez JA: Influence of asthma on sleep disordered breathing in children: a systematic review, *Sleep Med Rev* 18(5):393–397, 2014.
10. Callahan KA, Panter TM, Hall TM, Slemmons M: Peak flow monitoring in pediatric asthma management: a clinical practice column submission, *J Pediatr Nurs* 25(1):12–17, 2010.
11. Centers for Disease Control and Prevention: vital signs: asthma prevalence, disease characteristics, and self-management education: United States, 2001–2009, *MMWR Morb Mortal Wkly Rep* 60(17):547–552, 2011.
12. Cherniack RM, Cherniack L: *Respiration in health and disease*, ed 3, Philadelphia, 1983, WB Saunders.
13. Czinn SJ, Blanchard S: Gastroesophageal reflux disease in neonates and infants: when and how to treat, *Paediatr Drugs* 15(1):19–27, 2013.
14. Dean BB, Calimlim BM, Kindermann SL, et al.: The impact of uncontrolled asthma on absenteeism and health-related quality of life, *J Asthma* 46(9):861–866, 2009.
15. Deeb AS, Al-Hakeem A, Dib GS: Gastroesophageal reflux in children with refractory asthma, *Oman Med J* 25(3):218–221, 2010.
16. Fares MM, Alkhaled LH, Mroueh SM, Akl EA: Vitamin D supplementation in children with asthma: a systematic review and meta-analysis, *BMC Res Notes* 8:23, 2015.
17. Fletcher JM, Green JC, Neidell MJ: Long term effects of childhood asthma on adult health, *J Health Econ* 29(3):377–387, 2010.
18. Friend M, Morrison A: Interventions to improve asthma management of the school-age child, *Clin Pediatr (Phila)* 54(6):534–542, 2015.
19. Fuhlbrigge AL, Kelly HW: Inhaled corticosteroids in children: effects on bone mineral density and growth, *Lancet Respir Med* 2(6):487–496, 2014.
20. Goldstein NA, Aronin C, Kantrowitz B, et al.: The prevalence of sleep-disordered breathing in children with asthma and its behavioral effects, *Pediatr Pulmonol* 50(11):1128–1136, 2015.
21. Grad R, Morgan WJ: Long-term outcomes of early-onset wheeze and asthma, *J Allergy Clin Immunol* 130(2):299–307, 2012.
22. Greenough A, Alexander J, Boit P, et al.: School age outcome of hospitalisation with respiratory syncytial virus infection of prematurely born infants, *Thorax* 64(6):490–495, 2009.
23. Guide to Physical Therapist Practice, 3:0. Available at: URL: http://www.apta.org/Guide/.
24. Halbower AC, Barker PJ, et al.: Childhood obstructive sleep apnea associates with neuropsychological deficits and neuronal brain injury, *PLoSMed* 3(8):1391–1401, 2006.
25. Harmsen L, Ulrik CS, Porsbjerg C, et al.: Airway hyperresponsiveness and development of lung function in adolescence and adulthood, *Respir Med* 108(5):752–757, 2014.
26. Huffaker MF, Phipatanakul W: Pediatric asthma: guidelines-based care, omalizumab, and other potential biologic agents, *Immunol Allergy Clin North Am* 35(1):129–144, 2015.
27. Idrees M, FitzGerald JM: Vocal cord dysfunction in bronchial asthma. A review article, *J Asthma* 52(4):327–335, 2015.
28. Ivanova JI, Bergman R, Birnbaum HG, et al.: Effect of asthma exacerbations on health care costs among asthmatic patients with moderate and severe persistent asthma, *J Allergy Clin Immunol* 129(5):1229–1235, 2012.
29. Joseph-Bowen J, de Klerk NH, Firth MJ, Kendall GE, Holt PG, Sly PD: Lung function, bronchial responsiveness, and asthma in a community cohort of 6-year-old children, *Am J Respir Crit Care Med* 169(7):850–854, 2004.
30. Kase JS, Pici M, Visintainer P: Risks for common medical conditions experienced by former preterm infants during toddler years, *J Perinat Med* 37(2):103–108, 2009.
31. Kippelen P, Fitch KD, Anderson SD, et al.: Respiratory health of elite athletes—preventing airway injury: a critical review, *Br J Sports Med* 46(7):471–476, 2012.
32. Levy BD, Noel PJ, Freemer MM, et al.: Future Research Directions in Asthma: an NHLBI Working Group Report, *Am J Respir Crit Care Med* 192(11):1366–1372, 2015.
33. Lowhagen O: Diagnosis of asthma—new theories, *J Asthma* 52(6):538–544, 2015.

34. Lunardi AC, Marques da Silva CC, Rodrigues Mendes FA, et al.: Musculoskeletal dysfunction and pain in adults with asthma, *J Asthma* 48(1): 105–110, 2011.

35. Mahoney D: Treating kids' sleep apnea can improve brain function (according to Dr. Ann Halbower), *Chest Physician* 7(8):11, 2012.

36. Marcus CL, Brooks LJ, Draper KA, et al.: Diagnosis and management of childhood obstructive sleep apnea syndrome, *Pediatrics* 130(3):576–584, 2012.

37. Massery M: Musculoskeletal and neuromuscular interventions: a physical approach to cystic fibrosis, *J R Soc Med* 98(Suppl 45):55–66, 2005.

38. Metsala J, Kilkkinen A, Kaila M, et al.: Perinatal factors and the risk of asthma in childhood–a population-based register study in Finland, *Am J Epidemiol* 168(2):170–178, 2008.

39. Nabors LA, Meerianos AL, Vidourek RA, et al.: Predictors of flourishing for adolescents with asthma, *J Asthma* 1–9, 2015.

40. NIH: *Expert panel report 3: guidelines for the diagnosis and management of asthma, National Institutes of Health: National Heart, Lung, and Blood Institute,* 2007. Expert Panel Report 3.

41. Parish JM: Sleep-related problems in common medical conditions, *Chest* 135(2):563–572, 2009.

42. Patra S, Singh V, Chandra J, et al.: Gastro-esophageal reflux in early childhood wheezers, *Pediatr Pulmonol* 46(3):272–277, 2011.

43. Philpott JF, Houghton K, Luke A: Physical activity recommendations for children with specific chronic health conditions: juvenile idiopathic arthritis, hemophilia, asthma, and cystic fibrosis, *Clin J Sport Med* 20(3):167–172, 2010.

44. Reddel HK, Bateman ED, Becker A, et al.: A summary of the new GINA strategy: a roadmap to asthma control, *Eur Respir J* 46(3):622–639, 2015.

45. Ross KR, Storfer-Isser A, Hart MA, et al.: Sleep-disordered breathing is associated with asthma severity in children, *J Pediatr* 160(5):736–742, 2012.

46. Saravia J, You D, Shrestha B, et al.: Respiratory syncytial virus disease is mediated by age-variable IL-33, *PLoS Pathol* 11(10):e1005217, 2015.

47. Schmier JK, Manjunath R, Halpern MT, Jones ML, Thompson K, Diette GB: The impact of inadequately controlled asthma in urban children on quality of life and productivity, *Ann Allergy Asthma Immunol* 98(3):245–251, 2007.

48. Sonnenschein-van der Voort AM, Howe LD, Granell R, et al.: Influence of childhood growth on asthma and lung function in adolescence, *J Allergy Clin Immunol* 135(6):1435–1443, 2015. e1437.

49. Stanford RH, Gilsenan AW, Ziemiecki R, et al.: Predictors of uncontrolled asthma in adult and pediatric patients: analysis of the Asthma Control Characteristics and Prevalence Survey Studies (ACCESS), *J Asthma* 47(3):257–262, 2010.

50. Stocks J, Hislop A, Sonnappa S: Early lung development: lifelong effect on respiratory health and disease, *Lancet Respir Med* 1(9):728–742, 2013.

51. Teodorescu M, Broytman O, Curran-Everett D, et al.: Obstructive sleep apnea risk, asthma burden, and lower airway inflammation in adults in the Severe Asthma Research Program (SARP) II, *J Allergy Clin Immunol Pract* 3(4):566–575, 2015. e561.

52. Thakkar K, Boatright RO, Gilger MA, El-Serag HB: Gastroesophageal reflux and asthma in children: a systematic review, *Pediatrics* 125(4):e925–e930, 2010.

53. Umlawska W, Gaszczyk G, Sands D: Physical development in children and adolescents with bronchial asthma, *Respir Physiol Neurobiol* 187(1): 108–113, 2013.

54. Valet RS, Carroll KN, Gebretsadik T, et al.: Gastroesophageal reflux disease increases infant acute respiratory illness severity, but not childhood asthma, *Pediatr Allergy Immunol Pulmonol* 27(1):30–33, 2014.

55. Van Bever HP: Determinants in early life for asthma development, *Allergy Asthma Clin Immunol* 5(1):6, 2009.

56. van den Bemt L, Kooijman S, Linssen V, et al.: How does asthma influence the daily life of children? Results of focus group interviews, *Health Qual Life Outcomes* 8:5, 2010.

57. VanGarsse A, Magie RD, Bruhnding A: Pediatric asthma for the primary care practitioner, *Prim Care* 42(1):129–142, 2015.

58. Wandalsen GF, Chong-Neto HJ, de Souza FS, et al.: Early weight gain and the development of asthma and atopy in children, *Curr Opin Allergy Clin Immunol* 14(2):126–130, 2014.

59. Wertz DA, Pollack M, Rodgers K, Bohn RL, Sacco P, Sullivan SD: Impact of asthma control on sleep, attendance at work, normal activities, and disease burden, *Ann Allergy Asthma Immunol* 105(2):118–123, 2010.

SUGGESTED READINGS

Levy BD, Noel PJ, Freemer MM, et al.: Future Research Directions in Asthma: an NHLBI Working Group Report, *Am J Respir Crit Care Med* 192(11):1366–1372, 2015.

NIH: *Expert panel report 3: guidelines for the diagnosis and management of asthma: National Institutes of Health: National Heart, Lung, and Blood Institute. Expert Panel Report 3.* Available at: URL: http://www.nhlbi.nih.gov/health-pro/guidelines/current/asthma-guidelines/summary-report-2007.

Sonnenschein-van der Voort AM, Howe LD, Granell R, et al.: Influence of childhood growth on asthma and lung function in adolescence, *J Allergy Clin Immunol* 135(6):1435–1443, 2015.

28

Congenital Heart Conditions

Betsy Howell, Chris D. Tapley

Approximately 6 to 10 in 1000 children are born each year with moderate and severe forms of congenital heart defects.[88] Early detection, often prenatal, and improved medical and surgical management combine with the type of defect and the individual child characteristics to determine the impact. For example, two children, each diagnosed with a ventricular septal defect, may have entirely different histories. One child may go undiagnosed for several years, whereas the other child may require surgery in infancy. Many children are now diagnosed in utero—an especially important development for children with hypoplastic left heart syndrome (HLHS). In the past, most congenital heart defects were repaired when the child was at least 1 year old, often older. These surgeries are now being performed during the first days and months of life, which is likely to affect how children with congenital heart defects grow and develop. The likelihood of a physical therapist treating a child who has previously had open-heart surgery is greater now that more children survive open-heart surgery. The number of adults who have survived surgery in childhood for congenital heart defects continues to increase.

Physical therapists serving children with congenital heart conditions are encouraged to closely monitor and document the nature and extent of developmental differences that may result from surgical repair, as well as potential neurologic impairments related to the cardiac defect itself or to postoperative complications. To prepare therapists for this task, this chapter describes congenital heart defects; surgical repairs, including heart transplantation and mechanical assistive devices; acute and chronic physical impairments secondary to heart defects and surgery; and profound cyanosis or neurologic implications and complications. Physical therapy management following cardiac surgery and ongoing management of infants, children, and adolescents with congenital cardiac defects is presented.

BACKGROUND INFORMATION

Although embryologists can identify at what point during fetal development certain defects occur and what risk factors may contribute to their development, the cause of congenital heart defects remains largely unknown. The presence of more than one child with congenital heart defect in the same family or in the family history suggests a possible genetic component. Heart defects may be associated with Down syndrome, Turner syndrome, Williams syndrome, Marfan syndrome, Costello syndrome, DiGeorge syndrome, and the VATERL association, an acronym for the following characteristics: vertebrae, imperforate anus, cardiac anomalies, tracheoesophageal fistula, renal anomalies, and limb anomalies. The American

Heart Association published a lengthy statement on current knowledge of the genetic basis for congenital heart defects[167] that describes in detail many of the above syndromes and their chromosomal disorders and associated cardiac defects. The American Heart Association has also published a lengthy statement on noninherited risk factors linked to congenital heart defects.[98]

Infants of diabetic mothers also have an increased incidence of congenital heart disease (CHD). Other noninherited risk factors found to be associated with congenital heart defects are maternal phenylketonuria, rubella, maternal obesity, and many different medications.[98] Women who used a multivitamin supplement before or just after conception were reported to have a significant reduction in the incidence of cardiac defects in their children.[29]

Diagnosis of cardiac impairments may occur during prenatal life or at birth. Some congenital heart defects require immediate attention, and others may be followed by further evaluation. Even with improved diagnostic techniques, some infants with severe cyanotic disease are not diagnosed before they are discharged to home, but several weeks later they may be diagnosed with a heart defect when they develop symptoms of septic shock. Prenatal diagnosis is essential for some diagnoses, especially hypoplastic left heart syndrome. In a review of mortality rates and the number of cardiac cases performed each year by different institutions, those with smaller surgical programs had increased mortality rates when outcomes of the more severe defects were compared.[223] Other cardiac defects may not be diagnosed until much later, even as late as adolescence. For example, coarctation of the aorta is occasionally diagnosed during a sports physical examination when a large difference between upper and lower extremity blood pressures or an abnormally high upper extremity blood pressure is observed.

The infant with a congenital heart defect often has abnormal respiratory signs, including a labored breathing pattern and an increased respiratory rate. The infant may be diaphoretic and tachycardic. Symptoms may include edema around the eyes and decreased urine output (evidenced by dry diapers). Eating problems result from difficulty in coordinating sucking and swallowing with breathing at an increased rate. Irritability that is difficult to assuage may be noted. These symptoms of congestive heart failure can lead to the diagnosis of a cardiac defect or can provide evidence of worsening of a known defect.

Congenital heart defects are usually classified as acyanotic or cyanotic. With acyanotic conditions, the child is pink and has normal oxygen saturation. If mixing or shunting of blood occurs within the heart, the blood shunts from the left side of the heart to the right side, so oxygenated blood goes to the lungs

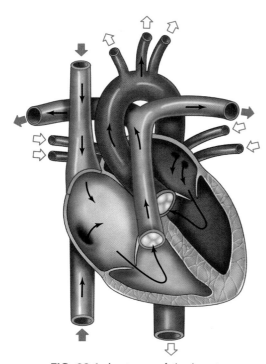

FIG. 28.1 Anatomy of the heart.

as well as to the body. Common acyanotic lesions include atrial septal defects (ASDs), ventricular septal defects (VSDs), patent ductus arteriosus (PDA), coarctation of the aorta, pulmonary stenosis, and aortic stenosis.

In cyanotic heart conditions, blood is typically shunted from the right side of the heart to the left side. Unoxygenated blood is then returned to the body, resulting in arterial oxygen saturation levels 15% to 30% below normal values. Common cyanotic lesions include tetralogy of Fallot, transposition of the great arteries, tricuspid atresia, pulmonary atresia, truncus arteriosus, total anomalous pulmonary venous return, and hypoplastic left heart syndrome.

Type and timing of intervention depend on the defect and the child's age. Some defects are repaired immediately, whereas others require a staged procedure, with the first of several surgeries being palliative rather than corrective. Some acyanotic defects are not repaired until the child is several years old.[140] Concerns regarding neurologic complications following surgery and their impact on long-term functional and cognitive development continue to be examined as an increasing number of infants survive earlier and more complex surgeries.[120] Acyanotic and cyanotic defects are further described in the next two sections and may be compared with normal anatomy of the heart (Fig. 28.1). Table 28.1 summarizes the common types of congenital heart defects, their typical surgical repair, and associated impairments and functional limitations described in the following sections.

TABLE 28.1   Summary of Congenital Heart Defects, Surgical Repair, and Associated Issues

Type of Defect	Surgical Repair	Associated Issues	Physical Therapy Issues
Atrial septal defect	Suture or patch closure/device closure		
Ventricular septal defect (VSD)	Dacron patch closure/device closure	Failure to thrive; pulmonary hypertension	Failure to thrive
Atrial ventricular septal defect/ endocardial cushion defect	Pericardial patch	Down syndrome; failure to thrive	Developmental delay
Coarctation of the aorta	Stent or subclavian patch/end-to-end anastomosis	Hypertension	Upper extremity range of motion
Pulmonary stenosis	Valvotomy		
Aortic stenosis	Valvotomy; aortic valve replacement; conduit		
Tetralogy of Fallot	VSD closed; right ventricular outflow tract resected	"Tet" spells	
Transposition of the great arteries (dextro)	Arterial switch operation	Edema; poor left ventricle function	Decreasing exercise tolerance with age
Pulmonary atresia (PA) with a VSD	Blalock-Taussig shunt (BT); VSD closed; right ventricle–to–pulmonary artery conduit	Developmental delay; poor oral intake	Developmental delay; feeding issues
Pulmonary atresia without a VSD	Valvotomy/BT shunt; right ventricular outflow tract patch, ASD closed, Fontan procedure	Very sick postoperatively, low oxygen saturations	Developmental delay
Total anomalous pulmonary venous return	Anomalous veins connected to left atrium; ASD closed	Failure to thrive	Failure to thrive
Tricuspid atresia	Atrial septostomy, BT shunt Bidirectional Glenn or hemi-Fontan procedure Fontan procedure	Low oxygen saturations	Failure to thrive
Truncus arteriosus	VSD closure, right ventricle–to–pulmonary artery conduit	Pulmonary hypertensive crisis	Developmental delay; failure to thrive
Hypoplastic left heart syndrome	Division of the main pulmonary artery; suture PA to the aorta; BT shunt and patent ductus arteriosus ligation; bidirectional Glenn or hemi-Fontan procedure; fenestrated Fontan procedure	Low oxygen saturations	Poor oral feeders; developmental delay; may not crawl; neurologic and behavioral issues; decreased exercise tolerance, especially with right-to-left shunt

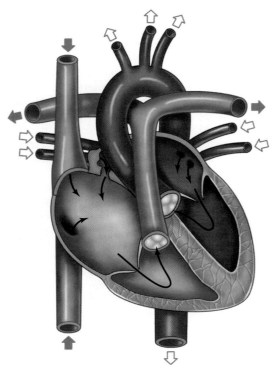

FIG. 28.2 Atrial septal defect.

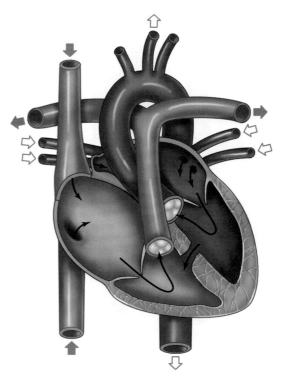

FIG. 28.3 Ventricular septal defect.

ACYANOTIC DEFECTS

Atrial Septal Defect

Atrial septal defect, one of the most common congenital heart defects, is an abnormal communication between left and right atria (Fig. 28.2). The defect is classified by its location on the septum. Blood is generally shunted from the left atrium to the right atrium. This defect generally does not require immediate repair because of slow progression of damage to the heart and lungs. The timing of surgery depends on the age of the child, when the diagnosis is confirmed, and how symptomatic the child is, but it typically occurs during the first 5 years of life. If a child has more severe symptoms, the defect is repaired sooner.[10] Some adults with signs of heart failure have a previously undiagnosed ASD. As medical technology advances, late diagnoses should become rare.

Closure of an ASD is usually done by placing a septal occluder or synthetic material to close the hole that is inserted via cardiac catheterization. Surgical repair may still occur if the ASD is in an unusual position, making it difficult to close via cardiac catheterization, or if the patient has other cardiac defects requiring repair. Surgery may be done through a median sternotomy incision; however, minimal-access techniques can be used, which can entail a smaller incision of approximately 4 cm.[10,103] Suture closure or, for larger defects, a patch closure is usually used to close the defect when surgery is necessary.[10,103] A longitudinal study of patients undergoing closure of an ASD during childhood reported excellent survival and low morbidity rates.[182]

Ventricular Septal Defect

VSD is the most common congenital heart defect, accounting for up to 40% of cardiac anomalies.[28] VSD can be present alone or in association with other defects such as tetralogy of Fallot and transposition of the great arteries. VSD alone is discussed here.

A VSD is a communication between the ventricles that allows blood to be shunted between them, generally from left to right (Fig. 28.3). The increase in blood flow through the right ventricle to the lungs may lead to pulmonary hypertension. In severe cases, in which pulmonary pressures exceed systemic pressures, shunting switches from right to left, which is often termed *Eisenmenger syndrome*.[142] A large defect may lead to early left ventricular failure. An infant with a large VSD has signs of severe respiratory distress, diaphoresis, and fatigability, especially during feeding, when the infant's endurance is stressed.[28] The infant's weight is dramatically affected in this situation. A child severely affected requires a much earlier surgical repair than a child who is asymptomatic.

Small defects may close spontaneously. Defects that compromise the clinical status of the patient must be surgically closed. The timing of surgery varies, depending on the child's tolerance of the defect. A child with a larger defect undergoes surgery earlier to diminish the negative effects on growth and the pulmonary system.

Surgical intervention is provided through a mediastinal approach and usually requires a synthetic patch closure.[28,142] Transcatheter devices are now being used with regularity and good success to close muscular VSDs but not as successfully as with perimembranous VSDs.[142]

Patent Ductus Arteriosus

The ductus arteriosus is a large vessel that connects the main pulmonary artery to the descending aorta (Fig. 28.4). It usually closes soon after birth but will dilate (remains patent) in response to hypoxia or prostaglandins E1 and E2. The ability to maintain patency of the ductus arteriosus becomes important in certain cyanotic heart defects (to be discussed later). Spontaneous closing of the ductus arteriosus can create a critical situation in the infant with an undiagnosed heart defect.[64] In some cases spontaneous closure does not occur. Reasons for

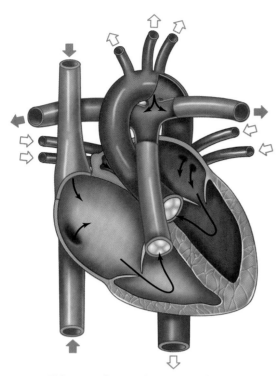

FIG. 28.4 Patent ductus arteriosus.

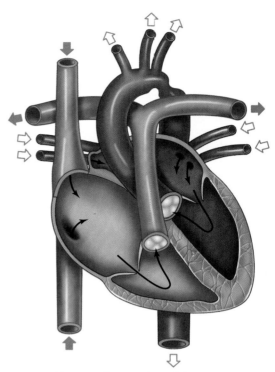

FIG. 28.5 Coarctation of the aorta.

nonclosure in the term infant are unclear but are thought to be due to ductal abnormalities, genetic factors, and some congenital infections. A high incidence of patency is found in premature infants because of respiratory distress syndrome and the resulting hypoxia.[152]

Several options are available if the PDA fails to close spontaneously or with medication. One option is video-assisted thoracoscopic surgery, which involves several small thoracostomies and results in no chest wall muscles being cut and no rib retraction.[152] Another option is transcatheter coil occlusion performed by cardiac catheterization, which can be an outpatient procedure. This is the preferred method of closure with all but the youngest children. Video-assisted and coil occlusion techniques are less traumatic, can reduce hospital stay,[64] and may decrease the risk of scoliosis, which is associated with thoracotomy. A left thoracotomy incision is the standard operative approach if video-assisted and coil occlusion cannot be performed. The ductus is ligated and sutured.

Coarctation of the Aorta

Coarctation of the aorta is defined as a narrowing or closing of a section of the aorta (Fig. 28.5). It may occur in isolation or in conjunction with other defects including bicuspid aortic valve, VSD, and in the neonatal population PDA.[116] Infants with a severe narrowing may develop cardiovascular collapse following closure of the ductus arteriosus. Early repair is necessary when a child is severely symptomatic.[9] The child or adult without symptoms may go undiagnosed until a routine physical examination reveals a hypertension.[9]

Surgical intervention is generally the method of treating coarctation of the aorta. Access to the aorta is gained through a left thoracotomy, after which the aorta is repaired with an end-to-end anastomosis, a subclavian flap, or a patch aortoplasty. The coarctation can also be treated via cardiac catheterization

using a balloon that is inflated in the constricted area, although this has been shown to have higher complications.[9]

Pulmonary Stenosis

Pulmonary stenosis, a narrowing of the right ventricular outflow tract, is classified by the location of the narrowing relative to the pulmonary valve. It often occurs in association with other heart defects. Timing of intervention depends on the severity of the narrowing and the degree of functional compromise, as well as on when pressure in the right ventricle becomes too high. Intervention is generally a balloon valvotomy that is performed via cardiac catheterization. Surgery when necessary is performed through a median sternotomy; the type of surgical procedure depends on the site of narrowing. A valvotomy may be performed, or, in severe cases, the valve may need to be replaced.[95]

Aortic Stenosis

Aortic stenosis, a narrowing of the left ventricular outflow tract, is classified by its relation to the aortic valve (supravalvular, valvular, or subvalvular) (Fig. 28.6). The narrowing will cause the left ventricle to work harder to pump blood through the narrowing. Depending on location and severity of obstruction surgical correction is indicated. Surgical technique will vary dependent on type and location of stenosis.[31]

CYANOTIC DEFECTS

Tetralogy of Fallot

Tetralogy of Fallot is the most common complex cardiac defect with an estimated incidence of 3.3 per 10,000 live births. The primary abnormalities that occur in the tetralogy of Fallot are a VSD, right ventricular outflow tract obstruction, an aorta that overrides the right ventricle, and hypertrophy of the right ventricle (Fig. 28.7).[155] Clinical manifestations depend on the

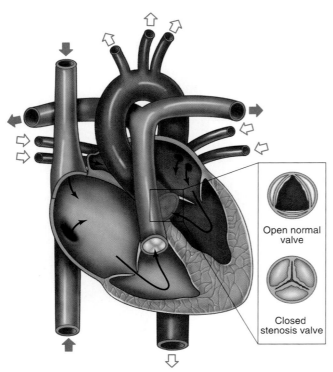

FIG. 28.6 Aortic stenosis.

Open normal
valve

Closed
stenosis valve

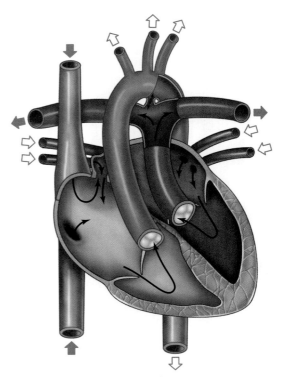

FIG. 28.8 Transposition of the great arteries.

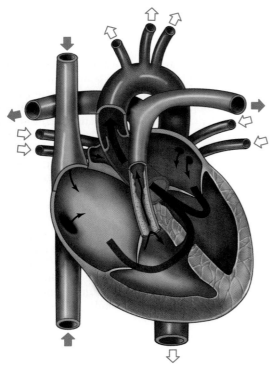

FIG. 28.7 Tetralogy of Fallot.

severity of obstruction of the right ventricular outflow tract. With increasing obstruction, an increase in cyanosis is observed over the first 6–12 months of life. Some children will develop hypercyanosis, or "tet spells," which are periods of profound systemic hypoxemia typically occurring in the context of crying, eating, or defecation. These spells are characterized by a marked

decrease in pulmonary blood flow and an increase in the right-to-left shunt across the VSD into the left ventricle and out the aorta and are characterized by dyspnea, syncope, and deepening cyanosis.[155] Cyanotic episodes can be relieved by squatting or by bringing the knees to the chest. These maneuvers are believed to increase systemic vascular resistance and ultimately to increase pulmonary blood flow. Medical management including increasing blood volume with fluid administration or transfusion, treating acidosis with bicarbonate, sedation, and use of medication to increase systemic vascular resistance may be necessary.[155]

Surgical intervention depends on the patient's symptoms and overall clinical picture. If possible, a complete repair is usually done early in life. Early palliation may be necessary if an infant is severely involved and would probably not survive corrective surgery. The palliative procedure used most often is a modified Blalock-Taussig (BT) shunt performed through a median sternotomy. The modified BT shunt involves a 3.5- or 4-mm Gore-Tex shunt being anastomosed end to side to the innominate artery and to the ipsilateral branch pulmonary artery, providing increased pulmonary blood flow while the infant gains more time to grow before undergoing corrective surgery.[205] Infants who receive early palliation continue to have cyanosis until complete repair is performed.

Corrective surgery involves closing the VSD and relieving the right outflow tract obstruction. After surgical repair a high incidence of ventricular and atrial arrhythmias has been seen and should be considered as activity is progressed.[205] Early (hospital) mortality rate following repair is reported to be between 1% and 5%.[155]

Transposition of the Great Arteries

In transposition of the great arteries, the pulmonary artery arises from the morphologic left ventricle, and the aorta arises from the right ventricle (Fig. 28.8).[50] In the absence of other defects, systemic blood returns to the body unoxygenated and pulmonary blood returns to the lungs fully oxygenated. This situation is not compatible with life unless the ductus arteriosus remains patent. Immediate intervention, usually with infusion of prostaglandin E1, is necessary to keep the ductus arteriosus open. An atrial septostomy is performed by a cardiac catheterization to keep the child alive until surgical intervention occurs.[141]

The preferred surgical technique for correction of transposition of the great arteries is the arterial switch procedure. Surgery during the first 2 to 4 weeks of life is desirable so that the left ventricle meets the systemic demands. Surgical repair occurs through a median sternotomy and involves transecting the aorta and pulmonary artery. The coronary arteries are excised with a wide button of aortic tissue and reimplanted in the old pulmonary arterial vessel; the great vessels are then switched and anastomosed so that the aorta connects to the left ventricle and the pulmonary artery connects to the right ventricle. The arterial switch procedure produces results that are free of the dysrhythmias and right ventricular failure associated with Mustard or Senning techniques.[141] Previously the Mustard or Senning techniques were used to redirect the venous return to the atria by baffles or flaps of atrial wall, respectively. These techniques leave the right ventricle as the pumping chamber for the system creating a physiologic but not anatomic correction.[141] The Mustard or Senning techniques are generally not used anymore due to complications including superior vena caval obstruction, baffle leak, atrial and ventricular arrhythmias, tricuspid valve insufficiency, and right ventricular failure.[141] Therapists may see teenage or young adult patients who have had this repair.

The Rastelli procedure is a surgical technique used when a severe left ventricular outflow tract obstruction and a VSD coexist. Repair usually occurs when the child is between 6 and 12 months old. A conduit diverts blood from the left ventricle through the VSD and the right ventricle to the aorta, a right ventricle–to–pulmonary artery conduit is formed, and any previous shunts are eliminated.[141]

Tricuspid Atresia

Tricuspid atresia is failure of development of the tricuspid valve, resulting in lack of communication between the right atrium and the right ventricle. Usually, an ASD or a VSD or both exist to allow pulmonary blood flow (Fig. 28.9). Right-to-left shunt allows mixing of unoxygenated and oxygenated blood, causing the child to be cyanotic. The right ventricle is frequently underdeveloped.[172]

Surgical repair is staged, with the initial operation shunting blood from the body to the lungs with a modified BT shunt. If the VSD is large and too much blood is going to the lungs, however, a band may be placed around the pulmonary artery to decrease blood flow to the lungs.[141] The child will remain cyanotic for several years. The next stage of surgical repair is often the Fontan procedure (or a modification thereof), performed through a median sternotomy in which the right atrium is attached to the pulmonary artery or directly to the right ventricle, using a conduit or baffle. The VSD may be surgically closed. In some institutions, a bidirectional Glenn procedure performed before the Fontan procedure leads to an improved outcome. In the Glenn procedure the superior vena cava is anastomosed to the right pulmonary artery. The child remains cyanotic but gains time for growth before undergoing the Fontan operation.[141]

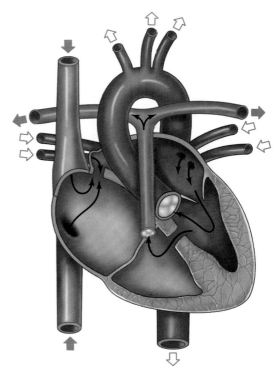

FIG. 28.9 Tricuspid atresia.

Pulmonary Atresia

Pulmonary atresia occurs when the pulmonary valve fails to develop, resulting in obstruction of blood flow from the right side of the heart to the lungs. Blood flow to the lungs is initially maintained by a PDA. An ASD or a VSD may also be present, allowing shunting of blood from the right to the left side of the heart and ultimately back to the body. The size of the right ventricle may vary, affecting later surgical decisions. Early intervention involves maintaining patency of the ductus arteriosus to increase blood flow to the lungs until surgery can be performed. Surgical repair will vary significantly depending on extent of right ventricle development and other malformations present.[83]

Truncus Arteriosus

Truncus arteriosus occurs when the aorta and the pulmonary artery fail to separate in utero and form a common trunk arising from both ventricles (Fig. 28.10). Four grades of the condition are differentiated, depending on the location of the pulmonary arteries. Early surgical intervention is necessary. Surgical repair is provided through a median sternotomy and involves removing the pulmonary arteries from the truncus, closing the VSD, and connecting the pulmonary arteries to the right ventricle by an extracardiac baffle. Hospital mortality rates range from 4.3% to 17% with most deaths occurring in the most complex forms.[24]

Total Anomalous Pulmonary Venous Return

Total anomalous pulmonary venous return (TAPVR) occurs when the pulmonary veins fail to communicate with the left atrium and instead connect to the coronary sinus of the right atrium or to one of the systemic veins. The ductus arteriosus often remains patent (Fig. 28.11). The increase in flow through the right side of the heart and into the lungs may lead to congestive heart failure. Anastomosis of the pulmonary veins to the

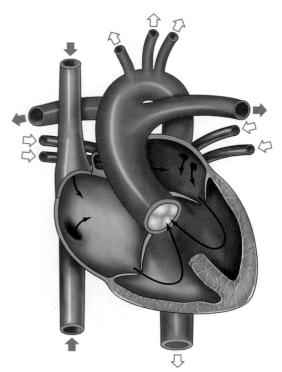

FIG. 28.10 Truncus arteriosus.

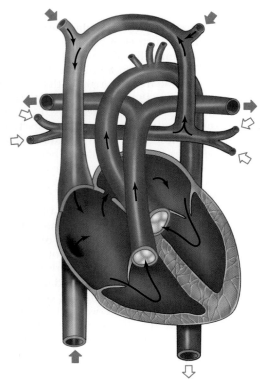

FIG. 28.11 Total anomalous pulmonary venous return.

left atrium through a median sternotomy is usually performed as soon as possible. Postoperative ventilation may be difficult because of stiffness and wetness of the lungs from the previous excessive blood flow. Mortality rates continue to improve with early and late mortality for simple TAPVR being 10% and 4%,

respectively.[164,216] There is one reported case of a 48-year-old patient who is 47 years postrepair for total anomalous pulmonary venous return.[42]

Hypoplastic Left Heart Syndrome

Hypoplasia (incomplete development or underdevelopment) or absence of the left ventricle and hypoplasia of the ascending aorta make hypoplastic left heart syndrome (HLHS) the most common form of a univentricular heart, often coexisting with severe aortic valve hypoplasia. A PDA provides systemic circulation until surgical intervention. Without surgical intervention, death is certain. Hospital survival rate (the percentage of children who leave the hospital alive after surgery for HLHS) still lags behind the rate for other congenital heart surgeries, but the surgical survival rate is now 90%.[168] Bove reported that the survival rate after second-stage palliation is now 97%, and the survival rate is 81% after the Fontan operation.[30] Five-year survival rates are between 69% and 71%, depending on the patient's anatomy,[30] and 10-year survival rates were observed to be at 55%.[16]

Prenatal diagnosis and care are essential for the parents to prepare for and to be counseled about prognosis and surgical options. They also enable the parents and medical staff to plan for delivery and the immediate postpartum period.[16] Tibballs observed that prenatal diagnosis led to termination of pregnancy at a rate of 44% to 71% in Europe and 18% to 45% in the United States.[210] It was observed by Mahle and colleagues that prenatal diagnosis was found to possibly decrease postoperative neurologic events when compared with those diagnosed postnatally.[128]

Three options are available to parents of infants diagnosed as having HLHS. One option is no surgical intervention. As a second option, the child's name may be placed on a waiting list for a heart transplant; as a third, the child may undergo a series of palliative procedures.[36]

The initial surgical procedure (Norwood I[30]) involves enlarging the ASD, transecting the main pulmonary artery and anastomosing it to the aorta, and reconstructing the aortic root. A BT or central shunt is placed to allow pulmonary blood flow. Some centers use a right ventricle (RV)–to–pulmonary artery (PA) conduit as the first stage.[16,127,168,193] This procedure may require the second stage to be performed sooner, and the potential long-term consequences of cutting into the right ventricle are not known.[30] A third technique for the child who is medically fragile is a hybrid technique that combines interventional cardiac catheterization with surgery. This involves an atrial septostomy and placing a pulmonary artery band to restrict pulmonary blood flow and a stent in the arterial duct to hold it open. The child does not need to go on cardiopulmonary bypass.[16] Before the second stage the child's oxygen saturation and activity level may start to decrease. Children may have more difficulty eating, especially with taking a bottle or nursing, which requires more energy. The second stage, generally completed between 4 and 10 months, is a hemi-Fontan or bidirectional Glenn procedure in which the superior vena cava is anastomosed to the pulmonary arteries and the BT shunt is ligated. The Fontan procedure is then performed between 18 and 24 months. This procedure provides continuity between the right atrium and the pulmonary artery, and pulmonary venous return is separated from the systemic system. As a result, the right ventricle pumps fully oxygenated blood to the body.[86]

HEART FAILURE

Pediatric heart failure can result from congenital heart defects, dilated cardiomyopathy, cardiomyositis, metabolic disorders, or from eventual failure of previous repairs or palliation.[184] The number of children with single-ventricle palliation is increasing with likely future increases in heart failure either as an older adolescent or young adult.[46] Management of these patients can be accomplished via pharmaceutical methods, surgical management including placement of mechanical assist devices, and in the worst cases orthotopic heart transplantation. This population tends to have frequent and often lengthy hospitalizations as well as ongoing functional deficits requiring acute and chronic rehabilitation efforts.[184] In this section we will present options for management and implications for the pediatric physical therapist.

Inotropic Support

Intravenous inotropic support is commonly used for end-stage congestive heart failure in the pediatric population.[23] Inotropic agents are drugs that increase or decrease the contractility of the heart during preload and afterload. These drugs include digoxin, dopamine, norepinephrine, epinephrine, isoproterenol, dobutamine, amrinone, and milrinone. Previously, these drugs have often been limited to in-hospital use because of the need for close monitoring and supervision.[23] There has been a trend to complete outpatient inotropic support with medications such as milrinone as a bridge to transplantation. Berg and colleagues reported the use of home inotropic support in 14 children with end-stage congestive heart failure and found minimal complications as well as substantial cost savings and improved family dynamics.[23] Birnbaum and colleagues[25] recently reported comparable results with a much larger study including 106 patients being supported at home with milrinone as a bridge to transplant: 85% of patients underwent transplantation, 8% of patients successfully weaned from support as outpatients, whereas 6% died.[25] McBride and associates also reported on the safety of a monitored exercise program for pediatric heart transplant candidates on multiple inotropic support.[143] They found that patients were able to engage in an aerobic and musculoskeletal conditioning program three times per week with no adverse episodes of hypotension or significant complex arrhythmias. Physical therapists need to be aware of the increased use of these medications in the home setting. As noted, studies are showing safety with activity while on inotropic support. Patients, however, still need to be carefully monitored when engaging in therapeutic activities while on inotropic support.

Technological Support

Extracorporeal Membrane Oxygenation

Extracorporeal membrane oxygenation (ECMO) may be used for cardiovascular and respiratory support in children after open-heart surgery. ECMO consists of an external circuit that moves venous blood through an artificial gas exchanger, which provides blood oxygenation and decarboxylation. ECMO support can be provided either in a veno-venous (VV) or veno-arterial (VA) setup. VV ECMO provides only respiratory support, bypassing the patient's lungs, while VA ECMO provides both respiratory and circulatory support, bypassing both heart and lungs.[195] The ECMO circuit takes over oxygenation and perfusion of the child's body while the heart and lungs are "rested." Indications for biventricular support by ECMO in the early postoperative period include progressive hypotension, increased ventricular filling pressures, poor peripheral perfusion, decreased urine output, and decreased mixed venous oxygen saturation.[57,107] ECMO is also used as a bridge to surgery or transplant in the severely compromised patient who is too ill to undergo repair immediately. Bautista-Hernandez and associates observed that 62% of their patients survived to discharge from the hospital—patients who probably would not have survived their initial surgery without EMCO first to stabilize them.[18] ECMO is capable of providing support for several days to at most a few weeks[11] and is associated with severe complications such as cerebral infarction, brain hemorrhage, renal failure, and multiorgan system failure.[93] Historically, patients on ECMO must remain intubated and sedated and therefore are unable to be mobilized while on support.[93] More recently, there is a push for early mobilization of patients on ECMO when medically appropriate. This has been used primarily in cases of VV ECMO and predominantly in settings of respiratory failure only.[115,169,212,231] As technology advances, early mobilization of children receiving other forms of ECMO may become possible. Early rehabilitation might improve outcomes. Therapists providing services to children with cardiac conditions in acute and outpatient settings should be aware of a history of ECMO due the high incidence of neurologic impairment and possible impact on developmental and functional outcomes.

Ventricular Assistive Devices

As previously noted, young children with the most severe heart failure are most often supported with ECMO.[93] An alternate approach uses ventricular assistive devices (VADs). VADs, circulatory pumps that supplement or completely replace the pumping function of one or both ventricles, have been used extensively in the adult population as a bridge to a transplant device or to a recovery device for many years. Their use in the pediatric population, however, has been limited because of limited availability of devices that meet pediatric physiology and cardiac flow needs.[11,180,208] Bastardi and colleagues and others have suggested that despite the lack of pediatric-specific devices, VADs are a viable option to be used as a bridge to transplant therapy or in some cases to recovery in the pediatric population.[17,35,84,180] In addition, Adachi et al. and Zafar et al. each showed significant decreases in heart transplant wait list mortality since more widespread use of pediatric VADs.[2,230]

Currently, a limited number of VADs are available for use in the pediatric population, especially in the infant and young pediatric population. The primary device used in the United States for this population is the Berlin Heart Excor (Berlin Heart AG, Berlin, Germany). This pneumatically driven, pulsatile VAD may be used as a left ventricular assistive device (LVAD) or as a biventricular assistive device (BiVAD). The Berlin Heart Excor supports a variety of blood pumps capable of delivering stroke volumes from 10 to 80 ml, making it suitable for use in children as small as 3 kg through full-size adults.[84,136,147,180,208] The Berlin Heart Excor is the only pediatric-specific device approved for use by the Food and Drug Administration (FDA).

Morales and associates[151] have reported their experience with use of the Berlin Heart Excor in a multicenter North American experience. Between June of 2000 and May of 2007, 73 patients underwent implantation at 17 different institutions with the Berlin Heart Excor system. Fifty-one patients (70%)

were successfully bridged to transplant, five patients (7%) were bridged to recovery, and 17 patients (23%) died.[151] Rockett and associates also reported their experience with the Berlin Heart Excor. Between April of 2005 and May of 2008, 17 patients underwent implantation with the Berlin Heart Excor System. Eleven of those patients went on to transplant, two patients underwent explantation due to recovery, three died while on support, and one patient remained on support at the time of publication of the study.[180] Malarisrie and colleagues reported similar findings with eight patients with the Berlin Heart Excor implanted.[134] Five patients survived until transplant, and three died while on support. Of note, in both reports a high incidence of neurologic complications was noted, with seven of 11 patients reported by Rockett[180] and five of eight patients reported by Malarisrie.[134] Despite the high level of neurologic complications in both studies, many children survived to transplant who would likely have died otherwise without use of a VAD system.

In addition to the Berlin Heart Excor there has been a recent increased use of VADs originally designed for use in adults in the older pediatric population. Most of these are continuous flow devices allowing smaller size and easier implantation. The HeartWare HVAD (HeartWare, Inc, Framingham, MA) has been implanted successfully in individuals with a body Surface Area (BSA) of > 0.7 m². [125,147] The HeartMate II (Thoratec Corp, Pleasanton, CA) has been successfully implanted in patients with a BSA of > 1.2 m². [125,148] Both devices have increased portability with the ability to discharge home as compared to the Berlin Heart Excor, which to date has not been amenable to discharge home.

Use of a VAD or other mechanical support system offers additional benefits as well. Most notably for physical therapists is the ability to mobilize and engage in aggressive physical therapy soon after implantation of a VAD in children of all ages.[178,180] Experience at multiple centers has shown the benefits and safety of mobilizing patients after VAD implantation.[63,91,178,180,163,198,203] During the immediate postoperative period, while patients remain intubated, the focus of physical therapy is positioning and prevention of contractures. After extubation, progression will depend on the age and medical status of the patient.

An important consideration is providing families education and support for handling and positioning their infants and toddlers for caregiving and development.[91,178] Many times, families are very hesitant to handle and care for their children after implantation of a VAD. Through education and support, parents and other family members gain comfort with handling and transferring the child as medically appropriate. All care needs to be provided in coordination with the medical and nursing team.

As the infant or toddler becomes more stable, it is essential to provide as much of a normalized routine as possible, incorporating physical therapy, occupational therapy, speech therapy, and school and activity staff as appropriate. Consideration must be given to device limitations, but, as able, children should be progressed through activities to facilitate achievement of developmental milestones. Each different device will present its own unique challenges, and collaboration and training among team members of all disciplines are required to provide the most comprehensive and appropriate care.[63,91,178]

For the older child and adolescent, many of the same considerations as noted for the infant and the toddler apply. A team approach should be implemented to normalize the daily schedule as much as possible. Physical therapy should focus on increasing the child's independence with activities of daily living

(ADLs), transfers, and mobility in early therapy sessions, with progression to higher-level functional activities and strengthening and endurance activities as the child's condition allows. The goal is to have the child at peak conditioning and level of fitness at the time of transplantation. It is also important to discuss device safety and limitations as appropriate.[91,178,203] If possible, children should be provided opportunities for physical activity and socialization off of the medical unit with appropriately trained staff and family. Continuous flow devices have enabled children return to school, community, and home settings.[163,198] Pediatric physical therapists in a variety of settings have a role in promoting and monitoring physical activity of children with VADs.

Children with a VAD have a high rate of neurologic complications.[17,35] The physical therapist may be the first member of the team to observe signs and symptoms of neurologic impairment, such as onset of muscle weakness, changes in level of arousal, balance impairments, and changes in speech. These "red flags" should be immediately shared with the medical team and addressed in treatment. Children have demonstrated significant functional recovery after neurologic complications, and their ability to participate in therapy plays a large role in that recovery.[180]

Because of the integral role that mechanical assistive devices have as a bridge to transplant in children, a focus of research is to create devices that can be used by children at various stages of development.[11,208] Pediatric therapists are likely to see increased numbers of children with a mechanical assistive device. Comprehensive rehabilitation programs and therapy management plans will be integral to participation of children with mechanical assistive devices in home, school, and community activities.

Heart Transplantation

Cardiac transplantation is a viable option for children with end-stage heart failure secondary to congenital malformations or for children with cardiomyopathy. Advances in surgical technique, immunosuppressive medications, and treatment for rejection have increased the median survival posttransplant to 20.6 years for infant transplant recipients, 17.3 years for children transplanted between the ages of 1 and 5 years, 14.6 years for children transplanted between the ages of 6 and 10 years, and 12.9 years for adolescents.[51,209]

In the past, the indication for transplantation in children was largely cardiomyopathy (62%). In recent years the number of transplants for congenital heart defects has surpassed that of cardiomyopathy. In infants, 55% of transplants are completed due to congenital heart disease while cardiomyopathy accounts for 41%. In other age groups percentages are similar with approximately 66% and 23% of the 11- to 17-year-old, 59% and 32% of the 6- to 10-year-old, and 54% and 40% of the 1- to 5-year old recipients having had transplant for cardiomyopathy and congenital heart disease, respectively.[51]

Lamour and colleagues conducted a review of the impact of age, diagnosis, and previous surgery on children undergoing heart transplantation, using data from the Pediatric Heart Transplantation Study and the Cardiac Transplant Research Database.[112] They found that morbidity was higher post–heart transplant in patients with CHD (86%) than in those with cardiomyopathy (94%). The 5-year survival rate was approximately 80% among children who received heart transplants between 1990 and 2002. Other variables related to increased morbidity included long ischemic times, history of Fontan pretransplant, and older recipient age. The mortality rate was less for those undergoing a cardiac transplantation after a Glenn procedure than after a Fontan.[97] Griffiths evaluated patients with failing Fontan physiology and their response to heart transplantation.[77] They found that patients who were transplanted because of impaired ventricular function had a lower mortality rate than those with preserved ventricular function but with secondary problems such as protein-losing enteropathy, plastic bronchitis, ascites, and edema. Overall, more than 50% of patients who underwent heart transplantation as a teenager were still alive 15 years later. This number is even higher for those who received heart transplantation as infants.[104]

Surgery is performed through a median sternotomy and involves removal of the recipient heart with residual atrial cuffs remaining. The atria are reanastomosed with the donor heart, and then the great arteries are connected.[185] Severing of the vagus nerve and the cervical and thoracic sympathetic cardiac nerves leaves the heart denervated.[160] The heart has an intrinsic control system, so it is not dependent on innervation for function. Cardiac impulse formation occurs because of spontaneous depolarization of the sinoatrial node. This results in a higher than normal resting heart rate and a decreased heart rate response.[160]

Primary control of increased heart rate with exercise occurs due to catecholamine release from the adrenal gland. Hormonal release takes several minutes to have an effect on heart rate and contractility. As a result, during the acute phase of rehabilitation it is generally advised that children perform several minutes of warm-up exercises before vigorous exercise. It also takes several minutes for the body to reduce the hormones to normal levels, so a cool-down period at the end of exercise is also advised. The resting heart rate is higher than usual in transplant recipients, and the peak heart rate is lower; both should be taken into account when transplant patients are exercising.[160] There is an ongoing debate on the most effective rehabilitation approach for children following heart transplantation. With evidence suggesting some level of reinervation,[160] some have suggested higher levels of exercise and possible interval training may be possible. The potential benefit of moderate or higher intensity exercise is unclear, and further research is needed.[160]

Antirejection treatment begins with triple drug immunosuppression with corticosteroids, a calcineurin inhibitor (e.g., cyclosporine or tacrolimus), and an antiproliferative agent (e.g., azathioprine or mycophenolate mofetil).[185] All serve to combat rejection of the donor heart. Rejection is an immune response to the donor heart. The resulting inflammation occurs through T-cell and humoral immune mechanism. Failure to control the inflammation can result in necrosis of the cardiac tissue and death. Rejection is the number one cause of death posttransplant.[4] Transplant recipients are often weaned from the use of steroids as soon as possible to minimize the detrimental effects of long-term steroid use.[4] Antirejection medicines can lead to bone loss, photosensitivity, thickening of the gums, muscle and bone weakness, headaches, increased potassium levels, nausea, and increased cholesterol levels.

Rejection is a concern for all children who receive heart transplantation. Signs and symptoms of rejection include: fever, malaise, poor appetite, weight gain, tachycardia, tachypnea, low urine output, complete heart block, pulmonary edema, and shock.[4,150] Symptoms associated with severe rejection have been observed in several adolescent transplant recipients after missing just one dose of immunosuppressive medicine.

Several complications from heart transplantation are common in children. Hypertension immediately posttransplant occurs frequently, and the cause may be multifactorial including persistent elevation in systemic vascular resistance, use of oversized donor organs, and corticosteroid treatment.[150] Other early posttransplant complications include impaired renal function due to nephrotoxic qualities of many of the immunosuppressive medications, infection due to immunosuppression, and severe muscular deconditioning due to pretransplant medical status.[150] Long-term complications include continued rejection with symptoms of weakness, fatigue, malaise, fever, and flulike symptoms. We have used the dyspnea index previously described to help patients know there may be a change in their cardiac status and they should call their cardiologists. A patient who has received heart transplantation can exercise and achieve normal endurance with a baseline dyspnea index of 1 breath to count out loud to 15. If he or she suddenly requires 2 breaths or more to count out loud to 15 he or she should contact his or her cardiologist. Other complications that can occur are: coronary allograft vasculopathy, chronic infections, continued renal dysfunction, hypertension, hyperlipemia, and development of posttransplant lymphoproliferative disease (PTLD). PTLD can present as a wide range of malignancies from benign tonsillar hyperplasia to life-threatening monoclonal lymphoma.[4,150] Therapists working with children with heart transplantation need to be aware of these potential complications as well as their signs and symptoms. Often therapists are the first to notice symptoms and bring this to the attention of the medical team. As more children survive successful initial cardiac transplant, the potential need for retransplantation increases. Availability of donors, long-term survival, and functional outcomes are factors that continue to be investigated.

FOREGROUND INFORMATION

MANAGEMENT FOLLOWING CARDIAC SURGERY

Most acute impairments after thoracic surgical procedures occur in the immediate or early postoperative period. Physical therapists play an important role in minimizing and helping to address these impairments. In this section management of pulmonary complications, pain, sedation, decreased mobility, and initiation of developmental care will be described. Considerations for physical therapy management following cardiac surgery are summarized in Box 28.1.

Pulmonary Management

One of the primary areas to be addressed after heart repair is the pulmonary status of the patient. Mechanical ventilation is common after open-heart surgery in the pediatric patient. Recent improvements in cardiopulmonary bypass, decreased operating time, and improved postoperative fluid management have allowed early extubation, often immediately after or within 4–6 hours of surgery.[206] This has led to decreased costs, early patient mobility, and fewer respiratory complications.

Following extubation, some patients are transitioned to noninvasive ventilation such as CPAP and BiPAP. Noninvasive ventilation has been shown to improve gas exchange, reduce work of breathing, and help to avoid intubation in children. It can be provided via a variety of interfaces including nasal prongs, nasal mask, or nasal mask, full facial mask, or helmet.

As well current noninvasive ventilators provide a wide range of settings.[206] In addition to CPAP and BiPAP, a nasal cannula may be used to deliver heated humidified high-flow nasal oxygen. High-flow oxygen delivery provides continuous positive airway pressure.[206] Inhaled nitric oxide can also be used with patients who have pulmonary hypertension postoperatively.

BOX 28.1 Considerations for Physical Therapist Management of Children with Congenital Cardiac Conditions

Postsurgical Management

Positioning and respiratory techniques (e.g., percussion, vibration, assisted cough) to mobilize secretions and increase aeration
Early mobilization including range of motion exercises and walking
Screening for neurologic impairments
Supporting the family to interact and care for their child
Facilitating age-appropriate activities and developmental play

Infancy and Early Childhood

Screening for and monitoring neurologic impairments
Screening and intervention for developmental and sensorimotor delays
Facilitating mutually enjoyable parent–child interactions
Assessing and educating on feeding difficulties and providing support as necessary
Encouraging the family to allow their child to self-limit activity and play, rather than parent-limited activity and play
Providing the family information to help them anticipate how the child's cardiac condition might influence development (e.g., crawling is often limited in infants with a cyanotic defect)

Childhood and Adolescence

Screening for and monitoring neurologic impairments
Assessing endurance as well as visual-perceptual, visual-motor, motor planning, and fine motor skills and adapting recommendations for physical activity including instruction and education as necessary
Establishing an exercise program to improve the child's endurance, strength, self-esteem, and to decrease parental anxiety
Supporting the child to engage in regular exercise including participation in desired recreational activities and addressing parental concerns

---

Although physical therapist intervention varies with the age of the child, the primary goals are to mobilize secretions, increase aeration, and increase general mobility (Fig. 28.12).

The child's position should be changed regularly to assist with effective ventilation and oxygenation. The full upright position is considered most beneficial and should be achieved as soon as possible. The supine position has been shown to cause diminished alveolar volume, functional residual capacity (FRC), and lung compliance; it thus interferes with the distribution of ventilation, respiratory muscle efficiency, and gas exchange; and promotes airway closure. Sidelying has been observed to be a better position than supine for improving oxygenation. In adults, oxygenation improved when the "good" lung was in the dependent position.[222] In children, however, the opposite was observed: namely, gas exchange improved with the good lung uppermost.[222] Sidelying with the best lung dependent may improve ventilation and perfusion matching but should be closely monitored for signs of distress or improvement.[222] Prone position has been associated with an improved ventilation and decreased work of breathing.[222] Positioning in prone may be beneficial in preventing respiratory difficulty in a child who is extubated.

Mucous transport is slowed after surgery, which can lead to atelectasis. Atelectasis also occurs secondary to an altered breathing pattern, prolonged positioning in supine, and possible diaphragmatic dysfunction in the early postoperative period.[222] Incentive spirometry is an effective tool for reducing the occurrence of atelectasis in the pediatric population. The primary emphasis with incentive spirometry or any other respiratory intervention should be prolonged slow inspiration to facilitate end-expiratory lung volume helping to decrease atelectasis.[206] Bubble blowing or blowing on a windmill can be used with young children (Fig. 28.13).[206] When performing these activities, children often take in a large inspiration before exhaling. Other respiratory techniques such as percussion and postural drainage, vibration, segmental expansion, and assisted cough techniques (Fig. 28.14) can be performed to mobilize secretions and increase aeration.[222]

Segmental lung expansion techniques may be performed to reduce postoperative complications and are used to

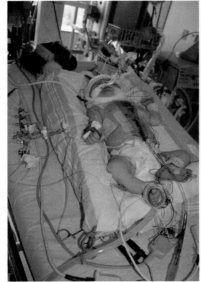 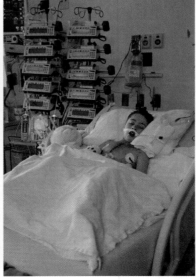

FIG. 28.12 Two examples of children 24 hours after open-heart surgery.

preferentially augment localized lung expansion. The goals are to increase and redistribute ventilation, improve gas exchange, aid in reexpansion of air spaces, mobilize the thoracic cage, and increase the strength, endurance, and efficiency of the respiratory muscles.[222]

Lung expansion techniques are performed by placing a hand over a particular segment and allowing it to move with the ventilator or respiratory cycle. Gentle pressure may be applied to the chest wall during exhalation at the end of the expiratory phase, just before the inspiratory phase. This facilitates airflow to the specific segment. When a specific lobe or segment has decreased aeration, this technique, used in conjunction with gentle sustained pressure on the opposite upper lobe, may increase aeration to the affected area.[222] This technique is particularly effective when the child is upset or does not tolerate percussion or other treatment techniques. It may decrease the respiratory rate and is especially useful with infants who cannot respond to the therapist's verbal cues for relaxation. We have used this technique with lung transplant recipients who are unable to cooperate or follow commands for deep breathing and coughing and found it effective in decreasing atelectasis

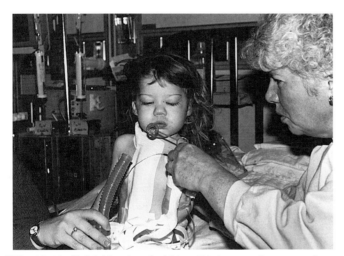

FIG. 28.13 Child blowing bubbles 24 hours after open-heart surgery.

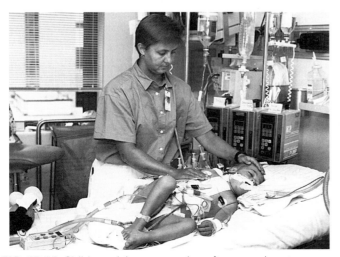

FIG. 28.14 Child receiving percussion after open-heart surgery.

and increasing oxygen saturation. Segmental expansion techniques performed before other respiratory techniques also may be beneficial.

Percussion may need to be performed to assist in removal of excess secretions. Percussion is defined as rhythmic clapping with cupped hands over the involved lung segment performed throughout the respiratory cycle, with the goal of mechanically dislodging pulmonary secretions.[222] Vibration also assists in mobilization of secretions. It is performed by creating a fine oscillating movement of the hand on the chest wall just before expiration and continuing until the beginning of inspiration.[222]

Both percussion and vibration techniques can be performed in conjunction with postural drainage. Optimal positions are described by Crane and are pictured in Frownfelter's text on chest physical therapy.[43] Positioning must be used with caution in the postoperative period. For example, the Trendelenburg position is often contraindicated after open-heart surgery. It is important to confirm with the nurse or the physician whether it is even suitable for the child to be flat in bed. Despite limitations, percussion and vibration can be performed in the positions available. It has been the authors' experience that children respond well to both percussion and vibration, even on the first postoperative day. Encouraging the child to tell you if the treatment hurts—because it should not be painful—often facilitates cooperation. It may also be helpful to coordinate the treatment with administration of pain medications. Percussion may be contraindicated when platelets are low, pulmonary artery pressures are too high, or the child becomes too agitated with treatment. Vibration can generally be safely used instead. Blood pressure and intracardiac pressures should be closely monitored throughout treatment because they are indicators of intolerance to treatment. The physician usually establishes parameters, set on an individual basis.

Massery described a counter rotation technique for altering respiratory rate in the neurologically impaired patient that has been safely used in children after open-heart surgery through a median sternotomy only.[222] The counter rotation technique has been used by the authors to slow the respiratory rate and increase expansion of the lateral segment. It generally relaxes children and increases their tidal volume. When the technique is used postoperatively following cardiac surgery, the therapist must take extreme caution to avoid disturbing chest tubes and other intravenous lines. This treatment is recommended only after intracardiac lines have been removed. The sternal incision has not been a problem: because it is stable, it does not undergo any mobilization during application of this technique. The counter rotation technique is performed with the child in sidelying and the therapist standing behind, near the child's buttocks. One hand is placed on the anterior iliac spine and the other hand is placed on the child's posterior shoulder. On inspiration the hand on the buttocks pulls down and posteriorly, while the hand on the shoulder gently pushes up and anteriorly. On expiration the therapist's hands and the child's body return to neutral. This is repeated several times in cycle with the child's breathing. It should be very relaxing and comfortable for the child.

The techniques described not only facilitate increased lung expansion but also mobilize secretions. Once mobilized, secretions act as an irritant in the airway when the child takes a deep breath, and a spontaneous cough usually occurs.[222] The child may require assistance to remove excess secretions, owing to

TABLE 28.2   FLACC Scale

	SCORING		
Categories	**0**	**1**	**2**
Face	No particular expression or smile	Occasional grimace or frown, withdrawn, disinterested	Frequent to constant quivering chin, clenched jaw
Legs	Normal position or relaxed	Uneasy, restless, tense	Kicking, or legs drawn up
Activity	Lying quietly, normal position, moves easily	Squirming, shifting back and forth, tense	Arched, rigid, or jerking
Cry	No cry (awake or asleep)	Moans or whimpers; occasional complaint	Crying steadily, screams or sobs, frequent complaints
Consolability	Content, relaxed	Reassured by occasional touching, hugging, or being talked to; distractible	Difficult to console or comfort

Merkel S: The FLACC: A behavioral scale for scoring postoperative pain in young children. *Pediatr Nurs* 23:293-297, 1997. Copyright 1997 by Jannetti Company, University of Michigan Medical Center.

lack of cooperation or to inability to cooperate secondary to age. This may be accomplished by coughing or airway suctioning.

Pain and Sedation Management

Pain management and level of sedation are extremely important for mobilization of children following cardiac surgery. Most institutions that perform cardiac surgery on children have pain management teams that assist the surgical team in monitoring and managing the child's postoperative pain because uncontrolled pain can be detrimental to the child's recovery. Monitoring and assessment of pain and level of sedation are critical components to an effective pain and sedation management regimen. The FLACC scale is often used to determine if the child is in pain (Table 28.2).

Opioids such as morphine and fentanyl are the primary medications employed for effective analgesia or pain relief. As with most medications they carry adverse side effects including respiratory depression and nausea and vomiting that must be monitored and balanced with appropriate pain relief.[175] In addition to pain relief, sedation management must also be considered. Sedation is often required to increase compliance and tolerance of treatment. In addition, it may be required to allow effective ventilation or support of cardiac function. Goals for sedation goals vary from mild calming to near anesthesia.[175] Several medications are used to achieve sedation; the two most common are dexmedetomidine and midazolam. Both medications provide appropriate levels of sedation without respiratory depression, though midazolam is not as well tolerated in the cardiac population.[175] Other techniques used to manage postoperative pain include regional anesthetic techniques and patient-controlled analgesia.[175]

Early Mobilization

Early mobilization and ambulation after surgery reduce both pulmonary and circulatory complications as well as demonstrate increases in functional outcomes and quality of life.[90,101,226] Early mobilization and physical therapy involvement in the adult ICU setting have been shown to have beneficial effects on muscle strength, physical function, health-related quality of life, ventilator-free days, and lengths of stay in the ICU and hospital.[101] Studies in the pediatric population are more limited but have shown similar results.[91,226] Postoperative immobility can lead to a variety of problems, including reduced ventilation and perfusion distribution, shallow breathing, fever, retention of secretions, fluid shifts, decreased muscle strength, and generalized discomfort from immobility.[219,222] The following section

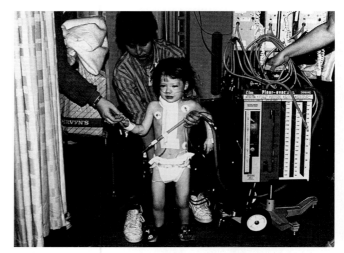

FIG. 28.15 A child walking 1 day after open-heart surgery.

reviews the importance of early mobilization and positioning and how to safely initiate both.

Range-of-motion (ROM) exercises should begin as soon as possible. Initially it may not be possible to attain full ROM because of discomfort or intravenous or arterial lines, but movement helps to mobilize the patient. ROM exercises are extremely important for the child with a thoracotomy incision because the incision tends to produce more guarding than is produced by a median sternotomy. Passive to active-assisted shoulder ROM to 90 degrees of flexion is usually tolerable. Discomfort often occurs when the arm is returned to a neutral position. The therapist may apply gentle resistance to the arm as the child attempts to return the arm to a neutral position because contraction of the arm muscles tends to minimize discomfort.

At our center, children are mobilized including ambulation as soon as atrial lines and groin lines are removed. Intubation with mechanical ventilation is not considered a reason not to initiate physical therapy intervention, though it may limit mobility. Children often ambulate for the first time with any or all of the following: central venous pressure line, peripheral intravenous line, arterial line, chest tubes, temporary pacemakers, and oxygen (Fig. 28.15). The first walk is often only for 5 to 10 feet and may be difficult for the child. Anxiety often plays as big role in the perceived difficulty as does the discomfort. It may be beneficial for the child to receive pain medication before the first walk. Children are often anxious, so the benefits of early

TABLE 28.3 Potential Limitations in Early Motor Development in Children With Congenital Heart Conditions

Age	Age-Expected Skills	Potential Limitations
0–3 months	Prone: lift head to 45 degrees, turn head to clear airway	Prone: lack of time and stimulation in prone
	Supine: reciprocal kicking, chin tuck, random upper extremity movement	Supine: prolonged period in supine, neck in hyperextension, arms restrained for IVs
	Sitting: head control 2–5 seconds, hands to surface for support	Sitting: limited time in upright/ being held and carried; arms not placed in flexion or weight-bearing position
	Standing: bear weight on lower extremities, hips not in line with trunk	Standing: limited to no time in supported standing
3–6 months	Prone: come up on extended upper extremities, arms beginning to be under shoulders	Prone: not encouraged to push with arms onto hands; lack of trunk strength due to not be carried
	Supine: bringing hands to mouth; starting to bring feet and knees to hands, rolling supine to prone	Supine: anterior incisions and prolonged supine weakens abdominal muscles so may have difficulty bringing hands to midline; feet to face and hands not encouraged; reaching across midline toward stimulation to roll is not encouraged or done
	Sitting: prop by 3–4 months with head steady, approaching independent by 6 months	Sitting: often not able to due to lack of opportunity, too much support, not carried on caregiver's hip
	Standing: in supported standing stands with hips in line with trunk	Standing: IV lines in groin may limit early lower extremity weight bearing; lack of time in prone limits time to strengthen hip extension against gravity
6–12 months	Prone: pivoting, coming up to 4-point, rocking in 4-point, creeping; rolling in and out of this position	Prone: Lack of prone time, upper extremity weight bearing and core stability; crawling and creeping may be too energy consuming, will move by rolling or scooting on back just not in 4-point, may desaturate if pushed
	Supine: fully function in and out of position	Supine: may have difficulty with segmental rolling due to lack of core strength
	Sitting: independent getting in and out of sitting, no support needed	Sitting: not willing to go into flexion to transition in and out of sitting to stand
	Standing: pulling to stand at surface, cruising, independent standing and early stepping	Standing: limited use of uppers and limited above head use of arms; toys brought to child instead of weight shifting and rotating to get toys
1–2 years	Independent walking progressing to low guard upper extremity position, running, throwing a ball underhand, weight shift to kick a ball	Delay in milestones, weak core and extremity proximal strength, lacks experience in standing, poor standing balance and trunk rotation
2–3 years	Climbing over objects and onto furniture; mature walking and running with arms down and reciprocal swing of arms; mature gait on stairs with reciprocal gait with one hand held; jumping with both feet off the ground; walking on heels and toes; kicking with some accuracy; throwing a ball overhand	Upper body weakness, lacks core strength, weakness of hip extensors and posture muscles; poor standing balance reactions; lack of experience with activity

ambulation should be explained to them with emphasis on the problems that can occur by remaining in bed.

Potential Effects of Cardiac Surgery on Early Motor Development

The potential effects of cardiac surgery on early motor development are summarized in Table 28.3. The infant who undergoes surgery within the first few days after birth experiences immediate disruption of all aspects of typical newborn life. The infant is often sedated, restrained, and intubated, all of which interfere with being held, bundled, and fed. The physical therapist provides the family information about sensory-motor activities the infant is unable to experience and instruction in ways to compensate for this deprivation. Encouraging parents, as well as nursing staff, to hold their child as soon as possible is recommended. Holding the infant prone on the parent's chest is beneficial to early development and bonding. The fact that their child is born with a congenital anomaly may impede the attachment process.[123] The therapist promotes parent-infant interaction by providing parents suggestions for engaging and calming their baby as well as positioning to minimize postoperative complications. We encourage therapists to involve parents in treatment as soon as possible.

Toddlers who have cardiac surgery often recover very quickly with little impairment. Anxiety over being left alone during the hospitalization may be the biggest problem interfering with function in this age group.[123] The child may feel abandoned and may react by becoming passive and apathetic or, conversely, by becoming aggressive. These behaviors are more commonly observed in the child who is in the hospital for the first time, such as the child with an ASD.

Toddlers are often limited more by restrictions imposed by their parents than by their own physical limitations.[40,123] Activity guidelines should be reviewed with parents on an ongoing basis; showing them by example may be even more helpful. Although it is beneficial to explain to the parents ahead of time what their child will experience, it may be helpful to wait to tell the toddler what is happening as it is happening. Connolly and colleagues evaluated children who underwent cardiac surgery at 5 to 12 years of age both preoperatively and postoperatively for posttraumatic stress disorder (PTSD) symptoms.[41] They found PTSD symptoms in 23% of the children, and 12% met criteria for PTSD. They also observed an increased number of symptoms correlated with an intensive care unit stay longer than 48 hours. The therapist can add "fun" to the postoperative activities to make it less threatening and ultimately more beneficial.

Adolescents who have cardiac surgery may need to be encouraged to move and may need to be assisted to become active. The parents are often more reluctant than the adolescent about early mobilization, including ambulation. They should be reassured that it is beneficial for their child to move as soon as possible. Adolescents may choose to assert their independence and try to do everything for themselves, or they may choose to become totally dependent on their parents and hospital staff. Whichever situation occurs, young people benefit from early education about how to move and what they should be doing. This helps them to realize what is expected of them. They should be informed of what they need to do and should not be given a choice when the task is not optional.[215]

Medical Complications

Several medical complications can affect postoperative function. Secondary to phrenic nerve palsy, some children may have a paralyzed diaphragm after surgery that affects their early postoperative course, as well as their long-term respiratory status and endurance.[206] Infants have horizontal ribs and lack the normal bucket handle movement, relying primarily on use of the diaphragm for respiration. Paralysis of the diaphragm by unilateral or bilateral phrenic nerve palsy can cause further respiratory problems, including difficulty in weaning from the ventilator.[206] Noninvasive positive-pressure ventilation has been successfully used for bilateral diaphragm paralysis until diaphragm function has returned.[109] In a study by Ross Russell and associates, phrenic nerve palsy was observed in as many as 20% of infants who underwent cardiac surgery, mechanical ventilation was at least an average of 72 hours in this group, and the risk of death before discharge from the hospital was greater than 10%.[188] The incidence was greater for those younger than 18 months of age, but two thirds of those with phrenic nerve palsy had fully recovered by 3 months postoperatively.

Prolonged mechanical ventilation is required for some children, especially infants, after surgery for congenital heart defects. Mechanical ventilation has been associated with nosocomial pneumonia, higher surgical risk, increased postoperative fluid, and low cardiac output.[201] Instances of children requiring a tracheostomy and/or gastrostomy after congenital heart surgery have been reported. Performing these procedures sooner may allow for earlier discharge from the hospital. The incidence of tracheostomy after surgery is fairly low at 1% or less,[186] but Kelleher and colleagues reported that 28% of their patients undergoing a Norwood operation required nasogastric tubes for feeding or placement of a gastrostomy tube at discharge from the hospital.[102] Guillemaud and associates found that at least 3% of all children with cardiac defects who underwent surgery had some type of airway problem, the most common being vocal cord paralysis.[79] This should be taken into account when an infant is having difficulty coming off the ventilator or when treating an infant with difficulty with oral feedings.

Neurologic Implications and Complications

Postoperative neurologic impairments were long thought to be largely due to prolonged surgical time, usually related to length of hypothermic arrest, low cardiac output, or arrhythmias after surgery.[58,224] Research on infants with congenital heart defects, however, has indicated that preoperatively brain maturation is delayed,[118] cerebral blood flow is diminished,[119] brain volumes are smaller,[121] and there is some incidence of mild ischemic lesions associated with periventricular leukomalacia.[119,130] Miller, et al.[149] observed that newborns with CHD had widespread brain abnormalities before cardiac surgery. Lynch et al.[126] studied neonates with HLHS and observed that earlier Norwood palliation may decrease acquired white matter injury. Neurodevelopment has also been noted to be affected postoperatively in children with repaired congenital heart defects possibly for several reasons, including how a child is rewarmed after surgery,[191] genetic factors,[68,232] seizures,[66] type of circulatory arrest,[20] and length of stay after surgery.[157] Seizures during the initial postoperative period are associated with a significant increase in abnormal neuromuscular findings. The mean Mental Developmental Index score on the Bayley Scales of Infant Development II was significantly lower for children with frontal lobe seizures compared to children with seizures in other areas of the brain.[66]

Hemodynamic instability and coagulation disturbances are risk factors for postoperative neurologic problems in infants as well. Thirty-five percent of premature infants weighing less than 2 kg who had open-heart surgery developed neurologic complications.[187] Neurologic consequences may be the result of an air embolus, a prolonged hypotensive period,[215] or complications of long-term cyanosis[5] as well as cerebral hypoxic-ischemic conditions.[87] Cerebral development may be deterred due to aortic-to-pulmonary collaterals that may develop in single-ventricle children and that can result in cerebral blood flow diminishing.[59] Choreoathetosis has been observed in some children after they have been on cardiopulmonary bypass. When a basal ganglia lesion is also seen, the prognosis is poor.[89] It is encouraging to note that of almost 700 children who underwent a Fontan operation, fewer than 3% had a stroke.[54]

In an attempt to reduce the risk of neurologic injury during surgery, some centers are using continuous regional cerebral perfusion, especially during aortic arch reconstruction.[30] Many centers are using near-infrared spectroscopy to monitor cerebral oxygenation in the perioperative period, but in a review of the literature on this topic, Hirsch and colleagues found little substantial evidence to support that the use of perioperative near-infrared spectroscopy has an impact on neurologic outcomes.[85] Multiple cardiac surgeries, longer hospital stays, poorer linear growth, and tube feeding were associated with worse neurologic outcomes in 131 children with CHD but without a known genetic defect.[153] Low regional cerebral oxygen saturation in the first 48 hours after the Norwood procedure was significantly correlated with an adverse outcome.[166]

Physical therapists are encouraged to seek opportunities to be involved in research to determine forms of cardiac monitoring that are associated with favorable postoperative neurologic outcomes. The child who has sustained a neurologic insult requires both early intervention and physical therapy following hospital discharge. A child with severe extensor tone may benefit from inhibitive casts on the lower extremities and hand splints to decrease the effects of increased tone and to maintain ROM. Parent education concerning the impact of a neurologic insult, including information on handling and positioning the child with increased muscle tone, appropriate stimulation, use of adaptive equipment, and long-term follow-up, should begin as soon as the diagnosis is confirmed. Box 28.2 summarizes characteristics of children with congenital cardiac conditions who are at highest risk for neurodevelopmental impairment

MANAGEMENT OF CHILDREN WITH CHRONIC ACTIVITY LIMITATIONS

Chronic Disabilities and Activity Limitations

Various disabilities and activity limitations occur as a result of primary impairments incurred by children with congenital heart defects (see Table 28.1). Considerations for physical therapy management are summarized in Box 28.1. The disabling process may start very early secondary to poor attachment between parent and infant.[75] Infants who had cardiac surgery showed less positive affect and engagement than typical babies, making it even more stressful for mothers who are already distressed.[65] Poor attachment can lead to poor social development.

The overprotection and excessive activity restrictions imposed by some parents may compound activity limitations. Parents have shared that they were afraid to permit physical activity in their child with CHD.[78] An important role of the physical therapist is to provide the family guidance in identifying physical activities that the child enjoys and has the physiologic capacity to safely perform. Maternal perceptions of their children's disease severity were a stronger predictor of emotional adjustment than was disease severity.[49] Emotional maladjustment may contribute to the poor self-esteem that is often noted in children with congenital heart defects. Limitations resulting from decreased activity, delayed development, poor self-esteem, overprotection by parents, and physical illness may lead to poor peer interactions and social participation. Concerns should be shared with parents and the child as early as possible to limit the potential effects on development.

Infancy

Recent research has been important in establishing the preoperative status of the brain, its development, and subsequent neurologic impairment in the infant with a congenital heart defect. Licht and associates assessed infants preoperatively with hypoplastic left heart syndrome and transposition of the great arteries.[118] Infants were found to have head circumferences that were smaller by a whole standard deviation, as well as brain development that lagged a full month behind their gestational age, thus indicating that in utero brain development is affected by the cardiac defect. This group of researchers also found that preoperative cerebral blood is diminished, which was sometimes associated with periventricular leukomalacia.[119] Thus children with congenital heart defects start off at a disadvantage neurologically and developmentally.

Infants with dextro-transposition of the great arteries who underwent a preoperative balloon atrial septostomy had an increased rate of embolic stroke compared with those who did not undergo balloon atrial septostomy.[113,157] Surveillance for this risk should be conducted when these infants are seen in the immediate postoperative period, or even later.

In children with CHD, several other contributing factors can lead to impairment and activity limitations in infancy. Common problems include poor feeding, poor growth, and developmental lag.[153] Owen et al.[162] found that infants with CHD showed poor behavioral state regulation leading them to become easily overwhelmed. This can add to parental anxiety. Parents must constantly watch for signs and symptoms of congestive heart failure in their infant at rest and while feeding. These signs include the onset of rapid breathing, changes in behavior, edema, excessive sweating, fatigue, vomiting, and poor feeding.[40] Parental frustration and stress can affect early attachment to the infant. It has been observed during the first year of life that securely attached infants showed greater improvements in health than did insecurely attached infants.[74] Gardner and associates observed infants with cardiac defects to be consistently less engaging with their mothers when compared with infants without defects.[65,67]

When compared with healthy infants and infants with cystic fibrosis, infants with CHD were the least attached to their mothers, and their parents were the most stressed.[75] Normal attachment may be difficult, particularly with the very sick infant who is frequently hospitalized. The health care team should begin working with the parents as early as possible on how they can interact with their infant to facilitate attachment and avoid overstimulating their infant. Positive gains were noted in feeding practices, parental anxiety, and worry as well as infant mental state when interventions were done to bolster mother–infant interaction, therapy, and parent skills training with infants with severe CHD and their mothers.[145]

It is not uncommon for infants with CHD to be poor feeders, which further increases parental stress. Infants with corrected cyanotic heart defects had a significantly delayed first feed when compared with those infants who had undergone correction for an acyanotic defect. They also had a longer duration from first feed to discharge.[94] The delay in being able to feed their infant followed by possible difficulty with feeding may add stress to the parents.

Many of the major centers that perform surgical repair for complex cardiac defects treat children from all over the world. It is important to be aware of the family's diet and foods that are available in their country, the size of the child's parents, and the issues surrounding the surgery when a child's nutritional state is evaluated. Vaidyanathan and colleagues studied the nutritional status of children in South India after surgical repair for congenital heart defects and found that persistent malnutrition was predicted by birth weight and initial nutritional status as well as by parental anthropometry.[214]

Infants expend most of their energy during eating. In normal infants, decreased ventilation is observed during feeding, creating a decrease in the partial pressure of oxygen and an increase in the partial pressure of carbon dioxide.[137,138] This decrease in ventilation may seriously compromise the child with CHD and is compounded by the increase in metabolic rate. Not only does the child not eat well, but he or she also requires more calories to thrive.[71] When studying infants with CHD after surgery, Nydegger and colleagues found that an increased resting energy expenditure before surgery persisted in infants repaired after 10 days of life; by 6 months of age, it was comparable to that in infants without CHD.[159] Abnormalities in mesenteric perfusion are documented in several studies, with mesenteric hypoperfusion noted after the Norwood operation.[47,82] This may lead to feeding intolerance in addition to difficulty in getting enough calories into the child's body.

Watching their child failing to thrive can be devastating to parents and increase their anxiety about feeding their child and trying to encourage adequate caloric intake.[71] The prolonged time the child needs to feed can be frustrating to parents and make them feel inadequate.[32,123] Dysphagia has been observed in 24% of infants with CHD who were studied postoperatively with 63% of those infants exhibiting aspiration on a videofluoroscopic swallow study.[228] If alternative feeding methods are used, such as nasogastric or gastrostomy tube feedings, parents should be educated not only on how to administer the feeding but also on how to hold and nurture their child during the feeding.[123] It may be helpful to tell parents that providing time for nonstressful interaction may improve the parent-infant attachment and ultimately may improve the health of their infant. It is helpful to inform parents that the overall time that supplemental feedings are necessary varies with each child. Some parents have stated that they were able to remove supplemental feedings within 1 week of leaving the hospital; others have stated that it took months for their child to take enough by mouth to be able to discontinue supplemental feedings. Many parents have stated to these authors that their infant ate better at home, where it was possible to eat on demand and to have a more routine day.

Physical therapy assessment is sometimes indicated to observe the infant feeding and parental interaction. Other problems unrelated to poor endurance may be exhibited by the infant with CHD. If oral-motor dysfunction exists, it should be addressed with parents as soon as possible. Some parents need assistance in how best to handle and support their child during feeding. It can be beneficial for parents to observe that their child does not feed well for anyone.

Poor growth is closely associated with poor feeding. It has been observed that infants with cyanotic heart disease have poor growth in height and weight, whereas infants with acyanotic heart disease, specifically those with a large left-to-right shunt, are severely underweight secondary to the marked increase in metabolism.[71] Growth improves after surgery, but the child may not achieve typical parameters. This lack of catch-up growth is especially remarkable in children with cyanotic defects with a right-to-left shunt.[71,183] Poor growth in height was associated with worse neurodevelopmental outcomes in infants with single ventricles.[174]

Functional and activity limitations, especially delayed achievement of basic motor skills, can be observed in the infant with cardiac disease. Schultz and associates assessed the development of infants with CHD who had undergone repair before 6 months of age and compared them with their twin siblings without CHD.[197] They found that infants with CHD had lower scores on the Psychomotor Developmental Index of the Bayley Scales of Infant Development II compared with the Mental Developmental Index and both indices were lower than those of their siblings without CHD. Infants with a univentricular heart were evaluated using the Alberta Infant Motor Scale and scored significantly lower than healthy infants especially in the prone and standing subscales; the infants with hypoplastic left heart syndrome were delayed in all subsets.[171] Many of the infants did not walk until almost 18 months. This is not that surprising considering most of these infants spent several months of their life in an ICU and experienced some level of hypoxia during this developing period.

Decreased nutrition and cardiac function may leave the infant too weak to expend the energy required for typical motor activity.[123] Some children with cyanotic heart defects preferentially scoot around on their buttocks and, even after extensive intervention at home, do not crawl. They often go on to walking without ever crawling,[99] probably because of the increased energy expenditure associated with use of both upper and lower extremities in crawling. Children with cyanotic heart defects tend to have an internal mechanism that permits them to do only what they are physically capable of doing, given their oxygen saturation.[40] They often rest without cueing and can rarely be pushed beyond what they are willing to do. Intervention may or may not improve the child's functional abilities; however, it may help relieve parental anxiety. The focus is on quality and efficiency of movement for exploration and play, instead of developmental delay. Therapists are encouraged to collaborate with parents to address concerns regarding physical activity and identify motor activities that promote positive parent–child interactions and can be incorporated into the family's daily routines, rather than one block of time.

The presence of congestive heart failure is associated with mental and motor developmental delay. Infants with congestive heart failure scored less well than expected on the Bayley Scales of Infant Development I as early as 2 months of age.[3] Haneda and associates observed a significant decrease in developmental quotient on the Gesell Developmental Schedules in infants and children who had circulatory arrest time greater than 50 minutes.[81] This information is useful when working with parents to help them understand that their child is demonstrating typical developmental skills for a child with CHD. This does not mean that intervention is not indicated. Resolution of neuromotor impairments by 15 months of age was reported for infants with CHD who had abnormal findings at 4–6 months of age and subsequently received physical therapy.[37] Therapists are encouraged to collaborate with families to promote motor development. If impairments in body functions and structures and activity limitations are minimized, the effects of reparative surgery may be dramatic.

Neurologic impairment and activity limitations may also occur from physiologic factors related to the surgical repair. Discrepancy exists regarding the effects of deep hypothermia and circulatory arrest on the psychomotor and intellectual development of infants.[26,80,146,187,200] Messmer and associates observed no delay in psychomotor and intellectual development in infants after deep hypothermia.[146] Kaltman and associates evaluated neurodevelopmental outcome in infants after an early repair for a VSD.[100] Mean mental and psychomotor indices were within the normal range for children who did not have a suspected or confirmed genetic syndrome. In another study, infants did not have neurologic impairments after surgery but did demonstrate mild developmental delays, most pronounced in infants with cyanotic heart defects.[80] Bellinger and associates observed that infants who had total circulatory arrest during the arterial switch operation scored lower on the Bayley Scales of Infant Development at 1 year of age than infants who had low-flow bypass.[21] These children were also observed to have expressive language difficulties at 2.5 years of age and exhibited more behavior problems.[21]

Deep hypothermic circulatory arrest greater than 40 minutes correlated with a greater occurrence of seizures postoperatively.[68] Clancy and associates observed seizures postoperatively in greater than 11% of infants in the immediate postoperative period.[39] All of the infants had undergone cardiopulmonary bypass during surgery.[39] The presence of a genetic syndrome was a strong predictor of lower scores on the Bayley Scales of Infant Development.[156] Gessler and associates performed neurologic examinations on infants preoperatively and postoperatively and reported mild asymmetries in muscle tone in one third of the infants preoperatively and in almost two thirds postoperatively.[69] They also found that the inflammatory response to cardiopulmonary bypass has an adverse effect on neuromotor outcome. Research by Sahu and associates indicates that weaning the infant off bypass at lower temperatures lowers the risk for postoperative neurophysiologic dysfunction more than weaning at slightly higher temperatures.[191] Parental report of their children's health-related quality of life at 1 year and 4 years after open-heart surgery was lower in the physical and cognitive dimensions especially if there was an underlying genetic defect or the infant was tube fed.[225]

There is a need for research to identify factors that are predictive of risk for neurologic impairments in young children after cardiac surgery.[211] In light of conflicting evidence, therapists should realize there is some uncertainty. Parents should be advised that their child might take longer than usual to accomplish developmental milestones. In a comprehensive review of the literature from the mid 1970s to the late 1990s, the overall long-term development of children after repair or palliation for CHD as infants was within the expected range for most standardized tests.[131]

Early Childhood

The young child (3–5 years of age) with chronic disabilities related to CHD has spent a lot of time in a medical environment. This familiarity with the environment may help to alleviate some of the child's and the parents' anxieties when surgery is imminent. Parental anxieties can be exacerbated during this period, however, as they begin to realize the impact that their child's cardiac disease has on growth and development. The child's symptoms could be worsening, and another surgery may soon be needed. Parent responses and interactions during this period are important; it should be recognized that parents already have the tendency to be overprotective of their child, and this may increase during the preschool period.

The emotional adjustment of the child has been observed to be affected by the mother's perception of the severity of the child's illness more than by its actual severity.[49] Among children with repaired CHD, increased parental stress was associated with behavior problems at 4 years of age.[218] In children with acyanotic heart defects, lower intelligence quotient was associated with poorer adjustment, greater dependence, and greater maternal pampering and anxiety.[173] These findings suggest that if a mother perceives her child's health challenges to be more severe than they are and limits the child accordingly, the child's physical development and social participation may be

affected. If this is a concern, we recommend that the therapist and parents discuss activities the child is capable of performing and observe whether the child self-limits physical activity when necessary.

Atallah and associates evaluated the mental and psychomotor developmental indices of children after the Norwood procedure and compared the traditional modified Blalock-Taussig shunt era with the newer right ventricle–to–pulmonary artery shunt era.[7] The mental development index did not differ between the two groups. Children who received the right ventricle–to–pulmonary artery shunt, however, had a psychomotor development index and more frequent sensorineural hearing loss.

Children with CHD have been reported to have developmental delays, especially those children with cyanotic disease.[21,56,135,173] Children with cyanosis scored significantly lower than children who were acyanotic and children without a cardiac condition on all subscales of the Gesell Developmental Schedules[81] and on Stanford-Binet and Cattell intelligence tests.[173] Children with cyanotic heart defects were observed to sit and walk later than children with acyanotic heart defects and children with typical development and were slower in speaking phrases than were children without disabilities.[56,173,202] Curtailment of physical activity in the child with severe cardiac dysfunction interferes with manipulation of objects, which facilitates sensorimotor processes.[173,202] When toddlers at 24 months of age (who had undergone open-heart surgery before 3 months of age) were assessed using the Peabody Developmental Motor Scale, gross motor quotients improved but fine motor quotients decreased significantly. All scores were less than average; fine motor quotients were greater than 1 standard deviation below the mean.[192] Despite concerns about the impact of limitations in amount of movement and manipulation of objects, intelligence and behavior are often within age expectations.[73] Activities of daily living are another area of development to consider.[120]

Educating parents about what their child is able to do is as important as teaching precautions. Children made significant improvement in gross motor advances during their second year of life when parental warmth was combined with a decrease in parental restrictions. It was also observed that children with CHD performed better on intelligence tests when their parents attempted to accelerate their children's development.[173] Parents should be informed that children with cardiac disease, particularly cyanotic disease, limit their own activity and stop and rest when needed.[40] Physical therapists can support the family in becoming more comfortable encouraging the child to initiate and sustain play within the limits of physical endurance. Children with Down syndrome and a cardiac defect were observed to score higher on developmental tests and achieve feeding milestones earlier if parents implemented therapy recommendations.[44]

Childhood

Cognitive function was not found to be affected in children who underwent an ASD repair between ages 3 and 17 years while on cardiopulmonary bypass.[204] However, children may be at risk for learning problems and academic issues independent of surgical closure or transcatheter closure.[194] This is an important finding because it has long been believed that this was a primary factor in neurologic problems after surgery for congenital heart defects. Children with an ASD, however, do not have the same associated risk factors, such as unstable hemodynamics, chronic hypoxemia, and metabolic acidosis, that children with other congenital heart defects have, particularly those with cyanotic heart defects. When comparing children who had an ASD closed surgically (using cardiac bypass) and children who had interventional closure by cardiac catheterization, Visconti and associates found that scores on the Wechsler Intelligence Scale for Children were significantly lower in the surgical closure group.[217] This was largely due to impairments in visual-motor and visual-spatial functions. Children who had interventional closure by cardiac catheterization, however, had significantly lower scores for sustained attention.

Bellinger and associates compared development and neurologic status of children who received hypothermic circulatory arrest during surgery compared with children who received low-flow cardiopulmonary bypass.[22] The two groups did not differ in IQ or overall neurologic status, but both groups had scores below age expectations for visual-spatial and visual-motor integration skills. Children with hypothermic circulatory arrest had lower scores on balance, nonlocomotor ability, and manual dexterity and more difficulty with speech, particularly with imitating oral movements and speech sounds. Bellinger and associates confirmed visual-perceptual motor deficits in another group of children who had undergone cardiac surgical repair as infants.[19] The findings were not associated with operative methods, but nevertheless the literature supports that all children undergoing surgical repair for a cardiac defect should be considered at risk for neurodevelopmental problems, especially visual-perceptual problems. Mahle and associates performed a similar study but did not find differences in verbal or performance IQ regardless of whether or not the child underwent cardiac bypass.[129] Along with congenital heart defects and subsequent surgery, children are at risk for lower IQ scores if they have other defects or a lower socioeconomic status.[60] Physical and psychosocial functioning were influenced negatively by lower family income.[144] Special attention should be given to children with congenital heart defects and a lower socioeconomic status.

School adjustment and peer interaction have been observed to be altered in children with CHD. In a study by Youssef, school absenteeism was high and proportionate to the severity of disability.[229] It has been observed that a child's adjustment to school is affected more by strain on the family than by the child's physical limitations related to the CHD.[34] Teachers have noted that children with CHD had more school problems; especially boys. Children with more behavior problems had lower self-esteem and more depression.[229] Some of the inability to focus and sustain attention on a task may be related to the surgery, the cardiac defect in and of itself, and frustration with the difficulty associated with visual-motor skills and completing fine motor tasks.[19,105] After surgical intervention, some of the behavioral problems may be alleviated; both missing school and diminished activity level should improve postoperatively.[122] Children may need rehabilitation after surgical repair, however, to learn how much they are capable of doing, to address limitations in visual-perceptual and fine motor tasks, and to help them manage activity limitations or inability to perform a task. This is critical due to the association between behavioral abnormalities and motor problems in children with CHD.[117]

Surgery to correct a cyanotic defect has a positive impact on the child's development. Improvement in IQ following surgery has been reported[122,161] and intellectual development was found to be essentially normal in children after the Fontan operation.[213]

Mahle and associates observed, however, that school-age children with hypoplastic left heart syndrome who had a seizure before their initial surgery scored lower on all IQ subsets.[132] Children with hypoplastic left heart syndrome were observed to have reduced exercise tolerance and more frequent education and behavioral concerns.[45] Self-confidence, social confidence, and general adjustment have been reported to improve after surgery.[122] Significant improvement in self-perception was observed in children after they had their heart defect repaired.[227] To the extent decreased experiences are a factor in developmental delay, a child whose activity is no longer limited by a cardiac defect should demonstrate an increased rate of development.

Parental overprotectiveness can continue to prove more limiting to a child's development than the defect itself. Parents were found to underestimate their child's exercise tolerance in 80% of the cases studied by Casey and associates.[33] Parents were also found to rate their child lower cognitively than the child scored on standardized neurologic testing administered by a professional.[129] Parental restriction generally begins with the advice of the physician and proceeds from there,[40,108] but parent perception of the physician's advice can be unclear. Longmuir and McCrindle evaluated the physical activity restrictions of children after the Fontan operation.[124] Twenty percent of children were being unnecessarily restricted in physical exertion by their parents. Yet only 40% of parents knew that their child should not participate in competitive sports, and 50% of parents did not understand that their child had body contact restrictions as a result taking anticoagulation medication.

Social and emotional maladjustment in children with cardiac disease can be due to maternal maladjustment and guilt.[108] Parental stress has been found to be correlated with IQ scores and with receptive language abilities, behavior scores, and socialization skills.[133] Psychosocial or family therapy interventions by professionals are sometimes recommended to facilitate positive parent–child interactions. Some improvement in maternal interaction and attitude was noted after surgical correction of the child's cardiac defect.[161] Interestingly, a study by Laane and associates found that children with congenital heart defects reported a higher quality of life than healthy children.[111] It was also observed that parents of children with hypoplastic left heart syndrome described their children's health, physical ability, and school performance as average or above.[132] When compared with healthy children, children with repaired pulmonary atresia had an overall equal quality of life.[55] It is important for therapists to keep these findings in mind when interacting with children with congenital heart defects and their families.

Adolescence

Adolescents who have CHD and physical limitations may have feelings of anxiety and impulsiveness.[110,154] Early professional intervention to assist the parents and child to cope best with the child's physical limitations may be helpful. It is also important to continue to monitor adolescents with CHD who underwent surgery as an infant. Studies are now finding diminished white matter, which may contribute to cognitive issues as well as decreased cortical grey matter.[181,220] Executive functions, perceptual reasoning, memory, visual perception, and visuomotor integration were found to be lower in adolescents with repaired CHD when compared to peers without CHD.[196,220]

A delay in the onset of puberty may further complicate social development and participation of adolescents with CHD. Body structure of adolescents with CHD was found to be different from adolescents with typical development.[6] Height and weight were significantly reduced in adolescents with CHD. Head, neck, and shoulder measurements were similar to those of healthy adolescents, but the thorax, trunk, pelvis, and lower extremities were significantly smaller. The anterior-posterior diameter of the pelvis was so reduced that it appeared almost flat. Physical differences of this magnitude can contribute to adolescents with CHD feeling different and low self-esteem.

Participation in physical activities, including guidelines on how to participate, may improve peer interaction and ultimately self-esteem of adolescents with CHD. Children who participated in an exercise program were observed to have improvement in their self-esteem as well as in their strength. Parents were found to be less restrictive and had less anxiety about their child after a formal exercise program.[52]

Exercise prescription for children with CHD should account for the type of cardiac defect and surgical intervention, as well as possible alterations in the child's response to exercise. The American Heart Association has published an extensive review of exercise testing in children, including recommendations for children with congenital heart defects.[96] Exercise testing performed on children 5 to 18 years after their operation for a Fontan revealed significantly lower maximal workload, maximal oxygen uptake, and maximal heart rate compared with peers without CHD. Children post Fontan surgery were also observed to have less efficient oxygen uptake during submaximal exercise.[179] Children post Fontan surgery who had a persistent right-to-left shunt were found to have decreased oxygen saturation levels during exercise.[207] This needs to be taken into account when any kind of therapy is provided to children who have a history of the Fontan procedure.

Children who participated in cardiac rehabilitation programs have made significant and beneficial changes in hemodynamics and improvement in exercise endurance and tolerance.[12,15,72,106,139,165,189] Following physical training, adolescents with CHD had near typical activity levels.[72] Children tested 10 years after an arterial switch procedure demonstrated excellent exercise capacity.[92] Psychological improvements may be noticeable and as important as physical improvements.[52,106,134]

Adolescents who have undergone heart transplantation are able to achieve an increase in cardiac output in response to exercise; however, they do not achieve the same peak workloads or maximal oxygen consumption as do adolescents without cardiac conditions.[38] During the early phase of rehabilitation, many children with transplanted hearts, lungs, or heart-lungs are so debilitated that they are unable to perform at an intensity that would raise their heart rate. The dyspnea index used as part of the Stanford heart transplant protocol is helpful in monitoring the child's physical tolerance during activity.[190] The child counts out loud to 15. The goal initially is to attempt to do this on one breath. At first, it may take three breaths to count to 15 while at rest. Exercise should increase the number of breaths to reach the count of 15 by only one or two breaths and should not be resumed until a return to resting baseline. Most children progress quickly, usually reaching 15 on one breath within 1 week of beginning exercise. The dyspnea index is an easily used measure for self-monitoring of exercise tolerance at home.[99] Children who underwent heart transplantation in infancy were found to have exercise capacities that were not different from those of children without cardiac conditions.[1] They did have a slightly lower peak heart rate, peak oxygen consumption, and a lower anaerobic threshold, but the respiratory exchange ratio was equal and the oxygen pulse index did not differ significantly.

Following heart, heart-lung, and lung transplants, children and youth often experience marked improvements after rehabilitation.[27] Following heart-lung transplantation, children have an increased ventilator response to exercise.[13,14,199] The dyspnea index is useful in monitoring physical tolerance to activity. The authors have found the dyspnea index highly beneficial for adolescents after transplant to change their lifestyle, as well as increase physical endurance. Quality of life often improves dramatically following heart transplantation with most children reported to be functioning at an age-appropriate level without developmental delays.[53,114,158]

In a systematic review of long-term survival and morbidity in the presence of CHD, Verheught and associates reported that survival is decreased in individuals with CHD when compared with the normal survival rate. Morbidity increased with more complex CHD. The review also concluded that supraventricular arrhythmias were prevalent in patients with ASD, transposition of the great arteries (TGA), and tetralogy of Fallot (TOF); ventricular arrhythmias were more prevalent in TOF, and CVAs were more common with TGA, ASD, and coarctation of the aorta. Heart failure, cyanosis, and complexity of lesions are predictors of increased mortality in adults with CHD. Increased ventilatory response or poor exercise capacity in adults 25 years after a Mustard or Senning operation for transposition of the great arteries increased risk for cardiac emergency or death.[70] Fredriksen and associates[61] found that patients who underwent surgical correction for TGA demonstrated a gradual decline in exercise performance with age and a significantly lower exercise capacity than healthy peers.[61] The International Society for Adult Congenital Heart Disease published an extensive report on the guidelines and management of adults with CHD.[221] Readers are referred to this resource for information on management of adults with repaired congenital heart defects.

SUMMARY

The physical therapist has an integral role in the habilitation and rehabilitation of children with congenital heart conditions. This chapter provided foundation knowledge for physical therapists on congenital heart conditions, surgical and medical management, and implications for physical activity and development. Because medical procedures and surgical interventions are occurring earlier, it has become increasingly important for physical therapists to monitor motor development and support parent–child interaction to promote socioemotional development. A major role of the physical therapist involves education and instruction to address parental concerns about physical activity. Knowledge of the physical capacity of children with congenital heart conditions is essential to promote motor development and for leisure and recreational activities.

Case Scenarios on Expert Consult

The case scenarios related to this chapter involve the following two topics: cardiomyopathy and complex cyanotic congenital heart disease. The first case looks at a 10-year-old child with a history of cardiomyopathy and a recent heart transplantation receiving physical therapy as an outpatient. The case includes a video that demonstrates exercising after heart transplantation. The second case looks at a child with complex cyanotic congenital heart disease. The child is presented from birth through age 26. Changes in physical capacity and physical therapy interventions at different ages are described.

REFERENCES

1. Abarbanell G, Mulla N, Chinnock R, Larsen R: Exercise assessment in infants after cardiac transplantation, *J Heart Lung Transplant* 23:1334–1338, 2004.
2. Adachi I, Khan MS, Guzmán-Pruneda FA, et al.: Evolution and impact of ventricular assist device program on children awaiting heart transplantation, *Ann Thorac Surg* 99(2):635–640, 2015.
3. Aisenberg RB, Rosenthal A, Nadas AS, Wolff PH: Developmental delay in infants with congenital heart disease, *Pediatr Cardiol* 3:133–137, 1982.
4. Ameduri R, Canter CE: Pediatric Heart Transplantation. In Mavroudis C, Backer C, editors: *Pediatric cardiovascular medicine*, ed 4, Hoboken, NJ, 2013, Blackwell, pp 1001–1120.
5. Amitia Y, Blieden L, Shemtove A, Neufeld H: Cerebrovascular accidents in infants and children with congenital cyanotic heart disease, *Isr J Med Sci* 20:1143–1145, 1984.
6. Angelov G, Tomova S, Ninova P: Physical development and body structure of children with congenital heart disease, *Hum Biol* 52:413–421, 1980.
7. Atallah J, Dinu IA, Joffe AR, et al.: Two-year survival and mental and psychomotor outcomes after the Norwood procedure, *Circulation* 118:1410–1418, 2008.
8. Reference deleted in proofs.
9. Backer CL, Kaushal S, Mavroudis C: Coarctation of the aorta. In Mavroudis C, Backer C, editors: *Pediatric cardiovascular medicine*, ed 4, Hoboken, NJ, 2013, Blackwell, pp 256–282.
10. Backer CL, Mavroudis C: Atrial septal defect, partial anomalous pulmonary venous connection, and scimitar syndrome. In Mavroudis C, Backer C, editors: *Pediatric cardiovascular medicine*, ed 4, Hoboken, NJ, 2013, Blackwell, pp 295–310.
11. Baldwin JT, Borovetz HS, Duncan BW, et al.: The National Heart, Lung and Blood Institute pediatric circulatory support program, *Circulation* 113:147–155, 2006.
12. Balfour IC, Drimmer AM, Nouri S, et al.: Pediatric cardiac rehabilitation, *Am J Dis Child* 145:627–630, 1991.
13. Banner N, Guz A, Heaton R, et al.: Ventilatory and circulatory responses at the onset of exercise in man following heart or heart-lung transplantation, *J Physiol* 399:437–449, 1988.
14. Banner NR, Lloyd MH, Hamilton RD, et al.: Cardiopulmonary response to dynamic exercise after heart and combined heart-lung transplantation, *Br Heart J* 61:215–223, 1989.
15. Bar-Or O: Physical conditioning in children with cardiorespiratory disease. In Terjung RL, editor: *Exercise and sport science review*, New York, 1985, Macmillan, pp 305–334.
16. Barron DJ, Kilby MD, Davies B, et al.: Hypoplastic left heart syndrome, *Lancet* 374:551–564, 2009.
17. Bastardi HJ, Naftel DC, Webber SA, et al.: Ventricular assist devices as a bridge to heart transplantation in children, *J Cardiovasc Nurs* 23:25–29, 2008.
18. Bautista-Hernandez V, Thiagarajan RR, Flynn-Thompson F, et al.: Preoperative extracorporeal membrane oxygenation as a bridge to cardiac surgery in children with congenital heart disease, *Ann Thorac Surg* 88:1306–1311, 2009.
19. Bellinger DC, Bernstein JH, Kirkwood MW, et al.: Visual-spatial skills in children after open-heart surgery, *J Dev Behav Pediatr* 24:169–179, 2003.
20. Bellinger DC, Jonas RA, Rappaport LA, et al.: Developmental and neurologic status of children after heart surgery with hypothermic circulatory arrest or low-flow cardiopulmonary bypass, *N Engl J Med* 332:549–555, 1995.
21. Bellinger DC, Rappaport LA, Wypij D, et al.: Patterns of developmental dysfunction after surgery during infancy to correct transposition of the great arteries, *J Dev Behav Pediatr* 18:75–83, 1997.
22. Bellinger DC, Wypij D, duPlessis AJ, et al.: Neurodevelopmental status at eight years in children with dextro-transposition of the great arteries: the Boston circulatory arrest trial, *J Thorac Cardiovasc Surg* 126:1385–1396, 2003.
23. Berg AM, Snell L, Mahle WT: Home inotropic therapy in children, *J Heart Lung Transplant* 26:453–457, 2007.
24. Bibevski S, Friedland-Little J, Ohye R, et al.: Truncus arteriosus. In Da Cruz EM, Ivy D, Jaggers J, editors: *Pediatric and congenital cardiology, cardiac surgery and intensive care*, London, 2014, Springer, pp 1983–2001.
25. Birnbaum BF, Simpson KE, Boschert TA, et al.: Intravenous home inotropic use is safe in pediatric patients awaiting transplantation, *Circ Heart Fail* 8(1):64–70, 2015.
26. Blackwood MJ, Haka-Ikse K, Steward DJ: Developmental outcome in children undergoing surgery with profound hypothermia, *Anesthesiology* 65:437–440, 1986.
27. Bolman RM, Shumway SS, Estrin JA, Hertz MI: Lung and heart-lung transplantation, *Ann Surg* 214:456–470, 1991.
28. Bonello B, Fouilloux V, Le Bel S, et al.: Ventricular septal defects. In Da Cruz EM, Ivy D, Jaggers J, editors: *Pediatric and congenital cardiology, cardiac surgery and intensive care*, London, 2014, Springer, pp 1455–1478.
29. Botto LD, Mulinare J, Erickson JD: Occurrence of congenital heart defects in relation to maternal multivitamin use, *Am J Epidemiol* 151:878–884, 2000.
30. Bove EL, Ohye RG, Devaney EJ: Hypoplastic left heart syndrome: conventional surgical management, *Semin Thorac Cardiovasc Surg Pediatr Card Surg Annu* 7:3–10, 2004.
31. Brink J, Brizard C: Sub-aortic stenosis. In Da Cruz EM, Ivy D, Jaggers J, editors: *Pediatric and congenital cardiology, cardiac surgery and intensive care*, London, 2014, Springer, pp 1599–1614.
32. Bruning MD, Schneiderman JU: Heart failure in infants and children. In Michaelson CR, editor: *Congestive heart failure*, St. Louis, 1983, Mosby, pp 467–484.
33. Casey FA, Craig BG, Mulholland HC: Quality of life in surgically palliated complex congenital heart disease, *Arch Dis Child* 70:382–386, 1994.
34. Casey FA, Sykes DH, Craig BG, et al.: Behavioral adjustment of children with surgically palliated complex congenital heart disease, *J Pediatr Psychol* 21:335–352, 1996.
35. Cassidy J, Haynes S, Kirk R, et al.: Changing patterns of bridging to heart transplantation in children, *J Heart Lung Transplant* 28:249–254, 2009.
36. Chang RK, Chen AY, Klitzner TS: Clinical management of infants with hypoplastic left heart syndrome in the United States, 1988-1997, *Pediatrics* 110:292–298, 2002.
37. Chock VY, Chang IJ, Reddy MV: Short-term neurodevelopmental outcomes in neonates with congenital heart disease: the era of newer surgical strategies, *Congenit Heart Dis* 7(6):544–550, 2012.
38. Christos SC, Katch V, Crowley DC, et al.: Hemodynamic responses to upright exercise of adolescent cardiac transplant patients, *J Pediatr* 121:312–316, 1992.
39. Clancy RR, Sahrif U, Ichord R, et al.: Electrographic neonatal seizures after infant heart surgery, *Epilepsia* 46:84–90, 2005.
40. Clare MD: Home care of infants and children with cardiac disease, *Heart Lung* 14:218–222, 1985.
41. Connolly D, McClowry S, Hayman L, et al.: Posttraumatic stress disorder in children after cardiac surgery, *J Pediatr* 144:480–484, 2004.
42. Cooley DA, Cabello OV, Preciado FM: Repair of total anomalous pulmonary venous return, *Tex Heart Inst J* 35:451–453, 2008.
43. Crane LD: The neonate and child. In Frownfelter DL, editor: *Chest physical therapy and pulmonary rehabilitation*, Chicago, 1987, Year Book, pp 666–697.
44. Cullen SM, Cronk CE, Pueschel SM, et al.: Social development and feeding milestones of young Down syndrome children, *Am J Ment Defic* 85:410–415, 1981.
45. Davidson J, Gringras P, Fairhurst C, et al.: Physical and neurodevelopmental outcomes in children with single-ventricle circulation, *Arch Dis Child* 100(5):449–453, 2015.
46. Davies RR, Pizarro C: Decision-making for surgery in the management of patients with univentricular heart, *Front Pediatr* 3:61, 2015.
47. Del Castillo SL, Moromisato DY, Dorey F, et al.: Mesenteric blood flow velocities in the newborn with single-ventricle physiology: modified Blalock-Taussig shunt versus right ventricle-pulmonary artery conduit. *Pediatr Crit Care Med* 7:132–137, 2006.

48. Reference deleted in proofs.

49. DeMaso DR, Campis LK, Wypij D, et al.: The impact of maternal perceptions and medical severity on the adjustment of children with congenital heart disease, *J Pediatr Psychol* 16:137–149, 1991.

50. Deshpande S, Wolf M, Kim D, Kirshbom P: Simple transposition of the great arteries. In Da Cruz EM, Ivy D, Jaggers J, editors: *Pediatric and congenital cardiology, cardiac surgery and intensive care*, London, 2014, Springer, pp 1919–1940.

51. Dipchand AI, Edwards LB, Kucheryavaya AY, et al.: The registry of the International Society for Heart and Lung Transplantation: seventeenth official pediatric heart transplantation report—2014; Focus theme: retransplantation, *J Heart Lung Transplant* 33(10):985–895, 2014.

52. Donovan EF, Mathews RA, Nixon PA, et al.: An exercise program for pediatric patients with congenital heart disease: psychological aspects, *J Cardiac Rehabil* 3:476–480, 1983.

53. Dunn JM, Cavarocchi NC, Balsara RK, et al.: Pediatric heart transplantation, at St. Christopher's Hospital for Children, *J Heart Transplant* 6:334–342, 1987.

54. duPlessis AJ, Chang AC, Wessel DL, et al.: Cerebrovascular accidents following the Fontan operation, *Pediatr Neurol* 12:230–236, 1995.

55. Ekman-Joelsson BM, Berntsson L, Sunnegardh J: Quality of life in children with pulmonary atresia and intact ventricular septum, *Cardiol Young* 14:615–621, 2004.

56. Feldt RH, Ewert JC, Stickler GB, Weidman WH: Children with congenital heart disease, *Am J Dis Child* 117:281–287, 1969.

57. Fenton KN, Webber SA, Danford DA, et al.: Long-term survival after pediatric cardiac transplantation and postoperative ECMO support, *Ann Thorac Surg* 76:843–847, 2003.

58. Ferry PC: Neurologic sequelae of open-heart surgery in children, *Am J Dis Child* 144:369–373, 1990.

59. Fogel MA, Li C, Wilson F, et al.: Relationship of cerebral blood flow to aortic-to-pulmonary collateral/shunt flow in single ventricles, *Heart* August 101(16):1325–1331, 2015.

60. Forbess JM, Visconti KJ, Hancock-Friesen C, et al.: *Circulation* 106 (Suppl I):I-95–I-102, 2002.

61. Fredriksen PM, Pettersen E, Thaulow E: Declining aerobic capacity of patients with arterial and atrial switch procedures, *Pediatr Cardiol* 30:166–171, 2009.

62. Reference deleted in proofs.

63. Furness S, Hyslop-St. George C, Pound B, et al.: Development of an interprofessional pediatric ventricular assist device support team, *ASAIO J* 54:483–485, 2008.

64. Garcia E, Granados M, Fittipaldi M, Comas J: Persistent arterial duct. In Da Cruz EM, Ivy D, Jaggers J, editors: *Pediatric and congenital cardiology, cardiac surgery and intensive care*, London, 2014, Springer, pp 1425–1437.

65. Gardner FV, Freeman NH, Black AM, Angelini GD: Disturbed mother-infant interaction in association with congenital heart disease, *Heart* 76:56–59, 1996.

66. Gaynor JW, Jarvik GP, Bernbaum J, et al.: The relationship of postoperative electrographic seizures to neurodevelopmental outcome at 1 year of age after neonatal and infant cardiac surgery, *J Thorac Cardiovasc Surg* 131:181–189, 2006.

67. Gaynor JW, Stopp C, Wypij D, et al.: Neurodevelopmental outcomes after cardiac surgery in infancy, *Pediatrics* 135(5):816–825, 2015.

68. Gaynor JW, Wernovsky G, Jarvik GP, et al.: Patient characteristics are important determinants of neurodevelopmental outcome at one year of age after neonatal and infant cardiac surgery, *J Thorac Cardiovasc Surg* 133:1344–1353, 2007.

69. Gessler P, Schmitt B, Pretre R, Latal B: Inflammatory response and neurodevelopmental outcome after open-heart surgery, *Pediatr Cardiol* 30:301–305, 2009.

70. Giardini A, Hager A, Lammers AE, et al.: Ventilatory efficiency and aerobic capacity predict event-free survival in adults with atrial repair for complete transposition of the great arteries, *J Am Coll Cardiol* 53:1548–1555, 2009.

71. Gingell RL, Hornung MG: Growth problems associated with congenital heart disease in infancy. In Lebenthal E, editor: *Textbook of gastroenterology and nutrition in infancy*, ed 2, New York, 1989, Raven Press, pp 639–649.

72. Goldberg B, Fripp RR, Lister G, et al.: Effect of physical training on exercise performance of children following surgical repair of congenital heart disease, *Pediatrics* 68:691–699, 1981.

73. Goldberg CS, Schwartz EM, Brunberg JA, et al.: Neurodevelopmental outcome of patients after the Fontan operation: a comparison between children with hypoplastic left heart syndrome and other functional single ventricle lesions, *J Pediatr* 137:646–652, 2000.

74. Goldberg S, Simmons RJ, Newman J, et al.: Congenital heart disease, parental stress, and infant-mother relationships, *J Pediatr* 119:661–666, 1991.

75. Goldberg S, Washington J, Morris P, et al.: Early diagnosed chronic illness and mother-child relationships in the first two years, *Can J Psychiatry* 55:726–733, 1990.

76. Reference deleted in proofs.

77. Griffiths ER, Kaza AK, Wyler von Ballmoos MC, et al.: Evaluating failing Fontans for heart transplantation: predictors of death, *Ann Thorac Surg* 88:558–564, 2009.

78. Gudermuth S: Mothers' reports of early experiences of infants with congenital heart disease, *Matern Child Nurs J* 4:155–164, 1975.

79. Guillemaud JP, El-Hakim H, Richards S, Chauhan N: Airway pathologic abnormalities in symptomatic children with congenital cardiac and vascular disease, *Arch Otolaryngol Head Neck Surg* 133:672–676, 2007.

80. Haka-Ikse K, Blackwood MA, Steward DJ: Psychomotor development of infants and children after profound hypothermia during surgery for congenital heart disease, *Dev Med Child Neurol* 20:62–70, 1978.

81. Haneda K, Itoh T, Togo T, et al.: Effects of cardiac surgery on intellectual function in infants and children, *Cardiovasc Surg* 4:303–307, 1996.

82. Harrison AM, Davis S, Reid JR, et al.: Neonates with hypoplastic left heart syndrome have ultrasound evidence of abnormal superior mesenteric artery perfusion before and after the modified Norwood procedure, *Pediatr Crit Care Med* 6:445–447, 2005.

83. Hazekamp M, Schneider A, Blom N: Pulmonary atresia with intact ventricular septum. In Da Cruz EM, Ivy D, Jaggers J, editors: *Pediatric and congenital cardiology, cardiac surgery and intensive care*, London, 2014, Springer, pp 1543–1555.

84. Hetzer R, Stiller B: Technology insight: use of ventricular assist devices in children, *Nat Clin Pract Cardiovasc Med* 3:377–387, 2006.

85. Hirsch JC, Charpie JR, Ohye RG, Gurney JG: Near infrared spectroscopy: what we know and what we need to know-A systematic review of the congenital heart disease, *J Thorac Cardiovasc Surg* 137:154–159, 2009.

86. Hirsch JC, Devaney EJ, Ohye RG, Bove EL: Hypoplastic left heart syndrome. In Mavroudis C, Backer C, editors: *Pediatric cardiovascular medicine*, ed 4, Hoboken, NJ, 2013, Blackwell, pp 619–635.

87. Hoffman GM, Brosig C, Mussatto K, et al.: Perioperative cerebral oxygen saturation in neonates with hypoplastic left heart syndrome and childhood neurodevelopmental outcome, *J Thorac Cardiovasc Surg* 146(5):1153–1164, 2013.

88. Hoffman JI, Kaplan S: The incidence of congenital heart disease, *J Am Coll Cardiol* 39:1890–1900, 2002.

89. Holden KR, Sessions JC, Cure J, et al.: Neurologic outcomes in children with post-pump choreoathetosis, *J Pediatr* 132:162–164, 1998.

90. Hollander SA, Callus E: Cognitive and psychologic considerations in pediatric heart failure, *J Card Fail* 20(10):782–785, 2014.

91. Hollander SA, Hollander AJ, Rizzuto S, et al.: An inpatient rehabilitation program utilizing standardized care pathways after paracorporeal ventricular assist device placement in children, *J Heart Lung Transplant* 33(6):587–592, 2014.

92. Hovels-Gurich HH, Kunz D, Seghaye M, et al.: Results of exercise testing at a mean age of 10 years after neonatal arterial switch operation, *Acta Paediatrica* 92:190–196, 2003.

93. Imamura M, Dossey AM, Prodhan P, et al.: Bridge to cardiac transplantation in children: Berlin Heart versus extracorporeal membrane oxygenation, *Ann Thorac Surg* 87:1894–1901, 2009.

94. Jadcherla SR, Vijayapal AS, Leuthner S: Feeding abilities in neonates with congenital heart disease: a retrospective study, *J Perinatol* 29:112–118, 2009.

95. Jaggers J, Barrett C, Landeck B: Pulmonary stenosis and insufficiency. In Da Cruz EM, Ivy D, Jaggers J, editors: *Pediatric and congenital cardiology, cardiac surgery and intensive care*, London, 2014, Springer, pp 1557–1576.

96. James FW, Blomqvist CG, Freed MD, et al.: Standards for exercise testing in the pediatric age group, *Circulation* 66:1377A–1397A, 1982.

97. Jayakumar KA, Addonizio LJ, Kichuk-Chrisant MR, et al.: Cardiac transplantation after the Fontan or Glenn procedure, *J Am Coll Cardiol* 44:2065–2072, 2004.

98. Jenkins KJ, Correa A, Feinstein JA, et al.: Noninherited risk factors and congenital cardiovascular defects: current knowledge. A scientific statement from the American Heart Association Council on cardiovascular disease in the young, *Circulation* 115:2995–3014, 2007.

99. Johnson BA: Postoperative physical therapy in the pediatric cardiac surgery patient, *Pediatr Phys Ther* 2:14–22, 1991.

100. Kaltman JR, Jarvik GP, Bernbaum J, et al.: Neurodevelopmental outcome after early repair of a ventricular septal defect with or without aortic arch obstruction, *J Thorac Cardiovasc Surg* 131:792–798, 2006.

101. Kayambu G, Boots R, Paratz J: Physical therapy for the critically ill in the ICU: a systematic review and meta-analysis, *Crit Care Med* 41(6):1543–1554, 2013.

102. Kelleher DK, Laussen P, Teizeira-Pinto A, Duggan C: Growth and correlates of nutritional status among infants with hypoplastic left heart syndrome after stage 1 Norwood procedure, *Nutrition* 22:236–244, 2006.

103. Kendall S, Karamichalis J, Karamlou T, et al.: Atrial septal defect. In Da Cruz EM, Ivy D, Jaggers J, editors: *Pediatric and congenital cardiology, cardiac surgery and intensive care*, London, 2014, Springer, pp 1439–1454.

104. Kirk R, Edwards LB, Aurora P, et al.: Registry of the International Society for Heart and Lung Transplantation: eleventh official pediatric heart transplantation report-2008, *J Heart Lung Transplant* 27:970–977, 2008.

105. Kirshbom PM, Flynn TB, Clancy RR, et al.: Late neurodevelopmental outcome after repair of total anomalous pulmonary venous connection, *J Thorac Cardiovasc Surg* 129:1091–1097, 2005.

106. Koch BM, Galioto FM, Vaccaro P, et al.: Flexibility and strength measures in children participating in a cardiac rehabilitation exercise program, *Phys Sports Med* 116:139–147, 1988.

107. Kolovos NS, Bratton SL, Moler FW, et al.: Outcome of pediatric patients treated with extracorporeal life support after cardiac surgery, *Ann Thorac Surg* 76:1435–1442, 2003.

108. Kong SG, Tay JS, Yip WC, Chay SO: Emotional and social effects of congenital heart disease in Singapore, *Aust Paediatr J* 22:101–106, 1986.

109. Kovacikova L, Dobos D, Zahorec M: Non-invasive positive pressure ventilation for bilateral diaphragm after pediatric cardiac surgery, *Interact Cardiovasc Thorac Surg* 8:171–172, 2009.

110. Kramer HH, Aswiszus D, Sterzel U, et al.: Development of personality and intelligence in children with congenital heart disease, *J Child Psychiatry* 30:299–308, 1989.

111. Laane KM, Meberg A, Otterstad JE, et al.: Quality of life in children with congenital heart defects, *Acta Paediatrica* 86:975–980, 1997.

112. Lamour JM, Kanter KR, Naftel DC, et al.: The effect of age, diagnosis, and previous surgery in children and adults undergoing heart transplantation for congenital heart disease, *J Am Coll Cardiol* 54:160–165, 2009.

113. Latal B, Kellenberger C, Dimitropoulos A, Beck I, et al.: Can preoperative cranial ultrasound predict early neurodevelopmental outcome in infants with congenital heart disease? *Dev Med Child Neurol* (7):639–644, 2015.

114. Lawrence KS, Fricker FJ: Pediatric heart transplantation: quality of life, *J Heart Transplantat* 6:329–333, 1987.

115. Lee H, Ko YJ, Suh GY, et al.: Safety profile and feasibility of early physical therapy and mobility for critically ill patients in the medical intensive care unit: beginning experiences in Korea, *J Crit Care* 30(4):673–677, 2015.

116. Lee M, Udekem Y, Brizard C: Coarctation of the aorta. In Da Cruz EM, Ivy D, Jaggers J, editors: *Pediatric and congenital cardiology, cardiac surgery and intensive care*, London, 2014, Springer, pp 1631–1646.

117. Liamlahi R, von Rhein M, Buhrer S, et al.: Motor dysfunction and behavioural problems frequently coexist with congenital heart disease in school-age children, *Acta Paediatrica* 103(7):752–758, 2014.

118. Licht DJ, Shera DM, Clancy RR, et al.: Brain maturation is delayed in infants with complex congenital heart defects, *J Thorac Cardiovasc Surg* 137:529–537, 2009.

119. Licht DJ, Wang J, Silvestre DW, et al.: Preoperative cerebral blood flow is diminished in neonates with severe congenital heart defects, *J Thorac Cardiovasc Surg* 128:841–850, 2004.

120. Limperopoulos C, Majnemer A, Shevell MI, et al.: Functional limitations in young children with congenital heart defects after cardiac surgery, *Pediatrics* 108:1325–1331, 2001.

121. Limperopoulos C, Tworetzky W, McElhinney DB, et al.: Brain volume and metabolism in fetuses with congenital heart disease: evaluation with quantitative magnetic resonance imaging and spectroscopy, *Circulation* 121(1):26–33, 2010.

122. Linde LM, Rasof B, Dunn OJ: Longitudinal studies of intellectual and behavioral development in children with congenital heart disease, *Acta Paediatrica* 59:169–176, 1970.

123. Loeffel M: Developmental considerations of infants and children with congenital heart disease, *Heart Lung* 14:214–217, 1985.

124. Longmuri PE, McCrindle BW: Physical activity restrictions for children after the Fontan operation: disagreement between parent, cardiologist and medical record reports, *Am Heart J* 157:853–859, 2009.

125. Lorts A, Zafar F, Adachi I, Morales DLS: Mechanical assist devices in neonates and infants, *Semin Thorac Cardiovasc Surg Pediatr Card Surg Ann* 17(1):91–95, 2014.

126. Lynch JM, Buckley EM, Schwab PJ, et al.: Time to surgery and preoperative cerebral hemodynamics predict postoperative white matter injury in neonates with hypoplastic left heart syndrome, *J Thorac Cardiovasc Surg* 148(5):2181–2188, 2014.

127. Maher KO, Pizarro C, Gidding SS, et al.: Hemodynamic profile after the Norwood procedure with right ventricle to pulmonary artery conduit, *Circulation* 108:782–784, 2003.

128. Mahle WT, Clancy RR, McGaurn SP, et al.: Impact of prenatal diagnosis on survival and early neurologic morbidity in neonates with the hypoplastic left heart syndrome, *Pediatrics* 107:1277–1282, 2001.

129. Mahle WT, Lundine K, Kanter KR, et al.: The short term effects of cardiopulmonary bypass on neurologic function in children and young adults, *Eur J Cardiothorac Surg* 26:920–925, 2004.

130. Mahle WT, Tavani F, Zimmerman RA, et al.: An MRI study of neurological injury before and after congenital heart surgery, *Circulation* 106(Suppl I):I-109–I-114, 2002.

131. Mahle WT, Wernovsky G: Long-term developmental outcome of children with complex congenital heart disease, *Clin Perinatol* 28:235–247, 2001.

132. Mahle WT, Wernovsky G, Moss EM, et al.: Neurodevelopmental outcome and lifestyle assessment in school age and adolescent children with hypoplastic left heart syndrome, *Pediatrics* 105:1082–1089, 2000.

133. Majnemer A, Limperopoulos C, Shevell M, et al.: Developmental and functional outcomes at school entry in children with congenital heart defects, *J Pediatr* 153:55–60, 2008.

134. Malaisrie SC, Pelletier MP, Yun JJ, et al.: Pneumatic paracorporeal ventricular assistive device in infants and children: initial Stanford experience, *J Heart Lung Transplant* 27:173–177, 2008.

135. Marino BS, Lipkin PH, Newburger JW, et al.: Neurodevelopmental outcomes in children with congenital heart disease: evaluation and management: a scientific statement from the American Heart Association, *Circulation* 126(9):1143–1172, 2012.

136. Mascio CE: The use of ventricular assist device support in children: the state of the art, *Artif Organs* 39(1):14–20, 2015.

137. Mathew OP: Respiratory control during nipple feeding in pre-term infants, *Pediatr Pulmonol* 5:220–224, 1988.

138. Mathew OP, Clark ML, Pronske ML, et al.: Breathing pattern and ventilation during oral feeding in term newborn infants, *J Pediatr* 106:810–813, 1985.

139. Mathews RA, Nixon PA, Stephenson RJ, et al.: An exercise program for pediatric patients with congenital heart disease: organizational and physiologic aspects, *J Cardiac Rehabil* 3:467–475, 1983.

140. Mavroudis C, Backer CL, Wiley Online Library (Online service): *Pediatric cardiac surgery*, Chichester, West Sussex, UK, 2013, Wiley Blackwell.

141. Mavroudis C, Backer CL: Transposition of the great arteries. In Mavroudis C, Backer C, editors: *Pediatric cardiovascular medicine*, ed 4, Hoboken, NJ, 2013, Blackwell, pp 492–529.

142. Mavroudis C, Backer CL, Jacobs JP, Anderson RH: Ventricular septal defect. In Mavroudis C, Backer C, editors: *Pediatric cardiovascular medicine*, ed 4, Hoboken, NJ, 2013, Blackwell, pp 311–341.

143. McBride MG, Binder TJ, Paridon SM: Safety and feasibility of inpatient exercise training in pediatric heart failure: a preliminary report, *J Cardiopulm Rehabi! Prev* 27:219–222, 2007.

144. McCrindle BW, Williams RV, Mitchell PD, et al.: Relationship of patient and medical characteristics to health status in children and adolescents after the Fontan procedure, *Circulation* 113:1123–1129, 2006.

145. McCusker CG, Doherty NN, Molloy B, et al.: A controlled trial of early interventions to promote maternal adjustment and development in infants born with severe congenital heart disease, *Child Care Health Dev* 36(1):110–117, 2010.

146. Messmer BJ, Schallberger Y, Gattiker R, Senning A: Psychomotor and intellectual development after deep hypothermia and circulatory arrest in early infancy, *J Thorac Cardiovasc Surg* 72:495–501, 1976.

147. Miller JR, Lancaster TS, Eghtesady P: Current approaches to device implantation in pediatric and congenital heart disease patients, *Expert Rev Cardiovasc Ther* 13(4):417–427, 2015.

148. Miller JR, Boston US, Epstein DJ, et al.: Pediatric quality of life while supported with a ventricular assist device, *Congenit Heart Dis* 10(4):E189–E196, 2015.

149. Miller SP, McQuillen PS, Hamrick S, et al.: Abnormal brain development in newborns with congenital heart disease, *N Engl J Med November* 357(19):1927–1938, 2007.

150. Miyamoto S, Campbell D, Auerbach S: Heart transplantation. In Da Cruz EM, Ivy D, Jaggers J, editors: *Pediatric and congenital cardiology, cardiac surgery and intensive care*, London, 2014, Springer, pp 2827–2850.

151. Morales DLS, Almond CSD, Jaquiss RDB, et al.: Bridging children of all sizes to cardiac transplantation: the initial multicenter North American experience with the Berlin Heart EXCOR ventricular assist device, *J Heart Lung Transplant* 30(1):1–8, 2011.

152. Mumtaz MA, Qureshi A, Mavroudis C, Backer CL: Patent ductus arteriosus. In Mavroudis C, Backer C, editors: *Pediatric cardiovascular medicine*, ed 4, Hoboken, NJ, 2013, Blackwell, pp 225–233.

153. Mussatto KA, Hoffmann R, Hoffman G, et al.: Risk factors for abnormal developmental trajectories in young children with congenital heart disease, *Circulation* 132(8):755–761, 2015.

154. Neal AE, Stopp C, Wypij D, et al.: Predictors of health-related quality of life in adolescents with tetralogy of Fallot, *J Pediatr* 166(1):132–138, 2015.

155. Nelson J, Bove E, Hirsch-Romano J: Tetralogy of Fallot. In Da Cruz EM, Ivy D, Jaggers J, editors: *Pediatric and congenital cardiology, cardiac surgery and intensive care*, London, 2014, Springer, pp 1505–1526.

156. Newberger JW, Sleeper LA, Bellinger DC, et al.: Early developmental outcome in children with hypoplastic left heart syndrome and related anomalies, *Circulation* 125:2081–2091, 2012.

157. Newberger JW, Wypij D, Bellinger DC, et al.: Length of stay after infant heart surgery is related to cognitive outcome at age 8 years, *J Pediatr* 143:67–73, 2003.

158. Niset G, Coustry-Degre C, Degre S: Psychosocial and physical rehabilitation after heart transplantation: 1-year follow-up, *Cardiology* 75:311–317, 1988.

159. Nydegger A, Walsh A, Penny DJ, et al.: Changes in resting energy expenditure in children with congenital heart disease, *Eur J Clin Nutrit* 63:392–397, 2009.

160. Nytroen K, Gullestad L: Exercise after heart transplantation: an overview, *World J Transplant* 3(4):78–90, 2013.

161. O'Dougharty M, Wright FS, Loewenson RB, Torres F: Cerebral dysfunction after chronic hypoxia in children, *Neurology* 35:42–46, 1985.

162. Owen M, Shevell MCM, Donofrio M, et al.: Brain volume and neurobehavior in newborns with complex congenital heart defects, *J Pediatr* 164(5):1121–1127e1, 2014.

163. Ozbaran M, Yagdi T, Engin C, et al.: New era of pediatric ventricular assist devices: let us go to school, *Pediatr Transplant* 19(1):82–86, 2015.

164. Patel P, Rotta A, Brown J: Partial and total anomalous pulmonary venous connections and associated defects. In Da Cruz EM, Ivy D, Jaggers J, editors: *Pediatric and congenital cardiology, cardiac surgery and intensive care*, London, 2014, Springer, pp 1885–1904.

165. Perrault H, Drblik SP: Exercise after surgical repair of congenital cardiac lesions, *Sports Med* 7:18–31, 1989.

166. Phelps HM, Mahle WT, Kim D, et al.: Postoperative cerebral oxygenation in hypoplastic left heart syndrome after the Norwood procedure, *Ann Thorac Surg* 87:1490–1494, 2009.

167. Pierpont ML, Basson DT, Benson DW, et al.: Genetic basis for congenital heart defects: current knowledge. A scientific statement from the American Heart Association Congenital Cardiac Defects Committee, Council on Cardiovascular Disease in the Young: endorsed by the American Academy of Pediatrics, *Circulation* 115:3015–3038, 2007.

168. Pizarro C, Malec E, Maher KO, et al.: Right ventricle to pulmonary artery conduit improves outcome after stage I Norwood for hypoplastic left heart syndrome, *Circulation* 108(Suppl II):II-155–II-160, 2003.

169. Polastri M, Loforte A, Dell'Amore A, Nava S: Physiotherapy for patients on awake extracorporeal membrane oxygenation: a systematic review, *Physiother Res Int*, 2015. [Epub ahead of print].

170. Reference deleted in proofs.

171. Rajantie IPT, Laurila MPT, Pollari KPT, et al.: Motor development of infants with univentricular heart at the ages of 16 and 52 weeks, *Pediatr Phys Ther* 25(4):444–450, 2013.

172. Rao PS: Tricuspid atresia. In Mavroudis C, Backer C, editors: *Pediatric cardiovascular medicine*, ed 4, Hoboken, NJ, 2013, Blackwell, pp 487–508.

173. Rasof B, Linde LM, Dunn OJ: Intellectual development in children with congenital heart disease, *Child Dev* 38:1043–1053, 1967.

174. Ravishankar C, Zak V, Williams IA, et al.: Association of impaired linear growth and worse neurodevelopmental outcome in infants with single ventricle physiology: a report from the pediatric heart network infant single ventricle trial, *J Pediatr* 162(2):250–256e2, 2013.

175. Rawlinson E, Howard R: Post-operative sedation and analgesia. In Da Cruz EM, Ivy D, Jaggers J, editors: *Pediatric and congenital cardiology, cardiac surgery and intensive care*, London, 2014, Springer, pp 705–719.

176. Reference deleted in proofs.

177. Reference deleted in proofs.

178. *Rehabilitation of patients on Berlin Heart EXCOR pediatric ventricular assist devices at Texas Children's Hospital*, Presented at Texas Children's Hospital, May 29, 2009.

179. Robbers-Visser D, Kapusta L, van Osch-Gevers L, et al.: Clinical outcome 5 to 18 years after the Fontan operation performed on children younger than 5 years, *J Thorac Cardiovasc Surg* 138:89–95, 2009.

180. Rockett SR, Bryant JC, Morrow WR: Preliminary single center North American experience with the Berlin Heart pediatric EXCOR device, *ASAIO J* 54:479–482, 2008.

181. Rollins CK, Newburger JW: Neurodevelopmental outcomes in congenital heart disease, *Circulation* 130(14):e124–e146, 2014.

182. Roos-Hesselink JW, Meijboom FJ, Spitaels SE, et al.: Excellent survival and low incidence of arrhythmias, stroke and heart failure long-term after surgical ASD closure at young age: a prospective follow-up study of 21-33 years, *Eur Heart J* 24:190–197, 2003.

183. Rosenthal A: Care of the postoperative child and adolescent with congenital heart disease. In Barness LA, editor: *Advances in pediatrics*, Chicago, 1983, Year Book, pp 131–167.

184. Rossano JW, Jang GY: Pediatric heart failure: current state and future possibilities, *Korean Circ J* 45(1):1–8, 2015.

185. Rossano JW, Morales D, Fraser CD: Heart transplantation. In Mavroudis C, Backer C, editors: *Pediatric cardiovascular medicine*, ed 4, Hoboken, NJ, 2013, Blackwell, pp 813–826.

186. Rossi AF, Fishberger S, Hannan RL, et al.: Frequency and indications for tracheostomy and gastrostomy after congenital heart surgery, *Pediatr Cardiol* 30:225–231, 2009.

187. Rossi AF, Seiden HS, Sadeghi AM, et al.: The outcome of cardiac operations in infants weighing two kilograms or less, *J Thorac Cardiovasc Surg* 116:29–35, 1998.

188. Ross Russell RI, Helms PJ, Elliot MJ: A prospective study of phrenic nerve damage after cardiac surgery in children, *Intensive Care Med* 34:727–734, 2008.

189. Ruttenberg HD, Adams TD, Orsmond GS, et al.: Effects of exercise training on aerobic fitness in children after open heart surgery, *Pediatr Cardiol* 4:19–24, 1983.

190. Sadowsky HS, Rohrkemper KF, Quon SYM: *Rehabilitation of cardiac and cardiopulmonary recipients: an introduction for physical and occupational therapists*, Stanford, CA, 1986, Stanford University Hospital.

191. Sahu B, Chauhan S, Kiran U, et al.: Neuropsychological function in children with cyanotic heart disease undergoing corrective cardiac surgery: effect of two different rewarming strategies, *Eur J Cardiothorac Surg* 35:505–510, 2009.

192. Sananes R, Manlhiot C, Kelly E, et al.: Neurodevelopmental outcomes after open heart operations before 3 months of age, *Ann Thorac Surg* 93(5):1577–1583, 2012.

193. Sano S, Ishino K, Kado H, et al.: Outcome of right ventricle-to-pulmonary artery shunt in first-stage palliation of hypoplastic left heart syndrome: a multi-institutional study, *Ann Thorac Surg* 78:1951–1958, 2004.

194. Sarrechia I, De Wolf D, Miatton M, et al.: Neurodevelopment and behavior after transcatheter versus surgical closure of secundum type atrial septal defect, *J Pediatr* 166(1):31–38e1, 2015.

195. Scaravilli V, Zanella A, Sangalli F, Patroniti N: Basic aspects of physiology during ECMO support. In Sangalli F, Patroniti N, Pesenti A, editors: *ECMO-extracorporeal life support in adults*, Milan, Italy, 2014, Springer-Vertag Italia, pp 19–36.

196. Schaefer C, von Rhein M, Knirsch W, et al.: Neurodevelopmental outcome, psychological adjustment, and quality of life in adolescents with congenital heart disease, *Dev Med Child Neurol December* 55(12):1143–1149, 2013.

197. Schultz AH, Jarvik GP, Wernovsky G, et al.: Effect of congenital heart disease on neurodevelopmental outcomes within multiple-gestation births, *J Thorac Cardiovasc Surg* 130:1511–1516, 2005.

198. Schweiger M, Vanderpluym C, Jeewa A, et al.: Outpatient management of intra-corporeal left ventricular assist device system in children: a multi-center experience, *Am J Transplant* 5(2):453–460, 2015.

199. Sciurba FC, Owens GR, Sanders MH, et al.: Evidence of an altered pattern of breathing during exercise in recipients of heart-lung transplants, *N Engl J Med* 319:1186–1192, 1988.

200. Settergren G, Ohqvist G, Lundberg S, et al.: Cerebral blood flow and cerebral metabolism in children following cardiac surgery with deep hypothermia and circulatory arrest: clinical course and follow-up of psychomotor development, *Scand J Thoracic Cardiovasc Surg* 16:209–215, 1982.

201. Shi SS, Zhao ZY, Liu XW, et al.: Perioperative risk factors for prolonged mechanical ventilation following cardiac surgery in neonates and young infants, *Chest J* 134:768–774, 2009.

202. Silbert A, Wolff PH, Mayer B, et al.: Cyanotic heart disease and psychological development, *Pediatrics* 43:192–200, 1969.

203. Staveski SL, Avery S, Rosenthal DN, et al.: Implementation of a comprehensive interdisciplinary care coordination of infants and young children on Berlin Heart ventricular assist devices, *J Cardiovasc Nurs* 26(3):231–238, 2011.

204. Stavinoha PL, Fixler DE, Mahony L: Cardiopulmonary bypass to repair an atrial septal defect does not affect cognitive function in children, *Circulation* 107:2722–2725, 2003.

205. Stewart RD, Mavroudis C, Backer CL: Tetralogy of Fallot. In Mavroudis C, Backer C, editors: *Pediatric cardiovascular medicine*, ed 4, Hoboken, NJ, 2013, Blackwell, pp 410–427.

206. Stigall W, Willis B: Mechanical ventilation, cardiopulmonary interactions, and pulmonary issues in children with critical cardiac disease. In Da Cruz EM, Ivy D, Jaggers J, editors: *Pediatric and congenital cardiology, cardiac surgery and intensive care*, London, 2014, Springer, pp 3147–3181.

207. Stromvall-Larsson E, Eriksson E, Holgren D, Sixt R: Pulmonary gas exchange during exercise in Fontan patients at a long-term follow-up, *Clin Physiol Funct Imaging* 24:327–334, 2004.

208. Throckmorton AL, Chopski SG: Pediatric circulator support: current strategies and future directions. Biventricular and univentricular mechanical assistance, *ASAIO J* 54:491–497, 2008.

209. Thrush PT, Hoffman TM: Pediatric heart transplantation-indications and outcomes in the current era, *J Thorac Dis* 6(8):1080–1096, 2014.

210. Tibballs J, Cantwell-Bartl A: Outcomes of management decisions by parents for their infants with hypoplastic left heart syndrome born with and without a prenatal diagnosis, *J Paediatr Child Health* 44:321–324, 2008.

211. Trittenwein G, Nardi A, Pansi H, et al.: Early postoperative prediction of cerebral damage after pediatric cardiac surgery, *Ann Thorac Surg* 76:576–580, 2003.

212. Turner DA, Rehder KJ, Bonadonna D, et al.: Ambulatory ECMO as a bridge to lung transplant in a previously well pediatric patient with ARDS, *Pediatrics* 134(2):e583–e585, 2014.

213. Uzark L, Lincoln A, Lamberti JJ, et al.: Neurodevelopmental outcomes in children with Fontan repair of functional single ventricle, *Pediatrics* 101:630–633, 1998.

214. Vaidyanathan B, Radhakrishnn R, Sarala DA, et al.: What determines nutritional recovery in malnourished children after correction of congenital heart defects. *Pediatrics* 124(2):e294–e299.

215. van Breda A: Postoperative care of infants and children who require cardiac surgery, *Heart Lung* 14:205–207, 1985.

216. Viola N, Caldarone CA: Total anomalous pulmonary venous connection. In Mavroudis C, Backer C, editors: *Pediatric cardiovascular medicine*, ed 4, Hoboken, NJ, 2013, Blackwell, pp 659–673.

217. Visconti KJ, Bichell DP, Jonas RA, et al.: Developmental outcome after surgical versus interventional closure of secundum atrial septal defect in children, *Circulation* 100(Suppl):II145–II150, 1999.

218. Visconti KJ, Saudino KJ, Rappaport LA, et al.: Influence of parental stress and social support on the behavioural adjustment of children with transposition of the great arteries, *J Dev Behav Pediatr* 23:314–321, 2002.

219. Vollman KM: Introduction to progressive mobility, *Crit Care Nurse* 30(2):S3–S5, 2010.

220. von Rhein M, Buchmann A, Hagmann C, et al.: Brain volumes predict neurodevelopment in adolescents after surgery for congenital heart disease, *Brain* 137(1):268–276, 2014.

221. Warnes CA, Williams RG, Bashore TM, et al.: ACC/AHA 2008 Guidelines for the Management of Adults with Congenital Heart Disease: a report of the American College of Cardiology/American Heart Association Task Force on Practice Guidelines (writing committee to develop guidelines on the management of adults with congenital heart disease), *Circulation* 118(23):e714–e833, 2008.

222. Watchie J: *Cardiovascular and pulmonary physical therapy: a clinical manual*, ed 2, St. Louis, 2009, Saunders.

223. Welke KF, O'Brien SM, Peterson ED, et al.: The complex relationship between pediatric cardiac surgical case volumes and mortality rates in a national clinical database, *J Thorac Surg* 137:1133–1140, 2009.

224. Wells FC, Coghill S, Caplan HL, Lincoln C: Duration of circulatory arrest does influence the psychological development of children after cardiac operation in early life, *J Thorac Cardiovasc Surg* 86:823–831, 1983.

225. Werner H, Latal B, Valsangiacomo Buechel E, et al.: Health-related quality of life after open-heart surgery, *J Pediatr* 164(2):254–258e1, 2014.

226. Wieczorek B, Burke C, Al-Harbi A, Kudchadkar SR: Early mobilization in the pediatric intensive care unit: a systematic review, *J Pediatr Intensive Care* 129–170, 2015.

227. Wray J, Sensky T: How does the intervention of cardiac surgery affect the self-perception of children with congenital heart disease? *Child Care Health Dev* 24:57–72, 1998.

228. Yi SH, Kim SJ, Huh J, et al.: Dysphagia in infants after open heart procedures, *Am J Phys Med Rehabil* 92(6):496–503, 2013.

229. Youssef NM: School adjustment of children with congenital heart disease, *Matern Child Nurs J* 17:217–302, 1988.

230. Zafar F, Castleberry C, Khan MS, et al.: Pediatric heart transplant waiting list mortality in the era of ventricular assist devices, *J Heart Lung Transplant* 34(1):82–88, 2015.

231. Zebuhr C, Sinha A, Skillman H, Buckvold S: Active rehabilitation in a pediatric extracorporeal membrane oxygenation patient, *PM R* 6(5):456–460, 2014.

232. Zetser I, Jarvik GP, Bernbaum J, et al.: Genetic factors are important determinants of neurodevelopmental outcome after repair of tetralogy of Fallot, *J Thorac Cardiovasc Surg* 135:91–97, 2008.

SUGGESTED READINGS

Almond CS, Thiagarajan RR, Piercey GE, et al.: Waiting list mortality among children listed for heart transplantation in the United States, *Circulation* 119:717–727, 2009.

Chock VY, Chang IJ, Reddy MV: Short-term neurodevelopmental outcomes in neonates with congenital heart disease: the era of newer surgical strategies, *Congenit Heart Dis* 7(6):544–550, 2012.

Kayambu G, Boots R, Paratz J: Physical therapy for the critically ill in the ICU: a systematic review and meta-analysis, *Crit Care Med* 41(6):1543–1554, 2013.

Majnemer A, Limperopoulos C, Shevell M, et al.: Developmental and functional outcomes at school entry in children with congenital heart defects, *J Pediatr* 153:55–60, 2008.

McCusker CG, Doherty NN, Molloy B, et al.: A controlled trial of early interventions to promote maternal adjustment and development in infants born with severe congenital heart disease, *Child Care Health Dev* 36(1):110–117, 2010.

Newburger JW, Bellinger DC: Brain injury in congenital heart disease, *Circulation* 113:183–185, 2006.

Verheugt CL, Uiterwaal C, Grobbee DE, Mulder BJM: Long-term prognosis of congenital heart defects: a systematic review, *Int J Cardiol* 131:25–32, 2008.

29

The Neonatal Intensive Care Unit

Beth McManus, Yvette Blanchard, Stacey Dusing

Providing services to high-risk infants and their families in the neonatal intensive care unit is a complex subspecialty of pediatric physical therapy requiring knowledge and skills beyond the competencies for entry into practice. Newborns in the neonatal intensive care unit (NICU) are among the most fragile patients that physical therapists treat, and therefore practice in the NICU requires a keen understanding of the influence of prematurity and medical fragility on the infant and family. To this end, pediatric physical therapists (PTs) need advanced education in areas such as early fetal and infant development; infant neurobehavior; family responses to having a sick newborn; the environment of the NICU, physiologic assessment, and monitoring; newborn pathologies, interventions, and outcomes; optimal discharge planning; and collaboration with the members of the health care team.[161]

This chapter describes the neonatal intensive care unit and the role of the physical therapist within this setting. In the Background section we describe conceptual models governing PT practice in the NICU. Next, we review the most common medical complications of the respiratory, neurologic, and gastrointestinal system for infants admitted to the NICU and implications for physical therapy interventions. The Foreground section describes examination and evaluation of infants in the NICU, including tests and measures most commonly administered by PTs. The current evidence base for PT interventions in the NICU is presented, including direct interventions (e.g., handling) as well as best practice for posthospital follow-up of NICU infants and their families. Two case scenarios on the Expert Consult apply knowledge to practice.

BACKGROUND INFORMATION

ADVANCES IN NEONATAL CARE

The NICU is designed to meet the needs of a wide range of infants, from the monitoring of apparently well infants at risk of serious illness to the intensive treatment of infants with acute illness. Since the 1970s the type and range of developmental interventions provided in the NICU for medically fragile infants have changed dramatically. As such, the role of the neonatal physical therapist has evolved tremendously over the last several decades. Two main, yet overlapping, factors have contributed to the evolution of the role of the physical therapist: 1) the evolution of special care nurseries and advances in medical technology in NICU care and 2) a paradigm shift in conceptual frameworks for therapeutic and developmental interventions in the NICU.

Dr. Julian Hess is credited with establishing the first special care nursery in the 1940s. At the time the main principles of neonatal care were support of body temperature, control of nosocomial infection, minimal handling, and provision of special nursing care. Interestingly, nurseries were quiet and lights were dimmed at night. Dr. Hess achieved a neonatal mortality rate for preterm infants of 20%, which was respectable for the time.[225] In response to the increased survival rate of premature infants reported by Hess, the previously mentioned principles of care were implemented in several areas across the United States.[170]

The increase in the availability of special care nurseries led to the development of centers for the care of preterm infants during the 1950s. At this time, management of the medically fragile infant involved transport to one of these regional special care nurseries, if available, while the mother of the baby remained at the birthing hospital under the care of her obstetrician.[87] By the late 1960s, medical advances in microlaboratory techniques for biochemical determinations from minute quantities of blood and the development of miniaturized monitoring equipment, ventilatory support systems, and means to conserve body heat improved the care of the neonate with serious illness. Expansion of neonatal pharmacology, widespread use of phototherapy for management of hyperbilirubinemia, and methods of delivery of high-caloric solutions parenterally when oral feeding was not possible also improved the chances for survival of the very sick neonate.[87]

Paralleling advances in special care medical technology, in 1975, the emergence of the subspecialties of neonatology and perinatology affirmed the need for practitioners skilled in the care of infants in the high-technology nursery.[87] As the field of neonatology and the number of special care nurseries grew, it was evident that separate nurseries with costly medical care were not a sustainable, cost-effective model of care. Rather, there was a need for a system for referrals to regional centers for medically fragile infants.[170] In an attempt to improve access to special care and expand regionalization, the National Health Planning Act of 1974 supported assessment of health service needs locally and at the state level, which fostered planning of activities to improve access to care. In particular, three states—Arizona, Massachusetts, and Wisconsin—were at the forefront of promulgating standards for maternity units and developed regional perinatal care centers.

These entailed early identification of high-risk pregnancies and allowed for the transfer of the mother to a regional perinatal center prior to delivery. In the 1970s, reports from these three states and several professional organizations, including the American Medical Association, the American College of Obstetricians and Gynecologists, the American Academy of Pediatrics, and the Academy of Family Physicians, stimulated the development of the regional organization of perinatal services.[87,170]

The March of Dimes report Toward Improving the Outcome of Pregnancy, published in 1976, articulated the concept of regionalized perinatal care with three levels of maternal and neonatal care.[69,170] A subsequent report restated the importance of regionalization and recommended changes in designations from levels I, II, and III to basic, specialty, and subspecialty with expanded criteria.[184] These designations were updated in 2004[18] and again in 2012 through an AAP policy statement titled Levels of Neonatal Care.[18] The three levels of neonatal care and capabilities within levels recommended by the American Academy of Pediatrics are presented in Box 29.1. Although difficult to accurately assess, recent estimates suggest there are approximately 3 NICU beds per 1000 live births across the United States.[170]

The newborn in the intensive care nursery transitions from the buoyant, warm, enclosed, and relatively quiet and dark environment of the womb to a bright, often noisy, technology filled, gravity-influenced environment and is subjected to procedures that often cause pain and discomfort. The newborn is extremely vulnerable to the environmental effects of the intensive care nursery. Over the last several decades, there has been an increase and an evolution in the research and recommendations to decrease NICU environmental effects and to facilitate the development of the infant in the NICU.

As mentioned previously, the first special care nurseries were dark and quiet environments.[1] The prevailing thought was that medically fragile neonates were overly sensitive to external environmental stimulation and that care should be taken to mimic the in-utero environment and limit the infant's exposure to environmental hazards such as light and sound. However, as the advancement of medical care occurred and opportunities to improve special care for preterm infants emerged, there was a shift toward providing sensory stimulation. Outcomes of preterm infants were still poor compared to their full-term counterparts, and the prevailing thought was that preterm infants experienced sensory deprivation as a result of preterm birth, and the developmental gaps between preterm and full-term infants could be addressed with sensory stimulation programs.[169]

In the 1980s, concern emerged that the typical nursery stay of several weeks may have detrimental effects on later behavior of the infant born at very low birth weight (less than 1500 g).[113] At that time, the neonatal intensive care nursery was characterized by bright lights both night and day, high noise levels, and the intrusive medical procedures characteristic of high-technology treatment.[54,98] Research ensued on the effects of different sensory inputs based on the premise that the neonatal care environment may impact development. Optimal care included modulation of the environment to facilitate development, recognition of infant distress and discomfort, and family-centered care.[256] As the field of neonatal therapy became more prevalent, psychologists, physical therapists, and occupational therapists took the lead in developing sensory stimulation programs. However, the success of such programs was limited and they did not appear to mitigate the disparities in developmental outcomes between preterm and full-term infants. Thus another paradigm shift occurred. The current conceptual framework supports individualized, developmentally supportive care, where sensory stimulation is matched to the unique needs, strengths, and vulnerabilities of the infant.[169,256]

During the past three decades, the availability of neonatal intensive care has improved outcomes for high-risk infants, including premature infants and those with serious medical or surgical conditions.[18] Improved survival for very low birth weight and extremely low birth weight infants has been continuously reported since 1988.[87,138,143,237] This improvement in survival is related to antenatal steroids, more aggressive resuscitation in the delivery room, and advanced treatments given in the special care nursery including surfactant therapy.[139] A recent March of Dimes report[163] suggests that, among the over 180,000 newborns studied, 14% had a neonatal care admission. Of the babies admitted for neonatal care, about half were born preterm (i.e., less than 37 weeks of gestation) and half were full term. Moreover, the study reports an average length of neonatal hospitalization as approximately 13 days.

Prematurity and Low Birth Weight

More than 500,000 infants are born prematurely (gestation of less than 37 weeks) in the United States every year.[102] Approximately 1% of live births are very preterm with

---

BOX 29.1 Hospital Perinatal Care Levels

Level I: Well-Baby Nursery

Provide neonatal resuscitation at every delivery.

Evaluate and provide postnatal care to stable term newborn infants.

Stabilize and provide care for infants born 35–37 wk gestation who remain physiologically stable

Stabilize newborn infants who are ill and those born at < 35 wk gestation until transfer to a higher level of care.

Level II: Special Care Nursery

Level I capabilities plus:

Provide care for infants born ≥ 32 wk gestation and weighing ≥ 1500 g who have physiologic immaturity or who are moderately ill with problems that are expected to resolve rapidly and are not anticipated to need subspecialty services on an urgent basis.

Provide care for infants convalescing after intensive care.

Provide mechanical ventilation for brief duration (< 24 h) or continuous positive airway pressure or both.

Stabilize infants born before 32 wk gestation and weighing less than 1500 g until transfer to a neonatal intensive care.

Level III: NICU

Level II capabilities plus:

Provide sustained life support.

Provide comprehensive care for infants born < 32 wk gestation and weighing < 1500 g and infants born at all gestational ages and birth weights with critical illness.

Provide prompt and readily available access to a full range of pediatric medical subspecialists, pediatric surgical specialists, pediatric anesthesiologists, and pediatric ophthalmologists.

Provide a full range of respiratory support that may include conventional and/or high-frequency ventilation and inhaled nitric oxide.

Perform advanced imaging, with interpretation on an urgent basis, including computed tomography, MRI, and echocardiography.

Level IV: Regional NICU

Level III capabilities plus:

Be located within an institution with the capability to provide surgical repair of complex congenital or acquired conditions.

Maintain a full range of pediatric medical subspecialists, pediatric surgical subspecialists, and pediatric anesthesiologists at the site.

Facilitate transport and provide outreach education.

From American Academy of Pediatrics Committee on Fetus and Newborn: Levels of neonatal care. Policy statement. *Pediatrics* 130:587-597, 2012.

gestational age younger than 32 weeks,[269] and 8% of live births (and 74% of all preterm births) are late preterm with gestational age between 34 weeks and 36 6/7 weeks.[154] Preterm birth is a leading cause of infant mortality and morbidity, accounting for over 70% of neonatal deaths and half of long-term neurologic disabilities such as cerebral palsy, cognitive impairment, and behavioral problems.[164,166] The current rate of preterm births in the United States is 12%.[102] Infants born prematurely or who are small for gestational age (SGA) are divided into three major categories: low birth weight (LBW), from 1501 to 2500 g; very low birth weight (VLBW), 1000 to 1500 g; and extremely low birth weight (ELBW), less than 1000 g.

The causes of preterm birth are not clear but seem to involve an interaction of multiple factors including genetic, social, and environmental factors. Spontaneous preterm delivery and birth have recently been described as a common complex disorder like heart disease, diabetes, and cancer.[269] Criteria for complex diseases include family history, recurrence, and racial disparities.[102] American black women have 1.5 times the rate of preterm birth and 4 times the rate of infant mortality because of preterm births compared with white women.[71] Approximately 40% of premature births are believed to be caused by intrauterine or systemic infections or both, which are not diagnosed until the onset of labor.[36] Pregnancy-specific stress is associated with smoking, caffeine consumption, and unhealthy eating, and it is inversely correlated with healthy eating, vitamin use, exercise, and gestational age at delivery.[153] Finally, infants born after assisted reproduction have a lower birth weight and gestational age when compared to matched controls.[158]

There has been a significant increase in survival of infants with VLBW and ELBW[139] as a result of more aggressive delivery room resuscitation, surfactant therapy, and a decreased rate of sepsis.[88,139,271] Approximately half of children surviving extremely low birth weight deliveries have subsequent moderate to severe neurodevelopmental disabilities.[139] Brain injury, retinopathy of prematurity, bronchopulmonary dysplasia, and neonatal infection increase the risk of mortality or neurosensory impairment (described later in this chapter).[32,164]

There is a national focus on preventing preterm birth spearheaded by the March of Dimes National Prematurity Campaign of 2003, recently extended to 2020.[163] The Prematurity Research Expansion and Education for Mothers who Deliver Infants Early (PREEMIE) Act (P.L. 109–450) was passed in 2006 with a subsequent Surgeon General's Conference on the Prevention of Preterm Birth in 2008.[177] The conference objectives were to (1) increase awareness of preterm birth in the United States; (2) review key findings on causes, consequences, and prevention of prematurity; and (3) establish an agenda for public and private sectors to address this public health problem. Conference recommendations included (1) increased research in medicine, epidemiology, psychosocial, and behavioral factors relating to prematurity; (2) professional education and training; (3) communication and outreach to the public; (4) addressing racial disparities; and (5) improvement of quality of care and health services.

ROLE OF THE PHYSICAL THERAPIST IN THE NICU

Newborn medicine changed rapidly with the advent of new drugs and technology. The NICU environment is cutting edge, fast paced, and high stress, but it affords the physical therapist incomparable learning opportunities because of the exceptional range of medical conditions and level of acuity of the infants,

numerous exchanges with health care professionals, and the opportunity to have a positive impact on this new family unit. This highly technical subspecialty area offers the opportunity for physical therapists to provide developmental services within a framework that is family centered and that views the infant as fully participating in the development process, principles that are central to pediatric physical therapy practice.

Neonates and infants in the NICU require specialized care due to the complexity of their medical conditions, their physiologic, neurologic, and developmental vulnerabilities, and the need to support the family during this stressful experience. Because of this complexity, physical therapists working in the NICU require specialized training through direct guidance from a highly skilled and experienced neonatal physical therapist or fellowship in neonatology. Clinical practice guidelines for physical therapists working in the NICU have been published in a two-part article series.[245,246] Part 1 articulates the path to professional competence and describes the clinical competencies for physical therapists, NICU clinical training models, and a clinical decision-making algorithm[245]; Part 2 presents the evidence-based practice guidelines, recommendations, and theoretical frameworks that support neonatal physical therapy practice.[246] The Practice Committee of the Section on Pediatrics of the American Physical Therapy Association has also published a Fact Sheet outlining recommendations for developing expertise in neonatal physical therapy practice (http://www.apta.org/NICU/). These sources clearly articulate that physical therapy practice in the NICU is not for the novice therapist.

Teamwork in the NICU

Similar to other areas of pediatric PT, teamwork and collaboration are a critical aspect of in the NICU practice. Teamwork and collaboration encompass "working together in a cooperative and coordinated way in the interest of a common cause."[185] Indeed, there are a number of medical, therapeutic and developmental, and support professionals working in the NICU. The medical team is principally concerned with infants' medical care and typically includes neonatologists, neonatal nurse practitioners, registered nurses, respiratory therapists, and registered dietitians. The organization of the medical team varies across institutions. For example, the presence and number of attending neonatologists, fellows, and neonatal nurse practitioners usually vary depending on whether the institution is an academic teaching, children's, or birthing hospital.[28,255]

The therapeutic and developmental care teams are principally concerned with providing individualized, developmentally supportive care in the NICU. The developmental team can include physical therapists, occupational therapists, speech and language pathologists, and developmental specialists. Typically, members of the therapeutic and developmental care team will receive physician or neonatal nurse practitioner orders to evaluate and treat infants being cared for in the NICU. These orders may be standing orders (e.g., all babies less than 32 weeks receive therapy services) or infant-specific (e.g., infant with tone abnormalities).[28,256] The roles of each developmental professional in the NICU may vary depending on their specialized training and expertise.

The role of the physical therapist in the NICU is multifaceted and includes: (1) the screening and examination of infants to determine the need for direct services in the NICU, referral for consultation by other health care professionals, and referral for developmental services postdischarge through early intervention or outpatient therapy services; (2) the design and implementation of individualized and developmentally appropriate interventions adapted to the infant's physiologic, motor, neurologic and developmental needs; (3) working in collaboration with other health care professionals to meet the needs of the infant and family members; (4) incorporating family members in the provision of care to best support the infant's developmental outcome. More detail about PT examination, evaluation, and intervention is presented later in the chapter.

The role of the occupational therapist in the NICU is to foster developmentally appropriate occupations, sensorimotor skills, and neurobehavioral organization. The provision of neonatal occupational therapy services includes: (1) caregiver communication, (2) appropriate use of NICU equipment, (3) administering formal assessment tools, (4) developing individualized developmentally supportive interventions, (5) monitoring the infant's response to intervention, (6) family collaboration, (7) providing thorough yet concise documentation, and (8) appropriate discharge planning.[28,255,256]

The role of the speech and language pathologist in the NICU is to assess and provide intervention with infants at risk or who are identified with communication, cognition, feeding, and/or swallowing disorders.[20,28,256] The provision of neonatal speech and language therapy services includes: (1) conducting communication, cognition, feeding/swallowing, and neurodevelopmental assessments; (2) conducting instrumental feeding/swallowing evaluation; (3) providing developmentally supportive, family-centered, evidence-based speech therapy interventions; (4) providing education, consultation, and support to NICU families and staff; (5) team and family collaboration and shared decision-making; (6) quality improvement and risk management; (7) discharge planning; and (8) participating in research, education and advocacy activities for NICU infants and their families.[20]

The role of the developmental specialist is to identify the infant's strengths and vulnerabilities and to: (1) partner with parents to identify and respond contingently to these infant behaviors (e.g., during caregiving episodes); (2) modify the caregiving environment to promote infants' strengths; and (3) promote optimal parent–infant interaction. The professional discipline and role of the developmental specialist will also vary across institutions and could be a physical, occupational, or speech therapist, registered nurse, or psychologist. Special care nurseries that are affiliated with the Newborn Individualized Developmental Care and Assessment Program (NIDCAP) Federation typically have a developmental specialist.[28,50,256]

In addition to the medical and developmental team members described above, there are a number of additional professionals who play a critical role in supporting families in the NICU. Certified lactation consultants provide breastfeeding support to NICU families, which can include assisting with accessing breast pumps, determining a pumping and breastfeeding schedule, and providing support, guidance, and direct interventions related to increasing maternal milk supply and infant feeding development. Social workers provide emotional support to families in the NICU and assist with accessing resources such as the Supplemental Nutrition Program for Women, Infants, and Children (WIC), Supplemental Nutrition Assistance Program (SNAP), or Medicaid. Finally, discharge planners may be social workers or nurses and their primary role is to assist families as they transition from the NICU. Although roles may vary across institutions, discharge planners help families to access home equipment (e.g., oxygen and feeding pumps), address concerns or problems related to health insurance, and coordinate follow-up services for families (e.g., follow-up specialist or pediatrician appointments).[28,256]

Given the wide range of professional disciplines and roles represented within the NICU, teamwork and collaboration are essential. A national expert panel was convened to determine the organizational culture and attributes of NICUs that were required for successful collaboration and quality improvement. The following characteristics of NICU were identified: (1) clear, shared purpose, (2) effective communication among team members, (3) management that leads by example, (4) trusting and respectful environment, (5) established standards of excellence, (6) competence and commitment among team members, and (7) commitment to conflict management.[185]

Models of Service Delivery

There is limited published literature to describe the type, frequency, and variability of NICU therapeutic models of service delivery.[28] However, models of service delivery commonly seen in pediatric rehabilitation are also applicable to the NICU. For example, in some NICUs, the therapeutic and developmental program is represented by only one professional discipline (e.g., physical therapy). In contrast, some NICUs have adopted a multidisciplinary model in which the therapeutic and developmental care team consists of more than one professional discipline (e.g., physical and occupational therapy) (Fig. 29.1). In this model, team members function in distinct but complementary roles.[28] For example, occupational therapists might be responsible for splinting, speech therapists address oral feeding development, and physical therapists focus on positioning and therapeutic handling or massage. Thus the determination of which professional discipline will perform the examination and intervention is guided by the infant's greatest area of need. In our experience the multidisciplinary model of care can foster a targeted use of resources and expertise when a primary infant need (e.g., splinting) is identified. However, as described later in the chapter, infants experience a variety of medical, neurobehavioral, and interactional vulnerabilities that require a multifaceted approach to examination and intervention. As such, a possible limitation to a multidisciplinary approach is that multiple therapists are working with the family, which has the

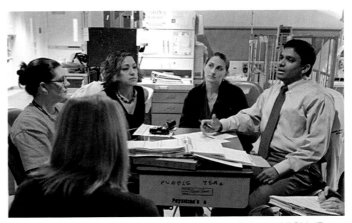

FIG. 29.1 Multidisciplinary patient care rounds in the NICU. (From Walden M, Elliott E, Gregurich MS: Delphi Survey of Barriers and Organizational Factors Influencing Nurses' Participation in Patient Care Rounds. *Newborn Infant Nurs* Rev 9(3):169-174, 2009.)

potential to create fragmentation, caregiver burden, and unnecessary handling of fragile infants.

To address potential limitations of a multidisciplinary model, a transdisciplinary model of care adopts a comprehensive and holistic view of the infant. As such, the transdisciplinary model requires that team members share professional roles such that the boundaries across disciplines become less distinct.[28,51] For example, all therapeutic and developmental care team members are competent in issues related to oral feeding, positioning, and neonatal massage. This model has a number of strengths such as reducing the number of providers handling the infant, allowing for a unified and integrated approach to care where "the role differentiation between disciplines is defined by the needs of the situation rather than by discipline-specific characteristics."[51] However, this amorphous role delineation can be problematic at times if therapists feel like a particular area of NICU intervention (e.g., oral feeding) is the purview of their professional discipline.[28] As such, the balance between a transdisciplinary model of care and professional role delineation is critical.

In addition to the model of service delivery, there are other important considerations for addressing the needs of infants and families in the NICU. Although therapists in other subspecialties within the hospital typically see 8 to 10 patients per 8-hour day (from 9 AM to 5 PM), physical therapists in the NICU are constrained by frequent medical procedures, strict feeding schedules, evening parental visiting schedules, and infection considerations for patients seen outside of the NICU. As such, the model of service delivery needs to be flexible with regard to productivity demands, work hours, and managing schedules of patients other than those in the NICU. The needs and realities of the rehabilitation department and ensuring equity of responsibility among all therapists are additional considerations.

Professional Role Delineation

Depending on NICU staff resources, organizational culture, and type of hospital, physical therapists may work closely with occupational therapists, speech language pathologists, and developmental specialists. As such, professional role delineations related to oral feeding, positioning, infant massage, and facilitation and handling may become blurred. According to the APTA, physical therapists are experts in examination and intervention of impairments in body functions and structures and motor activity limitations of the musculoskeletal and neuromuscular system.[245] To this end, this expertise may cross traditional professional boundaries, and physical therapists should work collaboratively with colleagues from other disciplines while advocating for the growth of their profession. Indeed, as described in the previous sections, the professional roles of each of the therapeutic and developmental care team members overlap. Yet, a unifying theme is developmentally supportive care.[28,256] In our experience, all therapeutic and developmental care team members should be competent in neurobehavioral evaluation and treatment in order to provide family-centered, individualized, developmentally supportive care across different contexts of NICU care (e.g., positioning, routine care, oral feeding, environmental modifications, and parent–infant interaction). Particular team members may choose to pursue advanced clinical practice training in NICU interventions (i.e., infant massage, oral feeding techniques) and can serve as valuable assets to the NICU therapeutic and developmental care team to provide expert consultation when necessary.

THEORETICAL FRAMEWORKS GUIDING PRACTICE IN THE NICU

Three theoretical frameworks for serving infants in the NICU are family systems, the International Classification of Functioning, Disability and Health (ICF) model, and the synactive theory. Those theoretical frameworks address the three main components of physical therapy intervention: communication and coordination, information sharing with parents, and procedural interventions (for more details, refer to Chapters 1 and 30).

Family Systems

Premature birth, followed by the intensity of the experience of the NICU, is highly stressful and sometimes traumatic not only for the baby but also for the parents and the whole family. The NICU experience for parents may vary depending on the severity of the infant's illness and the level of preparedness parents have prior to the infant's admission to the NICU.[180,256] Although prior knowledge of a possible premature or complicated birth may soften the intensity of the experience at first, all parents of premature infants are particularly vulnerable throughout their infant's neonatal period. The foremost concern is for survival. Once survival is certain, concern shifts to the quality of the infant's developmental outcome. The parents themselves can be considered to be "premature parents" and may be mourning the loss of the "imagined" or "wished-for baby" as they struggle to develop a bond with their "real baby."[52,133] Parents report that the NICU experience often leaves them with a temporary loss of their parental role and identity and that at time of discharge they may feel overwhelmed, worried, and even panicked, especially if their infant had required ventilation while in the NICU.[209] The phase immediately after discharge from the hospital is often one of anxious adjustment during which mothers express their lack of confidence and insecurity in caring for their preterm infant.[199] We encourage physical therapists to reflect on the impact of an early birth or birth of a sick infant on parents, on the sense of temporary loss of parental roles and identity, and feeling overwhelmed at time of discharge.

The length of stay for infants admitted to the NICU varies widely according to the severity of the condition leading to the admission. Some infants may spend as little as 1 day in the NICU (e.g., due to respiratory distress); others may spend months (e.g., due to extreme prematurity, short gut). Research on parental response to having their newborn admitted to the NICU has been fairly consistent in reporting a high level of parental stress and anxiety, which may lead to a posttraumatic stress reaction (PTSR). PTSR is a predictor of infant sleep and eating problems at 18 months.[200] The prevalence of postpartum depression (PPD) in mothers of newborns admitted to the NICU (45%) is higher compared to PPD in first-time mothers of healthy infants (8% to 15%).[33] On a more positive note a recent study reported that the implementation of the "parent friendly" changes as seen in most hospitals across the United States contributed to helping parents make a more successful adaptation to having an infant in the NICU.[62]

Admission of the newborn to the NICU happens at a critical time in the development of the family unit. For the infant, biobehavioral transition from intrauterine to extrauterine life occurs in the first months of life.[180] For the parents, the first months are a time when they search for "the goodness of fit" between themselves and their new baby.[249] The core challenge for parents is to engage with their baby in a way that is unique to them and fosters the baby's development.[234] Many factors may render the relationship between parents and their premature infant vulnerable. Premature infants have poor abilities to self-regulate physiologic rhythms, and attention is limited, which can disrupt the parent–infant synchrony so critical during interactive episodes.[89] Preterm infants are more irritable, smile less, and have facial signals that are less clear than full-term infants,[229] all of which affect the parents' ability to read and respond to their infant's cues.[89] Steinberg contended that posttraumatic stress reaction and depression interfere with the parents' ability to read their baby's cues and respond sensitively to the baby's needs.[233] Nevertheless, a number of studies have demonstrated that during this difficult hospital time, helping parents understand their baby's behavior appears to be critical in helping them maintain their role as parents and mitigate levels of stress.[141,156,210]

Physical therapists, with their unique skills in infant behavioral observation and developmental intervention, play an important role in the support offered parents during this difficult time. The physical therapist can help the parents read their baby's cues and provide feedback on their baby's responses. Several studies have reported long-term effects ranging from 9 months to 2 years of behaviorally based interventions on infant development, parent–infant interaction, maternal confidence and self-esteem, and paternal attitudes toward and involvement in caregiving.[73,97,192,208] Primarily derived from the Neonatal Behavioral Assessment Scale (NBAS) (described later in the chapter), behaviorally based intervention tools that have been developed to promote parent and child outcomes are summarized in Table 29.1 and may be useful resources of therapists working in the NICU.

Family-Centered Care

Family-centered care (FCC) was first defined in 1987 as part of former surgeon general Everett Koop's initiative for family-centered, community-based, coordinated care for children with special health care needs and their families. The American Academy of Pediatrics (AAP) recognizes the importance of FCC as an approach to health care[178] and stresses the importance of the role that families play in patient outcomes.[160] At the heart of family-centered care is the recognition that the family is the constant in a child's life. For this reason,

family-centered care is built on partnerships between families and professionals. The Institute for Family-Centered Care has identified eight core concepts of FCC that guide the delivery of services to families with children with health care needs: (1) respect, (2) choice, (3) information, (4) collaboration, (5) strengths, (6) support, (7) empowerment, and (8) flexibility (www.familycenteredcare.org).

Many medical institutions and NICUs across the country have instituted their own FCC guidelines and practices, but for the most part they all share the pursuit of being responsive to the priorities and choices of families. Cleveland published a systematic review of the literature to identify the needs of parents in the NICU and the type of nursing support most helpful during their stay in the NICU (see Table 29.1).[66] Parents need accurate information, to have contact with their infant, and to be fully included in their infant's care. Individualized care and knowing that the NICU staff is watching over and protecting their infant is also important to parents. The types of behaviors that best support parents in the NICU are those where they feel welcome at all times, are encouraged to participate in their child's care, and are engaged in a therapeutic relationship with the nursing staff. Parent-to-parent groups provide families with additional emotional support.[66,83] Parents report a preference for multiple presentations of different formats including hands on, written, and group sessions to learn how to support their infant's development as they prepare for NICU discharge.[83] The physical therapist can consider these recommendations in the implementation of family-centered interventions in the NICU. Readers are encouraged to reflect on the multiple ways physical therapists can support families of infants in the NICU.

International Classification of Functioning, Disability and Health

The International Classification of Functioning, Disability and Health, commonly referred to as the ICF, is a framework for understanding relationships between health and disability at both individual and population levels that is described in Chapter 1.[274] The ICF was developed to create a common language to improve communication among health care providers, researchers, policy makers, and people with disabilities and to provide a scientific basis for understanding and studying health and health-related states, outcomes, and determinants.[189] The health-related domains are classified from body, individual, and societal perspectives by means of two lists: a list of body functions and structures and a list of domains of activity and participation. Because an individual's functioning and disability occur in a context, the ICF also includes a list of environmental and personal factors (for more information, see www.who.int/classifications/icf/en).

The ICF provides a framework to guide the choice of examination procedures and intervention strategies for infants receiving services in the NICU. High-risk neonates frequently demonstrate impairments in muscle tone, range of motion, sensory organization, and postural reactions. These impairments in body functions and structures may contribute to limitations in activity such as difficulty in breathing, feeding, visual and auditory responsiveness, and motor activities such as head control and movement of hands to mouth. The interaction between impairments and activity limitations may contribute to restrictions in parent–infant interaction (participation). The ICF model also considers personal and environmental factors as relevant influences on body functions and structures, activity,

TABLE 29.1 Needs of Parents Who Have Infants in the NICU and the Types of Support That Are Most Helpful	
Needs of Parents	**Behaviors That Support Parents**
Accurate information	Emotional support
Contact with the infant	Parent empowerment
Inclusion in the infant's care	A welcoming environment with supportive unit policies
Vigilant watching-over and protecting the infant	Parent education with an opportunity to practice new skills through guided participation
Being positively perceived by the nursery staff	
Individualized care	
A therapeutic relationship with the nursing staff	

From Cleveland LM: Parenting in the neonatal intensive care unit. *J Obstet Gynecol Neonatal Nurs* 37:666-691, 2008.

and participation. Personal factors include an infant's health complications and temperament. Environmental factors range from levels of lighting and noise in the special care nursery to family and community support such as appropriate shelter and access to necessary food and supplies that will directly influence the infant's outcome and well-being (Table 29.2 shows an example of the ICF model adapted for the infant in the NICU).

Synactive Theory

Since the late 1980s, advances in perinatal and newborn intensive care have dramatically decreased the mortality rates of preterm and sick newborns at high risk for developmental problems. As premature infants have become younger in gestational age at birth (as young as 23 weeks of gestation) and smaller in birth weight (as little as 450 g), there has been a growing concern among health care professionals to not only ensure their survival but to optimize their developmental course and outcome. Better known as developmental care, the intervention model designed to address these issues focuses on the detailed observation of infant neurobehavioral functioning to design highly individualized plans of care and provide developmentally appropriate experiential opportunities for the newborn in the hospital setting and the provision of supportive care for the infant's family.[12] Recent research suggests that individualized developmental care may improve some medical complications and short-term outcomes such as length of stay, level of alertness, and feeding progression.[167,196]

Als's synactive theory provides a framework for the neurobehavioral functioning of the young infant.[5] Infant neurobehavioral functioning is understood as the unfolding of sequential achievements in four interdependent behavioral dimensions organized as subsystems.[5] The infant (1) stabilizes her autonomic or physiologic behavior, (2) regulates or controls her motor behavior, (3) organizes her behavioral states and her responsiveness through interaction with her social and physical environment, and (4) orients to animate and inanimate objects. Through maturation and experience, the infant is able to organize her behavior subsystems and actively participate in her social world including interactions with caregivers to meet her needs.[5,48] Competency in behavioral organization can be determined through the careful observation of the behaviors displayed by the infant within each of the behavioral dimensions. Als has categorized behaviors within each of the behavioral dimensions as either "approach/regulatory" or "avoidance/stress."[5] Regulatory behaviors indicate a state of well-being and are observed when an infant's self-regulatory abilities are able to support the social and environmental demands placed on her; she is then described as organized.[72] Stress behaviors indicate a state of exhaustion and are observed when the infant's threshold for self-regulation is exceeded by the demands placed on her; she is then described as disorganized.[72]

The application of neurobehavioral observations to clinical practice has been formalized with the Newborn Individualized Developmental Care and Assessment Program (NIDCAP).[8,9] The NIDCAP proposes a structured method of weekly observation and assessment of infant behavior by a NIDCAP-certified developmental specialist or physical therapist. Based on these observations and following consultations with the infant's family and medical team, an individualized care plan is developed and implemented. Intervention is aimed at facilitating prolonged periods of organization by reinforcing the infant's individual self-regulatory style while supporting families to nurture and care for their infant.[11,12,42] Research indicates that the NIDCAP is associated with reduced length of hospital stay and incidence of brain hemorrhage and improved long-term medical and developmental outcomes.[8,12,167]

MEDICAL COMPLICATIONS OF INFANTS ADMITTED TO THE NICU

Knowledge of medical complications common in infants admitted to the NICU is important for understanding how health conditions may affect the infant's capacity for handling and physical activity, growth and development, and the parents' experience in the NICU.

Respiratory System

Several pulmonary, neurologic, cardiac, and other health conditions in neonates are associated with increased risk for impairments in body functions and structures that affect cognitive,

---

TABLE 29.2 Application of the International Classification of Functioning, Disability, and Health for Infants in the Neonatal Intensive Care Unit

Health Condition (Includes disease or injury)

Examples: prematurity, respiratory distress, intraventricular hemorrhage, periventricular leukomalacia, arthrogryposis, spina bifida, failure to thrive, short gut, Down syndrome

Body Functions and Structures	Activities	Participation
Physiologic and Psychological Functions of Body Systems	**Execution of a Task or Action by an Individual**	**Individual's Involvement in NICU Life Situations**
Examples: muscle tone, postural reactions, range of motion, sensory organization, behavioral state control, neurobehavioral functioning, physiologic stability↓	Examples: breathing, sucking, crying, head control, hand to mouth, kicking, grasping, visual and auditory responsiveness↓	Examples: parent-infant interaction, communication, being held by parents, feeding, sleeping, growing↓
Impairments	**Activity Limitations**	**Participation Restrictions**
Examples: skeletal deformity, fluctuating tone, startles, deafness, decreased range of motion, behavioral disorganization	Examples: cannot breathe on own, tube fed, cannot locate sound, self-calm, brings hand to mouth	Examples: cannot be held or fed by parents because of the inability to maintain physiologic stability and neurobehavioral organization

Environmental Factors	Personal Factors
Physical, Social, and Attitudinal Features of the Family and NICU Setting	**Personal Characteristics of the Individual**
Examples: lighting and noise levels, maternity leave, family support, family's distance to travel to hospital, siblings	Examples: medical complications, temperament, sensitivity, preferences

motor, sensory, behavioral, and psychosocial development and may result in long-term activity limitations and participation restrictions.[139] The physical therapist providing services in the NICU should have a working knowledge of physiology of neonates, pathophysiology and associated impairments in body functions and structures, and how impairments affect the infant's behavior. Practice in the NICU is a complex subspecialty of pediatrics, and knowledge and skills should be obtained through advanced didactic and practical education. Clinical guidelines and clinical training models for neonatal physical therapy are outlined by Sweeney, Heriza, and Blanchard[245] and are described later in the chapter.

Respiratory Distress Syndrome

Respiratory distress syndrome (RDS), or hyaline membrane disease, is the single most important cause of illness and death in preterm infants and is the most common single cause of respiratory distress in neonates (Fig. 29.2).[236] RDS occurs in 10% of all premature infants in the United States. The percentage increases to 50% to 60% for infants born less than 29 weeks of gestational age.[19,65] The principal factors in the pathophysiology of RDS are pulmonary immaturity and low production of surfactant. Low surfactant production results in increased surface tension, alveolar collapse, diffuse atelectasis, and decreased lung compliance. These factors cause an increase in pulmonary artery pressure that leads to extrapulmonary right-to-left shunting of blood and ventilation-perfusion mismatching. Clinical manifestations of RDS include grunting respirations, retractions, nasal flaring, cyanosis, and increased oxygen requirement after birth. Prophylactic use of antenatal steroids to accelerate lung maturation in women with preterm labor of up to 34 weeks significantly reduced the incidence of RDS and decreased mortality.[65]

Treatment goals for RDS include improvement in oxygenation and maintaining optimal lung volume.[65] The type of intervention depends on the severity of the respiratory disorder and includes oxygen supplementation, assisted ventilation, surfactant administration, and extracorporeal membrane oxygenation (ECMO). Continuous positive airway pressure (CPAP) or positive end-expiratory pressure (PEEP) is applied to prevent volume loss during expiration. Nasal and nasopharyngeal prongs are used with positive end-expiratory pressure ventilators. Mechanical ventilation via tracheal tube is used in severe cases of RDS. (See Chapter 25 for a more detailed description of ventilators.) Mechanical ventilation may injure the lungs of premature infants through high airway pressure (barotrauma), large gas volumes (volutrauma), alveolar collapse and refill (atelectotrauma), and increased inflammation (biotrauma).[24]

The new generation of ventilators is equipped with microprocessors enabling effective synchronized (patient-triggered) ventilation.[130] High-frequency oscillatory ventilation (HFOV) was developed with the goal of decreasing complications associated with mechanical ventilation. Conventional intermittent positive-pressure ventilation is provided 30 to 80 breaths per minute, whereas HFOV provides "breaths" at 10 to 15 cycles per second or 600 to 900 per minute. At this time, evidence is insufficient to support the routine use of HFOV.[110]

Prophylactic use of surfactant for infants judged to be at risk of developing RDS (infants less than 30 to 32 weeks of gestation) has been demonstrated to decrease the risk of pneumothorax, pulmonary interstitial emphysema, and mortality.[236] Early administration of multiple doses of natural or synthetic surfactant extract results in improved clinical outcome and appears to be the most effective method of administration. When a choice of natural or synthetic surfactant is available, natural surfactant

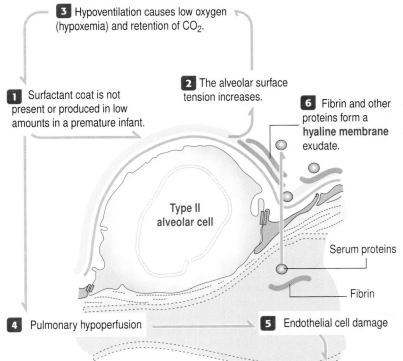

3 Hypoventilation causes low oxygen (hypoxemia) and retention of CO_2.

2 The alveolar surface tension increases.

1 Surfactant coat is not present or produced in low amounts in a premature infant.

6 Fibrin and other proteins form a **hyaline membrane** exudate.

Type II alveolar cell

Serum proteins

Fibrin

4 Pulmonary hypoperfusion

5 Endothelial cell damage

Surfactant deficiency

Surfactant is synthesized by type II alveolar cells after the 35th week of gestation. **Corticosteroids induce the synthesis of surfactant in the fetus.** **High levels of insulin** (diabetic mothers) **can antagonize the effect of corticosteroids.** Infants of diabetic mothers have a higher risk of developing **hyaline membrane disease.**

Surfactant reduces surface tension within the alveoli. Less pressure is required to keep alveoli open.

Surfactant also maintains alveolar expansion by modulating surface tension with alveolar size. In the newborn, **surfactant deficiency** causes the lungs to collapse (**atelectatic lung**) with each successive breath. A lack of O_2 impairs surfactant synthesis.

RDS in premature infants is complicated by a protein-rich, fibrin-rich exudation into the alveolar space, forming a **hyaline membrane** that leads to CO_2 retention.

FIG. 29.2 Neonatal respiratory distress syndrome (RDS) (From Kierszenbaum TL: *Histology and cell biology: an introduction to pathology.* 4th ed. Philadelphia: Saunders, 2016.)

shows greater early decrease in requirement for ventilatory support.[228,277] Newer synthetic surfactants include whole surfactant proteins or parts of the proteins (peptides). A clinical trial showed that these preparations decreased mortality and rates of necrotizing enterocolitis with other clinical outcomes being similar to those of natural surfactant preparations.[204] A pilot study showed that an inhaled steroid, budesonide, delivered intratracheally with surfactant administration to very low birth weight infants with severe RDS reduced mortality and chronic lung disease with no immediate adverse effects.[276]

ECMO is a technique of cardiopulmonary bypass modified from techniques developed for open-heart surgery that are used to support heart and lung function (for review of ECMO and implications for pediatric physical therapy, see[193]). In newborns with acute respiratory failure, the immature lungs are allowed to rest and recover to avoid the damaging effects of mechanical ventilation. Because of the need for systemic administration of heparin and the resultant risk of systemic and intracranial hemorrhage, ECMO is reserved for use with infants who are at least 34 weeks of gestational age, weigh more than 2000 g, have no evidence of intracranial bleeding, require less than 10 days of assisted ventilation, and have reversible lung disease.[240] ECMO is contraindicated for infants younger than 34 weeks of age because of high rates of intracranial hemorrhage, perhaps because of systemic anticoagulation necessary with ECMO or abnormal cerebrovascular pressures and flows accompanying ECMO. ECMO is used to manage intractable hypoxemia in near-term infants and newborns with meconium aspiration, RDS, pneumonia sepsis, and congenital diaphragmatic hernia.[65]

Although prognosis of infants with RDS is related to the severity of the original disease, the cause of infant mortality is most often complications of extreme prematurity such as infections, necrotizing enterocolitis, and intracranial hemorrhage rather than acute respiratory failure.[130] Infants who do not require assisted ventilation recover without developmental or medical sequelae, but the clinical course of the very immature infant may be complicated by air leaks in the lungs and BPD. Infants who survive severe RDS often require frequent hospitalization for upper respiratory tract infections and have an increased incidence of neurologic sequelae.[116]

Technologies for management of RDS include inhalation of nitrous oxide, liquid ventilation, or a hybrid of liquid and gas ventilation. The rationale for using liquid ventilation is to decrease alveolar surface tension by eliminating the air-liquid interface by filling the alveolus with liquid.[65] Inhalation of nitrous oxide helps decrease pulmonary artery resistance and cytokine-induced lung inflammation and increase gas exchange. Findings regarding the use of nitrous oxide (NO) and prevention of chronic lung disease and neurologic injury are inconclusive.[22] Inhaled nitric oxide for severe RDS is an experimental treatment that may decrease chronic lung disease and mortality. However, increase in intracranial hemorrhage caused a termination of a study in 2006.[114]

Bronchopulmonary Dysplasia and Chronic Lung Disease of Infancy

Very premature birth occurs during a stage of parenchymal development when oxygenation without support is not always feasible,[25] leading to the need for supplemental oxygenation and/or mechanical ventilation support. As a consequence, many preterm infants develop bronchopulmonary dysplasia (BPD) and are later diagnosed with chronic lung disease (CLD)

of infancy. The major predictors of BPD are lower gestational age and mechanical ventilation on day 7; however, the ability to identify infants at risk for BPD is imperfect at best.[123,263] The National Institute of Child Health and Human Development defines infants with mild BPD as requiring oxygen supplementation for 28 days but in room air at 36 weeks postmenstrual age (PMA), those with moderate BPD as requiring oxygen for first 28 days and oxygen < 30% at 36 weeks PMA, and those with severe BPD as requiring oxygen the first 28 days and oxygen > 30% and ventilatory support at 36 PMA.[124,239] Stoll and colleagues report rates of mild BPD as 27%, moderate as 23%, and severe as 18% in a cohort of 9575 infants born between 2003 and 2007.[239] The incidence of BPD increases as birth weight decreases, and infants with birth weights < 1250g constitute 97% of the population of infants with this condition.[262] CLD is diagnosed at 36 weeks of postmenstrual age if there is a continued need for supplemental oxygen, abnormal physical examination, and abnormal chest radiograph.

The cause of BPD is multifactorial but is primarily related to very premature birth and lung injury secondary to the ventilation and oxygen support provided to sustain these very premature infants.[25] The relationship between chorioamnionitis (antenatal infection) and BPD is unclear but may influence the infant's response to surfactant treatment.[123] Findings by Balinotti and his colleagues suggest that abnormal growth and development of the lung parenchyma occur even in clinically stable infants and toddlers with mild lung disease, and the degree of lung parenchyma development and gestational age at birth may be relevant factors in later alveolar development.[25] The lung tissue at 24 to 26 weeks is in the late canalicular stage of development and in the saccular stage between 30 to 32 weeks. During these phases, lung growth is marked with extensive vasculogenesis within the developing terminal saccules that then form secondary crests along with interstitial extracellular matrix loss and remodeling. Although alveoli are present in some infants at 32 weeks of gestation, they are not uniformly present until 36 weeks, during the alveolar stage of development. Thus premature birth and initiation of pulmonary gas exchange interrupts normal alveolar and distal vascular development.[68] The consistent lesion seen in BPD is alveolar simplification (decrease in alveolization) and enlargement, which results from an impairment, not an arrest, in postnatal alveolization in an extremely immature lung following preterm birth, an abnormal capillary morphology, and an interstitium with variable cellularity/fibrloproliferation.[67,68]

Because BPD is an evolving process of lung injury and recovery, the pathophysiology is likely to differ at different times.[262] Walsh and his colleagues propose three stages in the progression of BPD to guide the implementation of specific therapeutic modalities. Stage 1 is for the prevention of BPD and occurs during the perinatal (before birth and up to 4 days of age) and early postnatal (up to 7 days of age); stage 2 constitutes the phase of treatment of evolving BPD beginning at 7 to 14 days of age; stage 3 is for the treatment of established BPD beginning at 28 days of life. In stage 1 inflammation is the predominant issue needed to be addressed with anti-inflammatory treatments (e.g., antenatal corticosteroids, antioxidant therapies). In stage 2 the goal is to stop or minimize the development of the disease with therapies directed at controlling inflammation and lung water with systemic or inhaled corticosteroids, anti-inflammatory agents, and diuretics. In stage 3, where BPD is established, issues are related to overly reactive airways, lung fluid retention, and an oxygenation defect. Jobe advocates efforts to decrease the invasive nature of NICU care in general while empowering the premature infant to breathe spontaneously and grow.[123]

Meconium Aspiration Syndrome

Meconium aspiration syndrome (MAS) is defined as respiratory distress in an infant born through meconium-stained amniotic fluid whose symptoms cannot be otherwise explained.[87] It can be characterized by early-onset respiratory distress in term and near-term infants with symptoms of respiratory distress, poor lung compliance, and hypoxemia and radiographic findings of hyperinflation and patchy opacifications with rales and rhonchi on auscultation.[268] Because of the frequent occurrence of air leaks in these infants, positive-pressure ventilation is contraindicated. It is unclear whether the meconium itself causes pneumonitis severe enough to lead to the above symptoms or if the presence of meconium in the amniotic fluid is a result of other events such as stressed labor, postmaturity, and depressed cord pH that may have predisposed the fetus to severe pulmonary disease.[65] It is recommended that the infant with depressed physiologic function and meconium-stained fluid be suctioned endotracheally because pharyngeal suctioning does not reduce MAS.[251] Antibiotics are often given until bacterial infection is ruled out. The infant is hypersensitive to environmental stimuli and should be treated in the quietest environment possible. According to a Cochrane review in 2014, surfactant administration may reduce the severity of MAS and decrease the number of infants requiring ECMO.[85,224] Obstetric approaches to the prevention of MAS such as intrapartum surveillance, amnioinfusion, and delivery room management have not demonstrated a decrease in MAS.[275] Approximately 20% of infants with MAS demonstrated neurodevelopmental delays up to 3 years of age even though they responded well to conventional treatment.[34]

Cardiac System

Cardiac conditions common to neonates in the NICU include congenital heart defects such as patent ductus arteriosis (PDA), pulmonary atresia, tetralogy of Fallot (TOF), coarctation of the aorta (COA), and pulmonary atresia. Cardiac conditions are presented in Chapter 28.

Neurologic System

Intraventricular Hemorrhage and Periventricular Hemorrhage

Intraventricular hemorrhage (IVH) occurs in about 45% of infants with birth weights between 500–750 g and in about 20% of infants with birth weights < 1500 g.[121,270] Despite medical advances, IVH remains a major problem for the premature infant. Most hemorrhages occur within the first 48 hours after birth and are related to the fragility of the germinal matrix located on the head of the caudate nucleus and underneath the ventricular ependymal.[26] When the hemorrhage is substantial, the ependymal breaks and the blood spills into the ventricles.[26] Diagnosis is based on routine or symptom-driven screening through cranial ultrasound. Papile developed a four-level grading scale based on ultrasound scan to classify hemorrhages.[190] Grade I is a hemorrhage isolated to the germinal matrix; grade II is an IVH with normal-sized ventricles that occurs when hemorrhage in the subependymal germinal matrix ruptures through the ependyma into the lateral ventricles; grade III is an IVH with acute ventricular dilation; and, grade IV is a hemorrhage that spreads into the periventricular white matter. IVH is primarily associated with the fragility of the germinal matrix

vasculature, disturbances in the cerebral blood flow (CBF), and platelet and coagulation disorders.[26] Risk factors that can disturb CBF include vaginal delivery, low Apgar score, severe respiratory distress syndrome, pneumothorax, hypoxia, hypercapnia, seizures, patent ductus arteriosus, thrombocytopenia, infection,[26] and mechanical ventilation.[16]

The signs and symptoms of IVH may range from subtle and nonspecific to catastrophic. Clinical signs include abnormalities in the level of consciousness, movement, muscle tone, respiration, and eye movement. Catastrophic deterioration involves major acute hemorrhages with clinical signs of stupor progressing to coma, respiratory distress progressing to apnea, generalized tonic seizures, decerebrate posturing, generalized tonic seizure, and flaccid quadriparesis.[26]

Premature infants with grade I–II IVH are at risk for neurosensory impairment, developmental delay, cerebral palsy, and deafness at 2–3 years of age[44]; for those with more severe IVH, especially grade IV, the risk for cerebral palsy can be present in up to 39% of infants, hydrocephalus in up to 37% of infants with declines in cognitive functioning from a mental developmental index of 97 for grade I to 77.5 for grade IV.[206] Clearly, the occurrence of IVH in the premature infant has lifelong implications, even for those with lower-grade hemorrhages.

Efforts to prevent IVH directed at strengthening the germinal matrix vasculature with angiogenic inhibitors and stabilizing the CBF through the reduction of stimulation to the infants have met with varying degrees of success.[27] Prenatal care aiming at reducing premature birth includes preventive obstetric care for high-risk pregnancy, treatment of bacterial vaginosis, and prevention of preterm labor.[165] The use of antenatal steroids (betamethasone, dexamethasone) has been shown to reduce both the severity and incidence of severe IVH.[63] Indomethacin, commonly used to close patent ductus arteriosus, has been shown to prevent IVH as well.[27]

Interventions following IVH include close monitoring and management of ventricular dilation. Acute treatment includes physiologic support to maintain oxygenation, perfusion, body temperature, and blood glucose level. Physical handling is minimized. Management of ventricular dilation includes ventriculoperitoneal shunting or temporary ventricular draining.

Periventricular Leukomalacia

Periventricular leukomalacia (PVL) is a form of cerebral white matter injury consisting of periventricular focal necrosis, with subsequent cystic formation and diffuse cerebral gliosis in the surrounding white matter.[21,260] It is the leading known cause of cerebral palsy (CP) and commonly associated with cognitive impairment and visual disturbances.[260] It is more common in premature than term infants and occurs more frequently with decreasing gestational age and birth weight.[76] The pathogenesis of PVL is mainly linked to ischemia and inflammation in the preterm infant[131] and may occur with intraventricular and periventricular hemorrhage.[2] A case-control study conducted to examine the impact of potential risk factors other than prematurity on the incidence of PVL identified maternal obesity and chorioamnionitis as the only factors associated with PVL regardless of gestational age. Maternal age (> 35), preexisting and gestational diabetes, in vitro fertilization, severe preeclampsia, no prenatal steroids, vaginal delivery, and small for gestational age were not associated with PVL.[111]

PVL is caused by a cascade of events leading to a reduction in cerebral blood flow in the highly vulnerable periventricular region of the brain where the arterial "end zones" of the middle, posterior, and anterior cerebral arteries meet and is often associated with IVH.[260] Decreased cerebral blood flow leads to ischemia and a decrease in antioxidants. The resulting release of free oxygen radicals and glutamate toxicity primarily target premyelinated oligodendrocytes that predominate in the periventricular regions between 24–34 weeks of gestation.[126] The incidence of white matter damage increased in premature infants with decreased gestational age due to the added presence of an immature vascular supply and impairments in cerebral autoregulation.[132,260] PVL also affects subplate neurons that lie just below the developing cerebral cortex until programmed apoptosis (cell death). Subplate neurons play an essential role in axonal targeting of thalamocortical synapses, and their loss may contribute to motor, visual, and cognitive impairments.[76]

The area primarily affected by intraventricular or periventricular hemorrhaging includes the white matter through which long descending motor tracts travel from the motor cortex to the spinal cord. Because the motor tracts involved in the control of leg movements are closest to the ventricles and therefore more likely to be damaged, bilateral cerebral palsy with primary lower extremity involvement is the most common motor impairment. If the lesion extends laterally, the arms may be involved, resulting in bilateral cerebral palsy with both upper extremity and lower extremity involvement. Visual impairments may also result from damage to the optic radiations.[272]

Cranial ultrasonography (CUS) after birth is commonly used for routine screening of hemorrhaging lesions; later, CUS allows diagnosis of white matter abnormalities such as seen in PVL,[215] which can later be confirmed with magnetic resonance imaging. Later detection at or around term age of white matter abnormalities has the highest correlation with neuropathologic findings and subsequent neurodevelopmental outcome (cerebral palsy and cognitive impairments). Cerebral palsy occurs in more than 90% of infants who develop bilateral cysts larger than 3 mm in diameter in the parietal or occipital areas.[75]

Medical management focuses on prevention of events leading to decreased cerebral blood flow and IVH and includes prevention of intrauterine hypoxic or ischemic events, postnatal maintenance of adequate ventilation and perfusion, avoidance of systemic hypotension, and control of seizures.[260] Prevention of intrauterine hypoxic and ischemic events includes identification of high-risk pregnancies, fetal monitoring, fetal blood sampling, and cesarean section as indicated. Maintenance of adequate ventilation includes avoiding common causes of hypoxemia such as inappropriate feeding, inserting or removing ventilator connections, painful procedures and examinations, handling, and excessive noise. Adequate perfusion can be maintained with appropriate treatment if the infant exhibits apnea and severe bradycardia.

Hypoxic Ischemic Encephalopathy

Hypoxic ischemic encephalopathy (HIE) is the result of either hypoxemia or ischemia leading to the deprivation of oxygen and glucose to the neural tissue. Hypoxemia is a decrease in the amount of oxygen circulating in the blood while ischemia is a decrease in the blood flow able to perfuse the brain. Of the two, ischemia is the more problematic because delivery of glucose to the brain is decreased.[257] HIE is a type of neonatal encephalopathy diagnosed in infants who present with fetal abnormalities (fetal heart rate abnormalities, fetal distress), an acute event followed by a characteristic clinical presentation

(respiratory depression, abnormalities of tone, disturbance in cranial nerve function, and often, seizures), an arterial blood gas indicative of metabolic acidosis (pH < 7.0), depressed Apgar scores (≤ 5 at 5 and/or 10 minutes, need for respiratory support), and imaging findings consistent with hypoxic-ischemic disease.[259] Symptoms typically evolve over of period of 72 hours after birth. Ischemia appears to be the main cause of the brain lesions seen in HIE, typically located in the distribution of vascular end zones and border zones and involving neurons and premyelinating oligodendrocytes that are intrinsically vulnerable (e.g., to excitotoxicity).[260] The presence of hypoxia and ischemia leads to cellular energy failure, acidosis, glutamate release, intracellular accumulation of calcium, lipid peroxidation, and nitric oxide neurotoxicity, which in turn leads to the destruction of essential components of the cell, culminating in cell death.[257] The extent of the damage will be consistent with the timing, severity, and duration of the hypoxic-ischemic event leading to necrosis and neuronal cell death in the affected zones.

The incidence of HIE ranges between 1 and 8 per 1000 live births.[137] Causes of HIE are multiple and can occur from maternal (e.g., hypotension, insulin-dependent diabetes mellitus, cardiac arrest), uteroplacental (e.g., placental vasculopathy), intrapartum (e.g., prolapsed cord, abruption placentae, traumatic delivery with asphyxia), or fetal complications.[147] The Sarnat and Sarnat[216] staging of encephalopathy using clinical and electroencephalogram criteria, with classification into mild, moderate, and severe stages has been a useful tool in documenting the clinical progression of the severity of the injury and correlates well with neurodevelopmental impairment in infancy.[222] Predictors of neurologic and developmental outcome include abnormal neurologic examination, neonatal seizures, abnormal EEG and MRI with seizures highly correlated with poor developmental outcome at 1 year of age.[95] Neurodevelopmental outcome depends on the severity and extent of the cerebral lesions and is often profound and multisensorial.

Treatment of neonatal HIE includes the provision of adequate perfusion, ventilation, and oxygenation with control of seizures if present.[257] Whole body hypothermia to a target temperature of 33–34°C for 72 hours has been shown to reduce death or morbidity[222] but has not shown to completely resolve the adverse effects of HIE. Hypothermia is instituted within the first 6 hours of age to be most effective. The infant is placed on a precooled blanket and an esophageal temperature probe is inserted through the nose to a level of T6-9 to monitor body temperature for 72 hours.[257] Other neuroprotective interventions being studied include oxygen free radical scavengers and excitatory amino acid antagonists such as allopurinol and glutamate receptor antagonists.[257]

There is a 10% risk of death with moderate HIE, and up to 30% of infants manifest bilateral cerebral palsy with upper and lower extremity involvement and cognitive impairment resulting from cortical and subcortical injury in a parasagittal distribution.[260] In moderate HIE, the infant's initial clinical presentation includes lethargy, moderate feeding problems, high tone, and seizures. In severe HIE, mortality is 60% and the majority of all survivors will have long-term morbidity associated with damage to the thalami, basal ganglia, hippocampi, and mesencephalic structures. Long-term sequelae include cognitive impairment, spastic quadriparesis, seizure disorder, ataxia, bulbar and pseudobulbar palsy, atonic quadriparesis, hyperactivity, and impaired attention. The initial clinical presentation of the infant with severe HIE includes coma, ventilation support, severe feeding problems, flaccid tone, and seizures.[216]

Pain

Pain is defined as an unpleasant sensory and emotional experience associated with actual or potential tissue damage and is best described by self-report.[105] Obviously the neonate cannot report on pain but may express pain through specific pain behaviors, physiologic changes, changes in cerebral blood flow, and cellular and molecular changes in pain-processing pathways. Adverse sequelae may "include death, poor neurologic outcomes, abnormal somatization and response to pain later in life."[105] The peripheral nervous system is capable of responding to stimuli by 20 weeks postconception. Both the number and types of peripheral receptors are similar to those of adults by 20 to 24 weeks of gestation with a resulting increased density of receptors in the newborn as compared with adult. Spinal cord and brain stem tracts are not fully myelinated; therefore central nerve conduction is slow. There is evidence that pain pathways, cortical and subcortical centers of pain perception, and neurochemical systems associated with pain transmission are functional in premature neonates of 20 to 24 weeks of gestational age.[92]

Most nociceptive impulses are transmitted by nonmyelinated C fibers but also by A delta and A beta fibers, which transmit light touch and proprioception in adults.[105] However, the pain modulatory tracts, which can inhibit pain through release of inhibitory neurotransmitters such as serotonin, dopamine, and norepinephrine, are not developed until 36 to 40 weeks of gestation. As a consequence, the preterm infant is more sensitive to pain than term or older infants.[105,235] Painful stimuli resulting from medical conditions and medical procedures (such as heel sticks, intubation, ventilation, ocular exam, and IV placement) can lead to prolonged structural and functional alterations in pain pathways that may persist into adult life.[39,92] The infant also may associate touch with painful input, which can interfere with bonding and attachment.

Although it is difficult to assess pain in the neonate, the physical therapist working in the NICU should be aware of methods of examination and nonpharmacologic intervention to alleviate pain. Both physiologic and behavioral responses of the neonate to nociceptive or painful stimuli have been identified. Physiologic manifestations of pain include increased heart rate, heart rate variability, blood pressure, and respirations, with evidence of decreased oxygenation. Skin color and character include pallor or flushing, diaphoresis, and palmar sweating. Other indicators of pain are increased muscle tone, dilated pupils, and laboratory evidence of metabolic or endocrine changes.[207] Neonatal behavioral responses to nociceptive input include sustained and intense crying; facial expression of grimaces, furrowed brow, quivering chin, or eyes tightly closed; motor behavior such as limb withdrawal, thrashing, rigidity, flaccidity, fist clenching, finger splaying, and limb extension; and changes in behavioral state.[104] Pain may lead to poor nutritional intake, delayed wound healing, impaired mobility, sleep disturbances, withdrawal, irritability, and other developmental regression.[261]

Nonpharmacologic methods to alleviate pain include decreasing the number of noxious stimuli, decreasing stimulation, swaddling, nonnutritive sucking, tactile comfort measures, rocking, containment, and music.[261] Preterm neonates demonstrated a lower mean heart rate, shorter crying time, and shorter mean sleep disruption after heel stick with facilitated tucking (containing the infant with hands softly holding the infant's extremities in soft flexion) than without (Fig. 29.3).[70,265] Administration of breast milk, sucrose solution, and nonnutritive sucking may help decrease the pain response in newborn infants.[142,220] Sensorial stimulation, which includes subtle tactile, vestibular, gustative, olfactory, auditory, and visual modalities, was found to be effective in decreasing pain responses of premature infants receiving heel sticks.[35]

Other Complications
Gastroesophageal Reflux

Two thirds of otherwise healthy infants will have gastroesophageal reflux (GER) and seek advice from their pediatricians or other health care providers.[148] GER is defined as the passage of gastric contents into the esophagus and is distinguished from gastroesophageal reflux disease (GERD), which includes troublesome symptoms or complications associated with GER. GERD is far less common that GER.[254] GER, considered a normal physiologic process that occurs several times a day in infants, children, and adults, is generally associated with transient relaxations of the lower esophageal sphincter independent of swallowing, which permits gastric content to enter the esophagus.[148] GER typically occurs after meals and causes few or no symptoms. In infants, GER may be associated with regurgitation, spitting up, and even vomiting.[212] The content of the reflux is generally nonacidic and improves with maturation.[148]

GERD can be classified as either esophageal or extraesophageal and be further characterized by findings of mucosal injury on upper endoscopy.[148] Esophageal GERD conditions include vomiting, irritability, poor weight gain, dysphagia, abdominal or substernal pain, and esophagitis.[148] Extraesophageal conditions can include respiratory symptoms, including cough and laryngitis, as well as wheezing in infancy.[223] Dental erosions, pharyngitis, sinusitis, and recurrent otitis media can also be present as the child gets older. Children with neurologic impairment, certain genetic disorders, esophageal atresia, chronic lung disease, cystic fibrosis, and prematurity are at higher risk for GERD than other populations. The incidence of GERD is also lower in breastfed infants compared to formula-fed infants.[188]

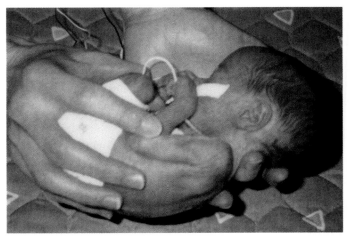

FIG. 29.3 Handling is slow and based on infant's cues. (From VandenBerg KA: Individualized developmental care for high risk newborns in the NICU: a practice guideline. *Early Hum Dev* 83(7):433-442, 2007.)

Diagnosis of GER is typically based on the infant's symptoms and physical examination. If the infant is growing and generally healthy, further testing is not indicated. Diagnostic tests for GERD include esophageal pH monitoring to measure the acidity of the infant's esophagus. A tube is inserted through the infant's nostril or mouth and left in place for 24 hours to monitor the frequency and duration of esophageal acid exposure.[148] X-rays may be needed if an obstruction is suspected, and an upper endoscopy may be done to rule out problems in the esophagus (stricture or inflammation). Upper GI tract contrast radiography is an option when infants are able to tolerate testing. A GERD behavioral scale questionnaire called the Infant Gastroesophageal Reflux Questionnaire (I-GERQ) has been shown to be valid and specific[134] and has been modified by Birch and Newell for premature infants.[40]

Management of GER is done through lifestyle modifications to minimize symptoms and does not require medication. Lifestyle modifications for both GER and GERD include a combination of feeding changes and positioning therapy. Modifying maternal diet in breastfed infants, changing formulas, reducing feeding volume while increasing frequency of feedings, and using thickened feedings are strategies shown to be effective in managing the symptoms of GER and milder symptoms of GERD.[254] Pharmacotherapeutic agents include acid suppressants, antacids, histamine 2 receptor antagonists (H2RAs), proton pump inhibitors (PPIs), and prokinetic agents. Surgical intervention is reserved for children with intractable symptoms or who are at risk for life-threatening complications of GERD. Surgical options include fundoplication, where the gastric fundus is wrapped around the distal esophagus, and total esophagogastric dissociation if fundoplication has failed.

Neonatal Abstinence Syndrome

Neonatal abstinence syndrome (NAS) or neonatal withdrawal is a term used to describe an array of signs and neurobehaviors seen in the newborn after abrupt termination of gestational exposure to substances taken by the mother during pregnancy, principally opioids.[122] Common substances and drugs include opioids such as heroin and methadone, prescription medications containing opioids such as hydrocodone or oxycodone, benzodiazepines, alcohol, antidepressants, and antipsychotics. These drugs are metabolized by the placenta and their metabolites cross the placental barrier through varied diffusion and transportation processes.[37] Further complicating the situation for the exposed infant is the possibility of polysubstance use, psychiatric co-morbidities, and other life factors such as violence, lack of prenatal care, and poor nutrition.[122]

Common clinical presentations in the neonate include high-pitched cry, irritability, sleep-wake disturbances, hyperactive primitive reflexes, transient tone alterations (tremors, hypertonicity), feeding difficulties, gastrointestinal disturbances (vomiting and loose stools), autonomic dysfunction (mottling, tachypnea, sweating, sneezing, nasal stuffiness, fever, yawning), failure to thrive, and seizures.[91] Symptoms of withdrawal usually occur within 72 hours after birth.[219]

The diagnosis of NAS is made based on maternal history, maternal and infant toxicology lab tests, and clinical examination of the infant. The severity of withdrawal or abstinence is commonly scored using the Finnegan Scoring System[91] on a list of 21 symptoms that are most frequently observed in opiate-exposed infants. Each symptom and its associated degree of severity are assigned a score, and the total abstinence score is determined by totaling the score assigned to each symptom over the scoring period. Neurobehavioral functioning and recovery can be assessed with the Neonatal Intensive Care Unit Network Neurobehavioral Scale (NNNs), which was designed to provide a comprehensive assessment of both neurologic integrity and behavioral functions.[144]

Infants with withdrawal symptoms may require admission to the NICU for close monitoring and pharmacologic treatment with closely monitored administration of opioid-containing medications (morphine, tincture of opium, or methadone) or buprenorphine, which is gradually weaned as withdrawal symptoms decline. Contingently to medication, supportive measures are offered to support the infant's ability to eat, sleep, and interact. Supportive therapeutic modalities include nonnutritive sucking, positioning/swaddling, gentle handling, demand feeding, minimal stimulation, and environmental modifications to promote a quiet and subdued environment for the infant.[135]

Necrotizing Enterocolitis

Necrotizing enterocolitis (NEC) is an acute inflammatory disease of the bowel that occurs most frequently in premature infants weighing less than 2000 g during the first 6 weeks of life.[99,157] Although the cause is not known, several factors appear to play a role in the pathogenesis of NEC. Many of these factors involve impaired blood flow to the intestine that results in death of mucosal cells lining the bowel wall making it permeable to gas-forming bacteria that invade the damaged area to produce pneumatosis intestinalis, air in the submucosal or subserosal surfaces of the bowel.[149]

Signs of obstruction of the bowels include vomiting, distention of the abdomen, increased gastric aspirates, passing of bloody stools, retention of stools, lethargy, decreased urine output, and alterations in respiratory status. Diagnosis of NEC is made by physical examination, laboratory tests, and radiography. Radiographic or abdominal ultrasonography is used to follow the course of the disease, with lucent bubbles appearing as the gas-forming bacteria enter the intestinal wall.[117] Medical treatment of NEC includes discontinuation of all oral feedings, abdominal decompression via nasogastric suction, administration of intravenous antibiotics, and correction of fluid and electrolyte imbalances.[45] Surgical intervention is indicated when there is radiographic evidence of fixed, dilated intestinal loops accompanied by intestinal distention, perforation, intestinal gangrene, and abdominal wall edema.

Retinopathy of Prematurity

Retinopathy of prematurity (ROP) is caused by proliferation of abnormal blood vessels in the newborn retina, which occurs in two phases. Phase I is delayed growth of retinal blood vessels after premature birth. Phase II occurs when the hypoxia created during phase I stimulates growth of new blood vessels.[162] The outcome of ROP varies from normal vision to total loss of vision if there is advanced scarring from the retina to the lens resulting in retinal detachment.[242] The incidence of ROP increases with lower gestational age, lower birth weight, and BPD.[162]

The classification system for ROP uses a standard description of the location of the retinopathy using zones and clock hours, the severity of the disease or stage, and presence of special risk factors.[119] The classification system was revised in 2005 to include a rapid progressive form of ROP.[120] Classification of ROP includes five stages.[241] Stage 1 is characterized by a visible line of demarcation between the posterior vascularized retina and the anterior avascular retina. Stage 2 is characterized by pathologic neovascularization that is confined to the retina and appears as a ridge at the vascular/avascular junction. Stage 3 includes new vascularization and migration into the vitreous gel. Stage 4 is characterized by a subtotal retinal detachment. Stage 5 is complete retinal detachment.

Hyperbilirubinemia

Hyperbilirubinemia, or physiologic jaundice, is the accumulation of excessive amounts of bilirubin in the blood. Bilirubin is one of the breakdown products of hemoglobin from red blood cells. This condition is seen commonly in premature infants who have immature hepatic function, an increased hemolysis of red blood cells as a result of high concentrations of circulating red blood cells, a shorter life span of red blood cells, and possible polycythemia from birth injuries. The pathogenesis of hyperbilirubinemia may be multifactorial and associated with late preterm gestational age, exclusive breastfeeding, and ABO hemolytic disease (blood incompatibility between mother and fetus).[266] The primary goal in treatment of hyperbilirubinemia is the prevention of kernicterus, which is the deposition of unconjugated bilirubin in the brain, especially in the basal ganglia, cranial nerve nuclei, anterior horn cells, and hippocampus. Phototherapy is administered via a bank of lights or fiberoptic blankets.

FOREGROUND INFORMATION

EXAMINATION AND EVALUATION

The purposes of the physical therapy examination and evaluation of infants in the NICU are to identify (1) impairments in body function and structure that contribute to activity limitations and participation restrictions, (2) the developmental status of the infant, (3) the infant's individualized responses to stress and self-regulation, (4) needs for skilled positioning and handling, and (5) environmental adaptations to optimize growth and development. The examination and evaluation must support goals aimed at the infant's participation in age-appropriate developmental activities (e.g., feeding, tucking, self-soothing, social interaction with caregivers) and interactions with the family (e.g., relationship-building, attachment).

Neurobehavioral Observation

The examination and evaluation of high-risk infants are best conducted using a combination of observation and handling techniques that occur over several sessions. Infants hospitalized in the NICU will often not tolerate a full standardized developmental examination. Rather, the physical therapist often formulates a neurobehavioral profile based on observation of the infant's behaviors. That is, the physical therapist describes the infant's successes and difficulties in achieving and maintaining self-regulation and identifies the strategies that best support the infant's own self-regulatory efforts and developmental level of the infant (Box 29.2).[42]

Physical therapy interventions must be appropriately timed and modulated to match the neurobehavioral profile of the infant because handling of medically fragile infants can impose physiologic stress. In accord with family-centered practice, examination and intervention should be in partnership with the family to assist with bonding, facilitate developmentally

---

> **BOX 29.2   Recommendations for Physical Therapist Examination and Evaluation of Infants in the NICU**
>
> Protect the infant's fragile neurobehavioral system, particularly for infants who may not tolerate handling or a standardized evaluation.
> Repeat observations over time.
> Partner with parents and members of the NICU team.
> Observe, interpret, and communicate infant behaviors to parents and members of the NICU team.

---

supportive positioning and handling, and allow for carryover of therapeutic strategies. Lastly, the physical therapist is part of an interdisciplinary team of health care providers. Consistent with the Guide to Physical Therapist Practice (http://guidetoptpractice.apta.org), effective communication and collaboration with professionals from all disciplines and accurate documentation are critical. In the next section, a neurobehavioral framework is presented for examination of the high-risk infant with examples of considerations for specific diagnoses.

Behavioral State

States of consciousness were originally proposed by Wolff and have been expanded to include six behavioral states: (1) deep sleep, (2) light sleep, (3) drowsy, (4) quiet awake, (5) active awake, and (6) crying.[273] Thus the terms *states of consciousness* and *behavioral states* are often used interchangeably by clinicians conducting neurobehavioral observations. That is, each state of consciousness is characterized by a set of associated behaviors. Als has expanded this paradigm to include 12 states to distinguish between the adaptive and maladaptive self-regulatory strategies of fragile infants.[8] As infants mature, they are able to transition smoothly and predictably between states. Important observations include: the range, clarity and robustness of behavioral states, the lability and transition patterns from state to state, and the ability to self-sooth. For example, an infant who is 25 weeks of corrected gestational age (CGA) will likely spend most of the day in a light sleep state and will have brief periods of quiet awake. Comparatively, an infant who is 40 weeks of CGA should have longer periods of quiet awake time, particularly before and following feedings. An infant's ability to achieve and maintain sleep and awake states will be compromised by her medical and neurodevelopmental status. The physical therapist plays a key role in educating parents and staff to identify state transitions and optimize the environment (e.g., modifications to light, sound, and interaction) to facilitate smooth transitions to and from sleep.

Infants with neonatal abstinence syndrome (NAS, described later in Common Diagnoses of Infants Hospitalized in the NICU) demonstrate difficulty with state organization.[217] During the examination of the infant with NAS, the PT should carefully observe the infant's state transition patterns, duration of each state, and self-soothing strategies. Before the examination, the infant's care team should be consulted to determine how NAS symptoms are being assessed (e.g., a standardized scoring method) and managed medically.

Autonomic System

During the examination of the autonomic system, the physical therapist obtains the infant's heart and respiratory rate from the cardiorespiratory monitor and observes the infant's breathing pattern, skin color, visceral signs, twitches, startles, and tremors. In the neonate, heart rates range from 120 to 180 beats per minute and respiratory rate ranges from 40 to 60 breaths per minute.[155] In addition, respiratory effort and digestive function during rest, routine care, handling, and social interaction should be noted. Irregular respirations or paling around the mouth, eyes, and nose; spitting up; straining; bowel movements; and hiccoughs indicate instability or difficulty in achieving self-regulation. Smooth respirations; even color; and minimal startles, tremors, and digestive instability indicate that the demands of the situation have not exceeded the infant's capacity for self-regulation.

Infants with chronic lung disease (CLD, described later in Common Diagnoses of Infants Hospitalized in the NICU) have limited endurance for functional activities. Changes in respiratory effort during the examination should be carefully observed. Costal retractions, head bobbing, and nasal flaring are evidence of increased work of breathing, and their presence, timing, and resolution should be carefully noted.[191] Collaboration with nursing and respiratory therapy staff to facilitate the developmental examination is necessary in order to coincide with optimal timing of diuretic therapy, how modification to oxygen therapy will be managed including the upper and lower parameters of oxygen, and whether the mode of oxygen therapy can be modified for the examination to allow for greater bedside mobility. The examination of the infant with CLD requires frequent breaks, appropriate pacing of activity, and modification of the environment (e.g., lighting, sound, and social interaction) to allow the infant to utilize strategies for self-regulation.

Motor System

Physical therapists are among the most highly qualified members of the health care team to examine the motor system of a fragile infant and interpret findings. Examination should include observation of the infant's muscle tone and posture at rest and active movements during quiet awake periods, routine care, social interaction, and feeding. Movements should be interpreted according to the progression of active flexion patterns that emerge with increasing gestational age. Typically these occur at 32 weeks for lower extremities, 35 weeks for upper extremities, and 37 to 39 weeks for head and trunk.[256] Thus the immature neuromotor system of the preterm infant often precludes independent antigravity flexion movements and predisposes the infant to "compensations," including retracted scapulae, externally rotated and abducted lower extremities, and extension and rotation postures of the cervical spine and trunk.[247] Applying the frameworks previously described, less emphasis is placed on testing reflexes. Rather, the physical therapist examination evaluates reflexes deemed more "functional" (e.g., suck, swallow, palmar and plantar grasp, and early righting responses).[176]

Infants with IVH are at risk for neuromotor impairments that range from mild to severe.[112,164] When examining an infant with IVH, the therapist should note asymmetries in postural muscles and active movements of the extremities, including absence of isolated distal or rotational movements. Clonus should be tested in both ankles. Muscle tone at rest and during active movement should be observed and changes documented. Flexor tone and antigravity movements should be evaluated and movement patterns observed when the infant is awake and alert because behavioral state influences motor system activity and hence infant motor control.

Social Interaction

Infants enter the world predisposed to socialize. While healthy, full-term infants can visually track faces or brightly colored objects and alert to familiar voices and orient to familiar voices,[39] preterm or medically fragile infants may be able to complete these tasks with support and facilitation from the caregiver or therapist.[8,41] A developmental examination may include presenting visual and auditory stimulation to an infant. Physical therapists should judiciously offer opportunities for the infant to socially interact because these complex tasks can be distressful and overwhelm the infant's capacity for self-regulation. The physical therapist plays a critical role in facilitating social interaction between infants and caregivers by modeling developmentally supportive interactions, modifying the environment as needed, and providing parents with anticipatory guidance about the progression of their infant's social interaction skills.[43]

TESTS AND MEASURES

Results of tests and measures are used to: (1) objectively document infant functioning over time, (2) justify the need for developmental interventions in the NICU, (3) evaluate intervention outcomes, and (4) identify the need for developmental follow-up and intervention after discharge from the NICU. Administration of tests to infants who are fragile and have medically complex conditions requires clinical judgment and constant monitoring of physiologic stability to determine whether the administration of the test is well tolerated by the infant and the results are representative of the infant's current abilities. Many infants will not have the physiologic stability required to withstand the stress of being handled during the administration of the test. For infants who are not physiologically stable, testing will have to be either postponed or done in multiple brief periods.

Most useful to the physical therapist are tests and measures of neurologic function, neurobehavioral functioning, motor behavior, and oral-motor function. The tests and measures used by physical therapists vary widely but the Test of Infant Motor Performance (TIMP), designed by and for physical therapists working with infants as young as 32 weeks of gestation, has become the most widely used assessment of infant functional motor behavior in the NICU.[179] Derived from traditional neurobehavioral assessments, the Newborn Behavioral Observation system NBO is a neurobehavioral relationship-building tool that supports the efforts of the physical therapist to establish a rapport with families and share with them developmental information about their infant in a positive context.[179] The Dubowitz, used to establish the gestational age of the infant at birth, provides physical therapists with an excellent opportunity to learn about neurologic maturity of infants in the weeks before term age.[81] Some tests such as the Newborn Individualized Developmental Care and Assessment Program (NIDCAP), Neonatal Behavioral Assessment Scale (NBAS), and the Assessment of Preterm Infant Behavior (APIB) require certification and take as long as 90 minutes to administer, score, and interpret. A team approach and sharing of information between professionals may help in addressing time and cost issues and improve coordination of care. Certification on the TIMP, NIDCAP, NBAS, or APIB will greatly enhance the clinical skills of physical therapists working with young infants. Table 29.3 provides a list of tests and measures commonly used by physical therapists in the NICU and described in this section.

TABLE 29.3 Tests and Measures Used to Assess Infants in the Neonatal Intensive Care Unit

Name	Domain(s) of the ICF Model Covered by the Test or Measure
Neurological Assessment of the Preterm and Full-Term Newborn Infant[a]	Body Structures and Functions Activities
Neonatal Behavioral Assessment Scale (NBAS)[b]	Body Structures and Functions Activities
Newborn Behavioral Observation System (NBO)[c]	Body Structures and Functions Activities Participation
Newborn Individualized Developmental Care and Assessment Program (NIDCAP)[d]	Body Structures and Functions Activities Participation
Assessment of Preterm Infant Behavior (APIB)[e]	Body Structures and Functions Activities
NICU Network Neurobehavioral Scale (NNNS)[f]	Body Structures and Functions Activities
Test of Infant Motor Performance (TIMP)[g]	Body Structures and Functions Activities
General Movement (GM) Assessment	Body Structures and Functions Activities
Neurobehavioral Assessment of the Preterm Infant (NAPI)	Body Structures and Functions Activities
Neonatal Oral-Motor Assessment Scale (NOMAS)[h]	Body Structures and Functions Activities
Nursing Child Assessment Feeding Scale (NCAFS)[i]	Body Structures and Functions Activities Participation
Early Feeding Skills Assessment (EFS)[j]	Body Structures and Functions Activities

[a]Dubowitz L, Dubowitz V: *The neurological assessment of the preterm and full-term newborn infant.* London: Heinemann, 1981.

[b]Brazelton TB, Nugent JK: *The Neonatal Behavioral Assessment Scale 4th ed.* Mac Keith Press, Cambridge, 2011.

[c]Nugent JK, Keefer CH, Minear S, et al.: *Understanding newborn behavior & early relationships: The Newborn Behavioral Observations (NBO) system handbook.* Baltimore: Brookes, 2007.

[d]Als H: A synactive model of neonatal behavioral organization: framework for the assessment of neurobehavioral development in the premature infant and for support of infants and parents in the neonatal intensive care environment. *Phys Occupat Ther Pediatr* 6(3/4):3-54, 1986.

[e]Als H, Lester BM, Tronick EZ, Brazelton TB: Manual for the assessment of preterm infants' behavior (APIB). In Fitzgerald HE, Lester BM, Yogman MW, editors: *Theory and research in behavioral pediatrics.* New York: Plenum Press, 1982. p. 65-132.

[f]Lester BM, Tronick EZ, Brazelton TB: The Neonatal Intensive Care Unit Network Neurobehavioral Scale Procedures. *Pediatrics* 113(3 Pt 2):641-667, 2004.

[g]Campbell SK, Hedeker D: Validity of the Test of Infant Motor Performance for discriminating among infants with varying risk for poor motor outcome. *J Pediatr* 139:546-551, 2001.

[h]Braun MA, Palmer MM: A pilot study of oral-motor dysfunction in "at-risk" infant. *Phys Occupat Ther Pediatr* 5(4):13-26, 1985.

[i]Barnard KE, Eyres SJ: *Child health assessment. Part 2: the first year of life.* (DHEW Publication No HRA79-25). Bethesda, MD: US Government Printing Office, 1979.

[j]Thoyre SM, Shaker CS, Pridham KF: The early feeding skill assessment for preterm infants. *Neonatal Netw* 24(3):7-16, 2005.

Neurological Assessment of the Preterm and Full-Term Newborn Infant

The Neurological Assessment of the Preterm and Full-Term Newborn Infant, commonly known as the Dubowitz, is a systematic, quickly administered, neurologic and neurobehavioral assessment developed to document changes in neonatal behavior in the preterm infant after birth, to compare preterm infants with newborn infants of corresponding postmenstrual age, and to detect deviations in neurologic signs and their subsequent evolution.[80,81] The assessment takes 15 minutes or less

to administer and is divided into six sections: (1) posture and tone, (2) tone patterns, (3) reflexes, (4) movements, (5) abnormal signs/patterns, and (6) orientation and behavior. Scoring is based on patterns of response rather than a summary or total score. Although the Dubowitz has a long tradition in the NICU, it is mostly used by physicians and medical residents to establish gestational age at birth by observation. For physical therapists working in the NICU, learning to administer the Dubowitz will contribute to the knowledge and expertise in evaluating the tone and posture of very young infants.

Neonatal Behavioral Assessment Scale

The Neonatal Behavioral Assessment Scale (NBAS) is the most commonly used assessment of infant neurobehavioral functioning in the world today.[47] Used extensively in research, the NBAS includes 28 behavioral items scored on a 9-point scale and 18 reflex items scored on a 4-point scale. The reflex items can be used to identify gross neurologic abnormalities but are not intended to provide a neurologic diagnosis. The NBAS also includes a set of seven supplementary items designed to summarize the quality of the infant's responsiveness and the amount of examination facilitation needed to support the infant during the assessment. These supplementary items were originally included to better capture the quality of behaviors seen in high-risk infants. Therefore the NBAS is well suited for use with the high-risk population. The NBAS is appropriate for use with term infants and stable high-risk infants near term age until the end of the second month of life postterm.

The NBAS has been used extensively in research to study and document the effects of prematurity; intrauterine growth retardation; and prenatal exposure to cocaine, alcohol, caffeine, and tobacco on newborn behavior.[182] The NBAS has also inspired others to develop scales for use with diverse populations. Examples include the Assessment of Preterm Infant Behavior for use with premature infants[10] and the NICU Network Neurobehavioral Scale for use with infants exposed to drugs in utero,[145] both described in this section. The NBAS's central focus on the facilitation of infant competence by a trained and sensitive examiner has also brought to light its powerful qualities as an intervention tool for use with a wide range of families. This subsequently led to the development of a number of NBAS-based relationship-building tools such as the Mother's Assessment of the Behavior of the Infant (MABI),[267] the Combined Physical Exam and Behavioral Exam (PEBE),[127] the Family Administered Neonatal Activities (FANA),[61] and most recently the Newborn Behavioral Observation (NBO) system described in this section.[180] More information on the NBAS is available at www.brazelton-institute.com.

Newborn Behavioral Observation System

As previously mentioned, the NBO is not an assessment tool but a relationship-building tool designed to help practitioners sensitize parents to their child's competencies and uniqueness, support the development of a positive and nurturing parent–infant relationship, and foster the development of the practitioner–parent relationship.[180] The NBO consists of 18 neurobehavioral items used to elicit infant competencies and make observations of newborn behavior, such as sleep behavior, the baby's interactive capacities and threshold for stimulation, motor capacities, crying, consolability, and state regulation.[180] Because it is conceptualized as an interactive behavioral observation, the NBO is administered in the presence of the family to provide a forum for parents and the practitioner to observe and discuss the newborn's behavior. The NBO takes 45 minutes or longer to administer and can be completed from term age (and in some cases in infants as young as 36 weeks corrected gestational age who are medically stable) to the end of the second month of life postterm. The NBO has been used in diverse settings such as routine pediatric postpartum exams in hospital, clinic, and home settings and is feasible to administer amidst the multiple demands placed on pediatric PTs because it can be easily incorporated into clinical practice settings. Research suggests that the NBO is effective in helping professionals support parents' confidence and competence in caring for their infant and promotes a collaborative relationship between parents and clinicians.[171,181,214] More information on the NBO is available at www.brazelton-institute.com.

Newborn Individualized Developmental Care and Assessment Program

The NIDCAP is a comprehensive approach to care for infants in the NICU that is developmentally supportive and individualized to the infant's goals and level of stability.[8,9] The NIDCAP is inclusive of families and professionals. Completion initially involves direct and systematic observation, without the observer manipulating or interacting, of the preterm or full-term infant in the nursery before, during, and after a caregiving event. Observation is guided by a behavioral checklist to record the caregiving event; positioning; environmental characteristics such as light, sound, and activity; and the infant's behaviors. The observation begins 10 minutes before care, to observe the infant's stability and behavioral reactions when undisturbed; observation continues until care is completed and for another 10 minutes thereafter or until the infant reaches preobservation stability levels. The behavior observation checklist is marked every 2 minutes for heart and respiratory rates, oxygen saturation levels, position of the infant, and the caregiving event taking place. The observation time can be minutes or hours depending on the caregiving event and the stability of the infant. Following this observation, a narrative is written that describes the caregiving event from the infant's perspective, highlighting in great detail the infant's behaviors in relationship with the caregiving and environmental events taking place simultaneously.

Suggestions for caregiving modifications to support the infant's physiologic maturation and strategies at self-regulation are developed from the narrative. A physical therapist trained and certified in the NIDCAP can share this information with the NICU team and provide suggestions for modifying the environment and caregiving activities. These suggestions may pertain to lighting, noise level, activity level, bedding, aids to self-regulation, interaction, timing of manipulations, and facilitation of transitions from one activity to another. The NIDCAP has been found to be most effective in influencing medical outcome,[11,12] and it is suggested to be a causative agent in altering brain function and structure.[6,7] More information and a list of NIDCAP training centers may be obtained at www.nidcap.org.

Assessment of Preterm Infant Behavior

The APIB is a comprehensive and systematic neurobehavioral assessment of preterm and high-risk infants[10,13,14] that is based on the Neonatal Behavioral Assessment Scale.[249] Also viewed as a neuropsychologic assessment, the APIB provides a detailed assessment of infants' self-regulatory efforts and thresholds to disorganization as viewed through the infant's behaviors. The exam proceeds through a series of maneuvers that increase in vigor as well as tactile and vestibular demands to determine the infant's self-regulatory abilities. The APIB may take up to an hour, depending on the level of stability of the infant, whereas scoring may take between 30 and 45 minutes. Writing the clinical assessment report from the APIB may take up to 3 hours, depending on the complexity of the medical history, developmental issues, and recommendations.[184] To be safely handled for the duration of the assessment, the infant must be physiologically stable and 32 weeks of postconceptional age or older. The APIB is appropriate for use with high-risk infants until approximately 44 to 48 weeks of postconceptional age. Training is extensive and available for clinicians and developmental professionals in the NICU and follow-up clinical settings. More information is available at www.nidcap.org.

NICU Network Neurobehavioral Scale

The NICU Network Neurobehavioral Scale (NNNs) is designed for the neurobehavioral assessment of medically stable drug-exposed and other high-risk infants, especially preterm infants between the ages of 30 and 46 to 48 weeks of postconceptional age.[145] The NNNs is used to document and describe developmental and behavioral maturation, central nervous system integrity, and infant stress responses. Although similar to the NBAS in content, the NNNs differs in the order of item administration. For example, items are skipped if the infant is not in the appropriate behavioral state, and deviations in administration are recorded. Additionally, the time required to administer the NNNs is shorter than the NBAS because the NNNs is less focused on infant best performance and the infant-examiner interaction. The NNNs comprises 115 items, 45 of which require specific manipulation of the infant, whereas the other 70 items are observed over the course of the examination. It is divided in three parts: (1) an Examination Scale that includes neurologic items that assess passive and active tone and primitive reflexes and items that reflect central nervous system integrity; (2) an Examiner Ratings Scale that includes behavioral items including state, sensory, and interactive responses; and (3) a Stress/Abstinence Scale that includes seven categories of items designed to capture behavioral signs of stress typical of high-risk infants and signs of neonatal abstinence or withdrawal commonly seen in drug-exposed infants.[145] The NNNs has been used to describe the neurobehavioral profile of infants exposed to methamphetamine,[194,227] cocaine,[213] and marijuana.[74]

Test of Infant Motor Performance

The TIMP is a test of functional motor behavior in infants for use by physical and occupational therapists and other professionals in the NICU and early intervention or diagnostic follow-up settings.[55] The TIMP can be used to assess the infants between the ages of 34 weeks of postconceptional age and 4 months postterm. The test examines postural and selective control of movement needed for functional motor performance in early infancy. The TIMP requires approximately 25 to 45 minutes for administration and scoring.[55] Spontaneous and elicited movements constitute separate subscales. The Observed Scale consists of 13 dichotomously scored items that assess the infant's spontaneous attempts to orient the body, to selectively move individual body segments, and to perform qualitative movements such as ballistic or oscillating movements.[57] Examples of observed behaviors include individual finger and ankle movements, reaching, and aligning the head in midline while supine.

The Elicited Scale consists of 29 items scored on a 5-, 6-, or 7-point hierarchic scale.[73] Elicited behaviors reflect the infant's response to positioning and handling in a variety of spatial orientations and to visual and auditory stimuli. Examples include rolling prone with head righting when the leg is rotated across the body and turning the head to follow a visual stimulus or to search for a sound in prone.

The TIMP has been shown to have excellent test-retest and rater reliability, good construct validity,[57,176] concurrent validity,[56] and predictive validity.[55,58,93,230] The TIMP can be used for the early identification of very young infants at risk for poor motor performance[58,93] and cerebral palsy as early as 2 months of adjusted age.[29,30] A shorter version used for screening purposes, the Test of Infant Motor Performance Screening Items (TIMPSI), is now available.[59] The TIMPSI takes half the time to administer when compared to the TIMP and is considered useful for fragile babies or for rapid screening that reduces the need for full TIMP testing in infants who do well on the TIMPSI. Users of the TIMPSI must have previous knowledge and training of the full TIMP in order to use it effectively. More information about the TIMP and TIMPSI can be found at www.timp.com. A video demonstrating administration of the TIMP is on Expert Consult.

General Movements Assessment

The General Movements (GM) Assessment is an assessment to identify movements and movement patterns that are predictive of cerebral palsy.[205] The underlying motor theory is that the emergence of typical movement patterns follows a predictable course whereby infants' movements can be characterized as writhing (from term to 8 weeks' postterm), fidgety, and voluntary (after 8 to 20 weeks' postterm). The purpose of the GM Assessment is to observe infant movement patterns for deviations from this theorized, typical trajectory. Examples of atypical movements include, in the prenatal period (i.e., until term): a limited movement repertoire or poor differentiation of movements; from term to 8 weeks' postterm: rigid and chaotic movements that lack smoothness and fluency (e.g., cramped synchronous movements); and from 6 weeks to 20 weeks' postterm: absent or abnormal fidgety movements. The GM Assessment is based upon observation or a video recorded while the infant is in an alert behavioral state, which makes it appropriate for even the most fragile NICU infants. It is particularly designed for infants at high-risk for cerebral palsy because the main purpose of the GM Assessment is to predict risk for cerebral palsy.[205]

The GM Assessment has been shown to have excellent (i.e., 90%) interrater reliability when assessed by trained examiners from videos. In addition, the persistence of cramped synchronous movements and the absence of fidgety movements are a valid predictor of cerebral palsy with 95% sensitivity and 96% specificity.[179,205] Both basic and advanced courses are available to learn the GM Assessment (http://general-movements-trust.info/46/invitation).

Neurobehavioral Assessment of Preterm Infant

The Neurobehavioral Assessment of the Preterm Infant (NAPI) is designed to monitor early infant development and evaluate the effects of interventions in the neonatal period. The NAPI is appropriate for infants 32 weeks to term age. The NAPI consists of seven domains: motor development, scarf sign, popliteal angle, attention and orientation, percent sleep, irritability,

and vigor of the infant's cry.[136] The NPAI has been shown to have good interrater reliability and stability of the domains over time. In addition, the NPAI has strong construct validity and detects changes over time in neonatal neurobehavioral development in response to intervention. However, the NAPI appears to be weakly correlated with neonatal physiologic measures.[179] More information about the NAPI can be found at: http://med.stanford.edu/NAPI/.

Oral-Motor Examination

Oral-motor examination is an advanced competency. Two useful measures are the Neonatal Oral-Motor Assessment Scale (NOMAS)[46,94] and the Nursing Child Assessment Feeding Scale (NCAFS).[31,244] The NOMAS measures components of nutritive and nonnutritive sucking. Variables assessed during sucking include rate, rhythmicity, jaw excursion, tongue configuration, and tongue movement. A pilot study determined cutoff scores for oral-motor disorganization and dysfunction. The NCAFS assesses parent–infant feeding interaction and evaluates the responsiveness of parents to their infant's cues, signs of distress, and social interaction during feeding. Both of those assessment tools require highly specialized training but provide an excellent diagnostic framework for fragile feeders. Neonatal physical therapists may also find useful the Early Feeding Skills Assessment (EFS) as a tool to assess infant readiness and tolerance for feeding and to identify a profile of an infant's specific skills relative to a developmental progression of oral feeding competencies.[250]

A systematic review of neuromotor and neurobehavioral assessment for preterm infants up to four months corrected gestational age identified GM Assessment, the TIMP, and the NAPI as having strong reliability and validity.[179] Specifically, the NNNs and APIB have strong reliability and validity and are very well suited for research. Similarly, the GM Assessment, TIMP, and NAPI are valid and reliable instruments and appear to be well suited and feasible for use in clinical settings. Finally, the results of the systematic review suggest that the GM Assessment is most accurate in prediction of cerebral palsy.[179]

With the variety of tests and measures available to pediatric PTs practicing in the NICU, the question often arises, What is the best assessment tool? In our experience the answer to this question depends on the purpose of administering the measure and the resources available to support use of the measure in clinical practice. For example, as noted above, tests and measures vary in their purpose from predicting CP (i.e., GM Assessment) to promoting the parent–infant relationship (i.e., NBO). If the primary purposes are to promote parent–infant bonding and to document the infant's self-regulatory behaviors, we often use the NBO in our clinical practice. If the primary purpose is to assess neuromotor skills, especially using a measure that can be repeated in a follow-up program, the TIMP is the choice we would make in our clinical practice. It is common for a combination of these tools to be used to describe the child's developmental abilities. However, as research scientist PTs in the NICU we typically use the TIMP because it has strong psychometric properties and is suited to the research questions we investigate on prediction of outcomes and efficacy of interventions.

Another important consideration in choice of measures is the monetary and time resources available to the PT or development and therapeutic team to choose a particular measure. For example, some measures require extensive resources not only to purchase the measure but also to train with an experienced clinician to become reliable in administering it (for example, NIDCAP and APIB require training by credentialed instructors). These measures also tend to be lengthy to administer, score, and document. Thus PTs must consider their productivity requirements and workload as well as the capacity of the therapeutic team to integrate lengthy evaluation tools into busy NICU practice. In our experience the PT who is the NICU's developmental specialist is typically trained in the NIDCAP and APIB and typically has the scheduling flexibility to administer these instruments. Moreover, the PT with expertise and mentoring in the NICU can learn to do the TIMP through continuing education courses and training DVDs followed by reliability checks. The TIMP can be included and billed as part of the clinical examination; administration may occur over two sessions, which typically aligns well with scheduling and productivity requirements. Thus the purpose of the assessment, training and resources of the PT, and time should also be considered in selecting clinical assessment tools.

PHYSICAL THERAPIST INTERVENTION

Developmental interventions in the NICU are designed to provide the infant: (1) sensory experiences that are individualized in type and intensity to the infant's developmental and physiologic capacity, (2) movement opportunities that promote positive movement experiences that may lead to adaptive neuroplasticity,[203,226] and (3) developmental support during the transition from the NICU to home provided by caregivers who have confidence and competency in caring for their infant.[83,84]

To the extent possible, developmental interventions should be integrated into the care and day/night routines of the infant. Cost-benefit is an important consideration. We recommend that physical therapist interventions be individualized, framed within a 24-hour care perspective, and part of an interdisciplinary team approach. Physical therapists should carefully assess and reflect on the relevance of all interventions provided in the NICU. Interventions of any kind, especially those based on theory, may in fact be harmful unless consideration is given to an infant's physiologic, sensory, and neurologic capacity and the environment. An infant whose sleep is interrupted numerous times during the day and night may benefit more from sleep protection than from sensory experiences and movement opportunities. Table 29.4 summarizes systematic reviews relevant to developmental interventions in the NICU. A summary of general recommendations for developmental care, direct interventions provided by physical therapists, and discharge planning presented in the following sections is provided in Table 29.5. It is important to note that research evidence is not sufficient to support specific interventions.

Developmental Care

Developmental care is a broadly defined term used in many NICUs and in research to describe the use of environmental interventions, such as sound and light reduction, along with sleep preservation or clustered care in order to support the infant's development.[248] Developmental care also encompasses an individualized developmental care plan followed by all members of the team including the physical therapist. As part of an interdisciplinary team providing developmental care in the NICU, physical therapists have an important role in coordination of care. This includes recommendations related to the NICU environment as a whole or for a specific infant.

The NIDCAP is a highly structured system of assessing the infant's behavioral responses to a caregiving event and subsequent design of an individualized developmental care plan. NIDCAP is typically implemented by an entire NICU with a developmental specialist or physical therapists providing the individualized assessments and recommendations. Although there have been no reports of adverse events or negative consequences from the use of the developmental care or NIDCAP, there is conflicting evidence on the short- and long-term outcomes. There is debate regarding the finding reported in a systematic review indicating that there was no significant difference in developmental outcomes for infants who had care provided with or without a NIDCAP approach.[15,107,186,187] Although some studies reported short-term improvements in developmental outcome, faster weight gain, and shorter length of stay in the NICU, other studies found no lasting gains. Other small studies found improved long-term developmental outcomes.[168] NIDCAP is a specific intervention approach, but many characteristics of NIDCAP are integrated in NICUs that do not specifically follow a NIDCAP approach with standardized assessment intervals. Thus the findings specific to NIDCAP should be considered as one component of developmental care, rather than being mutually exclusive.[107] Physical therapists who provide care in the NICU benefit from the NIDCAP training because it provides an outstanding opportunity to learn about the theoretical background of interaction with medically fragile infants.

Because physical therapists support the goals of developmental care or NIDCAP within a NICU, they must consider environmental factors including light, sound, and pain that are potential stressors for an infant in the NICU.[100,101,140,152,198] These factors need to be considered when the infant is at rest in an isolette or crib as well as during parent or therapist interactions with the infant. The recommendations for light and sound in the NICU are that (1) ambient light should be in the range of 10–600 Lux and (2) acoustic sound should not exceed 45 decibels.[152] Infants in the NICU are bombarded with sounds from the lifesaving equipment, staff, family, and other infants. Preterm birth results in the infant being exposed to sounds of greater than 250 Hz that are typically muted by the uterine walls throughout gestation. Thus the infant born preterm needs to cope with high-frequency sounds that may cause physiologic stress.[198] A Cochrane review on the use of sound-reduction interventions on growth and development of infants born very preterm identified only one study.[4] The single study reported that use of infant ear plugs in the NICU was associated with higher mental developmental index scores on the Bayley at 18 to 22 months. However, the Cochrane review reports the evidence is too limited to consider use in clinical practice.[1,4]

Environmental modification including the use of single infant or family rooms, rather than an open unit with multiple bed spaces, has been found to reduce environmental noise (Fig. 29.4).[151] However, other studies have raised concerns that the limited infant stimulation provided in single family rooms goes too far toward reducing stimulation and results in altered brain development and language delays at developmental follow-up.[202]

As part of general developmental care or environmental changes in the NICU, modification of lighting is common. However, there is debate on the best practices between the use of reduced lighting all day or the use of cycled lighting. Isolette covers or dimming room lights are common practices to reduce

TABLE 29.4   Systematic Reviews on Topics Relevant to Developmental Interventions of the High-Risk Infant in the NICU

Topic of Review	Conclusive Statement
Sound reduction in the NICU[a]	A Cochrane review on the use of sound reduction interventions on growth and development of infants born very preterm identified only one study that completed a RCT or quasi-RCT to determine if reduced sound impacted infant outcomes. The single study reports that use of infant ear plugs in the NICU were associated with higher mental developmental index scores on the Bayley at 18 to 22 months; however, the Cochrane review reports the evidence is too limited to consider use in clinical practice.
Developmental care[b]	The evidence suggests that these interventions may have some benefit to the outcomes of preterm infants; however, there continues to be conflicting evidence among the multiple studies. Therefore there is so far no clear evidence demonstrating consistent effects of developmental care interventions on important short- and long-term outcomes.
Developmental care[c]	No significant difference in developmental outcomes for infants who had care provided with or without a NIDCAP approach. Although some studies report short-term improvements in developmental outcome, faster weight gain, and shorter length of stay in the NICU, other studies find no lasting gains. The high cost of providing NIDCAP needs to be considered against these findings of limited to no developmental gains.
Cycled lighting[d]	A cycled light systematic review found that cycled light may be beneficial compared to continuous bright light. Infants in the cycled light groups may sleep more, have increased activity levels during the day, and demonstrate earlier feeding readiness or fewer days of ventilator support. However, this interpretation is based on few studies for each outcome measures and with limited comparison between reduced light and cycled light.
Light reduction in the prevention of retinopathy of prematurity[e]	Considerable research has been done on this, and the evidence suggests that bright light is not the cause of retinopathy of prematurity and it does not add to the problem.
Infant position during mechanical ventilation[f]	There is no clear evidence that body position during mechanical ventilation in newborn babies is effective in producing relevant and sustained improvement. However, putting infants on assisted ventilation in the face-down position for a short time slightly improves their oxygenation and infants in the prone position undergo fewer episodes of poor oxygenation.
Nonnutritive sucking[g]	The review of literature suggests that weight gain was similar with and without use of a pacifier. In two studies, preterm infants with pacifiers had shorter hospital stays (lower hospital costs), showed less defensive behaviors during tube feedings, spent less time in fussy and active states during and after tube feedings, and settled more quickly into sleep than those without pacifiers. Their transition to full enteral (by tube or mouth) or bottle feeds (three studies) and bottle-feeding performance, in general (one study), was easier. No negative outcomes were reported.
Physical activity programs for promoting bone mineralization and growth[h]	This review found that physical activity might have a small benefit on bone development and growth over a short term. There were inadequate data to assess long-term benefits and harms. Based on current knowledge, physical activity programs cannot be recommended as a standard procedure for premature babies.
Massage[i]	The review only included randomized controlled trials, studies in which a group of babies received massage or "still, gentle touch," in which nurses put their hands on babies but did not rub or stroke them. In most of these studies, babies were rubbed or stroked for about 15 minutes, three or four times a day, usually for 5 or 10 days. On average, the studies found that babies receiving massage, but not "still, gentle touch," gained more weight each day (about 5 g). They spent less time in the hospital, had slightly better scores on developmental tests, and had slightly fewer postnatal complications, although there were problems with how reliable these findings are. The studies did not show any negative effects of massage.
Early developmental intervention programs after hospital discharge[j]	The early developmental intervention programs in this review had to commence within the first 12 months of life, focus on the parent–infant relationship or infant development, and, although they could commence while the baby was still in hospital, they had to have a component that was delivered postdischarge from the hospital. A review of trials suggests those programs for preterm infants are effective at improving cognitive development in the short to medium term (up to preschool age). There is limited evidence that early developmental interventions improve motor outcome or long-term cognitive outcome (up to school age). The variability in the intervention programs limits the conclusions that can be made about the effectiveness of early developmental interventions.
Early developmental intervention programs after hospital discharge[k]	This update to the above study suggests that a little more evidence is present for the ability to intervention programs post NICU discharge to improve motor outcomes in the short term and cognitive outcomes through the preschool years.
Positioning for acute respiratory distress[l]	A total of 21 studies were assessed altogether. Three quarters of the 436 children were preterm babies and were mostly (71%) ventilated by machine. The prone position was better than supine for oxygenating the blood, but the difference was small. The increase in oxygen saturation on average increased by 2%. This finding was based on eight studies (183 children, 153 preterm and 95 ventilated) measuring this outcome. The rapid rate of breathing with respiratory distress was slightly lower in the prone position (on average four breaths/min lower) based on five studies (100 infants aged up to 1 month, 59 ventilated). There were no obvious differences with other positions. Note: It is important to remember that these children were hospitalized. Therefore given the association of the prone position with sudden infant death syndrome (SIDS), the prone position should not be used for children unless they are in hospital and where their breathing is constantly monitored.

Continued

TABLE 29.4 **Systematic Reviews on Topics Relevant to Developmental Interventions of the High-Risk Infant in the NICU—cont'd**

Topic of Review	Conclusive Statement
Kangaroo mother care to reduce morbidity and mortality in low birth weight infants[m,n]	Kangaroo mother care (KMC) involves skin-to-skin contact between mother and her newborn, frequent and exclusive or nearly exclusive breastfeeding, and early discharge from hospital. Compared with conventional care, KMC was found to reduce severe illness, infection, breastfeeding problems, and maternal dissatisfaction with method of care and improve some outcomes of mother-baby bonding. There was no difference in infant mortality. However, serious concerns about the methodologic quality of the included trials weaken credibility in these findings. More research is needed.

[a]Almadhoob A, Ohlsson A: Sound reduction management in the neonatal intensive care unit for preterm or very low birth weight infants. *Cochrane Database Syst Rev* 1: CD010333, 2015.

[b]Symington A, Pinelli J: Developmental care for promoting development and preventing morbidity in preterm infants. *Cochrane Database Syst Rev* 2:CD001814, 2006.

[c]Ohlsson A, Jacobs SE: NIDCAP: a systematic review and meta-analyses of randomized controlled trials. *Pediatrics* 131(3):e881-893, 2013.

[d]Morag I, Ohlsson A: Cycled light in the intensive care unit for preterm and low birth weight infants. *Cochrane Database Syst Rev* 8:CD006982, 2013.

[e]Phelps DL, Watts JL: *Cochrane Database Syst Rev* 1:CD000122, 2001.

[f]Balaguer A, Escribano J, Roqué M: *Cochrane Database Syst Rev* 4, CD003668, 2006.

[h]Schulzke SM, Kaempfen S, Trachsel D, Patole SK: Physical activity programs for promoting bone mineralization and growth in preterm infants. *Cochrane Database Syst Rev* 4:CD005387, 2014.

[i]Vickers A, Ohlsson A, J. B. Lacy JB, Horsley A: Massage for promoting growth and development of preterm and/or low birth-weight infants. *Cochrane Database Syst Rev* 2:CD000390, 2004.

[j]Spittle AJ, Orton J, Doyle LW, Boyd R: Early developmental intervention programs post hospital discharge to prevent motor and cognitive impairments in preterm infants. *Cochrane Database Syst Rev* 18(2):2007.

[k]Spittle AJ, Orton P, Anderson R, et al.: Early developmental intervention programmes post-hospital discharge to prevent motor and cognitive impairments in preterm infants. *Cochrane Database Syst Rev* 12:CD005495, 2012.

[l]Wells DA, Gillies D, Fitzgerald DA: *Cochrane Database Syst Rev* 2:CD003645, 2005.

[m]Conde-Agudelo A, Belizán JM: Kangaroo mother care to reduce morbidity and mortality in low birthweight infants. *Cochrane Database Syst Rev* 2:CD002771, 2003.

[n]Engmann C, Wall S, Darmstadt G, et al.: Consensus on kangaroo mother care acceleration. *Lancet* 382:e26-27, 2013.

TABLE 29.5 **General Recommendations for NICU Practice Based on the Authors' Interpretation of the Limited Evidence for Developmental Care and Physical Therapy in the NICU**

Developmental Care	Reduce light and noise Clustered care with limited interruptions during sleep Culture of parent participation in caregiving including use of kangaroo mother care/skin-to-skin holding, frequent visitation, and infant interaction Pain management
Direct Interventions	Positioning with extremities and head in midline, arms and legs flexed close to the body Massage ideally provided by parents in the form of firm touch Graded movement experience timed with infant's readiness for social engagement
Discharge Planning	Family support Education and readings on developmental cues and developmental supports available at home Referral to NICU follow-up programs and early intervention

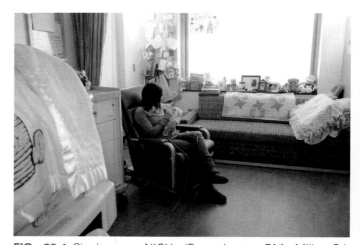

FIG. 29.4 Single-room NICU. (From Lester BM, Miller RJ, Hawes K, et al.: Infant neurobehavioral development. *Semin Perinatol* 35(1):8-19, 2011.)

light exposure. Cycled lights typically included low light levels for 12 hours at night and unrestricted light for 12 hours during the day. A systematic review found that cycled light may be beneficial compared to continuous bright light.[175] Infants in the cycled light groups may sleep more, have increased activity levels during the day, and demonstrate earlier feeding readiness or fewer days of ventilator support. However, this interpretation is based on few studies for each outcome measure and with limited comparison between reduced light and cycled light.[100]

Kangaroo Mother Care, or skin-to-skin holding, is an intervention provided by parents in which the infant is held by a parent, usually the mother, on the parent's bare chest (Fig. 29.5). The experience of kangaroo care has been shown to foster maternal attachment, improve maternal confidence in caring for her premature infant,[125] and improve the odds of breastfeeding at discharge from the NICU and into the first year of life.[108,183] A systematic review of kangaroo care suggested that mothers have reduced stress and depression following the use of kangaroo care.[23] In addition, mother–child interactions are improved in the NICU and some studies suggest through 6 months of age.[23] Feldman showed that preterm infants receiving kangaroo care in the NICU had more mature neurobehavioral profiles on the NBAS when compared to control infants.[89] Being held in the kangaroo position (on the mother's chest facing the mother with a cloth strip holding the infant in place for 8–12 hours per day) may also contribute to the development of increased trunk and leg flexion. One study showed increase surface electromyography activity following

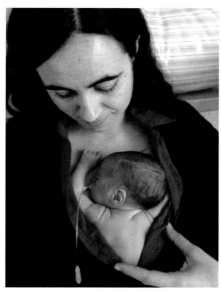

FIG. 29.5 Kangaroo mother care. (From Coughlin M: The Sobreviver (Survive) Project. *Newborn Infant Nurs Rev* 15(4):169-173, 2015.)

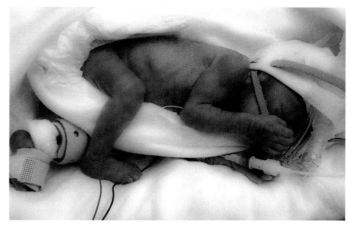

FIG. 29.6 Preterm infant placed in the left sidelying position. The arms and legs are in a flexed, midline position close to the body. (From Gouna G, Rakza T, Kuissi E, et al.: Positioning effects on lung function and breathing pattern in premature newborns. *J Pediatr* 162(6):1133-1137, 2013.)

96 hours of being positioned in the kangaroo care position.[77] The overwhelming data supporting the benefits and limited risks of kangaroo care lead to a 2013 consensus statement encouraging the international adoption of the standard use of kangaroo care in the care of all infants born preterm.[86] Although this practice has been adopted widely in NICUs, physical therapists can play an important role in encouraging kangaroo care as part of routine developmental care. In addition, physical therapists can work with families to engage them in caring for their infant and providing developmental support in the first weeks after birth.

Some NICUs have changed their environment from a large room with multiple beds to single-family or infant rooms based on recommendations for reduced sound, reduced or cycled light, and use of kangaroo care. Some studies suggest that single-family rooms increased family engagement and parents' sense of control and decreased maternal stressors and led to increased use of kangaroo care resulting in slight improvement in medical and developmental outcomes.[109,146] A systematic review of medical and development outcomes in single rooms suggested lower infection rates and possibly shorter length of stay.[221] While the majority of studies still suggest benefit, as noted earlier, other studies suggest that single-family rooms may be associated with delayed language.[101]

Direct Interventions by Physical Therapists

Infants in the NICU present with a wide range of conditions that have an impact on their later developmental outcome, including prematurity, neonatal seizures, intraventricular hemorrhage, stroke, hydrocephalus, respiratory distress syndrome, bronchopulmonary dysplasia, cystic fibrosis, spina bifida, arthrogryposis, and osteogenesis imperfecta. These conditions lead to impairments that affect the infant's activity levels and interactions with parents and caregivers. Physical therapists provide direct intervention and help parents learn how to provide movement experiences for their infant born preterm to address impairments in body functions or structures and/or

activity limitations. See the section on discharge planning for additional parent-therapist intervention approaches.

A review of the literature on interventions in the NICU indicates that interventions vary in focus and scope. It is difficult to reach consensus on effectiveness of any particular intervention because of the limited number of studies of well-defined interventions, the variety of outcome measures used, and heterogeneity of samples. We will provide a brief review of interventions focusing on positioning, massage, facilitated handling, physical activity to promote bone mineral density, and parent education because these interventions have more evidence than any others. Some consensus is available on these intervention modalities through systematic reviews, well-designed research trials, or reviews published by the Cochrane Collaboration, an international not-for-profit organization that provides up-to-date systematic reviews about the effects of health care (see Table 29.5).

Positioning

The musculoskeletal system of a preterm infant is very susceptible to positional deformities resulting from NICU positioning. In addition, infants born preterm may demonstrate instability of the autonomic nervous system in response to changes in position or a lack of postural support. Physical therapists have an important role in collaborating with the nursing team and parents on recommendations for positioning, especially for very preterm infants. Although some evidence exists for specific positioning devices or strategies,[128,159,252] there is not enough evidence to support a specific approach. As a result, physical therapists typically apply general positioning principles and work with nursing staff to implement positioning recommendations.[195]

Generally, the goals of positioning are to encourage midline head position, arms and legs flexed and close to the body. This simulates the intrauterine environment that contributes to typical skeletal alignment (Fig. 29.6). This position is often achieved with the use of blanket rolls or positioning aids to encourage alignment and aid in autonomic nervous system regulation.[103,159] Infants cared for with support of midline head position, flexed and supported extremities, had improved leg and shoulder alignment during functional tasks and improved quality of movement.[90,174]

When positioning a young infant who is medically fragile, skeletal alignment and the impact of the position on cerebral blood flow are important considerations. Infants who are medically fragile can have decreased jugular blood flow, decreased tissue oxygenation, and increased cerebral blood flow velocities when they are positioned in 90 degrees of cervical rotation. Use of midline head positioning and head elevation 30 degrees for 72 hours after delivery is considered as best practice to reduce the incidence of IVH.[161] After 3 days of age a variety of positions including prone, supine, and sidelying are recommended to promote skeletal alignment and reduce the likelihood of skeletal deformations including plagiocephaly and scaphocephaly.[253]

Although prone position has been thought to improve oxygenation, a 2012 Cochrane review found there is no evidence of improved apnea, oxygenation, or bradycardia in any position in infants who are breathing spontaneously.[49] However, there is some evidence that infants have better gastric emptying and reduced stress when positioned in prone.[60,64] Infants requiring phototherapy can receive adequate light exposure to reduce bilirubin positioned in either prone or supine.[38]

The AAP recommends that all infants sleep in supine to reduce the rate of sudden infant death syndrome. However, many infants are cared for in the NICU using a prone position. Although there is no evidence base to guide the time to transition preterm infants to supine, it must be done in the hospital before discharge to help the infant adjust to supine and facilitate the transition to home.[172] Hospitals with policies regarding transition to supine are more consistent in making the transition 1 week prior to discharge. Those without hospital policies are more likely to transition infants only 24 hours prior to discharge, which may add to the stress experienced by families during this difficult time.[173]

Massage

Massage for infants in the NICU ranges from light pressure with the hand staying still in the youngest infants to a kinesthetic program of providing full body infant massage, visual and vestibular input in infants nearing discharge. Massage is typically provided about 60 minutes before a feeding and, like all interactions, needs to be progressed in response to the infant's cues.

A Cochrane review and recent meta-analysis summarized the evidence on massage that included both tactile and kinesthetic stimulation in most of the studies. Massage with kinesthetic stimulation increased weight gain and decreased length of stay by 4.4 days but does not appear to impact NBAS scores.[258,264] No studies found negative effects of the massage interventions. Only a few studies have compared massage to other interventions. One found that massage and kangaroo care were equally effective in reducing length of stay and increasing weight in infants after 5 days of intervention 3 times per day. While additional research is needed on the effect of massage provided by staff versus parents, the similar results between massage and kangaroo care suggest that parents can support their infant's development through either intervention.

Physical Activity

Infants born preterm are at high risk for osteopenia, which may increase with limited physical activity in the NICU. Several studies have been conducted to determine the efficacy of physical activity programs to increase bone mineral density and weight gain. The physical activity programs typically consist of extension and flexion, range-of-motion exercises with end range holding in flexion to elicit pushing against resistance of the infant's upper and lower limb movement. Physical activity programs are administered for several minutes at a time several times a week for at least 2 weeks. A Cochrane review concluded that physical activity for hospitalized preterm infants may have small short-term but no long-term effects on bone mineralization and growth.[64] Physical activity programs are not recommended based on the evidence and high staff time commitment required.[218]

Facilitated Movement

Physical therapists and parents can play a role in supporting the development of infants born preterm during medical procedures. Facilitated tucking during suctioning has been found to reduce stress and pain in some studies while not in others.[3,106,197] Supporting an infant during painful or stressful caregiving procedures provides the physical therapist the opportunity to observe the infant's behavioral responses and identify individualized therapeutic strategies to enhance the infant's efforts at self-regulation. In addition, facilitation may promote movement patterns similar to those used by the infant while in utero and reduce maladaptive motor behaviors during caregiving.

Although the primary role of the physical therapist in the NICU is to support the development of the infant through a team-based intervention, there are times when direct intervention is warranted. However, direct therapy in the NICU needs to be based on the infant's readiness to interact and in support of the team and family goals to enhance development. Only a few studies have evaluated the outcomes from direct therapy intervention in the NICU, providing mixed results that are preliminary in nature.[53,84,96] Interventions that combine direct intervention and parent education in order to prepare the parent to provide the interventions are ideal.[231] Spittle et al. published a Cochrane review summarizing the findings of interventions that started in the NICU in most cases and continued into the home. Although additional research is needed, the review concluded that early intervention including parent and therapist interaction with the infant could improve cognitive outcomes at least in the short term.[231,232] Collaboration with parents will allow for the goal of daily positive motor and developmental experiences prior to NICU discharge and into the community.

Discharge Planning

Parents are a consistent presence in the lives of most infants born preterm and are best suited to support the infant's development. This process must start at the time of NICU admission and continue during the transition to home after NICU discharge. In the NICU, parents can play a role in many aspects of caregiving. As discussed previously, parents can provide support through kangaroo care, facilitated tucking, and incorporating sensory monitoring practices into their interaction. However, all NICU staff must be involved in this goal of engaging parents in the developmental care of their preterm infant.[82]

In preparation for the infant's discharge to home, parents may benefit from more focused education on ways to support development. Many parents report they are not sure how to support their infant's development in the first weeks and months at home.[83] Parent education programs on caregiving have been developed and implemented by nursing staff or developmental care teams in the NICU with a goal of reducing maternal stress or increasing mother–child interactions.[115,181,214] However, few interventions have focused on helping parents learn to support development through social interaction and age-appropriate play in the first months of life.[53,84] Physical therapists working in the NICU have an important role in helping parents prepare to support their infant's development during and after the transition to home. Physical therapists can help parents build a developmentally supportive relationship with their infant prior to discharge that will extend into the home environment. Working with parents to identify the infant's readiness cues for social interaction in the NICU will increase their ability to identify opportunities for tummy time, reaching, and other developmental play that support motor and cognitive development in the first year of life.

In addition to helping parents support their infants' development, physical therapists have a key role in helping to engage parents in NICU follow-up programs and community-based interventions. Although providers in the NICU may assume that all parents will seek developmental services after discharge, evidence suggests this is not always the case. In one study, the degree of parental developmental concerns and intent to access early intervention services were more related to maternal factors than infant factors, including the presence of IVH or white matter brain injury.[201] This suggests that prior to discharge NICU providers should open a dialogue about risk factors and parental beliefs and share any available evidence on time-sensitive interventions while recognizing the parents' right to opt in and out of developmental services during the transition to home.

Developmental Follow-up

For many high-risk infants and their families, life after discharge from the NICU may involve referrals to a number of medical specialists (e.g., pulmonary, neurology, neurosurgery, ear nose and throat, gastroenterology, craniofacial, orthopedics), a local early intervention program, and developmental follow-up to a hospital-based multidisciplinary clinic. Public law 108–446, known as the Individuals with Disabilities Education Improvement Act of 2004, or IDEA, ensures access to a free and appropriate public education to all children with disabilities. Part C of that law guarantees access to early intervention that may include physical therapy services in the home or other natural settings through local early intervention programs for children from birth up to age 3. Chapter 30 discusses early intervention services under IDEA.

In some states, infants born very preterm with neonatal brain injury or other conditions warranting care in an NICU are automatically eligible for early intervention services. In other states, infants are required to show developmental delays. For infants who are eligible, referral before NICU discharge can ease the process for parents. The physical therapist plays an important role in the transition of infants and families to early intervention services. It is vital that therapists know the local laws and policies, have access to educational materials, and understand the referral process. The physical therapist should communicate with the therapist or agency providing early intervention services to the infant and family. Ideally, providers from the local early intervention agency would meet the family before the infant's discharge from the NICU and thus ensure a smooth and less stressful transition into the family's community. When this situation is not possible, the physical therapist can make contact with the community therapist and provide as much information as possible on the infant's current development

and interventions while in the NICU. Medical and developmental documentation may be helpful or necessary during the process of determining eligibility for early intervention. For infants who are not eligible at NICU discharge but may be in the future, providing parents with an understanding of what early intervention is and when to contact their local program is recommended. Referral to early intervention can be a complicated process for NICU providers, parents, and families. As in many settings, a navigator to help families complete the enrollment process for early intervention prior to or following discharge from the NICU is recommended.[150]

Infants born preterm or with NICU stays are at risk for developmental delays and medical complications that require ongoing follow-up. The onus is on NICU staff to ensure that the parents of each infant have a clear understanding of the recommendations for both medical and developmental follow-up care.[78] The AAP and other organizations have outlined recommendations for follow-up of preterm infants.[17,78,118,263] Many level III and IV nurseries as well as hospitals with neonatology fellowship programs in medicine and physical therapy have a developmental or NICU follow-up clinic for high-risk infants. Clinics vary in staffing and criteria for follow-up care. Factors such as birth weight, gestational age, Apgar scores, time on a ventilator, IVH, seizures, and environmental factors such as maternal drug or alcohol use are commonly used criteria. These follow-up programs monitor the health outcomes of graduates of the NICU.[238]

Results of developmental assessments administered at the follow-up clinic are useful in determining whether specialized therapy services are necessary beyond the provision of general recommendations for development and parent education. Referrals for nutrition, audiology, and ophthalmology also are made when necessary. As a team member in the follow-up clinic or early intervention, the physical therapist plays an important role in the examination and monitoring of infant neuromotor development, provides parent education and anticipatory guidance, and assists the family with coordination of care and referrals to other professionals and community agencies when appropriate.

RESOURCES AND PROFESSIONAL DEVELOPMENT

According to the practice guidelines endorsed by the American Physical Therapy Association (APTA),[245] physical therapists in the NICU should meet a series of competencies across multiple domains of neonatal clinical practice ranging from theoretical frameworks to social policy governing practice involving high-risk infants. In addition, physical therapists should participate in a minimum of 6 months of precepting in the NICU. Many NICUs lack an established training program where experienced clinical specialists provide precepting and ongoing mentoring to physical therapists new to neonatal care. Physical therapists may need to advocate for education and training resources.

Fellowship and Residency Programs

Advanced training in neonatal physical therapy is available through pediatric residency and neonatal fellowship programs that are accredited by the American Physical Therapy Association (APTA). Currently, there are 17 APTA pediatric residencies offered across the United States. Although the focus of pediatric residencies is general pediatric physical therapy, many residencies offer opportunities for clinical practice in the NICU. More information about the APTA-accredited pediatric residency program can be found at: http://www.abptrfe.org/apta/abptrfe/Directory.aspx?navID=10737432672.

In addition, there are currently two APTA-accredited neonatology fellowship programs. The goal of the fellowships is to prepare physical therapists for evidence-based, ethical, and appropriate neonatal physical therapist practice. More information about the fellowships is available at http://www.abptrfe.org/apta/abptrfe/Directory.aspx?ProgramType=Fellowship&navID=10737432673.

NICU Special Interest Groups

An additional resource for physical therapists working in the NICU is the Neonatology Special Interest Group within the Section on Pediatrics of the APTA. Members can access resources such as clinical guidelines, APTA conference activities (e.g., Section on Pediatrics Annual Conference) related to neonatal physical therapist practice, and resources lists. There are also a number of opportunities to connect with other neonatal physical therapists either through social media and member groups. More information about the Neonatology Special Interest Group is available at: www.pediatricapta.org/special-interest-groups/neonatology/index.cfm.

Therapists Who Are New to the NICU

Many therapists who practice in the NICU have previous experience with infants in outpatient or early interventions settings and in working with critically ill children in the pediatric intensive care unit. Therapists who are considering providing care in the NICU are encouraged to start their training with a mentored experience in the NICU follow-up program. This provides the therapist with an understanding of the likely range of outcomes for infants in the NICU. Onsight mentorship from an experienced NICU therapist is vital. Beginning with observation and gradually transitioning to supervised and then independent interaction with infant is considered best practice. Therapists new to the NICU should begin working with the least medically fragile infants approaching discharge and gradually increase acuity. Therapists will also benefit from shadowing other health care disciplines in the NICU to gain an appreciation for the role of nursing, physicians, and respiratory therapists in the NICU.

Cases Scenarios on Expert Consult

The website includes three case scenarios. The first is a video demonstrating a physical therapy intervention in a Level II NICU. One written case is about an infant born extremely preterm who has significant respiratory difficulties, which affect his oral feeding development. The second is about an infant, born full-term, with Down syndrome. There is concern from the medical team that the infant's mother has not bonded with her daughter. The website also includes a video demonstrating administration of the Test of Infant Motor Performance (TIMP).

REFERENCES

1. Abou Turk C, Williams AL, Lasky RE: A randomized clinical trial evaluating silicone earplugs for very low birth weight newborns in intensive care, *J Perinatol* 29(5):358–363, 2009.
2. Al Tawil KI, El Mahdy HS, Al Rifai MT, et al.: Risk factors for isolated periventricular leukomalacia, *Pediatric Neurology* 26:149–153, 2012.
3. Peyrovi H, Alinejad-Naeini MP, Mohagheghi P, Mehran A: The effect of facilitated tucking during endotracheal suctioning on procedural pain in preterm neonates: a randomized controlled crossover study, *Glob J Health Sci* 6(4):278–284, 2014.
4. Almadhoob A, Ohlsson A: Sound reduction management in the neonatal intensive care unit for preterm or very low birth weight infants, *Cochrane Database Syst Rev* 1, 2015. CD010333.
5. Als H: Toward a synactive theory of development. Promise for the assessment and support of infant individuality, *Infant Ment Health J* 3:229–243, 1982.
6. Als H, Duffy FH, McAnulty G, et al.: NIDCAP improves brain function and structure in preterm infants with severe intrauterine growth restriction, *J Perinatol* 32:797–803, 2012.
7. Als H, Duffy FH, McAnulty G, et al.: Early experience alters brain function and structure, *Pediatrics* 113:846–857, 2004.
8. Als H: A synactive model of neonatal behavioral organization: framework for the assessment of neurobehavioral development in the premature infant and for support of infants and parents in the neonatal intensive care environment, *Phys Occupat Ther Pediatr* 6(3/4):3–54, 1986.
9. Als H, Butler S: Newborn individualized developmental care and assessment program (NIDCAP): changing the future for infants and families in intensive and special care nurseries, *Early Child Serv (San Diego)* 2:1–19, 2008.
10. Als H, Butler S, Kosta S, McAnulty GB: The Assessment of Preterm Infants' Behavior (APIB): furthering the understanding and measurement of neurodevelopmental competence in preterm and full-term infants, *Ment Retard Disabil Res Rev* 11:94–102, 2005.
11. Als H, Gilkerson L, Duffy FH, et al.: A three-center randomized controlled trial of individualized developmental care for very low-birth weight infants: medical, neurodevelopmental, parenting and caregiving effects, *J Dev Behav Pediatr* 24(6):399–408, 2003.
12. Als H, Lawhon G, Duffy FH, et al.: Individualized developmental care for the very low birthweight preterm infant. *JAMA* 272(111):853–885, 1994.
13. Als H, Lester BM, Tronick EZ, Brazelton TB: Manual for the Assessment of Preterm Infants' Behavior (APIB). In Fitzgerald HE, Lester BM, Yogman MW, editors: *Theory and research in behavioral pediatrics*, New York, 1982, Plenum Press, pp 65–132.
14. Als H, Lester BM, Tronick EZ, Brazelton TB: Toward a research instrument for the assessment of preterm infants' behavior. In Fitzgerald HE, Lester BM, Yogman MW, editors: *Theory and research in behavioral pediatrics*, New York, 1982b, Plenum Press, pp 35–63.
15. Als H: Re: Ohlsson and Jacobs, NIDCAP: a systematic review and meta-analyses, *Pediatrics* 132(2):e552–e553, 2013.
16. Aly H, Hammad TA, Essers J, Wumg JT: Is mechanical ventilation associated with intraventricular hemorrhage in preterm infants? *Brain Dev* 34:201–205.
17. American Academy of Pediatrics Committee on Fetus and Newborn: Policy statement. Hospital discharge of the high-risk neonate, *Pediatrics* 122:1119–1126, 2008.
18. American Academy of Pediatrics Committee on Fetus and Newborn: Levels of neonatal care. Policy statement, *Pediatrics* 130:587–597, 2012.
19. American Lung Association (ALA): Lung disease data at a glance: respiratory distress syndrome (RDS). Available at: URL: www.lungusa.org/site/pp.asp?c=dvLUK900E&b=327819.
20. American Speech-Language-Hearing Association: Knowledge and skills needed by speech-language pathologists providing services to infants and families in the NICU environment [Knowledge and Skills]. Available at: URL: www.asha.org/policy.
21. Andiman SE, Haynes RL, Trachtenberg FL, et al.: The cerebral cortex overlying periventricular leukomalacia: analysis of pyramidal neurons, *Brain Pathol* 20:803–814, 2010.
22. Arul N, Konduri GG: Inhaled nitric oxide for preterm neonates, *Clin Perinatol* 36:43–61, 2009.
23. Athanasopoulou E, Fox JR: Effects of kangaroo mother care on maternal mood and interaction patterns between parents and their preterm, low birth weight infants: a systematic review, *Infant Ment Health J* 35(3):245–262, 2014.

24. Attar MA, Donn SM: Mechanisms of ventilator-induced injury in premature infants, *Semin Neonatol* 7:353–360, 2002.

25. Balinotti JE, Chakr VC, Tiller C, et al.: Growth of lung parenchyma in infants and toddlers with chronic lung disease of infancy, *Am J Respir Crit Care Med* 181:1093–1097, 2010, http://dx.doi.org/10.1164/rccm.200908-1190OC.

26. Ballabh P: Intraventrical hemorrhage in premature infants: mechanism of disease, *Pediatr Res* 67(1):1–8, 2010.

27. Ballabh P: Pathogenesis and prevention of intraventricular hemorrhage, *Clin Perinatol* 41(1):47–67, 2014.

28. Barbosa VM: Teamwork in the neonatal intensive care unit, *Phys Occupat Ther Pediatr* 33(1):5–26, 2013.

29. Barbosa VM, Campbell SK, Berbaum M: Discriminating infants from different developmental outcome groups using the Test of Infant Motor Performance (TIMP) item responses, *Pediatr Phys Ther* 19:28–39, 2007.

30. Barbosa VM, Campbell SK, Smith E, Berbaum M: Comparison of Test of Infant Motor Performance (TIMP) item responses among children with cerebral palsy, developmental delay, and typical development, *Am J Occupat Ther* 59:446–456, 2005.

31. Barnard KE, Eyres SJ: *Child health assessment. Part 2: the first year of life*, Washington DC, 1979, (DHEW Publication No HRA79–25), Bethesda, MD. US Government Printing Office.

32. Bassler D, Stoll BJ, Schmidt B, et al.: Using a count of neonatal morbidities to predict poor outcome in extremely low birth weight infants: added role of neonatal infection, *Pediatrics* 123:313–318, 2009.

33. Beck C: Postpartum depression: stopping the thief that steals motherhood. AWHONN, *Lifelines* 3:41–44, 1999.

34. Beligere N, Rao R: Neurodevelopmental outcome of infants with meconium aspiration syndrome: report of a study and literature review, *J Perinatol* 28:S93–S101, 2008.

35. Bellieni CV, Buonocore G, Nenci A, et al.: Sensorial saturation: an effective analgesic tool for heel-prick in preterm infants, *Biol Neonate* 80:15–18, 2001.

36. Berghella V, editor: *Obstetric and maternal-fetal evidence-based guidelines* (Vol. 2). UK, 2007, Informa Healthcare. Thompson.

37. Bersani I, Corsello M, Mastandrea M, et al.: Neonatal abstinence syndrome, *Early Hum Dev* 89S4:S85–S97, 2013.

38. Bhethanabhotla SA, Thukral MJ, Sankar R, et al.: Effect of position of infant during phototherapy in management of hyperbilirubinemia in late preterm and term neonates: a randomized controlled trial, *J Perinatol* 33(10):795–799, 2013.

39. Bhutta AT, Anand KJ: Vulnerability of the developing brain: neuronal mechanisms, *Clin Perinatol* 29(3):357–372, 2002.

40. Birch JL, Newell SJ: Managing gastro-esophageal reflux in infants, *Arch Dis Child Fetal Neonatal* 47:134–137, 2009.

41. Blanchard Y: Using the Newborn Behavioral Observations (NBO) system with at-risk infants and families: United States. In Nugent JK, Brazelton TB, Patrauskas B, editors: *The newborn as a person: enabling healthy infant development worldwide*, Hoboken, NJ, 2009, John Wiley Sons, pp 120–128.

42. Blanchard Y, Mouradian L: Integrating neurobehavioral concepts into early intervention eligibility evaluation, *Infants Young Child* 13(2):41–50, 2000.

43. Blanchard Y, Øberg GK: Physical therapy with newborns: applying concepts of phenomenology and synactive theory to guide interventions, *Physiother Theory Pract* 31(6):377–381, 2015.

44. Bolisetty S, Dhawan A, Abdel-Latif M, et al.: Intraventricular hemorrhage and neurodevelopmental outcomes in extreme preterm infants, *Pediatrics* 133(1):55–62, 2014.

45. Bradshaw WT: Necrotizing enterocolitis: etiology, presentation, management, and outcomes, *J Perinat Neonat Nurs* 23:87–94, 2009.

46. Braun MA, Palmer MM: A pilot study of oral-motor dysfunction in "at-risk" infant, *Phys Occupat Ther Pediatr* 5(4):13–26, 1985.

47. Brazelton TB, Nugent JK: The Neonatal Behavioral Assessment Scale, ed 4, *Clin Dev Med* 190, 2011.

48. Brazelton TB: Crying in infancy, *Pediatrics* 29:579–588, 1962.

49. Bredemeyer SL, Foster JP: Body positioning for spontaneously breathing preterm infants with apnoea, *Cochrane Database Syst Rev* 6, 2012. CD004951.

50. Browne JV, VandenBerg K, Ross ES, Elmore AM: The newborn developmental specialist: definition, qualifications and preparation for an emerging role in the neonatal intensive care unit, *Infants Young Child* 11(4):65–78, 1999.

51. Bruder MB: Working with members of other disciplines: collaboration for success. In Wolery M, Wilbers JS, editors: *Including children with special needs in early childhood programs*, Washington, DC, 1994, National Association for the Education of Young Children, pp 45–70.

52. Bruschweiler-Stern N: Mère à terme et mère prématurée (The full-term and preterm mother). In Dugnat M, editor: *Le monde relationnel du bébé (The relational world of the newborn)*, France: ERES, 1997, Ramonville Saint-Agne, pp 19–24.

53. Cameron EC, Maehle V, Reid J: The effects of an early physical therapy intervention for very preterm, very low birth weight infants: a randomized controlled clinical trial, *Pediatr Phys Ther* 17(2):107–119, 2005.

54. Campbell SK: Organizational and educational considerations in creating an environment to promote optimal development of high-risk neonates, *Phys Occupat Ther Pediatr* 6(3/4):191–204, 1986.

55. Campbell SK, Hedeker D: Validity of the Test of Infant Motor Performance for discriminating among infants with varying risk for poor motor outcome, *J Pediatr* 139:546–551, 2001.

56. Campbell SK, Kolobe THA: Concurrent validity of the Test of Infant Motor Performance with the Alberta Infant Motor Scale, *Pediatr Phys Ther* 12:1–8, 2000.

57. Campbell SK, Kolobe THA, Osten ET, et al.: Construct validity of the Test of Infant Motor Performance, *Phys Ther* 75(7):585–596, 1995.

58. Campbell SK, Kolobe THA, Wright B, Linacre JM: Validity of the Test of Infant Motor Performance for prediction of 6-, 9-, and 12-month scores on the Alberta Infant Motor Scale, *Dev Med Child Neurol* 44:263–272, 2002.

59. Campbell SK, Swanlund A, Smith E. et al.: Validity of the TIMPSI for estimating concurrent performance on the Test of Infant Motor Performance, *Pediatr Phys Ther* 20:3–210, 2008.

60. Cândia MF, Osaku EF, Leite MA, et al.: Influence of prone positioning on premature newborn infant stress assessed by means of salivary cortisol measurement: pilot study, *Rev Bras Ter Intensiva* 26(2):169–175, 2014.

61. Cardone IA, Gilkerson L: Family administered neonatal activities: a first step in the integration of parental perceptions and newborn behavior, *Infant Ment Health J* 11:127–131, 1990.

62. Carter JD, Mulder RT, Bartram AF, Darlow BA: Infants in a neonatal intensive care unit: parental response, *Arch Dis Child Fetal and Neonatal Ed* 90:F109–F113, 2005.

63. Chawla S, Natarajan G, Rane S, et al.: Outcomes of extremely low birth weight infants with varying doses and intervals of antenatal steroid exposure, *J Perinat Med* 38:419–423, 2010.

64. Chen S-S, Tzeng Y-L, Gau BS, et al.: Effects of prone and supine positioning on gastric residuals in preterm infants: a time series with crossover study, *Int J Nurs Stud* 50(11):1459–1467, 2013.

65. Cifuentes J, Carlo W: Respiratory system. In Kenner C, Lott JW, editors: *Comprehensive neonatal care: an interdisciplinary approach*, ed 4, Philadelphia, 2007, Elsevier, pp 1–15.

66. Cleveland LM: Parenting in the neonatal intensive care unit, *J Obstetr Gynecol Neonatal Nurs* 37:666–691, 2008.

67. Coalson JJ: Pathology of new bronchopulmonary dysplasia, *Semin Neonatol* 8:73–81, 2003.

68. Coalson JJ: Pathology of bronchopulmonary dysplasia, *Semin Perinatol* 30:179–184, 2006.

69. Committee on Perinatal Health: *Toward improving the outcome of pregnancy: recommendations for the regional development of maternal and perinatal health services*, White Plains, NY, 1976, March of Dimes National Foundation.

70. Corff KE, Seidman R, Venkataraman PS, et al.: Facilitated tucking: a nonpharmacologic comfort measure for pain in preterm neonates, *J Obstetr Gynecol Neonatal Nurs* 24:143–148, 1995.

71. Culhane JF, Goldenberg RL: Racial disparities in preterm birth, *Semin Perinatol* 35(4):234–239, 2011.

72. D'Apolito K: What is an organized infant? *Neonatal Netw* 10(1):23–29, 1991.

73. Das Eiden R, Reifman A: Effects of Brazelton demonstrations on later parenting, *J Pediatr Psychol* 21(6):857–868, 1996.

74. De Moraes Barros MC, Guinsburg R, de Araujo Peres C, et al.: Neurobehavior of full-term small for gestational age newborn infants of adolescent mothers, *Journal of Pediatrics* 149(6):781–787, 2006.

75. De Vries LS, Van Haastert IL, Rademaker KJ, Koopman C, Groenendaal F: Ultrasound abnormalities preceding cerebral palsy in high-risk infants, *J Pediatr* 144:815–820, 2004.

76. Deng W, Pleasure J, Pleasure D: Progress in periventricular leukomalacia, *Arch Neurol* 65:1291–1295, 2008.

77. Diniz KT, Cabral-Filho JE, Miranda RM, et al.: Effect of the kangaroo position on the electromyographic activity of preterm children: a follow-up study, *BMC Pediatr* 13:79, 2013.

78. Doyle LW, Anderson PJ, Battin M, et al.: Long term follow up of high risk children: who, why and how? *BMC Pediatr* 14:279, 2014.

79. Reference deleted in proofs.

80. Dubowitz L, Dubowitz V: *The neurological assessment of the preterm and full-term newborn infant*, London, 1981, Heinemann.

81. Dubowitz L, Dubowitz V, Mercuri E: *The neurological assessment of the preterm and full-term newborn infant*, ed 2, London, 1999, McKeith.

82. Dusing SC, Van Drew CM, Brown SE: Instituting parent education practices in the neonatal intensive care unit: an administrative case report of practice evaluation and statewide action, *Phys Ther* 92(7):967–975, 2012.

83. Dusing SC, Murray T, Stern M: Parent preferences for motor development education in the neonatal intensive care unit, *Pediatr Phys Ther* 20(4):363–368, 2008.

84. Dusing SC, Brown SE, Van Drew CM, et al.: Supporting play exploration and early development intervention from NICU to home: a feasibility study, *Pediatr Phys Ther* 27(3):267–274, 2015.

85. El Shahed AI, Dargaville P, Ohisson A, Soll RF: Surfactant for meconium aspiration syndrome in full term/near term infants, *Cochrane Database Sys Rev* 2, 2014. CD002054.

86. Engmann CS, Wall G, Darmstadt B, et al.: Consensus on kangaroo mother care acceleration, *Lancet* 382(9907):e26–e27, 2013.

87. Fanaroff AA, Graven SN: Perinatal services and resources. In Fanaroff AA, Martin RJ, editors: *Neonatal-perinatal medicine: diseases of the fetus and infant*, St. Louis, 1992, Mosby, pp 12–21.

88. Fanaroff AA, Stoll BJ, Wright LL, et al.: Trends in neonatal morbidity and mortality for very low birthweight infants, *Am J Obstetr Gynecol* 196(147):e1–e8, 2007.

89. Feldman R: Parent-infant synchrony and the construction of shared timing: physiological precursors, developmental outcomes and risk conditions, *J Child Psychol Psychiatry* 48(3/4):329–354, 2007.

90. Ferrari F, Bertoncelli N, Gallo C, et al.: Posture and movement in healthy preterm infants in supine position in and outside the nest, *Arch Dis Child Fetal Neonatal Ed* 92(5):F386–F390, 2007.

91. Finnegan LP: Neonatal abstinence syndrome: assessment and pharmacotherapy. In Nelson N, editor: *Current therapy in neonatal-perinatal medicine*, ed 2, Ontario, 1990, BC Decker.

92. Fitzgerald M, Beggs S: The neurobiology of pain: developmental aspects, *Neuroscientist* 7(3):246–257, 2001.

93. Flegel J, Kolobe THA: Predictive validity of the Test of Infant Motor Performance as measured by the Bruininks-Oseretsky Test of Motor Proficiency at school age, *Phys Ther* 82:762–771, 2002.

94. Gaebler C, Hanzlik R: The effects of prefeeding stimulation program on preterm infants, *Am Occup Ther* 50:184–192, 1996.

95. Gieron-Korthals M, Colon J: Hypoxic-ischemic encephalopathy in infants: new challenges, *Fetal Pediatr Pathol* 24:105–120, 2005.

96. Girolami G, Campbell S: Efficacy of a neuro-developmental treatment program to improve motor control in infants born prematurely, *Pediatr Phys Ther* 6(4):175–184, 1994.

97. Gomes-Pedro J, de Almeida JB, Costa Barbosa A: Influence of early mother-infant contact on dyadic behavior during the first month of life, *Dev Med Child Neurol* 26:657–664, 1984.

98. Gottfried AW: Environment of newborn infants in special care units. In Gottfried AW, Gaiter JL, editors: *Infant stress under intensive care*, Baltimore, 1985, University Park Press, pp 23–54.

99. Grave GD, Nelson SA, Walker WA, et al.: New therapies and preventive approaches for necrotizing enterocolitis: report of a research planning workshop, *Pediatr Res* 62:510–514, 2007.

100. Graven SN: Sound and the developing infant in the NICU: conclusions and recommendations for care, *J Perinatol* 20(8):S88–S93, 2000.

101. Graven SN: Early neurosensory visual development of the fetus and newborn, *Clin Perinatol* 31(2):199–216, 2004.

102. Green NS, Damus K, Simpson JL, et al.: Research agenda for preterm birth: recommendations from the March of Dimes, *Am J Obstetr Gynecol* 193:626–635, 2005.

103. Grenier IR, Bigsby R, Vergara ER: Comparison of motor self-regulatory and stress behaviors of preterm infants across body positions, *Am J Occup Ther* 57(3):289–297, 2003.

104. Grunau E, Holsti L, Whitfield M, Ling E: Are twitches, startles, and body movements pain indicators in extremely low birth weight infants? *Clin J Pain* 16:37–45, 2000.

105. Hall R, Anand KJS: Physiology of pain and stress in the newborn, *Neo Rev* 6:e61–e68, 2005.

106. Hartley KA, Miller CS, Gephart SM: Facilitated tucking to reduce pain in neonates: evidence for best practice, *Adv Neonatal Care* 15(3):201–208, 2015.

107. Haumont D, Amiel-Tison C, Casper C: NIDCAP and developmental care: a European perspective, *Pediatrics* 132(2):e551–e552, 2013.

108. Heidarzadeh M, Hosseini MB, Ershadmanesh M: The effect of kangaroo mother care (KMC) on breast feeding at the time of NICU discharge, *Iran Red Crescent Med J* 15(4):302–306, 2013.

109. Heinemann AB, Hellstrom-Westas L, Hedberg Nyqvist K: Factors affecting parents' presence with their extremely preterm infants in a neonatal intensive care room, *Acta Paediatr* 102(7):695–702, 2013.

110. Henderson-Smart DJ, Cools F, Bhuta T, Offringa M: Elective high frequency oscillatory ventilation versus conventional ventilation for acute pulmonary dysfunction in preterm infants, *Cochrane Database Sys Rev* 18(3), 2007. CD000104.

111. Herzog M, Cerar LK, Srsen TP, et al.: Impact of risk factors other than prematurity on periventricular leukomalacia. A population-based matched case control study, *Eur J Gynecol Reprod Biol* 187:57–59, 2015.

112. Hintz SR, Kendrick DE, Vohr BR, et al.: Changes in neurodevelopmental outcomes at 18 to 22 months' corrected age among infants of less than 25 weeks' gestational age born in 1993-1999, *Pediatrics* 115:1645, 2005.

113. Hodgman JE: Introduction. In Gottfried AW, Gaiter JL, editors: *Infant stress under intensive care*, Baltimore, 1985, University Park Press, pp 1–6.

114. Hoehn T, Krause MF, Buhrer C: Metal-analysis of inhaled nitric oxide in premature infants: an update, *Klinische Pädiatrie* 218:57–61, 2006.

115. Holditch-Davis D, White-Traut RC, Levy JA, et al.: Maternally administered interventions for preterm infants in the NICU: effects on maternal psychological distress and mother-infant relationship, *Infant Behav Dev* 37(4):695–710, 2014.

116. Honrubia D, Stark AR: Respiratory distress syndrome. In Cloherty JP, Eichenwald EC, Stark AR, editors: *Manual of neonatal care*, ed 5, Philadelphia, 2004, Lippincott Williams Wilkins, pp 341-347.

117. Horton KK: Pathophysiology and current management of necrotizing enterocolitis, *Neonatal Netw* 24:37–46, 2005.

118. Hwang SS, Barfield WD, Smith RA: Discharge timing, outpatient follow-up, and home care of late-preterm and early-term infants, *Pediatrics* 132(1):101–108, 2013.

119. International Committee on Retinopathy of Prematurity (ICROP): An international classification of retinopathy of prematurity, *Pediatrics* 74:127–133, 1984.

120. International Committee on Retinopathy of Prematurity: The international classification of retinopathy of prematurity revisited, *Arch Ophthalmol* 123:991–999, 2005.

121. Jain NJ, Kruse LK, Demissie K, Khandelwal M: Impact of mode of delivery on neonatal complications: trends between 1997 and 2005, *J Matern Fetal Neonatal Med* 22:491–500, 2009.

122. Jansson LM, Velez M: Neonatal abstinence syndrome, *Curr Opin Pediatr* 24(2):252–258, 2012.

123. Jobe AH: The new bronchopulmonary dysplasia. *Curr Opin Pediatr* 23(2):167–172.

124. Jobe AH, Bancalari E: Bronchopulmonary dysplasia, *Am J Respir Crit Care Med* 163(7):1723–1729, 2001.

125. Johnson NN: The maternal experience of kangaroo holding, *J Obstetr Gynecol Neonatal Nurs* 36(6):568–573, 2007.

126. Kadhim H, Sebire G, Kahn A, et al.: Causal mechanisms underlying periventricular leukomalacia and cerebral palsy, *Curr Pediatr Rev* 1:1–6, 2012.

127. Keefer CH: The combined physical and behavioral neonatal examination: a parent-centered approach to pediatric care. In Brazelton TB, Nugent JK, editors: *Neonatal Behavioral Assessment Scale*, London, 1995, Mac Keith Press, pp 92–101.

128. Keller A, Arbel N, Merlob P, Davidson S: Neurobehavioral and autonomic effects of hammock positioning in infants with very low birth weight, *Pediatr Phys Ther* 15:3–7, 2003.

129. Reference deleted in proofs.

130. Keszler M: State of the art in conventional mechanical ventilation, *J Perinatol* 29:262–275, 2009.

131. Khwaja O, Volpe JJ: Pathogenesis of cerebral white matter injury of prematurity, *Arch Dis Child Fet Neonat Ed* 93(2):F153–F161, 2008.

132. Kinney HC: Human myelinization and perinatal white matter disorders, *J Neurol Sci* 228:190–192, 2005.

133. Klaus HH, Kennell JH, Klaus PH: *Bonding*. Reading, MA, 1995, Addison Wesley Longman.

134. Kleinman L, Rothman M, Strauss R, et al.: The infant gastroesophageal reflux questionnaire revised: development and validation as an evaluative instrument, *Clin Gastroenterol Hepatol* 4(5):588–596, 2006.

135. Kocherlakota P: Neonatal abstinence syndrome, *Pediatrics* 134(2): e547–e561, 2014.

136. Korner AF, Constantinou J, Dimiceli S, et al.: Establishing the reliability and developmental validity of a neurobehavioral assessment for preterm infants: a methodological process, *Child Dev* 62(5):1200–1208, 1991.

137. Kurinczuk JJ, White-Koning M, Badawi N: Epidemiology of neonatal encephalopathy and hypoxic-ischaemic encephalopathy, *Early Hum Dev* 86:329–338, 2010.

138. Lasswell SM, Barfield WD, Rochat RW, Blackmon L: Perinatal regionalization for very low-birth weight and very preterm infants: a meta-analysis, *JAMA* 304(9):992–1000, 2010.

139. Latal B: Prediction of neurodevelopmental outcome after preterm birth, *Pediatr Neurol* 40:413–419, 2009.

140. Lauderet S, Liu WF, Blackington S, et al.: Implementing potentially better practices to support the neurodevelopment of infants in the NICU, *J Perinatol* 27:S75–S93, 2007.

141. Lawhon G: Facilitation of parenting the premature infant within the newborn intensive care unit, *J Perinatal Neonatal Nurs* 16(1):71–83, 2002.

142. Leef KH: Evidence-based review of oral sucrose administration to decrease the pain response in newborn infants, *Neonatal Netw* 25:275–284, 2006.

143. Lemmons JA, Bauer CR, Oh W, et al.: Very low birth weight outcomes of the National Institute of Child Health and Human Development Neonatal Research Network, January 1995 through December 1996. NICHD Neonatal Research Network, *Pediatrics* 107(E1), 2001.

144. Lester BM, Tronick EZ, Brazelton TB: The Neonatal Intensive Care Unit Network Neurobehavioral Scale procedures, *Pediatrics* 113(3 Pt 2): 641–667, 2004.

145. Lester BM, Tronick EZ: *NICU Network Neurobehavioral Scale*, Baltimore, 2005, Brookes.

146. Lester B, Hawes K, Abar B: Single-family room care and neurobehavioral and medical outcomes in preterm infants, *Pediatrics* 134(4):754–760, 2014.

147. Levene MI, de Vries L: Hypoxic-ischemic encephalopathy. In Martin RJ, Fanaroff AA, Walsh MC, editors: *Neonatal-perinatal medicine*, Philadelphia, 2006, Mosby, pp 938–944.

148. Lightdale JR, Gremse DA: Section on gastroenterology, hepatology and nutrition: gastroesophageal reflux: management guidance for the pediatrician, *Pediatrics* 131(5):e1684–e1695, 2013.

149. Lin PW, Nasr TR, Stoll BJ: Necrotizing enterocolitis: recent scientific advances in pathophysiology and prevention, *Semin Perinatol* 32:70–82, 2008.

150. Little AA, Kamholz K, Corwin BK, et al.: Understanding barriers to early intervention services for preterm infants: lessons from two states, *Acad Pediatr* 15(4):430–438, 2015.

151. Liu WF: Comparing sound measurements in the single-family room with open-unit design neonatal intensive care unit: the impact of equipment noise, *J Perinatol* 32(5):368–373, 2012.

152. Liu WF, Laudert S, Perkins B, et al.: The development of potentially better practices to support the neurodevelopment of infants in the NICU, *J Perinatol* 27:S48–S74, 2007.

153. Lobel M: Pregnancy-specific stress, prenatal health behaviors, and birth outcomes, *Health Psychol* 27:604–615, 2008.

154. Loftin RW, Habli M, Snyder CC, et al.: Late preterm birth, *Rev Obstet Gynecol* 3(1):10–19, 2010.

155. Long T: *Handbook of pediatric physical therapy*, Baltimore, 2001, Lippincott, Williams, Wilkins.

156. Loo KK, Espinosa M, Tyler R, Howard J: Using knowledge to cope with stress in the NICU: how parents integrate learning to read the physiologic and behavioral cues of the infant, *Neonatal Netw* 22(1):31–37, 2003.

157. Louie JP: Essential diagnosis of abdominal emergencies in the first year of life, *Emerg Med Clin North Am* 25:1009–1040, 2007.

158. Ludwig AK, Sutcliff AG, Diedrich K, Ludwig M: Post-neonatal health and development of children born after assisted reproduction: a systematic review of controlled studies, *Eur J Obstet Gynecol Reprod Biol* 127:3–25, 2006.

159. Madlinger-Lewis L, et al.: The effects of alternative positioning on preterm infants in the neonatal intensive care unit: a randomized clinical trial, *Res Dev Disabil* 35(2):490–497, 2014.

160. Malusky SK: A concept analysis of family-centered care in the NICU, *Neonatal Netw* 24(6):25–32, 2005.

161. Malusky S, Donze A: Neutral head positioning in premature infants for intraventricular hemorrhage prevention: an evidence-based review, *Neonatal Netw* 30(6):381–396, 2011.

162. Mantagos IS, Vanderveen DK, Smith L: Emerging treatments for retinopathy of prematurity, *Semin Ophthalmol* 24:82–86, 2009.

163. March of Dimes Perinatal Data Center: *Special Care Nursery Admissions*. Available at: URL: https://www.marchofdimes.org/peristats/pdfdocs/nicu_summary_final.pdf, 2011.

164. Marlow N, Wolke D, Bracewell MA, Samara M: Neurologic and developmental disability at six years of age after extremely preterm birth, *N Engl J Med* 352(1):9–19, 2005.

165. Martin JB: Prevention of intraventricular hemorrhages and periventricular leukomalacia in the extremely low birth weight infant. *Newborn Infant Nurs Rev* 11(3):148–152.

166. Matthews TJ, Menacker F, MacDorman MF: Infant mortality statistics from the 2002 period. Linked birth-death data set, *Natl Vital Stat Rep* 53:1–29, 2004.

167. McAnulty GB, Duffy FH, Butler S, et al.: Individualized developmental care for a large sample of very preterm infants: health, neurobehaviour and neurophysiology, *Acta Paediatr* 98(12):1920–1926, 2009.

168. McAnulty G, Duffy FH, Kosta S, et al.: School-age effects of the newborn individualized developmental care and assessment program for preterm infants with intrauterine growth restriction: preliminary findings, *BMC Pediatr* 13:25, 2013.

169. McCormick MC, McManus BM: Cognitive and behavioral interventions. In Nosarti C, Murray R, Hack M, editors: *Preterm birth: long-term effects on brain and behaviours*, Cambridge, UK, 2010, Cambridge University Press, pp 237–250.

170. McCormick MC, Richardson DK: Access to neonatal intensive care, *Future Child* 5(1):162–175, 1995.

171. McManus BM, Nugent JK: A neurobehavioral intervention incorporated into state early intervention programming improves parent's social interaction with their high risk newborn, *J Behav Health Serv Res* 39:1–8, 2012.

172. McMullen SL: Transitioning premature infants supine: state of the science, *MCN Am J Matern Child Nurs* 38(1):8–12, 2013. quiz 13-14.

173. McMullen SL, Wu YW, Austin-Ketch T, Carey MG: Transitioning the premature infant from nonsupine to supine position prior to hospital discharge, *Neonatal Netw* 33(2):194–198, 2014.

174. Monterosso L, Kristjanson LJ, Cole J, Evans SF: Effect of postural supports on neuromotor function in very preterm infants to term equivalent age, *J Paediatr Child Health* 39(3):197–205, 2003.

175. Morag I, Ohlsson A: Cycled light in the intensive care unit for preterm and low birth weight infants, *Cochrane Database Syst Rev* 8, 2013. CD006982.

176. Murney ME, Campbell SK: The ecological relevance of the Test of Infant Motor Performance Elicited Scale items, *Phys Ther* 78:479–489, 1998.

177. National Institute of Child Health and Development: Surgeon General's Conference on the Prevention of Preterm Birth. Washington, DC. June 16-17, 2008. Available at: URL: www.nichd.nih.gov/about/meetings/2008/SG_preterm-birth/agenda.clm. Presentations can be accessed at http://videocast.nih.gov/PastEvents.asp?c=1.

178. Neff JM, Eichner JM, Hardy DR, et al.: Family-centered care and the pediatrician's role, *Pediatrics* 112(3):691–696, 2003.

179. Noble Y, Boyd R: Neonatal assessments for the preterm infant up 4 months corrected age: a systematic review, *Dev Med Child Neurol* 54:129–139, 2012.

180. Nugent JK, Keefer CH, Minear S, et al.: *Understanding newborn behavior early relationships: the Newborn Behavioral Observations (NBO) system handbook*, Baltimore, 2007, Brookes.

181. Nugent JK, Blanchard Y: Newborn behavior and development: implications for health care professionals. In Travers JF, Thies KM, editors: *The handbook of human development for health care professionals*, Sudbury, MA, 2005, Jones Bartlett, pp 79–94.

182. Nugent JK, Petrauskas BJ, Brazelton TB: *The newborn as a person*, Hoboken, NJ, 2009, Wiley Sons.

183. Nye C: Transitioning premature infants from gavage to breast, *Neonatal Netw* 27(1):7–13, 2008.

184. Oh W, Gilstrap I: *Guidelines for perinatal care*, ed 5, Old Grove Village, IL, 2002, American Academy of Pediatrics, American College of Obstetrician and Gynecologists.

185. Ohlinger J, Brown MS, Laudert S, et al.: Development of potentially better practices for the neonatal intensive care unit as a culture of collaboration: communication, accountability, respect, and empowerment. *Pediatrics* 111(4):e471–e481, 2003.

186. Ohlsson A, Jacobs SE: Authors' response: NIDCAP: a systematic review and meta-analyses of randomized controlled trials, *Pediatrics* 132(2):e553–e557, 2013.

187. Ohlsson A, Jacobs SE: NIDCAP: a systematic review and meta-analyses of randomized controlled trials, *Pediatrics* 131(3):e881–e893, 2013.

188. Orenstein SR, McGowan JD: Efficacy of conservative therapy as taught in the primary care setting for symptoms suggesting infant gastroesophageal reflux, *J Pediatr* 152(3):310–314, 2008.

189. Palisano RJ: A collaborative model of service delivery for children with movement disorders: a framework for evidence-based decision making, *Phys Ther* 86(9):1295–1305, 2006.

190. Papile LS, Burstein J, Burstein R: Incidence and evolution of the subependymal intraventricular hemorrhage: a study of infants with weights less than 1500 grams, *J Pediatr* 92:529–534, 1978.

191. Parad RB: Bronchopulmonary dysplasia/chronic lung disease. In Cloherty JP, Eichenwald EC, Stark AR, editors: *Manual of neonatal care*, ed 6, Philadelphia, 2008, Lippincott Williams Wilkins.

192. Parker S, Zahr LK, Cole JCD, Braced ML: Outcomes after developmental intervention in the neonatal intensive care unit for mothers of preterm infants with low socioeconomic status, *J Pediatr* 120:780–785, 1992.

193. Pax Lowes L, Palisano RJ: Review of medical and developmental outcome of neonates who received extracorporeal membrane oxygenation, *Pediatr Phys Ther* 7:215–221, 1995.

194. Paz MS, Smith LM, LaGasse LL, et al.: Maternal depression and neurobehavior in newborns prenatally exposed to methamphetamine, *Neurotoxicol Teratol* 31(3):177–182, 2009.

195. Perkins E, Ginn L, Fanning JK, Bartlett DJ: Effect of nursing education on positioning of infants in the neonatal intensive care unit, *Pediatr Phys Ther* 16:2–12, 2004.

196. Peters KL, Rosychuk RJ, Hendson L, et al.: Improvement of short- and long-term outcomes for very low birth weight infants: Edmonton NID-CAP trial, *Pediatrics* 124(4):1009–1020, 2009.

197. Peyrovi H, Alinejad-Naeini M, Mohagheghi P: The effect of facilitated tucking position during endotracheal suctioning on physiological responses and coping with stress in premature infants: a randomized controlled crossover study, *J Matern Fetal Neonatal Med* 27(15):1555–1559, 2014.

198. Philbin MK, Lickliter R, Graven SN: Sensory experience and the developing organism: a history of ideas and view to the future, *J Perinatol* 20 (8 Pt 2):S2–S5, 2000.

199. Phillips-Pula L, Pickler R, McGrath JM, et al.: Caring for a preterm infant at home: a mother's perspective, *J Perinatal Neonatal Nurs* 27(4):335–344, 2013.

200. Pierrehumbert B, Nicole A, Muller-Nix C, et al.: Parental post-traumatic reactions after premature birth: implications for sleeping and eating problems in the infant, *Arch Dis Child Fetal and Neonatal Ed* 88:400–404, 2003.

201. Pineda RG, Castellano A, Rogers C, et al.: Factors associated with developmental concern and intent to access therapy following discharge from the NICU, *Pediatr Phys Ther* 25(1):62–69, 2013.

202. Pineda RG, Neil J, Dierker D, et al.: Alterations in brain structure and neurodevelopmental outcome in preterm infants hospitalized in different neonatal intensive care unit environments, *J Pediatr* 164(1):52–60, 2014. e52.

203. Pineda RG, Neil J, Dierker D: Alterations in brain structure and neurodevelopmental outcome in preterm infants hospitalized in different neonatal intensive care unit environments, *J Pediatr* 164(1):52–60, 2014. e2.

204. Polin RA, Carlo WA: Committee on Fetus and Newborn. From the American Academy of Pediatrics Clinical Report Surfactant replacement therapy for preterm and term neonates with respiratory distress, *Pediatrics* 133(1):156–163, 2014.

205. Prechtl HFR: General movement assessment as a method of developmental neurology: new paradigms and their consequences. The 1999 Ronnie MacKeith Lecture, *Dev Med Child Neurol* 12:836–842, 2001.

206. Radic JAE, Vincer M, McNeely PD: Outcomes of intraventricular hemorrhage and posthemorrhagic hydrocephalus in a population-based cohort of very preterm infants born to residents in Nova Scotia from 1993 to 2010, *J Neurosurg Pediatr* 15:580–588, 2015.

207. Ranger M: Current controversies regarding pain assessment in neonates, *Semin Perinatol* 31:283–288, 2007.

208. Rauh V, Achenbach T, Nurcombe B, et al.: Minimizing adverse effects of low birthweight: four-year results of an early intervention program, *Child Dev* 59:S44–S553, 1998.

209. Redshaw ME: Mothers of babies requiring special care: attitudes and experiences, *J Reprod Infant Psychol* 15(2):109–121, 1997.

210. Reference deleted in proofs.

211. Reference deleted in proofs.

212. Rudolph CD, Mazur LJ, Liptak GS, et al.: Guidelines for evaluation and treatment of gastroesophageal reflux in infants and children: recommendations of the North American Society for Pediatric Gastroenterology and Nutrition, *J Pediatr Gastroenterol Nutr* 32(Suppl 2): S1–S31, 2001.

213. Salisbury AL, Lester BM, Seifer R, et al.: Prenatal cocaine use and maternal depression: effects on infant neurobehavior, *Neurotoxicol Teratol* 29(3):331–340, 2007.

214. Sanders LW, Buckner EB: The NBO as a nursing intervention. *Ab Initio*, Spring, 2009. Available at: URL: www.brazelton-institute.com/abinitio2009spring.

215. Sarkar S, Shankaran S, Laptook AR, et al.: Screening cranial imaging at multiple times points improves cystic periventricular leukomalacia detection, *Am J Perinatol* 32(10):973–979, 2015.

216. Sarnat HB, Sarnat MS: Neonatal encephalopathy following fetal distress, *Arch Neurol* 33, 1976: 696–675.

217. Schechner S: Drug abuse and withdrawal. In Cloherty JP, Eichenwald EC, Stark AR, editors: *Manual of neonatal care*, ed 6, Philadelphia, 2008, Lippincott Williams Wilkins, pp 213–227.

218. Schulzke S, Trachsel D, Patole S: Physical activity programs for promoting bone mineralization and growth in preterm infants, *Cochrane Database Syst Rev* 2, 2007. CD005387.

219. Serane VT, Kurian O: Neonatal abstinence syndrome, *Indian J Pediatr* 75:911–914, 2008.

220. Shah PS, Aliwalas L, Shah V: Breastfeeding or breastmilk to alleviate procedural pain in neonates: a systematic review, *Breastfeeding Med* 2:74–82, 2007.

221. Shahheidari M, Homer C: Impact of the design of neonatal intensive care units on neonates, staff, and families: a systematic literature review, *J Perinat Neonatal Nurs* 26(3):260–266, 2012. quiz 267-268.

222. Shankaran S, Laptook AR, Tyson JE, et al.: Evolution of encephalopathy during whole body hypothermia for neonatal hypoxic-ischemic encephalopathy. *J Pediatr* 160(4):567–572, 2012.

223. Sheikh S, Stephen T, Howell L, Eid N: Gastroesophageal reflux in infants with wheezing, *Pediatr Pulmonol* 28(3):181–186, 1999.

224. Short BL: Extracorporeal membrane oxygenation: use in meconium aspiration syndrome, *J Perinatol* 28:S279–S283, 2008.

225. Silverman WA: Incubator-baby side shows, *Pediatrics* 64:127–141, 1979.

226. Smith GC, et al.: Neonatal intensive care unit stress is associated with *Brain Dev* in preterm infants, *Ann Neurol* 70(4):541–549, 2011.

227. Smith LM, Lagasse LL, Derauf C, et al.: Prenatal methamphetamine and neonatal neurobehavioral outcome, *Neurotoxicol Teratol* 30(1):20–28, 2008.

228. Soll R, Morley CJ: Prophylactic versus selective use of surfactant in preventing morbidity and mortality in preterm infants, *Cochrane Database Syst Rev* 2, 2001. CD00510.

229. Spiker D, Ferguson J, Brooks-Gunn J: Enhancing maternal interactive behavior and child social competence in low birthweight, premature infants, *Child Dev* 64:754–768, 1993.

230. Spittle AJ, Doyle LW, Boyd RN: A systematic review of the clinometric properties of neuromotor assessments for preterm infants during the first year of life, *Dev Med Child Neurol* 50:254–266, 2008.

231. Spittle A, et al.: Early developmental intervention programmes posthospital discharge to prevent motor and cognitive impairments in preterm infants, *Cochrane Database Syst Rev* 12, 2012. CD005495.

232. Spittle AJ, et al.: Early developmental intervention programs post hospital discharge to prevent motor and cognitive impairments in preterm infants, *Cochrane Database Syst Rev* 18(2), 2007.

233. Steinberg Z: Pandora meets the NICU parent or whither hope? *Psychoanal Dialogues* 16(2):133–147, 2006.

234. Stern DN: *The motherhood constellation*, New York, 1995, Basic Books.

235. Stevens B, Franck L: Special needs of preterm infants in the management of pain and discomfort, *J Gynecol Neonatal Nurs* 24:856–861, 1995.

236. Stevens TP, Blennow M, Myers EH, Soll R: Early surfactant administration with brief ventilation vs. selective surfactant and continued mechanical ventilation for preterm infants with or at risk for respiratory distress syndrome, *Cochrane Database Syst Rev* 4, 2007. CD003063.

237. Stevenson DK, Wright LL, Lemons JA, et al.: Very low birth weight outcomes of the National Institute of Child Health and Human Development Neonatal Research Network, January 1993 through December 1994, *Am J Obstet Gynecol* 179:1632–1639, 1998.

238. Stewart J: Early intervention and follow-up programs for the premature infant. In Brodsky D, Ouellette MA, editors: *Primary care of the premature infant*, Philadelphia, 2008, Saunders, pp 285–288.

239. Stoll BJ, Hanse NI, Bell EF, et al.: Neonatal outcomes of extremely preterm infants from the NICHD Neonatal Research Network, *Pediatrics* 126:443–456, 2010.

240. Stork EK: Extracorporeal membrane oxygenation. In Fanaroff AA, Martin RJ, editors: *Neonatal-perinatal medicine: diseases of the fetus and infant*, St. Louis, 1992, Mosby, pp 876–882.

241. Stout AU, Stout JT: Retinopathy of prematurity, *Pediatr Clin North Am* 50:77–87, 2003.

242. Strodtbeck F: Opthalmic system. In Kenner C, Lott JW, editors: *Comprehensive neonatal care*, ed 4, Philadelphia, 2007, Saunders/Elsevier, pp 313–332.

243. Stroustrup A, Trasande L: Epidemiological characteristics and resource use in neonates with bronchopulmonary dysplasia, *Pediatrics* 126:291–297, 2010.

244. Sumner G, Spietz A: *NCAST caregiver/parent-infant interaction feeding manual*, Seattle, WA, 1994, NCAST Publications, University of Washington, School of Nursing.

245. Sweeney JK, Heriza HB, Blanchard Y: Neonatal physical therapy: clinical competencies and NICU clinical training models. Part I, *Pediatr Phys Ther* 21(4):296–307, 2009.

246. Sweeney JK, Heriza HB, Blanchard Y, Dusing S: Neonatal physical therapy. Part II: practice frameworks and evidence-based practice guidelines, *Pediatr Phys Ther* 2(1):2–16, 2010.

247. Sweeney J, Gutierrez T: Musculoskeletal implications of preterm infant positioning in the NICU, *J Perinatal Neonatal Nurs* 16(1):58–70, 2002.

248. Symington A, Pinelli J: Developmental care for promoting development and preventing morbidity in preterm infants, *Cochrane Database Syst Rev* 2, 2006. CD001814.

249. Thomas A, Chess S: *Temperament and development*, New York, 1977, Brunner-Maze.

250. Thoyre SM, Shaker CS, Pridham KF: The early feeding skill assessment for preterm infants, *Neonatal Netw* 24(3):7–16, 2005.

251. Vain NE, Szyld EG, Prudent LM, et al.: Oropharyngeal and nasopharyngeal suctioning of meconium-stained neonates before delivery of their shoulders: multicenter, randomized, controlled trial, *Lancet* 364:597–602, 2004.

252. Vaivre-Douret L, Golse B: Comparative effects of 2 positional supports on neurobehavioral and postural development in preterm neonates, *J Perinat Neonatal Nurs* 21(4):323–330, 2007.

253. Vaivre-Douret LK, Ennouri I, Jrad C, et al.: Effect of positioning on the incidence of abnormalities of muscle tone in low-risk, preterm infants, *Eur J Paediatr Neurol* 8(1):21–34, 2004.

254. Vandenplas Y, Rudolph CD, Lorenzo C, et al.: Pediatric gastroesophageal reflux clinical practice guidelines: joint recommendations of the North American Society for Pediatric Gastroenterology, Hepatology and Nutrition and the European Society for Pediatric Gastroenterology, Hepatology and Nutrition, *J Pediatr Gastroenterol Nutr* 49(4):498–547, 2009.

255. Vergara E, Anzalone M, Bigsby R, et al.: Specialized knowledge and skills for occupational therapy practice in the neonatal intensive care unit, *Am J Occupat Ther* 54:641–648, 2006.

256. Vergara ER, Bigsby R: *Developmental and therapeutic interventions in the NICIU*, Towson, MD, 2004, Brookes.

257. Verklan MT: The chilling details: hypoxic-ischemic encephalopathy, *J Perinatal Neonatal Nurs* 23(1):59–68, 2009.

258. Vickers A, et al.: Massage for promoting growth and development of preterm and/or low birth-weight infants, *Cochrane Database Syst Rev* 2, 2004. CD000390.

259. Volpe JJ: Neonatal encephalopathy: an inadequate term for hypoxic-ischemic encephalopathy, *Ann Neurol* 72(2):156–166, 2012.

260. Volpe JR: *Neurology of the newborn*, ed 5, Philadelphia, 2008, Saunders/Elsevier.

261. Walden M: Pain in the newborn and infant. In Kenner C, Lott JW, editors: *Comprehensive neonatal care*, Philadelphia, 2007, Saunders/Elsevier, pp 360–369.

262. Walsh MC, Szefler SS, Davis J, et al.: Summary proceedings from the bronchopulmonary dysplasia group, *Pediatrics* 117:S52–S56, 2006.

263. Wang CJ, McGlynn EA, Brook RH: Quality-of-care indicators for the neurodevelopmental follow-up of very low birth weight children: results of an expert panel process, *Pediatrics* 117(6):2080–2092, 2006.

264. Wang L, He JL, Zhang XH: The efficacy of massage on preterm infants: a meta-analysis, *Am J Perinatol* 30(9):731–738, 2013.

265. Ward-Larson C, Horn RA, Gosnell F: The efficacy of facilitated tucking for relieving procedural pain of endotracheal suctioning in very low birthweight infants, *Am J Matern Child Nurs* 29:151–156, 2004.

266. Watchko JF: Identification of neonates at risk for hazardous hyperbilirubinemia: emerging clinical insights, *Pediatr Clin North Am* 56:671–687, 2009.

267. Widmayer S, Field T: Effects of Brazelton demonstration on early interaction of preterm infants and their teenage mothers, *Infant Behav Dev* 3:79–89, 1980.

268. Wiedemann JR, Saugstad AM, Barnes-Powell L, Duran K: Meconium aspiration syndrome, *Neonatal Netw* 27:81–87, 2008.

269. Williamson D, Abe K, Bean C, et al.: Current research in preterm birth, *J Women Health* 17:1545–1549, 2008.

270. Wilson-Costello D, Friedman H, Minich N, et al.: Improved survival rates with increased neurodevelopmental disability for extremely low birth weight infants in the 1990s, *Pediatrics* 115:997–1003, 2005.

271. Wilson-Costello D, Friedman H, Minich N, et al.: Improved neurodevelopmental outcomes for extremely low birth weight infants in 2000-2002, *Pediatrics* 119:37–45, 2007.

272. Wiswell TE, Graziani LJ: Intracranial hemorrhage and white matter injury in preterm infants. In Spitzer AR, editor: *Intensive care of the fetus and neonate*, ed 2, St. Louis, 2005, Mosby (chapter 54).

273. Wolff PH: Observations on human infants, *Psychoanal Med* 221:110–118, 1959.

274. World Health Organization: *International Classification of Functioning, Disability and Health*, Geneva, 2001, WHO.

275. Xu H, Wei S, Fraser WD: Obstetric approaches to the prevention of meconium aspiration syndrome, *J Perinatol* 28:S14–S18, 2008.

276. Yeh TF, Lin HC, Chang CH, et al.: Early intratracheal instillation of budesonide using surfactant as a vehicle to prevent chronic lung disease in preterm infants: a pilot study, *Pediatrics* 121:e1310–e1318, 2008.

277. Yost CC, Soll RF: Early versus delayed selective surfactant treatment for neonatal respiratory distress syndrome, *Cochrane Database Syst Rev* 2, 2000. CD001456.

SUGGESTED READINGS

Als H: A synactive model of neonatal behavioral organization: framework for the assessment of neurobehavioral development in the premature infant and for support of infants and parents in the neonatal intensive care environment, *Phys Occupat Ther Pediatr* 6(3/4):3–54, 1986.

Blanchard Y, Øberg GK: Physical therapy with newborns: applying concepts of phenomenology and synactive theory to guide interventions, *Physiother Theory Pract* 31(6):377–381, 2015.

Brazelton TB, Nugent JK: The Neonatal Behavioral Assessment Scale. *Clin Dev Med 190*, ed 4, London, 2011, MacKeith Press.

Campbell SK: Use of care paths to improve patient management, *Phys Occupat Ther Pediatr* 33:27–38, 2013.

Spittle AJ, Orton P, Anderson R, et al.: Early developmental intervention programmes post-hospital discharge to prevent motor and cognitive impairments in preterm infants, *Cochrane Database Syst Rev* 12, 2012. CD005495.

Sweeney JK, Heriza HB, Blanchard Y, Dusing S: Neonatal physical therapy. Part II: practice frameworks and evidence-based practice guidelines, *Pediatr Phys Ther* 2(1):2–16, 2010.

Sweeney JK, Heriza HB, Blanchard Y: Neonatal physical therapy: clinical competencies and NICU clinical training models. Part I, *Pediatr Phys Ther* 21(4):296–307, 2009.

Symington A, Pinelli J: Developmental care for promoting development and preventing morbidity in preterm infants, *Cochrane Database Syst Rev* 2, 2006. CD001814.

Volpe JR: *Neurology of the newborn*, ed 5, Philadelphia, 2008, Saunders/Elsevier.

30

Infants, Toddlers, and Their Families: Early Intervention Services Under IDEA

Lisa Chiarello, Tricia Catalino

This chapter focuses on early intervention services in home and community settings under the US Individuals with Disabilities Education Improvement Act (IDEA) of 2004.[107] Part C of the IDEA authorizes federal assistance to states to implement a system of early intervention services for eligible infants and toddlers, from birth to 3 years of age, and their families. The law mandates family-centered services in natural environments to promote the child's development and participation in daily activities and routines. A relationship-based approach to early intervention in which the relationships among family members, providers, and administrators are valued as the foundation to effective care is recognized as best practice.[57] The organizational system climate for Part C can be challenging as the federal and state governments strive to fiscally support this program. Providing services in early intervention is complex but very rewarding as therapists advocate for quality care for young children and their families. Therapists practicing in early intervention truly have the opportunity to integrate the science and art of physical therapy. This chapter critiques theory, policy, and methods of service delivery and analyzes research. The role of the physical therapist in this service system is discussed, with an emphasis on both unique contributions and the team processes needed for collaborative decision making and service provision. This chapter describes the components of our conceptual framework for physical therapy practice in early intervention presented in Fig. 30.1. These components include the factors (policy, philosophy, and people) and processes (evidence-informed service delivery, family engagement, team collaboration, and service integration) that influence child and family outcomes in early intervention.

BACKGROUND INFORMATION

Early intervention is a multifaceted process to support infants and toddlers with developmental delay and disability and their families. Early intervention is predicated on the notion that early childhood is a sensitive period in development and families have the primary role of nurturing and providing early learning experiences for their children. The concept of sensitive period in early childhood refers to the significant influence the environment and experiences have on brain maturation during this time.[100] Shonkoff and Meisels[130] defined early intervention as follows:

> Multidisciplinary services … to promote child health and well-being, enhance emerging competencies, minimize developmental delays, remediate existing or emerging disabilities, prevent functional deterioration, and promote adaptive parenting

and overall family functioning. These goals are accomplished by providing individualized developmental, educational, and therapeutic services for children in conjunction with mutually planned support for their families. (pp xvii–xviii)

This definition embraces the concepts of prevention, remediation, experiential learning, individuality, and family centeredness and is consistent with the definition of early intervention in IDEA. IDEA defines early intervention as follows:

> Developmental services that are provided under public supervision, are provided at no cost except where federal or state law provides for a system of payments by families, including a schedule of sliding fees, and are designed to meet the developmental needs of an infant or toddler with disability in any one or more of the following areas: physical development; cognitive development; communication development; social or emotional development; or adaptive development.

In addition, IDEA stipulates that services are selected in collaboration with the parent. This definition emphasizes the service delivery aspect of early intervention; the primary premises are that services must be developmental and involve parent collaboration. Hebbeler and colleagues[70] have discussed that the Part C early intervention program is diverse in that it serves as both an intervention program to ameliorate the effects of disability for children with moderate to severe involvement and as a prevention and intervention program for children at risk for delay or with mild involvement who will attain skills comparable with their peers.

To be effective in early intervention, physical therapists must embrace responsibilities that go beyond technical knowledge and skill. Early intervention providers are required to partner with families and other providers, deliver services in multiple environments, comply with federal and state policy, and provide interventions informed by current evidence and principles of best practice. In addition to expertise in motor development, adaptive function, and self-care, it is essential that physical therapists have practical knowledge of family ecology and children's social, emotional, cognitive, communication, and language development.[89,131]

IDEA PART C: INFANTS AND TODDLERS

The Education of the Handicapped Act Amendments of 1986[108] provided for family-centered services for infants and toddlers from birth to 3 years of age. This law was subsequently reauthorized and amended as Part C of the Individuals with Disabilities

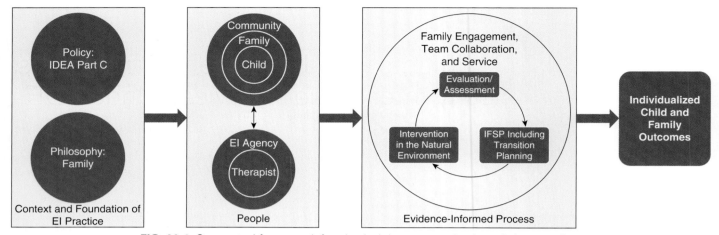

FIG. 30.1 Conceptual framework for physical therapy practice in early intervention.

Education Act Amendment (IDEA) of 1997[106] and Individuals with Disabilities Education Improvement Act (IDEIA) of 2004,[107] commonly referred to as IDEA. Part C mandates early intervention services based on the following declaration:

[That] Congress finds that there is an urgent and substantial need (1) to enhance the development of infants and toddlers with disabilities and to minimize their potential for developmental delay, and to recognize the significant brain development that occurs during a child's first 3 years of life; (2) to reduce the educational costs to our society, including our Nation's schools, by minimizing the need for special education and related services after infants and toddlers with disabilities reach school age; (3) to maximize the potential for their independently living in society; (4) to enhance the capacity of families to meet the special needs of their infants and toddlers with disabilities; and (5) to enhance the capacity of state and local agencies and service providers to identify, evaluate, and meet the needs of all children, particularly minority, low-income, inner-city, and rural children and infants and toddlers in foster care. (IDEIA, Part C, Sec. 631)

The legislation details the conditions that a state must meet in order to receive federal funding. In addition, Part C clearly articulates particular philosophies of care related to individualized family care, coordination of services, and services in natural environments.

Part C stipulates that early intervention services are designed to meet the developmental needs of an infant or toddler with a developmental delay or disability (or diagnosed physical or mental condition with high probability of resulting in developmental delay) in any one or more of the following areas: physical development, cognitive development, communication development, social or emotional development, and adaptive development. Each state has its own definition of developmental delay, and thus eligibility for early intervention varies from state to state.[70] In Alabama, children have to demonstrate a developmental delay of 25% in one of five areas; in the District of Columbia, children have to demonstrate a delay of 25% in two areas; and in Arizona, children have to demonstrate a delay of 50% in one area. The list of early intervention services identified in the legislation is provided in Box 30.1. Services are to be

> **BOX 30.1   Early Intervention Services Included in the Individuals With Disabilities Education Improvement Act**
>
> - Family training, counseling, home visits
> - Special instruction
> - Speech-language pathology and audiology services and sign language and cued language services
> - Occupational therapy
> - Physical therapy
> - Psychological services
> - Service coordination
> - Medical services only for diagnostic or evaluation purposes
> - Early identification, screening, and assessment services
> - Health services necessary to enable the infant or toddler to benefit from the other early intervention services
> - Social work services
> - Vision services
> - Assistive technology devices and services
> - Transportation and related costs necessary to receive early intervention services

provided by qualified personnel based on state licensing or certification requirements. Physical therapists are included under qualified personnel.

The components of service delivery identified in Part C are included in Box 30.2. The five major components are as follows:
- A public awareness program
- A central directory of information
- A comprehensive child find system
- Comprehensive evaluations and assessments
- An individualized family service plan (IFSP)

To receive funding under Part C, the states must comply with all provisions as detailed in IDEA. The law also states general guidelines on when, how, and where evaluations/assessments, IFSPs, and interventions must be planned, conducted, and implemented. For detailed information, therapists are advised to read the legislation and regulations, which can be accessed through several websites. The document *Providing Physical Therapy Services Under Parts B & C of the Individuals with Disabilities Education Act* (2nd edition) published by the American Physical Therapy Association[95] elaborates on the federal law and the role of the physical therapist.

FAMILY-CENTERED CARE

Although family-centered care is considered best practice in providing health care to all children, in early intervention this philosophy of care is essential because families are considered a direct recipient of services. Family-centered care is based on the premise that the family plays the central role in the life of a child. Parent self-efficacy beliefs have a direct influence on child development, adaptive behavior, and psychological well-being.[49,138] The underlying tenet is that optimal family functioning promotes optimal child development.[131] Family-centered care is a process that respects the rights and roles of family members while providing intervention to achieve child and family outcomes that promote well-being and quality of life. Family-centered care is a comprehensive approach to service that when individualized may include aspects of both child- and parent-centered approaches as therapists support the child's development and function and endeavor to address the concerns of the family.

Several definitions of family-centered intervention have been presented.[3,50,82,87,94] The common threads are that it is a philosophy and approach to service delivery based on core beliefs of (1) respect for children and families, (2) appreciation of the family's impact on the child's well-being, and (3) family-professional collaboration. The definition by Law et al.[87] is widely used:

> Family-centered service is made up of a set of values, attitudes, and approaches to services for children with special needs and their families. Family-centered service recognizes that each family is unique; that the family is the constant in the child's life; and that they are the experts on the child's abilities and needs. The family works with service providers to make informed decisions about the services and supports the child and family receive. In family-centered service, the strengths and needs of all family members are considered.

Perhaps the most important differences between family-centered and professional-driven approaches are that the professional's role is partly defined by the resources and priorities of each child and family and that service decisions are not based solely on the professional's knowledge and expertise. Initially, the less-defined role may be unsettling to professionals, whose education and expertise are biased toward addressing a child's impairments and activity limitations. In a review of early intervention approaches internationally, Dirks and Hadders-Algra[38] stated, "a major change in attitude and behavior is needed to implement family-centered services."

The key elements of family-centered care, proposed by the American Academy of Pediatrics and the Institute for Patient and Family-Centered Care,[3] influence provision of services to families and children. The elements are as follows:

- Listening to and respecting each child and family, honoring diversity, and including family preferences in service delivery.
- Having flexible organization systems to offer family choices and providing services that are responsive to family needs, beliefs, and cultural values.
- Sharing complete and honest information in useful ways so family can participate in decision making and care.
- Ensuring formal and informal support to the child and family.
- Promoting family-professional collaboration at all levels of health care.
- Appreciating and fostering strengths and building family capacity.

These elements appear to be common sense and often conceal the complexity of application to practice. Service providers may be inclined to regard family-centered care as not being different from what they have always practiced. Implicit in the family-centered approach is that the role of the family extends beyond involvement in the care of the child, to being beneficiaries of interventions.[48] The informational, educational, and health needs of the family are addressed in concert with those of the child based on the premise that supporting the family promotes the child's development.

Family-centered care is founded on a parent–professional partnership. Dunst, Trivette, and Snyder defined parent–professional partnership as follows[51]:

> Parents and other family members working together with professionals in pursuit of a common goal where the relationship between the family and the professional is based on shared decision-making and responsibility and mutual trust and respect.

Practitioners provide information and support to enable the family to make decisions and to enhance family competency in caring for and nurturing the child.[48] Information sharing is reciprocal and acknowledges that families know their children the best.[21] Families share valuable information about the child and family, priorities and concerns, and expectations of early intervention. Practitioners inquire about the child's health, development, daily activities and routines, and family resources and supports. Practitioners are responsive to the family's need for information about their child, community resources, and preparation for the future to enable families to effectively advocate for their children. As an example, therapists provide families information regarding their child's diagnosis and prognosis with honesty and collaborate to identify opportunities and supports so children can participate in life to their fullest potential. Dunst and Dempsey have found that a positive parent–professional partnership is related to parent's self-efficacy and sense of control.[46]

Parents value providers who are caring individuals with positive interpersonal and communication skills with families and children.[93] To provide family-centered care, physical therapists are encouraged to expand their knowledge to include understanding of the multidimensional aspects of the family including cultural values, interests, child-rearing practices, resources, and supports. It is important for the early intervention team to address the basic needs of the family.[127] Knowledge of the family is critical to avoid the concerns that with family-centered care professionals may be expecting too much from families, thus becoming a source of stress, as opposed to support.[88,93]

Effectiveness of Family-Centered Care

Several reviews support the effectiveness of family-centered care.[37,47,49,50,60,62,85] Similar to other areas of research in early intervention, a thorough synthesis of findings is challenging because studies vary in how family-centered care is defined, characteristics of families and children, service settings, and outcomes measured. For children with developmental disabilities, as noted in these reviews, family outcomes associated with family-centered care include knowledge of child development, perception of children's behavior, participation in intervention programs, satisfaction with services, developmental appropriateness of the home environment, parenting behaviors and competence, the parent–child relationship, enjoyment of parenting, family functioning, self-efficacy, sense of control, and empowerment. Family-centered care has also been associated with children's health, development, social-emotional competence, and functioning. Elements of family-centered care associated with these positive outcomes include communication, information sharing, collaboration, fostering family involvement and choice, building on strengths, and providing support. Despite the evidence, the complex and multidimensional nature of family-centered care and early intervention services under Part C of IDEA make it difficult to translate research into practice.

A meaningful understanding of the effectiveness of family-centered behaviors requires consideration of the characteristics of the child, family, therapists, intervention strategies, and service delivery systems.[43] Research on processes of family-centered care indicates that outcomes for children and families are mediated by parent self-efficacy.[37,47,49,138] Provider behaviors fostering parent involvement and choice are more strongly associated with positive outcomes than behaviors related to fostering the parent–professional relationship.[50]

Parent Self-Efficacy, Family Engagement, and Participation

As parental self-efficacy is a key mediator of family-centered care, it is important for services to focus on optimizing parents' beliefs that they (1) can access resources and supports and (2) have control and ability to take actions to ensure the outcomes they want for their family. We recommend that therapists have conversations with families to discuss whether family priorities and concerns are being addressed. It is also important to understand if families feel competent in nurturing their children's development. These conversations will enable therapists to learn how best to support the family, build on family strengths, enhance family competence,[48] and foster collaborative processes.

The family-centered approach, in addition to expanding the role of service providers, expands the role of the family, particularly parents. This might include learning and using skills related to advocacy, negotiation, collaboration, and intervention strategies. Because of the fragmented child health system, parents have to coordinate not only developmental services but

also services for primary health care, public health programs, specialized medical care, and behavioral health services. Some families may not be receiving the services they need and require assistance in accessing and utilizing services and community resources. Families experiencing difficulty in adapting to caring for a child with special needs may need more formal support from the early intervention team.[16]

We believe that it is important for families to be engaged in the early intervention process. King and Chiarello[82] have proposed that family engagement may also be a mediator between family-centered practices and outcomes. Family engagement refers to their active investment and involvement as a partner in the intervention.[83] Engagement reflects a family receptiveness and commitment to the process and their confidence with participating in the intervention. Engagement is a complex and dynamic process that involves a relationship between the family and the service providers. Engagement can vary over time and may be influenced by characteristics of the family, providers, intervention approach, and system of care. Three dimensions of engagement are affective, cognitive, and behavioral investment.[83] *Affective engagement* refers to emotional involvement including having a hopeful attitude and trusting in the process and provider. *Cognitive engagement* entails a commitment to the goals, a belief in the relevance of the intervention, and a willingness to invest time and effort. *Behavioral engagement* signifies confidence in being able and supported to participate in intervention tasks. "Client engagement requires a sharing of power and therapist skill in creating a therapeutic environment that is safe, open, and truly collaborative."[82]

As supported by research,[48,50,60,62] we encourage practitioners to provide opportunities for and support family involvement and choice in the early intervention process. The extent and type of participation will vary depending on factors unique to each family. The premise is that families have a right and responsibility to select the way in which they will be involved in early intervention services. Family involvement is viewed as a continuum rather than a hierarchy and may change over time. At times some parents may be minimally involved, either because of unfamiliarity with the service delivery system or because of the difficulty balancing work and family commitments. A family with a demanding work schedule may give permission for professionals to provide early intervention at a child's child care center but not at home. Parents may view the child care provider as an important person in the child's life who is helping support the family's goals for the child. It is important for practitioners to be flexible and responsive to family choices. Families may actively seek information from the professional team regarding the child's diagnosis, prognosis, and ideas on how to enhance their children's development. Collaboration and partnership are achieved when a family not only seeks information from professionals but also offers information and actively participates in the development and implementation of service plans. Service coordination and advocacy represent levels of family participation that involve management of services provided and educating others about children with special needs. Ongoing communication between the family and practitioners and revisiting family needs and participation are integral to family-centered services. Box 30.3 highlights reflections and considerations for engaging families in the intervention process. It is important for physical therapists to invite parents to participate, identify and discuss barriers, and provide supports to enable their participation.

BOX 30.3   Engaging Families: Reflections and Considerations

Therapists providing services in early intervention may experience a situation in which a parent watches TV, talks on the phone, or does a chore during the session. Instead of making a judgment about the parent, we encourage therapists to reflect on the situation and consider how they can respond.

Reflections

The parent may not understand or have a different perspective regarding family involvement.
The parent may need respite: time alone or to accomplish a task.

Considerations

- Share with the family the philosophy of early intervention and how much their role is valued.
- Discuss the various ways they can be involved during a session.
- Ask what they would like the focus of the session to be.
- Share how we can provide support to enable them to be involved.
- Be patient, share highlights of the session, find moments during the session to connect with the family, and continue to invite families to be involved.
- Incorporate watching TV and chores into the session activities and together develop strategies on opportunities to interact with the child or possibilities to have the child involved in self-play.
- Agree on a balance so the family has some time to rest or accomplish a task and some time to be involved in the session activities.
- Discuss family's interest in or need for respite resources.

EFFECTIVENESS OF EARLY INTERVENTION

Research on the benefits of early intervention are equivocal and vary across children and families.[25,61,65] This reflects the complex and multifaceted nature of early intervention services. Methodologic challenges have contributed to limited research and ability to generalize findings across children and settings. Research has focused on interventions for infants and toddlers experiencing delays who are at environmental or biologic risk. Interventions tend to be broad in scope with little detail on specific strategies and procedures, and the potential range of child and family outcomes has not been explored. Research is recommended to help therapists understand the complex influences, both direct and indirect, of child, family, environment, and service factors on meaningful outcomes for children and families.[17] Consequently, the knowledge of what interventions are most effective based on child and family characteristics remains unclear.

Physical therapists will find it particularly challenging to integrate and apply research findings on early intervention for three reasons: (1) a large proportion of the literature and research comes from the fields of medicine, psychology, sociology, and early childhood education and concentrates on health, cognition, and behavior; (2) the role of physical therapy as part of an early intervention team has seldom been addressed; and (3) well-designed studies with large samples, such as the Infant Health and Development Program,[18,110] have targeted "at-risk populations" of infants at risk for global developmental delay, speech and language disorders, or social-emotional maladjustment.[25,61]

Outcomes for children and families participating in Part C early intervention are generally positive. The National Early Intervention Longitudinal Study[69] found that infants and toddlers participating in Part C increased motor, social, and cognitive functioning and families felt competent in caring for their children's basic needs and felt they knew how to help their children learn and develop.[13] Data collected by states on child outcomes showed that 66% to 71% of the children receiving Part C early intervention had greater than expected growth in social relationships, use of knowledge and skills, and taking action to meet needs, and 59% to 61% exited early intervention functioning within age expectations in these areas.[56] The states also reported that 87% to 90% of families receiving Part C services know their rights, effectively communicate their children's needs, and help their children develop and learn.[55] A positive relationship among parents' perceptions of Part C services, state-collected data on family outcomes, and enhanced family quality of life has been reported.[58] Although results are encouraging, there are concerns about the quality of the data, as states continue to improve the reliability and validity of their data collection and reporting.

Empirical support for early intervention for children with physical disabilities and their families is inconclusive. Children with motor impairment have shown fewer functional gains compared to children with delays in other areas.[68] Findings for children with disabilities indicate that severity, not the type of physical disability, is a strong predictor of change; children with mild disabilities showed greater gains than children with severe disabilities, regardless of the intensity of services.[68] Norm-referenced developmental assessments are not responsive to changes that children with severe physical disabilities are capable of achieving.[99] Reviews and meta-analyses on the effectiveness of early intervention practices on motor outcomes include studies that are not specific to Part C,[20,65,98,102] define early intervention broadly to include interventions that take place in the neonatal intensive care unit or other program specific settings,[102] only include infants at risk for cerebral palsy,[65,98] or the interventions were heterogeneous making it difficult to generalize results.[20,65,98,102]

As an example, a systematic review of the effects of early intervention on motor development included studies with children both at high risk for or with developmental motor disorder.[20] This review did consider separate effects of interventions provided in the neonatal intensive care unit from interventions conducted later in infancy and early childhood. Among studies conducted following discharge from the neonatal intensive care unit, positive effects on motor development were found for what was categorized as specific or general developmental programs, whereas no support was found for interventions categorized as neurodevelopmental treatment or Vojta. It is challenging to translate this evidence to practice because of the variety of interventions considered as specific or general developmental programs, ranging from treadmill training to enhancing parent–infant interaction, and differences in method of service delivery including who provided the intervention. There is limited evidence on the effects of early intervention on adaptive function, participation in family and community life, ease of caregiving, and family functioning.

Keeping abreast of current research related to amounts and types of interventions for young children is important as therapists and families make decisions about early intervention services. However, evidence on the effects of specific procedural interventions and the amount of physical therapy services is hard to interpret and apply to early intervention. In early intervention, the team makes decisions regarding types and amount of services based on child and family needs. Studies on amount of services do not account for the confounding effects of practice and learning supported by family and other caregivers throughout a child's daily life. Research is needed to examine the effects of various schedules of service delivery in early intervention such as scheduling more frequent visits during team-identified periods when children are on the verge of learning a new activity or less frequent visits when families feel comfortable and confident implementing successful strategies with their children during daily routines.

FOREGROUND INFORMATION

PROVIDING EARLY INTERVENTION SERVICES

Role of the Physical Therapist

Part C of IDEA and the American Physical Therapy Association[122] support the role of physical therapists in early intervention. Acquisition of motor skills is a major part of early development, and young children are sensorimotor learners.[89] Physical therapists, as members of the early intervention team, provide interventions to promote children's activity and participation, including motor learning, environmental adaptations, assistive technology, family support, and education. As health care professionals recognized as movement specialists,[5] physical therapists have expertise in developing body functions and structures of the neuromuscular, musculoskeletal, cardiopulmonary, and integumentary systems and how impairments in these systems impact early development. This enables therapists to provide individualized recommendations for activities, activity adaptations, and environmental modifications that not only promote motor development but also enable exploration, social interactions, and play. Physical therapists also have a role in health promotion and prevention,[124] including discerning risk factors for secondary health complications (e.g., limitation in physical activity and obesity), fostering safety in the environment (e.g., use of outlet protectors, baby gates), and identifying signs and symptoms that indicate the need for referral to another health care professional[5] (e.g., lethargy, weight loss, persistent fever).

Even though physical therapists have a unique role in early intervention,[33] there is an overlap of expertise among service providers. Therefore communication and coordination among the team are crucial. Providers are encouraged to openly discuss the overlap in their areas of expertise and respect the contributions of all service providers. Physical therapists may experience overlap in roles and responsibilities with occupational therapy colleagues in the areas of motor and adaptive development as well as assistive technology. It is also important for physical therapists to collaborate with early childhood education specialists who have broad knowledge of early development and expertise in cognitive and social development.[39] Decisions on how each member of the team will contribute to the plan of care for a child and family are made based on who can best support the identified outcomes.

It is particularly valuable to consider the role of the physical therapist from the consumer perspective. Thirty-six parents of children with disabilities participated in focus groups to explore their perceptions of competent physical, occupational, and speech therapists in early intervention.[30,97] Parents discussed the skills and attributes of therapists that were important to them. The discussions were audiotaped, transcribed, and

analyzed for themes. The nine themes that emerged are described in Box 30.4. The themes reflect interactions among administration issues, expectations for "best practice," and the importance of the family–therapist relationship.

Elements of Early Intervention

This section presents the major elements of intervention included in Part C of IDEA. The elements are team collaboration, evaluation and assessment, the IFSP, providing services in natural environments, and transition. These elements are consistent with the recommendations for children from birth to 5 years of age with or at risk of developmental delays or disabilities developed by the Division for Early Childhood (DEC) of the Council for Exceptional Children.[40] It is through these elements of service provision that therapists implement family-centered care.

Team Collaboration

Team collaboration is the process of forming partnerships among family members, service providers, supervisors, administrators, systems of care, and the community with the common goal of enhancing the child's development and supporting the family.[104] "It is the sum of these interrelated relationships that create a web of support for children, their families, and those who support them."[57] At the systems level, federal legislation mandates interagency coordination to provide families with efficient and effective mechanisms to access and utilize services from multiple agencies.[107] The need for coordination of services among health care professionals, early intervention providers, and families has long been recognized.[22] The American Academy of Pediatrics advocates for collaboration between children's primary care and Part C early intervention services.[2] Care coordination is based on the assumption that integrated and coordinated services will result in improved outcomes, reduced costs, and more positive service experiences for children and families.[4] Part C of the IDEA

BOX 30.4   Families' Perspective of Desired Competencies of Early Intervention Therapists

Early intervention knowledge. Therapists have previously acquired or have access to general and disability-specific information relevant to family needs or requests related to their child.

Team coordination. Therapists actively support the coordination and planning among team members, including the family.

Family as part of therapy visits. Therapists are able to actively engage and include family members in therapy sessions.

Information sharing between the therapist and the family. Therapists share and support the use of therapy techniques throughout child and family daily routines and activities.

Commitment of the therapist. Therapists view their role as potentially impacting families and children, not simply as a job.

Flexibility of scheduling. Therapists are willing to juggle their schedules in order to work with families and children.

Respect for individual families. Therapists have respect for families in that they are sensitive to the family context and changes over time, use parent-friendly language, use active listening, and provide families with positive feedback.

Appreciation for the child. Therapists demonstrate appreciation for the child by using a strength-based intervention approach and have the ability to be "in tune" with the child.

Therapist as a person. Therapists possess a personality reflective of them as honest, patient, personable, creative, and humorous.

delineates that service coordinators are responsible for the implementation of the IFSP, coordination with other agencies, and assisting families with access to services.[107] Research supports the need for team collaboration and service coordination; interpersonal characteristics and organizational factors are interrelated and serve as either facilitators or barriers to team collaboration and service integration.[21,28,67,73,103]

Characteristics of team collaboration described by Briggs[23] and supported by the recommendations for early intervention by the Division for Early Childhood,[40] synthesis of literature on service integration,[103] and qualitative research[21] are summarized in Box 30.5. Team members demonstrate respect for each other by valuing cultural differences and acknowledging the expertise and competence each person brings to the team. Positive interpersonal relationships and clear behavioral expectations are important for effective collaboration. Opportunities for team members to share information and willingness to adapt to individual situations are viewed as important for collaboration.

Communication is an essential skill for effective collaboration.[111] Effective communication is the process of sharing knowledge and information among team members to facilitate coordination of services. Each member must be committed to keeping the team informed of important issues. Communication begins with listening, an essential process to understand and appreciate everyone's perspective, foster relationships,[81] and support parents' engagement and self-efficacy. It is important for practitioners to "listen mindfully, sensitively and with intent—to be authentic and present in the moment with the client."[81] King and colleagues[81] distinguished four types of listening skills: (1) receptive listening to attend to clients and be open to what they are saying, (2) exploratory listening to have a dialogue and facilitate deeper communication, (3) consensus-oriented listening to arrive at a shared understanding, and (4) action-oriented listening to establish decisions for a plan of care. To avoid miscommunication, it is helpful to restate what was heard to demonstrate understanding[81] and to ask for clarification or an example when information is not clear. Prompt follow-through communicates investment in the team. At the same time, being patient reflects an understanding of the group process. When discussing issues, it is essential to provide suggestions and options, a solution-focused versus problem-focused approach. A sense of humor helps to bring humanism to day-to-day team struggles.

BOX 30.5 Characteristics of Effective Teams and Collaborative Relationships

- In the developmental phase, team members take time to learn about each other.
- Members demonstrate honesty, trust, responsiveness, and mutual respect for each other.
- Membership is stable and all members demonstrate commitment and leadership.
- All share a common philosophy and goal.
- The group has a structure for interaction and organization.
- Open communication, exchange of information, meaningful discussion, and negotiation are practiced.
- Equal participation is encouraged, and partners contribute specific skills and strengths.
- Plans, priorities, and decisions are made together.
- Action plans with appropriate authority are used for implementing team recommendations.

A family-centered organizational culture enables the development and implementation of organizational structures and processes that support team collaboration.[21,67,73,103] The following strategies and practices are recommended to enhance collaboration[2,4,21,28,67,73,103]:
- Communication, teamwork, and advocacy training for families and providers
- Education on systems of care including the services and resources available
- Referral forms that establish ongoing collaboration including sharing of medical and development records
- Mechanisms and time for regular communication among team members including interagency systems
- Comprehensive policies, funding, and resources for care coordination services
- Documentation on the IFSP of all programs and services across the community and systems of care
- Determination of the service coordinator based on an appropriate match to support family's priorities and concerns
- Development of collaboration goals and action plans
- Maintenance of a list of services and resources for families
- Service options shared with families
- Flexibility in scheduling and staffing
- Options for service format including co-visits by team members, group and individual therapy, and center-based programs

At the system level, states lack policy and funding to support service coordination.[4,67,103,127] In regard to collaboration between medical and early intervention providers, family members and practitioners noted limited communication, lack of trust and understanding, and challenges in resolving differences in practice philosophies.[73] Families of young children with complex medical and developmental conditions expend considerable time and resources to coordinate care and meet their children's health, education, and development needs.[73] At the agency level, large caseloads, lack of consistency of staff, and problems with contracted employees have been cited as interfering with collaboration.[103] Although struggles may exist for "turf," power, or authority, more commonly problems appear to arise from a workplace structure that isolates service providers or one that does not have dedicated time or procedures in place for collaboration.[71,73,103] Providing services in natural environments requires time for travel and reduces direct contact among team members. It is important for administrators to support procedures and mechanisms for communication such as team meetings at a community-based center, electronic sharing of information, and time in the workload for phone calls and consultation.

Progressive leadership and administration at all levels are essential to discover solutions to barriers and to support practices that enable team collaboration.[40,41,57,86] Leaders establish interagency partnerships to foster service coordination.[40] Administrators need to set a tone that values and supports a deep level of teamwork, communication, and problem solving. Organizations need to secure funding to support the otherwise nonreimbursed time required for essential functions such as teamwork, planning, training, and supervision.[57] Despite a federal mandate for service coordination in early intervention and advances in the medical home, "a collective paradigm shift at the provider, agency, interagency, government and societal levels is necessary to provide coordinated care to families."[82] Partnership among policy makers, administrators, practitioners, and families is critical to influence system reform (e.g., funding, policies, and interdisciplinary education). Therapists

---

BOX 30.6 Addressing the Challenges in the Primary Service Provider Approach: Advocating for Meaningful Decision Making

The following is an example of how the team can advocate for individualized care when practicing the primary service provider approach.

Megan is a physical therapist working for a county early intervention system that uses the primary service provider approach. She values the approach and has found it beneficial for many children and families. Currently she serves as the primary service provider for Declan, a two-year-old boy with cerebral palsy, Gross Motor Functional Classification System level IV, and is collaborating with the family on adapting a powered-mobility ride toy. Megan is feeling overwhelmed in being able to support the child's communication and to prepare him for preschool. Her supervisor has approved a 1-hour consultation visit with the speech therapist but has indicated that only 1 hour is permitted for this 6-month period. During the visit, Megan, the family, and the speech therapist assess Declan's current receptive and expressive communication function and discuss strategies for a communication system. Megan is appreciative of the co-visit but does not feel that she has the competency to set up the system and teach Declan and his family without additional support. Megan, the speech therapist, and the parents hold an additional online audio-conference at night, on the therapists' personal time, to share and discuss options:

- The speech therapist has documented the consultation visit, which includes a recommendation for additional services by the speech therapist.
- Megan as the primary service provider will write a formal request for additional service visits by the speech therapist and a full team meeting. She notes that the full team meeting is needed to collaborate on this new strategy for communication as well as to receive further guidance from the early childhood education specialist and the occupational

therapist regarding supporting the IFSP outcome related to preparation for preschool.

- The family will investigate their medical insurance coverage for durable medical equipment and outpatient services.
- The speech therapist will contact the regional children's hospital to gather information on the augmentative communication clinic and outpatient services.
- The team will discuss the possibility of switching the primary service provider to the speech therapist in 3 months at the next IFSP review meeting. This 3-month period will provide Megan the opportunity to make sure that Declan and the family are confident with using the powered mobility ride toy.

Reflection on the primary service provider approach in action: Implementation of the primary service provider approach varies by state and may not encompass all of the teaming strategies explained by Rush and Shelden.[116] For example, in this vignette Megan used her personal time to communicate and coordinate with the team and family. In some states this teaming time is reimbursed, as it is essential to the approach and to carry out the strategies outlined in the IFSP. Another example that varies by state is the option to switch the primary service provider depending on the needs of the child and family. Therapists who work in states using the primary service provider approach are encouraged to advocate for the time and resources needed to implement the approach effectively. The American Physical Therapy Association Section on Pediatrics created a Fact Sheet that addresses common questions on the primary service provider approach and can be accessed on the section's website.[128]

---

are encouraged to embrace the interpersonal facilitators of team collaboration, advocate for implementation of system strategies, and participate in the leadership process[40,86] to enable coordinated care to become a reality.

Various approaches to team interaction exist in early intervention. In an *interdisciplinary approach*, team collaboration is necessary because multiple team members with various areas of expertise work together with the family to support one set of outcomes. However, a framework for team collaboration, specifically intensive team interactions, is an essential feature of the *transdisciplinary* approach to service delivery.[84,125] The transdisciplinary approach involves one primary service provider who implements the IFSP with the family with consultation from other team members. An advantage of the transdisciplinary approach is that the family and child interact primarily with one service provider but do have access to other team members as needed. The transdisciplinary approach is dependent on sharing of roles and crossing of disciplinary boundaries. Great variability exists in how this approach is actually implemented, and therapists may need to advocate for appropriate supports. If services are implemented without opportunities for consultation and supervision and do not include the option for additional team members to provide direct service when needed, then a child may not be receiving the services and strategies necessary to support the IFSP. Box 30.6 presents a vignette that highlights how a team can address challenges when implementing a primary service provider approach.

A specific approach to team interaction associated with the transdisciplinary care termed *coaching* has also been promoted in early intervention.[63,115,116] This approach advocates for family involvement in the intervention process, respects the family's strengths and expertise, and supports the family in expanding current abilities and learning new skills within their natural environments. Coaching is characterized as being

---

BOX 30.7 Supporting Families to Practice and Use Intervention Strategies

Therapists may find it helpful to share with families that trying a new intervention strategy was and at times still is not easy for them. Therapists can provide families with options on how they would best like to learn and practice the strategy:

- Would you like to try this together?
- What can I do to make it comfortable for you to try this strategy?
- Would you like me to try the strategy and you can first watch and ask me questions?
- Would you like to try the strategy and I can talk you through the steps?
- Would having a video of doing the strategy be helpful?
- Would you prefer to practice the strategy on your own this week?

Once a family has tried a strategy it is important to ask for feedback to ensure family members are confident using the strategy:

- What did you like best about trying the strategy?
- Do you feel comfortable using the strategy?
- Are there any parts of the strategy that are hard or difficult to do?
- What would make the strategy easier?
- Are there situations or circumstances when the strategy is easier or harder to use?

"consistent with adult learning, capacity building, non-directive, goal-oriented, solution focused, performance based, reflective, collaborative, context driven, and as hands on as it needs to be."[116] Rush and Shelden[116] synthesized the five critical processes: joint planning, observation, action, reflection, and feedback. After collaborative discussions and observations, the family and practitioner jointly select intervention strategies. The practitioner and family jointly interact with the child and practice the strategies together. Suggestions for asking families to practice strategies in ways that are family-centered and supportive are presented in Box 30.7. The family then implements the strategies throughout the child's daily routines. The practitioner follows up with the family to reflect on the strategies and whether they are having the intended effect. Collaboratively the practitioner and family determine whether modifications or changes are needed and, if the goal has been achieved, how to progress to the next step. During this process the practitioner may provide modeling, demonstration, and direct teaching as well as guidance and feedback when the family is practicing and mastering the intervention strategies.[63] This collaborative interactive process can be applied during all aspects of service delivery and can also be utilized during interactions with other team members.

Evaluation and Assessment

The IDEA addresses assessment of the child, family, and service needs. The IDEA specifies that assessment of the child is performed by qualified and trained personnel and includes review of the child's relevant medical records, observation of the child, informed opinion, and determination of the child's unique strengths and needs and functioning in five areas of development (physical, cognitive, communication, social or emotional, and adaptive). Comprehensive developmental tests and measures may be used for determining eligibility and documenting developmental progress; however, routines-based ecologic assessment of the child's functioning is also indicated to identify outcomes and guide interventions in natural environments.[8,10] The physical therapist synthesizes findings for motor development and adaptive function within the context of findings for all areas of development, social interactions, activities, and daily routines of the child and family. The assessment of the family includes a voluntary interview with the family to identify (1) their resources, priorities, and concerns and (2) the supports and services they need to strengthen their ability to meet their child's developmental needs.

Several key points on the evaluation and assessment process merit emphasis. Evaluation and assessment must be comprehensive and nondiscriminatory. A team approach supports a holistic view of the child. Information from multiple sources across various situations, including reports from families, is valued. Professional judgment of therapists and consensus decision making among parents and practitioners are important aspects of the evaluation and assessment process.[9] The team uses findings from child and family assessments to determine the child's initial and continued eligibility for early intervention. This determination cannot be made based on a single assessment procedure; however, medical records can be used to determine eligibility without additional assessment if they report information on the child's level of functioning in the five developmental areas. If a child is eligible for early intervention, the team evaluates the assessment information to determine the child's service needs.

Evaluation and assessment are to be provided in an individualized, strengths-based, and collaborative manner.[10,40] The purpose and process of the evaluation and assessment should be discussed in advance. Family input is requested in deciding *who* should attend, *what* activities and routines will be observed, *where* the evaluation or assessment should take place, and *when* the session will occur (date and time). Family members can take on many different roles during the evaluation and assessment. Some family members may elect to guide the process, interacting with their child in a variety of activities. Others may prefer to assist the therapist with activities. Another option for a family

member is to be a narrator, reflecting on the child's behaviors and providing commentary and elaboration to the other team members. Some families are comfortable with spontaneous exchange of ideas, and other families prefer to answer specific questions. At times, a family member may just want to observe and listen. Families can share photos, videos, and journals highlighting the child's performance in their daily life. At the end of the evaluation and assessment, it is important to ask the family to share their perspective on the process and whether the child's performance was representative of her or his current abilities.

To maximize the value of evaluation and assessment, consideration should be given to the information needed to make decisions on outcomes, the intervention plan, and how progress will be monitored and documented.[10] This process begins with the identification of child and family competencies that serve as a foundation for determining the child's readiness for learning new skills. In addition, an understanding of the family's culture and interests provides the framework for deciding on meaningful intervention strategies. This information is best gathered through the initial interview, ongoing conversation with the family, and systematic observation of the child and family during daily activities and routines.[10,77,78]

Family interview. An initial step in the process of evaluation and assessment is a family interview. The initial interview begins the process of developing a trusting relationship and partnership with the family and child.[15] The purpose of the interview is to learn from the family about the child's health, development, and personality; the child and family's daily routines and interests; the family's priorities and concerns; what resources and strategies are available to enhance the child's development; their perceptions about therapy; and their expectations of early intervention.[15,96,133] For some families, the interview process may be a new experience; therefore therapists encourage, support, and respect the various levels of involvement and value the information that families provide.[15] It is important for therapists to recognize and respect that families are being asked to share personal information.

An effective interview requires sufficient time and is characterized by the ability to have a conversation with the family, listen, acknowledge the child and family's strengths, expand the conversation with appropriate guiding questions, use friendly nonverbal communication, and demonstrate empathy.[15,96] A personable approach facilitates a comfortable environment, welcoming the family to share their thoughts. Inviting parents to share their story and use of open-ended questions fosters an informal, flexible approach that is acceptable to families.[15] This approach conveys to families that therapists are interested in learning and understanding the family's culture. For some families who have difficulty expressing themselves, it is important for therapists to provide guidance while being careful not to misrepresent the family's perspective.

Active listening is another key to effective interviewing and to establishing partnerships with families and collaboration on the IFSP. Active listening and acknowledging the family's concerns demonstrate respect and value for the family's priorities and help the therapist develop a deeper appreciation for the family's daily routines, opportunities for collaboration, how the family frames its resources, and the extent of the family's support network. Another effective interview strategy is the use of silence. There are times when silence is more helpful than questioning. Silence, with some nonverbal gesture of acceptance, may enable a family time to reflect and consider their response.

To support therapy in natural environments, a major component of the interview is gathering information on child and family daily routines in order to identify the context for intervention to promote children's participation in family and community life. Through conversations and open-ended questions, such as "tell me about your child" and "describe for me a typical day in your family," therapists gather information on family members' roles, interests, strengths, interactions, and daily experiences. Rosenbaum has advocated for a strengths-based approach that begins with asking families to share what they enjoy and are proud of regarding their child.[112] Therapists are encouraged to thoughtfully discuss with families their current routines related to play, self-care, and community outings. McWilliam and colleagues[96] emphasized the importance of identifying the needs of all family members and considering what the family would like to be able to do. Woods and Lindeman[144] discussed the importance of the interview being a reciprocal process where providers share information on the value of natural learning opportunities and families share information on daily activities and routines including child and family interests. The interview around daily routines is also an opportunity to begin collaborative problem solving with the family to discover the strategies and resources the family has to address challenges in caring for and promoting their child's development.[144] We believe the interview is a critical process, deserving of time and attention, in which the therapist and family are beginning a relationship, learning from each other, and setting the foundation for the family's engagement in early intervention.

Observation. The second step entails observations of the child within his or her natural environment. *Natural environment* is a broad construct referring to the everyday experiences that are part of the child's home and community settings. Observations in the natural environment may focus on family household routines, parent–child interaction, play, and other daily activities such as feeding, bathing, and dressing. Within the construct of the International Classification of Functioning, Disability and Health (ICF),[146] ecologic assessment encompasses the relationships among participation, activity, body function and structures, and environmental and personal factors.

The physical therapist's unique role as part of the team is to focus on postural control and mobility during play, exploration of the physical environment, self-care, and interactions with objects and people.[33] The family and therapist select the settings and activities that are most important for the therapist to observe. While observing, the therapist notes the following:

- What the child enjoys doing
- How the child interacts with others
- Opportunities for safe movement and sensorimotor exploration
- How often and under what circumstances the child moves
- Toys and materials that are available
- Areas of the home accessible to the child
- How much adult assistance or guidance is provided
- Abilities and resources the child needs to become more successful
- Musculoskeletal, neuromuscular, cardiopulmonary, integumentary and personal characteristics of the child that may facilitate or be a barrier to the child's participation

During the observation, the physical therapist engages in a conversation with the family members to learn about their perspective of the child's typical performance, abilities, strengths, and needs. Based on her or his observations, the therapist also shares information on the child's and family's strengths and may begin to discuss or try simple strategies to optimize the child's abilities. Information about the child's activity and participation in settings that are not observed can be gathered during the interview, or the therapist may elect to engage the child in an activity that is not the exact context of the daily routine.

The most meaningful observation occurs when watching a child do something enjoyable with a familiar adult or child. Parent–child interactions are sensorimotor experiences. Motor control, sensory integration, and muscle performance are part of parent–child interactions. In addition to looking at the motor components of the interaction, consideration is also given to social patterns of interaction between the child and caregiver. Kelly and Barnard[79] provided a comprehensive overview of assessment of parent–child interactions.

Play is the primary occupational behavior of childhood and is a naturally occurring situation during which children learn and develop new skills. In reference to observing play activities, it is important to look at both independent play as well as play with caregivers, siblings, and peers. Therapists gather information on what toys and play activities the child engages in (sensory/exploratory play, manipulative play, imaginative/dramatic play, or motor/physical play) and the child's likes and dislikes. Therapists consider the interplay between motor abilities and play skills. Is the child able to initiate play experiences? What positions can the child play in? Can the child freely move around to reach toys or play activities of interest? Further analysis considers if the child's movements are goal directed, the variability of movement to meet environmental demands, and the child's reaction to movement (i.e., level of enjoyment, safety, and body awareness). Lastly, a focus on the process of play provides valuable insights into the child's playfulness. Playfulness is concerned with a child's approach to an activity and includes observations related to the child's enjoyment, engagement, responsiveness, motivation, and locus of control.[101]

In addition to the family interview and ecologic observations, therapists use various tests and measures to evaluate motor development, function, and body functions and structures. These assessment tools are described in Chapter 2 and elsewhere.[90,123,137] An important consideration is that developmental measures normed on children without delay are valid for determining present level of development and eligibility but often are not valid for planning intervention and measuring change over time. Based on the top-down approach to service delivery,[141] considerations of body functions and structures are conducted after the team has a clear understanding of the family and child's goals and current abilities and relate to the team's hypothesis for impairments that may be a cause of limitations in activities and restrictions in participation. During observation and completion of standardized measures, the therapist notes impairments that appear to limit a child's activity and participation and, subsequently, screens for impairments in body functions and structures and determines when in-depth assessment is required. Therapists in early intervention may keep supplemental documentation of examination findings that are not included in the team report.[6]

Finally, therapists collaborate with the team to document the child's functioning related to three outcome areas of the national accountability system for Part C of IDEA.[69] These areas are "positive socio-emotional skills (including social relationships), acquisition and use of knowledge and skills (including early language/communication), and use of appropriate behaviors to meet their needs." These outcomes represent an integration of abilities across developmental domains and reflect a value for children's adaptive behavior, participation in meaningful activities, relationships with others, and self-determination. When children exit early intervention, data in aggregate form are collected to report the percentage of children who made improvements in these areas in relation to their same-age peers. This information is for progress monitoring of the early intervention system as a whole and is not meant to capture the individualized experience of a child.

Individualized Family Service Plan

The culmination of the evaluation and assessment process is the development of the individualized family service plan (IFSP). The principle underlying an IFSP is that families have diverse priorities and concerns based on their individual values and life situations. For intervention to be meaningful for the child, the individuality of each family must be recognized. The team members involved in the development of the IFSP include parents, caregivers, other family members, the family advocate, the service coordinator, practitioners involved with the assessment and evaluation, and, as appropriate, practitioners who will be providing the service.

The family should be provided with information that will enable them to make informed decisions and choices *before* the IFSP meeting in order to negotiate for the types of support they need and to ensure equal partnership and ownership in this process. This information may be shared face-to-face with the family during the information-gathering stages, in a meeting after the evaluation, or in writing in the form of an evaluation report. When feasible, questions the family may have pertaining to the evaluation results should also be addressed before the IFSP meeting so that questions related to the logistics of service provision can be fully discussed during the meeting. This will also help reduce the prolonged process that sometimes characterizes IFSP meetings. Another benefit to sharing the information before the IFSP meeting is that the family members can decide on whom they want to invite to the meeting, something that families consider to be a valuable form of support.

An initial IFSP must be developed in a timely manner at a meeting time and place convenient for the family. Logistics often make it difficult to arrange the meetings at nights or weekends, thus it is important to recognize that not all key family members may be able to attend and participate. If a service provider cannot attend, a representative or written information can be sent. Scheduling challenges are an area of concern and can be a barrier to the collaborative process when not all team members are present. In some regions, administrative efforts to comply with policies on nonbiased evaluations and timely initiation of services have resulted in long meetings where the evaluation and the development of the IFSP occur during the same visit by an independent team who will not then provide the services in the IFSP.[1] Although this practice meets legal requirements, it does not represent the spirit of the IFSP process. Parents often need to tend to their children during the meeting and have not had an opportunity to assimilate the evaluation findings. Another challenge is that when professionals are more occupied with completing paperwork for the IFSP, engagement and meaningful discussion with the family may be limited.[1,144]

Therapists working in states where evaluations are conducted by independent teams need to be sensitive to the issues that may arise. Therapists on the evaluation team recognize that although their relationship with the family is of short duration, it is still important to engage with the family in meaningful ways to support their active participation in the evaluation process. Therapists who are providers of service recognize that families now have to begin a relationship with another professional and that it may be challenging to have to tell their story again.

Although the federal law specifies the content of the IFSP (Box 30.8), it does not specify the format of the document or the process for its development. Typically the service coordinator leads the discussion and records the information. Family members can elect, however, to take the role of team leader. During the meeting, the team discusses the evaluation and assessment findings, shares information on the philosophy of early intervention to ascertain if this matches the family's expectations and priorities, and collaborates to develop the IFSP. The team promotes family participation, and decisions are made collaboratively. Applying federal law has been challenging, but reports indicate that families are participating in the development of the IFSP.[1,70] Aaron and colleagues however, reported that family involvement regarding decisions on the types and amounts of services was limited.[1] The findings from a study on quality indicators of IFSP documents were also mixed.[76] A high rating was noted for a focus on child strengths, and 86% of the outcomes were related to family concerns and priorities. However, IFSP documents contained technical jargon, and the family often had a limited role in the IFSP process.

Identification of IFSP outcomes that are family centered and participation based is essential for evidence-based early intervention supports and services. There are two types of outcomes: child focused and family focused. Child-focused outcomes are grounded in important routines or activities in the child's life that are meaningful to the family. Family-focused outcomes are based on the family's priorities and interests and support their access to community resources and supports.[92,128] Family-focused outcomes also increase capacity of the family to care for and support the child's development. Well-written IFSP outcome statements reflect real-life situations, cross developmental domains, are discipline- and jargon-free, emphasize

---

BOX 30.8   Content of the Individualized Family Service Plan

- Statement of present levels of development based on objective criteria: cognitive, communication, physical (motor, vision, hearing, health), social or emotional, adaptive
- Statement of the family's resources, priorities, and concerns related to enhancing the development of the child
- Statement of measurable outcomes expected with criteria, procedures, and timelines to determine progress
- Specific early intervention services based on peer-reviewed research needed to meet the needs of the child and family, including frequency, intensity, and method of delivery
- Statement of the natural environments in which services are to be provided (if services are not going to be provided in natural environments, a justification must be included)
- Determination of other services to enhance the child's development and a plan to secure such services through other public or private resources, such as medical resources
- Projected dates for the initiation of services and duration of services
- Identification of the service coordinator
- Transition plan: steps to be taken to assure smooth transition to preschool services or other suitable services if appropriate (at age 3)

the positive, and use active words.[92,128] IFSP teams often do not identify family-focused outcomes; however, there is some evidence that the routines-based interview (RBI) leads to more family-focused outcomes than traditional IFSP practices.[96]

The Early Childhood Outcomes Center, funded in 2003 by the US Department of Education, Office of Special Education Programs, has developed a family outcome measure for early intervention.[53] The global outcomes on this measure may assist providers in discussions with families to identify specific individualized family-focused outcomes to guide appropriate decisions about the supports and services they want or need. The global family outcomes[12] state that the family does the following:

- Understands their child's strengths, ability, and special needs
- Knows their rights and advocates effectively for their child
- Helps their child develop and learn
- Has support systems
- Can access desired services and activities in their community

Recognizing the importance of providing services that build family capacity[136] and self-determination, we encourage physical therapists to expand their knowledge to engage families in conversation of outcomes that are meaningful to them and support their autonomy (control and choice), relatedness (connected and supported), and competence (capable and confident).[105] However, identifying family-centered, participation-based outcomes can be challenging. Several issues often arise during this process. Table 30.1 outlines several situations that may be challenging and presents considerations and

recommendations for the team. We recommend the collaborative process described by Baldwin and colleagues[14] where the team honors the family's hopes for their child's future and engages them in a thoughtful conversation to develop outcomes and strategies together.

Teams might feel overwhelmed when numerous child and family needs are identified and then struggle to address all of the priorities in the IFSP outcome statements. Prioritizing a routine or activity that is important to the family might help the team create more cohesive and meaningful outcomes statements for the IFSP. For example, if the family identifies a current activity that is challenging and a high priority (e.g., visiting grandparents), the team might explore the reasons why the activity is challenging to address in one or more outcome statements. In this case, it might be reasonable to address challenges in communication, mobility, and self-help in an outcome statement about visiting grandparents. A case scenario highlighting the development and prioritization of IFSP outcomes is available on Expert Consult.

Identification of the types and amounts of services (frequency and length of early intervention sessions) to support the child's and family's outcomes requires an open discussion, team collaboration, an understanding of the expertise of various service providers, an appreciation of family preferences, and circumstances. This discussion also includes options for methods of service delivery, interagency collaboration, financial responsibilities, and transition planning for when the child turns 3 years old. Little is known about the types of supports and services that may be appropriate to address family-focused IFSP outcomes.[139] Family-directed service involves providing families with a range of supports including information, access to resources, care coordination, counseling, social work services, and respite care. Although the early intervention team is not expected to be able to provide all of the supports that a family may need, plans are made to assist families in accessing and coordinating appropriate community social services.

The discussion of supports and intervention strategies is essential to promote coordinated and complementary care. Mutually identified recommendations for strategies to address the child's and family's outcomes and to facilitate mobility, communication, adaptive behavior, self-care, and play enable all team members to contribute their knowledge and provide supports in a comprehensive manner. When selecting strategies, the team considers evidence-based practice and the provision of services in natural environments. For example, before suggesting a strategy of daily sessions of supported walking on a treadmill for an infant with Down syndrome,[140] we recommend that the team must consider the family's priorities, preferences, routines, and resources; the health of the infant; and other developmental needs.

The IFSP is not just a legal document; it is a process of collaboration between the family and practitioners to design a service plan that is acceptable to the family and addresses the child's needs. The IFSP serves as a means for coordinating services, a guide for intervention, and a standard for evaluating outcomes. The IFSP is reviewed every 6 months or more often at the request of a team member, and a formal meeting is held annually. Periodic IFSP reviews allow for renegotiations or revisions of the service plan, as well as monitoring of goal attainment. During an IFSP review, family satisfaction, effectiveness of the IFSP process, and status of the outcomes are discussed. If outcomes were not achieved, reflection of the appropriateness

TABLE 30.1 Considerations to Foster Development of Family-Centered Individualized Family Service Plan Outcomes

Situation	Considerations
Families look to the professionals for guidance in identifying outcomes	Avoid writing outcome statements that are based on therapist's priorities or are discipline specific Individualized family service plans that reflect what the practitioners determine to be the needs instead of what the family believes its needs are often do not include important family-focused outcomes, especially for families from diverse cultural backgrounds.[147] Review and discuss information gathered during the family interview to inform the identification of outcomes.[128] Knowledge of family beliefs, customs, and rituals not only helps teams to identify meaningful family-focused outcomes but also builds trust and communication.
Families prioritize skill-based outcomes that the child may not have the readiness or potential to achieve	Acknowledge family priorities. Explore why the outcome is important to the family. Discuss family insights about what their child may be ready to learn related to the outcome area they have identified. Share information about the child's condition to enable informed decision making.
Families express outcomes in ways that are not measurable	Ask family members to describe what the child will be doing in 6 months if everything goes well.[7]
Families focus on a child behavior they want to stop and state an outcome in negative terms	Probe for more information to determine routines and activities the child's behavior interferes with, and collaborate to create a positive outcome statement.

of the outcomes, service, and strategies is needed to effectively revise the IFSP.

Therapists practicing in early intervention require effective interpersonal and communication skills to be able to invite and support the family to contribute their insights, recommendations, and priorities. Anecdotal stories indicate that the IFSP process can be overwhelming and intimidating for families, especially when families do not believe that their opinions are valued. To make sure family's priorities and concerns are valued, any recommendation made by a therapist should align with information gathered during the family interview. Framing recommendations as questions allows the family the opportunity to agree or disagree. Additional strategies to make these experiences more positive include a focus on child and family strengths, use of lay language, and flexibility to allow informal conversation and sharing of ideas instead of rigidly following a predetermined format. Lastly, it is important to acknowledge that variability exists in how states have implemented the IFSP process. Therapists are encouraged to serve as an advocate to ensure that the spirit of family-centered care and individualization are honored.

Providing Services in Natural Environments

IDEA defines natural environments as "settings that are natural or normal for the child's age peers who have no disabilities." More meaningful is that natural environments are "a variety of settings where children live, learn, and play."[121] The *Mission and Key Principles for Providing Services in Natural Environments* of the National Early Childhood Technical Assistance Center (NECTAC) states that "early intervention builds upon and provides supports and resources to assist family members and caregivers to enhance children's learning and development through everyday learning opportunities."[145] The natural environment is not limited to the home but rather is defined as any place where children participate in activities and routines that provide learning opportunities that promote a child's behavior, function, and development. This includes child care settings, parks, grocery stores, YMCAs, and libraries.

Although natural environment implies a physical location, such as a playground, it goes beyond the physical place. It includes the people and relationships, the activities and routines the child and family typically engage in at that location, and the learning opportunities afforded by those activities. Dunst and colleagues[45] have identified common routines in a variety of family and community settings and present an approach for discussing with families activities and learning opportunities. These activities and learning opportunities include family routines (household chores and errands), caregiving routines (bathing, dressing, eating, grooming, bedtime), family rituals and celebrations (holidays, birthdays, religious events), outdoor activities (gardening, visits to the park/zoo), social activities (visiting friends, play groups), play activities (physical play and play with toys), and learning activities (listening to stories, looking at books/pictures). Physical therapists are encouraged to become familiar with the communities they serve including formal and informal leisure and recreational opportunities for families and young children.

Developmental frameworks and theories, such as the developmental systems theory,[64] the ecologic theory of human development,[24] and the transactional theory,[117] along with the ICF[146] are based on the assumption that the physical, social, and attitudinal environment is a mediator of child health, development,

and participation. Evidence suggests that the environment, especially related to socioeconomic status, is a determinant of early childhood development and therefore significantly related to health and well-being across the life span.[132] Shelter and food insecurity, lack of transportation, and community violence are factors that increase family stress and the ability to provide developmentally supportive caregiving. For example, a family's ability to establish consistent routines around eating, sleeping, and fitness is affected by the social and physical factors of their home and community environments. Families may struggle to engage in positive parent–child interactions when experiencing stress, therefore affecting infant mental health.[148] Understanding that the natural environment might not be optimal (home or community) for all children is essential when considering the factors that influence their development as well as the choices families make regarding their concerns and priorities. With this in mind, we recommend sensitivity to the family's personal situation when discussing, prioritizing, and implementing strategies—especially when optimizing outcomes for children requires optimizing their environment.

Natural environments match the purpose of early intervention: "support families in promoting their children's development, learning, and participation in family and community life."[121] This approach embraces family-centered care by recognizing that the family has a primary role in nurturing the child and fostering growth, development, and learning. Campbell and Sawyer found that when service is focused on natural learning environments, caregivers are actively participating in the session and interactions revolve around the caregiver–child dyad.[29] When providing interventions in natural environments, therapists can easily focus on the children's function, promote socialization with their family and friends, and "strengthen and develop lifelong natural supports for children and families"[121] (Fig. 30.2).

For infants and young children, self-determined behavior, the parent–child relationship,[80] and play form the foundation to support the child's role in the family and to prepare the child for interactions with peers and school (Fig. 30.3). Brotherson and colleagues[26] observed the families and home environments of 30 young children with disabilities and found that families provide a variety of opportunities in the home to

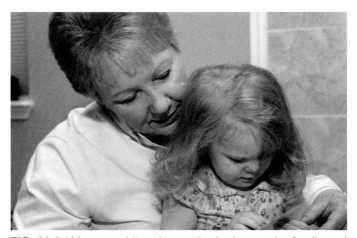

FIG. 30.2 When providing therapy in the home, the family and therapist may consider inviting the grandmother to participate in the visit to support her role as a resource for the family in nurturing her grandchild. (Copyright iStock.com.)

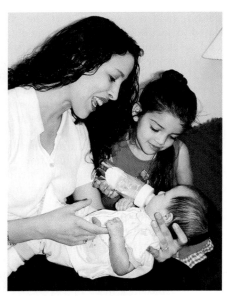

FIG. 30.3 Involvement of siblings in caregiving activities during therapy visits promotes family bonds and supports family routines. (From Hockenberry M, Wilson D: *Wong's nursing care of infants and children,* ed 10, St. Louis, MO, 2015, Mosby.)

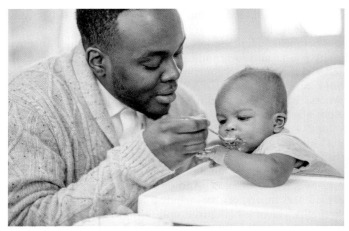

FIG. 30.4 It is important for therapists to partner with fathers and support their role in caregiving activities. (Copyright iStock.com.)

promote the development of their children's self-determination. The themes to describe these strategies included *choice and decision making, support of self-esteem, engagement with home environment and others,* and *control and regulation of the home environment.* Therapists can build on these strategies and reflect with parents on ways to support what the child does, what the family does, and what the environment affords to foster development of self-determination.[59] Chai and colleagues[34] identified socially and culturally based interactions as the common theme across various conceptual frameworks on natural environments. Therapists build a relationship with the family and provide support, feedback, and guidance to promote parent–child interactions that foster trust and competence.[80] Supporting play captures the essence of children in their daily lives. Therapists are encouraged to not simply address the physical components of play but rather to collaborate with the team to identify enjoyable play activities that incorporate all areas of development and involve parents, siblings, and friends to promote socialization.

Interventions for caregiving and self-care activities such as sleeping, feeding, bathing, dressing, and moving throughout the environment are essential (Fig. 30.4). Families of young children with cerebral palsy have identified self-care as their highest priority.[36] However, even in the natural environment, practitioners are more likely to employ teaching strategies in the context of toy play rather than naturally occurring routines and activities.[27] It is important for physical therapists to support feeding and nutrition needs, as this is a primary concern of families and critical for children's energy to move and grow.[143] As health care professionals, physical therapists have knowledge and skills in differential diagnosis, feeding disorders, pharmacology, oral-motor functioning, assistive technology, and community resources. Physical therapists also promote fitness, wellness, and injury/disease prevention of young children and families through parent education about daily age-appropriate physical activity and safety measures

such as use of car seats, baby-proofing the home, and healthy lifting for caregivers.

Providing services in natural environments is supported by principles of motor learning[141] and grounded cognition through perceptual-motor experiences.[89] Practice and repetition of activities in natural contexts and settings are more effective for learning and generalization. These places and activities are interesting and engaging and thus naturally motivating to children. This includes opportunities to learn by interacting with the people and objects in their environment[89] and through imitating peers and family members. Based on the family's daily life, therapists guide families on how to structure practice to promote learning of contextualized motor skills. Therapists help families to provide prompts and cues and, when necessary, physical assistance to enable the child to learn skills in self-care and mobility. Scales, McEwen, and Murray[118] found that although parents perceived benefits of instruction from providers, they noted that for some families, instruction may be a source of stress. Therapists are encouraged to collaborate with families to prioritize the activities and strategies and to support families in this process.

Therapists also collaborate with the family to adapt the physical environment, activities, and materials to enhance the child's participation in and access to learning opportunities. Examples include minor changes to the layout of a room or use of adapted toys or positioning and mobility devices. Assistive technology is an important component of intervention for children with severe physical disabilities.[135] Assistive technology, such as switches to activate toys, is underutilized for children under age 3.[42,91] Young children with physical disabilities can successfully learn to operate switches to produce meaningful outcomes.[32] Similarly, power wheelchair mobility or power adapted ride-on toys may afford infants and toddlers with limitations in mobility the opportunity for independence.[72,75,109] Planning forms and charts are available to guide the team in the decision-making process for designing and implementing adaptations.[31]

On one hand, consumers and professionals value services in natural environments. Research suggests that family routines provide the mechanism through which parents influence child outcomes.[133] Bernheimer and Weisner[19] gathered information on the daily lives of 102 families of children with disabilities and concluded, "If there is one message for practitioners from our parents and from our longitudinal studies, it is that no intervention, no matter how well designed or implemented, will have an impact if it cannot find a slot in the daily routines of an organization, family, or individual." In a national survey, families and providers identified critical outcomes of services in natural environments: child mastery, parent–child interactions, inclusion, and child learning opportunities.[43] Furthermore, learning opportunities characterized as being interesting, engaging, competence-producing, and mastery-oriented predicted positive child outcomes.[44]

On the other hand, challenges exist in providing services in natural environments, and therapists are encouraged to seek creative solutions.[66] Challenges include logistic concerns, such as the costs, safety, and time to travel to the child's natural environments as well as philosophic concerns that by mandating a particular approach to service delivery, the system may not be providing options to meet families' individualized needs and circumstances. It is important for agencies to develop and implement policies to ensure staff safety such as the use of cell phones, co-visits, and soliciting advocacy efforts from neighborhood child watch organizations. Visits can occur in a variety of community locations such as the library, town centers, and recreational facilities. When service is provided in a community child care setting, it is important to schedule periodic visits with the family as well as to collaborate with the child care providers. Information on child care regulations, philosophy, and early childhood curriculum will assist the therapist in partnering with child care providers (Fig. 30.5).

Implementation of intervention in natural environments requires insights and planning. The first step is to consider the family-identified priorities and IFSP outcomes. It is essential for there to be a match between the information from families regarding their concerns, priorities, and resources and the services provided. The next step is to discuss with the family the activities, routines, and people that are part of their daily life. Box 30.9 provides questions to consider when collaborating with families to identify activities. Therapists are encouraged to identify the functional learning opportunities that occur during each activity. If a child-focused IFSP outcome is for the child to be able to play at the park, riding a swing may be an activity to consider. The therapist may identify a variety of learning opportunities for the child, such as grasping with two hands, pumping with his or her legs, holding the head and trunk up, understanding high and low, and making sounds. Therapists integrate intervention strategies within the context of family activities and learning opportunities. Therapists are encouraged to balance adult-directed learning opportunities with child-directed activities to promote self-determination.[52] Therapeutic techniques are used to improve the body functions and structures necessary to achieve a functional ability and to prevent secondary complications related to the cardiopulmonary, musculoskeletal, and neuromuscular systems. When possible, therapists are encouraged to integrate impairment-focused interventions into practice of activities.[141] Therapists use their expertise to guide families and teach children through meaningful natural learning opportunities; however, they may struggle with providing interventions in natural environments. It is important for therapists to advocate for the support and training they need to be able to provide services in natural environments. A work group through the Office of Special Education Programs provides concrete guidelines on

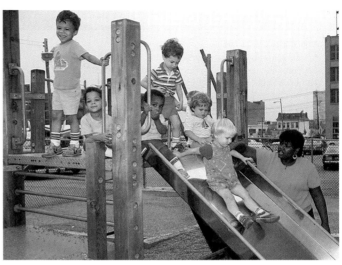

FIG. 30.5 Therapy at a child care setting can focus on promoting social interactions with peers and functional mobility to participate in activities on the playground. (From Hockenberry M, Wilson D: *Wong's nursing care of infants and children,* ed 10, St. Louis, MO, 2015, Mosby.)

BOX 30.9 **Questions to Discuss With Families When Establishing Activities for Services in Natural Environments**

- What activities make up your weekdays and weekends?
- What activities are going well, and which are not going well?
- What activities would you like to support for?
- What activities does the child prefer to participate in?
- What activities provide natural learning opportunities?
- What activities provide opportunities for child initiation?
- What activities provide opportunities for peer interaction?
- Are there new activities that you would like to try?

---

intervention practices that support natural environments.[145] Box 30.10 summarizes intervention strategies for physical therapists in early intervention.

The Transition Plan

The transition plan is part of the IFSP process that deserves special attention because of its essential role in assuring the child's progression in the educational system and participation in the community. The transition process is complex and can be a challenging experience for families. Child, family, program, and community characteristics influence the transition process,[113] and effective practices are comprehensive in order to address all dimensions.[114] Therapists, as early intervention team members, can take an active role in the transition process.

The first step is to become knowledgeable about how Part B Preschool Services (IDEA, 2004)[107] are implemented and about resources and service options in the community. IDEA provides for increased coordination between Part C and Part B programs. Parents may invite or permit one or more representatives from the Part C program to attend the initial Individualized Education Program (IEP) meeting when the child is transitioning to preschool services. In addition, IDEA provides states the flexibility to make Part C services

---

BOX 30.10 Intervention Strategies for Physical Therapists in Early Intervention

Team Collaboration

- Schedule periodic early intervention team meetings as needed.
- Conduct co-visits of early intervention team providers.
- Identify and access of community resources through community mapping.
- Establish interagency coordination plans as part of the IFSP.
- Visit or phone-conference with other health care professionals.
- Share documentation among early intervention team members and other agencies/practitioners serving the family.

Natural Environments

- Provide information and resources on family-identified concerns.
- Embed intervention strategies into the child's and family's daily life.

- Conduct visits when family members who are important in the child's life can participate.
- Conduct visits at community locations identified by the family.
- Provide intervention in different rooms in the home and outside to support a variety of daily activities and routines.
- Use the coaching process to engage families and children in the intervention process to foster self-determination and self-efficacy.
- Use family materials and toys, create simple objects with the family, and assist the family in accessing other toys and equipment to support IFSP outcomes.
- Implement adaptations, functional training, and restorative/preventive techniques to support self-regulation, adaptive behavior, parent-child interactions, self-care, mobility, play, and sibling/peer interactions.

---

available to children until they enter kindergarten or elementary school.

Second, it is important to make the commitment to collaborate with the early intervention and preschool teams. Focus groups have identified interagency relationships and communication as essential factors in the transition process.[114] This step includes an open discussion regarding the environmental characteristics that will support the child's learning and development including attention to the safety of the child in the new environment and during transportation. Therapists can offer, with the family's permission, to share information that will help the staff of the preschool program to meet the child's needs. The American Physical Therapy Association (APTA) Section on Pediatrics developed a transition worksheet to help share information between early intervention and school-based physical therapists.[126]

Third, therapists collaborate with families and provide them with resources, information, and support as they prepare for their child's transition. This support enables families to take an active role in the transition process. Most important, therapists serve as advocates, keeping in mind the family's dreams and vision for the child. Box 30.11 outlines strategies for collaborating with families.

Finally, therapists can focus on preparing children for the preschool environment and promote the development of school readiness skills. Awareness of early learning guidelines (ELGs)[119] and strategies to foster self-determination of young children[59,129] helps therapists collaborate with families to prepare young children for the preschool environment. Early learning guidelines are documents published by each state describing what children should know and be able to do before they start kindergarten. The five most common domains used in ELGs are health and physical development, social and emotional development, approaches to learning, language and communication development, and cognitive development.[120] Dimensions of self-determination such as self-awareness, self-regulation, engagement, self-initiation, making choices, problem solving, persistence, and self-efficacy can be nurtured in early childhood. Early intervention provides an opportunity to begin at a young age to influence children's self-esteem, ability to express themselves, make choices, and the belief that their actions have an impact on their world—competencies that are important for well-being and quality of life. Box 30.12 presents examples of strategies that physical therapists can incorporate during early intervention.

BOX 30.11 Strategies for Collaborating With Families to Support Transition From Early Intervention

- Listen to the family.
- Provide positive, but realistic, support for the preschool program:
  - Guide the family in gathering information without introducing your bias.
  - Provide the family with survey and interview guidelines for preschool programs.
  - Visit a program with the family and help orient the family and child to the new agency.
- Discuss separation from the child as a natural process.
- Celebrate graduation from early intervention with the family and child.
- Consider a follow-up communication with the family after transition.

BOX 30.12 Strategies to Prepare a Child for Preschool

- Provide the child with opportunities to play with other children (i.e., siblings, neighbors, play groups).
- Promote independent playtime.
- Encourage the child to participate in a variety of play experiences.
- Encourage self-care skills.
- Give the child an opportunity to practice following simple directions.
- Make the child responsible for small tasks, like putting away toys.
- Have the child make choices, and encourage the child to express wants and needs.
- Read stories about school.

PROGRAM EVALUATION

Program evaluation in early intervention determines the extent to which services are provided in an efficient and effective manner, including stakeholders' level of satisfaction and the degree to which child and family outcomes are achieved. Information from a program evaluation helps early intervention personnel at all levels (e.g., state and county lead agency administrators and practitioners) and families understand areas of strengths and, importantly, areas that need improvement. A four-tiered approach to program evaluation has been described.[74,142] Through the first tier, a needs assessment, the needs of the population being served are determined, policy or programs to meet the needs are proposed, and a monitoring system is developed to document progress. Through the second tier, monitoring and accountability, services are systematically documented to assist in program planning and decision making. Through the third tier, quality process, the quality of the services is judged to provide information for program improvement. Through the fourth tier, achieving outcomes, the extent to which IFSP outcomes are met and attributed to early intervention services is determined to provide information for program improvement and contribute to the knowledge base.

Program evaluation is recommended to determine how early intervention is actually implemented and to assess the outcomes for families and children. As previously discussed, a national accountability system is now in place to monitor the impact of early intervention on global child and family outcomes. However, individual programs are encouraged to engage in the program evaluation process to guide decisions on service delivery. Stuberg and DeJong[134] provided a useful example of how to implement a program evaluation for physical therapy service within early intervention and school settings. They reported that 91% of the children's individualized objectives were either achieved or progress was made. Children in early intervention and preschool had higher achievements than older children, and children with more severe disability had fewer achievements than children with less severe disability. These findings may guide program developers in how best to establish appropriate and meaningful individualized outcomes.

Bailey[11] proposed a framework for program evaluation in early intervention to assess family involvement and support. He discussed three levels of accountability: (1) providing what the legislation requires, (2) providing services that reflect current best practices, and (3) achieving family outcomes. Program evaluation is challenging secondary to the multiple dimensions of early intervention, the variability in the characteristics of children and families served, and the individualized needs of families and children. However, through program evaluation, facilitators, barriers to quality and effective services are identified and recommendations are provided for program improvements.

PROFESSIONAL DEVELOPMENT

Personnel preparation in early intervention (entry level and practice level) is an area of concern across disciplines and national efforts are under way to create integrated and comprehensive professional development models for practitioners who serve young children with disabilities and their families.[54] Physical therapists in early intervention are challenged to participate in ongoing professional development not only for licensure but to build their capacity to provide evidence-informed and family-centered services in natural environments.[33] Therapists are encouraged to participate in continuing education and implement new knowledge and skills during their interactions with children, families, and other practitioners. Reflecting on practice, creating a professional development plan, and seeking a mentor to discuss opportunities for professional growth are also recommended. Experienced and novice therapists, especially those new to early intervention, should strive to achieve the competencies for physical therapy early intervention practice.[35] The competencies are a valuable tool both to measure personal professional development and to identify the common and unique roles of the physical therapist on the early intervention team. Therapists are encouraged to use resources from the Early Childhood Personnel Center,[54]

the Division for Early Childhood,[40,41] and the APTA Section on Pediatrics website (www.pediatricapta.org) and to advocate for state- and agency-sponsored interdisciplinary professional development activities.

▌ SUMMARY

Physical therapists in early intervention support the implementation of IDEA by establishing collaborative partnerships with children, families, and practitioners from multiple disciplines to provide individualized, coordinated, and comprehensive care in natural environments. Physical therapists integrate their expertise of the movement system with knowledge of early childhood development, family ecology, and the environment to promote the child's development and participation in family and community life, as well as to support the family. This unique practice setting enables therapists to embrace the art of caring, prepare children for their roles in school, and foster health and well-being.

Case Scenarios on Expert Consult

Two case scenarios illustrate how the physical therapist, as a member of the early intervention team, provides family-centered services under the IDEA. The first case highlights Mateo, a 22-month-old with global developmental delay and failure to thrive, and his mother, Jenni. The process of discussing, writing, and prioritizing IFSP outcomes and strategies when multiple needs are identified is described. The second, a video-based case scenario, illustrates how intervention strategies for Andrew and his family are implemented through a collaborative, family-centered team approach in natural environments. The case scenario also includes a sample activity matrix to illustrate how intervention strategies can be integrated into family daily routines to support desired outcomes for the child.

REFERENCES

1. Aaron C, et al.: Relationships among parent participation, team support and intensity of services at the initial individualized family service planning meeting, *Phys Occup Ther Pediatr* 34:343–355, 2014.
2. Adams RC, Tapia C, the Council on Children with Disability, American Academy of Pediatrics: Early intervention, IDEA part C services, and the medical home: collaboration for best practice and best outcomes, *Pediatrics* 132:e1073–e1087, 2013.
3. American Academy of pediatrics, Committee on Hospital Care and Institute for Patient- and Family-Centered Care: patient- and family-centered care and the pediatrician's role, *Pediatrics* 129:394–404, 2012.
4. American Academy of Pediatrics, Council on Children with Disabilities and Medical Home Implementation Project Advisory Committee: Patient- and family-centered care coordination: a framework for integrating care for children and youth across multiple systems, *Pediatrics* 133:e1451–e1460, 2014.
5. American Physical Therapy Association: *Guide to physical therapist practice 3.0*, Alexandria, VA, 2014, Author. Retrieved from: http://guidetoptpractice.apta.org/.
6. American Physical Therapy Association: Defensible documentation: setting specific considerations: early intervention. Retrieved from: http://www.apta.org/Documentation/DefensibleDocumentation/.
7. An M, Palisano RJ: Family-professional collaboration in pediatric rehabilitation: a practice model, *Disabil Rehabil* 1–7, 2013.
8. Bagnato SJ: The authentic alternative for assessment in early intervention: an emerging evidence-based practice, *J Early Interv* 28:17–22, 2005.
9. Bagnato SJ, et al.: Valid use of clinical judgment (informed opinion) for early intervention eligibility: evidence base and practice characteristics, *Infants Young Child* 21:334–339, 2008.

10. Bagnato SJ, et al.: Identifying instructional targets for early childhood via authentic assessment: alignment of professional standards and practice-based evidence, *J Early Interv* 33:243–253, 2011.

11. Bailey DB: Evaluating parent involvement and family support in early intervention and preschool programs, *J Early Interv* 24:1–14, 2001.

12. Bailey DB, et al.: Recommended outcomes for families of young children with disabilities, *J Early Interv* 28:227–251, 2006.

13. Bailey DB, et al.: Thirty-six-month outcomes for families of children who have disabilities and participated in early intervention, *Pediatrics* 116:1346–1352, 2005.

14. Baldwin P, et al.: Solution-focused coaching in pediatric rehabilitation: an integrated model for practice, *Phys Occup Ther Pediatr* 33:467–483, 2013.

15. Banks RA, et al.: Discovering family concerns, priorities, and resources: sensitive family information gathering, *Young Exceptional Child* 6:11–19, 2003.

16. Barnett D, et al.: Building new dreams: supporting parents' adaptation to their child with special needs, *Infants Young Child* 16:184–200, 2003.

17. Bartlett DJ, Lucy SD: A comprehensive approach to outcomes research in rehabilitation, *Physiother Can* 56:237–247, 2004.

18. Beckman K, et al.: Summary of the infant health and development program. National Center for Children and Families. Teacher College Columbia University. Retrieved from: http://policyforchildren.org/wp-content/uploads/2013/08/IHDP-Final-5.11.10.pdf. Accessed May 11, 2010.

19. Bernheimer LP, Weisner TS: "Let me just tell you what I do all day …" The family story at the center of intervention research and practice, *Infants Young Child* 20:192–201, 2007.

20. Blauw-Hospers CH, Hadders-Algra M: A systematic review of the effects of early intervention on motor development, *Dev Med Child Neurol* 47:421–432, 2005.

21. Blue-Banning M, et al.: Dimensions of family and professional partnerships: constructive guidelines for collaboration, *Exceptional Child* 70:167–184, 2004.

22. Brewer EJ, et al.: Family-centered, community-based, coordinated care for children with special health care needs, *Pediatrics* 83:1055–1060, 1989.

23. Briggs MH: *Building early intervention teams: working together for children and families*, Austin, TX, 2005, Pro Ed.

24. Bronfenbrenner U: Ecology of the family as a context for human development research perspectives, *Devel Psychol* 22:723–742, 1986.

25. Brooks-Gunn J, et al.: Early childhood intervention programs: what about the family? In Shonkoff JP, Meisels SJ, editors: *Handbook of early childhood intervention*, New York, 2000, Cambridge University Press, pp 549–577.

26. Brotherson MJ, et al.: Understanding self-determination and families of young children with disabilities in home environments, *J Early Intervention* 31:22–43, 2008.

27. Campbell PH, Coletti CE: Early intervention provider use of child caregiver-teaching strategies, *Infants Young Child* 26:235–248, 2013.

28. Campbell P, Halbert J: Between research and practice: provider perspectives in early intervention, *Topics Early Child Spec Educ* 25:25–33, 2002.

29. Campbell P, Sawyer LB: Supporting learning opportunities in natural settings through participation-based services, *J Early Intervention* 29:287–305, 2007.

30. Campbell P, et al.: Preparing therapists as effective practitioners in early intervention, *Infants Young Child* 22:21–31, 2009.

31. Campbell P, et al.: Adaptation interventions to promote participation in natural settings, *Infants Young Child* 21:94–106, 2008.

32. Campbell P, et al.: A review of evidence on practices for teaching young children to use assistive technology devices, *Topics Early Child Spec Edu* 26:3–13, 2006.

33. Catalino T, et al.: Promoting professional development for physical therapists in early intervention, *Infants Young Child* 28:133–149, 2015.

34. Chai AY, et al.: Rethinking natural environment practice: implications from examining various interpretations and approaches, *Early Child Edu J* 34:203–208, 2006.

35. Chiarello L, Effgen S: Update of competencies for physical therapists working in early intervention, *Pediatr Phys Ther* 18:148–158, 2006.

36. Chiarello L, et al.: Family priorities for activity and participation of children and youth with cerebral palsy, *Phys Ther* 90:1254–1264, 2010.

37. Dempsey I, Keen D: A review of processes and outcomes in family-centered services for children with a disability, *Topics Early Child Spec Educ* 28:42–52, 2008.

38. Dirks T, Hadders-Algra M: The role of the family in intervention of infants at high risk of cerebral palsy: a systematic analysis, *Dev Med Child Neurol* 53(Suppl 4):62–67, 2011.

39. Division for Early Childhood: DEC position statement: the role of special instruction in early intervention. Retrieved from: http://dec.membership software.org/files/Position%20Statement%20and%20Papers/EI%20 Position%20Statement%206%202014.pdf, 2014.

40. Division for Early Childhood: DEC recommended practices in early intervention/early childhood special education 2014. Retrieved from: http://www.dec-sped.org/recommendedpractices, 2014.

41. Division for Early Childhood: DEC position statement: leadership in early intervention and early childhood special education. Retrieved from: http://dec.membershipsoftware.org/files/Position%20Statement%20and %20Papers/LdrshpPositionStatement_final_Mar%202015%20(1)(1).pdf, 2015.

42. Dugan LM, et al.: Making decisions about assistive technology with infants and toddlers, *Topics Early Child Spec Edu* 26:25–32, 2006.

43. Dunst CJ, Bruder MB: Valued outcomes of service coordination, early intervention, and natural environments, *Exceptional Child* 68:361–375, 2002.

44. Dunst CJ, et al.: Characteristics and consequences of everyday natural learning opportunities, *Topics Early Child Spec Educ* 21:68–92, 2001.

45. Dunst CJ, et al.: Natural learning opportunities for infants, toddlers, and preschoolers, *Young Exceptional Child* 4:18–25, 2001.

46. Dunst CJ, Dempsey I: Family-professional partnerships and parenting competence, confidence, and enjoyment, *Int J Disabil Dev Edu* 54:305–318, 2007.

47. Dunst CJ, et al.: Modeling the effects of early childhood intervention variables on parent and family well-being, *J Appl Quantitative Methods* 2:268–288, 2007.

48. Dunst CJ, Trivette CM: Capacity-building family-systems intervention practices, *J Fam Soc Work* 12:119–143, 2009.

49. Dunst CJ, Trivette CM: Meta-analytic structural equation modeling of the influences of family-centered care on parent and child psychological health, *Int J Pediatr* 2009:1–9, 2009.

50. Dunst CJ, et al.: *Research synthesis and meta-analysis of studies of family-centered practices*, Ashville, NC, 2008, Winterberry Press.

51. Dunst CJ, et al.: Family-professional partnerships: a behavioral science perspective. In Fine MJ, Simpson RL, editors: *Collaboration with parents and families of children and youth with exceptionalities*, ed 2, Austin, TX, 2008, Pro Ed, pp 27–48.

52. Dunst CJ, et al.: Contrasting approaches to natural learning environment interventions, *Infants Young Child* 14:48–63, 2001.

53. Early Childhood Outcomes Center: *Considerations related to developing a system for measuring outcomes for young children with disabilities and their families*, Washington, DC, 2004, Department of Education: U.S. Office of Special Education Programs.

54. Early Childhood Personnel Center: Mission. Retrieved from: http:// ecpcta.org, 2015.

55. ECTA Center: Family data: indicator C4 results and state approaches, FFY 2012. Retrieved from: http://ectacenter.org/eco/assets/pdfs/family outcomeshighlights.pdf, 2014.

56. ECTA Center: Outcomes for children served through IDEA's early childhood programs: 2012-13. Retrieved from: http://ectacenter.org/ eco/assets/pdfs/childoutcomeshighlights.pdf, 2014.

57. Edelman L: A relationship-based approach to early intervention. Resources and Connections, 3, retrieved from: http://www.cde.state .co.us/earlychildhoodconnections/Technical.htm, 2004.

58. Epley P, et al.: Family outcomes of early intervention: families' perceptions of needs, services, and outcomes, *J Early Interv* 33:201–219, 2011.

59. Erwin EJ, Brown F: From theory to practice: a contextual framework for understanding self-determination in early childhood environments, *Infants Young Child* 16:77–87, 2003.

60. Espe-Sherwindt M: Family-centered practice: collaboration, competency and evidence, *Support Learning* 23:136–143, 2008.

61. Farran DC: Another decade of intervention for children who are low income or disabled: what do we know now? In Shonkoff JP, Meisels SJ, editors: *Handbook of early childhood intervention*, ed 2, New York, 2000, Cambridge University Press, pp 510–548.

62. Forry ND, et al.: *Family-provider relationships: a multidisciplinary review of high quality practices and associations with family, child, and provider outcomes, Issue Brief OPRE 2011-26a*, Washington, DC, 2011, Office of Planning, Research and Evaluation, Administration for Children and Families, U.S. Department of Health and Human Services. Retrieved from: http://www.acf.hhs.gov/sites/default/files/opre/family_provider_multi.pdf.

63. Friedman M, et al.: Caregiver coaching strategies for early intervention providers, *Infants Young Child* 25:62–82, 2012.

64. Griffiths PE, Gray RD: Discussion: three ways to misunderstand developmental systems theory, *Biol Philos* 20:417–425, 2005.

65. Hadders-Algra M: Early diagnosis and early intervention in cerebral palsy, *Frontiers Neurol* 5:1–13, 2014.

66. Hanft EH, Pilkington KO: Therapy in natural environments: the means or end goal for early intervention? *Infants Young Child* 12:1–13, 2000.

67. Harbin GL, et al.: Early intervention service coordination policies: national policy infrastructure, *Topics Early Child Spec Educ* 24:89–97, 2004.

68. Hauser-Cram P, et al.: Children with disabilities: a longitudinal study of child development and parent well-being, *Monogr Soc Res Child Dev* 66:i–viii, 1–114, 2001.

69. Hebbeler K, Barton L: The need for data on child and family outcomes at the federal and state levels, *Young Exceptional Child* 9:1–15, 2007.

70. Hebbeler K, et al.: *Early intervention for infants and toddlers with disabilities and their families: participants, services and outcomes*, Menlo Park, CA, 2007, SRI International.

71. Hinojosa J, et al.: Team collaboration: a case study, *Qual Health Res* 11:206–220, 2001.

72. Huang H-H, Galloway J: Modified ride-on toy for early power mobility: a technical report, *Pediatr Phys Ther* 24:149–154, 2012.

73. Ideishi R, et al.: Therapist's role in care coordination between early intervention and medical health services for young children with special health care needs, *Phys Occup Ther Pediatr* 30:28–42, 2010.

74. Jacobs FH, Kapuscik JL: *Making it count: evaluating family preservation services*, Medford, MA, 2000, Tufts University.

75. Jones M, et al.: Effects of power wheelchairs on the development and function of young children with severe motor impairments, *Pediatr Phys Ther* 24:131–140, 2012.

76. Jung LA, Baird SM: Effects of service coordinator variables on individualized family service plans, *J Early Interv* 25:206–218, 2003.

77. Jung LA, Grisham-Brown J: Moving from assessment information to IFSPs: guidelines for a family-centered process, *Young Exceptional Child* 9:2–11, 2006.

78. Keilty B, et al.: Early interventionists' reports of authentic assessment methods through focus group research, *Topics Early Child Spec Educ* 28:244–256, 2009.

79. Kelly JF, Barnard KE: Assessment of parent-child interaction: implications for early intervention. In Shonkoff JP, Meisels SJ, editors: *Handbook of early childhood intervention*, New York, 2000, Cambridge University Press, pp 258–289.

80. Kelly JF, et al.: Promoting first relationships: a relationship-focused early intervention approach, *Infants Young Child* 21:285–295, 2008.

81. King GA, et al.: Development of a measure to assess effective listening and interactive communication skills in the delivery of children's rehabilitation services, *Disabil Rehabil* 34:459–469, 2012.

82. King G, Chiarello L: Family-centered care for children with cerebral palsy: conceptual and practical considerations to advance care and practice, *J Child Neurol* 29:1046–1054, 2014.

83. King G, Ziviani J: What does engagement look like? Goal-directed behavior in therapy. In Poulsen A, Ziviani J, Cuskelly M, editors: *Motivation and goal setting: engaging children and parents in therapy*, London, 2015, Jessica Kingsley, pp 70–79.

84. King G, et al.: The application of a transdisciplinary model for early intervention services, *Infants Young Child* 22:211–223, 2009.

85. King S, et al.: Family-centered service for children with cerebral palsy and their families: a review of the literature, *Semin Pediatr Neuro* 11:78–86, 2004.

86. LaRocco DJ, Bruns DA: It's not the "what," it's the "how": four key behaviors for authentic leadership in early intervention, *Young Exceptional Child* 16:33–44, 2013.

87. Law M, et al.: *What is family-centered services? FCS Sheet #1*, Can Child Centre for Childhood Disability Research, Hamilton, Ontario, 2003, McMaster University. http://www.canchild.ca/en/childrenfamilies/resources/FCSSheet1.pdf.

88. Leiter V: Dilemmas in sharing care: maternal provision of professionally driven therapy for children with disabilities, *Soc Sci Med* 58:837–849, 2004.

89. Lobo MA, et al.: Grounding early intervention: physical therapy cannot just be about motor skills anymore, *Phys Ther* 93:94–103, 2013.

90. Long T, Toscano K: *Handbook of pediatric physical therapy*, ed 2, Philadelphia, 2002, Lippincott Willliams & Wilkins.

91. Long T, et al.: Integrating assistive technology into an outcome-driven model of service delivery, *Infants Young Child* 16:272–283, 2003.

92. Lucas A, et al.: Enhancing recognition of high quality, functional IFSP outcomes. Retrieved from: http://www.ectacenter.org/~pdfs/pubs/rating-ifsp.pdf, 2014.

93. MacKean GL, et al.: Bridging the divide between families and health professionals' perspectives on family-centered care, *Health Expect* 8:74–85, 2005.

94. Maternal and Child Health Bureau: *Definition and principles of family-centered care*, Rockville, MD, 2005, Department of Health and Human Services.

95. McEwen I: *Proving physical therapy services under parts B & C of the Individuals with Disabilities Education Act (IDEA), Section on Pediatrics*, Alexandria, VA, 2000, American Physical Therapy Association.

96. McWilliam RA, et al.: The routines-based interview: a method for gathering information and assessing needs, *Infants Young Child* 22:224–233, 2009.

97. Milbourne S, et al.: *Competent therapist-reflective families: the crossroads of quality early intervention services*, Washington, DC, October 2003, Division for Early Childhood Conference.

98. Morgan C, et al.: Enriched environments and motor outcomes in cerebral palsy: systematic review and meta-analysis, *Pediatrics* 132:e735–e746, 2013.

99. National Research Council: *Early childhood assessment: why, what, and how*. Committee on Developmental Outcomes and Assessments for Young Children. In Snow CE, Van Hemel SB, editors: *Board on Children, Youth, and Families, Board on Testing and Assessment, Division of Behavioral and Social Sciences and Education*, Washington, DC, 2008, The National Academies Press.

100. National Scientific Council on the Developing Child: The timing and quality of early experiences combine to shape brain architecture: working paper #5. Retrieved from: http://www.developingchild.net, 2007.

101. Okimoto AM, et al.: Playfulness in children with and without disability: measurement and intervention, *Am J Occup Ther* 54:73–82.

102. Park H, et al.: Effects of early intervention on mental or neuromusculoskeletal and movement-related functions in children born low birthweight or preterm: a meta-analysis, *Am J Occup Ther* 68:268–276.

103. Park J, Turnbull AP: Service integration in early intervention: determining interpersonal and structural factors for its success, *Infants Young Child* 16:8–58, 2003.

104. Pilkington K, Malinowski M: The natural environment II: uncovering deeper responsibilities within relationship-based services, *Infants Young Child* 15:78–84.

105. Poulsen A, et al.: *Motivation and goal setting: engaging children and parents in therapy*, London, 2015, Jessica Kingsley.

106. Public Law 105-17: Individuals with Disabilities Education Act Amendments of 1997, 111 *Stat* 37–157.

107. Public Law 108-446: Individuals with Disabilities Education Improvement Act of 2004, 118 *Stat* 2647–2808.

108. Public Law 99-457: Education of the Handicapped Amendments of 1986, 100 *Stat* 1145–1177.

109. Ragonesi C, Galloway J: Short-term, early intensive power mobility training: case report of an infant at risk for cerebral palsy, *Pediatr Phys Ther* 24:141–148, 2012.

110. Ramey CT, et al.: Infant health and development program for low birth weight, premature infants: program elements, family participation, and child intelligence, *Pediatrics* 89:454–465, 1992.

111. Raver SA, Childress DC: Collaboration and teamwork with families and professionals. In Raver SA, Childress DC, editors: *Family-centered early intervention*, Baltimore, MD, 2015, Paul H. Brookes, pp 31–52.

112. Rosenbaum P: Communicating with families: a challenge we can and must address! *Phys Occup Ther Pediatr* 31:133–134, 2011.

113. Rous B, et al.: The transition process for young children with disabilities: a conceptual framework, *Infants Young Child* 20:135–148.

114. Rous B, et al.: Strategies for supporting transitions of young children with special needs and their families, *J Early Interv* 30:1–18.

115. Rush DD, et al.: Coaching families and colleagues: a process for collaboration in natural settings, *Infants Young Child* 16:33–47.

116. Rush D, Shelden M: *The early childhood coaching handbook*, Baltimore, MD, 2011, Paul H. Brookes.

117. Sameroff A: *The transactional model of development: how children and contexts shape each other*, Washington, DC, 2009, American Psychological Association.

118. Scales LH, et al.: Parents' perceived benefits of physical therapists' direct intervention compared with parental instruction in early intervention, *Pediatr Phys Ther* 19:196–202.

119. Scott-Little C, et al.: Infant-toddler early learning guidelines: the content that states have addressed and implications for programs serving children with disabilities, *Infants Young Child* 22:87–99.

120. Scott-Little C, et al.: Early learning guidelines resource: recommendations and issues for consideration when writing or revision early learning guidelines. Retrieved from: www.earlylearningguidelines-standards.org, 2010.

121. Section on Pediatrics of the American Physical Therapy Association: Natural learning environments in early intervention services. Retrieved from: https://pediatricapta.org/includes/fact-sheets/pdfs/Natural%20Env%20Fact%20Sheet.pdf, 2008.

122. Section on Pediatrics of the American Physical Therapy Association: Early intervention physical therapy: *IDEA Part C*. Retrieved from: https://pediatricapta.org/includes/fact-sheets/pdfs/IDEA%20EI.pdf, 2010.

123. Section on Pediatrics of the American Physical Therapy Association: List of pediatric assessment tools characterized by the ICF. Retrieved from: https://pediatricapta.org/includes/fact-sheets/pdfs/13%20Assessment&screening%20tools.pdf, 2012.

124. Section on Pediatrics of the American Physical Therapy Association: The role and scope of pediatric physical therapy in fitness, wellness, health promotion, and prevention. Retrieved from: http://pediatricapta.org/includes/fact-sheets/pdfs/12%20Role%20and%20Scope%20in%20Fitness%20Health%20Promo.pdf, 2012.

125. Section on Pediatrics of the American Physical Therapy Association: Using a primary service provider approach to teaming. Retrieved from: https://pediatricapta.org/includes/fact-sheets/pdfs/13%20Primary%20Service%20Provider.pdf, 2013.

126. Section on Pediatrics of the American Physical Therapy Association: Transition worksheet for early intervention and school-based physical therapy providers. Retrieved from: https://pediatricapta.org/includes/fact-sheets/pdfs/EI-SB%20Transition%20Worksheet%20for%20Ped%20PTs.pdf, 2014.

127. Shannon P: Barriers to family-centered services for infants and toddlers with developmental delays, *Soc Work* 49:301–308, 2004.

128. Shelden ML, Rush DR: IFSP outcomes made simple, *Young Exceptional Child* 17:15–27, 2014.

129. Shogren KA, Turnbull AP: Promoting self-determination in young children with disabilities: the critical role of families, *Infants Young Child* 19:338–352, 2006.

130. Shonkoff JP, Meisels SJ: *Handbook of early childhood intervention*, ed 2, New York, 2000, Cambridge University Press.

131. Shonkoff JP, Phillips DA: *From neurons to neighborhoods: the science of early childhood development*, Washington, DC, 2000, National Academy Press.

132. Siddiqi A, et al.: *Total environment assessment model for early child development: evidence report for the Commission on the Social Determinants of Health*, Geneva, Switzerland, 2007, World Health Organization, Commission on the Social Determinants of Health.

133. Spagnola M, Fiese BH: Family routines and rituals: a context for development in the lives of young children, *Infants Young Children* 20:284–299, 2007.

134. Stuberg W, DeJong SL: Program evaluation of physical therapy as an early intervention and related service in special education, *Pediatr Phys Ther* 19:121–127, 2007.

135. Sullivan M, Lewis M: Assistive technology for the very young: creating responsive environments, *Infants Young Child* 12:34–52, 2000.

136. Swanson J, et al.: Strengthening family capacity to provide young children everyday natural learning opportunities, *J Early Child Res* 9:66–80, 2011.

137. Tatarka ME, et al.: The role of pediatric physical therapy in the interdisciplinary assessment process. In Guralnick MJ, editor: *Interdisciplinary clinical assessment of young children with developmental disabilities*, Baltimore, 2000, Paul H. Brookes, pp 151–182.

138. Trivette CM, et al.: Influences of family-systems intervention practices on parent-child interactions and child development, *Topics Early Child Spec Educ* 30:3–19, 2010.

139. Turnbull AP, et al.: Family supports and services in early intervention: a bold vision, *J Early Interv* 29:187–206, 2007.

140. Ulrich D, et al.: Effects of intensity of treadmill training on developmental outcomes and stepping in infants with Down syndrome: a randomized trial, *Phys Ther* 88:114–122, 2008.

141. Valvano J, Rapport MJ: Activity-focused motor interventions for infants and young children with neurological conditions, *Infants Young Child* 19:292–307, 2006.

142. Warfield ME: *Early intervention program evaluation workshop*, Philadelphia, May 14, 2002, MCP Hahnemann University.

143. Washington State Department of Health: *Nutrition interventions for children with special health care needs*, ed 3, Washington State Department of Health, 2010. Retrieved from: http://here.doh.wa.gov/materials/nutrition-interventions/15_CSHCN-NI_E10L.pdf.

144. Woods JJ, Lindeman DP: Gathering and giving information with families, *Infants Young Child* 21:272–284, 2008.

145. Workgroup on Principles and Practices in Natural Environments: OSEP TA Community of Practice: part C settings/Agreed upon mission and key principles for providing early intervention services in natural environments. Retrieved from: http://ectacenter.org/~pdfs/topics/families/Finalmissionandprinciples3_11_08.pdf, March 2008.

146. World Health Organization: *ICIDH2: International Classification of Functioning, Disability and Health*, Geneva, 2001, World Health Organization.

147. Xu Y: Developing meaningful IFSP outcomes through a family-centered approach using the Double ABCX Model, *Young Exceptional Child* 12:2–19, 2008.

148. Zeanah G: *The handbook of infant mental health*, New York, 2009, Guilford Press.

SUGGESTED READINGS

Catalino T, et al.: Promoting professional development for physical therapists in early intervention, *Infants Young Child* 28:133–149, 2015. *Note: This article is part of a special edition of Infants & Young Children highlighting professional development for early intervention providers.*

Chiarello L, Effgen S: Update of competencies for physical therapists working in early intervention, *Pediatr Phys Ther* 18:148–158, 2006.

Division for Early Childhood: *DEC recommended practices in early intervention/early childhood special education 2014.* Available at: http://www.dec-sped.org/recommendedpractices, 2014.

Public Law 108-446: Individuals with Disabilities Education Improvement Act of 2004, 118 *Stat* 2647–2808. Available at: http://idea.ed.gov/explore/home.

31

The Educational Environment

Susan Effgen, Marcia K. Kaminker

Almost from the start of physical therapy in the United States, physical therapists have worked in educational environments. The civil rights movement of the 1960s and federal legislation of the1970s, however, marked the beginning of major changes in services for all children with special needs in school settings. As a consequence of continued federal and state mandates for the education of students with disabilities, the school system has become the practice setting that employs the greatest number of pediatric physical therapists. Since 1975, a generation of physical therapists has been instrumental in advocating for school-based practice and the development of standards for practice.[46] The educational setting is unique in emphasizing individualized outcomes for student participation in the education program and continues to present opportunities and challenges for pediatric therapists. This chapter reviews the history of the delivery of physical therapy in educational environments, in addition to discussing federal legislation and court cases that have changed how children with disabilities are educated and receive physical therapy. Key topics related to physical therapy in educational environments are presented, including inclusive education, models of team interaction, service-delivery models, the individualized educational program (IEP), and intervention strategies. Critical issues facing physical therapists working in educational settings are also highlighted.

BACKGROUND INFORMATION

Although the history of physical therapy in the United States is traced to "reconstruction aides" serving the injured of World War I, it can also be traced to the service of "crippled children," especially those with poliomyelitis. In major cities early in the 20th century, children with physical disabilities were served in hospitals and special schools. The children had a variety of diagnoses, including poliomyelitis and spastic paralysis,[23,56] cardiac disorders, "obstetric arms" (brachial plexus injuries), bone and joint tuberculosis, clubfeet, and osteomyelitis.[16,23,95] By the 1930s, numerous articles had been published describing the delivery of physical therapy in these special schools.[16,95,128,140] Epidemics of poliomyelitis increased the need for special schools and physical therapists. After the vaccine for poliomyelitis was developed in the 1950s, the need for special schools was temporarily reduced, until public awareness increased regarding the needs of children with other disabilities.

Historically, most children in special schools had normal or near-normal intelligence. Many schools required children to be toilet trained, and some required children to walk independently. This trend to serve only those with physical disabilities and normal intelligence continued in many areas of the United States until schools were federally mandated in 1975 to serve all children with disabilities by the enactment of Public Law (PL) 94-142, the Education for All Handicapped Children Act.[116]

FEDERAL LEGISLATION AND LITIGATION

A number of social and political events paved the way for the enactment of the Education for All Handicapped Children Act. In 1954, the historic US Supreme Court decision regarding segregated schools was handed down: Brown v. Board of Education of Topeka.[21] Separate-but-equal schools were found inherently unequal. This Supreme Court decision was to end the segregated education of African-American children, but the principles and foundation of this case could also apply to segregated schools for those with disabilities. The call for social equality had begun and would eventually include those with disabilities. President Kennedy's personal experience with his sister who had a disability expedited his establishment in 1961 of the President's Panel on Mental Retardation. Television documentaries exposed institutions in New York, and Blatt and Kaplan's book, *Christmas in Purgatory: A Photographic Essay on Mental Retardation*,[18] raised national concern for the care and treatment of individuals with disabilities. Leaders such as Wolfensberger[144] were influential proponents of deinstitutionalization and normalization. Cruickshank noted that "as is usually the case with major changes in social policy, the normalization trend is not based on empirical data showing greater effectiveness or efficiency of the changes proposed by its advocates".[31] Instead, it focused on the civil rights of individuals, a prevailing anti-institutional attitude—especially governmental institutions—and a commitment "to the democratic, the individualistic, and the humanitarian".[31] The federal Developmental Disabilities Assistance and Bill of Rights Act of 1975 (PL 94-103)[115] included a provision that states had to develop and incorporate a "deinstitutionalization and institutional reform plan".[20] Advocacy groups had gained power, and they used the judicial system to win their rights.

The Pennsylvania Association for Retarded Citizens (PARC) v. Commonwealth of Pennsylvania (1971)[103] was the historic, decisive court case establishing the uncompromising right to an education for all children with disabilities. This was a class-action suit on behalf of 14 specific children and all other children who were in a similar class to those with trainable mental retardation. In Pennsylvania, a child was excluded from public school if a psychologist or other mental health professional certified that attendance at school was no longer beneficial for that child. The local school board could refuse to accept or retain a child who had not reached the mental age of 5 years. Children classified as trainable mentally retarded, therefore, were unable to receive a public education in Pennsylvania. The court sided with the children.

In PARC *v.* Commonwealth of Pennsylvania, the court found that all children between 6 and 21 years of age, regardless of degree of disability, were to be given a "free and appropriate public education (FAPE)."[103] Children with disabilities were to be educated with children without disabilities in the least restrictive environment (LRE). The educational system was ordered to stop applying exclusionary laws, parents were to become involved in the child's program, and reevaluations were to be conducted. This landmark court case established many important principles that were later incorporated into the Education for All Handicapped Children Act. Simultaneous with the PARC case, other important court cases were being decided. Mills *v.* Board of Education of the District of Columbia (1972)[92] was filed on behalf of all children excluded by public schools for a disability of any kind, including behavioral problems. The major result of this case was that all children, no matter how severe their mental retardation, behavioral problem, or disability, were educable and must be provided for suitably by the public school system. Related services, including physical therapy, were to be part of their educational program.

In Maryland Association for Retarded Citizens *v.* Maryland (1972),[92] it was ruled that children have the right to tuition subsidies, the right to transportation, and the right to be educated with children who are not disabled. These cases and others across the nation began to establish the right of all children to a "free and appropriate public education." It was in this climate that PL 94-142 was enacted.

PL 94-142: EDUCATION FOR ALL HANDICAPPED CHILDREN ACT

Provisions

On November 29, 1975, the US Congress passed PL 94-142, the Education for All Handicapped Children Act.[116] The law included the elements won in individual court cases across the nation and provided for a "free and appropriate public education" for all children with disabilities from ages 6 to 21 years (age 5 years if a state provided public education to children without disabilities at age 5 years). The major provisions of PL 94-142, still in place today, concern the concepts of zero reject, education in the least restrictive environment, right to due process, nondiscriminatory evaluation, individualized educational program, parent participation, and the right to related services, which include physical therapy.

Zero Reject

All children, including children with severe or profound disabilities, are to receive an education. Initially these children were to receive priority for service because they probably were not receiving appropriate service at that time.

Least Restrictive Environment

Public agencies are to ensure the following:

> To the maximum extent appropriate, children with disabilities, including children in public or private institutions or other care facilities, are educated with children who are not disabled, and

special classes, separate schooling, or other removal of children with disabilities from the regular educational environment occurs only when the nature or severity of the disability of a child is such that education in regular classes with the use of supplementary aids and services cannot be achieved satisfactorily. [PL 108-446, 118 Stat. 2677, § 612 (a)(5)(A)][112]

Right to Due Process

The law provides parents with numerous rights. Parents have the right to an impartial hearing, the right to be represented by counsel, and the right to a verbatim transcript of a hearing and written findings. They can appeal and obtain an independent evaluation. Later, under PL 99-372, the Handicapped Children's Protection Act [1986, 20 USC § 1415(e)(4), (f)], parents would be able to be reimbursed for legal fees if they prevailed in a court case.[117]

Nondiscriminatory Evaluation

Several court cases had noted the discriminatory nature of the testing and placement procedures used in many school systems. Nondiscriminatory tests were to be administered, and no one test could be the sole criterion on which placement was based. Nondiscriminatory testing is critical in the cognitive and language domain; however, physical therapists, too, should be careful to determine that their tests are not biased. When possible, standardized tests that have norms for different racial and cultural groups should be used.

Individualized Educational Program

Every child receiving special education must have an individualized educational program (IEP). This is the comprehensive program outlining the specific special education, related services, and supports the child is to receive. It includes measurable annual goals. The IEP is developed annually at an IEP meeting.

Parent Participation

Active participation of parents is encouraged under PL 94-142. Parents are the individuals responsible for continuity of services for their child and should be the child's best advocates. Parents are major decision makers in the development of the IEP. They must give permission for an evaluation, they can restrict the release of information, they have access to their child's records, and they can request due process hearings.

Related Services

Related services, such as transportation, speech-language pathology, audiology, psychological services, physical therapy, occupational therapy, recreation, and medical and counseling services, are to be provided "as may be required to assist a child with a disability to benefit from special education" [PL 94-142, 89 Stat. 775, PL 108-446, 118 Stat. 2657, § 602 (26);].[111,116] This quotation from the law has been interpreted in many different ways. Physical therapy "to assist a child with a disability to benefit from special education" in some school systems is limited to only those activities that help the child write or sit properly in class. Other school systems more appropriately interpret the law to mean physical therapy that can help the child explore the environment, perform activities of daily living, improve function in school, prepare for vocational training, and improve physical fitness to be better prepared to learn and participate in a full life after school. This fulfills the purpose of IDEA, to prepare children "for further education, employment, and independent living [PL 108-446, Section 601 (d)(1)(A)].[112] Related service personnel are also now referred to as specialized instructional support personnel (SISP).

PL 99-457: EDUCATION OF THE HANDICAPPED ACT AMENDMENTS OF 1986; PL 102-119: INDIVIDUALS WITH DISABILITIES EDUCATION ACT AMENDMENTS OF 1991; PL 105-17: INDIVIDUALS WITH DISABILITIES EDUCATION ACT AMENDMENTS OF 1997; PL 108-446: INDIVIDUALS WITH DISABILITIES EDUCATION IMPROVEMENT ACT OF 2004

Congress must reauthorize the law at set intervals. At each reauthorization, the number of the public law changes to indicate which Congress is reauthorizing the law (the first number after PL) and which bill it is for that Congress (second number). In 1986, the reauthorization, PL 99-457, the Education of the Handicapped Act Amendments of 1986,[118] was particularly critical because this act extended services to infants, toddlers, and preschoolers with disabilities and their families. Services to infants and toddlers, now covered under Part C of the law, are discussed in Chapter 30. On October 7, 1991, PL 94-142 and PL 99-457 were reauthorized and amended as PL 102-119, the Individuals with Disabilities Education Act Amendments of 1991 (IDEA).[108] PL 105-17 was signed into law in June 1997,[109] and PL 108-446, the Individuals with Disabilities Education Improvement Act of 2004,[112] was signed on December 3, 2004. PL 108-446 was to be reauthorized in 2010, but this has been delayed. The reader is urged to check for information on the reauthorization and any new rules and regulations. The key elements of these reauthorizations, which comprise refinement and reorganization of the previous amendments, are described in this section.

Part A: General Provisions

Congress found the following:

> Disability is a natural part of the human experience and in no way diminishes the right of individuals to participate in or contribute to society. Improving educational outcomes for children with disabilities is an essential element of our national policy of ensuring equality of opportunity, full participation, independent living, and economic self-sufficiency for individuals with disabilities. [PL 108-446, 118 Stat. 2649, § 601(c)][112]

Critical to this policy is the recognition that education encompasses more than traditional academics and is also intended to prepare children for independent living and self-sufficiency. This expands the goals that can be considered "educationally relevant." Additionally, principles of universal design, which are part of the Assistive Technology Act of 1998,[110] have been added to IDEA 2004. These include the design of products that can be usable by all people, to the greatest extent possible, with minimal need for adaptations and accommodations. These elements strengthen the physical therapist's role in providing access to the educational environment and learning materials.

Part B: Assistance for Education of All Children With Disabilities

Part B outlines the right for all children 3 to 21 years of age to "a free appropriate public education [FAPE], that emphasizes special education and related services designed to meet their unique needs and prepare them for further education, employment, and independent living" [20 USC 1400. Sec. 601. (d)(1)(A)].[112] Children 3 to 5 and 18 to 21 years of age might not be served if inconsistent with state law. States are mandated to identify, locate, and evaluate all children with disabilities. Children considered eligible for special education and related services are those having one or more of the following disabilities:

> mental retardation [now referred to as intellectual impairment], hearing impairments (including deafness), speech or language impairments, visual impairments (including blindness), ... emotional disturbance, orthopedic impairments, autism, traumatic brain injury, other health impairments, or specific learning disabilities and who, by reason thereof, need special education and related services. (20 USC 1401. Sec. 602. (3)(A)(i)

At the discretion of the state, a child with a disability might also include those experiencing developmental delays at age 3 to 9 years.

Children 3 to 5 years of age are to have IEPs, as are school-age children; however, the 1991 reauthorization, PL 102-119,[108] allowed states the option of using individualized family service plans (IFSPs), required for infants and toddlers, for preschool-age children. The 2004 reauthorization also allows states the option to continue to provide early intervention services to children with disabilities until the child enters kindergarten or elementary school [PL 108-446, 118 Stat. 2746, § 632(5)(B)(ii)].[112] Some professionals believe that preschoolers and their families are better served by the family-centered approach embodied in early intervention.

Least Restrictive Environment

An ongoing area of national effort is the education of children with disabilities in the least restrictive environment (LRE). Children should be educated in their local schools to the maximum extent appropriate. The degree of inclusion in the local school and the general education classroom will vary based on what is appropriate for each child. Children are not merely to be *placed* in general education, but they are to participate fully and have goals related to their academic and social advancement. Since 1990, a significant reduction has occurred in the placement of children with disabilities in separate facilities and segregated classrooms, along with substantial increases in the amount of time they spend in regular classrooms.[138]

Transition

Transition planning was specifically addressed in IDEA 1997,[109] because this important service had often been neglected. Transition planning and required services must be included in the IFSP and IEP. Consideration must be given to transition from early intervention to preschool, from preschool to school, at critical points during school years, and especially from age 16 years to exit from school. Physical therapists and other related service personnel are to be involved in transition planning for post-school activities, as appropriate. Transition to adulthood is presented in Chapter 32.

Assistive Technology

Assistive technology devices and assistive technology services allow the child to benefit fully from the educational program:

> The term *"assistive technology device"* means any item, piece of equipment, or product system, whether acquired commercially off the shelf, modified, or customized, that is used to increase, maintain, or improve the functional capabilities of a child with a disability ... *"assistive technology service"* means any service that directly assists a child with a disability in the selection, acquisition, or use of an assistive technology device. [PL 108-446, 118 Stat. 2652, § 602(1)][112]

Assistive technology services include evaluation, selection, purchasing, and coordination with education and rehabilitation plans and programs. This is an important area, as physical therapists frequently provide assistive devices to improve a child's function and participation in school. Therapists adapt seating so children can function better and safely in the classroom. They assist other team members in devising communication systems, along with providing access to switching devices and computers. Physical therapists are generally the key related service providers involved in the choice and maintenance of mobility devices, including walkers, crutches, canes, and manual and power wheelchairs. These mobility devices allow children with disabilities to access the school building and grounds and thereby participate in all aspects of their education program. The extent of assistive technology services and the purchasing of devices vary among school systems. For additional information, see Chapter 33.

Early Intervening Services and Response to Intervention

Early intervening services (EISs) and response to intervention (RTI) are both new to IDEA 2004. An EIS focuses on children from kindergarten to grade 3 who would benefit from additional academic services and behavioral support to succeed in the general education environment.[112] RTI involves high-quality instruction/intervention, using the student's learning rate and level of performance for decision making. Important educational decisions are based on the student's response to instruction/intervention across multiple tiers.[10] RTI is an evaluation and intervention process used to monitor student progress and make data-based decisions about the need for and provision of instructional modification, evidence-based intervention, and increasingly intensified services for students having problems in school. The goal of RTI is to prevent over-identification of children for special education, especially those with potential learning disabilities. RTI is a departure from deficit-based assessments and focuses on possible successful interventions rather than "what is wrong" with the student. It is a multitiered service-delivery model with differentiated instruction to meet the individual needs of all students, not just those with specific disabilities.[4]

RTI holds many promises, in that collaboration and teaming are required to support implementation. RTI is defined by high-quality instruction and provides a curriculum structure that can be implemented in an inclusive setting.[70] RTI allows therapists to participate with the team to meet a student's needs *prior* to establishing eligibility for special education. Therapists may offer expertise in many areas, such as in modifying classrooms, suggesting learning strategies, providing adaptive equipment, or any necessary intervention. The goals incorporate what is required for the student to succeed in the curriculum with the fewest restrictions.

Questions often arise regarding RTI and the need for written parental approval to perform an evaluation, parental approval to provide services, and the extent of documentation necessary for evaluation and intervention. Answers to those questions will depend on individual state physical therapy practice acts and regulations[5]; however, it is usually appropriate to obtain written permission from parents for any form of evaluation and intervention. Documentation of interaction with a child is always an important element of ethical practice.

SECTION 504 OF THE REHABILITATION ACT

Section 504 of the Rehabilitation Act of 1973 (PL 93-112)[114] is a comprehensive antidiscrimination statute designed to ensure that federal funding recipients—including schools—provide equal opportunity to people with disabilities. It has been used to expand a student's eligibility for related services in school. Educational agencies that receive federal funds are not allowed to exclude qualified individuals with disabilities from participation in any program offered by the agency. The definition of qualified "handicapped person" under Section 504 is broader than it is in IDEA. Under Section 504, *"qualified handicapped person* means any person who (i) has a physical or mental impairment which substantially limits one or more major life activities, (ii) has a record of such an impairment, or (iii) is regarded as having such an impairment" [34CFR104.3(j)(1)].[114] "*Major life activities* means functions such as caring for one's self, performing manual tasks, walking, seeing, hearing, speaking, breathing, learning, and working" [34CFR104.3(j)(2)(ii)]. The Americans with Disabilities Amendments Act of 2008 (ADAAA)[113] includes a "conforming amendment" to Section 504, which means that the expanded coverage of ADAAA also applies to Section 504. The ADAAA retains the definition of disability under Section 504 but emphasizes that it should be interpreted broadly[139]:

> [The ADAAA] directs that the ameliorating effects of mitigating measures (other than ordinary eyeglasses or contact lenses) not be considered in determining whether an individual has a disability; expands the scope of "major life activities" by providing a non-exhaustive list of general activities and a non-exhaustive list of major bodily functions; clarifies that an impairment that is episodic or in remission is a disability if it would substantially limit a major life activity when active.[139]

Thus it is possible that a child who does not require special education according to the accepted definitions of disabilities under IDEA, but who is a *qualified handicapped person,* might be able to receive all the aids, services, and accommodations necessary to receive a free and appropriate public education through Section 504. Nationally, only 1.2% of public school students are Section 504 students, with the greatest numbers in middle and high school having attention deficit hyperactivity disorder.[64] The ADAAA means that more students will qualify for support under Section 504.[74] Interpretation of Section 504 varies among states and even among individual school districts; in some districts, students with 504 plans may receive direct physical therapy services or consultation, but in other districts they may not.

PL 101-336: AMERICANS WITH DISABILITIES ACT

The Americans with Disabilities Act (ADA) (PL 101-336)[107] was signed into law on July 26, 1990. It "extends to individuals with disabilities comprehensive civil rights protection similar to those provided to persons on the basis of race, sex, national origin, and religion under the Civil Rights Act of 1964." The regulations cover employment; public service, including public transportation, public accommodations, and telecommunications; and miscellaneous provisions. Although the law does not specifically address issues related to children in school, the provisions of ADA assist students with disabilities. The law is especially applicable to day care centers and transition to employment. Public buildings, including schools, must be accessible, and children should be able to use public transportation to get to school, work, and social activities. Children with disabilities should expect to use the skills learned at school in an accessible workplace. The ADA is also discussed in Chapter 32, Transition to Adulthood for Youth With Disabilities.

ELEMENTARY AND SECONDARY EDUCATION ACT

The Elementary and Secondary Education Act of 1965 (ESEA) was passed as part of the "War on Poverty." ESEA emphasizes equal access to education of all children and encourages high standards and accountability. The law provides federal funding for education programs that are administered by the states.

Congress amended and reauthorized ESEA as the No Child Left Behind Act of 2001 (NCLB) (PL 107-110).[112] This federal legislation was to ensure that all children, including those with disabilities, receive a high-quality education. To achieve this goal, all children were to demonstrate "adequate yearly progress" on standardized tests. There has been considerable criticism of this legislation. "Among these concerns are: over-emphasizing standardized testing, narrowing curriculum and instruction to focus on test preparation rather than richer academic learning, over-identifying schools in need of improvement, using sanctions that do not help improve schools, inappropriately excluding children with low-scores in order to boost test results, and inadequate funding."[97] In 2003, new federal provisions were announced, in recognition of the failure of NCLB to properly address the testing of children with disabilities and to meet annual yearly progress for closing the achievement gap. Under these provisions, local educational agencies (LEAs) have greater flexibility in meeting the requirements of NCLB.[50] Each state is now responsible for determining the definition of *significant cognitive disabilities*. To assist with the demands of NCLB, physical therapists working in school systems should ensure that children are properly positioned and have appropriate writing implements or computer access for testing situations. ESEA is being reviewed for reauthorization and the reader should seek information on how the reauthorized law might impact physical therapy service delivery.

CASE LAW

A law as comprehensive and complex as IDEA was bound to lead to some controversy. All possible situations could not be anticipated, and some issues were expected to be resolved by the courts. Disagreements that have led to due process hearings involving physical therapy have generally focused on (1) adequacy of physical therapy services, (2) qualifications and training of personnel, (3) need for services over the summer or during school breaks, (4) compensatory physical therapy, and (5) types of intervention provided.[73] As a result of due process disagreements, a number of state and federal court cases have helped define the scope of the law. Those of interest to physical therapists include cases involving related services, best possible education, extended school year (ESY), and LRE.

Related Services

Tatro v. Texas[84] was one of the early major cases involving PL 94-142. Amber Tatro had spina bifida and required clean intermittent catheterization several times during the school day. Her parents wanted assistance with catheterization at school. School officials refused, claiming that catheterization is a medical procedure, and Amber could not attend school unless her parents handled the procedure. The parents then initiated what turned out to be a 10-year legal battle. During the legal process, they were told that although catheterization was necessary to sustain Amber's life, it was not necessary to benefit from education; the school system, therefore, was not obligated to provide the service. After a complicated course through the court system, the US Supreme Court heard the case. Amber attempted to attend the proceedings, only to discover that the building was not wheelchair accessible. The Supreme Court ruled that clean intermittent catheterization was a related service that enabled the child to benefit from special education:

> A service that enables a handicapped child to remain at school during the day is an important means of providing students with the meaningful access to education that Congress envisioned. The Act makes specific provision for services, like transportation, for example, that do no more than enable a child to be physically present in class.[69]

This case led to the "bright-line" physician-nonphysician rule that a school district is not required to provide services of a physician (other than for diagnostic and evaluation purposes) but must offer those of a nurse or qualified layperson. This case is important to physical therapists because the realm of related services was expanded, as was the meaning of "required to benefit from special education."

Court cases have also involved related services and children who are medically fragile and require extensive services of a nurse and others. Some states advocate the use of an extent/nature test, in which decision making focuses on the individual case and considers the complexity of and need for services. The US Supreme Court in Cedar Rapids Community School District v. Garret F (1999)[27] reaffirmed that related services (in this case, nursing services) were not excluded medical services under IDEA and must be provided in schools, irrespective of the intensity or complexity of the services. This decision supported the right to an education for children with complex health care needs.

Best Possible Education

Board of Education of Hendrick Hudson Central School District v. Rowley[19] involved Amy Rowley, who was deaf. She had a special tutor, her teachers were trained in basic sign language, and she was provided with a sound amplifier. After experimenting with a sign language interpreter in a general education class, the school system decided she did not need the service. Her parents believed she needed the interpreter and went through due process to continue interpreter services. A district court held that Amy was not receiving a free and appropriate public education because she did not have "an opportunity to achieve her full potential commensurate with the opportunity provided to other children." The school district appealed, and the case eventually went to the US Supreme Court. The 1982 Supreme Court decision held that Congress did not intend to give children with disabilities the right to the best possible education (i.e., education that would "maximize their potential").[19] It rejected the standard used by the lower courts that children with disabilities are entitled to an educational opportunity "commensurate with the education available to nonhandicapped children." The decision set two standards: (1) a state is required to provide meaningful access to education for each child with a disability, and (2) sufficient supportive and related services must be provided to permit the child to benefit educationally from special education instruction.

When the Supreme Court applied these standards in Rowley, it found that Amy did not need interpreter services because she was making "exemplary progress in the regular education system" with the help of the extensive special services. The Supreme Court was careful to point out that merely passing from grade to grade does not mean a child's education is appropriate.

The Rowley decision has had a major impact on the provision of related services, including physical therapy. Unfortunately, in some school systems it has been used to limit the amount of physical therapy provided on the premise that schools are not obligated to provide the "best services." Therapists should recognize that "exemplary progress" may be a reason to terminate services unless an educational need for physical therapy can be substantiated.

Extended School Year

As children with special needs began to benefit from their educational programs, some parents realized that their children's skills were regressing during the summer and that it took several months to regain those skills when the children returned to school in the fall. Because the US Congress had realized that more than the traditional 12 years of schooling might be necessary for children with disabilities to reach their potential, perhaps it could be inferred that if a child regressed during the summer, extended school year services might be necessary.[84]

Several court cases addressed this issue. In both Battle v. Commonwealth of Pennsylvania (1981)[17] and Georgia Association of Retarded Citizens v. McDaniel (1981),[54] parents sought to extend the school year. In Pennsylvania, it was found that the state's policy of defining a school year as 180 days could not be used to prevent the provision of an extended school year. In Georgia, the court ruled that an extended school year must be based on individual cases. The child must show significant regression following school breaks, the extended year must be part of the IEP, and an extended year does not mean 5 days a week for 52 weeks but must be based on a program to attain goals.

Eligibility for extended school year (ESY) services is based on several criteria. These include "individual need, nature and severity of the disability, educational benefit, regression and recoupment, self-sufficiency and independence, and failing to meet short-term goals and objectives" (p 16).[124] The possibility of receiving services for the entire year has many implications for physical therapy. The children most likely to require ESY services are usually those with the most severe disabilities, often

requiring physical therapy. Some children may be deemed eligible for ESY academic services but not need ESY physical therapy services. One criterion used to qualify for ESY services is documentation of regression during vacations and the length of time it takes to recoup or relearn skills. It is therefore vital for physical therapists to do an examination and evaluation before and after school breaks. Documentation of regression, especially during short breaks, might enable a child to receive physical therapy during the summer. Using the child's status at the end of the summer as the basis for ESY physical therapy services might be confounded, however, if the child receives private physical therapy during the summer and regression is prevented.

An ethical dilemma can arise for some physical therapists over the ESY issue. Some school therapists provide private physical therapy during the summer and might prefer that the school system not provide the service. Others might not want the obligation of having to provide services during the summer, either through the school or privately. Therapists must be careful to recognize these potential conflicts of interest.

Least Restrictive Environment

The issue of LRE, also referred to as *inclusion,* has generated much discussion over the years; it has also generated many due process hearings and lawsuits. Outcomes have been mixed. During the early 1990s, the party seeking inclusion, usually the parent, prevailed in a series of court cases, the most noted being Oberti (3d Cir. 1993) and Daniel R.R. (5th Cir. 1989).[146] Later cases ruled against inclusive, general education placements as the LRE for students who were past elementary-school age and had severe disabilities. A rational approach must prevail in issues regarding inclusion. As discussed later in the chapter, options must exist for locations and types of services available to the child that can and should change over time.

EDUCATIONAL MILIEU

Although for many years, physical therapists have served children with disabilities in the general education setting, educational administrators and teachers vary in their perceptions of the role of physical therapy. Similarly, physical therapists have different perspectives of their role in the educational milieu. Hence, open communication and collaboration are essential. To create an effective working environment, physical therapists must take the time to develop relationships with administrators, teachers, and staff, and they need to understand the written and unwritten rules of the educational environment.

Least Restrictive Environment

Education of all children in the LRE, no matter how severe their disabilities, is the intent of the federal laws and is considered "best practice" (PL 105-17; PL 108-446).[91,136] The conceptual framework for education in the LRE started in the 1960s. Reynolds[125] advocated a continuum of placement options from most restrictive to least restrictive. Deno[36] named this the *cascade of educational placements.* The cascade of environments, from most to least restrictive, includes the residential setting, homebound services, special schools, special classes in neighborhood schools, general classes with resource assistance in neighborhood schools, and general classes in the neighborhood school without resource assistance. Taylor,[136] a longtime advocate for total integration of people with severe disabilities, proposed that the focus must change from expecting individuals to fit into existing programs to providing services and supports necessary for full participation in community life. Terminology used to describe LRE has evolved from *mainstreaming*, to *integrated*, to *inclusive*. The differences in terms are more than merely a change in language.

Inclusive education at its best involves the whole school where children with disabilities are served in the general education environment with the required "supplementary aids and services."[83] Models for meeting a student's needs in an inclusive setting include (1) general education and special education teachers co-teaching during all or part of the curriculum; (2) indirect, consultative support from the special education teacher; (3) material adaptation by the special education teacher; (4) including the special education teacher as a member of the team serving the child; and (5) a school-wide approach whereby the entire staff takes responsibility for all students.[83] As part of inclusive education, therapists are encouraged to provide services in the context of the student's education program with other students present.

Compliance with LRE requirements occurs to varying degrees across the nation. Physical therapists need to develop collaborative working relationships with all appropriate personnel for maximum communication and team effectiveness and for optimal student outcomes. Therapists must be prepared to work with administrators, teachers, and staff who may know little about children with disabilities and the role of the physical therapist in educational settings. This presents a challenging and potentially rewarding opportunity for therapists to share their knowledge about the health conditions of students with disabilities including activity accommodations, assistive technology, and environmental modifications to enable full participation in the education program. Interaction with other physical therapists is often limited when only a few children receive physical therapy services at each school. Therapists might also need to travel long distances to see a single child, and scheduling services and times to meet with teachers can be difficult. The reader is encouraged to examine other references for a more in-depth discussion of positive outcomes and aspects of inclusion.[25,28,57,86,121,127]

Models of Team Interaction

An evolution in the models of team interaction has occurred. The hierarchy of team interaction is presented in Box 31.1. A unidisciplinary model is not collaborative and should rarely, if ever, be used in school settings. The multidisciplinary model involves several professionals conducting independent evaluations and then meeting to discuss their evaluations and determine goals, objectives, and a plan of action. The meaning of *multidisciplinary* has changed since 1986 because of its usage in PL 99-457.[118] In the law, the term *multidisciplinary* is used to describe an interdisciplinary model, causing frequent confusion.

The definition and application of the transdisciplinary model are also ambiguous. For some, the continuous sharing of information across disciplines is sufficient for a transdisciplinary model. For others, there must be complete role release, which involves not just the sharing of information but also the sharing of performance competencies. Team members teach each other interventions so that all can provide greater consistency and frequency in meeting the child's needs. Occasionally in a transdisciplinary model, only one individual provides the intervention, thereby increasing consistency and allowing rapport to be established with the child and family.

As the team process has developed, several authors have advocated use of terms that describe the dynamics of team interaction and may include a combination of models based on the specific needs of educators, therapists, children, and families.[61,66,122,131] The defining characteristics of collaborative teamwork, as conceptualized by Rainforth and York-Barr,[122] are summarized in Box 31.2. Advantages of the collaborative model are derived from the diverse perspectives, skills, and knowledge available among individuals on the educational team. This combined talent is an enormous resource for problem solving and support. Collaborative teams are of vital importance when working with children with multiple disabilities or with those who are severely or profoundly disabled.

When joining a team, physical therapists should ask for clarification regarding models or expectations of team interaction. All individuals should have the same understanding to avoid miscommunication and conflict.

BOX 31.1 Models of Team Interaction

Unidisciplinary: Professional works independently of all others.

Intradisciplinary: Members of the same profession work together without significant communication with members of other professions.

Multidisciplinary: Discipline-specific roles are well defined and professionals work independently but recognize and value the contributions of other disciplines. There is little interaction among professionals. However, the Rules and Regulations (Federal Register, June 22, 1989, p 26313) for PL 99-457 redefine multidisciplinary to mean "the involvement of two or more disciplines or professions in the provision of integrated and coordinated services, including evaluation and assessment."

Interdisciplinary: Discipline-specific roles are well defined; however, individuals from different disciplines work together cooperatively on planning, implementation, and evaluation of services. Emphasis is on teamwork. Role definitions are relaxed.

Transdisciplinary: Professionals are committed to working across disciplines and sharing information. Role release occurs when a team member assumes the responsibilities of other disciplines for service delivery.

Collaborative: The team interaction of the transdisciplinary model is combined with the integrated service-delivery model. Professionals provide services across disciplinary boundaries as part of the natural routine of the school and community.

BOX 31.2 Characteristics of Collaborative Teamwork

- Equal participation in the team process by family members and service providers
- Consensus decision making in determining priorities for goals and objectives
- Consensus decision making about the type and amount of intervention
- All skills, including motor and communication skills, embedded throughout the intervention program
- Infusion of knowledge and skills from different disciplines into the design and application of intervention
- Role release to enable team members to develop the confidence and competence necessary to facilitate the child's learning

Adapted from Rainforth B, York-Barr J: *Collaborative teams for students with severe disabilities*, ed 2, Baltimore, 1997, Paul H. Brookes.

TABLE 31.1   Physical Therapy Service-Delivery Models in Educational Settings

	Direct	Integrated	Consultative	Monitoring	Collaborative	Relational Goal-Oriented[72]
Therapist's primary contact	Student	Student, teacher, parent, aide	Teacher, parent, aide, student	Student	Entire team, student	Entire team, student
Environment for service delivery	Distraction-free environment (may need to be separate from learning environment) Specialized equipment needed	Learning environment and other natural settings Therapy area if necessary for a specific child	Learning environment and other natural settings	Learning environment Therapy area if necessary for a specific child	Learning environment and other natural settings	Learning environment and other natural settings
Methods of intervention	Educationally related functional activities Specific therapeutic techniques that cannot safely be delegated Emphasis on acquisition of new motor skills	Educationally related functional activities Positioning Emphasis on practice of newly acquired motor skills in the daily routine	Educationally related activities Positioning Adaptive materials Emphasis on adapting to learning environment and generalization of acquired skills	Emphasis on ensuring that child maintains status to benefit from special education	Educationally related activities	Emphasis on overarching goals and desired outcomes that require relationship skills
Amount of actual service times	Regularly scheduled sessions, generally at least weekly	Routinely scheduled Flexible amount of time depending on needs of staff or pupil	Intermittent or as needed, depending on needs of staff or pupil	Intermittent, depending on needs of pupil, may be as infrequent as once in 6 months	Ongoing intervention Discipline-referenced knowledge shared among team members, so relevant activities occur throughout the day	Customized
Implementer of activities	PT, PTA	PT, PTA, teacher, parent, aide, OT, OTA	Teacher, parent, aide	PT	Team	Team
Individualized education program (IEP) objectives	Specific to therapy programs as related to educational needs	Specific to educational program	Specific to educational program	Specific to being able to maintain educational program	Organized around life domains in an ecologic curriculum	Short term to have positive child experience; mid-term to reduce impairment, optimize function, and enhance participation; long term to optimize adaptation and adjustment

IEP, individualized educational program; *OTA,* occupational therapist assistant; *OT,* occupational therapist; *PT,* physical therapist; and *PTA,* physical therapist assistant.
Adapted from Iowa Department of Education: *Iowa guidelines for educationally related physical services,* Des Moines, IA, 1996, State of Iowa, Department of Education.

Models of Service Delivery

Service-delivery models are frameworks that describe the format in which intervention is provided.[78] Common models include direct, integrated, consultative, monitoring, collaborative, and relational goal-oriented models. In their nationwide survey of school-based physical therapists, Kaminker and colleagues[76] found that therapists reported providing services most often through a combination of these models (Table 31.1). Effgen and colleagues found that most of the service was provided directly to the student without other students present[42] and separate from a school activity.[47]

Direct Model

In the direct model, the therapist is the primary service provider for the child. This is the most common model of physical therapy service delivery across practice settings. Direct intervention is provided when there is emphasis on acquisition of motor skills and when therapeutic techniques cannot be safely

delegated. It may take place in the context of the student's natural environment or, if necessary, in an isolated *pullout* setting; in either case, ongoing consultation with parents, teachers, and other team members is essential.[61] A child may receive direct intervention for one goal, whereas other models of service delivery are used to achieve other goals. A combination of several models of service delivery is consistent with the integrated and collaborative service-delivery models.

Integrated Model

The Iowa State Department of Education[63] defines the integrated model as one in which (1) the therapist interacts not only with the child but also with the teacher, aide, and family; (2) services are provided in the learning environment; and (3) several people are involved in implementation of the therapy program. Team collaboration is a key feature of the model. The integrated model frequently includes direct and consultative physical therapy services. Goals and objectives should be developed collaboratively, and all individuals serving the child should be instructed on how to incorporate objectives into the child's education program. Direct services, if appropriate, are provided in the least restrictive environment. Only when it is in the best interests of the child should the intervention be provided in a restrictive environment, such as a special room, because skills learned in one setting do not necessarily generalize to other settings.[22] Common examples of when therapy might be acceptable in a more restrictive environment are when the child is participating in academic courses, when extensive equipment is required, when the child is highly distractible, or when it is necessary for the child's safety.

Consultative Model

In the consultative model, the therapist interacts in the learning environment with appropriate members of the educational team, including the parents, who then implement the recommended activities. The physical therapist provides instruction and demonstration without direct intervention. Responsibility for the outcome lies with the individuals receiving the consultation.

Consultation may be provided for a specific child, as outlined in Table 31.1, but it might also include programmatic consultation with the education staff involving issues related to safety, transportation, architectural barriers, equipment, documentation, continuing education, and improvement of program quality.[82] Programmatic consultation should be the major activity of the therapist at the beginning of each academic year and may often be more important than child-specific goals and objectives. Once the environment is safe, the child is properly positioned throughout the day, and a safe means of mobility is determined, goals pertaining to skill development can be addressed.

Monitoring Model

In the monitoring model, the physical therapist shares information and provides instruction to team members, maintains regular contact with the child to check on status, and assumes responsibility for the outcome of the intervention. Similar to the consultative model, the therapist does not intervene directly. Monitoring is important for follow-up of children who have participation restrictions, activity limitations, or impairments that might become more pronounced over time. It also allows the therapist to check adaptive equipment and assistive devices. Monitoring may be an important way to determine whether a child is progressing as necessary for transition to the next level of educational or vocational services. It is useful for transition from direct or integrated services to discontinuation of services, and it provides the family, child, and therapist a sense of security that the child is being observed. If the need for direct services is identified, services are initiated because physical therapy is already listed on the IEP.

Collaborative Model

"School-based collaboration is an interactive team process that focuses student, family, education and related service partners on enhancing the academic achievement and functional performance of *all* students in school" (p 3).[61] Emphasis is on team operations and management and ways to seamlessly interact with team members to select and blend services. Collaboration should be part of all service-delivery models, although not everyone would consider it a model of service delivery.[61] However,

because collaboration is frequently defined as a combination of transdisciplinary team interaction and an integrated service-delivery model, it is discussed here as part of service delivery.[122] As noted in Box 31.2 and Table 31.1, services in a collaborative model are provided by all team members, as in an integrated model, but the degree of role release and crossing of disciplinary boundaries is greater. The team assumes responsibility for developing a consensus on the goals and objectives, as well as on implementation of program activities, which are educationally relevant and are conducted in the natural routine of the school and community. Theoretically, in the collaborative model, the amount of time the child practices an activity should be greater than in other models, because the entire team participates in the program. In reality, this might not be the case, because of the varied ability levels of team members, insufficient natural opportunities to practice skills, competing priorities in the student's schedule, and the student's difficulty in performing some activities. Research by Hunt and associates[66] suggests that for students with severe disabilities, collaborative teaming increases academic skills, engagement in classroom activities, interactions with peers, and student-initiated interactions. The researchers indicated that parents played a critical role in the development and implementation of the programs, and flexibility was essential to the practicality and applicability of suggestions.

In the past, many believed that state physical therapy practice acts prohibited other school personnel from performing procedures that are within the scope of physical therapy practice. Generally, this is not the case as long as the individual does not represent himself or herself as a physical therapist, does not bill for physical therapy, and does not perform a physical therapy evaluation.[120] In fact, a study by Rainforth[120] indicates few limitations on the delegation of procedures by others, especially of the nature likely to occur in an educational environment. Team members do not actually perform physical therapy but rather carry out activities that are recommended to assist the child to learn and practice motor skills in multiple environments.[89]

Relational Goal-Oriented Model

The relational goal-oriented model (RGM) of service delivery to children was developed by King[78] and builds on the framework of the life needs model of pediatric service delivery.[80] The life needs model addresses the "why" and "what" of service delivery, whereas the RGM focuses on the "how" of service delivery and incorporates relationship-based practice with goal orientation. The model consists of six elements: (1) overarching goals; (2) desired outcomes; (3) fundamental needs; (4) relational processes; (5) approaches, worldviews, and priorities; and (6) strategies. These elements are applied to client-practitioner and practitioner-organization relationships.

PROGRAM DEVELOPMENT

Eligibility for Physical Therapy

As noted previously, for school-age children, a motor delay or disability does not necessarily qualify a student for special education and related services. The child must have an educational need for special education. Once a child meets the criteria for special education, the related service needs are determined as "required to assist a child with a disability to benefit from special education" [PL 108-446, 118 Stat. 2657, § 602 (26)].[112] The requirements of federal law, state, and local regulations may include additional elements related to eligibility.

Many states have developed guidelines for school practice that can assist therapists in their decisions regarding both a student's need for physical therapy and service delivery. Generally, these guidelines can be found on the website of the state's Department of Education, the state's Physical Therapy Association, or both. For example, the document developed in Maryland (*Occupational and Physical Therapy Early Intervention and School-Based Services in Maryland: A Guide to Practice*),[85] published in December 2008, describes the process for determining the need for school-based occupational and physical therapy services as follows:

> Once the IEP team agrees on the present levels of the student's performance and IEP goals/objectives, the team then determines whether the unique expertise of an OT or PT is required for the student to be able to access, participate, and progress in the learning environment in preparation for success in his/her postsecondary life. Based on the individual needs of the student, the PLs [present levels], goals and objectives, the IEP team with recommendations from the OT or PT team member(s) determines necessary related services.[85]

The *Guidance of the Related Services of Occupational Therapy, Physical Therapy, and Speech/Language Therapy in Kentucky Public Schools* reminds therapists to ask a fundamental question: "Is an occupational therapist's, speech therapist's, or physical therapist's knowledge and expertise a necessary component of the student's educational program in order for him/her to achieve identified outcomes?"[77] Additional key questions regarding service determination listed in the Kentucky guidelines include the following:
- Does the challenge significantly interfere with the student's ability to participate in the general education curriculum and in preparation for employment and independent living?
- Does the challenge in an identified area appear to be caused by limitations in a motor, sensory, or communication area?
- Have the research-based instruction and intervention services successfully alleviated the concerns?
- Can the educational team manage the student's deficit areas without the expertise of an occupational, physical, or speech-language therapist?
- Does the student show potential to steadily progress without services?
- Can the student's deficit areas be managed through classroom accommodations or modifications?[77]

If a child is not eligible for special education, he or she may be eligible for related services under Section 504 of the Rehabilitation Act.[114] The need for related services must be based on the individual needs of the child. Some school districts have attempted to develop generalized exclusionary criteria such as *performance discrepancy criteria*, also called *cognitive referencing*. Performance discrepancy criteria limit services to children whose cognitive development is below their motor development.[24] Aside from the legal[119] and ethical questions, research does not support cognitive referencing.[14,29]

Evaluation

Results of the evaluation are used to make decisions about the need for school-based physical therapy services, IEP goals, frequency and duration of services, and ESY services. The elements of patient/client management in the *Guide to Physical Therapist Practice*[3] differ somewhat from those of federal education laws.

In the school setting, evaluations are conducted to "assist in determining whether the child is a child with a disability" [PL 108-446, 118 Stat. 27045, § 614(b)(2)][112]; they are also used to determine the educational needs of the child. The process of evaluation, therefore, is comparable with examination and evaluation in the *Guide*.

A comprehensive team evaluation should be conducted "at least every 3 years, unless the parent and the local educational agency agree that a re-evaluation is unnecessary" [PL 108-446, 118 Stat. 2704, § 614 (a)(2)].[112] It may be performed no more often than once a year, unless both parent and educational agency agree to more frequent evaluations. Physical therapy evaluation may need to be done more frequently according to the requirements of individual state practice acts and best practice guidelines. All therapists should be familiar with their state's requirements.

Physical therapy evaluation in the educational environment should be consistent with the framework of the World Health Organization's International Classification of Functioning, Disability and Health (ICF),[145] as discussed throughout this text, and is consistent with the 2014 revision to the *Guide*.[2] Evaluation should describe the student's participation (engagement in life situations), activities (tasks), and body functions (physiology) and structures (anatomy), with consideration of personal and environmental factors. These elements are reported from the perspective of access, participation, and progress in the educational program. Although the emphasis is on enablement, rather than disablement, the evaluation should incorporate participation restrictions (with required adaptations and assistance), activity limitations, and impairments in body functions and structures.[89] Evaluation should also make the distinction between capacity (what the student *can* do in controlled conditions) and performance (what the student actually *does* in the natural settings of daily life). Intervention strategies to reduce impairments of body functions and structures may be necessary to meet the student's educational needs. Examination should also include a review of body systems from the perspective of school function: musculoskeletal, neuromuscular, cardiovascular/pulmonary, and integumentary.[3]

IDEA 2004 mandates that goals and interventions be based on academic demands and functional performance within the educational setting.[112] However, many of the assessments currently used by occupational and physical therapists in school-based settings to create these goals and objectives focus on developmental skills as compared with those of same-age or same-grade peers.[35] These developmental assessments provide little information about the student's ability to participate in school-related tasks and reflect a conflict with the principles of IDEA 2004.[35] In addition, these measures do not provide information about performance in context and therefore are not appropriate outcome measures. Based on a model of inclusion for students with disabilities, assessments used in the educational setting should instead focus on participation and functional performance. They should identify to what extent the student requires assistance from an individual, accommodations, or modification of the environment to participate in the educational process.

Tests and measures should be technically sound and should be administered by trained and knowledgeable personnel, in accordance with instructions and in the child's native language without racial or cultural bias [PL 108-446, 118 Stat. 2705, § 614(b)(3)].[111] Selection of standardized tests should be based on professional judgment and dictated by the characteristics of the individual child. Therapists should collaborate with school personnel to identify appropriate tests and measures that gather relevant functional and developmental information. The child's abilities should be assessed in the natural environment when possible: in the classroom, hallway, playground, stairs, and other school settings.

The *School Function Assessment* (SFA), developed by Coster and coworkers,[30] is a standardized measure of participation in all aspects of the educational program for students in kindergarten through sixth grade. Findings may be used to identify IEP goals and develop the intervention plan, including the frequency and duration of services. The SFA measures skills that promote participation in the natural environmental settings of regular or special education, addressing both individual and contextual factors. It is a judgment-based, criterion-referenced measure that is both discriminative (identifies functional limitations) and evaluative (measures change over time). It assesses the student's levels of activity, required support, and performance in daily school routines; by contrast, other standardized assessments measure the student's capacity (optimal abilities under controlled conditions). Function is defined by the outcome of performance, not by the methods used; for example, travel over a designated distance is assessed by consistency of performance and level of assistance required, not by whether the student walks or uses a wheelchair, though those parameters are listed as well. The SFA comprises three major categories of student performance—participation, task supports, and activity performance—and includes 21 domains (12 physical tasks and 9 cognitive/behavioral tasks), with the required level of assistance and adaptations. Criterion cutoff scores are provided for children in grades K through 3 and grades 4 through 6, as are item maps that provide a visual (graphic) representation of scores. All members of the school team who are familiar with the student's levels of activity and performance in school-related tasks and environments can complete the SFA. It has high internal consistency (ranging from .92 to .98) and high test-retest reliability (Pearson *r* ranging from .80 to .99, and intraclass coefficients [ICC] ranging from .80 to .99); it is a valid instrument for use in school settings.[67]

For the student presented in the case scenario for this chapter, the five mobility domains of the SFA were completed collaboratively by the school physical therapist and the classroom teacher, both of whom are well acquainted with the student and her levels of performance. That process took about 20 minutes. Although the test is intended to be conducted in its entirety by staff members representing several disciplines, other staff members chose not to do so; it is not uncommon for some to be reluctant to participate in the full assessment, claiming that it is too time consuming. Perhaps, in time, the school physical therapist may be successful in persuading other members of the team to appreciate the value of information derived through the SFA. The Pediatric Evaluation of Disability Inventory Computer Adaptive Test (PEDI-CAT) is described in the discussion of measurement in Chapter 2.

The *School Outcomes Measure* (SOM) is another assessment developed specifically for the education setting.[11] The SOM is a minimal data set designed to measure outcomes of students who receive school-based occupational therapy and physical therapy. The SOM includes 30 functional status items that cover five general student ability areas traditionally addressed in school-based practice: self-care, mobility, assuming a student's role, expressing learning, and behavior. Data are recorded on student and therapist demographics, as are details on information from the student's IEP, therapy services provided, and therapeutic procedures used.[11] The SOM focuses on the measure of student functional status to enhance participation in the natural environments of school, home, and community. It allows teachers, parents, and others with knowledge of the student to provide information for any areas for which the therapist is not certain of the student's abilities.

Research supports the content validity, interrater reliability,[90] and test-retest reliability of the SOM for students who receive occupational and physical therapy.[11] The minimal data set was more responsive to children with mild/moderate functional limitations but less responsive to changes in children with severe disabilities.[12] Arnold and McEwen[11] reported that use of the SOM is suitable on an annual basis to evaluate outcomes for students, in conjunction with IEP goals, and that it is appropriate for use in outcomes research.

The SOM provides several advantages to the school-based therapist. The measure takes about 10 to 15 minutes to administer once a therapist is familiar with the student; this is clearly an asset for therapists attempting to balance caseload and essential evaluation/outcome data. Another asset is that the SOM requires no manipulatives or supplies.

The *Pediatric Evaluation of Disability Inventory* (PEDI)[59] is a judgment-based, criterion-referenced measure that preceded the SFA. It has been expanded to include children up to 20 years of age and is now a computer adaptive test (PEDI-CAT).[58] With the expanded age range, ease, and brevity of administration, the PEDI-CAT should be considered for use in the school setting. It provides a global assessment of daily activities, mobility, social/cognitive function, and responsibility. Wilson and colleagues[143] found fairly consistent concurrent validity between the SOM and the PEDI, indicating that motor performance was consistent across home and school environments. Other standardized tests and measures, as discussed throughout this text, may assist in determining the level of a child's physical functioning and assist in documenting student outcomes. The PEDI-CAT is described in Chapter 2.

Single-item measures such as the 6-minute walk test and timed up and go are described in Chapter 2 and may be useful for selected students.

Individualized Educational Program

The IEP is the document that guides the program of special education and related services for the school-age child, 5 to 21 years of age. It is also the document used in most states for the educational program of children ages 3 to 5 years attending preschool. The IEP is developed at a meeting involving the child's parents; at least one regular educator (if the child is or will be participating in the regular education environment); not less than one special education teacher; a representative of the local educational agency who is qualified to provide or supervise specially designed instruction and is knowledgeable about the general education curriculum and resources; an individual who can interpret the instructional implications of the evaluation; and "at the discretion of the parent or the agency, other individuals who have knowledge or special expertise regarding the child, including related services personnel as appropriate; and whenever appropriate, the child" [PL 108-446, 118 Stat. 2709, § 614(d)(1)(B)].[112] The physical therapist has a professional obligation to participate when decisions regarding physical therapy are being made. The physical therapist's contribution to the IEP must relate to the educational needs of the child. Individualized measurable annual academic and functional goals are developed at the IEP meeting. Short-term objectives are no longer required under IDEA 2004, except for those children who take alternate assessments; however, they are essential under "best practice" guidelines, and many school districts continue to expect them.[112] Even if the educational system does not require them, therapists should still develop short-term objectives to monitor and report intervention outcomes as required for the plan of care. Physical therapists must adhere to their state physical therapy practice acts, which may demand more documentation than the educational system requires, including a detailed plan of care. Table 31.2 describes the different elements of outcomes measures.

Attendance at IEP meetings may not be mandatory for all members of the team:

> If the parent of a child with a disability and the local educational agency agree that the attendance of such a member is not necessary because the member's area of curriculum or related services is not being modified or discussed .... [a] member of the IEP team may be excused ... if the parent and the local educational agency consent to the excusal; and the member submits, in writing to the parent and the IEP team, input into the development of the IEP prior to the meeting. [PL 108-446, 118 Stat. 2710, § 614(d)(1)(C)][112]

Therapists who are providing services for a child are now required to either attend the IEP meeting or receive approval not to attend and then submit their recommendations in writing. This new requirement of written input might encourage greater participation by therapists at IEP meetings.

Under IDEA 2004, the IEP document must include the following:

(I) a statement of the child's present levels of academic achievement and functional performance, including—

(aa) how the child's disability affects the child's involvement and progress in the general curriculum;

(bb) for preschool children, as appropriate, how the disability affects the child's participation in appropriate activities; and

(cc) for children with disabilities who take alternate assessments aligned to alternate achievement standards, a description of benchmarks or short-term objectives;

(II) a statement of measurable annual goals, including academic and functional goals, designed to—

(aa) meet the child's needs that result from the child's disability to enable the child to be involved in and make progress in the general curriculum; and

(bb) meet each of the child's other educational needs that result from the child's disability;

(III) description of how the child's progress toward meeting the annual goals…… … will be measured and when periodic reports on the progress the child is making toward meeting the annual goals (such as through the use of quarterly or other periodic reports, concurrent with the issuance of report cards) will be provided;

(IV) a statement of the special education and related services and supplementary aids and services, based on peer-reviewed research to the extent practicable, to be provided to the child, or on behalf of the child, and a statement of the program modifications or supports for school personnel that will be provided for the child—

(aa) to advance appropriately toward attaining the annual goals;

(bb) to be involved and progress in the general curriculum…… and to participate in extracurricular and other nonacademic activities; and

(cc) to be educated and participate with other children with disabilities and nondisabled children;

(V) an explanation of the extent, if any, to which the child will not participate with nondisabled children in the regular class;……

(VI) (aa) a statement of any individual accommodations that are necessary to measure the academic achievement and functional performance of the child on State and district wide assessments;……

(bb) if the IEP Team determines that the child shall take an alternate assessment… ….a statement of why the child cannot participate in the regular assessment……

(VII) the projected date for the beginning of services and modifications……and the anticipated frequency, location, and duration of those services and modifications; and

(VIII) beginning not later than the first IEP to be in effect when the child is 16, and updated annually thereafter—

(aa) appropriate measurable postsecondary goals based upon age appropriate transition assessments related to training, education, employment, and, where appropriate, independent living skills;

(bb) transition services (including courses of study) needed to assist the child in reaching these goals; and

(cc) beginning not later than 1 year before the age of majority under State law, a statement that the child has been informed of the child's rights under this title [PL 108-446, 118 Stat. 2707-2709, § 614(d)(1)(A)].[112]

TABLE 31.2 Elements of Outcome Measures

Measures	Part of Individualized Educational Program	Measurable	Time Frame	Dimension	Discipline Specific
Annual goals	Yes	Yes	School year	Participation Activities	No
Long-term objectives	Yes	Yes	School year	Participation Activities	No
Short-term objectives	Not required by federal law except for students who take alternate assessments*	Yes	Months, a grading period	Participation Activities Body functions and structures	Varies, some objectives might be within the domain of one discipline
Benchmarks	Yes, but not always	Yes	School year or months	Participation Activities	No, although objectives might be within the domain of one discipline

*Might be required by local educational agency or state physical therapist practice act as part of plan of care.

The IEP is a written commitment by the educational agency of the resources that will be provided to enable a child with a disability to receive necessary special education and related services. It also serves as a management, compliance, and monitoring tool and is used to evaluate a child's progress toward achievement of goals and objectives. IDEA does not require that teachers or other school personnel be held accountable if a child with a disability does not achieve the goals set forth in the IEP; however, calls for greater accountability are increasing.

In the past, the IEP could not be changed without initiating another IEP meeting; however, in IDEA 2004 there are provisions for making changes. The parent "and the local educational agency may agree not to convene an IEP meeting for the purposes of making such changes, and instead may develop a written document to amend or modify the child's current IEP" [PL 108-446, 118 Stat. 2712, § 614(d)(3)(D)].[112] This change could result in problems for both the child and service providers. For example, therapy services might be added or deleted without input from the therapist. Ongoing team communication and collaboration are essential to ensure that flexibility in modifying the IEP results in positive outcomes.

Developing Goals and Objectives

The physical therapist, as part of the collaborative team, assists in developing appropriate measurable annual goals, including academic and functional goals. For children requiring alternate assessment, short-term objectives must also be developed. Short-term objectives break down more global, comprehensive goals into manageable elements. They assist in determining whether the child is progressing in reasonable periods of time and help define criteria for the required progress reports. Short-term objectives also assist in clearly identifying when related services might be indicated. For example, instruction by a general or special education teacher might be considered sufficient for an annual goal regarding independently using the cafeteria or the library. A child who is just learning to use a walker around the school, however, may need the services of a physical therapist. General and special education teachers may not have the expertise to teach the child to use a walker and perform the task of opening the library and cafeteria doors, then entering and picking up a book or tray. Achievement of the annual goal might require a physical therapist to teach mobility activities and transfers, an occupational therapist to instruct in feeding activities, and a speech-language pathologist to work on communication in the food line or library.

For establishment of goals and objectives, the desired outcomes must first be identified. Determining desired outcomes might be as simple as merely asking the child, or it might require several team meetings. Outcome statements do not need to be measurable, but they should be functional. *Functional* in the federal regulations "refer to activities and skills that are not considered academic or related to a child's academic achievement."[49] Once the desired outcomes are selected, the IEP team must define the goals that are necessary for the student to achieve them. Goals should be context specific, defined by relevant life skills or academic tasks in a school setting.[88] Educational goals should also be discipline-free—that is, they are goals for the student, rather than goals for physical therapy or occupational therapy.[89] They must be measurable, reflecting best practice[3,81,88,123] and the requirements of IDEA 2004 (Public Law 108-446).[112] In an educational setting, goals are written to be achieved within the school year.

For students requiring alternate assessment and others, depending on state law, measurable short-term objectives are developed after desired outcomes and annual goals are identified. "Objectives are developed based on a logical breakdown of the major components of the annual goals, and can serve as milestones for measuring progress towards meeting the goals."[51] Objectives must relate to the educational program of the child, are based on a task analysis of the annual goal, and are not discipline specific (see Table 31.2). They should be functional and educationally relevant, and they might be written into the IEP. In some situations, a short-term objective for reduction of impairment is relevant, because that step is limiting the child's achievement of the annual goal. Short-term objectives for reducing impairments may be important to document progress toward achievement of the annual goal, but because they are not directly relevant to the educational program, they should not be part of the IEP.

To explain the relationships among impairments, activity limitations, and participation restrictions, a therapist might use reading as an analogy. Reading is a very important goal of education, and few teachers would dispute the importance of the child's first learning the prerequisite alphabet. The alphabet in itself has little value, just as complete knee range of motion has little value as an objective by itself. However, knowing the alphabet is critical for reading and writing, and knee range of motion is critical for walking and stair climbing. The ability to walk or climb stairs expands the child's ability to explore his environment, learn, and, most important, achieve the goal of IDEA of "independent living, and economic self-sufficiency for individuals with disabilities" [PL 108-446, 118 Stat. 2649, Part A, § 601(c)(1)].[112] Eliminating short-term objectives in the IEP is unfortunate, because they offer an excellent way of monitoring outcomes for progress reports, and they are often better indicators of the services required than are annual goals. Regardless of whether school districts continue to require short-term objectives, therapists might need to include them in their plans of care based on their state physical therapy practice act.

The physical therapist should participate in the IEP meeting to assist in determining the child's measurable annual goals for the next year. Consensus among experts in pediatric occupational and physical therapy indicates that outcomes should (1) relate to functional skills and activities, (2) enhance the child's performance in school, (3) be easily understood, (4) be free of professional jargon, and (5) be realistic and achievable within the time frame of the IEP.[37] These experts suggested that if a skill or activity cannot be observed or measured during the student's typical school day, then it might not be relevant to the student's educational needs and, therefore, may not be appropriate to include as an IEP goal. The therapists surveyed did not reach consensus on whether generalization of skills across settings is important. An example of a desired outcome and the objectives involving independent stair climbing is illustrated in Box 31.3. To climb stairs at school independently, a child should have 90 degrees of knee flexion and good strength in the quadriceps muscles. Educationally relevant objectives are included in the child's IEP, and the other short-term objectives, which may or may not be considered educationally relevant, are included in the therapist's plan of care. Documentation of progress toward achievement of each objective is important to share with the child and family. Attainment of short-term objectives should be recognized and rewarded in lieu of waiting, perhaps a long time, for achievement of the long-term goal.

BOX 31.3   Example of Desired Outcome, Annual Goal, and Short-Term Objectives

Desired Outcome

Jonathan says: "I want to be able to climb the steps to get into school."

Annual Goal (Long-Term Objective) That Is Measurable and Educationally Relevant

Jonathan will walk up and down the school stairs independently without using the railing.

Short-Term Objectives That Are Measurable and Educationally Relevant

1. Jonathan will climb up eight stairs to enter the school with standby supervision using a railing.
2. Jonathan will climb up eight stairs to enter the school with standby supervision without using a railing.
3. Jonathan will climb down eight stairs to enter the school with standby supervision using a railing.
4. Jonathan will climb down eight stairs to enter the school with standby supervision without using a railing.
5. Jonathan will climb up eight stairs to enter the school without supervision or using a railing.
6. Jonathan will climb down eight stairs to enter the school without supervision or using a railing.

Short-Term Objectives That Are Measurable but Not Directly Educationally Relevant

These objectives, which relate to impairments in body functions and structures, are necessary to achieve the educationally relevant short-term and annual goals and would be part of the therapist's plan of care but not in the individualized educational program.

1. Jonathan will progress from 30° to 50° of active flexion of his right knee.
2. Jonathan will progress from a poor (1/5) to a fair (3/5) muscle-strength grade in his left quadriceps.
3. Jonathan will achieve 90° of active flexion of his right knee.
4. Jonathan will achieve a good (4/5) muscle-strength grade in his left quadriceps.

TABLE 31.3   Example of Annual Goal Using Goal Attainment Scaling

−2 Baseline	When leaving 5 minutes ahead of class, Alicia walks using her walker from class to the playground (400 feet), 3 of the 5 days.
−1	When leaving 2 minutes ahead of class, Alicia walks independently using her walker from class to the playground (400 feet), 3 of the 5 days.
0 Desired level	When walking from class to the playground (400 feet), Alicia walks independently at end of line with her class using her walker, 3 of the 5 days.
+1	When walking from class to playground (400 feet), Alicia walks independently in middle of line with her class using her walker, 3 of the 5 days.
+2	When walking from class to playground (400 feet), Alicia walks independently as line leader using her walker, 3 of the 5 days.

provide lists of potential objectives should not replace professional judgment. In addition to the task variables, consideration should be given to the hierarchy of response competence.[1] A behavior is acquired and then refined as fluency or proficiency develops. The skill must then be maintained and then generalized or transferred to multiple environments, individuals, and equipment. *Acquisition, fluency, maintenance,* and *generalization of behaviors* are the terms used by educators that can be applied to motor learning. The concepts of efficiency, flexibility, and consistency have also been used to define skill components of goals. Use of this terminology is important when there is a need to convey the rationale for providing services past the acquisition phase.

Another option or format for writing short-term goals is the use of goal attainment scaling (GAS). GAS is an individualized criterion-referenced outcome measure that has demonstrated good content validity, reliability, and responsiveness in studies of children, as discussed in Chapter 2. It has been used to study school-based therapy practice[48,79] and is recommended as a useful tool to assess student outcomes for therapist performance appraisal. Table 31.3 provides an example of a student's GAS goal with a focus on participation.

Therapists are encouraged to consider using a prompting system as a strategy to achieve an objective and as a variable in writing the criteria for judging attainment of the objective (Fig. 31.1). Systematic delivery of levels of prompting assistance may be implemented in two ways. One is the "system of maximum prompts," and the other is the "system of least prompts."[1,39] The prompts are usually verbal or visual cues, demonstration or modeling, partial assistance or physical guidance, and maximum assistance. In the system of maximum prompts, the therapist initially provides maximum assistance and then gradually, over successive sessions, reduces the amount of assistance as the child achieves more independence. This is also referred to as *fading.* It is a common technique used by therapists and allows for maximal success during learning. This system is best suited for acquisition of skills, when it is important to avoid unsafe movement, and for a complex series of tasks such as some activities of daily living.

In the system of least prompts, the child is initially provided the least amount of assistance, usually a verbal or visual cue, and then progresses as necessary to model, guide, or maximal assistance. This approach allows the child to display

Measurable annual goals and objectives should contain a statement of the behavior to be achieved, under what conditions, and the criteria to be used to determine achievement.[39,81] "SMART" is a commonly used acronym that can guide the development of goals and objectives: specific, measurable, achievable, realistic, and time based.[133] When performing a task analysis and developing the short-term objectives, several variables should be considered: (1) changes in the behavior itself, (2) changes in the conditions under which the behavior is performed, and (3) changes in the criteria expected for ultimate performance.[1] Changes in behavior may reflect a progression from basic skills to more complex skills or to increasing levels of functional ability. Changes in conditions may range from simple to complex, such as walking in an empty hallway to walking in a hallway with other students.

Criteria for progression may be qualitative or quantitative. They might include the qualitative measure of perceived exertion during stair climbing or the quantitative measure of walking speed. Use of quantitative criteria, such as judgment by three of four trials, or 80% of the time, should be considered carefully for their practicability. Successfully crossing the street only 80% of the time can be fatal! Selection of the behavior, conditions, and criteria for judging attainment of each objective for each individual child must be based on sound professional judgment. Books, computer programs, and other materials that

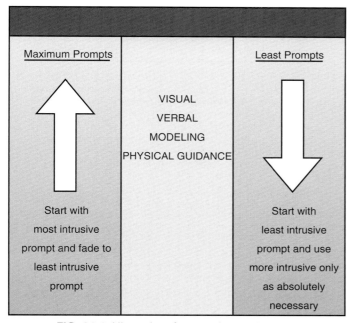

<table>
<tr><td>Maximum Prompts</td><td></td><td>Least Prompts</td></tr>
<tr><td></td><td>VISUAL
VERBAL
MODELING
PHYSICAL GUIDANCE</td><td></td></tr>
<tr><td>Start with
most intrusive
prompt and fade to
least intrusive
prompt</td><td></td><td>Start with
least intrusive
prompt and use
more intrusive only
as absolutely
necessary</td></tr>
</table>

FIG. 31.1 Hierarchy of prompting assistance.

his or her best effort before the therapist prematurely provides unnecessary assistance. The system of least prompts is best for tasks in which the child has some ability or is developing fluency or generalization to new settings, individuals, or equipment.

Therapists should incorporate other principles of motor learning into the development of short-term objectives and intervention sessions. Increasing muscle strength can contribute to improved motor control and function, particularly improved walking.[94] Practice of motor skills should be structured in ways to promote learning through consideration of part versus whole practice, use of contextual interference, blocked versus random practice, massed versus distributed practice, schedules of feedback, knowledge of performance, and knowledge of results.[129] Breaking down any of these elements into a progression of simpler to more complex skills can lead to achievement of objectives. In the education literature, this is referred to as *scaffolding* (see Chapter 3).

Frequency and Intensity of Intervention

At the IEP meeting, the frequency and intensity of all services should be determined by the entire team. The American Physical Therapy Association (APTA) Section on Pediatrics uses the terminology of *dosage* to refer to a combination of the frequency of intervention sessions, duration of each session, and length of an episode of care.[7] The physical therapist collaborates with other team members to determine the appropriate amount of physical therapy intervention, combined with the child's other interventions, the educational program, and recreational activities. Competing priorities need to be considered so that other areas of importance are not neglected for the child to receive therapy. An appropriate balance among education, therapy, and leisure (play) is an important issue for discussion with parents, particularly with those who believe that more is better. The availability of physical therapists should not be a factor in determining services. However, Kaminker and colleagues[75] found regional differences in frequencies of intervention provided

by school-based physical therapists, corresponding to ratios of available therapists to students.

The amount of the physical therapy services required to achieve a specific goal is neither well understood nor well documented.[13,68] Until sufficient peer-reviewed evidence is obtained, decisions on how much intervention is required to achieve a goal depend largely on professional judgment and consideration of the needs of the individual child. Numerous factors enter into decision making and include (1) potential for improvement, (2) critical period for skill development, (3) amount of training required to carry out an intervention (if anyone can assist with the intervention, then less therapist time is required), (4) significance of the problem for the child's education, (5) history of physical therapy intervention, and (6) medical status of the student.[68] Table 31.4 depicts a matrix of factors to consider when deciding on the extent of physical therapy services required. Guidance is provided on using four dosing intensities: intensive, frequent, periodic, and intermittent, based on a number of considerations.[7] On this scale, a student with several considerations indicating the need for intensive intervention would require more intervention than a student with predominant indications of periodic intervention.

Without the use of an accepted clinical reasoning tool or objective measure for establishing educational need, school-based physical therapists have difficulty making decisions that support the intent of IDEA while withstanding outside pressures. The *Considerations for Educationally Relevant Therapy for Occupational Therapy and Physical Therapy* (CERT)[53] and the *Determination of Relevant Therapy Tool* (DRTT)[26] are two examples of clinical reasoning models that provide objective data for school-based therapy decision making.

Therapists in Florida have been developing the CERT since the 1990s.[53] The CERT is not an assessment but rather "a summary of educational considerations based on a review of student records, evaluations, observations, progress notes, parent/teacher information and other data."[53] It includes a summary sheet, a student profile, and a therapy profile completed by the therapist. The student profile rates the student's abilities in personal care, mobility, gross motor skills, fine motor/visual motor skills, and sensory processing. The therapy profile indicates the number of years the student has received educationally relevant therapy, potential response to educationally relevant therapy, the student's learning environment, therapy services provided to the student, and support services provided to school staff or parents. Detailed information on the CERT is available at http://www.fldoe.org/ESE/cert.asp.

The DRTT was developed in Maryland to assist in occupational therapy and physical therapy service recommendations to the IEP team.[26] For therapists new to the educational setting, this method encompasses the range of roles and responsibilities of therapists and requires the user to consider all aspects of therapeutic and educational programming prior to decision making. For therapists who have experience in school practice, use of the DRTT provides a means to validate decisions related to models and delivery of services, beyond the use of clinical judgment alone. Consistent service delivery among therapists in any jurisdiction helps to alleviate the disputes between families and teams that may arise regarding service recommendations, as well as to support administration with appropriate staffing ratios to meet IEP needs, while managing therapist costs.

TABLE 31.4 **Factors to Consider When Determining the Intensity and Frequency (Dosage) of Physical Therapy (PT)**

Considerations	Intensive	Frequent	Periodic	Intermittent
	A highly concentrated amount of PT intervention provided over an episode of care. *Example:* Weekly sessions lasting 45 minutes or more or a frequency of 2× or more/week.	A moderate amount of PT intervention provided at consistent intervals over an episode of care. *Example:* Weekly or bimonthly sessions lasting less than 45 minutes.	A lower amount of PT intervention provided at regularly scheduled intervals for a specified number of minutes over an episode of care. *Example:* 1–2×/quarter for 20 minutes each session.	A low amount of PT intervention provided irregularly or when needed over an episode of care. Length of therapy session may vary. *Example:* 2–5×/year for a total of 60 minutes.
Participation Restrictions Student demonstrates restrictions of functional or foundational skills that limit participation.	Intensive PT intervention is needed to facilitate participation. Student is highly motivated and desires to participate.	Regular PT intervention is needed to facilitate ongoing participation.	Participation restrictions addressed by a physical therapist through periodic review.	Participation restrictions addressed through established accommodations, assistive technology devices, classroom programs, or adult assistance.
Chronologic Age/Readiness for Skill Acquisition The number of services must reflect the potential for skill acquisition during a critical period of development and the student's intrinsic desire to participate.	Extremely critical period when student is demonstrating emerging skills that require PT intervention for further development.	Critical period when student is demonstrating emerging skills, is experiencing a growth spurt, or is approaching a transitional period.	Outside a critical period but may have periodic challenges identified.	Not in critical period, based on age, and limited gains are expected through PT intervention.
Impact of PT Intervention The physical therapist makes decisions regarding the student's potential to benefit from PT intervention.	Student has potential for rapid progress toward established goals or has potential for rapid decline or loss of functional skills.	Student demonstrates motivation and continual progress toward established goals. Potential for regression or loss of skills could occur with service reduction.	Student demonstrates a reduced rate of goal attainment or shows decline solely due to the disease process.	Student demonstrates limited progress toward goal attainment or is near maximum benefit.
Support Available at School Considers the expertise and competency of other school-based providers who may support the student.	Student or staff requires extensive support of the physical therapist to assist the student's participation in the educational setting and progress toward goals.	Student requires regular PT support in the educational setting, where support staff is being trained to promote participation and progress toward goals. Other school staff is available and can contribute to meeting the specific areas of need.	Level of support in educational setting is adequate to maintain student's skills, meet new challenges, and allow participation in curriculum. Periodic review of required accommodations or modifications continues to be necessary.	Student is able to participate in educational program with assistance of support staff or specialized programs. Occasional monitoring may be needed to address modifications.
Transitions Student's transition to and present level of performance in a new program, placement, or environment are considered, as well as available supports.	Student requires the physical therapist to assist with acquisition of significant additional skills for access and participation related to the transition.	Student requires PT intervention for refinement or expansion of skills related to the transition.	Student's level of support in new program or environment is adequate to maintain skills, meet new challenges, and allow participation.	Student's level of support in new program or environment is adequate to allow participation, with intermittent PT services to review equipment, accommodations, or modifications.
Expertise, Clinical Decision Making, and Problem Solving Needed From a Physical Therapist Physical therapists are movement specialists who assist in optimizing movement for participation.	Student requires the clinical skills and problem solving of a physical therapist for a significant part of the educational program.	Student requires the clinical skills and problem solving of a physical therapist for part of the educational program, and other aspects can be safely performed by student or staff.	Student requires the clinical skills and problem solving of a physical therapist to periodically reassess student status and update educational program.	Classroom program can be safely performed by student or staff.
Previous Physical Therapy Intervention Considers the extent of and response to previous PT intervention.	Student continues to make significant progress with PT intervention.	Student has made steady progress with PT intervention.	Student has reached a plateau in skill acquisition. May need periodic examination for signs of readiness for new skill acquisition, generalization, or regression of skills.	Student has made limited progress despite PT intervention. May need intermittent examination for signs of regression or equipment/device management.

TABLE 31.4 Factors to Consider When Determining the Intensity and Frequency (Dosage) of Physical Therapy (PT)—cont'd

Considerations	Intensive	Frequent	Periodic	Intermittent
Health Condition A student who experiences a change in medical status may require modifications to school-based PT services.	Student with a significant change in health condition may initially require intensive PT intervention to address altered needs, training of school staff, and acquisition/fitting of assistive technology.	Student with moderate or ongoing changes in health condition that impact functional abilities may require frequent PT intervention.	Student with stable or gradual changes in health condition may require periodic PT intervention to monitor functional abilities, assistive technology, or training of staff.	Student with stable health condition or whose needs are appropriately managed by the student or school staff may require intermittent PT for monitoring.
Assistive Technology (AT) Intensity of PT services decreases as student/staff proficiency with AT increases.	Student requires intensive PT intervention for determination of complex AT needs. Staff requires extensive training with devices to ensure safe participation.	Student requires frequent PT intervention for determination of AT needs. Staff requires training with unfamiliar devices to ensure safe participation.	Student or staff use AT appropriately. Periodic PT intervention needed to monitor changes, safety, and maintenance.	Student or staff use all AT appropriately. Intermittent PT intervention needed to monitor devices/equipment.

Adapted from American Physical Therapy Association Section on Pediatrics. Dosage Considerations: recommending school-based physical therapy intervention under IDEA resource manual. Retrieved from: https://pediatricapta.org/includes/fact-sheets/pdfs/15%20Dosage%20Consideration%20Resource%20Manual.pdf; Bailes A, Reder R, Burch C: Development of guidelines for determining frequency of therapy services in a pediatric medical setting, *Pediatr Phys Ther* 20:194-198, 2008; Iowa Department of Education: *Iowa guidelines for educationally related physical therapy services*, Des Moines, IA, 2001, State of Iowa, Department of Education.

INTERVENTION

Intervention must be based on the needs of the child, not of the system or professionals. The content, goals, frequency, location, and intensity of intervention are decided collaboratively by the IEP team at the IEP meeting. Effective communication among team members is crucial for the planning, provision, and coordination of services and to avoid an overlap of services, missed services, and conflict.[89] The *Guide to Physical Therapist Practice*[3] describes three components of intervention, all of which are essential in the educational environment: coordination, communication, and documentation; patient/client-related instruction; and procedural interventions. The amount of time and effort devoted to each will depend on the needs of the child and may vary at different times during the school year.

Coordination, Communication, and Documentation

Coordination, communication, and documentation are particularly important in schools where the therapist is in the building only occasionally, and direct interaction with other team members is limited. Frequent communication with parents, teachers, and other related service personnel must be established and maintained. This may be accomplished through regularly scheduled meetings, informal conversation, and written progress reports, as well as by telephone and electronic communication.

Documentation must follow local, state, and national requirements for both education and physical therapy. This means that, although the education agencies might dictate that progress reports are provided to the family only at the same frequency as for children who do not have a disability, the state physical therapy practice act might require documentation after each intervention session. The APTA Defensible Documentation Resource[9] suggests the following: (1) documentation is required for every visit/encounter, (2) documentation should indicate cancellations, (3) documentation must comply with regulatory requirements, (4) entries must be made in ink and properly authenticated, (5) electronic entries should be secure, and (6) documentation in pediatrics should be aligned with family-centered care and should emphasize the functional abilities of the child. Specific to school settings, the physical therapist should "document all strategies, interventions, staff/student training and education, and communication with the student's parents/guardians or community based services."[9] In addition, although the IEP team might decide that physical therapy services are no longer required, discontinuation of physical therapy must be documented by the physical therapist in a final summary to close that episode of care. Services billed through Medicaid and other insurance providers usually require additional documentation. There is great variation across the country with regard to documentation of school-based physical therapy services; therapists must consult their state practice acts to ensure that they are in full compliance.

Child- and Family-Related Instruction

Child- and family-related instruction, along with instruction to other team members, is a critical area of practice in school settings. Practice is essential for the acquisition, fluency, and generalization of skills[32,141]; consequently, the family and the IEP team may be largely responsible for assisting the child in carrying out or practicing motor skills. Instruction of parents and appropriate staff members should be a major component of all intervention plans. Instruction should begin and continue as needed: at the start of every school year, at the initiation of physical therapy services, when a child enters a new school, and when a new staff member becomes involved in the care of the child.

In the integrated and collaborative service-delivery models, teachers, staff members, and parents participate in the delivery of some aspects of the intervention. Their involvement may be as simple as using proper positioning techniques or as complicated as handling procedures for transfers and mobility. These individuals must be instructed in proper positioning of the student, safe body mechanics of the caregiver, use of adaptive equipment, and ways to encourage selected motor activities. It is generally prudent for the physical therapist to provide the primary instruction at the initial acquisition stage of motor learning, relinquishing care to the classroom staff at the fluency and generalization stages.

The selection of activities to teach other caregivers is a professional decision that must be based on characteristics of the individual child, the specific activity, and the capabilities and interest of the other individuals. In a series of single-subject design studies, Prieto[106] found that teachers are more likely to encourage children to perform gross motor activities when they have been properly instructed. Soccio[132] compared the frequency of opportunities to practice specific gross motor skills during individual physical therapy sessions and group early intervention classes. There was no difference in the number of opportunities to practice head control when direct physical therapy was compared with integrated group sessions for a child with severe disabilities. Two children with cerebral palsy, however, had more opportunities to practice standing and ambulation activities during direct, individual physical therapy sessions than during integrated group sessions in the classroom. In studies of preschool classes, students sit for approximately 40 minutes of every hour and are in stability positions for about 50 minutes of every hour, which leaves very little time to practice their recommended mobility activities.[114,101] These results suggest that the opportunity to practice motor activities in the classroom varies, based on the type of movement and the class routines. Therapists must select carefully the activities they delegate to others because opportunities for active gross motor movement in classrooms may be very limited.[101]

Procedural Interventions

Procedural interventions in school settings are frequently not as important as the other two components of intervention. However, as noted in Table 31.4, some situations would suggest a need for direct intervention, such as (1) when a child is at a critical period of skill acquisition or regression, (2) when the interventions require the expertise of a physical therapist, and (3) when integrating therapy interferes with the educational program. Best practice, research, and federal law indicate that most, if not all, intervention should occur in the natural environment, with an emphasis on providing multiple opportunities to practice specific skills.[42,43,57,60,121,135] When gross motor skills are learned in isolated settings, such as a physical therapy department, there is little generalization to the more natural environments of the home, school, or recreational settings.[22]

Assessment of the school environment and safety considerations take precedence initially over direct interventions. The physical therapist should participate in the development of written plans for emergency evacuation from the school building and the school bus, in addition to instructing appropriate personnel on the implementation of these plans. The physical therapist should be present during evacuation drills and might assist in the practice of safe techniques using weighted dummies and different models of wheelchairs.

The physical therapist's assessment of the student's environment should begin with proper positioning on the bus and in classrooms. Safety of the aisles for walking or wheelchair mobility should be considered. Architectural barriers must be evaluated and appropriate actions taken to eliminate or lessen them. Teachers and family should be consulted regarding their concerns, and they should be instructed in proper handling, positioning, and use of body mechanics.

Direct intervention, if indicated, should start in the natural environment of the classroom. This is accomplished easily with preschoolers.[57] It is more difficult for children whose educational programs consist primarily of academic subjects that occur in the general education classroom. Physical therapy in the algebra class or school library, after the initial consultation, is generally inappropriate. Common sense must prevail. Perhaps therapy can be delivered during gross motor time in a preschool or during physical education. This is not always appropriate, however, because this might be the only time the child has to engage in free play and physical activity with peers. Taking this opportunity away from the child might affect motivation, cooperation, and the development of important social skills that occurs during these activities.

Merely moving traditional intervention from a special room to a more natural environment is also not in the spirit of best practice. The therapist must adjust intervention to the unique opportunities afforded by the natural environment. Available furniture or classroom items should be used, as opposed to bringing in special equipment. Use of these common objects increases the likelihood that the child might use them to practice and develop motor skills when the therapist is not present and allows the therapist to model their use for the parent or teacher. The specific type of intervention provided depends on the needs of the individual child and the education, training, and experience of the therapist. IDEA 2004 requires that interventions be provided "based on peer-reviewed research to the extent practicable" [PL 108-446, 118 Stat. 2707-2709, § 614(d)(1)(A)(IV)].[112] Although physical therapy intervention has been advancing toward evidence-based practice, many interventions are not supported by sufficient peer-reviewed research. Throughout this text, peer-reviewed research and evidence-based practice are presented when available. Effgen and McEwen[44,45] published systematic reviews of common interventions used in educational settings. Therapists must learn to search the literature for recent developments in research to support the interventions they use. If the appropriate intervention cannot be provided for a school-age child because it is not educationally relevant and is not related to the objectives in the IEP, the therapist has a professional obligation to inform the parents. Once the parents are aware of the focus of school-based physical therapy, they might obtain additional therapy elsewhere.

Careful monitoring of progress is critical in determining the effectiveness of and the need for continued intervention. David[34] outlined a measurement process that has been developed for use by collaborative educational teams. The system involves (1) defining the performance problem, (2) identifying the performance expected and outcome criteria, (3) developing a systematic, simple, and time-efficient measurement strategy, (4) creating a data-graphing system, (5) providing intervention, (6) monitoring progress, and (7) participating in systematic decision making and intervention changes. David stated that "monitoring without decision making is a waste of valuable time and effort."[34] A recommended tool is a simple but comprehensive system of data collection using self-graphing data-collection sheets.[39] The availability of laptop computers has also made data collection and its graphic presentation much easier for many therapists. Extensive documentation is necessary to support the need to increase, decrease, or discontinue intervention. Documentation of the child's status before and after short and long school breaks is important in determining the need for ESY services.

Physical therapy intervention is not a lifelong activity such as learning and fitness. Both therapists and parents must recognize that, after a period of service delivery with no measurable progress, intervention should be discontinued or the model should be changed to monitoring. A persistent desire for walking, for example, is not justification for continued therapy after due diligence in trying to achieve a goal. Therapists report that the most important factor in successful discontinuation of services is the child's achievement of functional goals.[40] Choosing to discontinue direct intervention when goals have not been met continues to be a challenging area of decision making, although tools like the CERT and DRTT should help in the process.

TRANSITION PLANNING

Change can be difficult for anyone, and the transition from one environment to another can be stressful for both children and their parents, especially for those students with a limited repertoire of response competence. Because all transitions are important, two critical times were identified in IDEA when attention must be paid to transition and the provision of transition services. These times include (1) when the child is preparing to move from family-centered early intervention services under Part C to preschool services under Part B[62] and (2) when the student is preparing to transition out of secondary school into the community.[52]

Although the transition from family-centered early intervention services to preschool services is intended to be seamless, the transition process is often difficult for both the child and the family. It is usually accompanied by a change in the state agency providing the services, which typically includes a change in the method of service delivery and in personnel. Family-centered services of early intervention are replaced by school-system services with reduced family involvement and with service providers focused on educational goals. Communication between parents and providers may also become more challenging. Physical therapists have not been as engaged as they should be in the transition process for children from early intervention to preschool. They rarely attend transition team meetings and have not received specialized training in transition, but they do report that they work with families during the transition process.[137] Greater involvement in the transition planning process includes practices supporting communication, collaboration, and strong, positive relationships with early intervention and preschool programs.[96] The School-Based Physical Therapy and the Early-Intervention Special Interest Groups of APTA's Section on Pediatrics collaborated in developing a worksheet to facilitate the communication of pertinent information from the early-intervention therapist to the school-based therapist.[6]

Under IDEA 2004, transition services for postsecondary education constitute

> a coordinated set of activities for a child with a disability that is designed within a results-oriented process that is focused on improving academic and functional achievement of the child with a disability to facilitate the child's movement from school to post-school activities, including postsecondary education, vocational education, integrated employment (including supported employment), continuing and adult education, adult services, independent living, or community participation; is based on the individual child's needs, taking into account the child's strengths, preferences, and interests; and includes instruction, related services, community experiences, the development of employment and other post-school adult living objectives, and, when appropriate, acquisition of daily living skills and functional vocational evaluation. [PL 108-446, 118 Stat. 2658, § 602(34)][112]

Transition assessments and services must begin no later than the first IEP to be in effect when the child is 16 years of age[112] or younger if determined appropriate by the IEP team.[49] Physical therapists should serve on transition teams for children with physical disabilities who are currently receiving services, as well as for those for whom services have been discontinued. A young adult may no longer have a school-related need for physical therapy, but the therapist can assist in evaluating and intervening to facilitate post-school planning and services.

All transition planning should be determined collaboratively by the school team along with both the student and the family. Emphasis should be placed on self-determination, person centeredness, and career orientation.[52] The role of the physical therapist in transition planning and in services for students with physical disabilities might include the following:
- Communication with the family and other transition team members regarding daily routines, physical expectations, and demands of the anticipated new environment
- Communication with the student's vocational rehabilitation counselor, occupational therapist, and teachers regarding preparation for mobility and functional activities in the new setting
- Onsite evaluation of the new physical environment and intervention to ensure the student's ability to physically maneuver throughout the setting
- Evaluation of the accessibility of required transportation systems and intervention as required
- Onsite consultation and education of the student, family, and staff related to the student's physical functioning in that environment
- Onsite assessment and identification of assistive technology needs of the student for the new environment
- Assistance in securing assistive technology and instruction in its use
- Attendance at IEP and other meetings, as appropriate
- Consultation throughout the transition process to ensure that recommendations are appropriate and that the student is successful[130]

Effective transition services can be impeded by issues related to collaboration and communication among team members. These include the following:
- Lack of shared information across agencies
- Follow-up data that could improve services
- Attention to health insurance and transportation
- Systematic transition planning with the agencies that will have responsibility for post-school services
- Anticipating the future needs of the student
- Effective management practices[72]

Although the physical therapist is usually not in a leadership role to make major changes in the transition service system, the therapist can provide assistance in several of the problem areas noted. The therapist has the ability to provide information on health insurance; evaluation of transportation needs; equipment for mobility, positioning, and self-care; and anticipation of the post-school physical demands required of the student. A therapist's knowledge of the physical demands of postschool settings, such as college or work environments, would help the team to assist the student in effective transitioning to those environments. Chapter 32, Transition to Adulthood for Youth with Disabilities, addresses the preparation of youth with disabilities for adult roles, including the use of transition services provided within the education and health care systems.

MANAGEMENT OF PHYSICAL THERAPY SERVICES

Successful management and service delivery in educational environments depend on an understanding of the importance of the team process. The physical therapist, as a member of the educational team, must collaborate effectively with the child, the family, and professionals of other disciplines to promote the child's total well-being through each phase of the educational process. Just as team leaders or case managers are important to intervention teams, a manager or director of physical therapy is also needed in school settings. A majority of directors of physical therapy services in school systems across the nation are not physical therapists or, indeed, any type of related-service personnel.[43] This has serious implications. To understand professional roles and responsibilities and how to nurture a professional, one must understand the profession. Many of the problems encountered in school systems could probably be prevented if an experienced therapist provided supervision. Therapist managers understand the profession and are able to address appropriately management issues. States such as Iowa and North Carolina, where therapists are employed by the state department of education, have become national leaders in setting policy for related-service providers. These therapists help to coordinate services throughout the state and educate both therapists and educators regarding the role of physical therapists in educational environments.

Therapists, unlike teachers, are educated to work in a wide variety of settings, but few have the opportunity to learn about school-based practice. Those who are new to practice in educational environments in general and those who are new to a particular school system should receive orientation, mentoring, and in-service education. The roles and responsibilities of the therapist and all support staff should be clearly identified in a detailed job description that complies with federal and state laws, as well as the state's physical therapy practice act. As part of a planned orientation program, therapists should be introduced to the entire team of professionals with whom they will be working at all sites. They need to know whom to ask for equipment, space, and other items necessary for successful intervention. Therapists need to know how referrals are received and handled; how workloads and caseloads are determined; how team meetings are planned and when they are scheduled; the written policies and procedures; how peer review or quality improvement is done; emergency procedures; and the policy for continuing education, to name but a few issues. These are not unusual requests, and they can be addressed easily and cost-effectively in any system.

After the therapist is properly introduced and oriented to the school district, administrators and therapists must continue to communicate regularly before problems arise, especially with therapists who are not school employees. Contracted therapists report rarely being included in school activities.[65] Frequent areas of discontent include too much travel among school buildings, as well as insufficient continuing-education opportunities, peer contact, a place to work, and time allotted for administrative tasks and meetings.[43,65] More time and effort should be spent on retention of physical therapists to reduce the need for recruitment and for continuity of care for the students.

All state physical therapy state practice acts in the United States now allow a therapist to examine and evaluate without a physician's referral, and most also permit therapists to provide intervention without a referral, though specific requirements vary by state.[10] In states where physician authorization is required for intervention, a system should be developed for obtaining referrals. The referral allows the therapist to determine and provide appropriate intervention. Depending on the complexity of the student's medical problems and the need for pertinent information, it might be prudent for the therapist to obtain a referral even when it is not legally required. Collaboration with physicians and all other members of the child's medical and educational team promotes optimal service delivery.

School districts need to develop guidelines to determine therapy workloads, as well as for decision making with regard to who should receive intervention and how much intervention should be provided. This can be a difficult task. The CERT, DRTT, and the APTA Section on Pediatrics fact sheet on dosage considerations (see Table 31.4) should assist in the decision-making process.[7,26,53] Children with critical needs for therapy require more intense intervention than do those with lesser needs. A therapist whose workload primarily includes children who require extensive therapy can serve fewer children than a therapist whose caseload mostly comprises children with minimal needs. A clear system of documentation is needed to support the complex, sensitive decisions regarding allocation of physical therapy services. The American Occupational Therapy Association, APTA, and the American Speech-Language-Hearing Association have produced a joint document on the workload approach for more effective service delivery and student outcomes.[2]

Through the American Recovery and Reinvestment Act of 2009 (ARRA), the Race to the Top Fund provided $4.35 billion in competitive-grant funding aimed at improving student achievement. A major component of that legislation focused on evaluating teacher effectiveness, based on both professional performance and student outcomes. In many states, related service providers, like physical therapists, are included in this initiative. Each state has established its own guidelines, and school districts within each state have chosen their own evaluation tools. Some states use modified versions of the Danielson[33] or Stronge[134] model. The School-Based Physical Therapy Special Interest Group of APTA's Section on Pediatrics developed a document that outlines an appropriate evaluation tool for physical therapists, based on the competencies described by Effgen, Chiarello, and Milbourne.[46]

ISSUES IN SCHOOL-BASED PRACTICE

Shortage of Pediatric Physical Therapists

Insufficient numbers of pediatric physical therapists with the skill set for serving children in the educational setting has been an ongoing problem. It may become worse as many of the therapists initially hired with the enactment of PL 94-142 begin to retire. Shortages of therapists may be attributed to relatively low pay, professional isolation, benefits of other areas of practice, and challenges of working with children. Solutions are numerous and sometimes complex, but one of the easiest is often neglected. An effective way to train and then recruit new physical therapists is to offer student clinical affiliations in educational settings.

Physical therapy is not the only school-based profession where shortages exist. The National Coalition on Personnel Shortages in Special Education and Related Services (NCPSSERS) notes that 49 states report shortages of special education teachers and specialized instructional support personnel.[98] The coalition represents 30 national, state, and local professional organizations from eight different disciplines. Its stated mission is "to sustain a discussion among all stakeholders on the need for and value of special education, related services, and early intervention; and to identify, disseminate, and support implementation of national, state, and local strategies to remedy personnel shortages and persistent vacancies for the benefit of all children and youth."[98]

Service-Delivery System

A dearth of qualified school-based physical therapists has affected the type of service-delivery system used and the roles assumed by school personnel. The literature supports integrated or collaborative service-delivery models.[61,122] There are obvious advantages to more frequent practice in natural settings with the support of all those who interact with the student. An appropriately administered therapy program in the natural environment might require more, not fewer, personnel. Training all staff members in an integrated or collaborative model requires a great deal of time for instruction and meetings.[55] There are those, however, who incorrectly think that these models can be used to decrease the time required for physical therapy. It should be noted that "Teams Take Time" (the three T's). Instead of direct intervention by a therapist, unqualified staff might perform activities without adequate supervised instruction, or a teacher might be forced to provide an intervention for which he or she is not properly trained. Instead of providing the intervention in a room with necessary equipment, a classroom or hallway is used in the name of natural environment. Rarely are empirical data sufficient to support any specific service-delivery system.

A national study, *Physical Therapy Related Child Outcomes in the Schools* (PT COUNTS),[41] found that students were seen for physical therapy an average of 26.8 minutes/week. The majority of physical therapy services were provided individually (average 23.3 minutes per week) and separate from school activities (average 19.6 minutes per week). Very little time was spent on activities within the context of school (average 9.5 minutes per week). Therapists spent approximately 13.2 minutes per week providing services on behalf of the student, which primarily included consultation, collaboration, and documentation. As measured on the School Function Assessment (SFA), students who were younger than 8 years of age with higher gross motor function improved more than students who were older and had lower gross motor function. There were statistically significant differences based on Gross Motor Function Classification[102] (GMFCS) levels; students at levels IV/V (lowest functional ability) made less improvement in all SFA subscales except *Travel*. On the individualized goal outcomes measured using GAS, on average, students achieved and slightly exceeded their expected goal attainment for their primary goal, as well as the goals categorized as *posture/mobility, recreation/fitness,* and *self-care*. The majority of students improved on their primary goal (75%), with 35% achieving goal expectations and 40% exceeding goal expectations. Goal attainment did not differ significantly for students by GMFCS level, diagnostic group, or between those receiving or not receiving outpatient physical therapy. Students 5 to 7 years of age had higher goal attainment for their primary goal compared to students 8 to 12 years of age. More minutes spent on services on behalf of the student (consultation/collaboration and documentation) were predictive of higher levels of goal attainment for *posture/mobility*. More minutes in self-care activities and services on behalf of the students were associated with exceeding goal expectations. An increase in 100 minutes of services on behalf of the student (5 minutes per week) increased the odds of exceeding goal expectations by 24%.[47] Consulting and collaborating with teachers, parents, and others were likely to have positively influenced student outcomes, probably by providing an understanding of the student's goals involving physical therapy and educating others on the importance of providing practice opportunities for fluency and generalization of skills. Documentation requires a thoughtful review of what was and what will be done with the student. This reflection might lead to more appropriate interventions with positive outcomes.

Professional Roles

In school systems with a full staff, professionals can collaborate to decide on the role of each team member. Overlap of professional roles is acknowledged, and divisions of responsibility are made that are best suited to the needs of the child, school system, and professional staff.[142] In general, the overlap in physical therapy, occupational therapy, and education is greatest when professionals from these disciplines are serving young children. For older children, less overlap in professional roles exists. Areas of frequent overlap between occupational therapy and physical therapy include programs for strength and endurance, body awareness, classroom positioning and adaptations, enhancement of motor experience, and sensory integration. Areas of overlap between physical therapists and educators might include advanced gross motor skills, endurance training, and transfers. In systems with a critical shortage of physical therapists, the breadth of roles assumed by other staff members increases, based on need and not necessarily on professional skill.

Educationally Relevant Physical Therapy

For decades, parents of children with disabilities, school administrators, teachers, and school-based physical therapists have debated the role of school-based physical therapy as compared with clinic-based services. In school districts with an adequate number of therapists, where there is a commitment to providing appropriate services for students with disabilities, the definition of educationally relevant physical therapy is comprehensive; it depends on the individual needs of the child, as addressed at the IEP meeting. IDEA clearly indicates that education is intended to prepare students for independent living and economic self-sufficiency, which have broad implications for the provision of physical therapy.[112]

Physical therapy is perceived as more educationally relevant when the entire IEP team mutually agrees upon goals and objectives. The educational system was never meant to provide for all of the child's therapy needs. Physical therapy may be provided outside of the educational system as needed; all therapists serving the child should collaborate and coordinate services. Therapists and parents must remember that therapy takes time away from other educational and social opportunities that are vital to the total well-being of the child. These competing priorities must be considered when making decisions regarding service delivery.[8] Educators and therapists alike must continually ask themselves if they are truly meeting the needs of each individual child.

Reimbursement for Services

The cost of providing related services in educational environments is a serious concern of program administrators. IDEA provides some federal funding to states, but it has never been sufficient to encompass the full spectrum of services needed by students in special education. To cover the costs of physical therapy, some school districts are charging third-party payers. This can be problematic because of the lifetime cap on many insurance policies, limited therapy coverage, and the possibility of losing insurance if bills are too high. Parents are not required to have their insurance company pay for these services, and they should not be intimidated into thinking that their child will not receive services without insurance payment. School districts may also bill Medicaid directly for physical therapy; however, reimbursement is usually based on direct services, and consultation, team intervention, and group services are discouraged. Medicaid rules and regulations are determined by each individual state, and therapists should be active at the state level to make certain that these rules and regulations facilitate and do not hinder appropriate school-based intervention.

Transportation

Transportation of children receiving special education is a required related service. Ensuring that they are transported safely and efficiently is the responsibility of the school district. Many individuals assist in the transportation process, and the National Highway Traffic Safety Administration[99] offers numerous resources that address the safe transportation of children. A physical therapist might be asked to assess the safety of seating of a student with a disability in a school bus seat or wheelchair, embarking and disembarking from the bus, emergency evacuation procedures, and the lifting techniques used by transportation personnel. Central to the therapist's role is an understanding of what makes a wheelchair appropriate for transportation, as well as how to tie down the wheelchair and use occupant-restraint systems. Team discussions regarding plans for emergency evacuation should include issues related to the student's size, weight, and height; implications of different medical diagnoses (e.g., osteogenesis imperfecta); orthopedic concerns; physical limitations; ability of the student to assist; whether a student stays in the wheelchair; and who gets off the bus first and last. Competence in transportation issues, which may be overlooked by some school-based therapists, is a critical component of service delivery.

Therapists New to the Educational Environment

Many school-based physical therapists begin their careers by working in adult or other pediatric settings. Upon entering the educational environment, those who are parents enjoy the benefit of having the same school hours and vacation schedules as their children. Therefore it is not uncommon for experienced therapists to seek employment in school settings with little or no background in pediatrics and lacking an understanding of the unique requirements of working under IDEA. Therapists who are new to school practice must immediately learn the rules and regulations of IDEA, as outlined in this chapter and as available from the suggested websites and references. In addition, they must be aware of individual state education laws, special education laws, and their state physical therapy practice act. It is the therapists' responsibility to be knowledgeable of the laws that govern practice in schools, just as they should know the rules for reimbursement and practice in hospital settings. In

this era of limited resources, administrators have been known to say that services are not appropriate for a child with a disability because they want to avoid paying for such a service. They might also say that because a therapist is not available, therapy cannot be recommended in the IEP. Of course, this is incorrect, but most parents and many therapists will not know that unless they are well versed in the laws.

School-based therapists need to become effective members of a team, using the various models described in this chapter. Those who have worked in other pediatric settings, such as early intervention and pediatric hospitals, may be accustomed to working with a team, as may therapists who have worked in rehabilitation settings. Therapists who have practiced in outpatient physical therapy settings, however, may not be adequately familiar with team functioning and the degree of role release and collaboration required in the school setting.

Intervention is also somewhat different from in educational environments than in other settings. As discussed in this chapter, goals and objectives must be educationally relevant. Intervention is based on the *Guide*,[3] including coordination, communication, and documentation, as well as patient/client-related instruction. For children who demonstrate a need for physical therapy as outlined in Table 31.4, procedural interventions might be provided. However, many students do not require direct intervention, and this change in focus can be difficult for some therapists who are accustomed to providing direct services.

Therapists new to school practice would be wise to seek an experienced mentor, either within or outside the school system. Many school therapists work in isolation, and they do not have access to the guidance and support provided in other clinical settings. They work frequently with teachers but not necessarily with other therapists who can evaluate their knowledge and skills and with whom they can discuss cases. School administrators need to recognize the effect of this professional isolation for both experienced therapists and those new to the school environment, and they should support the therapist in finding a mentor.

Therapists, especially new graduates and those new to educational environments, should strive to achieve the competencies for school-based physical therapists as outlined in Box 31.4.[46] For therapist performance appraisal, the APTA Section on Pediatrics has added competencies in advocacy and administration. These competencies may also be shared with administrators to help define the role of school-based physical therapy and to identify the resources necessary for effective service delivery. Therapists should continually read professional literature, participate in continuing education, take postprofessional courses, join journal clubs, and engage in dialogue with colleagues. The APTA Section on Pediatrics offers a wide variety of excellent resources for school-based therapists. Employers need to support therapists' efforts at ongoing professional development.

Physical Fitness for All Students

Although school-based physical therapists are usually employed to serve students with disabilities who have IEPs or Section 504 plans, some school districts are more inclusive and involve therapists in a broader range of services. This might include determination of architectural barriers, safe transportation, prevention of athletic injuries, and promoting developmentally appropriate motor programs. The national crisis regarding obesity and physical fitness of all students suggests that

BOX 31.4   Competencies for School-Based Physical Therapists

Content Area 1: The Context of Therapy Practice in Schools

1. Describe competencies for school-based physical therapists.
   a. Diagram the functional and supervisory organization of the education system served by the therapist.
   b. Identify the goals and outcomes of the educational curriculum from preschool through high school.
   c. Demonstrate an understanding of the eventual goals of independent living and working.
   d. Apply knowledge of the outcomes-based education curriculum.
2. Demonstrate knowledge of federal (for example, IDEA, Rehabilitation Act of 1973, ADA), state, and local laws and regulations that affect the delivery of services to students with disabilities.
   a. Discuss the implications of the laws (national, state, and local).
   b. Apply the guidelines of federal, state, and local regulations.
   c. Identify and use information sources for federal, state, and local legislation and regulation changes.
   d. Discuss and demonstrate professional behavior regarding ethical and legal responsibilities.
   e. Discuss professional competencies as defined by professional organizations and state regulations.
   f. Advocate to support services related to educational entitlements.
3. Apply knowledge of the theoretical and functional orientation of a variety of professionals serving students within the educational system.
   a. Initiate dialogue with colleagues to exchange professional perspectives.
   b. Disseminate information about the availability of therapy services, criteria for eligibility, and methods of referral.
   c. Describe evaluations and interventions commonly used by psychologists, diagnostic educators, classroom teachers, speech and language pathologists, adaptive physical educators, nurses, physical therapists, occupational therapists, and professionals in other education and health-related disciplines.
4. Assist students in accessing community organizations, resources, and activities.
   a. Demonstrate awareness of cultural and social differences that relate to family and student participation in the education program.
   b. In collaboration with the educational team, develop a plan for transition into community activities or adult services.
   c. Identify the need to make appropriate student referrals to community therapy and recreational services when school services are not able to meet all of the child's needs.
   d. Include the family in the educational process.
   e. Serve as a resource to family and other team members for information and appropriate community resources (medical, educational, financial, social, recreational, and legal).

Content Area 2: Wellness and Prevention in Schools

1. Implement school-wide screening program with school nurse, physical education teacher, and teachers.
   a. Apply knowledge of risk factors affecting growth, development, and learning.
   b. Identify the etiology, signs, symptoms, and classifications of common pediatric disabilities.
   c. Identify established biologic and environmental factors that affect children's development and learning.
   d. Select, administer, and interpret a variety of screening instruments and standardized measurement tools.
2. Promote child safety and wellness using knowledge of environmental safety measures.
   a. Maintain cardiopulmonary resuscitation (CPR) certification.
   b. Institute an environmental hazards and accident prevention plan.
   c. Recognize child neglect and abuse.

Content Area 3: Team Collaboration

1. Form partnerships and work collaboratively with other team members, especially the teacher to promote an effective plan of care.
   a. Demonstrate effective communication and interpersonal skills.
   b. Refer and coordinate services among family, school professionals, medical service providers, and community agencies.
   c. Implement strategies for team development and management.
   d. Develop mechanism for ongoing team coordination.
2. Function as a consultant.
   a. Identify the administrative and interpersonal factors that influence the effectiveness of a consultant.
   b. Implement effective consultative strategies.
   c. Provide technical assistance to other school team members, community agencies, and medical providers.
3. Educate school personnel and family to promote inclusion of the student within the educational experience.
   a. Assist school administrators with development of policy and procedures.
   b. Provide orientation to teachers and classroom aides.
   c. Conduct in-service sessions.
   d. Develop informational resources.
4. Supervise personnel and professional students.
   a. Apply effective strategies of supervision.
   b. Monitor the implementation of therapy recommendations by other team members.
   c. Establish a student clinical affiliation.
   d. Formally and informally teach or train therapy staff.
5. Serve as an advocate for students, families, and school.
   a. Attend public hearings.
   b. Serve on task force or decision-making committees.
   c. Provide necessary information to support student rights.
   d. Actively participate in the individualized educational program (IEP) process.

Content Area 4: Examination and Evaluation in Schools

1. Identify strengths and needs of student.
   a. Interview student, family, teachers, and other relevant school personnel.
   b. Gather information from medical personnel and records.
   c. Observe student in a variety of educational settings.
2. Collaboratively determine examination and evaluation process.
   a. Designate appropriate professional disciplines.
   b. Identify environments and student activities and routines.
   c. Select instruments.
   d. Establish format for conducting examination.
   e. Inform and prepare the student.
3. Determine student's ability to participate in meaningful school activities by examining and evaluating the following:
   a. Conduct of formal naturalistic observations to determine level of participation and necessary assistance and adaptations.
   b. Functional abilities, including gross motor, fine motor, perceptual motor, cognitive, social and emotional, and activities of daily living (ADLs).
   c. Impairments related to functional ability, including musculoskeletal status, neuromotor organization, sensory function, and cardiopulmonary status.
4. Utilize valid, reliable, cost-effective, and nondiscriminatory instruments for the following:
   a. Identification and eligibility.
   b. Diagnostic purposes.
   c. Individual program planning.
   d. Documentation of progress.

Content Area 5: Planning

1. Actively participate in the development of the IEP.
   a. Determine eligibility related to a student's educational program.
   b. Accurately interpret and communicate examination findings collaboratively with family, student, and other team members.
   c. Discuss prognosis of student performance related to curricular expectations.
   d. Discuss and prioritize outcomes related to student's educational needs based on current and future environmental demands and student and family preferences and goals.
   e. Offer appropriate recommendations for student placement and personnel needs in the least restrictive educational setting with intent to serve children in inclusive environments.

Continued

BOX 31.4   Competencies for School-Based Physical Therapists—cont'd

f. In collaboration with the team, determine how therapy can contribute to the development of an IEP, including the following:
   i. Meaningful student outcomes.
   ii. Functional and measurable goals and objectives.
   iii. Therapy service recommendations.
   iv. Specific intervention methods and strategies.
   v. Determination of frequency, intensity, and duration.
g. Develop mechanism for ongoing coordination and collaboration regarding the following:
   i. Implementation of the IEP.
   ii. Updates or modifications of IEP.
   iii. Transition planning and implementation of the transition plan.
   iv. Interagency activities.

Content Area 6: Intervention

1. Adapt environments to facilitate student access to and participation in student activities.
   a. Recommend adaptive equipment, assistive technology, and environmental adaptations.
   b. Monitor adaptive equipment, assistive technology, and environmental adaptations.
   c. Be able to instruct student and other team members in the appropriate use of adaptive equipment and assistive technology.
   d. Identify sources for obtaining, maintaining, repairing, and financing adaptive equipment, assistive technology, and environmental adaptations.
2. Use various types and methods of service provision for individualized student interventions.
   a. Employ direct, individual, group, integrated, consultative, monitoring, and collaborative approaches.
   b. Develop generic instruction plans and intervention plans that select and sequence strategies to meet the objectives listed on the student's IEP.
3. Promote skill acquisition, fluency, and generalization to enhance overall development, learning, and student participation.
   a. Use creative problem-solving strategies to meet the student's needs.
   b. Explain the basic motor learning theories, and relate them to therapy education programs.
   c. Address neuromuscular, musculoskeletal, sensory processing, and cardiopulmonary functions that support motor, social, emotional, cognitive, and language skills.
4. Embed therapy interventions into the context of student activities and routines.
   a. Implement appropriate positioning, mobility, environmental, and ADL strategies into curriculum, classroom schedule, and routines.
   b. Develop a matrix integrating objectives, routines and activities, and strategies.

Content Area 7: Documentation

1. Produce useful written documentation by doing the following:
   a. Writing reports in commonly understood and meaningful terms.
   b. Maintaining timely and consistent records.
   c. Concisely summarizing relevant information.
   d. Sharing records with family and other team members.
2. Collaboratively monitor and modify student's IEP.
   a. Establish a mechanism for and record ongoing communication with family and other team members.
   b. Establish a plan of action for reevaluation.
   c. Schedule preestablished team meetings to review student progress over the course of the school year.

3. Evaluate and document the effectiveness of therapy education programs.
   a. Establish baseline of student's level of participation and functional status.
   b. Collect ongoing data on the student's progress toward stated IEP outcomes.
   c. Summarize data to determine student's progress.

Content Area 8: Administrative Issues in Schools

1. Demonstrate flexibility, priority setting, and effective time management strategies.
2. Obtain resources and data necessary to justify establishing a new therapy program or altering an existing program.
3. Serve as a leader.
   a. Integrate knowledge of education, health, and social trends that affect therapy services.
   b. Identify and educate others on the overall roles, responsibilities, and functions of therapy services.
   c. Identify and differentiate characteristics of alternative approaches for resolving needs of therapy services.
   d. Identify the administrative needs of the therapy service within the school setting.
   e. Serve as a role model for other therapists regarding professional responsibilities.
4. Serve as a manager.
   a. Develop and analyze job descriptions for therapists.
   b. Implement a recruitment, orientation, mentorship, and professional development program for therapists and staff.
   c. Develop and implement policies and procedures to guide therapy services.
   d. Establish therapy caseloads [workloads], and staffing needs.
   e. Evaluate the performance of therapy personnel.
   f. Plan and implement a therapy quality assurance plan and program evaluation.
   g. Participate in the assessment of school facilities and educational activities.
   h. Make recommendations, especially related to ensuring accessibility and reasonable accommodations to school environments.
   i. Identify and use appropriate school, home, community, state, and national resources, especially funding sources.
   j. Demonstrate the ability to plan and manage a budget for the therapy component of services.

Content Area 9: Research

1. Demonstrate knowledge of current research related to child development, medical care, educational practices, and implications for therapy.
   a. Conduct a literature review.
   b. Seek assistance of experienced researchers in interpreting published research.
   c. Critically evaluate published research.
2. Apply knowledge of research to the selection of therapy intervention strategies, service delivery systems, and therapeutic procedures.
   a. Use objective criteria for evaluation.
   b. Justify rationale for clinical decision making.
   c. Expand clinical treatment case reports into single-subject studies.
3. Partake in program evaluation and clinical research activities with appropriate supervision.
   a. Identify research topics.
   b. Secure resources to support clinical research.
   c. Implement clinical research projects.
   d. Disseminate research findings.

From Effgen SK, Chiarello L, Milbourne S: Updated competencies for physical therapists working in schools, *Pediatr Phy Ther* 19:266-274, 2007.

school-based physical therapists should address these issues, in collaboration with physical educators.[87,93,104,126] Physical inactivity threatens not only physical but also cognitive health.[63] The evidence strongly supports physical activity programs for students with developmental disabilities to improve aerobic capacity, gross motor performance, and child/parent satisfaction.[71] A systematic review of studies of children and adults with intellectual disabilities also found that exercise interventions assist in decreasing challenging behaviors.[100] Additionally, physical activity has been shown to improve mental health and classroom performance in children with autism and attention deficit hyperactivity disorder.[105] The reader is encouraged to review the national website on Walk/Bike to School (www.walk-biketoschool.org) to learn about fun ways to encourage healthy habits and regular physical activity for all students. Evaluation and intervention for physical fitness are covered in Chapter 6, Physical Fitness During Childhood and Adolescence.

SUMMARY

In the United States, physical therapy is included as part of federally sponsored programs to serve infants, toddlers, children, and youth with disabilities. For preschool- and school-age children, physical therapy is a related service of the educational program under IDEA for children who require special education or under Section 504 of the Rehabilitation Act. The school setting is not the high-tech, health-focused environment of the modern hospital setting or the therapy-focused environment of the rehabilitation setting. Rather, the educational needs of students are the highest priority. To provide effective services and attain personal satisfaction, therapists must become knowledgeable of the educational milieu, including federal, state, and local laws, and regulations that govern physical therapy in the educational environment.

Physical therapists working in school settings witness firsthand the successes and struggles that students with special needs experience in their everyday lives as they participate in the school environment. As members of a team of professionals, physical therapists are asked to solve complex problems to enhance the ability of children to participate in educational programs. The educational environment is rewarding for physical therapists willing and able to meet the unique demands of this practice setting.

Case Scenario on Expert Consult

The case scenario related to this chapter includes a longitudinal case scenario and video on school-based physical therapy. Adrianna is presented. Her case highlights issues and challenges that are frequently encountered by physical therapists in school-based practice, including (1) promotion of the student's participation in the educational program in the least restrictive environment, (2) collaboration with other team members and physicians, (3) flexibility in selecting models of service delivery based on the student's goals, and (4) guidance for transition planning.

REFERENCES

1. Alberto PA, Troutman AC: *Applied behavior analysis for teachers*, ed 9, Boston, 2013, Pearson.
2. American Occupational Therapy Association, American Physical Therapy Association, American Speech-Language-Hearing Association: Workload approach: a paradigm shift for positive impact on student outcomes. Retrieved from: https://pediatricapta.org/special-interest-groups/SB/pdfs/APTA-ASHA-AOTA-Joint-Doc-Workload-Approach-.pdf, 2014.
3. American Physical Therapy Association: *Guide to physical therapist practice 3.0*, Alexandria, VA, 2014, American Physical Therapy Association. Retrieved from: http://guidetoptpractice.apta.org/.
4. American Physical Therapy Association, Section on Pediatrics: FAQs on response to intervention (RTI) for school-based physical therapists. Retrieved from: https://pediatricapta.org/includes/fact-sheets/pdfs/11%20FAQs%20for%20School%20PTs.pdf, 2011.
5. American Physical Therapy Association, Section on Pediatrics: School-based physical therapy: conflicts between Individuals with Disabilities Education Act (IDEA) and legal requirements of state practice acts and regulations. Retrieved from: https://pediatricapta.org/includes/fact-sheets/pdfs/14%20State%20Practice%20Acts%20IDEA.pdf, 2014.
6. American Physical Therapy Association, Section on Pediatrics: Transition worksheet for early intervention and school-based physical therapy providers. Retrieved from: https://pediatricapta.org/includes/fact-sheets/pdfs/EI-SB%20Transition%20Worksheet%20for%20Ped%20PTs.pdf, 2014.
7. American Physical Therapy Association, Section on Pediatrics: Dosage considerations: recommending school-based physical therapy intervention under IDEA resource manual. Retrieved from: https://pediatricapta.org/includes/fact-sheets/pdfs/15%20Dosage%20Consideration%20Resource%20Manual.pdf, 2015.
8. American Physical Therapy Association, Section on Pediatrics: Physical therapy for educational benefit. Retrieved from: https://pediatricapta.org/includes/fact-sheets/pdfs/15%20PT%20for%20Educational%20Benefit.pdf, 2015.
9. American Physical Therapy Association: Defensible documentation resource—an introduction. Retrieved from: http://www.apta.org, 2009.
10. American Physical Therapy Association: A summary of direct access language in state physical therapy practice acts. Retrieved from: http://www.apta.org/uploadedFiles/APTAorg/Advocacy/State/Issues/Direct_Access/DirectAccessbyState.pdf.
11. Arnold SH, McEwen IR: Item test-retest reliability and responsiveness of the school outcomes measure (SOM), *Phys Occup Ther Pediatr* 28:59–77, 2008.
12. Arnold SH, et al.: Assessing the discriminative ability and internal consistency of the School Outcomes Measure. ISRN rehabilitation, article ID 607416. Retrieved from: http://dx.doi.org/10.1155/2013/607416, 2013.
13. Bailes AF, et al.: Development of guidelines for determining frequency of therapy services in a pediatric medical setting, *Pediatr Phys Ther* 20:194–198, 2008.
14. Baker BJ, Cole, et al.: Cognitive referencing as a method of OT/PT triage for young children, *Pediatr Phys Ther* 10:2–6, 1998.
15. Reference deleted in proofs.
16. Batten HE: The industrial school for crippled and deformed children, *Phys Ther Rev* 13:112–113, 1933.
17. Battle v. Commonwealth of Pennsylvania, 629 F 269, 1981.
18. Blatt B, Kaplan F: *Christmas in purgatory: a photographic essay on mental retardation*, Boston, 1966, Allyn & Bacon.
19. Board of Education of Hendrick Hudson Central School District, Westchester County, et al. v. Amy Rowley, 347 U.S. 176, 1982.
20. Braddock D: *Federal policy toward mental retardation and developmental disabilities*, Baltimore, 1987, Paul H. Brookes, p 71.
21. Brown v. Board of Education of Topeka, 347 U.S. 488, 1954.
22. Brown DA, et al.: Performance following ability-focused physical therapy intervention in individuals with severely limited physical and cognitive abilities, *Phys Ther* 78:934–949, 1998.
23. Cable OE, et al.: The crippled children's guide of Buffalo, New York, *Phys Ther Rev* 16:85–88, 1938.
24. Carr SH: Louisiana's criteria of eligibility for occupational therapy services in the public school system, *Am J Occup Ther* 43:503–506, 1989.
25. Carter E, et al.: Peer interactions and academic engagement of youth with developmental disabilities in inclusive middle and high school classrooms, *Am J Ment Retard* 113:479–494, 2008.
26. Cecere SW, Williams JK: *Determination of relevant therapy tool (DRTT)*, unpublished manuscript, 2013.
27. Cedar Rapids Community School District v. Garret F., 526 U.S. 66, 1999.
28. Cole C, et al.: Academic progress of students across inclusive and traditional settings, *Ment Retard* 42:136–144, 2004.

29. Cole KN, et al.: Retrospective analysis of physical and occupational therapy progress in young children: an examination of cognitive referencing, *Pediatr Phys Ther* 3:185–189, 1991.

30. Coster W, et al.: *School function assessment*, San Antonio, TX, 1998, The Psychological Corporation.

31. Cruickshank WM: *Psychology of exceptional children and youth*, ed 4, Englewood Cliffs, NJ, 1980, Prentice-Hall, pp 65–66.

32. Damiano DL: Activity, activity, activity: rethinking our physical therapy approach to cerebral palsy, *Phys Ther* 86:1534–1540, 2006.

33. Danielson C: Danielson group: the framework. Retrieved from: http://danielsongroup.org/framework/, 2015.

34. David KS: Monitoring process for improved outcomes, *Phys Occup Ther Pediatr* 16:47–76, 1996.

35. Davies PL, et al.: Validity and reliability of the School Function Assessment in elementary school students with disabilities, *Phys Occup Ther Pediatr* 24:23–43, 2004.

36. Deno E: Special education as developmental capital, *Exception Child* 37:229–237, 1970.

37. Dole RL, et al.: Consensus among experts in pediatric occupational and physical therapy on elements of individualized education programs, *Pediatr Phys Ther* 15:159–166, 2003.

38. Reference deleted in proofs.

39. Effgen SK: Systematic delivery and recording of intervention assistance, *Pediatr Phys Ther* 3:63–68, 1991.

40. Effgen SK: Factors affecting the termination of physical therapy services for children in school settings, *Pediatr Phys Ther* 12:121–126, 2000.

41. Effgen SK, Chan L: Occurrence of gross motor behaviors and attainment of motor objectives in children with cerebral palsy participating in conductive education, *Physiother Theory Pract* 26:22–39, 2010.

42. Effgen SK, Kaminker MK: Nationwide survey of school-based physical therapy practice, *Pediatr Phys Ther* 26:394–403, 2014.

43. Effgen SK, Klepper S: Survey of physical therapy practice in educational settings, *Pediatr Phys Ther* 6:15–21, 1994.

44. Effgen SK, McEwen I: *Review of selected physical therapy interventions for school-age children with disabilities (COPSSE document Number OP-4)*, Gainesville, FL, 2007, University of Florida, Center on Personnel Studies in Special Education. Retrieved from: http://www.coe.ufl.edu/copsse/docs/PT_CP_090707_5/1/PT_CP_090707_5.pdf.

45. Effgen SK, McEwen I: Review of selected physical therapy interventions for school-age children with disabilities, *Phys Ther Rev* 13:297–312, 2008.

46. Effgen SK, et al.: Updated competencies for physical therapists working in schools, *Pediatr Phys Ther* 19:266–274, 2007.

47. Effgen SK, et al.: Executive summary: relationship of student outcomes to school-based physical therapy service. PT COUNTS. Retrieved from: http://www.mc.uky.edu/healthsciences/grants/ptcounts/docs/Executive%20Summary%203-23-15%20revised.pdf, 2015.

48. Effgen SK, et al.: The PT COUNTS study: an example of practice based evidence research, *Pediatr Phys Ther* 28:47–56, 2016.

49. Federal Register, Part II, Department of Education: 34 CFR Parts 300 and 301, Assistance to states for the education of children with disabilities and preschool grants for children with disabilities; and service obligations under special education. Personnel development to improve services and results for children with disabilities: final rule. Retrieved from: http://idea.ed.gov/download/finalregulations.pdf, August 14, 2006.

50. Federal Register, Part II, Department of Education: 34 CFR Part 200, Title I—Improving the academic achievement of the disadvantaged, final rule, vol 68, no 236, pp 68697–68708. Retrieved from: http://www.ed.gov/legislation/FedRegister/finrule/2003-4/120903a.html, December 9, 2003.

51. Federal Register, Part II, Department of Education: 34 CFR Parts 300 and 301: assistance to states for the education of children with disabilities program and preschool grants for children with disabilities, final rule, vol 57, no 189, September 29, 1992.

52. Flexer RW, et al.: *Transition planning for secondary students with disabilities*, ed 4, Upper Saddle River, NJ, 2012, Prentice-Hall.

53. Florida Department of Education: Exceptional Education & Student Services: considerations for educationally relevant therapy (CERT). Retrieved from: http://www.fldoe.org/ESE/cert.asp, 2009.

54. Georgia Association of Retarded Citizens v. McDaniel, 716 F. 2d 1565 (1981), ed 13 Law Rep. 609.

55. Giangreco MF, et al.: Providing related services to learners with severe handicaps in educational settings: pursuing the least restrictive option, *Pediatr Phys Ther* 1:55–63, 1989.

56. Givins EV: The spastic child in the classroom, *Phys Ther Rev* 18:136–137, 1938.

57. Guralnick MJ: *Early childhood inclusion*, Baltimore, 2001, Paul H. Brookes.

58. Haley SM, et al.: Pediatric Evaluation of Disability Inventory Computer Adaptive Test (PEDI-CAT). Retrieved from: http://pedicat.com/category/versions/, 2015.

59. Haley SM, et al.: *Pediatric Evaluation of Disability Inventory (PEDI)*, San Antonio, TX, 1992, The Psychological Corporation.

60. Hanft BE, et al.: *Coaching families and colleagues in early childhood*, Baltimore, 2004, Paul H. Brookes.

61. Hanft B, Shepherd J, editors: *Collaborating for student success: a guide for school-based occupational therapy*, Bethesda, MD, 2008, American Occupational Therapy Association.

62. Hanson MJ, et al.: Entering preschool: family and professional experiences in this transition process, *J Early Interv* 23:279–293, 2000.

63. Hillman CH: I. An introduction to the relation of physical activity to cognitive and brain health, and scholastic achievement, *Monogr Soc Res Child Dev* 79:1–6, 2014.

64. Holler RA, Zirkel PA: Section 504 and public schools: a national survey concerning "Section 504-only" students, *National Association of Secondary School Principals Bulletin* 92:19, 2008. Retrieved from: http://bul.sagepub.com/cgi/content/abstract/92/1/19.

65. Holt S, et al.: School-based physical therapists' perceptions of school-based practices, *Phys Occup Ther Pediatr* 35:381–395, 2015.

66. Hunt P, et al.: Collaborative teaming to support students at risk and students with severe disabilities in general education classrooms, *Exception Child* 69:315–332, 2003.

67. Hwang J, et al.: Validation of school function assessment with elementary school children, *Occupation Participation Health* 22:48–58, 2002.

68. Iowa Department of Education: *Iowa guidelines for educationally related physical therapy services*, Des Moines, IA, 2001, Author.

69. Irving Independent School District v. Tatro, 468 U.S. 883 (1984).

70. Jackson S, et al.: Response to intervention: implications for early childhood professionals, *Lang Speech Hear Serv Sch* 40:424–434, 2009.

71. Johnson CC: The benefits of physical activity for youth with developmental disabilities: a systematic review, *Am J Health Promot* 23:157–167, 2009.

72. Johnson DR, et al.: Current challenges facing secondary education and transition services: what research tells us, *Exception Child* 68:519–531, 2002.

73. Jones M, Rapport MJ: Court decisions, state education agency hearings, letters of inquiry, policy interpretation, and investigations by federal agencies related to school-based physical therapy. In McEwen IR, editor: *Providing physical therapy services under parts B & C of the Individuals with Disabilities Education Act (IDEA)*, Alexandria, VA, 2009, Section on Pediatrics, American Physical Therapy Association, pp 147–159.

74. Kaloi L, Stanberry K: Section 504 in 2009: broader eligibility, more accommodations, *National Center for Learning Disabilities*, 2009. Retrieved from: http://www.ncld.org/on-capitol-hill/federal-laws-aamp-ld/adaaa-a-section-504/section-504-in-2009.

75. Kaminker MK, et al.: Decision making for service delivery in schools: a nationwide analysis by geographic region, *Pediatr Phys Ther* 18:204–213, 2006.

76. Kaminker MK, et al.: Decision making for service delivery in schools: a nationwide survey of pediatric physical therapists, *Phys Ther* 84:919–933, 2004.

77. Kentucky Department of Education: Guidance of the related services of occupational therapy, physical therapy, and speech/language therapy in Kentucky Public Schools. Retrieved from: http://education.ky.gov/specialed/excep/documents/guidance%20documents/resource%20manual%20for%20educationally%20related%20ot%20and%20pt.pdf, 2012.

78. King G: A relational goal-oriented model of optimal service delivery to children and families, *Phys Occup Ther Pediatr* 29:384–408, 2009.

79. King GA, et al.: An evaluation of functional, school-based therapy services for children with special needs, *Phys Occup Ther Pediatr* 19:5–29, 1999.

80. King G, et al.: A life needs model of pediatric service delivery: services to support community participation and quality of life for children and youth with disabilities, *Phys Occup Ther Pediatr* 22:53–77, 2002.

81. Lignugaris-Kraft B, et al.: Writing better goals and short-term objectives or benchmarks, *Teach Exception Child* 34:52–58, 2001.

82. Lindsey D, et al.: Physical therapy services in North Carolina's schools, *Clin Manage Phys Ther* 4:40–43, 1980.

83. Lipsky DK: The coexistence of high standards and inclusion, *Sch Admin* 60:32–35, 2003.

84. Martin R: *Extraordinary children, ordinary lives: stories behind special education case law*, Champaign, IL, 1991, Research Press, pp 45–63.

85. Maryland State Steering Committee for Occupational and Physical Therapy School-Based Programs: Occupational and physical therapy early intervention and school-based services in Maryland: a guide to practice. Retrieved from: http://www.marylandpublicschools.org/nr/rdonlyres/954dfc2e-16d9-45fa-b5c4-e713b0134fea/19473/ot_pt_fulldocument_december11_final.pdf, 2010.

86. Mastropieri M, Scruggs T: *The inclusive classroom: strategies for effective differentiated instruction*, ed 4, Columbus, OH, 2010, Merrill.

87. McCambridge T, et al.: Active healthy living: prevention of childhood obesity through increased physical activity, *Pediatrics* 117:1834–1842, 2006.

88. McConlogue A, Quinn L: Analysis of physical therapy goals in a school-based setting: a pilot study, *Phys Occup Ther Pediatr* 29:154–169, 2009.

89. McEwen I, editor: *Providing physical therapy services under parts B & C of the Individuals with Disabilities Education Act (IDEA)*, Alexandria, VA, 2009, Section on Pediatrics, American Physical Therapy Association.

90. McEwen IR, et al., editors: Interrater reliability and content validity of a minimal data set to measure outcomes of students receiving school-based occupational therapy and physical therapy, *Phys Occup Ther Pediatr* 23:77–95, 2003.

91. Meyer LH, et al.: *Critical issues in the lives of people with severe disabilities*, Baltimore, 1991, Paul H. Brookes.

92. Mills v. Board of Education District of Columbia, 348 F. Supp. 866 (D. DC. 1972).

93. Mitchell LE, et al.: Habitual physical activity of independently ambulant children and adolescents with cerebral palsy: are they doing enough? *Phys Ther* 95:202–211, 2015.

94. Mockford M, Caulton JM: Systematic review of progressive strength training in children and adolescents with cerebral palsy who are ambulatory, *Pediatr Phys Ther* 20:318–333, 2008.

95. Mulcahey AL: Detroit schools for crippled children, *Phys Ther Rev* 16:63–64, 1936.

96. Myers CT, et al.: Factors influencing physical therapists' involvement in preschool transitions, *Phys Ther* 91:656–664, 2011.

97. National Center for Fair and Open Testing: Joint organizational statement on No Child Left Behind (NCLB) Act. Retrieved from: http://www.fairtest.org/joint%20statement%20civil%20rights%20grps%2010-21-04.html, 2009.

98. National Coalition on Personnel Shortages in Special Education and Related Services (NCPSSERS): About the shortage. Retrieved from: http://specialedshortages.org/about-the-shortage/, 2015.

99. National Highway Traffic Safety Administration: Proper use of child safety restraint systems in school buses. Retrieved from: http://www.nhtsa.dot.gov/people/injury/buses/busseatbelt/, 2015.

100. Ogg-Groenendaal M, et al.: A systematic review on the effect of exercise interventions on challenging behavior for people with intellectual disabilities, *Res Dev Disabil* 35:1507–1517, 2014.

101. Ott DAD, Effgen SK: Occurrence of gross motor behaviors in integrated and segregated preschool classrooms, *Pediatr Phys Ther* 12:164–172, 2000.

102. Palisano RJ, et al.: Content validity of the expanded and revised gross motor function classification system, *Dev Med Child Neurol* 50:744–750, 2008.

103. PARC v. Pennsylvania, 334 F. SuppK. 1257 (ED PA 1972).

104. Pate RR, et al.: Promoting physical activity in children and youth: a leadership role for schools. A Council on Nutrition, Physical Activity, and Metabolism (Physical Activity Committee) in Collaboration with the Councils on Cardiovascular Disease in the Young and Cardiovascular Nursing, *Circulation* 114:1214–1224, 2006.

105. Pontifex MB, et al.: VI. The role of physical activity in reducing barriers to learning in children with developmental disorders, *Monogr Soc Res Child Dev* 79:93–118, 2014.

106. Prieto GM: *Effects of physical therapist instruction on the frequency and performance of teacher assisted gross motor activities for students with motor disabilities, unpublished master's thesis*, Philadelphia, 1992, Hahnemann University.

107. Public Law 101-336: Americans with Disabilities Act, 42 *USC* §12101, 1990. Retrieved from: http://library.clerk.house.gov/reference-files/PPL_101_336_AmericansWithDisabilities.pdf.

108. Public Law 102-119: Individuals with Disabilities Education Act Amendments of, 105 587–608, 1991. Retrieved from: http://www.gpo.gov/fdsys/pkg/STATUTE-105/pdf/STATUTE-105-Pg587.pdf.

109. Public Law 105-17: Individuals with Disabilities Education Act Amendments of 1997, 111 Stat. 37–157. Retrieved from: http://www.gpo.gov/fdsys/pkg/PLAW-105publ17/pdf/PLAW-105publ17.pdf.

110. Public Law 105-394: Assistance Technology Act of 1998, 118 Stat. 1707. Retrieved from: http://www.gpo.gov/fdsys/pkg/PLAW-108publ364/html/PLAW-108publ364.htm.

111. Public Law 107-110: No Child Left Behind Act of, 115 Stat. 1425–2094, 2001. Retrieved from: http://www.ed.gov/policy/elsec/leg/esea02/107-110.pdf.

112. Public Law 108-446: Individuals with Disabilities Education Improvement Act of 2004, Retrieved from: http://www.copyright.gov/legislation/pl108-446.pdf.

113. Public Law 110-335: Americans with Disabilities Amendments Act, 42 *USC* §12101, 2008. Retrieved from: http://www.ada.gov/pubs/adastatute08.htm.

114. Public Law 93-112: Rehabilitation Act, 29 *USC Sec.* §794, 1973. Retrieved from: http://www.usbr.gov/cro/pdfsplus/rehabact.pdf.

115. Public Law 94-103: Developmental Disabilities Assistance and Bill of Rights Act, Stat. 89:486–507, 1975. Retrieved from: http://mn.gov/mnddc/dd_act/documents/75-DDA-USH.pdf.

116. Public Law 94-142: Education of All Handicapped Children Act, 89 Stat. 773–796, 1975. Retrieved from: http://www.gpo.gov/fdsys/pkg/STATUTE-89/pdf/STATUTE-89-Pg773.pdf.

117. Public Law 99-372: Handicapped Children's Protection Act, 20 USC §, 1986. 1415(e)(4)(f). Retrieved from: http://www.gpo.gov/fdsys/pkg/STATUTE-100/pdf/STATUTE-100-Pg796.pdf.

118. Public Law 99-457: Education of the Handicapped Act Amendments of 1986, 100 Stat. 1145–1177. Retrieved from: http://www.gpo.gov/fdsys/pkg/STATUTE-100/pdf/STATUTE-100-Pg1145.pdf.

119. Rainforth B: OSERS clarifies legality of related services eligibility criteria, *TASH Newsletter* 17:8, 1991.

120. Rainforth B: Analysis of physical therapy practice acts: implications for role release in educational environments, *Pediatr Phys Ther* 9:54–61, 1997.

121. Rainforth B, Kugelmass JW: *Curriculum instruction for all learners: blending systematic and constructivist approaches in inclusive elementary schools*, Baltimore, MD, 2003, Paul H. Brookes.

122. Rainforth B, York-Barr J: *Collaborative teams for students with severe disabilities*, ed 2, Baltimore, 1997, Paul H. Brookes.

123. Randall KE, McEwen IR: Writing patient-centered functional goals, *Phys Ther* 80:1197–1203, 2000.

124. Rapport MJ, Thomas SB: Extended school year: legal issues and implications, *J Assoc Pers Sev Handicaps* 18:16–27, 1993.

125. Reynolds M: A framework for considering some issues in special education, *Exception Child* 28:367–370, 1962.

126. Rowland JL, et al.: The scope of pediatric physical therapy practice in health promotion and fitness for youth with disabilities, *Pediatr Phys Ther* 15:2–15, 2015.

127. Ryndak DL, Fisher D: *The foundations of inclusive education: a compendium of articles on effective strategies to achieve inclusive education*, ed 2, Baltimore, MD, 2003, TASH.

128. Sever JW: Physical therapy in schools for crippled children, *Phys Ther Rev* 18:298–303, 1938.

129. Shumway-Cook A, Woollacott MH: *Motor control: translating research into clinical practice*, ed 4, Philadelphia, 2012, Lippincott Williams & Wilkins.

130. Smith J, Sylvester L: Transition. In McEwen I, editor: *Providing physical therapy services under parts B & C of the Individuals with Disabilities Education Act (IDEA)*, Alexandria, VA, 2009, Section on Pediatrics, American Physical Therapy Association.

131. Snell ME, Janney R: *Collaborative teaming*, Baltimore, MD, 2000, Paul H. Brookes.

132. Soccio CA: *Direct-individual versus integrated-group models of physical therapy service delivery*, unpublished master's thesis, Philadelphia, 1991, Hahnemann University.

133. Steenbeek D, et al.: Goal attainment scaling in paediatric rehabilitation: a report on the clinical training of an interdisciplinary team, *Child Care Health Dev* 34:521–529, 2008.

134. Stronge JH: Teacher effectiveness performance evaluation system. Handbook 2012-2013. Retrieved from http://fea.njpsa.org/documents/Stronge/Stronge%20NJ%20Training-district%20access/Tabs/Tab%205-Teacher%20Evaluation%20System%20Handbook.pdf, 2012.

135 TASH: *TASH resolution on inclusive quality education*, Baltimore, MD, 2000, Author.

136. Taylor SJ: Caught in the continuum: a critical analysis of the least restrictive environment, *J Assoc Pers Sev Handicaps* 13:41–53, 1988.

137. Teeters Myers C, Effgen SK: Physical therapists' participation in early childhood transitions, *Pediatr Phys Ther* 18:182–189, 2006.

138. U.S. Department of Education, Office of Special Education and Rehabilitative Services, Office of Special Education Programs: *30th annual report to Congress on the implementation of the Individuals with Disabilities Education Act, 2008*, Washington, DC, 2011, Author.

139. U.S. Department of Education: Civil rights discrimination. Retrieved from: http://ed.gov/policy/rights/guid/ocr/disability.html, 2009.

140. Vacha VB: History of the development of special schools and classes for crippled children in Chicago, *Phys Ther Rev* 13:21–26, 1933.

141. Valvano J, Fiss A: Neuromuscular system: the plan of care. In Effgen SK, editor: *Meeting the physical therapy needs of children*, ed 2, Philadelphia, 2013, FA Davis, pp 347–388.

142. Virginia Department of Education: *Handbook for occupational & physical therapy services in Virginia public schools*, Richmond, VA, 2010, Author. Retrieved from: http://www.doe.virginia.gov/special_ed/iep_instruct_svcs/related_services/handbook_occupational_physical_therapy.pdf.

143. Wilson RAA, et al.: Concurrent validity of the School Outcomes Measure (SOM) and Pediatric Evaluation of Disability Inventory (PEDI) in preschool-age children, *Phys Occup Ther Pediatr* 35:40–53, 2015.

144. Wolfensberger W: Will there always be an institution? The impact of new service models, *Ment Retard* 9:31–38, 1971.

145. World Health Organization (WHO: International Classification of Functioning, Disability and Health (ICF). Retrieved from: http://www.who.int/classifications/icf/en/, 2009.

146. Zirkel P: Inclusion: return of the pendulum? *Special Educator* 12(1):5, 1996.

SUGGESTED READINGS

American Occupational Therapy Association, American Physical Therapy Association, & American Speech-Language-Hearing Association: Workload approach: a paradigm shift for positive impact on student outcomes. Retrieved from: https://pediatricapta.org/special-interest-groups/SB/pdfs/APTA-ASHA-AOTA-Joint-Doc-Workload-Approach-.pdf.

Effgen SK, et al.: Updated competencies for physical therapists working in schools, *Pediatr Phys Ther* 19:66–274, 2007.

Hanft B, Shepherd J, editors: *Collaborating for student success: a guide for school-based occupational therapy*, Bethesda, MD, 2008, American Occupational Therapy Association.

Kentucky Department of Education: Guidance of the related services of occupational therapy, physical therapy, and speech/language therapy in Kentucky Public Schools. Retrieved from: http://education.ky.gov/specialed/excep/documents/guidance%20documents/resource%20manual%20for%20educationally%20related%20ot%20and%20pt.pdf, 2012.

Maryland State Steering Committee for Occupational and Physical Therapy School-Based Programs: Occupational and physical therapy early intervention and school-based services in Maryland: a guide to practice. Retrieved from: http://www.marylandpublicschools.org/nr/rdonlyres/954dfc2e-16d9-45fa-b5c4-e713b0134fea/19473/ot_pt_fulldocument_december11_final.pdf, 2010.

McEwen I, editor: *Providing physical therapy services under parts B & C of the Individuals with Disabilities Education Act (IDEA)*, Alexandria, VA, 2009, Section on Pediatrics, American Physical Therapy Association.

32

Transition to Adulthood for Youth With Disabilities

Nancy Cicirello, Antonette Doty, Robert J. Palisano

Transition to adulthood is a future-oriented process in which youth express their desires and goals and begin planning for adult roles and responsibilities.[19] The transition process is multifaceted and encompasses the health, psychosocial, and educational-vocational needs of adolescents as they move from child-oriented to adult-oriented lifestyles and systems.[146] Parent and youth priorities include functioning as independently as possible with appropriate supports, finding meaningful activities after high school, and establishing supportive social relationships.[113] Rutkowski and Riehie[118] shared the organizational vision of United Cerebral Palsy that people with cerebral palsy and other developmental disabilities will live and participate in their communities, have satisfying lives and valued social roles, have sufficient access to needed support and control over that support so that the assistance they receive contributes to lifestyles they desire, and be safe and healthy in the environments in which they live. The US Individuals with Disabilities Education Improvement Act (IDEA) of 2004 (PL 108-446) mandates transition planning to prepare youth with the knowledge and skills for adult roles. A consensus statement by the American Academy of Pediatrics (AAP), American Academy of Family Physicians, American College of Physicians, and American Society of Internal Medicine advocates a written health care transition plan for all youth with disabilities by age 14.[2] Implementation of comprehensive and coordinated health transition services and supports, however, has not been widely achieved.[2] Furthermore, young adults with intellectual or developmental disability are less likely to be employed, enroll in postsecondary education, and live independently after high school than peers with typical development.[104]

Transition to adulthood presents particular challenges for youth with disabilities, their families, health care professionals, and the broader health care system.[2,18,37,130] Blomquist et al. identified low expectations by parents and professionals, lack of knowledge of existing career and vocational education services, and lack of self-advocacy skills as particular challenges for youth with disabilities.[19] Similarly, Stewart identified lack of preparation, limited information, limited supports, lack of skills for adult roles, and disjointed adult services as potential barriers to successful transition.[126] In a national survey conducted by the PACER center, youth with disabilities identified job training, independent living skills, and college or vocational guidance as their most wanted transition services.[150] Only 45% reported that someone had discussed with them how to make medical decisions, and fewer than 50% had been asked about their work plans.[150] In another national survey, only 6% of families reported that their young adult child with special health care needs had achieved core outcomes for successful transition

to adulthood.[109] These findings underscore the need for innovative programs to prepare youth with disabilities for adult roles.

Preparing youth with disabilities for adult roles and meeting the needs of adults with childhood-onset conditions are emerging areas of physical therapy practice. Youth with disabilities often have needs for (1) personal assistance, (2) assistive technology, (3) instruction in self-advocacy, and (4) development of skills needed for postsecondary education and employment.[52,69,127,135] The International Classification of Functioning, Disability and Health (ICF),[149] described in Chapter 1, is a *biopsychosocial model* in which the interaction between the person and environment is critical for understanding health, health-related states, and participation outcomes. The transition experiences of youth across Canada support this perspective; the overall theme that emerged from interviews and focus groups was "complexities related to person-environment interactions."[129]

The objectives of this chapter are to (1) describe the transition process and challenges for youth with physical disabilities and families; (2) appraise transition approaches, services, supports, and outcomes; and (3) provide recommendations for the expanding role of the physical therapist in the transition process in and across educational, community, and hospital settings.

BACKGROUND INFORMATION

PREPARATION OF YOUTH WITH DISABILITIES FOR ADULT ROLES

Transition to adulthood encompasses new roles, responsibilities, and expectations and is influenced by a myriad of personal, familial, community, and societal factors. Havighurst identified tasks of adolescence including (1) forming new and more mature relations with age-mates of both sexes, (2) accepting one's physique and using one's body effectively, (3) achieving emotional independence from parents and other adults, (4) preparing for marriage and family life, (5) gaining economic independence, and (6) desiring and achieving socially responsible behavior.[57] Halfon et al.[53] proposed a lifecourse health development model in which health is conceptualized as an emergent set of developmental capacities that enables individuals to adapt to events and experiences and achieve life goals. Health development is sensitive to the timing and social structuring of environmental experience. These perspectives underscore person-environment transactions as critical to the transition process.

Youth with childhood-onset disabilities are consumers in the life tasks of finding meaningful work, accessing multiple physical environments, living independently or with self-chosen supports, and successful transition that is enabled by the community.[35] Rosenbaum and Rosenbloom[115] describe the intersection of social and medical systems for improving services to individuals with childhood-onset conditions. They encourage providers to partner with youth and families in advocating strengths-based approaches and participation roles for these youth.

Family Readiness

Collaboration among youth with disabilities, their families, and professionals is essential for successful transition.[8] A general expectation is that as adolescents mature, they will become more autonomous and assume adult roles and responsibilities. Families of youth with disabilities have expressed needs for future planning[107] and concerns about what will happen when they no longer are able to care for their adult child.[21,48,98] Parents of students with disabilities are not always involved in transition planning, even though they are often the primary support for their children after high school. McNair and Rush found that parents wanted more information regarding their child's skill level, work options, adult services, community living, and types of family support, and they desired more involvement in transition planning.[99] Parents of youth with intellectual or developmental disability associated successful transition with: "having an occupation or functional role in society," "moving out of home apart from parent or caregiver," "relationships with peers," and "skills required for success in daily functioning."[62] These findings reinforce the importance of addressing the family's priorities and concerns when transition planning.

Self-Determination

Self-determination is a desirable attribute of youth transitioning to adult roles.[43,92,127] Self-determination is defined as the "combination of skills, knowledge, and beliefs that enable a person to engage in goal directed, self-regulated, autonomous behavior."[44] Self-determination is both person centered and person directed and acknowledges the rights of people with disabilities to take charge of and responsibility for their lives.[73] Youth possessing self-determination are thought to have greater ability to take control of their lives and successfully assume adult roles. Youth with cerebral palsy identified being believed in, believing in yourself, and being accepted by others as important for success in life.[77] Social self-efficacy was associated with independence and persistence in a study of adolescents with physical disabilities.[78] Gall et al. have recommended that the transition process involves a gradual shift in responsibilities from the service provider to the parent/family and finally to the young person.[49]

In a systematic review on self-determination of students with disabilities, it was concluded that self-determination is teachable and outcomes are optimized by instructional or curricular interventions that contained multiple components.[30] Goal setting and self-management were the most frequent intervention strategies. Other components included decision making, planning, problem solving, learning and practicing skills, and self-advocacy. Evans et al. evaluated a multifaceted transition program provided through children's rehabilitation services that combined self-discovery, skill development, and community experiences.[43] Following participation in a 12-month program, youth and young adults with multiple disabilities demonstrated statistically and clinically important improvement in self-determination and their sense of personal control, spending significantly more time engaged in volunteer/work activities and community leisure activities. Adults with cerebral palsy shared that modeling, goal setting, self-awareness, supports from family, friends, and the community, and opportunities to experience and practice self-determination optimized the transition process while attitudinal barriers were often a greater challenge than physical barriers.[6]

Self-Management of Health Condition

To the fullest extent possible, youth with disabilities are encouraged to actively participate in the transition from a pediatric to an adult medical home. The ability to communicate with health care providers, including primary care physicians, specialty physicians, nurses, therapists, and dentists, is an important skill. For youth who require physical assistance for self-care, this includes the ability to instruct care providers. Equally important are skills for health promotion, injury prevention, and prevention of secondary impairments. Youth with disabilities may benefit from experience in coordination of services among their multiple health care providers. Learning to identify one's medical home provider and develop strategies for communicating and coordinating her/his specialty care such as maintaining a health status record and care are examples of outcomes for self-management. This may include a transition plan that is shared with each provider. The electronic medical record has potential to improve communication and coordination of care.

Wellness and Secondary Prevention

Healthy People 2020[140] is an initiative by the U.S. Department of Health and Human Services to promote health and disease prevention. Goals for people with disabilities include greater access to health, wellness, assistive technology, and treatment programs and a reduction in the proportion of people with disabilities who report encountering environmental barriers to participating in home, school, work, or community activities. Comprehensive and coordinated heath care, self-management of one's health condition, and physical activity are important for wellness and secondary prevention. In the Disability and Secondary Conditions section of *Healthy People 2020*, two new objectives are (1) reduce the proportion of people with disabilities reporting delays in receiving primary and periodic preventive care because of specific barriers and (2) increase the proportion of parents or other caregivers of youth with disabilities aged 12 to 17 years who report engaging in transition planning from pediatric to adult health care. The objectives reinforce the importance of introducing aging with disabilities and youth in transition into physical therapy education programs and service delivery.

Finding an Adult Medical Home

With medical advances over the past decades, many children with disabilities are now living into adulthood and facing new challenges in the areas of health and wellness.[14] Newacheck et al. reported that in the United States, 18% (12.6 million) of children and adolescents under 18 years of age have a chronic medical condition requiring health and related services beyond that required by children in general.[103] Ninety percent of youth with special health care needs reach their 21st birthday. An estimated 200,000 to 500,000 individuals with lifelong disabilities are over the age of 60, and this number is expected to double by 2030.[11]

An important outcome for youth with disabilities is continuous, comprehensive, and coordinated services in the adult health care system.[2,34,147] Presently, the health care system in the United States is not designed to facilitate the transition between pediatric and adult services, which results in a patchwork approach that is not likely to change in the near future.[14] Typically, people with a lifelong disability have less access to medical providers in the community than the general population. In addition, they have less preventive care, more emergency medical visits, less insurance coverage, and little to no experience managing their own health care. Forty-five percent of youth with special health care needs do not have a physician who is familiar with their health condition. Further, 30% of 18- to 24-year-olds in the United States lack a payment source for health care, and youth lack access to primary and specialty providers.[14]

Hepburn et al.[63] performed a scoping review of publicly available government documents on transition to adulthood and reported that, internationally, few jurisdictions address transition of care issues in either health or broader social policy documents. Most jurisdictions do not address the policy infrastructure required to support successful transitions or evaluate transition strategies. In the United States, the medical home model is an effort to improve coordination of services and reduce costs by identifying a primary care provider and coordination of health care and community services. The adult health care system, however, is lacking in primary care providers and the specialized health care and rehabilitation services needed by adults with childhood-onset chronic conditions such as cerebral palsy.[15,34,91,125] Lack of transition preparation of young people with disabilities and their families is thought to contribute to problems in transition to adult care.[114]

The American Academy of Pediatrics, American Academy of Family Physicians, American College of Physicians, and American Society of Internal Medicine published a consensus statement recommending that all youth with special health care needs have a written health care transition plan by age 14 years to identify appropriate health care professionals, provide guidelines for primary as well as preventive care, and ensure developmentally appropriate transition services.[2] A clinical report by these organizations advocates a well-timed, coordinated, and individualized plan for transition of youth between the ages of 18 and 21 years from child- to adult-oriented health care.[2] Transition plans should include: the expected age for transition to adult health care, the responsibilities of the youth, family, and/or caregiver, and the responsibilities of medical providers in preparing for transition. This process includes: (1) *Assessing* for transition readiness, (2) *Planning* a dynamic and longitudinal process for accomplishing realistic goals, (3) *Implementing* through education of all involved parties and empowerment of the youth in areas of self-care, and (4) *Documenting* to enable ongoing evaluation and sharing of information with adult care providers. The website for the American Academy of Pediatrics National Center for Medical Home Implementation includes resources for families, youth, and providers on finding a medical home and health care transition (https://medicalhomeinfo.aap.org/Pages/default.aspx). Resources for youth include transition notebooks, a portable medical record form, and videos on topics such as talking with your doctor and other health care professionals and planning for the future.

Tonniges and Roberts investigated health care and transition and found that youth with special health care needs spend more time on crisis management and less on typical life, fun, and activities.[138] Youth with special health care needs are said to live more as a patient and less as a young person, leading to missed school, interruptions in learning, functional declines, social isolation, and low expectations by adults about their abilities and future prospects. Youth express that they would like to live and work independently but often feel they are "treated like a child" and have a loss of control. Many youths feel they are not seen as unique individuals, separate from their condition, and health care providers often defer to their parents. Families of youth with special health care needs would like more information about resources, referrals to services, a written health transition plan, an advocate to assist and explain, and assistance from their medical home.[14]

Physical Activity

The importance of physical activity is a topic of education for youth with disabilities.[47] Promoting lifetime physical fitness is critical for prevention of secondary complications resulting from childhood-onset health conditions. A systematic review concluded that, across all ages and levels of motor function, children and youth with cerebral palsy participated in 13% to 53% less habitual physical activity than their peers. Levels of activity were approximately 30% lower than guidelines for physical activity, and sedentary times were twice the maximum recommended amount.[25] Maltais et al.[95] stress that low levels of physical activity might increase risk for related chronic diseases associated with poor health-related physical fitness. Based on research evidence, Maltais et al.[95] recommend that all children and youth with cerebral palsy engage in regular aerobic, anaerobic, and muscle-strengthening activities to the extent they are capable.

The health benefits of regular exercise include decreased risk of heart disease, cancer, age-related physiologic changes, obesity, and increased social well-being. The Surgeon General report stated that for people with chronic disabling conditions, regular physical activity can improve stamina, muscular strength, and quality of life and prevent disease.[141] The report identified a lack of available and accessible wellness and fitness programs and recommends implementing community-based programs with safe, accessible environments and including people with disabilities and their families in program planning.

Creating a habit of regular exercise is challenging for individuals with lifelong disabilities. Erson stated that fitness activities should be fun, goal oriented, and contribute to health and well-being in order for fitness to become a habit.[42] Exercise can improve academics, reduce maladaptive behaviors, and improve self-esteem and psychosocial functioning of adolescents with disabilities,[40,132] yet as youth advance through the education system, the amount of physical education often decreases.

Exposure to diverse recreation and leisure activities enables youth with disabilities to make informed choices. Making choices enhances self-determination and can decrease problem behavior.[131] Furthermore, preferred recreation and leisure activities are more likely to be enjoyable and sustained over time. Exposure to diverse activities enables youth to select alternative activities if initial choices do not work out. The Americans with Disabilities Act (ADA) legislates equitable access of community recreation programs for persons with disabilities. Participation of persons with disabilities in age-appropriate, community-based programs should increase public awareness that disability does not equate to ill health.

Physical fitness is addressed in detail in Chapter 6.

Community Living

The reauthorization of Individuals with Disabilities Education Act in 1997 included mandates to improve transition of youth from high school to other opportunities such as postsecondary education, employment, and community living. Johnson et al. suggested that transition challenges to community living and employment include (1) access to full spectrum of general education offerings and learning experiences; (2) education placement, curricular decisions, and diploma options that are based on meaningful indicators of learning and skills; (3) options for postsecondary education, community living, and employment; (4) participation of the student and family; and (5) interagency communication and collaboration.[71]

Young adults with disabilities desire options for community living other than the family home. These options may range in descending order of support from residential group homes (agency owned or operated), residential supported living (private housing with flexible supports such as attendant care), and independent living. Howe, Horner, and Newton evaluated supported community living versus residential group homes among 40 adults with cognitive impairments.[66] Howe et al. define supported living as developing supports needed to best match the individual's preferences and needs over time. The number of housemates for adults in supported independent living varied from 0 to 2, whereas the number of housemates for adults in residential living varied from 1 to 19. Housing provision costs were similar for both living arrangements. Young adults in supported living were either the owner of the residence or listed on the rental agreement, and housemates were identified as the preferred choice of each young adult with developmental disabilities. Young adults in supported living experienced significantly more variety in community activities and did preferred activities more frequently compared with young adults living in group homes.

The National Center for the Study of Postsecondary Educational Supports (NCSPES) has identified competencies for successful transition from secondary education.[102] Competencies include knowledge of self, including one's health condition, and the ability to access services and supports for community living. Life skill curricular content in secondary education such as identifying specific supports needed for living, postsecondary education, or work is recommended for students with special health care needs, regardless of cognitive ability. Curricular content could include accessibility, transportation, and skills for community living and work. Community living skills may include meal preparation, acquisition of food staples, paying bills, laundry, and/or the hiring, managing, or firing personal attendants. Skill sets for work might include the ability to interact with people providing attendant care and to describe and request necessary job accommodations including augmentative communication when needed. Physical therapists working in educational settings are encouraged to anticipate opportunities to be included in life skill programs for students with physical disabilities. Likewise, physical therapists in clinic and hospital practice settings are encouraged to communicate and coordinate with educators and professionals providing related services (transition coordinator, school-based therapists) and to interact with community organizations and agencies to address transition needs.

Postsecondary Education

Today more than ever students with disabilities are participating in postsecondary education. Postsecondary options include vocational/technical schools, community colleges, liberal arts colleges, and state or private universities. The number of students with disabilities applying and being admitted to institutions of higher education is increasing. The June 1999 National Center for Education Statistics: Statistical Analysis Report by Horn, Berktold, and Bobbitt concluded that students with disabilities, overall, fell behind their peers without disabilities in their high school academic preparation. This finding leads to these youth being less qualified for 4-year college admissions and less prepared for college-level courses.

Planning for postsecondary education begins early in high school with selection of coursework and academic requirements.[45] Hitchings, Retisch, and Horvath reported that students with disabilities are often not prepared for postsecondary education.[64] Transition plans of 110 students in grades 10 through 12 who attended two Illinois high schools were reviewed. Student interest in postsecondary education declined over a 3-year period from 77% to 47%. Only four students had 4-year transition plans preparing them for postsecondary education. Based on their findings, the authors stated the following recommendations for successful transition to postsecondary education: (1) students must be successful in general education classes to determine if they can learn academic content and meet teacher and workload requirements with or without accommodations, (2) transition planning should begin in the late elementary years and be sustained throughout high school, (3) students must be their own advocates, (4) students must actively engage in the career development process, and (5) educators and professionals providing related services must have knowledge of current policy for transition planning.

Getzel[51] and Madaus[93] both articulated that students with disabilities experience a significant shift of responsibility according to the legal rights afforded in secondary education under the IDEA as compared to legal rights in postsecondary education mandated by the Americans with Disabilities Act. Darrah et al.[36] examined community services for young adults with motor disabilities and described their thematic findings as a "paradox of services." These authors interviewed 76 individuals (mean age of 25 years, representative of all levels of gross motor function) for the purpose of determining their perceptions of programs and services in the spheres of education, employment, transportation, and assured income. Postsecondary education opportunities were limited in part due to "the fact that the educational programs designed to enrich their social experiences often restricted their future educational choices."

Two significant pieces of legislation support students with disabilities admitted to colleges or universities. Section 504 of the Rehabilitation Act of 1973 and the Americans with Disabilities Act (ADA, P.L. 101-336) ensure nondiscriminatory protection for students with disabilities on campuses of higher education. Section 504 stipulates that any institution that receives federal funding must ensure access for all persons with disabilities and specifically stipulates equal opportunity for "otherwise qualified handicapped individuals." The law also requires an "affirmative action obligation" on the part of institutions of higher education. Two purposes of the ADA are to provide "a national mandate for the elimination of discrimination against individuals with disabilities" and to provide strong "enforceable standards addressing discrimination against this population" (p 201).

The ADA mandates that all public and private businesses and institutions provide reasonable accommodations for persons with disabilities.[61] Federal legislation pertaining to youth with disabilities including the Individuals with Disabilities Education Improvement Act and the Americans with Disabilities Act is presented in Chapter 31.

College Admissions and Enrollment

Whereas education is a given opportunity for all children in the United States through high school, college is a self-chosen endeavor. The guarantees of a free and appropriate public education (FAPE), established under the auspices of IDEA for students with disabilities, do not extend to postsecondary institutions of learning. Instead, colleges and universities use the definition of disability in the ADA. The ADA defines a person with a disability as anyone who has a physical or mental impairment that substantially limits one or more major life activities, has a record of such impairment, or is regarded as having such impairment. Therefore a qualified student with a disability applying to postsecondary education is one who is able to meet a program's admission, academic, and technical standards either with or without accommodation.[136] Section 504 utilizes the term "otherwise qualified" in extending the same recognition to potential students. Rothstein raised the issues of what can be asked at preadmission and when students should disclose a disability.[116] For example, a student may not want to disclose a physical disability before a campus visit; however, by not disclosing this information, the campus personnel may be put at a disadvantage by not having lead time to make adjustments that could facilitate the visit.

Reasonable accommodations in higher education can include barrier-free design, academic modifications (waiver of certain courses, lighter course loads, and alternative methods of testing), and specific disability services such as translators, tutors, and readers. Important considerations are whether accommodations can be provided without altering the nature of the academic program, without jeopardizing the safety of the student of record or others, and without creating an undue burden of a financial or administrative nature.[116]

The ADA underscores the importance of preparing students with disabilities to articulate their specific needs. For high school students with disabilities, an annual goal could be to plan their individualized education plan (IEP) meeting, which would generalize to skills in articulating requests once enrolled in college. More specifically, students with disabilities could be encouraged to generate the accommodations needed to complete the IEP document as well as list the criteria that would indicate goal attainment. An IEP goal in a high school speech and communication class may be that a student develop a plan of action for requesting accommodations and participate in a mock student service meeting to articulate requests. Zadra suggested preregistration interviews between students with disabilities and college counselors as an excellent strategy for students to communicate their needs and counselors to gather accurate and meaningful information.

Campus Accessibility

Misquez, McCarthy, Powell, and Chu reported that the greatest impetus for making accessibility changes was having students with disabilities on college campuses.[101] Encouraging and supporting high school students with physical disabilities to take advantage of college campus visits serves a dual purpose. First, upon requesting to sit in on a college class, students can tour the campus grounds and visit university resource centers, libraries, and dormitories. Such visits provide perspective students with a better understanding of the spatial and temporal perimeters of college campus navigation as compared to a typically enclosed high school campus. Second, as more students with physical disabilities visit and attend institutions of higher education, college/university staff, faculty, and administrators will become more cognizant of accessibility barriers to their respective campus.

A specific IEP goal for the high school junior or senior may be to evaluate the accessibility of two college campuses using multiple resources (web page searches, telephone interviews, and onsite visitations). A student activity accessibility checklist developed by Roger Smith, Jill Warnke, and Dave Edyburn of the University of Wisconsin, Milwaukee, and Daryl Mellard, Noelle Kurth, and Gwen Berry of the University of Kansas is on the Expert Consult. The form provides a comprehensive list of questions for students with disabilities visiting, applying to, and attending a college or university.

Attending college means living away from home for many students. Typically, freshman and sophomore students experience their first extended period away from home living arrangements in college dormitories. Beds, desks, and dressers are standard features, with students bringing the various amenities such as computers, mini-refrigerators, and stereo systems. Students often share living quarters with another student or a group depending on the configurations of the dorm rooms. For the student with a physical disability, room accessibility can be a major challenge.

Physical therapists need to think long term when making recommendations about interventions with students in primary and secondary education that could generalize to college dormitory room independence. The terms *anticipatory guidance* and *future planning* refer to this process. Physical therapists should consider evaluation of dorm room and bathroom accessibility and the accompanying transfer skills to access beds, shower/tub, and toilets. If physical independence is not a feasible goal, the student's ability to direct an attendant in physical management would be a more appropriate goal. In a high school health or physical education class, a student's IEP goals may include competency in directing others for identified tasks where or when physical assistance is needed. Skills for advertising, interviewing, and hiring and firing of attendants are desirable. These skills could be practiced through role-play scenarios in a sociology or communication class.

Issues of Confidentiality

Unlike students with "hidden" disabilities such as a learning disability, students with physical disabilities are readily visible. Despite this, issues of confidentiality need to be respected and adhered to. High school students with disabilities need to know that institutions of higher education have policies regarding confidentiality. These policies should include (1) who can be informed, (2) who should be informed, (3) who must be informed, (4) who should not be informed, and (5) when and how any related waivers should be obtained.[116] High school educators and related services staff can assist students to be proactive in determining how they will disclose information. By being proactive, students with disabilities are demonstrating confidence, maturity, and self-esteem to college personnel.

Interaction With Instructors

Instructors in postsecondary education programs, with different expectations than high school teachers, understandably may exceed a student's comfort zone and create anxiety on the part of both the student and faculty. Amsel and Fichten compared interactions between college students with and without disabilities and their professors.[4] Students with disabilities were less likely to request or accept assistance. Paradoxically, students without disabilities and professors believed it is quite appropriate for students with disabilities to ask for accommodations. The authors concluded that it is imperative that students with disabilities not misperceive the appropriateness of requests for assistance.

Patrick and Wessel,[108] by means of a small qualitative study, concluded that first-year college students with disabilities experienced transitional issues and procured support through faculty mentorship. Postsecondary transitions included both academic and social transitions. The transition of physical separation from the students' families created a demand on becoming independent and making one's own decisions. Additionally, students interviewed shared experiencing inadequacies in taking on the responsibility for the accommodation process. Accommodations in the arenas of campus navigation, informing faculty and requesting academic accommodations, as well as utilizing attendants were new, given that many were accustomed to family members providing bathing, toileting, and dressing assistance. Positives of having established faculty mentorship included (1) advice, (2) awareness of campus resources, (3) getting to know faculty, and (4) individual support. Interviewed students reported faculty mentorship as being positive and that mentorship weaning over the course of their college experience was appropriate.

Employment

One of the major life roles of youth transitioning to adulthood is gaining economic independence.[57] Ninety percent of youth with special health care needs reach their 21st birthday, an age when most young adults are either employed are seeking employment.[20] In the National Longitudinal Transition study, 40% of individuals with childhood onset health conditions were employed 2 years after high school as compared to a 63% employment rate for same-age peers at large.[144] Nationally, 23,000 individuals with severe disabilities participated in supported employment in 1988; by 2002, 118,000 individuals participated.[70] Baker et al.[9] reported that according to the US Census Bureau's population employment survey, 22% of working-age Americans with disability were employed compared to 76% of same age Americans without a disability. It is unknown as to how inclusive the "disability" descriptor was. Though progress is slow, many youths with special health care needs continue wanting to work.

Darrah et al.[36] described an employment paradox for transitioning youth with disabilities. The paradox, as reported by participants in their study, was between solid employment preparation (skill development, job application, interview preparation) and minimal assistance in actual job finding and support once "training preparation" is completed. Employment opportunities, especially if linked to governmental programs, were time limited. Less attention to job accommodation was reported by several interview participants. Michelson et al.,[100] in a Danish study, reported that only 29% of 819 participants diagnosed with CP were competitively employed compared to 82% of controls. Rutkowski and Riehie[118] identified three functional areas vital to job identification and job performance: self-care, physical functioning/mobility, and communication. They also encouraged a paradigm shift of thinking of each individual as a "worker" rather than as a "patient" to emphasize employment potential.

Employment options for people with disabilities can be viewed on a continuum from least restrictive without supports (community based) to most restrictive (segregated programs with supports) (Fig. 32.1). In the 1960s through the 1980s, the primary employment options for people with severe disabilities were adult day programs and sheltered work programs. Supported employment is competitive work in integrated settings for individuals with disabilities for whom competitive employment has not traditionally occurred or for whom employment has been interrupted or intermittent because of a severe disability. These employees need ongoing support services to perform such work.[75] Supported employment includes the following: (1) provision of personalized job development, (2) on-the-job training, (3) ongoing support services, (4) individualized assessment (which is the opposite of norm-referenced assessment and placement), (5) person-centered job selection, which relies on the person's personal network, and (6) use assessment and activities that are meaningful and relevant.

Supported employment uses the services of job coaches and on-the-job training and long-term follow-along by an employment specialist following along if needed. Informal supports provided by friends, family, and coworkers are encouraged. Rusch and Braddock reported a stalled pattern of supported employment since 2000, with work settings limited to people with disabilities outnumbering work settings in the community at large.[117] Competitive employment with supports is a form of customized employment, although not a traditional category of employment. This type of service assists the students who have the ability to work independently but lack the job-seeking skills, interview skills, and organizational skills to obtain employment. With this type of career guidance, students can move on to more challenging careers and postsecondary training.[45]

Recommendations to improve employment of youth with disabilities include development of a national web-based system to coordinate entry into competitive employment, financial support availability through interagency partnerships, expanded guidance counseling services, and access to long-term support services.[117] Commentaries by Johnson[70] and Test[134] concur with Rusch and Braddock. Johnson concluded that improving

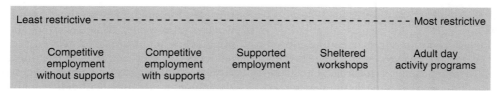

FIG. 32.1 Continuum of employment settings for people with disabilities.

graduation from postsecondary education or employment for students with disabilities outside sheltered workshops will depend on collaborative commitment from a wide base of constituents. Test suggested five strategies for achieving successful and meaningful economic independence: "(a) teach all students self-determination skills, (b) expand the mission of programs for 18- to 21-year-olds, (c) focus on interagency collaboration, (d) improve preparation of personnel, and (e) focus on the positive outcomes of supported employment" (p 248).[134]

Successful work transition is dependent on competencies in essential job functions and provision of appropriate supports or job modifications. Transition services that enable youth to learn essential job functions that are compatible with their abilities should advance individuals toward successful employment. Opportunities for development of work life skills should be incorporated in activities and routines. Examples of work life skills include getting ready for work, accessing transportation, keeping a schedule, learning appropriate work behavior and dress, developing communication with supervisors and work mates, eating and toileting, and directing attendants if and when necessary (Fig. 32.2).

Physical therapists can incorporate learning skills for work transition into therapeutic interventions. For example, a young person receiving physical therapy at an outpatient clinic could be encouraged to schedule or cancel his or her own therapy appointments. Learning how to direct others in physical management is fostered through having youth role play with the therapist in activities such as transfers in and out of a wheelchair, dressing, and donning and doffing orthotics. Youth can be supported to initiate communication with local employment agencies such as Vocational Rehabilitation. Consultation to employers is an unfamiliar area for pediatric physical therapists; however, many colleagues in adult practice have been involved with workplace reentry. Pediatric physical therapists are encouraged to expand their scope of practice to include consultation with community organizations and agencies, such as a job site where specific job-related activities can be observed,

analyzed, and solutions with or without accommodations developed. Pediatric therapists may also consider initiating transition to adult practitioner colleagues who are more versed in employment consultation. Darrah et al.[36] suggest that therapists encourage children with disabilities to actively participate in educational and employment opportunities. Additionally, these authors note that "coaching roles" go beyond health care concerns and thus demand therapists adopt the wider participation perspective of the ICF model.

One of the biggest employment challenges is the potential loss of an individual's Supplemental Security Income (SSI) and Social Security Disability Income (SSDI) if "too much" income is made. Requirements of limited income will keep individuals at or below the poverty line as well as sustaining a dependency rather than building on self-determination, which has been emphasized throughout the chapter as an important element of transition to adulthood. Transition to work must include a review of potential income sources to include supplemental security and work-related income. Youth must understand the delicate balance between benefits such as Medicaid or Medicare and work and optimize the benefits of both at appropriate times during the transition process. For some youth and families, exploring trusts for long-term security and support is a component of future planning. Therapists could consider developing their role and skills in advocacy for local, state, and federal policy development that facilitates continued SSI benefits for physical management support regardless of income earnings.

Transportation

Transportation is critical for all adult roles: education, work, adult living, and community participation. Youth with disabilities often lack reliable, cost-effective transportation options, which can limit social participation, friendships, and opportunities for work.[145] Gaining mobility transportation skills should be addressed as part of a student's IEP and transition plan or a patient's participation goal when therapy services are provided in a clinical setting. Skills such as using mobility devices independently and safely, accessing public transportation, identifying landmarks, and asking for directions can be developed as part of a community-based training program with assistance from the physical therapist, program staff, and family.[45] Lindsey[89] identified transportation as a significant predictor of employment for youth with disabilities transitioning to adulthood. Transportation barriers were identified by Schmidt and Smith[121] and Magill-Evans et al.[94] as well, which should direct therapists to pay greater attention to goals regarding independent mobility and community and workplace transportation negotiations.

Although the Americans with Disabilities Act mandates include public transportation accessibility, barriers still exist because of limited routes and may necessitate relocation to urban areas to increase transportation options. Students who use assistive walking devices or wheeled mobility may not be able to drive; therefore, they need to access alternative modes of transportation such as rides from coworkers or relatives, accessible public transportation, taxis, or program vans.[124] In 2004, President Bush released an executive order on Human Service Transportation Coordination to improve services for individuals with disabilities, older adults, and people with lower incomes. This was an effort to coordinate the 62 programs funding transportation, thereby reducing service duplication, consumer confusion, and service gaps. Partnership between the Coordinating

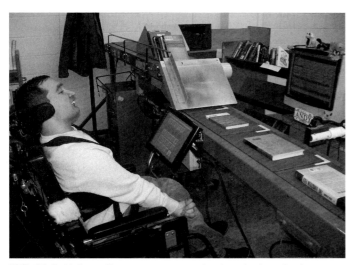

FIG. 32.2 Using a Dynavox communication device, Andy enters books into inventory and prices them for sale at Powell's Books. He hits his right head switch, sending a book onto the conveyor belt to be scanned. His right head switch controls the Dynavox, which acts as a keyboard, sending infrared signals to the store's computer, which causes a price label to be printed.

Council on Access and Mobility (CCAM) and United We Ride was established to provide coordination and common-sense solutions for everyone who needs transportation.[60] In some areas, transportation funding may be offered as part of state Medicaid waiver programs and as part of Impairment Related Work Expenses under the Social Security Administration.

TRANSITION MODELS AND APPROACHES

Transition planning involves communication and coordination among several systems and service providers. Within the health care system, the focus is on transition from the pediatric to the adult health care system. Within the education system, the focus is on preparing graduates for community living, postsecondary education, employment, and social and community participation. Children's rehabilitation services in a small number of communities have programs that address both aspects of transition. Cooperative collaboration amongst multiple systems and service providers is therefore imperative for successful transitions.

Contemporary approaches to preparing youth for life as an adult have an ecologic orientation that emphasizes the importance of real-world experiences, supports, and community accommodations.[76,80] King and colleagues appraised the literature to determine the main types of transition approaches and strategies for youth with disabilities, including those with chronic health conditions, and identified four approaches: skills training, prevocational and vocational guidance, youth- and family-centered approaches, and ecologic and experiential options. Transition programs were often guided by more than one approach and utilized multiple strategies.

The focus of *skills training* is to prepare youth for independence and success in chosen adult roles. Kingsnorth, Healy, and Macarthur performed a systematic review and identified six studies that included a comparison group.[82] Five reported short-term improvements in targeted skills such as social skills, assertiveness, and self-efficacy. The programs used a variety of strategies including goal setting, coaching, and experiential learning.

Prevocational and vocational guidance aim to enhance self-awareness strategies including planning and goal setting.[50] Emphasis is on support and guidance, job-seeking skills, and on-the-job skills training.[119] Research findings support the importance of involving youth in decisions about their transition-related goals[120] and teaching skills in real-world contexts.[28,29]

The focus of a *youth- and family-centered* approach is empowerment of youth and families through emotional support and knowledge of community resources and supports. There is evidence of the effectiveness of social support in facilitating positive outcomes and increasing self-esteem.[58] Research is needed on the effectiveness of youth- and family-centered transition approaches.

An *ecologic and experiential* approach is based on the principle that real-world opportunities and experiences optimize skill development.[10,23] The focus is on development of life skills, interpersonal relationships, environmental modifications, and task accommodations. Strategies include linking youth and family to community supports, enhancing knowledge of community opportunities, coaching and mentoring, creating individualized opportunities and experiences, and community education and advocacy. The results of the National

Longitudinal Transition study indicate that community-based work experience is more useful than school-based programs.[142] Students with and without disabilities who participated in work experiences in high school were twice as likely to have competitive employment 1 year after graduation compared with students without work experience.[13]

Service coordination and interagency collaboration are keys to all transition approaches. Within the education system, the interagency transition team should consist of the student, parents, educators, adult service professionals, employers, and community service agencies. Sharing information, expertise, and problem solving are encouraged among team members in order to meet a student's postsecondary goals. Collaborative practices are facilitated through interagency agreements that clearly define roles, responsibilities, and strategies of each community member. Potential barriers to collaboration include ineffective transition planning meetings, intimidating language, and the complexity of agency procedures.[84,85]

Access and accommodation technologies also referred to as assistive technology and assistive technology services are integral to transition services for youth with severe disabilities.[88,112] Assistive technology is defined as technology applied to people with disabilities to enable productivity, communication, self-care, and mobility; to reduce the need for personal assistance; and to promote self-advocacy.[83] The application of assistive technology requires a team approach that begins with a thorough examination that includes assessment of the individual's needs, abilities, preferences, and features of the environment.[26,65]

TRANSITION PLANNING IN THE EDUCATION SYSTEM

In 1983, Madeline Will, assistant secretary of the US Office of Special Education and Rehabilitation Services, proposed a *bridges model* for transition of youth from school to work that emphasizes linkages between school and post-school environments.[148] Three possible bridges were identified: (1) transition without special services, (2) transition with time-limited services, and (3) transition with ongoing services.[46] Subsequently, Halpern proposed *community adjustment* and *work preparation* models.[46] The *community adjustment* model is based on three pillars of community inclusion: employment, residential environments, and social networks. The *work preparation model* includes the four elements of transition services described in the Individuals with Disabilities Education Improvement Act (IDEA): (1) based on student needs, preferences, and interests, (2) a coordinated set of activities, (3) an outcome-oriented process, and (4) a progression from school to post-school activities.[46,72] Several promising practices for successful transition have been proposed by advocates, researchers, and policy makers.[83,110] These practices include (1) development of student self-efficacy and social skills, (2) community and paid work experiences, (3) technology to improve accessibility and accommodation, (4) secondary curricular reform, (5) vocational career education, (6) supports for postsecondary education, (7) service coordination and interagency collaboration, and (8) individualized backward planning in which the outcome is first identified and then a transition plan is developed.

The Individuals with Disability Act (IDA) of 1990 mandated an outcome-oriented process that included transition services, beginning at age 16. The statement of transition services, also known as the individualized transition plan (ITP), ensures that IEP activities help prepare the student for roles following secondary education. In most states the ITP is included as a page or section of a student's IEP. The plan is reviewed annually and includes coordinated activities that are based on a student's needs and preferences.[46] Activities might include instruction, community experiences, career development, daily living skills training, functional vocational evaluation, and linkages with adult services.[46] Reauthorization of IDA in 1997 lowered the age to begin transition services to 14 years. District and state testing were mandated in order to hold schools accountable for the student's progress in the general curriculum. Related services, including physical therapy, were added in the definition of transition services. The Perkins Technical and Vocational Act of 1998 (Public Law 105-332) emphasized the quality of vocational education and the need for supplemental services for individuals with special needs.

The Individuals with Disabilities Education Improvement Act of 2004 redefined the age of transition to 16 years and moved to a "results-oriented" process focusing on improving students' academic and functional achievement to promote post-school outcomes. Accountability was emphasized by requiring the transition plan to include appropriate measurable postsecondary goals. Transition services are defined as follows:

> *A coordinated set of activities for a student, with a disability, that: (A) is designed within a results oriented process, that is focused on improving the academic and functional achievement of the child with a disability to facilitate the child's movement from school to post-school activities, including postsecondary education, vocational education, integrated employment (including supported employment), continuing and adult education, adult services, independent living, or community participation; (B) is based on the student's needs, taking into account the student's strengths, preferences and interests; (C) includes instruction, related services, community experiences, the development of employment and other post-school objectives, and, when appropriate, acquisition of daily living skills and functional vocational evaluation. (Section 602, IDEA, 2004)*

Preparation of students with disabilities for postsecondary education, employment (including supported employment), independent living, and community participation must begin no later than 16 years of age under IDEA but can begin earlier. Goals must be measurable and progress tracked and reported. Local education agencies are required to provide students with a summary of their academic and functional performance along with recommendations for postsecondary environments upon exiting from school. Mandates for databased, coordinated transition planning and reporting of outcomes are ambitious and require considerable personnel development for implementation.[111]

Transition planning begins with determining the student's interests, abilities, strengths, and needs. The family and professionals should discuss future options with the student. The transition plan is completed at the IEP/ITP meeting. Post-school outcomes are identified and activities are coordinated within the school team and with external agencies and organizations. Students should be invited to the IEP/ITP meeting, actively participate, and lead the meeting when able. Representatives from adult service agencies often are present to assist the school team in planning services for students who are eligible for their

services. The team, which includes the student, determines the types of transition services (instruction, related services, community experiences, daily living skills, and functional vocational evaluation) necessary to promote movement to post-school environments. Finally, the transition plan includes measurable goals developed by the team. A transition plan for a student with severe disabilities who uses powered mobility and a communication device in vocational environments is included on Expert Consult.

Although in the past physical therapists have not always fully participated in the transition process, they have important roles. Physical therapists are encouraged to (1) prepare youth to be active participants and ideally leaders in developing their IEP; (2) participate in the transition planning process when invited by the student; (3) provide consultation and direct services, as needed, for seating, transfers, mobility, self-care, wellness and fitness, instruction for personal care attendants, assistive technology, and environmental modifications; and (4) work collaboratively with school personnel to ensure that health and physical function are adequately addressed in the school-based ITP. The transition plan on the Expert Consult illustrates services and activities that may be supported by a physical therapist.

Transition Outcomes in the Education System

Data from two National Longitudinal Transition Studies authorized by the US Congress identified areas for improvement of transition outcomes. Although the findings may not generalize to current transition outcomes due to the time frame of data collection, the issues identified are pertinent.

In 1983, Congress mandated and funded the first National Longitudinal Transition Study (NLTS). The NLTS was designed to gather data on experiences of students with disabilities during the first 3 to 5 years after high school. Interviews encompassing many facets of transition were completed with 1990 students and families. Although youth with disabilities made substantial progress, their employment rates, wages, postsecondary education, and residential independence were lower than peers without disabilities. Based on the findings, individualized transition planning that reflects the student's goals, strengths, needs, characteristics, and disability was recommended.[17]

Congress authorized a second National Longitudinal Transition Study (NLTS2) conducted from 2000 to 2005. The sample included 11,272 students from 501 local education agencies (LEA). Students 13 to 16 years old when the study began were receiving special education across 12 special education categories. Methods were similar to those of the NLTS. In the NLTS2, fewer students were classified with mental retardation (the current term is *intellectual disability*), whereas the number of students categorized as having other health impairments increased.[143] More youth with disabilities were living with at least one biologic parent, and the heads of households were less likely to be unemployed or high school dropouts. The number of students with intellectual disability or emotional disturbances living in poverty with an unemployed head of household increased between 1987 and 2001.

Parents in both National Longitudinal Transition Studies expected their children with disabilities to graduate from high school with a regular diploma. In the NLTS2, parents of youth with speech or hearing impairments had greater expectations for postsecondary education. Overall, 2-year colleges were considered more of an option in 2001 than in 1987, and employment expectations were higher. Parental expectations for employment of youth with intellectual disability, hearing impairment, other health impairments, and multiple disabilities increased.[143]

In the NLTS2, participation of students with disabilities in extracurricular activity remained lower than it did for their peers without disability. In 2001, significantly more youth with disabilities had paid jobs 1 year after graduation. The 1-year employment rate was 60%, which is similar to youth in the general population (63%). Youth had an increase in work-study jobs and pay but a decline in the average number of hours worked per week. In social adjustment, more youth with disabilities were suspended or expelled, fired from a job, or arrested in 2001 than in 1987.[143]

The 2010 Harris Poll by the Kessler Foundation and National Organization on Disability revealed that discrepancies in employment still exist. Of all working people, those with disabilities have a 21% employment rate when compared to 59% for the general population. The majority of companies interviewed stated that they had hired someone with a disability in the past 3 years, and most of these employees were recruited through the referral of friends or word of mouth. Finally, people with disabilities made up only 2% of the workforce in these companies, again demonstrating an employment gap.

Using a sample of 1510 students with orthopedic impairments (including cerebral palsy and spina bifida) from the NLTS 2, Bjornson et al.[16] investigated the relationship between occupational therapy and physical therapy services and postsecondary education and employment. At post–high school follow-up, 48% of the sample participated in postsecondary education and 24% had paid employment. Receiving therapy services at ages 13–16 years was significantly associated with enrollment in postsecondary education at 19–21 years. Social interactions and expressive language skills were significantly associated with employment, but high school therapy services were not.[16]

Several factors have been identified as predictors of postsecondary education and employment among students who receive transition services. Vocational education, attending a rural school, work-study participation, and having a learning disability (versus another condition) were predictors of full-time employment after graduation in a random sample of 140 graduates from special education programs interviewed 1 and 3 years following graduation.[7] Attending a suburban school and participating in general education curriculum were predictors of postsecondary education. Benz, Lindstrom, and Yovanoff reported that career-related work experience and completion of student-identified transition goals were associated with improved graduation and employment outcomes.[12] Students valued individualization of services and personalized attention. Halpern et al. identified the following predictors of success in postsecondary education: (1) high scores on a functional achievement inventory, (2) completing instruction successfully in relevant curricular areas, (3) participating in transition planning, (4) parent satisfaction with secondary education, (5) student satisfaction with secondary education, and (6) parent perception that the student no longer needed help in certain critical skill areas.[54] Critical skills that might pertain to physical therapy include community mobility, use of public transportation, use of restroom, positioning and mobility instruction for personal care attendants, positioning for work or postsecondary education activities, and proficiency with assistive technology.

COMMUNITY- AND HOSPITAL-BASED TRANSITION PROGRAMS

Community- and hospital-based transition programs are emerging and vary considerably in focus and scope. Research has identified needs and processes for service delivery. Outcomes have been described, but research is needed to generalize findings. A formidable challenge for community- and hospital-based transition programs is coordination of services with the education system and community organizations and agencies. Skill development, environmental supports, and an individualized approach were identified as important components of transition services in a systematic review by Stewart et al.[130] Binks et al. performed a systematic review of outcomes specific to the transition from child-centered to adult-centered health care for youth with cerebral palsy or spina bifida.[15] Elements associated with successful transition to adult-centered health care were (1) preparation, (2) flexible timing of transition programs with a suggested age of 14 to 16 years, (3) care coordination that includes an up-to-date transition plan, (4) transition clinic visits including a consult with both the child and adult health care providers, and (5) interested adult-centered health care providers.

The Life Needs Model[79] (Fig. 32.3) is a collaborative approach to service delivery designed to meet the long-term goals of community participation and quality of life for children and youth with disabilities. The Life Needs Model incorporates processes supported by research. Core values of community- and hospital-based transition programs for youth with physical disabilities are listed in Box 32.1. The following paragraphs describe characteristics of four innovative transition programs; each illustrates the importance of interagency collaboration.

The Center of Innovation in Transition & Employment (CITE) at Kent State University in Ohio provides leadership in graduate education and transition practices for youth 18 to 21 years old with disabilities (http://www.kent.edu/ehhs/centers/cite). Local high school students with disabilities participate in a continuum of job training, career exploration, and college experiences on the Kent State campus. Graduate students from several disciplines obtain practical experience in providing transition services. The objective of the collaborative is to prepare students with disabilities for competitive employment and postsecondary education by providing them opportunities for future planning, skill development, and self-advocacy and to prepare transition coordinators of the future. Since 1985, 20 to 40 high school students with severe disabilities have been provided career exploration and job training each year. In most cases, these students transition to supported employment and community living. More than 100 graduates have become transition leaders throughout the state and country.

Gillette Children's Specialty Healthcare in Minnesota (http://www.gillettechildrens.org) has a long-standing reputation for comprehensive services for children with physical disabilities. In response to the lack of services available to adults with childhood-onset physical disabilities and young adults who received services from Gillette as children continuing to return for care, the Lifetime Specialty Healthcare for Older Teens and Adults was created.[90] Transition services are available to prepare youth ages 16 and older who are eligible for care through Gillette Lifetime. Transition services include preparing youth to move from pediatric to adult health care, teaching them to manage their medical conditions to the best

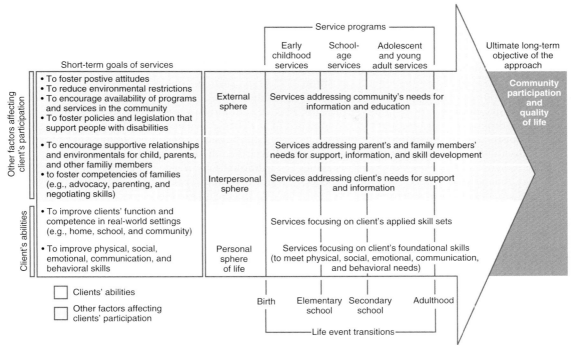

FIG. 32.3 Life needs model of service delivery.

BOX 32.1 Core Values of Community- and Hospital-Based Transition Programs for Youth With Physical Disabilities

Youth and family centered
Partnerships
Strengths based
Self-determination
Experiential learning

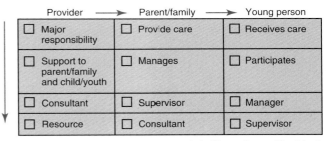

FIG. 32.4 Shared management model. (Data from Kieckhefer GM: Foundations for successful transitions: shared management as one critical component. Keynote presentation at the Hospital for Sick Children, Toronto, Canada, 2002.)

of their ability, and providing education and resources on legal, medical, and independent living. Gillette Lifetime extends services associated with the pediatric health care system to adults including specialty medical and surgical care, physical, occupational and speech therapy, orthotic and prosthetic services, and seating and adaptive equipment. Inpatient care and surgery are available until age 40. Linroth[90] describes the facilities and equipment for serving adults with childhood-onset disabilities and considerations for in-patient care.

Growing Up Ready is a multifaceted program at Holland Bloorview Kids Rehabilitation Hospital in Toronto, Ontario, Canada to help families understand the everyday experiences and skills their children need to become mature, confident adults and how to access them. The program is an outgrowth of a shared management approach to transition services for youth with disabilities by Gall, Kingsnorth, and Healy.[49] The shared management approach is based on the philosophy that development of a therapeutic alliance between youth, families, and health care providers is essential to allow young people with disabilities to develop into independent and healthy adults. As illustrated in Fig. 32.4, the therapeutic alliance is conceptualized as a dynamic relationship in which the roles change over time as the child grows and develops. A gradual shift in responsibilities occurs over time, and leadership is transitioned from

the health care provider and parents to the young person to the maximum extent possible. Youth are encouraged to use experiential learning to gain exposure to opportunities and develop life skills. Timetables and checklists of activities to achieve competencies at different ages are available on the program website: http://hollandbloorview.ca/programsandservices/ProgramsServicesAZ/Growingupready.

Holland Bloorview Kids Rehabilitation Hospital and the University Health Network-Toronto Rehabilitation partnered in 2008 to implement the LIFEspan (Living Independently and Fully Engaged) service designed to coordinate transfer of health care between pediatric and adult rehabilitation services. The program serves youth with cerebral palsy and acquired brain injury. Topics of discussion include: health care providers, school, funding, and community participation and knowledge of health care. Eleven clinical and three managerial staff in the LIFEspan program were interviewed regarding their perspective on service delivery.[55] Five service delivery themes were identified: (1) transition readiness and capacity; (2) shifting responsibility for health care management from parents to youth;

(3) determining services based on organizational resources; (4) linking pediatric and adult rehabilitation services; and (5) linking with multisector services. Participants expressed that a challenge to providing coordinated care was service integration with primary care, education, social, and community services. Recommendations included early introduction of transition information and opportunities to practice skills and establishment of formal partnership between agencies and systems.

The Youth En Route Program in London, Ontario, Canada was one of the first transition programs for youth and young adults with multiple disabilities to systematically evaluate processes and outcomes.[43] Jan Evans, a physical therapist, and Patricia Baldwin, an occupational therapist, were instrumental in development of the program. Youth and young adults 16 to 29 years with multiple disabilities who had completed secondary education were eligible for the program. The program was originally implemented through a partnership between Thames Valley Children's Centre and Hutton House, a community agency for adults with disabilities. The service model is based on self-determination and community participation (Fig. 32.5). A multifaceted approach is utilized that includes (1) self-discovery, (2) skill development, and (3) community experience. Self-determination is promoted through coaching and supporting youth to define, lead, and guide the services and supports they want as they learn more about themselves and their communities. Efforts are made to support youth goals for employment, education, voluntarism, and leisure with experiential opportunities within the community. The program evaluation consisted of a 1-year pre/posttest of 34 participants in the program. Statistical and clinically significant improvements were found in self-determination and sense of personal control. At posttest, youth reported spending more time on volunteer/work and community leisure activities. The authors emphasize the importance of a flexible, client-centered approach that offers youth opportunities for self-discovery, skill development, and community experiences. Thames Valley Children's Centre (http://www.tvcc.on.ca/) is one of 21 public funded children's rehabilitation centres in Ontario. Current programs based on model for Youth En Route include Youth Discovery Services and Youth for Youth.

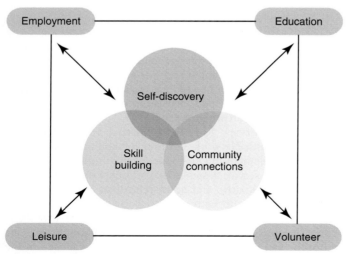

FIG. 32.5 Model for Youth En Route Program. (From Evans J, McDougall J, Baldwin P: An evaluation of the "youth en route" program. *Phys Occupat Ther Pediatr* 26[4]:63-87, 2006. Printed with permission of authors.)

FOREGROUND INFORMATION

ROLE OF THE PHYSICAL THERAPIST IN THE TRANSITION PROCESS

Preparing youth with physical disabilities for transition to the adult care system and postsecondary education, work, and community living is an emerging role of the physical therapist. In 1997, Campbell proposed that preparing individuals with physical disabilities to take personal responsibility for their health and physical fitness should begin at a young age.[24] Although physical therapists have worked in public schools for more than 30 years, the IDEA of 1997 was the first educational law to include related services as mandated services in transition. Several authors have suggested roles for physical therapists in the transition process including the following[3,24,39,68,122,155]:

- Assessing present or future environments utilizing an ecologic approach
- Assessing assistive technology needs and instruction of others in use of assistive technology
- Intervening for positioning, seating, transfers, mobility, and transportation
- Assisting with job development, coaching, and placement options
- Anticipating student needs for community living and work
- Promoting community leisure and health-related fitness activities
- Facilitating transition to adult health care services
- Collaborating with other professionals, staff, and community-based agencies to coordinate services

Physical therapists working in educational settings may provide consultative services during individualized education program (IEP/ITP) meetings. Therapists may provide direct services during times of the day when the student is on the job, at a postsecondary school, or participating in community recreation. Therapists also provide information and instruction of others including care providers, educators, and family members.[3,122] Though likely more challenging because of the nature of third-party payer systems, therapists working in noneducational practice settings are encouraged to consider these universally shared roles to facilitate youth-to-adult transitions.

The *Guide to Physical Therapist Practice* states that physical therapists should provide interventions across the life span in the following areas: (1) environmental barriers, (2) self-care and home management (including activities of daily living), (3) work (job/school/play), (4) community and leisure integration, and (5) orthotic, protective, and supportive devices.

A perspective on the role of the physical therapist in the continuum of care for individuals with childhood-onset disabilities endorsed by the American Physical Therapy Association summarizes issues and provides suggestions for practitioners.[106] The authors emphasize the need to improve transitions from pediatric to adult-oriented health care and adult health care systems that enable healthy living. Challenges experienced in health care transition are summarized, and recommendations are provided for physical therapy practice. An important challenge/barrier is that many physical therapists who serve adults feel ill prepared to provide services to adults with childhood-onset conditions. A recommendation for physical therapy education programs is to embed case studies of adults with childhood-onset developmental disabilities across body systems and clinical courses other than pediatrics so that students embrace the reality that children with developmental disabilities will be future adult clients who experience similar musculoskeletal and neuromuscular impairments as adults without developmental disabilities. Another recommendation is for physical therapists to consider providing consultation to fitness centers as a means to encourage participation of adults with childhood-onset disabilities at their neighborhood gyms. The authors highlight that adults with childhood-onset disabilities are not seeking services for their specific condition but rather to prevent or remediate secondary impairments that limit their ability to participate in meaningful community and life activities and to live a healthy lifestyle.

Physical therapist examination, evaluation, and intervention are driven by youth concerns, needs, and preferences and should occur in specific and relevant environments, present and future. Three environments that physical therapists are encouraged to consider during the transition years are (1) work or postsecondary education settings, (2) adult living environments, and (3) community settings for leisure or social participation. In addition, examination and intervention must be approached from a perspective of future inclusive community living and work rather than segregated living and work. Box 32.2 lists the types of interventions provided by physical therapists during the transition process. The phrase *student- or youth-related instruction* is preferred in the context of transition services.

Examination and Evaluation

The examination begins with identification of the youth's participation goals, reinforcing a person-centered approach. In the *Guide to Physical Therapist Practice,* this is part of the interview phase of the examination. We believe it is important for youth to express interest in self-discovery, experiential learning, and skill development and that families express a willingness to support and engage in activities to prepare their children for adult roles.

Next, task analysis is performed to identify what is necessary to accomplish the goals. The task analysis will guide the examination and evaluation of what the youth can do (strengths/capacity) and what problems, challenges, and barriers must be addressed for achievement of goals. The examination should be interactive with full participation of the youth and her or his family. Areas of examination by physical therapists are often directed toward optimization of health status, functional ability, and self-management. Evaluation involves interpretation of examination findings to identify participation restrictions, activity limitations, and contributing impairments in body functions and structures. The physical therapist's examination and evaluation contribute to the assessments performed by other members of the interprofessional team, including future planning, knowledge, skills, supports, and current participation in school and community activities related to transition to new environments. Box 32.3 includes considerations for examination and evaluation. Box 32.4 lists selected measures for transition planning focusing on student activity and participation roles. Some of these measures are team oriented and are best completed by the full educational team, including the physical therapist.

Goals and Plan of Care

The collaboration of youth, parent(s), and professionals leads to development of an ITP in the education environment in addition to the physical therapist's plan of care. This plan will include person-centered measurable long-term goals and short-term objectives. Therapists are encouraged to consider long-term, person-centered goals for activity and participation and short-term, person-centered objectives that address body functions and structures, personal, and environmental factors hypothesized to contribute to activity limitations and participation restrictions. The plan of care should include collaboration with community providers, organizations, and agencies. Combining the evaluations of all members of the transition team is essential for identifying youth-centered goals for activity and participation. It is unlikely that a participation goal would focus exclusively on a single domain (motor, cognitive, behavioral, self-help). Key activities, services, time frames, and individuals responsible for implementation should be documented. Therapists are encouraged to identify community collaborators who will provide the necessary support for transition plan goals. Whenever possible, therapists should involve the transitioning youth in this process to further support self-determination skills.

BOX 32.2 Considerations for Physical Therapist Interventions

Coordination, Communication, and Documentation

Participation in the IEP process
Collaboration with agencies: equipment suppliers, transportation agencies
Data collection to document change
Interdisciplinary teamwork (between schools, developmental disabilities agencies, vocational rehabilitation agencies)
Referrals to other professional sources (e.g., assistive technology vendors, orthotists)
Support youth to identify goals and engage in decision making

Student/Youth-Related Instruction

Instruction, education, and skill development of youth and caregiver regarding:
Knowledge of health condition
Enhancement of performance
Health wellness, fitness programs
Transitions across settings
Transitions to new roles (employment, adult living, community participation)
Opportunities for real-word experiences

Procedural Interventions

Positioning for prevention of secondary impairments in body functions and structures
Physical activity
Functional training in self-care, home management, and work (job/school)
Task adaptation for eating, dressing, grooming, toileting
Device use (such as power wheelchairs, communication devices, electronic calendars)
Travel training (public transportation and community mobility)
Shopping, meal preparation, scheduling activities and appointments
Job coaching
Safety across home, work, and postsecondary education environments
Leisure and recreational activities
Prescription, application, fabrication of devices and equipment
Environmental controls through use of assistive technology or rehabilitation engineering
Mobility devices, both ambulatory and powered mobility

BOX 32.3   Considerations for Physical Therapist Examination and Evaluation

What should physical therapists examine for transition planning?

Seating
Transfers
Mobility
Self-care
Leisure interests and activities
Device and equipment use

How should therapists examine students for transition planning?

Measures that describe and quantify
Checklists/scales
Logs, interviews (student interest/preferences survey)
Observations (ecologic assessment/task analysis)
Transportation assessments

Questionnaires
Video/pictures

Where should therapists evaluate students for transition planning?

Home
Community sites including recreation facilities
Postsecondary education environments including university and community
Job site

What data are generated from a physical therapy examination for transition planning?

Descriptions of environment and barriers
Student functioning in the environment
Ability to participate in environments
Need for equipment

BOX 32.4   Selected Measures for Transition Planning

Life Centered Career Education[22]
Canadian Occupational Performance Measure[86]
Children's Assessment of Participation and Enjoyment/Preferences for Activities of Children[81]
Enderle-Severson Transition Rating Scale[41]
Transition Planning Inventory[27]
Student Activity Accessibility Checklist[123]
Choose and Take Action[96]
Transition Assessment and Goal Generator (TAGG)[97]
Supports Intensity Scale (SIS) [137]
Keeping It Together for Youth[128]

Members of the educational interprofessional team will vary based on each youth's strengths, needs, program staff, and community resources. A transition coordinator ensures communication and coordination among team and external agencies and organizations. Although any team member may serve as the transition coordinator, knowledge of community resources and services is important. This knowledge enriches the services and support phase of the transition process. Youth and family learning styles and preferred methods of communication are important in determining formats for providing information, self-determination strategies, educational materials, and instruction. Therapists are encouraged to view their professional role as one that leads to greater independence of the youth with disability and/or his/her family. Guiding youth in this process, rather than becoming the "expert," should be fostered and thus become the emphasis of a therapist's role in transition.

Early communication with adult service providers such as vocational rehabilitation, developmental disability agencies, university disability services centers, and adult health care providers is a key to successful transition. Physical therapists can then direct and guide youth with disabilities and their families to each of these resources. Physical therapists can educate youth about maintaining optimal physical function by adopting a lifestyle that promotes health and wellness through activities and sports. Physical therapists in community and hospital settings can develop and utilize linkages with the school-based team and

other local resources to ensure effective communication and coordination of services.

The physical therapist may consult and provide interventions for positioning, transfers, mobility, self-care, transportation, recreation, and leisure activities. Environmental modifications, assistive technology, and task accommodations are important for household management, postsecondary education, and vocational training. Services are designed to optimize safety, efficiency, and independence in performance of functional tasks in real-life settings. Before youth leave the pediatric health care system, physical therapists can help them to identify therapy needs and services and to communicate with the adult health care providers they chose. Box 32.2 is a summary list of intervention areas to be considered by the physical therapist.

Four studies and case reports with transition-age students with cerebral palsy provide examples of involving/supporting youth as active participants in their individualized interventions. Hedgecock, Rapport, and Sutphin[59] described the improvements across the ICF continuum in both strength and functional activity, leading to mastery of participation in personal goals at school and in the community. The examination, intervention, and outcomes of a 3-month episode of physical therapy using functional training and progressive resistive exercise with an 18-year-old with cerebral palsy (GMFCS II) were described. The results included clinically significant improvements in functional strength, agility, and anaerobic power generation. Patient-defined participation increased as he mastered personal goals related to mobility at school and in the community, thereby preparing him for community activities in the postsecondary environment.

Although not part of a transition plan, a case report by Kenyon et al.[74] illustrates the importance of self-exploration and skill acquisition for an 18-year-old female with spastic quadriplegic cerebral palsy (GMFCS level V) and cortical blindness. Intervention included a 12-week power mobility training in an engaging environment focusing on specific skills. The student, who was previously unsuccessful in a onetime powered mobility trial with a standard joystick, now used a head switch to activate the power wheelchair trainer. The student's scores on a standardized measure of power mobility and the health index of life with disabilities improved after training. Improvements with purposeful driving included stop/go and direction-specific

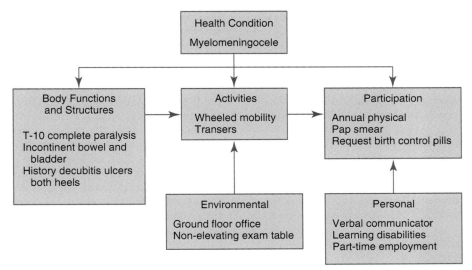

FIG. 32.6 ICF framework applied to an 18-year-old female accessing the adult health care system.

switch activations. Additionally, her mother noted that the participant was more aware of her surroundings. The participant did not achieve the level of driving ability to support funding for a power wheelchair, illustrating the importance of purposeful driving in real-world contexts as the desired long-term outcome.

Lephart and Kaplan[87] reported that that IEP goals for student-initiated communication and powered mobility were achieved through assistive technology for positioning and mobility in a 19-year-old with cerebral palsy (GMFCS level V) and scoliosis. A single-subject design was used to compare a standard planar wheelchair insert to a custom-molded back. The effects on oxygen saturation (SaO_2), heart rate (HR), respiratory rate (RR), body temperature, and processing time to activate switches, and response accuracy at school were assessed. When the student was positioned with the custom-molded back, SaO_2 changed from distressed to normal and fluctuations in HR, RR, and body temperature decreased. Processing time to activate switches decreased and accuracy increased. Student-initiated communication also increased because the student was more interactive when positioned in the custom-molded back. The finding that the custom-molded back not only improved activity and participation but also improved physiologic functions has important implications for seating comfort and endurance.

Sylvester et al.[133] investigated the effects of integrating self-determination strategies into physical therapy interventions and found this to benefit the mobility outcomes of young adults with intensive needs. Clinician-directed and client-directed approaches were compared when providing interventions for mobility skills. Although both interventions improved mobility skills, the client-centered approach using client-chosen goals proved more effective, especially during generalization and maintenance of skills. Findings indicated that clients preferred the self-determined sessions because they chose and were in control of intervention sessions.

The ICF framework is an additional lens from which physical therapists in collaboration with youth and their families can proceed through a transition planning meeting and goal setting. Using the ICF framework, three scenarios are presented for transition services in Figs. 32.6, 32.7, and 32.8. The first case involves a young woman accessing the adult health care system,

the second involves a young man attending a university, and the third involves a young man who has applied for a job. As suggested in Chapter 1, the arrows between the three components of health and environmental and personal factors are specific to each case.

Consider the following suggested instructions to apply the ICF framework to your thought processes on the role of the physical therapist in transition planning. Cover up all but the components of activity and participation. What are the environmental contexts for each example? Are the activity and participation entities adult or youth transition oriented? How often have you been future oriented and considered such examples? Now think about and list all the steps (task analysis) necessary to fully accomplish each activity. To avoid preconceived notions, do not look at the health condition of each youth. What physical therapy decisions would you make for each case? What additional information is needed to formulate a plan of care? What tests and measures would you consider administering for each case? What information is specific to physical therapy and what can be acquired through interprofessional collaboration?

Write a long-term goal and short-term objective for each case. Is the goal person/patient/client centered? Is the person/patient/student's goal measurable? Is it an activity or participation goal? Are the objectives toward meeting the long-term goal measurable? Are the measurement criteria appropriate? Based on the goal and objective written for each example, what are indicators that outcomes have been achieved?

What are the current barriers to you embracing this process? Were you able to proceed through this process using the examples in Figs. 32.6, 32.7, and 32.8 without focused attention to the individual health conditions? As an exercise, interchange the health conditions for each example. How does the process change, if at all?

Role of the Physical Therapist in Transition Processes

The extent to which and how physical therapists employed in educational settings participate in the transition planning and services are not well understood and even less so in other practice settings. Findings of earlier studies indicated that occupational therapists and physical therapists did not participate fully in the transition process for students with severe physical disabilities.[52,135] In reviewing the attendance at IEP meetings, Getzel and DeFur reported that occupational and physical therapists rarely participated in the meetings, although students received services such as material adaptations and assistive technology from these disciplines.[52] In related studies of occupational therapists' involvement in transition, Inge[67] and Anderson[5] found that therapists were minimally involved in transition planning and transition services.

Findings in a national survey investigating the scope of practice for physical therapists working with students in secondary education found more involvement than previously described.[38] More than 50% of the 1041 respondents had high school students on their caseload. Respondents reported more collaboration with school-related personnel in

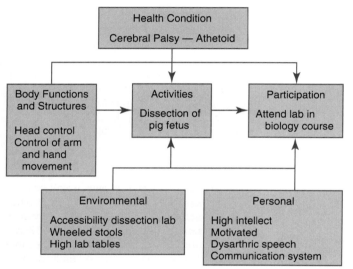

FIG. 32.7 ICF framework applied to a 21-year-old male enrolled in a university biology course.

transition planning than adult service agencies or universities and that they *sometimes* attend transition planning meetings. Respondents indicated that *most of the time* they used observation/narrative summaries and considered a student's preferences and interests. They *infrequently or never* used ecologic task analysis, observed students in the community, or used published checklist/tools. The most common practices in IEP/ITP development were providing input for goals/objectives, making decisions as a member of the educational team, and collaborating with teams about intervention ideas. Physical therapists were less involved with attending IEP meetings and completing the summary of performance. The authors concluded that physical therapists working in secondary transition programs need to: (a) complete more comprehensive evaluations across a variety of future environments with students who have intensive support needs; and (b) expand collaborative service delivery to include a student's local community and provide interventions in the community to promote generalizability of skills. Administrative support and in-service education were the strongest predictors of therapist involvement with transition-age students. Education in physical therapy, years of experience in school-based practice, and school-based practice with secondary age students were weak predictors of therapist involvement with transition-age students.

Physical therapists are encouraged to increase their involvement in transition planning and services because they have the expertise to intervene in areas that are often barriers to employment, independent living, and recreation for young adults with disabilities.[24,122] In James' qualitative study of five students with multiple disabilities transitioning to adulthood, students, families, and teachers stated that needs for assistive technology, use of transportation, and difficulties with toileting were insurmountable obstacles.[69] In a survey of pediatric physical therapists and occupational therapists, therapists identified themselves as practicing below an optimal level in promoting community recreation and leisure for children and adolescents

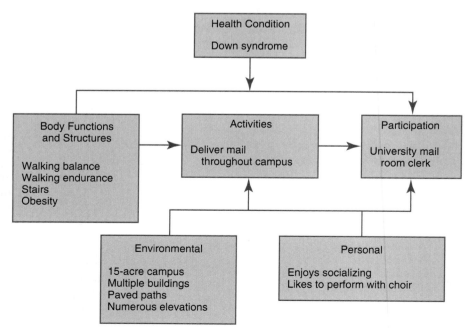

FIG. 32.8 ICF framework applied to work considerations for a young adult applying for a job.

with disabilities and their families.[135] For example, many therapists stated they were not discussing transportation options, barriers to accessing community facilities, or gathering information on social barriers.

Reasons why physical therapists are not routinely involved with transition services for students with physical disabilities in secondary education and the effects of physical therapist intervention on transition outcomes have not been investigated. Factors associated with professional preparation and cost of services may well impact on physical therapist involvement in transition planning and services in all practice settings (school, hospital, community). Professional education in pediatrics usually focuses on young children, with limited content on young and aging adults with developmental disabilities; physical therapists working with adults in hospitals or outpatient clinics are often not aware of issues common to adults with developmental disabilities.[31,32]

Practice settings often dictate the parameters for intervention. In contrast to hospitals and clinics, school-based practice is guided by federal and state legislation. Emphasis is on enhancing student participation in the education program. Transition is a natural part of the education process as the student advances through primary, middle, and secondary grades and schools. Interventions by physical therapists working in the hospital setting may focus on impairments in body functions and structures because of the acute nature of hospital admissions. Outpatient clinics, be they based in a hospital or private practice, generally do not have the typical real-world environment that is the context for activity and participation. Though professional organizations have embraced the ICF framework, the extent the ICF is applied in any of the practice environments is unknown. Communication between practitioners in any or all of these practice environments is especially critical at times of transitions.

ADULTS WITH CHILDHOOD-ONSET DISABILITIES

Demographics on adults with childhood-onset conditions underscore the importance of quality services to prepare youth with disabilities to transition to adulthood. Advances in health care since the late 1980s have increased the life span of individuals with childhood-onset conditions; 50% to 90% of adolescents with cerebral palsy, spina bifida, and acquired brain injury live into adulthood.[151] Approximately 200,000 individuals with developmental disabilities are over the age of 60, a number that is expected to double by 2030.[32] Further, more students with disabilities are pursuing postsecondary, higher education than ever before.[64]

As pediatric physical therapists strive to assist youth and young adults with physical disabilities in their transition to the adult health care system, a number of issues warrant consideration. Depending on the physical therapy education program attended and years since graduation, physical therapists whose practice is limited to adults may have limited knowledge of childhood-onset conditions. As a consequence, they may be uncomfortable providing interventions for secondary impairments such as pain, fatigue, and musculoskeletal contractures in adults with childhood-onset conditions. When referring youth who have aged out of the pediatric health care system, pediatric physical therapists are encouraged to enthusiastically offer consultation or shared intervention with their colleagues in adult practice settings. Proactively preparing youth to interact

with adult providers is encouraged. For some youth, this might entail creating a therapeutic/medical vocabulary for their augmentative communication systems in order to independently express concerns and respond to questions during the examination. We must continually ask ourselves how best to prepare young people with disabilities for transition to adulthood.

PROFESSIONAL RESOURCES FOR PHYSICAL THERAPISTS

Expert Consult includes a list of recommended websites with resources on transition for youth, family, and professionals. The websites include transition manuals, forms for screening and assessment, checklists, and transition activities. For the most part, the psychometric properties of measures and the utility of planning and activity resources have not been evaluated.

Adolescents and Adults with Developmental Disabilities Special Interest Group

The Adolescents and Adults with Developmental Disabilities Special Interest Group (AADD SIG) was established by the Section on Pediatrics of the American Physical Therapy Association (APTA) in 2001 to meet the professional development needs of therapists providing services to adolescents and adults with developmental disabilities. The goals are to provide a forum for therapists to meet, network, and promote quality care through education, research, and practice. The focus of the SIG includes (1) examination and prevention of impairments in adults with developmental disabilities to ensure maximum participation in society, (2) development of intervention guidelines for the adult with developmental disabilities, and (3) promotion of advocacy for adults with developmental disabilities through research and education.[33] The membership of the SIG and educational opportunities continue to grow and can be accessed through www.pediatricapta.org.

▌ S U M M A R Y

Transition to adulthood is a future-oriented process in which youth begin planning for adult roles and responsibilities including finding an adult medical home, living outside the family home, obtaining postsecondary education and employment, and participating in social and community activities. The transition process encompasses the health, psychosocial, and educational-vocational needs of adolescents as they move to adult-oriented lifestyles and systems.

Contemporary approaches to transition services are youth and family centered, involve youth as active participants, and emphasize real-world experiences, development of life skills, environmental supports, and community accommodations. Although transition planning and services are mandated for students with disabilities, physical therapists working in an educational setting have not fully participated in the transition process. Increasingly, community agencies and children's hospitals are providing transition services, although offering coordinated and comprehensive services for adults with childhood-onset disabilities is challenging.

Pediatric physical therapists are encouraged to embrace a lifecourse perspective and future-oriented process to help prepare youth with physical disabilities for adult roles. Complex person-environment issues challenge therapists to critically think beyond impairment-level interventions. This includes instruction of youth in self-management of their health conditions and instruction of others who provide care. Consultation and direct services are recommended, as needed, for seating, transfers, mobility, self-care, wellness and fitness, assistive technology, and environmental modifications. The very language practitioners are encouraged to use when writing goals and action plans, such as student, employee, resident, and athlete, rather than patient, should direct attention toward participatory outcome measures. Potential niche areas of practice include consultation to institutions of higher education, work environments employing persons with disabilities, health clubs interested in being more inclusive in membership recruitment, and adult-oriented physical therapists interested in serving adults with childhood-onset disabilities.

Case Scenarios on Expert Consult

The case scenarios for this chapter illustrate the application of knowledge to practice. One scenario focuses on the varied roles of the physical therapist as a member of the transition team during a student's last 2 years in secondary education. The second scenario describes the experiences and reflections of a pediatric physical therapist as she expands her practice knowledge to include transition of youth with physical disabilities. Additionally, Matt Freeman shares his thoughts on the transition process. Matt is a doctoral candidate in Rehabilitation Science at McMaster University and author of research on information needs of individuals with cerebral palsy and their families during the transition to adulthood and effective ways of delivering information. Matt has the lived experience as an individual with cerebral palsy.

REFERENCES

1. Reference deleted in proofs.
2. American Academy of Pediatrics, American Academy of Family Physicians, and American College of Physicians, Transitions Clinical Report Authoring Group: Supporting the health care transition from adolescence to adulthood in the medical home, *Pediatrics* 128(1):182–200, 2011.
3. American Physical Therapy Association: *Guide to physical therapist practice, 3.0*, 2014. Available at: URL: http://guidetoptpractice.apta.org/.
4. Amsel R, Fichten C: Interaction between disabled and nondisabled college students and their professors: a comparison, *J Postsecondary Educ Disabil* 8:125–140, 1990.
5. Anderson MA: *Survey of pediatric occupational therapists in the state of Oklahoma: is occupational therapy important for secondary level students to assist in successful transition into the community following graduation? Unpublished master's thesis*, Oklahoma City, 2000, University of Oklahoma.
6. Angell ME, Stoner JB, Fulk BM: Advice from adults with physical disabilities on fostering self-determination during the school years, *TEACHING Exceptional Children* 42:64–75, 2010.
7. Baer R, Goebel G, Flexer R, et al.: A collaborative followup study on transition, *Career Dev Except Individuals* 26(1):7–25, 2003.
8. Baer R, McMahan R, Flexer R: *Standards-based transition planning: a guide for parents and professionals*, Kent, OH, 2004, Kent State University.
9. Baker J, Mixner D, Harris D: *The state of disability in America: an evaluation of the disability experience by the life without limits project*, Washington, DC, 2009, United Cerebral Palsy.
10. Bandura A: *Social foundations of thought and action: a social cognitive theory*, Englewood Cliffs, NJ, 1986, Prentice Hall.
11. Barnhardt RC, Connolly B: Aging and Down syndrome: implications for physical therapy, *Phys Ther* 87(10):1399–1406, 2007.
12. Benz MR, Lindstrom L, Yovanoff P: Improving graduation and employment outcomes of students with disabilities: predictive factors and student perspectives, *Except Child* 66(4):509–529, 2000.
13. Benz MR, Yovanoff P, Doren B: School-to-work components that predict postschool success for students with and without disabilities, *Except Child* 63(2):151–166, 1997.
14. Betz C, Nehring W: *Promoting health care transitions for adolescents with special health care needs and disabilities*, Baltimore, 2007, Paul H. Brookes.
15. Binks JA, Barden WS, Burke TA, Young NL: What do we really know about the transition to adult-centered health care? A focus on cerebral palsy and spina bifida, *Arch Phys Med Rehabil* 88(8):1064–1073, 2007.
16. Bjornson K, Kobayashi A, Zhou C, Walker W: Relationship of therapy to postsecondary education and employment in young adults with physical disabilities, *Pediatr Phys Ther* 23(2):179–186, 2011.
17. Blackorby J, Wagner M: Longitudinal postschool outcomes of youth with disabilities: findings from the national longitudinal transition study, *Except Child* 62:399–413, 1996.
18. Blomquist KB: Healthy and ready to work-Kentucky: incorporating transition into a state program for children with special health care needs, *Pediatr Nurs* 32(6):515–528, 2006.
19. Blomquist KB, Brown G, Peersen A, Presler EP: Transitioning to independence: challenges for young people with disabilities and their caregivers, *Orthop Nurs* 17(3):27–35, 1998.
20. Blum RW: Transition to adult health care: setting the stage, *J Adolesc Health* 17(1):3–5, 1995.
21. Breslau N, Staruch KS, Mortimer Jr EA: Psychological distress in mothers of disabled children, *Am J Dis Child (1960)* 136(8):682–686, 1982.
22. Brolin DE: *Life Centered Education (version1.2)*, Arlington, VA, 2012, Council for Except Child.
23. Brollier C, Shepherd J, Markley KF: Transition from school to community living, *Am J Occup Ther* 48(4):346–353, 1994.
24. Campbell SK: Therapy programs for children that last a lifetime, *Phys Occup Ther Pediatr* 17(1):1–15, 1997.
25. Carlon SL, Taylor NF, Dodd KJ, Shields N: Differences in habitual physical activity levels of young people with cerebral palsy and their typically developing peers: a systematic review, *Disabil Rehabil* 35(8):647–655, 2013.
26. Chambers AC: *Has technology been considered? A guide for IEP teams*, Albuquerque, NM, 1997, Councils of Administrators in Special Education.
27. Clark GM, Patton JR: *Transition planning inventory*, ed 2, Austin, TX, 2014, PRO-ED.
28. Clark HB, Foster-Johnson L: Serving youth in transition into adulthood. In Stroul BA, editor: *Children's mental health: creating systems of care in a changing society*, New York, 1996, Brookes, pp 533–551.
29. Clement-Heist K, Siegel S, Gaylord-Ross R: Simulated and in situ vocational social skill training for youth with learning disabilities, *Except Child* 58:336–345, 1992.
30. Cobb B, Lehmann J, Newman-Gonchar R, Alwell M: Self-determination for students with disabilities: a narrative metasynthesis, *Career Dev Except Individuals* 32:108–114, 2009.
31. Compton-Griffith K, Cicirello N, Turner A: Clinicians' perceptions on incentives and barriers when providing physical therapy to adults with neuromotor disabilities: a preliminary study, *Phys Occup Ther Pediatr* 31(1):19–31, 2011.
32. Connolly B: Aging in individuals with lifelong disabilities, *Phys Occup Ther Pediatr* 21(4):23–47, 2001.
33. Connolly BH: Issues in aging in individuals with lifelong disabilities. In Connolly BH, Montgomery PC, editors: *Therapeutic exercise in developmental disabilities*, ed 3, Thorofare, NJ, 2005, Slack, pp 505–529.
34. Cooley WC: American Academy of Pediatrics Committee on Children with Disabilities: providing a primary care medical home for children and youth with cerebral palsy, *Pediatrics* 114(4):1106–1113, 2004.
35. Darrah J, Magil-Evans J, Adkins R: How well are we doing? Families of adolescents or young adults with cerebral palsy share their perceptions of service delivery, *Disabil Rehabil* 24(10):542–549, 2002.
36. Darrah J, Magil-Evans J, Galambos N: Community services for young adults with motor disabilities-a paradox, *Disabil Rehabil* 32(3):223–229, 2010.
37. Dornbush SM: Transitions from adolescence: a discussion of seven articles, *J Adolesc Res* 15:173–177, 2000.

38. Doty A, Flexer R, Barton L, et al.: *A national survey of school-based physical therapists and secondary transition practices.* Unpublished Doctoral Dissertation, Kent, Ohio, 2010, Kent State University.

39. Doty A, Hamilton E, O'Shea R: *The continuum of care for individuals with lifelong disabilities: exploring the issues and roles for physical therapists,* Presentation at the Annual Conference of the American Physical Therapy Association, June, 2008.

40. Dykens EM, Rosner BA, Butterbaugh G: Exercise and sports in children and adolescents with developmental disabilities: positive physical and psychosocial effects, *Child Adoles Psychiatr Clin N Am* 7(4):757–771, 1998.

41. Enderle J, Severson S: *Enderle-Severson Transition Rating Scale,* ed 3, Moorehead, MN, 2003, ESTR.

42. Erson T: *Gross motor activities for inclusive and special needs classrooms: the Courageous Pacers Program,* Framingham, MA, 2003, Therapro.

43. Evans J, McDougall J, Baldwin P: An evaluation of the "youth en route" program, *Phys Occupat Ther Pediatr* 26(4):63–87, 2006.

44. Field S, Martin J, Miller R, et al.: Self-determination for persons with disabilities: a position statement of the division on career development and transition, *Career Dev Except Individuals* 21(2):113–128, 1998.

45. Flexer RW, Baer RM: Transition planning and promising practices. In Flexer RW, Baer RM, Luft P, Simmons TJ, editors: *Transition planning for secondary students with disabilities,* ed 3, Upper Saddle River, NJ, 2008, Prentice-Hall, pp 3–28.

46. Flexer RW, Baer RM: Transition legislation and models. In Flexer RW, Baer RM, Luft P, Simmons TJ, editors: *Transition planning for secondary students with disabilities,* ed 3, Upper Saddle River, NJ, 2008, Prentice-Hall, pp 29–53.

47. Frey GC, Buchanan AM, Rosser Sandt DD: I'd rather watch TV: an examination of physical activity in adults with mental retardation, *Ment Retard* 43(4):241–254, 2005.

48. Friedrich WN, Greenberg MT, Crnic K: A short-form of the questionnaire on resources and stress, *Am J Ment Defic* 88(1):41–48, 1983.

49. Gall C, Kingsnorth S, Healy K: Growing up ready: a shared management approach, *Phys Occupat Ther Pediatr* 26(4):47–62, 2006.

50. Gaylord-Ross R: Vocational integration for persons with handicaps. In Gaylord-Ross R, editor: *Integration strategies for students with handicaps,* Baltimore, 1989, Brookes, pp 195–211.

51. Getzel E: Preparing for college. In Getzel E, Wehman P, editors: *Going to college: expanding opportunities for people with disabilities,* Baltimore, MD, 2005, Paul H. Brookes Publishing Co, pp 69–87.

52. Getzel E, deFur S: Transition planning for students with significant disabilities: implications for student centered planning, *Focus Autism Other Dev Disabil* 12(1):39–48, 1997.

53. Halfon N, Larson K, Lu M, et al.: Lifecourse health development: past, present and future, *J Matern Child Health* 18:344–365, 2014.

54. Halpern AS: Quality of life as a framework for evaluating transition outcomes, *Except Child* 59(6):486–498, 1993.

55. Hamdani Y, Jetha A, Norman C: Systems thinking perspectives applied to healthcare transition for youth with disabilities: a paradigm shift for practice, policy and research, *Child Care Health Dev* 37(6):806–814, 2011.

56. Reference deleted in proofs.

57. Havighurst R: *Developmental tasks and education,* ed 3, New York, 1972, D. McKay.

58. Heal LW, Khoju M, Rusch FR: Predicting quality of life of youths after they leave special education high school programs, *J Spec Ed* 31(3):279–299, 1997.

59. Hedgecock J, Rapport M, Sutphin A: Functional movement, strength, and intervention for an adolescent with cerebral palsy, *Pediatr Phys Ther* 27(2):207–214, 2015.

60. Helfer B: *United we ride and safe-T-Lu: new freedom transportation opportunities,* Baltimore, November, 2006, Presentation at Annual TASH Conference.

61. Helms L, Weiler K: Disability discrimination in nursing education: an evaluation of legislation and litigation, *J Prof Nurs* 9(6):358–366, 1993.

62. Henninger NA, Taylor JL: Family perspectives on a successful transition to adulthood for individuals with disabilities, *Intellect Dev Disabil* 52(2):98–111, 2014.

63. Hepburn CM, Cohen E, Bhawra J, et al.: Health system strategies supporting transition to adult care, *Arch Dis Child* 100(6):559–564, 2015.

64. Hitchings WE, Retisch P, Horvath M: Academic preparation of adolescents with disabilities for postsecondary education, *Career Dev Except Individuals* 28(2):26–35, 2005.

65. Holder-Brown L, Parette H: Children with disabilities who use assistive technology: ethical considerations, *Young Child* 47(6):73–77, 1992.

66. Howe J, Horner R, Newton J: Comparison of supported living and traditional residential services in the state of Oregon, *Ment Retard* 36(1):1–11, 1998.

67. Inge K: *A national study of occupational therapists in the public schools: an assessment of current practice, attitudes and training needs regarding the transition process for students with severe disabilities.* Unpublished dissertation, Richmond, 1995, Virginia Commonwealth University.

68. Inge K, Shepherd J: Occupational and physical therapy. In De Fur SH, Patton JR, editors: *Transition and school based services: interdisciplinary perspectives enhancing the transition process,* Austin, TX, 1999, Pro-ed, pp 117–165.

69. James S: *I was prepared to do nothing; I will do nothing: why students with multiple disabilities do not have jobs after leaving high school.* Unpublished master's thesis, Oklahoma City, 2001, University of Oklahoma.

70. Johnson D: Supported employment trends: implications for transition-age youth, *Res Pract Persons Severe Disabl* 29(4):243–247, 2004.

71. Johnson D, Stodden R, Emanuel E, et al.: Current challenges facing secondary education and transition services: what research tells us, *Except Child* 68(4):519–531, 2002.

72. Johnson J, Rusch F: Secondary special education and transition services: identification and recommendations for future research and demonstration, *Career Dev Except Individuals* 16(1):1–18, 1993.

73. Kennedy M, Lewin L: Fact sheet: summary of self-determination. Available at: URL: http://thechp.syr.edu/fs_selfdetermination.doc.

74. Kenyon L, Farris J, Bockway K, et al.: Promoting self-exploration and function through an individualized power mobility training program, *Pediatr Phys Ther* 27(2):200–206, 2015.

75. Kiernan W, Schalock R: *Integrated employment: current status and future directions,* Washington, DC, 1997, American Association of Mental Retardation.

76. King GA, Baldwin PJ, Currie M, Evans J: The effectiveness of transition strategies for youth with disabilities, *Child Health Care* 35(2):155–178, 2006.

77. King GA, Cathers T, Polgar JM, et al.: Success in life for older adolescents with cerebral palsy, *Qual Health Res* 10(6):734–749, 2006.

78. King GA, Shultz IZ, Steel K, et al.: Self-evaluation and self-concept of adolescents with physical disabilities, *Am J Occup Ther* 47(2):132–140, 1993.

79. King GA, Tucker MA, Baldwin PJ, LaPorta JA: Bringing the life needs model to life: implementing a service delivery model for pediatric rehabilitation, *Phys Occup Ther Pediatr* 26(1/2):43–70, 2006.

80. King G, Baldwin P, Currie M, Evans J: Planning successful transitions from school to adult roles for youth with disabilities, *Child Health Care* 34(3):193–216, 2005.

81. King G, Law M, King S, et al.: *Children's Assessment of Participation and Enjoyment (CAPE) and Preferences for Activities of Children (PAC),* San Antonio, TX, 2004, Harcourt Assessment.

82. Kingsnorth S, Healy H, Macarthur C: Preparing for adulthood: a systematic review of life skill programs for youth with physical disabilities, *J Adolesc Health* 41(4):323–332, 2007.

83. Kohler PD: Best practices in transition: substantiated or implied? *Career Dev Except Individuals* 16:107–121, 1993.

84. Kohler PD: Implementing a transition perspective of education: a comprehensive approach to planning and delivering secondary education and transition services. In Rusch FR, Chadsey J, editors: *Beyond high school: transition from school to work,* New York, 1998, Wadsworth, pp 179–205.

85. Kohler PD, Field S: Transition focused education: foundation for the future, *J Spec Educ* 37(3):157–163, 2003.

86. Law M, Baptiste S, Carswell A, et al.: *Canadian occupational performance measure,* ed 3, Toronto, 2005, Canadian Association of Occupational Therapists.

87. Lephart K, Kaplan S: Two seating systems' effects on an adolescent with cerebral palsy and severe scoliosis, *Pediatr Phys Ther* 27(3):258–266, 2015.

88. Lindsey JD: *Technology and exceptional individuals*, ed 3, Austin, TX, 2000, Pro-Ed.

89. Lindsey S: Employment status and work characteristics among adolescents with disabilities, *Disabil Rehabil* 33(10):843–854, 2011.

90. Linroth R: Meeting the needs of young people and adults with childhood-onset conditions: Gillette Lifetime Specialty Healthcare, *Dev Med Child Neurol* 51(Suppl 4):174–177, 2009.

91. Lotstein DS, McPherson M, Strickland B, Newacheck PW: Transition planning for youth with special health care needs: results from the national survey of children with special health care needs, *Pediatrics* 115(6):1562–1568, 2005.

92. Luther B: Age-specific activities that support successful transition to adulthood for children with disabilities, *Orthop Nurs* 20(1):23–29, 2001.

93. Madaus J: Navigating the college transition maze: a guide for students with learning disabilities, *Teaching Except Child* 37(3):32–37, 2005.

94. Magill-Evans J, Galambos N, Darrah J, Nickerson C: Predictors of employment for young adults with developmental motor disabilities, *Work* 31:433–442, 2008.

95. Maltais DB, Wiart L, Fowler E, et al.: Health-related physical fitness for children with cerebral palsy, *J Child Neurol* 29(8):1091–1100, 2014.

96. Martin JE, Marshall LH, Wray D, et al.: *Choose and take action: finding the right job for you*, Longmont, CO, 2004, Sopris West.

97. Martin J, Hennessey M, McConnell A, et al.: TAGG technical manual. Available at: URL: from https://tagg.ou.edu/tagg/.

98. McGavin H: Planning rehabilitation: a comparison of issues for parents and adolescents, *Phys Occup Ther Pediatr* 18:69–82, 1998.

99. McNair J, Rusch FR: Parental involvement in transition programs, *Ment Retard* 29(2):93–101, 1991.

100. Michelson S, Uldall P, Hansen T, et al.: Social integration of adults with cerebral palsy, *Dev Med Child Neurol* 48:643–649, 2006.

101. Misquez E, McCarthy B, Powell B, Chu L: *University students with disabilities are the chief on-campus accommodation ingredient*, Northridge, Conference, 1997, Paper presented at the Annual California State University.

102. National Center for the Study of Postsecondary Educational Supports (NCSPES): *Technical report: postsecondary education and employment for students with disabilities: focus group discussions on supports and barriers to lifelong learning*, Honolulu, 2000, University of Hawaii at Manoa.

103. Newacheck P, Strickland B, Shonkoff J, et al.: An epidemiologic profile of children with special health care needs, *Pediatrics* 102:107–123, 1998.

104. Newman L, Wagner M, Knokey A, et al.: *The post-high school outcomes of young adults with disabilities up to 8 years after high school. A report from the National Longitudinal Transition Study-2 (NLTS2) (NCSER 2011-3005)*, Menlo Park, CA, 2011, SRI International.

105. Reference deleted in proofs.

106. Orlin M, Cicirello N, O'Donnell A, Doty A: Continuum of care for individual with lifelong disabilities: role of the physical therapist, *Phys Ther* 94(7):1043–1053, 2014.

107. Palisano RJ, Almasri N, Chiarello L, et al.: Family needs of parents of children and youth with cerebral palsy, *Child Care Health Dev* 36(1):85–92, 2009.

108. Patrick S, Wessel R: Faculty mentorship and transition experience of students with disabilities, *J Postsecondary Educ Disabil* 26(2):105–118, 2013.

109. McPherson M, Weissman G, Strickland BB, et al.: Implementing community-based systems of services for children and youths with special health care needs: how well are we doing? *Pediatrics* 113(5):1538–1544, 2004.

110. Phelps LA, Hanley-Maxwell C: School-to-work transitions for youth with disabilities: a review of outcomes and practices, *Rev Educ Res* 67(2):176–226, 1997.

111. Powers KM, Gil-Kashiwabara E, Geenen SJ, et al.: Mandates and effective transition planning practices reflected in IEPs, *Career Dev Except Individuals* 28(1):47–59, 2005.

112. Raskind MH: A guide to assistive technology, *Their World*, New York, NY, 1997/1998, National Center for Learning Disabilities, pp 73–74.

113. Rehm RS, Fuentes-Afflick E, Fisher L, Chesla C: Parent and youth priorities during the transition to adulthood for youth with special health care needs and developmental disability, *ANS Adv Nurs Sci* 35(3):E57–E72, 2012.

114. Reiss JG, Gibson RW, Walker LR: Health care transition: youth, family, and provider perspectives, *Pediatrics* 115(1):112–120, 2005.

115. Rosenbaum PL, Rosenbloom L: *Cerebral palsy: from diagnosis to adult life*, London, 2012, Mac Keith Press.

116. Rothstein L: Students, staff, and faculty with disabilities: current issues for colleges and universities, *J Coll Univ Law* 17:471–482, 1991.

117. Rusch F, Braddock D, Adult day programs versus supported employment (1988-2002): spending and service practices of mental retardation and developmental disabilities state agencies, *Res Pract Persons Severe Disabil* 29(4):237–242, 2004.

118. Rutkowski S, Riehle E: Access to employment and economic independence in cerebral palsy, *Phys Med Rehabil Clin N Am* 20:535–547, 2009.

119. Ryder BE, Kawalec ES: A job-seeking skills program for persons who are blind or visually impaired, *J Vis Impair Blind* 89:107–111, 1995.

120. Sands DJ, Spencer KC, Gliner J, Swaim R: Structural equation modeling of student involvement in transition-related actions: the path of least resistance, *Focus Autism Other Dev Disabil* 14(1):17–27, 1999.

121. Schmidt M, Smith D: Individuals with disabilities perceptions on preparedness for the workforce and factors that limit employment, *Work* 28:13–21, 2007.

122. Simmons T, Flexer RW, Bauder D: Collaborative transition services. In Flexer RW, Baer RM, Luft P, Simmons TJ, editors: *Transition planning for secondary students with disabilities*, ed 3, Upper Saddle River, NJ, 2008, Prentice-Hall, pp 203–229.

123. Smith RO, Warnke J, Edyburn D, et al.: Student Activity Accessibility Checklist. Lawrence, KS: University of Kansas, Division of Adult Studies. Available at: URL: http://das.kucrl.org/materials/html/student-activity-accessibility-checklist.

124. Sowers J, Powers L: *Vocational preparation and employment of students with physical and multiple disabilities*, Baltimore, 1991, Paul H. Brookes.

125. Stein REK: Challenges in long-term health care for children, *Ambul Pediatr* 1(5):280–288, 2001.

126. Stewart D: Evidence to support a positive transition into adulthood for youth with disabilities, *Phys Occup Ther Pediatr* 26(4):1–4, 2006.

127. Stewart DA, Law MC, Rosenbaum P, Williams DG: A qualitative study of the transition to adulthood for youth with physical disabilities, *Phys Occup Ther Pediatr* 21(4):3–21, 2001.

128. Stewart D, Freeman M, Missiuna C, et al.: Keeping It Together™ for Youth. Hamilton, Ontario: CanChild Centre for Childhood Disability Research. Available at: URL: https://www.canchild.ca/en/research-in-practice/the-kit.

129. Stewart D, Law M, Young NL, et al.: Complexities during transitions to adulthood for youth with disabilities: person-environment interactions, *Disabil Rehabil* 36(23):1998–2004, 2014.

130. Stewart D, Stavness C, King G, et al.: A critical appraisal of literature reviews about the transition to adulthood for youth with disabilities, *Phys Occup Ther Pediatr* 26(4):5–24, 2006.

131. Strand J, Kreiner J: Recreation and leisure in the community. In Flexer RW, Simmons TJ, Luft P, Baer RM, editors: *Transition planning for secondary students with disabilities*, ed 2, Upper Saddle River, NJ, 2004, Prentice-Hall, pp 460–482.

132. Strong WB, Wiklmore JH: Unfit kids: an office-based approach to physical fitness, *Contemp Pediatr* 4:33–48, 1988.

133. Sylvester L, Martin J, Gardner J, et al.: *Comparison of clinician-directed and student-self-directed physical therapy interventions for youth with severe and multiple developmental disabilities*. Unpublished Doctoral Dissertation, Norman, Oklahoma, 2011, University of Oklahoma.

134. Test D: Invited commentary on Rusch and Braddock (2004): one person at a time, *Res Pract Persons Severe Disabil* 29(4):248–252, 2004.

135. Thomas AD, Rosenberg A: Promoting community recreation and leisure, *Pediatr Phys Ther* 15(4):232–246, 2003.

136. Thomas S: College students and disability law, *J Spec Educ* 33(4):248–258, 2000.

137. Thompson J, Bryant B, Campbell E, et al.: *Supports Intensity Scale—Adult*, Washington, DC, 2015, American Association on Intellectual and Developmental Disabilities.

138. Tonniges T, Roberts C: *Transitions: a lifelong process and everyone's responsibility.* Presentation for Oklahoma Health Sciences Center Grand Rounds, Oklahoma City, OK, 2007, Department of Pediatrics.
139. Reference deleted in proofs.
140. US Department of Health and Human Services: *Healthy people 2020.* Available at: URL: http://www.healthypeople.gov/.
141. US Department of Health and Human Services: *Surgeon General's report on physical activity and health,* Washington, DC, 1996, USDHHS.
142. Wagner M, Blackorby J, Cameto R, et al.: *The transition experiences of young people with disabilities: a summary of findings from the national longitudinal transition study of special education students,* Menlo Park, CA, 1993, SRI International.
143. Wagner M, Cameto R, Newman L: *Youth with disabilities: a changing population. A report of findings from the National Longitudinal Transition Study (NLTS) and the National Longitudinal Transition Study-2 (NLTS02),* Menlo Park, CA, 2003, SRI International.
144. Wagner M, Newman L, Cameto R, et al.: *An overview of findings from Wave 2 of the National Longitudinal Transition Study-2 (NLTS2).* National Center for Special Education Research, Menlo Park, CA, 2006, SRI International.
145. Wehman P: *Life beyond the classroom: transition strategies for young people with disabilities,* ed 4, Baltimore, 2006, Paul H. Brookes.
146. White PH: Success on the road to adulthood: issues and hurdles for adolescents with disabilities, *Rheum Dis Clin North Am* 23(3):697–707, 1997.
147. White PH: Transition: a future promise for children and adolescents with special health care needs and disabilities, *Rheum Dis Clin North Am* 28(3):687–703, 2002.
148. Will M: *OSERS programming for the transition of youth with disabilities: bridges from school to working life,* Washington, DC, 1983, US Department of Education, Office of Special Education and Rehabilitative Services (ERIC Document Reproduction Service No. ED 256 132).
149. World Health Organization: *International Classification of Functioning, Disability and Health (ICF),* Geneva, Switzerland, 2001, World Health Organization. Available at: URL: www.who.int/classifications/icf/en.
150. Wright B: Teens say job training their top need, *Point Depart* 2(2):8, 2001.
151. Young NL, McCormick A, Mills W, et al.: The transition study: a look at youth and adults with cerebral palsy, spina bifida, and acquired brain injury, *Phys Occup Ther Pediatr* 26(4):25–46, 2006.

SUGGESTED READINGS

American Academy of Pediatrics, American Academy of Family Physicians, and American College of Physicians, Transitions Clinical Report Authoring Group: Supporting the health care transition from adolescence to adulthood in the medical home, *Pediatrics* 128(1):182–200, 2011.

Bjornson K, Kobayashi A, Zhou C, Walker W: Relationship of therapy to postsecondary education and employment in young adults with physical disabilities, *Pediatr Phys Ther* 23(2):179–186, 2011.

Compton-Griffith K, Cicirello N, Turner A: Physical therapists' perceptions of providing services to adults with childhood neuromotor disabilities, *Phys Occup Ther Pediatr* 31(1):19–30, 2011.

Darrah J, Magil-Evans J, Galambos N: Community services for young adults with motor disabilities-a paradox, *Disabil Rehabil* 32(3):223–229, 2010.

Doty A, Flexer R, Barton L, et al.: *A national survey of school-based physical therapists and secondary transition practices.* Unpublished Doctoral Dissertation, Kent, Ohio, 2010, Kent State University.

King G, Baldwin P, Currie M, Evans J: Planning successful transitions from school to adult roles for youth with disabilities, *Child Health Care* 34(3):193–216, 2005.

Orlin M, Cicirello N, O'Donnell A, Doty A: Continuum of care for individual with lifelong disabilities: role of the physical therapist, *Phys Ther* 94(7):1043–1053, 2014.

Rosenbaum PL, Rosenbloom L: *Cerebral palsy: from diagnosis to adult life,* London, 2012, Mac Keith Press.

Stewart D, Law M, Young NL, et al.: Complexities during transitions to adulthood for youth with disabilities: person-environment interactions, *Disabil Rehabil* 36(23):1998–2004, 2014.

33

Assistive Technology

Roberta Kuchler O'Shea, Brenda Sposato Bonfiglio

Pediatric physical therapists have an important role in providing children and youth with impairments in body functions and structures with assistive technology to improve activity and participation. An assistive technology (AT) device is defined in federal legislation as any item, piece of equipment, or product system that increases, maintains, or improves an individual's functional status.[45] In contrast, an AT service is legally defined as any service, such as physical therapy, occupational therapy, or speech therapy, that directly assists someone with a disability in the selection, acquisition, or training of an AT device.[45] AT encompasses a vast range of materials, designs, and applications to enable adapted motor function when skill attainment is unrealistic or impossible.[39] Also referred to as enabling technology, AT can generate opportunities for social participation. Since the 1990s, there has been a virtual explosion in the number and type of assistive devices.

The creation of federally funded rehabilitation engineering centers in 1972 focused efforts on the research and development of new products, as well as on the delivery of services to the consumer.[13] This process brought together professionals from many disciplines including biomedical and rehabilitation engineering, physical therapy, occupational therapy, speech and language pathology, and special education. The Rehabilitation Engineering and Assistive Technology Society of North America (RESNA), an outgrowth of this shared interest, is an interdisciplinary association of professionals interested in applied technology for persons with activity limitations and participation restrictions.

Since 1975, many laws have been enacted to ensure the rights of people with disabilities to be included in natural education and work environments. These laws include Public Law 101-476, the Education of All Handicapped Children Act; the 1990 Amendment to the Individuals with Disabilities Education Act (IDEA); Public Law 101-47, the Technology-Related Assistance for Individuals with Disabilities Act of 1988 (TRAIDA/Tech Act); Public Law 93-112, the Rehabilitation Act; and Public Law 101-336, the Americans with Disabilities Act (ADA). These laws have helped to focus attention on and create a growing market for new technologies and products. Consumer demands for increased durability and performance have induced manufacturers to apply technologies created by the aerospace, medical, and information industries.

TRAIDA was the first federal legislation to define AT devices and services and to recognize the importance of technology in the lives of individuals with disabilities.[10] Grants awarded to states and territories provided funds for projects to improve access to technology and, subsequently, integration and inclusion of individuals with disabilities within the community and

workforce. Services currently offered vary from state to state and include information and referral services (databases, 800 numbers, and websites), centers for trying out devices and equipment, equipment exchange and recycling programs, funding resource guides, financial loan programs, mobile van outreach services, protection and advocacy services, and education programs on funding and self-advocacy. The Assistive Technology Act of 1998 provides for development of comprehensive technology-related programs. All states and territories are eligible for 10 years of federal funding, and states that have received 10 years of funding are eligible for an additional 3 years of funding. The 1997 Amendment to the IDEA advocates for consideration of AT devices and services for all individual education plans.

This chapter discusses the major elements of AT and the role of the physical therapist in selecting and obtaining appropriate equipment for children and their families. The five elements include adaptive seating and positioning, wheeled mobility, augmentative and alternative communication (AAC), computers, and electronic aids to daily living (EADLs). Research is appraised to provide evidence to inform the decision-making process.

ASSISTIVE TECHNOLOGY TEAM

Most technological devices require modification or customization in design, implementation, or attachment.[31,46] The complexity and expense of the AT required by individuals with severe physical impairments and activity limitations necessitate a thorough and careful process of selection and construction. All individuals who interact with the child and the equipment on a regular basis need to be considered part of the team. Professionals, the child, the family, and caregivers each contribute a particular area of knowledge and expertise. Lahm and Sizemore[30] contend that despite laws mandating AT assessment teams, the members of the team may have individual agendas. Many factors influence the assessment process, including the needs and preferences of the child and family, individual education and experience levels of team members, specialties represented on the team, and the approach advocated by each assessor. Teams need to be cognizant of their strengths and limitations. Are there members from several disciplines, or from just one or two? Are the child and family integral team members? An outcomes survey found that the professionals with the most experience (therapists) spent the least amount of time with the client and that the professionals with the least amount of training in disability studies (AT suppliers) spent the most time with the family.[30] Lahm and Sizemore advocate that professional education programs include more information on AT based on their findings that new graduates do not possess sufficient knowledge of AT and AT services.

The configuration of the AT team (Fig. 33.1) will vary depending on child and family needs and the setting in which services are provided. Central to the team are the child and family. Family-centered services emphasize the importance of engaging the child and primary caregivers in the goal-setting and decision-making process to ensure realistic and meaningful solutions.[45] The core team should include professionals with training and experience in the areas being examined (mobility, seating, augmentative and alternative communication, computers, and activities of daily living [ADLs]). The team usually includes some or all of the following professionals: physical therapist, occupational therapist, speech and language pathologist, rehabilitation engineer, and rehabilitation technology supplier.

In addition to the core team, other professionals, organizations, and agencies are involved in decision making and procurement of AT. Professionals involved in the child's education and health care often share roles with the core team and provide information that is essential for decision making. In the educational setting, this may include the physical therapist, occupational therapist, speech and language therapist, classroom teachers and aides, administrative personnel, psychologists, vocational counselors, and work supervisors. Goals and strategies must be coordinated with other service providers. Within the medical setting, the child's family physician, as well as other medical specialists and nurses, may need to be involved. Issues requiring collaboration with medical personnel include management of deformity and contractures, pressure sores, incontinence, self-injury, safety, and visual and other sensory impairments.

The issue of funding involves a third group of contributors that includes third-party payers, state-sponsored medical equipment programs, civic organizations, and other funding agencies. Many clinics employ a funding specialist to assist families in identifying and obtaining funding for prescribed technology. The team may also include other community and family members who engage in day-to-day interactions with the child or who provide special support services such as transportation or revision of architectural barriers.

Team makeup and setting are variable. For example, in many hospitals and rehabilitation centers with comprehensive technology service delivery programs, physicians

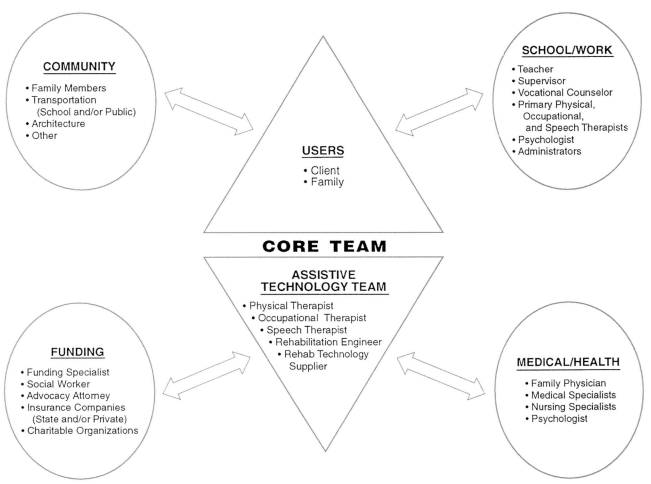

FIG. 33.1 Core team interactions are important for selecting and procuring assistive technology. Members and roles of each component may fluctuate, depending on specific client problems and settings.

(especially physiatrists and orthopedic surgeons) are an integral part of the core team. In schools and residential centers, one or more of the client's primary therapists, along with an equipment supplier, may function as the core team. The core team is responsible for imparting information regarding proper use, training, maintenance, responsibility, and safety relative to the prescribed devices to appropriate individuals.

Effective communication and coordination of care are essential components of intervention to ensure that once obtained, the technology is used. Abandonment of AT is costly for the family and child. There are financial costs of the equipment but also emotional and time costs that cannot be recuped.[26] Four factors were related to abandonment of AT: lack of consideration, ease of procurement, performance, and priorities.[26] Lack of consideration refers to the child's and family's opinion during the selection process. Ease of procurement was a second factor. Items purchased directly from a supplier (without team consultation) were the most likely to be abandoned. A third factor was poor device performance, which reflected the user's perception of the ability of the technology to enhance his or her performance in an easy, reliable, and comfortable manner. The fourth factor was change in users' needs and priorities over time, including functional changes, as well as changes in lifestyle and activities.

In 1995 RESNA began credentialing professionals in AT for the purposes of ensuring consumer safeguards and increasing consumer satisfaction. The credential indicates that the professional has specialized training and experience in AT and promotes a standard for recognizing qualifications and validating the broad-based knowledge required for safe and effective service in the field of AT. The activity technology professional (ATP) credential signifies a service provider who analyzes the needs of individuals with disabilities, assists in the selection of the appropriate equipment, and trains the consumer on how to properly use the specific equipment (see the RESNA website at www.resna.org/certification/index.php).

Professionals who provide AT services to individuals with disabilities should consider obtaining the activity technology professional credential. Professionals include but are not limited to physical therapists, occupational therapists, speech-language pathologists, rehabilitation engineers, special educators, and rehabilitation technology suppliers. The credential is extremely important for physical therapists working with children and adults with seating, positioning, and mobility needs. There is an increasing need for physical therapists who serve children with disabilities and their families to have specialized training and expertise in AT.

A rehabilitation technology supplier (RTS) is an individual who provides enabling technology in areas of wheeled mobility, seating and alternative positioning, ambulation assistance, environmental controls, and ADLs (note that communication systems and computers are not included). A National Registry of Rehabilitation Technology Suppliers (NRRTS) includes the names of suppliers whose qualifications have been verified through an evaluation process that includes work experience, references from professional associates, adherence to the Code of Ethics and Standards of Practice and Protocol, and commitment to continuing education. A certified RTS (CRTS) is a member in good standing of the NRRTS who has successfully completed the RESNA Assistive Technology Supplier examination.

INTERNATIONAL CLASSIFICATION OF FUNCTIONING, DISABILITY AND HEALTH FRAMEWORK FOR DECISION MAKING

Throughout the book, examples are provided of how AT is used to achieve child and family goals for activity and participation. AT devices are designed to improve users' participation in activities that may otherwise be limited by impairments in body structure and function. The International Classification of Functioning, Disability and Health (ICF)[60] is a useful framework to apply when making decisions about AT. Correctly prescribed and used, AT, especially positioning (adaptive seating), may help prevent secondary impairments such as skin breakdown, cardiopulmonary compromise due to scoliosis or slouched posture, and joint contracture or skeletal deformity due to inadequately supported body segments. Benefits of AT also may include reduction of muscle tone or excessive muscle activity and a decrease in nonvolitional movement. By providing a means for the child to compensate for impairments in postural stability and weight shifting, AT can reduce activity limitations in sitting, mobility, use of hands, and speech. AT also may increase the ability of the child to participate in daily activities and routines. A power wheelchair may allow independent access to school or work. Augmentative or alternative communication may facilitate interactions with peers and promote social skills. An EADL may make the difference between less restricted living in a supervised apartment and living in a nursing home or intermediate care facility.

Social policies and attitudes are important determinants of the availability and accessibility of AT. High product and service provider costs require evidence that technology improves the user's quality of life in ways that justify the costs. Reduction in costs of hospitalizations, surgical procedures, out of home residence, and attendant care are outcomes that would support the effectiveness of AT. Technology also has the potential to improve user appearance and visibility. This in turn could have a positive effect on social attitudes regarding the capabilities of people with severe disabilities.

Evaluation of AT is often based empirically on observation and clinical impressions. The literature is replete with descriptions of creative solutions for individual client problems. Less common are controlled studies of the effectiveness of AT intervention.

LIFE SPAN TECHNOLOGY

The needs of children with impairments in body functions and structures change with growth and development and, therefore, AT needs must be continually reevaluated. Careful selection, planning, and implementation of AT optimize child and family outcomes and efficient use of health care resources. During infancy, proper positioning helps to promote social interaction and development of early concepts such as cause and effect and object permanence. Prior to and during the preschool years, switch-activated toys and power-driven mobility toys can help children learn to self-initiate movement and interact with the environment. Children need a reliable way to indicate needs and make choices. The school-age child needs the postural support and comfort to enable learning and adaptive function. The adolescent needs to keep up with peers and be accepted socially. Adolescents should be included in the decision-making process regarding choice of mobility, seating, or communication options whenever possible. The young adult needs to be able to get to and from a job or day setting and rely as little as possible on others to achieve basic functions, such as position changes, communicating, eating, and toileting. Because individuals with severe limitations in mobility spend many more hours at a time in one position, hygiene and skin care become a priority.

Technology is quickly changing all facets of life. Things only dreamed about just a few years ago become a readily available reality very quickly. The personal digital assistant (PDA) was a handheld device that stored digital information. It is not unusual for academic institutions to utilize electronic versions of textbooks on laptops and tablets as well as Internet-based curriculum platforms. The use of technology is ubiquitous in classrooms today, benefiting all children regardless of abilities. Technology allows children to actively participate in their educational programs without the adult assistance that may have interfered with peer-to-peer and student-to-teacher interactions.[39]

SELECTION PROCESS

A person's environment refers to the surroundings or a setting in which he or she spends a great deal of time. Cooke and Polgar[13] described the human/activity/AT model (HAAT model). This model dovetails well with the International Classification of Functioning, Disability and Health. In the HAAT model, *human* represents someone doing something in some place. *Activity* is the process of doing something, the functional result of human performance. *AT* is the basis for how the human performance will be enhanced during an activity.[26] Thus translating the HAAT model into components of health, AT is designed to minimize impairments in body functions and structures and maximize activity and social participation. The selection process must consider all environments in which AT will be used. In addition, the wheelchair itself, with its adaptive seating and communication systems, is a microenvironment for many children with severe impairments.[14]

The elements of patient/client management in the *Guide to Physical Therapist Practice*[3] correspond with the process for selection and implementation of AT:

Step 1: Examination. Examination is the process of obtaining a history, performing systems reviews, and selecting and administering tests and measures to obtain relevant client information. The process begins with an interview to identify child/family goals and implication for AT. The team records relevant history and social information. The examination includes measurement of myotomes, dermatomes, skin, range of motion (ROM), muscle strength, and motor function, including sitting, transfers, and mobility.

Step 2: Evaluation. The team makes clinical judgments based on data gathered during the examination. Keeping in mind the information gathered in Step 1, the team considers options for AT.

Step 3: Diagnosis. The team makes a decision on the child's needs for AT.

Step 4: Prognosis. The team estimates the level of improvement that might be attained through AT and the amount of instruction and training required.

Step 5: Intervention. The child and family try out options for AT. The team selects the AT system and services to implement

a system that will provide maximal independence based on the child's diagnosis and prognosis. Funding is secured. The team may be responsible for gathering prescriptions and writing letters of medical need. The system is ordered, delivered, and fit to the user.

Step 6: Outcomes. Changes associated with the AT are documented, including activity and participation.

Step 7: Follow-up and reevaluation. The process described is usually only one of many repetitions of a cycle. Mechanical and electronic equipment wear out and break down, making repairs and replacement necessary. The child's problems and needs change with age, development of new skills, and change of environments. As technologies continue to improve, new solutions become available.

SEATING SYSTEMS

The purpose of the seating system is to provide external postural support for the child with activity limitations in sitting caused by impairments in body functions and structures. Seating is the interface between the child and the mobility device.[14] The goal is to enable the child to compensate for activity limitations, thereby maximizing participation in life activities. Seating systems can be classified into three categories: linear/planar, generically contoured/modular, and custom molded/custom contoured.

There are several desired outcomes when prescribing seating systems: comfort, neuromuscular management, improved postural control, and maintaining the integumentary system. Comfort is a desired outcome for all individuals using seating and mobility systems.[35] Outcomes for individuals with cerebral palsy (CP) or traumatic brain injury may include muscle tone management and improvement of upper body postural control to enhance head control and hand function. To achieve stable sitting, biomechanical forces and moments in all planes must be balanced.[14] Good positioning usually consists of an upright midline orientation of the entire body with a near-vertical alignment of the trunk and head. In children, the 90-90-90 rule often is used to maintain the hips, knees, and ankles at 90 degrees. As the child grows, it may not be reasonable, due to leg length, to maintain the knees at 90 degrees of flexion. In this case, the decision to go with a different angled front rigging must be made. Additionally, if the child has contractures of the legs or trunk, positioning in 90 degrees of hip, knee, and ankle flexion may not be possible.

Some professionals have questioned the rationale for static positioning, stating that it is unnatural and impedes function.[14] Individuals with abnormal tone may require dynamic components integrated with their wheelchair frames to accommodate for excessive movement. For example, a suspension assembly can be integrated at the seat-to-back angle junction to allow the back canes to move independently of the seat frame. This allows the wheelchair frame components to withstand the forces applied by the individual's extraneous movement. The components absorb the energy that would otherwise be transmitted into the wheelchair. Additionally, the stiffness of the elastomer part of the component can be matched to the force generated by the individual and can be adjusted as needed, minimizing or eliminating damage to the frame.

Research on therapeutic seating for children with neuromuscular disorders has focused on the effects of hip flexion angle (or seat-to-back angle) and orientation of the trunk and head (or angle-in-space). The former is achieved by independently changing the seat-back angle; the latter is achieved by tilting/rotating the entire system. There has been considerable interest in the anterior tipped (or forward-inclined) seat, in which the front edge of the seat is tilted downward, thus increasing the seat-to-back angle while maintaining a near-vertical back. Most clients with myelodysplasia or spinal cord injuries tolerate and function well in a typical upright position; however, sitting pressures are a concern and prevention of ulcerations a priority. Various types of sitting surfaces and adjustments to improve postural alignment have been studied in the attempt to reduce pressure and decrease the incidence of decubiti. In children with muscular dystrophy, prevention of spinal collapse, preservation of arm and hand function, and comfort are desirable outcomes of positioning. Washington and associates[59] reported that infants with neuromuscular impairments demonstrated better postural alignment and engagement with toys when seated on a contoured foam seat as compared to a regular highchair seat or highchair with a thin foam layer. Mothers of the infants reported that the contoured foam seat was feasible for use within their typical daily routines.

Effects of Adaptive Seating on Body Functions and Structures

Neuromuscular System

A long-standing assumption is that increased muscle tone, here defined as muscle activity at rest, can be reduced by altering seating angle. Seats are oriented either horizontally, wedged (front edge raised), or anterior tipped (front edge lowered). Backs are placed vertically, reclined, or forward inclined (closing the hip angle to more flexion). Several studies have examined the effect of seating angle on electromyographic (EMG) activity in children with CP. In a study that varied the hip angle by reclining the back or wedging the seat, lumbar muscle activity was lowest in vertical sitting, with a horizontal seat and a 90-degree hip angle.[14] Lumbar muscle activity was higher the more reclined the position regardless of the hip angle. Hip adductor activity was decreased when the back was vertical and the seat was wedged 15 degrees.[36]

In children with CP, as well as children without neuromuscular impairments, tilting the seating system 30 degrees posterior while maintaining the hip angle at 90 degrees increased electrical activity of paraspinal and hip adductor muscle groups.[36] The reclined position also resulted in increased electrical activity in the rectus femoris, adductor longus, biceps femoris, and gastrocnemius.[36] The addition of an abduction orthosis decreased leg muscle activity in all positions. For subjects with severe neuromuscular impairments, changes in EMG activity of back extensor and medial hamstring muscles to response to position changes were individualized.[36]

Children with CP who sat on anterior tilted seats without back support showed a decrease in midthoracic muscle activity and an increase in lumbar muscle activity,[36] indicating increased EMG activity of low back musculature relative to midback musculature. Myhr and von Wendt[40] advocate the use of anterior tilted seats, but they added an abduction orthosis and a cutout table for upper extremity support of forward leaning. When wearing the abduction orthosis, EMG activity of leg muscles was lower in the forward-leaning position compared with vertical or reclined sitting. The frequency of spastic or tonic reflex patterns (defined for each subject) was reduced in the anterior tilted sitting position compared with the subjects' own seating systems.[36]

Musculoskeletal System

The assumption that postural support systems prevent contractures and skeletal deformity in children with increased muscle tone has been examined.[33] In theory, maintenance of balanced forces to the trunk and lower extremities should prevent structural changes such as scoliosis and hip dislocation.[14] This theory may apply to young children with asymmetric postures that can be reduced through positioning. Maintenance of balanced forces through a postural control system may not be feasible for children with severely increased muscle tone, strong deforming muscle forces, and asymmetry.

Cardiovascular/Pulmonary System

Most studies have measured how pulmonary function is affected by seating position. Pulmonary function of children with spastic CP improved when the child was sitting in a modular seating system with adjustable support components compared to a wheelchair with standard sling seat and back.[14] The differences were attributed to (1) changes in the shape, structure, and capacity of the thorax and abdomen and (2) improved control of the respiratory muscles in the supported, upright position. Anterior tilted seating systems have potential to improve respiratory function in children with moderate CP.[14]

Integumentary System

Prevention of pressure sores is a goal for children who sit for long periods throughout the day. Insensate tissue compounds the problem of prolonged sitting. Pressure relief is also an important consideration for children with neuromuscular impairments who use wheeled mobility. Skeletal asymmetries, such as pelvic obliquity, hip dislocation, and scoliosis, predispose children who sit in wheelchairs to pressure problems.

Several factors contribute to the development of pressure sores including skin temperature, moisture, and shear and compressive forces.[18] Pressure (compressive force) has been the most-studied variable, because it has a clear relationship to the development of decubiti and is relatively easy to measure and manipulate during wheelchair seating. The risk of a pressure sore is directly related to the length of time soft tissue is compressed and inversely related to the area being compressed.

Pressure mapping devices (Fig. 33.2) are commonly used to study pressure distribution in individuals with and without motor impairment, reduction of seat interface pressure using various seat surfaces, and prevention of decubiti. Adults without physical impairments display even pressure distribution from side to side and a biphasic pattern of pressure concentration with a posterior concentration on the ischial tuberosities and a second but lesser concentration on the distal thighs.[21,29] Patients with "unbalanced sitting" due to pelvic obliquity or scoliosis showed a pronounced shift of pressure laterally and often posteriorly, thereby increasing pressure on the ischial tuberosity.[21,29]

For subjects without impairment, return to upright after a short period of recline in a wheelchair resulted in higher pressures and shear forces compared with the upright position.[27,36] When subjects leaned forward moving away from the backrest, forces returned to initial values. When the footrests were elevated, pressure under the ischial tuberosities increased. There was no difference in pressure under the ischial tuberosities between upright sitting and 10 degrees of recline in adults without impairment, but there was reduction of pressure in both positions when a lumbar support was added.[32] The reclined

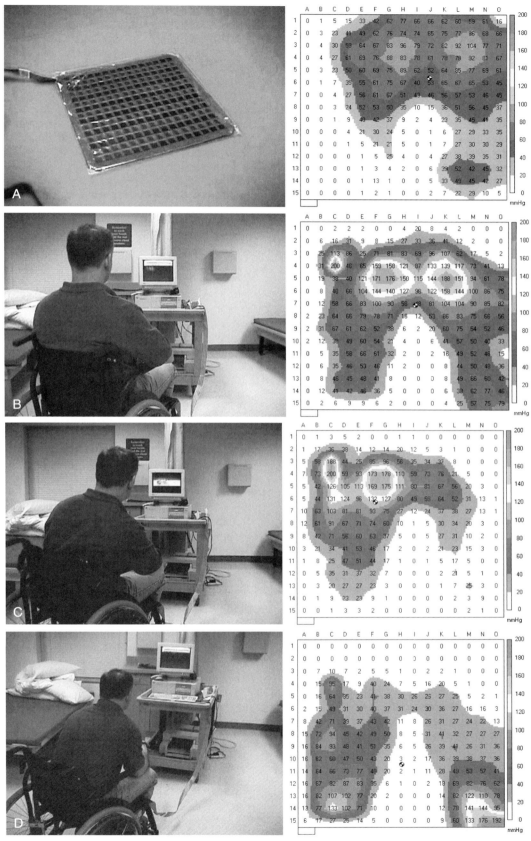

FIG. 33.2 Pressure mapping system and outputs. **A,** Pressure map *(left)* with computer screen output *(right)*. **B,** Individual seated in a wheelchair on a pressure map *(left)*. Output with symmetric sitting posture *(right)*. **C,** Output with individual leaning to the right while seated. **D,** Output with individual leaning forward, resting his elbows on his knees while seated.

position with lumbar support was recommended for individuals with spinal cord injury because they slide or rotate off the lumbar support in upright position due to tight hamstrings or weak trunk musculature.

Magnetic resonance imaging (MRI) has been used to evaluate soft tissue contours of the buttocks during loading. In a subject with paraplegia, less sitting pressure was required before soft tissue became compressed by a bony prominence and there was increased stiffness and lateral shifting of the gluteal muscle mass.[33] Foam cushions contoured to match the shape of the buttocks, as opposed to flat foam, improved the load transfer from buttocks to cushion because the total contact surface area was greater.[33] Foam stiffness is also a consideration in determining the seat contours, with dense foam having less deflection under the load. When clients with spinal cord injury were seated on flat versus contoured foam cushions of varying stiffness, pressures were lower on the contoured cushions than on the flat cushions, and they were lower on the more compliant foam than on the stiffer foam.[33] The buttocks were encompassed more on the contoured and softer cushion with less tissue distortion. The authors cautioned that foam that is too soft deforms too much and will "bottom out" quickly. In contrast, when subjects with paraplegia sat with the trunk bent laterally, the mean difference in pressure between the left and right ischial tuberosity was greater on a foam cushion than on a commercial air-bladder cushion.[27]

Several studies have compared sitting pressures, skin temperature, and relative humidity in subjects seated on commercially available cushions.[22,33,53] Findings indicate that no one cushion is effective for all clients and that a variety of cushion options are needed to meet individual needs.

Effect of Adaptive Seating on Activity and Participation
Postural Stability and Control in Sitting
Research has examined the effect of anterior tilted seats on the posture and stability of children with motor impairments using instrumented systems and rating scales. Two typical designs of anterior seats are (1) a flat bench with no trunk support, with feet flat on the floor, and (2) a forward-leaning system with an anterior trunk or upper extremity surface for support.

Children with CP and children with traumatic brain injury sat in a more upright position in an anterior tilted seat compared with a flat seat.[14] Postural sway also decreased in children with CP.[14] The position of the C7 spinous process was tracked to yield a radius of stability, with a smaller radius indicating reduced postural sway and thus increased stability. During quiet sitting on a flat bench, the postural sway of the children with neuromuscular impairments did not differ significantly from that of age-matched controls, although children with neuromuscular impairments demonstrated more variability. When positioned on a seat with a 10-degree anterior tilt, half of the children with CP (described as having spasticity with tight hamstrings) had a decrease in sway and a more upright posture (vertical measurement of C7 height). The other half of the children with CP (described as having low trunk tone and tight hamstrings) had an increase in sway on the anterior seat but also a more upright posture.

Interestingly, varying seat angle by 10 degrees did not affect the postural stability of children with motor impairments.[14] Trunk extension was greatest when children sat on an anterior tilted seat with a leg support to provide weight bearing through the knees and shins.[14] Additionally, postural of the head, trunk,

and feet improved when children sat on an anterior tilted seat.[14] Improvement in independent sitting ability, trunk posture in sitting, and powered mobility were observed in children after at least 3 years of using seating and power mobility system.[31,35] The critical features of the seating and mobility system (SAM) were a saddle-type seat, a solid anterior chest support, and a tray to support forward leaning.

Posture and arm movements of young children with CP improved when they were positioned on a seat with some anterior tilt, foot support, and no trunk support compared with sitting on a flat bench.[14,32] A more upright head and trunk and better alignment between body segments improved spinal extension.[14,35]

For most children, a seat-to-back angle of 90 degrees without any pitch (thus the seat is parallel to the floor) is most practical. If the child assumes a posterior pelvic tilt when sitting, anterior tilt of the seat may facilitate trunk extension. Hence the seat-to-back angle is increased or *opened*. For children with increased muscle tone, a seat with a posterior tilt, in which the front edge is relatively higher to the back edge, may reduce extensor spasms and enable a proper seated position. In this case, the seat-to-back angle is reduced or *closed*.

Arm and Hand Function
Wedging the seat did not improve functional hand function in children with marked extensor spasticity,[14] nor did it increase shoulder horizontal adduction movement time to trigger a switch in children with CP.[15] Movement time was fastest when children were positioned with their hips in a 90-degree position compared with in a wedged position and slowest with a hip angle of 50 degrees. When the hips were maintained at 90 degrees of flexion but the entire system tilted posterior 15 degrees or 30 degrees or anterior 5 degrees, performance on the shoulder adduction task was best in the upright position and worst in the anterior position.[14] Infants with neuromuscular impairments demonstrated improved posture and some improved arm use with contoured foam seating systems.[59]

Oral-Motor, Speech, and Communication
Very young children with impairments in multiple systems demonstrated improvements in oral-motor control during eating and drinking when positioned in individualized therapeutic seating devices; however, self-feeding and independent drinking did not improve.[14,34]

Mobility
Researchers have examined the effect of seating position on manual wheelchair propulsion.[14,31,58] Altering seat height, seat inclination, or anterior-posterior orientation for individual subjects improved upper extremity movement and wheeling efficiency. An individual's propulsion was optimized by adjusting the seating configuration in relation to the rear wheel position.[58] Additionally, an appropriate seating system and mobility base can decrease secondary complications and increase participation in the community and workplace.

Social Participation
Families reported increased social participation after their children or adults received adaptive seating equipment that included wheelchairs, travel chairs, and strollers, with custom adaptations as needed.[35] Changes reported following implementation of adapted seating and mobility included increased

ability to sit upright without leaning, more time spent in sitting and less time lying down, increased ability to grasp an object, and improved ability to eat with a spoon. Changes in social behavior reported included an increase in the number of community places visited and more time during the day spent with someone else.

Summary of Research Evidence

The variability in subject characteristics and responses support individualized decision making and the importance of postural support system simulation.[14,58] Research suggests that seating systems that provide external postural support improve pulmonary function in children with CP, reduce scoliosis when combined with a soft orthosis in children with muscular dystrophy, improve arm function in children with CP, and improve oral-motor skills, vocalizations, and social interaction in children with multiple disabilities.[14,58] More specifically, upright orientation is associated with decreased activity of extensor muscles in children with CP, improved pulmonary function in children with muscle weakness, improved upper extremity performance on a shoulder adduction task in children with CP, and an increase in adult-initiated interactions with students who have profound physical and cognitive impairments.[14,58]

Evidence of the effectiveness of an anterior tilted seat is inconclusive.[14] Previously it was thought that anterior tilted seats increase back extension and improve spinal alignment and upper extremity function; however, research has not supported this assumption. Current clinical thinking is that a neutral pelvic position is desirable.

There is evidence that contoured cushions improve pressure distribution as well as spinal support and posture.[59] The effectiveness of commercially available pressure relief cushions is variable; however, most manufacturers include blocks, foam pieces, or other additives to provide custom-contouring of their products.

Summary

Research is needed to identify the features and components of postural support systems that reduce impairment, improve activity, and increase the social participation of individuals with severe physical impairments.[58] More consistent reporting of the specific disorders and severity of impairments is necessary.[58] The impact of AT clinics and programs on the cost of health care has not been determined. Potentially, AT can reduce costs of hospitalizations due to secondary complications. In some cases, the cost of AT and vocational training may increase a client's employability but reduce his or her eligibility for Medicaid or other supplemental assistance. Regional centers that provide comprehensive and coordinated services may be the most effective way to deliver advanced technology to the greatest number of people; however, rural mobile vans may promote a broader range of access.

Principal Concepts in the Prescription of Seating Systems

Assistive seating technology is evolving rapidly, creating a confusion of terminology. RESNA has published a list of standardized terminology that is helpful in improving communication among research and service centers, professionals, clients, and funding sources.[31] It is imperative that the AT team possess knowledge of what components will accomplish child and family goals. If an inappropriate system is recommended, the child/

user may lose function and experience secondary musculoskeletal impairment, and financial resources may not be available for a new system.[14,58]

Examination and Evaluation

As part of the process of selecting a seating system, the physical therapist examines the child and evaluates the findings. The physical therapist applies knowledge of anatomy, kinesiology, biomechanics, and principles of neuromuscular control of posture and function when examining the child. Knowledge of biomechanics and movement are essential for assessing and recommending a therapeutic seating system.[14] The child is examined in both supine and sitting positions. ROM measurements at the hips, knees, ankles, trunk, shoulders, elbows, and wrists/hands are part of the examination process. Muscle tone and muscle strength also are examined. Anatomic linear measurements are taken. Precise measurement and documentation will help to determine the most appropriate size and type of the seating system, as well as assist in writing letters of medical necessity to third-party payers. Accurate documentation over time provides valuable information regarding a child's growth and development.

Pelvic alignment and an erect trunk are essential for optimal head control and arm and hand function. For many children, an erect trunk posture is achieved through neutral pelvic alignment. The assessment of posture in a seating system begins with the pelvis and its relationship to the trunk and lower extremities.[14,58] The orientation and range of mobility of the pelvis in all three planes will determine the alignment and support needed at the trunk, head, and extremities. The effect of hip flexion and knee extension ROM on the vertical orientation of the pelvis is among the most critical factors in selecting seating angles and components. If there are minimal contractures of the hamstrings, hip extensors, and hip flexors, passive mobility of the pelvis should be sufficient for vertical alignment of the trunk. If muscles are shortened, the pelvis may be immobile in either an anterior or a posterior tilt, or obliquity, and the child will require a more individualized solution.

Figs. 33.3 to 33.6 illustrate the linear measurements used to design and prescribe a well-fitting seating system. Measurements

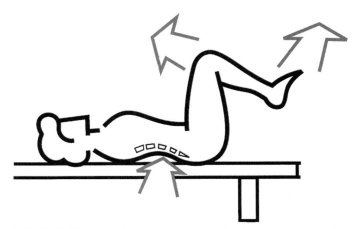

FIG. 33.3 The examiner must monitor the lumbar curve as the hips are flexed and the knees extended. (Redrawn with permission from Bergen AF, Presperin J, Tallman T: *Positioning for function: wheelchairs and other assistive technologies*, Valhalla, NY, 1990, Valhalla Rehabilitation Publications.)

taken with the child positioned in supine include hip and knee angles, thigh/hip length (Fig. 33.3), and calf length (Fig. 33.4). Measurements taken with the child sitting on a surface with a thin top and with feet supported, not dangling, are illustrated in Fig. 33.5. Measurements taken with the child in sitting include behind hips to popliteal fossa, popliteal fossa to heel, knee flexion angle, sitting surface to pelvic crest, sitting surface to axilla, sitting surface to shoulder, sitting surface to occiput, sitting surface to crown of head, sitting surface to hanging elbow, width across trunk, depth of trunk, width across hips, and heel to toe (Fig. 33.6).

Type and severity of deformity will influence selection of the seating system and components. Vertical and symmetrical head and trunk alignment can often be obtained for a *flexible*

deformity (one that can be manually corrected and maintained with a reasonable amount of force) with the appropriate support components. In contrast, *fixed deformity* (one that is not correctable without an undue amount of force) and severe joint contractures must be accommodated in the seating system. Seating systems are not intended to lengthen tight musculature or correct bony deformity. Efforts to do this invariably will compromise achieving the desired posture because the child will attempt to move and avoid the uncomfortable forces.

In the case of a fixed deformity, the seating system will accommodate and support the deformity. The back cushion can support the trunk in neutral alignment or in an alternative posture if there are fixed trunk asymmetries. For children with severe scoliosis and pelvic obliquity, neutral alignment of the pelvis is not always possible and does not result in acceptable trunk and head alignment. In such cases, it is better to start with a relatively vertical head and level shoulders and allow the pelvis to be tilted and rotated.

If a child is unable to be positioned with the hip flexed to 90 degrees, the seat-to-back angle will be determined based on hip ROM. In another scenario, if the child sits with the hips adducted but can achieve neutral hip alignment, the seating

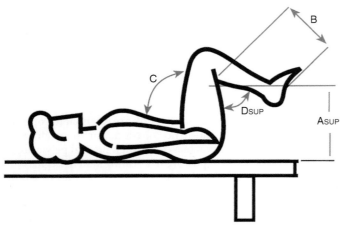

FIG. 33.4 Hip *(C)* angle, knee *(D_sup)* angle, thigh/hip *(A_sup)* length, and calf length *(B)* are measured first in supine. (Redrawn with permission from Bergen AF, Presperin J, Tallman T: *Positioning for function: wheelchairs and other assistive technologies,* Valhalla, NY, 1990, Valhalla Rehabilitation Publications.)

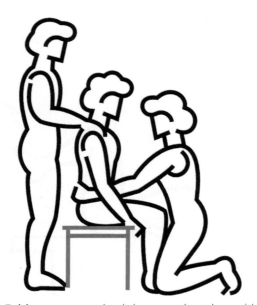

FIG. 33.5 Measurements in sitting must be taken with the client sitting on a surface with a thin top. This will allow the knees to flex as needed. (Redrawn with permission from Bergen AF, Presperin J, Tallman T: *Positioning for function: wheelchairs and other assistive technologies,* Valhalla, NY, 1990, Valhalla Rehabilitation Publications.)

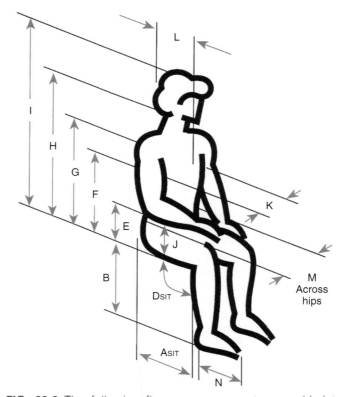

FIG. 33.6 The following figure measurements are added to those taken with the client in supine: *A_sit,* behind hips to popliteal fossa (right and left); *B,* popliteal fossa to heel (right and left); *D_sit,* knee flexion angle; *E,* sitting surface to pelvic crest; *F,* sitting surface to axilla; *G,* sitting surface to shoulder; *H,* sitting surface to occiput; *I,* sitting surface to crown of head; *J,* sitting surface to flexed elbow; *K,* width across trunk; *L,* depth of trunk; *M,* width across hips; *N,* heel to toe. (Redrawn with permission from Bergen AF, Presperin J, Tallman T: *Positioning for function: wheelchairs and other assistive technologies,* Valhalla, NY, 1990, Valhalla Rehabilitation Publications.)

system can hold the hips in an abducted position, or positioning components can be added to the seat to prevent adduction. Conversely, if the child has a tendency to maintain hips in extreme abduction, lateral supports can be used to position the lower extremities in a more neutral alignment. If knee ROM is limited, 60-degree hangers, instead of 90-degree hangers, may be used to accommodate for the loss of range. Modifications or supports are also used to accommodate for lack of ROM in the upper extremities.

In children at risk for skin breakdown, measurement of seat and back interface pressures should be included in the examination process. Pressure mapping systems are increasingly common in the clinic for comparing pressures while seated on various cushions. Variable-tilt and variable-recline features of manual and power wheelchairs can provide another source of pressure relief throughout a long day of sitting for some children.

Matching the Seating System With the Child's Needs

Seating systems and extrinsic positional components typically are classified into three levels: planar or linear, generically contoured, and custom molded/custom contoured. The first and least intensive level is the planar or linear system, which consists of a flat seat and back (Fig. 33.7). Children with good postural stability and sitting balance, a minimum of deformity, are most appropriate for this seating system. The seat and back consist of a solid base (plywood or high density plastic), covered by foam, and upholstered with vinyl or a fabric that stretches in all directions (e.g., Lycra or Dartex.) Trunk and pelvic supports may be added laterally. Many commercial linear systems are available, or a linear system can be constructed in the clinic. This system is easily changed and adapted and it is typically the least expensive.

The second level is the generically contoured or modular system, which provides external postural control by increasing the points of contact, especially laterally (Fig. 33.8). The seat and back surfaces are rounded by shaping layers of foam, air, or a viscous fluid to correspond to the curves of the body. Contours also help distribute pressures more evenly over the entire seat or back surface. A small amount of contouring often improves comfort and stability. A greater amount of contouring is often necessary for children with severe impairments. Today, nearly all generically contoured components are commercially available. Some generically contoured or modular systems include built-in growth capabilities for children.

The third level is the custom-contoured/custom-molded system. It provides an intimate fit by closely conforming to the shape of the child's body, thereby giving the most postural support (Fig. 33.9). Theoretically, when properly fabricated, the custom-molded system provides the greatest amount of pressure relief because it offers the greatest amount of contact surface area. The time and expense involved in the fabrication of custom-molded systems are considerable, and the molding process requires a great deal of skill. Production of the mold can involve a chemical reaction of liquid foams injected into a special bag, a vacuum consolidation method, or a computer digitization method. Several custom-molded systems are available, including those that can be completed on site and those that are sent to a central fabrication center.

Computer-aided design technology by mapping and digitizing body shape data directly using an instrumented simulator eliminates the need to make a mold. Information is transferred to a computer-driven carving machine that

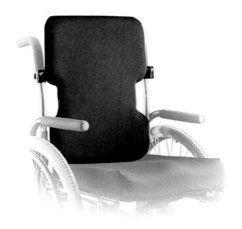

FIG. 33.7 Planar/linear back support. (Courtesy Invacare Corporation, Elyria, OH.)

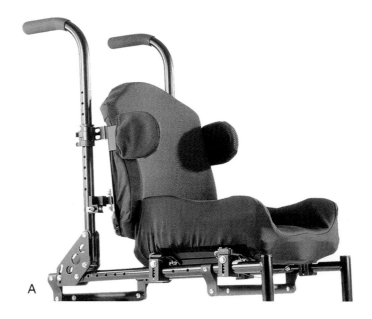

A

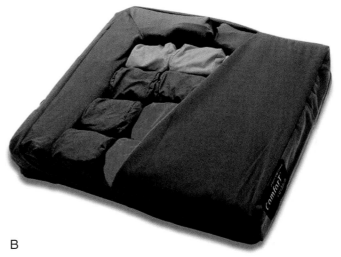

B

FIG. 33.8 Generic contour seating systems. A, Jay-fit adjustable contour system. B, ComforT cushion. (A, Courtesy Sunrise Medical, Boulder, CO. B, Courtesy Ottobock Health Care, Minneapolis, MN.)

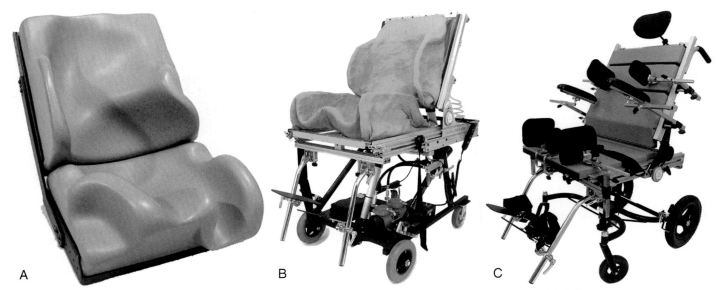

FIG. 33.9 **A,** Custom-molded cushion. **B,** Commercially available molding frame with fully powered tilt, recline and seat depth adjustment, built-in vacuum pump, and angle adjustable foot-rests. **C,** Commercially available linear seating simulator with multiple adjustable planar components and angles. (Courtesy Prairie Seating Corporation, Skokie, IL.)

produces the cushion. Typically, custom-molded systems do not allow for growth and cannot be modified. Additionally, if a child is not positioned properly within the molded cushion, pressure spots can develop and cause breakdown of underlying soft tissue.

In summary, the general rule of thumb in selecting a system is that less is better. If a child can control his or her head and trunk without supports or the use of minimal supports, has no history of skin breakdown, and can achieve independent pressure relief, a linear/planar seating system is generally acceptable. However, if the child cannot maintain proper positioning with supports and has a history of skin breakdown or is at risk for skin breakdown, a generic contour/modular seating system warrants consideration. Linear and generic contour systems can be changed and modified without great difficulty. The child with extensive positioning needs or who is at high risk for skin breakdown may benefit from a custom-molded seating system. The custom-molded systems are not adjustable or modifiable, so clinicians must take into account growth and musculoskeletal changes that may occur. Often, a hybrid system is recommended. The hybrid seating system includes components from different categories; for instance, a system might consist of a planar seat with a generically contoured back or a back that is custom molded exclusively along the paraspinal area and left flat on the periphery, which allows for the addition of adjustable lateral trunk supports.

Selection of a Seating System

The scope of this chapter and the rapidly evolving nature of technology preclude a thorough discussion of all options and features of postural support systems. Many excellent resources provide detailed descriptions, problem-solving lists, and charts.[14,44] Regardless of the level of postural support required, there are several important considerations to keep in mind. This section presents some of the most salient points in the decision-making process.

Seat cushions. The seat cushion is often the most critical element of the seating system. The seat cushion can be classified into the three previously mentioned categories: linear/planar, generically contoured, or custom contoured. The use of true planar seats is becoming less common because most therapists have found that a small amount of lateral contouring adds comfort and stability.[14] A number of commercially available cushions that include air or viscous fluid for pressure management have foam blocks and wedges that can be integrated to allow customization of cushion shape. Strategically placing commercial viscous fluid pads in a custom-made, contoured foam cushion can provide the extra, critical amount of pressure relief needed by some children. In antithrust seats, a block of high-density foam placed just anterior to the ischial tuberosities prevents the pelvis from sliding forward and equalizes pressure distribution along the thighs (Fig. 33.10). Antithrust seats can be added to planar as well as contoured systems, but they are thought to work best with deep lateral contours of the pelvis and lateral thigh supports (adductor pads).

Seat placement within the wheelchair frame is an important consideration. A thick cushion or inappropriate mounting hardware can place the seat too high and alter the child's center of gravity. This might reduce head and trunk stability and loss of independent transfers or wheeling. Forward or backward placement, especially in small children, can affect the knee angle required for foot placement on the footrests, access to the wheel rims for wheeling, and loading or unloading the front casters. For individuals who propel with their lower extremities, it is important to maintain a lower seat-to-floor height and a flat front edge of the seat cushion. These modifications relieve the pressure from the front edge of the seat and allow full knee flexion without irritating the hamstrings.

Back supports. Back supports also fall into three categories: linear/planar, generically contoured, and custom contoured. A back support with a gently curved surface can improve lateral trunk stability, posture, and comfort. Simple contouring and

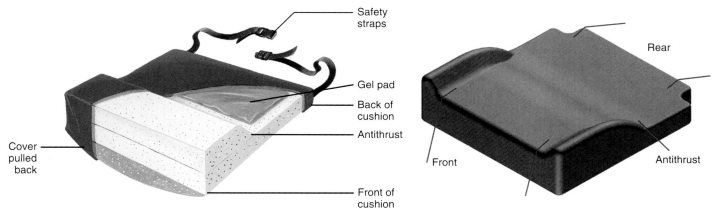

FIG. 33.10 An antithrust seat can help hold the pelvis back on the seat by blocking forward sliding of the ischial tuberosities (IT). (*Left,* Courtesy Skil-Care Corporation, Yonkers, NY; *right,* Courtesy Freedom Designs, Inc, Simi Valley, CA.)

lateral support can often be achieved within the integrity of the overall support. Many back supports are available with customized support options. More substantial contouring can be achieved using blocks/wedges of high-density foam. A custom-molded back should be considered for children with severe fixed spinal deformity. Some children who need contact and support along the paraspinal muscles, but who are still growing, benefit from a hybrid back support. A custom-molded back support can be contoured along the paraspinal region and then flatten laterally. Linear lateral trunk supports are then added to the contoured back. This allows for growth and maintains support along the spine.

Alignment of the spine in the sagittal plane has traditionally been adjusted using lumbar rolls; however, control of sagittal curves begins with the pelvis and sacrum rather than the lumbar spine.[14,58]

Pelvic stabilization. Techniques to improve pelvic control are largely a matter of clinical opinion and user preference. A pelvic support placed at a 45-degree angle at the seat-back junction is the most typical form of pelvic stabilization. Placement of the belt across the anterior thighs, just in front of the hips, allows more natural active trunk and pelvic mobility.[14,58] The pelvic positioning belt can use a two-point attachment system or a four-point attachment system. The four-point system allows for more control of pelvic alignment and greater distribution of pressure (Fig. 33.11). The subanterior superior iliac spine (sub-ASIS) bar is a form of rigid pelvic stabilization consisting of a padded bar attached to mounting plates lateral to the pelvis.[13] The pelvis must be maintained in a vertical orientation or the child will slide under the bar. Dynamic pelvic stabilization is achieved through the use of contoured pads that are placed around the pelvis, with a pivot mechanism allowing anterior-posterior tilting of the pelvis without loss of stability.[14,58] Adjustments are made to accommodate the deformity, control of direction and amount of tilting, and exert a dynamic force to return the pelvis to a neutral position.

Angles. There is no consensus as to the effects of seat and spatial angles on alignment and function. Factors to consider in determining seat angle include severity and type of impairment in muscle tone, joint contractures, skeletal deformities; postural control in sitting; and design and purpose of the mobility base. Although the concept of upright 90-90-90 sitting is theoretically

sound, it may not always be the best option. Slight anterior wedging of the seat may improve head alignment or keep very young children from sliding. Opening the hip angle (tipping the front seat edge) may be necessary when hip extension contractures are present. Allowing the knees to flex reduces the rotation force on the pelvis, minimizing the effect of tight hamstrings.

A seat with an anterior tilt has potential benefits for children with lower extremity muscle hypoextensibility but fair-to-good upper body control who "sacral sit" on a flat surface. A seat with an anterior tilt in a forward-lean position with a solid anterior chest support is also used for children with severe impairments. Good pelvic stabilization must be achieved to prevent sliding.

Variable seat-to-back angles allow adjustments of tilt and recline throughout the day. Tilt is useful for relieving pressure or trunk or neck fatigue, and it provides a combination of active sitting and rest positions. When in a tilt system, the seat-to-back angle does not change. Recline is useful for relief of fatigue, for hip or back pain, and if catheterization or other hygiene procedures must be performed in the chair. In a reclining seating system, the seat-to-back angle changes as the reclining position changes.

Dynamic or compliant seating systems are used for clients with severe and abrupt extensor spasms. Often the severity of tone or spasms is exacerbated by the rigidity of a conventional system. Dynamic or compliant devices use hinges, pivot points, and springs to allow movement of the seat or back with the child and provide a gentle returning force. Clients who used these systems exhibited a decrease in the severity of spasms or fluctuating tone over a period of weeks; comfort and ease of transfers also improved.

Upholstery. Upholstery for the seat cushion and back support can be made out of a variety of materials and is an important feature of the seating system. When choosing a covering, consideration must be given to whether the child is incontinent, if the child is typically hot, whether the child has allergies to specific fabrics, and who will care for the coverings. A fabric with a two-way stretch is ideal to allow for full benefit of the seat cushion and back support materials. Vinyl is a durable cushion covering; however, it can be hot and slippery and typically cannot be removed from the seating system. In addition, it is a very stiff fabric. As such, it typically does not allow for the full

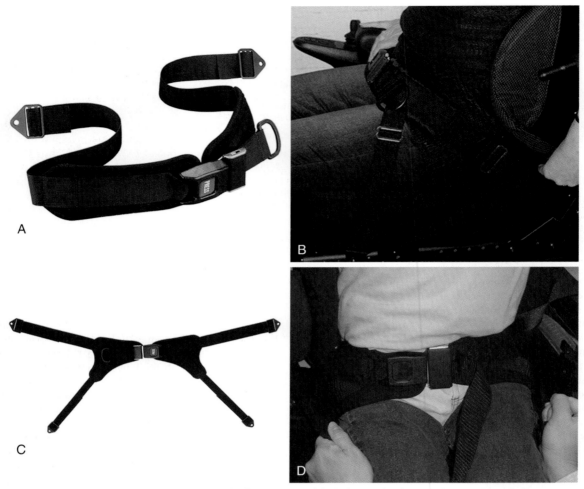

FIG. 33.11 *A,* Two-point pelvic belt. *B,* Two-point pelvic belt attached to seating system. *C,* Four-point pelvic belt. *D,* Four-point pelvic belt attached to seating system. (*A* and *C,* Courtesy Adaptive Engineering Labs, Milwaukee, WI. *B,* From Cook AM, Polgar JM: *Assistive technologies: principles and practice,* ed 4, St. Louis, 2015, Mosby.)

benefit of using different density foams or viscous fluid layers. Synthetic knit fabrics with waterproof backing are also a popular choice of covering. They are less slippery, thus decreasing shear, and can be removable for easy cleaning. Ideally, a child should have at least two sets of cushion covers, thus allowing one to be laundered while the other is being used.

Front riggings. Although a component of the mobility base, front riggings, or leg supports, are discussed in this section because of their direct influence on the entire seating system. Elevated leg rests are offset forward of the seat more than nonelevating leg rests and can contribute to forward sliding on the seat or poor positioning of the feet for weight bearing. Elevating leg rests should be ordered only when required, for instance, to control dependent edema or when the lower extremity is immobilized. Selection of footrests on small, pediatric chairs is often challenging because they may interfere with caster movement. Footplates that extend backward under the seat are helpful when clients have tight hamstrings. Footplates can be positioned parallel to the floor or angled to match foot/ankle position. Shoe holders and foot straps hold the feet in the desired location to assist with lower body stability and weight bearing. For clients with deformity or limited joint

movement, forcing the foot into neutral alignment on the footrest may impose undesirable stresses at the knees or hips. Children who are able to make postural adjustments during weight shifting and actively place their feet should not have their feet constrained. If the child is able or learning to transfer independently or actively assists in a sit-to-stand transfer, the front riggings and footplates should swing out to the sides. The child whose seating system has tapered front riggings and a fixed footplate will transfer by either stepping over the footplates or stepping onto the footplates and then stepping down. Alternatively, children carefully lower themselves onto the footplate and transfer from there.

Lateral and medial supports. Lateral trunk supports vary from simple, flat, padded blocks to contoured, wraparound supports. Swivel or swing-away mounting hardware allows the wraparound supports to fit properly, especially with varying seasonal clothing. In addition, the child is able to transfer into and out of the seating system without interference.

Contoured seats typically provide the most effective lateral thigh and pelvic support, as well as good pressure relief. Square or rectangular pads used as lateral thigh supports can maintain position of the legs and allow for growth. Medial thigh supports (abductor wedges or pommels) maintain hip alignment in neutral or slight abduction but do not stretch tight adductors or prevent forward sliding of the pelvis. Removable or swing-away pommels facilitate transfers and urinal or catheter use.

Anterior supports. Anterior trunk supports are designed to maintain the spine erect and upright over the pelvis. Anterior support can be gained via an H-harness or horizontal anterior chest strap. Butterfly-shaped supports should be used with caution as they present with extreme safety hazards. Typically, the lower straps are secured to the wheelchair seat frame or the back support itself. Then, the upper straps are used to adjust the tension of the fit, preventing the pad from sliding upward to the neck. Padded axillary straps, sometimes known as *Bobath straps* or *backpack straps,* also help maintain the trunk in an upright posture. They attach to the underside of the lateral thoracic support, are directed superiorly and medially over the front of the axilla, and attach at the top of the backrest, controlling shoulder protraction without crossing the chest. Trefler and Angelo[116] reported that the type of anterior chest supports used by children with CP did not influence performance on a switch activation task. They concluded that style of anterior chest support should be based on the child's needs and preference.

Headrest. Facilitating good head position in children who have poor voluntary control is challenging. In children with limited postural control, poor head positioning can make an otherwise effective postural support system fail. On the other hand, barium swallow studies suggest that some clients with the most severe physical and cognitive impairments may need to adopt a forward-hanging head position to cope with increased oral secretions or reflux.[12] For such clients, supporting the head in a position that "looks good" may increase the risk of aspiration or choking.[12]

Support under the occiput provides better head support than a flat contact on the back of the head. A pad with an occipital ledge and contoured head supports is available in several options. Some head supports can include a static or dynamic forehead strap to assist in maintaining an upright head position. Care must be taken that the head support does not unduly block the child's peripheral vision. Head supports can be the ideal mounting location for switches that control other AT such as augmentative communication systems.

Upper extremity supports. Trays are a common type of upper extremity support and can be designed for a multitude of special purposes. Posterior elbow blocks help to reduce the tendency to retract the arms and maintain the upper extremities in a forward position. Clients with severe dystonia often prefer wrist or arm cuffs to reduce unwanted movement of one or both arms.

WHEELED MOBILITY

The purpose of the mobility base depends on the child's level of function. For some, the primary purpose will be independent mobility, and the team must determine how best to achieve this. For others, the purpose of the base is to provide a means of being transported by a caregiver, and this must be accomplished in a safe, comfortable, and efficient manner. In either case, the base serves the additional role of supporting the seating system. Selection of a mobility base requires consideration of the seating system, the child's lifestyle, and the physical features of the environments in which the system will be used. Examination and evaluation for a new mobility base should be done concurrently with simulation for the postural support system, because the success of the entire system depends on all of the parts working together.

Excessive energy expenditure during locomotion is a common impairment of people with movement dysfunction. Persons with physical disability who walk with decreased speed and require an assistive device or who manually propel a wheelchair may prefer power mobility to reduce energy expenditure. Children with CP were reported to walk at nearly half the velocity of children without disability and consume more oxygen per kilogram of body weight per minute when walking.[7] Wheeled mobility is a more efficient mobility method than walking with braces and an assistive mobility device for children with myelomeningocele. Fifty percent of children with myelomeningocele who were ambulatory with braces stopped walking between ages 10 and 20 years.[49] Ambulation was 218% less energy efficient for children with myelomeningocele compared with children without disability. Children with muscle control at the L2 level or above expended energy equal to their maximal aerobic capacity when walking at slow speed, whereas children with muscle control at L3-L4 used 85% of their maximal aerobic capacity.[14] In contrast, wheelchair propulsion required 42% less energy than crutch walking at the same speed. Oxygen consumption during wheelchair propulsion was only 9% greater than the oxygen consumption of children without disability during walking.[49] Energy expenditure and speed of mobility during wheelchair propulsion of children with myelomeningocele were efficient and as fast as walking in children without disabilities.[44a] Fatigue associated with excessive energy expenditure during locomotion may adversely affect academic performance.[7] Academic performance (reading fluency, visual motor accuracy, and manual dexterity) was measured in three students with myelomeningocele attending middle school who alternated propelling their wheelchair or walking with assistive devices throughout the school day. Visual motor accuracy decreased for all three subjects when they walked. Manual dexterity decreased on days walked for one subject, and reading fluency did not change for any of the subjects.

Many factors affect the ability to manually propel a wheelchair, including physiologic capacities, such as strength and endurance, which are dependent on the user's diagnosis, age, sex, lifestyle, and build.[14,42,58] The position of the individual within the wheelchair, particularly in relation to the position of the rear wheels and access to the hand rims, determines the mechanical advantage of the user to propel the chair. Wheelchair factors that affect mobility are rolling resistance, control, maneuverability, stability, and movement dynamics. These factors are dependent on the quality and construction of the wheelchair, such as weight, rigidity of the frame, wheel alignment, mass distribution, and suspension. Wheelchair propulsion in children with spinal cord injury was similar to that in a neurologically matched group of adults.[54] The adults wheeled faster, but the children spent a similar proportion of the wheeling cycle in propulsion, and the angular changes in the kinematics of the elbow and shoulder were the same for both groups. Therefore, methods used to improve wheeling efficiency in adults may be applicable to children.

Self-mobility has important implications for development. The infant's experience with independent mobility impacts on perceptual, cognitive, emotional, and social processes.[42] For children who lack mobility, early provision of mobility aids has the potential to enhance development of spatial, cognitive, affective, and social functions. Prone scooters, caster carts, and walkers are alternatives for some young children with sufficient arm strength. For the child with more severe involvement, early power mobility offers the best choice and allows the child to increase his or her self-initiated movements during play.[16]

Historically, power mobility was considered a last mobility option put off until children reached their teens, when all attempts at effective ambulation were exhausted. Power wheelchairs were considered too expensive and too difficult for young children to learn to drive, and walking was too important a goal to give up. Research does not support this perspective. Studies indicate that children as young as 24 months can successfully learn independent power mobility within a few weeks.[9,24] A comprehensive evaluation is necessary to determine if a child is appropriate for powered mobility. The performance characteristics of the power base must be matched with the child's intended use, lifestyle, and comfort as part of the selection process.[46] The assessment should include an informative intake and a preliminary examination including an assessment of the child's performance in natural environments. Factors that influence a child's success or failure with power mobility include cognition, behavior, motor control, funding, family support, and transportation.[24] Benefits associated with power mobility include an increase in self-initiated behavior, including change in location, rate of interaction with objects, and frequency of communication.[46] Benefits to social participation that have been reported are increased peer interaction; increased interest in other forms of locomotion, including walking; increased family integration such as inclusion in outings; and decreased perception of helplessness by family members.[19] Major factors affecting performance of powered mobility were cognition, motor ability, driving as an activity, technology features of the mobility device, features of the environment, and a combination of these factors.[42] Instruction and training are important considerations in making decisions about power mobility devices for children. Inexperienced drivers improved their overall driving performance after simulator training.[46]

An interdisciplinary US Wheelchair Standards Committee, administered through RESNA and approved by the American National Standards Institute (ANSI), has produced a document on wheelchair standards. The standards represent a comprehensive approach to testing and disclosing information about wheelchairs. Manufacturers, suppliers, and consumers can use this information to improve their products, select chairs with the best performance for the cost, and identify chairs that meet performance needs.

Selection of a Mobility Base

The goal in selecting a mobility base is to provide an appropriate and efficient means of getting from one location to another. It is inappropriate to require someone to rely on his or her everyday mobility for exercise. Prohibiting children with limited ability to walk from using a manual wheelchair and children with limited ability to self-propel a wheelchair from using power mobility may compromise functional and academic performance due to excessive energy expenditure. A creative and structured fitness program is a more appropriate way of addressing strength and cardiovascular endurance goals.

It is generally agreed that the child's positioning needs are the most important factor when selecting a mobility system. At the same time, the design of the seating system should maximize potential for independent function in the wheelchair. This, in turn, influences chair modifications and the interface

hardware needed. For example, if a 3-inch thick modular foam seat cushion is necessary for positioning and pressure relief, yet the child has short extremities, as in myelodysplasia, both independent transfers and wheeling may be more difficult. A possible solution is to order a chair frame with a lower seat-to-floor height and without sling seat upholstery so that a solid seat board with drop brackets can be used to lower the cushion between the seat rails.

To assess driving skills and controller placement, a supportive trial seating system must be attached to a power base for evaluation. An attendant-held control can override the user's control, ensuring safety and appropriate feedback during assessment and training. The child should be provided the opportunity to test a variety of bases with appropriately simulated postural support.

The first step is to determine the type of mobility base desired. Mobility bases for children include strollers, manual wheelchairs and power wheelchairs. Manual wheelchairs can be configured for independent mobility (self-propulsion) or dependent mobility (another person pushes the chair) depending on the child's needs and abilities. Ideally, the selection is based on the potential level of independent mobility. However, other considerations that are often equally as important include the type of housing, method of transportation, availability of training or supervision, and availability of funding.

Once the mobility base is chosen, the next consideration is the style of the base. Within each type, there are several styles with different features and performance characteristics. Factors that influence this choice are the level and type of seating system required, the level of independence in transfers and ADLs, the environments in which the chair will be used, the method of transportation, and the needs of caregivers.

The size of the mobility device is based on the child's physical size, expected growth, the capability of the chair to accommodate growth, and the size and style of the seating system. Mobility bases designed for children are available in a variety of sizes and designs. The ability of mobility bases to expand and accommodate physical growth has improved as funding sources have demanded longer life from purchased items.

A final consideration is the model and manufacturer of the chair. Often the details of construction are important at this stage, such as the dimensions (seat width and depth) of the chair, angles, orientations, adjustability of parts such as footrests and armrests, and swing-away, detachment, or folding mechanisms. Other important factors are performance characteristics, styling, comfort, durability, availability of parts, service record, and cost. Regional preferences for various models and manufacturers are evident across North America.

Strollers

Stroller style mobility bases are appropriate for infants (0–3 years of age) and often preschool-age children (3–5 years of age) primarily because their designs are very similar to regular baby strollers. Basic models include sling seat and back upholstery with a 5-point safety harness (Fig. 33.12A). Models designed for the children with greater physical limitations include a supportive seat and back system along with a variety of positioning components that can be integrated to provide additional positioning support (Fig. 33.12B). These models also include an adjustable push handle that allows the child to face toward or away from the caregiver. For infants and young children, a stroller style mobility base is socially acceptable, is easy to fold

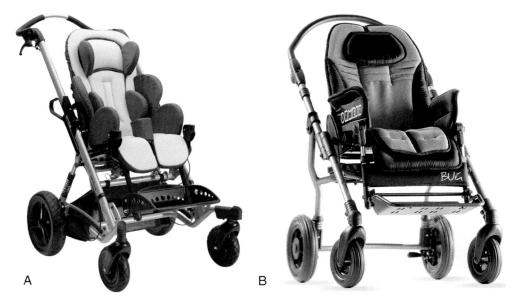

FIG. 33.12 **A,** Ottobock Kimba stroller base with modular positioning components. **B,** Ormesa Bug seating system on stroller base (jogger base and high-low base also available). (*A,* Courtesy Ottobock Rehab, Austin, TX. *B,* Courtesy ORMESA S.r.l., Foligno, Italy.)

for transport in an automobile, and is not perceived as medical equipment. By virtue of the design, stroller mobility bases include storage areas that can be used for items such as ventilators or suction equipment. In addition, some designs include the option of removing the seating system and attaching it to a high-low base for use in the home as a highchair and a floor sitter (Fig. 33.12C). Disadvantages of this style base are that it is not designed for independent propulsion and the child is not always at peer level. Also, for the 4- or 5-year-old, this style base can look childish, causing the child to appear younger than peers of the same age.

When selecting a mobility base for a stroller, it is imperative to consider the parents' preferences, as this can be an emotional decision. Consideration must also be given to how this base will transition with the child into a school-based program and be secured on school bus transportation. Strollers are considered a mobility device. Families and providers need to be cautious when using insurance dollars to purchase a stroller base, as this may impact coverage for a manual wheelchair within 5 years.

Manual Wheelchairs

The standard manual wheelchair has two large wheels, usually in back, for independent propulsion, and two small swiveling casters in front. Some models are specifically designed for the very young child (2–4 years of age) with low seat-to-floor heights to facilitate independent transfers along with wider tires that are easier for smaller hands to manipulate. In addition, the frame can be configured with the larger wheels in front instead of the back, often making it easier for young children to propel (Figs. 33.13A and B).

Pediatric styles often include designs and colors that are appealing to the young child (Fig. 33.13C). They can be configured for dependent mobility where a caregiver pushes the wheelchair or independent mobility where specific dimensions and features are critical to successful independent propulsion. For independent propellers, the 1980s and 1990s were the new

age of manual wheelchairs when lightweight chairs and chairs designed for recreational use and athletic competition became widely available. Lightweight and durable metals and fabrics, alternative wheel placement, improved frame dimensions and designs, adjustability, and adaptability to custom seating have all helped streamline the manual wheelchair to improve efficiency and control, ease of transfer, portability, and appearance. For the very active person, ultra-lightweight, high-performance chairs incorporate rigid frames and lightweight materials for optimal performance. The serious athlete can find specialized designs dedicated to performance needs that barely resemble the traditional concept of a wheelchair (Fig. 33.13D).

One-arm-drive wheelchairs are designed for individuals with functional limitation in one arm that prevents bimanual propulsion (Fig. 33.14). The classic style is the double hand rim on one side, with a linkage system to the other wheel. Styles that use a pumping action with a lever and ratchet system, although rarely used, are generally easier and more effective for wheeling and steering but create more problems in dependent wheeling by caregivers. It is imperative for a child to have the opportunity to try this style of base during the assessment process. Manipulation of the dual rim requires requisite cognitive capability as well as good unilateral upper extremity control. It is also important to observe the efficiency of propulsion and the occurrence of additional movement patterns. For children with impairments in muscle tone such as CP, operation of a one-arm-drive chair may exacerbate existing asymmetry.

Manual tilt-in-space (also referred to as rotational systems) and recline features are available on manual wheelchairs. For some children, a fixed angle of tilt or recline can be incorporated into the design of the seating system and its attachment to the wheelchair. Although this angle is not easily changed, it can enhance function. For others, the ability to vary the amount of tilt or recline throughout the day is critical for functional and physiologic reasons. In these cases, tilt-in-space or recline is integrated into the wheelchair frame design itself. Although the features have similar uses and benefits, it is important to note that they differ in design. Tilt-in-space frames maintain all seated angles throughout the rotational phase. This means that all positioning support achieved with the seating system components is preserved at all times. The angles at the hips, knees, and elbows remain constant while the weight is shifted off of the buttocks and thighs. Recliner frames incorporate the ability to change the seated angles by moving the wheelchair back canes backward in relation to the seat. This changes the hip and elbow angles while the overall weight is redistributed over a larger surface area. Seated pressures originally on the buttocks and thighs are now distributed

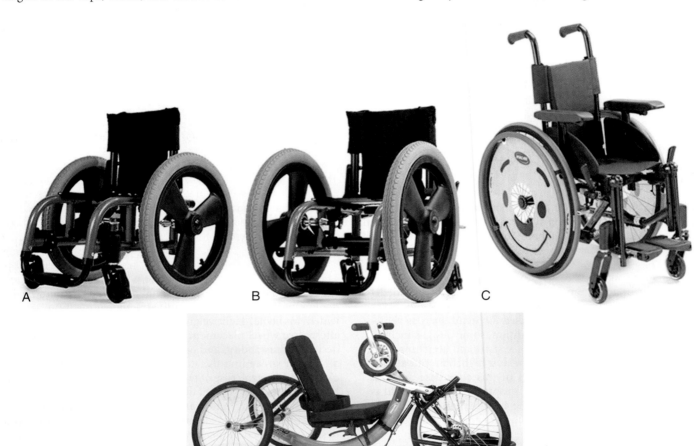

FIG. 33.13 A, Zippie Kidz in standard rear wheel. B, Zippie Kidz with reverse rear wheel configuration. C, Invacare MyOn Jr. pediatric manual wheelchair. D, Invacare TopEnd XLT Jr. handcycle. (A and B, Courtesy Sunrise Medical, Boulder, CO. C and D, Courtesy Invacare Corporation, Elyria, OH.)

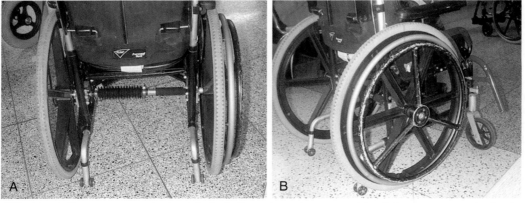

FIG. 33.14 One-arm manual wheelchair. A, Rear view of one-arm drive linkage on manual wheelchair. B, View of double hand rims for one-arm drive manual wheelchair.

over the buttocks, thighs, back, and back of the head. Recliner frames often include elevating leg rests to provide an alternate lower extremity position as well.

Both features provide a change in position relative to gravity that can increase tolerance for upright positioning post surgical or post injury, maintain good skin integrity to prevent pressure sores and decrease fatigue and discomfort. To unweight the buttocks and thighs sufficiently, the frame must be tilted a minimum of 45° from level in a tilt system. Similarly, in a recliner frame, the back canes must be reclined a minimum of 30° from fully upright to achieve adequate pressure relief. In addition, these features can facilitate access into and within a wheelchair-accessible van where clearances can become an issue as the child grows.

Each feature, on its own, can add significant functional benefits. Tilt-in-space can be essential to assist with transfers into and out of the wheelchair as well as aid in repositioning, allowing gravity to assist the process. Recline can also assist with transfers, dressing, and bowel/bladder management. It also provides passive range of motion at the hips, elbows, and knees (with use of elevating leg rests). Understanding the design features and functions is essential to match the benefits with the child's needs. For example, it is important to know that the child's relationship to the seating components will change when using the recliner, making use of custom-molded seats and back supports or modular components with significant contours problematic and not advisable. In addition, the recliner frame can trigger the atypical movement pattern for a child with strong tone, having a negative effect on the child's function.

The current technology design uses a weight-shifting rotational system rather than a gas spring tilt system. The weight-shifting system maintains the user's center of mass within the wheelbase during the tilt phase, resulting in a more stable system when the child is not upright. The wheelbase in this design is shorter than its gas spring tilt predecessor (Fig. 33.15).

Power Mobility

Four categories of function have been described in children using power mobility.[9] The first category includes children who do not walk or have a means of independent mobility other than use of a power device. The second category includes children with inefficient mobility—that is, they walk or use a manual wheelchair but with speed or endurance that is not sufficient to accomplish daily activities and routines. The third category includes children who have lost independent mobility through disease, brain injury, or spinal cord trauma. For this group, the developmental implications of independent mobility may be less important, but the acceptance of assisted mobility is a major issue. The fourth category includes children who require assisted mobility temporarily. This includes young children who are expected to walk as they get older, children who are recovering from surgery, and children who are recovering from an injury or trauma such as a brain injury.

Advances in technology have brought independent power mobility to a greater number of individuals with more severe disabilities than ever before. A wide variety of power bases and options are available, with more reliable and precise controls than ever before possible. The three main types of power wheelchairs are the conventional design with integral seat and chassis (evolved from the traditional, tubular manual wheelchair frame, rarely seen today), the power base or modular design with separate seat and chassis (typical designs found today), and scooters with either three- or four-wheeled platforms. Power chairs may be ordered with seats that tilt, backs that recline, units that recline and tilt, and units with seats and leg rests that elevate, all with the touch of a switch. Manufacturers have responded to an increased demand for child-sized power wheelchairs by producing wheelchairs that are lighter in weight, correctly proportioned for children, and have growth capabilities. Major advances in electronics have produced a greater variety of controls that are easier to access, more durable, and easier to adjust and customize. Power chairs are available in rear-wheel, mid-wheel, or front-wheel drive options. Each provides a different

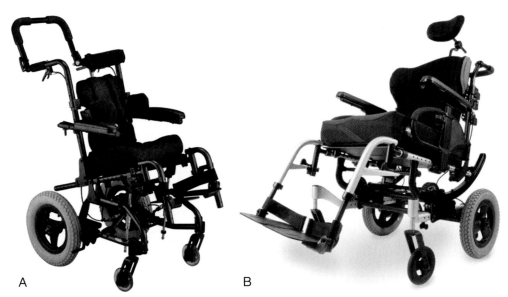

A   B

FIG. 33.15 **A,** Manual wheelchair with mechanical lock tilt-in-space mechanism. **B,** Manual wheelchair with weight-shifting, tilt-in-space mechanism. (*A,* Courtesy Invacare, Elyria, OH. *B,* Courtesy Sunrise Medical, Boulder, CO.)

sense of maneuverability. It is important that the individual have the opportunity to test-drive the different models before a final recommendation is made (Fig. 33.16A and B).

The style of power mobility base chosen will depend in part on the child's upper body control. Scooters are steered using a tiller that requires good sitting balance and arm active range of motion (Fig. 33.16C). The control functions are usually mounted on the tiller and require a grip-type action of the thumb or fingers. Scooters can be disassembled for transport in the trunk of a car and look least like a wheelchair. Although wheelchair bases are generally easy to adapt to a seating system, seating systems for scooters have limited adjustability and adaptability. Scooters are considered a power mobility device. As with strollers, families and providers need to be cautious of the timeline when using insurance dollars to purchase a scooter, as this may impact the insurance coverage decision in the future to fund a power wheelchair.

Today's power-base designs offer the greatest range of seating and control options. The entire seating unit can be removed from the pedestal mount of the modular base. The traditional belt-driven chair is obsolete. The direct-drive motors improve power, as well as control in turning. Front-, mid-, and rear-wheel drive designs offer different advantages and disadvantages in stability while driving and stopping, stability during recline or tilt, maneuverability in tight spaces, and the ability to climb curbs. The type of power wheelchair for a child must be as carefully selected as any other component of the wheelchair and seating system.

Power recline and power tilt capabilities offer excellent alternatives for children who require position changes throughout a long day of sitting to perform different functions or to prevent pain, fatigue, or pressure sores. The act of reclining, however, causes shearing of tissues due to the disproportionate movement between the child and the seating system. On returning

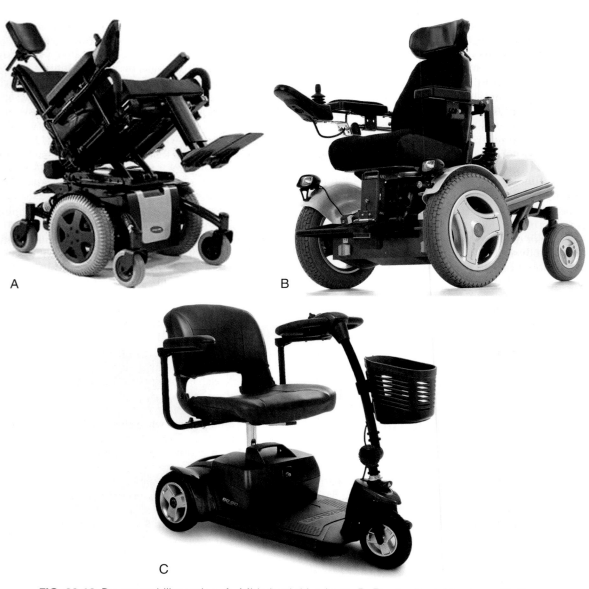

FIG. 33.16 Power mobility styles. **A,** Midwheel drive base. **B,** Front-wheel drive base. **C,** Three-wheeled scooter. (*A,* Courtesy Invacare Corporation, Elyria, OH. *B,* Courtesy Permobil, Timrå, Sweden. *C,* Courtesy Pride Mobility Products, Exeter, PA.)

to the upright position, most clients will have shifted position in the system, and the more complex the seating system, the more likely the position shift. Power recliners are available in reduced-shear models to help address these problems. Power tilt-in-space models work well for children with severe hypertonia or contractures who cannot tolerate having the seat-to-back angle opened up or who, once having done so, cannot return to an upright position without sliding.

Controls for power wheelchairs are available in two basic types: proportional and digital. The former has a proportional relationship between movement of the joystick and speed of the chair or sharpness of turning, whereas the latter has an on/off relationship to chair movement. An example of a proportional control is a standard joystick found on most power wheelchairs. It is customarily mounted on either the right or left armrest and will move in a 360-degree arc. The movement of the joystick controls the speed and the direction of the wheelchair. An alternative to the standard joystick is a joystick that is smaller and more compact. This feature allows a great deal of flexibility for joystick placement, provided sturdy mounting hardware is used. Proportional joysticks are also available in short-throw models that require less movement and force for activation and in heavy-duty models that can withstand a great deal of force. Head control joysticks are available for some wheelchairs.

An example of a digital multiple switch control system consists of four separate switches, with each switch controlling one direction—forward, reverse, left, and right. There are a variety of mechanical switches commercially available for selection of the most appropriate switch for a given individual. Use of digital switches during assessment allows for evaluation of different configurations. For example, the switches may be separated and set up in arrays to evaluate head control, or each of the four switches may be positioned at different body sites. The wafer board and arm-slot control are examples of alternative (switch) controls for wheelchair driving. Switch-driven chairs tend to be less precise and smooth while turning and changing directions because each direction is controlled by a separate switch.

With the recognition that age is no longer the determining factor in the successful use of power mobility has come the need to define selection criteria. Children under the age of 2 have successfully used power mobility independently as their primary means of mobility.[28] Furumasu, Tefft, and Guerette[20] developed an assessment to determine a child's readiness for powered mobility. This tool is based on Piagetian theories of development and evaluates the child on several learning domains. Furumasu, Tefft, and Guerette have also developed a 6-hour protocol for instruction of young children. The protocol is composed of activities performed in increasingly more complex environments ranging from free play in an open gym to activities performed in community environments such as the mall or clinic.

An alternative perspective is that children may learn spatial relationships implicitly through training in a power device. Jones et al.[28] provided a compelling argument for power mobility for very young children based on the importance of mobility rather than "readiness for driving" skills. She suggested that the child be allowed to explore movement in the device over a period of time, initially being restricted to a single turning direction in a small, safe environment. As the child's control over the power device improves and verbal labels for what she or he is doing are provided, the concept of independent mobility will develop. Joystick or switch-activated toys that are available

at local toy stores make an excellent inexpensive alternative for power training of young children when the devices can be suitably adapted for seating and control.

Simulators have proved to be successful training tools.[1] Hasdai and colleagues[47] found that inexperienced drivers following a simulator driving program improved their accuracy and performance. Whizz-Kidz in the United Kingdom provides a training program that includes basic, intermediate, and advanced training for manual and power chair users. The children are paired with a spotter and buddy to learn advanced skills that allow them to be safer and more independent in the community. The program information can be found at www.whizz-kidz.org.uk.

Virtual reality (VR) technology has enabled video gaming experiences to become wheelchair driver training experiences.[43,47] Harrison et al.[25] investigated the effectiveness of wheelchair training using virtual environments. All six participants demonstrated improved skills; however, they agreed that the VR wheelchair was more difficult to control than their own wheelchair. The authors recommended that a VR training environment is useful, although care must be taken not to make the environment overly complicated. Criteria for safe driving include the ability to turn the chair on and off, follow a straight course, turn both left and right, back the chair up, maneuver around objects and persons, and stop quickly.[15,48]

The *marginal driver* is one of any age who may show borderline cognitive or physical skills or whose visual-perceptual problems interfere with driving ability. With supervision, these individuals may do well driving in a familiar setting, such as their school, but are not successful in novel or unpredictable community settings. The value of a power chair in increasing self-esteem and promoting independence in specific skills must be carefully weighed against the expense and amount of training and supervision required.

Several practical considerations are essential for the selection of power mobility. Building accessibility and space will affect where and how the device is used. Often the power chair is kept and maintained at school and a manual base is used at home. Care and maintenance of a power chair are more complex than for manual systems. Transportation is also a more complicated issue. Some school districts refuse to transport certain types of power wheelchairs such as scooters. The family may need a van for transporting the chair, and a ramp or a lift may be required for loading and unloading. Funding options for more expensive power wheelchairs may be more restrictive. Usually a backup manual chair is also required, especially during maintenance or repair of the power system. Responsibility for supervision, training, and routine wheelchair maintenance should be determined prior to ordering the system.

The examination and evaluation process for a power mobility system are often more complicated than for other types of wheelchairs. First, a variety of power bases should be available for trial and preferably with capabilities to adjust speed, acceleration, deceleration, turning speed, sensitivity, and tremor dampening of the joystick. Children generally perform better in a child-sized wheelchair rather than an adult-sized wheelchair. Because proper support is critical to performance in a power wheelchair, the therapist needs access to a variety of seating components, supports, and straps to provide the stability that is necessary to optimize the child's motor function for operating the controls. A variety of controls and mounting options should be available for trial. Evaluation may take place over a period of several days to weeks and ideally in a variety of settings, especially for young and inexperienced drivers, who may require much practice with different options before making a decision.

A standard proportional control mounted on the armrest is preferred for children with some active control of arm and hand movements. This is the simplest and least expensive control. If a more midline position of the joystick is desired, placement of the control bracket on the inside of the wheelchair armrest is relatively easy.

Site options for the control increase with the use of a remote joystick and the proper hardware. Some possibilities include center mounting of the joystick close to the user to compensate for decreased range of motion or strength, mounting the joystick at arm's length on top of a lap tray to provide support and increased stability for children with dyskinetic movements or fluctuating muscle tone, or mounting the joystick for chin or foot operation. For children with limited functional movements and site options, an integrated control permits operation not only of the wheelchair but also of other equipment such as a communication aid, EADL, or computer equipment.

Transportation Safety

The US society is generally mobile and on the go. This includes children and adults who use wheeled mobility. RESNA and ANSI have set federal standards for using wheelchairs within vehicle transportation. Best practice dictates that, when at all possible, wheelchair users should transfer out of their wheelchair and into an age- or weight-appropriate vehicle seat and occupant restraint system that meets all the federal safety standards. The wheelchair should be stored and secured within the vehicle to prevent it from becoming a harmful projectile. Wheelchair occupants should ride in an upright position with back reclined less than 30 degrees. The headrest should be positioned to support the head and neck, and trays should be removed and secured.

If the occupant cannot transfer, a seating system is required that can be attached to a transit wheelchair frame. Transport wheelchairs meet ANSI/RESNA/WC19 standards, have been frontal crash tested, and have several advantageous features for use in vehicular transport compared with standard wheelchairs. A WC19 transport wheelchair can be secured at four crash-tested sites located on the floor of the vehicle, in less than 10 seconds per site, from areas accessible from one side of the wheelchair in an enclosed space. Transit wheelchairs have crashworthy frames, better accommodation of vehicle anchored belts, and proper instructions for use as a seat in a motor vehicle. It is imperative that the wheelchair and occupant face toward the front of the vehicle.

WC19 also set standards for lateral stability of a wheelchair in a forward-moving vehicle. This is due to the fact that wheelchair users are often injured when the wheelchair tips after the vehicle makes a quick stop or sharp turn. Effective in May 2002, regulations allow that a wheelchair occupant can use a crashworthy pelvic belt secured to the wheelchair frame, in which a separate vehicle-mounted shoulder belt could be inserted. This configuration may allow restraint systems to fit more securely. Information regarding WC19 can be found at the Rehabilitation Engineering Research Center on Wheelchair Transportation Safety website at www.rercwts.org.

If the occupant cannot transfer and cannot use the transport wheelchair, a wheelchair with a metal frame should be used with a wheelchair tie-down and occupant restraint system

(WTORS). Restraint systems that meet WTORS standards are labeled SAE J2249. Four tie-down straps are attached to strong places on the wheelchair frame such as the welded frame joints. Attachment points should be as high as possible but below the seat surface. Rear tie-down straps should maintain a 30- to 45-degree angle with the vehicle floor. The four-point tie-down system is considered the universal system. When used properly, the four-point system is effective and affordable. Tie-down straps should meet SAE J2249 standards.

Just as the wheelchair frame needs to be secured to the vehicle, the occupant needs to be secured with crashworthy lap and shoulder safety belts. Standard positioning belts and harnesses are not meant to restrain an occupant in a vehicle crash. Currently, most lap and shoulder belts anchor to the vehicle independent of the wheelchair user. Newer models of WC19 wheelchairs have crash-tested occupant restraints mounted directly to the frame and allow the vehicle-mounted shoulder belts to attach directly to the lap belt.[50]

EXAMINATION AND EVALUATION FOR OTHER ASSISTIVE TECHNOLOGY

Assistive technologies offer children with physical disabilities an opportunity to participate more fully and become more independent in their daily lives. In addition to manual or powered mobility and specialized seating, these technologies include specialized switches, communication devices, computers, and EADLs. Often the term *assistive technology* is used to designate these latter four types of electric or electronic devices, although the Tech Act and RESNA include all forms of mobility, positioning, and related devices in the definition of AT. The assessment and selection process for each type of AT tends to be similar.

The physical therapist, as a member of the AT team, is responsible for completing the physical skills examination needed for technology use. Regardless of impairment or functional limitations, children should be optimally positioned prior to completing an AT device evaluation. Proper positioning is essential for reducing fatigue, as well as for achieving optimal control of head, trunk, and upper extremity movements for selection of appropriate AT devices and services. A comprehensive physical examination includes but is not limited to ROM, muscle strength, muscle tone, endurance, gross and fine motor abilities, and sensory impairments. The therapist also examines postural control, righting and equilibrium reactions, and notes the presence of primitive reflexes. These data provide the team with information concerning a child's functional motor abilities such as head and trunk control, the variety and quality of active movements, and the ability to isolate one movement from another. For successful technology use, functional movements must be voluntary, reliable, repeatable, and in some cases sustainable. The child's movement patterns should not contribute to fatigue or pain nor should they elicit pathologic reflexes or increase postural tone.[14,23,39,44]

Collaboration among health professionals and agencies is important to prevent duplication of services and unnecessary expense to families and third-party payers. Recent examinations by the child's physical therapist should be shared with a consulting AT team. A detailed written report, video or still pictures, a telemedicine videoconference, and participation of the child's physical therapist in the examination process are examples of different ways in which recommendations for positioning can be shared and services coordinated.

The physical therapist, along with the other team members, also contributes information regarding the child's sensory, perceptual-motor, and cognitive abilities. Sensory skills needed for successful AT device use include visual and auditory discrimination and responses to tactile, kinesthetic, and proprioceptive input. Visual acuity allows a young child to focus on an image, such as a switch, joystick, or computer screen, and visual accommodation allows the eyes to adjust to near and far objects. Assessment of the child's visual field is necessary for placement of controls or displays. Tracking is the ability to follow a moving object with the eyes, and scanning is when the eyes move to find an object—these are necessary skills for successful technology use. Hearing impairments compromise a child's ability to receive auditory information, as well as the ability to produce and monitor speech output.[14] After members of the AT team are aware of how a child processes sensory information, they are able to select devices that are motivating and ensure success. Devices that provide a variety of sensory cues, such as auditory clicks or beeps, visual light displays, or tactile and proprioceptive cues such as textured or vibrating switches, can be highly motivating and may facilitate learning.

Knowledge of a child's cognitive function level and learning style is important for selection of appropriate access, feedback, application, and training with the various devices. During the assessment, the team directly observes a child's attention span; short-term memory; understanding of cause and effect; ability to follow directions, sequence, and problem solve; and intention and motivation for technology use.[17,26] Whenever possible, the child should participate in the decision-making process. This may be as simple as picking the color of his or her mobility device, cushion covers, or switches. In other words, the team should heed the "Nothing about me without me" saying.[56]

SWITCHES, CONTROLS, AND ACCESS SITES

Children with motor impairments may require special switches or controls to operate communication aids, computers, power wheelchairs, or EADLs. Switches are also called *control interfaces* and *input devices*. Switch technology can help teach cause and effect, encourage independent play, promote group participation, and give a child control over a part of his or her environment.

Typically, an access site (a body part that can produce a consistent movement) is selected, and then the switch or control to operate a device is chosen. If a child has purposeful, controlled movement of any body part, the team can identify a suitable switch site. A variety of switches and controls are available from manufacturers who specialize in technology aids for people with special needs. They vary in size, shape, cost, performance capabilities, and ways in which they are activated. Switches may be single (perform an on/off function), dual (perform on/off and a select function), or multiple (perform on/off and several functions). Examples of multiple-switch configurations are joysticks, wafer boards, slot controls, head arrays, and keyboards. Methods for activating switches include pressure (direct touch or breath) or signal transmission (infrared, Bluetooth, etc.). Switch activation can be timed (with use of a timer setting), latched (where the action begins with one touch and occurs until the switch is touched again, similar to a light switch), momentary (the action occurs only while the switch is activated and stops when the switch is released, similar to a doorbell), or

proportional (the speed generated relates directly to the amount of pressure applied to the switch, similar to a car gas pedal).[54]

Children as young as 6 months are capable of using hand or head switches for computer access.[54] Using the hands to activate switches is the typical mode for most children; however, switches can be operated by other body parts such as the head, chin, tongue, eyebrows, elbows, or lower extremities. At times, children will require additional support or extension devices to use a switch or control such as a head or chin pointer, a mouth stick, finger or hand splints, styluses, mobile arm supports, or overhead slings (Fig. 33.17).

Some switches have been specially designed to use with a certain body part such as an eyebrow switch, an eye blink switch, or a tongue touch keypad. Proximity switches will activate when a user gets near the switch, but actual physical contact is not required. A practical application of this technology is to imbed four proximity switches (one each for forward, reverse, right, and left) in a lap tray to operate a power wheelchair. Heavy-duty contact switches may be the most suitable choice for children with fluctuating muscle tone who have difficulty controlling the force of their movements, and tiny fiberoptic switches may be suitable for the user with limited range and strength. At one spinal cord treatment facility, switch evaluations are performed at bedside as soon as the patient is stable. Functional movements are examined, including use of tongue, lips, eyes, eyelids, eyebrows, and jaw.[4] Persons with high-level spinal cord injuries often use pneumatic breath control switches to operate AT devices, and many find that integrated control systems provide them with access to several types of technology.

An integrated control system is one in which several AT devices are operated/controlled using a single input device (e.g., switch, joystick). For example, a power wheelchair can be configured with an electronic controller that allows joystick use for driving the wheelchair, as well as for operation of a communication device, computer equipment, or environmental controls. Criteria to determine when an integrated control is the optimal choice include (1) the user has a single reliable access site; (2) the access method is the same for all devices used; (3) speed, accuracy, or endurance improve; and (4) the child or family has a preference.[4] There are also disadvantages to using integrated controls, including the higher cost of more sophisticated electronics required to perform several functions. In addition, because the individual uses the same input device for all of his or her technology, if the power wheelchair were to break down or need repair, the individual loses access to all of the technology. For this reason, it is extremely important that backup systems are in place for all of the individual's technologies.

AUGMENTATIVE AND ALTERNATIVE COMMUNICATION

In addition to spoken or verbal output, communication includes body language, gestures, facial expressions, and written output. Speech limitations in children may occur as a result of congenital or acquired dysarthria, developmental apraxia, developmental aphasia, congenital anomalies, cognitive impairments, autism, or hearing impairments.[44] When the ability to verbally communicate and interact is limited or absent, some form of AAC should be explored. Augmentative communication is any procedure or device that facilitates speech or spoken language. Alternative communication refers to the communication method used by a person without vocal ability.[2] Ideally, AAC

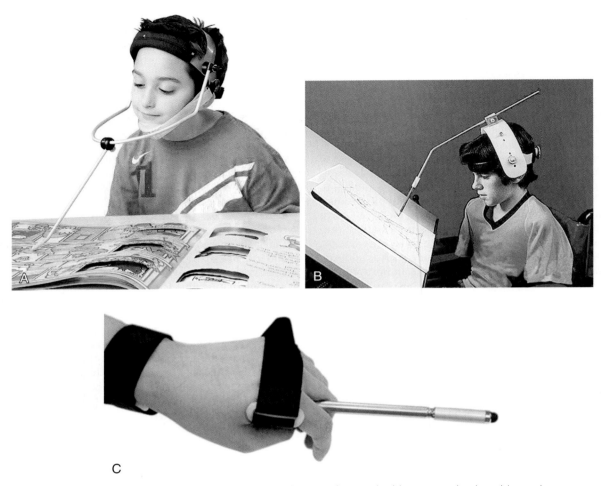

FIG. 33.17 Devices for pointing or indicating that may be used with communication aids or electronic aids to daily living (EADLs). Chin pointer (A), head stick (B), and adjustable stylus with velcro straps (C). (*A and B,* Courtesy Patterson Medical, Warrenville, IL. *C,* Courtesy Enabling Devices, Hawthorne, NY.)

should enable individuals to efficiently and effectively communicate in a variety of social situations.[37] Users of AAC include individuals with cognitive impairments, those requiring written augmentation, and individuals with a temporary limitation in expression due to illness or injury.

The speech and language pathologist along with the child and family members assume the lead roles in identifying the best choice for an AAC system. The physical therapist plays an important ongoing role in determining positions that optimize use of equipment for communication. Many classrooms contain a variety of chairs, corner chairs, prone or supine standers, and sidelyers, which require adjustment or adaptation for a particular child. The physical therapist instructs other team members in the proper use of positioning devices that enhance a child's communication. Therapists working in early intervention are in a unique position to influence the development of communication in infants and young children. Therapists should establish intervention goals that include allowing the child to indicate choices such as the ability to separate head and neck movements from eye movements. This provides the child a method of indicating needs. Additionally, family members are encouraged to talk to and read to their youngsters during daily activities and routines.

A number of techniques and devices for augmenting communication are available and classified as *high tech* and *low tech.* Low-tech equipment includes devices that are powered by batteries or electricity or nothing at all. High-tech equipment includes devices with adapted computers and switching systems.[44] Unaided techniques, such as eye gaze, signing, or gesturing do not require external devices or equipment but rely on the child's ability to physically respond in some consistent manner. Aided techniques include the use of an external device, which may or may not be electronic. A communication sheet or notebook (with pictures, symbols, or words) is an example of a nonelectronic communication aid.

Electronic communication aids offer a much greater range of capabilities and options for users. Simple devices may run less than $100; high-end devices cost several thousand dollars. Some low-cost durable devices play a single message or series of messages, whereas others offer four, eight, or more messages. Generally, the messages can be quickly changed as desired. New devices are continually evolving that are more compact, durable, lighter in weight, and easier to transport. The operation and programming of newer AAC devices have simplified over time. There are several downloadable applications that can be added to a smart phone or tablet. Given the ever-expanding variety of

AAC devices available, the AT team should be able to identify a device that meets the motor and cognitive abilities of each child.

At the high end of the spectrum are sophisticated, computer-based AAC devices that allow a variety of input methods (direct or scanning), high-quality voice output, storage capability for vocabulary and phrases, and the capability to operate computer-based software or EADLs through the device. Third-party payers may deny funding for these devices if they are viewed as educational equipment that the student's local education agency should provide.

The input, or selection, method for AAC devices and computers typically includes direct select or scanning. Direct selection is faster and often the preferred method to operate a communication system. Children with mild-to-moderate impairments often have sufficient motor control for direct selection. The child simply makes a choice from the options presented. For example, when a child touches a location on a communication device with a picture of a glass, the spoken response might be "May I have a drink please?"

Children with severe motor impairments may need to rely on scanning to operate their AAC or computer. The device runs through a sequence of choices (usually rows, then columns), repeating the sequence until the user makes a selection. The scanning rate is adjustable, which allows beginners ample time to become familiar with the new equipment and build confidence and accuracy before increasing speed. In most cases, the selection is made by using a special switch positioned to allow independent access. Examples include a pressure switch mounted on a lap tray and activated with the touch of the hand, a lever switch positioned near the side of the head and operated with lateral head movements, and a chin switch mounted on a collar and operated by flexion and extension movements of the head. Scanning can be both physically and cognitively demanding for some users because they must be able to wait for the appropriate selection, activate the switch at the right moment, release the switch, and repeat these steps for the next selection.

COMPUTER TECHNOLOGY

Computers are typically used for word processing to compose and edit the written word, data collection and storage, graphics for drawing and publishing, and communication via e-mail, the Internet, and social media as well as various educational and recreational activities. Typically, a computer is operated through a keyboard, the mouse, or both. Computers, as well as many computer-based devices such as communication aids, environmental controls, and power mobility controllers, are readily adaptable, can be customized as needed, and can be accessed using a variety of input methods. Voice activation, for example, allows individuals to use voice commands as an input to their electronic device. Typically voice activation systems require training to ensure consistent output accuracy. Hundreds of products are commercially available to adapt a computer for an individual with special needs. This variety is important for users whose needs may change. Input to computers and communication devices can be direct or indirect (scanning or Morse code), with direct access being faster and generally more intuitive.

Keyboard Adaptations and Alternatives

To successfully access the computer, the child with a disability may require some customized accessing method to interface with the computer. These interfaces are often provided by

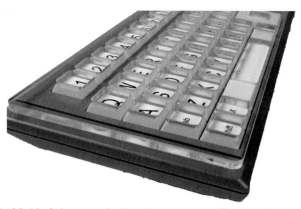

FIG. 33.18 A keyguard placed over a modified keyboard can eliminate unwanted keystrokes for individuals with poor fine motor control or accuracy. (Courtesy AbleNet, Inc, Roseville, MN.)

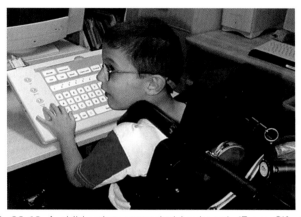

FIG. 33.19 A child using expanded keyboard. (From Cifu DX: Braddom's Physical Medicine and Rehabilitation, ed 5, Philadelphia, Elsevier, 2016.)

additional software or additional hardware for the computer. Software is available to decrease the need for additional keystrokes using word prediction capabilities, to minimize repetition of the same key, and to allow activation of more than one key at a time. Some computer systems have accessibility features built into the standard software package.

Many external options are available as well. A keyguard attached over a keyboard is used to prevent unwanted keystrokes when fine motor control or finger isolation is impaired (Fig. 33.18). Ergonomic keyboards or wrist-arm supports are used with children who require distal support or if tremor, pain, fatigue, or lack of endurance interferes with typing. Mobile arm supports and overhead slings may benefit users with muscle weakness.

Alternatives to the standard keyboard include mini-keyboards, expanded keyboards, and one-handed keyboards (Fig. 33.19). Mini-keyboards have advantages for children with muscular dystrophy who have fine motor control but limited ROM, decreased strength, or low endurance. Expanded or enlarged keyboards are helpful for children with poor coordination and the ability to isolate movement of a finger. These keyboards have up to 128 pressure-sensitive areas referred to as keys, and because the number, size, shape, and location of these keys can be modified, the possibilities for customization are numerous. For example, expanded keyboards could be set up to offer four choices with large contact areas, rather than 128 choices. Standard keyboards, mini-keyboards, and enlarged keyboards may be set up in the QWERTY (typical keyboard) pattern, in an alphabetic layout, or in a frequency-of-use layout. Keyboard patterns can be customized to place frequently used keys near the home row and are available in one-handed or two-handed models.[5]

Computers and tablets are available with integrated touch screens. Because touch screens use direct selection, they tend to be less cognitively demanding, which may be important to children being introduced to computer technology.[14]

Children with visual impairments require technology specific to their needs, such as software or hardware adaptations to provide auditory feedback, tactile keyboards, optical character recognition systems (screen readers that translate text to the spoken word), screen magnification systems, software that will enlarge the text, or Braille technology.

Mouse Alternatives

Mouse functions include moving the cursor on the screen, dragging a selected item on the screen, and clicking or double-clicking to select items and functions. Change in cursor size, color, or speed may make it easier for a child to locate the cursor on the computer screen. Keyboard functions using the arrow keys or the numeric keypad may assist a child who is unable to use a mouse effectively. Alternative mouse options are available, both on the general market and through manufacturers of special equipment, and include joysticks, trackballs, mouse pads, keypad mouse, and head-controlled mouse (Fig. 33.20). Therapists are encouraged to become familiar with commercially available input systems, as well as those developed for users with special needs, because they are often less expensive.

Virtual or onscreen keyboards display an image of a keyboard on the monitor, and the user moves the cursor to the desired key with a mouse, joystick, trackball, head-controlled mouse, or switch array. A selection is then made using a second switch or by dwelling on the key for a predetermined amount of time. Onscreen keyboards with scanning programs are commonly used by children who rely on a single or dual switch to access AT devices. Keyboard and mouse functions can also be achieved using light beams, Bluetooth, infrared, ultrasonic, and speech recognition technology.

Rate Enhancement

Therapists are encouraged not only to become familiar with different access and input methods but also to try them, because each access and input method requires different motor responses and cognitive processes. Consider that a trained typist without a disability is capable of transcribing text at an average of 100 words per minute. The same person typing while composing text averages 50 words per minute. Court reporters, using special keyboards, enter text at 150 words per minute. Contrast that with an average of 10 to 12 words per minute for a person typing with just one finger. The person using scanning usually averages 3 to 5 words per minute.[14] Overall speed of production, although not an issue for all users, can become an issue for students in regular education who are expected to produce a similar amount of written output as their classmates.

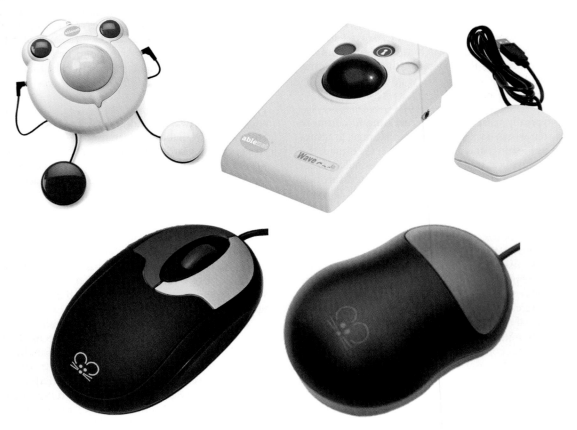

FIG. 33.20 Alternatives to a traditional mouse. (Courtesy AbleNet, Inc, Roseville, MN.)

Productivity also becomes an issue during transition planning if computer proficiency is a condition for employment.

When a computer or communication device is effortful and time consuming, use of macros, abbreviation expansion, or word prediction to enhance productivity should be investigated. Macro programs allow users to combine and automate tasks. Abbreviation expansion automatically types out an entire word or phrase when two or three letters have been typed. For example, a user can command the computer to type out "physical therapy" each time the user inputs the letters "PT." With word prediction software, a word is displayed after only two or three characters are entered. A list of likely choices appears on the screen and the correct number is selected.

ELECTRONIC AIDS TO DAILY LIVING

An electronic aid to daily living (EADL), previously known as an environmental control unit (ECU), is a device or system of devices that allows the operation of electrical appliances or equipment in a variety of ways and places. The purpose of an EADL is to apply technology to facilitate the user's control over the environment, to promote independent access to items required for daily living, and to improve the quality of life and participation in society.[32] Each of us encounters this technology on a daily basis in the form of energy- and time-saving devices such as electronic garage door openers, portable telephones, and remote controls for television and audio equipment. Many of these affordable, commercially available products require precise manual control, which often precludes their use by children with motor impairments; however, a range of environmental control devices are available from manufacturers of equipment for children and adults with physical challenges.

Control of the environment for an older child might include operating a blender with a head-activated switch to prepare treats at school or for a younger child or activating a pressure switch with the hand to operate a battery toy during free time (Fig. 33.21). A child may use a head stick to operate the television remote control to select a channel, control the volume, and turn off the set when done. Adapted phone equipment can be programmed to store several numbers, automatically dial a

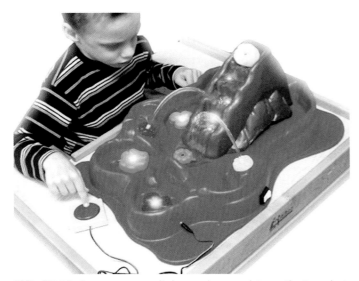

FIG. 33.21 A pressure switch can be used to activate a battery-operated toy. (Courtesy AbleNet, Inc, Roseville, MN.)

number, and answer calls with the touch of a switch, allowing the user to have access to important, age-appropriate socialization. These independent, functional activities help instill a sense of responsibility and independence from caregivers.

In young adults, EADLs may increase personal satisfaction, increased participation in life activities, possible employment, and possible reduction in cost for personal care attendants.[30] The use of EADLs in one residential facility to operate personal entertainment devices such as televisions, radios, and lights reduced the amount of nursing care required by about 2 hours per day per participant.[14] Both residents and nursing staff reported reduced frustration following the introduction of EADLs. Persons with spinal cord injuries who used EADLs used the telephone more often, were more inclined to travel, and spent more time in educational pursuits than nonusers.[33]

An EADL generally includes three parts: the main control unit (central processing unit), the switch (transducer), and any devices (peripherals) to be controlled or activated. Most EADLs emit some type of tactile, visual, or auditory feedback that indicates which function has been selected before the function is activated. Feedback can be an essential feature to the user.

The two basic types of EADLs are direct and remote. In a direct system, the devices to be controlled are plugged directly into the main control unit. In a remote system, the control unit acts as a transmitter, sending signals to remote receivers, which in turn activate the device. The remote system has the advantages of operating a number of devices or appliances from one location, such as a wheelchair or bed, and the absence of wires running from the unit to the device.[14]

Capabilities of systems vary from simply turning one device on and off to operating a whole-house configuration and integrated computer systems. Common functions include operation of a small electrical appliance, television, light fixture, door lock, intercom or call signal, electric bed, and telephone and computer equipment. EADLs can be activated through the wide variety of switches and controls described previously, through voice activation, or through the user's power wheelchair controller, electronic communication aid, or computer. Lange has produced several charts to assist practitioners in comparing the various features of popular EADLs that are commercially available. They include input options, what type of equipment can be controlled, what devices the EADL will interface with such as a computer or communication aid, whether battery backup is included, cost, and comments (http://www.atilange.com/Resources.html, accessed May 6, 2016).

EFFECTS OF MANAGED CARE ON ACQUISITION OF ASSISTIVE TECHNOLOGY

State-funded Medicaid programs, traditionally a major source of funding for children with disabilities, have contracted much of their coverage to private managed care insurance organizations, and in many cases this has affected accessibility to durable medical equipment and specialized devices.[12,24,52] Denials for requested items may increase, either because a narrower interpretation is used in determining medical necessity or because nonstandard or customized items do not fit the billing codes. The time between the initial request and approval may be prolonged if the reviewers are less experienced in the needs of children with physical disabilities and require more explanation, making repeated requests and justification necessary. Choice of products may be restricted because the amount that will be paid is often based on simpler adult equipment designs and does not cover the full cost of more expensive or more customized pediatric designs.

The capitation rate paid to medical equipment suppliers is often inadequate to cover actual expenses, thereby cutting profit margins and making it difficult to provide and service sophisticated or customized equipment. Medical and equipment needs of individuals with disabilities are much higher than what many private companies anticipate. If a managed care company discontinues its contract for state Medicaid patients, this could leave those individuals with little or no choice of coverage and may require a change of provider. There is often a struggle with reconciling the variety of devices that are available for achieving independent function with the increasing restrictions in funding and availability.

SUMMARY

Assistive technology (AT) is a critical component of intervention for children with impairments in body functions and structures and activity limitations in communication, mobility, and self-care. Five major areas for AT are seating and positioning, wheeled mobility, augmentative and alternative communication, computer accessing, and electronic aids to daily living. Current best practice involves a multidisciplinary team—which includes the child and family, AT specialists, and the child's service providers, including therapists, teachers, and medical staff—and a multilevel assessment. Although there is research evidence for AT, the needs and preferences of each child and family and the environments in which AT will be used are essential considerations for decision making. Additionally, funding is often a primary consideration. As a member of the team, the physical therapist should be knowledgeable of AT and aware that products are being improved and new technology is being developed. The potential impact of AT on a child's quality of life underlies the importance of evidence-based decision making that is individualized to the child, family, and environment and increases the child and young adult's ability to participate at home, school, and in their communities.

REFERENCES

1. Abellard P, et al.: Electric wheelchair navigation simulators: why, when, how? http://cdn.intechweb.org/pdfs/10190.pdf. Accessed June 5, 2015.
2. Accardo PJ, Whitman BY: *Dictionary of developmental disabilities terminology*, ed 2, Baltimore, 2002, Paul Brookes.
3. American Physical Therapy Association: *Guide to physical therapist practice*, Alexandria, VA, 2001, APTA.
4. Angelo J: Factors affecting the use of a single switch with assistive technology devices, *J Rehabil Res Dev* 37:591–598, 2000.
5. Bauer AM, Ulrich ME: I've got a Palm in my pocket: using handheld computers in an inclusive classroom, *Teach Excep Child* 35:18–22, 2002.
6. Reference deleted in proofs.
7. Bell KL, Davies PSW: Energy expenditure and physical activity of ambulatory children with cerebral palsy and of typically developing children, *Am J Clin Nutri* 92:312–319, 2010.
8. Reference deleted in proofs.
9. Butler C: Effective mobility for children with motor disabilities. www.global-help.org/publications/books/help_effectivemobility.pdf. Accessed June 7, 2015.
10. Cardon TA, Wilcox MJ, Campbell PH: Caregiver perspectives about assistive technology use with their young children with autism spectrum disorders, *Infants Young Child* 24:153–173, 2011.
11. Reference deleted in proofs.
12. Carlson SJ, Ramsey C: Assistive technology. In Campbell SK, Vander Linden DW, Palisano RJ, editors: *Physical therapy for children*, ed 2, Philadelphia, 2000, WB Saunders.
13. Cook A, Polgar JM: *Assistive technologies: principles and practice*, ed 4, St. Louis, 2015, Mosby.
14. Costigan FA, Light J: Functional seating for school-age children with cerebral palsy: an evidence-based tutorial, *Lang Speech Hear Serv Sch* 42:223–236, 2011.
15. Dawson DR, et al.: Power mobility indoor driving assessment (PIDA) manual. http://fhs.mcmaster.ca/powermobility/PIDA_Instructions_2006.pdf. Accessed June 7, 2015.
16. Deitz J, Swinth Y, White O: Powered mobility and preschoolers with complex developmental delays, *Am J Occup Ther* 56:86–96, 2002.
17. Desideri L, Mingardi A, Stefanelli B, et al.: Assessing children with multiple disabilities for assistive technology: a framework for quality assurance, *Technol Disabil* 159–166, 2013.
18. Dini V, Bertone MS, Romanelli M: Prevention and management of pressure ulcers, *Dermatol Ther* 19:356–364, 2006.
19. Effgen S, McEwen IR: Review of selected physical therapy interventions for school age children with disabilities, *Phys Ther Rev* 13:297–312, 2008.
20. Furumasu J, Tefft D, Guerette P: Pediatric powered mobility: readiness to learn, *Team Rehab* 29–36, 1996. Available at http://www.ranchorep.org/teamrehab.htm. Accessed March 20, 2010.
21. Gefen A: The biomechanics of sitting-acquired pressure ulcers in patients with spinal cord injury or lesions, *Int Wound J* 4:222–231, 2007.
22. Gil-Agudo A, De la Pena-Gonzalez A, Del Ama-Espinosa A, et al.: Comparative study of pressure distribution at the user-cushion interface with different cushions in a population with spinal cord injury, *Clin Biomechan* 24:558–563, 2009.
23. Goldstein DN, Cohn E, Coster W: Enhancing participation for children with disabilities: application of the ICF enablement framework to pediatric physical therapist practice, *Pediatr Phys Ther* 16:114–120, 2004.
24. Guerette P, Tefft D, Furumasu J: Pediatric powered wheelchairs: results of a national survey of providers, *Assist Technol* 17:144–158, 2005.
25. Harrison A, Derwent G, Enticknap A, et al.: The role of virtual reality technology in the assessment and training of inexperienced powered wheelchair users, *Disabil Rehabil* 24:599–606, 2002.
26. Hoppenbrouwers G, Stewart H, Kernot J: Assistive technology assessment tools for assessing switch use of children: a systematic review and descriptive analysis, *Technol Disabil* 26:171–185, 2014.
27. Jan YK, Jones MA, Rabadi MH, et al.: Effect of wheelchair tilt-in-space and recline angles on skin perfusion over the ischial tuberosity in people with spinal cord injury, *Arch Phys Med Rehabil* 91:1758–1764, 2010.
28. Jones M, McEwen I, Hansen L: Use of power mobility for a young child with spinal muscular atrophy, *Phys Ther* 83:253–262, 2003.
29. Lacoste M, Therrien M, Cote J, et al.: Assessment of seated postural control in children: comparison of a force platform versus a pressure mapping system, *Arch Phys Med Rehabil* 87:1623–1629, 2006.
30. Lahm EA, Nussbaum C: Factors that influence assistive technology decision making, *J Special Ed Technol* 17:15–26, 2002.
31. Lau H, Tam EWC, Cheng JCY: An experience on wheelchair bank management, *Disabil Rehabil Assist Technol* 3:302–308, 2008.
32. Makhsous M, Lin F, Bankard J, et al.: Biomechanical effects of sitting with adjustable ischial and lumbar support on occupational low back pain: evaluation of sitting load and back muscle activity, *BMC Musculoskelet Disord* 10:17, 2009.
33. McDonald R, Sawatzky B, Franck L: A comparison of flat and reamped, contoured cushions as adaptive seating interventions for children with neurological disorders, *Health Psychol Behav Med* 3:69–81, 2015.
34. McDonald R, Surtees R, Wirz S: The International Classification of Functioning, Disability and Health provides a model for adaptive seating interventions for children with cerebral palsy, *Br J Occup Ther* 67:293–302, 2004.
35. McDonald RL, Wilson GN, Molloy A, Franck LS: Feasibility of three electronic instruments in studying the benefits of adaptive seating, *Disabil Rehabil Assist Technol* 6:483–490, 2011.
36. McNamara L, Casey J: Seating inclinations affect the function of children with cerebral palsy: a review of the effect of different seat inclines, *Disabil Rehabil Assist Technol* 2:309–318, 2007.

37. McNaughton D, Bryen DN: AAC technologies to enhance participation and access to meaningful societal roles for adolescents and adults with developmental disabilities who require AAC, *Augment Altern Commun* 23:217–229, 2007.

38. Reference deleted in proofs.

39. Murchland S, Parkyn H: Using assistive technology for schoolwork: the experience of children with physical disabilities, *Disabil Rehabil Assist Technol* 5:438–447, 2010.

40. Myhr U, von Wendt L: Influence of different sitting positions and abduction orthoses on leg muscle activity in children with cerebral palsy, *Dev Med Child Neurol* 35:870–880, 1993.

41. Reference deleted in proofs.

42. Nicolson A, Moir L, Millsteed J: Impact of assistive technology on family caregivers of children with physical disabilities: a systematic review, *Disabil Rehabil Assist Technol* 7:345–349, 2012.

43. Oregon Research Institute: Applied Computer Simulation Labs. Accessed at: http://www.ori.org/~vr/, 2003.

44. O'Sullivan SB, Schmitz T: *Physical rehabilitation: assessment and treatment*, ed 4, Philadelphia, 2001, FA Davis. 2001. 87a.

44a. Ozek MM, Cinalli G, Maxiner WJ: Spina bifida: management and outcomes, Milan, Italy, 2008, Springler-Verlag.

45. Parette P, McMahon GA: What should we expect of assistive technology? *Teach Excep Child* 35:56–61, 2002.

46. Peterson BC: Considerations for power mobility: making most of your choices, *Excep Parent* 33:143–145, 2003.

47. Reid DT: The use of virtual reality to improve upper-extremity efficiency skills in children with cerebral palsy: a pilot study, *Technol Disabil* 14:53–61, 2002.

48. RESNA: *Position on the application of power wheelchairs for pediatric users*, Arlington, Virginia, 2008, RESNA Publications.

49. Rungsinee AL, Widman LM, Abresch RT, et al.: Body composition and resting energy expenditure in patients aged 11-21 years with spinal cord dysfunction compared to controls: comparison and relationships among the groups, *J Spinal Cord Med* 30:S105–S111.

50. Safe Transport for Children with Special Needs: Connecticut Children's Medical Center, Injury Prevention Center. Available at: www.ccmckids .org/training, 2004.

51. Reference deleted in proofs.

52. Seelman KD: Blueprint for the millennium: an analysis of regional hearings on assistive technology for people with disabilities. Available at: http://resnaprojects.org/nattap/library/blueprint.pdf. Accessed March 20, 2010.

53. Shechtman O, Hanson CS, Garrett D, Dunn P: Comparing wheelchair cushions for effectiveness of pressure relief: a pilot study, *Occupat Ther J Res* 21:29–48, 2001.

54. Sullivan M, Lewis M: Assistive technology for the very young: creating responsive environments, *Infants Young Child* 12:34–52, 2000.

55. Reference deleted in proofs.

56. Vaccarella B: Finding our way through the maze of adaptive technology, *Comput Libr* 21:44–47, 2001.

57. Reference deleted in proofs.

58. Walls G, Rosen A: Wheelchair seating and mobility evaluation, *PT Magazine Phys Ther* 11:28–31, 2008.

59. Washington K, Deitz JC, White OR, et al.: The effects of a contoured foam seat on postural alignment and upper extremity function in infants with neuromotor impairment, *Phys Ther* 82:1064–1076, 2002.

60. World Health Organization: *International Classification of Functioning, Disability and Health*, Geneva, 2001, World Health Organization. Retrieved July 2010 at: http://www.who.int/classifications/icf/en/.

Note: Page numbers followed by "*b*", "*f*" and "*t*" indicate boxes, figures and tables respectively.